Medical-Surgical Nursing

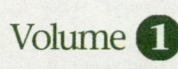

Assessment and Management of Clinical Problems

Volume 1

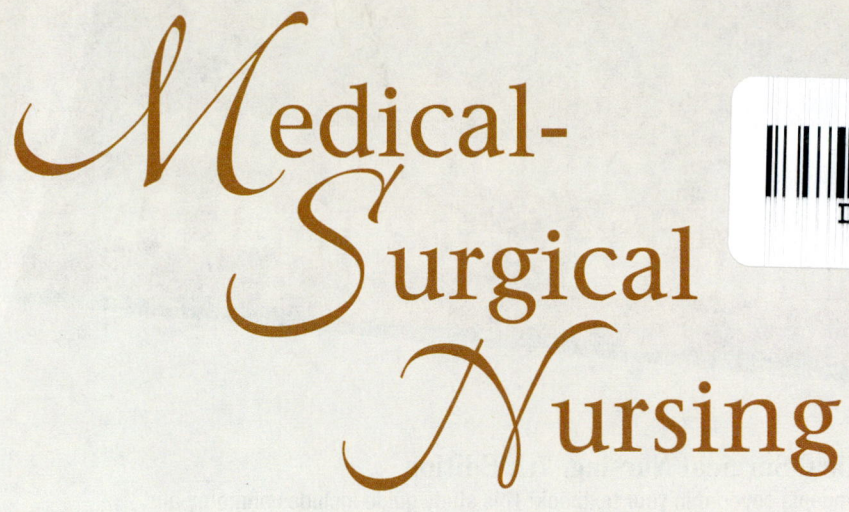

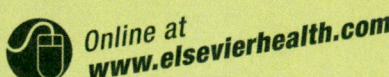

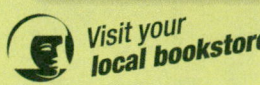

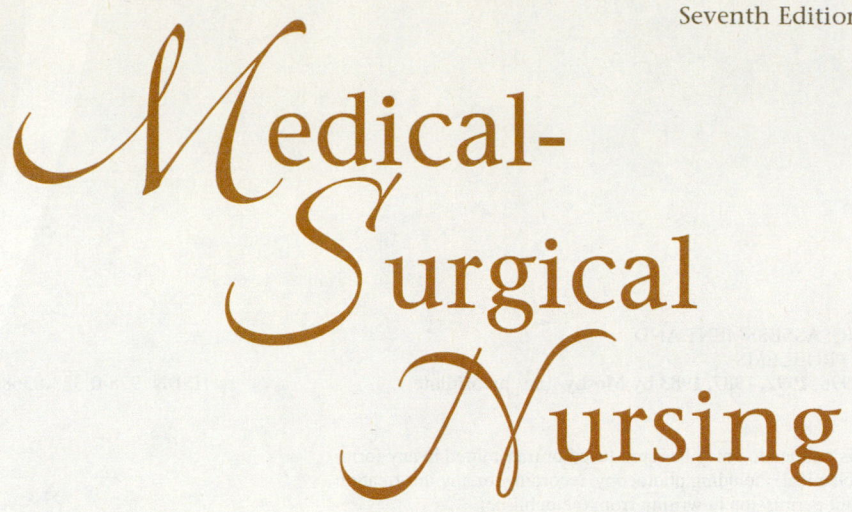

Seventh Edition

Medical-Surgical Nursing

Assessment and Management of Clinical Problems

Volume 1

Sharon L. Lewis, RN, PhD, FAAN
Professor, Schools of Nursing and Medicine
Castella Distinguished Professor in Nursing
University of Texas Health Science Center at San Antonio;
Clinical Nurse Scientist
Geriatric Research, Education, and Clinical Center
South Texas Veterans Health Care System
San Antonio, Texas

Margaret McLean Heitkemper, RN, PhD, FAAN
Professor and Chairperson, Biobehavioral Nursing and Health Systems
Elizabeth Sterling Soule Endowed Chair in Nursing
School of Nursing;
Adjunct Professor, Division of Gastroenterology
School of Medicine
University of Washington
Seattle, Washington

Shannon Ruff Dirksen, RN, PhD
Associate Professor, College of Nursing and Health Care Innovation
Arizona State University
Phoenix, Arizona

Patricia Graber O'Brien, APRN-BC, MA, MSN
Instructor, College of Nursing
University of New Mexico;
Clinical Research Coordinator
Lovelace Scientific Resources
Albuquerque, New Mexico

Linda Bucher, RN, DNSc
Associate Professor
School of Nursing
University of Delaware;
Nursing Research Facilitator
Christiana Care Health System
Newark, Delaware

MOSBY
ELSEVIER

MOSBY
ELSEVIER

11830 Westline Industrial Drive
St. Louis, Missouri 63146

MEDICAL-SURGICAL NURSING: ASSESSMENT AND MANAGEMENT OF CLINICAL PROBLEMS

ISBN: 978-0-323-03688-7

Notice

Knowledge and best practice in this field are constantly changing. As new research and experience broaden our knowledge, changes in practice, treatment and drug therapy may become necessary or appropriate. Readers are advised to check the most current information provided (i) on procedures featured or (ii) by the manufacturer of each product to be administered, to verify the recommended dose or formula, the method and duration of administration, and contraindications. It is the responsibility of the practitioner, relying on their own experience and knowledge of the patient, to make diagnoses, to determine dosages and the best treatment for each individual patient, and to take all appropriate safety precautions. To the fullest extent of the law, neither the Publisher nor the Authors assume any liability for any injury and/or damage to persons or property arising out or related to any use of the material contained in this book.

The Publisher

ISBN: 978-0-323-03688-7

Executive Publisher: Robin Carter
Acquisitions Editor: Kristin Geen
Senior Developmental Editor: Lauren Lake
Publishing Services Manager: Jeffrey Patterson
Senior Project Manager: Mary Stueck
Cover Design Director: Mark Oberkrom
Text Designer: Paula Ruckenbrod

Printed in China

Last digit is the print number: 9 8 7 6 5 4 3 2

About the Authors

SHARON L. LEWIS, RN, PhD, FAAN

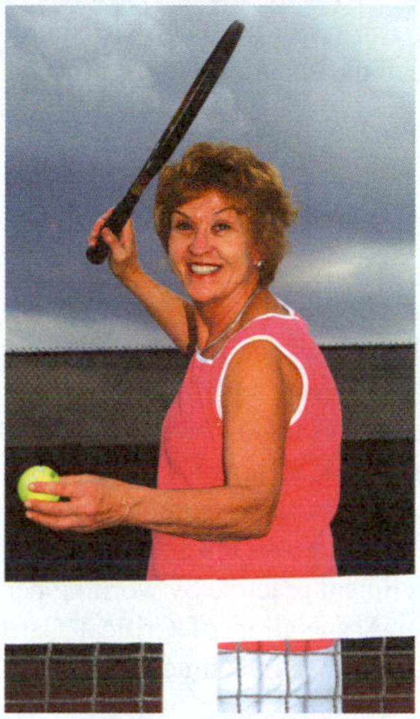

Sharon Lewis is Professor, Schools of Nursing and Medicine and Castella Distinguished Professor at the University of Texas Health Science Center–San Antonio and Clinical Nurse Scientist at the Geriatric Research, Education, and Clinical Center at the South Texas Veterans Health Care System. She received her Bachelor of Science in nursing from the University of Wisconsin-Madison, Master of Science in nursing with a minor in biological sciences from the University of Colorado-Denver, and PhD in immunology from the Department of Pathology at the University of New Mexico School of Medicine. She had a 2-year postdoctoral fellowship from the National Kidney Foundation. Her more than 35 years of teaching experience include inservice education and teaching in associate degree, baccalaureate, master's degree, and doctoral programs in Maryland, Illinois, Wisconsin, New Mexico, and Texas. Favorite teaching areas are pathophysiology, immunology, renal disease, and caregiving. She has been actively involved in clinical research for the past 25 years, investigating altered immune responses in various disorders. Her current research focus is on the newly emerging field of psychoneuroimmunology. At this time she is using biofeedback and immune parameters to study the effects of relaxation therapy and stress management for caregivers of patients with Alzheimer's and Parkinson's disease. Her free time is spent playing tennis, landscaping, and gardening.

MARGARET McLEAN HEITKEMPER, RN, PhD, FAAN

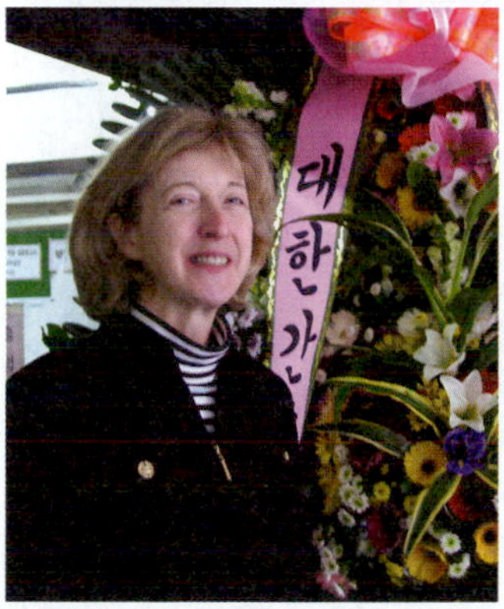

Margaret Heitkemper is Professor and Chairperson, Department of Biobehavioral Nursing and Health Systems at the School of Nursing, and Adjunct Professor, Division of Gastroenterology at the School of Medicine at the University of Washington. She is also Director of the National Institutes of Health–National Institute for Nursing Research–funded Center for Women's Health and Gender Research at the University of Washington. In the fall of 2006, Dr. Heitkemper was appointed the Elizabeth Sterling Soule Endowed Chair in Nursing. Dr. Heitkemper received her Bachelor of Science in nursing from Seattle University, a Master of Science in gerontologic nursing from the University of Washington, and a doctorate in Physiology and Biophysics from the University of Illinois at the Medical Center, Chicago. She has been on faculty at the University of Washington since 1981 and has been the recipient of three School of Nursing Excellence in Teaching awards and the University of Washington Distinguished Teaching Award. In addition, in 2002 she received the Distinguished Nutrition Support Nurse Award from the American Society for Parenteral and Enteral Nutrition (ASPEN), in 2003 the American Gastroenterological Association and Janssen Award for Clinical Research in Gastroenterology, and in 2005 she was the first recipient of the Pfizer and Friends of the National Institutes for Nursing Research Award for Research in Women's Health.

SHANNON RUFF DIRKSEN, RN, PhD

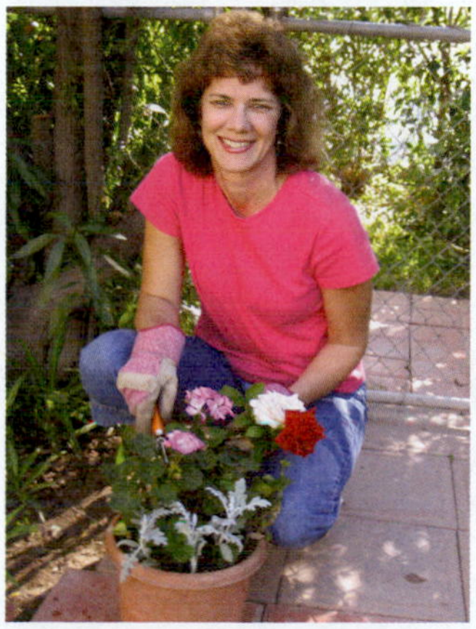

Shannon Dirksen is Associate Professor at the College of Nursing and Health Care Innovation, Arizona State University. She received her Bachelor of Science in nursing from Arizona State University, Master of Science in nursing from the University of Arizona, and doctorate in nursing with a minor in psychology from the University of Arizona. She has over 20 years of undergraduate and graduate teaching experience at the University of Arizona, Edith Cowan University (Western Australia), Intercollegiate College of Nursing–Washington State University, and University of New Mexico. She has been on the faculty at Arizona State University since 1996. She currently teaches management and leadership, and nursing research, including evidence-based practice. Her research focuses on cancer survivorship, with current studies examining behavioral interventions that positively impact insomnia, fatigue, mood, and quality of life in persons diagnosed with breast and prostate cancer. In her free time, she enjoys gardening, reading, and bicycling.

PATRICIA GRABER O'BRIEN, APRN-BC, MA, MSN

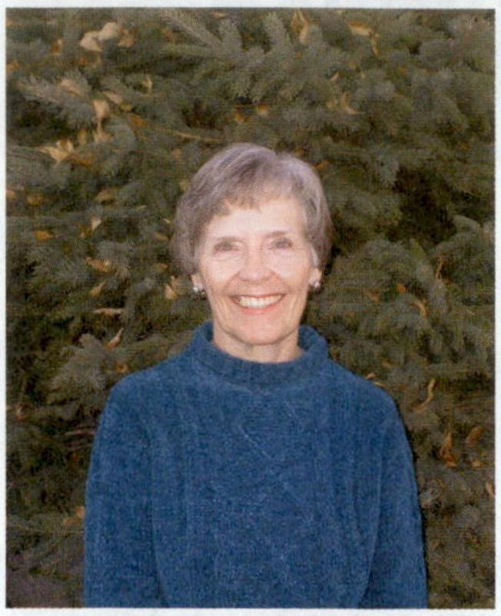

Patricia O'Brien retired from Albuquerque Technical-Vocational Institute, a community college, in 1993, and continues to teach part-time at the College of Nursing at the University of New Mexico. She is also employed part-time as a clinical research coordinator at Lovelace Scientific Resources in Albuquerque. She received her Bachelor of Science in nursing from the University of Kansas, Master of Arts in adult education from the University of New Mexico, and Master of Science in nursing with majors in medical-surgical nursing and nursing administration from the University of Texas at El Paso. During her nursing career, she has worked in medical-surgical nursing and home health care, but most of her experience is in nursing education. She is a certified clinical nurse specialist in medical-surgical nursing. She has directed and taught in nursing programs of all levels of basic nursing preparation for more than 30 years. Her primary interests in teaching include nursing process, pharmacology, and metabolic problems.

LINDA BUCHER, RN, DNSc

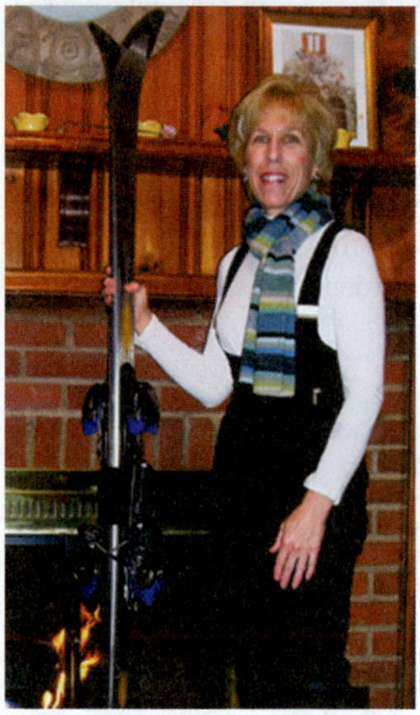

Linda Bucher has a joint appointment as an Associate Professor at the University of Delaware and a Nursing Research Facilitator at Christiana Care Health Services, both in Newark, Delaware. She received her Bachelor of Science in nursing from Thomas Jefferson University in Philadelphia, her Master of Science in adult health and illness from the University of Pennsylvania in Philadelphia, and her DNSc in nursing from Widener University in Chester, Pennsylvania. Her 26 years of nursing experience has spanned staff and patient education, and teaching in associate, baccalaureate, and graduate nursing programs in New Jersey, Pennsylvania, and Delaware. Her preferred teaching areas include cardiac and emergency nursing and research. She maintains her clinical practice by working per diem as an emergency nurse, is an active member of the American Association of Critical Care Nurses, and enjoys working as a volunteer nurse for Operation Smile. In her free time, she enjoys traveling and skiing with her family.

Contributors

Margaret M. Andrews, RN, PhD, CTN, FAAN
Professor of Nursing and Director, Department of Nursing
School of Health Professions and Studies
The University of Michigan
Flint, Michigan

Richard B. Arbour, RN, MSN, CCRN, CNRN
Staff Nurse/Clinical Researcher
Albert Einstein Healthcare Network
Philadelphia, Pennsylvania

Margaret Wooding Baker, RN, PhD
Assistant Professor, School of Nursing
Biobehavioral Nursing and Health Systems Department
University of Washington
Seattle, Washington

Bobbie Berkowitz, RN, PhD, FAAN
Alumni Endowed Professor of Nursing, School of Nursing
University of Washington
Seattle, Washington

Paula Blackwell, BS, MBA, MT(ASCP)
Senior Research Assistant
University of Texas Health Science Center at San Antonio
San Antonio, Texas

Audrey J. Bopp, RN, MSN, CNS
Assistant Professor of Nursing
University of Northern Colorado
Greeley, Colorado

Elisabeth G. Bradley, APRN-BC, MS, CCRN
Clinical Nurse Specialist, Cardiology/Critical Care
Christiana Care Health System
Newark, Delaware

Lucy Bradley-Springer, RN, PhD, ACRN, FAAN
Associate Professor of Medicine
University of Colorado Health Sciences Center;
Principal Investigator
Mountain Plains AIDS Education and Training Center
Denver, Colorado

Linda Bucher, RN, DNSc
Associate Professor
School of Nursing
University of Delaware
Nursing Research Facilitator
Christiana Care Health System
Newark, Delaware

Elizabeth Burkhart, RN, MPH, PhD
Assistant Professor
Marcella Niehoff School of Nursing
Loyola University–Chicago
Chicago, Illinois

Jormain Cady, ARNP, MS, AOCN
Nurse Practitioner
Department of Radiation Oncology
Virginia Mason Medical Center
Seattle, Washington

Sharon G. Childs, APRN-BC, MS, NP/CS, ONC
Adult, Acute Care Nurse Practitioner
The Sports Center
Baltimore, Maryland

Janet T. Crimlisk, RN, MS, NP-C, APRN-BC
Clinical Nurse Specialist
Boston Medical Center
Boston, Massachusetts

Paula Cox-North, RN, MN, NP-C
Advanced Registered Nurse Practitioner
Pacific Medical Centers
Seattle, Washington

Anne Croghan, ARNP, MN
Nurse Practitioner
Seattle Gastroenterology Associates
Seattle, Washington

Shannon Ruff Dirksen, RN, PhD
Associate Professor, College of Nursing and Health Care Innovation
Arizona State University
Phoenix, Arizona

Angela J. DiSabatino, RN, MS
Manager, Cardiovascular Research and Database
Christiana Care Health System
Newark, Delaware

Laura Dulski, RNC, MSN
Instructor
West Suburban College of Nursing
Oak Park, Illinois

Stephanie A. Elms, RN, MSN
Clinical Instructor, School of Nursing
Acute Care Department
University of Texas Health Science Center
San Antonio, Texas

Connie Engelking, RN, MS, OCN
President
The CHE Group, Inc
Mt. Kisco, New York

Mary Ersek, RN, PhD
Director of Research, Center for Nursing Excellence
Swedish Medical Center
Seattle, Washington

Ellen Fineout-Overholt, RN, PhD
Associate Professor of Clinical Nursing, College of Nursing and Health Care Innovation
Director, Center for the Advancement of Evidence-Based Practice
Arizona State University
Phoenix, Arizona

Hatice Y. Foell, ARNP-C, MSN
Nurse Practitioner
Diagnostic and Interventional Cardiology
Melbourne, Florida

Kathleen M. Geib, RN, DNSc
Associate Professor
Palm Beach Atlantic University
West Palm Beach, Florida

Shari Goldberg, RN, MS
Women's Health Nurse Practitioner;
Assistant Professor, Department of Nursing
Colby-Sawyer College
New London, New Hampshire

Peggi Guenter, RN, PhD, CNSN
Managing Editor for Special Projects
American Society for Parenteral and Enteral Nutrition
Silver Spring, Maryland

Elise F. Hazzard, ARNP-C, MS, ONC
Dermatology ARNP
Bloomingdale Medical Associates
Riverview, Florida

Margaret McLean Heitkemper, RN, PhD, FAAN
Professor and Chairperson, Biobehavioral Nursing and Health Systems
Elizabeth Sterling Soule Endowed Chair in Nursing
School of Nursing;
Adjunct Professor, Division of Gastroenterology
School of Medicine
University of Washington
Seattle, Washington

Sherry Garrett Hendrickson, APRN-BC, PhD
Assistant Professor of Clinical Nursing, School of Nursing
University of Texas at Austin
Austin, Texas

Mary Ann House-Fancher, ACNP, MSN, CCRN-CSC
Adult Acute Care Nurse Practitioner
Division of Cardio-Thoracic Surgery
University of Florida
Gainesville, Florida

Valerie Bender Howard, RN, MSN
Clinical Assistant Professor, Nursing
Robert Morris University
Moon Township, Pennsylvania

Gordon A. Irving, MD, MB, BS, FFA(SA), MMed, MSc, Diplomate ABA, ABPM, ABA Certificate in Pain Management
Clinical Associate Professor, Department of Anesthesiology
University of Washington School of Medicine;
Medial Director, Swedish Pain and Headache Center
Swedish Medical Center
Seattle, Washington

Vicki Y. Johnson, RN, PhD, CUCNS
Assistant Professor
University of Alabama School of Nursing at Birmingham
Birmingham, Alabama

Jane Steinman Kaufman, RN, MS, CS, ANP
Clinical Associate Professor, School of Nursing
University of North Carolina
Chapel Hill, North Carolina

Jack R. Kless, CRNA, MA, MSN
Instructor/Program Director
Frances Payne Bolton School of Nursing
Case Western Reserve University
Cleveland, Ohio

Judy A. Knighton, RegN, MScN
Clinical Nurse Specialist–Burns
Ross Tilley Burn Centre
Sunnybrook and Women's College
Health Sciences Centre
Toronto, Ontario, Canada

JoAnne Konick-McMahan, RN, MSN, CCRN
Staff Nurse–Respiratory Unit
Harrisburg Hospital, Pinnacle Health System
Harrisburg, Pennsylvania

Jennifer Kretzschmar, BBA
Senior Research Data Management Coordinator
University of Texas Health Science Center at San Antonio
San Antonio, Texas

Nancy Stoetzner Kupper, RN, MSN
Associate Professor of Nursing
Tarrant Community College
Fort Worth, Texas

Linda Laskowski-Jones, RN, MS, APRN-BC, CCRN, CEN
Vice President, Emergency, Trauma, and Aeromedical Services
Christiana Care Health System
Newark, Delaware

Sharon L. Lewis, RN, PhD, FAAN
Professor, Schools of Nursing and Medicine
Castella Distinguished Professor in Nursing
University of Texas Health Science Center at San Antonio;
Clinical Nurse Scientist
Geriatric Research, Education, and Clinical Center
South Texas Veterans Health Care System
San Antonio, Texas

Kathy Lucke, RN, PhD
Associate Dean for Academic Programs and Administration, School of Nursing
University of Texas Medical Branch
Galveston, Texas

Nancy J. MacMullen, RN, APN, CNS, PhD
Assistant Professor
Governors State University
University Park, Illinois

Linda Griego Martinez, RN, MSN, CCRN, APRN-BC
Clinical Nurse Specialist
Presbyterian Heart Group
Albuquerque, New Mexico

Terran R. Mathers, RN, DNS
Associate Professor, Division of Nursing
Spring Hill College
Mobile, Alabama

Cynthia Matthews WHNP, MSN
Nurse Practitioner
The Breast Center
Marietta, Georgia

De Ann Mitchell, RN, PhD
Professor of Nursing
Tarrant Community College
Fort Worth, Texas

Teri A. Murray, RN, PhD
Associate Director, School of Nursing
Doisy College of Health Sciences
Saint Louis University
St. Louis, Missouri

Sherry Neely, RN, MSN, CRNP
Assistant Professor
Butler County Community College
Butler, Pennsylvania

Janice A. Neil, RN, PhD
Associate Professor
East Carolina University
Greenville, North Carolina

Diane K. Newman, RNC, MSN, CRNP, FAAN
Co-Director
Penn Center for Continence and Pelvic Health, Division of Urology
University of Pennsylvania Medical Center
Philadelphia, Pennsylvania

Patricia Graber O'Brien, APRN-BC, MA, MSN
Instructor, College of Nursing
University of New Mexico;
Clinical Research Coordinator
Lovelace Scientific Resources
Albuquerque, New Mexico

Maureen Reilly, RN, PhD, MHS, CRNA
Associate Professor, United States Army Graduate Program in Anesthesia Nursing
University of Texas Health Science Center at Houston
Houston, Texas

Kathleen A. Rich, RN, DNSc, CCNS, CCRN, CEN, CNN
Cardiovascular Clinical Nurse Specialist
LaPorte Regional Health System
LaPorte, Indiana

Nancy C. Robbins, RN, MSN, CFNP, CDE
Family Nurse Practitioner
Virginia Beach Family Practice
Virginia Beach, Virginia

Dottie Roberts, MSN, MACI, RN, CMSRN, OCNS-C
Clinical Nurse Specialist
Rehabilitative and Medical Services
Palmetto Health Baptist Medical Center
Columbia, South Carolina

Sandra Irene Rome, RN, MN, AOCN
Clinical Nurse Specialist, Hematology/Oncology
Cedars-Sinai Medical Center
Los Angeles, California

Julie T. Sanford, RN, DNS
Associate Professor
College of Nursing
University of South Alabama
Mobile, Alabama

Marilee Schmelzer, RN, PhD
Associate Professor, School of Nursing
The University of Texas at Arlington
Arlington, Texas

Alyce Schultz, RN, PhD, FAAN
Clinical Professor, College of Nursing and Health Care Innovation
Associate Director, Center for the Advancement of Evidence-Based Practice
Arizona State University
Phoenix, Arizona

Maureen A. Seckel, RN, MSN, APRN-BC, CCNS, CCRN
Clinical Nurse Specialist, Medical Critical Care/Pulmonary
Christiana Care Health System
Newark, Delaware

Cory A. Shaw, MSTOM, L.Ac.
Laboratory Technical Assistant, Acute Nursing
University of Texas Health Science Center
Traditional Chinese Medicine Practitioner, Licensed Acupuncturist
San Antonio, Texas

Virginia Shaw, RN, MSN
Assistant Professor, School of Nursing
University of Texas Health Science Center
San Antonio, Texas

Brenda K. Shelton, RN, MS, AOCN, CCRN
Clinical Nurse Specialist
The Sidney Kimmel Comprehensive Cancer Center at Johns Hopkins
Baltimore, Maryland

Anita J. Shoup, RN, MSN, CNOR
Clinical Nurse Consultant
Regent Medical
Edmonds, Washington

Barbara Sinni-McKeehen, ARNP, MSN, DNC
Dermatology Nurse Practitioner/Clinical Administrator
Bay Pines VAMC
Bay Pines, Florida

Debra J. Smith, RN, MSN, CCRN
Instructor, College of Nursing
University of New Mexico
Albuquerque, New Mexico

Sarah C. Smith, RN, MA, CRNO
Advanced Practice Nurse/Educational Associate
Department of Ophthalmology
University of Iowa Healthcare
Iowa City, Iowa

Cheryl Ross Staats, RN, MSN, APRN-BC
Associate Professor/Clinical
Department of Acute Nursing Care
University of Texas Health Science Center at San Antonio
San Antonio, Texas

Colleen R. Walsh RN, MSN, ONC, CS, ACNP-BC
Faculty, Graduate Nursing, School of Nursing and Health Professions
University of Southern Indiana
Evansville, Indiana

Deirdre D. Wipke-Tevis, RN, PhD, BC
Associate Professor, Sinclair School of Nursing
University of Missouri-Columbia
Columbia, Missouri

Reviewers

Kathryn C. Anderson, RN, CEN, BA, AD, ACLS
Vernon, New Jersey

Lisa Anderson-Shaw, RN, DrPh
Chicago, Illinois

Margaret M. Andrews, RN, PhD, CTN
Flint, Michigan

Helen Wash Asbury, RN, ASN, BSHA, MSN, LNC
Albuquerque, New Mexico

Robert B. Babiak, RN, BSN, CWOCN
San Antonio, Texas

Martha C. Beeker, RN, PhD, CCRN, APRN
Springfield, Missouri

Marietta Bell-Scriber, MSN, APRN-BC, PhD
Big Rapids, Michigan

Nancy Mansueto Berg, RN, MSN, ANCC
Williston, Vermont

Mary-Liz Bilodeau, RN, MS, CCRN, CCNS, CS, BC
Boston, Massachusetts

Audrey J. Bopp, RN, MSN, CNS
Greeley, Colorado

Alexandra Bowen, RN, CGRN
Charleston, South Carolina

Josie M. Bowman, RN, DSN
Greenville, North Carolina

Caralee Brommé, RN, MSN, CCRN
Oakland, California

Janet Witucki Brown, RN, PhD
Knoxville, Tennessee

Karen R. Bruni, RN, MSN, NP, CVN
Albany, New York

Quincealea Brunk, RN, PhD
Valdosta, Georgia

Kathryn Bucks, RN, PhD
Columbia, Missouri

Teresa S. Burckhalter, RN, MSN, C
Beaufort, South Carolina

Barbara J. Burgel, RN, MS, COHNS, FAAN
San Francisco, California

Elizabeth Burkhart, RN, MPH, PhD
Chicago, Illinois

Jormain Cady, ARNP, MS, AOCN
Seattle, Washington

Susan Gallagher Camden, RN, PhD
Houston, Texas

Carolyn Carty, RN, MSN, CEN
Marlton, New Jersey

Sheila M. Choppala, RN, PhD
Vancouver, Washington

Phyllis L. Christianson, MN, ANCC, ARNP
Seattle, Washington

Maureen Chrzanowski, RN, MSN, CNM, FNP
Grand Rapids, Michigan

Mary Ciechanowski, RN, MSN, APRN-BC, CCRN
Newark, Delaware

Katherine M. Crawford, RN, MSN
Newark, Delaware

Virginia Crocker, RN, MS, CEN
Winchester, Massachusetts

Nancy Curry, RN, MSN
Shreveport, Louisiana

Judi Daniels, PhD, ARNP-BC
Lexington, Kentucky

Gayle H. Dasher, RN, PhD, CCRN, CNRN
San Antonio, Texas

Angele H. Davis, RN, MSN, CCRN
Thibodaux, Louisiana

Rhonda S. Davis, RN, MSN
Decatur, Alabama

David Derrico, RN, MSN
Gainesville, Florida

Louise Diehl-Oplinger, RN, MSN, CCRN, APRN-BC
Easton, Pennsylvania

Rose Ann DiMaria, RN, PhD, CNSN
Charleston, West Virginia

Angela J. DiSabatino, RN, MS
Newark, Delaware

Kelly Dodds, RN, MSN, APRN-BC
St Louis, Missouri

Cynthia L. Donell, RN, MSN
Reading, Pennsylvania

Penny Downer, APRN-BC, MSN,
Sidney, Michigan

MaryAnne Dudley, RN, MSN
Cheyenne, Wyoming

Sharon Dudley-Brown, APRN-BC, PhD, FNP
Washington, DC

Patti Eisenberg, APRN-BC, MSN
Indianapolis, Indiana

Marsha L. Ellett, RN, DNS, CGRN
Indiana Pohls, Indiana

Peggy Ellis, RN, PhD, FNP, ANP
St. Louis, Missouri

Coleen R. Elmers, RN, MSN
San Antonio, Texas

Stephanie A. Elms, RN, MSN
San Antonio, Texas

Christy H. Erickson, RN, MSN, NP, AOCN
Burlington, Vermont

Susan A. Ezzone, RN, MS, CNP
Columbus, Ohio

Kathryn Feigenbaum, CGRN, MSN
Bethesda, Maryland

Eleanor R. Fitzpatrick, RN, MSN, CRNP, CCRN
Philadelphia, Pennsylvania

Jan Foecke, RN, MS, ONC
Kansas City, Kansas

Karen Lee Fontaine, RN, MSN, ASSECT
Hammond, Indiana

Rebecca A. Fountain, RN, MSN
Tyler, Texas

John J. Gallagher, RN, MSN, CCNS, CCRN, RRT
Philadelphia, Pennsylvania

Cathy Garcia, RN-BC, CNA BC
Tyler, Texas

Beverly George-Gay, RN, MSN, CCRN
Richmond, Virginia

Eileen P. Geraci, MA, ANP-C, PhD(c)
Danbury, Connecticut

Shari Goldberg, RN, MS
New London, New Hampshire

Karen E. Greco, RN, MN, PhD, ANP
Portland, Oregon

Mary Ellen Grohar-Murray, RN, PhD
St. Louis, Missouri

Shelia Grossman, PhD, APRN-BC
Fairfield, Connecticut

Kathleen Halcomb, APRN-BC, MSN
Richmond, Kentucky

Margaret T. Haynes, RN, BSN, MN
Jackson, Mississippi

Judy Hendricks, MS, ANP, CDE
Newark, Delaware

Sherry Garrett Hendrickson, APRN-BC, PhD
Austin, Texas

Frank D. Hicks, RN, PhD
Chicago, Illinois

Doris Leal Hill, RN, PhD, CNOR
Bloomington, Minnesota

Janice J. Hoffman, RN, PhD
Baltimore, Maryland

Sandra Hoffman, APRN-BC, MSN
Chapel Hill, North Carolina

Linda M. Hoke, RN, PhD, CCRN
Philadelphia, Pennsylvania

M. Catherine Hough, RN, PhD
Jacksonville, Florida

Robert M. Hovis, CRNA
St. Louis, Missouri

Valerie M. Howard, RN, MSN
Pittsburgh, Pennsylvania

Sarah M. Howell, RN, MSN
Columbus, Mississippi

Donna Walker Hubbard, RN, MSN, CNN
Belton, Texas

Beth Hurley, BSN, CRNO, COE
Phoenix, Arizona

Patricia Jansen, APRN, CS, MS, BC
San Jose, California

Suzanne L. Jed, APRN-BC, MSN, FNP
Denver, Colorado

Ann-Marie John, RN, MS
Rochester, New York

Jane Steinman Kaufman, RN, MS, CS, ANP
Chapel Hill, North Carolina

Colleen Keller, RN, PhD, ANCC
Phoenix, Arizona

Mary Ellen Kern, RN, MSN, CCRN, APRN
Philadelphia, Pennsylvania

Jack R. Kless, CRNA, MA, MSN
Cleveland, Ohio

Paula Scharf Kohn, RN, PhD
Pleasantville, New Jersey

JoAnne Konick-McMahan, RN, MSN, CCRN
Harrisburg, Pennsylvania

Caroline Kuhlman, APRN-BC, MS, AOCN
Boston, Massachusetts

Kristine L. Kwekkeboom, RN, PhD
Iowa City, Iowa

Judy M. LaBonte, APRN-BC, MSN, FNP
Memphis, Tennessee

Linda LaCasse, RN, MSN
New Britain, Connecticut

Ann Marie Lagonegro, RN-C, MS, FNP
Rochester, New York

Linda Laskowski-Jones, RN, MS, APRN-BC, CCRN, CEN
Newark, Delaware

Canelia Layton, RN, MSN, PNP
Texas City, Texas

Kathleen Lopez-Bushnell, RNC (FNP), MPH, COHN-S, EdD
Albuquerque, New Mexico

Carolyn M. Lowe, RN, BSN, CDE
San Antonio, Texas

Joyce A. Marrs, APRN-BC, MS, AOCNP
Dayton, Ohio

Jeanne M. Martinez, RN, MPH, CHPN
Chicago, Illinois

Dorothy Mathers, RN, MSN
Williamsport, Pennsylvania

Terran R. Mathers, RN, DNS
Mobile, Alabama

Cynthia Matthews RN, MSN, NP
Kennesaw, Georgia

Barbara Maxwell, RNC, CNS, MSN
Stone Ridge, New York

Anthony W. McGuire, RN, MSN, CCRN, ACNP
Orange, California

Margaret A. Medvedev, RN, MSN
Carthage, Texas

Brenda Michel, RN, EdD
Springfield, Illinois

Douglas W. Mitchell, RN, MSN
Phoenix, Arizona

Diana King Mixon, RN, MSN
Boise, Idaho

Leigh W. Moore, RN, MSN, CNOR
Alberta, Virginia

Debra A. Morgan, RN, EdD
Wichita Falls, Texas

Mary L. Moser-Gautreauz, RN, EdD, CEN, CNS
Albuquerque, New Mexico

Anne C. Muller, RN, MSN, CRNP, CNS
Philadelphia, Pennsylvania

Claire Murphy-Marshall, (BScHons) RN
Perth, Western Australia

Teri A. Murray, RN, PhD
St. Louis, Missouri

Sherry Neely, RN, MSN, CRNP
Butler, Pennsylvania

Janice A. Neil, RN, PhD
Greenville, North Carolina

Geri B. Neuberger, RN, EdD
Kansas City, Kansas

Diane Newman, RNC, MSN, CRNP, FAAN
Philadelphia, Pennsylvania

Marian O'Rourke, RN, CCTC
New Orleans, Louisiana

Barbara Owens, RN, PhD, OCN
San Antonio, Texas

Judith A. Paice, RN, PhD, FAAN
Chicago, Illinois

Elizabeth A. Palmer, RN, PhD
Indiana, Pennsylvania

Barbara Pope, RN, MSN, CCRN, CCNS
Philadelphia, Pennsylvania

Renee Pozza, RN, PhD, CNS, CFNP
Azusa, California

Barbara D. Powe, RN, PhD
Atlanta, Georgia

Lola M. Prince, APRN-BC, PhD(c), FNP
Chicago, Illinois

Virginia E. Printz-Feddersen, RN, MSN, CNS
Albuquerque, New Mexico

Cynthia Zackrison Pritchett, RN, MSN
Mobile, Alabama

Dana Reeves, RN, MSN
Fort Smith, Arkansas

Darryl E. Reid, Sr., RN, MSN
San Antonio, Texas

Diane Reynolds, RN, MS, OCN
Brooklyn, New York

Donna Ricketts, RN, MSN
Richmond, Kentucky

Janet Riggs, RN, MSN, CCRN, CCNS
Philadelphia, Pennsylvania

Nancy C. Robbins, RN, MSN, CFNP, CDE
Virginia Beach, Virginia

Dana Rosdahl, RN, PhD, APRN-BC
Phoenix, Arizona

Kathleen Rourke, RN, BSN, ANP, ONC
Boston, Massachusetts

Judith L. Roy, RN, BSN, BC
Scarborough, Maine

Kathleen K. Salati, MSN, CCRN, NP-C
Newark, Delaware

Julie T. Sanford, RN, DNS
Mobile, Alabama

Bette A. Schans, PhD, RT(R)
Grand Junction, Colorado

Teri W. Scott, RN, MSN, FNP-C, COHN-S
Kansas City, Missouri

Lucinda Seidl, RN, MSN
Lincoln, Nebraska

Camille A. Servodidio, RN, MPH, CRNO, OCN
Hartford, Connecticut

Virginia Shaw, RN, MSN
San Antonio, Texas

Mary Shelkey, ARNP, PhD
Seattle, Washington

Brenda K. Shelton, RN, MS, CCRN, AOCN
Baltimore, Maryland

Tamara Shields, RN, MSN, CFNP
Lafayette, Indiana

Deborah Shows-Rushing, RN, MSN
Troy, Alabama

Barbara Sinni-McKeehen, ARNP, MSN, DNC
Bay Pines, Florida

Susan E. Sitter, RN, MSN
Edinboro, Pennsylvania

Diana Kristin Smith, RN, MSN, CDE, APRN-BC
Wilmington, Delaware

Julie S. Snyder, RN, MSN, BC
Norfolk, Virginia

Sheryl Sommer, RN, PhD
Chicago, Illinois

Debra Gartman Spring, RN, MS
Jackson, Mississippi

Darrell Spurlock, RN, MSN, CCRN, CEN
Columbus, Ohio

Susan K. Steele, RN, DNS, AOCN
New Orleans, Louisiana

Mary M. Sullivan-Whalen, RN, MSN, FNP
New York, New York

Suzanne Sutherland, RN, PhD, CCRN
Sacramento, California

Cheryl Swallow, RN, MSN
St. Louis, Missouri

Karen K. Swenson, RN, PhD(c), AOCN
St. Louis Park, Minnesota

Joanne Thanauaro, RN, MSN, CS, ANP
St. Louis, Missouri

Georgianna M. Thomas, RN, EdD
Oak Park, Illinois

Tamekia L. Thomas, RN, BSN
Newark, Delaware

Rosie Thompson, RN, MS, CS
Kansas City, Kansas

Cheryl L. Touhy, RN, MSN, FNP-C
Newark, Delaware

Sarah Reidunn Tvedt-Pool, RN, MS
Rochester, Minnesota

Pamela A. Van Bevern, MPAS
St. Louis, Missouri

Donna F. Wallner, RN, MS
St. Louis, Missouri

Colleen R. Walsh, RN, MSN, ONC, CS, ACNP-BC
Evansville, Indiana

Brian A. Weber, ARNP, PhD
Gainesville, Florida

Mary Ann Wehmer, RN, MSN, CNOR
Evansville, Indiana

Joyce E. Wenger, RN, MSN, CCRN
Lancaster, Pennsylvania

Elizabeth Wheeler, RN, DNS, WHNP
Staten Island, New York

Erlinda C. Wheeler, RN, DNS
Newark, Delaware

Christine L. Willis, RN, MSN, ANP-C
Durham, North Carolina

Anita K. Witzke, RN, CCRN
Newark, Delaware

Juvann M. Wolff, RN, MSN, ARNP
Seattle, Washington

Patricia Worthington, RN, MSN, CNSN
Philadelphia, Pennsylvania

Thomas Worms, RN, MSN
Chicago, Illinois

Kathleen R. Wren, CRNA, PhD
New Orleans, Louisiana

Nancy H. Wright, RN, BS, CNOR
Birmingham, Alabama

Julie A. Wubs, RN, MSN, CNP, CCRN
Chicago, Illinois

Mary Zaccagnini, RN, MS, AOCN
Minneapolis, Minnesota

Polly Gerber Zimmerman, RN, MS, MBA, CEN
Chicago, Illinois

To the
Profession of Nursing
and to the
Important People in Our Lives

Sharon: My husband, Peter, our sons and their wives, Marc and Heidi, Aaron and Roberta, Michael and Brianna, and Jeremy and Monica, and our grandchildren Malia Belle and Halle Gisele

Margaret: My husband, David, and our daughters Elizabeth and Ellen

Shannon: My husband, John, our children Marshall and Meaghan, and my mother, Marilyn

Pat: My husband, Lawrence, our daughter, Lisa, and the more than a thousand students who taught me so well

Linda: My mother, Charlotte, my siblings Millie, Janet, Barb, Rich, and Joanne, and my very good friend and hypnotherapist, Beth

Preface

The seventh edition of *Medical-Surgical Nursing: Assessment and Management of Clinical Problems* has been thoroughly revised to incorporate the most current medical-surgical nursing information in an easy-to-use format. More than just a textbook, this is a comprehensive resource containing essential information that students need to prepare for lectures, classroom activities, examinations, clinical assignments, and comprehensive care of patients. In addition to the readable writing style and full-color illustrations, the text includes many special features to help students learn medical-surgical nursing content, including patient and family teaching, gerontology, collaborative care, cultural and ethnic considerations, nutrition and drug therapy, home care, evidence-based practice, and much more.

The comprehensive and timely content, special features, attractive layout, and student-friendly writing style combine to make this the number one medical-surgical nursing textbook used in more nursing schools than any other medical-surgical nursing textbook.

The strengths of the first six editions have been retained, including the use of the nursing process as an organizational theme for nursing management. Numerous new features have been added to address some of the rapid changes in practice. Contributors have been selected for their acknowledged expertise in specific content areas; one or more specialists in the subject area have thoroughly reviewed each chapter to increase accuracy. The editors have undertaken final rewriting and editing to achieve internal consistency. All efforts have been directed toward building on the strengths of the previous edition while preparing an even more effective new edition.

ORGANIZATION

Content is organized into two major divisions. The first division, Section One (Chapters 1 through 12), discusses general concepts related to adult patients. The second division, Sections Two through Twelve (Chapters 13 through 69), presents nursing assessment and nursing management of medical-surgical problems.

The various body systems are grouped to reflect their interrelated functions. Each section is organized around two central themes: assessment and management. Chapters dealing with assessment of a body system include a discussion of the following:

1. A brief review of anatomy and physiology, focusing on information that will promote understanding of nursing care
2. Health history and noninvasive physical assessment skills to expand the knowledge base on which treatment decisions are made
3. Common diagnostic studies, expected results, and related nursing responsibilities to provide easily accessible information

Management chapters focus on the pathophysiology, clinical manifestations, diagnostic studies, collaborative care, and nursing management of various diseases and disorders. The nursing management sections are organized into assessment, nursing diagnoses, planning, implementation, and evaluation. To emphasize the importance of patient care in various clinical settings, nursing implementation of all major health problems is organized by the following levels of care:

1. Health Promotion
2. Acute Intervention
3. Ambulatory and Home Care

CLASSIC FEATURES

- **Patient and family teaching** is an ongoing theme throughout the text. Coverage includes a separate chapter (Chapter 5: Patient and Family Teaching) and 87 Patient and Family Teaching Guides throughout the text.
- **Home care/community-based care** is also emphasized. Coverage includes a separate chapter (Chapter 7: Community-Based Nursing and Home Care) and special Ambulatory and Home Care headings in the Nursing Implementation sections of the management chapters.
- **Collaborative care** is highlighted in special Collaborative Care sections in all management chapters and 90 Collaborative Care tables throughout the text.
- **Gerontology** is discussed in Chapter 6: Older Adults, and included throughout the text under Gerontologic Considerations and Effects of Aging headings and in Gerontologic Differences in Assessment tables.
- **Nutrition** is highlighted throughout the book. Nutritional Therapy tables summarize nutritional interventions and promote healthy lifestyles in patients with various health problems.
- **Nursing management** is presented in a consistent and comprehensive format, with headings for Health Promotion, Acute Intervention, and Ambulatory and Home Care. In addition, **56 Nursing Care Plans** appear in management chapters.
- A separate chapter on **complementary and alternative therapies** (CAT) addresses timely issues in today's health care settings related to these therapies. In addition, **Complementary and Alternative Therapies boxes** located in disorders chapters expand upon the information presented in the chapter, and summarize what nurses need to know about therapies such as herbal remedies, acupuncture, and biofeedback.
- **Cultural and ethnic health disparities** information is integrated into the text and appears in special boxes highlighting risk factors and other important issues related to the nursing care of various ethnic groups. A special **Culturally Competent Care heading** highlights expanded cultural and ethnic content as it relates to specific diseases and disorders.
- **Genetics in Clinical Practice boxes** highlight the genetic basis, genetic testing, and clinical implications for genetic disorders that affect adults.
- **Ethical Dilemmas boxes** promote critical thinking for timely and sensitive issues that nursing students may deal with in clinical practice—topics such as informed consent, advance directives, and confidentiality.

- **Emergency Management tables** outline the emergency treatment of health problems most likely to require emergency intervention.
- **Common Assessment Abnormalities tables** in assessment chapters alert the nurse to frequently encountered abnormalities and their possible etiologies.
- **Nursing Assessment tables** summarize the key subjective and objective data related to common diseases. Subjective data are organized by functional health patterns.
- **Health History tables** in assessment chapters present key questions to ask patients related to a specific disease or disorder.
- Student-friendly pedagogy includes:
  - **Learning Objectives** and **Key Terms** at the beginning of each chapter help students identify the key content for that body system or disorder.
  - **Electronic Resources** boxes included in each chapter opener alert students to supplemental content and exercises on the companion CD and Evolve website, making it easier than ever for students to integrate the textbook with media supplements such as animations, video and audio clips, and much more.
  - **NCLEX® Examination Review Questions** at the end of each chapter, which are matched to the learning objectives, help students learn the important points in the chapter. Answers are provided in an appendix so that the review questions serve as a self-study tool.
  - **Critical Thinking Exercises** appearing at the end of nursing management chapters include Case Studies with Critical Thinking Questions for clinical application.
  - **Resources** at the end of each chapter contain information about nursing and health care organizations that provide patient teaching and disease and disorder information. Resources include Internet sites to help students find current information online.

NEW FEATURES

- *New* **Chapter 2: Health Disparities** discusses differences in health status between groups of people as they relate to access to care, economic aspects of health care, gender and cultural issues, and disease risk in the context of overall health promotion and the government's *Healthy People* initiative.
- *New* **Chapter 41: Nursing Management: Obesity** discusses this increasingly common condition with which so many health risks are associated. It discusses weight reduction strategies, commonly used diets (Atkins, South Beach, Zone, etc.), bariatric surgical procedures, and metabolic syndrome.
- *New* **Gender Differences boxes** summarize how women and men are affected differently by conditions such as pain, irritable bowel syndrome, headaches, addiction, osteoporosis, stroke, coronary artery disease, multiple sclerosis, hypertension, and more.
- *New* **All nursing care plans** now incorporate **Nursing Interventions Classification (NIC)** and **Nursing Outcomes Classification (NOC)** in a way that clearly shows the linkages among NIC, NOC, and nursing diagnoses, and applies them to nursing practice.
- *New* **Drug Alerts** highlight important safety considerations applicable to key drugs throughout the management chapters.
- Each chapter has been carefully revised to ensure a **lower reading level** throughout the book making the content more reader-friendly and understandable than ever.
- *New* **Glossary** of key terms and definitions has been added to the book. It was developed in response to feedback from students. An expanded version of the glossary with audio pronunciations is included on the companion CD and Evolve website.
- *New* **Healthy People boxes** summarize government health care goals as they relate to specific disorders such as diabetes, obesity, cancer, and heart disease.
- The **Companion CD** packaged with this text has been completely revamped to include the following learning tools:
  - A completely unique **Stress-Busting Kit for Nursing Students** provides students with practical strategies for managing their patients' stress as well as their own. This includes imagery, breathing, yoga, meditation, and other relaxation strategies.
  - More than 50 **in-depth case studies** include state-of-the-art animations and a variety of interactive learning activities, which provide students with immediate feedback.
  - A dynamic collection of **Multimedia Supplements** includes animations, video clips, and audio clips.
  - A bank of **375 NCLEX® Examination Review Questions** allow for test preparation.
  - An expanded **glossary** provides pronunciations and definitions for the key terms in the book, and is available as one comprehensive glossary and organized by chapter.
- NCLEX Examination Review Questions in each chapter now include a **focus on prioritization of patient care.**
- **Evidence-Based Practice boxes** have been completely revamped to include updated material that provides synthesis of evidence for application to clinical practice.
- **Enhanced case studies** feature photos that "bring patients to life" and incorporate multiple disorders so that students learn how to **prioritize care and manage patients** in the clinical setting.
- *New* **content on organ transplant** covers organ donation, histocompatibility, rejection, and immunosuppressive therapy with new visual aids.
- **Chapter 9: Stress and Stress Management** replaces the former more theoretical and research-focused stress chapter with more practical information on basic stress management techniques (e.g., breathing, imagery, and meditation) and even self-care strategies for nurses.
- **Chapter 15: Infection and Human Immunodeficiency Virus Infection** now covers emerging infections, multi-resistant drugs, and the nursing care of patients with HIV.
- **Chapter 16: Cancer** reflects a new "healthy" focus on cancer survivors and their long-term care needs.
- **Chapter 18: Nursing Management: Preoperative Care** has been expanded with a new focus on ambulatory and outpatient surgery.
- **Chapter 34: Nursing Management: Coronary Artery Disease and Acute Coronary Syndrome** features expanded information on cardiac surgery and postoperative considerations.
- **Chapter 49 Nursing Management: Diabetes Mellitus** includes extensively revised and updated material with new figures and teaching materials.

- **Chapter 67: Nursing Management: Shock, Systemic Inflammatory Response Syndrome, and Multiple Organ Dysfunction Syndrome** has been completely rewritten for increased readability and student comprehension of this complex topic.
- **Chapter 69: Nursing Management: Emergency and Disaster Nursing** features expanded content on agents of terrorisms, and emergency and mass casualty incidents preparedness.

LEARNING SUPPLEMENTS FOR STUDENTS

- **Clinical Companion to *Medical-Surgical Nursing,* Seventh Edition,** presents approximately 200 common medical-surgical conditions and procedures in a concise, alphabetical format for quick clinical reference. Designed for portability, this popular reference includes the essential, need-to-know information for medical-surgical nursing practice. An attractive and functional two-color design highlights key information for quick, easy reference. This edition features a strong focus on treatments and procedures in which the nurse plays a major role. **Also available on Skyscape PDA!**
- An exceptionally thorough **Study Guide** contains over 500 pages of review material that has been thoroughly updated to reflect the revision of the textbook. Written by textbook coauthor Patricia O'Brien, it features a wide variety of clinically relevant exercises and activities, including fill-in-the-blank worksheets, anatomy identification review, true-false questions, critical thinking activities, crossword puzzles, case studies, matching exercises, word scrambles, and multiple-choice questions in NCLEX format. This edition features highlighted Alternate Item questions to better prepare students for the NCLEX exam. Answers to all questions are included in the back to provide students with immediate feedback as they study.
- **Evolve Student Resources** are available online at *http://evolve.elsevier.com/Lewis/medsurg/* and include the following valuable learning aids organized by chapter:
  - Content Updates
  - Audio Key Points summaries for each chapter that can be downloaded to a CD-ROM or iPod
  - Printable Key Points summaries for each chapter
  - Concept Map Creator
  - Key Term Flash Cards
  - Customizable Nursing Care Plans
  - 40 Patient and Family Instruction handouts in both English and Spanish that can be printed and distributed to patients
  - Physical Examination Video
  - Fluids and Electrolytes Tutorial
  - Electronic Calculators
  - WebLinks
  - Audio glossary of key terms, available as comprehensive alphabetical glossary and organized by chapter
- **Virtual Clinical Excursions 3.0** is an exciting learning tool that brings learning to life in a "virtual" hospital setting. Completely updated for easier use and more control, the VCE Pacific View workbook/CD-ROM package features textbook reading assignments that correspond with the CD-ROM and workbook activities. The workbook acts as a map, guiding students through the CD-ROM as they care for patients in the virtual hospital to help students make connections between what they experience through the CD-ROM and what they have learned in their textbook. Each virtual hospital visit allows the student to access realistic information resources essential to patient care resulting in a true-to-life, hands-on learning experience. Instructors receive an Implementation Manual with directions for using VCE as a teaching tool.

TEACHING SUPPLEMENTS FOR INSTRUCTORS

- The **Instructor's Electronic Resource with Integrated Lesson Plans on CD** remains the most comprehensive set of instructor's materials available, containing:
  - **Integrated Lesson Plans** with electronic resources organized by chapter to help instructors develop and manage the course curriculum. This exciting new resource includes:
    - Four-column lesson plans listing chapter outlines, classroom strategies, collaborative/active learning activities with critical thinking questions, and a "putting it all together" section that lists specific teaching resources available for each content section
    - Quizzes with answer guidelines
    - Case studies with answer guidelines
    - Learning objectives
    - Key terms with audio pronunciations

    This unique teaching aid includes links and cross-references to additional instructor and student materials for each chapter to help faculty "put it all together" and truly make the best use of all of the teaching/learning supplements. Included are links to the relevant content in the image collection, PowerPoint presentations, i-Clicker Question Suite, test bank, animation collection, content updates—as well as the related components of the companion CD and student Evolve resources. Also provided are quick-access links to resources useful for all chapters, including the concept map creator, electronic calculators, and much more.
  - The **ExamView® Test Bank** features approximately 1800 NCLEX® Examination test questions with text page references and answers coded for NCLEX Client Needs category, nursing process, and cognitive level. The 7th edition test bank has been revamped to include rationales, more application-based questions, additional questions in NCLEX alternate-item formats, and to incorporate prioritization and delegation content. The ExamView program allows instructors to create new tests; edit, add, and delete test questions; sort questions by NCLEX category, cognitive level, and nursing process step; and administer/grade online tests.
  - The **Image Collection** contains more than 800 full-color images from the text for use in lectures.
  - An extensive collection of **PowerPoint Presentations** is organized by chapter and includes over 8000 customizable slides for use in lectures. The presentations include applicable illustrations from the image collection and links to applicable animations.
  - A new **i-Clicker Question Suite** for each chapter developed especially for use with audience response systems.
- **Evolve Instructor Resources** are available online at *http://evolve.elsevier.com/Lewis/medsurg/* and feature the following valuable teaching aids:
  - Online access to the Integrated Lesson Plans, Test Bank, PowerPoint Presentations, Image Collection, and i-Clicker Question Suite

- A collection of additional "faculty only" state-of-the-art animations
- Course Management System
- Access to all student resources listed above

Evolve Select

This exciting new program is available to faculty who adopt a number of Elsevier texts, including *Medical-Surgical Nursing: Assessment and Management of Clinical Problems,* 7th edition. Evolve Select is an integrated electronic study center consisting of a collection of textbooks made available electronically in CD format. It is carefully designed to "extend" the textbook for an easier and more efficient teaching and learning experience. It includes study aids such as highlighting, e-note taking, and cut and paste capabilities. Even more importantly, it allows students and instructors to do a comprehensive search within the specific text or across a number of titles. Please check with your Elsevier sales representative for more information.

ACKNOWLEDGMENTS

The editors are especially grateful to many people at Elsevier who assisted with this major revision effort. In particular, we wish to thank the team of Kristin Geen, Lauren Lake, Mary Stueck, Jeff Patterson, and Paula Ruckenbrod. In addition, we want to thank the marketing team of Bob Boehringer and Tricia Schroeder.

A team of special persevering contributors put together our excellent ancillary package. These include Pat O'Brien (Study Guide and i-Clicker Question Suite), Barbara Bartz (Test Bank), Dorothy Mathers (Interactive Case Studies for Companion CD), and Jennie Shaw and Stephanie Elms (Instructor's Manual). Elizabeth Burkhart, Pat O'Brien, and Sara Doeberling revised the nursing care plans to incorporate NANDA nursing diagnoses, Nursing Interventions Classifications, and Nursing Outcomes Classifications.

Special thanks and appreciation go to Peter Bonner who assisted with many details of manuscript preparation. Our special assistants have earned our respect and thanks and include Cory Shaw, Alissa Calaway, Jennifer Kretzschmar, Brianna Chavez, Crystal Ninan, Bevin O'Connor, Kamilah Newland, Paula Blackwell, and Lisa Grabarec.

Ellen Fineout-Overholt and Alyce Schultz, Center for the Advancement of Evidence-Based Practice at the College of Nursing and Health Care Innovation, Arizona State University, Phoenix, Arizona, assisted with content on evidence-based practice.

Our exciting new Stress-Busting kit was a team effort of many people. Cory Shaw helped write and produce it. She and Allen Novian were our actors. Peter Bonner played guitar and contributed photos. Russ Keys played synthesizer. Our wonderful animations and illustrations were prepared by David Baker, Chris McKee, and Jeanne Robertson. The video, photography, and editing were done by Lester Rosebrock. Brian Luke Seaward was our narrator and contributed imagery scripts and photos. For additional information on stress management, see his website at *www.brianlukeseaward.net.*

We are particularly indebted to the faculty, nurses, and student nurses who have put their faith in our book to assist them on their path to excellence. The increasing use of this book throughout the United States, Canada, Australia, and other parts of the world has been gratifying. We appreciate the many users who have shared their comments and suggestions on the previous editions. All feedback is welcome.

We also wish to thank our contributors and reviewers for their assistance with the revision process. We sincerely hope that this book will assist both students and clinicians in practicing truly professional nursing.

Sharon Lewis
Margaret Heitkemper
Shannon Dirksen
Patricia O'Brien
Linda Bucher

Contents

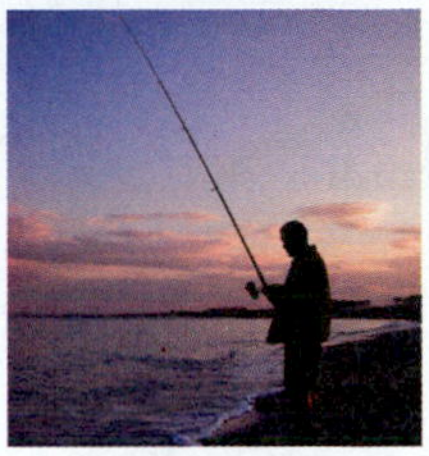

Section 1

CONCEPTS IN NURSING PRACTICE

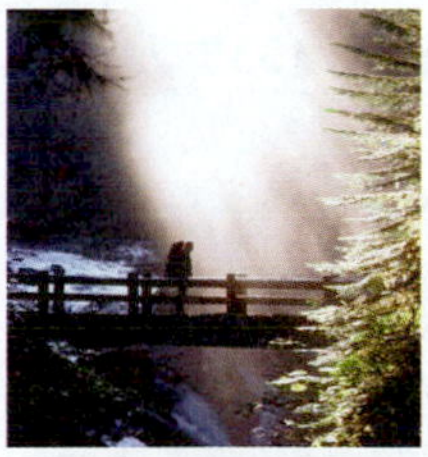

Section 2

PATHOPHYSIOLOGIC MECHANISMS OF DISEASE

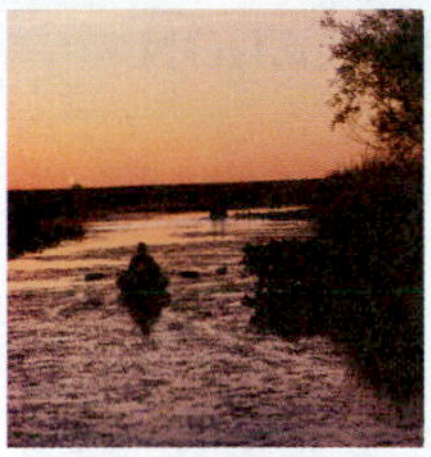

Section 3

PERIOPERATIVE CARE

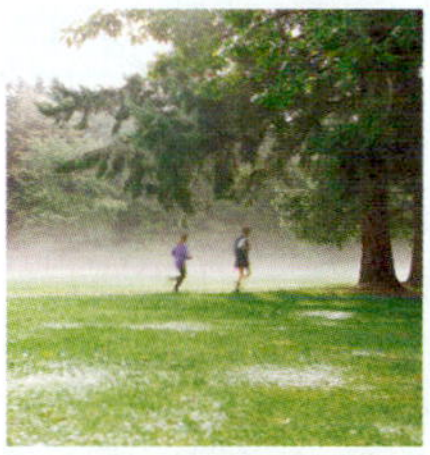

Section 4

PROBLEMS RELATED TO ALTERED SENSORY INPUT

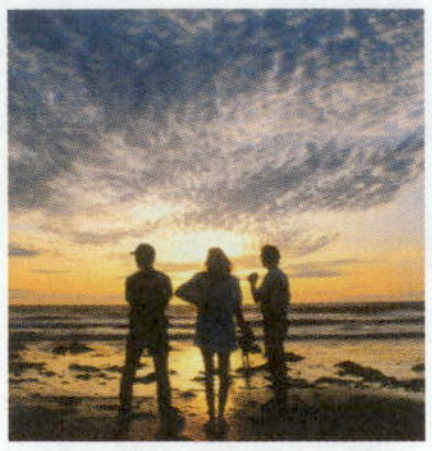

Section 5

PROBLEMS OF OXYGENATION: VENTILATION

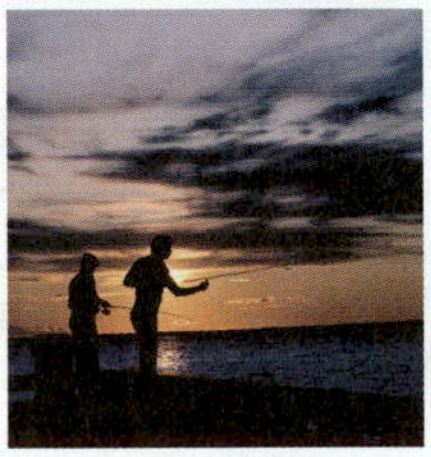

Section 6

PROBLEMS OF OXYGENATION: TRANSPORT

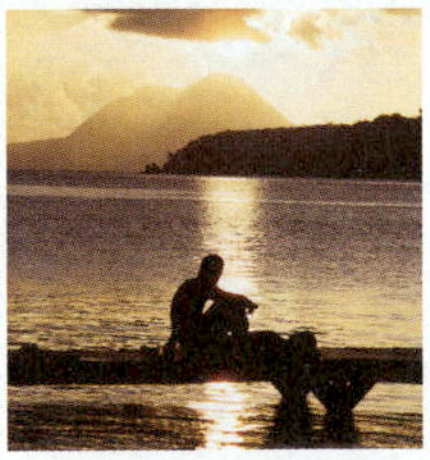

Section 7

PROBLEMS OF OXYGENATION: PERFUSION

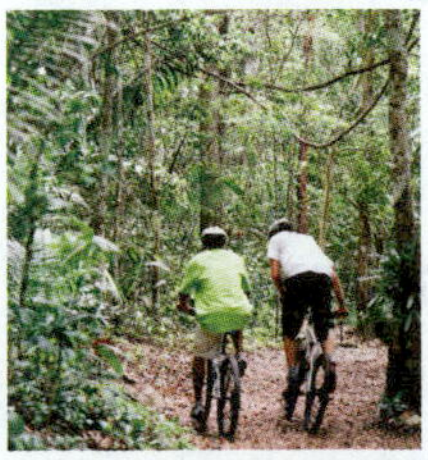

Section 8

PROBLEMS OF INGESTION, DIGESTION, ABSORPTION, AND ELIMINATION

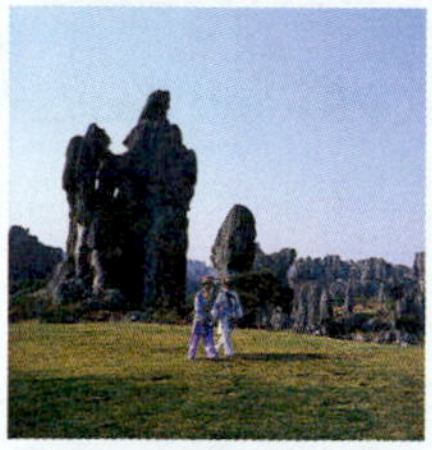

Section 9

PROBLEMS OF URINARY FUNCTION

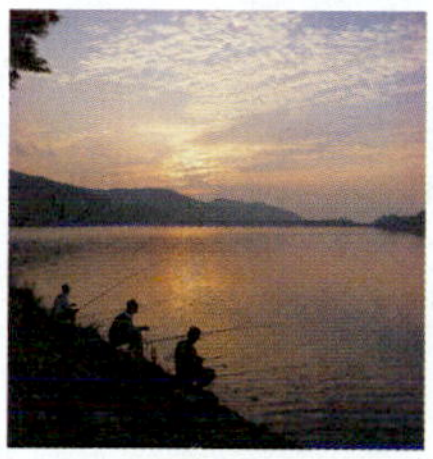

Section 10

PROBLEMS RELATED TO REGULATORY AND REPRODUCTIVE MECHANISMS

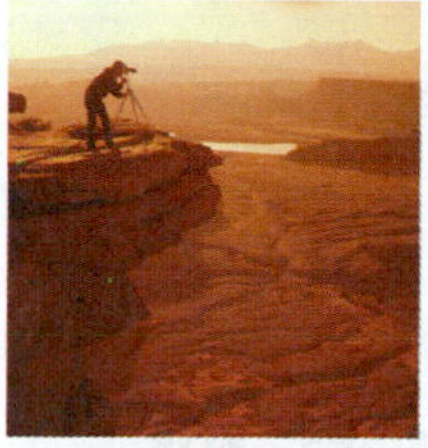

Section 11

PROBLEMS RELATED TO MOVEMENT AND COORDINATION

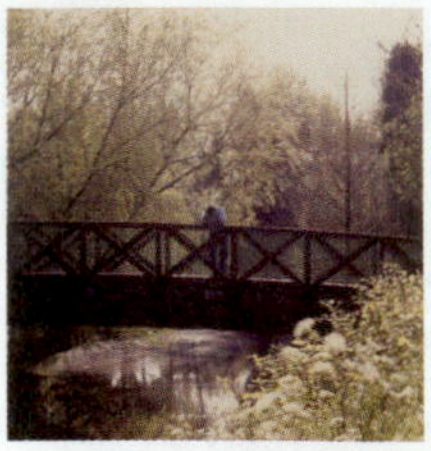

Section 12

NURSING CARE IN SPECIALIZED SETTINGS

Special Features

HEALTHY PEOPLE BOXES

GENDER DIFFERENCES BOXES

CULTURAL AND ETHNIC HEALTH DISPARITIES BOXES

COMPLEMENTARY AND ALTERNATIVE THERAPIES BOXES

EVIDENCE-BASED PRACTICE BOXES

GENETICS IN CLINICAL PRACTICE BOXES

ETHICAL DILEMMAS BOXES

COLLABORATIVE CARE TABLES

NUTRITIONAL THERAPY TABLES

PATIENT AND FAMILY TEACHING GUIDE TABLES

GERONTOLOGIC DIFFERENCES IN ASSESSMENT TABLES

EMERGENCY MANAGEMENT TABLES

NURSING CARE PLANS

COMMON ASSESSMENT ABNORMALITIES TABLES

DRUG THERAPY TABLES

Medical-Surgical Nursing

Volume 1

Assessment and Management of Clinical Problems

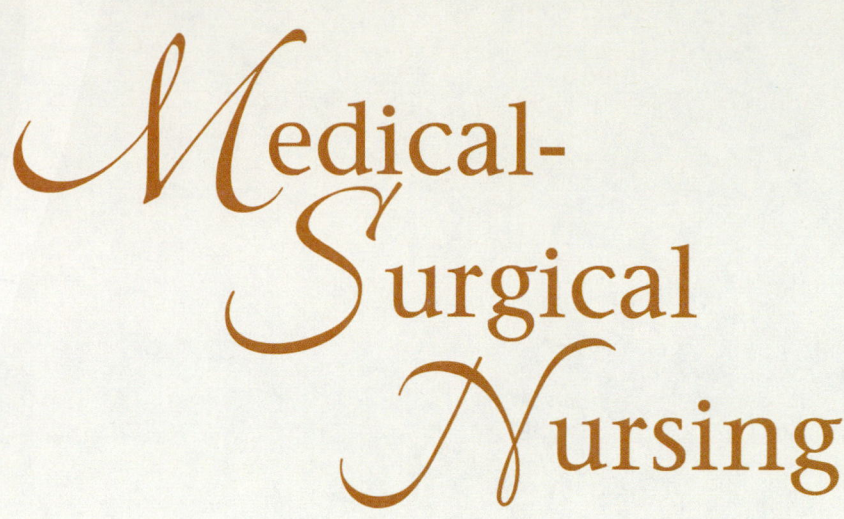

Section 1

Concepts in Nursing Practice

Section Outline

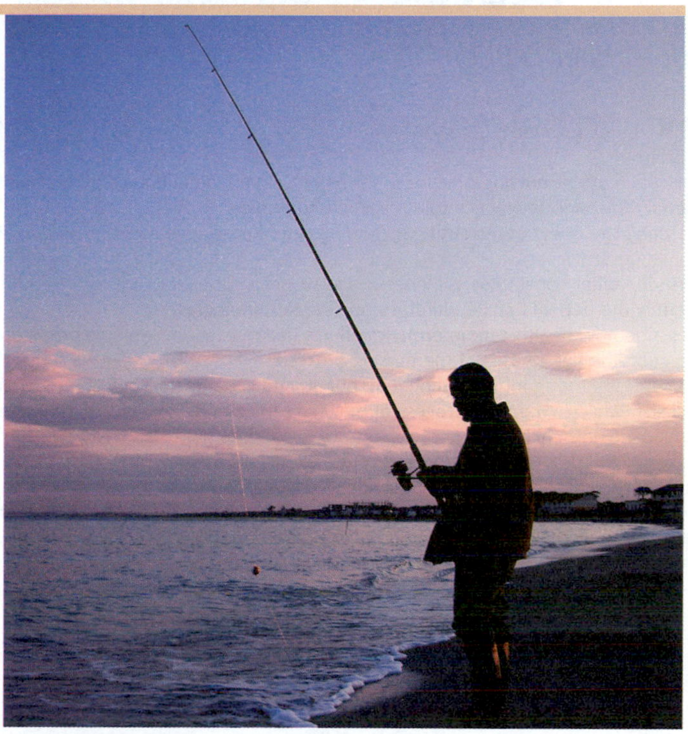

We cannot see tomorrow, but we have this day . . . to laugh, to hope, to love.

Susan Wheeler

1 Nursing Practice Today

Patricia Graber O'Brien

LEARNING OBJECTIVES

1. Describe current nursing practice in terms of domain, definitions, and recipients of care.
2. Identify the various practice roles available to nurses.
3. Describe the effect of increasing technology and knowledge and the *Healthy People* initiatives in future nursing practice.
4. Describe what constitutes evidence-based practice.
5. Identify the benefits of standardized nursing terminologies.
6. Describe how health care informatics affects health care and nursing practice.
7. Describe the five phases of the nursing process.
8. Distinguish among independent, dependent, and collaborative nursing functions.
9. Differentiate between the process of making a nursing diagnosis and a nursing diagnosis as a form of diagnostic nomenclature.
10. Describe the process of writing and selecting patient outcomes.
11. Identify the criteria for selecting nursing interventions.
12. Describe how standardized nursing terminologies for nursing diagnoses, patient outcomes, and nursing interventions can be linked to plan patient care.
13. Identify the places in the nursing process where evaluation is appropriate.

KEY TERMS

assessment, p. 9
clinical (critical) pathway, p. 16
collaborative problems, p. 12
concept map, p. 15
defining characteristics, p. 11
electronic health record (EHR), p. 8
evaluation, p. 9
evidence-based practice, p. 5
Healthy People, p. 5
implementation, p. 9
nursing, p. 3
nursing diagnosis, p. 9
nursing informatics, p. 9
nursing intervention, p. 13
nursing process, p. 9
patient outcomes, p. 12
planning, p. 9

Electronic Resources

Supplemental content related to Chapter 1 can be found . . .

Companion CD
- Stress-Busting Kit for Nursing Students
- NCLEX Examination Review Questions
- Comprehensive Glossary

Evolve Website
http://evolve.elsevier.com/Lewis/medsurg
- Content Updates
- Key Points (Printable and CD/MP3 Download)
- Concept Map Creator
- Expanded Audio Glossary
- Key Term Flash Cards
- Electronic Calculators
- Nursing Interventions Classification (NIC): Complete Listing
- Nursing Outcomes Classification (NOC): Complete Listing
- WebLinks

CURRENT NURSING PRACTICE

Domain of Nursing Practice

Nursing practice today is composed of a wide variety of roles and responsibilities necessary to meet the health care needs of society. Nurses are the frontline professionals of health care. They practice in virtually all health care settings and communities across the country. Never have nurses been more important to health care than they are today. Nurses offer skilled care to those recuperating from illness or injury, advocate for patients' rights, teach patients so that they can make informed decisions, support patients at critical times, and help them navigate the increasingly complex health care system (Fig. 1-1). Although the majority of nurses are employed in acute care facilities, many nurses practice in long-term care, home care, primary and preventive care, ambulatory clinics, and community health. Wherever nurses practice, recipients of their care include individuals, groups, families, or communities.

How the profession and society view nursing determines nursing's scope of practice. The social context from which nursing evolves determines what nursing skills and knowledge are needed or desired for the benefit of society.[1] A variety of professional and allied health care providers are concerned with the

Reviewed by Helen Wash Asbury, RN, ASN, BSHA, MSN, LNC, Nursing Instructor, Albuquerque (TVI) Community College, Albuquerque, N.Mex.

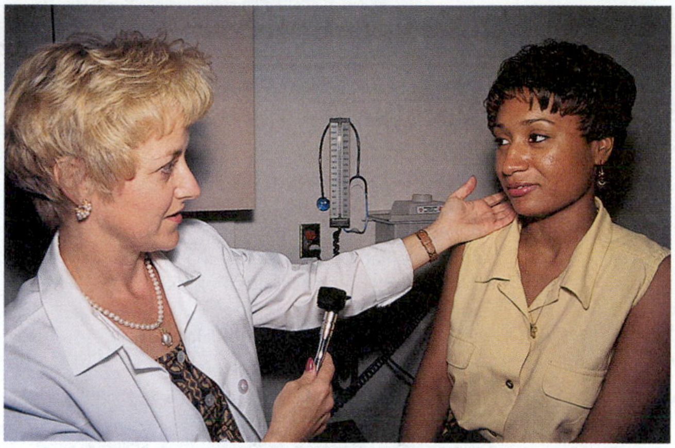

FIG. 1-1 Nurses are frontline professionals of health care.

health care needs of society. The unique focus of nursing is on the response of an individual or group to an actual or potential health problem or life process. For example, in caring for a person with a fractured hip, the nurse focuses on the patient's responses to immobility and pain. The physician's focus is the treatment and repair of the fracture. A physical therapist may provide treatments to restore mobility. However, the domain and scope of nursing practice are in a dynamic state. Nursing practice is continually evolving as society's needs change and knowledge and technology expand.

Definitions of Nursing

Several well-known definitions of nursing indicate that a basic theme of health, illness, and caring has existed since Florence Nightingale described nursing. Following are two such examples:

> **Nursing** is putting the patient in the best condition for nature to act (Nightingale).[2]
>
> The unique function of the nurse is to assist the individual, sick or well, in the performance of those activities contributing to health or its recovery (or to peaceful death) that he would perform unaided if he had the necessary strength, will, or knowledge. And to do this in such a way as to help him gain independence as rapidly as possible (Henderson).[3]

In 1980, the American Nurses Association (ANA) defined **nursing** as ". . the diagnosis and treatment of human responses to actual and potential health problems."[1] This widely accepted definition has been recently revised in the second edition of the ANA's *Nursing: A Social Policy Statement* to reflect the continuing evolution of nursing practice:

> **Nursing** is the protection, promotion, and optimization of health and abilities, prevention of illness and injury, alleviation of suffering through the diagnosis and treatment of human response, and advocacy in the care of individuals, families, communities, and populations.[1]

This definition reflects the increasing role of nurses in promoting health and wellness and advocating for the recipients of care.

Nursing's View of Humanity

Nursing's view of humanity must be considered when describing nursing. Although different terms have been used, there is widespread agreement among nursing theorists that an individual has physiologic (or biophysical), psychologic (or emotional), sociocultural (or interpersonal), spiritual, and environmental components or dimensions. In this text the human individual is considered "a biopsychosocial spiritual being in constant interaction with a changing environment."[4] The individual is composed of dimensions that are interrelated and not separate entities. Thus a problem in one dimension generally affects one or more of the other dimensions. Psychologic anxiety, for instance, affects the autonomic nervous system, a part of the biophysical dimension.

No two individuals are exactly alike. No one individual remains the same from moment to moment. Therefore each individual has value as an irreplaceable member of humanity. Inherent in this individuality is the right to develop one's unique potential according to a personal value system to the extent that the exercise of this right does not deny it to others.

The behavior of the individual is meaningful and oriented toward fulfilling needs, coping with stress, and developing one's self. At times, however, an individual needs help to meet these needs, to cope successfully, or to develop one's unique potential.

Nursing Roles

Entry-level nurses with an associate or baccalaureate degree in nursing are prepared to function as generalists. In this role nurses provide direct health care and focus on ensuring coordinated and comprehensive care to patients in a variety of settings. They work collaboratively with other health care providers to manage the needs of individuals and groups.[5] With continued experience and study, nurses may also specialize in an area of practice.

Professional recognition of expertise in a specialty area is obtained through **certification**. Certification in nursing specialties is offered through a variety of nursing organizations. It usually requires a certain amount of clinical experience and successful completion of an examination. Recertification usually requires ongoing clinical experience and some amount of continuing education. Nursing specialties include: ambulatory care; pain management; cardiovascular care; critical care; genetics nursing; and gerontologic, medical-surgical, perinatal, pediatric, psychiatric and mental health, and community health nursing.[6,7] An emerging specialty is forensic nursing, an area of nursing that addresses sexual assault, abuse, domestic violence, and death investigation.[8]

Additional formal education and experience can prepare nurses for advanced roles. An **advanced practice nurse** is a nurse with a master's degree in nursing, advanced education in pharmacology and physical assessment, and expertise in a specialized area of practice. Examples of advanced practice nurses are clinical nurse specialists, nurse practitioners, nurse midwives, and nurse anesthetists. In addition to managing and delivering direct patient care, advanced practice nurses have roles in health promotion, case management, administration, research, and multidisciplinary systems.[9] Table 1-1 identifies some specialty certifications available to both generalists and advanced practice nurses.

A new role for nurses has been introduced by the American Association of Colleges of Nursing (AACN) in response to patient care needs and in anticipation of competencies needed in the current and future health care system.[10] The new role is that of a clinical nurse leader (CNL). The clinical nurse leader is described as a generalist clinician with education at the master's degree level. The CNL oversees the care coordination of a distinct group of patients and actively provides direct patient care in complex situations. The CNL is different from other advanced

TABLE 1-1 Examples of Nursing Specialty Certifications

Certifications Requiring Valid Registered Nurse Licensure	Certifications Requiring Bachelor's Degree in Nursing or Related Field	Advanced Practice Certifications Requiring Master's or Higher Degree in Nursing
Addictions Nurse	First Assistant Nurse	**Nurse Practitioners (NPs)**
Ambulatory Care Nurse	Holistic Nurse	Acute Care NP (ACNP)
Ambulatory Perianesthesia Nurse	Home Health Nurse	Adult NP (ANP)
Cardiac/Vascular Nurse	Informatics Nurse	Adult Psychiatric and Mental Health NP
Critical Care Nurse	Nursing Administration	Advanced Diabetes Management NP
Diabetes Education Nurse	Nursing Professional Development	Family NP (FNP)
Dialysis Nurse	Occupational Health Nurse Specialist	Family Psychiatric and Mental Health NP
Emergency Nurse	Occupational Health Nurse Case Manager Specialist	Gerontological NP (GNP)
Flight Nurse	School Nurse	Palliative Care NP
Gastroenterology Nurse		Pediatric NP (PNP)
Gerontological Nurse		**Clinical Specialists (CSs)**
HIV/AIDS Nurse		CS in Adult Psychiatric and Mental Health Nursing
Hospice and Palliative Nurse		CS in Advanced Diabetes Management
Infection Control Nurse		CS in Child and Adolescent Psychiatric and Mental Health Nursing
Infusion Nurse		CS in Community Health Nursing
Inpatient Obstetric Nurse		CS in Gerontological Nursing
Low-Risk Newborn Nurse		CS in Home Health Nursing
Maternal Newborn Nurse		CS in Medical-Surgical Nursing
Medical-Surgical Nurse		CS in Palliative Care
Neonatal Intensive Care Nurse		CS in Pediatric Nursing
Nephrology Nurse		**Others**
Neuroscience Nurse		Advanced Nursing Administration
Nursing Case Management		Advanced Oncology Clinical Specialist
Occupational Health Nurse		Advanced Oncology NP
Occupational Health Nurse Case Manager		Advanced Practice Addictions Nurse
Oncology Nurse		Certified Nurse Midwife (CNM)
Ophthalmic Nurse		Clinical Nurse Leader
Orthopedic Nurse		Occupational Nurse Case Manager
Otorhinolaryngology Nurse		
Pain Management Nurse		
Pediatric Nurse		
Pediatric Oncology Nurse		
Perinatal Nurse		
Perioperative Nurse		
Plastic Surgical Nurse		
Postanesthesia Nurse		
Progressive Care Nurse		
Psychiatric and Mental Health Nurse		
Rehabilitation Nurse		
Sexual		
Assault		
Nurse Examiner Adult/Adolescent		
Telephone Nursing Practice		
Wound Ostomy Continence Nurse		

Sources: American Nurses Credentialing Center: *Specialty nursing practice certifications,* Washington, DC, 2003, The Center; Your guide to certification, *Am J Nurs 2005 Career Guide Supplement* 105(1):56, 2005.

practice nurses in that the CNL is a generalist in contrast with the specialized practice focus of clinical nurse specialists and nurse practitioners.

Delivery of Nursing Care

A variety of models have been used to deliver nursing care. *Team nursing* was the model of care used to provide inpatient care during the 1960s and 1970s. This model used a professional nurse as a *team leader*. The team leader planned and organized the care to be given to a group of patients by other professional nurses or nonprofessional health care workers such as licensed practical nurses and nursing assistants. Nursing shortages leading to the increased use of nonlicensed personnel have promoted the return of variations of this model in some care areas. *Primary nursing* was the model of the 1970s and 1980s. In this model one designated nurse was responsible for planning the patient's care and ensuring that all of the needs of the patient were met.

Managed care is the current health care delivery concept that evolved from the health care reform movement of the 1990s. Interdisciplinary or collaborative care is a component of managed care. Managed care involves *case management,* an approach that coordinates and links health care services to patients and their families. As a member of the interdisciplinary health care team, the nurse case manager coordinates the clinical care of the patient across care settings, from admission through discharge from the hospital, through other community agencies as needed, and back home in an effort to achieve optimal outcomes. (Case management is discussed in Chapter 7.) Today variations of different care delivery patterns are being used in view of nursing shortages, government-mandated nurse-patient ratios, and increased acuity of patient conditions.

INFLUENCES ON FUTURE NURSING PRACTICE

Expanding Knowledge and Technology

Rapidly changing technologies and dramatically expanding knowledge are increasing the responsibilities of nurses in a complex health care environment. Nurses are caring for patients with multiple health problems and widely diverse cultural and ethnic backgrounds in settings where there is a demand for high-quality, cost-effective care. Ethical dilemmas can be created by controversies regarding the use of new scientific knowledge and the inequality of access to technologically advanced health care. Access to the Internet allows patients to obtain information about their health problems and health care that may or may not be accurate and reliable. Nurses must be able to not only help patients find and use appropriate health care information, but also to evaluate information that relates to their own practice. In such a complex environment it is essential that nurses be able to think critically, problem solve, and make independent decisions that lead to the best outcomes for patients.

Critical thinking and methods to promote critical thinking have been subjects of concern for many professional practice fields affected by increasing technology and access to information. However, no standard definitions of critical thinking or methods of teaching and evaluating critical thinking have been accepted. One common definition of critical thinking developed by nurses states that **critical thinking** in nursing is an essential component of professional accountability and quality nursing care. Critical thinkers in nursing exhibit these habits of the mind: confidence, contextual perspective, creativity, flexibility, inquisitiveness, intellectual integrity, intuition, open-mindedness, perseverance, and reflection. Critical thinkers in nursing practice the cognitive skills of analyzing, applying standards, discriminating, information seeking, logical reasoning, predicting, and transforming knowledge.[11]

Whatever definition is accepted, critical thinking is a very important part of nursing practice. The complexity of care today requires the use of critical thinking to solve nursing problems for which there are no textbook answers or available resources. As greater demands are placed on the nursing profession by technology and information, only critical thinking will provide viable answers.

Healthy People Initiatives

Since 1979 the U.S. government has been active in establishing goals and objectives for promoting health and health care delivery for the nation. This activity is an initiative known as ***Healthy People.***[12] *Healthy People* is a broad-based program that involves government, private, public, and nonprofit organizations in preventing disease and promoting health. Individuals, groups, and organizations are encouraged to integrate *Healthy People* goals and focus areas into current programs, special events, publications, and meetings. These activities can further the health of all members of a community. The two overarching goals of the current *Healthy People* initiative are as follows:

Goal 1: Increase quality and length of healthy life

Goal 2: Eliminate health disparities[12]

Leading health indicators have been developed to measure and record progress toward the attainment of these goals. The 10 health indicators of *Healthy People 2010* reflect the major health concerns in the United States expected to be of importance in the first decade of the twenty-first century (Table 1-2). *Healthy People* boxes related to these leading health indicators and other areas of health outcomes are integrated throughout the book.

TABLE 1-2 Ten Major Health Issues for the Nation

1. Physical activity
2. Overweight and obesity
3. Tobacco use
4. Substance abuse
5. Responsible sexual behavior
6. Mental health
7. Injury and violence
8. Environmental quality
9. Immunization
10. Access to health care

Based on *Healthy People 2010: Leading Health Indicators.* Available at *www.healthypeople.gov*.

The *Healthy People* initiative is a big challenge for nursing. Both nursing education programs and clinical nursing practice must respond to the major trends in health care. Educational programs for entry-level nurses now require a greater emphasis on health promotion, maintenance, and cost-effective care that responds to the needs of culturally diverse groups and underserved populations. Evaluation of nursing programs must also measure the effectiveness of the program toward meeting the health objectives of the nation.[5] Today's nurses must address the identified health problems, developments in health care delivery, research outcomes, and new technologies. As a reflection of nursing's contract with society, nurses must be responsible for the improvement of the health status of the public and reduction of health disparities. (Health disparities are discussed in Chapter 2.)

Evidence-Based Practice*

If you could choose, would you rather have your health care based on the latest and best knowledge or would you rather be treated with traditional and ritualistic methods? Do you want to be a partner in the decisions made about your care or do you want someone else deciding what is best for you?

Evidence-based practice (EBP) is the conscientious use of the best evidence (i.e., findings from research, quality improvement and practice management initiatives, and patient assessment) in combination with clinician expertise and patient preferences and values in clinical decision making.[13] The expectation for high-quality, cost-effective care and the rapid expansion of easily accessible knowledge in a competing health care marketplace have driven the need for the daily use of evidence to improve point-of-service care (i.e., at the bedside). Regulatory and accrediting agencies (e.g., Joint Commission on Accreditation of Healthcare Organizations [JCAHO]) now require that practice be based on evidence. All of these factors have led to the need for all health care providers to gain knowledge and skill in EBP.

The impetus for EBP began when Archie Cochrane, a British epidemiologist, challenged health care providers' decision making regarding the management of women in preterm labor.[14] By carefully examining the results of a number of studies, Cochrane

*Material on evidence-based practice contributed by Ellen Fineout-Overholt, RN, PhD, and Alyce Schultz, RN, PhD, FAAN.

found that infant mortality rate was significantly decreased when corticosteroids were provided to high-risk women during labor. The synthesis of these research findings emphasized the ethical responsibility that all health care providers have to provide evidence-based care.[15]

EBP, in which synthesis of evidence is the key element, encompasses both research utilization and the conduct of research. In addition, EBP supports the appraisal, integration, and evaluation of both external evidence (i.e., generalizable studies) and internal evidence (i.e., population-specific data from quality improvement and practice management initiatives) to improve care. When there is no external evidence or the evidence is inconsistent or insufficient, health care providers need to partner with scientists to generate generalizable knowledge that supports best practice through the conduct of research.

Steps in the EBP Process. There are five steps in the EBP process (Table 1-3 and Fig. 1-2).

Step 1 of EBP. Step 1 of the EBP process is asking a clinical question in the PICO format. An example of a PICO question is, "In adult cardiac surgery patients (P) is morphine (I) or fentanyl (C) more effective in reducing postoperative pain (O)?" Formulating the clinical question is the most important and the most challenging step in the EBP process.[16] A clinical question that is searchable and answerable creates the context for integrating research findings, clinical judgment, and patient preferences. In addition, the question drives the search strategy and the type of evidence required to answer it.

Step 2 of EBP. Step 2 of the EBP process is an efficient search for and collection of evidence based on the question. The question directs the clinician to the databases that are the most appropriate. The search begins with the strongest external evidence to answer the question. Preappraised evidence such as systematic reviews and evidence-based guidelines are appropriate time-saving resources in the EBP process (Table 1-4). Systematic reviews of randomized controlled trials (RCTs) are considered the strongest level of evidence to answer questions about interventions (i.e., cause and effect). However, a limited number of systematic reviews are available to answer the many clinical questions. In addition, systemic reviews or meta-analyses may not always be the most appropriate to all clinically meaningful questions.

Evidence-based guidelines and reviews are an appropriate time-saving resource in the EBP process (see Table 1-4). If the clinical question is about how one experiences or copes with a health problem or lifestyle change, searching for a meta-synthesis of qualitative evidence may be the most appropriate approach. When there is insufficient research to guide practice, evidence from opinion leaders or authorities or reports from expert committees may be all that exist. This type of evidence should not be the sole substantiation for interventions. Care based on expert opinions requires diligent, ongoing, rigorous outcome evaluation to generate stronger evidence.

TABLE 1-3 Five Steps of the Evidence-Based Practice (EBP) Process

1. Ask the clinical question using the **PICO** format.
   P Patient population of interest
   I Intervention or area of interest
   C Comparison of interest or comparison group
   O Outcome(s) of interest
2. Collect the most relevant and best evidence.
3. Critically appraise and synthesize the evidence.
4. Integrate all evidence with one's clinical expertise, patient preferences, and values in making a practice decision or change.
5. Evaluate the practice decision or change.

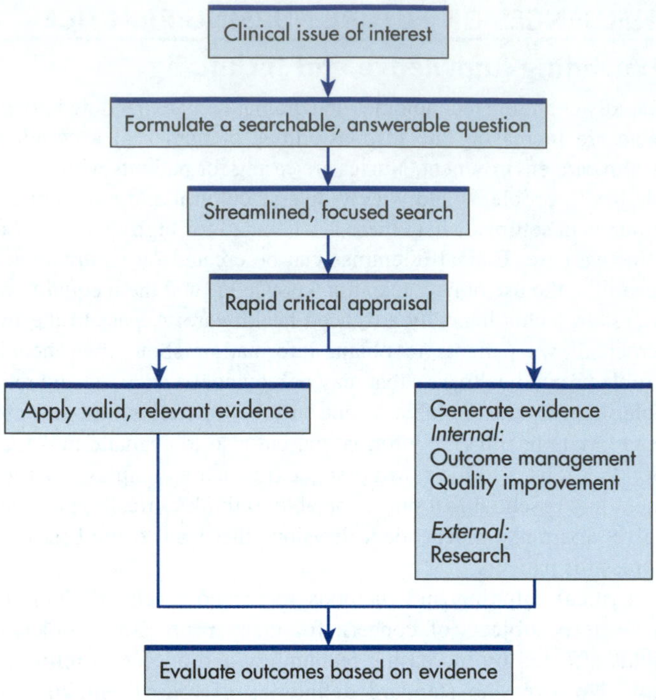

FIG. 1-2 Process of evidence-based practice.

Step 3 of EBP. Step 3 of the EBP process is critically appraising and synthesizing studies found in the search. A successful critical appraisal process focuses on three essential questions: (1) Are the results of the study valid? (2) What are the results? and (3) Are the findings clinically relevant to my patients? The purpose of critical appraisal is to determine the value of the research to practice and not only to examine the flaws of a study. Clinicians must determine the strength of the evidence and synthesize the findings related to the clinical question to conclude what is the best practice.

Step 4 of EBP. Step 4 of the EBP process may be different depending on the strength and breadth of the evidence to answer the question. Recommendations from sufficient, strong evidence (e.g., interventions with systematic reviews of well-designed RCTs) can be implemented into practice in combination with clinicians' expertise and patient preferences. Clinical judgment will influence how patient preferences and values are assessed, integrated, and entered into the decision-making process.[17] For example, although the evidence supports use of morphine as an effective analgesic, its use in a patient with renal failure may not be appropriate. In another example, although not supported by evidence, patients may be concerned about perceived addictive effects of morphine and prefer the use of fentanyl for their pain management. These types of decisions must be made with knowledge of the best available evidence, clinician judgment, and patients' perspective and values.

Without sufficient evidence, the fourth step would be to generate data to answer the question. Data can be gathered either through outcome management initiatives (i.e., internal evidence)

TABLE 1-4 Examples of Clinical Questions, Types of Evidence, and Where to Find It

Questions	Types of Evidence to Answer Question	Databases of Evidence
Therapy: In men with human immunodeficiency virus (HIV) infection, what is the effect of cognitive coping compared with emotional coping on mood, distress, and anxiety in response to worsening HIV symptoms?	Evidence-based guidelines Systematic review of randomized controlled trials (RCTs) Single RCT or group of RCTs	Cochrane Database of Systematic Reviews (CDSR) *(www.cochrane.org)* Database of Abstracts of Reviews of Effects (DARE) *(www.york.ac.uk/inst/crd/darehp.htm)* National Guideline Clearinghouse *(www.guideline.gov)*
Etiology: Are 30- to 50-year-old men who have high blood pressure at increased risk of stroke compared with men with normal blood pressure?	Cohort study	MEDLINE CINAHL
Diagnosis or diagnostic test: Is computed tomography (CT) scan more accurate than ultrasound in diagnosing appendicitis?	Randomized controlled trial Cohort study	Cochrane Database of Systematic Reviews (CDSR) Database of Abstracts of Reviews of Effects (DARE) National Guideline Clearinghouse MEDLINE CINAHL
Prevention: For obese women, does active involvement in an exercise support group reduce the risk of cardiovascular disease compared with participating in educational programs on lifestyle changes over a period of 5 years?	Prospective study RCT	MEDLINE CINAHL National Guideline Clearinghouse
Prognosis: Does dietary fat intake influence healthy weight maintenance (body mass index [BMI] <25 kg/m^2) in patients who have family history of obesity (BMI >30 kg/m^2)?	Cohort study Case-control studies	MEDLINE CINAHL
Meaning: How do women with children under 6 years of age with fibromyalgia perceive loss of motor function?	Qualitative study	MEDLINE CINAHL PsycINFO

Additional Resources for Evidence

Virginia Henderson Library *(www.nursinglibrary.org)*
Joanna Briggs Institute *(www.joannabriggs.edu)*
AHRQ Evidence-Based Practice Centers *(www.ahrq.gov)*
Registered Nurses Association of Ontario *(www.rnao.org)*

or through the conduct of rigorous research (i.e., external evidence). Clinicians need to partner with experts in research to achieve success in these endeavors.

Step 5 of EBP. Step 5 of the EBP process is evaluation of identified outcomes in the clinical setting. Outcomes must match the clinical project that has been implemented. For example, evaluating the cost of each medication when comparing effectiveness of morphine and fentanyl for pain control does not provide data about clinical effectiveness. Outcomes must reflect all aspects of the implementation and capture the interdisciplinary contributions elicited by the EBP process.

Implementation of EBP. To implement EBP, nurses must continuously seek scientific evidence that supports the care that they provide. The incorporation of evidence should be balanced with clinical expertise and should take into account the patient's unique circumstances and preferences. EBP closes the gap between research and practice, providing more reliable and predictable care than that which is based on tradition, opinion, and trial and error. It provides nurses with a mechanism to manage the explosion of new literature, introduction of new technologies, concern about health care costs, and increasing emphasis on quality and patient outcomes.

Throughout this book, evidence-based clinical practice guidelines are available for selected topics. The EBP boxes provide answers to specific clinical questions. The boxes contain the PICO question, critical appraisal of syntheses of evidence or primary studies, implications for nursing practice, and the source of the evidence. Evidence can support current practice and increase confidence that nursing care will continue to produce the desired outcome, or evidence may require a change in practice. In either case, it is important for nurses to be aware of the role of scientific evidence, their expertise and judgment, and patients' preferences and values in making clinical decisions about care.

Standardized Nursing Terminologies

The demands of the current health care system are challenging the nursing profession to define its practice and the impact that it has on the health and health care of individuals, families, and communities. The nursing profession is asking questions such as the following: What is it that nurses do? How do they do it? Does it make a measurable difference in the health of those they care for? How can nurses document care to identify what they do? What happens as a result of their care?

In response to these questions, nursing has moved toward standardizing nursing terminology. **Standardized nursing terminologies** are used to clearly define and evaluate nursing care. They can promote continuity of patient care and provide data that can support the credibility of the profession. Instead of using a wide variety of words and methods to describe the same patient problems and nursing care, a readily understood common language can improve communication among nurses. Standardized languages help identify the most effective nursing interventions as well.[18,19] Do the patient problems of pressure ulcer, decubitus ulcer, and skin breakdown all mean the same thing? Does turning the patient every 2 hours mean the same thing as repositioning the patient every 2 hours? And if the patient is turned or repositioned every 2 hours, what happens as a result? How are the results described? If a patient was placed on an air mattress, were the results different from one who was placed on a standard mattress and only turned? How do nurses know what works best? Using standardized languages, nurses can easily collect and analyze nursing data to identify the effectiveness of nursing interventions.

Standardized terminologies (also previously called *nomenclatures, languages, classification systems,* and *taxonomies*) offer ways to organize and describe nursing phenomena. Although philosophical debates exist concerning whether nursing needs one or more taxonomies considering the complexity of health care delivery, a number of classification systems are being developed. Table 1-5 lists the languages, or classification systems, recognized and approved by the ANA. The variety of languages that have been developed address different areas of nursing. The Omaha System and the Home Health Care Classification have been developed for community-based and home health care nursing, respectively. The Perioperative Nursing Dataset (discussed in Chapter 19) is used by perioperative nurses. The Nursing Management Minimum Data Set is available for use by nurse managers and administrators.

Three of the nursing terminologies recognized by the ANA are now available to consistently describe patient responses, nursing interventions, and patient outcomes: (1) NANDA International: Nursing Diagnoses, Definitions, and Classification; (2) the Nursing Interventions Classification (NIC); (3) and the Nursing Outcomes Classification (NOC). Each of these classification systems focuses on one component of the nursing process across all nursing specialties. Patients' responses or problems can be labeled using the nursing diagnoses classified and defined by NANDA.[20] Nursing interventions, or treatments, can be selected and implemented from NIC, which was developed by Dochterman and Bulechek at the University of Iowa College of Nursing.[21] Nursing-sensitive patient outcomes can be identified and evaluated by selecting appropriate NOC outcomes and indicators, which were identified and classified by Moorhead, Maas, and Johnson, also at the University of Iowa College of Nursing.[22] The use of these three classification systems in the nursing process and documentation are further described in this chapter and used throughout the text.

TABLE 1-5 ANA Recognized Nursing Terminologies

NANDA Nursing Diagnoses Definitions and Classifications 2005-2006
Nursing Interventions Classification (NIC)
Nursing Outcomes Classification (NOC)
Omaha System
Clinical Care Classification (CCC) (formerly Home Health Care Classification [HHCC])
Patient Care Data Set (PCDS)
Nursing Minimum Data Set (NMDS)
Nursing Management Minimum Data Set (NMMDS)
Perioperative Nursing Dataset (PNDS)
Systematized Nomenclature of Medicine Clinical Terminology (SNOMED CT®)
International Classification for Nursing Practice (ICNP®)
ABC codes
Logical Observation Identifiers Names and Codes (LOINC®)

Source: American Nurses Association: *Nursing information and data set evaluation center, ANA recognized terminologies that support nursing practice,* Washington, DC, 2005, American Nurses Association. Available at *www.nursingworld.org/nidsec/class1st.htm.*

Health Care Informatics

The current erratic and inconsistent use of paper records and computers to document, store, and retrieve patient care information is undergoing a major upheaval as federal initiatives promote the development of a uniform electronic health record. An **electronic health record (EHR)** is a computerized record of all of the health information related to an individual that can be electronically accessed by a variety of health care providers. The federal government currently plays a large part in the delivery and payment of health care for millions of Americans through Medicare, the armed services, and the Department of Veterans Affairs (VA). In an effort to provide one uniform health record to use throughout these services, the federal government is in the process of adopting EHR standards based on standards already used by the VA health care system.[23]

Patient records in the VA's electronic health system are fully electronic, portable, and readily accessible. The VA developed the EHR system to provide a single place for health care providers to review and update a patient's health record and to order medications, special procedures, x-rays, nursing orders, diets, and laboratory tests. All aspects of a patient's record are integrated, including active problems, allergies, current medications, laboratory results, vital signs, hospitalizations, and outpatient clinic history. The system also provides reminders, cautions, and remote data review. All electronic records require passwords to protect patient privacy.[23]

A national uniform EHR similar to the VA's health record has the potential of greatly reducing medical errors associated with traditional paper records and vastly improving patient safety and quality of care. It will allow all providers to more rapidly access patient-specific information and hopefully decrease the cost of health care. The goal of the government for EHRs is that uniform standards will be adopted throughout the health care industry that will lead to a national EHR for most Americans within the foreseeable future.

Part of a uniform EHR includes the use of a comprehensive, standardized medical vocabulary. One such standardized vocabulary is the Systematized Nomenclature of Medicine Clinical Terminology (SNOMED CT®) that is produced by the College of American Pathologists *(www.snomed.com).* In 2004 the federal government's licensure of SNOMED CT® made the vocabulary available, free of charge, to all health care providers through the National Library of Medicine.[24] Uses for SNOMED CT® include electronic medical records, intensive care monitoring, clinical decision support, medical research studies, clinical trials, computerized physician order entry, disease surveillance, and consumer health information services. The use of SNOMED CT® is of significant value to nursing in that SNOMED CT® includes the NANDA, NIC, and NOC terminologies of nursing.

Some current computer systems allow nurses to enter assessment data and interventions and record treatment and medication administration. However, with the use of SNOMED CT®, nursing diagnoses, interventions, and outcomes can be recorded with NANDA, NIC, and NOC (NNN) terminologies. It is possible to follow the links between diagnosis, interventions, and outcomes that will greatly advance EBP. For example, when choosing the NANDA diagnosis of *fatigue* on a computer, the code 00093 would be selected and entered into a database. Then the nurse would select the NOC outcome of *endurance* and the code 0001 would be incorporated into the database. The nurse would select the NIC interventions of *energy management (0180)* and *exercise promotion (0200)* and these codes would also be incorporated. The coded data can be separated from the patient's name, thus providing for the patient's anonymity and confidentiality.

Each piece of data that gets entered into the record can be tracked and reported on for many purposes. When nursing terminologies are used in information systems for documentation of nursing practice, nurses can track and report on the benefits of nursing care. This would serve not only to improve practice guidelines, but also to facilitate nursing research and easily demonstrate the effectiveness of nursing interventions. This will make nursing care visible while providing a continuing evaluation of nursing's efficacy.

Nursing Informatics. **Nursing informatics** is a nursing specialty integrating nursing science, computer science, and information science in identifying, collecting, processing, and managing data and information to support nursing practice, administration, education, research, and the expansion of knowledge.[25] This specialization in nursing allows for nurses to work within the information systems (IS) department so that nursing issues can be integrated at the beginning of computer projects rather than just evaluating the problems for nursing when a project is complete. Nursing informatics studies the structure and processing of nursing information to arrive at clinical decisions and to build systems to support and automate that processing. An informatics nurse has a diverse role that ranges from designing, developing, marketing, and testing to implementation, training, use, maintenance, evaluation, and enhancement of computer systems.

Nursing Process in Nursing Practice

The **nursing process** is an assertive, problem-solving approach to the identification and treatment of patient problems. It provides an organizing framework for the practice of nursing and the knowledge, judgments, and actions that nurses bring to patient care.[26] The nursing process requires cognitive (thinking, reasoning), psychomotor (doing), and affective (feelings, values) skills and abilities of the nurse.

Phases of the Nursing Process

The **nursing process** consists of five phases: assessment, diagnosis, planning, implementation, and evaluation (Fig. 1-3). These five phases of the nursing process are closely interrelated. For example, nurses may gather data about the wound condition (assessment) as they change a soiled dressing (implementation). There is, however, a basic order to the nursing process, beginning with assessment. **Assessment** is the collection of patient information on which to base the plan of care. Analysis of the assessment data and making a judgment about the nature of the assessment data usually follow immediately, resulting in a nursing diagnosis. **Nursing diagnosis** is the act of identifying and labeling human responses to actual or potential health problems/life processes. During **planning**, the nursing diagnosis directs the development of patient outcomes or goals and identification of nursing interventions to accomplish the outcomes. **Implementation** is the activation of the plan with the use of nursing interventions. Evaluation is a continuous activity in the nursing process. **Evaluation** determines if the patient outcomes have been met as a result of nursing interventions. If the outcomes were not met, a

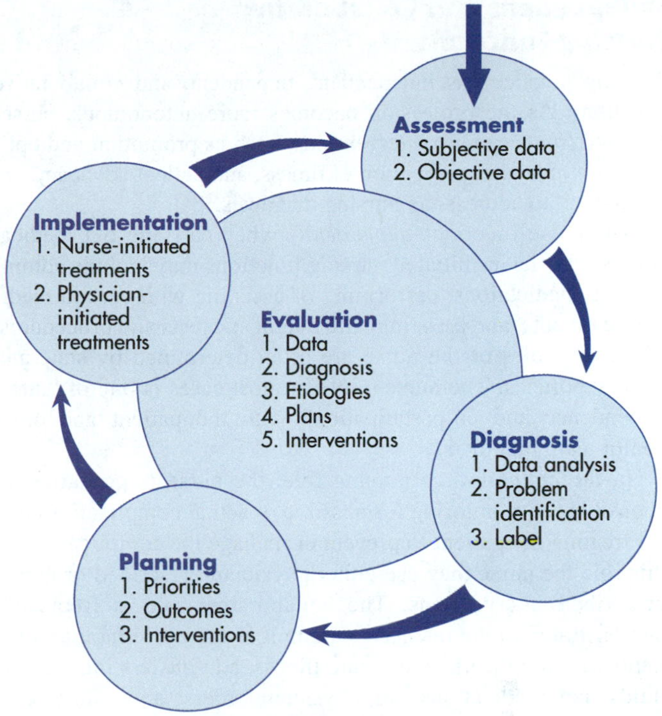

FIG. 1-3 Nursing process.

review of the steps of the process is necessary to determine why the outcomes were not met. Revision may be needed in the data collection method, the diagnosis, the patient outcomes, or the nursing interventions. Once begun, the nursing process is not only continuous but also cyclic in nature. There is no limit to the number of times the cycle can be reinitiated.

Application of the nursing process requires sound knowledge of the physical and behavioral sciences and a repertoire of intellectual, interpersonal, and technical skills. In the nursing process, the use of critical thinking skills is most important for the diagnosis phase. The interpretation of human responses is a complex undertaking and is frequently misjudged. Yet selection of the most appropriate nursing interventions based on the interpretation of human responses to achieve positive outcomes is the main reason people need and support nursing.

The nursing profession and the medical profession both use a problem-solving process in caring for a patient. The uniqueness of nursing's problem-solving approach stems from the goals of nursing and the means of accomplishing these goals. A comparison of the goals of medicine and nursing is made in Table 1-6.

TABLE 1-6 Comparison of Primary Goals: Nursing and Medicine

Nursing	Medicine
Determines responses to health problems, level of wellness, and need for assistance	Determines etiology of illness or injury
Provides physical care, emotional care, teaching, guidance, and counseling	Provides medical treatments and surgery
Interventions aimed at prevention and assisting the patient to meet his or her own needs	Interventions aimed at preventing and curing injury or illness

Independent and Collaborative Nursing Functions

Nursing practice has independent, dependent, and collaborative functions. As the profession becomes more autonomous, nurse-initiated *(independent)* interventions, such as promotion and optimization of health, prevention of illness, and patient advocacy, are carried out to address the nursing diagnosis.[21]

The nurse functions *dependently* when carrying out medical orders. Physician-initiated nursing functions may include administering medications, performing or assisting with certain medical treatments, and assisting with diagnostic tests and procedures. The exact roles of the nurse are often determined by state and agency policies. The nurse's role in most cases is one of "interdependence and co-participation" with the patient and other health team members.

In the *collaborative* nursing role, the nurse is primarily responsible for monitoring for possible or actual complications and for treating the patient to prevent or manage the complication. In this role the nurse may use either physician-prescribed or nurse-prescribed interventions. The collaborative role is frequently demonstrated in the intensive care unit as the nurse monitors patients for complications of acute illness, administers intravenous fluids and medications per physician orders, and implements nursing interventions such as providing emotional support or teaching about specific procedures.

ASSESSMENT PHASE

Data Collection

Accurate collection of data is the foundation for appropriate diagnosis, planning, and intervention (Fig. 1-4). A human being as a biopsychosocial spiritual being has needs and problems in all dimensions: biophysical, psychologic, sociocultural, spiritual, and environmental. A nursing diagnosis made without supporting data in all dimensions can lead to incorrect conclusions and depersonalized care. For example, a hospitalized patient who does not sleep all night may be mistakenly diagnosed as having a disturbed sleep pattern. In fact the patient may have worked nights his entire adult life and it is normal for him to be awake at night. Information concerning his sleep habits is necessary to individualize his care.

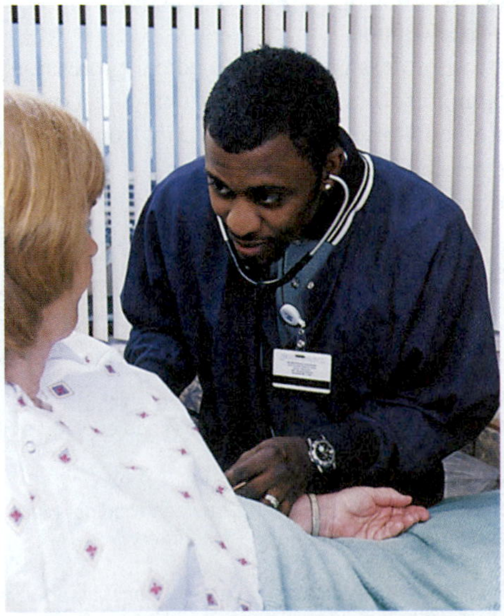

FIG. 1-4 Collection of data is a prerequisite to diagnosis, planning, and intervention.

Because nursing diagnoses and interventions are only as sound as the database on which they are formulated, it is critical that the database be accurate and complete. The use of a nursing database (discussed in Chapter 4) is recommended to facilitate the collection of data. When possible, information gained from sources such as the patient's record, other health care workers, the patient's family, and the nurse's observations should be validated with the patient. Likewise, when possible, questionable statements by the patient should be validated by a knowledgeable person.

DIAGNOSIS PHASE

Data Analysis and Problem Identification

The diagnosis phase begins with the clustering of information and ends with an evaluative judgment about a patient's health status. This evaluative judgment is reached after analysis of the assessment data. Analysis involves recognizing cues, sorting through and organizing or clustering the information, and determining patient strengths and unmet needs. The findings are then mentally compared with documented norms to determine whether anything is interfering or could interfere with the patient's needs or ability to maintain his or her usual health pattern. After a thorough analysis of all available information, the nurse makes a final judgment about the patient's health status. There may be no problems, needs, or life processes that require nursing intervention, or the patient may need nursing assistance to resolve a potential or an actual problem or life process. In addition, the patient may have an effective health status or function but expresses a desire for a higher level of wellness with which nursing can assist.

Nursing Diagnosis

Throughout this book, the term *nursing diagnosis* will mean (1) the process of identifying actual and potential health problems/life processes and (2) the label or concise statement that describes "a clinical judgment about an individual, family, or community response to actual or potential health problems/life processes. A nursing diagnosis provides the basis for the selection of nursing interventions to achieve outcomes for which the nurse is accountable."[20]

It is important to remember that not all conclusions resulting from data analysis lead to nursing diagnoses. Nursing diagnoses describe health states that nurses can legally diagnose and treat. Data may also point to collaborative problems that nurses treat with other health care providers. During the diagnostic process the nurse identifies both nursing diagnoses and collaborative problems that necessitate nursing intervention.

NANDA Nursing Diagnoses. NANDA International is a nursing organization that has been developing a standardized nursing terminology for identifying, defining, and classifying patients' actual or potential responses to health problems since 1973. The two main purposes of NANDA are to develop a diagnostic classification system *(taxonomy)* and to identify and accept nursing diagnoses. In selecting a nursing diagnosis for a patient from the NANDA list, the nurse labels the patient's responses in a language that specifically identifies and defines the patient's problem for other nurses and health care providers. In addition, the use of the standardized terminology of nursing diagnoses documents the analysis, synthesis, and accuracy required in making a nursing diagnosis. It verifies nursing's contribution to cost-effective, efficient, quality health care.

The current NANDA nursing diagnoses are listed in Appendix B. Each nursing diagnosis has an assigned code number facilitating its use in computerized documentation. The nursing diagnoses used in this textbook are NANDA approved. The NANDA list is continually evolving as research results are interpreted and as nurses identify new human responses. Revisions of accepted nursing diagnoses and new diagnoses may be submitted to NANDA by individual nurses or nursing groups. For information on submitting diagnostic material contact NANDA, 1211 Locust St., Philadelphia, Pennsylvania, 19107; 800-647-9002; also available at *www.nanda.org.*

Diagnostic Statements

Nursing diagnostic statements may be written as one-part, two-part, or three-part statements. One-part statements are used for *wellness* nursing diagnoses. A wellness diagnosis may be identified when an individual is in transition from a specific level of wellness to a higher level of wellness. A wellness diagnosis contains the label only. The label begins with "Readiness for enhanced," followed by the higher level wellness desired. An example of a wellness diagnosis is, "Readiness for enhanced nutrition." A two-part statement identifying only the problem and etiology is acceptable if the signs and symptoms data are easily accessible to other nurses caring for the patient. An example of this type of statement is, "Imbalanced nutrition: less than body requirements *related to* limited income for food purchases." *Risk* nursing diagnoses are also two-part statements because signs and symptoms are not present. An example is, "Risk for aspiration *related to* impaired swallowing." Use of a three-part statement is recommended during the learning process. The three-part statement identifies the critical thinking process that occurs in making the judgment about the patient's health status. When written as a three-part statement, the problem–etiology–signs and symptoms (PES) format is used.[26,27]

Problem (P): the nursing diagnosis label; the term that reflects the pattern of cues (e.g., pain)

Etiology (E): a brief description of the probable cause of the problem; contributing or related factors (e.g., related to surgical incision, localized pressure, edema)

Signs and symptoms (S): a list of the cluster of the objective and subjective data that lead the nurse to pinpoint the problem; critical, major, or minor defining characteristics (e.g., as evidenced by verbalization of pain, isolation, withdrawal)

It is important to remember that gathering the "S" comes first in the diagnostic process, even though the format has been described as PES.

Identifying the Problem. The nursing diagnoses accepted by NANDA International were originally organized as Taxonomy I using a modification of Gordon's functional health patterns (FHPs).[28] A new taxonomy, Taxonomy II, has been developed by NANDA International. Currently the NANDA, NIC, and NOC groups are working on one common organizing structure in which diagnoses, interventions, and outcomes can be placed together to facilitate their clinical use.[29] In this textbook, Gordon's 11 functional health patterns are used as a framework for nursing assessment and nursing diagnoses. Gordon's functional health patterns are discussed in Chapter 4 and compared with NANDA's Taxonomy II (see Table 4-3).

Taxonomy is simply the classification of things into an ordered system based on natural relationships. Scientists, informaticists, and database managers are the primary users of the taxonomic structure of nursing diagnoses, but the framework is useful to guide identification of problems or needs when clustering common patterns of responses. For example, assessment of a patient with heart failure reveals that the patient has dyspnea, shortness of breath, weakness, and increase in heart rate on exertion, and the patient says, "I feel too weak to do anything." These data are reflective of activity-rest and cardiovascular-pulmonary function. Nursing diagnoses classified in Gordon's activity-exercise FHP or NANDA Taxonomy II's domain of activity/exercise will probably be the most appropriate for this patient. In this case, the nurse could tentatively identify a nursing diagnosis label of activity intolerance, fatigue, or ineffective breathing pattern as the patient's response to the heart disease. To validate any of these nursing diagnoses the nurse should read, or be familiar with, the definitions and defining characteristics of the specific diagnoses to verify that the selected diagnostic labels match the descriptions provided.[20,26]

Etiology. The etiology of a nursing diagnosis is identified in the diagnostic statement. The etiology, or cause, of the problem provides direction for managing the problem. The etiology can be a pathophysiologic, maturational, situational, or treatment-related factor, but should be something that nursing can treat.[26,27] The etiology may be identified as secondary to a medical problem, but a medical diagnosis should not be the primary etiology. The etiology is written after the diagnostic label. These two components are separated by the phrase "*related to*." For example, in NCP 1-1 the nursing diagnosis is "Activity intolerance *related to* fatigue secondary to cardiac insufficiency and pulmonary congestion." The etiology directs the nurse to select the appropriate interventions to modify the factor of fatigue. The treatment of the cardiac insufficiency and pulmonary congestion is not within nursing's practice domain. When the etiology is not included in the diagnosis, the nurse is not able to plan the correct intervention to treat the specific cause of the problem.

When the etiology is unknown, the statement reads "*related to* unknown etiology." When identifying risk nursing diagnoses, the specific risk factors present in the patient's situation are identified as the etiology. Multiple etiologies become more common as expertise in the use of nursing diagnoses increases. There is often no single cause of a problem. Many nursing diagnoses presented in the nursing care plans of this book contain multiple etiologies. They can be used as a checklist of possible related factors to be considered when determining the nursing diagnosis specific to an individual patient.

Signs and Symptoms. Signs and symptoms, also called **defining characteristics,** are the clinical cues that, in a cluster, indicate the nursing diagnosis.[20] *Critical* defining characteristics must be present in the assessment data to make an accurate nursing diagnosis. *Major* defining characteristics are those signs or symptoms that are usually present when the diagnosis exists. At least one critical defining characteristic or one major defining characteristic must be present to have an actual nursing diagnosis. *Minor* defining characteristics have also been identified and are evidence of a possible nursing diagnosis. The signs and symptoms are included in the diagnostic statement using the phrase "as evidenced by." The complete nursing diagnostic statement in NCP 1-1 is, "Activity intolerance *related to* fatigue secondary to cardiac insufficiency and pulmonary congestion *as evidenced by* dyspnea,

NURSING CARE PLAN 1-1

Patient with Heart Failure*

NURSING DIAGNOSIS **Activity intolerance** *related to* fatigue secondary to cardiac insufficiency and pulmonary congestion *as evidenced by* dyspnea, shortness of breath, weakness, increase in heart rate on exertion, and patient's statement, "I feel too weak to do anything."

PATIENT GOAL Will achieve a realistic program of activity that balances physical activity with energy-conserving activities

OUTCOMES (NOC)

Activity Tolerance

(*Definition:* Physiologic response to energy-consuming movements with daily activities)

- Pulse rate with activity ___
- Oxygen saturation with activity ___
- Respiratory rate with activity ___
- Systolic BP with activity ___
- Diastolic BP with activity ___
- Electrocardiogram findings ___
- Skin color ___
- Ease of performing ADLs ___

Measurement Scale

1 = Severely compromised
2 = Substantially compromised
3 = Moderately compromised
4 = Mildly compromised
5 = Not compromised

INTERVENTIONS (NIC) and *RATIONALES*

Energy Management

(*Definition:* Regulating energy used to treat or prevent fatigue and optimize function)

- Encourage alternate rest and activity periods *to reduce cardiac workload.*
- Provide calming diversionary activities *to promote relaxation to reduce O_2 consumption and to relieve dyspnea and fatigue.*
- Monitor patient's oxygen response (e.g., pulse rate, cardiac rhythm, and respiratory rate) to self-care or nursing activities *to determine level of activity that can be performed.*
- Teach patient and significant other techniques of self-care *that will minimize oxygen consumption (e.g., self-monitoring and pacing techniques for performance of ADLs).*

Activity Therapy

(*Definition:* Prescription of and assistance with specific physical, cognitive, social, and spiritual activities to increase the range, frequency, or duration of an individual's activity)

- Assist to choose activities consistent with physical, psychologic, and social capabilities *to determine level of activity that can be performed.*
- Collaborate with occupational, physical, and/or recreational therapists *to plan and monitor activity/exercise program.*
- Determine patient's commitment to increasing frequency and/or range of activity *to provide patient with obtainable goals.*

ADLs, Activities of daily living; *BP,* blood pressure; *NIC,* Nursing Interventions Classification; *NOC,* Nursing Outcomes Classification.
*The complete nursing care plan for heart failure is NCP 35-1 on pp. 836 to 838).

shortness of breath, weakness, increase in heart rate on exertion, and patient's statement, 'I feel too weak to do anything.' "

Collaborative Problems

Collaborative problems are potential or actual complications of disease or treatment that nurses treat with other health care providers, most frequently physicians.[27] During the diagnosis phase of the nursing process, the nurse identifies these risks for physiologic complications in addition to nursing diagnoses. Identification of collaborative problems requires knowledge of pathophysiology and possible complications of medical treatment. For example, collaborative problems for the patient with heart failure in NCP 1-1 could include pulmonary edema, hypoxemia, dysrhythmias, and/or cardiogenic shock.[27] In the interdependent role, nurses use both physician-prescribed and nursing-prescribed interventions to prevent, detect, and manage collaborative problems.

Collaborative problem statements are usually written as "potential complication: _____" or "PC: ______" without a "*related to*" statement. An example is PC: pulmonary embolism. When potential complications are used in this textbook, "*related to*" statements have been added to increase understanding and relate the potential complication to possible causes.

PLANNING PHASE

Priority Setting

After the nursing diagnoses and collaborative problems are identified, the nurse must determine the urgency of the identified problems. Diagnoses of the highest priority require immediate intervention. Those of lower priority can be addressed at a later time. When setting priorities, the nurse should first intervene for life-threatening problems involving airway, breathing, or circulation (ABCs). Physical needs should be met before psychosocial needs.

It is also helpful to determine the patient's perception of what is important. When the patient's priorities are not congruent with the actual situation, the nurse may need to give explanations to help the patient understand the need to do one thing before another. Often it is more efficient to meet the patient's priority need before moving on to other priorities.

Identifying Outcomes

After priorities are established, outcomes for the patient are identified. **Patient outcomes** describe to what degree the patient's response identified in the nursing diagnosis should be prevented or changed as a result of nursing care. Moorhead, Johnson, and Maas of the Iowa Outcomes Project define a *nursing-sensitive patient outcome* as "an individual, family, or community state, behavior, or perception that is measured along a continuum in response to a nursing intervention(s). Each NOC outcome has an associated group of indicators that are used to determine patient status in relation to the outcome."[22] Outcomes should be set with the patient, if feasible, just as priorities of interventions are considered with the patient when possible (Fig. 1-5). In some practice areas the term *patient goals* may be substituted for *patient outcomes* to reflect the desired state of function or health. However, the setting of more specific outcomes with outcome indicators is necessary for systematic measurement of the patient's progress.

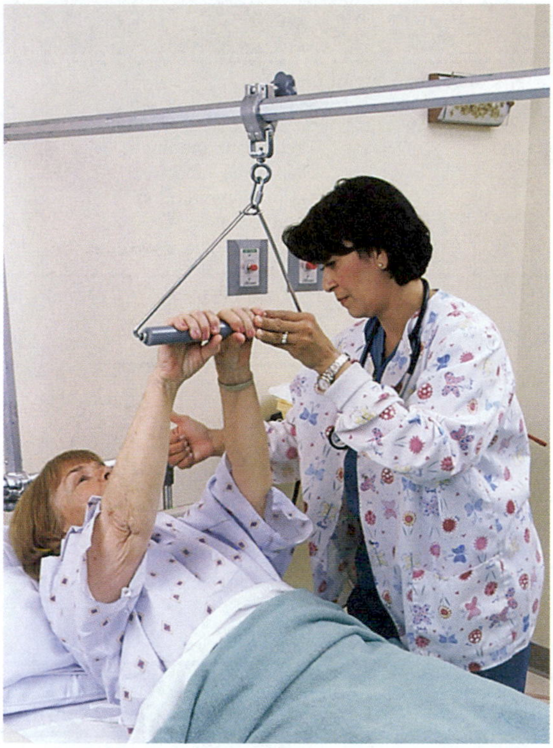

FIG. 1-5 Cooperation between the patient and the nurse is necessary in setting patient outcomes.

Outcomes may be developed using two methods: writing specific outcome statements or choosing outcomes from the Nursing Outcomes Classification (NOC). The nurse may write patient outcomes by describing desired, realistic, measurable patient behaviors to be accomplished by a specific date. For example, a short-term outcome for the patient in NCP 1-1 might be, "The patient will maintain normal vital signs in response to activity in 2 days," whereas a long-term expected outcome might be, "The patient will identify a realistic activity level to achieve or maintain by discharge." However, these statements provide no criteria by which to measure the patient's degree of progress from admission to discharge. If the outcomes are not met, the nurse has no way of knowing how close or how far the patient was from achieving the outcome. In addition, outcomes or patient goals written by individual nurses create nonstandardized data that cannot be used in research to determine what nursing interventions are most effective in reaching desired outcomes.[22]

Nursing Outcomes Classification (NOC). A research-based, standardized language for nursing outcomes, *Nursing Outcomes Classification (NOC),* has been developed to evaluate the effects of nursing interventions. NOC is a list of "concepts, definitions, and measures that describe patient outcomes influenced by nursing interventions."[22] Currently over 300 coded outcomes have been organized into 7 domains and 29 classes *(www.nursing.uiowa.edu/noc/).* Each outcome has a label, a definition, a set of specific indicators to be used in rating the outcomes, and a five-point scale for rating the overall outcome and the specific indicators.

For example, in NCP 1-1 the NOC *label* is activity tolerance and is *defined* as physiologic response to energy-consuming movements with daily activities.[22] The *indicators* describe the specific status of the patient in relation to the outcome. By choosing specific indicators that are listed with a given outcome, the nurse selects the criteria for evaluating the outcome and the effects of nursing interventions. Some indicators that might be appropriate to measure the outcome of activity tolerance for NCP 1-1 include pulse rate with activity, ease of breathing with activity, or walking pace. The five-point measurement scale to rate the outcome is as follows: 1 = severely compromised, 2 = substantially compromised, 3 = moderately compromised, 4 = mildly compromised, 5 = not compromised.

The measurement scale included with each outcome is constructed so that the fifth point of the scale is the most desirable condition relative to that outcome. Using the measurement scale, the nurse can rate each indicator for a particular patient at any given period of time. When a patient's baseline is established by an initial rating of the indicators, the nurse can monitor the overall progression of the patient over time. By going back after the interventions are applied and rating each indicator on the scale of 1 through 5, the nurse can evaluate the effect of the intervention on the outcome.

It is important to understand that NOC outcomes are *not* prescriptive. Because they are neutral labels, they are not expected patient outcomes. However, they can be individualized for a patient and translated into expected patient outcomes by identifying a desired state on the measurement scale. An example of a short-term expected outcome using NOC for the patient in NCP 1-1 might be, "Patient will have activity tolerance at a level of 3, moderately compromised, on all selected indicators in 2 days." A long-term expected outcome might be, "Patient will have activity tolerance at a level of 4, mildly compromised, on all selected indicators by discharge."

Determining Interventions

After patient outcomes are identified, nursing interventions should be planned. A **nursing intervention** is any treatment, based on clinical judgment and knowledge, that a nurse performs to enhance patient outcomes.[21] Nursing interventions include both direct and indirect care; nurse-initiated treatments resulting from nursing diagnoses; physician-initiated treatments resulting from medical diagnoses; and daily, essential activities that the patient cannot perform independently (Table 1-7). When choosing an intervention the nurse should consider the following:[21]

1. Desired patient outcomes
2. Etiology of the nursing diagnosis
3. Clinical practice guidelines developed from evidence-based summaries
4. Scientific principles from behavioral and biologic sciences
5. Feasibility of successfully implementing the intervention
6. Acceptability to the patient
7. Capability of the nurse

In addition, the nurse must use ingenuity, intuition, creativity, and past experience when tailoring a plan to meet a patient's needs. Factors such as availability of help and equipment must also be considered. The final selection of interventions should also include

TABLE 1-7 Examples of Nursing Interventions to Treat Health Care Problems

Intervention	Nursing Activities
Nurse-initiated treatments	Encourage patient to cough and deep breathe
Physician-initiated treatments	Administer medications
Essential activity patient cannot perform independently	Provide range-of-motion exercise

TABLE 1-8 Example of NANDA-NOC-NIC Linkage

NANDA Nursing Diagnosis: *Impaired skin integrity:* A state in which the individual has altered epidermis and/or dermis

NANDA-Related Factors	NOC Outcomes	NIC Interventions
Pressure	Tissue integrity: Skin and mucous membranes	Pressure management Skin surveillance
Nutritional deficit	Nutritional status: Food and fluid intake	Nutrition monitoring Nutrition therapy
Knowledge deficit	Knowledge: Illness care	Teaching: Disease process

NANDA, North American Nursing Diagnosis Association; *NIC,* Nursing Interventions Classification; *NOC,* Nursing Outcomes Classification.

the patient's choices when possible. The patient or the patient's family often has a wealth of information about measures that were successful or unsuccessful in the past. Significant time and effort are saved by asking the patient what has been tried and discarded as ineffective.

Nursing Interventions Classification (NIC). *Nursing Interventions Classification (NIC)* is the third standardized nursing terminology that focuses on the nursing process. NIC includes independent and collaborative interventions that nurses carry out, or direct others to carry out, on behalf of patients.[21] It includes treatments that nurses perform in all settings and in all specialties. NIC identifies both physiologic and psychosocial interventions, as well as interventions for health promotion, illness prevention, and illness treatment. It provides a common language for communication among nurses. Because each intervention has a coded number, the use of NIC interventions facilitates computer collection of standardized nursing data to evaluate the effectiveness of the interventions.

NIC includes over 500 interventions with a label name, a definition, and a set of activities for the nurse to choose from in order to carry out the intervention. The interventions are grouped into 7 domains and 30 classes *(www.nursing.uiowa.edu/nic).* Although over 500 interventions may seem overwhelming, nurses soon discover those interventions that are used most often in their particular specialty or with their patient population.[21] When planning care for a patient, the nurse chooses specific interventions from the domain or class that is appropriate for the patient based on the nursing diagnosis and patient outcomes. A group of activities is listed for each intervention, and the nurse can select the appropriate activities from the list to implement the intervention.

For example, in NCP 1-1 the *labels* of energy management and activity therapy are used to describe the interventions selected for the patient. Energy management is *defined* as regulating energy use to treat or prevent fatigue and optimize function. Activity therapy is *defined* as prescription of and assistance with specific physical, cognitive, social, and spiritual activities to increase the range, frequency, or duration of an individual's activity. From a set of 42 activities, 4 have been chosen to implement the intervention of energy management. From a set of 27 activities, 3 have been chosen to implement the intervention of activity therapy.

NIC does *not* prescribe interventions for specific situations. The nurse is responsible for making the important decision of when to use an intervention and for whom. Nurses need to select the appropriate intervention based on their knowledge of the patient and the patient's condition.

NANDA-NOC-NIC Linkages

NANDA, NOC, and NIC can be linked to illustrate how the three distinct nursing terminologies can be connected and used together when planning care for patients.[29] The determination of a nursing diagnosis, projection of a desired outcome, and selection of interventions to achieve the desired outcome may be assisted by use of the linkages. An example of a NANDA-NOC-NIC (NNN) linkage is found in Table 1-8. The integration of NANDA, NIC, and NOC into the nursing process is illustrated in Fig. 1-6.

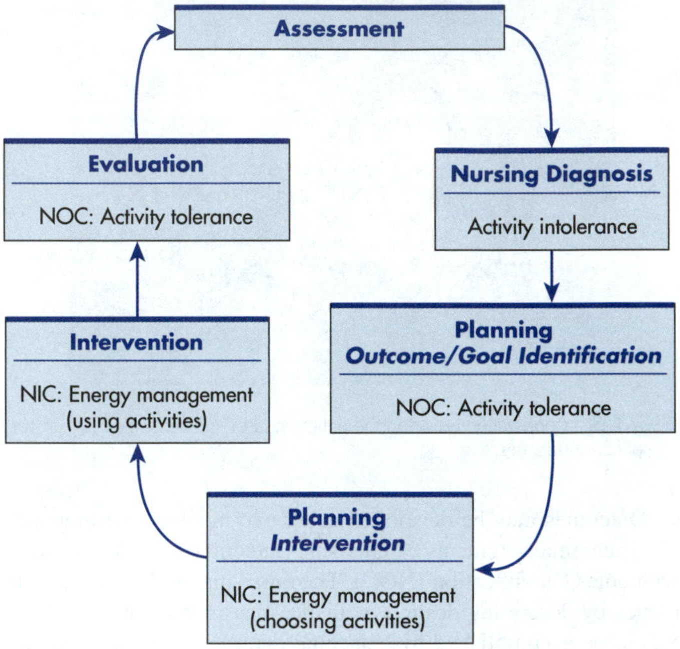

FIG. 1-6 Integration of NANDA, NIC, and NOC into the nursing process.

The linkages that have been developed are only guides for planning care. They do not alter the critical thinking that nurses must use in making decisions about patient care. The nurse must continually evaluate the situation and revise the diagnoses, outcomes, and interventions to fit each patient's unique needs. All of the nursing care plans throughout the text illustrate the NNN linkages.

IMPLEMENTATION PHASE

Carrying out the specific, individualized plan constitutes the implementation phase of the nursing process. The nurse performs the activities of interventions or may delegate activities and supervise others who are qualified to intervene. Delegation is the transfer of responsibilities for the performance of an activity from one person to another while retaining accountability for the outcome.[30]

Delegation of nursing interventions to licensed practical nurses/licensed vocational nurses (LPNs/LVNs) and unlicensed assistive personnel (UAP) is an important function of the professional nurse. LPNs/LVNs have a scope of practice and standards of practice that are defined by the state nursing practice act and regulated by state agencies. The professional nurse must know the local legal scope of practical/vocational nursing practice and delegate nursing functions appropriately. In most states LPNs/LVNs may administer medications, perform sterile procedures, and provide a wide variety of interventions planned by the professional nurse.

An **unlicensed assistive personnel (UAP)** is an unlicensed individual who is trained to function in an assistive role to the professional nurse. The term may include nursing aides, orderlies, assistants, attendants, or technicians. Professional nurses are responsible for defining and supervising the education, training, and use of UAP in providing direct patient care. It is also the responsibility of the professional nurse to use professional judgment to determine appropriate activities to delegate based on the needs of patients, the education and training of the nursing and assistive staff, and the extent of supervision required.[30] Nursing interventions that require independent nursing knowledge, skill, or judgment, such as assessment, patient teaching, and evaluation of care, cannot be delegated.

Throughout the implementation phase the nurse must evaluate the effectiveness of the method chosen to implement the plan. For example, in NCP 1-1, while implementing activity therapy, the nurse may find that the patient's pulse rate in response to activity has not changed since the initial assessment. The nurse may determine that a change in the interventions of activity therapy or in energy management may be necessary to meet the patient's outcomes.

Another example involves the evaluation of the use of a nursing assistant to help a patient perform postmastectomy exercises that were taught by the professional nurse. The nurse assumes the direct care of the patient when the evaluation finds that the patient is more depressed than anticipated and would benefit from care by the nurse who is knowledgeable about changes in body image. The exercise plan might remain the same, but the person implementing the plan would be different and would use different skills to carry out the plan. Referrals to other professionals, such as clinical nurse specialists, may also be made when the nurse anticipates that expertise in specialized areas is required to help the patient.

EVALUATION PHASE

The diagram of the nursing process (see Fig. 1-3) indicates that evaluation is continuous throughout the process and is essentially assessment at different points in time. When evaluation occurs as the last phase in the nursing process, the nurse determines if the patient's outcomes have been met. If not, the process is reviewed from the beginning. The nurse evaluates whether sufficient assessment data were obtained to support the identified nursing diagnosis. The diagnosis is, in turn, evaluated for accuracy. For example, was the pain actually related to the wound itself or related to pressure from a constricting dressing? Next the nurse evaluates whether the patient outcomes and nursing interventions were realistic, measurable, and achievable. If not, revision of patient outcomes and interventions is necessary. The effectiveness of each intervention and its contribution to progress toward the expected patient outcome is also evaluated. As a result of evaluation, the nurse determines whether the plan should be maintained, modified, discontinued, or referred to another health care professional.

DOCUMENTATION

Documentation provides evidence that nursing practice standards related to the nursing process have been maintained during care of the patient. Assessment, diagnosis, outcomes, interventions, and evaluation of the patient's response to care are a critical part of the patient's record. Many documentation methods and formats are used, depending on personal preference, agency policy, and regulatory standards such as those maintained by the Joint Commission on Accreditation of Healthcare Organizations (JCAHO).

Some examples of documentation formats that address the nursing process include SOAP (IER) charting, PIE charting, DAR (focus) charting, and charting by exception (CBE). Every method or combination of methods is designed to document the assessment of patient status, the implementation of interventions, and the outcome of interventions.

Nursing Care Plans

The nursing process is usually recorded and documented differently in nursing education and clinical nursing practice. In nursing education, the nursing process is frequently recorded in nursing care plans similar to those presented in this textbook. Student nurses practice and learn nursing process by collecting assessment data, identifying nursing diagnoses, and selecting patient outcomes and nursing interventions—all of which is recorded on specific forms. Rationales for the interventions that are selected are also identified. These plans may include specific directions for carrying out the planned interventions, including how, when, how long, how often, where, by whom, and with what resources the activities should be performed. These nursing care plans are used as teaching/learning tools.

In nursing practice areas, if written care plans are used, they are usually adapted for a particular setting and may include only nursing diagnoses, patient outcomes, and nursing interventions. Standardized care plans may be used in practice as guides for routine nursing care and as a basis for developing individualized care plans. When standardized care plans are used, they should be personalized and specific to the unique needs and problems of each patient. Nursing care plans may also be entered into computerized systems. As discussed earlier, health care informatics that include nursing terminologies will allow NNN linkages that will advance evidence-based nursing practice.

The nursing care plans presented throughout this book use the NANDA-approved nursing diagnoses with NOC outcomes and NIC interventions. When any of these care plans are used, they should be individualized for a specific patient. All of the nursing care plans for this text are available in electronic format on the Evolve website at *http://evolve.elsevier.com/Lewis/medsurg*.

Concept Maps

A **concept map** is another method of recording a nursing care plan. In a concept map care plan, the nursing process is recorded in a visual diagram of patient problems and interventions that illustrates the relationships among clinical data. Although the use of concept mapping is increasing in clinical areas, it is used primarily in nursing education to teach nursing process and care planning.

Various formats are used for concept maps, and a variety of shapes, colors, and connecting arrows are used to identify concepts and relationships. In one example, assessment data are used to identify the patient's primary reason for seeking health care. That health state (often a medical diagnosis) is positioned centrally on the map. Positioned around the reason for health care are nursing diagnoses that represent patient responses to the health state. Listed with each nursing diagnosis are the assessment data that support the nursing diagnosis. Diagnostic testing data, treatments, medications, and nursing interventions may be listed with the nursing diagnoses or may be identified in separate areas and con-

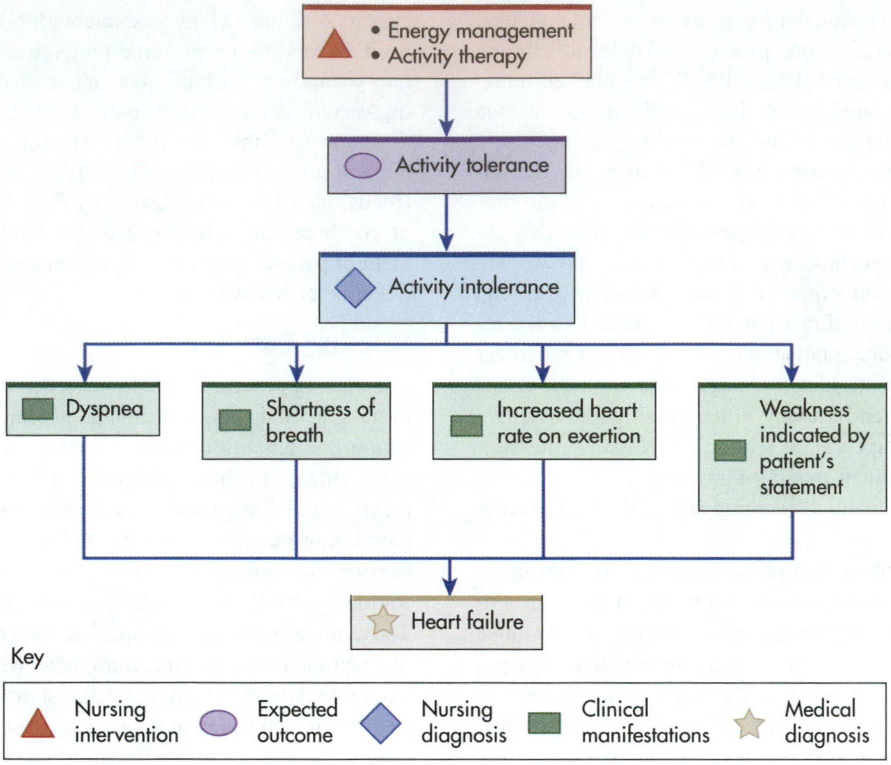

FIG. 1-7 Concept map.

nected to the nursing diagnoses with arrows.[31] Figure 1-7 includes a simplified version of a concept map for the patient with heart failure to compare with the care plan format in NCP 1-1. In addition, a concept map builder is available online on the Evolve website at *http://evolve.elsevier.com/Lewis/medsurg.*

Clinical (Critical) Pathways

Care related to common health problems experienced by many patients is delineated and documented using clinical (critical) pathways. A **clinical (critical) pathway** is a plan that directs the entire health care team in the daily care goals for select health care problems. It includes a nursing care plan, interventions specific for each day of hospitalization, and a documentation tool.[32] The case types selected for clinical pathways are usually those that occur in high volume and are highly predictable, such as myocardial infarction, stroke, and angina.

The clinical pathway describes the patient care required at specific times in the treatment. A multidisciplinary approach moves the patient toward desired outcomes within an estimated length of stay. The exact content and format of clinical pathways vary among institutions. If clinical pathways are used by an institution, they are usually specifically developed and used by that institution. In the clinical pathway, the nursing care plan is documented with the use of nursing diagnoses and evaluation of patient outcomes. Nurse-initiated and physician-initiated interventions designed to achieve the patient outcomes are identified throughout the pathway. The multidisciplinary approach can be seen in the referral to and consultation with other health professionals.

SUMMARY

Nursing roles continually evolve as our society changes and nurses learn to apply new technology. Although nursing is defined in different ways, past and current definitions of nursing have commonalities of health, illness, and caring. It is important that these concepts are carried into future definitions of nursing as greater demands are placed on the profession. Future use of the nursing process will continue to require the use of reasoning, critical thinking skills, and synthesis of rapidly expanding knowledge to assist others to maintain or attain optimal health.

Classification and electronic documentation of nursing's own terminologies will continue to legitimize nursing practice while at the same time an increased emphasis on accountability, assertiveness, persistence, risk taking, and decision making ensures that nursing meets the health care needs of society.

NCLEX® EXAMINATION REVIEW QUESTIONS

The number of the question corresponds to the same-numbered objective at the beginning of the chapter.

1. An example of a nursing activity that reflects the American Nurses Association's definition of nursing is
   a. establishing that the patient with jaundice has hepatitis.
   b. diagnosing that a patient with a feeding tube is at risk for aspiration.
   c. providing antianxiety drugs for a patient who has disturbed sleep patterns.
   d. identifying and treating dysrhythmias that occur in a patient in the coronary care unit.
2. To obtain certification in a specialty area of nursing, a nurse must at least
   a. have a bachelor's degree in nursing.
   b. belong to a nursing specialty organization.
   c. practice a specific period of time in the specialized area of nursing.
   d. acquire additional formal education beyond the basic nursing program.

3. In responding to the *Healthy People* initiatives, the nursing profession is expected to
   a. identify healthy people in the community to serve as role models for good health.
   b. teach patients to use the Internet to obtain information about health care problems.
   c. teach people healthy self-care behaviors related to the major health problems of the country.
   d. develop indicators to measure and record the progress of communities toward meeting the goals of *Healthy People*.
4. When using evidence-based practice, the nurse
   a. must use clinical practice guidelines developed by national health agencies.
   b. should use findings from randomized clinical trials to plan care for all patient problems.
   c. uses clinical decision making and judgment to determine what evidence is appropriate for a specific clinical situation.
   d. statistically analyzes the relationship of nursing interventions to patient outcomes to establish evidence that interventions are appropriate for the patient.
5. Standardized nursing terminologies benefit patient care in that
   a. patient problems and nursing care are clearly defined.
   b. nurses use the same terminology as physicians in delivery of patient care.
   c. a consistent, universal format is used to assess patient responses to health problems.
   d. established prescriptions for nursing care eliminate the need for time-consuming nursing care planning.
6. One advantage of the use of informatics in health care delivery is
   a. the ability to maintain high standards of care.
   b. increased patient anonymity and confidentiality.
   c. improved communication of the patient's health status to the health care team.
   d. access to standardized plans of care that are available for most types of health problems.
7. When the nurse determines that the patient's anxiety needs to be relieved before effective teaching can be implemented, the phase of the nursing process being used is
   a. assessment.
   b. diagnosis.
   c. planning.
   d. evaluation.
8. An example of an independent nursing intervention is
   a. administering blood.
   b. starting an intravenous fluid.
   c. teaching a patient about the effects of prescribed drugs.
   d. administering emergency drugs according to institutional protocols.
9. The process of making a nursing diagnosis differs from a diagnostic statement in that the diagnostic process involves
   a. stating what needs the patient has.
   b. analyzing assessment data to identify responses to health problems.
   c. identifying factors related to the pathophysiology of a disease process.
   d. writing the diagnosis, related factors, and signs and symptoms in PES format.
10. The nurse identifies the nursing diagnosis of risk for impaired skin integrity *related to* obesity and loss of skin elasticity for a patient. The most appropriate expected patient outcome related to this nursing diagnosis is that the
    a. patient's skin is intact.
    b. patient achieves a normal weight for height.
    c. patient changes position every 2 hours to prevent pressure areas.
    d. patient's linens will be changed if they become moist or wrinkled.
11. A patient has a nursing diagnosis of stress urinary incontinence related to overdistention between voidings. An appropriate nursing intervention for this patient related to this nursing diagnosis is to
    a. provide privacy for toileting.
    b. monitor color, odor, and clarity of urine.
    c. teach the patient to void at 2-hour intervals.
    d. provide the patient with perineal pads to absorb urine leakage.
12. Linkages of NANDA nursing diagnoses, NOC patient outcomes, and NIC nursing interventions can be used to
    a. evaluate patient outcomes.
    b. provide guides for planning care.
    c. predict the results of nursing care.
    d. shorten written care plans for individual patients.
13. The primary purpose of the evaluation phase of the nursing process is to
    a. assess the patient's strengths.
    b. describe new nursing diagnoses.
    c. implement new nursing strategies.
    d. identify patient progress toward outcomes.

REFERENCES

1. American Nurses Association: *Nursing: a social policy statement,* ed 2, Washington, DC, 2003, The Association.
2. Nightingale F: *Notes on nursing: what it is and what it is not, facsimile edition,* Philadelphia, 1946, Lippincott.
3. Henderson V: *The nature of nursing,* New York, 1966, Macmillan.
4. Roy S, Andrews H: *The Roy adaptation model,* ed 2, Stamford, CT, 1999, Appleton & Lange.
5. American Association of Colleges of Nursing: *Nursing education's agenda for the 21st century,* Washington, DC, 2002, The Association. Available at *www.aacn.nche.edu/Publications/positions/nrsgedag.htm* (accessed July 20, 2005).
6. Guide to nursing certification organizations, *Dimens Crit Care Nurs* 23:276, 2004.
7. American Nurses Credentialing Center: *Specialty nursing practice certifications*, Washington, DC, 2003, The Center. Available at *www.nursingworld.org/ancc/certification/cert/certs/specialty.html* (accessed July 20, 2005).
8. Burgess AW, Berger AD, Boersma RR: Forensic nursing, *Am J Nurs* 104(3):58, 2004.
9. American Nurses Credentialing Center: *Professional certification for advanced practice nurses*, Washington, DC, 2003, The Center. Available at *www.nursingworld.org/ancc/certification/cert/certs/specialty.html* (accessed July 20, 2005).
10. American Association of Colleges of Nursing: *The clinical nurse leader: developing a new nursing role,* Washington, DC, 2002, The Association. Available at *www.aanc.nche.edu/CNL/index.htm* (accessed July 20, 2005).
11. Scheffer BK, Rubenfeld MG: A consensus statement on critical thinking, *J Nurs Educ* 39:352, 2000.
12. US Department of Health and Human Services: *Healthy People 2010,* Washington, DC, 2004, US Department of Health and Human Services. Available at *www.healthypeople.gov* (accessed July 20, 2005).
13. Melnyk B, Fineout-Overholt E: *Evidence-based practice in nursing and healthcare: a guide to best practice*, Philadelphia, 2005, Lippincott Williams & Wilkins.
14. Cochrane AL: *Effectiveness and efficiency: random reflections on health services,* London, 1972, Nuffield Provincial Hospitals Trust. (Reprinted 1989 in association with the BMJ. Reprinted 1999 for Nuffield Trust by the Royal Society of Medicine Press, London.)
15. Schultz AA: Clinical scholars at the bedside: an EBP mentorship model for today *[http://www.nursingknowledge.org/Portal/Main.aspx?pageid=36&Sender=Primary&SKU=51102], Excellence in Nursing Knowledge* (accessed February 2005).
16. Sackett DL, Straus SE, Richardson WS, et al: *Evidence-based medicine: how to practice and teach EBM,* London, 2000, Churchill Livingstone.
17. Benner P, Leonard V: Patient concerns, choices, and clinical judgment in evidence-based practice. In Melnyk BM, Fineout-Overholt E, editors: *Evidence-based practice in nursing and healthcare: a guide to best practice,* Philadelphia, 2005, Lippincott Williams & Wilkins.
18. Simpson R: What's in a name? The taxonomy and nomenclature puzzle, part 1, *Nurs Manage* 34(6):14, 2003.
19. Simpson R: What's in a name? The taxonomy and nomenclature puzzle, part 2, *Nurs Manage* 34(8):12, 2003.

20. North American Nursing Diagnosis Association: *Nursing diagnoses: definitions and classification 2003-2004,* Philadelphia, 2003, The Association.
21. Dochterman JM, Bulechek GM: *Nursing interventions classification (NIC),* ed 4, St Louis, 2004, Mosby.
22. Moorhead S, Johnson M, Maas M: *Nursing outcomes classification (NOC),* ed 3, St Louis, 2004, Mosby.
23. US Department of Health and Human Services: Press release: VA's electronic health records system pushing national standards, Washington, DC, April 1, 2003, US Department of Health and Human Services. Available at *www.whitehouse.gov/omb/egov/press/CHI_April.htm* (accessed July 20, 2005).
24. College of American Pathologists: News release: HHH secretary Tommy G. Thompson announces access to SNOMED CT® through national library of medicine, Northfield, IL, May 6, 2004, College of American Pathologists. Available at *www.snomed.org/news/documents/050404_E_NLMPressRelease_Final_002.pdf* (accessed July 20, 2005).
25. Charters KG: Nursing informatics, outcomes, and quality improvement, *AACN Clin Issues* 14:282, 2003.
26. Ackley BJ, Ladwig GB: *Nursing diagnosis handbook: a guide to planning care*, ed 7, St Louis, 2006, Mosby.
27. Carpenito-Moyet L: *Nursing diagnosis: application to clinical practice,* ed 10, Philadelphia, 2003, Lippincott.
28. Gordon M: *Manual of nursing diagnosis*, ed 9, St Louis, 2000, Mosby.
29. Johnson M et al: *Nursing diagnoses, outcomes, and interventions: NANDA, NOC, and NIC linkages,* ed 2, St Louis, 2003, Mosby.
30. American Nurses Association: *Position statements: registered nurse utilization of unlicensed assistive personnel*, Washington, DC, 1997, The Association. Available at *http://nursingworld.org/readroom/position/uap/uapuse.htm*. Accessed August 2, 2005.
31. Schuster PM: *Concept mapping: a critical thinking approach to care planning*, Philadelphia, 2002, FA Davis.
32. Cannon CP: Critical pathways for acute myocardial infarction, *Rev Cardiovasc Med* 4:S47, 2003.

RESOURCES

American Nurses Association
800-274-4ANA
www.nursingworld.org

American Nursing Informatics Association (ANIA)
909-985-2811
www.ania.org

Canadian Nurses Association
613-237-2133
800-361-8404
www.cna-nurses.ca

Center for Nursing Classification
College of Nursing
University of Iowa
319-353-5414
www.nursing.uiowa.edu/cnc

Healthy People
www.healthypeople.gov

National Association of Hispanic Nurses
Email: TheHispanicNurses@earthlink.net
www.thehispanicnurses.org

National Black Nurses' Association, Inc.
301-589-3200
www.nbna.org

National Student Nurses' Association
718-210-0705
www.nsna.org

North American Nursing Diagnosis Association (NANDA)
215-545-8105
800-647-9002
Email: info@nanda.org
www.nanda.org

Sigma Theta Tau International
317-634-8171
888-634-7575
www.nursingsociety.org

For additional Internet resources, see the website for this book at *http://evolve.elsevier.com/Lewis/medsurg*.

Learning is not attained by chance, it must be sought for with ardor and attended to with diligence.
Abigail Adams

Health Disparities 2

Bobbie Berkowitz and Margaret McLean Heitkemper

LEARNING OBJECTIVES

1. Identify the key determinants of health.
2. Describe the primary factors that contribute to health disparities.
3. Determine how health disparities manifest themselves in different cultures and racial and ethnic minorities.
4. Differentiate disparities in health care access and disparities in health.
5. Describe the role of nursing in reducing health disparities.

KEY TERMS

determinants of health, p. 19
health disparities, p. 20
health care disparities, p. 20
health literacy, p. 22
health status, p. 20

Electronic Resources

Supplemental content related to Chapter 2 can be found . . .

Companion CD
- Stress-Busting Kit for Nursing Students
- NCLEX Examination Review Questions
- Comprehensive Glossary

Evolve Website evolve
http://evolve.elsevier.com/Lewis/medsurg
- Content Updates
- Key Points (Printable and CD/MP3 Download)
- Concept Map Creator
- Expanded Audio Glossary
- Key Term Flash Cards
- Electronic Calculators
- WebLinks

DETERMINANTS OF HEALTH

In the 1990s there was growing awareness and concern that wealthier citizens had "better" health outcomes than those who were poor and members of minority groups. As a result the National Institutes of Health began to focus on issues that accounted for those differences in health status or health disparities, as well as strategies to reduce them. Today, the reduction in health disparities is the goal of all health care professions, including nursing.

Why are there differences in the health status of the American people? How do these differences occur? The **determinants of health** are those factors that influence the health of individuals and groups[1] (Fig. 2-1). These factors influence health and illness and help explain why some people experience poorer health than others. Behavior is the major determinant of health today. An individual's behavior, both negative and positive, such as tobacco and illicit drug use, or the choice to engage in the recommended amount of physical activity (30 minutes of moderate activity most days per week), is highly linked to a number of health conditions (e.g., lung cancer, liver disease, and obesity). An individual's biologic makeup (e.g., genetics and family history of disease [e.g., heart disease]) can increase one's risk for specific diseases.

A person's social environment, including personal relationships, workplace, housing, transportation, and neighborhood violence, all contribute to health status. For example, the risk of youth homicide is much higher in neighborhoods with gang activity and high crime rates. The physical environment in which one lives, works, and plays exposes that individual to such risks as environmental hazards (workplace injuries), toxic agents (chemical spills and industrial pollution), and unsafe traffic patterns (absence of sidewalks).

These determinants of health can either improve a person's health status or put an individual at risk for disease, injury, and mental illness. The type and availability of medical care also contribute to an individual's health. For example, in some states health maintenance organizations are reducing the number of Medicaid patients that they will cover. There is a growing use of emergency departments for health care. Emergency departments are not set up to provide primary care or long-term follow-up.

Reviewed by Sheila M. Choppala, RN, PhD, Assistant Professor, Washington State University, Vancouver, Wash.

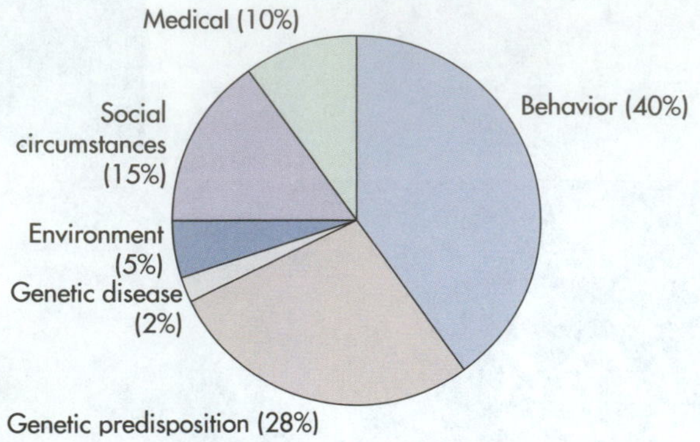

FIG. 2-1 Determinants of health.

Health status describes how healthy a person or a community is. For individuals, this means the sum of their current health problems plus their coping resources (e.g., family, financial resources). For a community, health status is the aggregate of health measures for all individuals living in the community. Health measures include birth and death rates, life expectancy, and morbidity and mortality rates of disease and injury. Many measures make up the concept of health status.

The *Healthy People 2010* report includes a number of measures that can be used to reflect the health status of the U.S. population.[2] *Healthy People 2010* identified many national health objectives and measures for which Americans are meeting or exceeding health status targets. However, for many Americans, meeting targeted goals for health improvement has been unattainable because of the lack of access to health-promoting activities. In addition, lack of adequate health care when ill and/or because of differences such as race, gender, ethnicity, disability, age, language, and culture can decrease the likelihood of achieving *Healthy People* goals. *Healthy People* boxes address these important issues throughout the book.

The *Healthy People 2010* objective for childhood obesity is to reduce obesity to 5% of children and adolescents between ages 6 and 19. Currently, 11% of children ages 6 to 19 are obese. However, certain minority groups, individuals with lower incomes, and people with disabilities have higher rates of obesity. Childhood obesity has been associated with hypertension later in adult life.[3]

HEALTH DISPARITIES

The number 2 goal of *Healthy People 2010* is to eliminate health disparities. **Health disparities** refer to the differences in measures of health status between different groups of people living in a community, a state, or the entire nation. Health disparities occur when one group of people has a higher incidence or mortality rate than another, or when survival rates are less for one group than another. Three additional definitions of health disparities are particularly useful for guiding the practice of nursing.

- *Health disparities* can be defined as the population-specific differences in the presence of disease, health outcomes, or access to health care.[4] This broad definition includes differences in prevalence of disease, outcomes of health care, and differences in the ability of an individual to obtain care based on a specific population type such as racial and ethnic minorities.
- The National Institutes of Health defines *health disparities* as differences in the incidence, prevalence, mortality, and burden of diseases and other adverse health conditions that exist among specific population groups in the United States.[5]
- The Institute of Medicine defines *health disparities* within the context of health care quality. **Health care disparities** are differences in the quality of health care that are not due to access-related factors or clinical needs, preferences, and appropriateness of the intervention but rather are due to stereotyping, biases, and prejudice.

Factors and Conditions That Lead to Health Disparities

Many factors and conditions can lead to the development of health disparities (Table 2-1). Health care provider attitudes and behaviors are one of the contributing factors to health disparities.

Race, Culture, and Ethnicity. Despite the dramatic improvements in treatments to prolong life and improve quality of life for most individuals, racial and ethnic minorities have benefited far less from these advances. Racial, ethnic, and cultural disparities are generally determined by comparing minority population groups with European Americans. In the United States, minority groups include African American, Asian, Pacific Islander, Hispanic and Latino, Native American, and Native Alaskan. Based on the last census, African Americans compose 12.3%, Hispanics or Latinos 12.6%, Asians 3.6%, Pacific Islanders 0.1%, and Native Americans and Native Alaskans 0.9% of the U.S. population. The percentages for most of these groups is expected to increase in the coming decades.[6]

Obesity and chronic illness rates for diabetes, hypertension, chronic obstructive pulmonary diseases, cancer, and stroke are higher among minority people. Minority adults are more likely to have health problems than whites. In addition, one of five Hispanics (22%), one of six African Americans (17%), and one of

HEALTHY PEOPLE

Health Impact of Access to Health Care

- Immunizations prevent the spread of many diseases
- Ready access to care decreases the impact of injury and illness
- Early prenatal care reduces the risks during pregnancy for both mother and child
- Routine checkups and screening greatly reduce the risk of preventable and treatable diseases

TABLE 2-1 Factors That Contribute to Health Disparities

- Race, culture, and ethnicity
- Geographic location
- Income
- Education
- Occupation
- Health literacy
- Gender
- Age
- Health care provider attitudes

TABLE 2-2 Impact of Health Disparities on Health Outcomes

Disease	Impact
Cancer	• African Americans have 35% higher mortality rates than whites. • Cancer screening in general is higher in whites than in minority groups.
Cervical cancer	• Vietnamese women in the United States have an incidence rate 5 times that of white women.
Lung cancer	• African American men have higher incidence than white men.
Colorectal cancer	• African Americans have higher rates than other ethnic groups.
Prostate cancer	• African American men have 50% higher mortality rate than white men.
Diabetes mellitus	• Minority groups make up 25% of people with type 2 diabetes. • Minority groups are 2-4 times more likely to have complications than whites. • African Americans with the disease are 7 times more likely to get amputations and develop renal failure than whites. • Low health literacy level is associated with long-term complications.
Obesity	• Affects 53% of African American women, 52% of Mexican American women, and 34% of white women.
Hypertension	• Racial and ethnic minorities have higher rates, develop at younger age, and are less likely to receive treatment.
Cardiovascular disease	• Death rates from heart disease are 40% higher in African Americans than whites. • Reduced rates of cholesterol screening in Mexican Americans, African Americans, and American Indians/Alaska Natives.
Stroke	• African Americans are more likely to die from stroke than other ethnic groups. • Particularly at risk to suffer a stroke if live in Southeast United States "stroke belt."
Infant mortality	• Whites have rate of 6/1000; African Americans 14.2/1000; American Indians 9/1000 live births.
Asthma	• Death due to asthma is 2-6 times more likely among African Americans than among whites.

six Asian Americans (17%) rate their health as fair or poor, compared with one of seven whites (14%).[7] Racial, ethnic, and cultural differences exist in health screening behaviors, treatments provided, and access to health care providers. For example, African American men are less likely to be offered intervention procedures for cardiovascular disease.[8] Hispanic women are less likely to have mammography for breast cancer screening.[9] Breast and cervical cancer mortality rates are higher in Hispanic women than in other American women. Differences in access to screening and treatment are important. When patient groups are given the same care, the treatment outcomes are similar across racial and ethnic groups.[10,11]

Disease risk and outcomes are also influenced by race and ethnicity (Table 2-2). For example, being African American is highly associated with dying early as a result of a stroke.[12,13] Cultural biases surrounding symptom tolerance and health care–seeking behavior can contribute to health disparities. In some cultures pain is considered something to be endured or ignored, and as a result the patient does not seek help. This delay in seeking health care services may explain some of the differences in mortality rates. For example, a survey of Native American women on three rural Indian reservations found that 32% would not take action if they experienced crushing chest pain lasting longer than 15 minutes.[14] In some cultures, diseases or problems may be viewed fatalistically; that is, there is no reason to seek treatment because it is believed to be unlikely to have benefit. In some cultures it may not be acceptable to see a health care provider who is not of the same gender or ethnic group. Such biases can result in delays in seeking health care and/or inadequate treatment.

Cultural differences exist in how well patients feel that they can communicate with their health care provider.[15] Communication issues include not understanding the health care provider, feeling that they are not listened to, and having questions but not asking them. In the United States, approximately 25% to 33% of minority patients have difficulty communicating with their care provider as compared with 16% of white Americans. Similarly, minority patients are less likely to have a regular health care provider as compared with white Americans[15] (Fig. 2-2). African Americans are more likely to receive outpatient care in the emergency department and have fewer physician visits.[16]

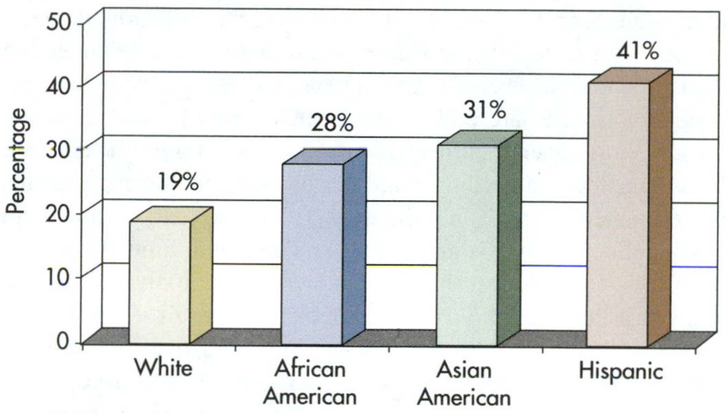

FIG. 2-2 Percent of adults (based on ethnicity) in the United States who have no regular doctor.

Historical trends may also contribute to reluctance to access health care services or to follow prescribed therapies. The Tuskegee experiment did little to decrease African Americans' tendency to be distrustful of the health care system. In that government-sponsored experiment, 399 African American men infected with syphilis were followed. They were asked to describe their symptoms and manifestations over a 40-year span. During this time the participants did not receive appropriate medical care, and many suffered painful and debilitating consequences of untreated syphilis. The "Tuskegee effect" has left many African Americans not only reluctant to participate in clinical research but also reluctant to use health care services.[17] Culture is discussed further in Chapter 3.

Geographic Location. Twenty-five percent of Americans live in rural areas (populations of ≤2500). Differences in access to health care services between rural and urban settings can create geographic health disparities. For example, Native Americans living on reservations may need to travel long distances to receive health care. This can result in inadequate or less frequent access to health care services. Some parts of the rural United States are considered "medically underserved" because of decreased numbers of health care providers per population. On average the ratio of patients to providers is higher in rural communities.

People living in rural areas have rates of cancer, heart disease, diabetes, and injury-related deaths that are higher than people living in urban areas. For example, in rural Appalachia the rates of lung, colon, cervical, and rectal cancer are higher than the national average.[18]

Rural populations have lower literacy rates and poorer health behaviors (e.g., increased smoking rates, increased substance abuse, and lower rates of physical activity). Generally the poorer and more isolated a community, the lower the health status and the more difficult it is to access quality health services.[18] Rural residents are also less likely to have health care insurance coverage.

Urban living centers may also predispose to health disparities. Lack of adequate income can reduce options for travel to health care settings even in urban environments. Concerns about personal safety (e.g., clinics located in high-crime neighborhoods) can make patients reluctant to visit health care providers.

Income, Education, and Occupation. Health care costs are one of the important health care system factors that contribute to health disparities. Persons of lower income, education, or occupational status experience worse health and die at a younger age than do those who are more affluent. Individuals who have no insurance or who are underinsured and those who lack financial resources to cover treatment for disease may forego health care visits and treatments. For example, blood lipid–lowering agents are estimated to cost approximately $2000 per year, putting them beyond the reach of the uninsured and those with limited financial resources. Patients who lack the knowledge to apply for government assistance programs (e.g., Medicaid) are also at risk. The number of uninsured Americans has increased over the past decade. In addition, hazardous work environments and occupations of laborers may also increase health risk and contribute to higher rates of illness, injury, and death.

Health literacy refers to a range of skills needed to prevent disease and promote health. These include the ability to read, comprehend, and analyze information; understand instructions; weigh risks and benefits; and ultimately make decisions and take action. Nearly half of all American adults have difficulty understanding and acting on health information.[15,18] Lack of language skills and illiteracy can serve as barriers to health care access and to obtaining appropriate disease treatment. Issues related to health literacy are more important today than ever before. On a daily basis, patients are expected to self-manage conditions such as diabetes and asthma. For example, patients with diabetes may not be able to maintain adequate blood glucose levels if they cannot read or understand the numbers on the home glucose monitoring system. Indeed, low health literacy level has been associated with poor glycemic control and subsequent adverse outcomes, including diabetic retinopathy.[19] The inability to read and understand medication labels can result in medications being taken at the wrong time or the wrong dose of medication being taken. Health literacy is discussed further in Chapter 5.

Gender. Health disparities between men and women start at the beginning of life, with fewer male infants surviving their first year. Adult women use health care services more than men. At the same time, women are less likely than men to have medical insurance. Studies suggest that women may not receive the same quality of care. For example, women are less likely to receive intervention procedures (e.g., cardiac catheterization) for cardiovascular disease.[20] When gender is combined with racial and ethnic differences, the disparities are even greater. For example, African Americans are less likely to participate in colorectal cancer screening, with African American women less likely than men.[21] (Gender boxes are presented throughout the book that highlight gender differences in disease risk and response to treatment.)

Age. The elderly are at risk for experiencing health disparities in number of diagnostic tests performed and aggressiveness of treatments used. Biases toward the elderly that affect their care, or *ageism,* are discussed in Chapter 6. Disparities related to race/ethnicity and economic factors continue to affect the elderly. Elderly persons who belong to minority groups are less likely than their white counterparts to receive screening for prostate and colorectal cancer.[21] Elderly women are less likely to be offered mammograms.[22] Elderly persons of low socioeconomic status experience greater disability, more limitations in activities of daily living, and more frequent and rapid cognitive decline.

Health Care Provider Attitudes. Certain behaviors and biases of the health care provider can contribute to health dispari-

ETHICAL DILEMMAS

Health Disparities

Situation

Elena, a 47-year-old Mexican American woman with type 2 diabetes mellitus, comes to the clinic to have her blood glucose measured. It has been 12 months since her last visit and at that time the nurse requested that she bring along her glucometer and strips to demonstrate how she checks her blood glucose because her serum glucose values were very high at her previous visits.

When the nurse checks Elena's equipment and glucose strips, it is clear that the strips are for a different machine and they had been expired for over 2 years. When the nurse inquires about the situation, Elena explains that she cannot afford to come to the clinic or to buy new equipment and supplies to check her blood glucose. During the day Elena cares for her three grandchildren so her daughter can work. Elena spends most of her income on food for her family so there is little money left over for her own health care.

Important Points for Consideration

- Ethnic minorities and other vulnerable or disadvantaged groups experience certain chronic illnesses at higher rates
- Socioeconomic status and access to health care are major contributors to health disparities.
- The diagnosis and treatment of some diseases may differ by ethnic group. These groups are at increased risk for morbidity and mortality from these diseases. These are issues that are considered in the broader context of social justice.
- According to the American Nurses Association Code of Ethics, nurses must not only work to improve the health of individual patients, but also the health of communities, the nation, and international communities.

Critical Thinking Questions

1. How could you work with Elena to help her obtain the necessary resources and knowledge to care for her diabetes?
2. What can you do to begin working on the problems of health disparities in your community?

ties. Factors such as stereotyping and prejudice can affect health care–seeking behavior in minority populations.[23] *Stereotyping* refers to viewing members of a specific culture or ethnic group as being alike or sharing the same beliefs. The stereotypes and general orientation (attitudes) that people bring to their interactions help organize and simplify complex or uncertain situations. Social stereotypes and attitudes tend to be systematically biased. For example, believing that the elderly are not compliant in maintaining a regular schedule of exercise may result in the provider neglecting to counsel her or his patient about the importance of physical activity in improving mobility in preventing osteoporosis. Health care providers may not recognize manifestations of prejudice in their own behaviors.

The health care system itself, such as the hospital, outpatient clinic, or public health department, may also contribute to the problem of health disparities. For example, a clinic located in an area with a large immigrant population of Vietnamese that does not provide translators or educational materials and financial forms in Vietnamese may limit the ability of immigrant families to understand how to access health care.

Discrimination and *bias* occur when there is a negative treatment based on race, ethnicity, gender, age, or sexual orientation. Sometimes discrimination is difficult to identify, especially when it occurs at the institutional level. Overt discriminatory behavior on the part of a health care provider may not be immediately evident to the patient and therefore may be difficult to confront. Although many policies exist to eliminate discrimination, it still exists in subtle forms.

Health Disparities' Impact on Health

Health disparities are most evident when rates of cancer, asthma, diabetes, and cardiovascular disease are examined. Examples of the impact of health disparities on health outcomes are shown in Table 2-2. All of these conditions are more prevalent in minority populations and those who live in poorer communities. More information is provided in specific chapters throughout the text.

NURSING MANAGEMENT
REDUCING HEALTH DISPARITIES

The causes of health disparities are not always easy to identify. Many times the solutions to reduce health disparities rest with the policy makers. Economic issues often dictate health care delivery. Access and public policy decisions dictate who is eligible for federal and state health insurance coverage. The nurse, along with the social worker, can help by identifying key resources in the community, including transportation services, reduced-fee screening programs, and appropriate federal and state offices for Medicaid and Medicare.

Although the problems associated with health disparities can seem overwhelming, a number of strategies are available to reduce and ultimately eliminate health disparities. These strategies include improving interpersonal communication, using disease management standards, increasing cultural competence, initiating quality improvement programs that monitor for disparities, advocating for workforce diversity, and participating in research related to understanding and reducing health disparities. Nurses play an important role in assessing patients who are vulnerable to reduced health care services because of limited access, inadequate resources, or illiteracy (Fig. 2-3). The nurse can serve as an advocate in finding and evaluating information on appropriate and individualized treatment and in navigating the health care system. Table 2-3 outlines seven areas where nurses can make a major contribution to the elimination of health disparities. Table 2-4 provides strategies for reducing health disparities in ethnically diverse populations. Chapter 3 addresses issues related to enhancing cultural competency.

Improving interpersonal skills is an important first step in reducing health disparities. Interpersonal skills such as active listening, relationship building, and communication skills are basic to the delivery of high-quality and equitable health care.[24] The nurse plays an important role in patient and family communication related to health promotion (e.g., screening), disease risk, and illness management.

Disease management strategies are important for reducing the burden of chronic disease and for ensuring that standards are applied

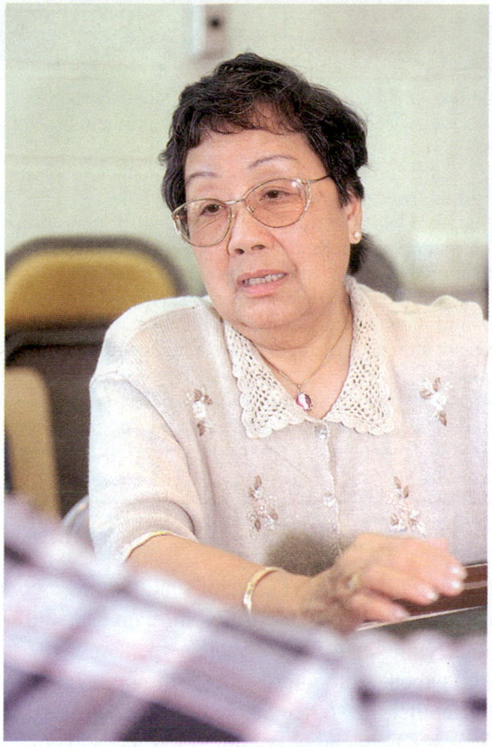

FIG. 2-3 Older Asian women are especially at risk for health disparities.

TABLE 2-3 Nursing Interventions to Eliminate Health Disparities

- Treat all patients equally
- Monitor your individual patients for their response to therapy
- Be a patient advocate regardless of cultural, language, or SES factors
- Design teaching materials to the specific needs and preferences of the patient
- Be aware of one's own biases or prejudices and work toward eliminating them
- Make sure the same standards of care are followed for all patients regardless of ethnicity
- Participate in research focused on understanding and improving care to ethnically diverse populations

SES, Socioeconomic status.

TABLE 2-4 Reducing Health Disparities for Ethnic Adults

- Inform ethnic adults about health care services available.
- Learn about services/programs that focus on specific ethnic groups.
- Identify health care practices and cultural practices that are important to an ethnic identity.
- Identify stereotypic attitudes toward an ethnic adult that may interfere with getting appropriate health care.
- Support the ethnic adult who is fearful about traveling outside the accepted neighborhood for health care services.
- Advocate for ethnic adults to receive health care services that provide special attention to language limitations and cultural health practices.
- Use strategies specific to an ethnic group. For example, African Americans may respond to themes such as "do it for your loved ones." Asian Americans may respond to fear of dependency themes.

equitably to all individuals. The use of standardized evidence-based care guidelines can reduce disparities in diagnosis and treatments. For example, guidelines for the management of hypertension are based on the patient's blood pressure, symptoms, history, and laboratory values rather than other characteristics such as gender, age, or culture. There are no racial or cultural differences in outcomes when the guidelines are followed.

Staff development programs within institutions and agencies need to collaborate to provide education on the existence and prevention of health disparities.[24,25] Cross-cultural education needs to be required at all educational levels. Academic settings, in particular, must ensure that culture and cultural sensitivity are common threads running through the curriculum. Health care providers at all levels should be able to demonstrate their skill in recognizing and reducing health disparities.

A powerful strategy for reducing health disparities is to increase the number of underrepresented populations in the health care professions (Fig. 2-4). Diversity of professionals within the health care system is likely to increase our awareness of the existence and impact of health disparities. It has been demonstrated that patients often feel more comfortable when care is provided by someone who shares their heritage and cultural values. A diverse nursing workforce is needed to assist in recognizing and responding to the health needs of diverse populations.

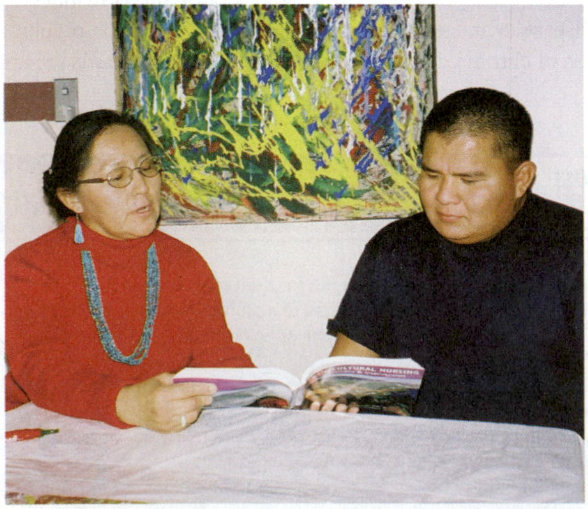

FIG. 2-4 A Navaho nurse instructs a Navaho patient.

CRITICAL THINKING EXERCISE

CASE STUDY

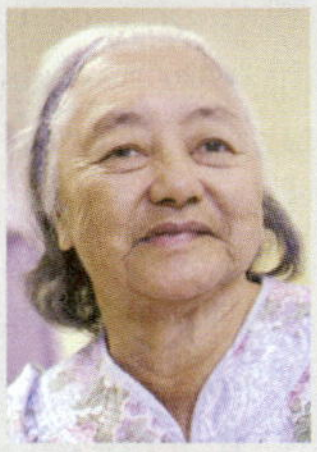

Anna Zyskowski is a 75-year-old woman who emigrated to the United States from Poland 10 years ago with her daughter, her son-in-law, and their five children. She has a number of health problems, including coronary artery disease and diabetes. Her daughter is the primary caregiver and frequently brings her to the rural community health clinic for a variety of health-related complaints. Recently Anna has been experiencing memory problems.

The visits to the clinic tend to be chaotic and time consuming for the clinic staff. The entire family comes to the health clinic with Anna. Because English is a second language for all of the adult family members, the staff relies on the oldest granddaughter to translate.

At this clinic visit Anna is complaining of shortness of breath. Via her granddaughter's translation, she tells the nurse that she is having trouble walking up the stairs in the house. The nurse does the history and assessment; checks her blood glucose, which is within normal limits; and advises that she get more exercise. Given Anna's memory problems and limited English, the nurse does not complete a 24-hour dietary recall or counsel her or the family about diabetes management. Anna is scheduled for an appointment with the cardiologist for an evaluation of her cardiac disease. Two weeks later, when Anna is seen by the cardiologist, her shortness of breath is much worse and she is having chest pain. She is hospitalized immediately.

Meanwhile, the clinic supervisor is completing a chart audit for their quality review program. She is reviewing Anna's chart and notices that although Anna has been a patient in the clinic for 3 years, she has never received instructions on blood glucose monitoring or general diabetes management. The clinic has a nurse diabetes educator who teaches individual patients and groups of patients with diabetes. The clinic manager reviews these findings with the nurse and asks why she has not recommended that Anna see the diabetes educator. The nurse stated that with all of the chaos in the family, Anna's memory problems, and the language barrier she just assumed that Anna would not benefit from the consultation.

Critical Thinking Questions

1. What type of health disparity has Anna experienced?
2. What factors led to Anna not receiving the standard of care?
3. What additional assessment should have been done at the initial visit?
4. What strategies might have worked to enhance patient education?
5. If you were the clinic manager, how would you recommend that the nurse improve her practice?

NCLEX EXAMINATION REVIEW QUESTIONS

The number of the question corresponds to the same-numbered objective at the beginning of the chapter.

1. Which of the following is the leading determinant of a patient's health?
   a. Behavior
   b. Family history of disease
   c. Home and work environment
   d. Type and quality of medical care received
2. In identifying patients at the greatest risk for health disparities, the nurse would note that
   a. patients who live in urban areas have readily available access to health care services.
   b. cultural differences exist in the ability of patients to communicate with their health care provider.
   c. a patient receiving care from a health care provider of a different culture would have decreased quality of care.
   d. men are more likely than women to have their cardiovascular disease symptoms ignored by their health care provider.
3. A 50-year-old Native American woman with type 2 diabetes mellitus living on a rural reservation has poor glycemic control. This situation may be related to all of the following factors *except*
   a. having a male Hispanic health care provider.
   b. eating fresh foods rather than prepackaged foods.
   c. geographic distance between home and health care facility.
   d. Native Americans' greater likelihood to have complications with diabetes than whites.
4. Disparities in health are related to a number of factors, including
   a. age: older adults have greater access to health care.
   b. geographic location: rural populations are more likely to have health insurance.
   c. occupation: laborers are more vulnerable to job-related injuries than white collar workers.
   d. race: African Americans tend to be more trusting of health care providers as compared with whites.
5. Nurses play an important role in reducing health disparities. One important mechanism to do this is to
   a. discourage use of evidence-based practice guidelines.
   b. insist that patients adhere to the *Healthy People 2010* guidelines.
   c. teach patients to use the Internet to find resources related to their health.
   d. engage in active listening and establish relationships with patients and families.

REFERENCES

1. McGinnis M, Williams-Russo P, Knickman J: The case for more active policy attention to health promotion, *Health Aff* 21:78, 2002.
2. US Department of Health and Human Services: *Healthy people 2010.* Available at *www.healthypeople.gov* (accessed April 23, 2006).
3. Lawlor DA, Smith GD: Early life determinants of adult blood pressure, *Curr Opin Nephrol Hypertens* 14:259, 2005.
4. Health Resources and Services Administration Workgroup for the Elimination of Health Disparities. US Department of Health and Human Services, Washington, DC. Available at *www.hrsa.gov/OMH/disparities* (accessed June 14, 2005).
5. First National Institutes of Health Work Group on Health Disparities. Available at *http://healthdisparities.nih.gov/whatare.html* (accessed June 14, 2005).
6. United States Census Bureau: Population estimates. Available at *www.census.gov/popest/estimates.php* (accessed June 14, 2005).
7. Minority Americans lag behind whites on nearly every measure of health care quality. Available at *www.cmwf.org/newsroom/newsroom* (accessed June 14, 2005).
8. Petersen LA, Wright SM, Peterson ED, et al: Impact of race on cardiac care and outcomes in veterans with acute myocardial infarction, *Med Care* 40:I86, 2002.
9. Li CI: Racial and ethnic disparities in breast cancer stage, treatment, and survival in the United States, *Ethn Dis* 15:S5, 2005.
10. Centers for Disease Control and Prevention (CDC): Disparities in screening for and awareness of high blood cholesterol—United States, 1999-2002, *Morb Mortal Wkly Rep* 54:117, 2005.
11. Martins D, Tareen N, Nicholas SB, et al: Education, motivation and medication for African Americans: bringing hypertension guidelines to practice, *Ethn Dis* 14:S2, 2004.
12. Shen JJ, Washington EL, Aponte-Soto L: Racial disparities in the pathogenesis and outcomes for patients with ischemic stroke, *Manag Care Interface* 17:28, 2004.
13. Stansbury JP, Jia H, Williams LS, et al: Ethnic disparities in stroke: epidemiology, acute care, and postacute outcomes, *Stroke* 36:374, 2005.
14. Struthers R, Savik K, Hodge FS: American Indian women and cardiovascular disease: response behaviors to chest pain, *J Cardiovasc Nurs* 19:158, 2004.
15. National Cancer Institute, Center to Reduce Cancer Health Disparities. Available at *http://crchd.nci.nih.gov/chd/disparities* (accessed June 15, 2005).
16. Massing MW, Foley KA, Carter-Edwards L, et al: Disparities in lipid management for African Americans and Caucasians with coronary artery disease: a national cross-sectional study, *BMC Cardiovasc Disord* 18:15, 2004.
17. Bates BR, Harris TM: The Tuskegee study of untreated syphilis and public perceptions of biomedical research: a focus group study, *J Natl Med Assoc* 96:1051, 2004.
18. Smedley B, Stith A, Nelson A: *Unequal treatment: confronting racial and ethnic disparities in healthcare,* Washington, DC, 2003, National Academy Press.
19. Thackeray R, Merrill RM, Neiger BL: Disparities in diabetes management practice between racial and ethnic groups in the United States, *Diabetes Educ* 30:665, 2004.
20. Harrold LR, Esteban J, Lessard D, et al: Narrowing gender differences in procedure use for acute myocardial infarction: insights from the Worcester heart attack study, *J Gen Intern Med* 18:423, 2003.

*21. Green PM, Kelly BA: Colorectal cancer knowledge, perceptions, and behaviors in African Americans, *Cancer Nurs* 27:206, 2004.

22. Morales LS, Rogowski J, Freedman VA, et al: Sociodemographic differences in use of preventive services by women enrolled in Medicare+Choice plans, *Prev Med* 39:738, 2004.
23. Rathore SS, Krumholz HM: Differences, disparities, and biases: clarifying variations in health care use, *Ann Intern Med* 19:635, 2004.
24. Burgess DJ, Fu SS, van Ryn M: Why do providers contribute to disparities and what can be done about it? *J Gen Intern Med* 19:1154, 2004.
25. Betancourt JR, Maina AW: The Institute of Medicine report "unequal treatment": implications for academic health centers, *Mt Sinai J Med* 71:314, 2004.

RESOURCES

Center to Reduce Cancer Health Disparities
301-496-8589
http://crchd.nci.nih.gov

Commonwealth Fund
212-606-3800
www.cmwf.org

Health Disparities Collaboratives
www.healthdisparities.net/hdc

National Center for Cultural Competence
800-788-2066
http://gucchd.georgetown.edu/nccc

National Center on Minority Health and Health Disparities
301-402-1366
http://ncmhd.nih.gov

National Council on Patient Information and Education (NCPIE)
301-656-8565
www.talkaboutrx.org

For additional Internet resources, see the website for this book at *http://evolve.elsevier.com/Lewis/medsurg.*

---

*Nursing research–based reference.

Remember that you are all people and that all people are you.

Joy Harjo

3 Culturally Competent Care

Cory A. Shaw and Margaret M. Andrews

LEARNING OBJECTIVES

1. Define the terms *culture, values, subculture, acculturation, assimilation, ethnicity, race, stereotyping, ethnocentrism, cultural imposition, transcultural nursing, cultural competency, folk healer,* and *culture-bound syndrome.*
2. Describe the potential effects of immigration on an individual's health.
3. Explain aspects of culture and ethnicity that may affect a person's physical and psychologic health.
4. Describe strategies for successfully communicating with a person who speaks a language that the nurse does not understand.
5. Identify physiologic and psychologic aspects of culture and ethnicity to consider when providing nursing care.
6. Identify ways that the nurse's own cultural background may influence nursing care when working with patients from different cultural and ethnic groups.
7. Identify strategies for incorporating cultural information in the nursing process when providing care for patients from different cultural and ethnic groups.

KEY TERMS

acculturation, p. 27
assimilation, p. 27
cultural competence, p. 28
cultural imposition, p. 28
culture, p. 27
culture-bound syndrome, p. 35
ethnicity, p. 28
ethnocentrism, p. 28
folk healers, p. 30
race, p. 28
stereotyping, p. 28
subcultures, p. 27
transcultural nursing, p. 28
values, p. 27

Electronic Resources

Supplemental content related to Chapter 3 can be found . . .

Companion CD

- Stress-Busting Kit for Nursing Students
- NCLEX Examination Review Questions
- Comprehensive Glossary

Evolve Website

http://evolve.elsevier.com/Lewis/medsurg

- Content Updates
- Key Points (Printable and CD/MP3 Download)
- Concept Map Creator
- Expanded Audio Glossary
- Key Term Flash Cards
- Electronic Calculators
- WebLinks

In today's increasingly multicultural environment nurses come in contact with patients, families, significant others, and members of the health care team from many different cultures during their professional careers. They find themselves in patient care situations that require an understanding of the patient's cultural beliefs and practices. This understanding is needed if nurses are to effectively participate in planning, providing, and evaluating culturally competent care. The demographics and cultural composition of the United States and other countries are changing. Therefore it is important for nurses to be aware of cultural differences in health care practices and of the potential differences in expectations of patients and health care providers.

Who are the nurses that provide care for this diverse population? Of the nation's 2.7 million registered nurses, 87% are white, 5% are African American, 4% are Asian/Pacific Islander, 2% are Hispanic, and 0.5% are American Indian/Alaska Native.[1] Although these nurses represent diversity in the workplace, their proportions do not match the patient population. Even when nurses provide care for patients from their own cultural background, the nurse may be from a different subculture than the patient. For example, considering that there are more than 550 federally recognized Native American tribes in the United States, it would be inappropriate to assume that a Native American nurse can give culturally appropriate care to a Native American patient when both may be from different tribes.

Reviewed by Doris Leal Hill, RN, PhD, CNOR, Department Chair—Nursing, Normandale College, Bloomington, Minn.

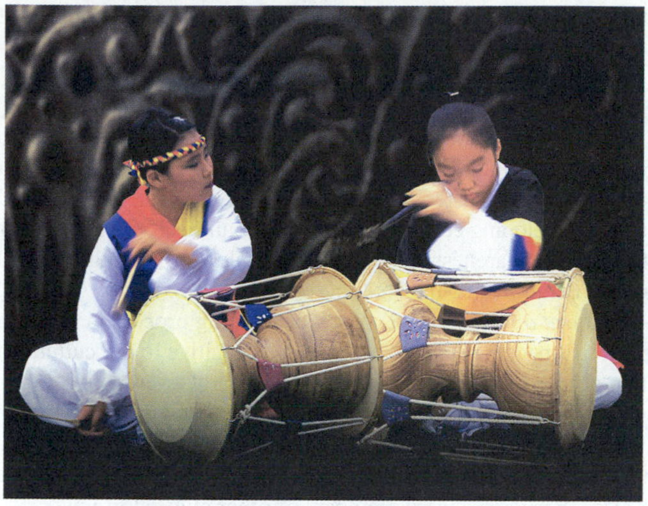

FIG. 3-1 These women express themselves through the customs of their culture.

CULTURE

There are many definitions of culture. In general, **culture** encompasses the knowledge, values, beliefs, art, morals, law, customs, and habits of the members of a society. Culture also includes the systems of technology, education, social structures, and political practices. Cultural patterns of behavior develop over time and are shared by members of the same cultural group and transmitted to the next generation (Fig. 3-1). Culture affects ways of perceiving, behaving, and evaluating the world, and serves as a guide for people's values, beliefs, and practices, including those related to health and illness.[2] The four classic characteristics of culture are described in Table 3-1.

Values are the sets of rules by which individuals, families, groups, and communities live. They are the principles and standards that serve as the basis for beliefs, attitudes, and behaviors. Although all cultures have values, the types and expressions of those values differ from one culture to another. These cultural values develop over time, guide decision making and actions, and may affect a person's self-esteem. Cultural values are often unconsciously developed as a child is assimilated into the culture, learning what is acceptable and unacceptable behavior. The extent to which a person's cultural values are internalized influences that person's tendency toward judging other cultures, while usually using his or her own culture as the accepted standard.[2,3] Table 3-2 illustrates some examples of different cultural values in America.

Although individuals within a cultural group will have many similarities through their shared values, beliefs, and practices, there is also diversity within groups. Each person is culturally unique. Such diversity may result from different perspectives and interpretations of situations. These differences may be based on age, gender, marital status, family structure, income, education level, religious views, and life experiences.

TABLE 3-1 Basic Characteristics of Culture

- *Dynamic* and ever-changing
- *Shared* by all members of the same cultural group
- *Adapted* to specific conditions such as environmental factors
- *Learned* through oral and written histories, as well as socialization

TABLE 3-2 Cultural Values of Different Ethnic Groups in America

Culture	Values
Native American	• Cultural rituals • Folk healing • Harmony with people and the environment • Pride in cultural heritage • Returning what is taken from nature • Respect for tribal elders and children • Spiritual guidance
Mexican American	• Cultural foods • Folk healing • Importance of extended family • Involvement of family in social activities • Less importance on exact time • Patriarchal • Religion/spirituality highly valued • Respect for elders and authority
African American	• Cultural foods • Family networks • Folk healing • Importance of religion • Interdependence with the ethnic group • Music and physical activities valued • Support and survival of the poor • Technology valued
Anglo American (mainly middle and upper class)	• Achievements and competition • Equal rights of genders • Generous in times of crisis • Independence and freedom valued • Less respect for elders • Materialistic • Science based • Self-reliance • Technology dependent • Youth and beauty valued

Adapted from Leininger MM, McFarland MR: *Transcultural nursing: concepts, theories, research, and practice,* ed 3, New York, 2002, McGraw-Hill.

Within any cultural group, there are smaller **subcultures** that may not hold all of the values of the dominant culture. These subcultures, including ethnic groups, have experiences that differ from the dominant group. These differences may be related to ethnic background, residence, religion, occupation, health-related characteristics, age, gender, education, or other factors that unite the group. Members of a subculture share certain aspects of culture that are different from the overall cultural group.[3] Religious subcultures include Catholics, Jews, Muslims, and other members of any of the 1200 recognized religions. Ethnic subcultures include groups who share common traits such as ancestry, language, or physical characteristics. These include African Americans, Hispanics, and Native Americans.

Cultural practices change over time through active or passive processes, including acculturation and/or assimilation. **Acculturation** is a process by which an individual or group learns how to take on many, but not all, values, beliefs, and practices of another culture. This process is usually gradual, and the changes that occur often result in increased similarities between the two cultures. **Assimilation** refers to the manner in which an individual or group from one culture adopts certain features of another culture, but does not embrace all of the other culture's features. Assimilation may be voluntary, or it may be forced on a group.

The meaning of the terms *ethnicity* and *race* continues to evolve and be debated. **Ethnicity** refers to groups whose members share a common social and cultural heritage. This heritage is passed on through the generations and involves identification with that group (Fig. 3-2). Members of an ethnic group may share a common language, history, education, lifestyle, and religion. They share a sense of identity, loyalty, and social belonging. The term **race** refers to divisions of humankind and is more closely related to people who share a common ancestry and physical characteristics such as skin color, bone structure, or blood group.

Stereotyping refers to viewing members of a specific culture, race, or ethnic group as being alike and sharing the same values and beliefs. This oversimplified approach does not take into account that individual differences exist within a culture. Being a member of a particular cultural, ethnic, or racial group does not make the person an expert on other members of that same group. Such stereotyping can lead to false assumptions and affect a patient's care. For example, it would be inappropriate to assume that just because a nurse is Mexican American, he or she would know how a Mexican American patient's beliefs may affect that patient's health care practices. A young nurse born and raised in a large city has assimilated a different culture than the elderly male patient who was born and raised in a rural area of Mexico.

Ethnocentrism refers to the belief that one's own ways are superior to those of others from different cultural, ethnic, or racial backgrounds.[4] Comparing others' ways to one's own can lead to seeing others as different or inferior. To avoid ethnocentrism, it is necessary to maintain an objective and nonjudgmental view of the values, beliefs, and practices of others. Failure to do this can result in ethnic stereotyping or cultural imposition.

Cultural imposition results when one's own cultural beliefs and practices are imposed on another person or group of people.[4] In health care it can result in disregarding or trivializing a patient's health care beliefs or practices. Cultural imposition may result when a health care provider is unaware of another person's beliefs and plans and implements care without taking into account the cultural beliefs of the patient.

The term **transcultural nursing** was coined by Madeleine Leininger in the 1950s. Transcultural nursing is a specialty that focuses on the comparative study and analysis of cultures and subcultures. The goal of transcultural nursing is the discovery of culturally relevant facts that can guide the nurse in providing culturally appropriate care.[4]

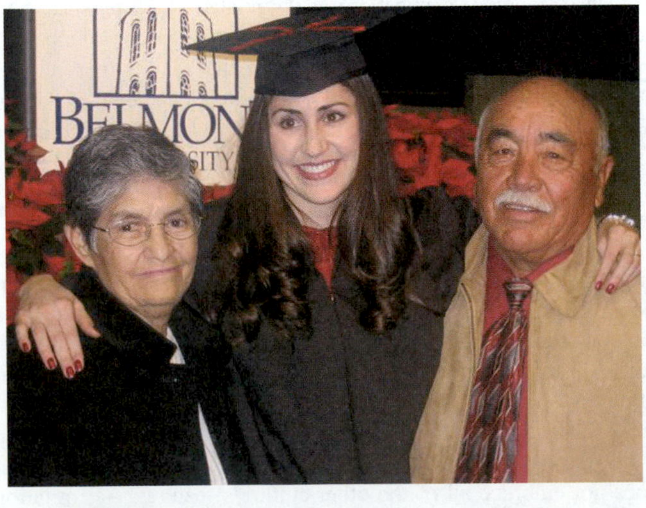

FIG. 3-2 Members of this family share a common heritage.

CULTURAL COMPETENCE

Cultural competence is a process that involves the integration of knowledge, attitudes, and skills that enhance cross-cultural communication and foster meaningful, respectful interactions with others. Developing cultural competence requires four components: (1) cultural awareness; (2) cultural knowledge; (3) cultural skill; and (4) cultural encounter[4] (Table 3-3).

Cultural awareness is a conscious learning process in which an individual becomes appreciative of and sensitive to the cultures of other people. A first step in developing cultural awareness is for the nurse to examine his or her own cultural biases toward people from different cultures. The nurse's biases may interfere with providing culturally appropriate health care because they have the potential to affect behavior toward members of other cultural groups.[5]

Cultural knowledge involves the process of understanding the key aspects of a group's culture, especially as it relates to health and health care practices. Cultural groups can have differences in (1) beliefs about the cause of illness and health, (2) the appropriate use of various treatments and healers, (3) beliefs about lengths of recovery or convalescence, and (4) sick role behavior.[5] Patients

TABLE 3-3 Processes Involved in Developing Cultural Competence

Cultural Awareness
- Identify one's own cultural background, values, and beliefs, especially as related to health and health care.
- Examine one's own cultural biases toward people whose cultures differ from one's own culture.

Cultural Knowledge
- Learn basic general information about predominant cultural groups in one's geographic area. Cultural pocket guides can be a good resource.
- Assess for presence or absence of cultural phenomena based on the understanding of generalizations about a cultural group.
- Do not make assumptions based on cultural background because the degree of acculturation varies among individuals.
- Read research studies that describe cultural differences.
- Read ethnic newspaper articles and novels.
- View documentaries about cultural groups.

Cultural Skill
- Be alert for unexpected responses with patients, especially as related to cultural issues.
- Become aware of cultural differences in predominant ethnic groups.
- Develop assessment skills to do a competent cultural assessment for any patient.
- Learn assessment skills for different cultural groups, including cultural beliefs and practices.

Cultural Encounter
- Create opportunities to interact with predominant cultural groups.
- Attend cultural events, such as religious ceremonies, significant life passage rituals, social events, and demonstrations of cultural practices.
- Visit markets and restaurants in ethnic neighborhoods.
- Explore ethnic neighborhoods, listen to different types of ethnic music, and learn games of various ethnic groups.
- Visit or volunteer at health fairs in local ethnic neighborhoods.
- Learn about prominent cultural beliefs and practices, and incorporate this knowledge into planning nursing care.

may use traditional or folk remedies that affect the treatment prescribed by the health care provider. Patients should be asked about "natural" or herbal substances that they take or actions they have taken to prevent or treat their condition.

Cultural skill refers to the ability to collect relevant cultural data regarding health histories and performing culturally specific assessments. Specific information is presented throughout this book to assist with developing an awareness of cultural differences and learning assessment skills for different cultural groups. Table 3-4 presents a cultural assessment instrument. Providing culturally competent care increases patient satisfaction, reduces health disparities, and prevents misunderstandings between nurses and patients. It also integrates cultural practices into Western biomedical interventions, and results in the provision of culturally appropriate care for patients from diverse cultures.

Cultural encounter is essential for the development of cultural competence and refers to direct cross-cultural interactions between people from culturally diverse backgrounds. Cultural competence requires extended contact with persons from different cultures and learning how their cultural beliefs and practices affect their health and health care practices. Through experience with members of a culture, the nurse can become more competent in caring for them.

TABLE 3-4 Cultural Assessment

Brief History of the Cultural Group with Which the Person Identifies

- With what cultural group(s) does the person affiliate (e.g., Hispanic, Polish, Navaho, or combination)? To what degree does the person identify with the cultural group (e.g., "we" concept of solidarity or as a fringe member)?
- What is the person's reported racial affiliation (e.g., African American, Native American, Asian American, and so on)?
- Where was the person born?
- Where has the person lived (country, city) and when (during what years)? NOTE: If a recent relocation to the United States, knowledge of prevalent diseases in country of origin will be helpful.

Values Orientation

- What are the person's attitudes, values, and beliefs about birth, death, health, illness, health care providers?
- How does the person view work, leisure, education?
- How does the person perceive change?

Cultural Sanctions and Restrictions

- How does the person's cultural group regard expression of emotion and feelings, spirituality, and religious beliefs? How are dying, death, and grieving expressed in a culturally appropriate manner?
- How is modesty expressed by men and women? Are there culturally defined expectations about male-female relationships, including the health care relationship?
- Does the person have any restrictions related to sexuality, exposure of body parts, certain types of surgery (e.g., amputation, vasectomy, hysterectomy)?
- Are there any restrictions against discussion of dead relatives or fears related to the unknown?

Communication

- What language does the person speak at home? What other languages does the person speak or read? In what language would the person prefer to communicate with you?
- Does the person need an interpreter? If so, is there a relative or friend whom he or she would like to interpret? Is there anyone whom the person would prefer did not interpret (e.g., member of the opposite sex, a person younger/older than the person, member of a rival tribe or nation)?
- How does the person feel about health care providers who are not of the same cultural background (e.g., African American, middle-class nurse and Hispanic of a different social class)? Does the person prefer to receive care from a nurse or doctor of the same cultural background, gender, and/or age?

Health-Related Beliefs and Practices

- To what cause(s) does the person attribute illness and disease (e.g., divine wrath, imbalance in hot/cold or yin/yang, punishment for moral transgressions, hex, soul loss)?
- What does the person believe promotes health (eating certain foods, wearing amulets to bring good luck, exercise, prayer, rituals to ancestors, saints, or intermediate deities)?
- What is the person's religious affiliation (e.g., Judaism, Islam, Pentecostalism, West African voodooism, Seventh-Day Adventism, Catholicism, Mormonism)?
- Does the person rely on cultural healers (e.g., curandero, shaman, spiritualist)? Who determines when the person is sick and when he or she is healthy? Who determines the type of healer and treatment that should be sought?
- In what types of cultural healing practices does the person engage (use of herbal remedies, potions, massage, wearing of talismans or charms to discourage evil spirits, healing rituals, incantations, prayers)?
- How are biomedical/scientific health care providers perceived? How does the person and his or her family perceive nurses or physicians? What are the expectations of nurses and nursing care?
- What is appropriate "sick role" behavior? Who determines what symptoms constitute disease/illness? Who decides when the person is no longer sick? Who cares for the person at home?
- How does the person's cultural group view mental disorders? Are there differences in acceptable behaviors for physical versus psychologic illnesses?

Nutrition

- What is the meaning of food and eating to the person? With whom does the person usually eat? What types of food are eaten? What does the person define as food? What does the person believe composes a "healthy" versus an "unhealthy" diet?
- How are foods prepared at home (type of food preparation, cooking oils used, length of time foods are cooked, especially vegetables, amount and type of seasoning added to various foods during preparation)?
- Do religious beliefs and practices influence the person's diet (e.g., amount, type, preparation or delineation of acceptable food combinations, such as kosher diets)? Does the person abstain from certain foods at regular intervals, on specific dates determined by the religious calendar, or at other times?
- If the person's religion mandates or encourages fasting, what does the term *fast* mean (e.g., refraining from certain types or quantities of foods, eating only during certain times of the day)? For what period of time is the person expected to fast?
- During fasting, does the person refrain from liquids/beverages? Does the religion allow exemption from fasting during illness? If so, does the person believe that an exemption applies to him or her?

Socioeconomic Considerations

- Who composes the person's social network (family, peers, and cultural healers)? How do they influence the person's health or illness status?
- How do members of the person's social support network define *caring* (e.g., being continuously present, doing things for the person, looking after the person's family)? What are the roles of various family members during health and illness?
- How does the person's family participate in his or her care (e.g., bathing, feeding, touching, being present)?

Data for spiritual considerations from Andrews MM, Hanson PA: Religion, culture, and nursing. In Andrews MM, Boyle JS, editors: *Transcultural concepts in nursing care,* ed 4, Philadelphia, 2003, Lippincott Williams & Wilkins. From Jarvis C: *Physical examination and health assessment,* ed 4, Philadelphia, 2004, Saunders.

Continued

TABLE 3-4 Cultural Assessment—cont'd

Socioeconomic Considerations—cont'd • Does the cultural family structure influence the person's response to health or illness (e.g., beliefs, strengths, weaknesses, and social class)? Is there a key family member whose role is significant in health-related decisions (e.g., grandmother in many African American families, eldest adult son in Asian families)? • Who is the principal wage earner in the person's family? What is the total annual income? (NOTE: This is a potentially sensitive question that should be asked only if necessary.) Is there more than one wage earner? Are there other sources of financial support (extended family, investments)? • What impact does economic status have on lifestyle, place of residence, living conditions, ability to obtain health care, discharge planning? **Organizations Providing Cultural Support** • What influence do ethnic/cultural organizations have on the person's receiving health care (e.g., Organization of Migrant Workers, National Association for the Advancement of Colored People [NAACP], Black Political Caucus, churches, schools, Urban League, community-based health care programs and clinics)? **Educational Background** • What is the person's highest educational level obtained? • Can the person read and write English, or is another language preferred? If English is the second language, are materials available in the primary language? • What learning style is most comfortable/familiar? Does the person prefer to learn through written materials, oral explanation, or demonstration?	**Religious Affiliation** • What is the role of religious beliefs and practices during health and illness? • Are there healing rituals or practices that the person believes can promote well-being or hasten recovery from illness? If so, who performs these? • What is the role of significant religious representatives during health and illness? Are there recognized healers (e.g., Islamic imams, Christian Scientist practitioners or nurses, Catholic priests, Mormon elders, Buddhist monks)? **Spiritual Considerations** • Does the person have religious objects in the environment? • Does the person wear outer garments or undergarments having religious significance? • Are get-well greeting cards religious in nature or from a religious representative? • Does the person appear to pray at certain times of the day or before meals? • Does the person make special dietary requests (e.g., Kosher diet; vegetarian diet; diet free from caffeine, pork, shellfish, or other specific food items)? • Does the person read religious magazines or books? • Does the person mention God (Allah, Buddha, Yahweh, or a synonym), prayer, faith, or other religious topics? • Is a request made for a visit by a member of the clergy or other religious representative? • Is there an expression of anxiety or fear about pain, suffering, death? • Does the person prefer to interact with others or to remain alone?

Data for spiritual considerations from Andrews MM, Hanson PA: Religion, culture, and nursing. In Andrews MM, Boyle JS, editors: *Transcultural concepts in nursing care,* ed 4, Philadelphia, 2003, Lippincott Williams & Wilkins. From Jarvis C: *Physical examination and health assessment,* ed 4, Philadelphia, 2004, Saunders.

CULTURAL DIVERSITY IN THE HEALTH CARE WORKPLACE

There is an alarming diversity gap when considering the ethnic composition of the health care workforce and the diversity of the overall population in the United States and Canada (Fig. 3-3). In the United States, for example, African Americans, Hispanic Americans, and Native Americans make up more than 25% of the population, but only 9% of the nation's nurses, 6% of its physicians, and 5% of its dentists. If trends continue, the health workforce of the future will resemble the U.S. and Canadian populations even less than it does today. "Unequal Treatment" was a landmark study conducted by the U.S. Institute of Medicine that documented the lower quality of health care and higher rates of illness, disability, and premature deaths among minority populations. These poorer health outcomes for minorities are linked to the shortage of minority health care providers, who have historically been underrepresented in the health professions.[6]

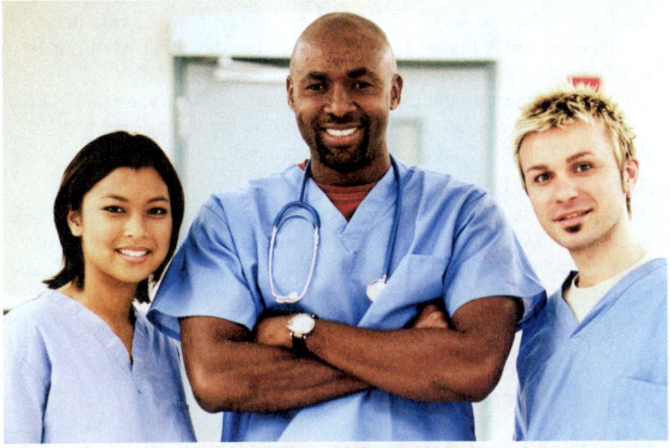

FIG. 3-3 Nurses working together in a multicultural health care environment.

When health care providers from different cultures and countries work together as members of the health care workforce, opportunities for miscommunication and conflict naturally ensue. The cultural origins of miscommunication and conflict in the workplace are often interconnected with cultural beliefs, values, and etiquette. Examples are the meaning, purpose, and value of work; family obligations; time orientation; gender/sexual orientation; and historic rivalries among groups.[7]

CULTURAL FACTORS AFFECTING HEALTH AND HEALTH CARE

Many culture-related factors affect the patient's health and health care. Several potential factors are presented in Table 3-5.

Folk Healers

Each culture has its own **folk healers,** which are also known as *traditional healers*. Most folk healers speak the person's native language and cost less than conventional health care providers. Among the many folk healers found worldwide, Hispanics may turn to a *curandero* (or *curandera*), African Americans may visit a *hougan*, Native Americans may seek help from a medicine man or *shaman,* and Asians may use the services of an acupuncturist. In addition to folk healers, some cultures involve lay midwives (e.g., parteras for Hispanic women) in the care of pregnant women.[3]

Folk medicine is a form of prevention and treatment that is culturally based and traditionally relies on oral transmission of

TABLE 3-5 Cultural Factors Affecting Health and Health Care

Time Orientation
- For some cultures it is more important to attend to a social role than to arrive on time for an appointment with a health care provider.
- Some cultures are future oriented; others are past or present oriented.

Language and Communication
- Patients may not speak English and may not be able to communicate with the health care provider.
- Even with interpreters, there may be difficulties with communication.

Economic Factors
- Patients may not get health care because they cannot pay for it or because of the costs associated with travel for health care.
- Refugee or illegal immigrant status may deter some patients from using the health care system.
- Patients may lack health insurance.

Health Care System
- Patients may not make or keep appointments because of the time lag between the onset of an illness and an available appointment.
- Hours of operation of health care facilities may not accommodate patients' need to work or use public transportation.
- Cumbersome requirements to access some types of care may discourage some patients from taking the steps to qualify for health care or health care payment assistance.
- Some patients have a general distrust of health care professionals and health systems.
- Lack of ethnic-specific health care programs may deter some individuals from seeking health care.
- Transportation may be a problem for patients who have to travel long distances for health care.
- Patients may not have a primary health care provider and may use emergency departments or urgent care centers for health care.
- Shortages of health care providers from specific ethnic groups may deter some people from seeking health care.
- Patients may have a lack of knowledge about the availability of existing health care resources.
- Facility policies may not be culturally sensitive (e.g., hospital policy may limit the number of visitors, which is problematic for cultures that value having many family members present).

Beliefs and Practices
- Care provided in established health care programs may not be perceived as culturally relevant.
- Religious reasons, beliefs, or practices may affect a person's decision to seek (or not seek) health care.
- Patients may delay seeking care because of fear or dependence on folk medicine and herbal remedies.
- Patients may stop treatment or discontinue visits for health care because the symptoms are no longer present, and there is the perception that further care is not required.
- Some patients associate hospitals and extended care facilities with death.
- The patient may have had a previous negative experience with culturally insensitive health care providers or discriminatory practices.
- Some people mistrust the majority population and institutions dominated by them.
- Some patients may feel apprehensive about unfamiliar diagnostic processes and treatment options.

healing techniques from one generation to the next. Much folk medicine is even practiced in the home without the guidance of a folk healer. For example, many European cultures will treat a sore throat with a hot tea made of honey and lemon or a warm gargle of salt water before visiting a medical professional.[8,9]

Spirituality and Religion

Spirituality and religion are aspects of culture that may affect a person's beliefs about health and illness. They may also play a role in nutrition and decisions related to health and ways that a person responds to or treats an illness.

Spirituality refers to a person's effort to find purpose and meaning in life.[10] It is influenced by a person's unique life experiences and reflects one's personal understanding of life's mysteries. Spirituality relates to the soul or spirit more than to the body, and it may provide hope and strength for an individual during an illness.[11]

Religion is a more formal and organized system of beliefs, including belief in or worship of God or gods. Religious beliefs include the cause, nature, and purpose of the universe and involve prayer and ritual(s). Religion is based on beliefs about life, death, good, and evil.[3]

The nurse can use several interventions to meet a patient's spiritual needs, including prayer, scripture, reading, listening, and referral.[10] Many patients find that rituals help them during times of illness.[11] Rituals help a person make sense of his or her life experiences and may take the form of prayer, meditation, or other rituals that the patient may create. The nurse needs to include spiritual assessment in the complete assessment of the patient and plan care based on that assessment. Table 3-6 summarizes health-related religious practices for selected religious groups.

Cross-Cultural Communication

Communication refers to an organized, patterned system of behavior that may be verbal or nonverbal (Fig. 3-4). Verbal communication includes not only the language or dialect, but also the voice tone, volume, timing, and one's ability to share thoughts and feelings.[2] More than 45 million people in the United States speak a language other than English in their home, with Spanish being the most common. A recent study by the Commonwealth Fund found that people of Hispanic background who do not speak English as their primary language report that they have greater communication problems with their health care providers than those for whom English was their primary language (53% versus 26%).[12]

Nonverbal communication may take the form of writing, gestures, body movements, posture, and facial expressions. Nonverbal communication also includes eye contact, use of touch, body language, style of greeting, and spatial distancing.[2] Eye contact varies greatly among cultures. Patients who are Asian, Arab, or Native American may avoid direct eye contact and consider direct eye contact as disrespectful or aggressive. Hispanic patients may expect the nurse to look directly at them, but may not return that direct gaze. Other variables to consider include the role of gender, age, acculturation, status, or position on what is considered to be appropriate eye contact. For example, Muslim-Arab women exhibit modesty when avoiding eye contact with men other than their husbands and when in public situations.

Silence is interpreted based on cultural experiences. Some people are comfortable with silence, whereas others become uncomfortable and may speak to decrease the silent times. Many Native Americans are comfortable with silence and interpret silence as essential for thinking and carefully considering a response. In these interactions,

TABLE 3-6 Health-Related Beliefs and Practices of Selected Religious Groups

Group	Remarks
Amish	• Alcoholic beverages and drugs prohibited unless prescribed by health care professional. • Abortion, artificial insemination, eugenics, and stem cell use prohibited. • Seldom purchase commercial health insurance.
Catholicism	• Fasting and abstaining from meat and meat products on Ash Wednesday and the Fridays of Lent. • Artificial contraception and direct abortion prohibited. Indirect abortion (e.g., treatment of cancerous uterus in a pregnant woman) may be morally justified. • Sacrament of the Sick includes anointing of sick with oil, blessing by a priest, and communion (unleavened wafer made of flour and water).
Church of Jesus Christ of Latter-Day Saints (Mormons)	• Strict dietary code called Word of Wisdom that prohibits all alcoholic beverages, hot drinks (nonherbal teas and coffee), tobacco, and illegal or recreational drugs. • Fasting for 24-hour periods occurs monthly on "Fast Sunday." • During hospitalization or serious illness, an elder anoints the ill person with oil while a second elder seals the anointing with a prayer and blessing (laying on of hands). • Abortion is prohibited except when the mother's life is in danger.
Hinduism	• Eating meat is prohibited because it involves harming a living creature. • Cremation is most common form of body disposal, but fetuses or newborns are sometimes buried.
Islam	• Fasting during daytime hours occurs during a month-long period called Ramadan. • Ritual cleansing with water before eating and before prayer is practiced. • Eating pork or taking medicines with pork derivatives is prohibited. • Drinking alcoholic or other intoxicating beverages is prohibited. • Artificial insemination is permissible only if from the husband to his own wife.
Jehovah's Witness	• Blood in any form and agents in which blood is an ingredient are not acceptable. Blood volume expanders are acceptable if they are not derivatives of blood. • Transplants that involve bodily mutilation are prohibited. • Therapeutic and on-demand abortions are prohibited. • Artificial insemination is prohibited for both donors and recipients.
Judaism	• Strictly observant Jews never eat pork, shellfish, or predatory fowl and never mix milk dishes and meat dishes. Fish with fins and scales are permissible. • Certain foods and drink are designated as *kosher,* which means "proper." All animals must be ritually slaughtered. • On the eighth day after birth, males are circumcised in a ritual called *brit milah* and females are given a dedication ceremony involving prayers and blessings. • Abortion is morally unacceptable except when the mother's life is in danger. • Organized support system for the sick includes a visit from the rabbi. The rabbi may pray with the sick person alone or in a *minyan,* a group of 10 adults over age 13. • If an autopsy is performed, all body parts must be returned for burial.
Seventh-Day Adventism	• Vegetarian diet encouraged. • Nonvegetarian members refrain from eating foods derived from any animal having a cloven hoof that chews its cud (e.g., pigs, goats). Eating fish with fins and scales is acceptable, but consuming shellfish is prohibited. • Consumption of alcoholic beverages is prohibited. • Fasting is practiced and involves abstaining from food or liquids by healthy members of the church.

Data from Andrews MM, Hanson PA: Religion, culture, and nursing. In Andrews MM, Boyle, JS, editors: *Transcultural concepts in nursing care,* Philadelphia, 2003, Lippincott Williams & Wilkins.

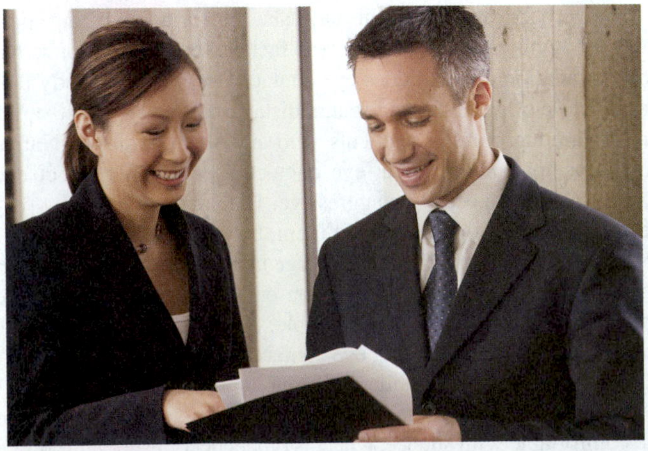

FIG. 3-4 Co-workers from different cultures communicate with verbal and nonverbal cues.

silence shows respect for the other person and demonstrates the importance of the remarks. In traditional Japanese and Chinese cultures, the speaker may stop talking and leave a period of silence for the listener to think about what has been said before continuing. Silence may be intended to show respect for the speaker's privacy, whereas in some cultures (e.g., French, Spanish, Russian) the person may interpret silence as meaning agreement. Asian Americans may use silence to demonstrate respect for elders, whereas African Americans may use silence as a response to what is perceived to be an inappropriate question.

Family Roles and Relationships

Family roles differ from one culture to another (Fig. 3-5). It is important for the nurse to determine who should be involved in communication and decision making related to health care. In some cultural groups there is an emphasis on interdependence rather than independence. For instance, in the United States and

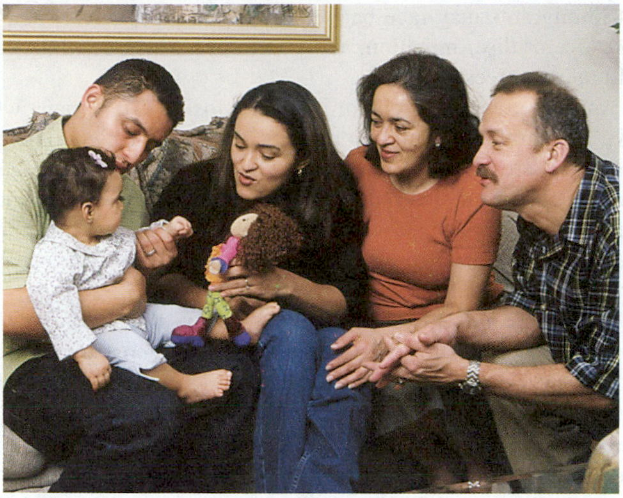

FIG. 3-5 Family roles and relationships differ from one culture to another.

Canada there are strong beliefs related to autonomy. In those countries an individual is expected to sign consent forms when receiving health care. In other cultural groups it may be another family member who is expected to make health care decisions. When the nurse encounters a family that values interdependence over independence, there may be conflicts on how decisions are made. There may be a delay in treatment while the patient waits for significant family members to arrive before giving consent for a procedure or treatment. In other instances, the patient may make a decision that is best for the family but may have negative or adverse consequences for the patient. Being aware of such values will better prepare the nurse to advocate for the patient.

There are also cultural differences related to expectations of family members in providing care. In some cultures, it is expected that family members will provide care for the patient even in the hospital. The patient may expect that the family, along with the health care providers, will provide all care. This view is the opposite of the predominant Western expectation that the patient will assume self-care as quickly as possible.

The nurse needs to ask about culturally relevant gender relationships. For example, in some cultures, such as many Arab groups, it is not appropriate for a man to be alone with a woman other than his wife nor for a woman other than a man's wife to provide physical care for him. The clinical implication of this cultural gender belief is that for many patients from Arab cultures, nurses cannot provide direct physical care for patients of the opposite gender. In some instances, procedures or treatments may be carried out for patients from the opposite gender but only if a third party is present.

Personal Space

Personal space zones refer to the preferred distances between two individuals. Personal space distances vary from culture to culture, as well as within a culture. For whites in the United States, the *intimate distance* ranges from 0 to 18 inches, and the *personal distance* ranges from 18 inches to 4 feet. The personal distance is the one experienced with friends. Social distance ranges from 4 to 12 feet, and public distance is 12 feet or more.[13] Nurses often interact with patients in the intimate or personal zones, which might be uncomfortable for the patient.

There is wide variation in the perception of appropriate distances when considering various cultural groups. Whereas a U.S. or Canadian nurse of European descent may be comfortable with a certain distance, a person from a Hispanic or Middle Eastern background may feel that the distance is too far and will move closer, perhaps causing the nurse to feel uncomfortable. If the nurse then moves away to a more comfortable distance, this may cause the other person to feel that the nurse is unfriendly, or the person may be offended. Personal space distance also varies within cultures. People from the United States, Canada, and the United Kingdom require more personal space than Latin Americans, Japanese, and Arabs.[9]

Touch

Physical contact with patients conveys various meanings depending on the culture. To do a comprehensive assessment, touching a patient is necessary. Many people of Asian and Hispanic heritage believe that touching a person's head is a sign of disrespect, especially because the head is believed to be the source of one's strength and/or soul. Numerous people in the world believe in the evil eye, or *mal ojo*. In this culture-bound syndrome it is believed that the person (usually a child or woman) may become ill as a result of excessive admiration by another person. In some cultures the proper way to ward against the evil eye is to touch the head. It is important for the nurse to ask permission before touching anyone, particularly if it is necessary to touch the person's head.

Nutrition

Food is an important part of cultural practices, including both the foods that are eaten and rituals and practices associated with food. Patients may be asked to make major changes in their diets because of health problems. It is important that the health care provider take into account ethnic and cultural practices and habits when helping a patient plan changes. Food pyramids have been developed for many different ethnic groups. They take into account food preferences of those cultures, while still indicating healthy nutritional practices.

When individuals and families immigrate to an area that is very different from their country of origin, they may be faced with unfamiliar foods, food-storage systems, and food-buying habits. They also may be arriving from countries that have limited food supplies because of poverty, wars, and poor sanitation. They may arrive with conditions such as general poor nutrition, hypertension, diarrhea, and/or dental caries. Other problems may develop after the person arrives in the new country. For example, second-generation Hispanic immigrants have a greater chance of becoming overweight than their first-generation counterparts. The rise in weight was found to be related to the degree of acculturation experienced by the immigrant.[14]

Disease Occurrence, Susceptibility to Disease, and Access to Health Care

The incidence of many diseases, injuries, and other health problems is disproportionately higher in some racial and ethnic populations in the United States and Canada. Such differences may be related to differences in genetic susceptibility and environmental influences that result in health disparities among cultural groups. For example, African Americans, Hispanics, Native Americans, and certain Pacific Islanders have higher incidences of diabetes than whites. Deaths from diabetes and related complications are higher among Native Americans and African Americans than among whites. Diabetes-associated renal failure is higher among Native Americans than among whites.[15] Health disparities are discussed in Chapter 2.

Differences in disease occurrence among ethnic groups presents a challenge for health care providers, but also an opportunity. When health disparities are understood, illness and death may be reduced and survival rates improved. Disparities among ethnic groups are discussed on the *Healthy People 2010* website.[16] This site gives the baseline incidences of several diseases and discusses reasons that these disparities may exist. Specific cultural and ethnic health disparities are discussed throughout this book.

Immigrants and Immigration

Indications show that global migration will accelerate throughout the twenty-first century. Migration is driven by a number of conditions, such as overcrowding, natural disasters, geopolitical conflict, persecution, and economic forces.[4] As a consequence of these migrations, a rich diversity of cultures can be found in many communities and countries today (Fig. 3-6). Nurses are expected to immediately provide culturally congruent and culturally competent care for all patients.

Recent immigrants may be at risk for physical and mental health problems for many reasons. Conditions in their countries of origin (e.g., poor nutrition, sanitation) may have resulted in chronic health problems. In addition, recent immigrants are at increased risk for health problems after arriving in a new area. Relocation is associated with many losses and can cause physical stress and mental distress.

As new immigrants go through the acculturation process, many immigrants experience cultural stress as they adjust to their new environment, especially if they have left relatives behind in their country of origin or are unable to return to their home country. Elderly immigrants are especially affected by changes in role and social position and may be come depressed.[9]

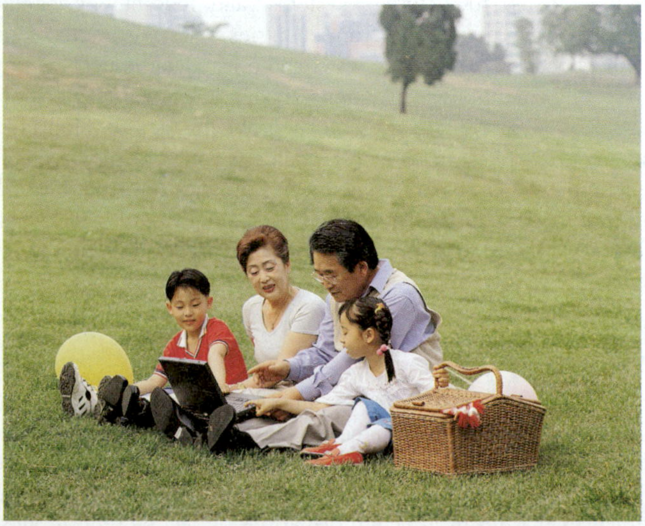

FIG. 3-6 Recently arrived immigrants participate in a common American tradition.

All immigrants may face barriers to social acceptance, such as prejudice or discrimination, and experience a lack of ethnic and cultural resources.

Another potential problem is tuberculosis (TB). Asians who have immigrated recently from areas that have a high endemic rate of TB are more likely to have TB. Compared with the general population of the United States, the TB rate is 112 times greater for newly arrived Vietnamese, 60 times greater for Filipinos, 37 times greater for mainland Chinese, and 28 times greater for Koreans.[3]

During the past 30 years, there has been a shift in the migration pattern of North America. Whereas once most immigrants came from Europe, now most immigrants originate from Asia, Latin America, and Africa. Additionally, there has been an increase in the number of first- and second-generation immigrants who have returned to their homeland in order to visit friends and relatives. These individuals are found to be at a higher risk for malaria, typhoid fever, cholera, and hepatitis A than native-born Americans.

As these immigration patterns continue, there are concerns for the future that will affect the health care environment. Many immigrants lack health insurance and rely on federal support for financing their health care. These individuals can create a burden on emergency departments and urgent care clinics, as they primarily obtain their health care in these settings.

Medications

Genetic differences among people from diverse ethnic or racial groups may explain differences in medication selection, dosage, or administration. For example, some medicines are more effective in certain ethnic groups than others. Side effects may vary among individuals from diverse backgrounds.[17] Table 3-7 highlights the ethnic differences in reaction to medications.

A study was conducted by the National Medical Association (NMA) and the National Pharmaceutical Council (NPC) titled "Racial and Ethnic Differences in Response to Medicines: Towards Individualized Pharmaceutical Treatment."[18] The study demonstrated that genetic variations can affect how the body processes a drug and the overall effect of selected drugs on the body. Although race and ethnicity are imprecise indicators of genetic differences, they can be helpful in anticipating variations in the response to a medicine. For example, there are differences in the characteristics of hypertension for African Americans and whites. Given that African Americans tend to retain more salt and have a higher incidence of salt-sensitive high blood pressure, diuretics used in combination with other blood pressure medications may be necessary to achieve targeted blood pressure levels among African Americans. Similarly, a medication used to treat heart failure (isosorbide dinitrate and hydralazine [BiDil]) is used only in African American patients.

Regardless of their cultural origins, many people use both cultural remedies and prescription drugs to treat their illnesses. Problems can result from interactions of these substances. For example, Chinese Americans who take ginseng as a stimulant and an antihypertensive drug may suffer adverse effects. Some Mexican Americans may treat gastrointestinal problems with preparations that contain lead. Many people now self-treat their depression with St. John's wort, which can result in adverse effects if prescription antidepressants are also taken.

TABLE 3-7 Ethnic Differences in Response to Drugs

Comparison Groups	Drug Class	Clinical Response
Chinese/whites	Benzodiazepines (diazepam [Valium], alprazolam [Xanax])	Chinese require lower doses of diazepam; more sensitive to sedative effects Whites have a higher clearance rate of alprazolam
Asians/whites Hispanics/whites African Americans/whites	Tricyclic antidepressants (e.g., amitriptyline, clomipramine, nortriptyline, imipramine, desipramine)	Asians and Hispanics require lower doses and have greater side effects African Americans show faster response but more side effects
Asians/whites African Americans/whites	Antipsychotics (e.g., haloperidol [Haldol], clozapine [Clozaril])	Asians require lower doses; develop more side effects at lower dose than whites African Americans' use is higher and they tend to receive higher doses
Asian Indians/whites	Analgesics (e.g., acetaminophen, codeine)	Asian Indians have greater clearance rates
Chinese/whites	Analgesics (e.g., codeine)	Chinese less able to metabolize; require increased doses to achieve therapeutic effects
African Americans/whites Chinese/whites	Antihypertensive agents (e.g., ACE inhibitors, β blockers, propranolol)	African Americans respond better to diuretics than whites Whites respond better to ACE inhibitors and β blockers than African Americans Chinese require lower doses of propanolol than whites
Asians/whites	Alcohol	Asians more sensitive to side effects
Native Americans/whites	Alcohol	Native Americans have faster metabolism and less tolerance

From Burroughs VJ, Maxey RW, Levy RA: Racial and ethnic differences in response to medicines: towards individualized pharmaceutical treatment, *J Natl Med Assn* 94(10 Suppl):1-26, 2002.
ACE, Angiotensin-converting enzyme.

Patients may avoid standard Western medicine until herbal and other remedies are ineffective or the illness becomes acute. The challenge for the nurse is to try to accommodate the patient's need for traditional aspects of care while also using scientific approaches as appropriate and as acceptable to the patient. Evaluating the safety and appropriateness of the traditional cultural healing therapies is an important part of this process.

Psychologic Factors

Symptoms are interpreted through a person's cultural norms and may vary from the recognized interpretations of Western medicine. All symptoms have meaning, and the meanings may vary from one culture to another.

Culture-bound syndromes are illnesses or afflictions that are recognized within a cultural group. The symptoms, course of the illness, and people's reactions to the illness are limited to specific cultures. Culture-bound syndromes have their origins in psychosocial characteristics of that culture. For instance, Hispanics may experience *empacho,* a condition described as food forming into a ball that clings to the stomach or intestines, causing pain and cramping. Empacho is treated by folk remedies such as strong massage over the stomach, use of medications, or gently pinching and rubbing the spine.[19] Another culture-bound syndrome is *susto,* which is found throughout Latin America. Susto, sometimes referred to as "fright sickness" or "soul loss," is a traumatic anxiety-depressive state that may result from a frightening experience, such as a loud sound or some threat. Susto can cause anxiety, insomnia, listlessness, loss of appetite, and social withdrawal. One treatment for susto is to have the affected person lie on the floor. The healer then sweeps indigenous herbs over the patient's body while praying to release the evil wind. See Table 3-8 for descriptions of other culture-bound syndromes.

TABLE 3-8 Culture-Bound Syndromes

Group	Syndrome	Description
Hispanics	*Bilis* or *colera*	Caused by strongly experienced anger or rage. Many Latino groups believe that anger affects the body balance of hot and cold. Symptoms include acute nervous tension, headache, trembling, screaming, stomach disturbances, and, in severe cases, loss of consciousness.
	Nervios	Brought on by difficult life experiences. Symptoms may include headaches or "brain aches," irritability, stomach and sleep disturbances, and an inability to concentrate.
Africans	Brain fag	Term describing brain "fatigue" caused by the challenges of school. Symptoms include difficulties in concentrating, remembering, and thinking.
	Thin blood	Affects the elderly, women, and children. Generally weakens an individual and increases susceptibility to illness.
Caribbean and Southern United States	Falling out	Characterized by a sudden collapse, which may sometimes be preceded by dizziness or "swimming" in the head. The person can hear but is unable to move.
Native Americans	Ghost sickness	Condition is sometimes associated with witchcraft and a preoccupation with death. Symptoms include bad dreams, weakness, feelings of fear, danger, futility, dizziness, and a sense of suffocation.
Chinese	*Shenjing shuairuo*	Characterized by physical and mental fatigue, headaches and other pains, dizziness, sleep disturbances, and concentration difficulties.

NURSING MANAGEMENT CULTURALLY COMPETENT CARE

■ *Nurse's Self-Assessment*

The first step in providing culturally competent care is for nurses to assess their own cultural background, values, and beliefs, especially those related to health and health care.[20] Many tools are available to assist in this process. Table 3-3 suggests ways to improve cultural competence. This information can help the nurse to better understand patients and provide more culturally competent care. Many other important aspects of culture related to health care are included in the Culturally Competent Care sections throughout this book.

■ *Patient Assessment*

A cultural assessment should be included in the nursing process. In some institutions, this assessment may involve a specific cultural assessment guide. An example of a cultural assessment guide is included in Table 3-4. It is important to determine (1) the patient's health beliefs and health care practices and (2) the patient's perspective of the meaning, cause, and preferred treatment of illness. When this is done, it will increase the likelihood of successful outcomes for the patient.

How is the nurse to be aware of the differences among ethnic groups? Using guides to cultural assessment will facilitate the nursing process when working with patients, families, or other groups who are from different cultures. Although pocket guides can assist in this process, nurses must be careful not to stereotype. Guides can be used to explore the degree to which patients share commonalities with the cultural information generally attributed to their cultural group.[15] Ultimately, it is most important to identify potential similarities and differences that can assist the nurse to deliver culturally relevant care.

■ *Nursing Implementation*

Communication. Effective communication is most likely to occur when meanings are mutually understood, whether that communication is through gestures, spoken words, or voice tones. To show respect for the patient, any communication should take into account the patient's usual communication style. For instance, a health history should start out in an unhurried manner, and it should include acceptable social and cultural amenities appropriate for the culture. In some cultures it is best to start with general rather than direct questions. For some cultures it is most effective to engage in "small talk," with the discussion including answers that may seem to be unrelated to the questions. If the nurse appears to be "too busy," communication may be impaired.

When meeting a patient or family members, it is appropriate for nurses to introduce themselves and indicate how the patient should address them. Indicate if the patient should use first names; Mr., Ms., or Mrs.; or a title, such as nurse. Also ask the patient how he or she prefers to be addressed. This shows respect and will assist the nurse to begin the relationship in a culturally appropriate manner.

If the nurse needs to gather personal information, it is important to understand the most effective approach to use. For instance, when talking with people from some cultural groups, it is imperative that the nurse takes time to establish trust and listen to the patient's responses to questions. There may be long (by American standards) silences as the person thinks about the question, taking time to show respect by giving the question the appropriate consideration before answering. In some cultures (e.g., Ojibwa and Western Apache) it would be acceptable to take a few days or weeks to properly answer a question. Clearly, most health care situations do not facilitate such answers. However, the nurse can take time to listen and help establish trust.

Silence has many meanings, and it is important for the nurse to understand the nature of the meaning of silence for different cultural groups. It is important to clarify what silence means in an interaction with a patient. Patients will sometimes nod their head, or say "yes" as if agreeing with the nurse or to indicate they understand, when actually they are doing this out of their culturally acceptable manner of showing respect, and may not understand at all.

Some cultures, such as the Hmong, rely primarily on oral communication. When working with patients who are from an oral culture, it would be important to include oral instructions during the teaching-learning process.[15]

The nurse must be cautious and not try to serve as an interpreter if he or she does not have a command of the language, because this could lead to misunderstandings. When the nurse cannot speak the patient's primary language, it is important to enlist the assistance of a person who is qualified to do medical interpretation (Table 3-9). Table 3-10 provides guidelines for communicating when no interpreter is available. With the large number of immigrants and the many different cultural groups in the United States and Canada, it is highly likely that the nurse will encounter patients who do not speak the dominant language.

Using a dictionary that translates from both the nurse's language and the patient's language is helpful (e.g., Spanish-English and English-Spanish dictionary). The nurse can look up questions and potential answers in several different languages using these types of dictionaries. One helpful approach would be to have these types of resources for those cultural groups who frequently use the health care facility. This would be especially beneficial for those instances when a qualified medical interpreter is not readily available and nurses need to learn important phrases in another language.

TABLE 3-9 Using a Medical Interpreter

Choosing an Interpreter

- Use an agency interpreter if possible.
- Interpreter should be a trained medical interpreter who knows how to interpret, has a health care background, understands patient's rights, and can help with advice about the cultural relevance or appropriateness of the health care plan and instructions.
- Use a family member if necessary. Be aware that there may be limitations if the family member does not understand medical terms, is younger or a different gender than the patient, or is not aware of the health care procedures or medical ethics.
- Interpreter should be able to do the following:
  - Translate the nonverbal as well as the literal translation.
  - Translate the message into understandable terms.
  - Act as a patient advocate to represent the patient's needs to the health care team.
  - Be culturally sensitive and understand how to provide teaching instructions.

Strategies for Working with an Interpreter

- If possible, the interpreter should meet with the patient ahead of time to establish rapport before the interpreting begins.
- Use simple language, using as few medical terms as possible.
- Speak in one to two sentences to allow for easier translation.
- Obtain feedback to be sure the patient understands.

TABLE 3-10 Guidelines for Communicating When No Interpreter Is Available

1. Be polite and formal.
2. Pronounce name correctly. If not sure, ask about the correct pronunciation of the name. Use proper titles of respect, such as "Mr.," "Mrs.," "Ms.," "Dr." Greet the person using the last or complete name.
   Gesture to yourself and say your name.
   Offer a handshake or nod. Smile.
3. Proceed in an unhurried manner. Pay attention to any effort by the patient or family to communicate.
4. Speak in a low, moderate voice and avoid excessive hand gestures. Remember that there is a tendency to raise the volume and pitch of your voice when the listener appears not to understand. The listener may perceive that you are shouting and/or angry.
5. Use any words that you might know in the person's language. This indicates that you are aware of and respect his or her culture.
6. Use simple words, such as "pain" instead of "discomfort." Avoid medical jargon, idioms, and slang. Avoid using contractions (e.g., don't, can't, won't). Use nouns repeatedly instead of pronouns.
   Example:
   Do not say: "He has been taking his medicine, hasn't he?"
   Do say: "Does Juan take medicine?"
7. Pantomime words and simple actions while you verbalize them.
8. Give instructions in the proper sequence.
   Example:
   Do not say: "Before you rinse the bottle, sterilize it."
   Do say: "First wash the bottle. Second, rinse the bottle."
9. Discuss one topic at a time. Avoid using conjunctions.
   Example:
   Do not say: "Are you cold and in pain?"
   Do say: "Are you cold (while pantomiming)? Are you in pain?"
10. Validate if the person understands by having him or her repeat instructions, demonstrate the procedure, or act out the meaning.
11. Write out several short sentences in English and determine the person's ability to read them.
12. Try a third language. Many Indochinese speak French. Europeans often know two or more languages. Try Latin words or phrases. Use English words that have Latin roots (e.g., use precipitation instead of rain).
13. Ask the person's family and friends who could serve as an interpreter.
14. Obtain phrase books from a library or bookstore, make or purchase flash cards, contact hospitals for a list of interpreters, and use both a formal and an informal network to locate a suitable interpreter.

From Jarvis C: *Physical examination and health assessment,* ed 4, Philadelphia, 2004, Saunders.

CRITICAL THINKING EXERCISE

CASE STUDY

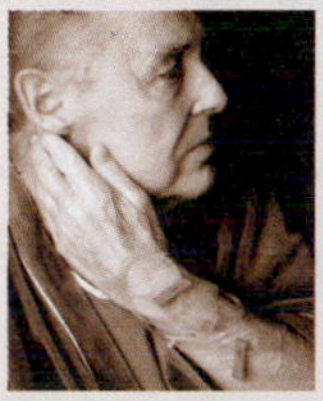

Mexican American Patient

Patient Profile. José, 72 years old, is a Mexican American man who was discharged from the hospital 4 days after a myocardial infarction. He and his wife live in an apartment 5 miles from the hospital. His case manager at the hospital referred him to the home health care agency for follow-up care. He has also been under the care of a curandero since his return home. Neither he nor his wife is able to drive. He is presently homebound because of weakness and shortness of breath. His son and sister live within a few miles of his home and stop in daily to check up on him. He is now unable to attend weekly church services because of his debilitated state and is depressed over his current condition.

Subjective Data

- Has history of hypertension
- Had myocardial infarction 3 years ago
- Cannot walk one block without getting short of breath
- Has swollen feet and cannot wear shoes
- Had fractured hip that was surgically repaired 6 months ago
- Is primarily Spanish speaking
- Immigrated to the United States from Mexico 5 years ago

Collaborative Care

- 2 g sodium diet
- Assessment of home environment
- Patient education program

Critical Thinking Questions

1. What are the initial priorities for the home health nurse?
2. What other members of the home health team should be involved in the care of José? What are their roles and responsibilities?
3. What type of patient education program should be implemented? What are the priority teaching goals? How would you assess José's English language skills? Written? Verbal?
4. What should the nurse consider in the nutrition assessment? How will the nurse address the cultural considerations related to his diet?
5. How would you assess José's religious and spiritual needs?
6. How can the nurse address José's coping skills and use community resources to intervene with his depression?
7. What types of medical equipment will José need? What teaching should accompany the use of this equipment?
8. José's wife inquires about an outpatient cardiac rehabilitation program. What would be an appropriate response from the home health nurse?
9. What are the long-term expected outcomes for José?

NCLEX EXAMINATION REVIEW QUESTIONS

The number of the question corresponds to the same-numbered objective at the beginning of the chapter.

1. Forcing one's own cultural beliefs and practices on another person is an example of
   a. stereotyping.
   b. ethnocentrism.
   c. cultural relativity.
   d. cultural imposition.
2. Immigration may potentially affect an individual's health in all of the following instances *except*
   a. Changes in role and cultural position may lead to depression
   b. The nurse might misinterpret silences during a nurse-patient interaction.
   c. Immigrants may be faced with unfamiliar foods, food-storage systems, and food-buying habits.
   d. Immigrants are rarely affected by changes when they move to an area that has a different physical environment.

3. Which of the following most accurately describes cultural factors that may affect health?
   a. Diabetes and cancer rates differ by cultural/ethnic groups.
   b. Most patients find that religious rituals help them during times of illness.
   c. There are limited ethnic variations in physiologic responses to medications.
   d. Silence during a nurse-patient interaction usually means that the patient understands the instructions.
4. When communicating with a patient who speaks a language that the nurse does not understand, it is important to first attempt to
   a. have a family member translate.
   b. use a trained medical interpreter.
   c. use specific medical terminology so there will be no mistakes.
   d. focus on the translation rather than nonverbal communication.
5. Which of the following accurately reflects a physiologic aspect of culture/ethnicity to consider when providing nursing care?
   a. Native Americans have a greater tolerance for alcohol than whites.
   b. African Americans have a greater response to β blockers than whites.
   c. Whites have a lower clearance rate of alprazolam than Chinese individuals.
   d. Asians may require a lower dose of tricyclic antidepressants and antipsychotics than whites.
6. Which of the following is the first step in developing cultural competence?
   a. Create opportunities to interact with a variety of cultural groups.
   b. Examine one's own cultural background, values, and beliefs about health and health care.
   c. Learn a multitude of folk medicines and herbal substances that different cultures use for self-care.
   d. Learn assessment skills for different cultural groups, including cultural beliefs and practices and physical assessments.
7. As part of the nursing process, cultural assessment is best accomplished by
   a. judging the patient's cultural values based on observations.
   b. using a cultural assessment guide as part of the nursing process.
   c. seeking guidance from a nurse from the patient's cultural background.
   d. relying on the nurse's previous experience with patients from that cultural group.

REFERENCES

1. USDHHS, Bureau of Health Professions, Division of Nursing: Registered nurse population. National sample survey of registered nurses. Final report, 2002, Bureau of Health Professions, Division of Nursing. Available at *http://bhpr.hrsa.gov/healthworkforce/reports/rnsurvey* (accessed April 20, 2006).
2. Giger JN, Davidhizar RE: *Transcultural nursing: assessment and intervention,* ed 4, St Louis, 2004, Mosby.
3. Jarvis C: *Physical examination and health assessment*, ed 4, Philadelphia, 2004, Saunders.
4. Leininger MM, McFarland MR: *Transcultural nursing: concepts, theories, research and practice,* ed 3, New York, 2002, McGraw-Hill.
5. Wells MI: Beyond cultural competence: a model for individual and institutional cultural development, *J Community Health Nurs* 17:189, 2000.
6. Sullivan Commission: Missing persons: minorities in the health professions. Report of the Sullivan Commission on diversity in the healthcare workforce, 2004. Available at *http://aacn.nche.edu/Media/pdf/SullivanReport.pdf* (accessed April 20, 2006).
7. Andrews MM: Cultural diversity in the healthcare workforce. In Andrews MM, Boyle JS, editors: *Transcultural concepts in nursing care,* Philadelphia, 2003, Lippincott Williams & Wilkins, pp 361-401.
8. Spector RE: *Cultural diversity in health and illness*, ed 6, Upper Saddle River, NJ, 2004, Prentice Hall Health.
9. Andrews MM, Boyle JS, editors: *Transcultural concepts in nursing care*, ed 4, Philadelphia, 2003, Lippincott Williams & Wilkins.
10. McEwan W: Spirituality in nursing: what are the issues? *Orthop Nurs* 23(5):321, 2004.
11. Taylor EJ: *Spiritual care: nursing theory, research, and practice*, Upper Saddle River, NJ, 2002, Prentice Hall Health.
12. Collins SC, Hughes DL, Doty MM, et al: Diverse communities, common concerns: assessing health care quality for minority Americans, 2002, Commonwealth Fund, pub no 523. Available at *www.cmfwf.org* (accessed April 20, 2006).
13. Hall E: Proxemics: the study of man's spatial relationships. In Gladstone I, editor: *Man's image in medicine and anthropology*, New York, 1963, New York International University Press.
14. Gordon-Larsen P, Harris KM, Ward DS, et al: Acculturation and overweight-related behaviors among Hispanic immigrants to the US: the National Longitudinal Study of Adolescent Health, *Soc Sci Med* 57(11):2023, 2003.
15. D'Avanzo CE: *Mosby's pocket guide to cultural health assessment*, ed 3, St Louis, 2003, Mosby.
16. *Healthy people 2010: understanding and improving health.* Available at *www.health.gov/healthypeople/Document/tableofcontents.htm#partb* (accessed April 16, 2006).
17. Munoz C, Hilgenberg C: Ethnopharmacology: understanding how ethnicity can affect drug response is essential to providing culturally competent care, *Am J Nurs* 105(8):41, 2005.
18. Burroughs VJ, Maxey RW, Levy RA: Racial and ethnic differences in response to medicines: towards individualized pharmaceutical treatment, *J Natl Med Assoc* 94(10):1, 2002. Available at *www.npcnow.org* (accessed April 20, 2006).
19. Ludwig-Beymer PA: Transcultural aspects of pain. In Andrews MM, Boyle JS, editors: *Transcultural concepts in nursing care,* Philadelphia, 2003, Lippincott Williams & Wilkins, pp 405-431.
20. Odom-Forren J: Cultural competence: a call to action, *J Perianesth Nurs* 20(2):79, 2005.

RESOURCES

Bioethics Resources on the Web: Culture and Ethnicity in Medicine
301-496-4000
www.nih.gov/sigs/bioethics/culturalcomp.html

Center for Cross-Cultural Research
360-650-3574
www.ac.*wwu.edu/~culture*

Cross Cultural Health Care Program
206-860-0329
www.xculture.org

Diversity Rx
www.diversityrx.org

EthnoMed
206-731-3000
http://ethnomed.org

Minority Health
520-626-6241
www.ahsl.arizona.edu/weblinks/resources_by_topic.cfm?name=Minority%20Health

National Center for Cultural Competence
202-687-5000
http://gucchd.georgetown.edu/ncc/documents

Transcultural C.A.R.E. Associates
www.transculturalcare.net

Transcultural Nursing Society
888-432-5470
www.tcns.org

For additional Internet resources, see the website for this book at *http://evolve.elsevier.com/Lewis/medsurg.*

The most important practical lesson that can be given to nurses is to teach them what to observe.
Florence Nightingale

Health History and Physical Examination

4

Patricia Graber O'Brien

LEARNING OBJECTIVES

1. Explain the purpose, components, and techniques related to a patient's health history and physical examination.
2. Obtain a nursing history using a functional health pattern format.
3. Describe the appropriate use and techniques of inspection, palpation, percussion, and auscultation.
4. Differentiate between a screening physical examination and a focused examination in terms of indications, purposes, and components.
5. Record a nursing history and physical examination using a standard format.

KEY TERMS

auscultation, p. 48
functional health patterns, p. 43
general survey statement, p. 46
inspection, p. 47
objective data, p. 40
palpation, p. 47
percussion, p. 47
subjective data, p. 40

Electronic Resources

Supplemental content related to Chapter 4 can be found . . .

Companion CD

- Stress-Busting Kit for Nursing Students
- NCLEX Examination Review Questions
- Comprehensive Glossary

Evolve Website evolve

http://evolve.elsevier.com/Lewis/medsurg

- Content Updates
- Key Points (Printable and CD/MP3 Download)
- Concept Map Creator
- Expanded Audio Glossary
- Key Term Flash Cards
- Electronic Calculators
- Physical Examination Video
- WebLinks

Obtaining a patient's health history and performing a physical examination are activities completed by the nurse during the assessment phase of the nursing process. The information obtained during this phase contributes to a database that identifies the patient's current and past health status and provides a baseline against which future changes can be evaluated. The purpose of the nursing assessment is to enable the nurse to make a clinical judgment or diagnosis about the patient's health status.[1] Although assessment is identified as the first step of the nursing process, it is performed continuously throughout the nursing process to validate diagnoses, evaluate the patient's response to nursing interventions, and determine the extent to which patient outcomes and goals have been met.

DATA COLLECTION

Collection of data about the patient is not solely the nurse's responsibility. The **database** is all the health information about a patient. It includes the nursing history and physical examination, the physician's history and physical examination, results of laboratory and diagnostic tests, and information contributed by other health professionals. The nurse and physician both perform a patient history and physical examination, but they use different formats and analyze the data differently because of each discipline's focus.

Medical Focus

A **medical history** is a standard format designed to collect data to be used primarily by the physician to determine risk for disease and diagnose a medical condition (Table 4-1). The medical history is usually collected by a member of the medical team (physician, resident, physician's assistant, or medical student) or a nurse practitioner. The physician's physical examination and laboratory and diagnostic tests assist in establishing a medical diagnosis and evaluating specific medical therapy. The information collected and reported by the physician is also used by nurses and other health care providers, but within the focus of their care. For example, the

Reviewed by Dorothy Mathers, RN, MSN, Associate Professor, Nursing, Pennsylvania College of Technology, Williamsport, Pa.; and Colleen R. Walsh, RN, MSN, ONC, CS, ACNP-BC, Faculty Graduate Nursing, University of Southern Indiana School of Nursing and Health Professions, Evansville, Ind.

TABLE 4-1 Medical History Format

- Demographic data
- Chief complaint
- History of present illness
- Past health history
- Family health history
- Review of systems

abnormal results of a neurologic examination by a physician may assist in the diagnosis of a brain lesion, but the nurse may use those same results to identify a nursing diagnosis of risk for falls. A physical therapist may also use the information to plan therapy involving exercise, splints, or ambulatory aids.

Nursing Focus

The focus of nursing care is the diagnosis and treatment of human responses to actual or potential health problems or life processes. The information obtained from the **nursing history** and physical examination is used to determine the strengths of the patient or responses the patient exhibits, or could potentially exhibit, as a result of a health problem. In the patient with a medical diagnosis of diabetes mellitus, one of the patient's responses may be anxiety or a lack of knowledge for self-management of the condition. The patient may also experience the physical response of fluid volume deficit because of the abnormal fluid loss caused by hyperglycemia. These human responses to the condition of diabetes can be diagnosed and treated by nurses. During the nursing history interview and physical examination, the nurse obtains the necessary data to support the identification of nursing diagnoses.

Types of Data

The database includes both subjective and objective data. **Subjective data** are collected by interviewing the patient during the nursing history. It includes information that can only be described or verified by the patient. It is what the person tells the nurse about himself or herself either as spontaneously offered information or as a response to direct questioning. Subjective data are also referred to as *symptoms.* Knowledgeable others, such as family members and caregivers, can also contribute subjective data about the patient.

Objective data are data that can be observed and measured. This type of data is obtained using inspection, palpation, percussion, and auscultation during the physical examination. Objective data are also provided by other health care providers and diagnostic testing. Objective data are also called *signs.* Usually subjective data are obtained by interview and objective data are obtained by physical examination. However, it is common for the patient to provide subjective data while the nurse is performing the physical examination and for the nurse to observe objective signs while interviewing the patient during the history. The term **clinical manifestations** may be used to describe the objective and subjective data obtained from a patient that are commonly associated with a clinical problem.

Approaches to Data Collection

Numerous approaches and formats are used to gather information about the patient. The amount and organization of data collected depend on the needs of the patient, the health care setting, and the clinical situation. A *comprehensive database* is obtained at the onset of care in a primary care setting and on admission to a hospital or a long-term care facility. It includes information related to the patient's health status, health maintenance behaviors, individual coping patterns, support systems, current developmental tasks, and any risk factors or lifestyle changes. For the ill patient, the database also includes a description of the health problem, the patient's perception of the illness, functional ability or patterns of living, and response to health problems.[1]

Shorter, more focused databases are more commonly compiled. An *episodic or problem-centered assessment* is performed when a problem of limited scope is identified. It is used in all health care settings and includes a history and examination related to one problem, such as an upper respiratory infection, a minor injury, or specific abnormal findings in a hospitalized patient. A *follow-up database* is an assessment to evaluate the status of previously identified problems. In an emergency situation, an *emergency database* may be obtained by rapid, specific questioning of the patient while performing assessment and maintenance of vital functions.

Interviewing Considerations

The purpose of the patient interview is to obtain a health history—subjective data about the patient's past and present health state. Effective communication is a key factor in the interview process. Creating a climate of trust and respect is critical to establishing a therapeutic relationship.[2] The nurse must communicate acceptance of the patient as an individual by using an open, responsive, nonjudgmental approach. Individuals communicate not only through language but also in their manner of dress, gestures, and body language. Modes of communication are learned through one's culture, influencing not only the words, gestures, and posture one uses, but also the nature of information that is shared with others (see Chapter 3). In addition to understanding the principles of effective communication, each nurse must develop a personal style of relating to patients. Although no single style fits all people, wording specific questions in certain ways will increase the probability of eliciting the needed information. Ease at asking questions, particularly those related to sensitive areas such as sexual functioning and economic status, comes with experience.

The amount of time needed to complete a nursing history may vary with the format used and the experience of the nurse. It may be completed in one or several sessions, depending on the setting and the patient. In the case of an older adult patient with a low energy level, several short sessions may need to be scheduled. It is important to allow time for the patient to volunteer information about particular areas of concern. When a patient is unable to provide the necessary data (e.g., is unconscious or aphasic), the nurse should ask the person who has assumed responsibility for the patient's welfare to provide as much information as possible.

Before beginning the nursing history, the nurse should explain to the patient that the purpose of a detailed history is to collect information that will provide a health profile for comprehensive health care, including health promotion. This detailed information is collected during entry into the health care system, and subsequently, only updates are needed. The nurse should explain that personal and social data are needed to individualize the plan of care. This explanation is necessary because the patient may not be accustomed to sharing personal information and may need to know the purpose of such questioning. Patients should also be informed that federal legislation affects the electronic exchange, privacy, and security of an individual's health information. When the Health Insurance Portability and Accountability Act (HIPAA) was enacted in 1996 to protect health insurance coverage for workers and their families when they change or lose their jobs, one provision of the law was the "Privacy Rule." The Privacy Rule addresses the use and disclosure of an individual's health information to ensure that such information is properly protected while also allowing the flow of the information needed to provide and promote high-quality health care.

Most health plans, health care providers, and health care clearinghouses that transmit health information in electronic form are subject to the Privacy Rule. Although most patients receive written information about their privacy rights on initial contact with a health care entity, the nurse must know and be able to explain the provisions of the law. Patients should be informed that they can see and get a copy of their health records, that they can have corrections added to their health information, and that they can decide whether to give their permission before their information can be used or shared for certain purposes. (Detailed information about HIPAA and the Privacy Rule is provided in fundamental and legal textbooks and at *www.hhs.gov/ocr/hipaa*.)

To obtain factual, easily categorized information a direct interview technique can be used. Closed questions such as "Have you had surgery before?" that require brief, specific responses are used. When asking sensitive personal and social questions, the nurse can communicate the acceptance or normalcy of behaviors by prefacing questions with phrases such as "most people" or "frequently." For example, stating, "Many people taking antihypertensive drugs have concerns about sexual functioning; do you have any you would like to discuss?" shows the patient that a particular situation may not be unique to that patient. Another method of putting the patient at ease is to word the question so that an affirmative answer appears expected. An example of this technique is to ask, "What do you like to drink at a party?" instead of, "Do you drink?" These questions are open ended, encouraging the patient to discuss the issue in the patient's own words and at his or her own pace.[2]

The nurse must judge the reliability of the patient as a historian. An older adult may give a false impression about his or her mental status because of a prolonged response time or visual and hearing impairments. The complexity and long duration of health problems may also make it difficult for an older adult to be an accurate, orderly historian.

It is important that the nurse determine the patient's priority concerns and expectations from the present encounter. Often there is a lack of congruency between the priorities of the patient and the nurse. For example, the nurse's priority may be to obtain needed information and complete necessary documentation, whereas the patient is interested only in getting relief from symptoms. Until the patient's priority need is met, the nurse will probably be unsuccessful in obtaining complete data.

The nurse must make a judgment about the amount of information that should be collected on initial contact with the patient. In interviews with older adult patients, patients with long-term chronic disease, patients with pain, and patients in emergency situations, the nurse may choose to ask only those questions that are pertinent to a specific problem and to defer the complete history interview until a more appropriate time.

Symptom Investigation

At any time during assessment the patient may relate a symptom such as pain, fatigue, or weakness. Because symptoms are directly experienced by the patient and not observable to the nurse, the symptom must be investigated. Table 4-2 lists eight areas that should be investigated if a symptom is present. The information that is obtained may help determine the cause of the symptom. For example, if a patient states that he has "pain in his leg at times," the nurse would obtain and record the following information:

> Has right midcalf pain (location), described as "like being stabbed with a knife" (quality). Pain is so severe that it is not possible for the patient to continue walking (quantity). Onset is abrupt, lasting for 1 to 2 minutes; it occurs once or twice daily, and it last occurred on 1/30/07 (chronology). Generally occurs at work when climbing stairs after lunch, but last occurred when cutting lawn (setting). Pain is alleviated by rest for 2 to 3 minutes. The patient has been salting his food "more heavily" than he used to, but "it doesn't help" (alleviating factor). Leg pain is at times accompanied by chest pain that causes some nausea (associated manifestations). The patient has not altered his lifestyle because of the intermittent pain. He thinks it is caused by "muscle cramps from lack of salt" (personal meaning).

TABLE 4-2 Investigation of a Symptom

Location	
Ask	"Where do you feel it? Where is it located?"
Record	Region of the body Local or radiating, superficial or deep
Quality	
Ask	"What does it (feel, look) like?"
Record	The patient's analogy (e.g., "Like being burned")
Quantity	
Ask	"How often do you have this feeling? How bad is it? How much is it? How big is it?"
Record	Frequency (mild, moderate, severe), volume, size, extent, number
Chronology	
Ask	"When was the first time it occurred? Any particular time of day, week, month, or year?"
Record	Time of onset, duration, periodicity and frequency, course of symptoms
Setting	
Ask	"Where are you when this occurs? What are you doing?"
Record	Where patient is when symptom occurs, what patient is doing, if symptom is related to anything
Aggravating or Alleviating Factors	
Ask	"What makes it better? Worse? Is there any activity that seems to cause it? What have you done for it? Did it help? Was there some reason you didn't do anything about it?"
Record	Influence of physical and emotional activities, patient's attempts to alleviate (or treat) the symptom
Associated Manifestations	
Ask	"What other things do you see or feel when it occurs? Has it affected your appetite? Elimination? Sleeping?"
Record	Other symptoms
Meaning of the Symptom to the Patient	
Ask	"How has it affected your life? Why have you sought care now? What do you think may be the cause?"
Record	Patient's statements about the effect of the symptom and the cause of the symptom

TABLE 4-3 Comparison of Functional Health Patterns and NANDA International Taxonomy II

Functional Health Patterns	Taxonomy II Domains
Health Perception–Health Management	**Health Promotion**
Perception of health status and relevance to activities and plans	Awareness of normal function and well-being
Health risk management	Identifying and using activities to maintain health and well-being
General health care behavior	
Adherence to health promotion activities, medical or nursing prescriptions, and follow-up care	
Nutritional-Metabolic	**Nutrition**
Usual food and fluid intake; appetite	Taking food or nutrients into the body
Daily eating times	Using nutrients for tissue maintenance, tissue repair, and production of energy
Recent weight change and reason	Taking in and absorption of fluids and electrolytes
Food restrictions or preferences, diet supplements	
Swallowing, chewing, eating problems, food allergies	
Skin lesions and general ability to heal	
Condition of skin, hair, nails, mucous membranes, and teeth	
Temperature, height, weight	
Elimination	**Elimination**
Bowel	Secretion and excretion of waste products from the body: urine, bowel waste products, skin excretion, and by-products of metabolic processes from the lung
Usual pattern of excretory function	
Changes in frequency, quality, quantity	
Use of routines or laxatives	
Assistive devices	
Bladder	
Usual frequency, quality, quantity	
Problems with control	
Assistive devices	
Skin Condition	
Excess perspiration, odor problems	
Turgor, edema, pruritus	
Activity-Exercise	**Activity-Rest**
Exercise, activity, leisure, and recreation	Production, conservation, expenditure, or balance of energy resources
Type, quantity, and quality of exercise	Sleep and rest; doing work and moving body
Factors that interfere with desired patterns	State of harmony between intake and expenditure of resources
Limitations in activities of daily living	Cardiopulmonary mechanisms that support activity/rest
Sleep-Rest	
Usual sleep/rest patterns	
Perception of quality and quantity of sleep	
Aids, including medications and routines	
Cognitive-Perceptual	**Perception-Cognition**
Sensory adequacy: hearing, sight, smell, touch, taste	Mental readiness to notice or observe
Prosthetic devices (glasses, hearing aids)	Awareness of time, place, and person
Pain perception/management	Receiving and comprehending information through the senses
Heat or cold sensitivity	Uses of memory, learning, thinking, judgment, problem solving, insight, language
Language, judgment, memory abilities	Sending and receiving verbal and nonverbal information
Self-Perception–Self-Concept	**Self-Perception**
Self-description/perception	Perceptions of total self
Attitudes about self	Assessment of one's own worth, capability, significance, and success
Perception of abilities, body image, identity, self-esteem	Mental image of one's own body
Posture, eye contact, voice and speech patterns	
Role-Relationship	**Role-Relationships**
Life roles and responsibilities	Caregiving roles by nonprofessionals providing care
Satisfaction or dissatisfaction in family, work, and social relationships	Family relationships and associations
Responsibilities related to roles	Role functioning in expected behavior patterns
Sexuality-Reproductive	**Sexuality**
Patterns of satisfaction or dissatisfaction with sexuality	Sexual identity
Adequacy of sexual knowledge	Capacity or ability to participate in sexual activities
Reproductive pattern/state (female: premenopausal or postmenopausal)	Reproduction of new people

Sources: Gordon M: *Manual of nursing diagnosis,* ed 10, St Louis, 2002, Mosby; NANDA International: *Nursing diagnoses: definitions and classification 2005-2006*, Philadelphia, 2005, NANDA International.
NANDA, North American Nursing Diagnosis Association.

TABLE 4-3 Comparison of Functional Health Patterns and NANDA International Taxonomy II—cont'd

Functional Health Patterns	Taxonomy II Domains
Coping–Stress Tolerance General coping strategies Stress tolerance, stress reduction behaviors Support systems Ability to manage situations	**Coping–Stress Tolerance** Reactions to physical or psychologic trauma Managing environmental stress Nerve and brain function evidenced by behavioral responses
Value-Belief Values, goals, beliefs that are basis for decisions Important factors in life; quality of life Perceived conflicts in health-related values or beliefs Spiritual practices	**Life Principles** Identification and ranking of preferred modes of conduct or end states Acts or customs that are true or have intrinsic worth Balance between values, beliefs, and actions
	Safety-Protection Response to infection, bodily harm, or hurt Potential for violence, environmental hazards Defensive processes; thermoregulation
	Comfort Sense of physical, environmental, and social well-being or ease
	Growth and Development Increases in physical dimensions; maturity of organ systems Attainment, lack of attainment, or loss of developmental milestones

Data Organization

Assessment data must be systematically obtained and organized in such a manner that they can be readily analyzed to make a judgment about the patient's health status and any health problems. Some assessment forms are organized to ask the patient about symptoms and problems associated with body systems. Although this information is helpful to nurses, it is incomplete because areas such as health promotion behaviors, sleep, coping, and values are not addressed.

Functional health patterns, developed by Gordon,[3] constitute the framework used throughout this textbook for obtaining a nursing history. This format includes an initial collection of important health information followed by assessment of 11 areas of health status or function (Table 4-3). Data organized in this format promotes the identification of areas of wellness (or positive function), as well as health problems.[2]

NANDA International has also developed Taxonomy II, a classification system for nursing diagnoses, that is similar to Gordon's functional health patterns.[4] This format includes 13 domains of function that cluster data related to specific nursing diagnoses. Because of its broad overview, Taxonomy II may also be used to organize assessment data. Table 4-3 compares Gordon's functional health patterns with NANDA International's Taxonomy II.[3,4]

CULTURALLY COMPETENT CARE
ASSESSMENT

The process of obtaining a health history and performing a physical examination is a very intimate experience for both the nurse and the patient. As noted earlier in the chapter, one's culture influences patterns of communication, as well as what information is shared with others. During interviewing and physical assessment, the nurse must be sensitive to issues of eye contact, space, modesty, and touching, as discussed in Chapter 3. Adhering to cultural codes related to male-female relationships and gender identification is especially important during physical examination. To avoid violating any culturally based practices, the nurse should ask the patient about cultural aspects of male-female relationships and if the patient would like to have a friend or family member present during the history and/or physical examination.[1]

NURSING HISTORY: SUBJECTIVE DATA

Important Health Information

Important health information provides an overview of past and present medical conditions and treatments. Past health history, medications, and surgery or other treatments are included in this part of the history.

Past Health History. The past health history provides information about the patient's prior state of health. The patient is specifically asked about major childhood and adult illnesses, injuries, hospitalizations, operations, therapeutic regimens, travel, habits, and the use of supportive devices. Specific questioning is more effective than simply asking if the patient has had any illness or health problems in the past.

Medications. Specific details related to past or present medications are obtained. This includes the use of prescription drugs, over-the-counter drugs, vitamins, herbal products, and dietary supplements. Patients frequently do not consider herbal products and dietary supplements as drugs. Because they can interact adversely with existing medications, it is important to specifically ask about their use. (See Complementary and Alternative Therapies box on p. 44.) Examples of specific prescription and over-the-counter medications to ask about include corticosteroids, birth control pills, antibiotics, diuretics, aspirin, antacids, and laxatives. Older adult patients, in particular, should be questioned about medication routines. Changes in absorption, metabolism, reaction to drugs, and elimination of drugs, as well as surgery and concurrent disease, make drug-related concerns a serious potential problem for older adults.[5]

Surgery or Other Treatments. All injuries, hospitalizations, and surgeries are recorded along with the date of the event, the treatment, and the outcome. The outcome includes whether the problem was completely resolved or if there are residual effects. Blood transfusions received by the patient also are noted.

COMPLEMENTARY AND ALTERNATIVE THERAPIES

Assessment of Use of Herbal Products and Dietary Supplements

- Herbal products and dietary supplements may have side effects and/or may interact adversely with existing medications.
- Most patients do not tell health care providers that they are using herbal preparations and dietary supplements. They may fear health care professionals will disapprove of their use.
- Available forms include pills, capsules, tinctures, powders, teas, ointments, and suppositories.
- Patients at high risk for drug-herb interactions include those taking anticoagulant, antihypertensive, or immune-regulating therapy and patients receiving anesthesia for surgery.
- Nurses should create an accepting and nonjudgmental environment when assessing use of or interest in herbal products or dietary supplements.
- Use open-ended questions such as "What types of herbs, vitamins, or supplements do you take?" and "What effects have you noticed from using them?"
- Respond to patients with comments that invite an open-minded discussion.
- Avoid using the expression "alternative therapy" because patients may not consider what they are doing to be alternative.
- Many herbal preparations contain a variety of ingredients. Therefore the nurse may need to ask the patient or family members to bring labeled containers to the health care site to determine the composition of the products.
- Documentation of any herbal product(s) or dietary supplements used should be recorded in the patient database.

Functional Health Patterns

The nurse assesses the patient's functional health patterns to identify positive functions and to determine if dysfunctional health patterns and/or potential dysfunctional patterns exist. Dysfunctional health patterns result in nursing diagnoses, and potential dysfunctional patterns identify risk conditions for problems. In addition, the nurse may identify patients with effective function who express a desire for a higher level of wellness. Examples of specific questions appropriate to ask the patient related to the functional health patterns are presented in Table 4-4.

Health Perception–Health Management Pattern. Assessment of the health perception–health management functional health pattern focuses on the patient's perceived level of health and well-being and on personal practices for maintaining health. This includes preventive screening activities, such as breast and testicular examinations; colorectal cancer, hypertension, and cardiac disease risk screening; Papanicolaou (Pap) test; and immunizations such as tetanus, pneumonia, hepatitis, and flu vaccines. The nurse should ask about the type of health care provider that the patient uses. Culture may play a role in who is the patient's primary health care provider. For example, if the patient is Native American, a medicine man may be considered as the primary health care provider. If the patient is of Hispanic origin, a curandero (Hispanic healer who uses folk medicine, herbal products, and/or magic to treat patients) may be the primary health care provider (see Chapter 3).

There are several ways to identify the patient's perceived level of health and well-being. First, when questioning the patient, the nurse determines the patient's feelings of effectiveness at staying healthy by asking what helps and what hinders. Next, the patient is asked to describe personal health and any concerns about it. This information should be recorded in the patient's own words. It often is useful to determine whether the patient considers his or her health to be excellent, good, fair, or poor.

The questions for this pattern also seek to identify risk factors by obtaining a family history, history of health habits (e.g., smoking, alcohol, drug use), and exposure to environmental hazards. The patient is asked about a family history of major problems, such as cardiovascular disease, hypertension, cancer, diabetes mellitus, psychiatric illness, and genetic disorders. Information about sexual abuse, violence, and drug and alcohol use/abuse should also be obtained.

If the patient is hospitalized, expectations of this experience should be determined. A description of the patient's understanding of the current health problem, including a description of its onset, course, and treatment, should be obtained. Determining what the patient does when ill is important. These questions elicit information about a patient's knowledge of the health problem, awareness of what should be done, and ability to use appropriate resources to manage the problem.

Nutritional-Metabolic Pattern. The processes of ingestion, digestion, absorption, and metabolism are assessed in this pattern. A 24-hour dietary recall should be obtained from the patient. From this information the nurse can evaluate the quantity and quality of foods and fluids consumed. If a problem is identified, the nurse may request that the patient keep a 3-day food diary for a more careful analysis of dietary intake. Food frequency questionnaires based on weekly intake are also available to obtain information from the person. Metabolism is evaluated by questioning the patient regarding weight gain, weight loss, energy level, and skin lesions or dryness.

The impact of psychologic factors such as depression, anxiety, and self-concept on nutrition is assessed. For example, "How is your appetite affected by anxiety?" is an appropriate question. Socioeconomic and cultural factors such as food budget, who prepares the meals, and food preferences are also assessed.

Determining how the patient's present condition has interfered with eating and appetite is important. If the patient's present condition has produced symptoms such as nausea, intestinal gas, or pain, the effect of these symptoms on appetite should be determined. Food allergies and the need for a special or restricted diet should be noted. Food allergies should be differentiated from food intolerances, such as lactose intolerance. Additional information about the person's nutritional status can be determined by asking specific questions such as the following:

"How many fruits and vegetables do you eat a day?"
"Give me an example of your usual intake of meat."
"How well do you heal from a wound?"

Elimination Pattern. The nurse assesses bowel, bladder, and skin function in this pattern. The nurse asks about the frequency of bowel and bladder activity. A description of consistency, amount, color, and unusual odor of urine and stools should be elicited. The patient should be asked if loss of control or pain is associated with defecating or urinating. If laxatives or enemas are used, the frequency, type, and results should be noted. If any collecting devices are used, such as catheter or colostomy equipment, the nurse asks about their use and care.

The skin is assessed again in the elimination pattern in terms of its excretory function. The patient should be asked about the condition of his or her skin and whether edema, pruritus, or excessive perspiration is problematic.

Activity-Exercise Pattern. The patient's usual pattern of exercise, activity, leisure, and recreation is assessed by the nurse. The patient should be questioned about his or her ability to perform activities of daily living. Table 4-4 includes the grading scale for self-care abilities under the activity-exercise pattern. If the patient is unable to perform activities of daily living, such as toileting, eating, and moving independently, the specific problems that limit an activity should be noted. Chest pain, dyspnea, dizziness, intermittent claudication, musculoskeletal pain, fatigue, and weakness are problems that commonly result in some degree of self-care deficit.

TABLE 4-4 Nursing History: Functional Health Pattern Format

Demographic Data
Name, address, age, occupation
Culture and ethnicity

Important Health Information
Past health history
Medications/Supplements
Surgery or other treatments

Functional Health Patterns

Health Perception–Health Management Pattern
1. Reason for visit?
2. General state of health?
3. Number of colds in past year?
4. Most important things done to keep healthy? Breast self-examination? Testicular self-examination? Other routine screening?
5. Health compliance problems?
6. Cause of illness? Action taken? Results?
7. Things important to you while here?
8. Family health history?
9. Illness and injury risk factors: use of cigarettes, alcohol, drugs?
10. Allergies? Immunizations?

Nutritional-Metabolic Pattern
1. Typical daily food intake (describe)? Supplements?
2. Typical daily fluid intake (describe)?
3. Weight loss or gain (amount, time span)?
4. Desired weight?
5. Appetite?
6. Food or eating: Discomfort? Diet restrictions?
7. Change in appetite with anxiety?
8. Heal well or poorly?
9. Skin problems: Lesions? Dryness?
10. Dental problems?
11. Food preferences?
12. Food allergies?

Elimination Pattern
1. Bowel elimination pattern (describe): Frequency? Character? Discomfort? Laxatives? Enemas?
2. Urinary elimination pattern (describe): Frequency? Problem in control? Diuretics?
3. Any external devices?
4. Excess perspiration? Odor problems? Itching?

Activity-Exercise Pattern
1. Sufficient energy for desired or required activities?
2. Exercise pattern? Type? Regularity?
3. Spare time (leisure) activities?
4. Dyspnea? Chest pain? Palpitations? Stiffness? Aching? Weakness?
5. Perceived ability for (code for level):

Feeding ____	Cooking ____	Grooming ____
Bed mobility ____	Bathing ____	Dressing ____
Toileting ____	Shopping ____	General mobility ____

Functional Levels Code
Level 0: Full self-care
Level I: Requires use of equipment or device
Level II: Requires assistance or supervision from another person
Level III: Is dependent and does not participate

Sleep-Rest Pattern
1. Generally rested and ready for daily activities after sleep?
2. Sleep onset problems? Aids? Dreams (nightmares)? Early awakening?
3. Usual sleep rituals?
4. Usual sleep pattern?

Cognitive-Perceptual Pattern
1. Hearing difficulty? Hearing aids?
2. Vision? Wear glasses? Last checked?
3. Any change in taste? Any change in smell?
4. Any recent change in memory?
5. Easiest way to learn things?
6. Any discomfort? Pain? How managed?
7. Ability to communicate?
8. Understanding of illness?
9. Understanding of treatments?

Self-Perception–Self-Concept Pattern
1. Self-description? Self-perception?
2. Effect of illness on self-image?
3. Relieving factors?

Role-Relationship Pattern
1. Live alone? Family? Family structure diagram?
2. Difficult family problems?
3. Family problem solving?
4. Family dependence on you for things? How managing?
5. Family's and others' feelings about illness/hospitalization?*
6. Problems with children? Difficulty handling?*
7. Belong to social groups? Have close friends? Feel lonely (frequency)?
8. Work satisfaction (school)? Income sufficient for needs?*
9. Feel part of or isolated from neighborhood where living?

Sexuality-Reproductive Pattern
1. Any changes or problems in sexual relations?*
2. Effect of illness?
3. Use of contraceptives? Problems?
4. When menstruation started? Last menstrual period? Menstrual problems? Gravida? Para?†
5. Effect of present condition or treatment on sexuality?
6. Sexually transmitted diseases?

Coping–Stress Tolerance Pattern
1. Tense a lot of the time? What helps? Use any medicines, drugs, alcohol?
2. Have someone to confide in? Available to you now?
3. Recent life changes?
4. Problem-solving techniques? Effective?

Value-Belief Pattern
1. Satisfied with life?
2. Religion important in your life?
3. Conflict between treatment and beliefs?

Other
1. Other important issues?
2. Questions?

Modified from Gordon M: *Manual of nursing diagnosis*, ed 10, St Louis, 2002, Mosby.
*If appropriate.
†For women.

Sleep-Rest Pattern. This pattern describes the patient's pattern of sleep, rest, and relaxation in a 24-hour period. The individual's perception of the effectiveness of sleep and relaxation is pertinent. This information can be elicited by asking, "Do you feel rested when you wake up?" Most people take sleep for granted unless they have a problem with sleeping.

The patient's usual activities related to bedtime and the usual sleep pattern should be determined. Particular routines, position, medications, and environmental factors used to foster sleep should also be elicited.

Cognitive-Perceptual Pattern. Assessment of this pattern involves a description of all senses (vision, hearing, taste, touch, and smell) and the cognitive functions such as communication, memory, and decision making. In addition, pain is assessed as a sensory perception in this pattern. (See Chapter 10 for details on pain assessment.) The patient should be asked about any sensory deficits that affect the ability to perform activities of daily living. Routine eye care, including the date of the last examination, should be elicited. Ways in which the patient compensates for any sensory-perceptual problems should be discussed and noted. Patients should be asked how they communicate best and about their understanding of their illness and treatment. This information is used by the nurse in planning patient teaching.

Self-Perception–Self-Concept Pattern. This pattern describes the patient's self-concept, which is critical in determining the way the person interacts with others. Included are attitudes about self, perception of personal abilities, body image, and general sense of worth. The nurse should ask the patient for a self-description and how the health condition affects self-attitude. Expressions of hopelessness or loss of control by the patient frequently reflect an inability to care for oneself.

Role-Relationship Pattern. This pattern describes the roles and relationships of the patient, including major responsibilities. It also examines the patient's self-evaluation of his or her performance of the expected behaviors related to these roles.

The patient should be asked to describe family, social, and work relationships. The nurse should determine if patterns in these relationships are satisfactory or if strain is evident. The nurse should note the patient's feelings about his or her role in these relationships and the effect the present condition has on his or her role and relationship.

Sexuality-Reproductive Pattern. This pattern describes satisfaction or dissatisfaction with personal sexuality and describes the reproductive pattern. Assessing this pattern is important because many illnesses, surgical procedures, and medications affect sexual function. A patient's sexual and reproductive concerns may be expressed, teaching needs and treatable problems may be identified, and normal growth and development may be monitored through information obtained in this pattern.

The interview should be appropriate to the gender, age, and developmental stage of the patient. For example, a 40-year-old widowed female patient might be asked if she has any problems related to her genital area, such as vaginal discharge. She also should be asked whether she is sexually active and, if so, whether she uses a condom or requires her partner to use a condom. A 25-year-old male patient might be asked about his knowledge and use of condoms.

Specifically, the nurse should determine if there is a lack of knowledge in relation to sexuality and reproduction. Whether the patient perceives a problem in the area of sexuality should also be determined. The effect of the patient's present condition or treatment on personal sexuality should be noted.

Obtaining information related to sexuality often is difficult for the nurse. However, it is important to take a health history and screen for sexual function and dysfunction. Based on the complexity of the problem, the nurse may be able to provide limited information or refer the patient to a more experienced professional.

Coping–Stress Tolerance Pattern. This pattern describes the patient's general coping pattern and the effectiveness of the coping mechanisms. Assessment of this pattern involves analyzing the specific stressors or problems that confront the patient, the patient's perception of the stressor, and the patient's response to the stressor.

The major losses or changes experienced by the patient in the previous year are important to document. Current major stressors confronting the patient are also important. The strategies used by the patient to deal with stressors and relieve tension should be noted. Individuals and groups who make up the patient's social support networks should be recorded.

Value-Belief Pattern. This pattern describes the values, goals, and beliefs (including spiritual) that guide health-related choices.[3] The patient's ethnic background and the effects of culture and beliefs about health and illness on health practices should be documented. The patient's wishes about continuation of religious practices and the use of religious articles should be noted and honored. The possibility of a conflict in values or beliefs can be determined by asking a question such as, "Does your plan of care cause any conflict in your value or belief system?"

PHYSICAL EXAMINATION: OBJECTIVE DATA

General Survey

Following the nursing history, a **general survey statement** is made. The general survey is a statement of the provider's general impression of a patient, including behavioral observations. This initial survey is considered a scanning procedure and begins with the provider's first encounter with the patient and continues during the health history interview.

Although the provider may include other data that seem pertinent, the major areas usually included in the general survey statement are (1) body features, (2) state of consciousness and arousal, (3) speech, (4) body movements, (5) obvious physical signs, (6) nutritional status, and (7) behavior. Vital signs and the body mass index (BMI) that is calculated from height and weight are often included in the general survey statement. Observations of these areas provide the data for the general survey statement. The following is a sample of a general survey statement:

> Mrs. H. is a 34-year-old Hispanic woman, BP 130/84, P 88, R 18. No distinguishing body features. Alert but anxious. Speech rapid with trailing thoughts. Wringing hands and shuffling feet during interview. Skin flushed, hands clammy. Overweight relative to height. Sits with eyes downcast and shoulders slumped and avoids eye contact.

Physical Examination

The **physical examination** is the systematic assessment of the physical and mental status of a patient, and findings are considered objective data. Throughout the physical examination, any positive findings are explored using the same criteria as the investigation of a symptom during the nursing history (see Table 4-2). A **positive finding** indicates that the patient has or had the particular problem or sign under discussion (e.g., if the patient with jaundice has an enlarged liver, it is a positive finding). Relevant information about this problem should then be gathered.

Negative findings may also be significant. A **pertinent negative** is the absence of a sign or symptom usually associated with a problem. For example, peripheral edema is common with advanced liver disease. If edema is not present in a patient with advanced liver disease, this should be specifically noted as "no peripheral edema."

Types. There are two types of physical examinations: the screening physical examination and a focused or problem-centered examination. The **screening physical examination** is performed for screening situations, health surveillance, and health maintenance purposes. It is an organized, purposeful check of major body systems to detect any possible problems. If a problem is detected in the course of the screening physical examination, a more detailed focused examination of the involved system should be done.

A **focused** (problem-centered) **examination** is a more detailed assessment of a particular body system. The patient's clinical manifestations should alert the nurse to the appropriate focused examination. For example, abdominal pain indicates the need to do a focused examination of the abdomen. Some problems necessitate more than one focused examination. A complaint of headache may indicate the need to do musculoskeletal, neurologic, and head and neck examinations.[6] Focused examinations are frequently used to assess the progress of a specific problem identified during a screening examination.

Techniques. Four major techniques are used in performing the physical examination: inspection, palpation, percussion, and auscultation. The physical assessment techniques are usually performed in the sequence of inspection, palpation, percussion, and auscultation. The only exception to this sequence is for the abdominal examination. In this situation the sequence is inspection, auscultation, percussion, and palpation. Palpation and percussion of the abdomen before auscultation can alter bowel sounds and produce false findings. Every assessment area does not require the use of all four assessment techniques (e.g., assessment of the musculoskeletal system requires only inspection and palpation).

Inspection. Inspection is the visual examination of a part or region of the body to assess normal conditions or deviations from normal. Inspection is more than just looking. This technique is deliberate, systematic, and focused. The nurse needs to compare what is seen with the known, generally visible characteristics of the body part being inspected. For example, most 30-year-old men have hair on their legs. Absence of hair may indicate a vascular problem and signals the need for further investigation, or it may be normal for a patient of a particular ethnicity. For example, Native American men have very little body hair.

Palpation. Palpation is the examination of the body through the use of touch. The use of light and deep palpation can yield information related to masses, pulsations, organ enlargement, tenderness or pain, swelling, muscular spasm or rigidity, elasticity, vibration of voice sounds, crepitus, moisture, and differences in texture.[7] Different parts of the hand are more sensitive for specific assessments. For example, the tips of the fingers are used to palpate lymph nodes, the dorsa of hands and fingers are used to assess temperatures, and the palmar surface is best suited for feeling vibrations (Fig. 4-1).

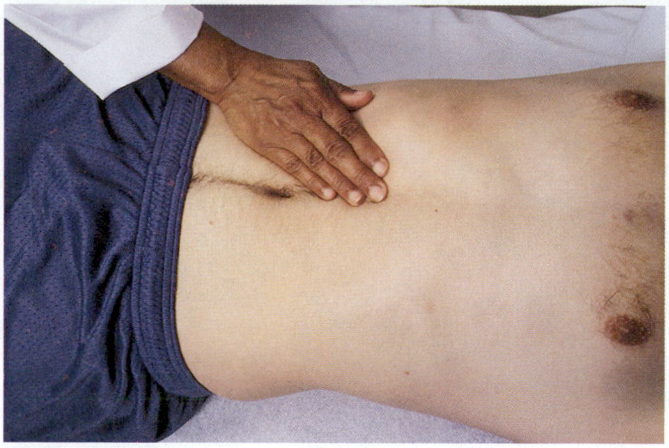

FIG. 4-1 Palpation is the examination of the body through the use of touch.

Percussion. Percussion is an assessment technique involving the production of sound to obtain information about the underlying area. The percussion sound may be produced directly or indirectly. Direct percussion is performed by directly tapping the body with one or two fingers to elicit a sound. Indirect, or mediated, percussion is the more common percussion technique. The middle finger (pleximeter) of the nondominant hand is placed firmly against the body surface. The nondominant finger is usually hyperextended to prevent excess pressure on the region being percussed, thus dampening resonance. The tip of the middle finger of the dominant hand (plexor) strikes the distal phalanx or the distal interphalangeal joint of the pleximeter finger (Fig. 4-2). A relaxed wrist and rapid strike produce the best sounds. The sounds and the vibrations produced are evaluated relative to the underlying structures. Deviation from an expected sound may indicate a problem. For example, the usual percussion sound in the right lower quadrant of the abdomen is tympany. Dullness in this area may indicate a problem that should be investigated.

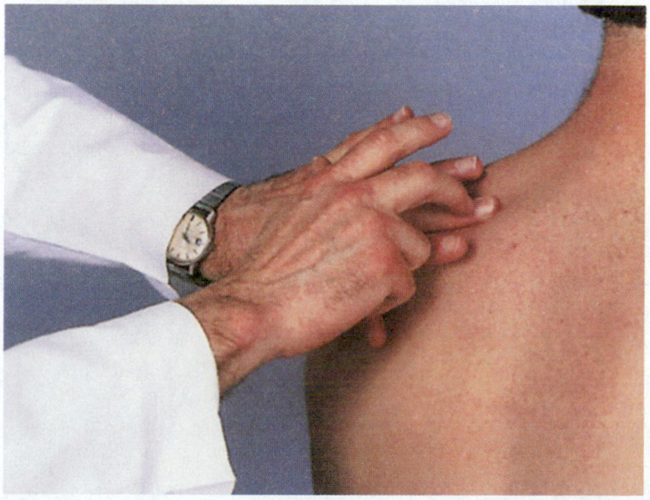

FIG. 4-2 Percussion technique. Tapping the interphalangeal joint. Only the middle finger of the nondominant hand should be in contact with the skin surface.

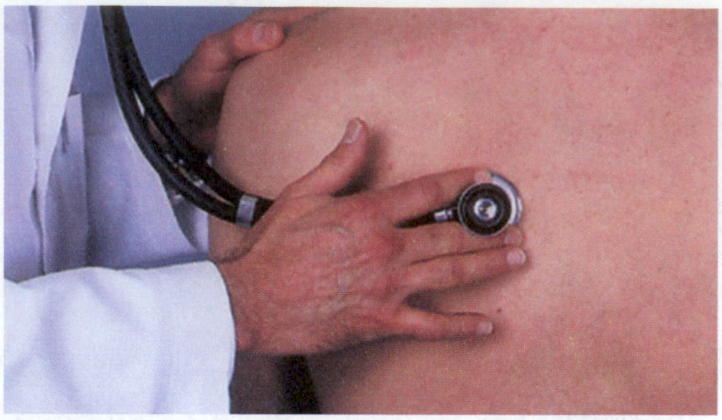

FIG. 4-3 Auscultation is listening to sounds produced by the body to assess normal conditions and deviations from normal.

TABLE 4-5 Equipment for Screening Physical Examination

• Stethoscope (with bell and diaphragm, tubing 15-18 in [38-46 cm])	• Pocket flashlight
• Wristwatch (with second hand or digitalized)	• Tongue blades
• Blood pressure cuff	• Cotton balls
• Ophthalmoscope/otoscope set	• Percussion hammer
• Eye chart (wall chart or Snellen pocket eye card)	• Tuning fork
	• Alcohol swabs
	• Patient gown
	• Paper cup with water
	• Examining table or bed

(Specific percussion sounds of various body parts and regions are discussed in the appropriate assessment chapters.)

Auscultation. Auscultation is listening to sounds produced by the body to assess normal conditions and deviations from normal. Auscultation is usually indirect, using a stethoscope to clarify sounds by blocking out extraneous sounds (Fig. 4-3). The bell of the stethoscope is more sensitive to low-pitched sounds. The diaphragm of the stethoscope is more sensitive to high-pitched sounds. Auscultation is particularly useful in evaluating sounds from the heart, lungs, abdomen, and vascular system. (Specific auscultatory sounds and techniques are discussed in the appropriate assessment chapters.)

Equipment. The equipment needed for the physical examination should be easily accessible during the examination (Table 4-5). Organizing equipment before the examination saves the time and energy of the patient and the nurse. (The uses of specific pieces of equipment are discussed in the appropriate assessment chapters.)

Organization of the Examination. The physical examination should be performed systematically and efficiently. Explanations should be given to the patient as the examination proceeds. The factors to be considered are the nurse's efficiency and the patient's comfort, safety, and privacy. The examiner is less likely to forget a procedure, a step in the sequence, or a portion of the body if the same sequence is followed every time. Table 4-6 presents an outline for the screening physical examination that is organized, logical, and complete. Adaptations of the physical examination often are useful for the older adult patient, who may have age-related problems such as decreased mobility, limited energy, and

TABLE 4-6 Outline for Screening Physical Examination

1. General Survey *Observe general state of health (patient is seated):* • Body features • State of consciousness and arousal • Speech • Body movements and carriage • Physical appearance • Nutritional status • Stature **2. Vital Signs** *Record vital signs:* • Blood pressure—both arms for comparison • Radial pulse • Respiration • Temperature • Record height and weight • Body mass index (BMI) **3. Integument** *Inspect and palpate skin for the following:* • Color • Lesions • Scars • Bruises • Edema • Moisture • Texture • Temperature • Turgor • Vascularity	*Inspect and palpate nails for the following:* • Color • Lesions • Size • Flexibility • Shape • Angle • Capillary refill time **4. Head and Neck** *Inspect and palpate head for the following:* • Shape and symmetry of skull • Masses • Tenderness • Hair • Scalp • Skin • Temporal arteries • Temporomandibular joint • Sensory (CN V, light touch, pain) • Motor (CN VII, shows teeth, purses lips, raises eyebrows) • Looks up, wrinkles forehead (CN VII) • Raises shoulders against resistance (CN XI) *Inspect and palpate (occasionally auscultate) neck for the following:* • Skin (vascularity and visible pulsations) • Symmetry • Postural alignment • Range of motion • Pulses and bruits (carotid) • Midline structure (trachea, thyroid gland, cartilage)

AP, Anterior-posterior; *CN,* cranial nerve; *CVA,* costovertebral angle.

TABLE 4-6 Outline for Screening Physical Examination—cont'd

4. Head and Neck—cont'd

- Lymph nodes (preauricular, postauricular, occipital, mandibular, tonsillar, submental, anterior and posterior cervical, infraclavicular, supraclavicular)

Inspect and palpate eyes for the following:

- Visual acuity
- Eyebrows
- Position and movement of eyelids (CN VII)
- Visual fields
- Extraocular movements (CN III, IV, VI)
- Cornea, sclera, conjunctiva
- Pupillary response (CN III)
- Red reflex
- Eyeball tension

Inspect and palpate nose and sinuses for the following:

- External nose: shape; blockage
- Internal nose: patency of nasal passages; shape; turbinates or polyps; discharge
- Frontal and maxillary sinuses

Inspect and palpate ears for the following:

- Placement
- Pinna
- Auditory acuity (Weber's or Rinne, whispered voice, ticking watch) (CN VIII)
- Mastoid process
- Auditory canal
- Tympanic membrane

Inspect and palpate mouth for the following:

- Lips (symmetry, lesions, color)
- Buccal mucosa (Stensen's and Wharton's ducts)
- Teeth (absence, state of repair, color)
- Gums
- Tongue for strength (asymmetry, ability to stick out tongue, side to side, fasciculations) (CN XII)
- Palates
- Tonsils and pillars
- Uvular elevation (CN IX)
- Posterior pharynx
- Gag reflex (CN IX and X)
- Jaw strength (CN V)
- Moisture
- Color
- Floor of mouth

5. Extremities

Observe size and shape, symmetry and deformity, involuntary movements

Inspect and palpate arms, fingers, wrists, elbows, shoulders for the following:

- Strength
- Range of motion
- Crepitus
- Joint pain
- Swelling
- Fluid
- Test reflexes:
  - Biceps
  - Triceps
  - Brachioradialis
  - Patellar
  - Achilles
  - Plantar

Inspect and palpate legs for the following:

- Strength of hips
- Edema
- Hair distribution
- Pulses (dorsalis pedis, posterior tibialis)

6. Posterior Thorax

Inspect for muscular development, respiratory movement, approximation of AP diameter

- Palpate for symmetry of respiratory movement, tenderness of CVA, spinous processes, tumors or swelling, tactile fremitus
- Percuss for pulmonary resonance
- Auscultate for breath sounds
- Auscultate for egophony, bronchophony, and whispered pectoriloquy

7. Anterior Thorax

- Assess breasts for configuration, symmetry, dimpling of skin
- Assess nipples for rash, direction, inversion, retraction
- Initiate teaching or review of breast self-examination
- Inspect for apical impulse, other precordial pulsations
- Palpate the apical impulse and the precordium for thrills, lifts, heaves, tenderness
- Inspect neck for venous distention, pulsations, waves
- Palpate axillae
- Palpate breasts
- Auscultate for rate and rhythm, character of S_1 and S_2 in the aortic, pulmonic, Erb's point, tricuspid, mitral areas; bruits at carotid, epigastrium; breath sounds at RML

8. Abdomen

- Inspect for scars, shape, symmetry, bulging, muscular position and condition of umbilicus, movements (respiratory, pulsations, presence of peristaltic waves)
- Auscultate for peristalsis, bruits
- Percuss border of liver, four abdominal quadrants
- Palpate to confirm positive findings; check liver (size, surface contour, tenderness); spleen; kidney (size, contour, consistency, tenderness); urinary bladder (distention); femoral pulses; inguinofemoral nodes; and abdominal aorta

9. Completion of Examinations of Extremities

Observe the following:

- Range of motion of hips, knees, ankles, feet
- Crepitus
- Joint pain
- Swelling
- Fluid
- Muscle development
- Coordination (heel to shin)
- Homans' sign
- Proprioception (position sense of great toe)

10. Neurologic

Motor status observations:

- Gait
- Toe walk
- Heel walk
- Drift

Coordination:

- Finger to nose
- Romberg sign
- Heel to opposite shin
- Spine (scoliosis)

11. Genitalia*

Male External Genitalia

- Inspect penis, noting hair distribution, prepuce, glans, urethral meatus, scars, ulcers, eruptions, structural alterations
- Inspect epidermis of perineum, rectum
- Inspect skin of scrotum; palpate for descended testes, masses, pain

Female External Genitalia

- Inspect hair distribution; mons pubis, labia (minora and majora); urethral meatus; Bartholin's, urethral, Skene's glands (may also be palpated, if indicated); introitus
- Assess for presence of cystocele, prolapse
- Inspect perineum, rectum

RML, Right middle lobe; S_1 and S_2, heart sounds.

*If the nurse has the appropriate training, the speculum and bimanual examination of women and the prostate gland examination of men should be performed after this inspection.

TABLE 4-7 GERONTOLOGIC DIFFERENCES IN ASSESSMENT
Adaptations in Physical Assessment Techniques

General Approach
Keep patient warm and comfortable, because loss of subcutaneous fat decreases ability to stay warm. Adapt positioning to physical limitations. Avoid unnecessary changes in position. Perform as many activities as possible in the position of comfort for the patient.

Skin
Handle with care because of fragility and loss of subcutaneous fat.

Head and Neck
Provide a quiet environment free from distraction because of possible sensory deficits (e.g., decreased vision, touch, hearing).

Extremities
Use nonvigorous movements and reinforcement techniques. Avoid having patient hop on one foot or perform deep knee bends because of patient's limited range of motion of the extremities, decreased reflexes, and diminished sense of balance.

Thorax
Adapt examination for changes due to decrease in force of expiration, weakened cough reflex, and shortness of breath.

Abdomen
Use caution in palpating patient's liver because it is readily accessible because of a thinner, softer abdominal wall. The older adult patient may have diminished pain perception in abdominal wall.

Genitalia
Use a well-lubricated, smaller speculum for vaginal examination because dryness and atrophy of the female genitalia may cause discomfort.

perceptual changes.[5] An outline listing some of the useful adaptations is found in Table 4-7.

Recording the Screening Physical Examination. Only abnormal findings should be recorded during the actual examination. This prevents needless interruptions in the examination to write lengthy normal findings. At the conclusion of the examination, the nurse should combine the normal and abnormal findings in a carefully recorded physical examination. Table 4-8 is an example of how to record a screening physical on a healthy adult. See Table 6-3 for the age-related assessment findings in each assessment chapter for helpful references in recording age-related assessment differences.

PROBLEM IDENTIFICATION AND NURSING DIAGNOSES

After completing the history and physical examination, the nurse clusters and analyzes the data to develop a list of nursing diagnoses and collaborative problems. Fig. 4-4 illustrates the problem identification phase of the nursing process. (Chapter 1 explains the process of establishing nursing diagnoses.)

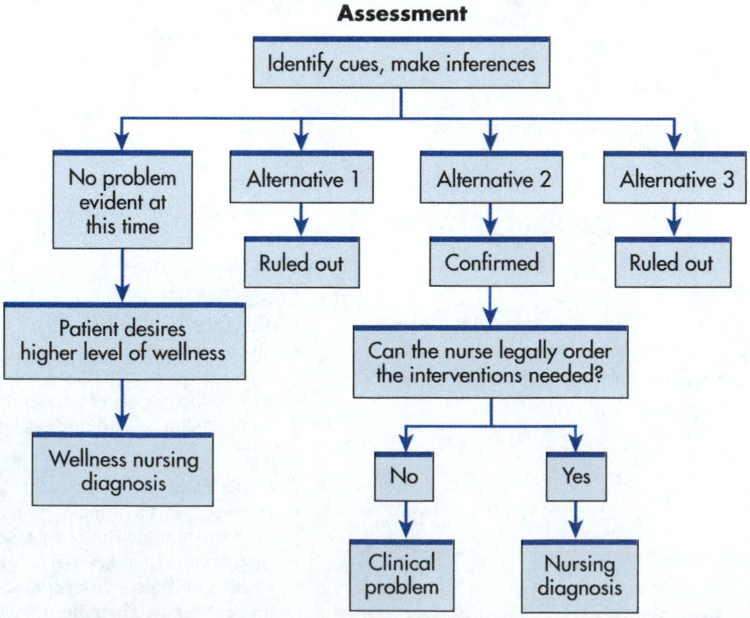

FIG. 4-4 Problem identification phase of the nursing process.

TABLE 4-8 Documentation of Normal Findings on a Screening Physical Examination

Patient's Name ______________________

Age ______________________

General Status
Well-nourished, well-hydrated, well-developed white (woman) or (man) in NAD, appears stated age, looks pleasant, smiles readily, speech clear and evenly paced; is alert and oriented ×3; cooperative, calm

Skin
Clear s̄ lesions, warm and dry, trunk warmer than extremities, turgor returns quickly, no ↑ vascularity, no varicose veins

Nails
Well-groomed, round 160-degree angle s̄ lesions, nail beds pink, nails flexible

Hair
Thick, brown, shiny, normal (male, female) distribution

Head
Normocephalic, sinuses nontender

Eyes
Visual fields intact on gross confrontation

VA:	Right eye	20/20
	Left eye	20/20
	Both eyes	20/20
	s̄ glasses	

EOM: Intact on all gazes s̄ ptosis, nystagmus

Fundi: Red reflex present bilat no opacities, fundi: optic disc has clear margins and appropriate cup size, vessels taper with no indentation or displacement

Pupils: PERRLA, negative cover and uncover tests, negative Hirschberg test

Ears
Pinna intact, in proper alignment; external canal patent; small amount cerumen present; TMs intact; pearly gray LM, LR visible, not bulging; Rinne: AC>BC; Weber's: does not lateralize, whisper heard at 3 ft

Nose
Patent bilaterally; turbinates pink, no swelling

Mouth
Moist and pink, soft and hard palates intact, uvula rises midline on "ahh," 24 teeth present and in good repair

Throat
Tonsils surgically removed, no redness

Tongue
Moist, pink, size appropriate for mouth

Neck
Supple, s̄ masses, s̄ bruits, lymph nodes nonpalpable and nontender

Thyroid: Palpable, smooth, not enlarged

ROM: Full, intact strong

Trachea: Midline, nontender

Breasts
Soft, nonpendulous, s̄ venous pattern, s̄ dimpling, puckering

Nipples: s̄ inversion, point in same direction, areola dark and symmetric, no discharge, no masses, nontender

Axilla
Hair present, shaved, no lesions, nontender

Thorax and Lungs
AP < transverse diameter, resp rate 18, reg rhythm, no ↑ in tactile fremitus, no tenderness, lungs resonant throughout, diaphragmatic excursion 4 cm bilaterally, chest expansion symmetric, lung fields clear throughout

Heart
Rate 82, reg rate and rhythm; no lifts, heaves

Apical impulse: 5th ICS at MCL; no palpable thrills; S_1, S_2 louder, softer in appropriate locations; no S_3, S_4; no murmurs, rubs, clicks

Carotid, femoral, pedal, and radial pulses present; equal, 2+ bilaterally

Abdomen
No pulsations visible, rounded, active bowel sounds, no bruits or CVA tenderness, no palpable masses

Liver
Lower border percussed at costal margin, smooth, nontender; approx 9 cm span

Spleen
Nonpalpable, nontender

Neurologic System
Cranial nerves I-XII intact

Motor (drift, toe stand) intact

Coord (FN, Romberg) intact

Reflexes: *See diagram*

Grading Scale

0	No response
1 +	Diminished
2 +	Normal
3 +	Increased
4 +	Hyperactive

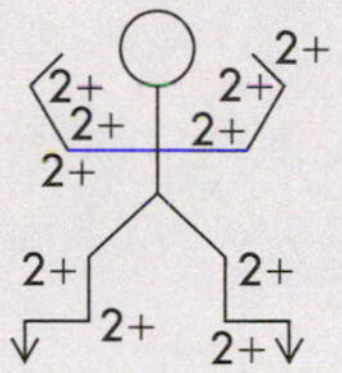

Sensation (touch, vibration, proprioception) intact

Musculoskeletal System
Well developed, no muscle wasting; s̄ crepitus, nodules, swelling

ROM: Full, intact, and equal bilaterally; no scoliosis

Strength: Equal, strong bilaterally 5/5

Gait: Walks erect 2-foot steps, arms swinging at side s̄ staggering

Female Genitalia*
External genitalia: No swelling, redness, tenderness in BUS; normal hair distribution, no cysts

Vagina: No lesions, discharge; bulging, pink

Cervix: Os closed; pink, no lesions, erosions, nontender

Uterus: Small, firm, nontender

Adnexa: No enlargement; nontender

Rectovaginal: Sphincter intact; confirms above findings

Male Genitalia
Normal male hair distribution, negative inguinal hernia

Penis: Urethral opening patent; no redness, swelling, discharge; no lesions, structural alterations

Scrotum: Testes descended; no redness, masses, tenderness

Rectal*: No lesions, redness; sphincter intact; prostate small, nontender

Psychologic Status
Affect appropriate; eye contact

Orientation: Oriented ×3

Mood: Pleasant, appropriate

Thought content: Intelligent, coherent

Memory: Remote and recent intact

Serial sevens: Not done or intact

Signature ______________________

AC>BC, Air conduction greater than bone conduction; *AP,* anterior-posterior; *BUS,* Bartholin's gland, urethral meatus, Skene's duct; *coord,* coordination; *CVA,* costovertebral angle; *EOM,* extraocular movements; *FN,* finger to nose; *ICS,* intercostal space; *LM,* landmarks; *LR,* light reflex; *MCL,* midclavicular line; *NAD,* no acute distress; *PERRLA,* pupils equal, round, reactive to light and accommodation; *ROM,* range of motion; *s̄,* without; S_1, S_2, S_3, and S_4, heart sounds; *TM,* tympanic membrane; *VA,* visual acuity.

*These data would be obtained from an examination of the genitalia if the nurse has the appropriate training.

NCLEX EXAMINATION REVIEW QUESTIONS

The number of the question corresponds to the same-numbered objective at the beginning of the chapter.

1. The nursing history provides information to assist the nurse primarily in
   a. diagnosing a medical problem.
   b. investigating a patient's symptoms.
   c. classifying subjective and objective data.
   d. supporting identification of nursing diagnoses.
2. The nurse would place information that the patient revealed about his concern that his illness is threatening his job security in which of the following functional health patterns?
   a. Role-relationship
   b. Cognitive-perceptual
   c. Coping–stress tolerance
   d. Health perception–health management
3. To examine the skin of a patient who has a full-thickness burn, the nurse primarily uses the technique of
   a. inspection.
   b. palpation.
   c. percussion.
   d. auscultation.
4. A focused examination is performed when
   a. the patient denies a health problem.
   b. a baseline health maintenance examination is required.
   c. a specific problem is identified during physical examination.
   d. the medical diagnosis directs attention to a specific problem area.
5. After performing a screening history and physical, the first information the nurse records is the
   a. health history.
   b. general survey.
   c. patient symptoms.
   d. abnormal findings.

REFERENCES

1. Jarvis C: *Physical examination and health assessment*, ed 4, St Louis, 2004, Saunders.
2. Wilson S, Giddens J: *Health assessment for nursing practice,* ed 3, St Louis, 2005, Mosby.
3. Gordon M: *Manual of nursing diagnosis,* ed 10, St Louis, 2002, Mosby.
4. NANDA International: *Nursing diagnoses: definitions and classification 2005-2006*, Philadelphia, 2005, NANDA International.
5. Eliopoulos C: *Gerontological nursing,* ed 6, Philadelphia, 2004, Lippincott.
6. Seidel H et al: *Mosby's guide to physical examination,* ed 6, St Louis, 2006, Mosby.
7. Weber J, Kelley J: *Health assessment in nursing,* ed 2, Philadelphia, 2003, Lippincott.

For additional Internet resources, see the website for this book at *http://evolve.elsevier.com/Lewis/medsurg.*

Education is light, lack of it, darkness.

Russian Proverb

5 Patient and Family Teaching

Patricia Graber O'Brien

LEARNING OBJECTIVES

1. Identify four specific goals of patient and family teaching.
2. Describe teaching implications related to adult learning principles.
3. Describe specific skills that enhance the nurse's role as teacher.
4. Identify strategies to manage barriers to nurse-teacher effectiveness.
5. Discuss the role of the family in patient teaching.
6. Explain the basic steps in the teaching-learning process.
7. Identify physical, psychologic, and sociocultural characteristics of the patient that affect the teaching-learning process.
8. Describe the components of a correctly written learning objective.
9. Identify the advantages, disadvantages, and uses of various teaching strategies.
10. Describe common methods of short- and long-term evaluation.

KEY TERMS

facilitator, p. 61
health literacy, p. 58
learning, p. 54
learning needs, p. 59
learning objectives, p. 60
literacy, p. 58
peer teaching, p. 61
stages of behavioral change, p. 55
teaching, p. 54
teaching plan, p. 54
teaching process, p. 57

Electronic Resources

Supplemental content related to Chapter 5 can be found . . .

Companion CD

- Stress-Busting Kit for Nursing Students
- NCLEX Examination Review Questions
- Comprehensive Glossary

Evolve Website

http://evolve.elsevier.com/Lewis/medsurg

- Content Updates
- Key Points (Printable and CD/MP3 Download)
- Concept Map Creator
- Expanded Audio Glossary
- Key Term Flash Cards
- Electronic Calculators
- WebLinks

ROLE OF PATIENT AND FAMILY TEACHING

Patient and family teaching is a critical part of nursing care and is one of the most challenging roles that nurses have today. Although offering patient and family education is required by accrediting agencies and institutional regulations, constraints on time and resources may limit the nurse's ability to provide education. As a result, teaching is frequently a neglected nursing intervention even though its omission can have devastating consequences for patients and their families. Teaching patients about their health care can be the one nursing intervention that most often makes a difference in the patient's quality of life.

Nurses provide patient and family education to help patients and their families maintain health and cope with acute and chronic health problems. More specific goals of education include health promotion, prevention of disease, management of illness, and appropriate selection and use of treatment options. Health promotion and disease prevention facilitate high levels of wellness throughout the life span. Teaching can help people make informed decisions about health practices and treatment choices. In patients with acute health problems, teaching can prevent complications and promote recovery. For those patients with chronic illnesses, teaching can promote self-care and independence. Seventy percent of the deaths in the United States are due to chronic illnesses, illnesses with which patients often live for many years.[1] Whether patients adequately manage their chronic illnesses and maintain quality of life depends primarily on what they are taught and learn about their conditions.

Teaching may occur wherever nurses work, including the community, schools, industry, ambulatory care centers, hospitals, long-term care facilities, and homes. Although institutions may employ

Reviewed by Sarah Reidunn Tvedt-Pool, RN, MS, Nursing Education Specialist, Mayo Clinic, Rochester, Minn.

clinical nurse specialists and patient educators to establish and oversee patient education programs, all nurses in any setting are responsible for patient and family teaching. Every interaction the nurse has with patients or family members is an opportunity to provide teaching that can dramatically affect their lives.

Much patient teaching is incidental and is incorporated into nursing interventions that promote health and/or prevent complications of illness. Teaching a patient with asthma how to use a peak flow meter or teaching a surgical patient how to use a patient-controlled analgesia (PCA) machine do not require formal teaching plans. However, when a patient has specific learning needs about health promotion, risk reduction, or management of a health problem, a teaching plan should be developed and implemented with the patient. A **teaching plan** includes assessment of the patient's ability, need, and readiness to learn and identification of problems that can be resolved with teaching. The nurse then determines objectives with the patient, delivers educational interventions, and evaluates the effectiveness of the teaching. This chapter describes the steps involved in providing patient and family education and discusses factors that contribute to successful educational experiences.

TEACHING-LEARNING PROCESS

Teaching is not just imparting information. Learning is not just experiencing instruction. **Learning** occurs when there is an internal mental change characterized by rearrangement of neural pathways.[2] It can result in a temporary or persistent change in behavior. Observation of this behavior is an indication that learning has occurred. Learning may also result in a potential or capability to change behavior. This is seen in a patient who understands the instruction and is fully informed, but chooses not to change behavior. In this case, teaching gives the patient the capability to make a decision to change behaviors, but the decision is the patient's. The patient learns the necessary information to make an informed choice, and the choosing is the behavior that is observed.

Teaching is a process of deliberately arranging external conditions to promote the internal transformation that results in a change in behavior. It can be a planned or incidental experience that uses a combination of methods such as instruction, counseling, and behavior modification to influence the patient's knowledge and behavior. The teacher is the one who plans and manages the external conditions to promote learning.[3] Learning may occur without teaching, but teaching can organize information and skills to make learning more efficient. The challenge for the nurse is to identify and use strategies that promote patient learning that results in behaviors that are beneficial for health.

In patient education, the teaching-learning process involves the patient, the nurse, and the patient's family and/or social support system. The complex nature of each of these variables must be taken into account when planning and implementing the education process.

Adult Learner

Adult Learning Principles. Understanding how and why adults learn is important for the nurse to effectively teach patients. Educational research and theory development specifically about adults have identified adult learning principles and characteristics that differentiate adult education from education of children. These concepts provide a foundation for effectively teaching adults. Many of the theories of adult learning have risen from the work of Malcolm Knowles, who identified seven principles of *androgogy* (adult learning) that are essential for the nurse to consider when teaching adults.[4] These principles and implications for patient teaching are presented in Table 5-1. Additional characteristics of adult learners that should be considered by nurses teaching adults[5] are identified in Table 5-2.

TABLE 5-1 Principles of Adult Education Applied to Patient Teaching

Principles	Teaching Implications for the Nurse
Adults are independent learners.	• Teacher is a facilitator to direct the patient to resources, not the source of all information. • Patients expect to make decisions about their own lives and learning experiences and take responsibility for those decisions. • Respect for the patient's independence can be reflected in statements such as, "What do you think you need to learn about this topic?"
Readiness to learn arises from life's changes.	• Patients see life processes as problems to be solved. • Readiness and motivation to learn are high when facing new tasks. • Crises in health are "teachable moments."
Past experiences are resources for learning.	• Patients have had many life experiences and have engaged in informal learning for years. • Motivation is increased when patients feel that they already know something about the subject from past experiences. • Identification of past knowledge and experiences can help find familiar ground to increase patients' confidence.
Adults learn best when the topic is of immediate value.	• Patients need to apply learning immediately. • Long-term goals may have little appeal. • Short-term, realistic goals should be provided. • Focus education on information that the patient views as being needed right now.
Adults approach learning as problem solving.	• Patients seek out various resources for specific learning to help them deal with a problem. • Information that is not relevant to the problem is not readily learned. • When relevancy is not recognized by the patient, explanations of the value of the learning should be offered. • Teaching should target the specific problem or circumstance.
Adults see themselves as doers.	• Patients learn better by doing. • Demonstrations, computer activities, and practice of skills should be offered when appropriate.
Adults resist learning when conditions are incongruent with their self-concepts.	• Patients do not learn when they are treated as children and told what they must do. • Patients need control and self-direction to maintain their sense of self-worth.

TABLE 5-2 Characteristics of the Adult Learner

- Likes to have choices.
- Adjusts less easily to distractions.
- Suffers more from being deprived of success.
- Has a variety of learning styles and preferences.
- Needs to have abilities and achievements honored.
- Has greater difficulty in remembering isolated facts.
- Is more rigid in thinking and has a set pattern of behavior.
- Does best in an environment where feels safe, accepted, and respected.
- Requires a longer time to perform learning tasks although capacity to learn is unchanged.

From Baker D: Principles of adult learning: application to clinical teaching, 2005. Available at *www.med.fsu.edu/education/FacultyDevelopment/PowerPoint_Presentations/AdultLearningPrinciplesforweb.htm*.

Motivation of Adult Learners. Motivation and readiness to learn depend on multiple factors, such as need, attitude, beliefs, stimulation, and reinforcement.[6] When teaching adults, it is important to identify what is valued by the person to enhance motivation. If the person perceives a need for information to enhance health or avoid illness, or has a belief that a behavior change has health value, motivation to learn is increased. Although humans like what is familiar and often resist change, they also search for and respond to novelty. Motivation to learn is increased when topics and learning activities are new and stimulating to the patient and/or family members.

Reinforcement is a strong motivational factor for maintaining behavior. Positive **reinforcement** involves rewarding a desired behavior with a positive stimulus such as money or awards to increase its occurrence. Removal or avoidance of an aversive situation is the process of negative reinforcement. Behavior may be strengthened by negative reinforcement when the behavior removes a negative consequence, such as pain or illness symptoms.[6]

When a change in health behaviors is recommended, patients and their families may progress through a series of steps before they are willing or able to accept a change in health behaviors. Six stages of change have been identified in the Transtheoretical Model of Health Behavior Change developed by Prochaska and Velicer.[7] The **stages of behavioral change** and the implications for patient teaching are described in Table 5-3. It is important to note that individuals progress through these stages at their own pace and that progression through the stages is often nonlinear and cyclic, going through periods of relapse and restarting the process. Assessment of the patient's stage of change will help the nurse guide the patient through one stage to the next.

Nurse as Teacher

Required Skills

Knowledge of Subject Matter. The scope and setting of nursing practice is large and diverse. Although it is impossible to be an expert in all areas, the nurse can develop confidence as a teacher by developing a thorough knowledge of the subject that is to be taught. Additional study of health risks, diseases, and appropriate self-care in textbooks, journals, and other resources may be necessary if the nurse has limited experience with or knowledge of the subject. For example, if a nurse is teaching a patient about management of hypertension, the nurse must be able to explain what hypertension is, why it is important to control the disease, and what the patient needs to know about exercise, diet, and expected and untoward effects of medication. The nurse should be able to teach the patient to use blood pressure equipment to monitor the blood pressure and to identify situations that should be reported to health care providers. In addition, the nurse should provide the patient with sources of additional information, such as written brochures, appropriate websites, and support organizations (e.g., American Heart Association).

It is not unusual for the patient to ask questions that the nurse may not be able to answer. If the nurse is not sure of an answer, the patient should be told and the nurse should follow through by seeking additional information to answer the question.

Communication Skills. Patient education is an interactive process. It is dependent on communication between the nurse and the patient or family member. During the teaching process the nurse should use basic communication skills as described in Chapter 4. Some specific communication skills that are particularly important in teaching are discussed next.

Medical jargon is inherently intimidating and frightening to most patients and their families. Patients can feel alienated when large, complex medical terms are used in their presence without an understanding of what the terms mean. The nurse should begin by defining the medical words or terms that are necessary to understanding the content to be taught. For example, if a patient is told that he has thrombocytopenia, he most likely will need the nurse to interpret this diagnosis in words that mean something to him. The nurse can

TABLE 5-3 Stages of Change in the Transtheoretical Model

Stage	Patient Behavior	Nursing Implications
1. Precontemplation	Is not considering a change; is not ready to learn	Provide support, increase awareness of condition; describe benefits of change and risks of not changing
2. Contemplation	Thinks about a change; may verbalize recognition of need to change; says "I know I should" but identifies barriers	Introduce what is involved in changing the behavior; reinforce the stated need to change
3. Preparation	Starts planning the change, gathers information, sets a date to initiate change, shares decision to change with others	Reinforce the positive outcomes of change, provide information and encouragement, develop a plan, help set priorities, and identify sources of support
4. Action	Begins to change behavior through practice; tentative and may experience relapses	Reinforce behavior with reward, encourage self-reward, discuss choices to help minimize relapses and regain focus, help patient plan to deal with potential relapses
5. Maintenance	Practices the behavior regularly; able to sustain the change	Continue to reinforce behavior; provide additional education on the need to maintain change
6. Termination	Change has become part of lifestyle; behavior no longer considered a change	Evaluate effectiveness of the new behavior; no further intervention needed

Adapted from Prochaska J, Velicer W: The transtheoretical model of health behavior change, *Am J Health Promot* 12:38, 1997.

use word roots, explaining that *thrombocyte* refers to a clotting cell, a platelet, and that *penia* means deficiency. A one-sentence interpretation that explains that the patient has a deficiency of platelets, the blood cells responsible for clotting, enhances the patient's learning.

The importance of nonverbal communication in the teaching process is pivotal. To provide positive nonverbal messages it is important for the nurse to sit in an open, relaxed position facing the patient with their eyes level (Fig. 5-1). In a hospital setting this may necessitate elevating the patient's bed or having the nurse sit in a chair at the bedside. Open body gestures communicate interest and a willingness to share.

It is also important for the nurse to develop the art of active listening. This means paying attention to what is said, as well as observing the patient's nonverbal cues. The nurse concentrates on the patient as a communicator of vital information and allows the patient full hearing by not interrupting. Nodding in response to the patient's statements and rephrasing and reflecting what the patient is saying will help clarify communication. To allow time for listening without appearing in a hurry requires thoughtful organization and planning on the part of the nurse. Attentive listening allows the nurse to obtain important information needed for the assessment phase of the teaching process.

Empathy. Empathy can be defined as having the courage to enter into the world of another in a manner that does not judge, sympathize, or correct, but in a manner where the goal is creative understanding. Empathy means putting aside one's own self for a moment and stepping into the shoes of the patient. With regard to patient teaching, empathy means holistically assessing the patient's needs before implementing teaching. For example, the nurse who is working in a busy outpatient clinic is asked to teach a newly diagnosed diabetic patient the symptoms of hypoglycemia. The nurse enters the room with the packet of written information and finds the patient sitting very still, with gaze fixed and mouth slightly ajar. The empathetic approach to this situation may include entering the room, sitting down in a chair next to the patient, and discussing the patient's responses to the new diagnosis before starting the discussion of diabetes complications.

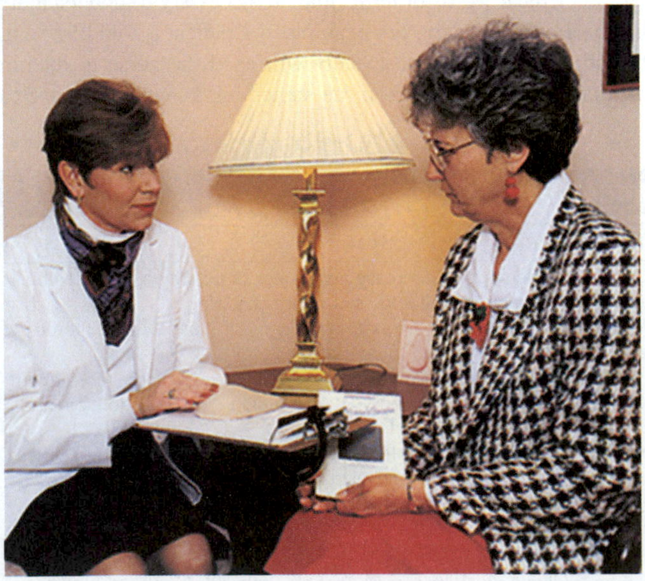

FIG. 5-1 Open, relaxed positioning of patient and nurse at eye level promotes communication in teaching and learning.

Barriers to Nurse-Teacher Effectiveness. Lack of time is a major barrier that detracts from the effectiveness of the teaching effort. Teaching often is not as instantly rewarding to the nurse as other interventions and therefore may not be given priority when time is limited. When time is limited, the nurse should tell the patient at the beginning of the interaction how much time the nurse can devote to the session. To make the most of limited time it is critical that the nurse and patient set priorities of the patient's learning needs so that important teaching can be done during any contact with the patient or family.

An additional barrier to the nurse's effectiveness as a teacher is insecurity about the nurse's own knowledge and competence, as discussed earlier in this chapter. Also, disagreement between nurse and patient regarding the expectations of teaching can be a barrier. The nurse must accept that some patients or families may not be willing to talk about the health problem or its implications. The patient or family may be in denial or hold ideas and values that are in conflict with conventional health care. The nurse may face hostility or resentment but must respect the patient's response to the health problem.

Another important barrier for the nurse who is attempting to provide patient education is the current health care system. Shortened lengths of hospitalizations have resulted in patients being discharged into the community with only the basic elements of educational plans established. At the same time health care is offering more and complex treatment options, increasing the educational needs of the patient and family. Patients and families also have more difficulty using resources as the complexity of the health care system increases. Strategies that can be used to help manage or overcome these barriers are presented in Table 5-4.

TABLE 5-4 Suggested Approaches to Overcoming Barriers to Nurse-Teacher Effectiveness

Barrier	Approaches
Lack of time	Preplan. Set realistic goals. Use time with patient efficiently, using all possible opportunities for teaching, such as when bathing or changing a dressing. Break teaching and practice into small time periods. Advocate for time for patient teaching. Carefully document what was taught and the time spent teaching in order to emphasize that it is a primary role of nursing and that it takes time.
Lack of knowledge	Broaden knowledge base. Read, study, ask questions. Screen teaching materials, participate in other teaching sessions, observe more experienced nurse-teachers, attend classes.
Disagreement with patient	Establish agreed-on, written goals. Develop a plan and discuss with patient before teaching begins. Introduce a role model to help illustrate therapeutic expectations. Enlist the aid of family and significant others. Revise expectations; learn to be satisfied with small achievements.
Powerlessness, frustration	Recognize personal reaction to barriers. Develop a support system. Rely on friends and family for positive encouragement. Network with other nurses, health professionals, and community leaders to change the situation. Become proactive in legislative processes affecting health care delivery.

Family and Social Support

Support provided by the family is important to a patient's sense of physical, psychologic, and spiritual well-being. Because it has been shown that family members can promote the patient's self-care and prevent complications, it is important for the nurse to identify and include family members in the teaching plans for the patient.[8]

In the family support model, the patient's ultimate well-being is composed of his or her ability to perform self-care activities in and through both formal and informal support systems. In this model no part of the system is an independent agent because the well-being of the individual depends on support from family, community resources, and the health care system.[9] Identifying patients with minimal support and working collaboratively with other health care professionals to develop networks for these patients have been shown to improve the patients' long-term outcomes.[10,11]

Patients and families may have different educational needs. For example, the first priority of an elderly diabetic patient with a large ulcer on the back of his leg may be to learn how to rise from a chair in the least painful manner. On the other hand, family members may be most concerned about learning the technique for dressing changes. Both the patient's and the family's learning needs are important. The patient and family may also have differing or conflicting views of the illness and of treatment options. Frequently the health problem has effects on family roles and functions. Developing a successful teaching plan requires the nurse to view the patient's needs within the context of the family's needs. For instance, the nurse may teach a patient with right-sided *paresis* (weakness) self-feeding techniques with special implements, but at a home visit the nurse finds the patient being fed by the spouse. On questioning, the spouse reveals that it is too difficult to watch the patient struggle with feeding, it takes too long, and it is easier to do it for the patient. This is an example of a situation where both the patient and the spouse need additional teaching about the goals of self-care.

PROCESS OF PATIENT EDUCATION

Many different models and approaches are used in the process of patient education. The nurse may find that some institutions or programs may adopt specific models. Examples include the ASSURE model,[12] the empowerment approach,[13] and Leventhal's self-regulation model.[14] However, the approach used most frequently by nurses is actually a parallel of the nursing process. The **teaching process** and the nursing process both involve development of a plan that includes assessment, diagnosis, setting patient outcomes or objectives, intervention, and evaluation. The teaching process, like the nursing process, may not always flow in sequential order, but the steps serve as checkpoints to ensure that the relevant variables that affect the teaching-learning activity have been considered.

Assessment

During the general nursing assessment the nurse gathers data that determine if the patient has learning needs that teaching can meet. For example, what does the patient know about the health problem and how does he or she perceive the present problem? If a learning need is identified, a more refined assessment of need is made and that problem is addressed with the teaching process. The general nursing assessment also identifies many variables that affect the teaching-learning process, such as the patient's physical and mental state of health and sociocultural characteristics. Assessment can also include the family members or caregivers to determine their abilities to care for the patient at home. An assessment that is performed for the purpose of developing a teaching plan includes physical, psychologic, and sociocultural characteristics that specifically affect learning and the patient's characteristics related to the teaching-learning process. Key questions addressing each of these areas are included in Table 5-5.

Physical Characteristics. The age of the patient is an important factor to consider in the teaching plan. The patient's experiences, rate of learning, and ability to retain information are affected by age. The effects of increased age are often obvious, but the inexperience of younger individuals can also affect learning. For example, a man in his twenties who has never thought about his own mortality may be unable to grasp the long-term implications of an unhealthy behavior, such as smoking.

Sensory impairments, such as hearing or vision loss, decrease sensory input and can alter learning. Magnifying glasses and bright lighting may help the patient with impaired vision read teaching materials. Hearing loss can be helped with hearing aids and teaching techniques that use more visual stimuli. Central nervous system (CNS) function may be affected by disorders of the

TABLE 5-5 Assessment of Characteristics That Affect Patient Teaching

Characteristics and Key Questions
Physical
• What is the patient's age and gender?
• Is the patient acutely ill?
• Is the patient fatigued? In pain?
• What is the primary diagnosis?
• Are there additional medical problems?
• What is the patient's current mental status?
• What is the patient's hearing ability? Visual ability? Motor ability?
• What drugs does the patient take? Do they affect learning?
Psychologic
• Does the patient appear anxious, afraid, depressed, defensive?
• Is the patient in a state of denial?
• What is the patient's level of self-efficacy?
Sociocultural
• Is the patient employed?
• What is the patient's present or past occupation?
• How does the patient describe his or her financial status?
• What is the patient's educational experience and reading ability?
• What is the patient's living arrangement?
• Does the patient have family or close friends?
• What are the patient's beliefs regarding his or her illness or treatment?
• What is the patient's cultural/ethnic identity?
• Is proposed teaching consistent with the patient's cultural values?
Educational
• What does the patient already know?
• What does the patient think is most important to learn first?
• What prior learning experiences establish a frame of reference for current learning needs?
• What has the patient's health care provider told the patient about the health problem?
• Is the patient ready to change behavior or learn?
• Can the patient identify behaviors and habits that would make the problem better or worse?
• How does the patient learn best? Through reading, listening, doing things?
• In what kind of environment does the patient learn best? Formal classroom? Informal setting, such as home or office? Alone or among peers?
• In what way should the family be involved in patient education?

nervous system, such as stroke and head trauma, but also by other diseases, such as renal disease, liver impairment, and cardiovascular failure. Patients with alterations in CNS function have difficulty learning and may require small amounts of information repeated frequently. Manual dexterity is needed to perform procedures such as self-administration of injections or blood pressure monitoring. Problems performing manual procedures might be resolved by using adaptive equipment.

Pain, fatigue, and certain medications also influence the patient's ability to learn. No one can learn effectively when in severe pain. When the patient is experiencing pain, the nurse should provide only brief explanations and follow-up with more detailed instruction when the pain has been managed. A fatigued and weakened patient cannot learn effectively because of the inability to concentrate. Sleep disruption is common during hospitalization, and patients are frequently exhausted at the time of discharge. Drugs that cause CNS depression, such as opioids and sedatives, cause a general decrease in mental alertness. Many chemotherapeutic agents cause nausea, vomiting, and headaches that also affect the patient's ability to assimilate new information. The nurse must adjust the teaching plan to accommodate these factors by setting high-priority goals that are need-based and realistic in expectations. Teaching methods should also be adjusted to accommodate for limitations in the patient's ability to learn at any given time. The patient may need follow-up teaching and referral to someone who can answer questions that arise after discharge.

Psychologic Characteristics. Psychologic factors have a major influence in the patient's ability to learn. Anxiety and depression are common reactions to illness. Although mild anxiety increases the learner's perceptual and learning abilities, moderate and severe anxiety limit learning. Both anxiety and depression can negatively affect the patient's motivation and readiness to learn. For instance, the newly diagnosed diabetic patient who is depressed about the diagnosis may not listen or respond to instructions about blood glucose testing. Discussions with the patient about these concerns or referring the patient to an appropriate support group may enable the patient to learn that management of diabetes is possible.

Patients also respond to the stress of illness with a variety of defense mechanisms, such as denial, rationalization, or even humor. A patient who denies having cancer will not be receptive to information related to treatment options. A patient using rationalization will imagine any number of reasons for avoiding change or for rejecting instruction. For example, a patient with cardiovascular disease who does not want to change dietary habits will relate stories of persons who have eaten bacon and eggs every morning for years and lived to be 100 years of age. Humor is also used by some patients to filter reality or decrease anxiety. Laughter may be used to escape from the experience of facing threatening situations. A common example of the use of humor is seen when patients assign a name and personality characteristics to an altered body structure or even a drainage device. Humor in the teaching process is important and useful, but the nurse must determine when humor is used excessively to avoid reality.

One important psychologic determinant of successful adoption of new behaviors is the patient's sense of self-efficacy. **Self-efficacy** is a person's belief in his or her ability to successfully cope with and manage a situation. An individual's belief in his or her capability to produce and regulate events in life affects motivation, thought patterns, behavior, and emotions.[5] There is a strong relationship between self-efficacy and outcomes of illness management.[15,16] Self-efficacy increases when a person gains new skills in managing a threatening situation, but decreases when the individual experiences repeated failure, especially early in the course of events. These findings have significant implications for patient and family teaching. The nurse should plan easily attainable objectives early in the teaching sessions, proceeding from simple content to more complex, to establish a positive feeling of success. The use of role play to rehearse new behaviors and peer learning are teaching strategies that also can increase self-efficacy in patients and family members.

Sociocultural Characteristics. The patient's sociocultural characteristics influence his or her perception of health, illness, health care, life, and death. Social elements include the patient's lifestyle, status within a family, occupation, income, education, housing arrangement, and living location. Cultural elements include dietary and sleep patterns, exercise, sexuality, language, values, and beliefs.

Occupation and Income. Knowing the patient's present or past occupation may assist the nurse in determining the vocabulary to use during teaching. For example, an auto mechanic might understand the volume overload associated with heart failure as flooding of an engine. An engineer may understand the principles of physics associated with gravity and pressures when discussing vascular problems. This technique of teaching requires creativity but can promote a patient's understanding of pathophysiologic processes.

The patient's occupation will also give the nurse an idea about the patient's financial status or availability of health insurance. Management of chronic health problems is very expensive, and the cost of care should be addressed with the patient or family. In a time when there is a growing number of uninsured, the nurse may need to use different teaching resources or improvise materials based on the patient's ability to afford supplies and equipment.

Literacy and Health Literacy. Literacy is the ability to use printed and written information to function in society. The recent focus on the literacy rates of the U.S. population and their effects on health and health care have major implications for patient and family education. The last published findings of literacy surveys in the United States indicated that approximately 40 million Americans could not read or write, and another 50 million had only marginal literacy skills. The average reading level in the United States was between the eighth and ninth grades, and one quarter of the population was functionally illiterate (read below the fifth-grade level). New surveys are being planned, but it is believed that the literacy rate is approximately the same as, or even lower than, it was in 1993.[17]

Assessment of literacy is challenging because patients rarely admit they have difficulty reading, due to feelings of inadequacy and low self-esteem. Many individuals use a variety of methods to conceal their illiteracy, such as asking others to read for them or "forgetting" their glasses. Determining the patient's level of formal education may be helpful in identifying appropriate methods and vocabulary to use when teaching, but research findings are not consistent regarding the relationship between level of education and reading ability.[18]

Health literacy is defined as the degree to which individuals have the capacity to obtain, process, and understand basic health information and services needed to make appropriate health decisions.[19] As the health care environment has become more complex, individuals with limited literacy have increasing trouble understanding and acting on health information, leading to limited health literacy. Even patients with higher general literacy can have low health literacy when faced with trying to understand complicated health information. In 2004 the Institute of Medicine reported that nearly half of the adult population in the United States may be health illiterate.[20] Many recent studies indicate that functional health illiteracy results in poor patient outcomes, nonadherence with treatment plans, limited self-management skills, and increased health disparities.[21-23]

No formal standardized methods for assessing a patient's health literacy are currently available. Two tools, the Rapid Estimate of Adult Literacy in Medicine (REALM)[24] and the Test of Functional Health Literacy in Adults (TOFHLA),[25] have been widely used in research but require too much time to be useful in most clinical situations. Until quick, accessible assessment tools are available, it is recommended that assessment focus on the patient's subtle cues that reflect illiteracy. In addition, patient education materials should be written at the fifth- to sixth-grade reading level.[26]

Housing Arrangement and Living Location. The patient should be asked about living arrangements that can affect the teaching-learning process. Whether the patient lives alone, with friends, or with family will influence who else is included in the teaching process. If the patient lives in another city or a rural area at a distance from the site of teaching, the nurse may need to make arrangements for continued teaching in those areas. Modifications of instructions may need to be made if the patient does not have access to electricity, phones, or modern plumbing.

Cultural Considerations. Learning is closely related to the wider culture and the subculture to which a patient belongs. Health practices, beliefs, and behavior vary by religious, ethnic, and family group. Many factors affecting patient teaching are included in the cultural assessment in Table 3-4. To prevent stereotyping patients according to cultural group, it is important to simply ask if there is a cultural group or practice with which the patient identifies. Patients may also be asked to describe their beliefs regarding health and illness.

One cultural element that specifically affects the teaching-learning process is a conflict between the patient's cultural beliefs and values and the behaviors promoted by teaching. For example, a patient who values a trim figure can be taught to diet and exercise to retain that figure while at the same time improving blood pressure control. However, in another patient's culture, being heavy is valued as a sign of financial success and sexuality. This patient may have more difficulty accepting the need for diet and exercise unless the importance of blood pressure control is understood.

The nurse must also assess the patient's use of cultural remedies and folk healers. For teaching to be effective, cultural health practices must be incorporated into the teaching plan. Consideration should also be given to cultural remedies that may interfere with or are contraindicated in the treatment plan being taught. In addition, it is important to know who has authority in the patient's culture. The patient may defer to the authority, such as an elder, a spiritual leader, or a folk healer, for decisions. In this case, the nurse will also need to identify and work with the decision makers in the patient's cultural group.

Educational Characteristics. Finally, the nurse should assess those patient characteristics that are directly related to the development of the teaching plan. These factors include the patient's learning needs, readiness to learn, and learning style.

Learning Needs. Learning needs are the new knowledge and skills that an individual must have to be able to meet an objective or a goal. The assessment of learning needs should first determine what the patient already knows, if the patient has misinformation, and any history of past experiences with health problems. Patients with long-standing health problems have different learning needs than those patients with newly diagnosed health problems. The nurse then identifies the information, behaviors, or skills known to improve patient outcomes that should be included in the teaching plan. For example, a patient who has had a myocardial infarction should be given information regarding the condition, risk factors, medications, diet, psychologic concerns, activities, stress management, and symptoms so that the condition can be managed and informed decisions about potential lifestyle changes can be made.

It may appear on the surface that it is obvious what a patient should learn about managing an illness or what behaviors should be changed to promote health. However, there is often a large difference between what health care professionals think is important for patients to learn and what patients want to know. Remembering that adults learn best when teaching provides information that they view as being needed immediately, the nurse should prioritize what patients see as the most critical information when developing the teaching plan.

To individualize learning needs for a particular patient, the nurse may give the patient a list of the recommended topics and ask the patient to number the topics in order of importance. Another method includes writing each topic in question format on a single card and asking the patient to sort the cards in priority. Examples of the questions on the cards for a patient with heart failure include, "What are the side effects of my medications?" and "How will I know when I should call my health care provider?"[27] Blank cards could also be provided so the patient could identify any other needs. By allowing a patient to prioritize his or her own learning needs, the nurse can begin with the patient's most important needs and end with the least important. When information regarding life-threatening complications is a factor, the nurse can promote the patient's priority of learning this content by explaining why the information is a "need to know." Individualization of learning needs helps ensure that the most important topics are addressed when time limits the comprehensive discussion of all topics.

Readiness to Learn. Before implementing the teaching plan, the nurse should determine where the patient is in the stages of change process (see Table 5-3). If the patient is only in the precontemplation stage, the nurse may just provide support and increase the patient's awareness of the problem until the patient is ready to consider a change in behavior. Nurses in outpatient settings and home health care may continue to evaluate the patient's readiness to learn and implement the teaching plan as the patient moves through the stages of change.

Learning Style. Each person has a distinct style of learning that is as individual as his or her personality. The three learning styles are (1) visual (reading), (2) auditory (listening), and (3) physical (doing things). People often use more than one learning style. To assess a patient's learning style, the nurse might ask how the patient learns best, if reading or listening is the preferred method to gain information, and how the patient has learned in the past. During assessment of the patient's learning style the nurse may be able to identify the patient who does not read. For example, the patient may tell the nurse that he or she does not read much, but likes to learn from television programs, the radio, or illustrations. Auditory methods should always be used when patients specifically identify them as learning styles.

Diagnosis

Information obtained from the assessment related to what the patient knows, believes, and is able to do is compared with what the patient wants to know, needs to know, and needs to be able to do.

Identifying the gap between the known and unknown helps determine the nursing diagnosis, or the deficiency that can be corrected with teaching. A common nursing diagnosis for learning needs is that of deficient knowledge. This refers to the state in which the individual experiences an absence or a deficiency of cognitive knowledge related to a specific topic. Another nursing diagnosis commonly identified when patients have learning needs is that of ineffective health maintenance. This diagnosis refers to an inability to identify, manage, and/or seek out help to maintain health.

If deficient knowledge is identified, it is important to specify the exact nature of the deficit so that the objectives, strategies, implementation, and evaluation relate to the identified problem. For example, the nursing diagnosis of deficient knowledge related to inability to recognize symptoms of drug toxicity provides the nurse with a clear direction for the teaching-learning process.

Planning

Following the assessment and the identification of a nursing diagnosis, the next step in the education process is setting goals, determining objectives for the learner, and planning the learning experience. The patient and nurse mutually prioritize the patient's learning needs and agree on learning objectives. If the physical or psychologic condition of the patient interferes with his or her participation, the patient's family or significant other can assist the nurse in the planning phase.

Writing clear, specific, attainable, and measurable learning objectives is important. Learning objectives describe the intended result of the learning process, guide the selection of teaching strategies and materials, and help evaluate patient and teacher progress. Learning objectives are parallel to patient outcomes in the nursing care plan and are written using the same criteria. Objectives should be in writing and made readily available to all members of the health care team, including the patient and family.

Writing Specific Learning Objectives. **Learning objectives** are written statements that define exactly how patients demonstrate their mastery of the content. The objectives contain the following four elements:

1. Who will perform the activity or acquire the desired behavior?
   Examples: I (the patient) will
   I (the spouse) will
   We (the patient's family) will
2. The actual behavior that the learner will exhibit to demonstrate mastery of the objective.
   Examples: List the symptoms
   Self-administer an insulin injection
   Identify from a hospital menu
3. The conditions under which the behavior is to be demonstrated.
   Examples: In front of the nurse
   Select from a random list
   Choose from a restaurant menu
4. The specific criteria that will be used to measure the patient's success, such as time and degree of accuracy.
   Examples: With 100% accuracy
   Using correct technique
   Within 3 minutes

Note that well-written learning objectives have precise descriptions using terms with few interpretations. When writing objectives the nurse uses verbs such as "identify," "list," "describe," "demonstrate," "name," "recognize," and "compare and contrast." Vague, ambiguous terms, such as "appreciate," "learn," "understand," "enjoy," "feel," or "value," cannot be measured and should be avoided.

An example of a poorly written learning objective is, "The patient will appreciate the importance of foot care." In this objective it is not clear how the patient will demonstrate that he "appreciates" the importance of foot care, when and to whom he will demonstrate this behavior, or what criteria will be used to determine whether the objective has been met.

The following are examples of well-written learning objectives:

- The patient will demonstrate to the nurse the correct technique for changing his colostomy bag.
- In front of the nurse, the patient will administer a subcutaneous injection of insulin to herself using correct technique.
- The patient will select breakfast, lunch, and dinner menus keeping within a 2000 mg sodium diet for 3 consecutive days with 90% accuracy.
- Given a list of symptoms of heart failure, the patient will identify the early symptoms of heart failure with 80% accuracy before discharge from the hospital.

When learning objectives are clear and specific and when they are written down and available in the patient record, all members of the health care team can work together to accomplish the same objectives. Once the objectives are clearly stated, the nurse, patient, and patient's family should choose the strategy or strategies that are most appropriate to meet the objectives of the learning process.

Selecting Teaching Strategies. Selecting a particular strategy is determined by at least three factors: (1) patient characteristics (e.g., age, educational background, nature of illness, culture); (2) subject matter; and (3) available resources. Frequently, several teaching strategies are used together to enhance learning (Fig. 5-2). A discussion of some teaching strategies that can be employed to achieve learning objectives follows. Each has advantages and disadvantages that make it more or less suitable to a particular patient and learning situation (Fig. 5-3).

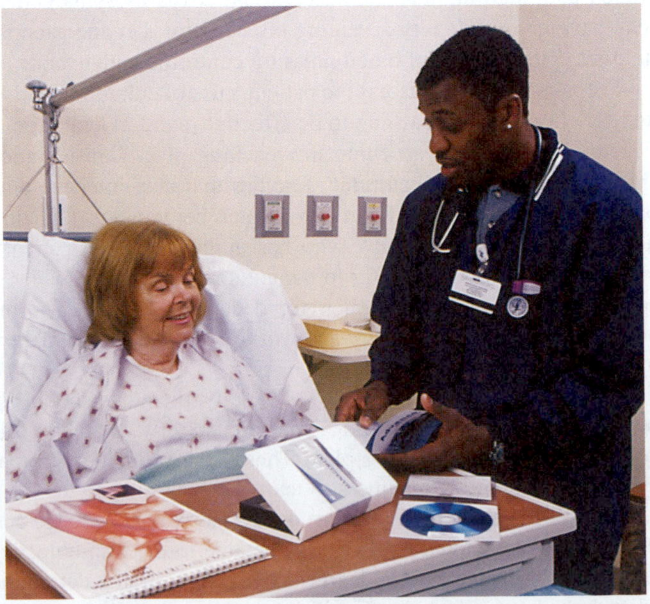

FIG. 5-2 Effective teaching using a variety of materials.

Patient A
Learning style
Prefers direct, straightforward approach; dislikes formal classroom environment
Task oriented; good talker

Educational background
High-school graduate; took several vocational courses; above average grades

Subject matter
Post-MI instruction

Facilities
A major urban hospital with extensive resources

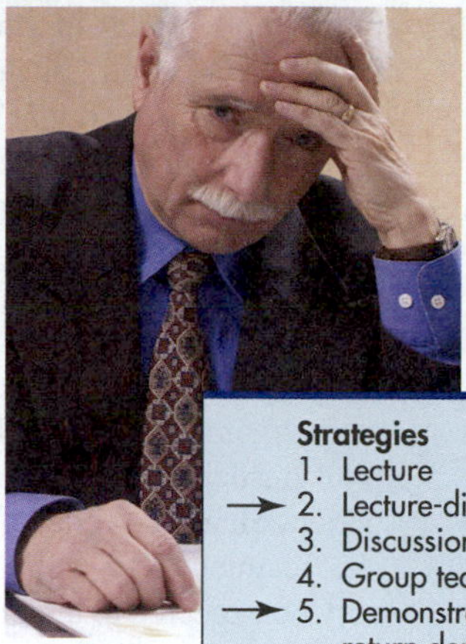

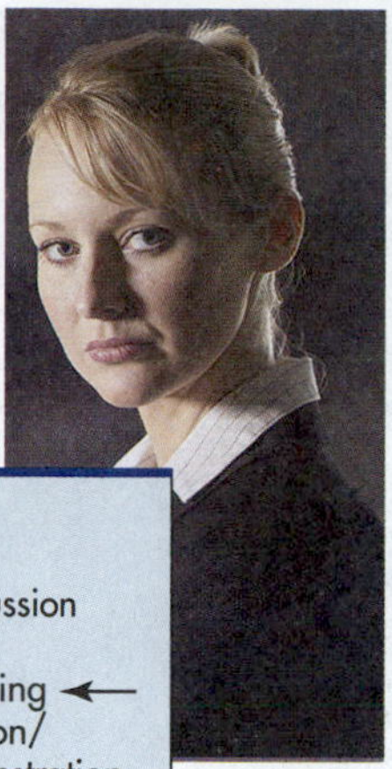

Patient B
Learning style
Works well with other adults
Enjoys sharing ideas

Educational background
One year of college; majored in elementary education

Subject matter
Breast self-examination
Patient fearful and depressed

Facilities
Meeting rooms in local women's resource center

Strategies
1. Lecture
2. Lecture-discussion ←
3. Discussion
4. Group teaching ←
5. Demonstration/return demonstration ←
6. Role playing
7. Audiovisuals ←

FIG. 5-3 Selecting teaching strategies. *MI,* Myocardial infarction.

Lecture. The lecture format is an efficient, versatile, and economical teaching strategy that can be used when the amount of time is limited or when a group of patients and family members can benefit from a core of basic information. The nurse presents a series of related ideas or facts to one person or to a group. Usually, the lecture is short, from 15 to 20 minutes, and some visual reinforcement, such as an outline or illustration, emphasizes key points. It is important to remember that the average adult learner can remember five to seven points at a time. Disadvantages of the lecture format are that it often has negative "school learning" connotations, and individual learning is difficult to evaluate. The nurse is active, but the patients are passive unless they are allowed to participate or ask questions.

Lecture-Discussion. The lecture-discussion can overcome some of the disadvantages of the lecture only. With this strategy, the nurse presents specific information by using the lecture technique, followed by a period during which patients and their families ask questions and exchange points of view with the nurse. This strategy assists the patient in becoming an active participant in the learning process and creates a more informal give-and-take learning environment.

Discussion. The purpose of discussion may be to exchange points of view concerning a topic or to arrive at a decision or conclusion. The nurse can discuss content with an individual or with a group, keeping the specific learning objectives in mind and clarifying information as needed. Participants' questions can also help the nurse identify and correct inaccurate information. This strategy is a good choice when the patient or patients have previous experience with a subject and have information to share, such as smoking cessation, post–coronary artery bypass surgery, or preoperative teaching classes. The discussion allows the patient or family members to actively participate and to apply their own experiences and observations to the learning process. The informal sharing and nonthreatening environment of discussions are positive factors, but this format usually requires more time depending on the topic and the number of participants.

Group Teaching. There are two kinds of group teaching. In the first, the nurse acts as a **facilitator,** or helper, for group sharing about a common problem. Fig. 5-4 shows the nurse acting as a facilitator in small group discussion. As a facilitator, the nurse participates by keeping information moving among all group members. The nurse may introduce the patient to an existing group or may form a group of patients with similar problems, such as women who are caregivers.

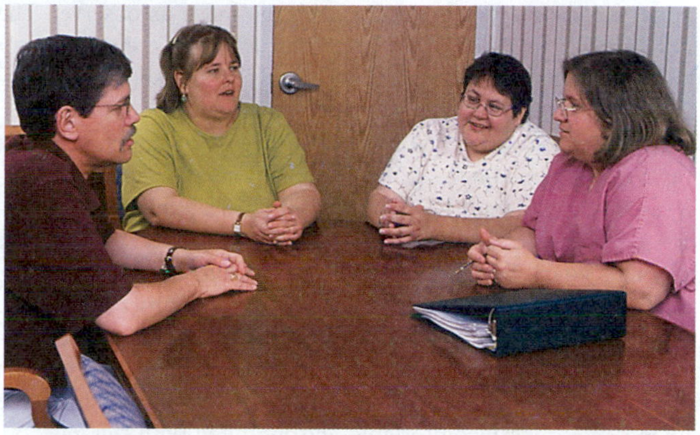

FIG. 5-4 Nurse acts as a facilitator in a small group discussion.

A second kind of group teaching involves **peer teaching** as found in support groups. A support group is a self-help organization that can provide continuing information, shared experiences, acceptance, understanding, and useful suggestions about a problem or concern. Patients with problems such as impotence, cancer, alcoholism, Parkinson's disease, compulsive overeating, diabetes, or heart surgery can benefit from peer teaching. The nurse should actively look for opportunities to refer a patient or family to a support group. This action should be taken in addition to, not instead of, the nurse's planned teaching sessions.

Demonstration/Return Demonstration. The demonstration/return demonstration is a common strategy used by the nurse. The purpose is to show how to perform a motor skill, such as a dressing change, an injection, or a blood pressure measurement (Fig. 5-5). The focus is on correct procedure and application. To handle this strategy correctly, the nurse tells the patient the purpose of the demonstration and makes sure that the patient can see and hear clearly. Then the nurse presents the demonstration in an informal manner, defines unfamiliar terms, and watches for signs of confusion from the patient. The nurse clarifies and repeats as needed, and then the

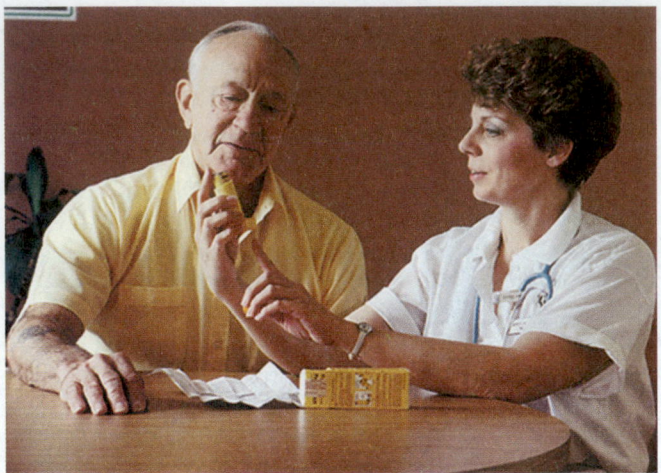

FIG. 5-5 Careful teaching using demonstration and return demonstration increases the possibility of successful learning by the patient.

patient returns the demonstration with the nurse as observer. The entire process should last no more than 15 to 20 minutes. Motor skills take practice to achieve, and the procedure should be practiced by the patient between teaching sessions.

Role Play. Role play is another strategy that the nurse might employ depending on teaching objectives. This format is most often used when patients need to examine their attitudes and behaviors, when they need to understand the viewpoints and attitudes of others, or when they need to practice carrying out ideas or decisions. The nurse gives information and clear instructions to role players and observers and provides time for feedback and evaluation. Role playing requires maturity, confidence, and flexibility on the part of the participants. It is important to remember that some patients may feel uncomfortable and inhibited with this method. Role playing takes time, which must be factored into the teaching plan. An example of the use of role playing is a wife who needs to rehearse how to talk with her husband about his need to quit smoking. In this case, "play acting" or practicing the discussion with the nurse ahead of time may be a helpful strategy.

Audiovisual Materials. Audiovisual materials, including videotapes, slides, posters, computer-based programs, charts, audiotapes, or simple transparencies, are commonly used to supplement other teaching strategies. These materials can enhance the presentation of information because they promote learning through both visual and auditory stimulation. To use this strategy, the nurse must know what materials are available within the facility, from support agencies, and from professional groups. These materials must be previewed and evaluated for accuracy, completeness, and appropriateness to the learning objectives before being shown to the patient and family. Audiotapes and CDs are relatively easy to use and can be inexpensive. The use of videotapes and DVDs can be extremely beneficial, particularly when teaching content that is largely visual, such as the steps and processes of procedures (e.g., dressing changes, injections, hemodialysis). Increasingly available are interactive computer-based programs designed to present specific health information for patient education.[28,29]

Printed Materials. Printed educational materials are extensively used for the purpose of teaching patients and families. These materials are most often used in combination with previously presented teaching strategies. For instance, following a lecture on the physiologic effects of smoking, the nurse distributes a pamphlet from the American Cancer Society that reviews and reinforces the topic. Or the nurse might select a book or magazine article written by a woman who has had a mastectomy and suggest that the patient read this material to prepare for other teaching sessions. Written materials are always recommended for patients whose preferred learning style is reading.

Written materials must be appropriate for the reading level of the patient. The Joint Commission on Accreditation of Healthcare Organizations (JCAHO)[30] standards and the American Hospital Association's Patient's Bill of Rights[31] both mandate that a patient obtain current information concerning his or her diagnosis, treatment, and prognosis in terms that the patient can reasonably be expected to understand. This means that written materials must be appropriate for the patient's reading level. Because of the extent of health illiteracy, it is now recommended that all patient education materials be written at the fifth- to sixth-grade reading level.

Before written materials are used with patients, the nurse should evaluate the readability level if it is not indicated on the materials. Many different formulas have been developed to assess the readability of written materials, but one that is easy to use and has been used for many years is the SMOG formula.[32] The steps to use the SMOG formula are as follows:

1. Choose 10 consecutive sentences at the beginning, middle, and end of the document (30 total sentences).
2. Count every word in these sentences that has three or more syllables. If a word is repeated, count the repetition. Proper nouns with three or more syllables should be counted. Hyphenated words are considered one word.
3. Calculate the square root of the total number of words with three or more syllables.
4. Add 3 to the square root.
5. The result is the SMOG readability level.

For example, if there are 94 words with 3 or more syllables in the 30 sentences, the square root of 94 is 9.7, plus 3, equals a reading level of 12.7. This is too high for the average adult in the United States, who reads at the eighth-grade level, and is out of reach for those who are functionally illiterate.

When writing teaching materials the nurse can use several techniques to reduce the reading level, including the following: (1) give key information first using bold or italics; (2) use short, common words of one or two syllables; (3) define medical words in simple language if they must be used; (4) keep sentences under 10 words if possible, and 15 at the most; (5) use pictures or drawings; and (6) use an active voice in the manner you would say something.[33]

Major resources for acquiring relevant printed material include the hospital or care facility library, pharmacy, public library, federal and state agencies, universities, voluntary organizations, research centers, and websites. Written materials, including computer-based programs, should be reviewed by the nurse before being used. In addition to reading level, the following criteria for review are suggested: (1) accuracy, (2) completeness, (3) whether the material meets specific learning goals, (4) use of pictures and diagrams to stimulate interest, (5) use of one main idea or concept per pamphlet or program, (6) whether the material contains information the patient would like to know, and (7) whether the material is culture and gender sensitive and appropriate.[3] In addition, materials that promote specific commercial or proprietary products should be avoided.

Internet. The use of the Internet by patients to obtain health information is increasing at a phenomenal rate. Many patients use their own computers or those available at public libraries to access desired information. In addition to a wealth of information available to all users, the Internet also offers established education programs and online support groups for specific learners. Examples include the use of a computer website for preoperative teaching and a Web-based intervention for persons with traumatic brain injury.[34,35] However, use of the Internet as a source of information is a double-edged sword. It offers a large number of high-quality health resources and poses seemingly unlimited opportunities to inform, teach, and connect health professionals and patients alike. On the other hand, much Internet information is incomplete, misleading, or inaccurate.

Not surprisingly, older patients use the Internet less frequently for health information than younger patients.[36] However, several computer education programs for older adults have been developed. Organizations dedicated to improving the quality of life for older adults are promoting user-friendly websites and publishing guides to help older adults evaluate health information on the Internet (available at *www.nlm.nih.gov/pubs/checklist.pdf*).

The nurse is challenged by several factors when using the Internet as a teaching strategy. The nurse must have adequate computer competency to review and evaluate information and programs available on the Internet. Evaluations of specific websites are gradually being published in professional literature, but assessments of most websites are not readily available. In that a new website is added to the Internet about every 30 minutes and there are over 10,000 health-related websites, nurses are advised to learn website evaluation to guide patients to the best resources. Criteria for website evaluation developed by the Health Information Technology Institute (HITI) have been endorsed by the American Public Health Association as a standard for development and evaluation of Internet health information.[37] These criteria can be found online at *http://hitiweb.mitretek.org/docs/criteria.html.* In addition to completion of evaluation criteria, the reading level of the information at the website should also be determined.

Personal computer competency is also necessary to teach patients and families unfamiliar with computers how to access information, especially older adults. All patients who use the Internet must also be taught how to identify reliable and accurate information. The nurse should encourage patients to use sites established by the government, universities, or reputable medical or health-related associations (e.g., American Medical Association, American Diabetes Association, American Heart Association, National Institutes of Health, National Library of Medicine, or U.S. Food and Drug Administration). Resources at the end of the chapter identify selected reliable patient education websites for the nurse to review and use for patient referral.

Implementation

During the implementation phase the nurse uses the planned strategies to present information and demonstrations. Verbal and nonverbal communication skills, active listening, and empathy are incorporated into the process. Based on the assessment of the patient's physical and psychologic condition, the nurse can determine how much active participation the patient can assume.

In implementing the teaching plan the nurse should remember the principles and characteristics of the adult learner. Reinforcement and reward are important, but the nurse should be aware that phrases such as "Very good" or "Aren't you doing well?" in the tone one would use with a child can be very condescending to adult learners. Techniques to enhance the teaching process with adults are presented in Table 5-6.

Evaluation

Evaluation is the final step in the learning process and is a measure of the degree to which the patient has mastered the learning objectives. The nurse monitors the performance level of the patient so that changes can be made as needed. The nurse may find that the patient has achieved the goals. However, if certain goals are not reached, the nurse may need to reassess the patient and alter the teaching plan. If the patient has developed new needs, the nurse then plans new objectives, content, and strategies.

For example, an elderly man with diabetes mellitus entered the hospital with a blood glucose level of 550 mg/dl (30.53 mmol/L). When the student nurse began to prepare his insulin injection, the nurse asked, "Are you going to have him give his own insulin and observe his technique?" "Oh, no," replied the student nurse, "He has been a diabetic for 20 years!" The assumption was that a patient with diabetes would know how to perform this task correctly. The two nurses returned to the patient's room and asked him to prepare an insulin injection. The patient filled the syringe with 20 units of insulin and 20 units of air, instead of 40 units of insulin. After correcting the dosage and questioning the patient more fully, the nurses concluded that the patient could not accurately see the markings on the syringe and that the patient may have been administering insufficient insulin to himself for a long period of time. The patient's vision was not as good as it had been 20 years ago, and special equipment was now necessary for him to safely and accurately administer the insulin.

Evaluation techniques may be short-term or long-term. Short-term evaluation techniques are used to quickly evaluate the patient's mastery of a concept, skill, or behavior change and can be accomplished in the following ways:

1. *Observe the patient directly.* "Show me how you will change your dressing." "Let me see how you administer your injection." By observation, the nurse determines if a task has

TABLE 5-6 Techniques to Enhance Patient Learning

- Remember that simple is best.
- Keep the physical environment relaxed and nonthreatening.
- Maintain a respectful, warm, and enthusiastic attitude.
- Let the patient's expressed needs direct what information is provided.
- Focus on "must-know" information.
- Save "nice-to-know" information if time allows.
- Involve the patient and family in the process; emphasize active participation.
- Be aware of and take into consideration the patient's previous experiences.
- Emphasize the relevancy of the information to the patient's lifestyle and suggest how it may provide an immediate solution to a problem.
- Schedule and pace learning experiences according to the patient's needs and abilities.
- Individualize the teaching plan even if standardized plans are used.
- Emphasize helping the patient to learn and not just transmitting subject matter.
- Review written materials with the patient.
- Ask for frequent feedback.
- Affirm progress with rewards valued by the patient to reinforce desired behaviors.

been mastered, if further instruction is needed, or if the patient is ready for new or additional content.

2. *Observe verbal and nonverbal cues.* If the patient asks the nurse to repeat instructions, asks questions, shakes his or her head, loses eye contact, slumps or droops in the chair or bed, becomes restless and fidgety, or otherwise expresses doubt about understanding, the patient may be indicating that further instruction is needed or an alternative approach should be taken.
3. *Ask direct questions.* "What are the major food groups?" "How often must you change your dressing?" "What should you do if you develop chest pain after returning home?" Open-ended questions will provide more information about the patient's understanding than questions that require a "yes" or "no" answer.
4. *Use a written measurement tool, graded for accuracy.* Paper-and-pencil tests may increase anxiety in patients. Adults may "freeze" when given a test, or "go blank" when asked to write something that will be graded. Assess the patient's comfort and learning style before using this method of evaluation.
5. *Talk with a member of the patient's family or support system.* "Is he eating regularly?" "How is he handling the walker?" "When is she taking her medications?" Because the nurse cannot be with the patient 24 hours a day, use other people who have contact with the patient.
6. *Seek the patient's self-evaluation of progress.* What evidence does the patient have that the objectives are being met? Is the patient confident or unsure? Is the patient ready to go forward with new material? It is important to remember that self-direction is important in adult learning. By seeking out a patient's opinion the nurse is allowing the patient input into the evaluation process.

Long-term evaluation requires follow-up by the nurse, outpatient clinic, or outside agency. The nurse's role is to explain to the patient the positive outcomes associated with regular reevaluation by someone familiar with the patient's needs. The nurse should set up a schedule of visits for the patient before the patient leaves the hospital or clinic, or otherwise refer the patient to the proper agencies. The nurse keeps written documentation of follow-up telephone calls or mailed, written reminders to urge the patient to maintain the follow-up schedule. The patient's family or support person should be familiar with the follow-up plan, so that everyone is involved in the patient's long-term progress.

Documentation is an essential component of the entire teaching-learning transaction. The nurse records everything from the assessment through short- and long-term plans for evaluation. As mentioned, the documentation should be forwarded to the agency or health professional providing long-term follow-up. Because many different members of the health care team will use these records in different places and for different reasons, the teaching objectives, content, strategies, and evaluation results should be written clearly and completely.

Standardized teaching plans are often included in care maps and clinical pathways and have become an accepted method of developing a teaching plan. Standardized teaching plans contain widely accepted knowledge and skills that a patient and family need to know concerning a specific health problem or procedure. However, the nurse should always individualize these plans to meet the patient's specific needs.

NCLEX EXAMINATION REVIEW QUESTIONS

The number of the question corresponds to the same-numbered objective at the beginning of the chapter.

1. The nurse is teaching a middle-aged Hispanic woman in a clinic about various methods to relieve the patient's symptoms of menopause. The goal of this teaching would be to
   a. prevent disease.
   b. maintain health.
   c. alter the patient's cultural belief regarding the use of herbs.
   d. provide information for selection and use of treatment options.
2. When planning teaching with consideration of adult learning principles, the nurse would
   a. present material in an efficient, lecture format.
   b. recognize that adults enjoy learning regardless of the relevance to their personal lives.
   c. provide opportunities for the patient to learn from other adults with similar experiences.
   d. postpone practice of new skills until the patient can independently practice the skill at home.
3. A necessary skill of the nurse in the role of teacher is the ability to
   a. determine when patients are too distressed physically or psychologically to learn.
   b. assure the patient that the nurse understands what is necessary for the patient to learn.
   c. develop standardized teaching plans for use with all patients to save time and overcome time constraints.
   d. present information in medical language to increase the patient's vocabulary and understanding of pathophysiology.
4. When the nurse finds only a limited time available for patient teaching, a strategy that might be used is
   a. setting realistic goals that have high priority for the patient.
   b. referring the patient to a nurse educator in private practice for teaching.
   c. observing more experienced nurse-teachers to learn how to teach faster and more efficiently.
   d. providing reading materials for the patient instead of discussing information the patient needs to learn.
5. The nurse includes family members in patient teaching primarily because
   a. they provide most of the care for patients.
   b. patients have been shown to have better outcomes when families are involved.
   c. the patient may be too ill or too stressed by the situation to understand teaching.
   d. they might feel rejected and unimportant if they are not included in the teaching.
6. When the nurse, the patient, and the patient's family decide together what strategies would be best to meet the learning objectives, the step of the teaching process that is involved is
   a. planning.
   b. evaluation.
   c. assessment.
   d. implementation.
7. A patient characteristic that enhances the teaching-learning process is
   a. high anxiety.
   b. high self-efficacy.
   c. being in the precontemplative stage of change.
   d. being able to laugh about the health problem that is present.
8. Which of the following is an example of a correctly written learning objective?
   a. The patient will lose 25 pounds in 6 weeks.
   b. The patient should understand the implications of the condition.

c. The patient will read two pamphlets on the subject of breast self-examination.
d. The patient's spouse will demonstrate to the nurse how to correctly change a gastrostomy bag before discharge.

9. A patient tells the nurse that she enjoys talking with others and sharing experiences, but easily falls asleep when reading. In planning teaching strategies with the patient, the nurse recognizes that the patient would probably learn best with
a. role play.
b. group teaching.
c. lecture-discussion.
d. discussion supplemented with computer programs.

10. Short-term evaluation of teaching effectiveness includes
a. observing the patient and asking direct questions.
b. following the patient for 3 to 6 months after the teaching.
c. monitoring for the behavior change for up to 6 weeks following discharge.
d. asking the patient what he or she found helpful about the teaching experience.

REFERENCES

1. National Center for Chronic Disease Prevention and Health Promotion: *Chronic diseases overview,* Washington, DC, 2004, Centers for Disease Control and Prevention.
2. Smith MK: Learning theory: the encyclopedia of informal education, 2003. Available at *www.infed.org/biblio/b-learn.htm* (accessed June 10, 2005).
3. Redman BK: *The practice of patient education,* ed 9, St Louis, 2001, Mosby
4. Knowles M: *The adult learner: a neglected species,* ed 4, Houston, 1990, Gulf Publishing.
5. Baker D: Principles of adult learning: application to clinical teaching, 2005. Available at *www.med.fsu.edu/education/FacultyDevelopment/PowerPoint_Presentations/AdultLearningPrinciplesforweb.htm* (accessed April 22, 2006).
6. Kearsley G: Explorations in learning and instruction: the theory into practice database, 2004. Available at *http://tip.psychology.org/motivate.html* (accessed April 22, 2006).
7. Prochaska JO, Velicer WF: The transtheoretical model of health behavior change, *Am J Health Promot* 12:38, 1997.
8. Guinn MJ: A daughter's journey promoting geriatric self-care: promoting positive health care interactions, *Geriatr Nurs* 25(5):267, 2004.
9. Boise L, Heagerty B, Eskenazi C: Facing chronic illness: the family support model and its benefits, *Patient Educ Couns* 27:75, 1996.

*10. Winslow BW: Family caregivers' experiences with community services: a qualitative analysis, *Public Health Nurs* 20(5):341, 2003.

*11. Lorig KR, Ritter PL, Gonzalez VM: Hispanic chronic disease self-management: a randomized community-based outcome trial, *Nurs Res* 52(6):361, 2003.

12. Heinich F, Molenda M, Russell JD: *Instructional media and the new technologies of instruction,* ed 4, New York, 1992, Macmillan.
13. Feste C, Anderson RM: Empowerment: from philosophy to practice, *Patient Educ Couns* 26:139, 1995.
14. Leventhal H, Meyer D, Nerenz D: The common sense representation of illness danger. In Rachman S, editor: *Contributions to medical psychology,* New York, 1980, Permagon.

*15. Farrell K, Wicks MN, Martin JC: Chronic disease self-management improved with enhanced self-efficacy, *Clin Nurs Res* 13(4):289, 2004.

*16. Resnick B: A longitudinal analysis of efficacy expectations and exercise in older adults, *Res Theory Nurs Pract* 18(4):331, 2004.

17. Kirsch I, Jungeblut A, Jenkins L, Kolstad A: *Adult literacy in America: a first look at the results of the national adult literacy survey,* Washington, DC, 1993, National Center for Education Statitistics, US Department of Education.
18. Boswell C, Cannon S, Aung K, Eldridge J: An application of health literacy research, *Appl Nurs Res* 17(1):61, 2004.
19. Davis TC, Wolf MS: Health literacy: implications for family medicine, *Fam Med* 36(8):595, 2004.
20. Institute of Medicine: *Health literacy: a prescription to end confusion,* Washington, DC, 2004, National Academies Press.

*21. Rothman R et al: The relationship between literacy and glycemic control in a diabetes disease-management program, *Diabetes Educ* 30(2):263, 2004.

*22. Wolf MS et al: Health literacy and patient knowledge in a southern US HIV clinic, *Int J STD AIDS* 15(11):747, 2004.

*23. Kennen EM et al: Tipping the scales: the effect of literacy on obese patients' knowledge and readiness to lose weight, *South Med J* 98(1):15, 2005.

24. Davis TC et al: Rapid estimate of adult literacy in medicine: a shortened screening instrument, *Fam Med* 36(8):582, 2004.
25. Parker RM, Baker DW, Williams MV, Nurss JR: The test of functional health literacy in adults: a new instrument for measuring patients' literacy skills, *J Gen Intern Med* 10:537, 1995.
26. Bass L: Health literacy: implications for teaching the adult patient, *J Infus Nurs* 28(1):15, 2005.
27. Luniewski M, Reigle J, White B: Card sort: an assessment tool for the educational needs of patients with heart failure, *Am J Crit Care* 8:297, 1999.
28. Alemagno SA, Niles SA, Treiber EA: Using computers to reduce medication misuse of community-based seniors: results of a pilot intervention program, *Geriatr Nurs* 25(5):281, 2003.
29. Neafsey PJ: Interactive personal technology education program decreases adverse medication events, *Home Healthc Nurse* 21(10):697, 2003.
30. Joint Commission on Accreditation of Healthcare Organizations: *Comprehensive accreditation manual for hospitals: the official handbook,* Oakbrook Terrace, Ill, 2005, The Commission.
31. American Hospital Association: *Patient's bill of rights,* Chicago, 1992, The Association.
32. McLaughlin GH: SMOG grading—a new readability formula, *J Reading* 12:639, 1969.
33. Aldridge MD: Writing and designing readable patient education materials, *Nephrol Nurs J* 31(4):373, 2004.

*34. Hering K et al: The use of a computer website prior to scheduled surgery (a pilot study): impact on patient information, acquisition, anxiety level, and overall satisfaction with anesthesia care, *AANA J* 73(1):29, 2005.

35. Rotondi AJ, Sinkule J, Spring M: An interactive Web-based intervention for persons with TBI and their families: use and evaluation by female significant others, *J Head Trauma Rehabil* 20(2):173, 2005.
36. Pew Internet and American Life, 2003. Available at *www.pewinternet.org/reports/index.asp* (accessed June 10, 2005).
37. Oermann MH, Gerich J, Ostosh L, Saleski S: Evaluation of asthma websites for patient and parent education, *J Pediatr Nurs* 18(6):389, 2003.

RESOURCES

Medline Plus Health Information
U.S. National Library of Medicine
www.nlm.nih.gov/medlineplus

Healthfinder
Office of Disease Prevention and Health Promotion, U.S. Department of Health and Human Resources
www.healthfinder.gov

Health Information Online
(Sources of reliable Internet health information)

U.S. Food and Drug Administration
www.fda.gov/fdac/features/596_info.html

Centers for Disease Control and Prevention
404-639-3311
http://www.cdc.gov

Office of Disease Prevention and Health Promotion
Office of Public Health and Science, Office of the Secretary
240-453-8280
Fax: 240-453-8282
www.odphp.osophs.dhhs.gov

Clinical and Patient Education
Medical University of South Carolina
(Reading grade level [RL] indicated on material)
www.musc.edu/medcenter/pted

For additional Internet resources, see resources at the end of specific chapters and the website for this book at *http://evolve.elsevier.com/Lewis/medsurg.*

*Nursing research–based references.

The longer I live, the more beautiful it becomes.

Frank Lloyd Wright

6 Older Adults

Margaret Wooding Baker and Margaret McLean Heitkemper

LEARNING OBJECTIVES

1. Describe the effects of ageism on the care of older adults.
2. List the major biologic theories of aging.
3. Describe the needs of special populations of older adults.
4. Describe nursing interventions to assist chronically ill older adults.
5. Describe common problems of older adults related to hospitalization and acute illness and the role of the nurse in assisting them with selected care problems.
6. Describe challenges and concerns related to the caregiving role.
7. Identify care alternatives to meet patient-specific needs of older adults.
8. Identify the legal and ethical issues related to older adults.
9. Identify the role of the nurse in health screening and promotion and disease prevention for older adults.

KEY TERMS

ageism, p. 67
elder abuse, p. 73
elder neglect, p. 73
ethno-geriatrics, p. 72
frail elderly, p. 71
nonstochastic theory, p. 68
old-old adult, p. 67
polypharmacy, p. 80
stochastic theory, p. 68
young-old adult, p. 67

Electronic Resources

Supplemental content related to Chapter 6 can be found . . .

Companion CD

- Stress-Busting Kit for Nursing Students
- NCLEX Examination Review Questions
- Comprehensive Glossary

Evolve Website evolve

http://evolve.elsevier.com/Lewis/medsurg

- Content Updates
- Key Points (Printable and CD/MP3 Download)
- Concept Map Creator
- Expanded Audio Glossary
- Key Term Flash Cards
- Electronic Calculators
- WebLinks

Gerontologic nursing is the care of older adults based on the specialty body of knowledge of gerontology. The nurse approaches the older adult patient with a whole-person (physical, psychologic, socioeconomic) perspective. This chapter presents specific information about older adults that will assist the nurse in providing care to individuals or groups. Care of older adults presents challenges to nurses that require skilled assessment and creative adaptations of nursing interventions.

DEMOGRAPHICS OF AGING

In the last three decades the older adult population (those 65 years of age and older) has grown twice as fast as the rest of the population. About 36 million people, or 12% of the population, are age 65 or older.[1] Approximately 4.9 million citizens are over age 85. Similarly, in Canada approximately 13% of the population is over age 65. In 2003 in the United States, 17% of persons over age 65 were minorities, including 8% African Americans, 3% Asians or Pacific Islanders, and less than 1% American Indians or Native Alaskans. Persons of Hispanic origin (who may be of any race) represented 6% of the older population. Several factors have led to the overall increase in the older population. The large post–World War II immigrant population has now grown older. Common diseases of the early 1900s that killed many older adults, such as influenza and diarrhea, are now less common, and people are living longer. Drug therapies, including antibiotics and chemotherapy, and earlier detection of diseases have contributed to the increase in life span.

This growth in the older population is expected to continue during this century, and by 2030 there will be 71.5 million older adults

Reviewed by Mary Shelkey, ARNP, PhD, Geriatric Specialist and Director of Nursing Research, Virginia Mason Medical Center, Seattle, Wash.

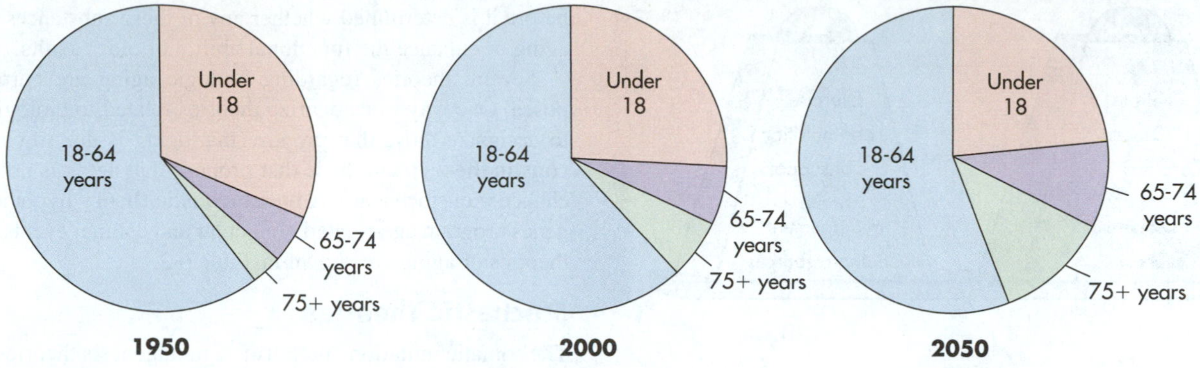

FIG. 6-1 Age distribution of total U.S. population based on U.S. Census Bureau, 1950 and 2000 censuses and 2050 population projections.

representing 20% of the population. Figure 6-1 shows a comparison of the U.S. population in 1950 and 2000 with that projected for 2050. Within the next 3 to 4 years, the "baby boomers" will begin to turn 65, placing greater demands on health care. Minority populations are projected to represent 26.4% of the elderly population by 2030. A child born in the United States in 2002 could expect to live 77.3 years, about 30 years longer than a child born in 1900. The U.S. Census Bureau predicts life expectancy to continue to increase for both men and women. In 2002, persons reaching age 65 had an average life expectancy of 83.2 years (84.5 years for women and 81.6 years for men).[2,3] For Canadians a female child born in 2002 has a life expectancy of 83.2 years and a male child 77.2 years.[4]

The most rapidly increasing age group is composed of those persons 85 years of age and older. Since the 1960s, this group has increased 250%. The terms **young-old adult** (55 to 75 years of age) and **old-old adult** (85 years of age and older) were introduced in 1978. These two groups represent chronologic ranges that often present different characteristics and needs. The old-old adult is usually a widowed woman dependent on family or kinship support. Many have outlived children, spouses, and siblings. The old-old adult is often characterized as a hardy, elite survivor. Because the old-old adult has lived so long, she or he may have become the family icon, the symbol of family tradition and legacy. Approximately 18% of individuals 85 or older live in long-term care or similar institutions.[1] The term *frail elderly* has been suggested to represent those 75 years of age and older with a variety of ongoing and accumulating health concerns.[5] (Frail older adults are discussed later in this chapter.)

ATTITUDES TOWARD AGING

Who is old? The answer to this question often depends on the age and attitude of the respondent. It is important that the nurse maintains the position that aging is normal and is not related to disease. Age is a date in time and is influenced by many factors, including emotional and physical health, developmental stage, socioeconomic status, culture, and ethnicity.

As people age, they are exposed to more and different life experiences. The accumulation of these differences makes older adults more diverse than any other age group. As the nurse assesses the older adult, it is important to consider this diversity. The nurse should assess the patient for perceptions of age. Older adults with poor health report a higher perceived age and lower sense of psychologic well-being as compared with healthy older adults.[6] Age is important, but it may not be the most relevant factor for determining appropriate care of an individual older adult patient.

Myths and stereotypes about aging, found throughout society, are often supported by media reports of problematic older adults. Myths and stereotypes regarding aging provide the basis of commonly held misconceptions that may lead to errors in assessments and unnecessary limitations to interventions. For example, if the nurse thinks that all old people are rigid, new ideas will not be presented to the patient.

Ageism is a negative attitude based on age. It leads to discrimination and disparities in the care given to the older adult. The nurse who demonstrates negative attitudes may fear his or her own aging process or be misinformed about aging and the health care needs of the older adult. The nurse may benefit from gaining knowledge about normal aging and increasing contact with the healthy, independent older adult.

BIOLOGIC AGING THEORIES

From a biologic view, *aging* is defined as the progressive loss of function. This age-related decrease occurs along with decreasing fertility and increased mortality. The exact etiology or cause of biologic aging remains to be determined. Biologic aging is clearly a multifactorial process involving genetics, oxidative stress, diet, and environment.[7,8] In part, biologic aging can be viewed as a balance of positive factors such as healthy diet, regular exercise, and coping resources and negative factors such as obesity, unhealthy lifestyle (smoking), chronic illness, and stress that exceeds the individual's coping resources (Fig. 6-2).

With regard to biologic aging, research efforts are directed at increasing both the average life span and the quality of life of older adults. It is hoped that new antiaging therapies will be developed to slow down or reverse age-related changes that result in chronic illness and disability. Based on numerous laboratory studies in rodents, caloric restriction (reducing dietary intake by 25% to 50%) has been most consistently shown to significantly extend the life span.[7] Caloric restriction in rodents results in a decrease in metabolic activity, but whether this accounts for the increase in longevity is not known. It may be that caloric restriction results in changes in body composition, metabolism, and hormones that are conducive to long life.[8,9] However, whether this is also true for humans remains to be determined. Some of

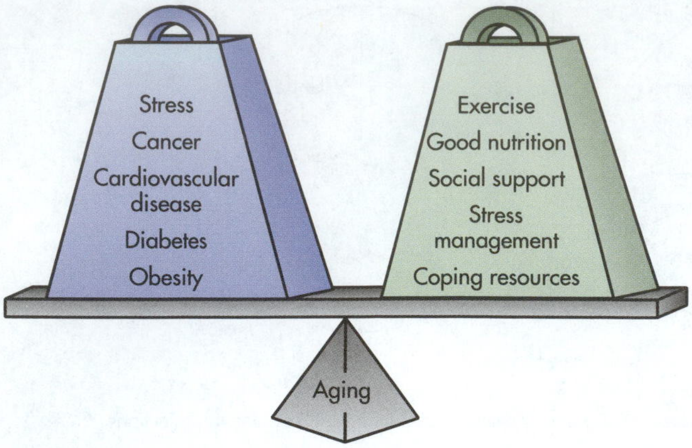

FIG. 6-2 The aging process can be viewed as a balance between negative and positive factors.

the antiaging strategies that are currently under investigation are presented in Table 6-1.

There has long been an interest in slowing down or reversing the effects of aging. A number of nutrients have been examined and tested for their potential benefits in reducing the impact of aging. Examples include vitamin A (retinol), β-carotene, selenium, ginkgo, and chromium.[10] However, much more research is needed before it is determined whether any of these substances will delay aging or enhance the functional ability of older adults.

Several theories regarding biologic aging are currently proposed. One way to categorize theories related to biologic aging is to designate those that propose that aging is due to chance (**stochastic theory**) and those that propose that aging is not related to chance (nonstochastic). A **nonstochastic theory** hypothesizes that genes program age-related molecular and cellular events. Proposed theories of aging are shown in Table 6-2.

Stochastic Theories

The somatic mutation and intrinsic mutagenesis theories postulate that aging is a result of lifelong genetic damage. This damage may include the progressive accumulation of errors in the cell's information-containing molecules. According to *somatic mutation theory,* body cells develop spontaneous mutations in the same way germ cells do. Subsequent cell divisions perpetuate the mutations until organs become inefficient and ultimately fail. The *intrinsic mutagenesis theory* suggests that the increase in mutational cells occurs because of a breakdown of genetic regulatory mechanisms. The basic premise is that the genetic regulatory mechanisms decrease throughout life. Thus more mutations occur with aging and these will ultimately result in functional failure. Although both theories are attractive, little evidence exists to support or deny them.

TABLE 6-1 Current Strategies for Slowing or Reversing Aging

Antiaging Strategies	Scientific Basis and Examples of Findings
Caloric restriction	• Increase in mean and maximum life span and delay in appearance of biologic aging markers in laboratory rodents (mice, rats) and nonhuman primates on >25% calorie-restricted diets. • Humans who have low caloric intake or low body mass index have lower overall mortality rates. • Unknown mechanism but may be related to decreased rate of cell division and/or decreased free radical production.
Cell-based therapies	• Studies done using cell transplantation techniques. • Include clinical procedures such as stem cell transplants used in the treatment of diseases. • Potential to help with age-related diseases (e.g., Parkinson's disease) is under investigation. • Unknown effect on mean life span.
Hormone therapy	• Hormones with anabolic effects decrease some biologic aspects of aging. • Women treated with hormone therapy during the postmenopausal period have decreased incidence of osteoporosis. • Results from clinical trials with androgens and growth hormone to determine effects on muscle mass and physical stamina are inconclusive at this time.
Genetic manipulation	• Laboratory studies to identify the "aging" genes, as well as age-related changes in DNA and RNA. • Potential ability to manipulate select genes to prolong life span or decrease incidence of age-related diseases.

TABLE 6-2 Summary of Biologic Theories of Aging

Theory	Dynamics
Stochastic Theories	
Error	Faulty synthesis of DNA, RNA, or both.
Somatic	Alteration in RNA/DNA; protein or enzyme synthesis causes defective structure or function.
Transcription	Failure of transcription or translation between cells; malfunctions of RNA or related enzymes.
Free radical	Oxidation of fats, proteins, and carbohydrates creates free electrons that attach to other molecules, altering cellular function.
Cross-link	Lipids, proteins, carbohydrates, and nucleic acid react with chemicals or radiation to form bonds that cause an increase in cell rigidity and instability.
Nonstochastic Theories	
Programmed	Biologic clock triggers specific cell behavior at specific time. Organism capable of specific number of cell divisions and specific life span.
Neuroendocrine	Control mechanisms (pituitary and hypothalamus) regulate interplay between various organs and tissues; efficiency of signals between mechanisms is altered or lost.
Immunologic/ autoimmune	Alteration of B and T cells leads to loss of capacity for self-regulation; normal or age-related cells recognized as foreign matter; system reacts by forming antibodies to destroy these cells.
Telomere-telomerase hypothesis	With aging there is a loss of telomeres (repeated sequences at the ends of DNA). This loss limits the number of times cells can divide.

The *free radical theory* was initially proposed in 1956 by Harman and remains a focus of ongoing research.[8] A free radical is a highly reactive atom or molecule that carries an unpaired electron and thus seeks to combine with another molecule, causing an oxidative process. This process, also called *oxidative stress*, can ultimately disrupt cell membranes and alter DNA and protein synthesis. Common diseases such as atherosclerosis and cancer are associated with oxidative stress.[7] Cellular integrity, function, and regeneration mechanisms are injured. Free radicals are natural byproducts of many normal cellular processes and are also created by such environmental factors as smog, tobacco smoke, and radiation. There are numerous natural protective mechanisms in place to prevent oxidative damage. Recent research has focused on the roles of various antioxidants, including vitamins C and E, β-carotene, and selenium, to slow down the oxidative process and ultimately the aging process.[10] However, optimal doses of these substances have not been established. These substances are being investigated for their usefulness in preventing diseases related to aging, such as oral, esophageal, and reproductive cancers; coronary artery disease; and cataracts.

Another stochastic theory is the *cross-link theory,* which postulates that over time and as a result of exposure to chemicals and radiation in the environment, cross-links form between lipids, proteins, and carbohydrates, as well as nucleic acids. These cross-links result in decreased flexibility and elasticity, and this increases rigidity in tissues (e.g., blood vessels). Such changes in cell structure may explain the observable cosmetic changes associated with aging, such as wrinkles of the skin and decreased distensibility of arterial blood vessels. However, it is unlikely that such changes account for all of the detrimental physical events associated with aging.

Nonstochastic Theories

For many years it was believed that cells had the capability to reproduce for an infinite amount of time. However, in the 1950s Hayflick in a series of classic experiments found that cultured skin fibroblasts would reproduce or divide a finite number of times. From these observations rose the *programmed theory of cell death.* In this theory it is proposed that there is an impairment in the ability of the cell to continue dividing. A more recent theory of aging is the *telomere-telomerase hypothesis.*[11] Telomeres are specialized repeated sequences that are present at the ends of DNA strands. Telomerase is the enzyme that synthesizes these repeat sequences. With aging there is loss of these strands and a decrease in telomerase activity, both of which affect the number of times a cell can divide. It has also been hypothesized that shortening of the DNA is associated with cancer development in older adults.[11,12]

The *neuroendocrine theory* proposes that aging occurs because of functional decrements in neurons and associated hormones.[13] It suggests that neural and endocrine changes may be pacemakers for many cellular and physiologic aspects of aging. This approach relates aging to the organism's loss of responsiveness of neuroendocrine tissue to various signals. In some cases this is a result of a loss of receptors, but in others, it is caused by changes in neurotransmission beyond the receptors. An important focus of this theory is the functional changes of the hypothalamic-pituitary system. These changes are accompanied by a decline in functional capacity in other endocrine organs, such as the adrenal and thyroid glands, ovaries, and testes.[14] In particular, researchers have looked at the age-related declines in the adrenal hormones dehydroepiandrosterone (DHEA), dehydroepiandrosterone sulfate (DHEAS), and growth hormone as markers of neuroendocrine dysfunction with aging.[15]

The *immunologic theory* proposes declining functional capacity of the immune system as the basis for aging.[16] It suggests that aging is not a passive wearing out of systems but an active self-destruction mediated by the immune system. This theory is based on observing an age-associated decline in T cell functioning, accompanied by a decrease in resistance and an increase in autoimmune diseases with aging. Whether the immunologic changes are genetically determined, regulated by environment, or influenced by endocrine factors remains to be defined. However, some studies of cell division suggest that the cells of the immune system become more diversified with age and demonstrate a progressive loss of self-regulatory patterns. The result is an autoimmune phenomenon in which cells normal to the body are mistaken as foreign and are attacked by the person's own immune system.

TABLE 6-3 Gerontologic Differences in Assessment Tables

System	Table Number	Page
Visual	21-1	401
Auditory	21-7	410
Integumentary	23-1	452
Respiratory	26-4	517
Hematologic	30-4	672
Cardiovascular	32-1	744
Gastrointestinal	39-5	933
Urinary	45-2	1141
Endocrine	48-5	1242
Reproductive	51-3	1331
Nervous	56-5	1454
Musculoskeletal	62-1	1619

AGE-RELATED PHYSIOLOGIC CHANGES

Age-related changes affect every body system. These changes are normal and occur as people age. However, the age at which specific changes become evident differs from person to person and within the same person. For instance, a person may have gray hair at age 45 but relatively unwrinkled skin at age 80. The nurse should assess for these age-related changes. Table 6-3 presents a list of tables where specific age-related assessment findings can be found throughout the book.

SPECIAL OLDER ADULT POPULATIONS

Older Adult Women

For the aging woman, the impact of an aging body and being a woman is considered a double jeopardy.[17,18] Many factors have a significant negative impact on the health of the older woman (see Gender box). Many of these are directly related to reduced financial resources and the greater longevity experienced by women. Thus older women often experience disparities, including unequal access to quality health care. (Health disparities are discussed in Chapter 2.) The nurse is in an excellent position to be an advocate for equity for the older woman in the health care system and federal research funding. Advocacy organizations, such as the Older Women's League (OWL) and the Society for Women's Health Research, can be helpful in this process.

GENDER DIFFERENCES
Older Adults

Men	Women
• More likely to be living with spouse. • More likely to have health insurance. • Higher income after retirement. • Less likely to be involved in caregiving activities. • Generally have fewer chronic health problems than women.	• More likely to live alone. • Loss of spouse more common. • Less likely to have health insurance. • Disproportionately higher number of women than men live in poverty. • Minority women have highest poverty rates. • Lack of formal work experience leads to lower income. • More women rely on social security as major source of income. • More likely to be caregiver of ill spouse. • Have a higher incidence of chronic health problems such as arthritis, hypertension, strokes, and diabetes.

Cognitively Impaired Older Adults

For the majority of healthy older adults, there is no noticeable decline in mental abilities. The older adult may experience a memory lapse or benign forgetfulness that is significantly different from cognitive impairment. This is often referred to as age-associated memory impairment. Table 6-4 presents the effects of aging on adult mental functioning.

The older adult who is forgetful should be encouraged to use memory aids to attempt recall in a calm and quiet environment, and actively engage in memory improvement techniques. Memory aids include clocks, calendars, notes, marked pillboxes, safety alarms on stoves, and identity necklaces or bracelets. Memory techniques include word association, mental imaging, and mnemonics.

Declining physical health is an important factor that influences cognitive impairment. The older adult who experiences sensory loss or cerebrovascular disease may show a decline in cognitive functioning. An appropriate cognitive assessment includes functional ability, memory recall, orientation, use of judgment, and appropriate emotional state. Standard mental status examinations and behavioral descriptions provide data for determining cognitive status. Cognitive impairment and dementia are discussed in Chapter 60.

TABLE 6-4 GERONTOLOGIC DIFFERENCES IN ASSESSMENT
Effects of Aging on Adult Mental Functioning

Function	Effect of Aging
Fluid intelligence	Declines during middle age
Crystallized intelligence	Improves
Vocabulary and verbal reasoning	Improves
Spatial perception	Constant or improves
Synthesis of new information	Declines during middle age
Mental performance speed	Declines during middle age
Short-term recall memory	Declines during old age
Long-term recall memory	Constant

Rural Older Adults

Persons over age 65 are less likely to live in metropolitan areas than younger persons. Approximately 50% of older persons live in the suburbs and 27% live in cities. The remaining 23% live in nonmetropolitan areas.[1]

Rural older adults face special challenges. Because of geographic isolation and a higher poverty level, the rural older adult is often stressed by changing financial resources and declining self-care abilities.[19] Particularly vulnerable are rural, minority elders who have even less access to health care providers.[20] Although the rural older adult fears dependence on others, symptoms of ill health are greater than those found in urban peers. In addition, the rural older adult is less likely to engage in health-promoting activities, and rural communities are often underserved by health care workers.

The nurse working with the rural older adult must clearly define the lifestyle values and practices of rural life (Fig. 6-3). Health care providers should consider transportation as a possible barrier to service. Alternative service approaches such as computer-based Internet sources and chat rooms, videotapes, radio, community centers, and church social events should be used to promote healthful practices or to conduct health screening. The development of telehealth devices for monitoring patients in their home environments has enhanced the ability to provide care to isolated individuals. Innovative models of nursing practice must continue to be developed to assist the rural older adult.[21]

Homeless Older Adults

In areas where homelessness is increasing, the older adult is at additional risk because many aging network services are not designed to reach out to homeless persons. It is estimated that between 14% and 50% of homeless persons are older adults.[22] The older homeless person is less likely to use shelters or meal sites. The low-income older adult often becomes homeless because of a

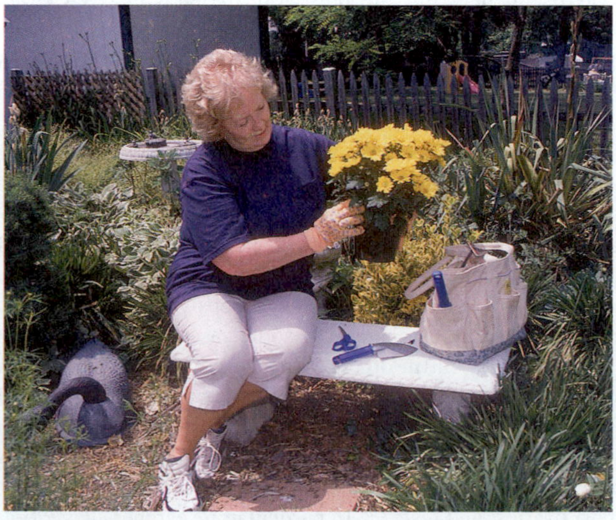

FIG. 6-3 Many older adults enjoy outdoor activities.

lack of affordable housing. Key factors that are associated with homelessness include (1) having a low income, (2) reduced cognitive capacity, and (3) living alone. Long-term care placement is often an alternative to homelessness, especially when the person is cognitively impaired and alone. Fear of institutionalization may explain the reason that the older homeless adult does not use shelter and meal site services. The older homeless person needs affordable housing. Homelessness among the elderly requires more research related to risk factors, as well as solutions.

Frail Older Adults

The **frail elderly** is a term used to identify those older adults who, because of declining physical health and resources, are most vulnerable. Frailty is not directly related to age per se, although age is a risk factor. Old age is just one element of frailty. *Frailty* has been defined as the presence of three or more of the following: unplanned weight loss (≥10 lb in last year), weakness, poor endurance and energy, slowness, and low activity.[5] Risk factors include disability, multiple chronic illnesses, and dementia. The old-old population (85 years of age and older) is most at risk for frailty, although many in this age group remain healthy and robust.

The frail older adult has difficulty coping with declining functional abilities and decreasing daily energy. When stressful life events (e.g., the death of a pet) and daily strain (e.g., caring for an ill spouse) occur, the frail individual often cannot cope with the effects of stress and, as a result, may become ill. Common health problems of the frail older adult include mobility limitations, sensory impairment, cognitive decline, falls, and increasing frailty.

The frail older adult is at particular risk for malnutrition and problems with hydration status. Malnutrition and dehydration are related to sociopsychologic factors such as living alone, depression, and low income. Physical factors such as declining cognitive status, inadequate dental care, sensory decreases, physical fatigue, and limited mobility also add to the risks of malnutrition and dehydration. Because many frail older adults have multiple drug regimens, their nutritional state may be altered. It is important for the nurse to monitor the frail older adult for adequate calorie, protein, iron, calcium, vitamin D, and fluid intake.

Assessment tools that include a focus on physical, social, and environmental risk factors (Table 6-5) have been developed to assess the risk factors for poor nutritional status in older adults. Once the older adult's nutritional needs are identified, common interventions include home-delivered meals, dietary supplements, food stamps, dental referrals, and vitamin supplements.

The nurse should remember that the frail older adult tires easily, has little physical reserve, and is at risk for disability, elder mistreatment, and institutionalization. This older adult is dependent on a network of family, individual, and social support that should be respected and supported.

TABLE 6-5 Nutritional Assessment of Older Adults

The acronym SCALES can remind the nurse to assess important nutritional indicators:

- **S**adness, or mood change
- **C**holesterol, high
- **A**lbumin, low
- **L**oss or gain of weight
- **E**ating problems
- **S**hopping and food preparation problems

Chronically Ill Older Adults

Daily living with chronic illness is a reality for many older adults. Although persons of all ages have chronic health problems, chronic illness is most common in the older adult.[1] The incidence of chronic illness triples after age 45. Most persons 65 years of age and older have at least one chronic condition and many have multiple conditions.[1] The most common chronic conditions present in the older adult are hypertension, arthritis, heart disease, cancer, sinusitis, and diabetes. Other common chronic conditions include vision loss, deafness and hearing impairment, Alzheimer's disease, osteoporosis, hip fractures, urinary incontinence, stroke, Parkinson's disease, and depression.

Often, chronic illness is composed of multiple health problems that have a protracted, unpredictable course. Diagnosis and the acute phase of a chronic illness are often managed in a hospital. All other phases of a chronic illness are usually managed at home. The management of a chronic illness can profoundly affect the lives and identities of the patient, family caregiver, and family.

Although health status refers to acute and chronic illness, it also includes an individual's level of daily functioning. Functional health includes activities of daily living (ADLs), such as bathing, dressing, eating, toileting, and transfer. Instrumental ADLs (IADLs), such as using a telephone, shopping, preparing food, housekeeping, doing laundry, arranging transportation, taking medications, and handling finances, are also included in a functional health assessment.

As age increases, a pattern of declining functional health and increasing disability is seen. The nurse caring for the older adult can advocate accurate, comprehensive assessment in which health and disease states are diagnosed accurately and can actively teach health promotion strategies.[23]

Disease in the older adult may be difficult to accurately diagnose. The older adult may underreport symptoms and treat these symptoms by altering functional status. The older adult eats less, sleeps more, or "waits it out." The older adult often attributes a new symptom to "old age" and will ignore it.

Disease in the older adult may vary greatly. As one disease is treated, another may be affected. For example, the use of a drug with anticholinergic properties such as a tricyclic antidepressant may cause urinary retention (e.g., amitriptyline [Elavil]). In the older adult, disease symptoms are often atypical, and complaints of "aching in the joint" may actually be a broken hip. Silent asymptomatic pathology frequently occurs. Cardiac disease may be diagnosed when the patient is being treated for a urinary tract infection. Pathologies with similar symptoms are often confused. Depression may be misdiagnosed and treated as dementia. A *cascade disease pattern* may occur. An example of cascade disease pattern would occur when the patient who experiences insomnia treats the condition with a hypnotic medication, becomes lethargic and confused, falls, breaks a hip, and subsequently develops pneumonia.

Tasks required for daily living with chronic illness are multiple (Table 6-6). Both the patient and the nurse must practice behaviors different from those required of patients with an acute illness if the older adult is to accomplish the tasks necessary to deal with a chronic disease.

TABLE 6-6 Helping Older Adults Manage Chronic Illness

Older adults living with chronic illness need to do the following:
- Prevent social isolation
- Control symptoms of the chronic illness
- Attempt to normalize interactions with others
- Adjust to changes in the course of the disease
- Prevent and manage the episodes of acute illness
- Carry out prescribed therapies for the chronic illness
- Use technology to enhance function, independence, and safety

CULTURALLY COMPETENT CARE
OLDER ADULTS

The term **ethno-geriatrics** is used to describe the specialty area of providing culturally competent care to ethnic elders.[5] The older adult who identifies with a certain ethnic group presents a particular challenge to the nurse (Fig. 6-4). Ethnic identity can be determined by asking the following questions:

1. Does this person identify with an ethnic or racial group?
2. Do others identify this person with an ethnic or racial group?
3. Does this person show behavioral patterns that are unique to the ethnic group?

Ethnic identity is often found in certain religious groups, nations, and minorities. As American society changes, ethnic institutions and neighborhoods may be altered. For the older adult with strong ethnic roots, the loss of friends who speak the "mother tongue," the loss of the church that supports social ethnic activities, and the loss of stores that carry desired ethnic foods may present situational crises that emphasize and diminish a sense of self-worth and personhood. This loss of self is increased when children and others deny or ignore ethnic practices and behaviors. Support for the ethnic older adult is most frequently found in family, religious practices, and isolated geographic or community ethnic clusters. In the old-old population, ethnic group members often live with extended family and often continue to speak their native language.

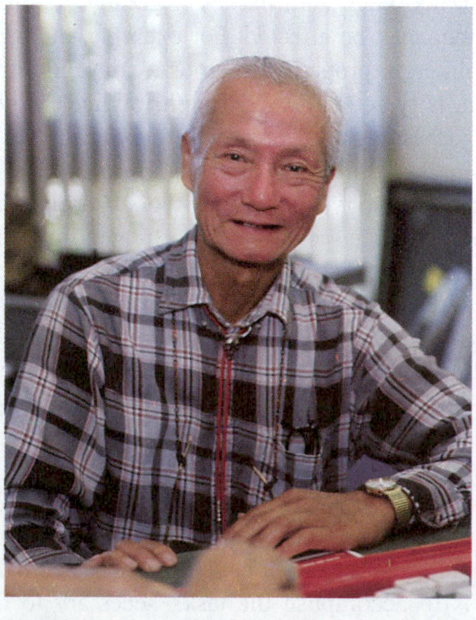

FIG. 6-4 Ethnic older adults need special consideration.

TABLE 6-7 Assessment of Ethnic Older Adults

Questions to ask ethnic older adults about health-related practices include the following:
1. What makes people ill?
2. When do you know someone is sick?
3. What helps people get better?
4. Who can assist people to get well?
5. Do you believe this drug or treatment will help you get well?

The ethnic older adult is faced with specific problems. Because the ethnic older adult often lives in older neighborhoods, physical security and personal safety related to crime become a concern. Because the individual with an ethnic identity often has a disproportionately low income, Medicare deductibles or drugs needed to treat chronic illnesses may not be affordable. Perceptions of health also differ by ethnic group. In 2003, only 38.6% of noninstitutionalized older adults assessed their health as excellent or very good (compared with 66.6% for all persons ages 18 to 64). In the older adult group, fewer African Americans and Hispanics rated their health as excellent or good as compared with older white adults.[1]

For the nurse to be effective with the ethnic older adult, a sense of respect and clear communication are critical. The nurse must identify self-behaviors that could be interpreted as noncaring or disrespectful, such as a refusal to allow a patient to display an item considered important for healing. Nursing interventions to assist in meeting the needs of the ethnic older adult are described in Table 2-4. Additional assessment questions of the ethnic older adult are shown in Table 6-7.

American culture is changing. For some older adults, ethnic identity is also changing. The nurse should not assume that ethnic identity is or is not of value to the patient and the patient's family. The nurse must assess each older adult's ethnic orientation.[5,23] (Culturally competent care is discussed in Chapter 3.)

SOCIAL SUPPORT AND THE OLDER ADULT

Social support for the older adult occurs at three levels. Family and kinship relations are the first and preferred providers of social support. Second, a semiformal level of support is found in clubs, churches, neighborhoods, and senior citizen centers. Last, the older adult may be linked to a formal system of social welfare agencies, health facilities, and government support. Generally, the nurse is part of the formal support system.

Caregivers

Approximately 6 to 7 million Americans provide care to a family member or friend over age 65 with a chronic or long-term illness. Of the 3 million Americans with Alzheimer's disease living at home, the majority receives care from their family members or friends. A **caregiver** is someone who provides supervision and direct care and coordinates services. The tasks of caregiving include (1) assisting with ADLs and IADLs, (2) providing emotional and social support, and (3) managing health care. A caregiver is usually a married woman who is often old herself, has chronic diseases and disabilities, and is often poor. Ethnic background influences the type of caregiving network. Italian American, Polish American, Irish American, Asian American, African American, and Latino people most commonly use extended family networks for caregiving.

TABLE 6-8 Caregiver Challenges

- Lack of respite or relief from caregiving
- Conflict in the family unit related to decisions about caregiving
- Lack of understanding of the time and energy needed for caregiving
- Inability to meet personal self-care needs, such as socialization and rest
- Inadequate information about specific tasks of caregiving, such as bathing or drug administration
- Financial depletion of resources as a result of a caregiver's inability to work and the increased cost of health care

Caregiver concerns change as the intensity of the caregiving role changes. For example, a caregiver may need to adjust work schedules to accommodate patient health care appointments, or the caregiver may need to be available to monitor the cognitively impaired patient's safety 24 hours a day, seven days a week (Table 6-8).

The intensity and complexity of caregiving place the caregiver at risk for high levels of stress. The caregiver may develop a sense of being overwhelmed with feelings of inadequacy and powerlessness.[24] The stress of caregiving may result in emotional problems such as depression, anger, and resentment.[25] Although most older adults deny loneliness even when they spend much time alone, the caregiver often lacks sufficient social interaction. The primary caregiver is often at risk for social isolation. The burden of caregiving separates the individual from others who provide social, emotional, and interactional involvement. Time commitments, fatigue, and, at times, socially inappropriate behaviors of the dependent older adult contribute to social isolation. The socially isolated caregiver needs to be identified, and plans should be designed to meet the needs for social support and interaction. The burden of caregiving may result in the nursing diagnosis of caregiver role strain.

Many family members involved in direct caregiving activities also identify rewards associated with this role. Positive aspects of caregiving include (1) knowing that their loved one is receiving good care (often in a home environment), (2) learning and mastering new tasks, and (3) finding opportunities for intimacy. At the same time, the tasks involved in caregiving often provide opportunities for family members to gain greater insights into each other and strengthen their relationships.

The nurse should consider the caregiver as a patient and plan behaviors to reduce caregiver role strain. The nurse should communicate a sense of empathy to the caregiver while allowing discussion about the burdens and joys of caregiving. The caregiver can be taught about age-related changes and diseases and specific caregiving techniques. The nurse should encourage attendance at a support group. The nurse can also assist the caregiver in seeking help from the formal social support system regarding matters such as respite care, housing, health coverage, and finances. Finally, the nurse should monitor the caregiver for indications of declining health, emotional distress, and caregiver role strain.

Elder Mistreatment/Abuse

The term **elder mistreatment** (EM) is used to describe acts of commission **(elder abuse)** or omission **(elder neglect)** that harm or threaten to harm an older adult's health or welfare. Elder mistreatment may be intentional or unintentional and occur in the community (domestic EM) or in an institution (institutional EM). Elder mistreatment includes physical, sexual, and psychologic abuse and/or neglect, as well as financial and/or material exploitation[26] (Table 6-9). Up to 70% of cases involve neglect.[26] Elders who have been mistreated have a three times higher risk of death than elders who have not been mistreated. The primary causes of death are cardiovascular diseases, ill-defined conditions, and cancer, indicating that stress may play a role in the shortened survival of mistreated elders.[27]

Domestic EM affects approximately 32 out of 1000 adults in the United States and 4% of adults over age 65 in Canada.[26] Because they account for the majority of the older population, the majority of victims are women. When women are mistreated, they suffer more serious abuse (i.e., physical and/or emotional harm) than men. Overall EM is an underreported problem. It has been estimated that for every case of EM that is reported, there may be five that are not reported.[26] Lack of reporting by victims often stems from the older adult's isolation; impaired cognitive or

TABLE 6-9 Types of Elder Mistreatment

Types	Characteristics	Manifestations
Physical abuse	Slapping; striking, restraining; incorrect positioning; oversedation with medications	Bruises, bilateral injuries (ankles, wrists), repeated injuries in various stages of healing, oversedation; utilization of several emergency departments
Physical neglect	Withholding of food, water, medications, clothing, hygiene; failure to provide physical aids such as dentures, eyeglasses, hearing aid; failure to ensure safety	Pressure ulcers on sacral area, heels; loss of body weight; laboratory values showing dehydration (e.g., ↑ Hct, ↑ serum sodium), malnutrition (↓ serum protein); poor personal hygiene
Psychologic abuse	Berating verbally; harassment; intimidation; threats of punishment or deprivation; childlike treatment; isolation	Depression, withdrawn behavior; agitation; ambivalent attitude toward caregiver/family member
Psychologic neglect	Failing to provide social stimulation; leaving alone for long periods of time; failing to provide companionship	Depression, withdrawn behavior; agitation; ambivalent attitude toward caregiver/family member
Sexual abuse	Touching inappropriately; forcing sexual contact	Unexplained vaginal or anal bleeding; bruised breasts; unexplained STDs or genital infections
Financial abuse	Denying access to personal resources, stealing money or possessions; coercing to sign contracts or durable power of attorney; making changes in will or trust	Living situation is below level of personal resources; sudden change in personal finances; sudden transfer of assets
Violation of personal rights	Denying right to privacy or right to make decisions regarding health care or living environment; forcible eviction	Sudden inexplicable changes in living situation; confusion

Hct, Hematocrit; *STDs,* sexually transmitted diseases.

physical function; feelings of shame, embarrassment, guilt, or self-blame; fear of reprisal; pressure from family members; fear of losing their home and independence; and cultural norms. Lack of reporting by health care providers may be due to lack of confidence in identifying or reporting victims of EM; perceived inability to successfully intervene; and desire to avoid responsibility for further action.[27,28]

Family members are the perpetrators in about 9 out of 10 proven cases of domestic elder abuse and neglect.[26,27] The primary risk factors for EM are the characteristics of the abuser. Abusers tend to be adult children who are dependent on the parent for housing and financial means. They also tend to (1) have a history of violence and/or antisocial behavior; (2) be unemployed; and (3) be disabled because of substance abuse and/or mental illness.[27] Victim characteristics, such as frailty, also add to the risk of mistreatment. Frailty increases the likelihood that an elder is unable to seek help or defend herself or himself. Alcohol abuse can also place the elder at risk in that an older person who abuses alcohol is 10 times more likely to be mistreated. Elders who live alone have a lower risk of mistreatment.[27]

The different types of abuse are characterized in Table 6-9. Nurses should assess the elder for the presence of dehydration, malnutrition, pressure ulcers, poor personal hygiene, and lack of compliance with the medical regimen. It is important for the nurse to examine the patient's sacral area and feet for pressure ulcers. These areas are often hidden by clothing, but may be the only findings.

It is mandatory for nurses to report cases of abuse or neglect in most states. Nurses should know their legal responsibility by checking the laws in their state. Appropriate nursing interventions are listed in Table 6-10.

Institutional elder mistreatment is mistreatment that occurs in long-term care facilities, boarding homes, and adult family homes. Although the prevalence of institutional EM is unknown, the problem is thought to be widespread. The types of EM that can occur in institutions are the same as those described in Table 6-9. In addition, failure to follow the plan of care is considered a form of abuse. For example, unauthorized use of physical or chemical restraints and use of medication or isolation as punishment are considered abuse. Individual risk factors for mistreatment of residents include frailty, dementia, and immobility. Elders who are institutionalized are also at risk for mistreatment if they do not have regular visitors or out-of-facility contacts. System issues can also contribute to the risk faced by institutionalized elders. These include insufficient resources, staffing and supervision problems, and larger societal issues, such as ageism.[29]

TABLE 6-10 Nursing Management
Elder Mistreatment

- Mandatory report to the appropriate state agency and/or law enforcement on the suspicion of abuse or neglect
- Thorough assessment with precise documentation (including photographic documentation taken before the victim is washed or treated)
- Collection and preservation of any and all physical evidence (e.g., dirty or bloody clothing, bandages, sheets)
- Social services consultation
- If the elder is in immediate danger, consider implementing a safety plan (e.g., hospital admission)

The nursing approach to a suspected victim should be a very careful medical history and screening for mistreatment. It is imperative that victims be interviewed alone, because they may not disclose accurate information in the presence of the person who accompanied them to the facility, particularly if that person is the abuser. Nurses should follow the facility's written EM diagnostic and intervention protocol. If one does not exist, tools available for use by clinicians include the Elder Assessment Instrument and the American Medical Association's Diagnostic and Treatment Guidelines on Elder Abuse and Neglect.[27] Key assessment findings include explanations (e.g., about the cause of injuries) that are not consistent with what is observed or contradictory explanations between the patient and caregiver.

Nursing assessment of the institutionalized individual is similar to that of a community-dwelling adult. In addition, the resident should be examined for unexplained bruising or injuries; recurrent infections; poor hygiene and dirty clothing; weight loss or lack of interest in meals; and recurrent or worsening pressure ulcers. The nurse should be especially alert for vague excuses for missing activities or therapies or complaints about evening or night shift staff. It is on these shifts when supervision is lowest and the risk for mistreatment highest. The elder should also be assessed for recurring problems despite treatment that, if given as ordered, should be effective. Last, the elder should be assessed for new onset of psychiatric or behavior problems, bowel or bladder incontinence, or sleep problems.[30] Specific nursing interventions to minimize the risk for mistreatment of institutionalized elders include developing and monitoring the patient's plan of care; avoiding orders for restraints or antipsychotic drugs for behavioral modification or control; and monitoring systems reports carefully, such as those sent by the pharmacist after Drug Utilization Review.[31]

SOCIAL SERVICES FOR OLDER ADULTS

A network of services supports the older adult both in the community and in health care facilities. Most older adults are involved in at least one social or governmental service. This is true in both Canada and the United States. To understand the older adult situation, the nurse should know the government structures that fund and regulate the older adult programs.

In the United States, the Department of Health and Human Services is the responsible federal agency for many older adult programs. In 1958, interest in health and welfare of older citizens inspired the formation of the President's Council on Aging. From this beginning, the current Administration on Aging (AoA) has evolved. The general goal of AoA is to include older people wherever programs exist by cooperating and consulting with other agencies or organizations. There are several major grant programs under AoA. Title III of the Older Americans Act funds comprehensive, community-based service systems. Title IV funds the training of persons who are employed or preparing for employment in the field of aging. Funding from the AoA is funneled to state and local Area Agencies on Aging.

In Canada, the Department of National Health and Welfare is the responsible federal agency for many older adult programs. The policies of the federal and provincial governments cannot be easily separated. Policy often results in an intermingling of activities through shared jurisdiction and cost sharing. Since 1950 a wide range of federal and provincial programs have evolved. The role of the government has changed from that of regulator to provider.

MEDICARE

Almost all U.S. citizens older than 65 years of age have Medicare coverage. **Medicare** is a health insurance program for people 65 years of age and older, as well as for some people with disabilities under age 65 and for people with end-stage renal disease requiring dialysis or a transplant. Medicare was designed for acute illness care. Reimbursement is based on daily documentation that indicates a patient is improving in function. This nursing documentation process is complex and critical for adequate reimbursement of services.

Medicare is composed of two parts, A and B. Part A covers inpatient hospital care. Medicare Part A pays reasonable charges on the basis of the diagnosis, not on the length of stay. Skilled nursing facility care in a hospital or long-term care facility is paid if the stay results in an improved or rehabilitated condition. However, these skilled nursing benefit days are limited. The percentage of coverage changes each year. Medicare Part A pays for home care if it requires skilled nursing or rehabilitation intervention and is needed on a part-time basis. The patient must be homebound, meaning that it must take considerable effort to leave the home. Durable medical equipment used daily is covered, but home safety equipment is not. Hospice care is covered under Medicare Part A. When hospice care is elected, the patient no longer qualifies for the condition to be treated in the standard Medicare program.

Medicare Part B covers outpatient treatment and physician's services. Medicare Part B is voluntary and has a monthly premium and an annual deductible before payment begins. Medicare Part B covers a one-time physical examination if the examination is completed within 6 months of enrolling in Part B. Medicare Part B also covers screening examinations, such as cardiovascular screening; cancer tests (mammograms, Papanicolaou [Pap] test and pelvic examinations, colorectal cancer screening, and prostate cancer screening); immunizations (flu shots, hepatitis B, and pneumococcal); diabetes screening, supplies, and self-management training; and glaucoma tests.

Medicare beneficiaries who are covered by Medicare Part A or Part B may join the Medicare Prescription Drug Benefit Program. This plan is known as Medicare Part D. Members pay a yearly deductible, a monthly premium, and a copayment. People with lower incomes and limited assets will qualify for extra help to pay for prescriptions.[32] Medicare does not cover long-term care, custodial ADLs or IADLs care, dental care or dentures, routine foot care, hearing aids, or eyeglasses. (More information is available at *www.Medicare.gov.*)

These costs, plus the Medicare deductible costs, account for the fact that most older adults pay for 50% of all acquired health care costs yearly. Analysis of chronic health care needs in the United States continues to indicate widespread unmet needs.

CARE ALTERNATIVES FOR OLDER ADULTS

Housing

Many older adults stay in their place of residence and do not move to a different home or geographic location (Fig. 6-5). Most do not move or return to the geographic location of childhood when health becomes frail. The community becomes important to the older adult as an environment that is safe from crime and accidents. The older adult needs privacy and companionship, as well as a sense of belonging. The community should be accessible. The older adult may need housing assistance through property tax relief, assistance with home repair, and fuel payment. A variety of subsidized, low-income housing arrangements are available for older adults in many areas.

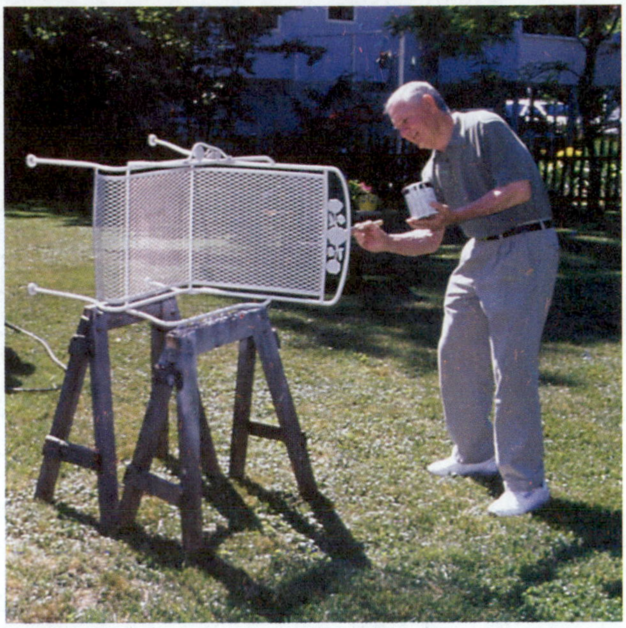

FIG. 6-5 Home maintenance is part of an older adult's independent lifestyle.

For the older adult who chooses to remain in the home as functional abilities decline, home adaptations and modifications can be made. Homes can be made wheelchair accessible. Lighting can be increased and adjusted. Safety devices can be installed in bathrooms and kitchens. Alarms and assistive listening devices can be used.

Retirement communities may be an option for some older adults. These communities are age-segregated, self-contained developments and provide social activities, security, and recreational facilities. When retirement communities offer expanded health care and social support services, including long-term care, they become *continuing care retirement communities* (CCRCs). The CCRCs require an entrance fee and monthly fees for continuing care. (See Chapter 7 for discussion of community-based care settings.)

Congregate housing provides services to the older adult at two levels: independent and assisted living. Independent living facilities provide housing and congregate meals, but no supervision. Other home maintenance and care services can be purchased from these facilities. Board and care homes provide housing and meals in small congregate home environments.

Assisted-living facilities are designed to provide housing and personalized health care. Because over half of community-based older adults require assistance with ADLs or IADLs, this is the most rapidly developing area of long-term care. Services vary from state to state. Nurses provide care to or manage assisted-living facilities and services. Nurses working in this area are challenged by questions related to regulations, use of unlicensed assistive workers, assessment to ensure safe "fit of resident to facility," and shared resident decision making.

Creative housing options are being developed by home sharing, the use of "granny flats," and apartment rentals in established older homes. The nurse can play a role in meeting the housing needs of older adults by identifying housing preferences and by advocating community housing changes that create a safe, livable community.

Community-Based Older Adults with Special Needs

Older adults with special care needs include homeless persons, persons who need constant assistance with ADLs, persons who are homebound, and persons who can no longer live at home. The older adult may be served by adult day care, home health care, and long-term care.

Adult Day Care Programs. *Adult day care (ADC) programs* provide daily supervision, social activities, and ADLs assistance for two major groups of older adults—persons who are cognitively impaired and persons who have problems with ADLs. The services offered in the ADC programs are based on patient needs. Restorative programs for persons with problems of ADLs offer health monitoring, therapeutic activities, one-to-one ADLs training, individualized care planning, and personal care services. Programs designed for the cognitively impaired offer therapeutic recreation, support for family, family counseling, and social involvement. Patient characteristics in the cognitively impaired group include a high number of persons with Alzheimer's disease.

Day care centers provide relief to the caregiver, allow continued employment for the caregiver, and delay institutionalization for the patient. Centers are regulated and standards are set by the state. Medicare does not cover costs. Adult day care is tax deductible as dependent care. Appropriate placement in a day care program that matches the patient's needs is important. The nurse can assist by knowing the available day care services and assessing the needs of the patient. The nurse is then in a position to aid the patient and family in making a good placement decision. The caregiver and the patient are often uninformed about day care and its services as an alternative care option.

Home Health Care. Home health care can be a cost-effective care alternative for the older adult patient who is homebound, has health needs that are intermittent or acute, and has supportive caregiver involvement. Home health care is not an alternative for the patient in need of 24-hour ADLs assistance or continuous safety supervision. Home health care services require physician recommendation and skilled nursing care for Medicare reimbursement. Unless these requirements are met, assistance by a home health aide for ADLs management or assistance by a homemaker for IADLs management will not be paid by Medicare. (Home health care is discussed in Chapter 7.)

Long-Term Care Facilities

Long-term care facilities are a placement alternative for the older adult who can no longer live alone, who needs continuous supervision, who has three or more ADLs disabilities, or who is frail. The cost of long-term care facilities is high. These costs are paid privately for 50% of all patients and by state-funded public assistance programs (Medicaid) for 40% of all patients. When patients receive Medicaid, they contribute all their personal income to pay their expenses, except for a small amount per month kept as a personal needs allowance. (Long-term care is discussed in Chapter 7.)

Three factors appear to precipitate placement in a long-term care facility: (1) rapid patient deterioration, (2) caregiver inability to continue care as a result of "burnout"—too much and too long, and (3) an alteration in or loss of family support system. Changes in orientation (e.g., increased confusion), incontinence, or a major health event (e.g., stroke) can accelerate placement.

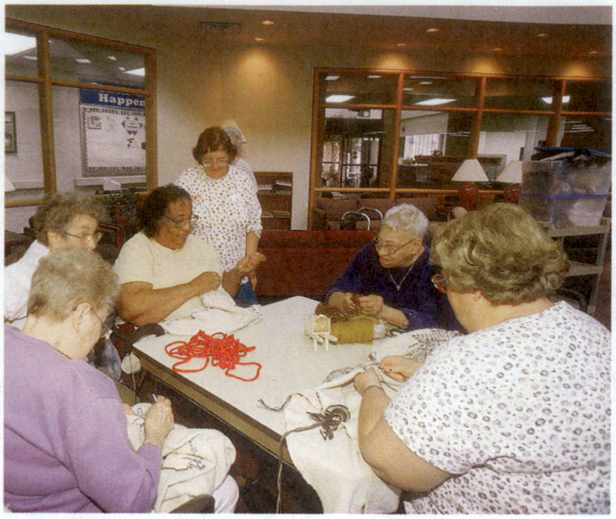

FIG. 6-6 Social interaction and acceptance is important for older adults.

The conflicts and fears faced by the family and patient make placement a transition time. Common caregiver concerns include the following: (1) process of admission will be resisted by the patient; (2) level of care given by staff will be insufficient; (3) patient will be lonely; and (4) financing of nursing care will not be adequate.

This time of disruption is increased by the physical relocation of the patient. The nurse should anticipate that the process of physical relocation results in adverse health effects for the older adult.[33] Appropriate interventions to reduce the effects of relocation should be used. Whenever possible, the older adult should be involved in the decision to move and should be fully informed about the location. The caregiver can share information, pictures, or a videotape of the new location. New health personnel can send a welcome message. On arrival, the new resident can be greeted by a staff member to orient the older adult. To bridge the relocation, the new resident can be "buddied" with a seasoned resident.

The satisfied resident in a long-term care facility tends to show a variety of behaviors indicating adjustment (Fig. 6-6). The resident is assertive and self-reliant; keeps active, follows a routine, keeps mentally involved, and is sociable; maintains family interaction; and shows a level of acceptance. The satisfied resident also expresses a determined, positive perspective. The satisfied resident uses coping strategies that increase control and management of her or his life. The nurse can encourage and enable the use of these strategies.

Case Management

Matching older adult social support services to the needs of the older adult is complex. For family members who live out of town and cannot provide direct caregiving, the use of a case manager may be helpful. This is a new and developing role that the nurse is well suited to assume. The case manager supervises and manages care to ensure continuity of care for the older adult. The process of locating and organizing older adult services is time consuming. A written directory of nationwide services *(A National Eldercare Directory of Information and Referral)* is available from the National Association of Area Agencies on Aging (see Resources at end of chapter).

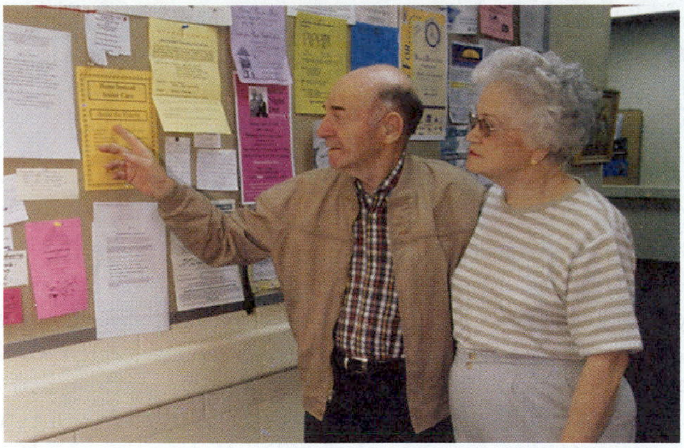

FIG. 6-7 Bulletin board at a senior center showing times that legal help is available.

LEGAL AND ETHICAL ISSUES

Legal assistance is a concern for many older adults. Legal concerns center on advance directives, estate planning, taxation issues, and appeals for denied services. Legal aid is available to the low-income older adult by contacting a local multipurpose senior center (Fig. 6-7). This service is supported by funds authorized through Title III of the Older Americans Act.

The Patient Self-Determination Act of 1991 mandates advance directives on admission to a health care facility. Advance directives are written statements of a person's wishes regarding medical care. The first advance directive was known as a living will. However, this term has now been replaced with more specific directives known as *natural death acts*. Natural death acts include directives to physicians (DTPs), durable power of attorney for health care (DPAHC), and medical power of attorney. These acts allow patients to more specifically direct their own care at end of life. These acts are discussed in greater detail in Chapter 11. Discussion of estate planning, taxation issues, and appeals for denied services is beyond the scope of this text.

The nurse who works with the older adult identifies areas of ethical concern that influence practice. This nurse identifies that these issues include the following: (1) to restrain or not restrain and (2) to evaluate the patient's ability to make decisions. Other ethical concerns related to (1) resuscitation, (2) treatment of infections, (3) issues of nutrition and hydration, and (4) transfer to more intensive treatment units are all a part of long-term care.

These situations are often complex and emotionally charged. The nurse can assist the patient, family, and other health care workers by acknowledging when an ethical dilemma is present by (1) keeping current on the ethical implications of new biotechnology and (2) advocating for an institutional ethics committee to help in the decision-making process.

NURSING MANAGEMENT
OLDER ADULTS

Nursing Assessment

As with all age groups, assessment of the older adult provides the database for the rest of the nursing process. It is important to remember that the older adult may face a health problem with fear and anxiety. Health care workers may be perceived as helpful, but institutions may be perceived as negative, potentially harmful places. The nurse can communicate a sense of concern and care by use of direct and simple statements, appropriate eye contact, direct touch, and gentle humor. These actions assist the older adult to relax in this stressful situation.

Before beginning the assessment process the nurse should attend to primary needs first, for example, ensuring that the patient is pain free and does not need to urinate. All assistive devices, such as glasses and hearing aids, should be in place. The interview should be short so the patient is not fatigued. The interviewer should allow adequate time to give information, as well as to respond to questions. The older adult and caregiver should be interviewed separately unless the patient is cognitively impaired or specifically requests the caregiver's presence. Medical history may be lengthy. The nurse must determine what is relevant information. Medical records should be obtained and available for review.

The focus of a comprehensive geriatric assessment is to determine appropriate interventions to maintain and enhance the functional abilities of the older adult. The comprehensive geriatric assessment is interdisciplinary and at a minimum includes the medical history, physical examination, functional abilities assessment, and social resources. The comprehensive geriatric assessment is often conducted at a geriatric evaluation unit by an interdisciplinary geriatric assessment team. The interdisciplinary team may include many disciplines, but the minimum components include the nurse, the physician, and the social worker. After the assessment is complete, the interdisciplinary team meets with the patient and family to present the team's findings and recommendations. These assessment centers are often affiliated with large medical complexes.

Elements in a comprehensive nursing assessment include a history using a functional health pattern format (see Chapter 4), physical assessment, mood assessment, assessment of ADLs and IADLs, mental status evaluation, and a social-environmental assessment. Evaluation of mental status is particularly important for the older adult because results of this evaluation often determine the patient's potential for independent living. Evaluation of the results of a comprehensive nursing assessment helps determine the service and placement needs of the older adult patient. A good match between needs and services should be the goal of the assessment. The nurse also collects data regarding community resources that are needed to assist the older adult and his or her family to maintain maximal functioning.

The comprehensive nursing assessment should be based on instruments that are reliable, valid, and specific to the older adult population.[23] Interpretation of laboratory results can be problematic because many values change with age, and parameters are not well defined for the older adult, particularly the old-old patient. An appropriate reference book should be consulted for the correct ranges of laboratory values for the older adult. The nurse is in an important position to recognize and correct inaccurate interpretation of laboratory tests (Fig. 6-8).

Cure is often not possible because of the complexity and chronicity of the health problems that commonly affect the older adult. Consequently, the nurse directs the planning and implementation of those actions that assist the older adult in remaining as functionally independent as possible.

Nursing Diagnoses

With few exceptions the same nursing diagnoses apply to the older adult as to a younger person. Often, however, the etiology and defining characteristics are related to age and unique to the older

Patient name______________ Date______________

SPICES	EVIDENCE
Sleep disorders	
Problems with eating or feeding	
Incontinence	
Confusion	
Evidence of falls	
Skin breakdown	

FIG. 6-8 SPICES.

adult. Table 6-11 lists nursing diagnoses that are seen in older adults as a result of age-related changes. The identification and management of nursing diagnoses result in improved patient function and quality patient care for the older adult.

Planning

When setting goals with the older adult, it is helpful to identify the strengths and abilities that the patient demonstrates. Caregivers should be included in goal development. Personal characteristics such as hardiness, persistence, and the ability to laugh and learn are positive factors in goal setting. Individualized care is the standard of practice with older adults. The older adult who perceives increasing dependence and learned helplessness as an appropriate response may be resistant to self-care. Priority goals for the older adult might include gaining a sense of control, feeling safe, and reducing stress.

Nursing Implementation

When carrying out a plan of action, the nurse may need to modify the approach and techniques used on the basis of the physical and mental status of the elderly patient. Small body size, common in the frail older adult, may necessitate the use of pediatric equipment (e.g., blood pressure cuff). Bone and joint changes often require transfer assistance, altered positioning, and use of gait belts and lift devices. The older adult with declining energy reserves may require additional time to complete tasks. A slower approach, restricted scheduling, and the use of a bedside commode or other adaptive equipment may be necessary.

Cognitive impairment, if present, requires the nurse to offer careful explanations and a calm approach to avoid producing anxiety and resistance in the patient. Depression can result in apathy and poor cooperation with the treatment plan.

Health Promotion. Health promotion and prevention of health problems in the older adult are focused on three areas: reduction in diseases and problems, increased participation in health promotion activities (Fig. 6-9), and increased targeted services that reduce health hazards. The nurse places a high value on health promotion and positive health behaviors. Programs have been successfully developed for screening for chronic health conditions, smoking cessation, geriatric foot care, vision and hearing screening, stress reduction, exercise programs, drug usage, crime prevention, elder mistreatment, and home hazards assessment. The nurse can carry out and teach the older adult about the need for specific preventive services.

Health promotion and prevention can be included in nursing interventions at any location or level where the nurse and the older adult interact. The nurse can use health promotion activities to strengthen self-care, increase personal responsibility for health, and increase independent functioning that will enhance the well-being of the older adult. The nurse interested in older adult health promotion can contact the Health Promotion Institute, the National

TABLE 6-11 NURSING DIAGNOSES Associated with Age-Related Physiologic Changes

Cardiovascular System	**Reproductive System**
Activity intolerance	Disturbed body image
Decreased cardiac output	Ineffective sexuality patterns
Fatigue	Sexual dysfunction
Respiratory System	**Gastrointestinal System**
Impaired gas exchange	Constipation
Ineffective airway clearance	Imbalanced nutrition
Ineffective breathing pattern	Impaired oral mucous membrane
Risk for aspiration	**Nervous System**
Risk for infection	Disturbed thought processes
Integumentary System	Disturbed sensory perception
Impaired skin integrity	Hyperthermia
Urinary System	Hypothermia
Deficient fluid volume	Insomnia
Impaired urinary elimination	**Senses**
Musculoskeletal System	Disturbed body image
Impaired physical mobility	Impaired verbal communication
Chronic pain	Social isolation
Risk for injury	**Immune System**
Self-care deficit	Risk for infection
Sedentary lifestyle	

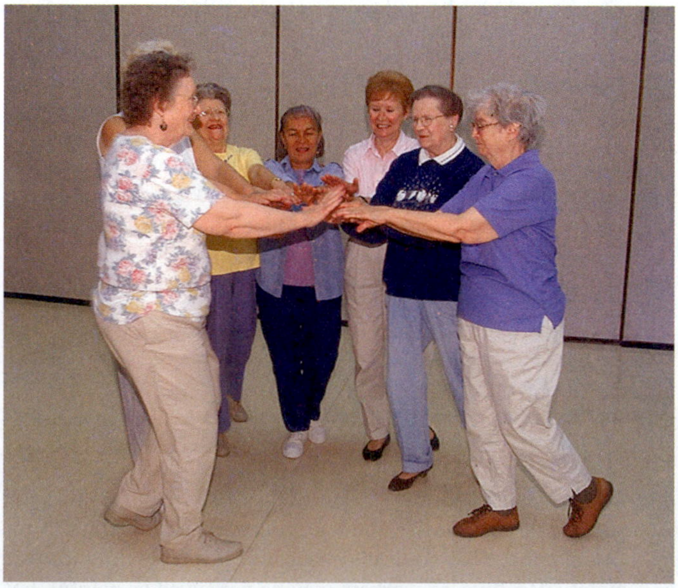

FIG. 6-9 Dancing is an example of a health promotion activity for older adults.

TABLE 6-12 *PATIENT AND FAMILY TEACHING* Older Adults

Challenges with Older Adults	Specific Strategies
• Time needed to learn is increased • New learning must relate to the patient's actual experience • Anxiety and distractions decrease learning • Lack of risk taking and cautiousness decrease motivation to learn • Sensory-perceptual deficits and cognitive decline require modified teaching techniques	• Present material at a slower rate • Use visual aids when possible • Use peer educators when appropriate • Encourage participation of a spouse or family member • Use simple phrases or sentences and provide for repetition • Support the belief that change in behavior is both helpful and worth the effort • Emphasize that a person is never too old to learn new things

Institute on Aging, or the local Area Office on Aging (see Resources at end of chapter).

Teaching Older Adults. The nurse is involved in teaching the older adult self-care practices to enhance health and modify disease processes (Table 6-12). (Patient teaching is discussed in Chapter 5.)

Acute Care. Frequently the hospital is the first point of contact for the older adult and the formal health care system. In 2002, over 12.5 million older adults in the United States were discharged from hospitals. This was three times the rate of persons ages 45 to 64.[1] The hospitalized older adult is often experiencing multisystem failure. Illnesses that most commonly result in hospitalization include dysrhythmias, heart failure, stroke, fluid and electrolyte imbalances (e.g., hyponatremia, dehydration), pneumonia, and hip fractures. The complexity of the acute situation often results in a loss of the whole-person perspective and focuses care on the diseased part. Because the nurse provides an integrated approach, care that is individualized and helpful to the older adult can be reestablished.

When caring for the hospitalized older adult, both patient and caregivers are assisted when the nurse performs a variety of functions (Table 6-13). The outcome of hospitalization for the older adult varies. Of particular concern are the problems of high surgical risk, acute confusional state, nosocomial infection, and premature discharge with an unstable condition. Each of these is described later in the book with special attention to the older adult patient.

Hospital Discharge. At the time of hospital discharge, many older adults are considered to be in an unstable condition. The frail older adult and the old-old patient are particularly vulnerable. Most of these patients are discharged under Medicare regulations that require a registered nurse or qualified person to develop a plan for discharge. The discharge plan should be periodically reassessed, and caregivers and patients must be counseled to prepare the patient for posthospital care.

The nurse can use screening tools to identify high-risk patients. The postdischarge assistance needed by high-risk patients includes bathing, taking medications, housekeeping, shopping, preparing meals, and making satisfactory transportation arrangements. Risk of unstable discharge increases in the patient who experiences greater length of stay and who is dependent on others for meals. Early hospital discharge is most successful when patients have had little change in functional status or are returning to a place with a high level of assistance, such as a long-term care facility.

Geriatric Rehabilitation. Geriatric rehabilitation interventions are focused on adapting to or recovering from disability. With proper training, assistive equipment, and attendant personal care, the patient with disabilities can often live an independent life. The older adult, primarily through Medicare reimbursement, can receive rehabilitative assistance through inpatient rehabilitation (limited days) and home care programs (Fig. 6-10).

The nurse needs to understand physical disability in the older adult. The older person with cerebrovascular disease, arthritis, and coronary artery disease has a risk of becoming functionally limited. Hip fracture, amputation, and stroke occur at higher rates in the older adult population. These disabilities lead to increased mortality rates, decreased life span, and increased rates of institutionalization. Reducing disability through geriatric rehabilitation is important to the quality of life of the older adult.

Often, the older adult has specific fears and anxieties related to falling. The older adult is limited in the rehabilitation process by sensory-perceptual deficits, other disease states, slowed cognition, poor nutrition, and financial problems. Nurse and caregiver encouragement, support, and acceptance can assist the older adult in remaining motivated for the hard work of rehabilitation.

TABLE 6-13 Care of the Hospitalized Older Adult

- Identify the frail and old-old patients at risk for *iatrogenic* (due to medical/surgical treatment) effects.
- Consider discharge needs early in the hospital stay, especially assistance with ADLs, IADLs, and medications.
- Encourage the development and use of interdisciplinary teams, special care units, and individuals who focus on the special needs of gerontologic patients.
- Develop standard protocols to screen for at-risk conditions commonly present in the hospitalized older adult patient, such as urinary tract infection and delirium.
- Advocate for referral of the patient to appropriate community-based services (see Chapter 7).

ADLs, Activities of daily living; *IADLs*, instrumental activities of daily living.

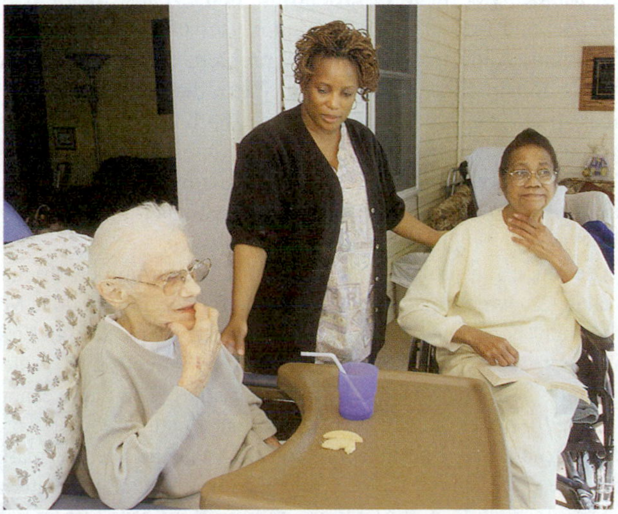

FIG. 6-10 The nurse assists two patients in the geriatric rehabilitation facility.

Rehabilitation of the older adult is influenced by several factors. First, the older patient shows greater initial variability in functional capacity than an adult at any other age. Preexisting problems associated with reaction time, visual acuity, fine motor ability, physical strength, cognitive function, and motivation affect the rehabilitation potential of the older adult.

Second, the older adult often loses functioning because of inactivity and immobility. This deconditioning can occur as a result of unstable acute medical conditions, environmental barriers that limit mobility, and a lack of motivation to stay in condition. The effect of inactivity clearly leads to "use it or lose it" consequences. The older adult can improve flexibility, strength, and aerobic capacity even into very old age. The nurse must use passive and active range-of-motion exercises with all older adults to prevent deconditioning and subsequent functional decline.

Last, the goal of geriatric rehabilitation is to strive for maximal function and physical capabilities considering the individual's current health status. When a patient demonstrates suboptimal health, the nurse screens and evaluates for risk behaviors. For example, a woman with osteoporosis should be given a fall-risk appraisal. The older adult patient with diabetes should receive a geriatric foot assessment and appropriate follow-up care.

Assistive Devices. The use of assistive devices should be considered as an intervention for the older adult. Using appropriate assistive devices such as dentures, glasses, hearing aids, walkers, wheelchairs, adult briefs or protectors, adaptive utensils, elevated toilet seats, and skin protective devices can diminish disability. These tools and devices should be included in the patient's care plan when appropriate. Both the nurse and caregivers are critical to the success of these modifications.

Computer technology will continue to affect the evaluation and care of older adults. Electronic monitoring equipment can be used to monitor heart rhythms and blood pressure, as well as to locate the wandering person in the home or long-term care facility. Computerized assistive devices can be used to help patients with speech difficulties following stroke, and small electronic devices can serve as memory aids.

Safety. Environmental safety is crucial in the health maintenance of the older person. With normal sensory changes, slowed reaction time, decreased thermal and pain sensitivity, changes in gait and balance, and medication effects, the older adult is prone to accidents. Most accidents occur in or around the home. Falls, motor vehicle accidents, and fires are the common causes of accidental death in older adults. Another environmental problem arises from the older person's impaired thermoregulation system that cannot adapt to extremes in environmental temperatures. The body of an older adult can neither conserve nor dissipate heat as efficiently as younger adults. Therefore both hypothermia and heat prostration (hyperthermia) occur more readily. This age group accounts for the majority of deaths during severe cold spells and heat waves.

The nurse can provide valuable counsel regarding environmental changes, which may improve safety for the older adult. Measures such as stronger lighting, colored step strips, tub and toilet grab bars, and stairway handrails can be effective in "safety-proofing" the living quarters of the older adult. The nurse can also advocate for home fire and security alarms. Uncluttered floor space, railings, increased lighting and night-lights, and clearly marked stair edges are some of the easiest and most practical adaptations.

The older adult in an inpatient or long-term care setting needs a thorough orientation to the environment. The nurse should repeatedly reassure the patient that he or she is safe and attempt to answer all questions. The unit should foster patient orientation by displaying large-print clocks, avoiding complex or visually confusing wall designs, clearly designating doors, and using simple bed and nurse-call controls. Lighting should be adequate while avoiding glare. Environments that provide consistent caregivers and an established daily routine assist the older adult patient.

Medication Use. Medication use in the older adult requires thorough and regular assessment and care planning. The use and abuse of medication by the older adult is supported by the following facts:

1. On average, a 70-year-old takes seven different medications.[34,35]
2. Individuals age 85 and over take an average of 12 prescribed drugs.
3. The frequency of adverse drug reactions increases as the number of prescribed drugs increases.
4. Twelve percent of older adult hospital admissions occur because of drug reactions.
5. After discharge from a hospital, even one unnecessary medication may put the older adult at risk for an adverse drug reaction.

Age-related changes alter the pharmacodynamics and pharmacokinetics of drugs. Drug-drug, drug-food, and drug-disease interactions all influence the absorption, distribution, metabolism, and excretion of drugs. Fig. 6-11 illustrates the effects of aging on drug metabolism. The most dramatic changes with aging are related to drug metabolism and clearance. Overall, by age 75 to 80 there is a 50% decline in the renal clearance of drugs. Hepatic blood flow decreases markedly with aging, and the enzymes largely responsible for drug metabolism are decreased as well. Thus the drug half-life is increased in the older as compared with a younger patient.[34,35]

In addition to changes in the metabolism of drugs, the older adult may have difficulty as a result of cognitive decline, altered sensory perceptions, limited hand mobility, and the high cost of many prescriptions. Common reasons for drug errors made by the older adult are listed in Table 6-14. **Polypharmacy** (the use of multiple medications by one patient who has more than one health problem), overdose, and addiction to prescription drugs are recognized as major causes of illness in the older adult.[34,35]

To accurately assess drug use and knowledge, many nurses ask their older adult patients to bring to the health care appointment all medications (over-the-counter, prescription, and herbal remedies) that they take regularly or occasionally. The nurse can then accurately assess all medications that the older adult is taking, including drugs that the patient may have omitted or thought unimportant. Additional nursing interventions to assist the older adult in following a safe medication routine are listed in Table 6-15.

Depression. Approximately 15% of the community-dwelling older population has symptoms of depression. Depression is the most common mood disorder in older adults. Rates of depressive symptoms in institutionalized older adults are high. Depression is associated with being female, being divorced or separated, low socioeconomic status, poor social support, and a recent adverse and unexpected event.[36] Depression in the older adult tends to arise from a loss of self-esteem and may be related to life situations, such as retirement or loss of a spouse. Problems such as hypochondriac complaints, insomnia, lethargy, agitation, decreased memory, and inability to concentrate are common. Depression is an underrecognized problem for many older adults.

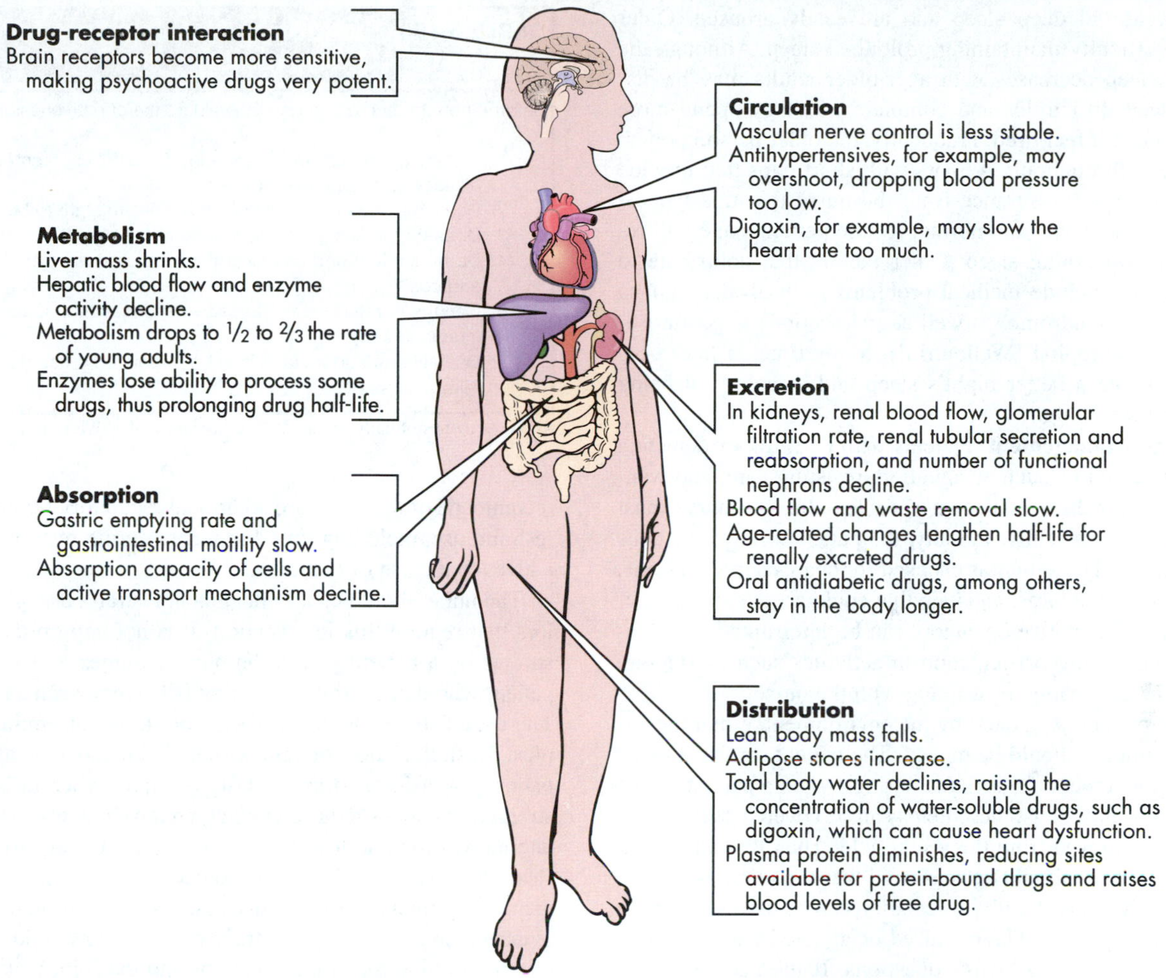

Drug-receptor interaction
Brain receptors become more sensitive, making psychoactive drugs very potent.
Circulation
Vascular nerve control is less stable.
Antihypertensives, for example, may overshoot, dropping blood pressure too low.
Digoxin, for example, may slow the heart rate too much.
Metabolism
Liver mass shrinks.
Hepatic blood flow and enzyme activity decline.
Metabolism drops to 1/2 to 2/3 the rate of young adults.
Enzymes lose ability to process some drugs, thus prolonging drug half-life.
Excretion
In kidneys, renal blood flow, glomerular filtration rate, renal tubular secretion and reabsorption, and number of functional nephrons decline.
Blood flow and waste removal slow.
Age-related changes lengthen half-life for renally excreted drugs.
Oral antidiabetic drugs, among others, stay in the body longer.
Absorption
Gastric emptying rate and gastrointestinal motility slow.
Absorption capacity of cells and active transport mechanism decline.
Distribution
Lean body mass falls.
Adipose stores increase.
Total body water declines, raising the concentration of water-soluble drugs, such as digoxin, which can cause heart dysfunction.
Plasma protein diminishes, reducing sites available for protein-bound drugs and raises blood levels of free drug.

FIG. 6-11 The effects of aging on drug metabolism.

TABLE 6-14 DRUG THERAPY
Common Causes of Medication Errors by Older Adults

- Poor eyesight
- Forgetting to take drugs
- Use of nonprescription over-the-counter drugs
- Use of medications prescribed for someone else
- Lack of financial resources to obtain prescribed medication
- Failure to understand instructions or the importance of drug treatment
- Refusal to take medication because of undesirable side effects such as nausea and impotence

TABLE 6-15 DRUG THERAPY
Medication Use by Older Adults

1. Emphasize medications that are essential.
2. Attempt to reduce medication use that is not essential for minor symptoms.
3. Screen medication use using a standard assessment tool, including over-the-counter drugs, eyedrops and eardrops, antihistamines, and cough syrups.
4. Assess alcohol use.
5. Encourage the use of written or medication-reminder systems.
6. Monitor drug dosage strength; normally the strength should be less than that of a younger person.
7. Encourage the use of one pharmacy.
8. Work with health care providers and pharmacists to establish routine drug profiles on all older adult patients.
9. Advocate (with drug companies) for low-income prescription support services.

Late-life depression often occurs together with medical illness such as heart disease, stroke, diabetes, and cancer.[36] Depression can exacerbate medical conditions by affecting compliance with diet, exercise, or drug regimens. It is important that assessment include physical examination and laboratory testing for physical disorders that may have symptoms similar to depression (thyroid disorders, vitamin deficiencies).

The older adult who exhibits depressive symptoms should be encouraged to seek treatment. Because a patient with depression may feel unworthy, withdraw, and become isolated, the nurse may need the support of the family to assist in helping the older adult seek treatment. The depressed older adult who is involved in caregiving should seek respite and reevaluate the caregiving role.

Of all suicides, older adults commit 18% in the United States and 12.6% in Canada.[37,38] In the United States, elderly men have the highest rate of suicide.

Sleep. Adequacy of sleep is often a concern of the older adult because of altered sleep patterns. Older people experience a marked decrease in deep sleep and are easily aroused. Older adults have difficulty maintaining prolonged sleep. Although the demand for sleep decreases with age, older adults may be disturbed by sleep difficulties and complain that they spend more time in bed but still feel tired. Frequently, the older person prefers to spread sleep throughout 24 hours with short naps that provide adequate rest. Often, assurance from the nurse that this type of sleep pattern is adequate and normal for the patient's age will reduce anxiety concerning sleep. Other factors that contribute to sleep difficulties include medical problems such as sleep apnea and restless legs syndrome, as well as medications (e.g., furosemide [Lasix], bupropion [Wellbutrin]). Many times a later bedtime will promote a better night's sleep and a feeling of being refreshed on awakening.

Behavioral Management. Patients with delirium or dementia may display behaviors such as agitation, resisting care, and wandering. As these behaviors become problematic, the nurse must plan interventions carefully. Initially, the patient's physical status must be assessed. The patient is checked for changes in vital signs, urinary and bowel patterns, and pain that could account for behavioral problems. Disruptive behaviors can be interrupted and redirected by encouraging participation in activities such as singing, playing music, exercising, or walking with the nurse.

When the patient is agitated by the environment, either the patient or the stimulus should be moved. The patient can be assisted to call family members if this is reassuring. When a patient resists or pulls tubes or dressings, these items can be covered with stretch tube gauze or removed from the visual field. The older adult with behavioral problems should be reassured that the nurse is present to keep him or her safe. Reality orientation can be used to orient to time, place, and person. The confused or agitated patient should not be asked challenging "why" questions. If the patient cannot verbalize distress or the confusional state is irreversible (e.g., Alzheimer's disease), his or her mood should be validated. The patient's emotional state should be closely observed. The patient's statement can be rephrased to validate its meaning.

When dealing with the difficult patient, the nurse's frustration should be acknowledged. The nurse should not threaten to restrain the patient or threaten to call the physician. A calming family member can be requested to stay with the patient until the person becomes calmer. The patient should be monitored frequently, and all interventions should be documented. The use of positive nurse actions can reduce the use of physical and chemical (drug therapy) restraints.

Use of Restraints. Physical restraints are devices, materials, and equipment that physically prevent the individual from moving freely (by choice) in the environment.[5] This includes preventing the person from walking, standing, lying, transferring, or sitting. Common devices include seat belts, "geri-chairs," and jacket vests. The individual who is being physically restrained cannot remove the device. The Omnibus Budget Reconciliation Act (OBRA) of 1987 stated that restraints could be used only to ensure the person's safety or the safety of others. Furthermore, there must be a written order from a physician for physical restraints to be applied to long-term care patients. Since the passing of this Act, there has been a marked reduction in the use of physical restraints in long-term care facilities. Chemical and physical restraints should be a last resort in the care of the older patient. If a physical restraint device is to be used in the hospital or long-term care setting, it requires a physician or an independent licensed nurse practitioner to make the recommendation. There are additional regulatory requirements for restraint use, including time limit, care during restraint, and alternatives to the use of restraints.

TABLE 6-16 Evaluating Nursing Care for Older Adults

Information the nurse can use to evaluate the effectiveness of patient care:

1. Is there an identifiable change in ADLs, IADLs, mental status, or disease signs and symptoms?
2. Does the patient consider his or her health state to be improved?
3. Does the patient think the treatment is helpful?
4. Do the patient and caregiver think the care is worth the time and cost?
5. Can the nurse document positive changes that support interventions?
6. Does change adequately meet the required mandates for reimbursement?

ADLs, Activities of daily living; *IADLs,* instrumental activities of daily living.

The nurse should clearly document restraint use and the behaviors that require this intervention. It is not appropriate to use restraints on a patient whom the nurse assumes will fall or on the patient who demonstrates irritating behaviors, such as calling out. The use of restraints makes care more time consuming and complex. Restraints do not reduce falls,[39] but do increase potential patient confusion and the severity of injury when falls occur. Restraint alternatives require vigilant, creative nursing care. Restraint alternatives include low beds, body props, and electronic devices (bed alarm signaling). The nurse can avoid chemical restraint by using early interventions as discussed in the section on behavioral management. The use of restraints must follow rigid and explicit criteria. Long-term care regulations and the Joint Commission on Accreditation of Healthcare Organizations set standards for restraint usage. The movement to "restraint-free" environments is supporting a decline in the use of restraints.

Evaluation

The evaluation phase of the nursing process is similar for all patients. Evaluation is ongoing throughout the nursing process. The results of evaluation direct the nurse to continue the plan of care or revise as indicated. Often the change in health status is not as dramatic in the older adult as it is in the younger patient. Because of this, the nurse needs to be cautious in changing plans prematurely.

When evaluating nursing care with the older adult, the nurse should focus on functional improvement rather than cure. Useful questions to consider when evaluating the plan of care for an older adult are included in Table 6-16.

NCLEX EXAMINATION REVIEW QUESTIONS

The number of the question corresponds to the same-numbered objective at the beginning of the chapter.

1. Ageism is characterized by
   a. denial of negative stereotypes regarding aging.
   b. positive attitudes toward the elderly based on age.
   c. negative attitudes toward the elderly based on age.
   d. negative attitudes toward the elderly based on physical disability.

2. Autoimmune diseases increase with aging. This is consistent with which of the following theories of aging?
   a. immune theory of aging
   b. programmed theory of aging
   c. neuroendocrine theory of aging
   d. intrinsic mutation theory of aging
3. An ethnic older adult may experience a loss of self-worth when the nurse
   a. informs the patient about ethnic support services.
   b. allows a patient to rely on ethnic health beliefs and practices.
   c. has to use an interpreter to provide explanations and teaching.
   d. emphasizes that a therapeutic diet does not allow ethnic foods.
4. An important nursing action helpful to a chronically ill older adult is to
   a. avoid discussing future lifestyle changes.
   b. assure the patient that the condition is stable.
   c. treat the patient as a competent manager of the disease.
   d. encourage the patient to "fight" the disease as long as possible.
5. When older adults become ill they are more likely than younger adults to
   a. complain about the symptoms of their problems.
   b. refuse to carry out lifestyle changes to promote recovery.
   c. seek medical attention because of limitations on their lifestyle.
   d. alter their daily living activities to accommodate new symptoms.
6. An important fact for the nurse to know about caregivers is that they
   a. may need nurses to assist them in reducing caregiver strain.
   b. are usually trained health care workers who do not live with the patient.
   c. are generally strong and healthy but need teaching to carry out care activities.
   d. are often reluctant to share the burden of caregiving with other family members.
7. An appropriate care choice for an older adult living with an employed daughter but who requires assistance with activities of daily living is
   a. adult day care.
   b. long-term care.
   c. a retirement center.
   d. an assisted-living home.
8. A natural death act is an advance directive that
   a. is legally binding.
   b. encourages the use of artificial means to prolong life.
   c. allows a person to direct his or her health care in the event of terminal illness.
   d. designates who can act for the patient when the patient is unable to do so personally.
9. Nursing interventions directed at health promotion in the older adult are primarily focused on
   a. disease management.
   b. controlling symptoms of illness.
   c. teaching positive health behaviors.
   d. teaching regarding nutrition to enhance longevity.

REFERENCES

1. Administration on Aging: A profile of older Americans: 2003. Available at *www.aoa.gov/prof/Statistics/profile/2003/profiles2003.asp* (accessed June 14, 2005).
2. Projections of the total resident population by 5 year age groups, race, and Hispanic origin with special age categories: middle series, 1999 to 2000. US Census Internet update, March 2004. Available at *www.census.gov/main/www/cen2000.html* (accessed April 27, 2006).
3. Stotts N, Deitrich C: The challenge to come: the care of older adults, *Am J Nurs* 104:40, 2004.
4. Life expectancy and death statistics in Canada. Available at *http://canadaonline.about.com/od/statistics/a/lifedeathstats.htm* (accessed June 14, 2005).
5. Ebersole P, Hess P: *Geriatric nursing and healthy aging,* ed 2, St Louis, 2005, Mosby.
6. Turvey CL et al: Attitudes about impairment and depression in elders suffering from chronic heart failure, *Int J Psychiatry Med* 33:117, 2003.
7. Harper ME et al: Ageing, oxidative stress, and mitochondrial uncoupling, *Acta Physiol Scand* 182:321, 2004.
8. Hughes KA, Reynolds RM: Evolutionary and mechanistic theories of aging, *Annu Rev Entomol* 50:421, 2005.
9. Robine JM, Michel JP: Looking forward to a general theory on population aging, *J Gerontol A Biol Sci Med Sci* 59:M590, 2004.
10. Mayne ST: Antioxidant nutrients and chronic disease: Use of biomarkers of exposure and oxidative stress status in epidemiologic research, *J Nutr* 133:933S, 2003.
11. Shay JW, Wright WE: Senescence and immortalization: role of telomeres and telomerase, *Carcinogenesis* 26:867, 2005.
12. Lue NF: Adding to the ends: what makes telomerase processive and how important is it? *Bioessays* 26:955, 2004.
13. Fabris N: Neuroendocrine-immune interactions: a theoretical approach to aging, *Arch Gerontol Geriatr* 12:219, 1991.
14. Bjornerem A et al: Endogenous sex hormones in relation to age, sex, lifestyle factors, and chronic diseases in a general population: the Tromso Study, *J Clin Endocrinol Metab* 89:6039, 2004.
15. Traustadottir T, Bosch PR, Matt KS: The HPA axis response to stress in women: effects of aging and fitness, *Psychoneuroendocrinology* 30:392, 2005.
16. Boren E, Gershwin ME: Inflammation-aging: autoimmunity, and the immune-risk phenotype, *Autoimmun Rev* 3:401, 2004.
17. Fleming KC: A history of old age in America. In Legato M, editor: *Principles of gender-specific medicine,* San Diego, 2004, Elsevier Academic Press.
18. Roberts B: Gender-specific aspects of the experience of coronary artery disease. In Legato M, editor: *Principles of gender-specific medicine,* San Diego, 2004, Elsevier Academic Press.
19. Wilcox S et al: Psychosocial and perceived environmental correlates of physical activity in rural and older African American and white women, *J Gerontol B Psychol Sci Soc Sci* 58:P329, 2003.
20. Borders TF: Rural community-dwelling elders' reports of access to care: are there Hispanic versus non-Hispanic white disparities? *J Rural Health* 20:210, 2004.
21. Stromberg A: The crucial role of patient education in heart failure, *Eur J Heart Fail* 16:363, 2005.
22. Stergiopoulos V, Herrmann N: Old and homeless: a review and survey of older adults who use shelters in an urban setting, *Can J Psychiatry* 48:374, 2003.
23. AACN, John A Hartford Foundation Institute for Geriatric Nursing: Older adults: recommended baccalaureate competencies and curricular guidelines for geriatric nursing care. Available at *www.aacn.nche.edu/Education/gercomp.htm* (accessed June 15, 2005).

*24. Given B et al: Burden and depression among caregivers of patients with cancer at the end of life, *Oncol Nurs Forum* 16:1105, 2004.

25. Pinquart M, Sorensen S: Associations of caregiver stressors and uplifts with subjective well-being and depressive mood: a meta-analytic comparison, *Aging Ment Health* 8:438, 2004.
26. National Academies of Sciences, Bonnie R, Wallace R, editors: *Elder abuse: abuse, neglect and exploitation in an aging American,* Washington, DC, 2002, National Academies Press.
27. Lachs MS, Pillemer K: Elder abuse, *Lancet* 364 (9441):1263, 2004.
28. Fulmer T, Peveza G: Neglect in the elderly patient, *Nurs Clin North Am* 33:457, 1998.
29. Hawes C, editor: *Elder abuse in residential long-term care settings: what is known and what information is needed?* Washington, DC, 2003, National Academies Press.
30. Dyer CB et al: The high prevalence of depression and dementia in elder abuse or neglect, *J Am Geriatr Soc* 48:205, 2000.
31. Fulmer T: Elder abuse and neglect assessment, *J Gerontol Nurs* 29:4, 2003.
32. Centers for Medicare and Medicaid Services: Medicare and you: 2006. Available at *www.medicare.gov/publications/pubs/pdf/10050.pdf* (accessed April 27, 2006).
33. Hodgson N et al: Biobehavioral correlates of relocation in the frail elderly: salivary cortisol, affect, and cognitive function, *J Am Geriatr Soc* 52:1856, 2004.

*Nursing research–based reference.

34. Hajjar ER et al: Adverse drug reaction risk factors in older outpatients, *Am J Geriatr Pharmacother* 2:82, 2003.
35. Klarin I, Wimo A, Fastbom J: The association of inappropriate drug use with hospitalisation and mortality: a population-based study of the very old, *Drugs Aging* 22:69, 2005.
36. Edwards M: Assessing for depression and mood disturbance in later life, *Br J Community Nurs* 9:492, 2004.
37. Juurlink DN et al: Medical illness and the risk of suicide in the elderly, *Arch Intern Med* 164:1179, 2004.
38. Bruce ML et al: Reducing suicidal ideation and depressive symptoms in depressed older primary care patients: a randomized controlled trial, *JAMA* 291:1081, 2004.
39. Hamers JP, Gulpers MJ, Strik W: Use of physical restraints with cognitively impaired nursing home residents, *J Adv Nurs* 45:246, 2004.

RESOURCES

Administration on Aging
800-677-1116 (Eldercare Locator—to find services for an older person in his or her locality)
202-619-0724 (AoA National Aging Information Center for technical information and public inquiries)
202-401-4634 (Office of the Assistant Secretary for Aging)
www.aoa.dhhs.gov

Alliance for Retired Americans
202-974-8222
www.*retiredamericans.org*

American Association of Homes and Services for the Aging
202-738-2242
www.aahsa.org

American Association for International Aging
202-293-2856
www.unm.edu/~aging/AAIAwelc.html

American Association of Retired Persons (AARP)
888-687-2277
www.aarp.org

American Geriatrics Society
212-308-1414
www.americangeriatrics.org

American Society on Aging
415-974-9600
Email: info@asaging.org
www.asaging.org

Canadian Association on Gerontology
613-271-1083
Email: cagacg@igs.net
www.cagacg.ca

Centers for Medicare and Medicaid Services
410-786-3000
www.cms.hhs.gov

ElderWeb
309-451-3319
www.elderweb.com

Gerontological Society of America
202-842-1275
www.geron.org

Geroweb
Institute of Gerontology
Wayne State University
313-577-2297
www.iog.wayne.edu/IOGlinks.html

Health Promotion Institute
National Council on the Aging
www.ncoa.org

International Federation on Aging
514-396-3358

International Senior Citizens Association, Inc.
213-625-5008

Meals on Wheels America
703-548-5558
www.mowaa.org

National Advisory Council on Aging (NACA)
613-957-1968
Email: info@naca-ccnta.ca
www.naca.ca

National Association of Area Agencies on Aging
202-872-0888
www.n4a.org

National Association for Hispanic Elderly
Asociacion Nacional por Personas Mayores
626-564-1988
www.anppm.org

National Caucus and Center on Black Aged
202-637-8400
www.ncba-aged.org

National Center on Elder Abuse
202-898-2586
Email: ncea@nasua.org.
www.elderabusecenter.org/default.cfm

National Council on the Aging, Inc.
202-479-1200
www.ncoa.org

National Gerontological Nursing Association
850-473-1174
800-723-0560
Email: ngna@puetzamc.com
www.ngna.org

National Hispanic Council on Aging
202-429-0787
www.nhcoa.org

National Indian Council on Aging
505-292-2001
www.nicoa.org

National Institute on Aging
301-496-1752
www.nia.nih.gov

Older Women's League (OWL)
202-783-6686
800-825-3695
www.owl-national.org

For additional Internet resources, see the website for this book at *http://evolve.elsevier.com/Lewis/medsurg.*

I am an old man and have known a great many troubles, but most of them never happened.

Mark Twain

Community-Based Nursing and Home Care 7

Teri A. Murray

LEARNING OBJECTIVES

1. Describe how the factors changing the health care delivery system are influencing the shift of patient care from hospitals to community-based settings.
2. Differentiate community-based nursing from community-oriented population-focused nursing.
3. Compare community-based patient care settings and the services provided in these settings.
4. Describe the roles and challenges of nurses working in community-based settings.

KEY TERMS

Electronic Resources

Supplemental content related to Chapter 7 can be found . . .

Companion CD

- Stress-Busting Kit for Nursing Students
- NCLEX Examination Review Questions
- Comprehensive Glossary

Evolve Website

http://evolve.elsevier.com/Lewis/medsurg

- Content Updates
- Key Points (Printable and CD/MP3 Download)
- Concept Map Creator
- Expanded Audio Glossary
- Key Term Flash Cards
- Electronic Calculators
- WebLinks

Major changes in nursing practice and patient care are occurring as a result of numerous factors affecting the health care system. Social, economic, technologic, and health factors are driving the delivery of health care from hospitals to community-based settings. In response to these factors, the practice of professional nursing has moved from an almost exclusively hospital-based practice to practice opportunities in community health settings. Nurses are providing patient care in a wide variety of health care settings outside of the hospital. A national survey of nurses found that in 1980 approximately 66% of employed registered nurses (RNs) worked in hospitals. By 2000 the proportion had declined to 59%. Between 1980 and 2000 the number of nurses employed in public health and community settings increased by 155% and those employed in ambulatory care settings increased by 127%.[1]

Nursing practice that occurs in the community has taken on a variety of meanings, creating confusion among terms such as *community-based nursing, community-oriented nursing, public health nursing,* and *population-focused practice*.[2] Community-based nursing practice is different from community-oriented, population-focused nursing. The focus of **community-based nursing** is illness-oriented care of individuals and families throughout the life span. Its goal is to help individuals and families manage acute or chronic health conditions in community and home settings as opposed to hospital settings. **Community-oriented, population-focused nursing** practice involves the engagement of nursing in promoting and protecting the health of populations. It is focused on the whole and reaches out to help not only those seeking care, but also those not seeking care. Population-focused practice (1) examines the health needs of specific groups or aggregates within the population; (2) seeks to identify patterns or trends related to the health needs of the particular group; and (3) identifies, implements, and evaluates strategies aimed at improving the health of the group as a whole. *Public health nursing* is a specialty practice of community-oriented, population-focused practice that involves assessment of the health

Reviewed by Paula Scharf Kohn, RN, PhD, Associate Professor, Pace University, Pleasantville, N.J.

conditions, risks, and resources of various groups within the population, especially those deemed high risk.[2]

This chapter presents an overview of the changing health care system and discusses nursing care in community-based settings rather than community-oriented, population-focused practice. Although long-term care and rehabilitation facilities are not typically considered community-based settings, they are included in this chapter.

CHANGING HEALTH CARE SYSTEM

Factors Influencing Change

Socioeconomic Considerations. The changes in health care have been largely initiated by the continued efforts of the government, employers, insurance companies, and regulating agencies to provide health care in the most cost-effective manner. Historically, the most notable event related to changing reimbursement patterns was the institution of prospective payment systems and the use of Diagnosis Related Groups (DRGs) in the Medicare program. With these changes, hospitals were no longer reimbursed for all costs. Instead, payment for hospital services to Medicare patients was based on flat fees per admission based on DRGs. In many instances the implementation of DRGs has shifted patient care from acute care settings to community and home settings. The prospective payment system has been and continues to be one of the most significant factors affecting health care. These policies and recent advances in technology allow nurses to care for increasingly complex patients in community and home settings.

Private and other public health care systems eventually followed the prospective payment system established by the Medicare program. **Health maintenance organizations (HMOs)*** and **preferred provider organizations (PPOs)**† evolved as a means of offering cost-effective health care delivery.[3] In these managed care systems, charges are negotiated in advance of the delivery of care using predetermined reimbursement rates or capitation fees for medical care, hospitalization, and other health care services. Like the Medicare program, these organizations have caused a shift in the delivery of care from the acute care hospital setting to less expensive community settings.

Changing Demographics. Twelve percent of the total U.S. population (36 million people) are over age 65.Within the twentieth century, the population age 65 and older grew from 3 million to 35 million people.[4] By 2050, the U.S. Census Bureau projects that the population age 65 or over will be between 80 and 90 million people. The growth of the population age 65 and over affects all aspects of society and particularly challenges health care providers to meet the needs of an aging society. Aging Americans may have disabilities that compromise their ability to remain functional in their own homes without supportive community or professional help. The elderly may also have complex medical and health care needs, experiencing multiple chronic conditions that compromise their ability to remain independent. Physical and functional problems, dementia, fixed incomes, and limited family or community support put the elderly at an increased need for social and health care assistance. (Health care needs of the older adult are discussed further in Chapter 6.)

Immigrants, particularly nondocumented immigrants and refugees, often lack the resources necessary to access health care. Inability to pay for health care is associated with a tendency to delay seeking care, resulting in more serious illnesses. The need to identify and meet health care needs of this population requires reaching into the community where these individuals live and work. (Cultural factors affecting health care are discussed further in Chapter 3.)

Nature and Prevalence of Illness. The increased life expectancy of the population and lifestyle factors contribute to increases in the number, severity, and duration of chronic conditions. Chronic diseases are responsible for 70% of deaths in the United States. The four leading causes of death from chronic diseases, including cardiovascular disease, cancer, diabetes, and chronic obstructive pulmonary diseases, are related to lifestyle behaviors.[5] Tobacco use, lack of physical activity, and poor nutrition (including obesity) are the major contributors to cardiovascular disease and cancer.[5] The focus of health care is now shifting from intervention in the acute phase of diseases toward health promotion and disease prevention. Nursing practice directed toward the prevention and management of chronic illness occurs in community-based settings through (1) promotion of regular screening, (2) education about the effects of lifestyle choices and their relationship to health and illness, and (3) assisting individuals and families to manage chronic illness in the home.

Technology. Surgical innovations, such as advances in cardiac surgery, and medical interventions, such as new drugs for cancer treatment, have allowed individuals to live longer, shifting both acute and long-term care to community-based settings. New technology has improved diagnostic procedures and management of patient care. Computers, lifesaving drugs, and telehealth interventions have simplified diagnosis and treatment and shortened hospital stays.

Patient care has moved to outpatient settings such as surgical centers, providing services that have been traditionally delivered only in hospitals. Complex patient care treatments, such as intravenous (IV) antibiotic therapy and total parenteral therapy, are increasingly being delivered through home infusion services. Evolving technology, the focus on reducing rapidly increasing health care costs, and patient preference to be at home have stimulated the movement to provide health care in the community and home settings.

Increasing Consumerism. Health care is becoming a more consumer-focused business. Patients are becoming more interested and active participants in their health care. Many patients eagerly seek out information about their health from the media and Internet sources. They also expect that information will be provided so that they may collaborate with health care providers in making the appropriate decisions about their health care. In addition, the public has come to view health care as an entitlement or a human right. Health care legislation emphasizes equal access to health care services, regardless of the ability to pay. As increasing demands are made on scarce and costly health care resources, nurses are becoming more active partners with patients in promoting self-care through education and advocacy.

*An HMO consists of an association of health care professionals and facilities that provide a specified package of health care for a fixed sum of money paid in advance for a specified period of time. The HMO contracts with health care professionals and facilities to provide the specified care. Generally a patient cannot seek care outside of the health care providers and/or hospitals under contract with the HMO.

†A PPO is a group of health care professionals and/or hospitals who contract with an employer, insurance company, or third-party payer to provide medical care to a specified group of potential patients. The services offered are not prepaid or fixed. There is typically more choice in a PPO than in an HMO, and thus it is more costly.

Case Management

Case management is a collaborative process that involves assessing, planning, facilitating, and advocating for health services to meet an individual's or family's needs through communication and use of available resources to promote cost-effective quality outcomes.[6] Although health care agencies or organizations may define and practice case management in various ways, the concept of case management involves managing the patient's care across multiple settings and levels of care.[2] The goals of case management are to provide quality care along a continuum, decrease fragmentation of care across many settings, enhance the patient's quality of life, and contain costs.

The case manager often assesses the needs of an individual or family, coordinates services for them, makes referrals as appropriate, and evaluates progress to ensure that short- and long-term goals are met in a cost-effective manner.[7] For example, a patient with severe coronary artery disease may be assigned a nurse as a case manager in an outpatient clinic. When the patient is hospitalized for coronary bypass surgery, the same case manager coordinates care so that all health care providers understand the patient's unique needs. When the patient is discharged, the case manager determines whether home health care or other services are necessary for the patient.

The goal of case management is to deliver cost-effective services for individuals while achieving wellness and autonomy through advocacy, communication, education, identification of service resources, and service facilitation.[8]

COMMUNITY-BASED CARE

Continuum of Patient Care

Depending on an individual's health status and the cost of care required, patients can move among different health care settings. There is a continuum of care whereby different settings accommodate the varying needs of the patient. Within this continuum, many persons today are cared for in community-based settings that include home health care. For example, a person may be hospitalized in a trauma unit following a motor vehicle accident. After the person is stabilized, he or she may be transferred to a general medical-surgical unit and then to an acute rehabilitation facility. After a period of rehabilitation, the person may be discharged to his or her home to continue with outpatient rehabilitation and to be followed by home health care nurses and/or cared for in an outpatient clinic.

The continuum of care does not always include hospitalization. Most patients receive community-based care without experiencing an acute problem requiring hospitalization. Health problems may be identified in a variety of outpatient settings. In addition, individuals or families may seek specific assistance from health care resources in the community.

For example, a patient may be screened for diabetes mellitus in a community-based screening program and, when indicated, referred to a clinic where a diagnosis of diabetes can be established. A diabetes clinical nurse specialist may function as a case manager to coordinate the diabetes management team consisting of diabetic educators, nurses, dietitians, pharmacists, physicians, and other health care professionals. Services may include care and education at a variety of settings, as well as follow-up by home health care nurses.

Patients can be treated in a multitude of settings, opting for the one most appropriate for their health care needs but within the constraints of health care insurance plans and the cost of care. Today health care is increasingly constrained by third-party payer cost containment efforts. At the same time third-party payers are demanding outcome-based quality care. Although the hospital remains the mainstay for acute care interventions, settings such as extended care facilities, assisted living centers, and home health care offer patients the opportunity to live or recover in settings that maximize their independence and preserve human dignity.

Community-Based Nurses

Nurses practicing in community-based settings care for acutely or chronically ill individuals where they reside, work, or go to school.[8] Nursing roles include home health care nurses, school nurses, occupational nurses, and nurses working in outpatient clinics and ambulatory care centers. Nurses in nurse-managed clinics provide direct care to patients in an ambulatory setting. Parish, or congregational, nurses practice holistic health care within a faith community, em-

TABLE 7-1 Characteristics of Ambulatory Care Settings

- Provide health care services on an outpatient basis.
- Include physician and nurse practitioner offices, clinics, outpatient surgical or diagnostic centers, churches, schools, day care centers, and occupational or work sites.
- Nurses in ambulatory care settings assess patients' problems, evaluate need for resources and information, and provide appropriate interventions that allow patients to care for themselves.
- Patient teaching and telephone follow-up are routine practices.

TABLE 7-2 Practice Settings for Transitional Care

Setting	Characteristics
Subacute care	• Postacute care designed for patients who need a greater intensity of care than generally provided in a skilled nursing facility but no longer require acute care. • Typical patients requiring subacute care are chronically ill, ventilator dependent, or those needing specialized monitoring, equipment, and nursing care.
Acute rehabilitation	• Postacute level of care specializing in therapies for patients with neurologic or physical injuries, such as those with head trauma, spinal cord injury, or stroke. • May be in separate units of a hospital or in freestanding facilities in the community. • Patient may receive several hours of exercise and other rehabilitative training or therapy daily. • Patients learn to use assistive devices and need time and encouragement to perform activities of daily living and other aspects of self-care. • Patients may need weeks to months of rehabilitative care before they can return home.
Long-term acute care	• Settings are distinct units of a hospital or may be a separate facility designed to care for patients who require acute care that may extend to 30 days. • Individuals may be ventilator dependent or require extensive and complicated dressing changes or combinations of multiple medical and nursing interventions. • Discharge planning is focused on discharge to home or long-term care settings.

TABLE 7-3 Practice Settings for Long-Term Care

Setting	Characteristics
Skilled nursing facilities	• Provide care for patients who require 24-hr nursing supervision, many of whom are confined to bed for some portion of the day or are incontinent (Fig. 7-1). • Offer treatment under the supervision of licensed practical nurses and at least one RN who must be on duty during the day. • Licensed by state licensing authorities. • Medicare pays for a small portion of care.
Long-term home health care programs (LTHHCP)	• Coordinated plans of medical, nursing, and rehabilitative care provided at home to disabled persons who would otherwise be placed in a skilled nursing facility. • Programs offer patients an alternative to institutionalization. • Services may include all those available in an institution, but care costs are less than those of a skilled nursing facility.
Intermediate care facilities	• Provide convalescent care and regular medical, nursing, social, and rehabilitative services in addition to room and board for people not capable of independent living (Fig. 7-2). • Offer a mix of medical care, nursing and rehabilitative care, and personal and residential care services. • *Special care units* in these facilities have been developed for individuals with cognitive impairments (e.g., Alzheimer's disease) who may require special assistance. • Although these units are appropriate for patients with early- to middle-stage dementia, they may not be appropriate for those in advanced stages of dementia.
Continuing care retirement community (CCRC)	• Blend of several options, including housing complex, activity center, and health care system. • CCRCs differ from other retirement options by providing a continuum of housing, services, and health care. • Written agreement or contract between the resident and the CCRC that is generally intended to last the resident's lifetime or for a specific period of time.
Residential care facilities	• Supervisory care homes or assisted living arrangements. • Both settings are generally licensed by the state to ensure that quality living, safety, and health care standards are met. • Residents generally must be able to care for themselves and move about without the help of another person. • Residents often live in care homes to obtain additional assistance for their ADLs, such as grooming and meal preparation, or supervision with their medications. • Many of these facilities also have a skilled nursing facility. • Enables residents who temporarily need skilled nursing care to receive it until they can return to their own residence.

ADLs, Activities of daily living.

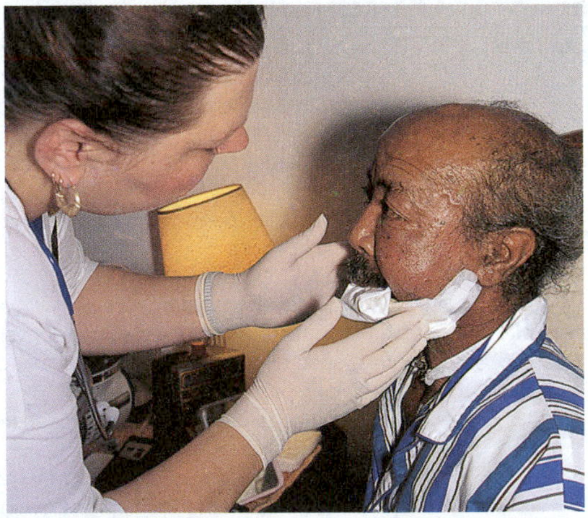

FIG. 7-1 Nurse providing care in a skilled nursing care facility.

phasizing the relationship between spiritual faith and health. Parish nurses complement the work of other health care workers, acting as a liaison with congregational and community resources.[9]

Community-based settings where nursing care is provided include **ambulatory care** (Table 7-1), transitional care, and long-term care. **Transitional care** refers to intermediary care between the acute care setting and the home. Various practice settings for this type of care are described in Table 7-2. **Long-term care** refers to the care of patients for a time period greater than 30 days. It may be required for individuals who are severely developmentally disabled, are mentally impaired, or have physical deficits requiring continuous medical or nursing management, such as those who are ventilator dependent or those with Alzheimer's disease. Long-term care facilities include **skilled nursing facilities, intermediate care facilities,** retirement communities, and **residential care facilities** (Table 7-3).

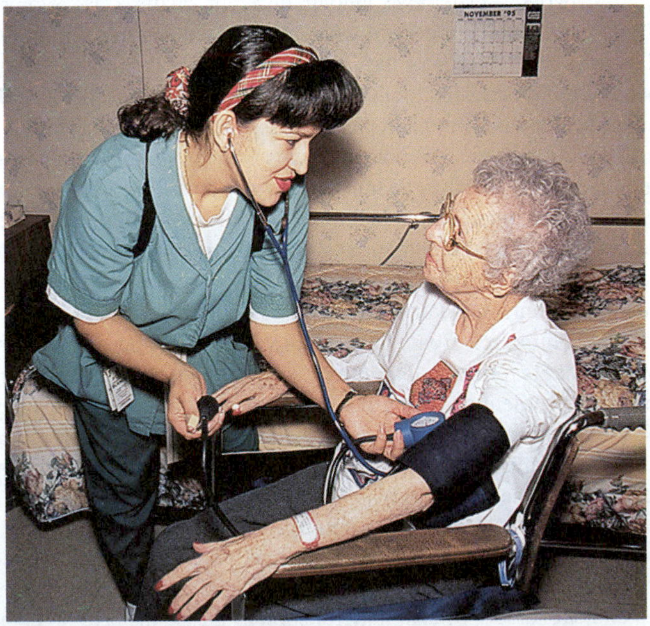

FIG. 7-2 Nurse taking blood pressure for patient in an intermediate care facility.

As noted at the beginning of the chapter, some of these settings are not typically considered community-based settings. However, they do include areas where nurses practice outside of the hospital and constitute many of the less expensive community settings used in managed care.

TABLE 7-4 Funding Mechanisms for Home Health Care

1. Title programs under the Social Security Act of 1965
   - Medicare or Title XVIII
   - Medicaid or Title XIX
2. Title program under the Social Services Amendment of the Social Security Act of 1975
   - Title XX for homemaking and chore service for low-income persons
3. Older Americans Act of 1965
   - Title III, governed by the Area Agencies on Aging, for homemaker services, home health aide, nutrition, home-delivered meals, legal services
   - Title IV, research and demonstration projects for frail elderly who are at risk for institutionalization
4. Title V provides maternal, child health, and crippled children services
5. Private or commercial insurance
6. Managed care arrangements, such as through preferred provider organizations (PPOs) or health maintenance organizations (HMOs)
7. Veterans benefits through the Veterans Administration
8. Private payment or out-of-pocket payment
9. No-fault insurance
10. Charity organizations and foundations, such as the United Way

HOME HEALTH CARE

Home health care refers to health care delivered in the home setting. The National Association for Home Care (NAHC) defines *home care* as the broad spectrum of health care and social services provided in the home environment to recovering, disabled, or chronically ill patients.[10] Home health care may include health maintenance, education, illness prevention, diagnosis and treatment of disease, palliative care, and rehabilitation. Care may be delivered in assisted living situations when no other skilled nursing professionals are available for patient care needs. Patients receiving home health care may require intermittent services or full-time, 24-hours-a-day assistance.

In the past decade there has been an explosive growth in home health care services, coupled with a steady decline in hospital bed occupancy and length of hospital stay. The growth in home health care has been stimulated by DRGs, the increase in managed care, and the patient's preference to be cared for at home. Home health care is one of the most rapidly growing segments in health care today, with the primary motivation being to shift health care to less costly services.[3] However, the Balanced Budget Act of 1997 (P.L. 105-33) affecting Medicare reimbursement for home health care has created a financial crisis in many home health care agencies. This is a direct result of several factors, including a reduction in the reimbursement for visits, the implementation of mandated monitoring and outcomes documentation, and limitations on what was considered as reimbursable skilled nursing. In 2000 prospective payment for Medicare home health care patients was instituted, and in 2001 further reductions in Medicare reimbursements were made.[12] This restrictive legislation has resulted in serious consequences for home health care agencies and their ability to provide patient care in the home. Home health agencies may be licensed by state licensing bureaus and certified to receive reimbursement for care to Medicare beneficiaries.[11] Forms of insurance coverage for payment of home health care can be found in Table 7-4.

Nurses and home health aides provide most home health care services. Registered nurses are the coordinators of patient care, being accountable both for the supervision of personal care services by home health aides and for case management services, including all aspects of care in the home. Other services commonly provided by home health agencies include physical therapy, occupational therapy, and social worker services.

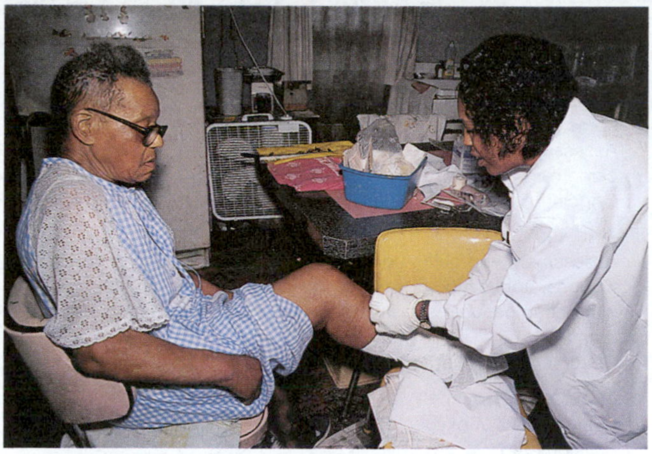

FIG. 7-3 Nurse providing wound care in the home.

Patient Care in the Home

Frequently seen diagnoses for home care patients are diabetes mellitus, hypertension, heart failure, osteoarthritis, stroke, acute and chronic wounds, chronic obstructive pulmonary disease, heart disease, and cancer. Skilled nursing care may include observation, assessment, management, evaluation, teaching, training, administration of medications, wound care (Fig. 7-3), tube feedings, catheter care, and behavioral health interventions (Table 7-5). Commonly performed treatments in the home include administration of infusion therapy (e.g., antibiotic administration), patient-controlled analgesia for pain control, enteral feedings, parenteral nutrition, chemotherapy, and hydration therapy. The nurse and a rehabilitation team member may also provide medical equipment in the home to facilitate medical treatment and safety. These may include electrical beds, wheelchairs, commodes, walkers, and other assistive devices.

Patients have benefited from sophisticated technology in the home care setting. The miniaturization of infusion pumps makes it possible for patients to go to work while receiving antibiotics, parenteral nutrition, or chemotherapy. The use of central venous catheter devices and peripherally inserted central catheters has eliminated many problems associated with short-term and less reliable IV therapy. Tabletop ventilators allow patients who are dependent on mechanical ventilation to be cared for in the home setting, allowing for even greater mobility when the equipment is strapped to the back of a wheelchair. Oxygen delivery in a variety of forms is also frequently provided in the home (see Chapter 29).

Concerns of patients requiring home health care are presented in Table 7-6. Examples of nursing diagnoses for patients requiring home health care are presented in Table 7-7.

Although the patient is the focus of care and visit reimbursement is based on what is done for the patient, nursing care in the home must be family centered. An illness experienced by one family member will affect the entire family and alter family interactions. Families often provide care for ill members and assist in decision making about the type and extent of care provided. Care provided by health professionals is usually episodic, leaving the

TABLE 7-5 Examples of Home Health Care Nursing Activities

Assessment
- Performance of in-depth holistic assessment of patient, family, and home environment.
- Assessment of community services as a source of referral for patient/caregiver needs.
- Ongoing evaluation of patient's progress.

Wound Care
- Assessment and culture of wounds, debridement and irrigation of wounds, application of wound care products, dressing change.
- Instructing patients and families in wound care management and nutrition.
- Documentation (written and photographic).

Respiratory Care
- Management of oxygen therapy, mechanical ventilation, chest physiotherapy.
- Suctioning and care of tracheostomies.

Vital Signs
- Measuring blood pressure and pulse, assessment of cardiopulmonary status.
- Teaching patients and families to take blood pressure and pulse.
- Teaching patients and families signs and symptoms to monitor and emergency measures to take if signs and symptoms are exhibited.

Elimination
- Assistance with colostomy irrigation and skin care procedures.
- Insertion of urinary catheters, irrigation, and evaluation of signs and symptoms of infection.
- Instruction of patient and family in intermittent catheterization and insertion, replacement, and irrigation of urethral and suprapubic catheters.
- Bowel and bladder training.

Nutrition
- Assessment of nutrition and hydration status.
- Nutritional counseling, teaching, reinforcement about prescribed therapeutic diet.
- Administration of nasogastric and percutaneous tube feedings, including gastrostomy and jejunostomy tubes, and teaching families about tube feedings.
- Placement and replacement of tubes and ongoing management and evaluation.

Rehabilitation
- Teaching patients and families to use assistive devices, range-of-motion exercises, ambulation, and transfer techniques.
- Referral of patients for physical therapy and occupational therapy services.

Medications
- Teaching patients and families about administration and side effects of medications.
- Evaluating adherence to drug regimen and effectiveness of prescribed drugs.
- Administration of and teaching about injectable medications (e.g., cobalamin [vitamin B_{12}]).
- Weekly preparation of medications that are self-administered (e.g., insulin, oral medications).

Intravenous Therapy
- Assessment and management of dehydration.
- Administering antibiotic drugs, parenteral nutrition, blood products, and analgesic and chemotherapeutic agents.
- Flushing peripheral and central lines and changing dressings.

Pain Management
- Assessment of pain, including location, characteristics, precipitating factors, and impact on life.
- Teaching patient and family about nonpharmacologic techniques (e.g., relaxation, imagery) for pain management.
- Providing optimal pain relief with prescribed analgesics.

Selected Laboratory Studies
- Drawing blood for studies related to monitoring disease processes or therapy (e.g., drug levels).

TABLE 7-6 Concerns of Patients Requiring Home Health Care Organized by Functional Health Patterns

Health Perception–Health Management Pattern
Ability to care for self
Risk factors for potential health problems
Effect and understanding of prescribed therapy

Nutritional-Metabolic Pattern
Chewing, swallowing, and eating problems
Skin and hair integrity
Diet restrictions or modifications

Elimination Pattern
Bowel and bladder patterns
Bowel and bladder control
Need for assistive devices

Activity-Exercise Pattern
Endurance during activities
Impairments in mobility
Energy for home maintenance

Sleep-Rest Pattern
Altered sleep patterns
Sleep/activity asynchrony

Cognitive-Perceptual Pattern
Need for sensory prosthetic devices
Memory and learning capability
Acute and/or chronic pain
Sensory impairments

Self-Perception–Self-Concept Pattern
Effects of illness on self
Body image and esteem disturbances
Feelings of powerlessness

Role-Relationship Pattern
Changes in living arrangements
Capability for vocation/employment
Social contact and involvement
Altered family responsibilities

Sexuality-Reproductive Pattern
Changes in sexuality patterns
Alternative means of sexual activity

Coping–Stress Tolerance Pattern
Perception and management of stress
Dealing with change and loss
Exhaustion of adaptive abilities
Sources of formal and informal support

Value-Belief Pattern
Maintenance of the human spirit
Holistic well-being
Value or belief conflict

family with the burden of care day in and day out. In some situations, an elderly patient may be cared for by a spouse of similar age who also has chronic illnesses. In other situations an elderly parent needing care may live with a busy middle-aged family with young children. In any home care situation it is common for caregivers to become physically, emotionally, and economically overwhelmed with the responsibilities and demands of caring for a family member. The home health nurse needs to help family members understand and cope with changing roles, responsibilities, and stresses. Referral to various support groups in the community or on the Internet is one way that the nurse can help family members cope with the experience of providing home care.

Teaching needs to involve both the patient and the family. Family members who are providing care should learn how to administer treatments and manage equipment. For example, diet modification is a cornerstone of diabetes management. Although an elderly diabetic person may be the patient, it may be the patient's spouse or daughter who does the grocery shopping and cooking. Dietary teaching that does not include the family may not be successful.

Nursing in the home involves a very different set of dynamics than that of care provided in the hospital. In the hospital, the health care team has the dominant role and the environment is controlled. In the home, the family and/or the patient plays the dominant role, and the nurse is a visitor in the health care setting. Home health care is delivered within the context of the family's and the patient's cultural values and beliefs. In the home, the nurse is more likely to encounter the patient's use of healing practices arising from cultural beliefs and the use of home remedies and complementary and alternative therapies. The home care nurse must be knowledgeable about cultural practices and complementary and alternative therapies to guide the patient and family in their safe and effective use. (Culture is discussed in Chapter 3, and complementary and alternative therapies are discussed in Chapter 8.)

Patients seen by home health care nurses are most often discharged from hospital settings. However, they may also be referred directly from a physician's office or nursing care facilities, or the patient may request this service. Coverage for home health care varies depending on whether the patient is covered by Medicare, an HMO, or other types of insurance.[13] In general, to qualify for coverage, patients must be confined to the home or require a considerable and taxing amount of effort to leave the home for brief periods. This is known as "homebound status." In addition, the patient must be in need of intermittent professional skilled care such as nursing.[3] Depending on the needs of the patient, home health visits may be as frequent as twice daily or as infrequent as once a month. Visits may be extensive and require significant time, such as the initial visit, or they may be shorter in length, such as visits to assess cardiopulmonary status. These visits may be characterized by a predetermined routine or treatment regimen, such as prefilling insulin syringes, prepouring oral medications, administering injected cobalamin (vitamin B_{12}), or performing wound care and dressing changes.

Home Health Care Team

The home health care team includes many members, including the patient, family, nurses, physician, social worker, physical therapist, occupational therapist, speech therapist, home health aide, pharmacist, respiratory therapist, and dietitian (Table 7-8). The mem-

TABLE 7-7 NURSING DIAGNOSES
Patients Requiring Home Care

- **Acute pain** *related to* tissue damage, therapy, decreased joint mobility
- **Caregiver role strain** *related to* 24-hour care responsibilities, marginal coping patterns, unrealistic expectations
- **Chronic pain** *related to* actual or potential tissue damage, disease progression
- **Constipation** *related to* decreased fluid intake, lack of mobility, narcotic analgesics
- **Deficient fluid volume** *related to* inadequate nutrition and hydration, dysphasia, and confusion
- **Fatigue** *related to* disease process and therapy
- **Imbalanced nutrition: less than body requirements** *related to* inability to ingest or digest food, inability to absorb nutrients
- **Impaired home maintenance** *related to* decreased mobility, decreased endurance
- **Impaired skin integrity** *related to* physical immobility, radiation, pressure
- **Risk for aspiration** *related to* enteral tube feedings, impaired gag reflex or swallowing, inability to expectorate sputum
- **Risk for infection** *related to* inadequate primary or secondary defenses, impaired immune status, malnutrition
- **Risk for injury** *related to* altered mobility, confusion, fatigue
- **Self-care deficit** (any combination of the following):
  - **Bathing/hygiene, dressing/grooming, feeding, or toileting** *related to* pain, musculoskeletal impairment, decreased endurance
- **Social isolation** *related to* physical immobility, alteration in physical appearance

TABLE 7-8 Roles of Additional Members of the Home Care Team

Team Member	Description of Services Provided
Physical therapist (PT)	Will work with patients on strengthening and endurance, gait training, transfer training, and developing a patient education program. Physical conditions or diagnoses that may trigger a referral to a physical therapist include orthopedic conditions, such as hip or knee surgeries or neuromuscular deterioration commonly seen with multiple sclerosis, amyotrophic lateral sclerosis, and stroke.
Occupational therapist (OT)	May assist patient with fine motor coordination, performance of the activities of daily living, cognitive-perceptual skills, sensory testing, and the construction or use of assistive or adaptive equipment.
Speech therapist	Focuses on various speech pathologies for those who have suffered speech or swallowing disorders seen in patients with stroke, laryngectomy, or progressive neuromuscular diseases.
Social worker	Assists patients with coping skills, caregiver concerns, securing adequate financial resources or housing assistance, or making referrals to social service or volunteer agencies.
Home health aide	Assists patients with their personal care needs, such as bathing, dressing, hair washing, or some homemaking activities (e.g., meal preparation or light housekeeping).
Pharmacist	Prepares medications and infusion products.
Respiratory therapist	May assist with oxygen therapy in the home.
Dietitian	Is available for dietary consultation.

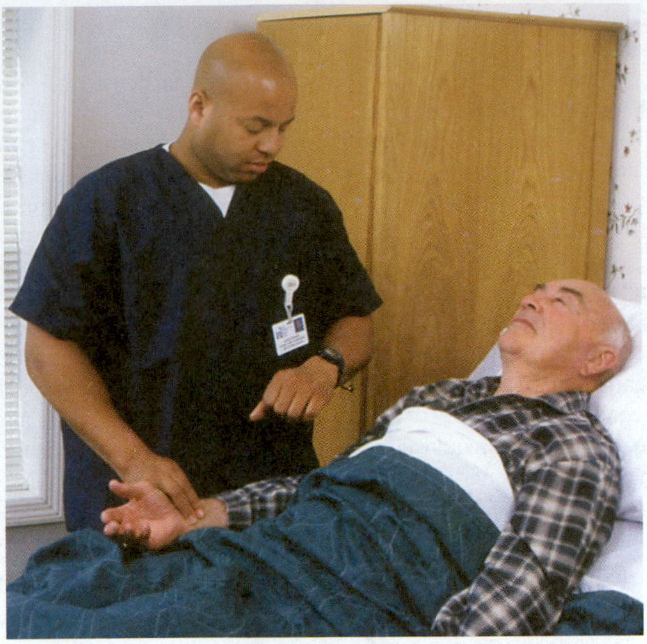

FIG. 7-4 Nursing care can be effectively provided in a home setting.

TABLE 7-9 Skills Essential to Effective Delivery of Home Care Nursing

- Organizational skills
- Independent decision-making abilities
- Prioritization and clinical decision-making skills
- Responsiveness to problems
- Adaptability and flexibility
- Time management
- Case management
- Effective communication
- Nursing process skills
- Resource identification
- Teaching
- Discharge planning
- Technologic competence
- Outcomes management
- Documentation for reimbursement
- Advocacy
- Improvisation

bers of the home health care team work collaboratively with the home health care nurse to plan and evaluate the patient's progress. This is done on a regular basis with a significant emphasis placed on teaching and counseling. Nursing care is one of the primary services in the home setting (Fig. 7-4). Skills essential to effective delivery of nursing care in the home environment can be found in Table 7-9. Home care nurses focus on empowering the patient and family to meet their own needs so they can feel in control of their lives. Goals aim for long-term rather than short-term results. Decision making and priority setting become shared activities among the patient, family, and nurse.

Hospice

Hospice exists to provide support and care for people in the last phases of incurable diseases so that they might live as fully and as comfortably as possible. Hospice is not a place but a concept of care that provides compassion, concern, and support for the dying.[14] Hospice care represents a return to previous times when dying individuals were helped to remain at home and to die at home, if possible, surrounded by familiar sights, sounds, and smells and by the love of those who care.

Many people choose to die at home in the comfort of their own home and surrounded by family and friends. Terminally ill patients may die in dignity at home without the heroic measures commonly seen in acute care settings. (Hospice and end-of-life care are discussed in Chapter 11.)

SUMMARY

Many changes are occurring in the health care delivery system. Patient care settings are becoming highly diversified. The evolving structure of health care is in flux, but it is becoming more focused on providing patient care in the community and home. The increasing number of home health care settings allows patients to receive technical nursing care, education, and support in the home environment.

Nursing is diversifying, adapting, and moving into a variety of patient care settings. As nurses' roles expand, patients are expecting advanced clinical skills and complex health care within a variety of environments, including community-based settings. Nurses need to (1) develop and maintain clinical proficiency and critical thinking skills and (2) become proficient in problem solving, teaching, and management to promote wellness for patients in all settings along the continuum of patient care.

NCLEX EXAMINATION REVIEW QUESTIONS

The number of the question corresponds to the same-numbered objective at the beginning of the chapter.

1. A patient tells the nurse that she has had to change her primary physician four times in the past 3 years because of changes in her health insurance at work and asks what is happening to health care. The best response by the nurse includes the information that
   a. patients are becoming more demanding in their expectations from health care providers.
   b. the federal government is controlling access to health care through Medicare and Medicaid.
   c. an increasing aging society requires more financial and service resources than can be met with Medicare.
   d. prospective payment systems and preferred provider organizations are used to provide more cost-effective health care.
2. In providing community-based patient care, nurses
   a. assess the needs of the community for illness prevention programs.
   b. determine how the health status of individuals and groups affects the community as a whole.
   c. provide coordinated and continuous care for ill patients and their families where they are in the community.
   d. deliver personal health services to individuals, families, and groups to promote and maintain the health of the community.
3. A patient has exhausted the DRG days and is to be discharged from the hospital's acute unit with an open infected abdominal wound requiring intravenous antibiotics and dressing changes. The nurse case manager plans transfer of this patient to a
   a. subacute care unit.
   b. skilled nursing facility.
   c. acute rehabilitation unit.
   d. intermediate care facility.

4. At an initial visit to a patient in the home, the nurse explains that the patient and family can expect the nurse to
   a. perform all health and personal care required by the patient.
   b. teach the family to be able to eventually provide all the care the patient will need.
   c. coordinate services provided by all members of the home care team needed by the patient.
   d. visit the home as often as necessary to evaluate the performance of the members of the home care team.

REFERENCES

1. US Department of Health and Human Services: *The registered nurse population—March 2000: findings from the National Sample Survey of Registered Nurses*, Washington, DC, 2001, Division of Nursing, Bureau of Health Professions, Health Resources and Services Administration. Available at *http://bhpr.hrsa.gov/healthworkforce/reports/rnsurvey/rnss1.htm* (accessed June 15, 2005).
2. Murray T: Distinguishing population-focused practice from community-based care. In Murray T, Ellis P, editors: *Community and public health nursing: a population-based perspective*, Philadelphia, in press; Lippincott Williams & Wilkins.
3. Maurer F, Smith C: *Community/public health nursing practice: health for families and populations*, St Louis, 2005, Elsevier Science.
4. Federal Interagency Forum on Aging Related Statistics: *Older Americans 2004: key indicators of well-being*, Washington, DC, 2004, US Government Printing Office.
5. Centers for Disease Control and Prevention: *The burden of chronic diseases and their risk factors*, Washington, DC, 2002, The Centers. Available at *www.cdc.gov/nccdphp/burdenbook2002/01_tables.htm* (accessed June 15, 2005).
6. Case Management Society of America [CMSA]: *Definition of case management*, 2005, The Society. Available at *www.cmsa.org* (accessed June 15, 2005).
7. Allender J, Spradley B: *Community health nursing: promoting and protecting the public's health*, Philadelphia, 2004, Lippincott Williams & Wilkins.
8. Stanhope M, Lancaster J: *Community and public health nursing*, St Louis, 2004, Mosby.
9. National Health Ministries: *Parish nursing*, 2004. Available at *www.pcusa.org/health/usa/parishnursing* (accessed June 15, 2005).
10. National Association for Home Care: *What is home care?* No date. Available at *www.nahc.org* (accessed June 15, 2005).
11. National Association for Home Care: *State licensure and certificate of need survey*, Washington, DC, 2003, The Association.
12. National Association for Home Care: *Basic statistics about home care*, Washington, DC, 2001, The Association.
13. Turner CH, Floyd LM: Reimbursement. In Neal L, Harris MD, editors: *Core curriculum for home health nursing. Section 1. Program management*, Washington, DC, 2001, Home Care University.
14. American Nurses Association: *Scope and standards of hospice and palliative nursing practice*, Washington, DC, 2002, American Nurses Publishing.

RESOURCES

Accreditation Association for Ambulatory Health Care, Inc.
847-853-6060
www.aaahc.org

American Academy of Ambulatory Care Nursing
856-256-2350
www.aaacn.org

American Association of Homes and Services for the Aging
202-783-2242
www.aahsa.org

American Association of Managed Care Nurses, Inc.
804-747-9698
www.aamcn.org

American Association of Occupational Health Nurses, Inc.
770-455-7757
www.aaohn.org

Association of Rehabilitation Nurses
800-229-7530
847-375-4710
www.rehabnurse.org

Canadian Gerontological Nurses Association
www.cgna.net

Canadian Home Care Association
613-569-1585
www.cdnhomecare.on.ca

Home Healthcare Nurses Association
202-546-4754
www.hhna.org

National Association for Home Care
202-547-7424
www.nahc.org

National Gerontological Nursing Association
850-473-1174
800-723-0560
www.ngna.org

For additional Internet resources, see the website for this book at *http://evolve.elsevier.com/Lewis/medsurg.*

Within you there is a stillness and sanctuary to which you can retreat at any time and be yourself.
Hermann Hesse

8 Complementary and Alternative Therapies

Virginia Shaw

LEARNING OBJECTIVES

1. Compare and contrast the Western biomedical model and the integrative model for health care.
2. Describe commonly used complementary and alternative therapies.
3. List indications for the use of Traditional Chinese Medicine (TCM).
4. Describe the general types of herbal therapy and indications for use.
5. List concepts to be included in patient teaching regarding herbal supplements.
6. Describe the practice of holistic nursing.
7. Describe the process of assessing patients' use of complementary and alternative therapies.
8. Describe the roles of the nurse when integrating complementary and alternative therapies into nursing practice.

KEY TERMS

acupuncture, p. 96
complementary and alternative therapies, p. 95
herbal therapy, p. 100
holistic nursing, p. 107
massage therapy, p. 103
prayer, p. 100
Traditional Chinese Medicine, p. 96

Electronic Resources

Supplemental content related to Chapter 8 can be found . . .

Companion CD

- Stress-Busting Kit for Nursing Students
  - Take a Yoga Break
- NCLEX Examination Review Questions
- Comprehensive Glossary

Evolve Website

http://evolve.elsevier.com/Lewis/medsurg

- Content Updates
- Key Points (Printable and CD/MP3 Download)
- Concept Map Creator
- Expanded Audio Glossary
- Key Term Flash Cards
- Electronic Calculators
- WebLinks

Historically wellness has been viewed as incorporating the physical, emotional, mental, and spiritual realms. Hippocrates, the father of medicine, advised a daily aromatic bath and fragrant massage for the maintenance of health. Florence Nightingale believed that nursing is putting patients in the best condition for nature to act on them. The concepts of holism and balance guided the belief that the body heals itself and works to maintain homeostasis. The concepts of spirituality and harmony with nature were inseparable from the concepts of health and wellness.

This view of "wholeness" began to change with the works of Rene Descartes (1596–1650) and Sir Isaac Newton (1642–1727). They postulated a "reductionistic approach" whereby the body is seen as a series of parts that can be broken down and studied. This mechanistic approach views the body as a machine. In this approach whatever part is broken is analyzed and then repaired, without regard for other aspects of the person involved.[1] The Western biomedical model of health care is based on this approach. Health focuses on the physical body to the exclusion of the mind and the spirit. Emphasis is placed on what can be seen, measured, and quantified.

This Western biomedical model has guided American health care for over 100 years. In the 1980s Americans began to explore health care therapies that were outside this biomedical model. This consumer-led movement fostered development of a new model of health care, a more "integrative" model. In this model consumers combine the use of complementary and alternative therapies with conventional therapies. The biomedical and integrative health care models are compared in Table 8-1.

The new integrative model focuses on (1) personal responsibility for health, (2) joining of mind-body-spirit, and (3) use of natural, less invasive modalities. This model promotes health and wellness, not just the treatment of disease. Consumers have demonstrated a

Reviewed by Karen Lee Fontaine, RN, MSN, ASSECT, Professor of Nursing, School of Nursing, Purdue University of Calumet, Hammond, Ind.

TABLE 8-1 Comparison of Biomedical and Integrative Health Care Models

Biomedical Health Care Model	Integrative Health Care Model
Focus on physical body	Focus on mind-body-spirit
Focus on treatment of symptoms using medications and surgery	Focus on self-healing of the body using herbs, exercise, nutrition, stress management
Health care provider directs care	Individual directs care; personal responsibility for health encouraged
Focus on disease states	Focus on health and wellness
Technologic, invasive	Noninvasive
Increasing cost	Lower cost
Little focus on prevention	Focus on prevention

desire for more involvement in their health care decisions. They desire modalities that are more natural, less costly, and safer. The rise of chronic diseases and stress-related disorders has also led to consumers' interest in complementary and alternative therapies.

COMPLEMENTARY AND ALTERNATIVE THERAPIES

Complementary and alternative therapies are defined as a "broad domain of resources that encompasses health systems, modalities, and practices and their accompanying theories and beliefs, other than those intrinsic to the dominant health system of a particular society or culture in a given historical period."[2] This definition highlights that what might be considered "complementary and alternative" in one country or at one period of history might be considered "conventional" in another place or time. Because complementary and alternative therapies fall outside the Western biomedical model, many American health care providers have not received training related to these therapies. Yet these therapies have been used for years in other cultures and in other parts of the world. Most are safe and effective. As Americans realize the limitations of the biomedical health care model, they seek out other therapies.

Terms frequently used to describe health-related approaches that are outside the dominant system of health care include *alternative, complementary,* and *integrative.* Initially the term *alternative therapies* was used. Use of this term signified that these therapies were used instead of Western medicine. Most Americans, however, were using complementary and alternative therapies in conjunction with Western medicine. The terms *complementary* and *integrative* better describe this combined use. Other terms used include *holistic, natural, nontraditional,* and *integral.* The term *integral* expands the concept further by its focus on restoring wholeness, healing, and awareness of consciousness. *Integral medicine* identifies the need for wholeness of both the patient and provider, and emphasizes body, mind, and spirit as related to self, nature, and culture.[3]

Complementary and alternative therapies are harmonious with many of the values of nursing. These include a view of humans as holistic beings, an emphasis on healing, recognition that the provider-patient relationship should be a partnership, and a focus on health promotion and illness prevention. In 1980 the American Holistic Nurses' Association was established to facilitate care for the "whole" person and significant others through focusing on holistic principles of health, preventive education, and the integration of caring-healing modalities.[4]

Health care professionals have raised important questions about the effectiveness and safety of complementary and alternative approaches in the face of their increased use by consumers. In response to this need, the National Center for Complementary and Alternative Medicine (NCCAM) was established *(www.nih.nccam.gov).* A branch of the National Institutes of Health (NIH), the NCCAM serves as the federal government's lead agency for scientific research on complementary and alternative therapies. The primary functions include the study of complementary and alternative modalities using rigorous scientific methods, the education of complementary and alternative researchers, and the dissemination of authoritative information to the public and professionals.[5] In collaboration with the NCCAM, the Cochrane Collaboration provides a focus on complementary and alternative approaches, providing a valuable source for synthesized evidence on this topic.[6]

Since the 1990s, multiple studies have revealed that 29% to 62% of Americans are using some form of complementary and alternative therapy.[7-11] Figure 8-1 shows the results of one study. Consumers often "self-select" therapies, using these therapies without professional supervision. Nearly half of the users of these therapies do not consult an alternative and complementary practitioner or disclose such use to their traditional health care provider.[10] Health care providers typically have little knowledge regarding these therapies, and may be prejudiced against their use.[12] Yet the consumer-driven movement continues to grow, with the yearly number of visits to a complementary and alternative provider surpassing the number of visits to a traditional medical provider.[9]

A large study conducted by NCCAM and the Centers for Disease Control and Prevention (CDC) investigated the types of complementary and alternative therapies used (Fig. 8-2). The study showed that 62% of adults had used some form of complementary and alternative therapy during the prior 12 months, when the definition of complementary and alternative therapies included prayer for health reasons. When prayer was excluded, 36% of adults had used these therapies. Reasons for use were as follows: (1) 55% said they believe it helps them when used in conjunction with conventional medical treatments, (2) 50% said it would be interesting to try, (3) 28% said conventional medicine did not help them, (4) 26% were following the advice of a conventional health care provider, and (5) 13% said it offered a cheaper alternative. Not surprisingly, rates of use of complementary and alternative therapies were high among those with life-threatening illness and those with chronic pain.[13]

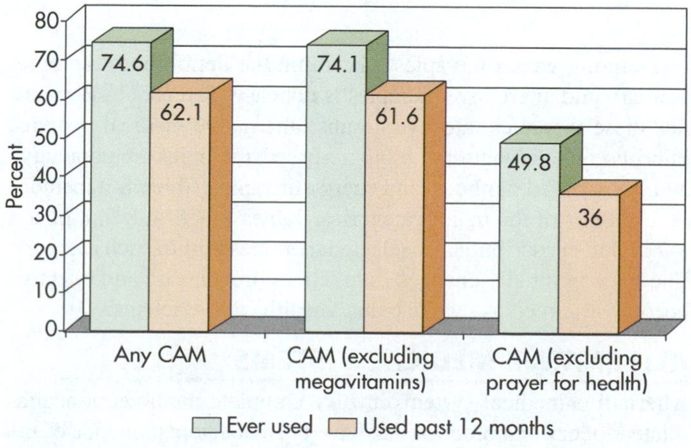

FIG. 8-1 Percentage of Americans using complementary and alternative therapies.

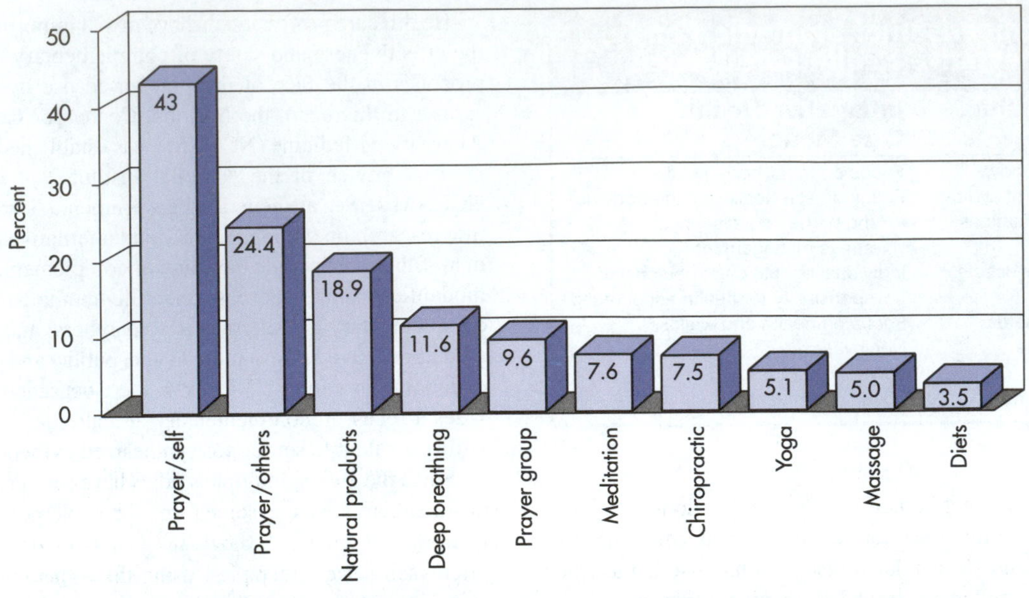

FIG. 8-2 Most commonly used complementary and alternative therapies.

TABLE 8-2 NCCAM Categories of Complementary and Alternative Therapies

Category	Description
Alternative medical systems	Complete systems of health care, apart from the conventional biomedical system used in the United States (see Table 8-3).
Mind-body interventions	Therapies that use the mind's ability to affect the physical body. Science of psychoneuroimmunology demonstrates the strength of this mind-body connection (see Table 8-4).
Biologic-based therapies	Therapies that use substances found in nature for their impact on health and well-ness (see Table 8-5).
Manipulative and body-based methods	Therapies that manipulate or move one or more parts of the body (see Table 8-6).
Energy therapies	Therapies that use or manipulate energy fields (see Table 8-7).

NCCAM, National Center for Complementary and Alternative Medicine.

Defining which therapies fall within the definition of complementary and alternative therapies is not easy. The NCCAM classifies these therapies into five groups: alternative medical systems, mind-body interventions, biologic-based therapies, manipulative and body-based methods, and energy therapies. Table 8-2 includes descriptions of the major categories. Tables 8-3, 8-4, 8-5, 8-6, and 8-7 include descriptions of selected therapies within each category. The list continually changes as practices proven safe and effective become accepted as "mainstream" health care practices.

ALTERNATIVE MEDICAL SYSTEMS

Alternative medical systems involve complete methods of health-related theory and practice that have been developed outside of the Western biomedical model. Many are traditional systems that are practiced by individual cultures throughout the world. Traditional Chinese Medicine is one of the subcategories that NCCAM has identified.

Traditional Chinese Medicine

Traditional Chinese Medicine (TCM) is a complete system of medicine capable of treating a full spectrum of complaints and problems. Over the past several thousand years, it has evolved based on cultural and philosophic developments, as well as extensive clinical observation and testing. The principle of yin and yang is a core tenet of Chinese art, philosophy, and science, as well as TCM. *Yin* and *yang* are viewed as dynamic, interacting, and interdependent energies, neither of which can exist without the other, each containing some part of the other within it (Fig. 8-3). These energies are a part of everything in nature and must be maintained in a harmonious state of balance to achieve optimal health. Various states are associated with yin (cold, heavy, moist, negative) and yang (hot, dry, light, positive) energies. Imbalance is associated with illness. TCM modalities work to restore balance between yin and yang energies.

Strengths of TCM include its individualized system of diagnosis and treatment, as well as its focus on prevention. Assessment tools include a comprehensive health history, tongue diagnosis, and pulse diagnosis. Traditional Chinese Medicine includes an array of modalities, with the most common choices being acupuncture and Chinese herbal medicine. These modalities are used together to replenish and soothe the flow of Qi throughout the body. **Qi** is a form of energy found in all life; when it is disrupted, illness and pain can occur. **Acupuncture** involves the insertion of fine needles into the circulation of Qi underneath the skin's surface (Fig. 8-4). Specific points are selected based on the diagnosis and nature of the complaint. With proper point selection and manipulation, acupuncture corrects disruptions in the flow of Qi.

Chinese herbs are used to supplement the effects of an acupuncture treatment. Taken regularly over time, Chinese herbal formulas strengthen the body's ability to correct its own imbalance so that regular treatments are no longer necessary. Herbs are selected based on specific assessment findings and on complaint history;

TABLE 8-3 Alternative Medical Systems

Examples	Description
Traditional Chinese Medicine (TCM)	Based on restoring and maintaining the balance of vital energy *(Qi)*. Interventions include acupressure, acupuncture, Chinese herbology, cupping, moxibustion, nutrition, meditation, Tai Chi, and Qi gong. One of the world's oldest, most complete medical systems.
Ayurveda	Based on the balance of mind, body, and spirit. Developed in India. Views disease as an imbalance between a person's life force *(prana)* and basic metabolic condition *(dosha).* Interventions include breathing exercises, nutrition, detoxification, herbs, meditation, and yoga.
Native American health care	Based on a spiritual domain whereby all things have "spirit." Community is valued and plays a role in the healing process. Gratitude and harmony with nature are central themes. Medicine men and women use herbs and natural medicines, spiritual rituals, and ceremony.
Hispanic health care	Based on a blend of Native American and Spanish cultural beliefs. The healer is the curandero/curandera. Interventions include herbalism, spiritualism, mysticism, faith healing, and energy medicine.
Homeopathy	Based on "like cures like." Remedies are specially prepared from the same substance that causes the symptom or problem. Extremely small amounts of the substance are used for the remedy. The remedies are generally safe and free from interactions with other medications. Remedies are believed to work through an energy transfer.
Naturopathy	Based on promotion of health rather than symptom management. Focuses on enhancing the body's natural healing response using a variety of individualized interventions such as nutrition, herbology, homeopathy, physical therapies, and counseling. Naturopathic physicians are graduates of accredited naturopathic medical schools, and licensing varies by state.

TABLE 8-4 Mind-Body Interventions

Examples	Description
Relaxation breathing	Uses slow diaphragmatic breathing to elicit the relaxation response. See Chapter 9 for further information.
Prayer	Involves communication with the Creator or the Sacred. Found in all cultures. A frequently used therapy. Nurses may incorporate prayer into their practice.
Meditation	State of being with increased concentration and awareness. Focuses one's attention and increases self-awareness. Two branches exist: (1) inclusive, mindfulness; (2) exclusive, concentrative. Mindfulness meditation focuses on "living in the moment" without judgment. Concentrative meditation involves "moving inward"—often initiated by concentrating on the breath, a mantra, or an object. Outcomes may include relaxation, spiritual growth, and personal healing.
Biofeedback	Involves a method of learned control of physiologic responses of the body.[1] Information about physiologic function(s) is received, interventions are used, and a feedback loop allows for voluntary control of certain functions.
Imagery	Uses one's mind to generate images that have a calming effect on the body. Involves use of vision, sound, smell, and taste, as well as the senses of movement, position, and touch.[14] Outcomes may include reduction of anxiety, relaxation, enhanced immunity, and changes in hormonal responses.
Hypnosis	Involves a state of attentive, focused concentration with suspension of some peripheral awareness.[14] May be effective in promoting healing, decreasing pain, managing chronic illness, and preparing for surgery and other procedures.[1]
Music therapy	Includes listening to music and creating music. Type of music used is individually determined. Outcomes may include relaxation, decreased anxiety, and decreased pain.
Art therapy	Involves creative expression through a variety of artistic mediums. May be used to facilitate expression of emotions, memories, and conscious and unconscious concerns. Outcomes may include decreased stress, as well as facilitation of healing from past distress or trauma.
Journaling	Involves writing down one's feelings, thoughts, perceptions, personal events, or memories. Outcomes may include stress reduction, as well as personal development through self-reflection.
Animal-assisted therapy (AAT)	Uses specifically trained animals to assist in attainment of health care goals. An example is hippotherapy (use of horseback riding) to meet physical therapy and rehabilitation goals. Animal-assisted activities (AAAs) include use of trained animals for motivational, educational, and/or recreational objectives. An example is placement of animals in assisted-living facilities.

TABLE 8-5 Biologic-Based Therapies

Examples	Description
Herbal therapy	Involves use of unrefined plant-based products to treat, prevent, or cure disease. Effects are slow and less dramatic than effects of pharmaceutical drugs.
Nutraceuticals	Involves use of vitamin and mineral supplements. Best source of vitamins and minerals is a well-balanced diet. Yet many Americans take supplements regularly.
Nutritional therapy	Involves special diets for health promotion. Popular diets come and go. Special diets must be studied for potential benefit.
Aromatherapy	Involves use of plants' essential oils for their beneficial effect. Americans seek out this therapy primarily for stress reduction, and use these oils via inhalation or topically. In other cultures, essential oils are used more comprehensively in health care.

TABLE 8-6 Manipulative and Body-Based Methods

Examples	Description
Chiropractic therapy	Restores and maintains health by properly aligning the spine using a variety of adjustment and manipulation techniques. Correct spinal alignment facilitates self-healing and improves health and well-being.
Acupressure	Involves the use of applied finger and hand pressure to specific areas of body (acupoints defined by charts of energy meridians) to improve energy flow, relieve pain, and stimulate the body's innate healing abilities.
Massage therapy	Involves manipulation of soft tissues to improve health and promote healing. Outcomes include relaxation, reduced tension, improved immune function, increased flexibility, and pain relief.
Yoga	Includes mental and physical exercises, ethical principles, and guidelines for healthy living. Part of the Ayurveda medical system. Americans use yoga more for its physical benefits and for stress reduction.

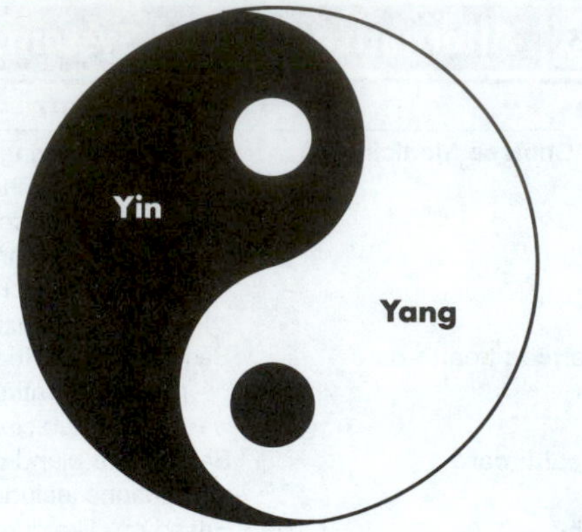

FIG. 8-3 Yin/yang symbol. The circle representing the whole is divided into yin and yang. The small circles of opposite shading illustrate that within the yin there is yang and within the yang there is yin. The dynamic curve dividing them indicates that yin and yang are continuously merging. Thus yin and yang create each other, control each other, and transform into each other. When yin and yang are in balance, *Qi,* or the fundamental life force, flows evenly through the body, leading to good health.

TABLE 8-7 Energy Therapies

Examples	Description
Therapeutic Touch	Involves the use of the practitioner's hands to assess and balance the patient's energy field. Healing intent is incorporated. Based on the belief that healing is facilitated when the human energy field is in balance.
Healing Touch	Includes Therapeutic Touch, as well as other energy healing modalities. Primarily used by nurses.
Reiki	A Japanese therapy that involves use of the hands to affect the human energy field with the intent to heal.
Magnet therapy	Uses the principle that every animal, plan, and mineral has an electromagnetic field that allows other objects to interact as part of one unified energy system.[1] Magnets are frequently used to reduce pain, relieve swelling and inflammation, and promote healing of soft tissue and bone.

formulas are individually created to match the patient's needs. Other TCM interventions include acupressure, moxibustion, cupping, Chinese massage, meditative physical exercise (e.g., Tai Chi and Qi gong), and nutrition counseling. Tai Chi and Qi gong are slow movement exercises that require focused breathing.

Clinical Applications of Acupuncture. **Acupuncture** is the primary treatment modality used by TCM practitioners. It is the most common complementary therapy recommended by U.S. physicians. In regard to benefit coverage by health insurance, it is the second most covered complementary therapy, with chiropractic therapy being the first.

Clinical studies have indicated that acupuncture is effective in treating adult postoperative and chemotherapy-associated nausea and vomiting, as well as postoperative dental pain. Other conditions for which acupuncture may be useful include addiction, stroke rehabilitation, menstrual cramps, fibromyalgia, osteoarthritis, and myofascial pain.[15-18] See Table 8-8 for a more complete listing of the uses of acupuncture.

Acupuncture is considered a safe therapy when the practitioner has been appropriately trained and the practitioner uses disposable needles. Patients should review the credentials of their practitioner. The practitioner should have at least a master's degree in Oriental Medicine and be registered to practice acupuncture in that state. The practitioner should have passed the National Commission of the Certification of Acupuncture and Oriental Medicine examinations. In addition, some medical doctors (MDs) practice medical acupuncture. Patients should ensure that MD acupuncturists are qualified to do so *(www.medicalacupuncture.org).*

Acupressure (described in Table 8-6) is a natural, hands-on healing therapy based on the same principles as acupuncture. Finger pressure is applied along the body's energy meridians. Acupressure works by accessing and releasing blocked or congested energy in the body. Acupressure can be used for many conditions. It is a technique that can be easily learned by nurses. Requirements for use include (1) study of meridians and indications for use of specific acupoints, (2) explanation to patients of acupressure and its proposed benefits, and (3) the patient's consent to receive acupressure.

Two commonly used acupressure points are Neiguan (PC6) and Hegu (LI4). Neiguan is indicated for the treatment of nausea, including postoperative nausea and chemotherapy-induced nausea. The point is located on the medial forearm, roughly two thumb-widths from the carpal wrist and between the tendons of the flexor radialis and palmaris longus. Pressure should be applied with the thumb using gentle yet firm pressure for 2 to 3 minutes (Fig. 8-5, *A*). Another acupressure point, Hegu is indicated for the treatment of all types of headaches, including migraine and sinus headaches. It is located on the dorsum of the hand between the first and second metacarpal bones and at the midpoint of the second metacarpal. Pressure should be applied by pressing the point between the thumb and forefinger for 2 to 3 minutes (Fig. 8-5, *B*).

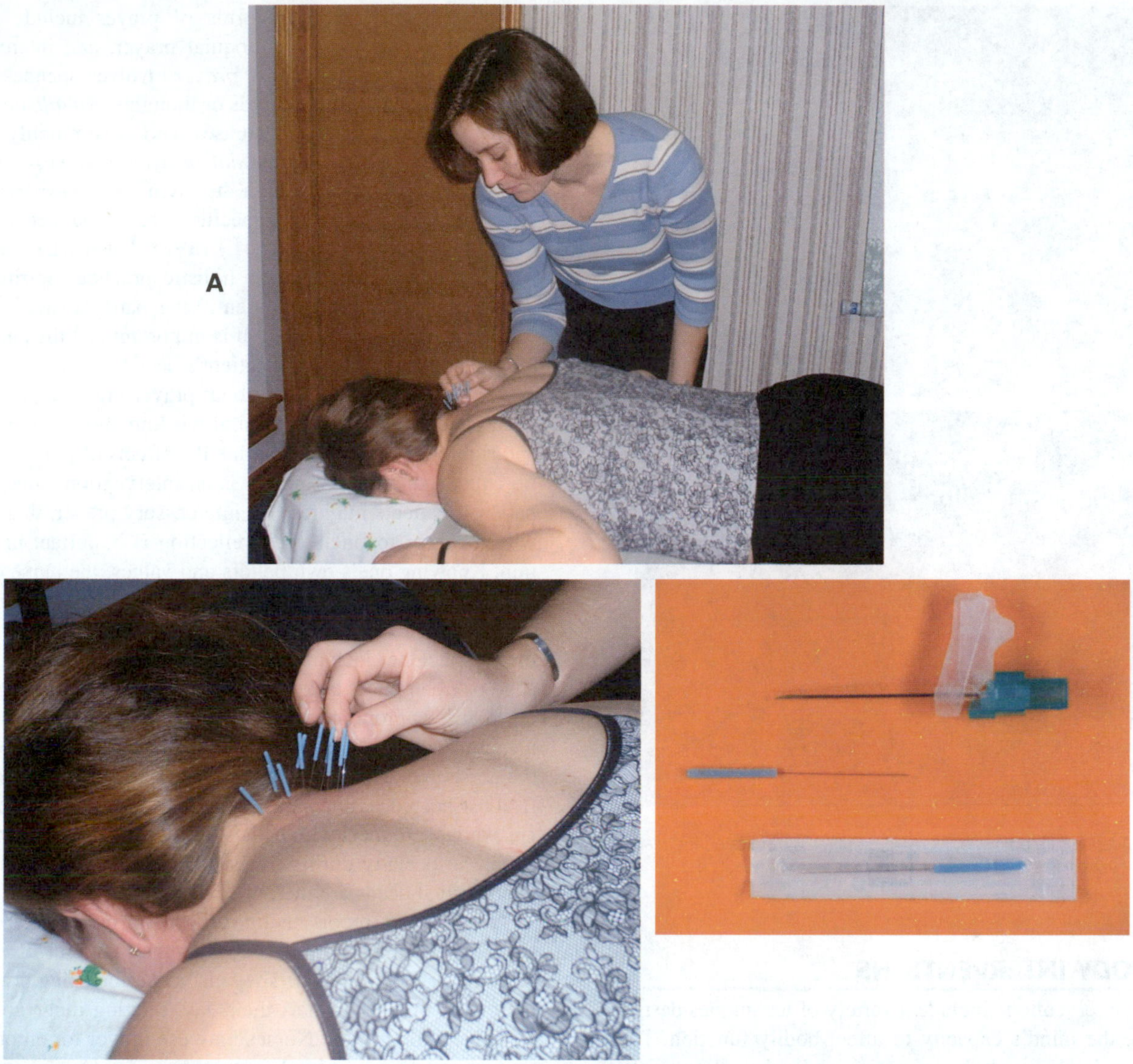

FIG. 8-4 Acupuncture. **A,** TCM practitioner placing acupuncture needles. The needles are placed along the meridians to balance the flow of Qi. **B,** Acupuncture treatment for numbness in arms related to damage of neck vertebrae. **C,** Comparison of injection needles and acupuncture needles. Injection needles are larger and hollow in the center. Acupuncture needles are very thin and solid. They are so flexible that a guide tube is used during insertion.

TABLE 8-8 Conditions That May Benefit from Acupuncture

Pain Management	**Chemotherapy-Induced Nausea**	**Asthma**
Low back pain	**Neurologic Disorders**	**Gastrointestinal Conditions**
Headache pain	Acute stroke	Irritable bowel syndrome
Osteoarthritis	Stroke rehabilitation	Chronic constipation
Cervical neck pain	**Gynecologic and Obstetric Conditions**	**Substance Abuse**
Musculoskeletal and myofascial pain	Induction of labor	Smoking cessation
Fibromyalgia	Infertility	Opioid dependence
Surgical Analgesia	Menopausal symptoms	
Procedural analgesia	Dysmenorrhea	
Postoperative pain		
Postoperative nausea and vomiting		

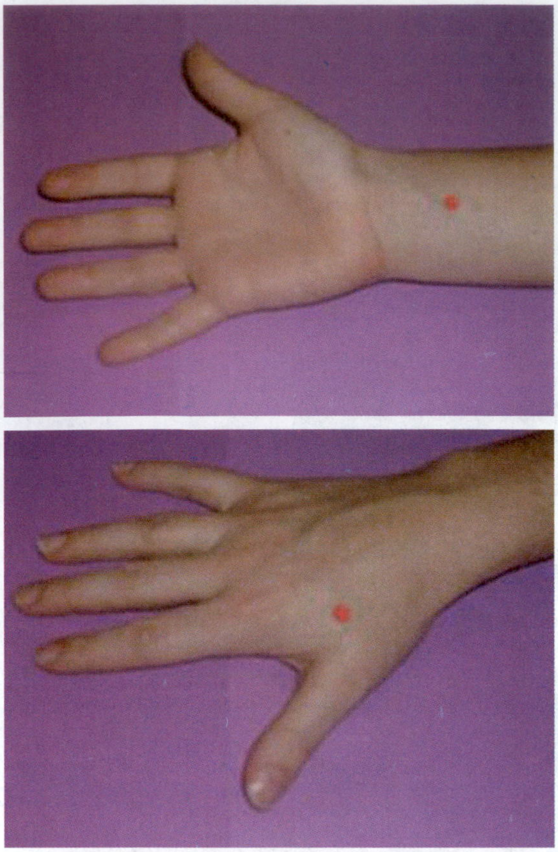

FIG. 8-5 Acupressure points. **A,** Neiguan point *(PC6).* Indicated for treatment of nausea. **B,** Hegu point *(L14).* Indicated for treatment of headaches.

MIND-BODY INTERVENTIONS

Mind-body interventions include a variety of techniques designed to facilitate the mind's capacity to affect bodily function. These include behavioral, psychologic, social, and spiritual approaches to health. Specific examples are included in Table 8-4. It should be noted that in behavioral approaches such as psychotherapy, certain uses of hypnosis and biofeedback are considered "mainstream" within the category of mind-body methods. Nurses can use many of these mind-body approaches.

Prayer

Prayer (described in Table 8-4) is one of the mind-body interventions used most commonly by Americans. Ninety percent of Americans believe in prayer, 72% to 82% have prayed for personal healing, and 87% have prayed for the healing of others.[19] Yet prayer is difficult to define. Viewed globally, prayer can be described as connecting with the sacred. An ancient healing practice, prayer has recently been acknowledged in health care literature. Terms such as *distant healing, mental healing,* and *spiritual healing* are used, as researchers attempt to study the outcomes of prayer. The term *theosomatic medicine* has been developed to describe the study of health as related to an apparent connection between God/Spirit and the human body. In exploring this connection, religious involvement has been found to be generally associated with lower levels of illness and higher levels of wellness. Prayer has been linked to the prevention of illness and the healing of disease.[20]

Forms of Prayers. Forms of prayer include meditative prayer, ritualistic prayer, colloquial prayer, and intercessory (or petitionary) prayer. *Meditative prayer* involves openness to the divine and does not require words or thoughts. *Ritualistic prayer* involves repeated words and phrases, and is commonly associated with formal liturgy. *Colloquial prayer* involves spontaneous thought and conversation with the divine. *Intercessory prayer* involves making a request for specific needs to be met.

Clinical Applications of Prayer. Nurses are committed to spiritual care as part of their holistic practice. Spiritual assessments can guide nurses in identifying patients' needs. Different formats or tools may be used. It is important that the nurse be nonjudgmental and open to the patient's needs.

Nurses need "knowledge about prayer practices, awareness of what patients want, cross-cultural wisdom about how people pray and rigorous research to examine the effects of prayer."[21] Nursing literature indicates that prayer is an intervention valued by many patients. Patients may request intercessory prayer, that is, to pray with them, or for them. Self-reflection is important in this situation. Knowing one's own beliefs and values, the nurse can decide to meet the patient's request directly. However, many nurses feel uncomfortable praying with their patients. Barriers to praying with patients include "lack of time, personal discomfort, lack of knowledge or experience, lack of private space, and difficulty ascertaining if it is appropriate."[19] For whatever reason, if the nurse feels uncomfortable or is unable to address the patient's request directly, the nurse may consult with a spiritual director or religious leader. In most hospitals, chaplains of various faiths and denominations are available to meet with patients. Since patients find prayer comforting, especially during times of illness, nurses need to ensure that spiritual needs are met.

Nurses also report using prayer in more personal ways. Nurses who are hesitant to pray with their patients often say they do pray for their patients. They also describe using prayer before their shift or as they start their day, seeking inner guidance for effective nursing care. Nurses may use prayer for emotional support, motivation, spiritual awareness, or enhanced professional performance.[22]

BIOLOGIC-BASED THERAPIES

Biologic-based therapies include herbal therapies (phytotherapy), aromatherapy, special diet therapies, and dietary supplements.

Herbal Supplements. **Herbal therapy** is the use of individual herbs or combinations of herbs for therapeutic benefit (see Table 8-5). An herb is a plant or plant part (bark, roots, leaves, seeds, flowers, or fruit) that produces and contains chemical substances that act on the body. It is estimated that approximately 25,000 plant species are used medicinally throughout the world and approximately 30% of modern prescription drugs are derived from plants. Botanical medicine is the oldest form of medicine; archaeologic evidence suggests that Neanderthals used plant-based remedies 60,000 years ago. Today about 80% of the world's population relies extensively on plant-derived remedies.

Over the past 30 years a resurgence of interest in herbal therapy has occurred in countries whose health care is dominated by the biomedical model. Interest in herbal products is related to several factors, including the high cost and potential for side effects associated with prescription drugs. Herbal remedies are considered "natural" and are often viewed as safer. They are directly available to consumers, allowing individuals to assume more autonomy regarding their health care. Advantages of herbal supplements include (1) fewer side effects, (2) amenable to self-care, and (3) lower cost. Disadvantages of herbs include (1) longer period of time to onset of action, (2) possible drug-herb interactions, (3) inconsistent manufacturing practices, and (4) information available to consumers is not always reliable.

The practice of phytotherapy is regulated in many parts of the world. For example, in France all phytotherapists are also credentialed physicians, and in Germany 70% of all general medical practitioners prescribe herbal remedies to their patients. The governments of China and Japan officially support herbal therapies within their national health care system. Regulating agencies in Germany, France, the United Kingdom, and Canada enforce standards of quality and safety assessments on manufacturers.

In contrast, in the United States herbs are considered dietary supplements as defined by the U.S. Dietary Supplement Health and Education Act of 1994 (DSHEA). This law states that dietary supplements can be marketed without proven safety or efficacy and without consistent manufacturing practices. In March 2003 the U.S. Food and Drug Administration (FDA) published proposed rules on good manufacturing practice regulations for dietary supplements. In November 2004 the FDA announced major initiatives to further implement DSHEA. These initiatives include the following objectives: (1) to improve the evidentiary base the FDA uses to make safety and enforcement decisions about dietary ingredients and dietary supplements; (2) to seek public comment on the type, quantity, and quality of evidence manufacturers should provide to the FDA in a new dietary ingredient notification; and (3) to ensure product quality by establishing industry-wide standards on manufacturing of dietary supplements.

The amount of scientific research data on herbal supplements is growing. However, these reports often have limitations that make it difficult for any provider to make specific recommendations to patients. For example, studies frequently involve one active ingredient of the plant, yet commercial products use parts of the entire plant. Some studies do not list the actual chemical makeup of the product studied. Variation among brands and manufacturing practices add inconsistency. Research must be analyzed in detail, and caution is advised about generalizing results to patient use.

Clinical Applications of Herbal Therapy. Medicinal plants work in much the same way as drugs; both are absorbed and trigger biologic effects that can be therapeutic. Many have more than one physiologic effect and thus have more than one condition for which they can be used. The range of action of herbs is extensive.

Overall the use of herbal products continues to increase. Also, the pattern of use has changed, with 95% of herbal use now being self-care based.[23] Decisions to use herbs are based on individual needs and individual responses to the herb; that is, more on subjective information than on objective information. If a patient experiences symptomatic relief or a subjective change in health care status, the patient will continue to use the product. If the product does not appear to help the problem, the patient will discontinue it. Most patients do not include data from scientific studies in their decision making.

Although most herbal therapies can safely be used without professional assistance, side effects and interactions with prescription drugs have been described. There is concern that side effects resulting from the use of herbal remedies are underreported, thus promoting the impression that herbal remedies are completely safe to use. Because consumers tend not to share their use of herbal therapies with their primary health care provider, herb-drug interactions may also be underreported. For example, patients who are scheduled for surgery should be advised to stop taking herbal remedies 2 to 3 weeks before surgery. Herbal products that interfere with surgery are discussed in Chapter 18. Patients who are being treated with conventional drug therapy should be advised to discontinue herbal remedies with similar pharmacologic effects, because the combination may lead to an excessive reaction or to unknown interaction effects. General patient teaching guidelines related to herbal therapy use are presented in Table 8-9.

TABLE 8-9 PATIENT AND FAMILY TEACHING GUIDE
Herbal Therapies

- Ask the patient about use of herbal therapies. Take a complete history of herbal use, including amounts, brand names, and frequency of use. Ask the patient about allergies.
- Investigate whether herbs are used instead of or in addition to traditional medical treatments. Find out whether herbal therapies are used to prevent disease or to treat an existing problem.
- Instruct the patient to inform health care provider before taking any herbal treatments.
- Make the patient aware of the risks and benefits associated with herbal use, including drug reactions when taken in combination with other drugs.
- Advise the patient using herbal therapies to be aware of any side effects while taking herbal treatments and to immediately report them to health care provider.
- Make the patient aware that moisture, sunlight, and heat may alter the components of herbal treatments.
- Inform the patient of the need to be aware of the reputation of the manufacturers of herbal products and the safety of the product before buying herbal treatments.
- Encourage the patient to read labels of herbal therapies carefully. Advise the patient not to take more of an herb than is recommended.
- Inform the patient that most herbal therapies should be discontinued at least 2-3 weeks before surgery.
- Inform the patient that the employees of health food stores are not trained health care professionals.

Patients should be advised that if they take herbal therapies, they should adhere to the suggested dosage. If herbal preparations are taken in high doses, they can be toxic. The potency of a particular herbal remedy can vary widely because of factors such as where and how it was grown, as well as harvesting and processing methods. Herbal medicines should be purchased only from reputable manufacturers. Because of the potential for adverse effects, herbal products should be used with caution in pregnant women, nursing mothers, and older adults with liver or cardiovascular disease.

Commonly used herbs are presented in Table 8-10. Some common herbs are shown in Fig. 8-6. Complementary and Alternative Therapy boxes related to specific diseases are found throughout the book (see also the box on p. 103). Commonly used dietary supplements are found in Table 8-11.

MANIPULATIVE AND BODY-BASED METHODS

Manipulative and body-based methods include interventions and approaches to health care that are based on manipulation or movement of the body. Examples include chiropractic therapy, yoga, massage, acupressure, and other forms of body work. Yoga (Fig. 8-7) is one of the fastest growing complementary and alternative therapies among Americans.[23] Massage therapy is one of the body-based methods commonly used by nurses.

TABLE 8-10 Commonly Used Herbs*

Name	Examples of Common Uses	Comments
Aloe	Constipation† Genital herpes, psoriasis vulgaris‡	Use no longer than 7 days for constipation May cause electrolyte imbalances May lower blood glucose
Bilberry	Cataracts, retinopathy§ Peripheral vascular disease§ Varicose veins§ Diabetes mellitus§	May lower blood glucose May increase risk of bleeding
Black cohosh	Menopausal symptoms‡	Generally safe when used for up to 6 months in healthy, nonpregnant women
Chamomile	Common cold§ Gastrointestinal disorders§ Sleep aid/sedation§	Contraindicated with known sensitivity to members of the ragweed family May cause drowsiness May increase risk of bleeding
Echinacea	Treatment of upper respiratory infections‡ Prevention of upper respiratory infections§ Immune system stimulation§	Use with caution in patients with conditions affecting the immune system May lead to liver inflammation Short-term use (10-14 days) is recommended
Evening primrose	Eczema, skin irritation‡	Contraindicated in individuals with seizure disorders
Feverfew	Migraine headache prevention‡ Rheumatoid arthritis§	May increase risk of bleeding Long-term users may experience withdrawal symptoms
Garlic	Hyperlipidemia‡ Hypertension§	Use with caution in patients with bleeding disorders Do not use in large amounts
Ginger	Nausea and vomiting of pregnancy‡ Nausea and vomiting (postoperative or chemotherapy-induced)§ Motion sickness§	Use with caution in patients with bleeding disorders Use in pregnancy should not exceed 1 g/day Supervision by health care provider is recommended for pregnant women considering use of ginger
Ginkgo biloba	Claudication (peripheral vascular disease)† Dementia treatment (multi-infarct and Alzheimer's type)† Cerebral insufficiency‡	Generally well tolerated in recommended dosages for up to 6 months May increase risk of bleeding May affect blood glucose
Ginseng (panax species, including Asian and American ginseng)	Improve mental performance‡ Lower blood glucose in type 2 diabetes mellitus‡	Use with caution in diabetic patients Use with caution in patients taking medications, herbs, supplements that affect BP or heart rhythm Generally safe when used for up to 3 months
Goldenseal	Heart failure§ Immunostimulant§ Infectious diarrhea§ Upper respiratory tract infection§	Should not be used for longer than 2-3 weeks Use with caution in patients with cardiovascular disease May increase risk of bleeding
Hawthorn	Heart failure† Coronary artery disease§	May have additive effect with digoxin or with medications that lower BP
Kava	Anxiety†	Should be used only under the supervision of a health care practitioner May cause hepatotoxicity May increase risk of bleeding
Milk thistle	Hepatitis (chronic)‡ Cirrhosis‡	Generally safe in recommended dosages for up to 4-6 years Use with caution in diabetic patients
Peppermint	Antispasmodic (gastric spasm)§ Indigestion§ Irritable bowel syndrome§	Use peppermint oil in small dosages only May interfere with liver's cytochrome P450 system
St. John's wort	Depressive disorder (mild to moderate)† Anxiety§	Generally well tolerated for up to 1-3 months Interacts with many herbs, supplements, medications Advise patients to consult a health care practitioner before using with any herb/medication
Saw palmetto	Benign prostatic hyperplasia (BPH)†	Generally well tolerated for up to 3-5 years May increase risk of bleeding May increase BP
Turmeric	Dyspepsia§ Osteoarthritis§	May cause upset stomach when used in high doses or if taken over a long period of time May increase risk of bleeding
Valerian	Insomnia‡ Anxiety disorder§	Generally safe in recommended dosages for up to 4-6 weeks Chronic use may result in insomnia

From Ulbricht CE, Basch EM: *Natural standard herb and supplement reference: evidence-based clinical reviews*, St Louis, 2005, Mosby. Available at *www.naturalstandard.com*.
*Advise patients who are pregnant or lactating to consult a health care practitioner before using any herbs. There is limited scientific evidence for the use of most herbs during pregnancy or lactation.
†Strong scientific evidence exists for this use.
‡Good scientific evidence exists for this use.
§Unclear scientific evidence exists for this use.

A B C D

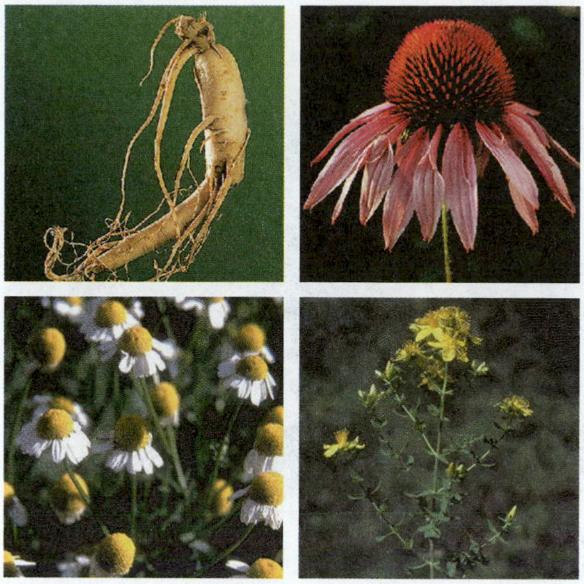

FIG. 8-6 Herbs. **A,** Ginseng. **B,** Echinacea. **C,** Chamomile. **D,** St. John's wort.

TABLE 8-11 Commonly Used Dietary Supplements*

Name	Examples of Common Uses	Comments
Chondroitin sulfate	Osteoarthritis†	Often combined with glucosamine
Coenzyme Q_{10}	Hypertension‡	Can reduce insulin requirements
Dehydroepi-androsterone (DHEA)	Osteoporosis§	Long-term safety unknown
Fish oil/omega-3 fatty acids	Hypertension† Hypertriglyceridemia† Cardiovascular disease prevention† Rheumatoid arthritis‡	Use product free of toxins
Glucosamine	Knee osteoarthritis† Osteoarthritis (in general)‡ Rheumatoid arthritis§	Use with caution in individuals with allergy to shellfish
Green tea	Cancer prevention§ High cholesterol§ Weight loss§	Contains caffeine, which is a stimulant of the central nervous system May add to effects of other stimulants May reduce effectiveness of warfarin
Melatonin	Jet lag† Insomnia in the elderly‡	Generally safe in recommended dosages for short-term use May increase risk of bleeding May lower BP

From Ulbricht CE, Basch EM: *Natural standard herb and supplement reference: evidence-based clinical reviews*, St Louis, 2005, Mosby. Available at *www.naturalstandard.com.*

*Advise patients who are pregnant or lactating to consult a health care practitioner before using any supplements. There is limited scientific evidence for use during pregnancy or lactation.

†Strong scientific evidence exists for this use.

‡Good scientific evidence exists for this use.

§Unclear scientific evidence exists for this use.

COMPLEMENTARY AND ALTERNATIVE THERAPIES

Complementary and Alternative Therapies Boxes Throughout the Book

Information related to various complementary and alternative therapies can be found in the following boxes throughout the book.

Massage Therapy

Massage therapy includes a range of techniques that manipulate the soft tissues and joints of the body. Involving touch and movement, massage is typically delivered with the hands, although elbows, forearms, or feet may be used. Massage techniques are used in body-work, sports training, physical therapy, nursing, chiropractic therapy, osteopathy, and naturopathy. Benefits of massage relate to its effects on the musculoskeletal, circulatory, lymphatic, and nervous systems. Massage also positively affects mental and emotional states. Massage therapy continues to grow in popularity, with most people using massage therapy as a means to reduce stress.

Clinical Applications of Massage Therapy. Until the 1970s nurses were taught to perform "PM care," which consisted of a back rub and other measures to promote relaxation and sleep. After that time PM care and back rubs became the exception rather than the rule. Yet today, with the increased focus on providing holistic care, nurses are again recognizing the benefits of massage. Massage is a form of touch and also a form of caring, communication, and comfort. The role of the nurse regarding massage differs from that of the registered massage therapist. Whereas massage

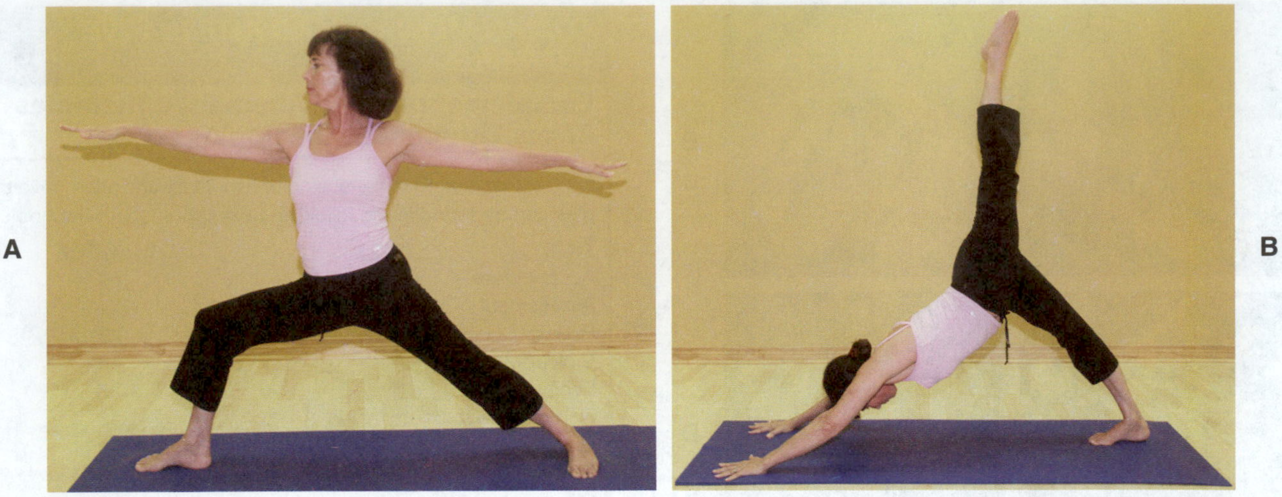

FIG. 8-7 Yoga postures promote strength, flexibility, and diaphragmatic breathing. **A,** Warrior pose strengthens the legs, ankles, and groin. **B,** Downward-facing dog variation stretches the shoulders, hamstrings, calves, arches, and hands.

therapists can provide more comprehensive massage therapies, nurses can use specific massage techniques as part of nursing care, when indicated by the nursing diagnosis or patient assessment. For example, a back massage can be used to help promote sleep. For a bedridden patient, gentle massage can stimulate circulation and help prevent skin breakdown.

When a nurse identifies that massage may be indicated in meeting a patient goal, the nurse must first assess the patient's preference regarding touch and massage. The nurse should consider cultural and social beliefs, and discuss potential benefits with the patient. The indicated plan of care (e.g., hand massage, back massage) can then be implemented, with reassessment following the massage.

Massage Techniques. Nursing use of massage typically begins with *effleurage,* or gliding strokes, to promote relaxation. Stroking is done from distal to proximal, along the long axis of the muscle (Fig. 8-8, *A*). After relaxing the muscles with effleurage, *petrissage,* or a "kneading" stroke, may be used to gently lift and knead the muscle (Fig. 8-8, *B*). Gently scented lotions or diluted essential oils may be included in the massage.

A simple hand massage (Fig. 8-9) can be used to have a calming and relaxing effect, especially for patients who are anxious or agitated. When a patient is frustrated or agitated, a hand massage can distract a person and return him or her to a calm state.

Family members can be taught to perform massage on their loved one, providing a way for family members to participate in patient care. This can be therapeutic for both the patient and the family, even when the loved one is mentally ill or unresponsive. Massage is beneficial throughout the life continuum. During the end-of-life process, hospice nurses may incorporate massage into their nursing care, as the massaging touch can lessen pain and restlessness.

Massage is contraindicated in patients who have recent injuries or trauma, recent surgery, open wounds, deep vein thrombosis, inflammation or infections, bleeding, edema, or decreased sensation. Massage therapy is also contraindicated when someone has used alcohol or recreational drugs.

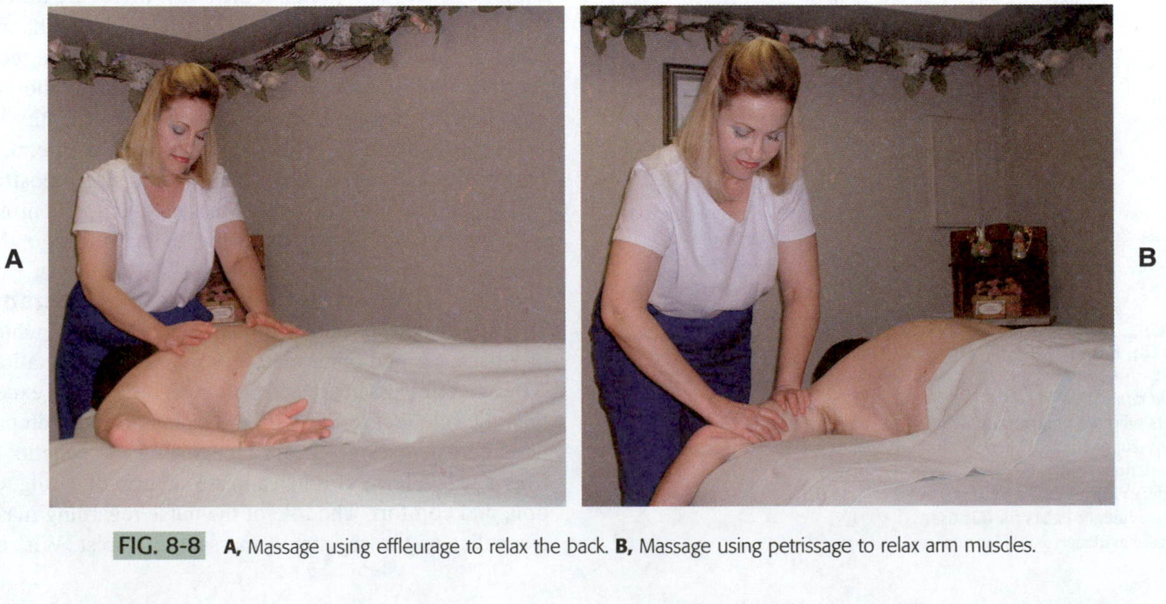

FIG. 8-8 **A,** Massage using effleurage to relax the back. **B,** Massage using petrissage to relax arm muscles.

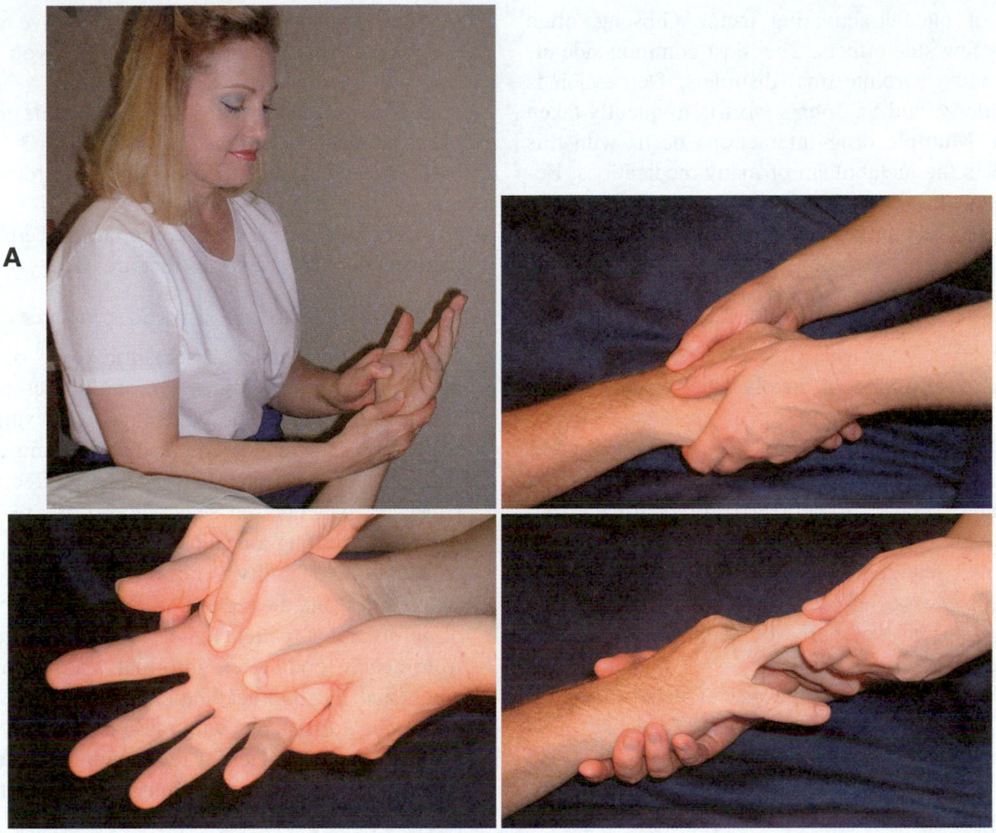

FIG. 8-9 **A,** Hand massage. **B,** Technique of hand massage: Bend the wrist backward and forward to relax the wrist, then massage the wrist and top of the hand, using circular movements. **C,** Massage the palm of the hand with the cushions of the thumbs, using circular movements. **D,** Massage each finger from the base to the tip.

ENERGY THERAPIES

Energy therapies are those that involve the manipulation of energy fields. They focus on energy fields originating within the body (biofields) or those from other sources (electromagnetic fields). Examples of biofield therapies include Therapeutic Touch, Healing Touch, and Reiki. Biofield therapies are based on the theory that energy systems in the body need to be balanced to enhance healing. Some forms of energy therapy manipulate biofields by placing the hands in, or through, these fields.

Therapeutic Touch

Therapeutic Touch (TT) is a method of detecting and balancing human energy (see Table 8-7). It involves the conscious use of the hands to direct or modulate human energy fields. It is a contemporary interpretation of several ancient healing practices. TT was developed in the 1970s by a nurse, Dolores Krieger, and a traditional healer, Doris Kunz. TT is based on the assumptions that a human being is an open energy system, a balanced flow of energy underlies good health, and illness is a reflection of an imbalance in an individual's energy field.

Clinical Applications of Therapeutic Touch. During the actual treatment, nurses use their hands to assess the patient's energy field. Hands are positioned 2 to 6 inches from the body. The energy field is assessed for bilateral similarities or differences in the flow of energy. The next step is clearing and balancing the energy field. Nurses then redirect energy through their own intentionality. The session ends with a smoothing of the energy. TT is not a diagnostic tool, but is used as a form of treatment in conjunction with a biomedical treatment plan.

The North American Nursing Diagnosis Association has accepted the nursing diagnosis "energy field disturbance," for which TT is an appropriate intervention. Research has been conducted on the effectiveness of TT for a wide range of conditions, including wound healing; sleep promotion; enhancement of immune function; and the reduction of anxiety, agitation, postoperative pain, tension headache, and stress. The findings are inconclusive and indicate the need for further research.

Specialized instruction is needed to perform TT. Some individuals are able to "feel" the energy field more readily than others. However, with patience, determination, and a desire to help others, anyone (including families) can learn to use TT.

GERONTOLOGIC CONSIDERATIONS
COMPLEMENTARY AND ALTERNATIVE THERAPIES

Older adults with non–life-threatening, chronic conditions are most likely to use complementary and alternative therapies. They report satisfaction with these therapies, relating improvements in both mental and physical health. They value the ability to make treatment decisions themselves, and they regard their practitioner as a partner in their care. Trust is a critical part of the patient-provider relationship and correlates with patient satisfaction with these therapies.[24]

One common complementary and alternative therapy used by older adults is herbal therapy. Herbs commonly used include ginkgo biloba, ginseng, St. John's wort, saw palmetto, and echinacea. Gingko is often used to prevent deterioration in cognitive function. Older adults need to be monitored for bleeding due to gingko's inhibition of platelet-activating factor. Ginseng, often used for fatigue, has few side effects. The most common side effects are headache and gastrointestinal disorders. Depression is widespread in the elderly, and St. John's wort is frequently taken for mild depression. Multiple drug interactions occur with this herb, because it affects the metabolism of many medications. Before an older adult uses St. John's wort, it is important to determine if any of the medications that the patient is taking will interact with the herb. Saw palmetto is usually well tolerated and can reduce the symptoms of benign prostatic hyperplasia (BPH) in older men. Echinacea, commonly used for upper respiratory infections, is usually well tolerated.[25]

For the older adult, safety concerns involve age-related changes and polypharmacy. Age-related changes, such as osteoporosis or fragile skin, may affect the use of manipulative or manual therapies. Decreased renal or liver function may slow metabolism and excretion of herbs and dietary supplements. Polypharmacy (described in Chapter 6) addresses multiple medications taken by one patient. Clearly this may lead to herb-drug or dietary supplement–drug interactions. This is especially problematic because patients often do not disclose the use of herbs or supplements to their health care provider.

Socioeconomic factors can affect the use of these therapies. Older adults report that the requirement for out-of-pocket payments is frequently a barrier to the use of these therapies. With the rising cost of health care, patients may select herbs or dietary supplement in place of prescription drugs.

Most older adults would welcome a better integration of conventional medicine with complementary and alternative therapies. Better education about complementary and alternative therapies and how to safely use them is needed for all adults, especially the elderly.

NURSING MANAGEMENT COMPLEMENTARY *and* ALTERNATIVE THERAPIES

The role of the nurse with respect to complementary and alternative therapies is evolving. Roles of the nurse may include (1) assessing a patient's use of complementary and alternative therapies and the possible risk of complications or adverse interactions with conventional therapies, (2) promoting safety and serving as a resource, (3) providing holistic self-care and holistic nursing care, (4) serving as a provider, and (5) participating in research.

Nursing Assessment

It is important for the nurse to collect data on patients' use of complementary and alternative therapies. This is especially important because most patients do not voluntarily tell their health care provider about their use of these therapies. However, they will usually share this information with a nurse when asked. Nurses need to ask general open-ended questions, while remaining nonjudgmental and respectful of the patient's response.

Examples of assessment questions include the following:

1. What are you doing to maintain or improve your health and wellness?
2. How involved are you in planning and carrying out your health-related care?
3. What is your view of the ideal relationship between yourself and your health care provider(s)?
4. Do you have any conditions that have not responded to conventional medicine? If so, have you tried any other approaches?
5. Are you using any vitamin, mineral, dietary, or herbal supplements?
6. Are you interested in obtaining information about alternative or complementary approaches?

Along with assessing use, the nurse needs to document the effectiveness of interventions that are used.

Promoting Safety and Serving as a Resource

The American Nurses Association Code of Ethics states: "The nurse promotes, advocates for, and strives to protect the health, safety, and rights of the patient." A wide variety of therapies fall within the category of complementary and alternative therapies, and some of these therapies may be ineffective or even harmful. However, patients self-select use of these therapies, generally without consulting a health care professional. Safety concerns encompass the reliability of information, the safety and effectiveness of therapies, and the regulation of practitioners. Regarding sources of information, patients most commonly get their information from health food stores, informal word of mouth, books, magazines, and the Internet. Patients need to be encouraged to seek professional assistance with these decisions.

Also, there is a lack of regulation of some types of providers. In most states, for example, massage therapists and acupuncturists are licensed by the state. However, this practice varies by state. Practitioners of some other modalities are more loosely regulated. Along with facing the challenge of obtaining accurate information, patients may be unable to assess the competency of practitioners. The nurse can serve as a resource to guide patients in the safe use of therapies and in the safe choice of health care practitioners.

Serving as a patient advocate, the nurse provides information on both conventional therapies and complementary and alternative therapies. Patients should be advised that complementary therapies do not replace conventional therapies, but can often be used in combination with conventional therapies. By providing information for the patient, the nurse fosters informed decision making.

To serve as a resource for patients, nurses must first develop their own knowledge base. Even if specific information about complementary and alternative therapies is not provided in basic nursing programs, nurses are educated as critical thinkers and problem solvers. Thus nurses are prepared to seek ongoing education regarding complementary and alternative therapies and to continue to read and critique research conducted about these therapies.

Providing Holistic Self-Care and Holistic Nursing Practice

Some individuals choose to become nurses because they want to care for others—to be a caregiver for their patients. This is a compelling reason to choose nursing. Yet many nurses fail to recognize that "caring for others" can occur only when one's values and practices include "care for self." In their careers nurses eventually learn that "they can offer their best selves, their best vitality and caring, only when their own cup is full."[26] *Self-care* (caring for one's own general level of health and well-being) is essential on both a personal and professional level. On a *personal* level self-care involves commitment to maintaining one's own level of wellness. Keeping one's mind, body, and spirit healthy is required so that one has the strength to care for others. On a *professional* level self-care is important because nurses are role models. They are role models for family, friends, patients, health care professionals, and the community. By demonstrating self-care practices, nurses motivate others to achieve greater health and wellness.

Learning about complementary and alternative therapies can be one road to self-care. Initially, nurses are eager to learn about complementary and alternative therapies so that they can provide better patient care and be holistic practitioners. Yet nurses often find that these therapies can be used personally to enhance their own level of health and wellness. Since many different therapies are included as part of complementary and alternative therapies, each individual nurse should be able to find ways to promote personal well-being. Examples of therapies commonly used by nurses for personal well-being include relaxation breathing, meditation, prayer, yoga, massage, and music. It is essential that the "caregiver" first care for him- or herself.

Professional nursing from its onset included care of the whole person, which is the concept of mind-body-spirit. However, the Western biomedical model, with its focus on the physical body, resulted in nursing moving its practice to a more "medical" model. The recent growth of the use of complementary and alternative therapies provides an opportunity for nursing to return to its origin and a focus on holistic nursing practice. **Holistic nursing** incorporates mind-body-spirit principles into the development of a caring-healing relationship with patients. Core concepts of holistic nursing include the following: (1) the nurse accepts patients as they are, without judgment and with compassion; (2) the nurse's care is based on holism and integrates mind-body-spirit principles; (3) the nurse serves as a facilitator, recognizing the patient's capacity for self-healing; (4) the nurse incorporates self-care and self-responsibility, recognizing the greater interconnectedness of all individuals; and (5) the nurse's practice is guided by holistic education and research.[27]

Nursing interventions include therapeutic listening and empathy. The nurse also promotes a therapeutic environment and honors cultural diversity. The holistic nurse may also choose to integrate complementary and alternative therapies as part of nursing practice, recognizing the value of both conventional and complementary and alternative therapies.

Serving as a Provider

Nursing has a long history of providing therapies that have been considered complementary and alternative. These include massage, relaxation therapy, music therapy, and Therapeutic Touch, as well as other strategies to promote comfort, reduce stress, improve coping, and promote symptom relief (Table 8-12). Although these therapies are generally included within the scope of nursing practice, they are not specifically addressed in some U.S. state nursing practice acts. Similarly, practice acts in the United Kingdom and Australia address nurses' accountability for their own actions and their responsibility to know their limitations and function within those limits.

Some of these therapies require additional education and/or supervision. The nurse must check with the Board of Nursing/Practice Act to determine what therapies fall within the nursing domain in a specific state. The nurse is always expected to obtain the necessary additional education and experience in order to be competent to use a selected therapy. Institutional or workplace policies must be in place, supporting the use of these therapies.

TABLE 8-12 Complementary and Alternative Therapies That Can Be Integrated Into Nursing Practice

• Acupressure	• Massage
• Acupuncture	• Meditation
• Animal-assisted therapy	• Music
• Aromatherapy	• Prayer
• Healing Touch	• Relaxation breathing
• Humor	• Reiki
• Imagery	• Therapeutic Touch
• Journaling	

Nurses are responsible for ensuring that the patient has given consent for a given therapy. The patient must be aware of the proposed benefit and any potential risks involved. The nurse needs to document the effectiveness of the interventions. A mechanism needs to be in place to evaluate the outcomes of care.

Participating in Research

Nurses are responsible for critiquing research and applying relevant research findings to their practice, as well as participating in the identification of researchable problems. Using summaries of research evidence on complementary and alternative therapies is one strategy for developing evidence-based practice. Practicing with a questioning mind can facilitate identification of research questions that can be investigated with research-trained health care professionals. In the Western biomedical model, research is conducted using randomized controlled trials (RCTs). This is considered the "gold standard" of clinical research studies. However, challenges arise when researchers attempt to use RCTs to study complementary and alternative therapies. Difficulties include the following: (1) the individualized treatments of complementary and alternative therapies can make findings difficult to generalize; (2) the aim of complementary and alternative therapies is often to promote health, rather than treat disease; (3) the outcomes of complementary and alternative therapies may take months, even years, to achieve; (4) the effects of the treatments are often subtle and difficult to quantify; (5) complementary and alternative therapies are often used in combination; and (6) the widespread use of these therapies has led to a general belief that they are effective.[2]

Other questions that arise include the following: What about the patient's relationship with the health care provider? What about the placebo effect? New innovative study designs are being developed to scientifically examine these therapies. Examples of such designs include observational and cohort studies, case-control studies, and studies of combinations of therapies.[2]

Patient interest and participation in complementary and alternative therapies is increasing. Therefore it is important for nurses to be knowledgeable of the multiple therapies available and to develop effective strategies to document the use of these therapies. It is also important for nurses to know about the current research being done in this area to provide accurate information to both patients and other health care professionals. Nurses are well positioned to become the "link" between conventional therapy and complementary and alternative therapies.

INTEGRATIVE NURSING PRACTICE

Scripps Center for Integrative Medicine in La Jolla, California

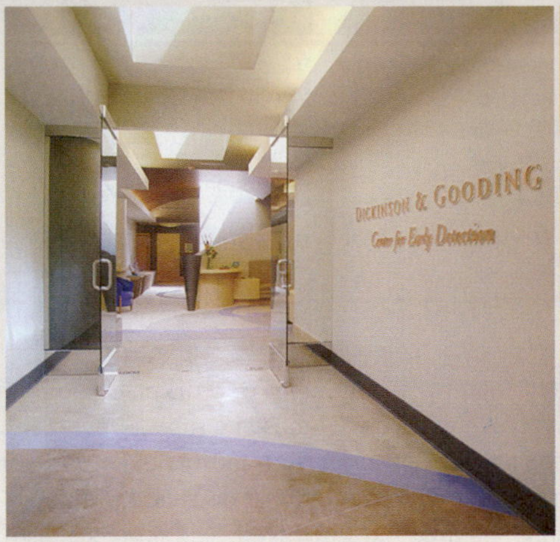

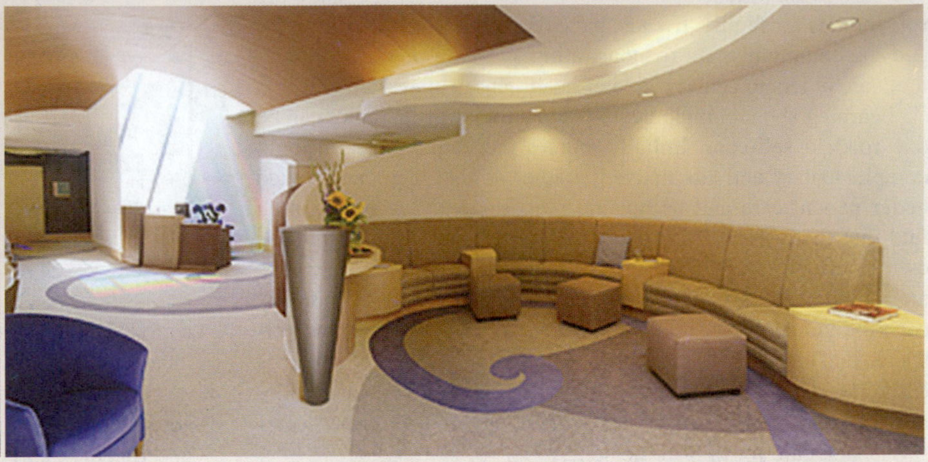

The Scripps Center for Integrative Medicine is a place where people come to find healing for their body, mind, and spirit. The Center is part of Scripps Health, a five-hospital system in San Diego, California. The Center overlooks the Pacific Ocean and the world-famous Torrey Pines Golf Course. The setting contributes to the Center's healing environment. The Center's architecture was designed to elicit a calm, peaceful state of mind. The healing environment is based on principles of sacred geometry.

Features

The Center blends a combination of conventional health care with complementary therapies to support health and healing. The focus is on physical, emotional, mental, and spiritual healing. A full spectrum of care is provided, from prevention to treatment and rehabilitation.

Complementary Therapies

Biofeedback, acupuncture, Healing Touch, osteopathic manipulation, homeopathic remedies, herbal therapies, and massage, as well as classes on yoga, meditation, stress management, music therapy, and spirituality, are offered.

Case Study

Charles H., a 56-year-old newly diagnosed cardiac patient, comes to the Scripps Center emergency department with chest pain. He is rushed to the cardiac catheterization laboratory for an interventional procedure including angioplasty and stent placement. These procedures are extremely stressful for him, as well as his loved ones. He is not only in physical crisis but in emotional, mental, and spiritual crisis as well. With the use of complementary therapies, the team is able to assist him with his nonphysical needs.

After 1 week he is scheduled for bypass surgery after the stent does not alleviate his chest pain. The Center's protocol for open-heart surgery patients is to have a complementary therapy services coordinator (a nurse) see the patient before surgery if possible. Charles receives a Healing Touch treatment to balance his energy system for the best possible outcome. Charles receives guided imagery CDs, which helps to prepare him emotionally, mentally, and spiritually for the procedure. When he arrives in the intensive care unit after surgery, he receives Healing Touch again. At that point he receives a guided imagery CD that focuses on pain management.

The Center's patient outcome surveys show that patients' pain and anxiety decrease with the use of Healing Touch and guided imagery. The Center's vision of "healing people and changing lives through science and compassion" forms the basis for all of the care provided.

Provided by Rauni Prittinen King, RN, BSN, HNC, CHTPP/I, Founder and Manager of the Center.

NCLEX EXAMINATION REVIEW QUESTIONS

The number of the question corresponds to the same-numbered objective at the beginning of the chapter.

1. One characteristic of the integrative model of health care is
   a. a focus on physical disease states.
   b. an integration of mind-body-spirit.
   c. that the plan of care is directed by the health care provider.
   d. that American consumers' interest in this model is decreasing.
2. Complementary and alternative therapies can be described as therapies
   a. used as a primary form of treatment.
   b. that contradict the values of nursing.
   c. based on extensive scientific research.
   d. outside the Western biomedical model.
3. Which of the following patients is most likely to benefit from treatment by a Traditional Chinese Medicine practitioner?
   a. A patient with pneumonia
   b. A patient with mental illness
   c. A patient with chronic back pain
   d. A postoperative patient with low blood pressure
4. A common complication of the use of garlic, ginkgo, ginseng, and ginger is
   a. allergic reactions.
   b. clotting alterations.
   c. skin photosensitivity.
   d. increased blood pressure.
5. Which of the following concepts should be included in patient teaching regarding use of herbal products?
   a. All herbal products are safe to use.
   b. Herbal products are effective immediately.
   c. Herbal products' labels give all essential information.
   d. Use of herbal products needs to be reported to the patient's health care provider.
6. Which of the following statements describes holistic nursing?
   a. Holistic nursing focuses on physical health.
   b. Holistic nursing is practiced only by experienced nurses.

c. Holistic nursing promotes self-care and self-responsibility.
d. Holistic nursing is based on the biomedical model of health care.

7. In assessing a patient's use of complementary and alternative therapies, it is important that the nurse do all of the following *except*
   a. assess the patient's use and frequency of use of these therapies.
   b. determine the patient's knowledge of the therapies that he or she is using.
   c. use the term "alternative therapies" when assessing the patient's use of these therapies.
   d. create an open and nonjudgmental environment where the patient will be comfortable to discuss use of these therapies.
8. Roles of the nurse regarding complementary and alternative therapies include
   a. caring for patients rather than caring for self.
   b. prescribing the appropriate herbal therapies for a patient.
   c. serving as a resource to guide patients in the safe use of therapies.
   d. advocating for use of complementary and alternative therapies instead of conventional health care.

REFERENCES

1. Fontaine K: *Complementary and alternative therapies for nursing practice,* ed 2, Upper Saddle River, NJ, 2005, Prentice Hall.
2. Institute of Medicine: *Complementary and alternative medicine in the United States,* Washington, DC, 2005, National Academies Press.
3. Schlitz M, Amorok T, Micozzi M: *Consciousness and healing: integral approaches to mind-body medicine,* St Louis, 2005, Elsevier.
4. Frisch N, et al: *AHNA standards of holistic nursing practice: guidelines for caring and healing,* Gaithersburg, Md, 2000, Aspen.
5. National Center for Complementary and Alternative Medicine. Available at *www.nccam.nih.gov* (accessed February 27, 2005).
6. Ezzo J, Berman BM, Vickers AJ, et al: Complementary medicine and the Cochrane Collaboration, *JAMA* 280:1628, 1998.
7. Astin J: Why patients use alternative medicine: results of a national study, *JAMA* 279:1548, 1998.
8. Eisenberg DM, Kessler RC, Foster C, et al: Unconventional medicine in the United States, prevalence, costs and patterns of use, *N Engl J Med* 328:246, 1993.
9. Eisenberg DM, Davis RB, Ettner SL, et al: Trends in alternative medicine use in the United States, 1990-1997: results of a follow up study, *JAMA* 280:1569, 1998.
10. Eisenberg DM, Kessler RC, Van Rompay MI, et al: Perceptions about complementary therapies relative to conventional therapies among adults who use both: results from a national survey, *Ann Intern Med* 135:344, 2001.
11. Ni H, Simile C, Hardy A: Utilization of complementary and alternative medicine by United States adults: results from the 1999 National Health Interview Survey, *Med Care* 40:353, 2002.
12. Parkman C: CAM therapies and nursing competency, *Journal for Nurses in Staff Development* 18:61, 2002.
13. National Center for Complementary and Alternative Medicine: The use of complementary and alternative medicine in the United States. Available at *www.nccam.nih.gov/news/camsurvey* (accessed February 27, 2005).
14. Freeman L: *Complementary and alternative medicine: a research based approach,* St Louis, 2004, Mosby.
15. Berman B, Lao L, Langenberg P, et al: Effectiveness of acupuncture as adjunctive therapy in osteoarthritis of the knee, *Ann Intern Med* 141:901, 2004.
16. Birch S, Hesselink JK, Jonkman FA, et al: Clinical research on acupuncture (part 1): what have reviews of the efficacy and safety of acupuncture told us so far, *Journal of Alternative and Complementary Medicine* 10:468, 2004.
17. Weil A: Focus on therapy, stick with acupuncture, *Self Healing, Creating Natural Health for Your Body and Mind Newsletter,* February 8, 2004.
18. White P, Lewith G, Prescott P, et al: Acupuncture versus placebo for the treatment of chronic mechanical neck pain, *Ann Intern Med* 141:911, 2004.
19. Taylor E: Prayer's clinical issues and implications, *Holistic Nursing Practice* 17:179, 2003.
20. Levin J: *God, faith, and health: exploring the spirituality-healing connection,* New York, 2001, Wiley.
21. Ameling A: Prayer: an ancient healing practice becomes new again, *Holistic Nursing Practice* 14:40, 2000.
22. Cavendish R, Konecny L, Luise BK, et al: Nurses enhance performance through prayer, *Holistic Nursing Practice* 18:26, 2004.
23. Tindle H, Davis RB, Phillips RS, et al: Trends in use of complementary and alternative medicine by US adults: 1997-2002, *Alternative Therapies* 11:42, 2005.
24. Willison K, Andrews G: Complementary medicine and older people: past research and future directions, *Complementary/Therapies in Nursing and Midwifery* 10:80, 2004.
25. Albrecht C: Botanical and diet-based biological therapies and their use by older persons: part 1, *Clinical Geriatrics* 13:26, 2005.
26. Andrus V: Caring for self, becoming a healing presence, *AHNA Beginnings* 25:1, 2005.
27. Dossey B, Keegan L, Guzzetta C: *Holistic nursing: a handbook for practice,* Sudbury, Mass, 2005, Jones & Bartlett.

RESOURCES

Acupuncture Today
www.acupuncturetoday.com

American Association of Oriental Medicine
www.aaom.org

American Botanical Council
www.herbalgram.org

American Holistic Nurses Association
www.ahna.org

American Massage Therapy Association
www.amtamassage.org

Association for Applied Psychophysiology and Biofeedback
303-422-8436
800-477-8892
Email: aapb@resourcenter.com
www.aapb.org
www.biofeedback.org

Center for Food Safety and Applied Nutrition
www.cfsan.fda.gov

Center for Spirituality and Healing at the University of Minnesota
www.csh.umn.edu

Consumer Labs
www.consumerlabs.com

Dr. Andrew Weil
Director of Program in Integrative Medicine
University of Arizona
www.drweil.com

George Washington Institute for Spirituality and Health
www.gwish.org

Healing Touch International
www.healingtouch.net

Healthfinder, a Service of the National Information Center
U.S. Department of Health and Human Services
www.healthfinder.gov

MedlinePlus—Alternative Medicine
U.S. National Library of Medicine
www.nlm.nih.gov/medlineplus/alternativemedicine.html

National Center for Complementary and Alternative Medicine (NCCAM)
National Institutes of Health
www.nccam.nih.gov

Natural Standard
www.naturalstandard.com

Office of Dietary Supplements
National Institutes of Health
www.ods.od.nih.gov

Therapeutic Touch
NH-PAI, Inc.
www.therapeutic-touch.org

The most wasted of all days is that on which one has not laughed.

Nicolas-Sebastien Chamfort

9 Stress and Stress Management

Sharon L. Lewis and Cory A. Shaw

LEARNING OBJECTIVES

1. Differentiate between the terms *stressor* and *stress.*
2. Explain the role of coping in managing stress.
3. Describe the role of the nervous and endocrine systems in the stress process.
4. Describe the effects of stress on the immune system.
5. Discuss the effects of stress on health.
6. Describe the coping and relaxation strategies that can be used by a nurse or patient experiencing stress.
7. Describe the nursing assessment and management of a patient experiencing stress.

KEY TERMS

coping, p. 116
imagery, p. 118
meditation, p. 117
psychoneuroimmunology, p. 114
relaxation (abdominal) breathing, p. 117
stress, p. 110
stressors, p. 111

Electronic Resources

Supplemental content related to Chapter 9 can be found . . .

Companion CD
- Stress-Busting Kit for Nursing Students
  - Take a Yoga Break
- NCLEX Examination Review Questions
- Comprehensive Glossary

Evolve Website
http://evolve.elsevier.com/Lewis/medsurg
- Content Updates
- Key Points (Printable and CD/MP3 Download)
- Concept Map Creator
- Expanded Audio Glossary
- Key Term Flash Cards
- Electronic Calculators
- WebLinks

What goes on in one's mind influences every part of the body. Stress has a powerful effect on the mind and therefore a significant effect on one's health and well-being.

Stress is linked to leading causes of death, including heart disease, cancer, accidents, and suicide. Chronic stress can double a person's risk of having a myocardial infarction. Seventy-five percent of visits to doctor's offices concern stress-related ailments.[1] Thus the study of stress is very important in understanding its role in relationship to physical and emotional health.

Our current understanding of stress began with Hans Selye, who did his research at McGill University in Montreal about 70 years ago. He conceptualized stress as a response to an environmental demand or stressor. He identified stress as a nonspecific response of the body to any demand made on it. Selye referred to these stress-inducing demands as *stressors.*[2]

Although much of his original research focused on physiologic stressors or what Selye called "diverse nocuous agents," extensive research since that time has shown that stress can also be caused by a wide variety of emotional and psychologic events. Nurses can have a very important role in helping patients manage stressful events. Therefore the primary focus of this chapter is on emotional/psychologic stress.

DEFINITION OF STRESS

Stress occurs when individuals perceive that they cannot adequately cope with the demands being made on them or with the threats to their well-being[3] (Fig. 9-1). Circumstances or events are stressful only if the person perceives them as a stressor. What is emotionally or psychologically stressful to one person may not be stressful to another. In humans there can be great variability among

Reviewed by Virginia Shaw, RN, MSN, Certified in Holistic Stress Management, Clinical Assistant Professor, School of Nursing, University of Texas Health Science Center—San Antonio, San Antonio, Tex.

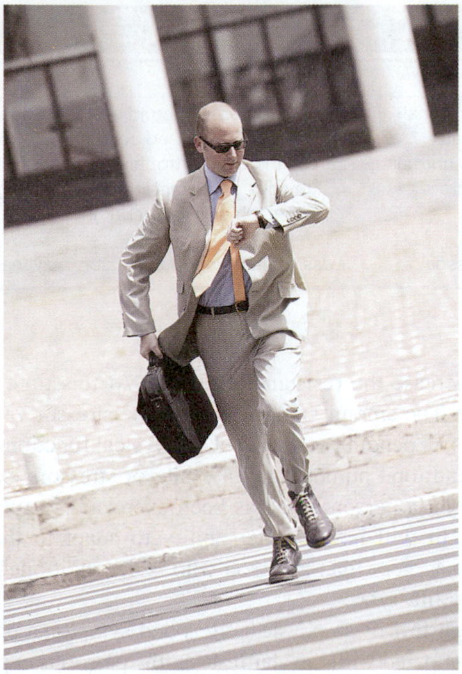

FIG. 9-1 During stressful situations, the demands seem to exceed the resources, such as the amount of time in a day.

individuals in response to the same stressor. Stress perception and personal meaning attached to a potential stressor influence the way an individual responds to a stressor. This is demonstrated in the following examples.

> A nurse may be surprised by a woman's response to a laparoscopic hysterectomy when she becomes very depressed following surgery and refuses to participate in normal self-care activities. In this situation the removal of her uterus is a great stressor because the woman perceives it as a loss of her womanhood and femininity.
>
> In another situation the nurse is surprised when a patient who is told she has type 2 diabetes reacts with a smile. The nurse is perplexed, thinking that this diagnosis would be very stressful for the patient. However, the patient is relieved because for weeks she has been very stressed worrying that her symptoms were related to terminal cancer.

Many different events, factors, or stimuli can be called **stressors.** They can be physiologic or emotional/psychologic (Table 9-1). The emotional/psychologic stressors can be positive or negative. The key aspect of stressors is that they require an individual to adapt.[3] In addition, there are differences in the behavioral and physiologic adaptive responses to a stressor based on the duration of a stressor (acute or chronic) and intensity of a stressor (mild, moderate, or severe). For example, an individual dealing with the chronic stress of caring for a loved one may also be exposed to a multitude of acute episodic stressors (e.g., car accident, influenza). Therefore the type, duration, and intensity of a stressor are important variables that can influence an individual's adaptive response.

TABLE 9-1 Examples of Stressors

Physiologic	Emotional/Psychologic
Skin burn	Diagnosis of cancer
Chronic pain	Marital problems
Hypothermia	Failing an examination
Infectious disease	Inadequate financial resources to meet needs
Excessive noise	Grieving the loss of a family member
Starvation	Caring for a disabled child
Running a marathon	Winning or losing an athletic event
Birth of a baby	Winning the lottery

FACTORS AFFECTING RESPONSE TO STRESS

Why do people respond so differently to stress? Why do some people cope better with stress than others? Interestingly, some individuals experience significant adverse life events but do not succumb to the effects of stress. Factors that affect an individual's response to stress include internal and external influences (Table 9-2). These factors indicate the importance of using a holistic approach when assessing the impact of stress on an individual.

In attempting to understand why some individuals do not have negative consequences from stress, researchers have identified key personal characteristics, such as hardiness, sense of coherence, resilience, and attitude, as possible factors that buffer the impact of stress. *Hardiness* is believed to be a mediating factor in the relationship between stress and illness.[4] The hardy person has (1) a clear sense of personal values and goals, (2) a strong tendency toward interaction with the environment, (3) a sense of meaningfulness, and (4) an internal rather than external locus of control. An *internal locus of control* means that the hardy person perceives that her or his life is self-determined as opposed to being directed by outside/external events or luck/chance (an *external locus of control*).

Sense of coherence (SOC), a concept closely related to hardiness, is believed to be a more powerful mediator of stress and illness than hardiness and is a key determinant of health.[5,6] In general, SOC refers to how an individual sees the world and one's life in it. The three components of SOC are comprehensibility (stimuli derived from one's internal and external environments are structured, predictable, and explorable), manageability (resources are available to meet the demands posed by these stimuli), and meaningfulness (demands are challenges worthy of investment and engagement). An individual with a strong SOC has an enduring tendency to see one's life as ordered, predictable, and manageable. On

TABLE 9-2 Factors Affecting an Individual's Response to Stress

Internal	External
Age	Cultural and ethnic influences
Health status	Socioeconomic status
Personality characteristics	Social support
Previous experience with stressors	Religious/spiritual influences
Genetic background	Timing of stressors
Hardiness	Number of stressors already experiencing
Sense of coherence	
Resilience	
Attitude	
Nutritional status	
Sleep status	

TABLE 9-3 Stages of the General Adaptation Syndrome

Alarm	Resistance	Exhaustion
Increased secretion of corticosteroids and resultant changes Increased activity of sympathetic nervous system Increased norepinephrine secretion by adrenal medulla "Fight-or-flight" syndrome changes (see Fig. 9-5)	Corticosteroid secretion returns to normal Sympathetic activity returns to normal Norepinephrine secretion returns to normal "Fight-or-flight" syndrome disappears	Increased corticosteroid secretion but eventually marked decreased secretion Stress triad (hypertrophied adrenals, atrophied thymus and lymph nodes, bleeding ulcers in stomach and duodenum)
Low resistance to stressor	*High resistance (adaptation) to stressor*	*Loss of resistance to stressor; may lead to death*

Adapted from Thibodeau GA, Patton KT: *Anatomy and physiology,* ed 6, St Louis, 2007, Mosby.

the other hand, individuals with a weaker SOC are more likely to interpret stressors as threatening or anxiety provoking.[7]

Resilience is another characteristic that is believed to moderate or buffer the negative effects of stress. **Resilience** is defined as being resourceful, being flexible, and having an available source of problem-solving strategies. Individuals who possess a high degree of resilience are not as likely to perceive an event as stressful or taxing.[8]

Attitude can also affect the way stress affects a person. People with positive attitudes view situations differently from those with negative attitudes. How stress is managed also depends on a person's attitude. To some extent positive emotional attitudes can prevent disease and prolong life.[9]

Optimists are able to cope more effectively with stress. Optimism also reduces a person's chances of developing stress-related illnesses. When optimistic people do become ill, they tend to recover more quickly. Pessimists are likely to deny the problem, distance themselves from the stressful event, focus on stressful feelings, or allow the stressor to interfere with achieving a goal. People with a more pessimistic attitude tend to report poorer health compared to people with optimistic attitudes.[10-12]

Characteristics such as hardiness, sense of coherence, resilience, and attitude may help explain why some people remain healthy despite enduring significant stress in their lives. Individuals who are hardy, are resilient, have a strong sense of coherence, and have a positive attitude are more likely to effectively cope with life's stressors.

GENERAL ADAPTATION SYNDROME

Selye's early research using animals showed that stressors from different sources produced a similar physical response. He termed this physical response to stress the **general adaptation syndrome** (GAS).[2] The GAS is composed of three stages: alarm reaction, stage of resistance, and stage of exhaustion (Table 9-3). Once the environmental event or stressor stimulates the central nervous system, multiple responses occur because of activation of the hypothalamic-pituitary-adrenal axis and the autonomic nervous system.

The first stage of the stress response is the *alarm reaction* of the GAS, in which the individual perceives a stressor physically or mentally and the *fight-or-flight response* is initiated. When the stressor is of sufficient intensity to threaten the steady state or homeostasis of the individual, it leads to a series of physiologic changes that promote adaptation. This temporarily decreases the individual's resistance and may even result in disease or death if the stress is prolonged and severe.

Ideally the individual quickly moves from the alarm reaction to the *stage of resistance,* in which physiologic reserves are mobilized to increase the resistance to stress. At this time adaptation may occur. The amount of resistance to the stressor varies among individuals, depending on the level of physical functioning, coping abilities, and total number and intensity of stressors experienced. For example, a person who has been exercising regularly and is physically fit will have greater ability to adapt to the stress of emergency surgery than a person who is deconditioned and leads a sedentary lifestyle.

Although few overt physical signs and symptoms occur in this stage as compared with the alarm stage, the person is expending energy in an attempt to adapt. The resources available to the individual limit this adaptive energy. These resources include not only the individual's internal physical and psychologic reserves, but also external resources such as social support from family, friends, and health care workers. When resources are adequate, the individual may successfully recover from a stressor such as surgery and return to his or her baseline (presurgery) state. If adaptation does not occur, the person may move to the next phase of the GAS.

The *stage of exhaustion* is the final stage of the GAS. It occurs when all of the energy for adaptation has been expended (Fig. 9-2). Physical symptoms of the alarm reaction may briefly reappear in a final effort by the body to survive. A terminally ill person who becomes alert and has stronger vital signs shortly before death exemplifies this. The individual in the stage of exhaustion usually becomes ill and may die if assistance from outside sources is not available. This stage can often be reversed by external sources of adaptive energy, such as medication.

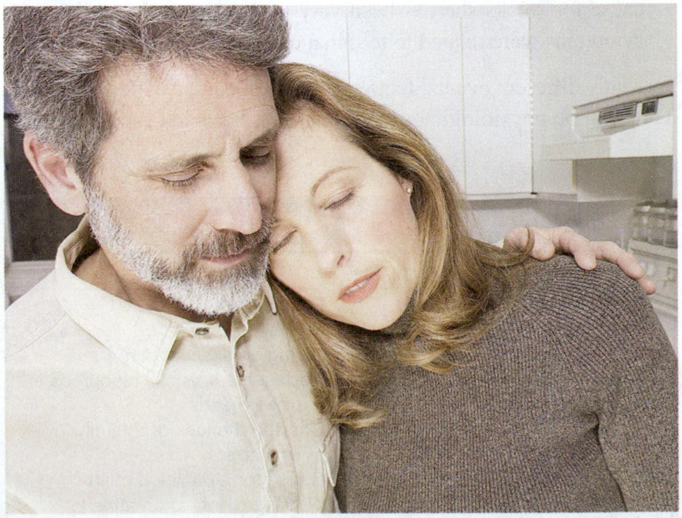

FIG. 9-2 This couple has reached the stage of exhaustion after multiple repeated stressors in their lives.

Selye's research indicated that there is a predictable, uniform pattern in the physiologic response to various stressors. This is due in part to the fact that Selye used animal models that were not capable of representing complex psychologic processing of a stressor.

PHYSIOLOGIC RESPONSE TO STRESS

The following discussion is divided into the roles of the nervous, endocrine, and immune systems. However, these systems are interrelated, and thus the physiologic response of the person to stress reflects the interrelationship of the three systems (Fig. 9-3). Further, stress activation of these systems affects other systems, such as the cardiovascular, respiratory, gastrointestinal, renal, and reproductive systems.

The complex process by which an event is perceived as a stressor and by which the body responds is not fully understood. A person's response to a stressor determines the impact that stress will have on the body. In addition, the body responds physiologically to both actual and potential stressors.

Nervous System

Cerebral Cortex. The cerebral cortex evaluates the emotional/psychologic event (stressor) in light of past experiences and future consequences, and thus plans a course of action. These functions are involved in the perception of a stressor.

Limbic System. The *limbic system* lies in the inner midportion of the brain near the base of the brain. The limbic system is an important mediator of emotions and behavior. When the limbic system is stimulated, emotions, feelings, and behaviors can occur that ensure survival and self-preservation.

Reticular Formation. The *reticular formation* is located between the lower end of the brainstem and the thalamus. It contains the *reticular activating system* (RAS), which sends impulses contributing to alertness to the limbic system and to the cerebral cortex. When the RAS is stimulated, it increases its output of impulses, leading to wakefulness. Stress usually increases the degree of wakefulness and can lead to sleep disturbances.[13]

Hypothalamus. The hypothalamus, which lies at the base of the brain just above the pituitary gland, has many functions that assist in adaptation to stress. Stress activates the limbic system, which in turn stimulates the hypothalamus. Because the hypothalamus secretes neuropeptides that regulate the release of hormones by the anterior pituitary, it is central to the connection between the nervous and endocrine systems in responding to stress (Fig. 9-4).

The hypothalamus plays a primary role in the stress response by regulating the function of both the sympathetic and parasympathetic branches of the autonomic nervous system. When an individual perceives a stressor, the hypothalamus sends signals that initiate both the nervous and endocrine responses to the stressor. It does this primarily by sending signals via nerve fibers to stimulate the sympathetic nervous system (SNS) and by releasing corticotropin-releasing hormone (CRH), which stimulates the pituitary to release adrenocorticotropic hormone (ACTH)[14] (see Chapter 48).

Endocrine System

Once the hypothalamus is activated in response to stress, the endocrine system becomes involved. The SNS stimulates the adrenal medulla to release epinephrine and norepinephrine (catecholamines). The effect of catecholamines and the SNS, including the response of the adrenal medulla, is referred to as the *sympathoadrenal response.* Epinephrine and norepinephrine prepare the body for the *fight-or-flight response* (Fig. 9-5).

Stress activates the hypothalamic-pituitary-adrenal (HPA) axis. In response to stress, the hypothalamus releases CRH, which stimulates the anterior pituitary to release proopiomelanocortin (POMC). Both ACTH (a hormone) and β-endorphin (a neuropeptide) are derived from POMC. Endorphins have analgesic-like effects and blunt pain perception during stress situations involving pain stimuli. ACTH, in turn, stimulates the adrenal cortex to synthesize and secrete corticosteroids (e.g., cortisol) and, to a lesser degree, aldosterone.

Corticosteroids are essential for the stress response. Cortisol produces a number of physiologic effects that include increasing blood glucose levels, potentiating the action of catecholamines on blood vessels, and inhibiting the inflammatory response. Cortico-

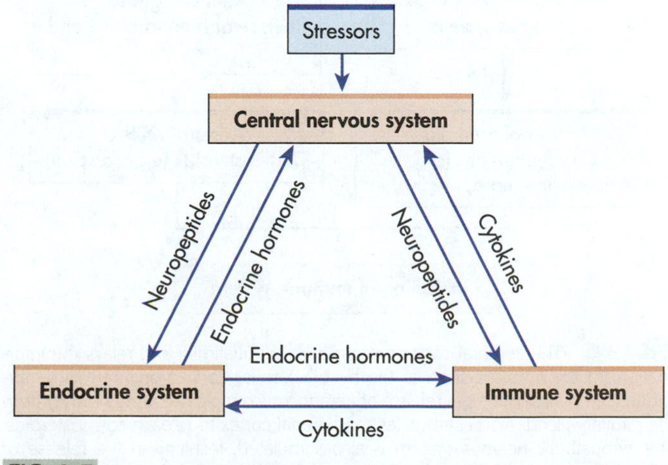

FIG. 9-3 Neurochemical links among the nervous, endocrine, and immune systems. The communication among these three systems is bidirectional.

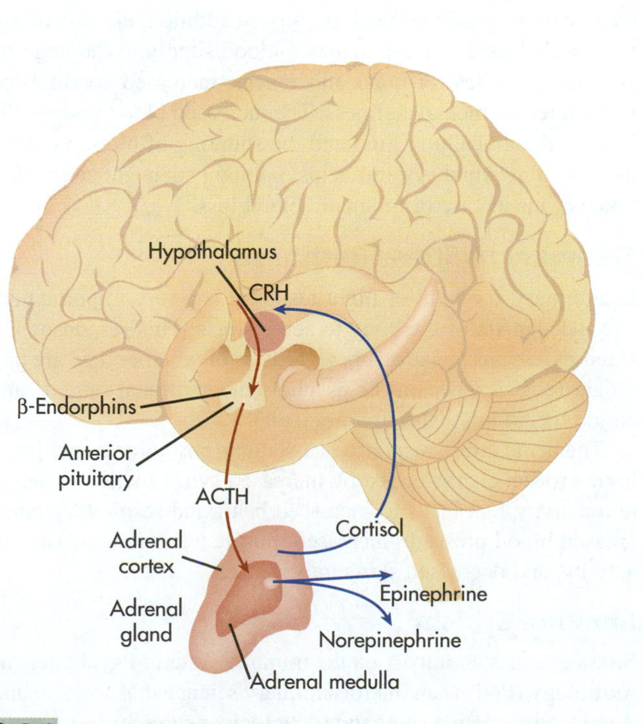

FIG. 9-4 Hypothalamic-pituitary-adrenal axis. *ACTH,* Adrenocorticotropic hormone; *CRH,* corticotropin-releasing hormone.

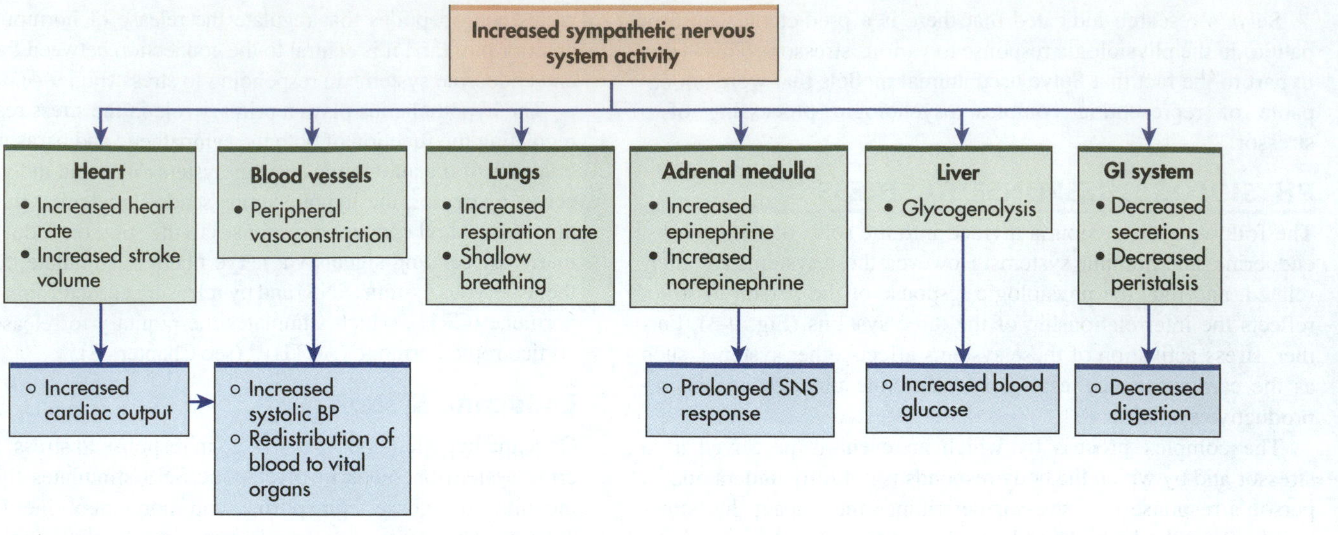

FIG. 9-5 "Fight-or-flight" reaction. Alarm reaction responses resulting from increased sympathetic nervous system activity. *SNS,* Sympathetic nervous system.

steroids play an important role in "turning off" or blunting aspects of the stress response, which if uncontrolled can become self-destructive. This is best exemplified by the ability of corticosteroids to suppress the release of proinflammatory mediators, such as the cytokines tumor necrosis factor (TNF) and interleukin-1 (IL-1). The persistent release of such mediators is believed to initiate organ dysfunction in conditions such as sepsis. Hence, corticosteroids act not only to support the adaptive response of the body to a stressor, but also act to suppress an overzealous and potentially self-destructive response.[15]

The increased cardiac output (resulting from the increased heart rate and increased stroke volume), increased blood glucose levels, increased oxygen consumption, and increased metabolic rate make the responses possible (see Fig. 9-5). In addition, dilation of skeletal muscle blood vessels increases blood supply to the large muscles and provides for quick movement; increased cerebral blood flow increases mental alertness. The increased blood volume (from increased extracellular fluid and the shunting of blood away from the gastrointestinal system) helps maintain adequate circulation to vital organs in case of traumatic blood loss.

Summary of Stress Response

In summary, the fight-or-flight response is a very important adaptive mechanism of the body to acute stress. This response is activated in response to stressors regardless of whether they are physiologic (e.g., acute pain) or psychologic/emotional (e.g., death of child, loss of home through fire, fear).

The acute stress response is a state of physiologic and psychologic arousal characterized by increased sympathetic nervous system activity that leads to increased heart and respiratory rate, increased blood pressure, increased muscle tension, increased brain activity, and decreased skin temperature.

Immune System

Stress also has an impact on the immune system. **Psychoneuroimmunology** (PNI) is an interdisciplinary science that seeks to understand the interactions among psychologic, neurologic, and immune responses.[16,17] Because it is now known that the brain is connected to the immune system by neuroanatomic and neuroendocrine pathways, stressors have the potential to lead to alterations in immune function (Fig. 9-6). Nerve fibers extend from the nervous system and synapse on cells and tissues (i.e., spleen, lymph nodes) of the immune system. In turn, the cells of the immune system have receptors for many neuropeptides and hormones, which permit them

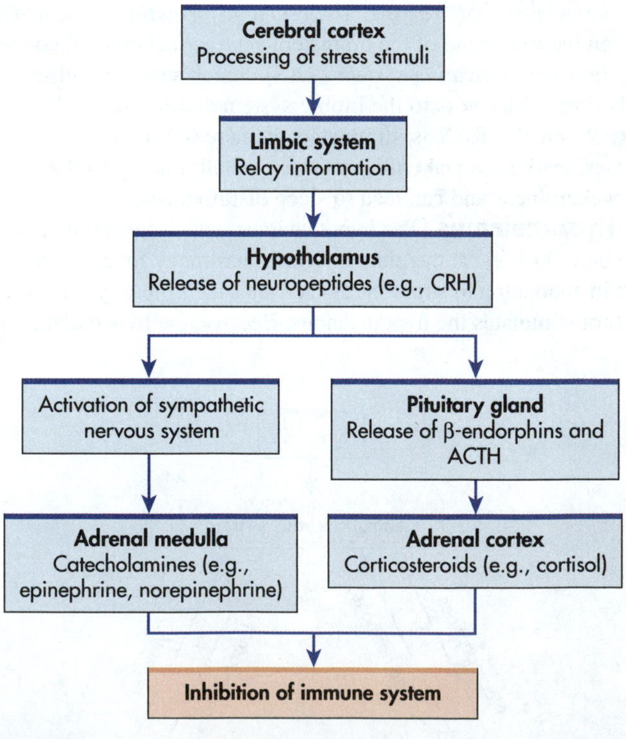

FIG. 9-6 The cerebral cortex processes stressful stimuli and relays the information via the limbic system to the hypothalamus. Corticotropin-releasing hormone (CRH) stimulates the release of adrenocorticotropic hormone (ACTH) from the pituitary gland. ACTH stimulates the adrenal cortex to release corticosteroids. The sympathetic nervous system is also stimulated, resulting in the release of epinephrine and norepinephrine from the adrenal medulla. The end result is the inhibition of the immune system.

to respond to nervous and neuroendocrine signals. As a result, the mediation of stress by the central nervous system leads to corresponding changes in immune cell activity. Both acute and chronic stress can affect immune function, including decreased number and function of natural killer cells; altered lymphocyte proliferation; decreased production of *cytokines* (soluble factors secreted by white blood cells and other cells), such as interferon and interleukins; and decreased phagocytosis by neutrophils and monocytes (reviewed by Segerstrom and Miller[18]). Most of these studies show that chronic stress induces immunosuppression. (Natural killer cells, lymphocytes, and cytokines are discussed in Chapter 14.)

Importantly, the network that links the brain and immune system is bidirectional (see Fig. 9-3). Signals from these systems travel back and forth. This allows for communication among these systems. Consequently, not only do emotions modify the immune response, but products of immune cells send signals back to the brain and alter its activity. Many of the communication signals sent from the immune system to the brain are mediated by cytokines, which are central to the coordination of the immune response. For example, IL-1 (a cytokine made by monocytes) acts on the temperature regulatory center of the hypothalamus and initiates the febrile response to infectious pathogens (see Fig. 13-6).

EFFECTS OF STRESS ON HEALTH

Acute stress leads to physiologic changes that are important to the adaptive survival of the individual. However, if stress is excessive or prolonged, these same physiologic responses can be maladaptive and lead to harm and disease. When a person sustains chronic, unrelieved stress, the body's defenses can no longer keep up with the demands. Over time stress takes its toll (Fig. 9-7). Therefore stress plays a role in the development or progression in the diseases of adaptation, or stress-related illnesses (Table 9-4).

Stress can have effects on cognitive function, including poor concentration, memory problems, distressing dreams, sleep disturbances, and impaired decision making. In addition, stress can also cause a wide variety of changes in behavior. These include people withdrawing from others, becoming very quiet or unusually talkative, changing eating habits, drinking alcohol excessively, or becoming irritable.

Chronic and intense stress may have profound effects on brain structure and function, especially the hippocampus.[19,20] The hippocampus plays an important role in long-term memory and is also important for cognitive functions, such as spatial learning. The release of corticosteroids in response to stress appears to act in concert with certain neurotransmitters to produce stress-induced hippocampal damage. In humans, magnetic resonance imaging (MRI) studies of the brain have shown that individuals who have endured prolonged stress (3 to 4 years) or have experienced traumatic events (violence, rape, war, natural disasters) also have selective atrophy of the hippocampus. These changes are accompanied by memory impairments.[19]

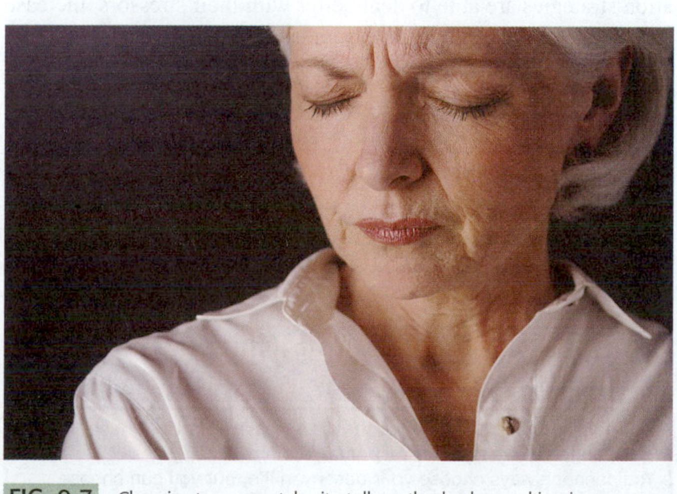

FIG. 9-7 Chronic stress can take its toll on the body, resulting in poor concentration and memory problems.

TABLE 9-4 Examples of Disorders and Diseases with a Stress Component

• Depression	• Hypertension
• Dyspepsia	• Insomnia
• Eating disorders	• Irritable bowel syndrome
• Erectile dysfunction	• Low back pain
• Fatigue	• Menstrual irregularities
• Fibromyalgia	• Peptic ulcer disease
• Headaches	• Sexual dysfunction

Long-term exposure to catecholamines resulting from excessive activation of the sympathetic nervous system may increase the risk of cardiovascular diseases such as atherosclerosis and hypertension.[21] Other conditions that are either precipitated or aggravated by stress include migraine headaches, irritable bowel syndrome, and peptic ulcers.[22] Control of metabolic conditions, such as diabetes mellitus, is also affected by stress. Behavioral interventions aimed at stress reduction and relaxation have been successful in helping to manage these diseases in conjunction with standard medical therapy.

The central nervous system is capable of influencing the function of the immune system. Stress-induced immunosuppression may exacerbate or increase the risk of progression of immune-based diseases such as multiple sclerosis, asthma, rheumatoid arthritis, and cancer.[17,18,23,24] Stressful life events can make a person more susceptible to infection. For example, psychologic stress may increase one's risk for developing the common cold. In a landmark study, healthy volunteers were inoculated intranasally with low doses of upper respiratory tract viruses. The subjects underwent psychologic testing to determine the occurrence of stressful events in their lives and their reactions to such stresses. The results showed that both the rates of viral infection and clinical colds increased with the degree of psychologic stress. In this study social support buffered the harmful effects of stress.[25]

The link between stress and susceptibility to infectious disease has also been demonstrated in a study of elderly individuals caring for a spouse with Alzheimer's disease. The chronic stress of caregiver burden in these individuals was associated with an impaired immune response to influenza vaccine. The results of this study suggest that chronic stress may increase an elderly person's vulnerability to influenza.[26]

Many questions about stress and the immune response remain unanswered. For example, it is not known how much stress is needed to cause these changes or how much of an alteration in the immune system is necessary before disease susceptibility occurs. A current challenge for researchers in the field of PNI is to study stress-induced immune changes and their relationship to health and to illness outcomes.

COPING

Coping is a person's cognitive and behavioral efforts to manage specific external or internal stressors that seem to exceed available resources.[3] Coping can be either positive or negative. Positive coping includes activities such as exercise and use of social support. Negative coping may include substance abuse and denial.

The availability of coping resources affects an individual's ability to cope with stressful situations. *Coping resources* are characteristics or actions drawn on to manage stress and include factors within the person or the environment. These may include (1) health status, (2) belief systems, (3) problem-solving skills, (4) social skills, (5) social support, and (6) financial resources. In a clinical setting, knowledge of a patient's resources will assist the nurse in supporting existing resources and developing strategies to expand the patient's coping resources.

Coping strategies can be divided into two broad categories: emotion-focused coping and problem-focused coping. **Emotion-focused coping** involves managing the emotions that an individual feels when a stressful event occurs. Examples of emotion-focused coping include discussion of feelings with a friend or taking a hot bath. **Problem-focused coping** attempts to find solutions to resolve the problems causing the stress. For example, setting priorities or collecting information and seeking advice would be considered problem-focused coping.

Both forms of coping strategies can be used to cope with stressors. Combinations of both strategies can be used to cope with the same stressors. Table 9-5 provides examples of emotion- and problem-focused coping when applied to the same stressful situation. When a situation is unchangeable or uncontrollable, emotion-focused coping may predominate. A primary purpose of emotion-focused coping is to help decrease negative emotions. Emotion-focused coping strategies (e.g., having the patient share her feelings about the loss of the uterus) help create a feeling of well-being. Although it may not seem to be working toward a solution, emotion-focused coping is a valid and appropriate way to deal with different stressful situations.

If a problem can be changed or controlled, problem-focused coping is the most helpful coping strategy. Problem-focused coping strategies allow an individual to look at a challenge objectively, take action to address the problem, and thereby reduce the stress.

A key concept to successful coping is the use of *coping flexibility.* Coping flexibility involves the ability to change and adapt coping strategies over time and across different stressful conditions. Stressful circumstances are handled best when an individual uses coping flexibility because certain strategies work more effectively than others depending on the circumstances.

TABLE 9-5 Examples of Problem- and Emotion-Focused Coping

Stressor	Problem-Focused Coping	Emotion-Focused Coping
Failing an examination	Obtaining a tutor	Going for a run
Being diagnosed with diabetes	Attending diabetic education classes	Getting a massage
Receiving questionable mammogram results	Scheduling follow-up testing for ultrasound	Expressing feelings of anxiety to friends and nurse

TABLE 9-6 Examples of Coping Strategies

Strategy	Description
Social support	May take the form of organized support and self-help groups, relationships with family and friends, and professional help.
Exercise	Can take the form of any form of movement, especially aerobic movement. Results in improved circulation, increased release of endorphins, and an enhanced sense of well-being.
Journaling	Allows an individual to express self in written form. This may include such things as personal events, thoughts, feelings, memories, and perceptions. May allow individual to reduce stress, enhance coping, and increase self-awareness.
Art therapy	Allows an individual to nonverbally express and communicate feelings, emotions, and thoughts. Can assist an individual to reduce stress, relax, and process experiences. Based on the belief that creative process is healing and life enhancing.
Humor	Can take the form of laughter, cartoons, funny movies, videos, riddles, comic books, and joke books. Humor carts have been set up in many clinical settings to be used by patients and families.

Specific coping strategies, such as journaling or art therapy, may be used to help manage stress. Brief descriptions of a variety of coping strategies can be found in Table 9-6.

RELAXATION STRATEGIES

The *relaxation response* is a state of physiologic and psychologic deep rest. It is the opposite of the stress response and is characterized by decreased SNS activity, which leads to decreased heart and respiratory rate, decreased blood pressure, decreased muscle tension, decreased brain activity, and increased skin temperature.[27]

The relaxation response can be elicited through a variety of relaxation strategies, including relaxation breathing, meditation, imagery, muscle relaxation, prayer (see Chapter 8), and physical exercise. The most common relaxation strategies (Table 9-7) are described here. Regular elicitation of the relaxation response has been proven to be an effective treatment for a wide range of stress-related disorders, including chronic pain, insomnia, and hypertension.[28]

Some common principles underlying stress management are presented in Table 9-8. Individuals who regularly engage in relaxation strategies are able to deal better with their stressors, increase their sense of control over stressors, and reduce their tension.[29]

TABLE 9-7 Relaxation Strategies

- Relaxation breathing
- Meditation
- Imagery
- Music for relaxation
- Muscle relaxation
  - Progressive
  - Passive
- Massage

TABLE 9-8 Principles Underlying Stress Management

You may not be able to change the stressors in your life, but you can change your reaction or response to them.

You cannot always choose your destiny in life, but you can choose how you cope with it.

Relaxation Breathing

The way one breathes affects every aspect of one's life. When a person is stressed, muscles tense and breathing becomes shallow and rapid. Therefore one of the simplest and most effective ways to stop the stress response is to breathe deeply and slowly. It is difficult to maintain tension when breathing in a slow, deep, and relaxed pattern.

Relaxation (abdominal) breathing can be performed while sitting, standing, or lying down. It is especially useful during a stressful or anxious situation to reduce stress. Relaxation breathing forms the basis for most relaxation strategies.

Before practicing relaxation breathing it is important to assess one's normal breathing pattern (Table 9-9). Chest breathing, which involves the upper chest and shoulders, is associated with inefficient breathing. This type of breathing is often associated with the type of breathing during anxiety and distress. Relaxation breathing, which involves the diaphragm, is natural for newborns and sleeping adults. It is associated with efficient breathing.

Relaxation breathing involves the primary use of the diaphragm and less use of the upper chest and shoulders to assist in each breath. In this type of breathing the abdomen gently moves in and out during exhalation and inhalation. The breaths should be slow, steady, and deep.

One basic technique for relaxation breathing is as follows: (1) Inhale slowly and deeply, pushing the abdomen out with each breath in, thinking about breathing in peace. (2) Exhale slowly, letting the abdomen come in, letting all the muscles relax. (3) Repeat these deep breaths 10 times without interruption. As with any breathing exercise, if a light-headed feeling arises, stop for 30 seconds and then start again. A common method used to teach relaxation breathing is the 4 × 4 technique (Table 9-10). The relaxing sigh is another good breathing technique that can be used for quick stress relief (see Table 9-10).

Initially, relaxation breathing may feel unusual. With practice it becomes easier, and its relaxing benefits are soon obvious. For use in a clinical setting, the nurse should personally learn to use relaxation breathing before teaching it to patients. Once it has been learned, relaxation breathing can be easily taught to patients in a variety of settings. Relaxation breathing is very important to use when patients are undergoing stressful and painful procedures.

TABLE 9-9 Breathing Assessment

- Begin by placing one hand gently on your abdomen below your waistline.
- Place the other hand on the center of your chest on the sternum.
- Without changing the normal breathing pattern, take several breaths. During inhalation notice which hand rises the most.
- When relaxation breathing is performed properly, the hand on the abdomen should rise more than the hand on the chest.

TABLE 9-10 Relaxation Breathing Techniques

4 × 4 Technique
- Sit up straight with your back flushed to the support of the chair and your feet flat on the floor.
- Rest your arms on your lap, thighs, or arms of the chair.
- Take in a deep breath through your nose to a count of four (1…2…3…4).
- Hold your breath to a count of four (1…2…3…4).
- Release your breath through your mouth to a count of four (1…2…3…4).
- Rest for a count of four (1…2…3…4).
- Repeat the cycle four times.

Relaxing Sigh
- Sit up straight.
- Sigh deeply, letting out a sound of deep relief as the air rushes out.
- Do not think about inhaling—just let the air come in naturally as you breathe deeply.
- Take 6 to 8 of these relaxing sighs very slowly. Repeat as needed.

Meditation

Meditation is the oldest type of relaxation strategy. In all cultures **meditation** is a state of being with increased concentration and awareness. Meditation can be used to create a sustained period of time in which one focuses attention and increases self-awareness. For many, meditation is sought out in response to a deep human need for something transcendental or beyond everyday experiences. However, meditation can also be used as a way to reduce stress.

Three basic ways to practice meditation include (1) concentration methods, (2) guided meditation, and (3) mindfulness practices. The *concentration technique* (e.g., Zen meditation) directs the mind to a single focus, such as the breath, an object, or a *mantra* (Table 9-11). A *guided meditation* is similar to a guided imagery (described below) where the mind and imagination are focused toward a conscious goal. *Mindfulness practices* (e.g., transcendental meditation) are not restricted to any one object but rather attend to any and all sensations, perceptions, cognitions, and emotions as they arise moment to moment in the field of awareness.

Although meditation can be performed anywhere, it is best to practice meditation in a quiet place, free of distractions. Table 9-11 provides some basic guidelines on how to meditate. Meditation is often practiced while seated, and it is important to maintain a comfortable posture (Fig. 9-8). Meditation can also be performed while walking in which the focus is on a single action such as the move-

TABLE 9-11 Basic Guide to Meditation

You can teach yourself the basics of meditation by following a few simple steps:
- Find a quiet place.
- Make sure there are no distractions.
- Sit in a comfortable position.
- Close your eyes.
- Shut out the world so your brain can stop processing information coming from your senses.
- Pick a word or phrase; find a word or phrase that means something to you, whose sound or rhythm is soothing when repeated (e.g., one, peace, shalom, the Lord is my shepherd, Hail Mary full of grace).
- Breathe slowly and practice relaxation breathing.
- Say the word or phrase again and again.
- Try saying the word or phrase silently to yourself with every exhalation.
- The monotony will help you focus.
- Do not be concerned when other thoughts come to mind; just acknowledge them and return calmly to your word or phrase.
- Continue for 10 to 20 minutes, but even 5 minutes can leave you feeling calm and refreshed.
- Rise slowly.

Practice once or twice daily.

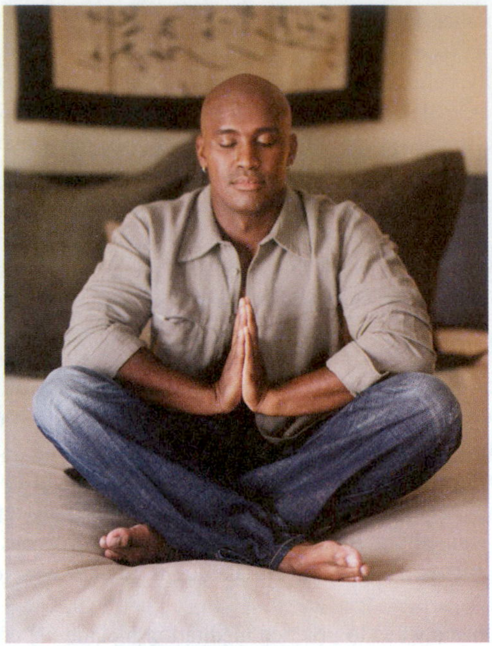

FIG. 9-8 Meditation should be performed in a comfortable setting and position. Although this man is sitting in a traditional meditation pose, meditation can be performed in any lying or sitting position.

ment of the feet. In the beginning individuals typically start with just 5 to 10 minutes of meditation at a time and often increase the time as the practice becomes more comfortable.

In people who meditate regularly, the brain is reoriented from a stressful fight-or-flight mode to one of acceptance, a shift that increases contentment.[30] There are many positive health benefits of meditation. These include reversal of coronary artery disease, decreased levels of cortisol, decreased cholesterol levels, increased airflow to the lungs, and promotion of wound healing.[31]

Imagery

Imagery is the use of one's mind to generate images that have a calming effect on the body. It involves the use of a focused mind and incorporates all the senses to create physiologic and emotional changes. It is a simple relaxation technique that requires no equipment other than an active imagination. *Guided imagery* is a variation of imagery in which images are suggested by another person (either live or on CD or tape).

Imagery can be used in many clinical settings for stress reduction and pain relief. Benefits of imagery include anxiety reduction, decreased muscle tension, improved comfort during medical procedures, immune system improvement, decreased recovery time following surgery, and reduction in sleeping problems.[32-34] Nurses may use imagery in their own lives or use guided imagery with their patients. One of the uses of imagery is to create a safe and special place that can become a place of mental retreat to elicit the relaxation response. Table 9-12 describes the steps involved in creating a special place.

When imagery is performed, it is best to find a comfortable position. Slow, deep breaths should be taken. Focus should involve all senses (sight, hearing, touch, smell). For example, one can use an image such as Figure 9-9 for imagery. As one focuses on this image, all senses should be engaged. Feel the wind on your face, hear the sounds of the ocean, and smell the seawater.

TABLE 9-12 Imagery: Creating Your Special Place

- Begin by closing your eyes and taking several slow, deep breaths.
- Imagine a place where you feel completely comfortable and peaceful. It may be a real place or one you imagine; one from your past or some place you have always wanted to go.
- Allow this special place to take form, slowly. As it takes form, look around, to your left, to your right. Enjoy the scenery: the colors, the texture, the shapes.
- Listen carefully to the sounds of your place. What do you hear?
- Is there a gentle breeze or sunshine warming your face? Pick up or touch some favorite objects from your special place.
- Take in a deep breath through your nose, and notice the rich smells around you. Perhaps your favorite flower is in bloom, or you smell the scents of the ocean.
- Take another deep breath and relax. Enjoy the peace, comfort, and safety of your special place.
- This is your special place. You relax and feel thankful that you are here, in your special place.
- You can return to this place any time that you wish.

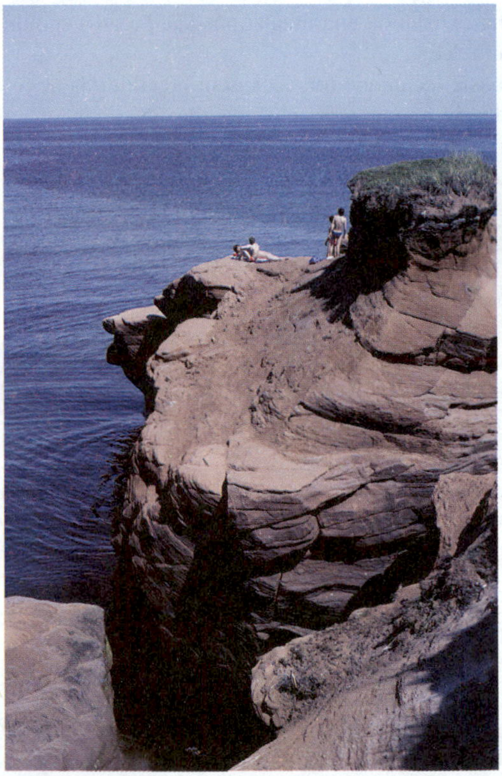

FIG. 9-9 Imagery. Special places should be created involving all the senses, such as a place where waves can be heard, seawater is smelled, wind is felt, and a relaxing landscape is seen.

Imagery can also be used to specifically target a disease, problem, or stressor. Table 9-13 describes some suggestions for using imagery in specific diseases or disorders.

Imagery can also be used to enhance performance or process stressful or difficult tasks. For example, it can be used to help an athlete or anyone achieve greater success. Imagery allows one an opportunity to mentally rehearse the difficult or challenging situation. It can be used to help a fearful nurse start an IV or perform a difficult procedure. It can also be used with a patient who is

TABLE 9-13 Examples of Imagery

Imagery can be used to relieve stress and promote health and healing in conjunction with regular medical care. Special images can be created to alleviate symptoms or treat diseases/disorders. The image should be strong and vivid for the person, using many senses to create the image. Below are some examples that some people have found useful.

Disease/Disorder	Images
Infection	White blood cells with flashing red sirens arrest and imprison harmful germs
Cancer	Shark gobbles up cancer cells Radiation or chemotherapy treatments enter the body like healing rays of light; they destroy cancer cells
Coronary artery disease	Water flows freely through a wide, open river
Weakened immune system	White blood cells rapidly multiply like millions of seeds bursting from ripe seed pod
Asthma	Tiny elastic rubber bands that constrict the airways pop open
Depression	Troubles and feelings of sadness are attached to big colorful helium balloons and are floating off into a clear blue sky
Pain	Pain is washed away by a cool calm river flowing through the entire body

Adapted from Sobel DS, Ornstein R: *Healthy mind, healthy body*, New York, 1996, Patient Education Materials, Time Life.
Additional information on guided imagery is available at *www.healthjourneys.com*.

afraid to have a stressful procedure performed (e.g., radiation therapy).

Imagery tapes and CDs are available commercially (see *www.healthjourneys.com*). Another way to create an imagery audiotape or CD is to personally record an imagery script of one's own voice, possibly using background music. Then a person can listen to his or her own voice while doing imagery.

Music for Relaxation

Music can help achieve relaxation and bring about healthy changes in emotional and/or physical states. Listening to relaxing music may act as a diversion to refocus one away from a stressful situation. In addition, healing vibrations from music can return the mind and body to a deeper level of balance.

Music has been used in many clinical settings. Music decreases anxiety and pain, and it evokes the relaxation response.[35] In the perioperative setting it has been successful in decreasing anxiety and heart rate, providing distraction, and increasing the pain threshold; thus patients have required fewer pain medications.[35-38]

Music that contains approximately 60 to 80 beats per minute is considered to be soothing. Low-pitch tones and music without words is recommended for relaxation. Mozart's music is the most popular form of music used for relaxation. On the other hand, fast-tempo music can stimulate and uplift a person. However, each person considers different music to be relaxing, so it is important to find the music that best matches the needs of the individual person. To achieve the optimal relaxation, all interruptions should be minimized and a comfortable posture should be found while listening to the music.

Music can be incorporated into clinical practice. It is noninvasive, safe, inexpensive, and easy to use. First it is important to establish the purpose and benefit of using music with the patients in a given clinical setting. Then it is important to assess each individual patient's interest and preference in music. A listening environment needs to be created, encouraging the patient to be in a comfortable position. Headphones or earphones and a CD or tape player can be used. Music can be played for 20 to 30 minutes per day at least twice a day. The patients' response to the music should be evaluated by asking them how it sounds and how it makes them feel.

Another form of using music for relaxation is simply creating one's own music. Singing a song, humming a tune, or playing a musical instrument can be a very uplifting experience during stressful times. Music can also be played in the background as a person performs chores, such as housework or office work, to help induce relaxation.

Muscle Relaxation

Muscle tension is a universal reaction to stress. As the stress response sets in, muscles of the entire body tend to tighten. Therefore muscle relaxation is a common method of eliciting the relaxation response. There are two types of muscle relaxation: progressive and passive.

Progressive muscle relaxation (PMR) involves the tensing and relaxing of muscles. The use of this tension/relax method is intended to help differentiate between when a muscle is tensed and when it is relaxed. This recognition will allow an individual to reduce muscle tension when it occurs during stress. PMR is based on the principle that when the muscles are relaxed, the mind will relax. Typically a session of PMR will begin at the extremities and gradually move across the whole body. An example of PMR can be found in Table 9-14. Patients with muscle or connective tissue damage or those having low back pain should not use PMR. In addition, PMR should not be used by patients with increased intracranial pressure, uncontrolled hypertension, or severe coronary artery disease.

TABLE 9-14 Progressive Muscle Relaxation Exercise

- Lie down in a quiet place where you will not be disturbed.
- Relax your entire body as much as possible, allowing it to feel heavy.
- Take a few slow, deep relaxation breaths.
- Imagine the tension flowing out with each breath.
- Now contract the muscles of your feet as you inhale.
- Hold the contraction briefly.
- Then relax as you breathe out, still imagining the tension flowing out with the exhalation.
- Notice the feel of the muscles as they are contracted and then relaxed.
- Move up the body, contracting and then relaxing in turn the muscles of the calf, thigh, buttocks, abdomen, and so on, including the arms and hands.
- End with the face by tensing and then relaxing the muscles of the mouth, jaw, eyes, and scalp.
- Lie still for a few minutes, experiencing the relaxed muscles.
- Continue to breathe slowly and deeply, feeling tension flow out and relaxation get deeper and deeper with each breath.
- When you are ready to get up, count backward from 4 to 1 and slowly rise.

COMPLEMENTARY AND ALTERNATIVE THERAPIES

Ginseng

Ginseng refers to several species of the genus Panax. Herbs commonly used are Asian ginseng *(Panax ginseng)* and American ginseng *(Panax quinquefolius L)*.

Clinical Uses

- Improve mental performance, lower blood glucose in type 2 diabetes mellitus*
- Reduce symptoms of coronary heart disease, improve stamina, lower BP, enhance immune system, improve sense of well-being†

Effects

Is well tolerated in most people when used at recommended doses. Serious side effects appear to be rare. May lower blood glucose, with the effect being greater in patients with diabetes than in nondiabetic patients. May cause headache, tremors, mania, or insomnia if used in combination with monoamine oxidase (MAO) inhibitors. May alter effects of BP or cardiac medications.

Nursing Implications

Use with caution in patients taking medications, herbs, and supplements that affect BP or heart rhythm. Use with caution in diabetic patients. In these patients, blood glucose must be closely monitored and medication dosages may need adjusting. Contraindicated during pregnancy or lactation. Can generally be used for up to 3 months with a repeated course of therapy possible.

From Ulbricht CE, Basch EM: *Natural standard herb and supplement reference: evidence-based clinical reviews,* St Louis, 2005, Mosby. Available at *www.naturalstandard.com.*
*Good scientific evidence exists for their use.
†Unclear scientific evidence exists for their use.

Passive muscle relaxation, on the other hand, has the mind focus only on relaxation of the muscles. It works similarly to PMR, moving from one extremity to the rest of the body, with the exception that the muscles are never tightened. Passive muscle relaxation simply puts the mind's focus on relaxing each muscle group separately. This form of muscle relaxation may be used more frequently in individuals who have chronic pain that may be exacerbated by the tension involved during PMR.

Massage

Massage is another important relaxation strategy. It involves the systematic manipulation of the soft tissue of the body to reduce tension and enhance health and healing. It also adds an essential human need—touch. Massage can be implemented as back rubs for patients.[39] Massage is discussed in more detail in Chapter 8.

NURSING MANAGEMENT STRESS

Nursing Assessment

Nurses are in a key position to assess stress in patients and families, to assist them to identify high-risk periods for stress, and to implement stress management strategies that can prevent the negative consequences of stress on their health. The number of stressors, the duration of these stressors, and the previous experience with similar demands should be assessed. An assessment of the personal meaning attached to the stressful situation will provide useful insight for planning stress management strategies with the patient. Family responses to the demands on the patient should also be assessed.

The patient faces many potential stressors that can have health consequences. The nurse must be aware of situations that are likely to result in stress and must also assess the patient's perception of these situations (Fig. 9-10). In addition to the stressor itself, specific coping strategies have health consequences and therefore must be included in the assessment.

Although the manifestations of stress may vary from person to person, the nurse should assess the patient for the signs and symptoms of the stress response. Responses may include an increased heart rate and blood pressure, hyperventilation, sweating, headache, musculoskeletal pain, gastrointestinal upset, loss of appetite, skin disorders, insomnia, and fatigue. In addition, the patient may exhibit some of the stress-related illnesses or diseases of adaptation (see Table 9-4).

Behavioral manifestations may include inability to concentrate, accident proneness, impaired speech, anxiety, crying, frustration, and irritability. Work-related behaviors related to stress may include absenteeism or tardiness at work, decreased productivity, and job dissatisfaction. Cognitive responses include self-reports of inability to make decisions and forgetfulness. Some of these responses may also be apparent to significant others.

Another major source of stress relates to illness experienced by a patient, which often also causes stress for family members. The nurse should assess what aspects of the illness are the most stressful for the patient. These may include the patient's physical health, job responsibilities, finances, and children. This information is valuable because it gives the nurse the patient's perspective of the stressors. Knowledge of stressors, the feelings these stressors invoke, and the psychologic sequelae they can produce will assist nurses to identify potential and actual sources of stress, as well as the impact these stressors have on the patient.[40]

Nursing Diagnoses

Key nursing diagnoses emphasize the importance of stress and coping in providing patient care. A coping–stress tolerance pattern has been identified as 1 of 11 functional health patterns.[41] This pattern includes the diagnoses presented in Table 9-15. Assessment of the health pattern results in a description of the coping–stress

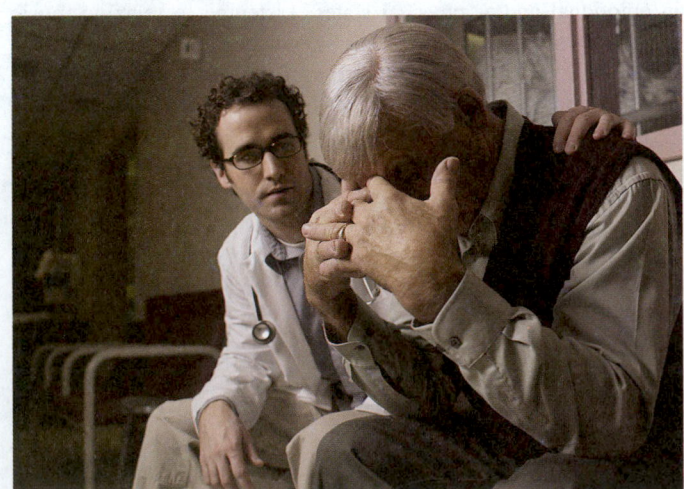

FIG. 9-10 The nurse needs to be aware of situations that are stressful to the patient and assess their impact on the patient's life.

COMPLEMENTARY AND ALTERNATIVE THERAPIES

St. John's Wort

Clinical Uses

- Wound healing (external)*
- Depressive disorder (mild to moderate)†
- Anxiety disorder, severe depressive disorder, obsessive-compulsive disorder, perimenopausal symptoms, premenstrual syndrome, seasonal affective disorder‡
- Human immunodeficiency virus infection§

Effects

Generally well tolerated at recommended doses for up to 1 to 3 months. May interact with medications metabolized by the cytochrome P450 system (e.g., birth control pills, cyclosporine, nifedipine [Procardia]). The U.S. Food and Drug Administration recommends that patients with HIV infection avoid St. John's wort.

Nursing Implications

Interacts with many herbs, supplements, over-the-counter drugs, and prescription drugs. Patients are advised to consult a health care professional before using St. John's wort in combination with any other medication. Contraindicated in pregnancy. Depression is a serious illness. Advise patients to consult with a health care practitioner before self-medicating with St. John's wort.

From Ulbricht CE, Basch EM: *Natural standard herb and supplement reference: evidence-based clinical reviews,* St Louis, 2005, Mosby. Available at *www.naturalstandard.com*.

*Uses based on tradition, theory, or limited scientific evidence.

†Strong scientific evidence exists for its use.

‡Unclear scientific evidence exists for their use.

§Fair scientific evidence exists against its use.

HIV, Human immunodeficiency virus.

tolerance patterns of a patient. Stressors can be identified at the individual, family, or community level.

Two specific nursing diagnoses have been identified related to stress: ineffective coping and compromised family coping. *Ineffective coping* is defined as the inability to form a valid appraisal of the stressors, inadequate choices of practiced responses, and/or inability to use available resources. Potential etiologies include inadequate level of confidence in ability to cope, uncertainty, inadequate social support, inadequate resources, and high degree of threat. *Compromised family coping* refers to the usually supportive primary person (family member or close friend) providing insufficient, ineffective, or compromised support, comfort, assistance, or encouragement, which may be needed by the patient to manage or master adaptive tasks related to the health challenge.[41]

TABLE 9-15 Nursing Diagnoses: Coping–Stress Tolerance Pattern

• Caregiver role strain	• Readiness for enhanced family coping
• Compromised family coping	• Relocation stress syndrome
• Defensive coping	• Risk for caregiver role strain
• Disabled family coping	• Risk for other-directed violence
• Ineffective community coping	• Risk for self-directed violence
• Ineffective coping	• Risk for self-mutilation
• Ineffective denial	• Risk prone health behavior
• Posttrauma syndrome	• Stress overload
• Rape-trauma syndrome	

COMPLEMENTARY AND ALTERNATIVE THERAPIES

Yoga

Yoga includes a set of practices that include gentle stretches, posture, breathing practices, progressive deep relaxation, and meditation. The goal of yoga is attainment of physical and mental well-being through mastery of the body achieved through exercise, holding of postures, proper breathing, and meditation.

Clinical Uses

Yoga's primary emphasis is on general well-being. Although yoga has been shown to be beneficial in a variety of conditions, it is not considered a therapy for specific diseases. Rather, yoga employs a broad holistic approach that focuses on teaching people a new lifestyle and way of thinking. In the process it is also found to have healing effects.

Effects

Yoga gives elasticity to the spine, firms up the skin, removes tension from the body, strengthens muscles, and corrects poor posture. Other benefits include decreasing nervousness and irritability and improving depression and mental fatigue.

Nursing Implications

Yoga can provide benefits to people at many different levels. It is important to assess why an individual is interested in yoga and provide information on the different types of yoga. Regardless of the type of yoga, deep abdominal relaxation breathing is a main component and helps one to focus on the inner self and promotes the relaxation response. Additional information on yoga can be found at *www.yogasite.com*.

Nursing Implementation

The first step in managing stress is to become aware of its presence. This includes identifying and expressing stressful feelings. The role of the nurse is to facilitate and enhance the processes of coping and adaptation. Nursing interventions depend on the sever-

COMPLEMENTARY AND ALTERNATIVE THERAPIES

Kava

Clinical Uses

- Anxiety*

Effects

Moderately effective in treatment of anxiety. Hepatotoxicity has been reported. The U.S. Food and Drug Administration has issued warnings to consumers and physicians regarding increased risk of liver toxicity. Short-term use (1 to 2 months) is recommended.

Nursing Implications

Inadequate scientific information exists to determine kava's safety. Should be used only under the supervision of a health care provider and only in recommended doses. Should be avoided by patients with liver problems and patients taking medications that affect the liver.

From Ulbricht CE, Basch EM: *Natural standard herb and supplement reference: evidence-based clinical reviews,* St Louis, 2005, Mosby. Available at *www.naturalstandard.com*.

*Strong scientific evidence exists for its use.

The healing environment that nurses create is important to both the body and the mind.

Florence Nightingale

The attitude you take toward problems and difficulties is far and away the most important factor in controlling and mastering them.

Norman Vincent Peale

ity of the stress experience. In the person with multiple trauma, the person expends energy in an attempt to physically survive. The nurse's efforts are directed to life-supporting interventions and to the inclusion of approaches aimed at the reduction of additional stressors for the patient. For example, an individual who has endured multiple trauma is much less likely to adapt or recover if faced with additional stressors such as sleep deprivation or an infection.

Coping resources and strategies that are used should be adaptive and not a source of additional stress for the patient. Coping resources and strategies were previously discussed in this chapter.

The nurse can assume a primary role in implementing stress management strategies. Tips for handling stress are presented in Table 9-16. Ideas for how to incorporate stress management strategies into nursing practice are presented in Table 9-17. Although some may require additional training, many stress management strategies are within the scope of nursing practice, including relaxation breathing, imagery, music for relaxation, passive and progressive muscle relaxation, exercise, massage, meditation, art therapy, and journaling. (Additional resources are available at the end of the chapter and on the CD that accompanies this book.)

Before teaching stress management strategies to patients, the nurse needs to personally become familiar with them. Most relaxation strategies can be taught in 10 to 15 minutes. To prepare for a relaxation training session, have the patient wear loose-fitting clothing and ensure that the setting is private, comfortable, and free from distractions or noises. Choose a relaxation strategy to best suit the patient and the situation. Give directions calmly and slowly in short, simple sentences. End the session gradually so as to not disrupt the relaxation that was just elicited. Say a phrase such as, "I am going to count backwards from five to one. With each number, you will feel more alert, but still feel at peace." After counting backwards, instruct the patient to slowly open his or her eyes.

Effective stress management provides an individual a sense of control of the stressful situation. As stress management practices are incorporated into daily activities, the individual is able to increase his or her confidence and self-reliance and limit the emotional response to the stressful circumstances. Possessing a sense of control is an important characteristic that can deter the harmful effects inherent in the stress response.

Nurses are in an ideal situation to take the lead in integrating stress management in their practice. Nurses are also well equipped to develop and test the effectiveness of new approaches to manage stress and promote positive health outcomes. However, it is important for the nurse to recognize when the patient or family needs to be referred to a professional with advanced training in counseling.

TABLE 9-16 Tips for Handling Stress

- Be realistic.
- Do not try to be superhuman.
- Learn to "let go" of things that are outside of your control.
- Learn to adapt.
- Be flexible.
- Learn acceptance of yourself.
- Exercise regularly.
- Share your feelings.
- Keep a sense of humor; laugh often.
- Learn relaxation breathing.
- Use imagery.
- Meditate or pray.
- Live a healthy lifestyle.
- Develop hobbies.
- Take time for yourself to relax every day.
- If needed, get professional counseling.

TABLE 9-17 How to Implement Stress Management in Clinical Practice

- Learn relaxation breathing.
- It is the easiest method of relaxation to use.
- Practice teaching relaxation breathing.
- First practice with peers before teaching to patients.
- Pick coping strategies (see Table 9-5) and stress management strategies that are appropriate for your clinical area.
- Make a commitment to learn the strategies.
- Practice using the strategy yourself. It becomes easier with time.
- Be confident in your ability to learn the strategies and teach patients.
- Anticipate setbacks. They provide feedback about what you are doing wrong. Do NOT quit!
- Take advantage of opportunities to teach coping and relaxation strategies to patients.
- Attend seminars and workshops on stress management to learn more.

CRITICAL THINKING EXERCISE

CASE STUDY

Stress Associated with Cancer Diagnosis and Treatment

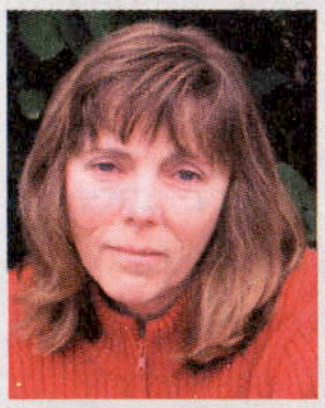

Case Study photo ©iStockphoto.com/ Rosemarie Colombraro.

Patient Profile. Mrs. Z., a Russian immigrant, was diagnosed with stage IIB breast cancer at age 44. Her treatment plan included lumpectomy followed by a regimen of chemotherapy and then radiation therapy. She attributed her breast cancer to her depression, which developed while she cared for her mother, who suffered from Alzheimer's disease. Her mother died 6 months before her breast cancer diagnosis.

After completion of her lengthy breast cancer therapy, Mrs. Z.'s depression worsened. She no longer had her frequent visits to the breast cancer center, and she missed the interaction with the nurses and other patients. In addition, Mrs. Z. expressed fears to her nurse that her cancer would recur and she worried that she would "pass it on" to her two teenage daughters. She would not discuss her fears with her husband or daughters because she did not want to burden them. She began to lose weight and constantly felt fatigued. She felt "alone" with her cancer and lost interest in other aspects of her life. She thought about joining a cancer support group but was embarrassed by her Russian accent.

Critical Thinking Questions

1. Consider Mrs. Z.'s situation and describe the physiologic and psychologic/emotional stressors with which she is dealing. Describe the possible effects of these stressors on her health.
2. What specific nursing interventions can be included in Mrs. Z.'s management that will enhance her coping strategies?
3. What resources are available to Mrs. Z. to help her cope with her fears related to her cancer diagnosis?
4. Should Mrs. Z. join a cancer support group? If so, how might this benefit her?
5. Review the assessment data provided and write two or more nursing diagnoses. Are there any collaborative problems?

NCLEX EXAMINATION REVIEW QUESTIONS

The number of the question corresponds to the same-numbered objective at the beginning of the chapter.

1. Determination of whether an event is a stressor is based on a person's
   a. tolerance.
   b. perception.
   c. adaptation.
   d. stubbornness.
2. The nurse recognizes that a patient with newly diagnosed cancer of the breast is using an emotion-focused coping process when she
   a. joins a support group for women with breast cancer.
   b. considers the pros and cons of the various treatment options.
   c. delays treatment until her family can take a weekend trip together.
   d. tells the nurse that she has a good prognosis because the tumor is small.
3. The nurse would expect which of the following findings in a patient as a result of the physiologic effect of stress on the reticular formation?
   a. An episode of diarrhea while awaiting painful dressing changes
   b. Refusing to communicate with nurses while awaiting a cardiac catheterization
   c. Inability to sleep the night before beginning to self-administer insulin injections
   d. Increased blood pressure, decreased urine output, and hyperglycemia following a car accident
4. The nurse utilizes knowledge of the effects of stress on the immune system by encouraging patients to
   a. sleep for 10 to 12 hours per day.
   b. avoid exposure to upper respiratory infections.
   c. receive regular immunizations when they are stressed.
   d. use emotion-focused rather than problem-focused coping strategies.
5. The nurse recognizes that a person who is subjected to chronic stress could be at higher risk for
   a. osteoporosis.
   b. colds and flu.
   c. low blood pressure.
   d. high serum cholesterol.
6. During a stressful circumstance that is uncontrollable, which type of coping strategy is the most effective?
   a. Avoidance
   b. Coping flexibility
   c. Emotion-focused coping
   d. Problem-focused coping
7. An appropriate nursing intervention for a hospitalized patient who has a nursing diagnosis of ineffective coping related to inadequate psychologic resources is
   a. controlling the environment to prevent sensory overload and promote sleep.
   b. encouraging the patient's family to offer emotional support by frequent visiting.
   c. arranging for the patient to phone family and friends to maintain emotional bonds.
   d. asking the patient to describe previous stressful situations and how she managed to resolve them.

REFERENCES

1. National Mental Health Association: Available at *www.nmha.org* (accessed May 9, 2006).
2. Selye H: The stress concept: past, present, and future. In Cooper CL, editor: *Stress research: issues for the eighties,* New York, 1983, Wiley.
3. Lazarus R, Folkman S: *Stress, appraisal, and coping,* New York, 1984, Springer.
4. Ford-Gilboe M, Cohen JA: Hardiness: a model of commitment, challenge, and control. In Rice VH, editor: *Stress, coping, and health,* Thousand Oaks, Calif, 2000, Sage.
5. Antonovsky AA: *Unraveling the mystery of health: how people manage stress and stay well,* San Francisco, 1987, Jossey-Bass.
6. Williams SJ: The relationship among stress, hardiness, sense of coherence, and illness in critical care nurses, *Medical Psychotherapy* 3:171, 1990.
7. Wolff AC, Ratner PA: Stress, social support, and sense of coherence, *West J Nurs Res* 21:182, 1999.
8. Wagnild GM, Young HM: Development and psychometric evaluation of the resilience scale, *J Nurs Meas* 1:165, 1993.
9. Danner DD, Snowden DA, Friesen WV: Positive emotions in early life and longevity: findings from the nun study, *J Pers Soc Psychol* 80:804, 2001.
10. Kubzansky LD, Sparrow D, Vokonas P, et al: Is the glass half empty or half full? A prospective study of optimism and coronary heart disease in the normative aging study, *Psychosom Med* 63:910, 2001.
11. Carver CS, Pozo-Kaderman C, Harris SD, et al: Optimism versus pessimism predicts the quality of women's adjustments to early stage breast cancer, *Cancer* 73:1213, 1994.
12. Robinson-Whelen S, Cheongtag K, MacCallum RC, et al: Distinguishing optimism from pessimism in older adults: is it more important to be optimistic or not be pessimistic? *J Pers Soc Psychol* 73:1345, 1997.
13. Thibodeau GA, Patton KT: *Anatomy and physiology,* ed 6, St Louis, 2007, Mosby.
14. Lovallo WR: *Stress and health: biological and psychological interactions,* ed 2, Thousand Oaks, Calif, 2005, Sage.
15. McCance KL, Huether SE: *Pathophysiology: the biologic basis for disease in adults and children,* ed 5, St Louis, 2006, Mosby.
16. Glaser R: Stress-associated immune dysregulation and its importance for human health: a personal history of psychoneuroimmunology, *Brain Behav Immun* 19:3, 2005.
17. Daruna JH: *Introduction to psychoneuroimmunology*, Burlington, Mass, 2004, Elsevier.
18. Segerstrom SC, Miller GE: Psychological stress and the human immune system: a meta-analytic study of 30 years of inquiry, *Psychol Bull* 130:601, 2004.
19. McEwen BS: Effects of adverse experiences for brain structure and function, *Biol Psychiatry* 48:721, 2000.
20. Sandi C: Stress, cognitive impairment, and cell adhesion molecules, *Nature Reviews Neuroscience* 12:917, 2004.
21. Ramachandruni S, Handberg E, Sheps DS: Acute and chronic psychological stress in coronary disease, *Curr Opin Cardiol* 19(5):494, 2004.
22. Maunder RG: Evidence that stress contributes to inflammatory bowel disease: evaluation, synthesis, and future directions, *Inflammatory Bowel Disease* 6:600, 2005.
23. Vedhara K, Irwin M: *Human psychoneuroimmunology*, New York, 2005, Oxford Press.
24. Reiche E, Nunes S, Morimoto H: Stress, depression, the immune system, and cancer, *Lancet Oncology* 5:617, 2004.
25. Cohen S, Tyrrell DA, Smith AP: Psychological stress and susceptibility to the common cold, *N Engl J Med* 325:606, 1991.
26. Kiecolt-Glaser JK, Glaser R, Gravenstein S, et al: Chronic stress alters the immune response to influenza virus vaccine in older adults, *Proc Natl Acad Sci U S A* 93:3043, 1996.

27. Benson H: *The relaxation response,* New York, 1975, Avon.
28. Benson H: *Timeless healing: the power and biology of belief,* New York, 1996, Scribner.
29. Seaward BL: *Managing stress: principles and strategies for health and well-being,* ed 5, Boston, 2006, Jones & Bartlett.
30. Davidson RJ, Kabat-Zinn J, Schumacher J, et al: Alterations in brain and immune function produced by mindfulness meditation, *Psychosom Med* 65:564, 2003.
31. Canter PH: The therapeutic effects of meditation, *BMJ* 326:1049, 2003.
32. Gruzeiler JH: A review of the impact of hypnosis, relaxation, guided imagery and individual differences on aspects of immunity and health, *Stress: The International Journal of the Biology of Stress* 2:147, 2002.
33. Scherwitz LW, McHenry P, Herrero R: Interactive guided imagery therapy with medical patients: predictors of health outcomes, *Journal of Alternative and Complementary Medicine* 1:69, 2005.
34. Halpin LS, Speir AM, CapoBianco P, et al: Guided imagery in cardiac surgery, *Outcomes Manag* 3:132, 2002.
35. Hanser SB, Mandel SE: The effects of music therapy in cardiac healthcare, *Cardiology in Review* 1:18, 2005.
36. Good M, Anderson GC, Ahn S, et al: Relaxation and music reduces pain following intestinal surgery, *Res Nurs Health* 28:240, 2005.
37. Dunn K: Music and the reduction of postoperative pain, *Nurs Stand* 36:33, 2004.
38. Voss JA, Good M, Yates B, et al: Sedative music reduces anxiety and pain during chair rest after open-heart surgery, *Pain* 12:197, 2004.
39. Richards KC, Gibson R, Overton-McCoy AL: The effects of massage in acute and critical care, *AACN Clin Issues* 11(1):77, 2000.
40. Casey A, Benson H: *Mind your heart: a mind body approach to stress management, exercise, and nutrition for heart health,* New York, 2004, Simon & Schuster.
41. NANDA International: *Nursing diagnoses: definitions and classifications 2005-2006,* Philadelphia, 2005, North American Nursing Diagnosis Association.

RESOURCES

Academy for Guided Imagery
www.academyforguidedimagery.com

American Institute of Stress
Email: stress124@earthlink.net
www.stress.org

Centre for Stress Management
www.managingstress.com/index.html

International Stress Management Association
www.isma.org.uk

Job Stress Help
www.jobstresshelp.com

Medline Plus: Stress Resources
www.nlm.nih.gov/medlineplus/stress.html

Music Therapy
www.musictherapy.org

National Institute for Occupational Safety and Health (NIOSH) Stress at Work
800-35-NIOSH
www.cdc.gov/niosh/tropics/stress

Sidran Traumatic Stress Institute
410-825-8888
Fax: 410-337-0747
www.sidran.org

Stress Information Electronic Book
www.teachhealth.com

Stress Management Resources
www.mentalhealth.about.com/cs/stressmanagement

Stress Management Website
812-855-4011
www.indiana.edu/~health/stres.html

World Wide Web Virtual Library
www.clas.ufl.edu/users/gthursby/stress

For additional Internet resources, see Chapter 8 and the website for this book at *http://evolve.elsevier.com/Lewis/medsurg*.

It would be good for us to remember that one of the greatest gifts we can share with others in pain, despair, or confusion is a clear sense of our peace and knowledge that we are loved.

Robert J. Wicks

Pain 10

Mary Ersek and Gordon A. Irving

LEARNING OBJECTIVES

1. Define pain.
2. Describe the neural mechanisms of pain and pain modulation.
3. Differentiate between nociceptive and neuropathic types of pain.
4. Explain the physical and psychologic effects of unrelieved pain.
5. Interpret the subjective and objective data that are obtained from a comprehensive pain assessment.
6. Describe effective multidisciplinary pain management techniques.
7. Describe pharmacologic and nonpharmacologic methods of pain relief.
8. Explain the nurse's role and responsibility in pain management.
9. Discuss ethical and legal issues related to pain and pain management.
10. Evaluate the influence of one's own knowledge, beliefs, and attitudes about pain assessment and management.

KEY TERMS

analgesic ceiling, p. 135
breakthrough pain, p. 132
dermatomes, p. 128
equianalgesic dose, p. 140
neuropathic pain, p. 128
nociception, p. 127
pain, p.126
patient-controlled analgesia, p. 142
suffering, p. 127
trigger point, p. 143

Electronic Resources

Supplemental content related to Chapter 10 can be found . . .

Companion CD

- Stress-Busting Kit for Nursing Students
- Interactive Case Study: Pain
- NCLEX Examination Review Questions
- Comprehensive Glossary

Evolve Website evolve

http://evolve.elsevier.com/Lewis/medsurg

- Content Updates
- Key Points (Printable and CD/MP3 Download)
- Concept Map Creator
- Expanded Audio Glossary
- Key Term Flash Cards
- Electronic Calculators
- WebLinks

PAIN

Pain is a complex, multidimensional experience. For many people, it is a major problem that causes suffering and reduces quality of life. Pain is one of the major reasons that people seek health care. A thorough understanding of the physiologic and psychosocial dimensions of the pain is important for effective assessment and management of patients with pain.

Pain occurs in all clinical settings and among many different groups of patients. Nurses have a central role in pain assessment and management. Components of the nursing role include (1) assessing pain and communicating this information to other health care providers, (2) ensuring the initiation and coordination of adequate pain relief measures, (3) evaluating the effectiveness of these interventions, and (4) advocating for people with pain. This chapter presents current knowledge about pain to enable nurses to assess and manage pain successfully in collaboration with other health care providers.

MAGNITUDE OF THE PAIN PROBLEM

Acute pain and chronic pain are major health problems that affect millions of North Americans every year. (See p. 131 for definitions of acute pain and chronic pain.) Acute pain is the most common reason for health care visits. Specific conditions for which patients seek health care include musculoskeletal and gastrointestinal (GI) pain, angina and other types of chest pain, headache, and injuries. Chronic pain occurs at epidemic levels in the United States and Canada. Over 50 million people are affected with back pain, arthritis, and migraine headache, which are the most common causes of

Reviewed by Judith A. Paice, RN, PhD, FAAN, Director, Cancer Pain Program, Research Professor of Medicine, Northwestern University, Chicago, Ill.

chronic pain. Many people with chronic pain have experienced it for more than 5 years.[1-3]

The financial impact of pain is staggering. Unrelieved and inadequate management of pain costs an estimated $100 billion each year as a result of longer hospital stays, rehospitalizations, and visits to outpatient clinics and emergency departments.[1] Many people have pain that leads to disability, resulting in economic losses. Lost productive time from common pain conditions (i.e., headache, back, and musculoskeletal pain) costs the U.S. economy over $61 billion each year.[4]

Despite the high prevalence and costs associated with acute and chronic pain, many studies document inadequate pain management across care settings and patient populations. For example, families report that over 24% of dying persons did not receive any or enough help with pain relief. This failure to manage pain adequately was highest among patients in nonhospice home care and nursing home settings but also occurred in hospitals and hospice home care.[5] Cancer pain, which occurs in 28% of newly diagnosed patients, 50% to 70% of patients undergoing active therapy, and 64% to 80% of those with advanced disease, is frequently undertreated.[6] Up to 75% of patients experience moderate to severe pain at some point during hospitalization.[7] Procedural pain also is often inadequately treated; in one study over half of adults undergoing painful procedures received no analgesics before the procedure.[8] Persistent, inadequately treated pain also is a problem among institutionalized elderly.[9]

Consequences of untreated pain include unnecessary suffering, physical and psychosocial dysfunction, impaired recovery from acute illness and surgery, immunosuppression, and sleep disturbances.[1,10] In the acutely ill patient, unrelieved pain can result in increased morbidity as a result of respiratory dysfunction, increased heart rate and cardiac workload, increased muscular contraction and spasm, decreased GI motility and transit, and increased catabolism[11] (Table 10-1).

The reasons for the undertreatment of pain are varied. Among health care providers, frequently cited explanations include (1) inadequate knowledge and skills to assess and treat pain; (2) unwillingness of providers to believe patients' report of pain; (3) lack of time, expertise, and perceived importance of conducting regular pain assessments; and (4) inaccurate and inadequate information regarding addiction, tolerance, respiratory depression, and other side effects of opioids.[1,12,13] In addition, some health care providers fear that aggressive pain management may hasten or cause death.[14] Clinicians and researchers also cite legal and systems-level barriers, including restrictions in the use of controlled substances, failure of health care organizations to provide clear standards of pain management practices, lack of standardized institutional pain management policies and procedures, and lack of accountability for pain management practices.[1,13,15] Among patients and family caregivers, attitudes toward pain and opioids play a major role in the underreporting and undertreatment of pain.[1,7,16] Fear of addiction, tolerance, and side effects often makes patients reluctant to report pain or comply with a regimen that involves opioid drugs. Other hindrances include the belief that pain is inevitable and a result of worsening disease and the expectation that the drugs will not relieve pain. The belief that pain is inevitable and the desire to be a "good" patient who does not complain are also given as patient-related reasons. Such attitudes are particularly common among older adults.

TABLE 10-1 Harmful Effects of Unrelieved Pain

System	Response	Possible Clinical Consequences
Endocrine/metabolic	↑ Adrenocorticotropic hormone (ACTH) ↑ Cortisol ↑ Antidiuretic hormone (ADH) ↑ Epinephrine, ↑ norepinephrine ↑ Renin, ↑ aldosterone ↓ Insulin Gluconeogenesis Glycogenolysis Muscle protein catabolism	Weight loss (from ↑ catabolism) Increased respiratory and heart rate Shock Glucose intolerance Hyperglycemia Fluid overload Hypertension Urinary retention, ↓ urine output
Cardiovascular	↑ Heart rate ↑ Cardiac output ↑ Peripheral vascular resistance ↑ Myocardial oxygen consumption ↑ Coagulation	Hypertension Unstable angina and myocardial infarction Deep vein thrombosis
Respiratory	↓ Tidal volume Hypoxemia ↓ Cough and sputum retention	Atelectasis Pneumonia
Genitourinary	↓ Urinary output Urinary retention	Fluid imbalance Electrolyte disturbance
Gastrointestinal	↓ Gastric and bowel motility	Constipation Anorexia Paralytic ileus
Musculoskeletal	Muscle spasm Impaired muscle function	Immobility Weakness and fatigue
Neurologic	Impaired cognitive function	Confusion Impaired ability to think, reason, and make decisions
Immunologic	↓ Immune response	Infection Sepsis

DEFINITIONS AND DIMENSIONS OF PAIN

Over 35 years ago, Margo McCaffery, a nurse and pioneer in pain management, defined **pain** as "whatever the person experiencing the pain says it is, existing whenever the person says it does."[17] The International Association for the Study of Pain (IASP) defines **pain** as "an unpleasant sensory and emotional experience associated with actual or potential tissue damage, or described in terms of such damage."[18] Note that these definitions emphasize the subjective nature of pain, in which the patient's self-report is the most valid means of assessment. Although understanding the patient's experience and relying on his or her self-report is essential, this stance is problematic in many patients. For example, patients who are comatose or who suffer from dementia, patients who are mentally disabled, and patients with expressive aphasia possess varying ability to report pain. In these instances, the nurse must incorporate nonverbal information such as behaviors into their pain assessment.

In defining pain as a human experience, successful pain assessment and treatment must incorporate multiple dimensions. The multidimensional nature of pain includes the physiologic, affective, cognitive, behavioral, and sociocultural influences on pain perception and expression.

The *physiologic* dimension, which is described in greater detail in the section on pain mechanisms, includes the genetic, anatomic, and physical determinants of pain. These physical components influence how painful stimuli are recognized and described.

The *affective* component of pain is the emotional response to the pain experience. These affective responses include anger, fear, depression, and anxiety. Negative emotions impair the patient's quality of life. Studies of depression and pain consistently demonstrate a link between these two conditions, with a negative effect on function.[1] Treating depression and anxiety in patients with chronic pain cannot only relieve depressive symptoms, but can also relieve the pain. It is important for nurses to recognize this cycle and intervene quickly and effectively.

The emotional and existential distress of pain can cause suffering. **Suffering** is defined as the state of severe distress associated with events that threaten the intactness of the person.[19] When suffering occurs, people can experience spiritual distress. Achieving pain relief is one essential step in relieving suffering. In addition, the assessment of ways in which a person's spirituality influences and is influenced by pain is important.

The *behavioral* component of pain refers to the observable actions used to express or control the pain. For example, facial expressions such as grimacing may reflect pain or discomfort. People who are unable to communicate verbally, such as those with advanced dementia, may demonstrate changes in behavior, such as becoming less physically active or more socially withdrawn. They also may become agitated or combative when they experience pain. People often use behavioral strategies such as decreasing their activity level, exercising, taking medications, or using relaxation techniques to manage the pain.

The *cognitive* component of pain refers to beliefs, attitudes, memories, and meaning attributed to the pain. The meaning of the pain to the patient can be particularly important. For example, a woman in labor may experience severe pain, but can manage it without analgesics because for her it is associated with a joyful event. Moreover, she may feel control over her pain because of the training she received in prenatal classes and the knowledge that the pain is self-limited. In contrast, a woman with chronic, undefined musculoskeletal pain may be plagued by thoughts that her pain is "not real," is uncontrollable, or is caused by her own actions. These cognitions will influence the ways in which a person responds to the pain and must be incorporated into the comprehensive treatment plan.

The cognitive dimension also includes pain-related beliefs and the cognitive coping strategies that people use. For example, some people cope with pain by distracting themselves, whereas others convince themselves that the pain is permanent, untreatable, and overwhelming. Research has shown that people who believe that their pain in uncontrollable and overwhelming are more likely to have poorer clinical outcomes.[20]

Cognitions about the pain also determine a patient's goals for and expectations about pain relief and treatment outcomes. Moreover, factors that affect cognition, such as sedation, dementia, delirium, and mental disability, alter the response to pain and make it more difficult for the observer to assess it.

Finally, the *sociocultural* dimension of pain encompasses factors such as demographics (e.g., age, gender, education, socioeconomic status), support systems, social roles, and culture. Age, gender, and education can influence pain perception, beliefs, and coping strategies.[21] Age and gender also influence nociceptive processes and responses to opioids[22] (see Gender box). Families and caregivers influence the patient's response to pain through their beliefs and behaviors. For example, families may discourage the patient from taking opioids because they fear the patient will become addicted. For patients who are unable to care for themselves, family or professional caregivers may act as gatekeepers and administer inadequate doses of analgesics.[23] Culture also affects the experience of pain, specifically pain expression, medication use, and pain-related beliefs and coping. The cultural determinants of pain must be assessed without stereotyping patients based on ethnic background.

GENDER DIFFERENCES
Pain

Men
- Men are less likely to report pain than women.
- Men report more control over pain.
- Men are less likely than women to use alternative treatments for pain.

Women
- 46% of American women report daily pain.
- Women are more likely to report headache, back pain, arthritis, and foot ache.
- Women identify stress as a cause of pain.

Pain Mechanisms

Nociception is the physiologic process by which information about tissue damage is communicated to the central nervous system (CNS).[1] Learning about the neurophysiologic mechanisms of pain is necessary to understanding the guidelines for pain assessment and treatment. Nociception involves four processes: (1) transduction, (2) transmission, (3) perception, and (4) modulation (Fig. 10-1).

Transduction. **Transduction** is the conversion of a mechanical, thermal, or chemical stimulus into a neuronal action potential. The transduction of pain signals occurs at the level of the peripheral nerves, in particular the free nerve endings, or nociceptors. Noxious (tissue-damaging) stimuli, including thermal (e.g., sunburn), mechanical (e.g., surgical incision, pressure), or chemical (e.g., toxic substances) injuries cause the release of numerous chemicals into the area surrounding the peripheral nociceptors. This "biologic soup" of chemicals includes hydrogen ions, substance P, and adenosine triphosphate (ATP). Other chemicals, including serotonin, histamine, bradykinin, and prostaglandins, are released from mast cells. Macrophages attracted to the inflamed area release bradykinin, interleukins, nerve growth factor, and tumor necrosis factor. These chemicals activate or sensitize nociceptors to excitation. Activation results in an action potential, which is carried from the nociceptors to the spinal cord primarily via small, rapidly conducting, myelinated A-delta fibers and unmyelinated, slowly conducting C fibers.

Understanding the chemical milieu surrounding nociceptors is important to understanding the transduction of chemical, thermal, or mechanical stimuli into a neural impulse (action potential). Inflammation and the subsequent release of chemical mediators increase the likelihood of transduction. This increased susceptibility is called *peripheral sensitization.* For example, a sunburn in which there is inflammation secondary to thermal injury can result in the sensation of pain or discomfort when the affected skin is lightly

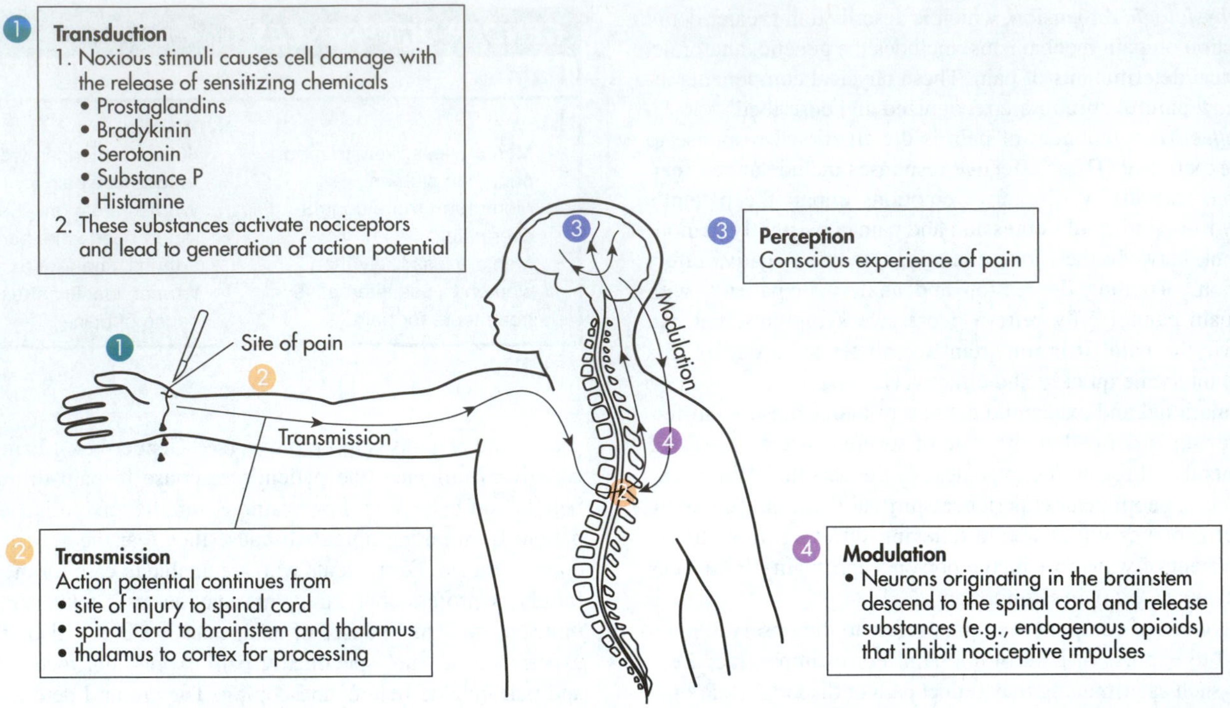

1 Transduction
1. Noxious stimuli causes cell damage with the release of sensitizing chemicals
• Prostaglandins
• Bradykinin
• Serotonin
• Substance P
• Histamine
2. These substances activate nociceptors and lead to generation of action potential
3 Perception
Conscious experience of pain
Modulation
1 Site of pain
2
Transmission
3
4
2 Transmission
Action potential continues from
• site of injury to spinal cord
• spinal cord to brainstem and thalamus
• thalamus to cortex for processing
4 Modulation
• Neurons originating in the brainstem descend to the spinal cord and release substances (e.g., endogenous opioids) that inhibit nociceptive impulses

FIG. 10-1 Nocioceptive pain originates when the tissue is injured. *1,* Transduction occurs when there is release of chemical mediators. *2,* Transmission involves the conduct of the action potential from the periphery (injury site) to the spinal cord and then to the brainstem, thalamus, and cerebral cortex. *3,* Perception is the conscious awareness of pain. *4,* Modulation involves signals from the brain going back down the spinal cord to modify incoming impulses.

touched. Several chemicals such as leukotrienes, prostaglandins, and substance P are involved in this process of sensitization.

The pain produced from activation of peripheral nociceptors is called **nociceptive pain.** There is a second source of pain-related action potentials arising from abnormal processing of stimuli by the nervous system. This kind of pain is called **neuropathic pain.** Both types of pain are described later in the chapter.

Therapies that alter either the local environment or sensitivity of the peripheral nociceptors can prevent transduction and initiation of an action potential. Decreasing the effects of chemicals released at the periphery is the basis of several drug approaches to pain relief. For example, nonsteroidal antiinflammatory drugs (NSAIDs), such as ibuprofen (Advil, Motrin) and naproxen (Naprosyn, Aleve), and corticosteroids, such as dexamethasone (Decadron), exert their analgesic effects by blocking pain-sensitizing chemicals. NSAIDs block the action of cyclooxygenase, thereby interfering with the production of prostaglandins. Corticosteroids block the action of phospholipase, thereby reducing the production of both prostaglandins and leukotrienes (see Chapter 13, Fig. 13-5). Drugs that stabilize the neuronal membrane and inactivate peripheral sodium channels inhibit production of the nerve impulse. These medications include local anesthetics (e.g., injectable or topical lidocaine, bupivacaine [Sensorcaine]), and antiseizure drugs (e.g., carbamazepine [Tegretol], oxcarbazepine [Trileptal], and lamotrigine [Lamictal]).

Transmission. **Transmission** is the movement of pain impulses from the site of transduction to the brain (see Fig. 10-1). Three segments are involved in nociceptive signal transmission: (1) transmission along the peripheral nerve fibers to the spinal cord, (2) dorsal horn processing, and (3) transmission to the thalamus and the cerebral cortex.

Transmission to the Spinal Cord. The first-order neuron extends the entire distance from the periphery to the dorsal horn of the spinal cord with no synapses. For example, an afferent fiber from the great toe travels from the toe through the fifth lumbar nerve root into the spinal cord; it is one cell. Once generated, an action potential travels all the way to the spinal cord unless it is blocked by a sodium channel inhibitor (e.g., local anesthetic) or disrupted by a lesion at the central terminal of the fiber (e.g., by a dorsal root entry zone [DREZ] lesion).

The manner in which nerve fibers enter the spinal cord is central to the notion of spinal dermatomes. **Dermatomes** are areas on the skin that are innervated primarily by a single spinal cord segment. The distinctive pattern of the rash caused by herpes zoster (shingles) across the back and trunk is determined by dermatomes. Fig. 10-2 illustrates different dermatomes and their innervations.

Dorsal Horn Processing. Once the nociceptive signal arrives in the CNS, it is processed within the dorsal horn of the spinal cord. This processing includes the release of neurotransmitters from the afferent fiber into the synaptic cleft. These neurotransmitters bind to receptors on nearby cell bodies and dendrites of cells that may be located elsewhere in the dorsal horn. Some of these neurotransmitters produce activation (e.g., glutamate, aspartate, substance P), whereas others inhibit activation of nearby cells (e.g., γ-aminobutyric acid [GABA], serotonin, norepinephrine). In this area exogenous and endogenous opioids also play an important role by binding to opioid receptors and blocking the release of neurotransmitters, particularly substance P. Endogenous opioids, which include enkephalin and β-endorphin, are chemicals that are synthesized and secreted by the body. They are capable of producing analgesic effects similar to those of exogenous opioids such as morphine. When enhanced excitability occurs in spinal neurons, it is termed *central sensitization.* Peripheral

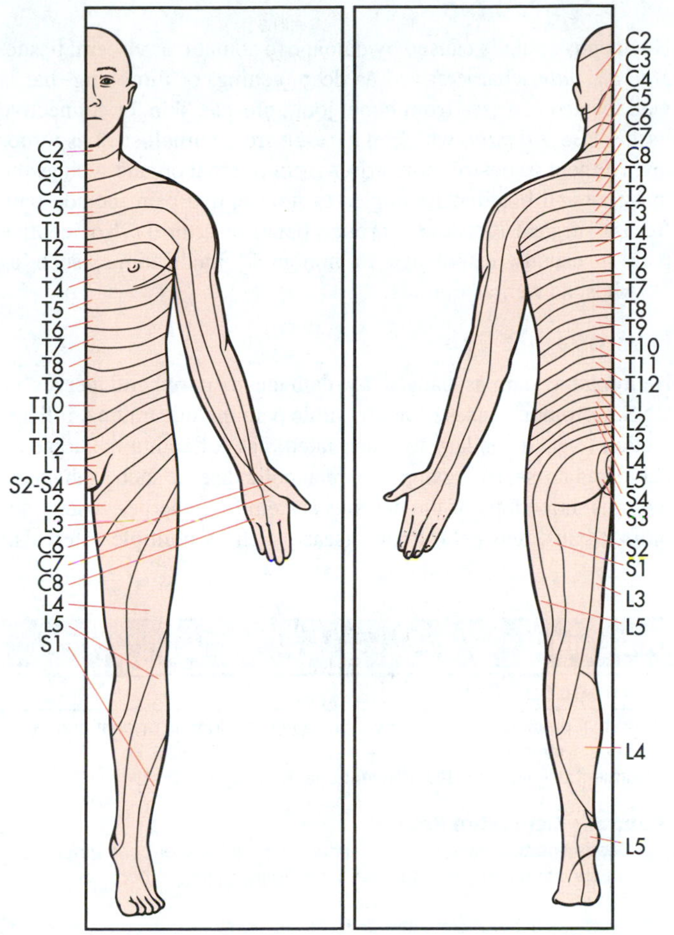

FIG. 10-2 Spinal dermatomes representing organized sensory input carried via specific spinal nerve roots. *C,* Cervical; *L,* lumbar; *S,* sacral; *T,* thoracic.

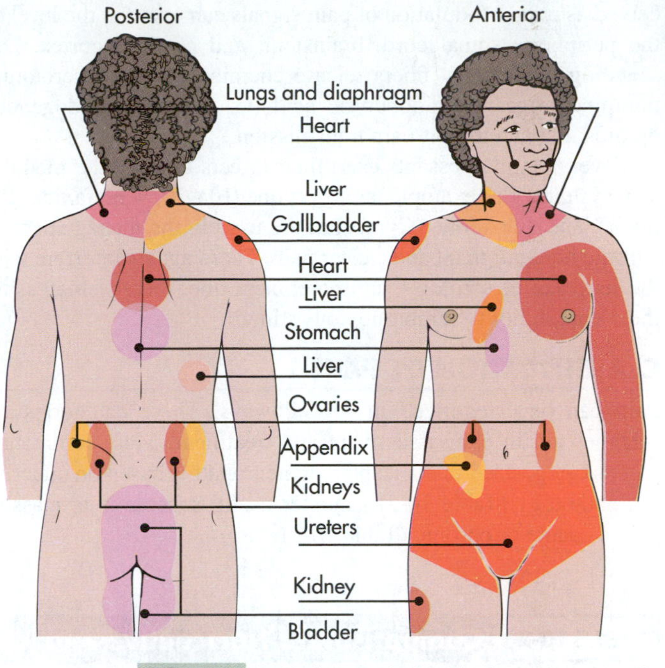

FIG. 10-3 Typical areas of referred pain.

tissue damage or nerve injury can cause central sensitization, and continued nociceptive input from the periphery is necessary to maintain it.[1] With ongoing stimulation of slowly conducting unmyelinated C-fiber nociceptors, firing of specialized dorsal horn neurons gradually increases. This process is known as "windup" and is dependent on the activation of *N*-methyl-D-aspartate (NMDA) receptors. Therefore NMDA receptor antagonists are promising agents that can potentially block central sensitization.

Glial cells act both as the structural support cells in the spinal cord and as immune-modulating cells. There are increasing data to suggest that glial cells may play an important role in central pain modulation, especially in chronic pain states. For example, cyclooxygenase-2 (COX-2) is produced by glial cells.[24]

Clinically, the central sensitization of the dorsal horn results in (1) increased responses to noxious stimuli (also known as *hyperalgesia*); (2) painful responses to normally innocuous stimuli (termed *allodynia*); (3) prolonged pain after the original noxious stimulus ends (called *persistent pain*); and (4) the spread of pain to uninjured tissue *(referred pain).*[1]

Referred pain must be considered when interpreting the location of pain reported by the person with injury to or disease involving visceral organs. The location of a tumor may be distant from the pain location reported by the patient (Fig. 10-3). For example, pain from liver disease is located in the right upper abdominal quadrant, but it frequently is referred to the anterior and posterior neck region and to a posterior flank area. If referred pain is not considered when evaluating a pain location report, diagnostic tests and therapy could be misdirected.

Transmission to Thalamus and Cortex. From the dorsal horn, nociceptive stimuli are communicated to the *third-order neuron,* primarily in the thalamus, and several other areas of the brain. Fibers of dorsal horn projection cells enter the brain through several pathways, including the spinothalamic tract (STT) and spinoreticular tract (SRT). Distinct thalamic nuclei receive nociceptive input from the spinal cord and have projections to several regions in the cerebral cortex, where the perception of pain is presumed to occur.

Perception. **Perception** occurs when pain is recognized, defined, and responded to by the individual experiencing the pain. In the brain, nociceptive input is perceived as pain. There is no single, precise location where pain perception occurs. Instead, pain perception involves several brain structures. For example, it is believed that the reticular activating system (RAS) is responsible for warning the individual to attend to the pain stimulus; the somatosensory system is responsible for localization and characterization of pain; and the limbic system is responsible for the emotional and behavioral responses to pain. Cortical structures also are thought to be crucial to constructing the meaning of the pain. Therefore behavioral strategies such as distraction and relaxation strategies are effective pain-reducing therapies for many people. By directing attention away from the pain sensation, patients can reduce the sensory and affective components of pain. For example, blood flow to the anterior central gyrus, an area intimately involved with the perception of the unpleasantness of pain, can be altered by hypnosis.[25]

The brain is necessary for pain perception; however, much is unknown about how and where pain is perceived. Until it is clearly understood where pain is perceived, it is important that nursing care involves treatment of any noxious stimulus as potentially painful, even in the cognitively impaired or comatose patient.

Modulation. **Modulation** involves the activation of descending pathways that exert inhibitory or facilitatory effects on the transmission of pain (see Fig. 10-1). Depending on the type and degree of modulation, nociceptive stimuli may or may not be perceived as pain. Modulation of pain signals can occur at the level of the periphery, spinal cord, brainstem, and cerebral cortex. Descending modulatory fibers release chemicals such as serotonin, norepinephrine, γ-aminobutyric acid (GABA), and endogenous opioids that can inhibit pain transmission.

Several antidepressants exert their effects through the modulatory systems. For example, amitriptyline (Elavil), venlafaxine (Effexor), and duloxetine (Cymbalta) are used in the management of chronic nonmalignant and cancer pain. These agents interfere with the reuptake of serotonin and norepinephrine, thereby increasing their availability to inhibit noxious stimuli.

CLASSIFICATION OF PAIN

Pain can be categorized in several ways. These categorization schemes aid in pain assessment and treatment. Most commonly, pain is categorized as nociceptive or neuropathic based on underlying pathology (Table 10-2). Another useful scheme is to classify pain as acute or chronic (Table 10-3).

Nociceptive Pain

Nociceptive pain is caused by damage to somatic or visceral tissue. *Somatic pain,* characterized as deep, aching, or throbbing that is well localized, arises from bone, joint, muscle, skin, or connective tissue. *Visceral pain,* which may result from stimuli such as tumor involvement or obstruction, arises from internal organs such as the intestine and bladder. Examples of nociceptive pain include pain from a surgical incision, a broken bone, or arthritis. Nociceptive pain is usually responsive to nonopioid medications, such as NSAIDs, as well as opioids.

Neuropathic Pain

Neuropathic pain is caused by damage to peripheral nerves or CNS. Common causes of neuropathic pain include trauma, inflammation (e.g., secondary to a herniated disk inflaming the adjacent nerve and dorsal root ganglion), metabolic disease such as diabetes mellitus, infections of the nervous system (e.g., herpes zoster), tumors, toxins, and neurologic disease such as multiple sclerosis.[1]

TABLE 10-2 Comparison of Nociceptive and Neuropathic Pain

	Nociceptive Pain	Neuropathic Pain
Definition	Normal processing of stimulus that damages normal tissue or has the potential to do so if prolonged. Usually responsive to nonopioid and/or opioid drugs.	Abnormal processing of sensory input by the peripheral or central nervous system. Treatment usually includes adjuvant analgesics.
Types	**Somatic Pain** Arises from bone, joint, muscle, skin, or connective tissue; usually aching or throbbing in quality and is well localized. **Visceral Pain** Arises from visceral organs, such as the GI tract and bladder. Can be further subdivided into the following: • Tumor involvement of the organ capsule that causes aching and fairly well-localized pain. • Obstruction of hollow organ that causes intermittent cramping and poorly localized pain.	**Centrally Generated Pain** • Deafferentation pain. Injury to either the peripheral or central nervous system (e.g., phantom pain may reflect injury to peripheral nerve). • Sympathetically maintained pain. Associated with dysregulation of the autonomic nervous system (e.g., reflex sympathetic dystrophy). **Peripherally Generated Pain** • Painful polyneuropathies. Pain is felt along the distribution of many peripheral nerves (e.g., diabetic neuropathy, alcohol-nutritional neuropathy, Guillain-Barré syndrome). • Painful mononeuropathies. Usually associated with a known peripheral nerve injury, and pain is felt at least partly along the distribution of the damaged nerve (e.g., nerve root compression, trigeminal neuralgia).

Adapted from McCaffery M, Pasero C: *Pain: clinical manual*, ed 2, St Louis, 1999, Mosby.

TABLE 10-3 Differences Between Acute and Chronic Pain

	Acute Pain	Chronic Pain
Onset	Sudden	Gradual or sudden
Duration	<3 months or as long as it takes for normal healing to occur	>3 months; may start as acute injury or event but continues past the normal time for recovery
Severity	Mild to severe	Mild to severe
Cause of pain	Generally can identify a precipitating event or illness (e.g., illness, surgery)	May not be known; original cause of pain may differ from mechanisms that maintain the pain
Course of pain	↓ Over time and goes away as recovery occurs	Typically pain does not go away; characterized by periods of waxing and waning
Typical physical and behavioral manifestations	Manifestations reflect sympathetic nervous system activation: • ↑ Heart rate • ↑ Respiratory rate • ↑ Blood pressure • Diaphoresis/pallor • Anxiety, agitation, confusion • Urine retention	Predominantly behavioral manifestations: • Flat affect • ↓ Physical movement/activity • Fatigue • Withdrawal from others and social interaction
Usual goals of treatment	Pain control with eventual elimination	Pain control to the extent possible; focus on enhancing function and quality of life

Deafferentation pain (injury to either the peripheral nervous system or CNS) and *sympathetically maintained pain* (associated with dysregulation of the autonomic nervous system) are considered centrally generated pain. Painful peripheral neuropathies (pain felt along the distribution of multiple peripheral nerves) and painful mononeuropathies (pain felt along the distribution of a damaged nerve) are considered peripherally generated pain. Examples of neuropathic pain include postherpetic neuralgia, phantom limb pain, diabetic neuropathies, and trigeminal neuralgia.

Typically described as numbing, burning, shooting, stabbing, or electrical in nature, neuropathic pain can be sudden, intense, short-lived, or lingering. Neuropathic pain often is not well controlled by opioid analgesics alone, and treatment often includes the use of adjuvant therapies, including antidepressants (e.g., amitriptyline [Elavil], venlafaxine [Effexor], buproprion [Wellbutrin]), antiseizure drugs (e.g., gabapentin [Neurontin]), and α_2-adrenergic agonists (e.g., clonidine [Catapres]).

Acute and Chronic Pain

Table 10-3 shows the classification of pain as acute or chronic. Acute pain and chronic pain are different as reflected in their cause, course, manifestations, and treatment. Examples of *acute pain* include postoperative pain, labor pain, pain from trauma (e.g., lacerations, fractures, sprains), infection (e.g., dysuria from cystitis), and angina. For acute pain, treatment includes analgesics for symptom control and treatment of the underlying cause (e.g., splinting for a fracture, antibiotic therapy for an infection). Normally, acute pain diminishes over time as healing occurs. However, acute pain that persists can ultimately become chronic pain. In some cases, however, acute pain evolves into a chronic state. For example, pain associated with herpes zoster (shingles) subsides as the acute infection resolves, usually within a month. However, sometimes the pain persists and develops into a chronic pain state called *postherpetic neuralgia.*

Chronic pain, or *persistent pain,* lasts for longer periods, often defined as longer than 3 months or past the time when an expected acute pain or acute injury should subside. Whereas acute pain functions as a signal, warning the person of potential or actual tissue damage, chronic pain does not appear to have any adaptive role. Chronic pain can be disabling and often is accompanied by anxiety and depression.[1,11]

Sometimes, chronic pain is further subdivided into cancer pain and noncancer pain. Chronic cancer-related pain arises from many causes, including disease progression, diagnostic procedures, anticancer therapies, and infection.[6] Cancer pain is often considered separate from noncancer pain because its cause can be determined, its course differs from noncancer pain (cancer pain often worsens with documented disease progression), and treatment strategies can be different from noncancer pain. However, despite these differences, there is little evidence to support this distinction, and the American Pain Society has stated that pain should simply be classified as acute or chronic.[1]

PAIN ASSESSMENT

Assessment is an essential, though often overlooked step, in pain management. Many local and national initiatives have aimed to ensure timely and consistent pain assessment. Several of these efforts urge clinicians to designate pain as the "fifth vital sign."[26]

The key to accurate and effective pain assessment is to conduct the evaluation in accordance with core principles established by several organizations.[1,2,26] These principles are listed in Table 10-4. Note that these basic tenets underscore the right of *all* patients to have their pain appropriately evaluated and treated.

The goals of a nursing pain assessment are (1) to describe the patient's multidimensional pain experience for the purpose of identifying and implementing appropriate pain management techniques and (2) to identify the patient's goal for therapy and resources for self-management. Often it is the nurse who is responsible for (1) gathering and documenting assessment data and (2) making collaborative decisions with the patient and other health care providers about pain management.

Elements of a Pain Assessment

Most components of a pain assessment involve direct interview or observation of the patient. Diagnostic studies and physical examination findings complete the initial assessment. Although the assessment will differ according to the clinical setting, patient popu-

TABLE 10-4 Core Principles of Pain Assessment

Principle	Nursing Implication
Patients have the right to appropriate assessment and management of pain.	Pain should be assessed in all patients.
Pain is always subjective.	The patient's self-report of pain is the single most reliable indicator of pain. The nurse needs to accept and respect this self-report unless there are clear reasons for doubt.
Physiologic and behavioral (objective) signs of pain (e.g., tachycardia, grimacing) are not sensitive or specific for pain.	Observations should not replace patient self-report unless the patient is unable to communicate.
Pain is an unpleasant sensory and emotional experience.	Assessment should address physical and psychologic aspects of pain.
Assessment approaches, including tools, must be appropriate for the patient population.	Special considerations are needed for obtaining assessment data for patients with difficulty communicating. Family members should be included in the assessment process, when possible.
Pain can exist even when no physical cause can be found.	Pain without an identifiable cause should not be attributed to psychologic causes.
Different patients experience different levels of pain in response to comparable stimuli.	A uniform pain threshold does not exist.
Patients with chronic pain may be more sensitive to pain and other stimuli.	Pain tolerance varies among and within individuals depending on various factors (e.g., heredity, energy level, coping skills, prior experience with pain).
Unrelieved pain has adverse physical and psychologic consequences.	Nurses should encourage patients to report pain, especially those who are reluctant to discuss pain, deny pain when it is likely present, or fail to follow through on prescribed treatments.

lation, and point of care (i.e., whether the assessment is part of an initial workup or a reassessment of pain following therapy), the evaluation of pain should always be multidimensional.

Before beginning any assessment, the nurse needs to recognize that patients may use words other than "pain." For example, older adults may deny that they have pain, but respond positively when asked if they have soreness or aching. The specific words that the patient uses to describe pain need to be documented, and the patient should be consistently asked about pain using those words.

Pain Characteristics. Basic pain characteristics include the following elements: onset, duration and pattern of the pain, location, intensity, quality, associated symptoms, and factors that increase or relieve the pain.[1]

Pattern of Pain. Pain *onset* involves finding out when the pain started. Patients with acute pain resulting from injury, acute illness, or treatment (e.g., surgery) typically will know exactly when the pain started. Those with chronic pain resulting from a failure of the body to heal properly or from a chronic progressive illness may be less able to identify when the pain started. Establishing how long the pain has lasted, or its *duration,* helps to determine if the pain is acute or chronic and assists in identifying the etiology of the pain. For example, a patient with advanced cancer who also has chronic low back pain from spinal stenosis reports a sudden, severe pain in the back that began 2 days ago. Knowing the onset and duration can lead to a diagnostic workup that may reveal new metastatic disease in the spine.

Pain pattern also provides clues about the cause of the pain and directs treatment. Many types of chronic pain wax and wane over time; for example, this pattern is typical of arthritis pain. A patient may have pain all the time (constant, around-the-clock pain), as well as discrete periods of intermittent pain. **Breakthrough pain** is a transient, moderate to severe pain that occurs beyond the pain treated by current analgesics. Many patients with cancer experience breakthrough pain. It is usually rapid in onset and brief in duration, with highly variable intensity and frequency of occurrence. Episodic, procedural, or incident pain is a transient increase in pain that is caused by a specific activity or event that precipitates the pain. Examples include dressing changes, movement, eating, position changes, and procedures such as catheterization.

Fig. 10-4 shows one method that can be used for the patient to document the pain pattern. This method allows the patient to report how pain intensity changes with time. A similar method can be used to document the changes in the area or nature of the pain.

Area of Pain. The area or *location* of pain assists in identifying possible causes and treatment. Some patients may be able to specify the precise location(s) of their pain, whereas others may describe very general areas, or comment that they "hurt all over." The location of the pain may also be referred from its origin to another site (see Fig. 10-3). Pain may also radiate from its origin to another site. For example, angina pectoris is known to radiate from the chest to the jaw or down the left arm. *Sciatica* is pain that follows the course of the sciatic nerve. It may originate from joints or muscles around the back or from compression or damage to the sciatic nerve. The pain is projected along the course of the peripheral nerve, causing painful shooting sensations down the back of the thigh and inside of the leg to the foot.

Typically, information about the location of pain is elicited by asking the patient to (1) describe the site(s) of pain, (2) point to painful areas on the body, or (3) mark painful areas on a pain map (Fig. 10-5). Because many patients have more than one site of

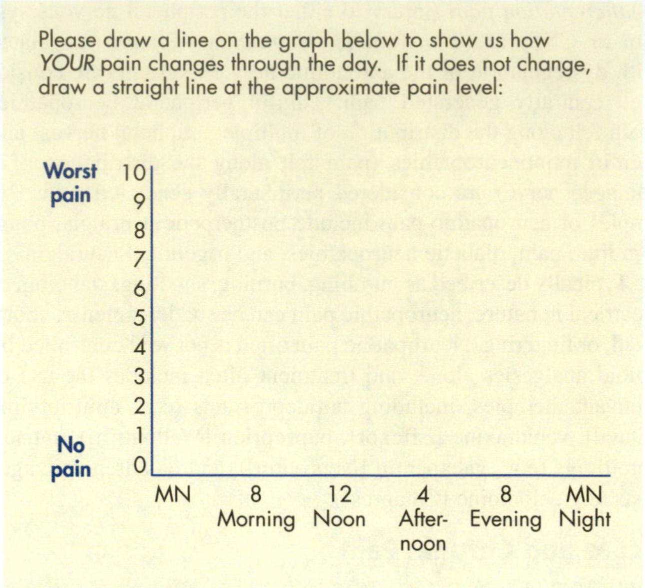

FIG. 10-4 A method of tracking pain over time.

pain, it is important to make certain that the patient describes every location.

Intensity of Pain. Assessing the severity, or *intensity,* of pain provides a reliable measure that is used to determine the type of treatment, as well as its effectiveness. Pain scales are useful tools to help the patient communicate pain intensity. Scales must be adjusted to age and cognitive development. Most adults can rate the intensity of their pain using numeric scales (e.g., 0 = no pain and 10 = the worst pain), verbal descriptor scales (e.g., none, a little, moderate, and severe), or visual analog scales (a 10-cm line with one end labeled "no pain" and the other end labeled "worst possible pain") (Fig. 10-6).

For nonverbal patients, such as comatose patients and those with advanced dementia, observational tools should be used to detect behaviors that are associated with pain. Several observational tools have been developed to provide valid and reliable assessment data.[27-29]

Pain Quality. The pain *quality* refers to the nature or characteristics of the pain. For example, patients typically describe neuropathic pain as a burning, numbing, shooting, stabbing, or itchy sensation. Nociceptive pain may be described as sharp, aching, throbbing, and cramping.

Associated Symptoms. Associated symptoms such as anxiety, fatigue, and depression may exacerbate or be exacerbated by pain. The nurse should ask about activities and situations that increase or alleviate pain. For example, musculoskeletal pain often is exacerbated with movement and ambulation. In contrast, resting or immobilizing a painful body part can decrease pain.

Management Strategies. As people experience or live with pain, they try different strategies to manage it. Some are successful whereas others are not. To maximize the effectiveness of the pain treatment plan, it is important to ask patients what they are using now to control pain and what they have used in the past. Strategies include prescription and nonprescription drugs and nondrug therapies such as hot and cold applications, complementary and alternative therapies (e.g., herbal products, acupuncture), and relaxation strategies (e.g., imagery). All strategies must be documented, both those that work and those that are ineffective.

Initial Pain Assessment Tool

Date ____________

Patient's Name ________________________ Age ________ Room ________

Diagnosis ________________________ Physician ________________________

Nurse ________________________

1. LOCATION: Patient or nurse mark drawing.

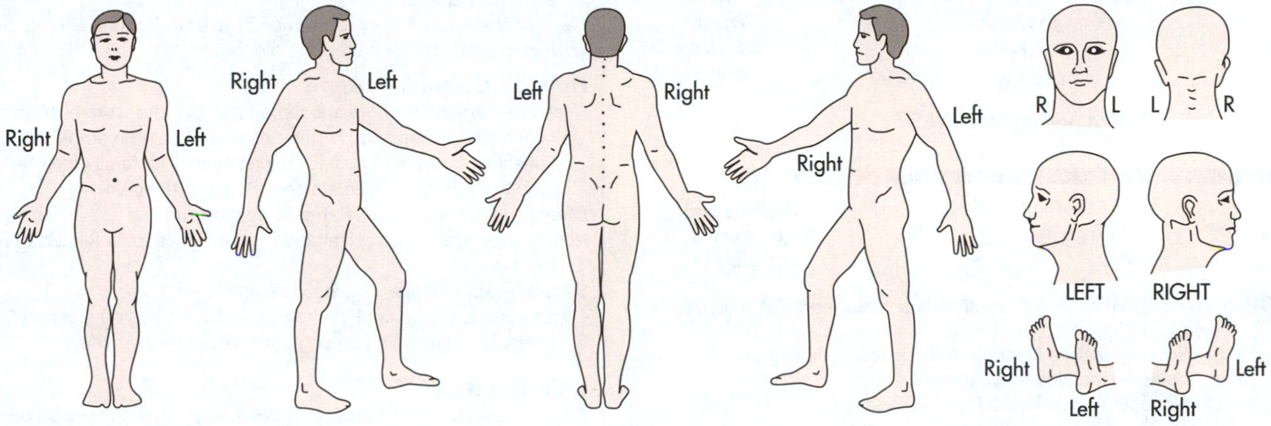

2. INTENSITY: Patient rates the pain. Scale used ________________________

Present: ________________________

Worst pain gets: ________________________

Best pain gets: ________________________

Acceptable level of pain: ________________________

3. QUALITY: (Use patient's own words, e.g., prick, ache, burn, throb, pull, sharp) ________________________

4. ONSET, DURATION, VARIATIONS, RHYTHMS: ________________________

5. MANNER OF EXPRESSING PAIN: ________________________

6. WHAT RELIEVES THE PAIN? ________________________

7. WHAT CAUSES OR INCREASES THE PAIN? ________________________

8. EFFECTS OF PAIN: (Note decreased function, decreased quality of life.)

Accompanying symptoms (e.g., nausea) ________________________

Sleep ________________________

Appetite ________________________

Physical activity ________________________

Relationship with others (e.g., irritability) ________________________

Emotions (e.g., anger, suicidal, crying) ________________________

Concentration ________________________

Other ________________________

9. OTHER COMMENTS: ________________________

10. PLAN: ________________________

FIG. 10-5 Initial pain assessment tool. *(May be duplicated for use in clinical practice. From McCaffery M, Pasero C: Pain: clinical manual, ed 2, St Louis, 1999, Mosby. Copyright © 1999, Mosby.)*

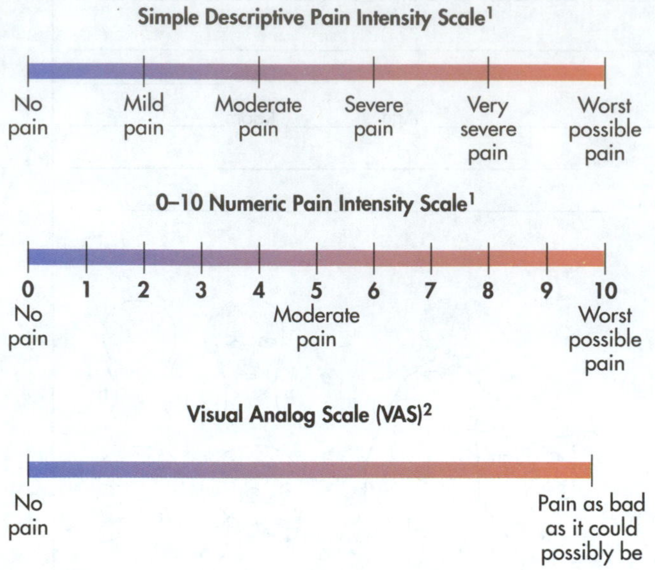

FIG. 10-6 Simple descriptive word tool and visual analog scale (VAS) used to assess patient's pain.
[1]If used as a graphic rating scale, a 10-cm baseline is recommended.
[2]A 10-cm baseline is recommended for VAS scales.
(From Acute Pain Management Guideline Panel, 1992.)

TABLE 10-5 NURSING ASSESSMENT
Pain

Subjective Data

Important Health Information

Health history: Pain history includes onset, location, intensity, quality, patterns, and expression of pain; coping strategies; past treatments and their effectiveness; pain triggers; review of health care utilization related to the pain problem (e.g., emergency department visits, treatment at pain clinics, visits to primary health care providers and specialists)

Medications: Use of any prescription or over-the-counter, illicit, or herbal products for pain relief; alcohol use

Functional Health Patterns

Health perception–health management: Social and work history; mental health history; smoking history; effects of pain on emotions, relationships, sleep, and activities; interviews with family members; records from psychiatric treatment related to the pain

Elimination: Constipation related to opioid drug use

Activity-exercise: Fatigue, limitations in activities, pain related to muscle use

Sexuality-reproductive: Decreased libido

Coping–stress tolerance: Psychologic evaluation using standardized measures to examine coping style, depression, anxiety

Objective Data

Physical examination, including evaluation of functional limitations
Psychosocial evaluation

Affective, Behavioral, Cognitive, and Sociocultural Components

Impact of Pain. Pain can have profound influences on a patient's quality of life and functioning. Pain that is persistent can have a profound, negative impact on a person's life. Assessment should include the effect of the pain on the patient's ability to sleep, enjoy life, interact with others, perform work and household duties, and engage in physical and social activities. One should also assess the impact of pain on the patient's mood.

Patient's Beliefs, Expectations, and Goals. Patient and family beliefs, attitudes, and expectations influence responses to pain and pain treatment. The nurse assesses attitudes and beliefs that may hinder effective treatment, such as the belief that opioid use will result in addiction. Patients are asked about their expectations and goals for pain management.

In an acute care setting, time limitations may dictate an abbreviated assessment of the affective, behavioral, cognitive, and sociocultural dimensions of pain. At a minimum, the effects of the pain on the patient's sleep and daily activities, relationships with others, physical activity, and emotional well-being should be assessed. In addition, the ways in which the patient describes the pain and the strategies that the patient has used to accept and control the pain should be included.

In some clinical settings, additional assessment information is necessary to ensure effective treatment. This is particularly true when working with chronic pain patients. Initial evaluation for this patient population typically includes items shown in Table 10-5. This comprehensive assessment involves a multidisciplinary pain team, including physicians, nurses, psychologists, and physical and occupational therapists.

Documentation of the pain assessment is critical to ensure effective communication among team members and appropriate care planning and implementation. Many health care facilities and agencies have adopted specific tools to record an initial pain assessment, treatment, and reassessment. One example of an initial pain assessment tool appears in Fig. 10-5. There also are many multidimensional pain assessment tools. Examples include the Brief Pain Inventory, the Memorial Pain Assessment Card, and the Neuropathic Pain Scale.[30, 31]

Reassessment of pain also is critical and should occur at appropriate intervals. For example, reassessment for a postoperative patient should be within 30 minutes of an intravenous dose of an analgesic. In a long-term care facility, residents with persistent pain should be reassessed at least quarterly or with a change in condition or functional status.[32] Frequency and scope of reassessment are guided by factors such as pain severity, physical and psychosocial comorbidities, and institutional policy.

PAIN TREATMENT

Basic Principles

All pain treatment is guided by the same underlying principles. Although treatment regimens range from the relatively simple, short-term management of postoperative pain to multimodal, long-term therapy required for patients with chronic pain syndromes, all treatment should follow the same basic standards. The following are basic principles in treating pain.

1. *Follow the principles of pain assessment.* These guidelines are listed in Table 10-4. Remember that pain is a subjective experience. Thus the patient is not only the best judge of his or her own pain, but also is the expert on the effectiveness of each pain treatment.
2. *Every patient deserves adequate pain management.* Many patient populations, including racial minorities, the elderly, and people with past or current substance abuse, are at risk for inadequate pain management. Health care providers need to be aware of their own biases and ensure that all patients are treated respectfully.

3. *Base the treatment plan on the patient's goals.* Discussion about the patient's goals for pain treatment should occur at the initial pain assessment. Although this goal can be described in terms of pain intensity (e.g., the desire for average pain to decrease from an "8/10" to a "3/10"), in chronic pain conditions functional goal setting should be encouraged (e.g., a person sets a goal of performing certain daily activities, including socializing and hobbies). Over the course of prolonged therapy, these goals should be reassessed, and progress toward meeting them should be documented. The patient, rather than the health care team, determines new goals. If the patient has unrealistic goals for therapy, such as wanting to be completely rid of all chronic arthritis pain, the nurse should work with the patient to establish a more realistic goal.
4. *Use both drug and nondrug therapies.* Although medications are often considered the mainstay of therapy, particularly for moderate to severe pain, nondrug therapies should be incorporated to increase the overall effectiveness of therapy and to allow for the reduction of drug dosages to minimize adverse drug effects.[1,10]
5. *Address pain using a multidisciplinary approach.* It is difficult to address all dimensions of the pain experience without incorporating multiple disciplines. These disciplines frequently include clinical psychology, physical and occupational therapy, pharmacy services, spiritual care, and multiple medical specialties such as neurology, pain and palliative care, oncology, surgery, and anesthesiology. Some pain services also include complementary therapy practitioners such as massage therapists, acupuncturists, and art therapists.
6. *Evaluate the effectiveness of all therapies to ensure that they are meeting the patient's goals.* Therapy must be individualized for each patient. Achievement of an effective treatment plan often requires trial and error. Adjustments in drug, dosage, or route are common to achieve maximal benefit while minimizing adverse effects. This trial-and-error process can become frustrating for the patient and family. They need to be reassured that pain relief, if not pain cessation, is possible and that the health care team will continue to work with them to achieve adequate pain relief.
7. *Prevent and/or manage medication side effects.* Side effects are a major reason for treatment failure and nonadherence. Side effects are managed in one of several ways,[33] as described in Table 10-6. The nurse plays a key role in monitoring for and treating side effects, as well as patient and family teaching to minimize adverse effects.

TABLE 10-6 DRUG THERAPY
Managing Side Effects of Pain Medications

- Changing the dosing regimen to maintain relatively constant blood levels
- Changing to a different medication in the same class
- Adding a drug to counteract the adverse effect of the analgesic (e.g., initiating a bowel regimen using a gentle stimulant laxative and a stool softener for patients experiencing opioid-induced constipation)
- Using an administration route that minimizes drug concentrations at the site of the side effect (e.g., intraspinal administration of opioids is sometimes used to minimize high drug levels that produce sedation, nausea, and vomiting)

8. *Incorporate patient and family teaching throughout assessment and treatment.* Content should include information about the cause(s) of the pain, pain assessment methods, treatment goals and options, expectations of pain management, instruction regarding the proper use of drugs, side effect management, and nondrug and self-help pain relief measures. Teaching should be documented, and both patient comprehension and family comprehension of the teaching are evaluated.

Drug Therapy for Pain

Pain medications generally are divided into three categories: nonopioids, opioids, and co-analgesic or adjuvant drugs. The pain treatment plan may include medications from one or more of these groups. Mild pain often can be relieved using nonopioids alone. Moderate to severe pain usually requires an opioid. Certain types of pain, such as neuropathic pain, often require a co-analgesic and adjuvant drug. Pain caused by specific medical conditions, such as cancer and rheumatoid arthritis, may be treated with curative or disease-modifying therapies (e.g., chemotherapy for cancer; tumor necrosis factor antagonists such as etanercept [Enbrel] for rheumatoid arthritis), as well as pain medications.

Nonopioids. Nonopioid analgesics include acetaminophen, aspirin and other salicylates, and NSAIDs (Table 10-7). These agents are characterized by the following: (1) there is an **analgesic ceiling** to their analgesic properties; that is, increasing the dose beyond an upper limit provides no greater analgesia; (2) they do not produce tolerance or physical dependence; and (3) many are available without a prescription. It is important to monitor over-the-counter (OTC) analgesic use to avoid serious problems related to drug interactions, side effects, and overdose.

Aspirin is effective for mild pain but its use is limited by its common side effects, including gastric upset, platelet dysfunction, and bleeding. Other salicylates such as choline magnesium trisalicylate (Trilisate) cause fewer GI disturbances and bleeding abnormalities. Like aspirin, acetaminophen (Tylenol) has analgesic and antipyretic effects, but unlike aspirin, it has no antiplatelet or antiinflammatory effects. Although acetaminophen is well tolerated, it is metabolized by the liver, and doses of greater than 3 to 4 g/day, acute overdose, or use by patients with alcoholism or liver disease can result in severe hepatotoxicity. Recent studies suggest that acetaminophen may not be as safe on the stomach or kidneys as first thought, and recommendations by some are that the daily maximum dosage should be 3 g or less, particularly in older adults.[34]

The NSAIDs represent a broad class of drugs with varying efficacy and side effects. All NSAIDs inhibit the enzyme cyclooxygenase (COX), the enzyme that converts arachidonic acid into prostaglandins and related compounds. The COX enzyme is found in all tissues and helps regulate multiple processes, such as inflammation, protection of gastric mucosa, platelet aggregation, and maintenance of renal blood flow.

***Drug Alert** - Nonsteroidal Antiinflammatory Drugs (NSAIDs)*
- *NSAIDs (except aspirin) have been linked to a higher risk for increased cardiovascular events such as stroke and myocardial infarction.*
- *Patients who have just had heart surgery should not take NSAIDs.*

There are two forms of the enzyme, COX-1 and COX-2. COX-1 is found in almost all tissues and is responsible for several protective physiologic functions. In contrast, COX-2 is produced mainly at the sites of tissue injury, where it mediates inflammation (Fig. 10-7).

TABLE 10-7 DRUG THERAPY
Comparison of Selected Nonopioid Analgesics

Drug	Analgesic Efficacy Compared to Standards	Nursing Considerations
acetaminophen (Tylenol)	Comparable to aspirin	Rectal suppository available; sustained-release preparations available; maximum daily dose of 3-4 g Doses above 3 g per day may cause gastric irritation and bleeding Acute overdose: acute liver failure Chronic overdose: liver toxicity
Salicylates		
aspirin	Standard for comparison	Rectal suppository available; sustained-release preparations available Possibility of upper GI bleeding
choline magnesium trisalicylate (Trilisate)	Longer duration than aspirin	Unlike aspirin and NSAIDs, does not increase bleeding time
Nonsteroidal Antiinflammatory Drugs (NSAIDs)		
ibuprofen (Motrin, Nuprin, Advil)	Superior at 200 mg to aspirin 650 mg	Concern regarding the potential for upper GI bleeding
indomethacin (Indocin)	25 mg comparable to aspirin 650 mg	Not routinely used because of high incidence of side effects; rectal, IV, and sustained-release oral forms available
ketorolac (Toradol)	30 mg equivalent to 6 mg morphine	Limit treatment to 5 days; may precipitate renal failure in dehydrated patients
diclofenac K (Cataflam)	50 mg superior in efficacy and analgesic duration to aspirin 650 mg	Available in oral, ophthalmic, topical preparations
Cyclooxygenase-2 (COX-2) Inhibitors		
celecoxib (Celebrex)	Similar to other NSAIDs	Cause fewer GI side effects, including bleeding, than other NSAIDs but risk still present; are more costly than other NSAIDs

Inhibition of COX-1 causes many of the untoward effects of NSAIDs, such as impairment of renal function, bleeding tendencies, and GI upset and ulceration. Inhibition of COX-2 is associated with the therapeutic, antiinflammatory effects of NSAIDs.

Older NSAIDs, such as ibuprofen, inhibit both forms of COX and are referred to as nonselective NSAIDs. In the late 1990s, NSAIDs that selectively inhibit COX-2 were introduced. These medications, which include celecoxib (Celebrex), are called COX-2 inhibitors. Although these drugs initially were marketed as effective and safe, concerns about increased risk of adverse cardiovascular effects, including myocardial infarction, strokes, and heart failure, have raised questions about the future of these agents. Two COX-2 inhibitors, rofecoxib (Vioxx) and valdecoxib (Bextra), have been removed from the market. Whether or not the class of COX-2 inhibitors as a whole carries the same risks remains a matter of debate. However, patients with a history of cardiac problems or stroke should be prescribed these medications cautiously, for as short a time as possible, if at all.[35]

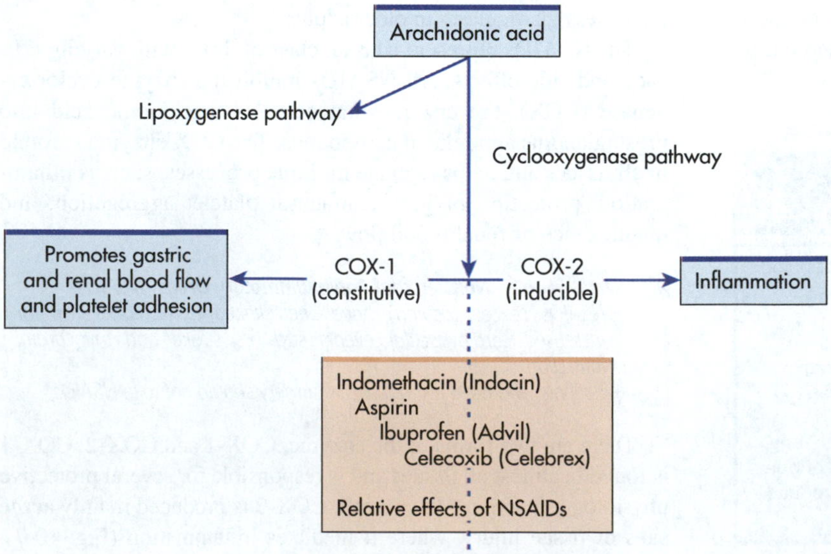

FIG. 10-7 Arachidonic acid is oxidized by two different pathways: lipoxygenase and cyclooxygenase. The cyclooxygenase pathway leads to two forms of the enzyme cyclooxygenase: COX-1 and COX-2. COX-1 is known as "constitutive" (always present) and COX-2 is known as "inducible" (meaning its expression varies markedly depending on the stimulus). NSAIDs differ in their actions, with some having more effects on COX-1 and others more on COX-2. Indomethacin acts primarily on COX-1, whereas ibuprofen is equipotent on COX-1 and COX-2. Celecoxib primarily inhibits COX-2.

Some NSAIDs possess equal analgesic efficacy as aspirin, whereas others have higher efficacy.[33] Patients vary greatly in their responses to a specific NSAID, so when one NSAID does not provide relief, another should be tried. NSAIDs are associated with many side effects, including bleeding tendencies secondary to decreased platelet aggregation and GI problems ranging from dyspepsia to ulceration and hemorrhage. Renal insufficiency and CNS dysfunction also occur. Serious side effects of NSAIDs result in thousands of hospitalizations every year. Thus the use of NSAIDs should be limited in those at highest risk for adverse effects, including the elderly and patients with a history of peptic ulcer disease.[10]

Opioids. Opioids (Table 10-8) produce their effects by binding to receptors in the CNS. This results in (1) inhibition of the transmission of nociceptive input from the periphery to the spinal cord; (2) altered limbic system activity; and (3) activation of the descending inhibitory pathways that modulate transmission in the spinal cord. Thus opioids act on several nociceptive processes.[1]

Types of Opioids. Opioids are categorized according to their physiologic action (i.e., agonist and antagonist) and binding at specific opioid receptors (e.g., mu, kappa, and delta).[1] Since most opioids used clinically bind to mu receptors, discussion will focus on two groups of opioids: pure agonists and agonist-antagonists/partial agonists. Naloxone (Narcan), an opioid antagonist, is used to reverse the respiratory sedation accompanying acute overdoses of opioids and to ameliorate other opioid side effects.

Opioid agonists are used for acute and chronic pain. Nociceptive pain appears to be more responsive to opioids than neuro-

TABLE 10-8 *DRUG THERAPY* Opioid Analgesics

Drug	Routes of Administration	Nursing Considerations
Mu Agonists		
morphine (Roxanol, MSContin, Avinza, Kadian, Epimorph, MSIR, Oramorph SR)	PO (immediate-release and sustained-release forms), rectal, IV, subcutaneous, epidural, intrathecal, sublingual	Standard comparison for opioid analgesics Indicated for moderate to severe pain Can stimulate histamine release
hydromorphone (Dilaudid)	PO, rectal, IV, subcutaneous, epidural, intrathecal	Slightly shorter duration than morphine
methadone (Dolophine)	PO, IM	Good oral potency; 24-36 hr half-life Accumulates with repeated dosing Use with caution in older adults
levorphanol (Levo-Dromoran)	PO, IV, IM, subcutaneous	Plasma half-life 12-16 hr; accumulates with repeated dosing
fentanyl (Sublimaze, Duragesic, Actiq)	IV, epidural, intrathecal, oral transmucosal, transdermal	Immediate onset after IV route; 7-8 min after IM route; 5-15 min after transmucosal route; onset may take several hours after transdermal route IV fentanyl often combined with benzodiazepines for procedural analgesia and sedation Very potent—dosages are in micrograms (mcg)
oxycodone (Percocet, Percodan, Endocet, Tylox, Roxicodone, OxyContin, Combunox)	PO (immediate-release and sustained-release forms)	Immediate-release and sustained-release preparations Available as single entity and in combination with a nonopioid Can be used like oral morphine for severe pain Often combined with a nonopioid for acute, moderate pain
hydrocodone (Lortab, Vicodin, Zydone)	PO (currently only available in combination with acetaminophen, aspirin, or ibuprofen)	Available in combination with nonopioid Hydrocodone plus acetaminophen for moderate or moderately severe pain Hydrocodone plus ibuprofen combination product indicated for short-term (generally <10 days) management of acute pain (e.g., trauma, musculoskeletal)
codeine (Tylenol #3)	PO, subcutaneous	Associated with higher incidence of nausea and constipation than other mu agonists Many codeine preparations are combined with acetaminophen
Mixed Agonist-Antagonists		
pentazocine (Talwin)	Formulated in combination with acetaminophen, aspirin, ibuprofen; some preparations include naloxone to discourage parenteral abuse	May cause psychotomimetic effects (e.g., hallucinations) and may precipitate withdrawal in opioid-dependent patients
butorphanol (Stadol)	Not available orally; not scheduled under Controlled Substance Act	Psychotomimetic effects lower than with pentazocine May precipitate withdrawal in opioid-dependent patients
Partial Agonists		
buprenorphine (Buprenex) buprenorphine plus naloxone (Suboxone)	Lower abuse potential than morphine; does not produce psychotomimetic effects Suboxone used as a sublingual preparation for opioid addict maintenance or for easier withdrawal when necessary to taper from opioids	May precipitate withdrawal in opioid-dependent patients; not readily reversed by naloxone

IM, Intramuscular; *IV*, intravenous; *PO*, per os (orally).

pathic pain, although opioids are used in both types of pain. Pure opioid agonists include morphine, oxycodone (Oxycontin), hydrocodone, codeine, methadone, hydromorphone (Dilaudid), and levorphanol (Levo-Dromoran) (see Table 10-8). These drugs are effective for moderate to severe pain because they are potent, have no analgesic ceiling, and can be administered through several routes. Morphine is the standard of comparison for all other opioid analgesics.

Drug Alert - *Morphine*
- *May cause respiratory depression.*
- *If respirations are ≤12 per minute, withhold medication and contact health care provider.*

When opioids are prescribed for moderate pain, they are usually combined with a nonopioid analgesic such as acetaminophen (e.g., codeine plus acetaminophen [Tylenol #3], hydrocodone plus acetaminophen [Vicodin], or ibuprofen [Vicoprofen]). Addition of acetaminophen or NSAIDs limits the total daily dose that can be given.

Mixed *agonist-antagonists* (e.g., pentazocine [Talwin], butorphanol [Stadol]) bind as agonists on the kappa receptor and as weak antagonists or partial agonists on the mu receptor. Because of this difference in binding, mixed agonist-antagonists produce less respiratory depression than drugs that act at only mu receptors (mu agonists). However, they also cause more dysphoria and agitation. In addition, opioid agonist-antagonists have an analgesic ceiling and can precipitate withdrawal if used in a patient who is physically dependent on mu agonist drugs. Partial opioid agonists (e.g., buprenorphine [Buprenex]) bind weakly to mu and kappa receptors, which decreases their analgesic efficacy. Agonist-antagonists and partial agonists currently have limited availability and clinical value in pain management.[1]

Opioids to Avoid. There is growing consensus that some opioids should be avoided because of limited efficacy and/or toxicities. For example, propoxyphene (Darvon) is only as effective as 600 mg of aspirin and produces a toxic metabolite that can cause seizures. Thus it generally is not recommended in analgesic guidelines.[10] Another opioid with limited usefulness is meperidine (Demerol, Pethidine). This drug is associated with neurotoxicity (e.g., seizures) caused by accumulation of its metabolite, normeperidine. Meperidine is contraindicated for patients with acute pain lasting more than 2 days and for those in whom large doses (more than 600 mg per 24 hours) are needed.[33] It should not be used in treating chronic pain. A hyperpyrexic syndrome with delirium, which can cause death, can occur if meperidine is given to patients taking monoamine oxidase inhibitors.[33]

Side Effects of Opioids. Common side effects of opioids include constipation, nausea and vomiting, sedation, respiratory depression, and pruritus. With continued use, many side effects diminish; the exception is constipation. Less common side effects include urinary retention, myoclonus, dizziness, confusion, and hallucinations.

Constipation is the most common opioid side effect. Because tolerance to opioid-induced constipation does not occur, a bowel regimen should be instituted at the beginning of opioid therapy and continue for as long as the person takes opioids. Although dietary roughage, fluids, and exercise should be encouraged to the extent possible, these measures may not be sufficient by themselves. Thus most patients should begin immediately on a gentle stimulant laxative (e.g., senna) plus a stool softener (e.g., docusate sodium [Colace]). Other agents (e.g., milk of magnesia, bisacodyl [Dulcolax], polyethylene glycol [MiraLax], or lactulose [Constulose]) can be added if necessary. Left untreated, constipation may not only increase the individual's pain but can lead to impaction and paralytic ileus that can be difficult to differentiate from obstruction.

Nausea often is a problem in opioid-naive patients. The use of antiemetics such as metoclopramide [Reglan], transdermal scopolamine [Transderm-Scop], hydroxyzine [Vistaril], or a phenothiazine (e.g., prochlorperazine [Compazine]) can prevent or minimize opioid-related nausea and vomiting until tolerance develops, which usually occurs within 1 week. Metoclopramide is particularly effective when a patient reports a feeling of gastric fullness. Opioids delay gastric emptying, and this effect can be reduced by metoclopramide. If nausea and vomiting are severe and persistent, changing to a different opioid may be necessary.

Concerns about sedation and respiratory depression are two of the most common fears associated with opioids. Sedation usually is seen in opioid-naive patients. However, for most patients, sedation resolves with the development of tolerance. Persistent sedation with chronic opioid use can be effectively treated with psychostimulants such as caffeine, dextroamphetamine (Dexedrine), methylphenidate (Ritalin), or the newer anticataleptic drug modafinil (Provigil).[36]

Clinically significant respiratory depression is rare in opioid-tolerant patients and when opioids are titrated to analgesic effect. Patients at risk for respiratory depression include those who are opioid naive, are elderly, have underlying lung disease, or are receiving other CNS depressants (e.g., sedatives, benzodiazepines, antihistamines). Clinically significant respiratory depression cannot occur in patients who are awake. Thus level of consciousness should be monitored in addition to the respiratory rate.[1,37]

If severe respiratory depression occurs and stimulation of the patient (calling and shaking patient) does not reverse the somnolence or increase the respiratory rate and depth, naloxone (Narcan, 0.4 mg in 10 ml saline), an opioid antagonist, can be administered intravenously or subcutaneously in 0.5-ml increments every 2 minutes. However, if the patient has been taking opioids regularly for more than a few days, naloxone should be used judiciously and titrated carefully because its use can precipitate severe, agonizing pain, profound withdrawal symptoms, and seizures. Because naloxone's half-life (60 to 90 minutes) is shorter than most opiates, nurses should monitor the patient's respiratory rate because it can drop again 1 to 2 hours after naloxone administration.[37] A continuous infusion of low-dose naloxone may be appropriate until the original opioid is cleared by metabolism.

Pruritus (itching) is another common side effect of opioids and occurs most frequently when opioids are administered via intraspinal (i.e., epidural, intrathecal) routes. An antihistamine such as diphenhydramine (Benadryl) often is effective but causes drowsiness. Changing to a different opioid may be necessary. If other measures are ineffective, a low-dose opioid antagonist (e.g., naloxone) or mixed agonist-antagonist can be used, but the patient must be carefully assessed for reversal of analgesia and withdrawal.[33]

Adjuvant Analgesic Therapy. These medications, sometimes referred to as *co-analgesics*, are drugs used in conjunction with opioid and nonopioid analgesics. Generally, these agents were developed originally for other purposes (e.g., antiseizure, antidepressants) and found later to be effective for pain. Commonly used analgesic adjuvants are listed in Table 10-9.

Antidepressants. Tricyclic antidepressants enhance the descending inhibitory system by preventing the cellular reuptake of

TABLE 10-9 DRUG THERAPY
Adjuvant Drugs Used for Pain Management

Drug	Specific Indication	Nursing Considerations
Corticosteroids	Inflammation	Avoid high dose for long-term use
Antidepressants		
amitriptyline (Elavil) doxepin (Sinequan) imipramine (Tofranil-PM) nortriptyline (Pamelor)	Neuropathic pain	Monitor for anticholinergic adverse effects Monitor blood levels during chronic therapy
Antiseizure Drugs		
carbamazepine (Tegretol) gabapentin (Neurontin)	Neuropathic pain	Start with low doses, increase slowly; *carbamazepine:* check liver function tests, renal function, and blood counts at baseline and at 2 and 6 wk; *gabapentin:* monitor for idiosyncratic side effects (e.g., ankle swelling [more common in the elderly and at doses >1800 mg/day], ataxia)
Muscle Relaxant		
Baclofen (Lioresal)	Neuropathic pain, muscle spasms	Monitor for weakness, urinary dysfunction; avoid abrupt discontinuation because of CNS irritability
α_2-Adrenergic Agonist		
clonidine (Duraclon)	Particularly useful for neuropathic pain when administered intrathecally	Side effects include sedation, orthostatic hypotension, dry mouth; often combined with anesthetics (e.g., bupivacaine [Sensorcaine])
Anesthetics: Systemic or Oral		
mexiletine (Mexitil)	Diabetic neuropathy; neuropathic pain	Monitor for side effects; high incidence of nausea, dizziness, perioral numbness, paresthesias, tremor; can cause seizures, dysrhythmias, and myocardial depression at high doses; avoid in patients with preexisting cardiac disease
Anesthetics: Local		
Topical EMLA (eutectic mixture of local anesthetics): lidocaine 2.5% + prilocaine 2.5%	Local skin analgesic before venipuncture or incision; possibly effective for postherpetic neuralgia	Must be applied under an occlusive dressing (e.g., Tegaderm, DuoDerm, or on an anesthetic disk); absorption from the genital mucosa more rapid and onset time shorter (5-10 min) than after application to intact skin; common adverse effects include mild erythema, edema, skin blanching
capsaicin (Zostrix)	Pain associated with arthritis, postherpetic neuralgia, diabetic neuropathy	Apply very sparingly onto affected area; use gloves or wash hands with soap and water after application; side effects include skin irritation (burning, stinging) at the application site, as well as cough

serotonin and norepinephrine. Higher levels of serotonin and norepinephrine in the synaptic cleft inhibit the transmission of nociceptive signals in the CNS. Other potential beneficial actions of tricyclic antidepressants include sodium channel modulation, α_1-adrenergic antagonist effects, and a weak NMDA receptor modulation. They appear to be effective for a variety of pain syndromes, especially neuropathic pain syndromes.[38]

Doses of antidepressants required for pain relief often are lower than those necessary for depression. Anticholinergic side effects (dry mouth, urinary retention, sedation, and orthostatic hypotension) often decrease patient compliance and adherence. Weight gain and sexual dysfunction are two additional reasons why patients stop taking antidepressant medications. The usefulness of selective serotonin reuptake inhibitors (e.g., paroxetine [Paxil], sertraline [Zoloft], and fluoxetine [Prozac]) in treating pain has not been demonstrated in large, randomized, controlled trials. At this time, they are recommended only in the treatment of psychologic distress (e.g., depression, anxiety) associated with chronic pain.[39]

Antiseizure Drugs. Antiseizure or antiepileptic drugs (AEDs) affect both peripheral nerves and the CNS in several ways, including sodium channel modulation, central calcium channel modulation, and changes in excitatory amino acids and other receptors. AEDs are effective for neuropathic pain and prophylactic treatment of migraine headaches.[38,40]

α_2-Adrenergic Agonists. Currently, clonidine (Catapres) and tizanidine (Zanaflex) are the most widely used α_2-adrenergic agonists. They are thought to work on the central inhibitory α-adrenergic receptors. These agents may also decrease norepinephrine release peripherally. They are used for chronic headache and neuropathic pain. Common side effects are sedation, dry mouth, and orthostatic hypotension. Hypotension and dry mouth may be milder with tizanidine than with clonidine.

Corticosteroids. These drugs, which include dexamethasone [Decadron], prednisone, and methylprednisolone [Medrol], are used for management of acute and chronic cancer pain, pain secondary to spinal cord compression, and inflammatory joint pain syndromes. Mechanisms of action are unknown but may be due to the ability of corticosteroids to decrease edema and inflammation. They also may decrease activation of an inflamed neuron. Because of this effect, corticosteroids are useful when injected epidurally for acute or subacute disk herniations. Corticosteroids have many side effects, especially when given chronically in high doses. Adverse effects include hyperglycemia, fluid retention, dyspepsia and GI bleeding, impaired healing, muscle wasting, osteoporosis, adrenal suppression, and susceptibility to infection. Because they act through the same final pathway as NSAIDs, corticosteroids should not be given at the same time as NSAIDs.

Local Anesthetics. Oral, parenteral, and topical applications of local anesthetics are used to interrupt transmission of pain signals to the brain. Local anesthetic injections are used for acute pain resulting from surgery or trauma. Chronic neuropathic pain also can be controlled with local anesthetics. A gel patch containing 5% lidocaine (Lidoderm) has been approved by the Food and Drug Administration (FDA) for the pain of postherpetic neuralgia and may work in other focal neuropathic pain states.[41]

Side effects of systemically administered local anesthetics include dizziness, paresthesia (especially around the mouth), and seizures (at high doses). Incidence and severity of side effects depend on dose and route of administration. These agents also affect cardiac conductivity, thereby causing dysrhythmias and myocardial depression.[1,38]

GABA Receptor Agonists. Baclofen (Lioresal), an analog of the inhibitory neurotransmitter GABA, can interfere with the transmission of nociceptive impulses, and is mainly used for muscle spasms. It crosses the blood-brain barrier poorly and is much more effective for spasticity when delivered intrathecally.

NMDA Receptor Antagonists. These agents include a variety of drugs, including the anesthetic ketamine (Ketalar) and dextromethorphan, which is an ingredient in cough and cold products. These drugs have limited clinical usefulness because of debilitating CNS side effects. Amantadine, a noncompetitive NMDA antagonist, is in clinical studies for the treatment of peripheral neuropathic pain.[38] Several other NMDA receptor antagonists are in development.[1]

Mixed Mu Agonist Opioid and NE/5-HT Reuptake Inhibitors. Tramadol (Ultram) is a weak mu agonist and also inhibits the reuptake of norepinephrine and serotonin. It has approximately the same efficacy as Tylenol #3. Trials have shown efficacy in low back pain, osteoarthritis, diabetic peripheral neuropathic pain, polyneuropathy, and postherpetic neuralgia.[1,42] Combined with acetaminophen, additional benefit has been reported in patients suffering fibromyalgia.[43] The most common side effects are similar to those of other opioids, including nausea, constipation, dizziness, and sedation. As with other medications that increase serotonin and norepinephrine, this agent should be avoided in patients with a history of seizures because it lowers seizure threshold.[1]

Administration

Scheduling. Appropriate analgesic scheduling focuses on prevention or control of pain rather than the provision of analgesics only after the patient's pain has become severe. A patient should be premedicated before painful procedures and activities that are expected to produce pain. Similarly, a patient with constant pain should receive analgesics around the clock rather than on an "as needed" (prn) basis. These strategies control pain before it starts and usually result in lower analgesic requirements. Fast-acting drugs should be used for incident or breakthrough pain, whereas long-acting analgesics are more effective for constant pain. Examples of fast-acting and sustained-release analgesics are described later in this section.

Titration. Analgesic **titration** is dose adjustment based on assessment of the adequacy of analgesic effect versus the side effects produced. There is wide variability in the amount of analgesic needed to manage pain, and titration is an important strategy in addressing this variability.[33,44] An analgesic can be titrated upward or downward, depending on the situation. For example, in a postoperative patient the dose of analgesic generally decreases over time as the acute pain resolves. On the other hand, opioids for chronic, severe cancer pain may be titrated upward many times over the course of therapy to maintain adequate pain control. The goal of titration is to use the smallest dose of analgesic that provides effective pain control with the fewest side effects.

Equianalgesic Dosing. The term **equianalgesic dose** refers to a dose of one analgesic that is equivalent in pain-relieving effects compared with another analgesic. This equivalence permits substitution of analgesics in the event that a particular drug is ineffective or causes intolerable side effects. Generally, equianalgesic doses are provided for opioids and are important because there is no upper dosage limit for many of these drugs. Equianalgesic charts and conversion programs are widely available in textbooks, in clinical guidelines, in health care facility pain protocols, and on the Internet. They are useful tools, but health care providers need to understand their limitations. Equianalgesic dosages are estimates, and some are based on small, single-dose studies on healthy volunteers.[33,45] Differences exist among different published charts. For these reasons, all changes in opioid therapy must be carefully monitored and adjusted for the individual patient. When possible, health care providers should use equianalgesic conversions that have been approved for their facility or clinic and, if concerned, should consult a pharmacist before making changes.

Administration Routes. Opioids and other analgesic agents can be delivered via many routes. This flexibility allows the health care provider to (1) target a particular anatomic source of the pain, (2) achieve therapeutic blood levels rapidly when necessary, (3) avoid certain side effects through localized administration, and (4) provide analgesia when patients are unable to swallow. The following discussion highlights the uses and nursing considerations for analgesics delivered through a variety of routes.

Oral. Generally, oral administration is the route of choice for the person with a functioning GI system. Most pain medications are available in oral preparations, such as liquid and tablet formulations. For opioids, larger oral doses are needed to achieve the equivalent analgesia as doses administered intramuscularly or intravenously. For example, 10 mg of parenteral morphine is equivalent to approximately 30 mg of oral morphine.[33] The reason larger doses are required is related to the *first-pass effect* of hepatic metabolism. This means that oral opioids are absorbed from the GI tract into the portal circulation and shunted to the liver. Partial metabolism in the liver occurs before the drug enters systemic circulation and becomes available to peripheral receptors or can cross the blood-brain barrier and access CNS opioid receptors, which is necessary to produce analgesia. Oral opioids are as effective as parenteral opioids if the dose administered is large enough to compensate for the first-pass metabolism.

Some opioids (morphine, oxycodone) are available in short-acting (immediate-release) and long-acting (sustained-release) oral preparations. Immediate-release products are effective in providing rapid, short-term pain relief. Sustained-release preparations generally are administered every 8 to 12 hours. Onset of action is about 2 hours. As with other sustained-release preparations, these products should not be crushed, broken, or chewed. Long-acting preparations of morphine (Kadian, Avinza, MSContin) are sustained-release formulations that are administered every 12 to 24 hours. Oxycodone also comes in sustained-release formulations (OxyContin, Oxycodone SR). Approximately one third of oxycodone in the OxyContin preparation is released as the immediate-release, short-acting form. Patients should not take their "breakthrough" medications at the same time as their Oxycodone SR.

Sublingual and Buccal. Opioids can be administered under the tongue or held in the mouth and absorbed into systemic circulation, which would exempt them from the first-pass effect. Although morphine is commonly administered to persons with cancer pain via the sublingual route, little of the drug is actually absorbed from the sublingual tissue. Instead, most of the drug is dissolved in saliva and swallowed, making its metabolism the same as that of oral morphine.

Fentanyl citrate (Actiq) is administered *transmucosally.* The fentanyl dose is embedded in a flavored lozenge on a stick. The drug is absorbed by the permeable buccal mucosa after being rubbed actively over it (not sucked as a lollipop), allowing for the drug to enter the bloodstream and travel directly to the CNS. Approximately 25% to 50% of the dose gets absorbed by the buccal route. Pain relief typically occurs within 5 to 7 minutes after administration. Duration of action ranges from 2.5 to 5 hours. Actiq is FDA approved for use before surgery and procedures and for the treatment of cancer-related breakthrough pain.[33]

Intranasal. Intranasal administration allows delivery of medication to highly vascular mucosa and avoids the first-pass effect. Butorphanol (Stadol) is one of the few intranasal analgesics available in the United States; it is not available in Canada. This drug is indicated for acute headache and other intense, recurrent types of pain.

Rectal. The rectal route is often overlooked but is particularly useful when the patient cannot take an analgesic by mouth, such as those patients with severe nausea and vomiting. Analgesics that are available as rectal suppositories include hydromorphone, oxymorphone, morphine, and acetaminophen.[33]

Transdermal. Fentanyl (Duragesic) is available as a transdermal patch system for application to nonhairy skin. This delivery system is useful for the patient who cannot tolerate oral analgesic drugs. Absorption from the patch is slow, and it takes 12 to 17 hours to reach full effect with the first application. Therefore transdermal fentanyl is not suitable for rapid dose titration but can be effective if the patient's pain is stable and the dose required to control it is known. Patches may need to be changed every 48 hours rather than the recommended 72 hours based on individual patient responses. Rashes caused by the adhesive of the patch may be reduced by preparing the skin 1 hour before placement with a weak corticosteroid cream. Bio-occlusive dressings are available if the patch keeps falling off because of excessive sweating.

Drug Alert *- Fentanyl Patches*

- *Fentanyl patches (Duragesic) may cause death from overdose.*
- *Signs of overdose include trouble breathing or shallow respirations; tiredness, extreme sleepiness, or sedation; inability to think, talk, or walk normally; and feeling faint, dizzy, or confused.*

A 5% lidocaine impregnated transdermal patch (Lidoderm patch) is used for postherpetic neuralgia. The patch, placed directly on the intact skin in the area of postherpetic pain, is left in place for up to 12 hours. Topical local anesthetics are generally well tolerated and cause few systemic side effects, even with chronic use. They can even be used in patients with cardiovascular disease.[1]

Currently, creams and lotions containing 10% trolamine salicylate (Aspercreme, Myoflex cream) are available for joint and muscle pain. This aspirin-like substance is absorbed locally. This route of administration avoids gastric irritation, but the other side effects of high-dose salicylate are not prevented.

Ointments, lotions, gels, liniments, and balms (most of which are OTC products) are sometimes applied to the skin to achieve pain relief. Common ingredients include methyl salicylate combined with camphor and/or menthol. On application, these agents usually produce a strong hot or cold sensation and should not be used after massage or a heat treatment when blood vessels are already dilated. Skin testing is advisable when the patient has not used the particular agent before because the strengths of the agents vary and different intensities of sensation are produced. These products are indicated for arthralgia, bursitis, myalgia, and tendinitis.

Other topical analgesic agents, such as capsaicin (e.g., Icy-Hot, Zostrix) and a eutectic (easily melted) mixture of prilocaine plus lidocaine (eutectic mixture of local anesthetics [EMLA]), also provide analgesia. Derived from red chili pepper, capsaicin acts on the vanilloid heat receptors of the C fibers. If used regularly three or four times a day for 4 to 6 weeks it will cause the C nociceptor fibers to become inactive because of excessive calcium entering the nerve cell. The result is neuronal resistance to painful stimuli. Capsaicin can control pain associated with postherpetic neuralgia, diabetic neuropathy, and arthritis. EMLA is useful for control of pain associated with venipunctures, ulcer debridement, and possibly postherpetic neuralgia. The area to which EMLA is applied should be covered with a plastic wrap for 30 to 60 minutes before beginning a painful procedure.

Parenteral Routes. The parenteral route includes subcutaneous, intramuscular (IM), and intravenous (IV) administration. Single, repeated, or continuous dosing (subcutaneous or IV) is possible via parenteral routes. Although it is frequently used, the IM route is not recommended because injections cause significant pain, result in unreliable absorption, and with chronic use can result in abscesses and fibrosis. Onset of analgesia following subcutaneous administration is slow and thus the subcutaneous route rarely is used for acute pain management. However, continuous subcutaneous infusions are effective for pain management at the end of life. This route is especially helpful for people with abnormal GI function and limited venous access. Intravenous administration is the best route when immediate analgesia and rapid titration are necessary. Continuous IV infusions provide excellent steady state analgesia through stable blood levels.

Intraspinal Delivery. Intraspinal (epidural or intrathecal) opioid therapy involves inserting a catheter into the subarachnoid space *(intrathecal delivery)* or the epidural space *(epidural delivery).* Analgesics are injected either by intermittent bolus doses or continuous infusion (Fig. 10-8).

Percutaneously placed temporary catheters are used for short-term therapy (2 to 4 days), and surgically implanted catheters are used for long-term therapy. Although the lumbar region is the most common site of placement, epidural catheters may be placed at any point along the spinal column (cervical, thoracic, lumbar, or caudal). The tip of the epidural catheter is placed as close to the nerve supplying the painful dermatome as possible. For example, a thoracic catheter is placed for upper abdominal surgery and a high lumbar catheter is used for lower abdominal surgery. To ensure correct placement of the catheter, fluoroscopy is needed. However, fluoroscopy is usually not used for the placement because of lack of time and/or equipment.

Intraspinally administered analgesics are highly potent because they are delivered close to the receptors in the spinal cord dorsal horn. Thus much smaller doses of analgesics are needed when compared with other routes, including IV. For example, 1 mg of intrathecal morphine is approximately equivalent to 10 mg of epidural morphine, 100 mg of IV morphine, and 300 mg of oral morphine. Drugs that are delivered intraspinally include morphine, fentanyl, sufentanil (Sufenta), hydromorphone (Dilaudid), ziconotide (Prialt) (a calcium channel receptor modulator for use in neu-

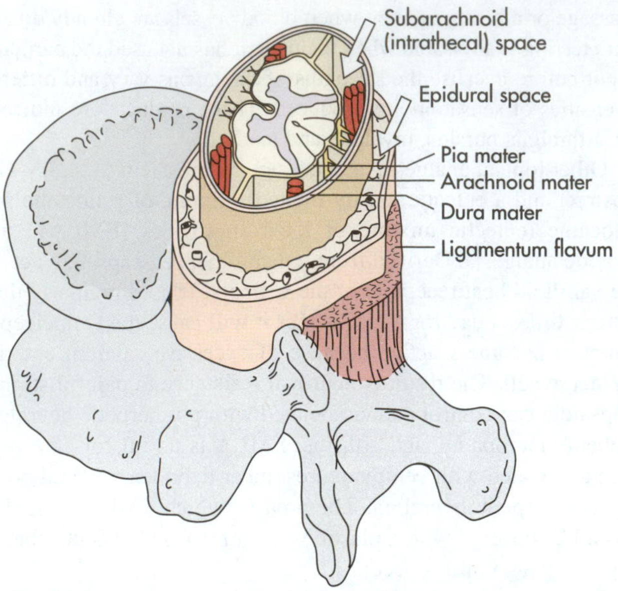

FIG. 10-8 Spinal anatomy. The spinal cord extends from the foramen magnum to the first or second lumbar vertebral space. The subarachnoid space (intrathecal space) is filled with cerebrospinal fluid that continually circulates and bathes the spinal cord. The epidural space is a potential space filled with blood vessels, fat, and a network of nerve extensions.

ropathic pain syndromes), and clonidine. Nausea, itching, and urinary retention are common side effects of intraspinal opioids. Intraspinal clonidine can cause significant hypotension. Common adverse effects of ziconotide include dizziness, ataxia, nausea, confusion, and headache.

Placement of an epidural catheter may be complicated by an initial "wet tap" where the needle goes across the dura. Cerebrospinal fluid (CSF) escapes out the needle. A lumbar puncture headache often results from a wet tap, especially in the younger patient. The patient describes a severe headache only when sitting or standing that rapidly resolves when lying flat.

Complications of intraspinal analgesia include catheter displacement and migration, accidental infusions of neurotoxic agents, and infection. Clinical manifestations of catheter displacement or migration depend on catheter location and the drug being infused. A catheter that migrates out of the intrathecal or epidural space will cause a decrease in pain relief with no improvement, even with additional boluses or increase in the infusion rate. If an epidural catheter migrates into the subarachnoid space, an increase in side effects will become quickly apparent. Somnolence, confusion, and an increased anesthesia (if the infusate contains an anesthetic) occur. Correct placement of an intrathecal catheter can be checked by aspirating CSF. Migration of a catheter into a blood vessel may cause an increase in drug side effects because of systemic drug distribution.

A number of drugs and chemicals are highly neurotoxic when administered intraspinally. These include many preservatives such as alcohol and phenol, antibiotics, chemotherapy agents, potassium, and parenteral nutrition. To avoid inadvertent injection of IV drugs into an intraspinal catheter, the catheter should be clearly marked as an intraspinal access device, and only preservative-free drugs should be injected.

Infection is a rare but serious complication of intraspinal analgesia. The skin around the exit site should be carefully assessed for inflammation, drainage, or pain. Signs and symptoms of an intraspinal infection include diffuse back pain, pain or paresthesias during bolus injection, and unexplained sensory or motor deficits in the lower limbs. Fever may or may not be present. Acute bacterial infection (meningitis) is manifested by photophobia, neck stiffness, fever, headache, and altered mental status. If infection is suspected, magnetic resonance imaging (MRI) is often done on an urgent basis to assess if an epidural abscess requiring surgical intervention is present. Infection is avoided by providing regular, meticulous wound care and using sterile technique when caring for the catheter and injecting drugs.

Long-term epidural catheters may be placed for terminal cancer patients or patients with certain pain syndromes that are unresponsive to other treatments. If a long-term indwelling epidural catheter is used, double bacterial filters are recommended. Because the highest infective risk occurs when the medication bags are changed, the concentration and volume in the infusing bag should be optimized to reduce the number of bag changes.

Implantable Pumps. Intraspinal catheters can be surgically implanted for long-term pain relief. The surgical placement of an intrathecal catheter to a subcutaneously placed pump and reservoir allows the delivery of drugs directly into the intrathecal space. The pump, which is normally placed in a pocket made in the subcutaneous tissue of the abdomen, may be programmable or fixed. Changes are made by either reprogramming the pump or changing the mixture or concentration of drug in the reservoir. The pump is refilled every 30 to 90 days depending on flow rate, mixture, and reservoir size.

Patient-Controlled Analgesia. A specific type of IV delivery system is **patient-controlled analgesia** (PCA), or demand analgesia. It can also be connected to an epidural catheter (patient-controlled epidural analgesia [PCEA]). With PCA, a dose of opioid is delivered when the patient decides a dose is needed. PCA uses an infusion system in which the patient pushes a button to receive a bolus infusion of an analgesic. PCA is used widely for the management of acute pain, including postoperative pain and cancer pain. The addition of a continuous infusion to a PCA regimen may improve nighttime pain relief and promote sleep.

Use of PCA begins with patient teaching. The patient needs to understand the mechanics of getting a drug dose and how to titrate the drug to achieve good pain relief. The patient should be taught to self-administer the analgesic before pain intensity is greater than the patient's desired pain intensity goal. The patient also needs to be assured that he or she cannot "overdose" because the pump is programmed to deliver a maximum number of doses per hour. Pressing the button after the maximum dose is administered will not result in additional analgesic. If the maximum doses are inadequate to relieve pain, the pump can be reprogrammed to increase the amount or frequency of dosing. In addition, bolus doses can be given by the nurse if they are included in the physician's orders. To make a smooth transition from infusion PCA to oral drugs, the patient should receive increasing doses of oral drug as the PCA analgesic is tapered.

Interventional Therapy

Therapeutic Nerve Blocks. Nerve blocks generally involve one-time or continuous infusion of local anesthetics into a particular area to produce pain relief. These techniques also are referred to as *regional anesthesia.* Nerve blocks interrupt all afferent and efferent transmission to the area, and thus are not specific to nociceptive pathways. They include local infiltration of anesthetics into a surgical area (e.g., excision of a breast lump, inguinal hernia surgery, intraarticular after joint surgery) and injection of anesthetic into a specific nerve (e.g., occipital or pudendal nerve) or nerve plexus (e.g., brachial or celiac plexus).[46] Nerve blocks often are used during and after surgery to manage pain. For longer-term relief of chronic pain syndromes, local anesthetics can be administered via a continuous infusion.

For intractable chronic pain, neuroablative nerve blocks with phenol or alcohol may be used. For example, a neurolytic celiac plexus block may be performed for pain caused by pancreatic cancer, or an intercostal neurolytic block may be performed for post-thoracotomy pain. Many neurolytic procedures that use heat or microwaves produce nerve tissue destruction.[46]

Neuroablative Techniques. *Neuroablative interventions* are performed for severe pain that is unresponsive to all other therapies. Neuroablative techniques destroy nerves, thereby interrupting pain transmission. Destruction is accomplished by surgical resection or thermocoagulation, including radiofrequency coagulation. Neuroablative interventions that destroy the sensory division of a peripheral or spinal nerve are classified as *neurectomies, rhizotomies,* and *sympathectomies.* Neurosurgical procedures that ablate the lateral spinothalamic tract are classified as *cordotomies* if the tract is interrupted in the spinal cord, or *tractotomies* if the interruption is in the medulla or the midbrain of the brainstem. Fig. 10-9 identifies the sites of neurosurgical procedures for pain relief. Both cordotomy and tractotomy can be performed with the aid of local anesthesia by a percutaneous technique.

Neuroaugmentation. *Neuroaugmentation* involves electrical stimulation of the brain and the spinal cord. Spinal cord stimulation (SCS) is performed much more often than deep brain stimulation. Recent advances have allowed the use of multiple leads and multiple electrode terminals so as to stimulate large areas. In the United States and Canada the most common use of SCS is for chronic back pain secondary to nerve damage that is unresponsive to other therapies.

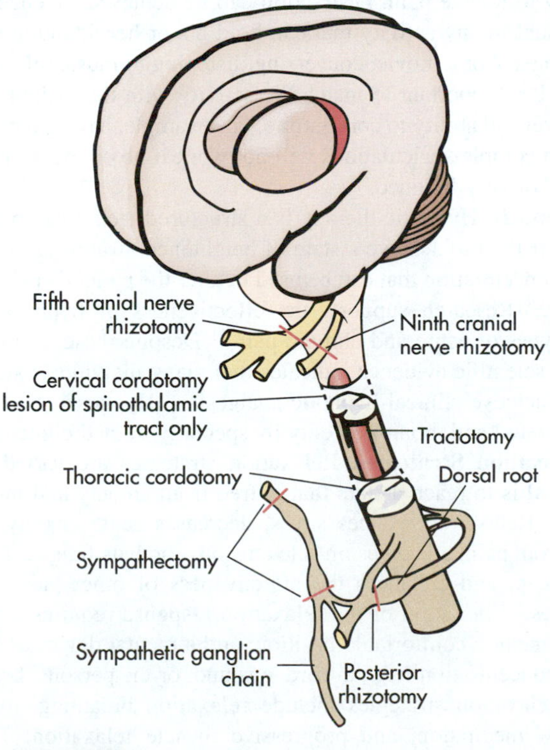

FIG. 10-9 Sites of neurosurgical procedures for pain relief.

Potential complications include those related to the surgery (bleeding and infection), migration of the generator (which usually is implanted in the subcutaneous tissues of the upper gluteal or pectoralis area), and nerve damage. Stimulation of deep brain structures (e.g., thalamus) was performed in the 1970s and 1980s to achieve pain control but rarely is done today.

Nondrug Therapies for Pain

Nonpharmacologic pain management strategies can reduce the dose of an analgesic required to relieve pain and thereby minimize side effects of drug therapy. They also can increase patients' sense of personal control about managing their pain and bolster their coping skills. Some strategies are believed to alter ascending nociceptive input or stimulate descending pain modulation mechanisms. Nonpharmacologic pain relief methods can be categorized as physical or cognitive strategies (Table 10-10).

Physical Pain Relief Strategies

Massage. Massage is a common therapy for pain. Many different massage techniques exist. Examples include moving the hands or fingers over the skin slowly or briskly with long strokes or in circles (superficial massage) or applying firm pressure to the skin to maintain contact while massaging the underlying tissues (deep massage). Another example is trigger point massage. A **trigger point** is a circumscribed hypersensitive area within a tight band of muscle that is caused by acute or chronic muscle strain. Several common trigger points have been identified on the neck, back, and arms. Trigger point massage is performed either by applying strong, sustained digital pressure, deep massage, or gentler massage with ice followed by muscle heating. (Massage is discussed in Chapter 8.)

Exercise. Exercise is a critical part of the treatment plan for patients with chronic pain, particularly those with musculoskeletal pain. Research supports the effectiveness of many types of exercise for a variety of painful conditions.[47] Many patients become physically deconditioned as a result of their pain, which in turn leads to more pain. Exercise acts via many mechanisms to relieve pain. It enhances circulation and cardiovascular fitness, reduces edema, increases muscle strength and flexibility, and enhances physical and psychosocial functioning. An exercise program should be tailored to the physical needs and lifestyle of the patient and should include aerobic exercise, stretching, and strengthening

TABLE 10-10 Nonpharmacologic Therapies for Pain

Physical Therapies
Acupuncture
Application of heat and cold (see Table 10-11)
Exercise
Massage
Percutaneous electrical nerve stimulation (PENS)
Transcutaneous electrical nerve stimulation (TENS)
Cognitive Therapies
Distraction
Hypnosis
Imagery
Relaxation strategies (see Chapter 9)
• Relaxation breathing
• Imagery
• Meditation
• Art therapy
• Music therapy
• Progressive muscle relaxation

exercises. The program also should be supervised by trained personnel (e.g., exercise physiologist, physical therapist). Examples of exercise programs include yoga, Tai Chi, and water aerobics. (Tai Chi is discussed in Chapter 8.)

Transcutaneous Electrical Nerve Stimulation. *Transcutaneous electrical nerve stimulation* (TENS) involves the delivery of an electric current through electrodes applied to the skin surface over the painful region, at trigger points, or over a peripheral nerve. A TENS system consists of two or more electrodes connected by lead wires to a small, battery-operated stimulator (Fig. 10-10). Usually, a physical therapist is responsible for administering TENS therapy, although nurses can be trained in the technique.

TENS may be used for acute pain, including postoperative pain and pain associated with physical trauma. The effects of TENS on chronic pain are less clear but may be effective for some chronic pain patients.[48]

Percutaneous Electrical Nerve Stimulation. Percutaneous electrical nerve stimulation (PENS) stimulates deeper peripheral tissues through the insertion of a needle to which a stimulator is attached near a large peripheral or spinal nerve. The amount of electric current is regulated to provide maximum pain relief. If the PENS successfully reduces the patient's pain, a permanent peripheral nerve stimulator is surgically implanted. PENS has been shown to be effective in the treatment of some types of musculoskeletal pain.[49]

Acupuncture. Acupuncture is a technique of Traditional Chinese Medicine in which very thin needles are inserted into the body at designated points. Acupuncture is applied to many, varied pain problems, including musculoskeletal conditions, repetitive strain disorders, myofascial pain syndrome, postsurgical pain, postherpetic neuralgia, peripheral neuropathic pain, and headaches.[50] (Acupuncture is discussed in Chapter 8.)

Heat Therapy. Heat therapy is the application of either moist or dry heat to the skin. Heat therapy can be either superficial or deep. Superficial heat can be applied using an electric heating pad (dry or moist), a hot pack, hot moist compresses, warm wax (paraffin), or a hot water bottle. For exposure to large areas of the body, patients can immerse themselves in a hot bath, shower, or whirlpool. Physical therapy departments provide deep-heat therapy through such techniques as short-wave diathermy, microwave diathermy, and ultrasound therapy. Patient teaching regarding heat therapy is described in Table 10-11.

Cold Therapy. Cold therapy involves the application of either moist or dry cold to the skin. Dry cold can be applied by means of

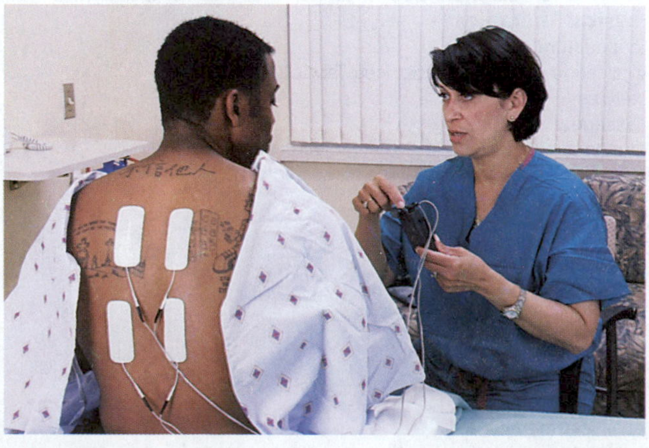

FIG. 10-10 Initial TENS treatment being given by a physical therapist to assess value in pain relief.

TABLE 10-11 ***PATIENT AND FAMILY TEACHING GUIDE*** **Heat and Cold Therapy**

When patients use superficial heating techniques, they should be taught the following:

- Do not use heat on an area that is being treated with radiation therapy, is bleeding, has decreased sensation, or has been injured in the past 24 hours.
- Do not use any menthol-containing products (e.g., Ben-Gay, Vicks, Icy Hot) with heat applications because this may cause burns.
- Cover the heat source with a towel or cloth to prevent burns.

When patients use superficial cold techniques, they should be taught the following:

- Cover the cold source with a cloth or towel.
- Do not apply cold to areas that are being treated with radiation therapy, have open wounds, or have poor circulation.
- If it is not possible to apply the cold directly to the painful site, try applying it right above or below the painful site, or on the opposite side of the body on the corresponding site (e.g., left elbow if the right elbow hurts).

an ice bag, moist cold by means of towels soaked in ice water, cold hydrocollator packs, or immersion in a bath or under running cold water. Icing with ice cubes or blocks of ice made to resemble Popsicles is another technique used for pain relief. Cold therapy is believed to be more effective than heat for a variety of painful conditions, including acute pain from trauma or surgery, acute flare-ups of arthritis, muscle spasms, and headache.

Cognitive Therapies. Techniques to alter the affective, cognitive, and behavioral components of pain include a variety of cognitive strategies and behavioral approaches. Some of these techniques require little training and often are adopted independently by the patient. For others, a trained therapist is necessary.

Distraction. Distraction involves redirection of attention onto something and away from the pain. It is a simple but powerful strategy to relieve pain. Distraction can be achieved by engaging the patient in any activity that can hold his or her attention (e.g., watching TV or a movie, conversing, listening to music, playing a game). It is important to match the activity with the patient's energy level and ability to concentrate. For example, having a patient perform complex calculations will not work if he or she is "math-phobic" or very fatigued.

Hypnosis. Hypnotic therapy is a structured technique that enables a patient to achieve a state of heightened awareness and focused concentration that can be used to alter the patient's pain perception.[25] Research supports the effectiveness of hypnosis for many types of acute and chronic pain.[51] Despite these promising results, scientific evidence indicates that many individuals are unable to achieve clinical hypnotic analgesia.[51] Hypnosis should be administered and monitored only by specially trained clinicians.

Relaxation Strategies. Relaxation strategies are varied, but their goal is to reach a state that is free from anxiety and muscle tension. Relaxation reduces stress, decreases acute anxiety, distracts from pain, alleviates muscle tension, combats fatigue, facilitates sleep, and enhances the effectiveness of other pain relief measures.[1] Elicitation of the relaxation response requires a quiet environment, a comfortable position, and a mental device as a focus of concentration (e.g., a word, a sound, or the person's breathing). Relaxation strategies include relaxation breathing, music, imagery, meditation, and progressive muscle relaxation. These strategies are described in Chapters 8 and 9.

NURSING *and* COLLABORATIVE MANAGEMENT PAIN

The nurse is an important member of the multidisciplinary pain management team. The nurse acts as planner, educator, patient advocate, interpreter, and supporter of the patient in pain and the patient's family. Because pain can be present in any patient in a wide variety of care settings, the nurse must be knowledgeable about current therapies and flexible in trying new approaches to pain management. The extent of the nurse's involvement depends on the unique factors associated with the patient, the setting, and the cause of the pain. Many nursing roles have been described earlier, including conducting pain assessments, administering therapies, monitoring for side effects, and teaching patients and families. However, the success of these actions depends on the nurse's ability to establish a trusting relationship with the patient and family and to address the concerns that they have regarding pain and its treatment.

Effective Communication

Because pain is a subjective experience, patients need to feel confident that their reporting of pain will be believed and will not be perceived as "complaining." The patient and the family also need to know that the nurse considers the pain significant and understands that pain may profoundly disrupt a person's life. The nurse needs to communicate concern about the patient and assure the patient that he or she is committed to helping the patient obtain pain relief and cope with any unrelieved pain. Pharmacologic and nonpharmacologic interventions should be incorporated into the treatment plan. The patient should be supported through the period of trial and error that may be necessary to implement an effective therapeutic plan. It also is important to clarify responsibilities in pain relief. The nurse should help the patient understand the role of the members of the health care team, as well as the roles and expectations of the patient.

In addition to addressing specific aspects of pain assessment and treatment, the nurse evaluates the total impact that the pain may have on the lives of the patient and family. Thus other possible nursing diagnoses must be considered. Table 10-12 lists possible nursing diagnoses that may be appropriate for the patient in pain. Table 10-13 addresses teaching needs of patients and families related to pain management.

Barriers to Effective Pain Management

Pain is a complex, subjective experience, and its management is influenced greatly by psychosocial, sociocultural, and legal-ethical factors. These factors include emotions, behaviors, beliefs, and attitudes of patients and family members about pain and use of pain therapies. Achieving effective pain management requires careful consideration of these factors.

TABLE 10-12 *NURSING DIAGNOSES* Pain

• Activity intolerance	• Hopelessness
• Acute pain	• Ineffective coping
• Anxiety	• Ineffective role performance
• Chronic pain	• Insomnia
• Constipation	• Interrupted family processes
• Disturbed thought processes	• Powerlessness
• Fatigue	• Risk for self-mutilation
• Fear	• Social isolation

TABLE 10-13 *PATIENT AND FAMILY TEACHING GUIDE* Pain Management

The goals of teaching related to pain management include that the patient and family member understand the following:

- Negative consequences of unrelieved pain
- Need to maintain a record of pain level and effectiveness of treatment
- No need to wait until pain becomes severe to take drugs or use nondrug therapies for pain relief
- Medication will stop working after it is taken for a period of time, and dosages may need to be adjusted
- Potential side effects and complications associated with therapy/therapies; side effects can include nausea and vomiting, constipation, sedation and drowsiness, itching, urinary retention, sweating
- Need to report when pain is not relieved to tolerable levels

Concerns regarding tolerance, dependence, and addiction are common barriers. Patients, family members, and health care providers often share these concerns. It is important for the nurse to understand and to be able to explain the differences among these various concepts.

Tolerance. *Tolerance* occurs with chronic exposure to a variety of drugs. In the case of opioids, tolerance is characterized by the need for an increased opioid dose to maintain the same degree of analgesia. The incidence of clinically significant opioid tolerance in chronic pain patients is unknown. If dosage needs do increase in cancer patients, it usually is the result of disease progression rather than tolerance.[52] Although tolerance is not as common as once thought, it is essential to assess for increased analgesic needs in patients on long-term therapy. If manifestations of possible tolerance appear, appropriate evaluations should be made to rule out other causes of increased analgesic needs, such as disease progression or infection. Although an increased opioid dose may be indicated, recent evidence suggests that high opioid use may actually contribute to hyperalgesia; thus increasing the dose may be ineffective and result in higher pain levels. If tolerance to opioids is considered to be a concern, opioid rotation to another type of opioid is recommended.[53]

Physical Dependence. Like tolerance, physical dependence is an expected physiologic response to ongoing exposure to pharmacologic agents that is manifested by a withdrawal syndrome that occurs when blood levels of the drug are abruptly decreased. Symptoms of opioid withdrawal are listed in Table 10-14. When opioids are no longer needed to provide pain relief, a tapering schedule should be used in conjunction with careful monitoring. A typical tapering schedule begins with calculating the 24-hour dose used by the patient and dividing by 2. Of this decreased amount, 25% is given every 6 hours. After 2 days, the daily dose is reduced by an additional 25% every 2 days until the 24-hour oral dose is 30 mg (morphine equivalent) per day. After 2 days on this minimum dose, the opioid is then discontinued.[52]

Addiction. *Addiction* is a complex neurobiologic condition characterized by a drive to obtain and take substances for other than the prescribed therapeutic value (see Chapter 12). Tolerance and physical dependence are not indicators of addiction. Rather they are normal physiologic responses to chronic exposure to certain drugs, including opioids.

TABLE 10-14 Manifestations of Withdrawal from Short-Acting Opioids

	Early Response (6-12 hr)	Late Response (48-72 hr)
Psychosocial	Anxiety	Excitation
Secretions	Lacrimation Rhinorrhea Diaphoresis	Diarrhea
Other	Yawning Piloerection Shaking chills Dilated pupils Anorexia Tremor	Restlessness Fever Nausea and vomiting Abdominal cramping pain Hypertension Tachycardia Insomnia

The risk of developing addiction may be greater in specific patient populations, such as those on long-term opioid therapy for chronic noncancer pain or patients with a history of addiction.[54] The risk of addiction, however, should not prevent clinicians from using opioids to treat moderate to severe acute and chronic pain. Several professional organizations and government agencies have issued joint statements about the roles and responsibilities of health care professionals in the appropriate use of opioids in the treatment of pain.[55]

In addition to the fears about addiction, physical dependence, and tolerance, other barriers hinder effective pain management. These include concern about side effects, difficulties remembering to take drugs, desire to be stoic about pain, and not wanting to distract the health care provider from treating the disease. Table 10-15 lists these and other barriers and includes strategies to address the barriers.

TABLE 10-15 *PATIENT AND FAMILY TEACHING GUIDE* Reducing Barriers to Pain Management

Barrier	Nursing Considerations
Fear of addiction	• Provide accurate definition of addiction. • Explain that addiction is uncommon in patients taking opioids.
Fear of tolerance	• Provide accurate definition of tolerance. • Teach that tolerance is normal physiologic response to chronic opioid therapy. If tolerance does develop, the drug may need to be changed (e.g., morphine in place of oxycodone). • Teach that there is no upper limit to pure opioid agonists (e.g., morphine). Dosages can be increased indefinitely, and patient should not save drugs for when his or her pain is worse. • Teach that tolerance develops more slowly to analgesic effects of opioids than to many side effects (e.g., sedation, respiratory depression). Tolerance does not develop to constipation; thus a regular bowel program should be started early.
Concern about side effects	• Teach methods to prevent and to treat common side effects. • Emphasize that side effects such as sedation and nausea decrease with time. • Explain that different drugs have unique side effects and other pain drugs can be tried to reduce the specific side effect. • Teach nondrug therapies to minimize the dose of drug needed to control pain.
Fear of injections	• Explain that oral medicines are preferred. • Emphasize that even if oral route becomes unusable, transdermal or indwelling parenteral routes can be used rather than injections.
Desire to be a "good" patient	• Explain that patients are partners in their care and that the partnership requires open communication of both the patient and nurse. • Emphasize to patients that they have a responsibility to keep the nurse informed about their pain.
Desire to be stoic	• Explain that although stoicism is a valued behavior in many cultures, failure to report pain can result in undertreatment and severe, unrelieved pain.
Forgetting to take analgesic	• Provide and teach use of pill containers. • Provide methods of record keeping for drug use. • Recruit family members as appropriate to assist with the analgesic regimen.
Fear of distracting the health care provider from treating the disease	• Explain that reporting pain is important in treating both the disease and its symptoms.
Concern that pain signifies disease progression	• Explain that increased pain or analgesic needs may reflect tolerance. • Emphasize that new pain may come from a non–life-threatening source (e.g., muscle spasm, urinary tract infection). • Institute pharmacologic and nonpharmacologic strategies to reduce anxiety. • Ensure that the patient and family members have current, accurate, comprehensive information about the disease and prognosis. • Provide psychologic support.
Sense of fatalism	• Explain that research has shown that pain can be managed in most patients. • Explain that most therapies require a period of trial and error. • Emphasize that side effects can be managed.
Ineffective medication	• Teach that there are multiple options within each category of medication (e.g., opioid, NSAIDs) and another medication from the same category may provide better relief. • Emphasize that finding the best treatment regimen often requires trial and error. • Incorporate nondrug approaches in treatment plan.

Adapted from Ersek M: Enhancing effective pain management by addressing patient barriers to analgesic use, *J Hospice Palliat Nurs* 1:87, 1999.
NSAIDs, Nonsteroidal antiinflammatory drugs.

INSTITUTIONALIZING PAIN EDUCATION AND MANAGEMENT

Besides patient and family barriers, other major barriers to effective pain management are inadequate health care provider education and lack of organizational support. Traditionally, medical and nursing school curricula have spent little time teaching future physicians and nurses about pain and symptom management. This lack of emphasis contributed to the problem that health care providers lacked the knowledge and skills to treat pain adequately. Moreover, pain assessment and treatment were not priorities in clinical practice, and health care providers also were likely to have misconceptions about pain and pain medications.

Over the past decade, some improvements have been made in overcoming these barriers. Medical and nursing schools now devote more time to addressing pain, and many educational programs have enhanced professional expertise in varied clinical settings.[1] In addition, numerous professional organizations have published evidence-based guidelines for assessing and managing pain in many patient populations and clinical settings.[1,10,26,32,33] Although progress has been made, there is still room for improving knowledge and expertise.

Health care institutions also have been remiss in their support of pain management. In the past decade, researchers and health care providers have documented the central role that institutional commitment and practices have in changing clinical practice. Without institutional support, pain outcomes are unlikely to change.[1] One major step in institutionalizing pain management is the development and adoption of the Joint Commission on Accreditation of Healthcare Organizations (JCAHO) guideline on pain.[26] JCAHO is the accrediting body for most U.S. health care facilities (hospitals, nursing homes, and health care clinics). Under the standards, health care facilities are required to (1) recognize the patient's rights to appropriate assessment and management of pain; (2) identify pain in patients during their initial assessment and as needed, during ongoing, periodic reassessments; (3) educate health care providers in pain assessment and management and ensure competency; and (4) educate patients and their families about pain management.

ETHICAL ISSUES IN PAIN MANAGEMENT

Fear of Hastening Death by Administering Analgesics

It is common for the health care professional, patient, and family members to be concerned that providing sufficient drug to relieve pain will precipitate the death of a terminally ill person. Despite the fear, however, there is no scientific evidence that opioids can hasten death, even among patients at the very end of life.[14] Several nursing organizations have emphasized nurses' moral obligation to use aggressive pain relief strategies at the end of life.[14,56] They remind nurses that the bioethical principle, the rule of double effect, provides ethical justification for administering analgesics despite the possibility of hastening death. This rule states that if an unwanted consequence (i.e., hastened death) occurs as a result of an action taken to achieve a moral good (i.e., pain relief), the action is justified because the nurse's intent is to relieve pain and not to hasten death.[57]

Requests for Assisted Suicide

Unrelieved pain is one of many reasons that patients make requests for assisted suicide; aggressive pain management may decrease the number of requests. Assisted suicide is a complex issue that extends beyond pain and pain management. The American Nurses Association (ANA) has carefully described the role of nurses in providing end-of-life care and symptom management. This role does not include active participation in assisted suicide or euthanasia.[58] Currently, Oregon is the only place in North America where assisted suicide is legal. To address the legal and ethical issues confronting nurses in this unique situation, the Oregon Nurses Association prepared a position paper on this topic.[59]

Use of Placebos in Pain Assessment and Treatment

Although their use has declined recently, placebos still are sometimes used to assess and to treat pain. Using a placebo involves deceiving patients by making them believe that they are receiving an analgesic (usually an opioid) when in fact they are typically receiving an inert substance such as saline. The use of placebos to assess or treat pain is uniformly condemned by several professional organizations.[33,60]

GERONTOLOGIC CONSIDERATIONS
PAIN

Chronic nonmalignant pain is a common problem in the elderly. It is often associated with significant physical disability and psychosocial problems. Estimates of the prevalence of chronic pain problems among community-dwelling older adults have ranged from 58% to 70%. Among the elderly living in nursing homes, the estimated prevalence is 45% to 80%.[10] The most common painful conditions among older adults are musculoskeletal conditions such as osteoarthritis, low back pain, and previous fracture sites. Chronic pain often results in depression, sleep disturbance, decreased mobility, increased health care utilization, and physical and social role dysfunction. Despite its high prevalence, pain in the elderly often is inadequately assessed and treated.[10]

There are several barriers to pain assessment in the older patient. In general, the barriers discussed earlier in the chapter are more prevalent among elderly patients. Thus older patients often believe that pain is a normal, inevitable part of aging. They may also believe that nothing can be done to relieve the pain. Older adults may not report pain for fear of being a "burden" or a "bad patient." They may have greater fears of taking opioids than other age groups. Also, older patients are more likely to use words such as "aching," "soreness," or "discomfort" rather than "pain." For all these reasons, nurses must be persistent in asking older adults about pain. The assessment process should be carried out in an unhurried, supportive manner.

Another barrier to pain assessment in older adults is the relatively high prevalence of cognitive, sensory-perceptual, and motor problems that interfere with a person's ability to process information and to communicate. Examples of these problems include dementia and delirium, post-stroke aphasia and paraplegia, and language barriers. Also, hearing and vision deficits may complicate assessment. Therefore pain assessment tools may need to be adapted for older adults. For example, it may be necessary to use a large-print pain intensity scale. Although there is some concern that older adults have difficulty using pain scales, it has been documented that many older adults, even those with mild-to-moderate cognitive impairment, can use quantitative scales accurately and reliably. Older adults may prefer numeric rating scales and verbal descriptor scales[61] (see Fig. 10-6).

In older patients with chronic pain, a thorough physical examination and history should be performed to identify causes of pain, possible therapies, and potential problems. Because depression and functional impairments are common among elderly persons with pain, these also must be assessed.[10]

Treatment of pain in the elderly is complicated by several factors. First, older adults metabolize drugs more slowly than younger patients and thus are at greater risk for higher blood levels and adverse effects. For this reason, the adage "start low and go slow" is applied to analgesic therapy in this age group. Second, the use of NSAIDs in the elderly is associated with a high frequency of serious GI bleeding. For this reason, acetaminophen should be used whenever possible. Third, older people often are taking many drugs for one or more chronic conditions. The addition of analgesics can result in dangerous drug interactions and increased side effects. Fourth, cognitive impairment and ataxia can be exacerbated when analgesics such as opioids, antidepressants, and antiseizure drugs are used. This requires that health care providers titrate drugs slowly and monitor carefully for side effects.[10]

Treatment regimens for older adults must incorporate nonpharmacologic modalities. Exercise and patient teaching are particularly important nonpharmacologic interventions for older adults with chronic pain. Family and paid caregivers also should be included in the treatment plan.

SPECIAL POPULATIONS

Cognitively Impaired Individuals

Although patient self-report is the gold standard of pain assessment, severe cognitive impairment often prevents patients from communicating clearly regarding their pain. For these persons, behavioral and physiologic changes may be the only indicators that they are in pain. Therefore the nurse must be astute at recognizing behavioral symptoms of pain.

Several scales have been developed to assess pain in cognitively impaired elders.[27] Typically, these scales assess pain based on common behavioral indicators such as the following:

- Vocalization: Moans, grunts, cries, sighing
- Facial expressions: Grimacing, wincing, frowning, clenched teeth
- Breathing: Noisy, labored
- Body movements: Restlessness, rocking, pacing
- Body tension: Clenched fist, resistance to movement
- Consolability: Inability to be consoled or distracted

Because it is not possible to validate the meaning of the behaviors, nurses should rely on their own knowledge of the patient's usual behavior. If the nurse does not know the patient's baseline behaviors, she or he should obtain this information from other caregivers, including family members. When pain behaviors are present, empirical pain therapy should be instituted, and patients should be carefully reassessed to evaluate treatment effectiveness.

Patients with Substance Abuse Problems

Approximately 19.5 million Americans (over 8% of those 12 years and older) regularly use illicit drugs. Over 21 million Americans are classified as having problems with substance dependence or abuse (9.1% of the total population age 12 and older). Of these, 3.8 million are dependent on or abuse illicit drugs, 14.8 million are dependent on or abuse alcohol, and 3.1 million are dependent on or abuse both illicit drugs and alcohol.[62] The nurse is faced with the challenge of assessing and providing pain relief to individuals with the dual diagnosis of pain and substance abuse disorder.

Individuals with a past or current substance abuse disorder have the right to receive effective pain management. A comprehensive pain assessment is imperative, including a detailed history, physical examination, psychosocial assessment, and diagnostic workup to determine the cause of the pain. The use of screening tools to determine the possible risk of addiction has been described.[63] The goal of the pain assessment is to facilitate the establishment of a treatment plan that will relieve the individual's pain effectively, as well as prevent and/or minimize withdrawal symptoms.

Opioids may be used effectively and safely in patients with substance dependence when indicated for pain control. Withholding opioids from chemically dependent patients with pain has not been shown to increase the likelihood of recovery from addiction. Opioid agonists-antagonists (e.g., pentazocine [Talwin], butorphanol [Stadol]) should not be used in this population because they may precipitate withdrawal. The use of "potentiators" and psychoactive drugs that do not have analgesic properties should be avoided. In individuals who are tolerant to CNS depressants, larger doses of opioids or increased frequency of drug administration is necessary to achieve pain relief.

Pain management for people with addiction is challenging and requires a multidisciplinary team approach. Team members need to be aware of their own attitudes and misconceptions about people with substance abuse problems, which may result in undertreatment of pain.

CRITICAL THINKING EXERCISE

CASE STUDY

Pain

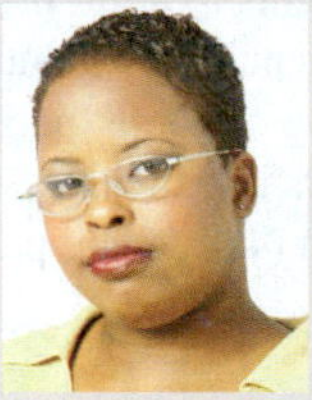

Patient Profile. Mrs. C. is a 280 lb (112 kg) 43-year-old African American woman admitted for an incision and drainage of a right renal abscess. She is being discharged on her third postoperative day. Her married daughter will assist with dressing changes at home.

Subjective Data

- RN for 20 years
- Lives alone
- Desires 0 pain but will accept 1 to 2 on a scale of 0 to 10
- Reports incision area pain as a 2 or 3 between dressing changes and as a 6 during dressing changes
- States sharp pain persists 1 to 2 hr after dressing change
- Reports pain between dressing changes controlled by one or two Percocet tablets

Objective Data

- While in the hospital received intravenous morphine for pain before dressing changes
- Requires qid dry-to-dry dressing changes for 1 week
- For discharge, Percocet (two tablets q4hr for pain prn) is prescribed.

Critical Thinking Questions

1. Describe the assessment data that are important for determining whether Mrs. C. has adequate pain management.

CRITICAL THINKING EXERCISE—cont'd

2. How long should the daughter wait after the Percocet is given to begin the dressing change?
3. What additional pain therapies might the nurse plan to help Mrs. C. through the dressing change?
4. What side effects might Mrs. C. experience because of her pain medication? How can these be managed?
5. Based on the data presented, write one or more appropriate nursing diagnosis. Are there any collaborative problems?

NCLEX EXAMINATION REVIEW QUESTIONS

The number of the question corresponds to the same-numbered objective at the beginning of the chapter.

1. Pain is best described as
   a. a creation of a person's imagination.
   b. an unpleasant, subjective experience.
   c. a maladaptive response to a stimulus.
   d. a neurologic event resulting from activation of nociceptors.
2. A neurotransmitter known for its involvement in pain modulation is
   a. dopamine.
   b. acetylcholine.
   c. prostaglandin.
   d. norepinephrine.
3. Which of the following words is most likely to be used to describe neuropathic pain?
   a. Dull
   b. Mild
   c. Aching
   d. Burning
4. Unrelieved pain is
   a. expected after major surgery.
   b. expected in a person with cancer.
   c. dangerous and can lead to many physical and psychologic complications.
   d. an annoying sensation, but it is not as important as other physical care needs.
5. A cancer patient who reports ongoing, constant moderate pain with short periods of severe pain during dressing changes
   a. is probably exaggerating his pain.
   b. should be referred for surgical treatment of his pain.
   c. should be receiving both a long-acting and a short-acting opioid.
   d. should receive regularly scheduled short-acting opioids plus acetaminophen.
6. An example of distraction to provide pain relief is
   a. TENS.
   b. music.
   c. exercise.
   d. biofeedback.
7. An appropriate nonopioid analgesic for mild pain is
   a. oxycodone.
   b. ibuprofen (Advil).
   c. lorazepam (Ativan).
   d. codeine with acetaminophen (Tylenol #3).
8. An important nursing responsibility related to pain is to
   a. leave the patient alone to rest.
   b. help the patient appear to not be in pain.
   c. believe what the patient says about the pain.
   d. assume responsibility for eliminating the patient's pain.
9. Providing opioids to a dying patient who is experiencing moderate to severe pain
   a. may cause addiction.
   b. will probably be ineffective.
   c. is an appropriate nursing action.
   d. will likely hasten the person's death.
10. A nurse believes that patients with the same type of tissue injury should have the same amount of pain. This statement reflects
    a. a belief that will contribute to appropriate pain management.
    b. an accurate statement about pain mechanisms and an expected goal of pain therapy.
    c. a premise that the nurse's belief will have no effect on the type of care provided to people in pain.
    d. the nurse's lack of knowledge about pain mechanisms, which is likely to contribute to poor pain management.

REFERENCES

1. *www.ampainsoc.org* (accessed May 20, 2006).
2. American Pain Foundation: Pain facts: an overview of American pain surveys. Available at *www.painfoundation.org* (accessed May 20, 2006).
3. Chronic Pain Association of Canada: *Pain facts*. Available at *www.chronicpaincanada.com* (accessed May 20, 2006).
4. Stewart WF, Ricci JA, Chee E, et al: Lost productive time and cost due to common pain conditions in the US workforce, *JAMA* 290:2443, 2003.
5. Teno JM, Clarridge BR, Casey V, et al: Family perspectives on end-of-life care at the last place of care, *JAMA* 291:88, 2004.
6. Cherny NI: Cancer pain: principles of assessment and syndromes. In Berger AM, Protenoy RK, Weissman DE, editors: *Principles and practice of palliative care and supportive oncology,* ed 2, Philadelphia, 2002, Lippincott Williams & Wilkins.
7. Maroney CL, Litke A, Fischberg D, et al: Acceptability of severe pain among hospitalized adults, *J Palliat Med* 7:443, 2004.

*8. Puntillo KA, Wild LR, Morris AB, et al: Practices and predictors of analgesic interventions for adults undergoing painful procedures, *Am J Crit Care* 11:415, 2002.

9. Won AB, Lapane KL, Vallow S, et al: Persistent nonmalignant pain and analgesic prescribing patterns in elderly nursing home residents, *J Am Geriatr Soc* 52:867, 2004.
10. American Geriatrics Society: The management of persistent pain in older persons, *J Am Geriatr Soc* 50(suppl 6):1, 2002.
11. Pasero C, Paice JA, McCaffery M: Basic mechanisms underlying the causes and effects of pain. In McCaffery M, Pasero C, editors: *Pain: clinical manual,* ed 2, St Louis, 1999, Mosby.

*12. Tarzian AJ, Hoffmann DE: Barriers to managing pain in the nursing home: findings from a statewide survey, *J Am Med Dir Assoc* 5:82, 2004.

*13. Herr K, Titler MG, Schilling ML, et al: Evidence-based assessment of acute pain in older adults: current nursing practices and perceived barriers, *Clin J Pain* 20:331, 2004.

14. Hospice and Palliative Nurses Association: Position statement: providing opioids at the end of life, 2004. Available at *www.hpna.org/positions.asp* (accessed May 14, 2006).
15. Goldstein DH, Ellis J, Brown R, et al: Recommendations for improved acute pain services: Canadian collaborative acute pain initiative, *Pain Res Manag* 9:123, 2004.

*16. Letizia M, Creech S, Norton E, et al: Barriers to caregiver administration of pain medication in hospice care, *J Pain Symptom Manage* 27:114, 2004.

17. McCaffery M: *Nursing practice theories related to cognition, bodily pain and man-environmental interactions*, Los Angeles, 1968, UCLA Students Store.
18. Merskey H, Bugduk N: *Classification of chronic pain, descriptions of chronic pain syndromes and definitions of pain terms,* ed 2, Seattle, 1994, IASP Press.
19. Cassell EJ: The nature of suffering and the goals of medicine, *N Engl J Med* 306:639, 1982.
20. Keefe FJ, Rumble ME, Scipio CD, et al: Psychological aspects of persistent pain: current state of the science, *J Pain* 5:195, 2004.
21. Myers CD, Riley JL, Robinson ME: Psychosocial contributions to sex-correlated differences in pain, *Clin J Pain* 19:225, 2003.

*Nursing research–based references.

22. Sarton E, Romberg R, Dahan A: Gender differences in morphine pharmacokinetics and dynamics, *Adv Exp Med Biol* 523:71, 2003.
23. Ferrell BR: Pain observed: the experience of pain from the family caregiver's perspective, *Clin Geriatr Med* 17:595, 2001.
24. Watkins LR, Milligan ED, Maier SF: Spinal cord glia: new players in pain, *Pain* 93:201-205, 2001.
25. Barber J: Hypnosis. In Loeser JD et al, editors: *Bonica's management of pain,* ed 3, Baltimore, 2001, Lippincott Williams & Wilkins.
26. Joint Commission on Accreditation of Health care Organizations: Pain: current understanding of assessment, management and treatments, effective 2001. Available at *www.jcaho.org* (accessed May 20, 2006).
27. Herr K, Decker S, Bjoro K: State of the art review of tools for assessment of pain in nonverbal older adults, 2004. Available at *www.cityofhope.org/prc/elderly.asp* (accessed May 20, 2006).
28. Fuchs-Lacelle S, Hadjistavropoulos T: Development and preliminary validation of the pain assessment checklist for seniors with limited ability to communicate (PACSLAC), *Pain Management Nurs* 5:37, 2004.
*29. Warden V, Hurley AC, Volicer L: Development and psychometric evaluation of the pain assessment in advanced dementia (PAINAD) scale, *J Am Med Dir Assoc* 4:9, 2003.
30. Chapman CR, Syrjala KL: Measurement of pain. In Loeser JD et al, editors: *Bonica's management of pain*, ed 3, Baltimore, 2001, Lippincott Williams & Wilkins.
31. Galer BS, Jensen MP: Development and preliminary validation of a pain measure specific to neuropathic pain: the neuropathic pain scale, *Neurology* 48:322, 1997.
32. American Medical Directors Association: Pain management in the long-term care setting: clinical practice guideline, 2003. Available at *www.amda.com* (accessed January 27, 2006).
33. American Pain Society: *Principles of analgesic use in the treatment of acute and cancer pain*, ed 5, Glenview, Ill, 2003, American Pain Society. Available at *www.ampainsoc.org/pub/principles.htm* (accessed May 20, 2006).
34. Rahme E, Pettitt D, LeLorier J: Determinants and sequelae associated with utilization of acetaminophen versus traditional nonsteroidal antiinflammatory drugs in an elderly population, *Arthritis Rheum* 46:3046, 2002.
35. Juni P, Nartey L, Reichenbach S, et al: Risk of cardiovascular events and rofecoxib: cumulative meta-analysis, *Lancet* 364:2021, 2004.
36. Webster L, Andrews M, Stoddard G: Modafinil treatment of opioid-induced sedation, *Pain Med* 4:135, 2003.
37. University of Wisconsin Hospital and Clinics: Fast facts: respiratory depression from opioids, 2003. Available at *www.cityofhope.org/prc/pdf/RespiratoryDepression%20Fast%20Fact.pdf* (accessed January 27, 2006).
38. Namaka M, Gremlich CR, Ruhlen D, et al: A treatment algorithm for neuropathic pain, *Clin Ther* 26:951, 2004.
39. Fishbain D: Evidence-based data on pain relief with antidepressants, *Ann Med* 32:305, 2000.
40. Dworkin RH, Backonja M, Rowbotham MC, et al: Advances in neuropathic pain: diagnosis, mechanisms, and treatment recommendations, *Arch Neurol* 60:1524, 2003.
41. Barbano R, Herrmann DN, Hart-Gouleau S, et al: Effectiveness, tolerability and impact of quality of life for the 5% lidocaine patch in diabetic polyneuropathy, *Arch Neurol* 61:914, 2004.
42. Boureau F, Legallicier P, Kabir-Ahmadi M: Tramadol in post-herpetic neuralgia: a randomized, double-blind, placebo-controlled trial, *Pain* 104:323, 2003.
43. Bennett RM, Kamin M, Karim R, et al: Tramadol and acetaminophen combination tablets in the treatment of fibromyalgia pain: a double-blind, randomized, placebo-controlled study, *Am J Med* 114:537, 2003.
44. American Society for Pain Management Nursing and American Pain Society: Consensus statement: the use of "as needed" range orders for opioid analgesics in the management of acute pain, 2004. Available at *www.ampainsoc.org/advocacy/range.htm* (accessed May 20, 2006).
45. Gammaitoni AR, Fine P, Alvarez N, et al: Clinical application of opioid equianalgesic data, *Clin J Pain* 19:286, 2003.
46. Buckley FP: Regional anesthesia with local anesthetics. In Loeser JD et al, editors: *Bonica's management of pain*, ed 3, Baltimore, 2001, Lippincott Williams & Wilkins.
47. Busch A, Schachter CL, Peloso PM, et al: Exercise for treating fibromyalgia syndrome, *Cochrane Database Syst Rev* 3:CD003786, 2002.
48. Chabal C: Transcutaneous electrical nerve stimulation. In Loeser JD et al, editors: *Bonica's management of pain*, ed 3, Baltimore, 2001, Lippincott Williams & Wilkins.

*Nursing research–based references.

49. Weiner DK, Ernst E: Complementary and alternative approaches to the treatment of persistent musculoskeletal pain, *Clin J Pain* 20:244, 2004.
50. Birch S, Hesselink JK, Jonkman FA, et al: Clinical research on acupuncture: what have reviews of the efficacy and safety of acupuncture told us so far? *J Altern Complement Med* 10:468, 2004.
51. Patterson DR, Jensen MP: Hypnosis and clinical pain, *Psychol Bull* 129:495, 2003.
52. Inturrisi CE: Clinical pharmacology of opioids for pain, *Clin J Pain* 18(4 suppl):S3, 2002.
53. Ballantyne J, Mao J: Opioid therapy for chronic pain, *N Engl J Med* 349:1942, 2004.
54. Nedeljkovic SS, Wasan A, Jamison RN: Assessment of efficacy of long-term opioid therapy in pain patients with substance abuse potential, *Clin J Pain* 18(4 suppl):S39, 2002.
55. American Pain Society: Promoting pain relief and preventing abuse of pain medications: a critical balancing act, 2004. Available at *www.ampainsoc.org/advocacy/promoting.htm* (accessed May 7, 2006).
56. American Nurses Association: Position statement on pain management and control of distressing symptoms in dying patients. Available at *www.nursingworld.org/readroom/position/ethics/etpain.htm* (accessed May 7, 2006).
57. Beauchamp TL, Childress JF: *Principles of biomedical ethics,* ed 5, New York, 2001, Oxford University Press.
58. American Nurses Association: ANA's position on assisted suicide, *Am Nurse* 28:9, 1996. Available at *www.nursingworld.org/readroom/position/ethics/etsuic.htm* (accessed May 7, 2006).
59. Oregon Nurses Association: Position paper on the death with dignity act, 1995. Available at *www.oregonrn.org/associations/3019/files/AssistedSuicide.pdf* (accessed May 5, 2006).
60. Hospice and Palliative Nurses Association: Position statement on pain, 2003. Available at *www.hpna.org/pdf/Pain_position_Statement_PDF.pdf* (accessed May 7, 2006).
61. Ardery G, Herr KA, Titler MG, et al: Assessing and managing acute pain in older adults: a research base to guide practice, *Medsurg Nurs* 12:7, 2003.
62. Department of Health and Human Services: Overview of findings from the 2003 national survey on drug use and health. Available at *http://oas.samhsa.gov/NHSDA/2k3NSDUH/2k3OverviewW.pdf* (accessed May 28, 2006).
63. Butler SF, Budman SH, Fernandez K, et al: Validation of a screener and opioid assessment measure for patients with chronic pain, *Pain* 112:65, 2004.

RESOURCES

American Academy of Pain Management
209-533-9744
www.aapainmanage.org

American Academy of Pain Medicine (AAPM)
847-375-4731
Email: aapm@amctec.com
www.painmed.org

American Chronic Pain Association
800-533-3231
www.theacpa.org

American Pain Society
847-375-4715
Email: info@ampainsoc.org
www.ampainsoc.org

American Society of Pain Management Nursing
888-342-7766
www.aspmn.org

City of Hope Pain/Palliative Care Resource Center
Email: prc@coh.org
www.cityofhope.org/prc/web

International Association for the Study of Pain (IASP)
206-547-6409
Email: IASP@locke.hs.washington.edu
www.iasp-pain.org/:index.html

Pain.com
www.pain.com

PainLink
www.edc.org/PainLink

For additional Internet resources, see the website for this book at *http://evolve.elsevier.com/Lewis/medsurg*.

Should you shield the canyons from the wind storms, you would never see the true beauty of their carvings.

Elisabeth Kübler-Ross

11 End-of-Life and Palliative Care

Margaret McLean Heitkemper and Cheryl Ross Staats

LEARNING OBJECTIVES

1. Describe the physical manifestations at the end of life.
2. Relate the common psychologic manifestations at the end of life.
3. Explain the process of grief at the end of life.
4. Examine the cultural and spiritual issues related to end-of-life care.
5. Discuss ethical and legal issues in end-of-life care.
6. Discuss the purpose of palliative care and hospice.
7. Describe the nursing management for the dying patient.
8. Explore the special needs of family caregivers in end-of-life care.
9. Discuss the special needs of the nurse who cares for dying patients and their families.

KEY TERMS

bereavement, p. 153
brain death, p. 153
Cheyne-Stokes respiration, p. 152
death, p. 152
end of life, p. 151
end-of-life care, p. 151
grief, p. 153
hospice, p. 156
palliative care, p. 156

Electronic Resources

Supplemental content related to Chapter 11 can be found . . .

Companion CD

- Stress-Busting Kit for Nursing Students
- NCLEX Examination Review Questions
- Comprehensive Glossary

Evolve Website

http://evolve.elsevier.com/Lewis/medsurg

- Content Updates
- Key Points (Printable and CD/MP3 Download)
- Concept Map Creator
- Expanded Audio Glossary
- Key Term Flash Cards
- Electronic Calculators
- WebLinks

Life and death have intrigued humankind throughout history. Artists, writers, philosophers, scientists, religious leaders, and many others have pondered the meaning of life and death. Traditionally, mortality and the death experience are difficult and awkward topics to discuss and accept in Western society. Before the 1960s patients who were not expected to survive were placed in isolated hospital areas, were given less than quality care, and died without appropriate medical care.

Today, as a result of the "graying of America" and the increasing number of persons with chronic diseases, terminal illness and dying have received greater attention. At this time 75% of Americans live past age 65 and 83% of Americans die while covered by Medicare. Most individuals will have a long period of serious illness before dying, with the onset months or years before death. For example, approximately half of all patients diagnosed with cancer will die from their disease within a few years.[1,2] In the United States the majority of deaths each year are due to natural causes, with less than 6% resulting from accidents, suicide, or homicide. Of those who die, death is due to one or more preexisting conditions such as heart disease, stroke, cancer, chronic lung disease, dementia, or chronic liver disease.[3] The special needs of the dying and the terminally ill are now acknowledged and integrated into care. Nurses spend more time with patients near the end of life than any other health care professionals.[1]

End-of-life care (EOL care) is the term currently used for issues related to death and dying, as well as services provided to address these issues. The Institute of Medicine defines **end of life** as the period of time during which an individual copes with declining health from a terminal illness or from the frailties associated with advanced age even if death is not clearly imminent.[1,2] The time from diagnosis of a terminal illness to death varies considerably depending on the patient's diagnosis and extent of disease. EOL care focuses on physical and psychosocial needs at the end of life for the patient and the patient's family. The goals for EOL care are

Reviewed by Jeanne M. Martinez, RN, MPH, CHPN, Quality and Education Specialist, Northwestern Memorial Home Health Care, Chicago, Ill.

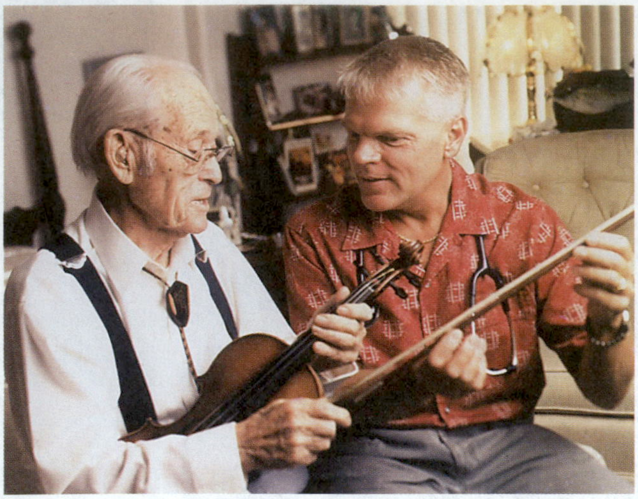

FIG. 11-1 One goal of end-of-life care is to improve the quality of the patient's remaining life.

to (1) provide comfort and supportive care during the dying process, (2) improve the quality of the remaining life, and (3) help ensure a dignified death (Fig. 11-1).

PHYSICAL MANIFESTATIONS AT END OF LIFE

Death occurs when all vital organs and systems cease to function. **Death** is the irreversible cessation of circulatory and respiratory function or the irreversible cessation of all functions of the entire brain, including the brainstem. Trauma and disease processes can affect physical manifestations at the end of life. As death approaches, metabolism is reduced and the body gradually slows down until all function ends. Generally, respirations cease first. Then the heart stops beating within a few minutes. Physical manifestations of approaching death are listed in Table 11-1.

Sensory Changes

With decreased oxygenation and circulation to the brain, there are alterations in the interpretation of sensory input. Sensory changes can include blurred vision, decreased sense of taste and smell, and decreased pain and touch perception. The blink reflex is eventually lost, and the patient appears to stare. The sense of touch decreases first in the lower extremities because of circulatory alterations. Hearing is commonly believed to be the last sense to remain intact at the end of life.

Circulatory and Respiratory Changes

With decreased oxygenation and altered circulation causing metabolic changes, the heart rate slows and weakens and the blood pressure falls progressively. Body temperature may be elevated related to a disease process and changes in hypothalamic function. Respirations may be rapid or slow, shallow, and irregular. Breath sounds may become wet and noisy, both audibly and on auscultation. Noisy, wet-sounding respirations, termed the **death rattle,** are due to mouth breathing and accumulation of mucus in the airways. **Cheyne-Stokes respiration** is a pattern of breathing characterized by alternating periods of apnea and deep, rapid breathing. This type of breathing is usually seen as a person nears death.

There is decreased circulation, especially noticeable on the skin. The extremities become pale, mottled, and cyanotic. The skin feels cool to the touch, first in the feet and legs, then progressing to the hands and arms, and finally progressing to the torso. The skin may feel warm because of an elevated body temperature related to an underlying disease process.

TABLE 11-1 Physical Manifestations of Approaching Death

System	Manifestations
Sensory system	
Hearing	• Usually last sense to disappear
Touch	• Decreased sensation • Decreased perception of pain and touch
Taste and smell	• Decreased with disease progression
Sight	• Blurring of vision • Sinking and glazing of eyes • Blink reflex absent • Eyelids remain half-open
Integumentary system	• Mottling on hands, feet, arms, and legs • Cold, clammy skin • Cyanosis on nose, nail beds, knees • "Waxlike" skin when very near death
Respiratory system	• Increased respiratory rate • Cheyne-Stokes respiration (pattern of respiration characterized by alternating periods of apnea and deep, rapid breathing) • Inability to cough or clear secretions resulting in grunting, gurgling, or noisy congested breathing (death rattle) • Irregular breathing, gradually slowing down to terminal gasps (may be described as guppy breathing)
Urinary system	• Gradual decrease in urinary output • Incontinent of urine • Unable to urinate
Gastrointestinal system	• Slowing of gastrointestinal tract and possible cessation of function (may be enhanced by pain-relieving drugs) • Accumulation of gas • Distention and nausea • Loss of sphincter control may produce incontinence • Bowel movement may occur before imminent death or at time of death
Musculoskeletal system	• Gradual loss of ability to move • Sagging of jaw resulting from loss of facial muscle tone • Difficulty speaking • Swallowing can become more difficult • Difficulty maintaining body posture and alignment • Loss of gag reflex • Jerking seen in patients on large amounts of opioids
Cardiovascular system	• Increased heart rate; later slowing and weakening of pulse • Irregular rhythm • Decrease in blood pressure • Delayed absorption of drugs administered intramuscularly or subcutaneously

Loss of Muscle Tone

As death becomes imminent, metabolic changes cause the muscular system to gradually weaken, leading to sluggish functional abilities. Facial muscles lose tone, causing the jaw to sag. Decreased muscle coordination leads to difficulty in speaking. Swallowing becomes increasingly difficult, and the gag reflex is eventually lost. Gastrointestinal (GI) motility and transit diminish, leading to constipation, gas accumulation, distention, and nausea. Pain-relieving drugs may exacerbate these GI manifestations. The ability of the urinary system to function and produce urine decreases. Loss of sphincter control can lead to fecal and urinary incontinence.

Brain Death

The diagnosis of death is based on brain or cerebral death. In the United States **brain death** is defined as irreversible loss of all brain functions, including the brainstem. Brain death is a clinical diagnosis, and it can be made in patients whose hearts continue to beat and who are maintained on mechanical ventilation in the intensive care unit.[4,5] Brain death occurs when the cerebral cortex stops functioning or is irreversibly destroyed. The cerebral cortex, or the higher brain, is responsible for voluntary movement and actions, as well as for cognitive functioning.

Since the development of technology that assists in supporting life, controversies have arisen related to an exact definition of death. Questions and discussions have developed around whether brain or cerebral death occurs when the whole brain (cortex and brainstem) ceases activity or when cortical function alone stops. In 1995 the Quality Standards Subcommittee of the American Academy of Neurology recommended diagnostic criteria guidelines for clinical diagnosis of brain death in adults.[6] These criteria for brain death include coma or unresponsiveness, absence of brainstem reflexes, and apnea. Specific assessments by a physician are required to validate each of the criteria.[5,6]

Currently, legal and medical standards require that all brain function must cease for brain death to be pronounced and life support to be disconnected by the physician. Diagnosis of brain death is of particular importance when organ donation is an option. In some states, under specific circumstances registered nurses are legally permitted to pronounce death. Policies and procedures may vary from state to state, among the Board of Nurse Examiners for Registered Nurses in each state, and among institutions.

PSYCHOSOCIAL MANIFESTATIONS AT END OF LIFE

A variety of feelings and emotions affect the dying patient and family at the end of life. Specific psychosocial manifestations are listed in Table 11-2. Most patients and families struggle with a terminal diagnosis and the realization that there is no cure. Time may be needed to process the impending death and to formulate emotional responses. The patient and the family feel overwhelmed, fearful, powerless, and fatigued. The patient's needs and wishes must be respected. Patients need time to ponder their thoughts and express their feelings. Response time to questions may be sluggish because of fatigue, weakness, and confusion.

TABLE 11-2 Psychosocial Manifestations of Approaching Death

- Altered decision making
- Anxiety about unfinished business
- Withdrawal
- Decreased socialization
- Fear of loneliness
- Fear of meaninglessness of one's life
- Fear of pain
- Helplessness
- Life review
- Peacefulness
- Restlessness
- Saying goodbyes
- Unusual communication
- Vision-like experiences

GRIEF

Bereavement is an individual's emotional response to the loss of a significant person. It is important to note that bereavement may begin before death occurs. Bereavement is a natural and needed reaction to a loss. Bereavement is associated with a time of intense personal suffering for the majority of people. It is a result of the individual's sorrow over the loss, the feelings of loneliness, and impact of the loss of a lifetime of shared experiences. While loss is universal, a person's reaction to the loss is unique to the individual.

Grief develops from bereavement and is a dynamic psychologic and physiologic response following the loss. It is the lived experience in reaction to the loss. Grief is one of the most powerful emotional states and affects all aspects of a person's life. Grieving related to loss from death is a complex and intense emotional experience. It encompasses thoughts, feelings, and behaviors.

Grief is manifested in a variety of ways. Every loss is as different as each person is unique. There are no guidelines to predict grief reactions. Individuals experience different aspects of the grieving process at different times. The individual's cultural beliefs, religious influences or spiritual beliefs, and value system influence grief reactions. The intensity of grief is driven by an individual's personality, the nature of the relationship with the dying person, concurrent life crises, coping resources, and the availability of support systems.[7]

Manifestations of grieving can be classified into four different areas: (1) feelings, including despair, guilt, loneliness, sadness, anger; (2) behaviors, including crying spells, social withdrawal, agitation; (3) thoughts, including preoccupation with thinking about the dead person, hopelessness, helplessness, problems with memory and concentration; and (4) physical manifestations, including not eating, insomnia, fatigue, headaches, excess alcohol intake, and heart palpitations.

Kübler-Ross, Martocchio, and Rando have each identified stages of grief.[8-10] A comparison among the three is listed in Table 11-3. Kübler-Ross identified denial, anger, bargaining, depression, and acceptance as the five stages of grieving.[8] These stages are not necessarily sequential stages. People can move from one stage to another and then back again or skip a stage as they attempt to deal with the loss.

Martocchio presented five clusters of grief to include (1) shock and disbelief; (2) yearning and protest; (3) anguish, disorganiza-

TABLE 11-3 Comparison of Stages of Grieving

Kübler-Ross (1969)[8]	Martocchio (1985)[9]	Rando (1993)[10]
Denial	Shock and disbelief	Avoidance
Anger/bargaining	Yearning and protest	Confrontation
Depression	Anguish, disorganization, and despair	
	Identification of bereavement	
Acceptance	Reorganization and restoration	Accommodation

A nurse does not strive only to alleviate physical pain or render physical care—she ministers to the person. The nurse cares for the individual, not a body part. The existence of suffering whether physical, mental, or spiritual is the proper concern of the nurse.

From Allen-Shelly J, Fish S: *Spiritual care: the nurse's role,* ed 3, Downers Grove, Ill, 1988, InterVarsity Press.

tion, and despair; (4) identification of bereavement; and (5) reorganization and resolution.[9] Rando refined three phases of responses to grieving that were identified as avoidance, confrontation, and accommodation.[10]

Working through the grief process helps adapt to the loss. The process of resolution in normal grief may take months to years. *Pathologic grief* can manifest as chronic grief when the intensity does not wane after the first year. The bereaved person becomes "bogged down" in the grieving process. Grief can manifest as *conflicted grief* when the person has not resolved ambivalent feelings toward the deceased. Grief can manifest as *absent grief* when the bereaved person appears to be coping and carrying on as if nothing has happened.

Grief that is prolonged, unresolved, or disruptive may be termed *maladaptive* or *dysfunctional grief.* Grief that is delayed or exaggerated may be identified as dysfunctional. Dysfunctional grieving may relate to a real loss or a perceived loss. It may occur when grief is not resolved from a prior experience or when the expression of grief is blocked in some way. With dysfunctional grief, feelings and behaviors may become exaggerated and disruptive to a person's usual lifestyle.

Grief that is helpful or that assists the person in accepting the reality of death is called *adaptive grief.* Adaptive grief is a healthy response. It may be associated with grieving before a death actually occurs or when the reality that death is inevitable is known.

The grieving process takes time, energy, and work. Goals for the grieving process include resolving emotions, reflecting on the dying person, expressing feelings of loss and sadness, and valuing what has been shared.

VARIABLES AFFECTING END-OF-LIFE CARE

People experiencing the inevitability of death are in need of caregivers who are knowledgeable about personal issues and attitudes that affect the end-of-life experience. The attitudes of the dying person, family and significant others, and nurses affect the death experience.

Health care professionals must be aware of cultural differences as they care for patients and families.[11] An adequate understanding of spiritual, cultural, and familial influences is beneficial when focusing on the dying person's and family's needs, wants, and fears. Although there may be influences from spirituality, culture, and family, the uniqueness of each person will lead to varied responses.

The nurse, along with other members of the health care team, identifies the cultural needs of the patient and family. This includes assessing and documenting the patient's cultural background, concerns, health practices, and attitudes about suffering. Open-ended questions related to the patient's perspectives on his or her illness, as well as the patient's expectations of care, can be used. This assessment is then used to guide the patient's plan of care and evaluation. It can also be used to suggest or plan grief and bereavement counseling for family members. At the same time, accommodations need to be made related to language, diet, and ritual practices for the patient. When appropriate, medical interpreter services should be accessed and used so that the patient's wishes are known.

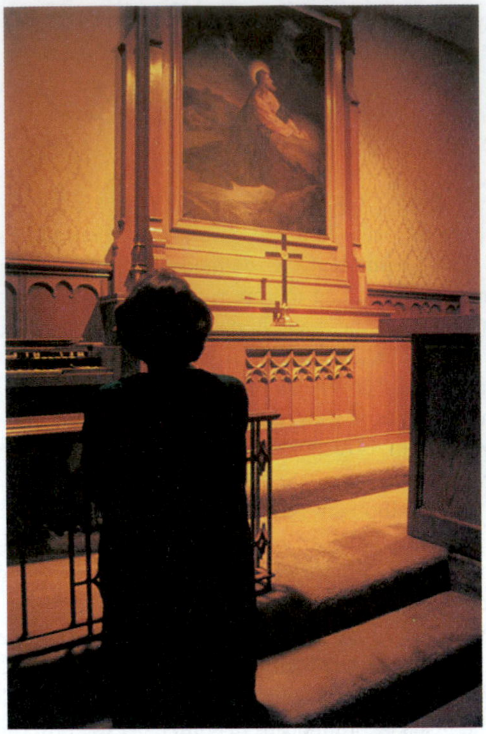

FIG. 11-2 Spiritual needs are an important consideration in end-of-life care.

Spiritual Needs

Assessment of spiritual needs in EOL care is a key consideration (Fig. 11-2). Spiritual needs do not necessarily equate to religion. A person may be of no particular faith but have a deep spirituality. Many times at the end of life, patients question their beliefs about a higher power, their own journey through life, religion, and an afterlife. Some patients may choose to pursue a spiritual path. Some may not. Their individual choice needs to be respected. The patient's and family's preferences related to spiritual guidance or pastoral care services should be noted.

Deep-seated spiritual beliefs may surface for some patients when they deal with their terminal diagnosis and related issues. Spiritual distress may occur, with a challenge to and questioning of beliefs and values surrounding the past, present, and future.[12]

Spirituality has been associated with decreased despair in patients at the end of life. Some dying patients are secure in their faith about the future. It is common to observe patients relinquishing material values of life and focusing on values they believe will lead them on to another place.[13]

CULTURALLY COMPETENT CARE
END OF LIFE

Both spiritual and cultural beliefs affect a person's understanding of and reaction to death or loss. Frequently, beliefs and attitudes are interrelated between spirituality and culture. The Western work ethic is closely related to the American ethic, which emphasizes independence, self-reliance, hard work, and rugged individualism. With these attitudes many people believe that privacy is imperative. Death and dying tend to be private matters shared only with significant others. Often feelings are repressed or internalized. People who believe in "toughing it out" or "being strong" may not express themselves when they are experiencing a tragic loss.

Some cultural groups, such as African Americans and Hispanics, may express their feelings and emotions more easily.[14] Kinship tends to be very strong in the Hispanic culture. In this culture, family members, both immediate and extended, provide support for one another. Expressing feelings of loss is encouraged and accepted easily.

Culture should be considered throughout the end-of-life process. If palliative or hospice care is recommended, certain cultural groups are less likely to use this as a resource. For example, within the Mexican American culture, hospice care is used less often because many Mexican Americans live in close-knit communities and they often prefer to care for their own family members. The decision to use palliative care or hospice services may be perceived as "giving up" or receiving second-rate care. Such attitudes are best approached by clear and open discussions with the patient and the family about the philosophy and services of palliative and hospice organizations.

Culture affects decision making with regard to life support and withholding and withdrawing of treatments. In some cultures, such as the Filipino American, it is appropriate to first discuss a terminal diagnosis with the family before informing the patient, and then the family will decide if the patient should be told the information.[14]

Family involvement is integral to providing culturally competent care. In certain cultures, if a family member is dying, the family may want to keep constant vigil with the patient or in the waiting area. For example, Jewish Americans believe that the spirit should not be alone when it leaves the body at the time of death. Therefore someone who is terminally ill should never be left alone. Once a death has occurred, some cultures, such as the Puerto Rican American culture, may want to kiss and touch the body after death has occurred in order to say goodbye.

Cultural variations in symptom expression (e.g., pain expression) and use of health care services also exist. It is known that ethnic minority groups are often undertreated in terms of pain medications. This is critically important with regard to palliative care management. Providing culturally competent care requires greater attention to assessment of nonverbal cues such as grimaces, body position, and decreased or guarded movements. Issues related to pain assessment and management are discussed in Chapter 10.

Differences among spiritual and cultural beliefs and values are innumerable. Nursing assessments of beliefs and preferences should be made on an individual basis to avoid stereotyping individuals with different spiritual and cultural belief systems.[14] (Culturally competent care is discussed in Chapter 3.)

LEGAL AND ETHICAL ISSUES AFFECTING END-OF-LIFE CARE

Patients and families struggle with many decisions during the terminal illness and dying experience. Many people decide that the outcomes related to their care should be based on their own wishes. The decisions may involve the choice for (1) organ and tissue donations, (2) advance directives (e.g., medical power of attorney, living wills), and (3) resuscitation.

Organ and Tissue Donation

Persons who are legally competent may choose organ donation. Any body part or the entire body may be donated. The decision to donate organs or to provide anatomic gifts may be made by a person before death. The decision to donate organs may be made by immediate family members following death. Family permission must be obtained at the time of donation.

Some people carry donor cards. Some states allow for organ donation to be marked on drivers' licenses. The names of agencies that handle organ donation will vary by locale. Common names for such an agency might be the organ bank, organ-sharing network, and organ sharing alliance. Both organ and tissue donations follow specific legal guidelines. Legal requirements and facility policies for organ or tissue donation must be followed. The physician must be notified immediately when organ donation is intended because some tissues must be used within hours after death.[15]

Legal Documents Used in End-of-Life Care

In 1991 the Omnibus Reconciliation Act of 1990 became effective. It is frequently known as the Patient Self-Determination Act.[16] This act requires all institutions that participate in Medicare to provide written information to patients concerning their right to accept or refuse treatment. This information should include the right to initiate advance directives. **Advance directives** are written statements of a person's wishes regarding medical care. The first advance directive was known by laypersons as a *living will.* It was developed by the Euthanasia Education Council. **Advance care planning** is focused on anticipated challenges that the patient and family will face because of illness, medical treatment, and other concerns.[17]

Most states have replaced the idea of living wills with *natural death acts.* Within many of these acts are specific aspects related to the individual's wishes. *Directives to physicians* (DTP), *durable power of attorney for health care* (DPAHC), and *medical power of attorney* (MPOA) may be included in the natural death acts. Under the natural death acts an individual can tell the physician exactly what treatment is or is not desired. Each state has its own unique requirements. Table 11-4 identifies common legal and ethical documents used in EOL care.

Copies of state-specific forms can be obtained from local medical associations and the Internet. However, a person may write his or her wishes without special forms. Verbal directives may be given to physicians with specific instructions in the presence of two witnesses. Attorneys and notaries may not necessarily be required. In the event that the person is not capable of communicating his or her wishes, the surrogate decision maker and the physician can agree on what measures will or will not be taken. The physician should record the family's decision.

Resuscitation

In the past 35 years cardiopulmonary resuscitation (CPR) has become common practice in health care. Patients who suffered respiratory or cardiac arrest have been given CPR unless a *do-not-resuscitate (DNR) order* was given by the physician. Many times patients and families have had no choice as to whether CPR was used.

In recent years, much has been written concerning the right to die and the right to choose. Many people believe that the patient or the patient's family has the right to decide whether CPR will be used. It is no longer the sole decision of the physician. The Ameri-

TABLE 11-4 Common Documents Used in End-of-Life Care

Document	Description	Special Considerations
Advance directive	A general term used to describe documents that give instructions about future medical care and treatments and who should make them in the event the person is unable to communicate.	• Should comply with guidelines established by state of residence.
Directive to physicians	A written document specifying the patient's wish to be allowed to die without heroic or extraordinary measures.	• Specific measures to be used or withheld are indicated.
Do not resuscitate (DNR)	A written physician's order instructing health care providers not to attempt CPR; often requested by family; must be signed by a physician to be valid.	• Any specific measures to be used or withheld must be indicated.
Durable power of attorney for health care	A term used by some states to describe a document used for listing the person or persons to make health care decisions should a patient become unable to make informed decisions for self.	• May be the same as medical power of attorney. • Specific measures to be used or withheld are indicated.
Living will	A lay term used frequently to describe any number of documents that give instructions about future medical care and treatments or the wish to be allowed to die without heroic or extraordinary measures should the patient be unable to communicate for self.	• Specific documents must be identified.
Medical power of attorney	A term used by some states to describe a document used for listing the person or persons to make health care decisions should a patient become unable to make informed decisions for self.	• May be the same as durable power of attorney for health care, health care proxy, or appointment of a health care agent or surrogate. Specific measures to be used or withheld are specified. • Person appointed may be called a health care agent, surrogate, attorney-in-fact, or proxy.

can Nurses Association (ANA) supports the patient's right to self-determination and believes that nurses will and must play a primary role in implementation of the law.[18]

A physician's order should be written to include the information concerning the patient's or family's wishes for the use of CPR. Several different types of CPR decisions can be made. Complete and total heroic measures, which may include CPR, drugs, and mechanical ventilation, can be referred to as a *full code.* Some people choose variations of the full code. A *chemical code* involves the use of drugs for resuscitation without the use of CPR. A "no code" or a DNR order allows the person to die with comfort measures only and without the interference of technology.[19] Some states have implemented a form called *out-of-hospital DNR* for use by terminally ill patients who wish to have no heroic measures used to prolong life after they leave an acute care facility.[20]

A new term being used to replace "no code" or DNR is the term *allow natural death (AND).* This term more accurately conveys what actually happens. It is also sometimes referred to as "comfort code" status, meaning that all comfort measures associated with pain control and symptom management are carried out. However, the natural physiologic progression to death is not delayed or interrupted.

Withholding or withdrawing treatments must be included in an advance directive. What is to be done and what is not to be done must be included in clear terms. The ANA position statements on foregoing nutrition and hydration and active euthanasia from 1992 and 1994, respectively, recognize that honoring the refusal of treatments that a patient does not desire, are disproportionately burdensome to the patient, or will not benefit the patient can be ethically and legally permissible. Additionally, the decision to withhold artificial nutrition and hydration should be made by the patient or surrogate with the health care team.[21,22]

The nurse needs to be aware of legal issues and the wishes of the patient.[19] Advance directives and organ donor information should be located in the medical record and identified on the patient's record and/or the nursing care plan. All caregivers responsible for the patient need to know the patient's wishes. Additionally, the nurse is responsible for becoming familiar with state, local, and agency procedures in EOL care documentation.

PALLIATIVE CARE AND HOSPICE

The World Health Organization defines **palliative care** as the active total care of patients whose disease is not responsive to curative treatment.[1,2] Palliative care focuses on controlling pain and other symptoms, as well as reducing psychologic, social, and spiritual distress for the patient and the family. Six major skill sets make up palliative care: communication, decision making, management of complications of treatment and disease, symptom control, psychosocial care of patient and family, and care of the dying. Palliative care is the framework for hospice care. Palliative care can start much earlier in a disease process, whereas hospice traditionally is limited to the projected last 6 months of life.

Hospice is not a place but a concept of care that provides compassion, concern, and support for the dying (Fig. 11-3). Hospice

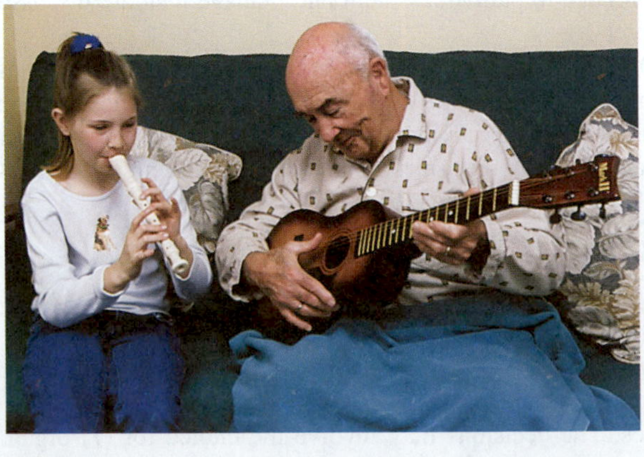

FIG. 11-3 Hospice care is designed to provide compassion, concern, and support for the dying.

You matter because you are you and you matter to the last moment of your life. We will do all we can not only to help you die peacefully, but to live until you die.

From Clark D: *Cicely Saunders, founder of the modern-day hospice movement,* New York, 2002, Oxford University Press.

and palliative care are frequently used interchangeably. Hospice exists to provide support and care for persons in the last phases of incurable diseases so that they might live as fully and as comfortably as possible. Hospice programs provide multidisciplinary care at the end of life with emphasis on symptom management, advance care planning, spiritual care, and family support, including bereavement.[23]

During the 1970s the concept of hospice was introduced into health care in the United States, and by the end of the decade, every state had hospice programs. In 1982 the Medicare hospice benefit was created, which provided families with the resources to care for their dying loved one at home. In 2003 approximately 950,000 patients were admitted to one of the 3300 programs in the United States. Of these patients, 49% had a cancer diagnosis, 11% end-stage heart disease, 9.6% dementia, 6.8% lung disease, 3% end-stage kidney disease, and 1.6% end-stage liver disease. Of those admitted to hospice, 37% died within 7 days.[24] Like home health care, hospice programs are organized under a variety of models. Some are hospital-based programs, others are part of existing home health care agencies, and others are freestanding or community-based, volunteer-intensive programs. However, regardless of their organization, all hospices emphasize palliative rather than curative care.

Hospice care is generally provided in the home, with inpatient care reserved for acute pain management or respite care for families or caregivers in need of a break. Home care is provided on a part-time, intermittent, on-call, regularly scheduled, or continuous basis. Hospice services are available 24 hours a day and 7 days a week to provide help to patients and families in their homes. The inpatient hospice settings have been deinstitutionalized to make the atmosphere as relaxed and homelike as possible (Fig. 11-4). Staff and volunteers are available to the patient and family. A multidisciplinary team approach often provides holistic health care.

A medically supervised interdisciplinary team of professionals and volunteers provides hospice services. The hospice nurse is an integral part and plays a pivotal role in coordination of the hospice team. Hospice nurses work collaboratively with hospice physicians, pharmacists, dietitians, physical therapists, social workers, certified nursing assistants, clergy, and volunteers to provide care and support to the patient and family members. Hospice nurses are educated in pain control and symptom management. As with home health care, hospice care requires excellent teaching skills, compassion, flexibility, and adaptability to patient needs.

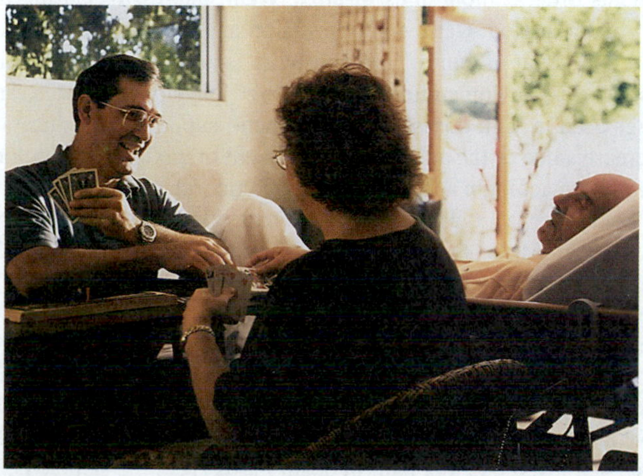

FIG. 11-4 Inpatient hospice settings have been deinstitutionalized to make the atmosphere as relaxed and homelike as possible.

The decision to begin hospice care is difficult. Several reasons for this exist. Patients, families, and physicians may lack information about hospice care. Physicians may be reluctant to give referrals because they sometimes view a patient's decline as their personal failure. Some patients or family members see it as giving up. The hospice requirement of a "6-month" prognosis is applicable to Medicare and Medicaid hospice benefit patients. Because of the difficulty of predicting a prognosis, Medicare does allow for hospice care beyond 6 months as long as the patient still meets hospice criteria.

Admission to a hospice program has two criteria. First, the patient must desire the services; second, a physician must certify that the patient has 6 months or less to live. For Medicare and Medicaid patients, two physicians must certify that the patient is terminally ill with less than 6 months to live. After this initial certification, only one physician (e.g., the hospice medical director) is needed to recertify the patient. Studies are being conducted to determine if these criteria meet the needs of chronically ill and dying patients. Patients with terminal conditions related to cancer, acquired immunodeficiency syndrome, chronic obstructive pulmonary disease, and end-stage cardiovascular or renal disease may qualify for hospice care. In addition, patients with disease processes such as Alzheimer's disease and other dementias, amyotrophic lateral sclerosis (ALS), Parkinson's disease, and liver disease may qualify for hospice care.

Bereavement counseling is an important aspect of hospice programs. The objective of a bereavement program is to provide support and to assist survivors in the transition to a life without the deceased person. Grief support is incorporated into the plan of care for family members and significant others during the patient's illness, as well as after the death.

NURSING MANAGEMENT
END OF LIFE

Nursing care of terminally ill and dying patients is holistic and encompasses all aspects of psychosocial and physical needs. Nursing care focuses on the psychosocial manifestations and the grieving process, as well as the physical changes that are associated with dying. The patient and the family need to be the focus of nursing care. Respect, dignity, and comfort are important for the patient and for the family.[25] In addition, nurses and other care providers must recognize their own needs when dealing with grief and dying.

Nursing Assessment

Assessment of the terminally ill or dying patient varies with the patient's condition and proximity of approaching death. In general, the assessment is limited to essential data. The nurse documents the specific event or change that brought the patient into the health care agency. The patient's medical diagnoses, medication profile, and allergies are recorded. If the patient is alert, a brief review of the body systems to detect important signs and symptoms should be completed. Discomfort, pain, nausea, and dyspnea are carefully assessed so that prompt interventions can be implemented.

The functional assessment of activities of daily living elicits information about the patient's abilities, food and fluid intake, patterns of sleep and rest, and response to the stress of terminal illness. Coping abilities of the patient and family should also be assessed.

The physical assessment is abbreviated and focuses on changes that accompany terminal illness and the specific disease process. The frequency of assessment depends on the patient's stability but is done at least every 8 hours in the institutional setting. For patients cared for in their homes by hospice programs, assessment may occur weekly. As changes occur, assessment and documentation need to be done more frequently.

As death approaches, neurologic assessment is especially important and includes level of consciousness, presence of reflexes, and pupil responses. Evaluation of vital signs, skin color, and temperature indicates changes in circulation. Respiratory status, character and pattern of respirations, and the characteristics of breath sounds are monitored and described. Monitoring nutritional and fluid intake, urinary output, and bowel function provides assessment data for renal and gastrointestinal functioning. Skin condition must be assessed on an ongoing basis because skin becomes fragile and may easily break down.

It is important to be sensitive and not to impose repeated, unnecessary assessments on the dying patient. Health history data that are available in the chart should be used when available rather than tiring the patient with an interview. However, it is important to assess the patient's status frequently.

Nursing Diagnoses

Several nursing diagnoses dealing with psychosocial manifestations (Table 11-5) and physical manifestations (Table 11-6) are associated with EOL care.

Planning

Planning for EOL care uses a holistic approach. Coordination of care must focus on both the patient's needs and the needs of the family members and significant others. Education, counseling, advocacy, and support for the patient and the family are priorities.

TABLE 11-5 NURSING DIAGNOSES
Psychosocial Manifestations at the End of Life

- Acute confusion
- Chronic confusion
- Chronic sorrow
- Complicated grieving
- Compromised family coping
- Death anxiety
- Disturbed thought processes
- Fear
- Grieving
- Hopelessness
- Impaired religiosity
- Impaired social interaction
- Impaired verbal communication
- Ineffective coping
- Ineffective denial
- Insomnia
- Interrupted family processes
- Readiness for enhanced spiritual well-being
- Risk for complicated grieving
- Risk for loneliness
- Risk for spiritual distress
- Risk prone health behavior
- Social isolation
- Spiritual distress

TABLE 11-6 NURSING DIAGNOSES
Physical Care at the End of Life

- Acute pain
- Bowel incontinence
- Chronic pain
- Constipation
- Decreased cardiac output
- Diarrhea
- Fatigue
- Imbalanced nutrition: less than body requirements
- Impaired bed mobility
- Impaired comfort
- Impaired gas exchange
- Impaired oral mucous membrane
- Impaired physical mobility
- Impaired skin integrity
- Impaired swallowing
- Impaired tissue integrity
- Impaired urinary elimination
- Ineffective airway clearance
- Ineffective breathing pattern
- Ineffective thermoregulation
- Ineffective tissue perfusion
- Nausea
- Risk for aspiration
- Risk for imbalanced fluid volume
- Risk for infection
- Risk for injury
- Self-care deficit
- Urinary incontinence

Psychosocially, nursing goals center on the patient's abilities to express and share feelings with others. Nursing care goals during the last stages of life involve comfort measures and physical maintenance care.[11,26]

Education of both the patient and family is an important part of the nurse's planning in EOL care. Families need ongoing information on the disease, the dying process, and any care that will be provided. They need information on how to cope with many issues during this period of their lives. Denial and grieving may be barriers to learning and understanding at the end of life for both the patient and family members. Nurses must take the time to develop a comprehensive plan to support, educate, and evaluate patients and families in EOL care issues.

Nursing Implementation

Nursing interventions for the dying patient focus on comfort and improving the quality of life. Psychosocial care and physical care are interrelated for both the dying patient and the family members or significant others.

Psychosocial Care

Anxiety and Depression. Anxiety is the most common distress symptom near the end of life. Anxiety is an uneasy feeling whose cause is not easily identified. Anxiety is frequently related to fear. Patients often exhibit signs of anxiety and depression during the end-of-life period. Causes of depression and anxiety may include pain that is out of control, psychosocial factors related to the disease process or impending death, altered physiologic states, and drugs used in high doses. Encouragement, support, and education decrease some of the anxiety. Management of anxiety may include both pharmacologic and nonpharmacologic interventions.

Fear. Fear is a typical feeling associated with dying. The nurse needs to assist the dying person to cope with fears. Four specific fears associated with dying are fear of pain, fear of shortness of breath, fear of loneliness and abandonment, and fear of meaninglessness.

Fear of Pain. There is a tendency to associate death with pain. Common sayings such as "on pain of death" or "a violent death" have influenced the way that death is perceived. A dying person who has lost a loved one to a painful death may expect the same type of experience. Subsequently many people assume that pain always accompanies death. Physiologically, there is no absolute indication

ETHICAL DILEMMAS
End-of-Life Care

Situation

A terminally ill 50-year-old woman with metastatic breast cancer has developed severe bone pain that is not adequately controlled by her present dose of IV morphine. She moans at rest and verbalizes severe pain from any movement to reposition her. Even though she appears to sleep at intervals, she requests pain medicine frequently and her family is demanding additional pain medicine for her. At the team conference the nurses have discussed the need for more effective pain control, but are concerned that additional pain medicine could hasten her death.

Important Points for Consideration

- Adequate pain relief is an important outcome for all patients but in particular for patients who are terminally ill. The *principle of beneficence* means that care is provided to benefit patients.
- When the goal of treatment of the terminally ill is providing adequate pain control to alleviate suffering, the goal is based on the *principle of nonmaleficence:* preventing or reducing harm to the patient. The secondary effect of hastening the patient's death is ethically justified; this is known as the concept of *double effect.*
- *Euthanasia*, the deliberate act of hastening death, is not morally acceptable.
- Adequate pain relief at the end of life continues to be a major concern of health care professionals and consumers.

Critical Thinking Questions

1. What type of discussions need to occur among members of the health care team, patient, and family as this phase of care is approached in the terminally ill?
2. Distinguish between assisted suicide and euthanasia, and between promotion of comfort and relief of pain in dying patients. (Use the American Nurses Association position statements at *www.ana.org*.)

that death is always painful. Psychologically, pain may occur based on the anxieties and separations related to dying. Terminally ill patients who do experience physical pain should have pain-relieving drugs available. The patient and the family need assurance that drugs will be given promptly when needed and that side effects of drugs can and will be managed. Patients can participate in their own pain relief by discussing pain relief measures and their effects. Most patients want their pain relieved without the side effects of grogginess or sleepiness. Pain relief measures such as drugs need not deprive the patient of the ability to interact with others.

Fear of Shortness of Breath. Respiratory distress and shortness of breath (dyspnea) are common near the end of life. The sensation of air hunger results in anxiety for the patient and family members. Currently there are no clinical practice guidelines for its management in EOL care. Current therapies involve the use of opioids, bronchodilators, and oxygen, depending on the cause of the dyspnea. Anxiety-reducing agents (e.g., anxiolytics) may help produce relaxation.

Fear of Loneliness and Abandonment. Most terminally ill and dying people do not want to be alone and fear loneliness. Many dying patients are afraid that loved ones who are unable to cope with the patient's imminent death will abandon them. Dying patients typically want someone whom they know and trust to stay with them (Fig. 11-5). It may be a loved one or a caregiver. The

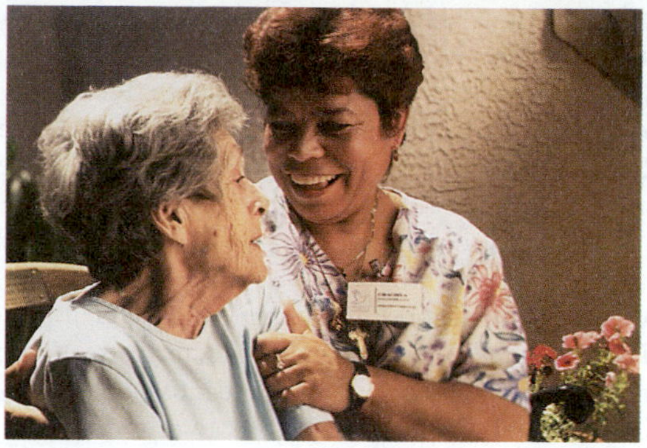

FIG. 11-5 Dying patients typically want someone whom they know and trust to stay with them.

simple presence of someone provides support and comfort. Neither words nor actions are necessary unless the patient requires something. Holding hands, touching, and listening are considered to be high-quality nursing responses. Simply providing companionship allows the dying person a sense of security.

Fear of Meaninglessness. Fear of meaninglessness leads most people to review their lives. They review their intentions during life, examining actions and expressing regrets about what might have been. *Life review* helps patients recognize the value that their lives have held. Patients need to look at positive aspects of their lives. Nurses and family members can help patients review their lives. The worth of the dying person needs to be expressed. The nurse can assist patients and their families in identifying the positive qualities of the patient's life. The sharing of thoughts and feelings may provide comfort for the patient. The nurse needs to respect and accept the practices and rituals associated with the patient's life review while remaining nonjudgmental.

Communication. Communication among the health care provider, patient, and family is seen as a key ingredient for quality care at the end of life. Therapeutic communication is an important nursing intervention used to assist the dying patient and family (Fig. 11-6). Empathy and active listening are essential communication components in EOL care. *Empathy* is the identification with and understanding of another's situation, feelings, and/or motives. Listening is an active process required in the development of empathy toward another's feelings.

Patients and families need to be allowed time to express their feelings and thoughts. They may have difficulties expressing them-

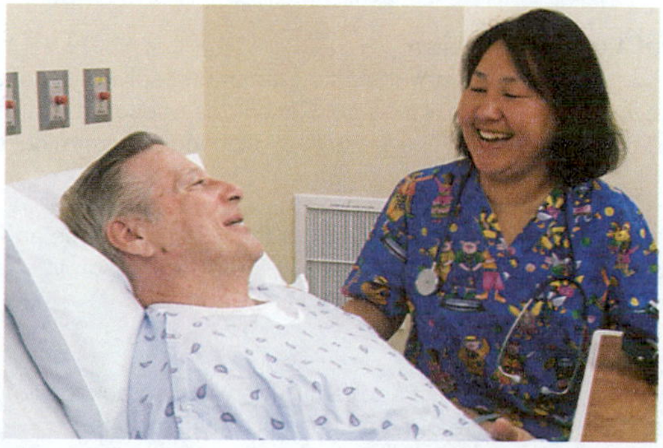

FIG. 11-6 Therapeutic communication is an important aspect of end-of-life nursing care.

selves emotionally. Making time to listen and interact in a sensitive way enhances the relationship among the nurse, patient, and family. Listening is essential. There may be silence. Frequently silence is related to the overwhelming feelings experienced at the end of life. Silence can also allow time to gather thoughts. Listening to the silence sends a message of acceptance and comfort. Communication also needs to consider the patient's ethnic, cultural, and religious backgrounds.

Unusual communication by the patient may take place at the end of life. Frequently, near the end of life, the patient's communication may become what is oftentimes identified as confused, disoriented, or garbled. Patients may speak to or about family members or others who have predeceased them, give instructions to those who will survive them, or speak of projects yet to be completed. Active, careful listening allows for the identification of specific patterns in the dying person's communication and decreases the risk for inappropriate labeling of behaviors.

Grief. Resolution of grief is the primary focus for anticipatory and dysfunctional grieving. Interventions are similar for these two types of grieving, and therefore they are addressed together. Specific interventions are planned for the specific stage of the grief process or the specific feelings expressed by the patient or family. Goals for grief resolution include patient expression of feelings related to grief, acknowledgment of the impending loss, and demonstrations of behaviors that reflect progress in grief resolution.

Priority interventions for grief must focus on providing an environment that allows the patient to express feelings. Open discussion of feelings helps both the patient and family work toward resolution of the grief process. The patient should be free to express feelings of anger, fear, or guilt without judgment on the part of the nurse. The patient and family need to know that the grief reaction is normal. Respect for the patient's privacy and need or desire to talk (or not to talk) is important. Honesty in answering questions and giving information is essential. Families and patients need encouragement to continue their usual activities as much as possible. They need to discuss their activities and maintain some control over their lives. At times it helps to discuss what can and cannot change. Assistance with planning for the future or for the funeral may be needed based on the patient's or family's coping abilities.

Anger is a common and normal response to grief. It is important to understand that the grieving person cannot be forced to accept the loss. The surviving family members may be angry at the dying loved one who is leaving them. There is a need to acknowledge and encourage the expression of feelings but at the same time realize how difficult it is to come to terms with grief. Nurses are sometimes the target of the anger, and must understand what is happening and not react on a personal level.

Feelings of hopelessness and powerlessness are common at the end of life. The nurse needs to encourage realistic hope within the limits of the situation. The patient and the family should be allowed to identify and to deal with what is within their control and to recognize what is beyond their control. Patient-identified goals can be encouraged to restore some sense of power. Decision making about care can also foster a sense of power and control for the patient.

Evaluation of the specific coping skills demonstrated and expressed by the patient or the family will assist in planning care. Outcome criteria for goal achievement include verbalization of specific feelings, expression that the loss is real, and identification of specific progress in the grief work. The nurse facilitates the patient's choice of where to die and how to finish life tasks. The criteria are evaluated based on specific behaviors and verbalizations exhibited by the patient or the significant others.

As death approaches, the nurse should encourage the family to respond appropriately to the patient's psychosocial manifestations at the end of life. Table 11-7 discusses management of psychosocial manifestations near death.

Physical Care. Nursing management related to physical care at the end of life deals with symptom management and caring rather than treatment for curing a particular disease or disorder. Meeting the patient's physiologic and safety needs is the priority. Physical care focuses on the needs for oxygen, nutrition, pain relief, mobility, elimination, and skin care. People who are dying deserve and require the same physical care as people who are expected to recover. Table 11-8 delineates the physical care at the end of life.

TABLE 11-7 Nursing Management: Psychosocial Care at End of Life

Characteristic	Nursing Management
Withdrawal	
Patient near death may seem to be withdrawn from the physical environment, maintaining the ability to hear while not able to respond.	Converse as if the patient is alert, using a soft voice and gentle touch.
Unusual Communication	
Unusual communication may indicate that an unresolved issue is preventing the dying person from letting go. Patient may become restless and agitated or perform repetitive tasks (may also indicate terminal delirium).	Encourage the family to talk with and reassure the dying person. Encourage visit by appropriate spiritual care service provider, chaplain, or family members.
Vision-like Experiences	
Patient may talk to persons who are not there or see places and objects not visible. Vision-like experiences assist the dying person in coming to terms with meaning in life and transition from it.	Affirm the dying person's experience as a part of transition from this life.
Saying Goodbyes	
It is important for the patient and family members to acknowledge their sadness, mutually forgive one another, and say goodbye.	Encourage the dying person and family members to verbalize their feelings of sadness, loss, forgiveness; to touch, hug, cry. Allow the patient and family privacy to express their feelings and comfort one another.

TABLE 11-8 Nursing Management: Physical Care at End of Life

Characteristic	Nursing Management
Pain • Pain may be a major symptom associated with terminal illness and the one most feared. • Pain can be acute or chronic. • Physical and emotional irritations can aggravate pain.	• Assess pain thoroughly and regularly to determine the quality, intensity, location, and contributing factors. • Minimize possible irritants such as skin irritations from wetness, heat or cold, and pressure. • Administer medications around the clock in a timely manner and on a regular basis to provide constant relief rather than waiting until the pain is unbearable and then trying to relieve it. • Provide complementary and alternative therapies such as guided imagery, massage, acupressure, heat and cold, Therapeutic Touch, distraction, and relaxation techniques as needed (see Chapters 8 and 9). • Evaluate effectiveness of pain relief measures frequently to ensure that the patient is on a correct, adequate drug regimen. • Do not delay or deny pain relief measures to a terminally ill patient.
Delirium • A state characterized by confusion, disorientation, restlessness, clouding of consciousness, incoherence, fear, anxiety, excitement, and often hallucinations. • May be misidentified as depression, psychosis, anger, or anxiety. • Use of opioids and/or corticosteroids in end-of-life care may cause delirium. • Underlying disease process may contribute to delirium. • Generally considered a reversible process.	• Perform a thorough assessment for reversible causes of delirium, including pain, constipation, and urinary retention. • Provide a room that is quiet, well lighted, and familiar to reduce the effects of delirium. • Reorient the dying person to person, place, and time with each encounter. • Administer ordered benzodiazepines and sedatives as needed. • Stay physically close to frightened patient. Reassure in a calm, soft voice with touch and slow strokes of the skin. • Provide family members with emotional support and encouragement in their efforts to cope with the behaviors associated with delirium. • Encourage the family to participate in the care of the patient.
Restlessness • May occur as death approaches and cerebral metabolism slows.	• Assess for spiritual distress as a cause of restlessness and agitation. • Do not restrain. • Use soothing music; slow, soft touch and voice. • Limit the number of persons at the bedside.
Dysphagia • May occur because of extreme weakness and changes in level of consciousness.	• Identify the least invasive alternative routes of administration for drugs needed for symptom management. • Suction orally as needed.
Dehydration • May occur during the last days of life. • Hunger and thirst are rare in the last days of life. • As the end of life approaches, patients tend to take in less food and fluid.	• Assess condition of mucous membranes frequently to prevent excessive dryness, which can lead to discomfort. • Maintain complete, regular oral care to provide for comfort and hydration of mucous membranes. • Do not force the patient to eat or drink. • Encourage consumption of ice chips and sips of fluids or use moist cloths to provide moisture to the mouth. • Use moist cloths and swabs for unconscious patients to avoid aspiration. • Apply lubricant to the lips and oral mucous membranes as needed. • Reassure family that cessation of food and fluid intake is a natural part of the process of dying.
Dyspnea • Subjective symptom. • Accompanied by fear of suffocation and anxiety. • Underlying disease process can exacerbate dyspnea. • Coughing and expectorating secretions become difficult.	• Assess respiratory status regularly. • Elevate the head and/or position on side to improve chest expansion. • Use a fan or air conditioner to facilitate movement of cool air. • Administer supplemental oxygen as ordered. • Administer drugs such as opioids, sedatives, diuretics, antibiotics, corticosteroids, and bronchodilators as ordered to relieve congestion and coughing and to decrease apprehension. • Suction as needed to remove accumulation of mucus from the airways. Suctioning is used cautiously in the terminal phase.
Weakness and Fatigue • Expected at the end of life. • Metabolic demands related to disease process contribute to weakness and fatigue.	• Assess the patient's tolerance for activities. • Time nursing interventions to conserve energy. • Assist the patient to identify and complete valued or desired activities. • Provide support as needed to maintain positions in bed or chair. • Provide frequent rest periods.

Continued

TABLE 11-8 Nursing Management: Physical Care at End of Life—cont'd

Characteristic	Nursing Management
Myoclonus	
• Mild to severe jerking or twitching sometimes associated with use of high dose of opioids. • Patient may complain of involuntary twitching of upper and lower extremities.	• Assess for the initial onset, the duration, and any discomfort or distress experienced by patient. • If myoclonus is distressing or becoming more severe, discuss possible drug therapy modifications with the physician. • Changes in opioid medication may alleviate or decrease myoclonus.
Skin Breakdown	
• Skin integrity is difficult to maintain at the end of life. • Immobility, urinary and bowel incontinence, dry skin, nutritional deficits, anemia, friction, and shearing forces lead to a high risk for skin breakdown. • Disease and other processes may impair skin integrity. • As death approaches, circulation to the extremities decreases and they become cool, mottled, and cyanotic.	• Assess the skin for signs of breakdown. • Implement protocols to prevent skin breakdown by controlling drainage and odor and keeping the skin and any wound areas clean. • Perform wound assessments as needed. • Follow appropriate nursing management protocol for dressing wounds. • Follow appropriate nursing management protocol for a patient who is immobile, but consider realistic outcomes of skin integrity vs. maintenance of comfort. • Follow appropriate nursing management to prevent skin irritations and breakdown from urinary and bowel incontinence. • Use blankets to cover for warmth; never apply heat. • Prevent the effects of shearing forces.
Bowel Patterns	
• Constipation can be caused by immobility, use of opioid medications, lack of fiber in the diet, and dehydration. • Diarrhea may occur as muscles relax or from a fecal impaction related to the use of opioids and immobility.	• Assess bowel function. • Assess for and remove fecal impactions. • Encourage movement and physical activities as tolerated. • Encourage fiber in the diet if appropriate. • Encourage fluids if appropriate. • Use suppositories, stool softeners, laxatives, or enemas if ordered.
Urinary Incontinence	
• May result from disease progression or changes in the level of consciousness. • As death becomes imminent, the perineal muscles relax.	• Assess urinary function. • Use absorbent pads for urinary incontinence. • Follow the appropriate nursing protocol for the consideration and use of indwelling or external catheters. • Follow appropriate nursing management to prevent skin irritations and breakdown from urinary incontinence.
Anorexia, Nausea, and Vomiting	
• May be caused by complications of disease process. • Drugs contribute to nausea. • Constipation, impaction, and bowel obstruction can cause anorexia, nausea, and vomiting.	• Assess the patient for complaints of nausea and/or vomiting. • Assess possible contributing causes of nausea or vomiting. • Have family members provide the patient's favorite foods. • Discuss modifications to the drug regimen with the health care provider. • Provide antiemetics before meals if ordered. • Offer and provide frequent meals with small portions of favorite foods. • Offer culturally appropriate foods. • Provide frequent mouth care, especially after vomiting.

The provision of nursing care is done in collaboration with other health care team members. To meet the holistic needs of the patient the nurse collaborates with the social worker, chaplain, physical therapist, occupational therapists, certified nursing assistants, and volunteers as dictated by the individual needs of the patient.

Postmortem Care. After the patient is pronounced dead, the nurse prepares or delegates preparation of the body for immediate viewing by the family with consideration for cultural customs and in accord with state law and agency policies and procedures. In some cultures and in some types of death, it may be important to allow family members to prepare or assist in preparing the body. In general, the nurse closes the patient's eyes, replaces dentures, washes the body as needed (placing pads under the perineum to absorb urine and feces), and may remove tubes and dressings. The body should be straightened, leaving the pillow to support the head and prevent pooling of blood and discoloration of the face. The family should then be allowed privacy and as much time as they need with the deceased person. In the case of an unexpected or unanticipated death, preparation of the body for viewing or release to a funeral home depends on state law and agency policies and procedures.

SPECIAL NEEDS OF CAREGIVERS IN END-OF-LIFE CARE

Special Needs of Family Caregivers

Family caregivers are important to meeting the person's physical and psychosocial needs. The role of caregiver includes working and communicating with the patient, supporting the patient's concerns, helping the patient resolve any unfinished business, working with other family members and friends, and dealing with the caregiver's own needs and feelings. Families often face emotional, physical, and economic consequences as a result of caring for a family member. It is important to note that caregiver responsibilities often do not end when the person is admitted to a hospital or nursing home.

An understanding of the grieving process as it affects both the patient and the family caregivers is of great importance. Being present during a family member's dying process can be highly stressful. Recognizing signs and behaviors among family members who may be at risk for abnormal grief reactions is an important nursing intervention. These may include dependency and negative feelings about the dying person, inability to express feelings, concurrent life crises, a history of depression, difficult reactions to previous losses, perceived lack of social or family support, low self-esteem, multiple previous bereavements, alcoholism, and/or substance abuse.

Family caregivers and other family members need encouragement to continue their usual activities as much as possible. They need to discuss their activities and maintain some control over their lives. At times it helps to discuss what can and cannot change.

Grieving relatives, friends, and significant others can provide emotional support for one another. Health care providers need to be sensitive to the importance of significant others who are not necessarily relatives. Resources such as community counseling and local support may assist some people in working through their grief. Generally, simply allowing the involved people to express their feelings helps to resolve the grief. Caregivers should be encouraged to facilitate the building of a support system of extended family members, friends, faith community, and clergy. The caregivers should have access to people whom they can call on at any time to express any feelings that they are experiencing. Caregivers and family members should also allow time to be alone.

Family caregivers need to be encouraged to take care of themselves. Keeping a journal can help the caregiver express feelings that may be difficult to express verbally. Eating a balanced diet at regular times will provide for the caregiver's well-being. Nourishing the spirit as well as the body is important for the caregiver to consider. Physical contact with others provides emotional support and acknowledgment of the caregiver's own need for physical comfort. Exercise often relieves stress. Maintenance of regular activities and interests is also important to help the caregiver. Humor is important, and its use from time to time in some situations can provide distraction and relieve stress-filled situations.

Special Needs of Nurses

Many nurses who care for dying patients do so because they are passionate about providing quality EOL care. However, caring for dying patients is intense and emotionally charged. A bond or connection develops among the patient, family, and nurse. Nurses need to be aware of how grief affects them personally. The nurse who is responsible for the care of terminally ill or dying patients is not immune to feelings of loss. It is common for nurses to feel helpless and powerless when dealing with death. Feelings of sorrow, guilt, and frustration need to be expressed.

There are interventions that help to ease physical and emotional stress for the nurse. It is necessary for the nurse to recognize and acknowledge what can and cannot be controlled. Recognizing personal feelings allows openness in exchanging feelings with the patient and family. Realizing that it is okay to cry with the patient or family during the grief process is essential to the nurse's well-being.

Interventions focusing on personal needs will assist in alleviating stress for the nurse. Involvement in hobbies or other interests, scheduling time for oneself, maintaining a peer support system, and developing a support system beyond the workplace will benefit the nurse. Crises and grief result in varying forms of stress for nurses. Hospice agencies can provide care of their team members with professionally assisted groups, informal discussion sessions, and flexible time schedules.

Terminal illness and dying are extremely personal events that affect the patient, the family, and health care providers. Providing care for patients and their families at the end of life is a challenging and rewarding experience. EOL care offers an opportunity to apply the skills and personal commitments that nurses bring to their profession.

> The loss of a loved person is one of the most intensely painful experiences any human being can suffer.

From Bowlby J: *Notes on symptom control in hospice and palliative care,* rev ed, Essex, 2000, Hospice Education Institute.

> What we leave behind is not what is engraved in stone monuments, but what is woven into the lives of others.

Pericles, fifth-century Greek statesman

NCLEX EXAMINATION REVIEW QUESTIONS

The number of the question corresponds to the same-numbered objective at the beginning of the chapter.

1. Mr. Garcia is in the terminal stages of lung cancer. On assessment it is noted that he has rapid, audibly noisy respirations with an associated grunting sound. The correct terminology to use in documenting the assessment data would be to specify that he is experiencing:
   a. tachypnea.
   b. death rattle.
   c. guppy breathing.
   d. Cheyne-Stokes respirations.
2. Mrs. Johnson has inoperable pancreatic cancer. Until recently she has been very active in her neighborhood association. Her husband is concerned because his wife is "not herself." Which common end-of-life psychologic manifestation is she demonstrating?
   a. Decreased socialization
   b. Decreased disease progression
   c. Decreased sense of helplessness
   d. Decreased perception of pain and touch
3. Tom has repeatedly asked his mother to donate his deceased father's belongings to charity, but his mother has refused. She sits in the bedroom closet, crying and talking to her long-dead husband. What type of grief is Tom's mother experiencing?
   a. Adaptive
   b. Disruptive
   c. Anticipatory
   d. Dysfunctional
4. While caring for his dying wife, Mr. Smith states that his wife is a devout Roman Catholic but he is a Baptist. Who is considered the most reliable source for spiritual preferences concerning EOL care for Mrs. Smith?
   a. A priest
   b. Mr. Smith
   c. Mrs. Smith
   d. Hospice staff
5. The family attorney informed Mr. Wilson's adult children and wife that he did not have an advance directive after he suffered a serious

stroke. Who is responsible for identifying end-of-life measures to be instituted when the patient cannot communicate his or her specific wishes?
a. Adult children
b. Notary and attorney
c. Physician and family
d. Physician and nursing staff

6. The primary purpose of hospice is to:
a. allow patients to die at home.
b. provide better quality of care than the family can.
c. coordinate care for dying patients and their families.
d. provide comfort, support, and care of dying patients and their families.

7. Mrs. Alejandro, who has end-stage cardiac disease and is not a candidate for a heart transplant, is medicated with morphine. Recently she has been having chest pain and expressing concern that she may have another heart attack and die in pain. The nurse can decrease the psychosocial impact of physical symptoms of such pain by:
a. referring Mrs. Alejandro to a community agency.
b. evaluating the side effects of Mrs. Alejandro's drugs.
c. encouraging pain relief measures that cause sleepiness.
d. evaluating the pain relief and the effects of the relief measures.

8. When Mr. Washington was diagnosed with renal failure, his new wife asked his children from a previous marriage to help with their father's care. Each of the children refused to help. Mrs. Washington cared for her husband without help until his death. The behaviors of the children indicate that they may be at risk for abnormal grief reactions related to:
a. maintenance of negative feelings.
b. development of new relationships.
c. maintenance of current relationships.
d. development of independent behaviors.

9. Sue Vale has been working full time as a nurse with terminally ill patients for 3 years. She has been experiencing irritability and mixed emotions when expressing sadness since four of her patients died on the same day. To optimize the quality of her nursing care she should examine her own:
a. full-time work schedule.
b. past feelings toward death.
c. patterns for dealing with grief.
d. demands for involvement in care.

REFERENCES

1. Lunney J, Foley KM, Smith TJ: *Describing death in America: what we need to know,* Washington, DC, 2003, National Academy Press.
2. Field M, Cassel C: *Approaching death: improving care at the end of life,* Washington, DC, 1997, National Academy Press.
3. Kochanek KD, Smith BL: Deaths: preliminary data for 2002, *National Vital Statistics Reports,* 52(13):1, 2004.
4. Siminoff LA, Burant C, Youngner SJ: Death and organ procurement: public beliefs and attitudes, *Soc Sci Med* 59:2325, 2004.
5. Henneman EA, Karras GE: Determining brain death in adults: a guideline for use in critical care, *Mass Crit Care Nurse* 24:50, 2004.
6. American Academy of Neurology: Practice parameters: determining brain death in adults. Available at *http://aan.com/professionals/practice/pdfs/pdf1995_thru_1998/1995.45.1012.pdf* (accessed October 15, 2005).
7. Rich S: Providing quality end-of-life care, *J Cardiovasc Nurs* 20:141, 2005.
8. Kübler-Ross E: *On death and dying,* New York, 1969, MacMillan.
9. Martocchio BC: Grief and bereavement healing through hurt, *Nurs Clin North Am* 20:327, 1985.
10. Rando TA: *Treatment of complicated mourning,* Champaign, Ill, 1993, Research Press.
11. Coyle N, Ferrell BR: *Textbook of palliative nursing,* New York, 2005, Oxford University Press.
12. Hinshaw DB: Spiritual issues in surgical palliative care, *Surg Clin North Am* 85:257, 2005.
13. McClain-Jacobson C, Rosenfeld B, Kosinski A, et al: Belief in an afterlife, spiritual well-being and end-of-life despair in patients with advanced cancer, *Gen Hosp Psychiatry* 26:484, 2004.
14. Giger JN, Davidhizar RE: *Transcultural nursing*, St Louis, 2004, Mosby.
15. Roark DC: Overhauling the organ donation system, *Am J Nurs* 200:44, 2000.
16. Omnibus Reconciliation Act, Title IV 4206, 1990, *Cong Rec* 12638.
17. Tulsky JA: Beyond advance directives: importance of communication skills at the end of life, *JAMA* 294:359, 2005.
18. American Nurses Association, ANA Position Statements: *Nursing and the patient self-determination act,* Washington, DC, 2003, American Nurses Association.
19. American Nurses Association, ANA Position Statements: *Nursing care and do-not-resuscitate decisions,* Washington, DC, 2003, American Nurses Association.
20. Cherry MJ, Engelhardt HT: Informed consent in Texas: theory and practice, *J Med Philos* 29:237, 2004.
21. American Nurses Association, ANA Position Statements: *Foregoing nutrition and hydration,* Washington, DC, 1992, American Nurses Association.
22. American Nurses Association, ANA Position Statements: *Active euthanasia,* Washington, DC, 1994, American Nurses Association.
23. Lorenz KA, Asch SM, Rosenfeld KE, et al: Hospice admission practices: where does hospice fit in the continuum of care? *J Am Geriatr Soc* 52:725, 2004.
24. Hospice facts and figures, National Hospice and Palliative Care Organization. Available at *www.nhpco.org/files/public/Hospice_Facts_110104.pdf* (accessed October 14, 2005).
25. Chochinov HM, Hack T, Hassard T, et al: Dignity and psychotherapeutic considerations in end-of-life care, *J Palliat Care* 20:134, 2004.
26. National consensus project: Clinical practice guidelines for palliative care, 2004. Available at *www.Nationalconsensusproject.org* (accessed May 11, 2006).

RESOURCES

Americans for Better Care of the Dying
Email: info@abcd-caring.org
www.abcd-caring.org

Association for Death Education and Counseling
847-509-0403
www.adec.org

Coalition on Donation
804-782-4920
http://shareyourlife.org

Compassion and Choices
800-247-7421
www.compassionindying.org

End-of-Life Nursing Education Consortium (ELNEC)
American Association of Colleges of Nursing
202-463-6930 ext. 238
www.aacn.nche.edu/elnec/

End of Life Physician Education Resource Center (EPERC)
www.eperc.mcw.edu/

Hospice Education Institute
207-255-8800
www.hospiceworld.org/

Hospice Foundation of America
800-854-3402
www.hospicefoundation.org

Hospice and Palliative Nurses Association
412-787-9301
www.hpna.org

National Association for Home Care and Hospice
202-547-7424
www.nahc.org

National Consensus Project for Quality Palliative Care
Palliative Care Clinical Practice Guidelines
www.nationalconsensusproject.org/

National Hospice and Palliative Care Organization
703-837-1500
www.nhpco.org

Palliative Care Educational Resource Team (PERT)
Educational resources for delivering end-of-life care in nursing homes
www.swedishmedical.org/PERT/links.htm

For additional Internet resources, see the website for this book at *http://evolve.elsevier.com/Lewis/medsurg.*

The one thing a clenched fist cannot do is to accept the helping hand.

Frederick Buechner

Addictive Behaviors 12

Patricia Graber O'Brien

LEARNING OBJECTIVES

1. Define *addiction, addictive behavior, substance misuse, substance abuse, dependence, tolerance, withdrawal, craving, abstinence,* and *detoxification.*
2. Describe the neurophysiology of addiction.
3. Identify the major health complications of substance abuse and dependence.
4. Recognize the effects of the use of stimulants, depressants, hallucinogens, and inhalants.
5. Identify nursing interventions for tobacco and smoking cessation.
6. Describe the nursing management of patients who experience intoxication, overdose, or withdrawal from stimulants, depressants, or hallucinogens.
7. Describe nursing management of the surgical patient who abuses drugs.
8. Discuss the nursing management of pain in the patient who is dependent on central nervous system depressants.
9. Describe the use of motivational interviewing to initiate behavior change in patients with addictions.
10. Describe substance abuse and dependence in the older adult.

KEY TERMS

addiction, p. 166
addictive behaviors, p. 166
craving, p. 166
cross-tolerance, p. 178
dependence, p. 166
detoxification, p. 178
motivational interviewing, p. 188
opioids, p. 179
physiologic dependence, p. 168
psychologic dependence, p. 168
substance abuse, p. 166
substance dependence, p. 166
tolerance, p. 166

Electronic Resources

Supplemental content related to Chapter 12 can be found . . .

Companion CD

- Stress-Busting Kit for Nursing Students
- NCLEX Examination Review Questions
- Comprehensive Glossary

Evolve Website evolve

http://evolve.elsevier.com/Lewis/medsurg

- Content Updates
- Key Points (Printable and CD/MP3 Download)
- Concept Map Creator
- Expanded Audio Glossary
- Key Term Flash Cards
- Customizable Nursing Care Plan: Alcohol Withdrawal
- Patient and Family Instruction Guide in English and Spanish: Smoking and Tobacco Use Cessation
- Electronic Calculators
- WebLinks

Addiction and substance abuse are serious problems affecting the health care system and society today. Addictions to chemical substances usually include dependence on psychoactive agents that result in pleasure or modify thinking and perception. These include legal substances such as alcohol and tobacco and drugs with therapeutic value such as analgesics, sedative-hypnotics, tranquilizers, and amphetamines. (Although the use of alcohol and tobacco is illegal for minors, these substances are not considered illicit.) Illegal substances most commonly used in the United States include, in descending order, marijuana/hashish, cocaine, hallucinogens, and heroin.[1] Addictions also include some compulsive behaviors such as eating disorders, gambling, computer gaming and interacting, and even strenuous exercising. Although addiction to illegal substances is commonly thought to be the major problem, dependence on alcohol, tobacco, food, and gambling is responsible for more illness and death than is the use of illicit drugs. Exact prevalence of substance abuse and addictions is difficult to determine because of underreporting, but it is estimated that 35.7 million Americans are nicotine dependent, 18 million are dependent on alcohol, and 3.5 million are dependent on illicit drugs.[1]

Individuals who abuse substances use the health care system more than those who do not abuse substances. All nurses care for

Reviewed by Kathleen Lopez-Bushnell, RNC (FNP), MPH, COHN-S, EdD, Clinical Nurse Researcher, University of New Mexico Hospital, Albuquerque, N.Mex.

TABLE 12-1 Terminology of Substance Abuse

Term	Definition
Abstinence	• Avoidance of substance use.
Addiction	• Compulsive, uncontrollable dependence on a substance, behavior, or practice to such a degree that cessation causes severe emotional, mental, or physiologic reactions.
Addictive behavior	• Behavior associated with maintaining an addiction.
Craving	• Subjective need for a substance, usually experienced after decreased use or abstinence. Cue-induced craving is stimulated in the presence of experiences previously associated with drug taking.
Dependence	• Reliance on a substance that has reached the level that absence of it will cause an impairment in function.
Physical	• Altered physiologic state from prolonged substance use; regular use is necessary to prevent withdrawal.
Psychologic	• Compulsive need to experience pleasurable response from the substance.
Detoxification	• Process of removing the substance and its effects from the individual's body.
Relapse	• Return to substance use after a period of abstinence.
Substance	• Drug, chemical, or biologic entity that is self-administered. The words "drug," "substance," and "chemical" are often used interchangeably.
Substance abuse	• Overindulgence of a substance that has a negative impact on psychologic, physiologic, and/or social functioning of an individual.
Substance misuse	• Use of a drug for purposes other than those for which it is intended.
Tolerance	• Decreased effect of a substance that results from repeated exposure. It is possible to develop cross-tolerance to other substances in the same category.
Withdrawal	• Combination of physiologic and psychologic responses that occur when there is abrupt cessation or reduced intake of a substance on which an individual is dependent.

patients dependent on substances, whether they are identified as dependent or not, simply because of the prevalence of substance abuse and its association with health problems. In every health care setting the nurse has a responsibility to identify and intervene with patients who are abusing or addicted to substances.

Substance abuse and **substance dependence** (defined in Table 12-1) are specific psychiatric diagnoses.[2] Comprehensive discussions of addictive behaviors and substance abuse are provided in psychiatric resources. Long-term management of addiction is most often provided in specialized treatment facilities and mental health clinics that provide both pharmacologic and behavioral therapies. This chapter is limited to addressing the nursing role in identifying and managing the addicted or substance-abusing patient in the general ambulatory or acute care setting. Eating disorders are discussed in Chapter 40, and health problems related to addictive behaviors are discussed throughout the text.

OVERVIEW OF ADDICTIVE BEHAVIORS

Terminology of Addictive Behavior

A lack of standard terminology for addiction and substance abuse problems makes defining various terms difficult. Different psychiatric, social, and philosophic viewpoints lead to preference of one term over another by professional groups and laypeople. In this chapter, **addiction** is defined as a compulsive, uncontrollable **dependence** on a substance, behavior, or practice to such a degree that cessation causes severe emotional, mental, or physiologic reactions. Those behaviors that are associated with maintaining an addiction are referred to as **addictive behaviors** (see Table 12-1).

Neurobiology of Addiction

Addiction is a complex disorder that is a treatable, chronic, relapsing disease. Current research indicates that most addictive drugs, and possibly certain compulsive behaviors, appear to increase the availability of dopamine in the "pleasure" area of the mesolimbic system of the brain. This area has been identified as the **brain reward system** and is a system that creates the sensation of pleasure for certain behaviors necessary for survival, such as eating and sexual behavior.[3]

Normally dopamine is released at a slow rate by neurons in the mesolimbic system, producing normal affect or mood. Both endogenous and exogenous opiates have been found to increase the firing rate of dopaminergic neurons. Cocaine has been shown to decrease the reuptake of dopamine at the synapse, thereby decreasing its breakdown and increasing the amount of available dopamine. Nicotine, alcohol, marijuana, amphetamines, and caffeine also increase dopaminergic neuron activity. The resulting increase in mesolimbic dopamine leads to mood elevation and euphoria, factors that provide strong motivation to repeat the experience. Many addictive drugs also increase the availability of other neurotransmitters, such as serotonin and γ-aminobutyric acid (GABA), but dopamine's effect on the reward system appears to be strongly related to the addictive process.

Addiction results from the prolonged effects of addictive drugs or behaviors on the brain. Repeated use of addictive drugs causes synaptic remodeling and reduces the responsiveness of dopamine receptors. This decreased responsiveness leads to **tolerance,** the need for a larger dose of a drug to obtain the original effect, and also reduces the sense of pleasure from experiences that previously resulted in positive feelings. Without the substance or behavior the individual experiences depression, anxiety, and irritability. To even feel normal, the individual must take the drug or perform the behavior.[4]

Drug **craving** is another characteristic of addiction. An important type of craving experienced by addicts, **cue-induced craving,** occurs in the presence of people, places, or things that have been previously associated with drug taking. The strength of craving appears to depend on the balance of the excitatory neurotransmitter glutamate and the inhibitor neurotransmitter GABA in the brain. Cue-induced craving may occur after long periods of abstinence and is a common cause of **relapse** (see Table 12-1).

Contributing Factors to Addiction

It is important that addiction not be perceived simply as a physical disease but as a biobehavioral disorder. It is a disease that is expressed in behavioral ways and within a social context. Once addiction occurs, it changes the brain, perpetuating itself. But it starts with the voluntary act of taking drugs. If drugs are never used, addiction does not occur. No single factor has been identified to determine whether an individual might abuse a substance, nor is it understood why some people become addicted and others do not. Some contributing factors include those typically associated with drug abuse: drug availability, peer influences (Fig. 12-1), environment, psychiatric illnesses, adverse social conditions, and cultural influences. Increasing evidence also indicates that genetics plays a significant role in alcoholism and nicotine use. In addition, there are significant gender differences in addictive behaviors[5,6] (see Gender box).

Sociocultural factors also affect the incidence of substance abuse and are often related to other factors such as unemployment, poverty, or adverse social conditions. Although the rates of drug use are similar among white, African American, and Hispanic populations, much higher rates of alcoholism and other drug dependence are present in Native Americans.[1] Current assessment and treatment of addictions in minority populations must become more culturally sensitive, addressing cultural values and practices.

Health Complications of Addictions

Health problems related to substance abuse and dependence lead to more immediate, extensive, and long-lasting problems than the social disruptions caused by addictions. Almost every drug of abuse harms some tissue or organ in addition to the brain. Some health problems are caused by the effects of specific drugs, such as liver damage related to alcohol use and chronic obstructive pulmonary disease (COPD) related to smoking. Other health problems result from the behaviors of addiction, such as injecting drugs and neglecting nutrition. Common health complications of substance abuse are identified in Table 12-2.

Treatment of Addictions

Rehabilitation and sustained abstinence are the primary long-term treatment goals of substance abuse and dependence. Treatment of addictions focuses heavily on behavioral therapies to control substance use. In addition, advances in scientific knowledge about the brain and the effects of addicting substances on the brain have led to the development and testing of new drugs to control addictions. These agents decrease craving, block the effects of addicting substances, or stimulate the development of antibodies against specific

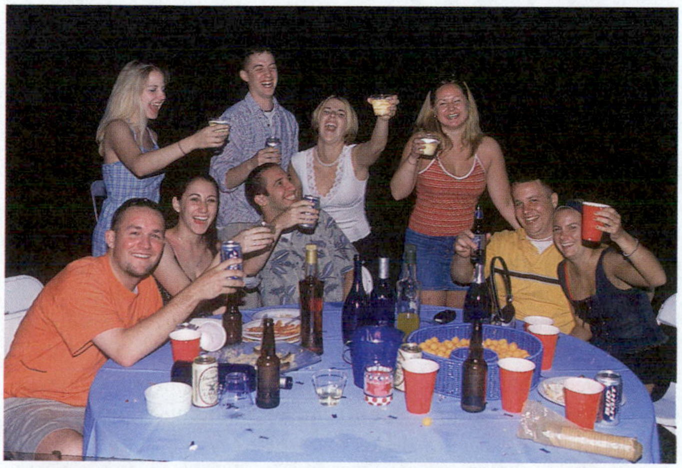

FIG. 12-1 Peer influence can contribute to alcohol abuse in young adults.

GENDER DIFFERENCES
Addictive Behaviors

Men	Women
• More likely to have opportunities to use abused substances. • More likely to abuse alcohol and marijuana. • Relapse in men is associated with anxiety and positive feelings. • Men with a genetic mutation that inhibits nicotine metabolism in the brain are less likely to become addicted to nicotine and find it easier to quit smoking. • In all age groups, more men smoke than women. • Men are almost twice as likely to have a problem with substance dependence or abuse.	• Women are as likely to use drugs when given the opportunity. • Women are more likely to abuse sedatives and tranquilizers. • Relapse in women is triggered by depression and negative feelings. • A genetic mutation that inhibits nicotine metabolism in the brain does not affect women's smoking. • Women are less successful in quitting smoking than men. • Women who smoke have almost double the risk for myocardial infarction. • Women smokers have nearly double the risk of lung cancer. • Drug abuse is nearly twice as likely to be associated with AIDS in women. • Women have less stomach metabolism of alcohol, resulting in higher blood alcohol concentrations for longer periods of time.

AIDS, Acquired immunodeficiency syndrome.

drugs. Some drugs currently approved by the Food and Drug Administration (FDA) for other purposes are also being evaluated for their role in addiction treatment. Current FDA-approved drugs are discussed in this chapter, but it is expected that in the near future a number of drugs will be approved as adjuncts to addiction treatment.

Stimulants

NICOTINE

Characteristics

The addictive behavior that the nurse is most likely to encounter in a patient is tobacco use. Nicotine is the alkaloid in tobacco that causes dependence and it is the most rapidly addicting of the drugs of abuse. It is estimated that 22.5% of adults and 26% of high school seniors smoke.[1] Cigarette smoking is the predominant form of tobacco abuse in the United States.

Effects of Use

Nicotine is rapidly absorbed into the blood through the lungs in smoking, and more slowly through the buccal mucosa in chewing and through the nasal mucosa in snuffing. When absorbed, it acts on nicotinic receptors in the central and peripheral nervous sys-

TABLE 12-2 Common Health Problems Related to Substance Abuse and Dependence

Substance	Health Problems*
Nicotine and smoking	• Chronic obstructive pulmonary disease (COPD) • Cancers of the lung, mouth, larynx, esophagus, stomach, pancreas, bladder, prostate, cervix • Coronary artery disease, peripheral artery disease • Peptic ulcer disease, GERD
Cocaine	• Nasal sores, septal necrosis or perforation • Chronic sinusitis • "Crack lung" pneumonia • Cardiac dysrhythmias, myocardial ischemia and infarction • Stroke • Psychosis
Amphetamines	• Cardiac dysrhythmias, myocardial ischemia and infarction • Death of brain cells • Syndrome of uncontrollable tremors
Caffeine	• Gastrointestinal irritation, peptic ulcer disease, GERD • Anxiety, sleep disruption • Elevated blood pressure
Alcohol (see Table 12-9)	• Gastritis, peptic ulcer disease • Cirrhosis of the liver, pancreatitis • Cancers of esophagus, stomach, head and neck, lung • Dementia • Decreased bone density • Hypertension
Sedative-hypnotics	• Possible memory impairment • Respiratory depression • Risk for falls and fractures
Opioids	• Sexual dysfunction • Gastric ulcers • Glomerulonephritis
Cannabis	• Bronchitis, chronic sinusitis • Memory impairment • Impaired immune function • Reproductive dysfunction
Behaviors	**Health Problems**
Injecting drugs	• Blood clots, phlebitis, skin infections • Hepatitis B and C • HIV/AIDS • Other infections: endocarditis, tuberculosis, pneumonia, meningitis, tetanus, bone and joint infections, lung abscesses
Snorting drugs	• Nasal sores, septal necrosis or perforation • Chronic sinusitis
Risky sexual behavior	• HIV/AIDS • Hepatitis B and C • Other sexually transmitted diseases
Personal neglect	• Malnutrition, impaired immunity • Accidental injuries

Source: National Institute on Drug Abuse: *Medical consequences of drug abuse,* Bethesda, Md, 2005, National Institute on Drug Abuse, National Institutes of Health. Available at *www.drugabuse.gov/index.html.*

GERD, Gastroesophageal reflux disease; *HIV/AIDS,* human immunodeficiency virus/acquired immunodeficiency syndrome.

*The health problems related to substance abuse and dependence are discussed in the appropriate chapters throughout the text where addictive behaviors are identified as risk factors for these problems.

tems. Effects include stimulation of the cardiovascular system with increased myocardial oxygen consumption, general central nervous system (CNS) stimulation, and gastrointestinal (GI) stimulation. Nicotine also causes changes in the endocrine system, including release of prolactin, growth hormone, vasopressin, endorphins, and adrenocorticotropic hormone (ACTH) with a subsequent increase in cortisol.[7] Although nicotine abusers report that nicotine use causes a depressant effect with relaxation and relief of anxiety, it is thought that these effects actually occur when periodic nicotine withdrawal is relieved by further nicotine. The effects of nicotine are listed in Table 12-3.

The strong **psychologic dependence** (see Table 12-1) associated with nicotine use occurs by nicotine's activation of the pleasure-producing mesolimbic area of the brain.[8] **Physiologic dependence** (see Table 12-1) occurs with regular use and is evidenced by increased tolerance and withdrawal symptoms following attempts to stop smoking. Tolerance develops to some of nicotine's effects, but not to the cardiovascular effects. Smokers continue to experience increased blood pressure and increased cardiac workload when they smoke. Because nicotine has a half-life of 1 to 2 hours, withdrawal symptoms may occur within the first few hours of abstinence (see Table 12-3). Symptoms peak in 24 to 48 hours and may last from a few weeks to several months.[7] After withdrawal subsides, cue-induced craving may cause smoking relapse.

Complications

The complications of nicotine dependence are related to the dose and the method of ingestion. Smoking cigarettes is the most deleterious method of nicotine use. Cigarette smoke contains hundreds of chemicals and gases, including at least 45 cancer-causing or tumor-promoting agents and a number of hydrocarbons or solvents. Although nicotine is not believed to be carcinogenic, it is the addictive substance.

The chronic respiratory irritation caused by exposure to cigarette smoke is the most important risk factor in the development of lung cancer and COPD. The toxic gases inhaled in cigarette smoke constrict the bronchi, paralyze the cilia, thicken the mucus-secreting membranes, dilate the distal airways, and destroy the alveolar walls.

Chronic irritation from smoke and tar also is a factor in the increased incidence of cancer of the mouth, larynx, and esophagus in smokers. Carcinogens absorbed into the blood from tobacco smoke may be responsible for the increased incidence of cancers of the bladder, prostate, and pancreas in those who smoke.

Carbon monoxide is also a component of cigarette smoke. Its effects, combined with those of nicotine, increase the risk for coronary artery disease. Carbon monoxide has a high affinity for hemoglobin and combines with it more readily than oxygen, reducing oxygen-carrying capacity. Smokers also inhale less oxygen when smoking, adding to the decreased available oxygen. Together with the increased myocardial oxygen consumption that nicotine causes, carbon monoxide significantly decreases the oxygen available to the myocardium. The result is an even greater increase in heart rate and myocardial oxygen consumption that may lead to myocardial ischemia.[9]

Passive, involuntary, or secondhand smoking occurs when nonsmokers are exposed to cigarette smoke. Children whose parents smoke have a higher prevalence of respiratory symptoms and respiratory disease. In adults secondhand smoking is associated with

TABLE 12-3 Effects of Addictive Substances

Substance	Physiologic and Psychologic Effects	Effects of Overdose	Withdrawal Symptoms
Stimulants			
Nicotine	Increased arousal and alertness; performance enhancement; increased heart rate, cardiac output, and blood pressure; cutaneous vasoconstriction; fine tremor, decreased appetite; antidiuretic effect; increased gastric motility	Rare: nausea, abdominal pain, diarrhea, vomiting, dizziness, weakness, confusion, decreased respirations, seizures, death from respiratory failure	Craving, restlessness, depression, hyperirritability, headache, drowsiness/insomnia, decreased BP and heart rate, increased appetite
Cocaine Amphetamines: dextroamphetamine (Dexedrine), methamphetamine (Desoxyn), methylphenidate (Ritalin), phentermine (Adiphex-P)	*Early:* Euphoria, excitation, restlessness, talkativeness; tachycardia, hypertension, angina, dysrhythmias, palpitations; dyspnea, tachypnea, chest pain; sexual arousal, delayed orgasm; anorexia *Long-term:* Depression, hallucinations, tremors, seizures; hypotension, myocardial infarction, heart failure, cardiomyopathy; congestion of lungs; rhinorrhea; loss of interest in sexual activity; depression or suicidal thoughts	Agitation; increased temperature, pulse, respiratory rate, blood pressure; cardiac dysrhythmias, myocardial infarction, hallucinations, seizures, possible death	Severe craving, severely depressed mood, exhaustion, prolonged sleep, apathy, irritability, disorientation
Caffeine	Mood elevation, increased alertness, nervousness, jitteriness, irritability, insomnia; increased respirations, heart rate, and force of myocardial contraction; relaxation of smooth muscle, diuresis	Rare: hyperstimulation, nervousness, confusion, psychomotor agitation, anxiety, dizziness, tinnitus, muscle twitching, elevated blood pressure, tachycardia, extrasystoles, increased respiratory rate	Headache, irritability, drowsiness, fatigue
Depressants			
Alcohol Sedative-hypnotics • Barbiturates: secobarbital (Seconal), phenobarbital (Luminal), pentobarbital (Nembutal), amobarbital (Amytal) • Benzodiazepines: diazepam (Valium), chlordiazepoxide (Librium), alprazolam (Xanax) • Nonbarbiturates-nonbenzodiazepines: methaqualone (Quaalude), chloral hydrate (Somnote)	Initial relaxation, emotional lability, decreased inhibitions, drowsiness, lack of coordination, impaired judgment, slurred speech, hypotension, bradycardia, bradypnea, constricted pupils	Shallow respirations; cold, clammy skin; weak, rapid pulse; hyporeflexia, coma, possible death	Anxiety, agitation, weakness, nausea and/or vomiting, muscle cramps, increased reflexes, tremors, delirium, seizures, possible respiratory and cardiac arrest
Opioids: heroin, morphine, opium, codeine, fentanyl (Sublimaze), meperidine (Demerol), hydromorphone (Dilaudid), pentazocine (Talwin), oxycodone (Percodan), methadone (Dolophine)	Analgesia, euphoria, drowsiness, detachment from environment, relaxation, constricted pupils, constipation, nausea, decreased respiratory rate, slurred speech, impaired judgment, decreased sexual and aggressive drives	Slow, shallow respirations; clammy skin; constricted pupils; coma; possible death	Watery eyes, dilated pupils, runny nose, yawning, tremors, pain, chills, fever, diaphoresis, nausea, vomiting, diarrhea, abdominal cramps
Cannabis			
Marijuana Hashish	Relaxation, euphoria, lack of motivation, slowed time sensation, sexual arousal, abrupt mood changes, impaired memory and attention, impaired judgment, reddened eyes, dry mouth, lack of coordination, tachycardia, increased appetite	Fatigue, paranoia, panic reactions, hallucinogen-like psychotic states	None except for rare insomnia, hyperactivity

Continued

TABLE 12-3 Effects of Addictive Substances—cont'd

Substance	Physiologic and Psychologic Effects	Effects of Overdose	Withdrawal Symptoms
Hallucinogens			
Lysergic acid diethylamide (LSD) Psilocybin (mushrooms) Dimethyltryptamine (DMT) Diethyltryptamine (DET) 3,4-methylenedioxyamphetamine (MDMA, Ecstasy) Mescaline (peyote) Phencyclidine (PCP)	Perceptual distortions, hallucinations, delusions (PCP), depersonalization, heightened sensory perception, euphoria, mood swings, suspiciousness, panic, impaired judgment, increased body temperature, hypertension, flushed face, tremor, dilated pupils, constricted pupils (PCP), nystagmus (PCP), violence (PCP)	Prolonged effects and episodes, anxiety, panic, confusion, blurred vision, increases in blood pressure and temperature	Abrupt withdrawal of hallucinogens generally does not result in withdrawal symptoms
Inhalants			
Aerosol propellants Fluorinated hydrocarbons Nitrous oxide (in deodorants, hair spray, pesticide, whipped cream spray, spray paint, cookware coating products) Solvents (gasoline, kerosene, nail polish remover, typewriter correction fluid, cleaning solutions, lighter fluid, paint, paint thinner, glue) Anesthetic agents (nitrous oxide, chloroform) Nitrites (amyl nitrite, butyl nitrite)	Euphoria, decreased inhibitions, giddiness, slurred speech, illusions, drowsiness, clouded sensorium, tinnitus, nystagmus, dysrhythmias, cough, nausea, vomiting, diarrhea; irritation to eyes, nose, mouth	Anxiety, respiratory depression, cardiac dysrhythmias, loss of consciousness, sudden death	Abrupt withdrawal of inhalants generally does not result in withdrawal symptoms

decreased pulmonary function, increased risk for lung cancer, and increased mortality rates from coronary artery disease.[9]

Women appear to be at greater risk than men for smoking-related diseases (see Gender box). Smoking in women is associated with greater menstrual bleeding and duration of dysmenorrhea, as well as early menopause and infertility. Smoking is the primary cause of lung cancer. Lung cancer now has surpassed breast cancer as the leading cause of cancer death among women. In addition, there is also some evidence that the risk for breast and cervical cancer may be increased among women who smoke.[10]

Although those who use smokeless tobacco (snuff, plug, and leaf) have less risk of lung disease compared with smokers, the use of smokeless tobacco is not without complications. Holding tobacco in the mouth increases the risk of cancer of the mouth, cheek, tongue, and gingiva nearly 50-fold.[11] Smokeless tobacco users also experience the systemic effects of nicotine on the cardiovascular system, thus increasing the risk for cardiovascular disease.

All users of nicotine in any form may develop complications that are directly related to the effects of nicotine itself. Such complications may include an increased risk for peripheral arterial disease, delayed wound healing, peptic ulcer disease, and gastroesophageal reflux disease (GERD).[7] Common health problems associated with tobacco use are presented in Table 12-2.

Collaborative Care

Prevention of Tobacco Use. Prevention of tobacco use in children and adolescents is the emphasis of substance abuse prevention. Most current adult smokers began daily smoking by age 16, and it is estimated that 3000 minors in the United States begin smoking each day. Recently there has been a general decline in tobacco use after age 25, but the highest rates of smoking are in young adults ages 18 to 25.[1] Of particular concern are the findings that adolescent smokers are more likely than adult smokers to become dependent on nicotine. In addition, young smokers are more likely than their non-smoking peers to abuse other drugs.[12] If tobacco use is not started and maintained during childhood and adolescence, there is a much better chance that other drugs will not be abused as the person ages. An emphasis on the health hazards of tobacco use, as well as on those of other addictive substances, should be part of the total curriculum beginning in elementary schools.

Tobacco Cessation. Because tobacco use is the leading cause of preventable illness and death in the United States, much attention is currently focused on treatment of nicotine addiction and methods to promote tobacco cessation.[13] A combination of medications, behavioral approaches, and support is believed to be most effective in long-term tobacco cessation. A variety of nicotine replacement products can be used to reduce the amount of the craving and withdrawal symptoms associated with tobacco cessation (Table 12-4). These agents enable a smoker to reduce nicotine previously obtained from cigarettes with a system that provides slower delivery of the drug and elimination of the carcinogens and gases associated with tobacco smoke. Nicotine replacement therapy is not generally recommended for pregnant women and persons who have recently experienced an acute myocardial infarction, have unstable angina, or have life-threatening dysrhythmias.

Non-nicotine drugs may also be used in smoking cessation. Bupropion (Zyban) is an antidepressant approved as an aid to quit smoking. It is a relatively weak inhibitor of neuronal uptake of norepinephrine, serotonin, and dopamine. It reduces the urge to smoke, reduces some symptoms of withdrawal, and helps prevent weight gain associated with smoking cessation. Varenicline (Chantix) is a new drug used to aid smoking cessation. Varenicline is unique in that it has both agonist and blocking actions at nicotinic receptors. Its

TABLE 12-4 Agents Used for Smoking Cessation*

Agents	Side Effects	Considerations
Nicotine Gum (OTC) Nicorette 2 mg, 4 mg; use 12 weeks or more	Hiccups, mouth ulcers, indigestion, nausea, jaw pain	Specific 30-minute chewing regimen with periods of holding the gum between cheek and teeth; food and drink should be avoided 15 minutes before or during use.
Nicotine Lozenge (OTC) Commit 2 mg, 4 mg; use 8-12 weeks or more	Nausea and indigestion, hiccups, headache, cough, mouth soreness, flatulence	Dissolves in the mouth in 20-30 minutes; chewing and swallowing the lozenge increases GI side effects; food and drink should be avoided during use.
Nicotine Patch (OTC) NicoDerm CQ Nicotrol Nicotine transdermal system • 18 or 24 hr doses • Use 8 weeks or more	Skin rash at patch site, headache, dizziness, weakness, indigestion, diarrhea, sleep disturbances with 24-hr patch	Differs from other agents in that it helps prevent craving; cannot be used by those with adhesive allergies.
Nicotine Nasal Spray Nicotrol NS • Use up to 6 months	Nose and throat irritation, sneezing, rhinitis, watery eyes, cough	
Nicotine Inhaler Nicotrol nicotine inhalation system • Delivers 4 mg • Use up to 6 months	Cough; nose, mouth, and throat irritation; heartburn and nausea	Requires a prescription; simulates smoking with mouthpiece and nicotine cartridge; may not be advisable for those with asthma or pulmonary disease.
Bupropion (Zyban) 150 mg daily for 3 days, then 150 mg twice a day • Use 12 weeks; can use up to 6 months or longer	Insomnia, irritability; constipation, nausea, vomiting, anorexia	Contraindicated with history of seizures or eating disorders.
Varenicline (Chantix) 0.5 mg daily for 3 days, 0.5 mg bid for 4 days, then 1 mg bid • Use 12 weeks; additional 12 weeks recommended for those who stop smoking to increase chance of long-term abstinence	Nausea, sleep disturbances, constipation, flatulence, vomiting, headache	If taken concurrently with nicotine replacement therapy, incidence of nausea, headache, vomiting, dizziness, dyspepsia, and fatigue is increased, but nicotine pharmacokinetics not affected.
Nortriptyline (Aventyl)† 25-75 mg/day • Use 12 weeks, longer if depressed	Dry mouth, blurred vision, drowsiness, constipation, hypotension	Must have stable ECG; do not use immediately after MI.
Clonidine (Catapres)† 0.1 mg q6hr prn for craving	Dry mouth, drowsiness, constipation, hypotension	Used to control craving; change position slowly to prevent postural hypotension.

ECG, Electrocardiogram; *MI,* myocardial infarction; *OTC,* over-the-counter.
*Additional information and patient instructions are available from the American Lung Association at *www.lungusa.org*.
†Nortriptyline and clonidine are not approved by the Food and Drug Administration for treatment of smoking cessation but have been used successfully for this purpose.

agonist activity at one subtype of nicotinic receptors provides some nicotine effects to ease the withdrawal symptoms. It also blocks the effects of nicotine and prevents stimulation of the mesolimbic dopamine system by blocking another subtype of nicotinic receptors. Thus it provides some nicotine effects to ease the withdrawal symptoms and it blocks the effects of nicotine from cigarettes if a person resumes smoking.[14] Nortriptyline (Aventyl), clonidine (Catapres), and mecamylamine (Inversine) are not approved by the FDA for use in smoking cessation, but are used in some cases to reduce withdrawal symptoms and promote cessation.[7]

Participation in tobacco cessation programs is recommended in conjunction with nicotine replacement therapy. Behavioral approaches teach patients to avoid high-risk situations for smoking relapse, such as those that promote cue-induced craving. Tobacco cessation programs also promote development of other coping skills, such as cigarette refusal skills, assertiveness, alternative activities to cope with stress, and use of peer support systems.

Helping individuals to stop smoking or using tobacco is one intervention in which every nurse has a professional role. Unfortunately, it is a role that has been largely ignored. It has been reported that 70% of smokers say they would like to quit, but only half of those are encouraged to do so by health care providers.[15] Because fewer than 5% of smokers are successful on their first attempt at quitting and the average smoker requires multiple attempts before being successful, some health care providers have become cynical with regard to counseling their patients to abstain from tobacco use. However, smoking a few cigarettes during a cessation attempt (a *slip*) is much different than resuming the full smoking habit (a *relapse*). One goal of the current *Healthy People* initiative is to decrease the incidence of tobacco use in the U.S. population from 25% to 12% or less.[16] To help meet this goal and put an end to the thousands of unnecessary cases of chronic illness and death, the nurse must be proactive, identifying and talking with tobacco users to provide them with information on ways to stop the use of tobacco.

The Agency for Healthcare Research and Quality (AHRQ) has developed the *Clinical Practice Guideline: Treating Tobacco Use and Dependence* for use by clinicians, including nurses, to aggressively motivate smokers and other tobacco users to quit.[17] The guideline identifies the "five *A*s" of brief clinical interventions that should be used at each patient encounter. These interventions are designed to identify tobacco users, encourage them to quit, determine their willingness to quit, assist them in quitting, and arrange for follow-up to prevent relapse. If a tobacco user is unwilling to quit, a motivational intervention using the "five *R*s" provides the nurse an opportunity to educate, reassure, and motivate tobacco users to quit at each contact. These interventions are presented in Table 12-5 and Fig. 12-2. A patient and family teaching guide (Table 12-6) expands on the fourth brief strategy, "Assist—aid the patient in quitting."

Research into tobacco use behaviors, drug therapy for nicotine addiction, and strategies effective in promoting tobacco cessation is ongoing. Many factors are recognized as being important in the initiation and continuation of tobacco use, such as peer pressure, rebelliousness, curiosity, self-image, environmental cues, and psychologic needs. One cessation program is not necessarily the best for every tobacco user. Tobacco cessation programs may involve hypnosis, acupuncture, behavioral interventions, aversion therapy, group support programs, individual therapy, and self-help options. Some smokers are able to stop tobacco use "cold turkey." Except

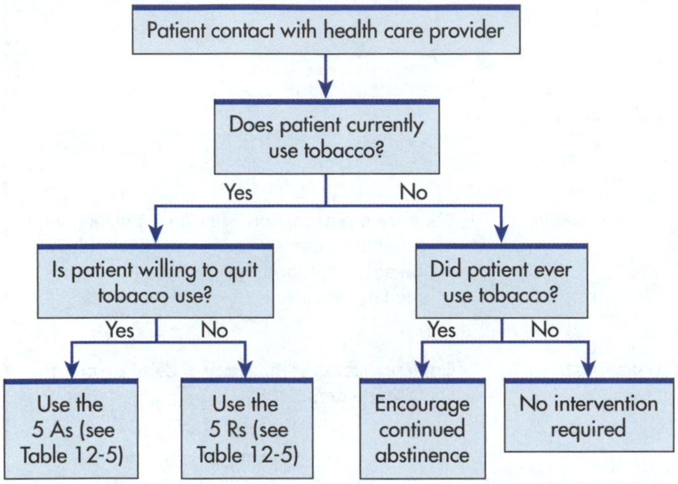

FIG. 12-2 Clinical practice guidelines: treating tobacco use and dependence.

TABLE 12-5 Clinical Practice Guideline: Treating Tobacco Use and Dependence

The Five *A*s for Individuals Who Desire to Quit	The Five *R*s for Individuals Unwilling to Quit
1. **Ask:** identify all tobacco users at every contact	1. **Relevance:** ask the patient to indicate why quitting is personally relevant (e.g., family, health)
2. **Advise:** strongly urge all tobacco users to quit	2. **Risks:** ask the patient to identify negative consequences of tobacco use (e.g., cough, shortness of breath)
3. **Assess:** determine willingness to make a quit attempt	3. **Rewards:** ask the patient to identify potential benefits of stopping tobacco use (e.g., saving money, feeling better)
4. **Assist:** aid the patient in developing a plan to quit	4. **Roadblocks:** ask patiet to identify barriers or impediments to quitting (e.g., weight gain, partner smokes)
5. **Arrange:** schedule follow-up contact	5. **Repetition:** repeat process every clinic visit

Source: US Department of Health and Human Services: *Clinical practice guideline: treating tobacco use and dependence,* Washington, DC, 2000, US Public Health Service.

EVIDENCE-BASED PRACTICE

Which Nicotine Replacement Therapy Is the Most Effective to Assist with Smoking Cessation?

Clinical Question

Among cigarette smokers (P), which form of nicotine replacement therapy (I) (chewing gum, transdermal patches, nasal sprays, inhalers, or tablets) (C), is most effective at achieving a reduction in cigarettes smoked (O)?

Best Available Evidence

Systemic review of randomized controlled trials (RCTs)

Critical Appraisal and Synthesis of Evidence

- Meta-analysis of 123 RCTs ($n = 35{,}600$) comparing nicotine replacement therapy (NRT) and placebo or non-NRT control group.
- No strong evidence was found to support combinations of NRT being more effective than use of single NRT.
- Wearing the patch only during waking hours (16 hours a day) was as effective as wearing it for 24 hours a day.

Conclusions

- The five forms of NRT were all significantly more effective than placebo or no NRT in helping smokers achieve abstinence.
- All commercially available forms of NRT increase the odds of quitting approximately 1.5 to 2 times.

Implications for Nursing Practice

- Present information about NRT to patients (see Table 12-4).
- Helping individuals to stop smoking is an important nursing role.

Reference for Evidence

Silagy C, Lancaster T, Stead L, et al: Nicotine replacement therapy for smoking cessation, Cochrane Tobacco Addiction Group *Cochrane Database of Systematic Reviews* 4, 2005.

PICO: P, patient population of interest; *I,* intervention or area of interest; *C,* comparison of interest or comparison group; *O,* outcome(s) of interest (see p. 6).

in special circumstances, nicotine replacement therapy is recommended for all tobacco users in addition to other approaches. Research has found that clinical advice alone will help only 2% of patients quit smoking, whereas the addition of nicotine replacement therapy results in a quit rate of 11% in 1 year.[17]

The advice and motivation of health care professionals can be a powerful force in smoking cessation. A nurse who uses tobacco must try to stop before serving as a role model for the patient who wants to quit tobacco use. A national program called "Tobacco Free Nurses" is focused on helping nurses and student nurses to stop smoking. The program's website at *www.tobaccofreenurses.org* provides nurses with smoking cessation information, smoking research, international links, and information about trying to quit. This website is a valuable tool for nurses who want to help their patients quit smoking and nurses who want to quit smoking themselves.

TABLE 12-6 ***PATIENT AND FAMILY TEACHING GUIDE***
Smoking and Tobacco Use Cessation

The following interventions are methods that work for quitting tobacco use. Patients have the best chance of quitting if they use more than one method.

Develop a Quit Plan

- Set a quit date, ideally within 2 weeks.
- Tell family, friends, and co-workers about quitting and request understanding and support.
- Anticipate withdrawal symptoms and challenges when quitting.
- Before quitting avoid smoking in places where you spend a lot of time (work, car, home).
- Throw away all tobacco products on the quit date.
- Do not take even a single puff or dip after the quit date. Total abstinence is essential.

Use Approved Nicotine Replacement Systems

- Learn about agents that can be used for smoking cessation (see Table 12-4).
- Do not use other forms of tobacco when using nicotine replacement systems.

Dealing with Urges to Use Tobacco

- Be aware of things that may cause you to want to smoke or use other tobacco, such as being around other smokers, being under time pressure, getting into an argument, feeling sad or frustrated, and drinking alcohol (alcohol should be avoided or used only in moderation).
- Avoid difficult situations while you are trying to quit. Try to lower your stress level.
- Exercise, such as walking, jogging, or bicycling, can help.
- Distract yourself from thoughts of smoking and the urge to use tobacco by talking to someone, getting busy with a task, or reading a book.
- Drink a lot of water.
- Take a shower or soak in the tub.

Support and Encouragement

- If you have tried to stop using tobacco before, identify what helped and what hurt in previous quit attempts.
- Counseling can help you learn how to live life as a nonuser. You may want to join a quit-tobacco program.
- If you get the urge for tobacco, call someone to help talk you out of it—preferably an ex-user.
- Do not be afraid to talk about how you feel while quitting, especially fears of not being able to quit for good. Ask your spouse/partner, friends, and co-workers to support you. Self-help materials and hot lines are also available:
  - American Lung Association: 800-586-4872; *www.lungusa.org*
  - American Cancer Society: 800-227-2345; *www.cancer.org/tobacco*
  - Cancer Information Service: 800-422-6237; *www.nci.nih.gov*
  - Smoking Cessation Consumer Tool Kit: 800-358-9295; *www.ahrq.gov*
  - Smoking, Tobacco, and Health: 800-CDC-1311; *www.cdc.gov/tobacco*
  - Try To Stop, Massachusetts Department of Public Health: 800-TRY TO STOP; *www.trytostop.org*

Avoiding Relapse

Most relapses occur within the first 3 months after quitting. Do not be discouraged if you start using tobacco again. Remember, most people try several times before they finally quit. Explore different ways to break habits. You may have to deal with some of the following triggers that cause relapse.

- *Change your environment.* Get rid of cigarettes, tobacco (in any form), and ashtrays in your home, car, and place of work. Get rid of the smell of cigarettes in your car and home.
- *Alcohol.* Consider limiting or stopping alcohol use while you are quitting tobacco.
- *Other smokers at home.* Encourage housemates to quit with you. Work out a plan to cope with others who smoke, and avoid being around them.
- *Weight gain.* Tackle one problem at a time. Work on quitting tobacco first. You will not necessarily gain weight, and increased appetite is often temporary.
- *Negative mood or depression.* If these symptoms persist, talk to your health care provider. You may need treatment for depression.
- *Severe withdrawal symptoms.* Your body will go through many changes when you quit tobacco. You may have a dry mouth, cough, or scratchy throat, and you may feel irritable. The patch or gum may help with cravings (see Table 12-4).
- *Thoughts.* Get your mind off tobacco. Exercise and do things you enjoy.
- *Keep a list.* Keep a list of "slips" and near-slips, what caused them, and what you can learn from them.
- *Focus on the benefits of quitting:*
  1. At 20 minutes after you quit, blood pressure decreases, pulse rate drops, and the body temperature of your hands and feet increases.
  2. At 8 hours, the carbon monoxide level in your blood drops to normal and the oxygen level in your blood increases to normal.
  3. At 24 hours, your chance of a heart attack decreases.
  4. At 48 hours, nerve endings start regrowing and the ability to smell and taste is enhanced.
  5. At 2 weeks to 3 months, your circulation improves; walking becomes easier; lung function increases; and coughing, sinus congestion, fatigue, and shortness of breath decrease.
  6. At 1 year, your risk of heart disease is decreased to half that of a smoker.
  7. By 10 to 15 years, your risk of stroke, lung and other cancers, and early death returns to nearly the level of people who have never smoked.

Sources: US Department of Health and Human Services: *Clinical practice guideline: treating tobacco use and dependence,* Washington, DC, 2000, US Public Health Service; *You can quit smoking: consumer guide,* June 2000, US Public Health Service. Available at *www.surgeongeneral.gov/tobacco/consquits.htm; Freedom from Smoking Online,* New York, 2004, American Lung Association. Available at *www.lungusa.org/; You can quit smoking: tips for the first week,* March 2001, US Public Health Service. Available at *www.surgeongeneral.gov/tobacco/1stweek.htm.*

ETHICAL DILEMMAS
Impaired Health Care Providers

Situation
The nurses on the surgical unit know that one of their colleagues has undergone treatment for prescription drug addiction. She seemed to be doing well until recently when she has been totally focused on her separation and subsequent divorce. Her colleagues suspect that she is using drugs again and worry that it will affect her patient care.

Important Points for Consideration
- Nurses have an ethical obligation to prevent harm from coming to patients.
- Nurses are responsible for documenting the observed behaviors, possibly confronting their colleague, and reporting their observations to their supervisor and to the State Board of Nursing.
- In most states, mandatory reporting of substance abuse is required and whistle-blowing protection is provided under the Nurse Practice Act.
- Greater benefit may also result for the nurse suspected of substance abuse when the opportunity for treatment is provided under provisions of the state Nurse Practice Act, rather than ignoring the problem.

Critical Thinking Questions
1. How should the nurses handle this situation?
2. What are the provisions of your state's Nurse Practice Act regarding impaired nurses?

The nurse must have a thorough knowledge of the physiologic changes that are encountered with tobacco cessation and consistently provide facts and support to help a tobacco user quit. The nurse also needs to be aware of resources in the community to assist the individual who is motivated to quit. Local chapters of the American Lung Association and the American Cancer Society have information on available programs.

Women are less successful than men in quitting smoking. Some of the reasons include concern about weight gain, less responsiveness to nicotine replacement therapy, variability in mood and withdrawal as a function of the menstrual cycle, inadequate emotional support from others, and the possibility that smoking-associated environmental cues may be more influential in smoking behavior in women than men.[10] The identification of gender differences in smoking cessation suggests that women who use nicotine replacement do better with nicotine inhalers than the nicotine patch and that women can increase their chances for quitting by timing their attempt to coincide with the first half of their menstrual cycles. A new anticraving drug in development (rimonabant) that helps curb both appetite and nicotine craving might be able to promote smoking cessation in women who are reluctant to quit because of resultant weight gain.

COCAINE

Characteristics
Cocaine is the most potent of the abused stimulants. Although its use is not as high today as at its peak in 1983, the annual number of new users of any form of cocaine is increasing in youths ages 12 to 17 years.[1] "Crack," a cocaine alkaloid that gets its name from the popping sound the crystals make when heated, is also popular because it is less expensive, is readily available, is easy to use, and has an increased purity over cocaine.

Effects of Use
Cocaine's effects have been extensively studied, and it serves as the prototype of an addictive stimulant substance. All stimulants work in part by increasing the amount of dopamine in the brain, producing euphoria and increasing energy and alertness. This action on the brain reward system magnifies pleasure and leads to rapid dependence. In addition to stimulation of the CNS, cocaine and other stimulants also cause adrenalin-like effects in the peripheral nervous system and the cardiovascular system.[3,7] Physical and psychologic effects are presented in Table 12-3.

The most common method of administration of cocaine is intranasal (snorting) (Fig. 12-3), but it may be smoked as "crack" cocaine or in "freebase" form, injected intravenously (IV), taken orally, or absorbed through mucous membranes. Smoking and intravenous (IV) methods result in the fastest absorption and the highest "rush."

Cocaine withdrawal is characterized by intense craving and cocaine-seeking behavior for the first 9 hours to 14 days. Marked agitation, subtle muscular aches and pains, feelings of depression, exhaustion, and a need to sleep may occur (see Table 12-3). Eventually mood becomes more normal, but a desire to return to the drug, especially prompted by cue-induced craving, remains for an indefinite period of time.[7]

Complications
Health problems resulting from administration of cocaine intravenously, intranasally, or by smoking are identified in Table 12-2. A *stimulant psychosis* may occur with the chronic use of cocaine. A cocaine psychosis usually progresses from paranoid delusions to visual hallucinations of "snow lights" (colored lights when cocaine is administered) and tactile hallucinations of bugs crawling under the skin. Skin excoriations from scratching; needle marks; and elevated blood pressure, heart rate, and temperature are findings that help differentiate a stimulant psychosis from schizophrenia.[3]

Acute cocaine toxicity may be manifested by cardiac palpitations, tachycardia, increased respiratory rate, and fever. At high

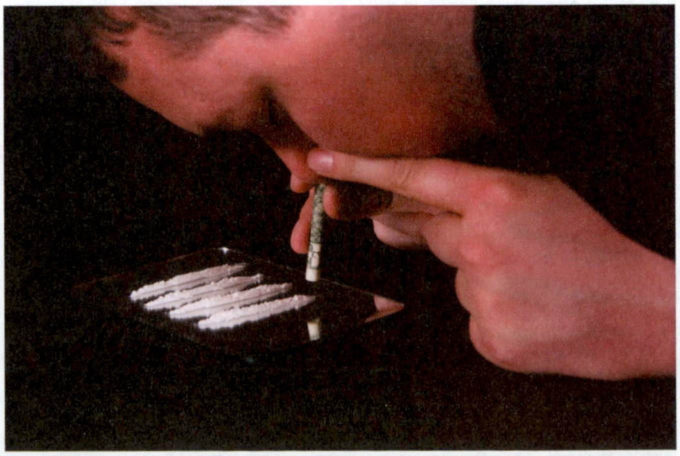

FIG. 12-3 Snorting cocaine is the most widespread method of using this common stimulant.

TABLE 12-7 EMERGENCY MANAGEMENT
Cocaine and Amphetamine Toxicity

Etiology	Assessment Findings	Interventions
Intranasal, inhalation, parenteral, oral, vaginal, rectal, or sublingual administration of cocaine Oral or parenteral administration of amphetamines	**Cardiovascular** Palpitations Tachycardia Hypertension Dysrhythmias Myocardial ischemia or infarction **Central Nervous System** Feeling of impending doom Euphoria Agitation Combativeness Seizures Hallucinations Confusion Paranoia Fever **Other** Track marks Consumption of bags of cocaine	**Initial** Ensure patent airway Anticipate need for intubation if respiratory distress evident Establish IV access and initiate fluid replacement as appropriate Obtain a 12-lead ECG Treat ventricular dysrhythmias as appropriate with lidocaine, bretylium (Bretylol), or procainamide (Pronestyl) Anticipate the need for propranolol (Inderal) or labetalol (Normodyne) for hypertension and tachycardia Severe hypertension may require administration of nitroprusside (Nipride) or phentolamine (Regitine) Aspirin may be administered to lower the risk of myocardial infarction Administer IV diazepam (Valium) or lorazepam (Ativan) for seizures Administer IV antipsychotic drugs for psychosis and hallucinations Naloxone (Narcan) IV should be given if CNS depression is present and concurrent opiate use is suspected **Ongoing** Monitor vital signs, level of consciousness, cardiac rhythm Use restraints only if needed to protect the patient and staff

CNS, Central nervous system; *ECG,* electrocardiogram; *IV,* intravenous.

levels of overdose, seizures, hypertension, and dysrhythmias or myocardial ischemia can occur. The patient experiences restlessness, paranoia, agitated delirium, confusion, and repetitive stereotyped behaviors. Death is often related to stroke, fatal dysrhythmias, or myocardial infarction.[7]

Collaborative Care

An individual who is addicted to cocaine frequently does not seek treatment for drug abuse but rather for problems with sleep, appetite, depression, sinusitis, respiratory infections, chest pain, or headaches. The nurse should have a high degree of suspicion of stimulant drug abuse in any patient seeking health care who has dilated pupils, tachycardia, hyperactivity, fever, or behavioral abnormalities.

Emergency management of cocaine intoxication will depend on the patient findings at the time of treatment and may be complicated by the possibility that the patient has combined the use of cocaine with heroin, alcohol, or phencyclidine hydrochloride (PCP). A specific antidote for cocaine toxicity is not available. Emergency management of cocaine toxicity is presented in Table 12-7.

AMPHETAMINES

Characteristics

Amphetamine with its derivatives and similar stimulants is strictly regulated for therapeutic use. Specific drugs classified as amphetamines are identified in Table 12-3. Because amphetamines may be prescribed for treatment of narcolepsy, attention deficit disorders, and weight control, abuse may occur from slowly increasing the prescribed dose. However, they are also initially used as the "poor man's cocaine." Methamphetamine (crank) and smokable methamphetamine crystals (crystal meth, ice) are easily produced illegally in clandestine laboratories using inexpensive over-the-counter ingredients. Methamphetamine abuse is becoming the dominant drug problem in many sections of the United States, including rural areas where the incidence of drug abuse has traditionally been low.

Effects of Use

Amphetamines are similar to cocaine and stimulate the central and peripheral nervous systems and the cardiovascular system. Initial use results in increased alertness, improved performance, relief of fatigue, and anorexia. As with cocaine use, amphetamines used over time may lead to irritability, anxiety, paranoia, and hostile and violent behaviors[18] (see Table 12-3).

Amphetamines are usually taken orally. Rapid effects are obtained by smoking, snorting, or IV injection. Amphetamines have a longer half-life than cocaine and, because they are more often taken orally, have a longer effect. Withdrawal symptoms of amphetamines are similar to those of cocaine use[3] and are presented in Table 12-3.

Complications

Toxic reactions to amphetamines are similar to those of cocaine. Increased levels of stimulation, sometimes described as "overamping," may result in amphetamine psychosis, paranoia, seizures, and death (see Table 12-3). Without medical intervention, death may occur as a result of dysrhythmias, myocardial infarction, hyperthermia, or cerebral hemorrhage.

Collaborative Care

Patients often seek treatment for complications of amphetamine abuse such as panic reactions or temporary psychosis related to intoxication, overdose, or withdrawal. Emergency management of amphetamine toxicity is the same as that for cocaine and is presented in Table 12-7.

CAFFEINE

Characteristics

Caffeine is the most widely used psychoactive substance in the world.[19] Its use to promote alertness and alleviate fatigue is safe in most people. Although weaker than other stimulant drugs, caffeine shares characteristics of intoxication, tolerance, and withdrawal symptoms in some individuals. Approximately 80% of Americans report a regular intake of caffeine, and 20% of those using caffeine consume doses larger than 350 mg, enough to cause clinical symptoms and dependence. Depending on preparation methods, one cup of coffee contains approximately 90 to 100 mg of caffeine, one cup of tea averages 30 to 100 mg of caffeine, and traditional cola soft drinks average 25 to 50 mg of caffeine.[7] Popular commercial "energy" beverages contain two to three times the amount of caffeine found in a can of soda. In addition to beverages, caffeine is found in foods and numerous prescription and over-the-counter analgesics, stimulants, appetite suppressants, and cold and flu preparations.

Effects of Use

Caffeine is a relatively weak CNS stimulant. It is a diuretic and a myocardial stimulant. Caffeine also relaxes smooth muscles, enhances contraction of skeletal muscles, and increases gastric acid secretion. Caffeine causes peripheral vasodilation but constricts vessels in the CNS. Chronic or heavy intake of 500 mg or more per day is known to cause intoxication manifested by CNS and cardiovascular stimulation. Ingestion of a lethal dose (10 g) is extremely rare.[7] The effects of caffeine are presented in Table 12-3.

Physical and psychologic dependence on caffeine has been found with chronic use of more than 500 mg/day. However, dependence may occur in some individuals at lower doses. The most commonly reported withdrawal symptoms are listed in Table 12-3. Caffeine withdrawal may be responsible for some cases of headache that occur after general anesthesia. It is thought that weekend headaches may be related to caffeine withdrawal because caffeine consumption in many individuals is higher at work than at home.[20]

Complications

Chronic and heavy use of caffeine may cause GI upset, including abdominal pain, diarrhea, and heartburn. Heavy users are reported to have slightly higher blood pressure, heart rates, and basal metabolic rates (see Table 12-2). Because symptoms of chronic use develop gradually, most people with caffeine dependence do not link sleep disruption, anxiety, and other symptoms with caffeine intake. In toxic doses, caffeine influences behavior patterns and may precipitate panic states in addition to CNS and cardiovascular stimulation.

Collaborative Care

Management of the patient with symptoms of caffeine dependence includes assisting the patient to gradually reduce or stop the intake of caffeine. A list of caffeinated products with their dosages may be needed by the patient who quits coffee only to substitute other foods and beverages containing caffeine. Substituting decaffeinated beverages may also help. Toxic reactions to caffeine and lethal doses of caffeine are managed symptomatically, with attention to maintaining respirations and controlling hypertension, dysrhythmias, and seizures.

Depressants

Drugs classified as depressants have common physiologic and psychologic effects. Drugs in this category include alcohol, sedative-hypnotics, and opioid narcotics. With the exception of alcohol and some federally regulated drugs, most CNS depressants are medically useful. These drugs are also widely recognized for their rapid development of tolerance and dependence and medical emergencies involving overdose and withdrawal.

ALCOHOL

Characteristics

Alcohol is consumed by almost half of Americans ages 12 and older. Most people use alcohol in moderation, with some positive cardiovascular effects. However, it is estimated that alcoholism, or alcohol dependence, affects 10% of the population.[1] Alcohol abuse and/or dependence can lead to significant health, social, legal, and interpersonal problems. Alcoholism is currently viewed as a chronic progressive, potentially fatal disease if untreated. Alcohol dependence generally occurs over a period of years and may be preceded by heavy social drinking (Fig. 12-4).

Effects of Use

Alcohol affects almost all cells of the body and has complex effects on the neurons in the CNS. Alcohol, like other addictive substances, causes increased levels of dopamine, but it also depresses all areas and functions of the CNS.[4] Alcohol is absorbed directly from the stomach and small intestine. Alcohol is primarily metabolized in the liver, although a small amount is metabolized in the stomach. In a moderate drinker, the metabolism of alcohol occurs at a relatively constant rate of approximately one drink (7 g of alcohol) per hour. One drink is equal to 12 ounces of beer, 5 ounces of wine, or 1 ounce of distilled spirits. Because women have significantly lower rates of stomach metabolism, they have higher blood alcohol levels than men after the same amount of alcohol intake.[7]

The effects of alcohol are related to the concentration of alcohol and individual susceptibility to the drug. The concentration of alcohol in the body can be determined by assessing the blood alcohol concentration (BAC). Alcohol may be measured in the blood

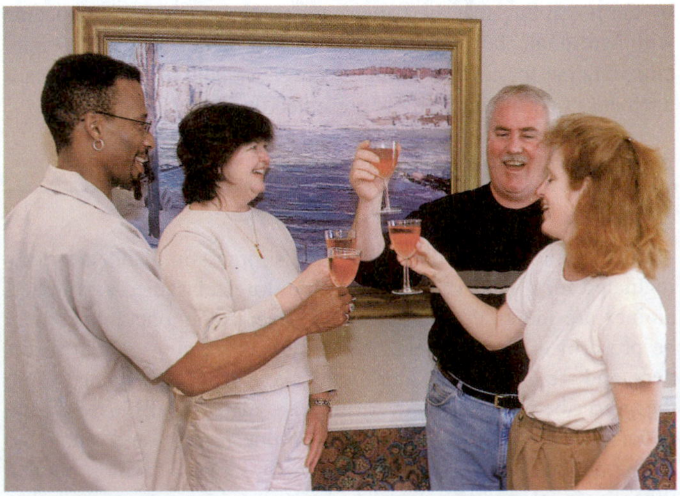

FIG. 12-4 Alcohol abuse is not easy to identify in our society.

within 15 to 20 minutes of ingestion, peaks in 60 to 90 minutes, and has a duration of 12 to 14 hours. BAC is affected by the amount consumed, drinking rate, body size and composition, drink concentration, and hormones. For the nondependent drinker, the BAC is generally predictable of alcohol's effects (Table 12-8). The relationship between BAC and behavior is different in a person who has developed tolerance to alcohol and its effects. This individual is commonly able to drink large amounts without obvious impairment and perform complex tasks without problems at BAC levels several times higher than levels that would produce obvious impairment in the nontolerant drinker.[20]

TABLE 12-8 Blood Alcohol Concentration (BAC) and Related Effects

BAC* mg/dl (mg%)	Psychophysiologic Effect
20 (0.02)	Light and moderate drinkers begin to feel some effects. Approximate BAC is reached after one drink.†
40 (0.04)	Most people begin to feel relaxed.
60 (0.06)	Judgment is mildly impaired. People are less able to make rational decisions about their capabilities (e.g., driving skills).
80 (0.08)	Definite impairment of muscle coordination and driving skills occurs. Person is legally intoxicated in some states.
100 (0.10)	Clear deterioration of reaction time and control is observed. Person is legally intoxicated in most states.
120 (0.12)	Vomiting occurs unless this level is reached slowly.
150 (0.15)	Balance and movement are impaired. Equivalent of one half pint of whiskey is circulating in the bloodstream.
300 (0.30)	Many people lose consciousness.
400 (0.40)	Most people lose consciousness, and some die.
450 (0.45)	Breathing stops; person eventually dies.

*Blood alcohol concentration (BAC) is generally recorded in milligrams of alcohol per deciliter (mg/dl) of blood or milligrams percent (mg%). Percentage is used for legal definitions of intoxication. BAC is dependent on how much alcohol is consumed, how fast it is consumed, and the person's weight.
†One drink is 12 oz beer, 5 oz wine, or 1 oz distilled spirits, all of which provide approximately the same amount of alcohol.

Alcohol intoxication is evidenced with an increasing BAC and results in behavioral and physical changes described in Tables 12-3 and 12-8. Disturbances in memory and blackouts may occur in dependent drinkers.

After withdrawal from excessive drinking, nondependent individuals experience hangovers manifested by malaise, nausea, headache, thirst, and a general feeling of fatigue. In alcoholics, sudden withdrawal may have life-threatening effects. Withdrawal should be anticipated if the individual reports consumption of over 10 drinks every day for a period of 2 weeks.[7]

Withdrawal symptoms may occur within 4 to 6 hours after the last drink, peak at 24 to 28 hours, and may last up to 5 days or more. Characteristic symptoms are presented in Table 12-3. Seizures are most likely to occur 7 to 48 hours after the last drink. *Alcohol withdrawal delirium* is a serious complication that may occur from 30 to 120 hours after the last drink. Delirium components include disorientation, visual or auditory hallucinations, and increased hyperactivity without seizures. Death may be caused by hyperthermia, peripheral vascular collapse, or cardiac failure.[7]

Complications

Acute alcohol toxicity may occur with binge drinking or the use of alcohol with other CNS depressants. Alcohol-induced CNS depression leads to respiratory and circulatory failure manifested by depressed respirations, hypotension, hypothermia, and a decreased level of consciousness (see Table 12-3).

Individuals who abuse alcohol have many health problems. Physical complications of chronic alcohol abuse are outlined in Table 12-9 and are frequently the reasons that alcohol-dependent individuals seek health care.

One complication of chronic alcohol abuse is **Wernicke's encephalopathy,** an inflammatory, hemorrhagic, degenerative condition of the brain. Wernicke's encephalopathy is caused by a thiamine deficiency resulting from poor diet and alcohol-induced

TABLE 12-9 Effects of Chronic Alcohol Abuse

Body System	Effects
Central nervous system	Alcoholic dementia; Wernicke's syndrome (confusion, nystagmus, paralysis of ocular muscles, ataxia); Korsakoff's psychosis (confabulation, amnesic disorder); impairment of cognitive function, psychomotor skills, abstract thinking, and memory; depression, attention deficit, labile moods, seizures, sleep disturbances
Peripheral nervous system	Peripheral neuropathy including pain, paresthesias, weakness
Immune system	Increased risk for tuberculosis and viral infections; increased risk for cancer of oral cavity, pharynx, esophagus, liver, colon, rectum, and possibly breast
Hematologic system	Bone marrow depression, anemia, leukopenia, thrombocytopenia, blood clotting abnormalities
Musculoskeletal system	Painful, tender, swelling of large muscle groups; painless progressive muscle weakness and wasting; osteoporosis
Cardiovascular system	Elevated pulse and blood pressure; decreased exercise tolerance; cardiomyopathy (irreversible); increased risk for hemorrhagic stroke, coronary artery disease, hypertension, sudden cardiac death
Hepatic system	Steatosis*—nausea, vomiting, hepatomegaly Alcoholic hepatitis*—anorexia, nausea, vomiting, fever, chills, abdominal pain Cirrhosis Cancer
Gastrointestinal system	Gastritis, gastroesophageal reflux disease (GERD), peptic ulcer, esophagitis, esophageal varices, enteritis, colitis, Mallory-Weiss tear, pancreatitis
Nutrition	Decreased appetite, indigestion, malabsorption, vitamin deficiencies (especially thiamine)
Urinary system	Diuretic effect from inhibition of antidiuretic hormone
Endocrine and reproductive systems	Altered gonadal function, testicular atrophy, decreased beard growth, decreased libido, diminished sperm count, gynecomastia, glucose intolerance
Integumentary system	Palmar erythema, spider angiomas, rosacea, rhinophyma

*In the early stages of the disease this is reversible if the person quits drinking.

TABLE 12-10 Clinical Manifestations of Alcohol Withdrawal and Suggested Drug Treatment

Clinical Manifestations	Suggested Drug Treatment
Minor Withdrawal Syndrome	
Tremulousness, anxiety	Benzodiazepines (e.g., lorazepam [Ativan], diazepam [Valium], chlordiazepoxide [Librium]) to stabilize vital signs, reduce anxiety, and prevent seizures and delirium
Increased heart rate	Thiamine (prevents Wernicke's encephalopathy)
Increased blood pressure	Multivitamins (folic acid, B vitamins)
Sweating	Magnesium sulfate (if serum magnesium is low)
Nausea	IV glucose solution
Hyperreflexia	Thiamine and other vitamins and minerals may be administered in glucose solution
Insomnia	
Increased hyperactivity without seizures	
Major Withdrawal Syndrome	
Visual/auditory hallucinations	Continue use of benzodiazepines
Gross tremors	Carbamazepine (Tegretol) or phenytoin (Dilantin) to prevent or treat seizures
Seizures	Antipsychotic agents (e.g., chlorpromazine [Thorazine], haloperidol [Haldol]) if psychosis persists after benzodiazepine administration
Alcohol withdrawal delirium	

suppression of thiamine absorption. This syndrome is readily reversible with administration of thiamine. Untreated or progressive Wernicke's encephalopathy may lead to **Korsakoff's psychosis,** an irreversible form of amnesia characterized by loss of short-term memory and an inability to learn.[7]

Complications may also arise from the interaction of alcohol with commonly prescribed or over-the-counter drugs. Drugs that interact with alcohol in an additive manner include antihypertensives, antihistamines, antianginals, and salicylates (aspirin). Alcohol taken with aspirin may cause or exacerbate GI bleeding. Alcohol taken with acetaminophen may increase the risk of liver damage. Potentiation and cross-tolerance with other CNS depressants also may occur. **Potentiation** occurs when an additional CNS depressant is taken with alcohol, increasing the effect. **Cross-tolerance,** requiring an increased dose for effect, occurs when an alcohol-dependent individual is alcohol free and receives other CNS depressants.[7]

Collaborative Care

Initial treatment of alcohol intoxication or overdose requires **detoxification** (defined in Table 12-1) as necessary and stabilization of the patient's condition. Supportive measures are used to promote ventilation and circulation until the alcohol is metabolized. Alcohol-induced hypotension cannot be corrected with vasoconstrictors. No antidote for alcohol is available, and stimulants should not be given. The patient who is intoxicated with rising BACs should not be given other depressants because of their additive effects.

Because Wernicke's encephalopathy is potentially preventable and reversible, IV thiamine may be administered during alcohol intoxication. Patients with alcohol intoxication may also experience hypoglycemia, decreased serum magnesium levels, and other signs of malnutrition. Glucose solutions may precipitate Wernicke's encephalopathy in a previously unaffected patient. For this reason, thiamine should be administered before or with IV glucose solutions. A premixed IV solution of 5% dextrose in 0.45% sodium chloride containing 2 g of magnesium sulfate, 1 ml of folate, and 100 mg of thiamine is frequently administered for alcohol intoxication.[21]

Management of alcohol withdrawal frequently includes the use of a variety of drugs.[7] Anticipating withdrawal syndrome in patients is important because alcohol withdrawal delirium can usually be prevented by administration of benzodiazepines, such as lorazepam (Ativan). An evidence-based guideline developed from a review of alcohol withdrawal delirium treatments demonstrated that sedative-hypnotic agents such as benzodiazepines and barbiturates lower the risk of death and shorten the duration of delirium during alcohol withdrawal.[22] Table 12-10 presents the clinical manifestations of alcohol withdrawal and suggested drug treatment.

Although cessation of drinking is the short-term goal that is accomplished through detoxification, sustained abstinence is the primary long-term goal of alcohol dependency. Patients should be referred to inpatient or intensive outpatient programs for treatment. Treatment includes behavioral therapy and may also include a variety of drugs. Naltrexone (ReVia, Trexan) is an opioid antagonist that decreases craving and blocks the desired effects of alcohol. A monthly injectable form of naltrexone (Vivitrol) is available for people who are not actively drinking. Disulfiram (Antabuse) is an agent that discourages drinking by causing aversive consequences when alcohol is consumed, such as a throbbing headache, nausea, vomiting, chest pain, and tachycardia. Acamprosate (Campral) is a new FDA-approved drug that decreases craving and distress during abstinence from alcohol.[23] Because it is not substantially metabolized (inactivated) in the liver, it can be used in alcoholics with liver disease. Currently several drugs approved for other uses are under study for alcohol treatment. These include the antiseizure drugs topiramate (Topamax) and gabapentin (Neurontin) and the antiemetic ondansetron (Zofran).

SEDATIVE-HYPNOTICS

Characteristics

Commonly abused sedative-hypnotic agents include barbiturates, benzodiazepines, and barbiturate-like drugs. Benzodiazepines have largely replaced barbiturates for medical treatment of anxiety and insomnia because they are safer in terms of risk of overdose and toxicity. Barbiturates are preferred as recreational drugs because they more frequently produce euphoric effects.

Two patterns of abuse and dependence have been recognized with sedative-hypnotic drugs. The first pattern begins with prescription use for the treatment of anxiety or insomnia. Subsequently, the patient may become tolerant to the effects and increase

TABLE 12-11 EMERGENCY MANAGEMENT
Overdose of Depressant Drug

Etiology	Assessment Findings	Interventions
Ingestion, inhalation, or injection of CNS depressants—accidental or intentional	Aggressive behavior Agitation Confusion Lethargy Stupor Hallucinations Depression Slurred speech Pinpoint pupils Nystagmus Seizures Needle tracks Cold, clammy skin Rapid, weak pulse Slow or rapid shallow respirations Decreased O_2 saturation Hypotension Dysrhythmia ECG changes Cardiac or respiratory arrest	**Initial** Ensure patent airway Anticipate intubation if respiratory distress evident Establish IV access Obtain temperature Obtain 12-lead ECG Obtain information about substance (name, route, when taken, amount) Obtain specific drug levels or comprehensive toxicology screen Obtain a health history, including drug use and allergies Administer antidotes as appropriate Perform gastric lavage if necessary Administer activated charcoal and cathartics as appropriate **Ongoing** Monitor vital signs, temperature, level of consciousness, O_2 saturation, cardiac rhythm

CNS, Central nervous system; *ECG,* electrocardiogram; *IV,* intravenous.

the dose and frequency of use without medical advice or indication. The second and more common pattern involves illegal sources, which often begins with intermittent use by teenagers or young adults at parties and leads to daily use to achieve effects.

Effects of Use

Sedative-hypnotic drugs act primarily on the CNS, causing sedation at low doses and sleep at high doses. Excessive amounts produce an initial euphoria and an intoxication that resembles that of alcohol. Although benzodiazepines are believed to have a wide margin of safety, they are not without adverse reactions, including *rebound anxiety* and insomnia with short-acting drugs and confusion and memory loss with long-acting drugs. The drugs are usually taken orally, but barbiturates and benzodiazepines may be injected intravenously.[7] The effects of sedative-hypnotics are presented in Table 12-3.

Tolerance develops rapidly to the drugs' effects, requiring higher doses to achieve euphoria. Tolerance may not develop to the brainstem-depressant effects so an increased dose may trigger hypotension and respiratory depression, resulting in death.

Withdrawal from sedative-hypnotics can be very serious. Common symptoms of withdrawal syndrome are identified in Table 12-3. After 24 hours the patient is craving the drug and may experience delirium, seizures, and respiratory and cardiac arrest. Symptoms of withdrawal peak on the second or third day for short-acting drugs (e.g., alprazolam [Xanax], secobarbital [Seconal], pentobarbital [Nembutal]) and on the seventh or eighth day for long-acting drugs (e.g., diazepam [Valium], chlordiazepoxide [Librium], phenobarbital [Luminal]).

Complications

An overdose of a sedative-hypnotic may cause death as a result of respiratory depression. Symptoms of overdose are listed in Table 12-3. Complications associated with IV use of the drugs (e.g., blood-borne infections) can also occur.

Collaborative Care

Overdoses of benzodiazepines are treated with flumazenil (Romazicon), a specific benzodiazepine antagonist. It must be used with caution because in some cases it has not completely reversed respiratory depression. It can cause seizures with physical dependence on benzodiazepines. There are no known antagonists to counteract the effects of barbiturates or other sedative-hypnotic drugs. Emergency life support measures must be taken in cases of overdose. Table 12-11 presents emergency management of CNS depressant overdose. Treatment of an individual dependent on a sedative-hypnotic requires gradual withdrawal of the drug. Hospitalization is recommended during drug withdrawal for individuals who have been abusing large amounts of barbiturates to safely manage their symptoms.[7]

OPIOIDS

Characteristics

Opioids include the naturally occurring **opiates** derived from opium in addition to the many semisynthetic and synthetic narcotic agents used as analgesics. Commonly abused opioids are identified in Table 12-3. Opioid antagonists include naloxone (Narcan) and naltrexone.

Individuals dependent on opioids include those who use illegal drugs sold on the street and those who misuse opioids in a medical setting. Heroin and fentanyl (Sublimaze) are commonly used street drugs, but recently the IV use of controlled-release oxycodone (OxyContin) has become epidemic. Street use of opioids is found in younger people, who often began their substance abuse problems with tobacco and alcohol and then progress to marijuana and other drugs of abuse. Although the rates of opioid dependency are lower than for other illegal drugs, their use is associated with high levels of crime, violence, human immunodeficiency virus (HIV) infection, and death from overdose. In a medical setting, some people misuse prescribed analgesics. These individuals tend to be middle-class and older than those using street drugs. A significant group in the medical setting includes health care professionals, who may have the highest rate of opioid abuse and dependence of any middle-class population.[7] Meperidine (Demerol) is frequently used by health care professionals. Ready access to drugs, stresses of caring for other people's problems, and long hours that interfere with family life are considered contributing factors in health care professionals.

Effects of Use

By acting on opiate receptors and neurotransmitter systems in the CNS, opioids cause CNS depression and a major effect on the brain reward system.[7] As drugs of abuse, they are taken orally, sniffed, smoked, or injected subcutaneously ("skin-popping") or intravenously ("mainlining") (Fig. 12-5).

The primary effects of opioids are identified in Table 12-3. Opioid use leads to rapid tolerance and physical dependence after short-term use. Cross-tolerance among the opioids is common, but cross-tolerance to other CNS depressants does not occur. However, additive effects of other CNS depressants may cause increased CNS depression.

Signs of overdose of opioids include pinpoint pupils, clammy skin, depressed respiration, coma, and death, if not treated (see Table 12-3). Unintentional overdose frequently occurs with recreational use of the drugs because of the unpredictability in potency and purity.

Withdrawal from opioids occurs with decreased amounts or cessation of the drug after prolonged moderate to heavy use. The administration of an opioid antagonist, such as naloxone, will cause withdrawal symptoms in dependent individuals. Symptoms may include craving, abdominal cramps, diarrhea, nausea, and vomiting. Additional symptoms are presented in Table 12-3.

Complications

Opioids are usually injected IV, increasing the user's risk for HIV infection, acquired immunodeficiency syndrome (AIDS), hepatitis B virus (HBV) infection, and hepatitis C virus (HCV) infection. Sharing and reuse of syringes and injection paraphernalia that have been used by infected individuals is a primary source of infectious diseases among drug users. Injection drug users represent the highest risk group for acquiring HCV infection. In addition, drug abuse by any route of administration increases the risk of contracting HIV because of the tendency of substance abusers to engage in risky sexual behaviors in exchange for drugs or money or because of lack of inhibition.[24]

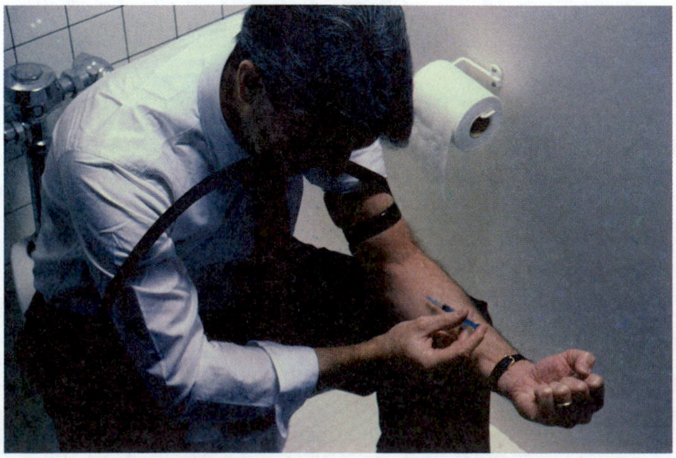

FIG. 12-5 Injecting or "mainlining" heroin.

Other complications occur as a consequence of injecting drugs or neglect of health and hygiene. These include a variety of infections, as well as damage to the kidneys, electrolyte abnormalities, and dysrhythmias. Health problems associated with opioid use are presented in Table 12-2.

Collaborative Care

Overdose of opioids can precipitate a medical emergency. Table 12-11 outlines interventions for overdose of depressant drugs. A toxicologic blood or urine screen may be helpful to identify the specific drug. An opioid antagonist such as naloxone should be given as soon as life support is instituted. The patient should be monitored closely because opioid antagonists have a shorter duration of action than most opioids. It is also possible the patient may have a mixed drug ingestion that does not respond to opioid antagonists.

Treatment of opioid withdrawal is symptom based and does not always require the use of medications. Withdrawal is acutely uncomfortable but is not usually life threatening, as is withdrawal from other CNS depressants. Methadone (Dolophine) in decreasing doses is the drug used most often during detoxification to decrease symptoms. Some patients experience relief of withdrawal symptoms with the use of clonidine (Catapres), a centrally acting α_2-adrenergic agonist.[7]

The most promising available treatment for IV opioid addiction involves the use of opioid agonists, opioid antagonists, or mixed opioid agonists-antagonists combined with education, counseling, and vocational training programs. Methadone may also be used for long-term treatment in addition to its use in detoxification. By substituting oral methadone for the abused opioid, withdrawal syndrome can be avoided and the euphoria that leads to craving can be prevented. Although methadone is an addictive drug, its use in maintenance programs alters the drug-using lifestyle, reduces exposure to infections, and controls drug use.

A less successful treatment of opioid dependence involves the use of naltrexone (Trexan, ReVia), an opioid antagonist. Voluntarily taken orally each day, naltrexone prevents opioid-induced euphoria, but does not stop opioid craving. Buprenorphine is an opioid agonist-antagonist that can be used for detoxification and maintenance therapy. For treatment of withdrawal symptoms it is available in a sublingual tablet marketed as Subutex, and for long-term maintenance buprenorphine is combined with naltrexone in a sublingual tablet marketed as Suboxone. In this preparation, naltrexone is added to the buprenorphine to prevent users from injecting the tablets IV, which would cause intense withdrawal symptoms in opioid-addicted individuals.[25]

Other Drugs of Abuse

CANNABIS

Characteristics

Cannabis, or marijuana, is the most widely used illicit drug in North America. Because it is usually the first illegal drug used by young people, it is considered a "gateway" drug to more addicting drugs. Patterns of use are similar to alcohol in that there is occasional use, misuse resulting in temporary problems, and abuse or dependence associated with a high potential for future problems.

In the United States cannabis is usually sold as marijuana. The key active ingredient in cannabis responsible for most of the psychoactive effects is tetrahydrocannabinol (THC). Although a number of potential benefits of THC have been reported, the only approved THC preparation is dronabinol (Marinol). Dronabinol is available by prescription to control nausea and vomiting resulting from cancer chemotherapy and to stimulate the appetite in patients with AIDS.[7]

Effects of Use

At low to moderate doses, THC produces fewer physiologic and psychologic alterations than do other classes of psychoactive drugs, including alcohol. Although its mechanism of action is uncertain, THC affects dopamine and other neurotransmitter activity and a variety of receptors in the brain. When marijuana is smoked, effects usually occur in about 20 to 30 minutes and may last up to 7 hours. Because it is stored in body fat, it is eliminated slowly, resulting in a half-life of 2 to 7 days.[3]

Marijuana produces three principal effects: euphoria, sedation, and hallucinations. The most commonly affected organs are the brain and the cardiovascular and respiratory systems. Decreased sperm production and decreased reproductive hormones in both men and women may occur. Signs of intoxication are presented in Table 12-3. Problems of chronic use include impaired short-term memory, decreased motor coordination, tremors, and increased heart and respiratory rates. A condition known as amotivational syndrome characterized by apathy, dullness, and disinterest may also occur.[7]

Complications

Complications of marijuana use are generally mild and transient. Heavy use may cause health problems identified in Table 12-2. It may precipitate seizures in persons with epilepsy, psychotic episodes in persons with schizophrenia, and ketoacidosis in persons with diabetes mellitus. Marijuana may also complicate preexisting conditions in persons with heart disease.[7]

Collaborative Care

Acute reactions, including intoxication and withdrawal, are usually mild and time limited. An individual may be treated for toxic reactions to a combination of drugs that includes marijuana or may seek treatment for panic reactions. Treatment is directed toward relief of symptoms, and the administration of sedative drugs is avoided if possible.

PSYCHEDELIC AGENTS

Psychedelic agents, or hallucinogens, produce a change in level of consciousness and induce hallucinations and mental states that resemble psychosis. They are able to activate mechanisms that produce dreaming without causing unconsciousness.[7] Common agents and their effects are identified in Table 12-3. Although it was originally thought that d-lysergic acid diethylamide (LSD) could provide a model for the study of psychosis, no legitimate or therapeutic use of any of the psychedelic agents has been found. Currently 3,4-methylenedioxymethamphetamine (MDMA), or "Ecstasy," is the most commonly used psychedelic. It is a popular drug among adolescents and young adults at nightclubs and all-night dance parties known as "raves." It also has been used as a date-rape drug.

Physical and psychologic effects of psychedelic agents are identified in Table 12-3. Although most effects are psychologic, cardiovascular and neurologic toxicity can occur. Seizures, cardiac stimulation, and hyperthermia are treated symptomatically. Panic attacks may be treated with an antianxiety agent such as diazepam (Valium) and a nonthreatening environment.

INHALANTS

Inhalation is the major route of ingestion for a number of common household and industrial volatile substances. Forms of use include sniffing, huffing, bagging, and spraying. Because inhalants are readily accessible, are inexpensive, and produce a rapid high, their use among preadolescents and adolescents is high.

There are four main classes of inhalants: volatile solvents, aerosols, anesthetic agents, and nitrites. They act as CNS depressants but are also extremely damaging to the cardiovascular and respiratory systems. Common agents and their effects are presented in Table 12-3. Users may develop peripheral neuropathies and exhibit tremors and weakness. Treatment of toxicity is symptomatic. Sudden death may result from direct toxic effects, aspiration of gastric contents, trauma, and/or suffocation.[3]

NURSING MANAGEMENT
ADDICTIVE BEHAVIORS

■ *Nursing Assessment*

It is not an easy task to identify drug-dependent individuals who seek health care for problems other than treatment of the addiction. Yet early recognition and identification of a patient with substance dependence is crucial to successful treatment outcomes for any health problem. Possible behaviors and physical complaints suggesting substance dependence are listed in Table 12-12, but these behaviors are not all-inclusive. Because the nurse may fail to recognize signs and symptoms of abuse in a patient who does not fit the stereotype of an "addict" and because most patients will underreport or deny substance abuse, an assessment of drug and alcohol use should be performed for all patients. The history should include questioning about the use of all substances, including prescribed medications, over-the-counter drugs, herbal and homeo-

TABLE 12-12 Symptoms and Behaviors That May Suggest Dependence on Substances

- Fatigue
- Insomnia
- Headaches
- Seizure disorder
- Changes in mood
- Anorexia, weight loss
- Vague physical complaints
- Overabundant use of mouthwash or toiletries
- Appearing older than stated age, unkempt appearance
- Leisure activities that involve alcohol and/or other drugs
- Sexual dysfunction, decreased libido, erectile dysfunction
- Trauma secondary to falls, auto accidents, fights, or burns
- Driving while intoxicated (more than one citation suggests dependence)
- Failure of standard doses of sedatives to have a therapeutic effect
- Financial problems, including those related to spending for substances
- Frequent references to alcohol or alcohol use indicating preoccupation with and importance of alcohol in the person's life
- Problems in areas of life function (e.g., frequent job changes; marital conflict, separation, and/or divorce; work-related accidents, tardiness, absenteeism; legal problems, including arrest; social isolation, estrangement from friends and/or family)

pathic products, caffeine, tobacco, alcohol, and recreational drugs. During the assessment the nurse should be aware of patient behaviors that influence history taking such as denial, avoidance, underreporting or minimizing substance use, or giving inaccurate information. Asking questions in a way that lets the patient know that you find a behavior normal or at least understandable is also helpful. The nurse might ask, "Given your situation, I wonder if you have been using anything to help relieve your stress?"

Although a variety of screening tools are available, one culturally sensitive tool that is easily used by nurses to identify alcohol dependence is the Alcohol Use Disorders Identification Test (AUDIT) (Table 12-13). A score of 8 points or less is considered nonalcoholic, whereas 9 points or above indicates alcoholism. Another instrument frequently used is the CAGE questionnaire (Table 12-14). In addition, if the patient provides information concerning drug use that is inconsistent with assessment findings, the nurse should question the patient further.

Physical assessment also reveals clues about substance abuse. The nurse must be alert to signs and symptoms of the many health problems associated with addictive behaviors that may be apparent during the physical examination. Assessment of the patient's general appearance and nutritional status and examination of the abdomen, skin, and the cardiovascular, respiratory, and neurologic systems often reflect problems associated with substance abuse.

TABLE 12-13 Alcohol Use Disorders Identification Test (AUDIT)

Please answer each question by checking one of the circles in the second column.

		Score
1. How often do you have a drink containing alcohol?	❍ Never	(0)
	❍ Monthly or less	(1)
	❍ 2-4 times per month	(2)
	❍ 2-4 times per week	(3)
	❍ 4+ times per week	(4)
2. How many drinks containing alcohol do you have on a typical day when you are drinking?	❍ 1 or 2	(0)
	❍ 3 or 4	(1)
	❍ 5 or 6	(2)
	❍ 7 to 9	(3)
	❍ 10 or more	(4)
3. How often do you have six or more drinks on one occasion?	❍ Never	(0)
	❍ Less than monthly	(1)
	❍ Monthly	(2)
	❍ Weekly	(3)
	❍ Daily or almost daily	(4)
4. How often during the last year have you found that you were not able to stop drinking once you had started?	❍ Never	(0)
	❍ Less than monthly	(1)
	❍ Monthly	(2)
	❍ Weekly	(3)
	❍ Daily or almost daily	(4)
5. How often in the last year have you failed to do what was normally expected of you because you were drinking?	❍ Never	(0)
	❍ Less than monthly	(1)
	❍ Monthly	(2)
	❍ Weekly	(3)
	❍ Daily or almost daily	(4)
6. How often during the last year have you needed a first drink in the morning to get yourself going after a heavy drinking session?	❍ Never	(0)
	❍ Less than monthly	(1)
	❍ Monthly	(2)
	❍ Weekly	(3)
	❍ Daily or almost daily	(4)
7. How often during the last year have you had a feeling of guilt or remorse about drinking?	❍ Never	(0)
	❍ Less than monthly	(1)
	❍ Monthly	(2)
	❍ Weekly	(3)
	❍ Daily or almost daily	(4)
8. How often during the last year have you been unable to remember what happened the night before because you had been drinking?	❍ Never	(0)
	❍ Less than monthly	(1)
	❍ Monthly	(2)
	❍ Weekly	(3)
	❍ Daily or almost daily	(4)
9. Have you or someone else been injured as a result of your drinking?	❍ No	(0)
	❍ Yes, but not in the last year	(2)
	❍ Yes, during the last year	(4)
10. Has a relative, friend, doctor, or other health worker been concerned about your drinking or suggested that you cut down?	❍ No	(0)
	❍ Yes, but not in the last year	(2)
	❍ Yes, during the last year	(4)

Scoring for AUDIT: Questions 1 through 8 are scored 0, 1, 2, 3, or 4. Questions 9 and 10 are scored 0, 2, or 4 only. The minimum score (nondrinkers) is 0 and the maximum possible score is 40. A score of 9 or more indicates hazardous or harmful alcohol consumption.

Source: Saunders JB et al: Development of the Alcohol Use Disorders Identification Test (AUDIT), WHO collaborative project on early detection of persons with harmful alcohol consumption. II, *Addiction* 88:791, 1993. Available at *www.niaaa.nih.gov/publications/audit.htm.*

TABLE 12-14 CAGE Questionnaire Adapted to Include Drugs (CAGEAID)

Have you felt you ought to cut down on your drinking *(or drug use)*?
_____ Yes _____ No
Have people annoyed you by criticizing your drinking *(or drug use)*?
_____ Yes _____ No
Have you felt bad or guilty about your drinking *(or drug use)*?
_____ Yes _____ No
Have you ever had a drink *(or used drugs)* first thing in the morning to steady your nerves or get rid of a hangover (or to get the day started)?
_____ Yes _____ No

From Fleming MF, Barry KL: *Addictive disorders,* St Louis, 1992, Mosby; Ewing JA: Detecting alcoholism: the CAGE questionnaire, *JAMA* 252:1905, 1984.
NOTE: **Boldface** text shows the original CAGE question; ***boldface italic*** text shows modifications of CAGE questions used to screen for drug disorders. In general population, two or more positive answers indicate a need for a more in-depth assessment.

Even if a patient does not acknowledge substance abuse or dependence, if there is any indication of alcohol or other CNS depressant use when a patient is hospitalized, the nurse should always question when the patient last used the substance. This information will help the nurse anticipate drug interactions or the time of possible onset of withdrawal symptoms if the patient is indeed dependent on a substance. Urine drug screening may also be performed in some situations to determine drug use.

The history should be taken in a setting that ensures privacy and avoids interruption. The patient is unlikely to discuss any substance problems in the presence of accompanying family members or friends from whom it is hidden. It is also important for the nurse to explain why the information is needed and how it will be used to provide appropriate care. Telling the patient that complete honesty is necessary to avoid drug interactions or manage withdrawal symptoms is critical. The substance-abusing patient may also be afraid of losing control of drug administration and may be concerned that substance use will be reported to legal authorities. The patient should be informed that federal privacy laws prohibit nurses and other health care providers from disclosing any treatment of substance abuse without the specific written consent of the patient. The nurse should reassure the patient that all information will remain confidential and will be used only to provide safe care.

A critical factor in obtaining accurate information from the patient during assessment is the ability of the nurse to promote open and nonjudgmental communication with the patient. The nurse must be aware of personal feelings and attitudes about substance abuse and be able to express concern for the patient without criticism or rejection.

Nursing Diagnoses

Nursing diagnoses for the patient in alcohol withdrawal may include, but are not limited to, those presented in NCP 12-1. In addi-

NURSING CARE PLAN 12-1

Patient in Alcohol Withdrawal

NURSING DIAGNOSIS **Ineffective protection** *related to* sensorimotor deficits, seizure activity, and confusion *as evidenced by* altered level of consciousness and disorientation

PATIENT GOALS
1. Experiences no injury during alcohol withdrawal
2. Demonstrates decrease in tremors and psychomotor activity

OUTCOMES (NOC)

Neurologic Status

- Consciousness___
- Communication appropriate to situation___
- Rest-sleep pattern___
- Blood pressure___
- Apical pulse rate___
- Radial pulse rate ___
- Cognitive orientation___
- Cognitive ability___

Measurement Scale

1 = Severely compromised
2 = Substantially compromised
3 = Moderately compromised
4 = Mildly compromised
5 = Not compromised

- Seizure activity___

Measurement Scale

1 = Severe
2 = Substantial
3 = Moderate
4 = Mild
5 = None

INTERVENTIONS (NIC) and *RATIONALES*

Environmental Management: Safety

- Create a safe environment for the patient.
- Identify the safety needs of the patient based on level of physical and cognitive function and history of behavior *to plan appropriate preventive measures.*
- Remove environmental hazards (e.g., loose rugs and small, movable furniture) *to minimize hazards and risks.*
- Safeguard with side rails/side-rail padding *to physically limit mobility or access to harmful situations.*

Substance Use Treatment: Alcohol Withdrawal

- Monitor vital signs during withdrawal to identify extreme autonomic nervous system response.
- Administer anticonvulsants or sedatives to prevent alcohol withdrawal delirium and relieve other symptoms during withdrawal.
- Administer vitamin therapy to prevent Wernicke's syndrome.
- Provide emotional support to patient/family to decrease anxiety.

Seizure Precautions

- Keep suction, ambu bag, and oral or nasopharyngeal airway at bedside *to establish respiratory function after seizure activity.*
- Use padded side rails and keep side rails up *to prevent injury during seizure activity.*

Continued

NURSING CARE PLAN 12-1

Patient in Alcohol Withdrawal—cont'd

NURSING DIAGNOSIS **Sensory/perceptual alterations: visual, auditory, and tactile** *related to* neurochemical imbalance *as evidenced by* visual distortions, disorientation, and hallucinations

PATIENT GOALS
1. Is oriented to person, place, and time
2. Experiences no hallucinations

OUTCOMES (NOC)

Distorted Thought Self-Control
- Asks for validation of reality___
- Reports decrease in hallucinations or delusions___
- Perceives environment accurately___
- Exhibits logical thought flow patterns___
- Exhibits reality-based thinking ___
- Exhibits appropriate thought content ___

Measurement Scale
1 = Never demonstrated
2 = Rarely demonstrated
3 = Sometimes demonstrated
4 = Often demonstrated
5 = Consistently demonstrated

INTERVENTIONS (NIC) and *RATIONALES*

Delirium Management
- Monitor neurologic status on an ongoing basis *to determine appropriate interventions.*
- Verbally acknowledge the patient's fears and feelings to *decrease anxiety.*
- Provide patient with information about what is happening and what can be expected to occur in the future *to assist in reality orientation.*
- Maintain a well-lit environment that reduces sharp contrasts and shadows *to reduce external stimuli.*
- Remove stimuli, when possible, that create misperception in a particular patient (e.g., pictures on the wall or television) *to reduce misinterpretation of environment.*
- Inform patient of person, place, and time *to promote orientation.*
- Use environmental cues (e.g., signs, pictures, clocks, calendars, and color coding of environment) *to stimulate memory, reorient, and promote appropriate behavior.*

NURSING DIAGNOSIS **Ineffective health maintenance** *related to* inadequate coping mechanisms and resources *as evidenced by* abuse of alcohol

PATIENT GOALS
1. Acknowledges a substance abuse problem
2. Identifies positive coping mechanisms and resources to use during alcohol abstinence

OUTCOMES (NOC)

Risk Control: Alcohol Use
- Acknowledges personal consequences associated with alcohol misuse___
- Recognizes changes in general health status___
- Develops effective alcohol use control strategies___
- Commits to alcohol use control strategies___

Measurement Scale
1 = Never demonstrated
2 = Rarely demonstrated
3 = Sometimes demonstrated
4 = Often demonstrated
5 = Consistently demonstrated

INTERVENTIONS (NIC) and *RATIONALES*

Substance Use Treatment
- Encourage patient to take control over own behavior *to change undesired behaviors.*
- Discuss with patient the impact of substance use on medical condition or general health *to promote acknowledgment of consequences of use.*
- Identify constructive goals with patient *to provide alternatives to the use of substances to reduce stress.*
- Assist patient to learn alternative methods of coping with stress or emotional distress *to reduce substance use.*
- Identify support groups in the community for long-term substance abuse treatment *to promote continued abstinence.*

tion, other nursing diagnoses for an individual with substance abuse may include, but are not limited to, the following:
- Ineffective denial *related to* inability to acknowledge substance abuse or dependence
- Disturbed thought processes *related to* drug or alcohol effects
- Risk for infection *related to* increased environmental exposure to pathogens and risk-taking behavior
- Imbalanced nutrition: less than body requirements *related to* lack of nutritional intake
- Ineffective health maintenance *related to* lack of knowledge of progression of substance abuse and its effects
- Risk for other-directed violence *related to* substance withdrawal
- Disabled family coping *related to* substance abuse by significant member with unexpressed feelings of guilt, hostility, and despair by family members

Planning

The overall goals are that the patient with addictive behaviors will (1) have normal physiologic functioning, (2) acknowledge a substance abuse problem, (3) explain the psychologic and physiologic effects of substance use, (4) abstain from the use of addicting substances, and (5) cooperate with a proposed treatment plan.

Nursing Implementation

Health Promotion. Prevention of substance abuse problems and addictive behaviors includes primary, secondary, and tertiary prevention. Primary prevention targets primarily adolescents and young adults with education about effects and negative outcomes of continued use of addictive substances. Secondary prevention focuses on early detection of substance abuse, interventions through peer or employee assistance programs, and continuing education about substance-free alternatives and stress management techniques. Tertiary prevention occurs when individuals have established dependence and includes motivating individuals to enter addiction treatment and referral to treatment and relapse prevention programs.

Acute Intervention. Acute care situations precipitated by substance abuse involve acute intoxication, overdose, or withdrawal (see Table 12-3). Intoxication responses usually last less than 24 hours and are directly related to the ingestion of psychoactive drugs. Intoxication effects are generally dose related, and symptoms usually include the desired effects of using the drug. Overdose leads to toxic reactions that may include respiratory and circulatory arrest and other life-threatening complications. Overdose occurs with the ingestion of an excessive dose of one drug or when a combination of similarly acting drugs is used. The nurse should be aware that intoxication and overdose may occur in a hospitalized patient dependent on substances if visitors provide the substances. Table 12-15 presents a timeline of commonly abused substances and routes to assist in anticipating intoxication, overdose, and withdrawal manifestations.

Alcohol Intoxication. Acute alcohol intoxication may manifest as an emergency primarily because of the narrow range between the intoxicating, the anesthetic, and the lethal doses of this drug. It is important to obtain as accurate a history as possible, using collateral information as necessary, and assess for injuries, trauma, diseases, and hypoglycemia. The basic principles of airway, breathing, and circulation (the ABCs) must be implemented. Vital signs and level of consciousness should be monitored. Generally the heart rate is normal in uncomplicated intoxication but elevated in withdrawal.

To identify Wernicke's encephalopathy in the patient with chronic alcoholism, the nurse should assess the patient for ocular abnormalities, including nystagmus and paralysis of the lateral rectus muscles, as well as ataxia and a global confusion state. Because the patient who is intoxicated may have symptoms similar to

HEALTHY PEOPLE
Health Impact of Avoiding Substance Abuse

- Reduces risk of sexually transmitted and blood-borne diseases, including HIV
- Reduces risk of heart and liver disease, cancer, and pancreatitis
- Lowers risk of accidental death from overdose, motor vehicles, and drowning
- Decreases risk of depression, abuse, teen pregnancy, suicide, and homicide
- Prevents many complications during pregnancy, including fetal alcohol syndrome

HIV, Human immunodeficiency virus.

HEALTHY PEOPLE
Health Impact of Avoiding Smoking and Environmental Tobacco Smoke

- Lowers incidence of asthma, emphysema, and chronic bronchitis
- Decreases risk of injuries and death from accidental fires
- Decreases incidence of miscarriage and premature delivery
- Reduces risk of heart disease and stroke
- Reduces risk of lung cancer and cancer of the bladder, prostate, and pancreas
- Lowers incidence of cancer of the mouth, larynx, and esophagus
- Reduces the risk of secondhand smoke exposure to family and friends

TABLE 12-15 Onset, Peak, Duration, and Withdrawal Onset of Abused Substances

Substance/Route	Onset	Peak	Duration	Onset of Withdrawal Symptoms
Inhaled				
Nicotine	Immediate	5 min	5-15 min	3-4 hr
Marijuana	5-20 min	30-60 min	3-7 hr	—
Cocaine	Immediate	5-30 min	60 min	9 hr
Inhalants	Immediate	10-15 min	20-45 min	—
Intravenous				
Cocaine	Immediate	10-20 min	20-30 min	2 hr
Opioids	Immediate	60-90 min	2-4 hr	8-10 hr
Amphetamines	Immediate	10-20 min	20-30 min	2 hr
Oral				
Alcohol	15-20 min	60-90 min	12-14 hr	10-12 hr
Amphetamines	10-30 min	60-90 min	2-4 hr	8-10 hr
Sedative-hypnotics	15-30 min	2-4 hr	4-12 hr	12-16 hr
Caffeine	10-20 min	30 min	3-7 hr	12-24 hr
Opioids	30 min	2 hr	4-8 hr	8-10 hr
Intranasal				
Cocaine	3-5 min	5-30 min	2-4 hr	4 hr
Amphetamines	3-5 min	5-20 min	45 min	2 hr
Buccal				
Nicotine	10-15 min	20-30 min	30-60 min	1-2 hr

those of encephalopathy, and because untreated encephalopathy may progress to Korsakoff's psychosis, the nurse should expect to administer IV thiamine followed by IV glucose solution to all intoxicated patients.[17]

The nurse should stay with the patient as much as possible, orienting to reality as necessary. Agitation and anxiety are common, and the patient should be assessed for increasing belligerence and a potential for violence. The patient is also at risk for injury because of lack of coordination and impaired judgment, and protective measures should be used. It is critical to continue assessment and interventions until the BAC has decreased to at least 100 mg/dl (0.10 mg%) and until any associated disorders or injuries have been ruled out. A BAC of 100 mg/dl is usually reached within 6 to 10 hours after the last intake of alcohol.

Cannabis and Hallucinogen Intoxication. In acute intoxication with marijuana or hallucinogens, the nurse should perform a physical examination, a toxicology screen, and a thorough history. The approach is basically the same for treating panic, flashbacks, and toxic reactions related to the use of marijuana or hallucinogens. An individual with cannabis intoxication or acute problems related to use of hallucinogens is seldom hospitalized. The main interventions are to provide a quiet environment and to support and reassure the patient by explaining what is happening. The patient should understand that the level of intoxication may fluctuate over several days as metabolites are released.

Overdose. A drug overdose is an emergency situation, and management is based on the type of substance involved. Drug overdose can be accidental or intentional. If multiple substances have been ingested, a complex and potentially confusing clinical picture can result. Serum and urine drug screens may be helpful in identifying the type and amounts of drugs present in the body. The first priority of care in overdose is always the patient's ABCs. Continuous monitoring of neurologic status, including level of consciousness, and respiratory and cardiovascular function is critical until the patient is stable. Vital signs and intake and output should be monitored. Emergency management of overdose and toxicity of CNS stimulants and CNS depressants is presented in Tables 12-5 and 12-9.

Pharmacologic agents are administered as ordered to counteract toxic effects of drugs. Naloxone (Narcan) and flumazenil (Romazicon) may be administered when a depressant effect is present but the ingested drug is unknown. Naloxone rapidly reverses the effects of opioids, and flumazenil reverses the effects of benzodiazepine overdose. The effects of these antagonists require frequent monitoring because these drugs have a short half-life and may need to be repeated after the initial reversal of toxic effects. Specific antagonists are not available for other drugs of abuse, but a variety of other medications may be used to control symptoms.[7]

The patient who has overdosed on sedative-hypnotics other than benzodiazepines must be treated aggressively. Dialysis may be required to decrease the drug level and to prevent irreversible CNS depressant effects and death. Gastric lavage and administration of activated charcoal may be instituted if the drug was taken orally within 4 to 6 hours. CNS stimulants are not used in the treatment of depressant drug overdose.

As soon as the patient is stable, a thorough history and physical examination must be completed. When the patient is unwilling or unable to give a history, a collateral history should be obtained from the patient's significant others. Important information to obtain includes recent drug use, including the type, amount, and time of use, and the presence of any chronic illnesses. A patient who intentionally overdosed should not be allowed to return home until seen by a psychiatric professional.

Withdrawal. In general, withdrawal signs and symptoms are opposite in nature from the direct effects of the drug (see Table 12-3). Because abused substances are psychoactive, changes are consistently noted in the neurologic system. These changes often manifest as acute anxiety and protracted depression. Withdrawal from CNS depressants, including alcohol, is the most dangerous withdrawal syndrome and may be life threatening. The nurse must be alert to the possibility of withdrawal in any patient who has a history of substance abuse.[26] In withdrawal from all abused substances, nursing management includes monitoring physiologic function, ensuring safety and comfort, preventing the progression of symptoms, providing reassurance and orientation, and motivating the patient to engage in long-term treatment.

Alcohol Withdrawal. A patient with alcohol dependence who is hospitalized for other illnesses, health conditions, or trauma can develop alcohol withdrawal syndrome when the ingestion of alcohol is abruptly stopped. The greater the patient's dependence on alcohol, the greater is the risk of serious withdrawal symptoms. The onset of signs and symptoms of alcohol withdrawal is variable depending on the patient's drinking pattern, but initial symptoms may occur 4 to 6 hours after the last drink and symptoms may last for 3 to 5 days[27] (see Tables 12-8 and 12-15).

Symptoms of alcohol withdrawal can be minimized and progression of symptoms to alcohol withdrawal delirium can be prevented by administration of benzodiazepines, such as lorazepam (Ativan). Thiamine and multiple vitamins are important to prevent or reverse Wernicke's encephalopathy to prevent progression to the irreversible Korsakoff's psychosis. Benzodiazepines and other drugs used to facilitate alcohol withdrawal[7] are identified in Table 12-8. A quiet, calm environment is important to prevent exacerbation of symptoms. The use of restraints and IV lines should be avoided whenever possible. Supportive care is needed to ensure adequate rest and nutrition. The nursing care plan for the patient in alcohol withdrawal is presented in NCP 12-1 on pp. 183 to 184.

Withdrawal from Other CNS Depressants. Withdrawal from sedative-hypnotics can be highly variable, and the severity and onset of symptoms depend on many factors, including the drug, the pattern of use, the dose and duration of use, and the presence of concurrent alcohol use. Symptoms may begin 12 hours after cessation of a short-acting drug and more than 100 hours after cessation of a long-acting drug. Withdrawal from high doses is potentially life threatening and requires close monitoring in an inpatient setting. Management of withdrawal from sedative-hypnotic agents is symptomatic and includes a gradual reduction in drug dosage. Long-acting agents such as diazepam (Valium), chlordiazepoxide (Librium), clonazepam (Klonopin), or phenobarbital may be substituted for the drug and tapered after stabilization. Mild to moderate symptoms can persist for 2 to 3 weeks after a 3- to 5-day period of acute symptoms.

Although withdrawal from opioids is not life threatening, symptoms are dramatic, temporarily disabling, and painful. Symptoms result from rebound excitability in those organs that were previously depressed by the use of opioids, and their onset and intensity depend on the pattern of use and the duration of the drug (see Table 12-15). Specific nursing approaches include careful monitoring of symptoms and providing comfort, nutrition, and hygiene. Methadone or other opioids may be administered in decreasing amounts over a period of 2 weeks to control withdrawal symptoms. Nonopioids such as benzodiazepines or clonidine (Catapres) may also be administered to reduce opioid withdrawal symptoms.[7]

Stimulant Withdrawal. Withdrawal from cocaine and amphetamines may cause very few physical symptoms, but fatigue, prolonged sleep, and depression do occur in some individuals. Craving for the drug is intense during the first hours to days of drug cessation and may continue for weeks (see Table 12-15). It is unusual for an individual dependent on stimulants to be hospitalized for management of withdrawal symptoms. However, the nurse may identify withdrawal symptoms in a patient dependent on cocaine or amphetamines who is hospitalized for other health problems. Nursing management of withdrawal symptoms is supportive and includes measures to decrease agitation and restlessness in the early phase and allowing the patient to sleep and eat as needed in later phases. Mild symptoms (e.g., headache) of stimulant withdrawal can also be experienced by the patient dependent on caffeine when meals and fluids are withheld before diagnostic testing or during a surgical experience. Withdrawal symptoms are also experienced by patients dependent on nicotine when smoking restrictions are applied. A nicotine replacement agent should be provided for tobacco users to control symptoms of withdrawal when they are hospitalized.

Perioperative Care. An individual who abuses substances is more likely to have accidents and injuries that require surgery. All trauma victims must be carefully assessed for signs and symptoms of substance overdose and withdrawal that could lead to adverse drug interactions with analgesics or anesthetics. During elective surgery in both inpatient and outpatient surgical settings, the patient dependent on substances is at risk for postoperative complications and death. Preoperative assessment must include a thorough health history and assessment of substance use, including questions related to nicotine and caffeine use. Respiratory changes in smokers make introduction of endotracheal and suction tubes more difficult and increase the risk for postoperative respiratory problems. Postoperative headaches may be caused by caffeine withdrawal in heavy users. During the patient's surgical recovery period, the nurse should be alert for signs and symptoms of drug interactions with pain medications or anesthesia or for signs of withdrawal. Special nursing considerations for the substance-abusing patient undergoing surgery are presented in Table 12-16.

TABLE 12-16 Considerations for Substance-Abusing Patients Undergoing Surgery

- Standard amounts of anesthetic and analgesic drugs may not be sufficient if patient is cross-tolerant.
- Increased doses of pain medications may be required if patient is cross-tolerant.
- Anesthetic agents may have a prolonged sedative effect if the patient has liver dysfunction. This situation requires an extended observation period.
- Patients have an increased susceptibility to cardiac and respiratory depression.
- Patients have an increased risk for bleeding, postoperative complications, and infection.
- Withdrawal symptoms from substances may be delayed for up to 5 days because of effects of anesthetics and pain medications.
- Dosage of pain medications must be reduced gradually.

Special precautions must be taken for the patient who is alcohol intoxicated or dependent and requires surgery. Alcohol use may be overlooked in an accident victim if there are injuries that cause CNS depression. Many persons are undiagnosed as alcoholics at the time of admission for elective surgery. Optimally, health problems such as malnutrition, dehydration, and infection should be treated before surgery is performed. The patient who is alcohol dependent but is not currently drinking usually requires an increased level of anesthesia because of cross-tolerance. The intoxicated individual needs a decreased level of anesthesia because of the synergistic effect of the alcohol.[17]

Whenever possible, surgery is postponed in intoxicated individuals until the BAC is less than 200 mg/dl. Synergistic effects occur with anesthesia when BAC is over 150 mg/dl. A patient with a BAC over 250 mg/dl has significantly increased surgical and mortality risks. Acute alcohol withdrawal delirium may be triggered by surgery and the cessation of alcohol consumption. Surgery should be delayed for at least 48 to 72 hours, if possible. Alcohol interferes with pulmonary function, and decreased liver function affects metabolism of many drugs. The medical problems associated with alcohol use may affect the outcome of surgery. Vital signs, including body temperature, must be closely monitored to identify signs of withdrawal, possible infections, and respiratory or cardiac problems. Anesthetics and pain medications used in the acute period can delay withdrawal symptoms for up to 5 days postoperatively.[26]

Pain Management. Nurses and physicians have historically been reluctant to administer opioids to substance-abusing patients for fear of promoting or enhancing addictions. However, there is no evidence that providing opioid analgesia to these patients in any way worsens their addictive disease. In fact, the stress of unrelieved pain may contribute to relapse in the recovering patient or increased drug use in the patient who is actively using or abusing drugs. Guidelines for pain management in patients with addictive disease have been established by the American Society of Pain Management Nurses. These guidelines reflect the nurse's role in a multimodal team approach to treatment of addiction in which patients with addictive disease and pain have the right to be treated with dignity, respect, and the same quality of pain assessment and management as all other patients.[28]

If the patient acknowledges opioid use, it is important to determine the types and amounts of drugs used. It is best to avoid exposing the patient to the drug of abuse, and effective equianalgesic doses of other opioids may be determined if daily drug doses are known. If a history of drug abuse is unknown, or if the patient does not acknowledge substance abuse, the nurse should suspect abuse when normal doses of analgesics do not relieve the patient's pain. Aggressive behavior patterns and signs of withdrawal may also occur. Withdrawal symptoms can exacerbate pain and lead to drug-seeking behavior or illicit drug use. Toxicology screens may be helpful in determining recently used drugs. Discussing these findings with the patient may help gain the patient's cooperation in pain control.

Severe pain should be treated with opioids, and at much higher doses than those used with drug-naive patients. The use of one opioid is preferred. A mixed opioid agonist-antagonist such as butorphanol (Stadol) or a partial agonist such as buprenorphine (Buprenex) should be avoided because these may precipitate withdrawal symptoms. Nonopioid and adjuvant analgesics and nonpharmacologic pain relief measures may also be used as appropriate. To maintain opioid blood levels and prevent withdrawal symptoms, analgesics should be provided around the clock. Supplemental doses should be used to treat breakthrough pain. Patient-controlled analgesia (PCA) may be considered to improve pain control and reduce drug-seeking behavior.

A written agreement or treatment plan that describes the pain management should be developed with the patient. The plan should ensure that pain will be treated based on the patient's perception and report of pain. In addition, the plan should clearly outline the gradual tapering of the analgesic dose, with eventual substitution of parenteral analgesics with long-acting oral preparations, and possibly cessation of opioids by the time of discharge.[28]

Motivational Interviewing for Addictive Behaviors. The nurse is in a unique position to motivate and facilitate addictive behavior change while caring for patients in primary and acute care settings. Recognition of the health problems associated with substance abuse and the effects of chronic alcohol abuse identified in Tables 12-2 and 12-7 can help nurses identify patients with addictive behaviors. When patients seek care for health problems related to substance abuse or when hospitalization interferes with the patient's usual pattern of substance use, the patient's awareness of problems associated with addictive behaviors is increased. Intervention by nurses at this time can be a crucial factor in promoting behavior change.

A current Treatment Improvement Protocol (TIP), *Enhancing Motivation for Change in Substance Abuse Treatment,* is a best practice guideline provided by the Substance Abuse and Mental Health Services Administration's Center for Substance Abuse Treatment.[29] This protocol describes the use of motivational interviewing developed by Miller and Rollnick.[30] **Motivational interviewing** uses nonconfrontational interpersonal communication techniques to motivate patients to change behavior. The techniques are linked to the stages of change as identified by Prochaska and DiClemente in the transtheoretical model of change.[31] The stages of change identified in the **transtheoretical model of change** include precontemplation, contemplation, preparation, action, maintenance, and termination, as described in Chapter 5. The first five stages are applied in motivational interviewing. The stages are not viewed as linear, but rather as a cycle through which patients move back and forth. During the process of change, relapse and recycling is an expected finding. Patients who do not change behaviors or who return to substance use after a period of cessation are often labeled "noncompliant" and "unmotivated." However, this may reflect a predictable relapse or may indicate that the interventions used do not consider the patient's stage of change.[32] Therefore it is important for the nurse to identify the patient's current stage of readiness for change and the stage to which the patient is moving. Patients who are in the early stages of change need and use different kinds of motivational support than patients at later stages of change.

Motivational interviewing includes the use of any intervention that enhances the patient's motivation for change. The interventions are those that respect the patient's autonomy and establish a nonjudgmental, collaborative relationship.[29] The key aspects of successful motivational interviewing are presented in Table 12-17.

A substance-abusing patient who seeks care for a medical problem or is hospitalized is often in the *precontemplation* or *contemplation* stage of change. In the precontemplation stage patients are not concerned about their substance use and are not considering changing their behavior. An example is when a patient is asked if he thinks his smoking contributes to his shortness of breath and he replies that he does not think so because he has never had it before during years of smoking. During this stage it is most important for the nurse to help the patient increase awareness of risks and problems related to the current behavior and to create doubt about the use of substances.[29] Asking the patient what he or she thinks could happen if the behavior is continued, providing evidence of the problem such as abnormal laboratory values, and offering factual information about the risks of substance abuse are indicated. Although patients may not be ready to change behavior while experiencing an acute health problem, the seeds of doubt can be sown. In other cases, such as when a patient experiences a life-threatening condition, there may be an immediate awareness of the problem and motivation to change.

TABLE 12-17 Key Aspects of Successful Motivational Interviewing

- Listen rather than tell.
- Adjust to, rather than oppose, patient resistance.
- Express empathy through reflective listening.
- Focus on the positive; do not "put a person down."
- Gently persuade, with the understanding that change is up to the patient.
- Focus on the patient's strengths to support the hope and optimism needed to make changes.
- Avoid argument and direct confrontation, which can cause defensiveness and a power struggle.
- Help the patient recognize the "gap" between where he or she is and where he or she hopes to be.

A patient in the *contemplation* stage of change often experiences ambivalence. The patient understands that the behavior is a problem and that change is necessary. However, he feels that change is too difficult or that the pleasures of using the behavior are worth the risks. This can be seen in the patient who says, "I know that I have to stop drinking. This car accident almost killed me. And one more traffic ticket while I'm intoxicated means I'll lose my license. But all my friends drink, and it is the only way I can relax. I don't think I can stop." During this stage of change the nurse should help the patient thoughtfully consider the positive and negative aspects of his or her substance use, gently trying to tip the balance in favor of beneficial behavior. Helping the patient discover internal motivators in addition to those external motivators (e.g., accidents, traffic tickets, legal and health problems, costs) that push the patient toward change can move the patient from contemplating change to preparation and action. Summarizing the patient's concerns and affirming the patient's ambivalence are useful techniques. Throughout this process, the patient's personal choices and responsibilities for change should be emphasized.[29]

As the patient moves from contemplation to *preparation,* a commitment to change can be strengthened by helping the patient develop self-efficacy. *Self-efficacy* in this case is the patient's optimism that substance-use behaviors can be changed, and the nurse should support even the smallest effort to change. Movement through action and maintenance stages of change requires continued support to increase the patient's involvement and participation in treatment. A comprehensive discussion of motivational interviewing throughout the entire change process is presented in the Treatment Improvement Protocol available at *www.ncbi.nlm.nih.gov/books/bv.fcgi?rid=hstat5.chapter.61302.*

The resolution of acute health problems or discharge from the hospital often occurs before the patient moves to the preparation and action stages of change. It is critical that, as the patient develops readiness to change in the contemplative stage of change, support of the change process be continued by referral to appropriate community and outpatient resources.

Ambulatory and Home Care. Before treatment and rehabilitation for addiction are considered, acute health problems must be resolved. Many of the patients with substance abuse problems that the nurse encounters in hospitals and primary care centers seek care because of health problems associated with substance abuse, not to receive care for the addiction. It is the nurse's responsibility, in collaboration with a multidisciplinary team composed of physicians, social workers, and addiction specialists, to address the patient's substance problem and motivate the patient to change behaviors and seek treatment for the addiction. Although the nurse working in the medical-surgical setting is not usually involved in long-term treatment of patients with addictive behaviors, it is the nurse's responsibility to identify the problem, increase the patient's awareness of the problem, and be able to refer the patient to inpatient and outpatient programs in the community that provide treatment and rehabilitation. Failure to confront the patient's addiction, thus enabling the patient's addictive behavior, is a breach of professional responsibility.

GERONTOLOGIC CONSIDERATIONS
ADDICTIVE BEHAVIORS

Substance misuse, abuse, and dependence in older adults are much less likely to be recognized by nurses and other health care providers than in younger adults. Older adults do not fit the image that most people in today's society have of those who abuse substances. In addition, patterns of substance use in older adults are different from those in younger and middle-age adults. Because alcohol and substance abuse among older adults is often mistaken for other conditions (e.g., neuropathy, anemia, mental status changes) associated with the aging process, the problem is often undiagnosed and untreated.

Although illicit drug use is minimal in older adults except for long-term addicts, older adults have the highest use of over-the-counter (OTC) and prescription drugs.[33] The prescription drugs used by older adults are primarily psychoactive in nature, including sedative, hypnotic, anxiolytic, and opioid agents. Older women are more likely than men to become dependent on prescription drugs, especially benzodiazepines.[34] Simultaneous use of OTC drugs, prescription drugs, and alcohol occurs in many older adults. This presents a pattern of drug misuse and abuse that is not commonly seen in younger populations.

The effects of alcohol and other psychoactive substances increase with aging. Age-related decreases in circulation, metabolism, and excretion slow the body's detoxification of drugs, potentiate tolerance, and accelerate physical dependence on addictive substances. Physiologic changes that accompany aging may lead to intoxication at levels that may not have been a problem earlier in life.[34]

The adverse effects of interaction of alcohol and other drugs also increase with aging. When taken with alcohol, sedative-hypnotic drugs, minor tranquilizers, and CNS depressants have additive and synergistic effects. Misuse and abuse of psychoactive agents, either alone or in combination, by older adults may cause confusion, disorientation, delirium, memory loss, and neuromuscular impairment. The effects of alcohol and drug use can also be mistaken for medical or psychiatric conditions common among older adults, such as insomnia, depression, poor nutrition, heart failure, and frequent falls. Withdrawal symptoms also occur in the older adult when alcohol, opioids, or sedative-hypnotics are abruptly stopped and may be more severe than in younger individuals. Because of the possibility of alcohol use in older adults, the nurse should always consider that behavior changes in the older patient may be caused by alcohol use or withdrawal.

Identification of substance misuse, abuse, and dependence in the older patient presents a challenge. Family members who are concerned about a patient's possible problem are important sources of information. Evidence of addictive disorders is not always obvious in the older adult, and manifestations may be similar to those caused by common health problems of the elderly. As with all patients, it is important for the nurse to discuss all drug and alcohol use with older patients, including OTC, herbal, and homeopathic drug use. The patient's knowledge of medications that are currently being taken should be assessed.

Questionnaires customarily used to screen for alcoholism may be inappropriate for the older adult, who may not exhibit the social, legal, and occupational consequences of alcohol abuse generally used to diagnose problem drinkers. However, the AUDIT questionnaire described earlier has been found to be appropriate for screening older adults for alcoholism.[35] Screening for warning signs such as unexplained falls; neglect of personal hygiene; and complaints of mood, sleep, or memory problems is important.

Smoking and other tobacco use is also an issue in older adults. Older adults who have been chronic smokers for decades can feel unable to stop, or may feel that there is no benefit to stopping at an advanced age. However, smoking contributes to and exacerbates many chronic illnesses found in the older population, and smoking cessation at any age is beneficial. In fact, many older adults want to quit smoking and have proven to be more successful in their attempts at quitting than younger populations.[36] The clinical practice guideline on treating tobacco use and dependence discussed earlier is appropriate for helping older adults with smoking cessation (see Tables 12-4, 12-5, and 12-6).

Patient education for the older adult includes teaching about the desired effects, possible side effects, and appropriate use of prescribed and OTC drugs. The nurse should recommend that the patient use only one pharmacy because many pharmacies maintain a drug profile that may prevent problems with drug interactions. Patients should be advised not to drink alcohol when using prescribed and OTC drugs. Where there is no medical condition or possible drug interactions that would preclude the use of alcohol, older patients should be advised to limit their alcohol intake to one drink per day.

Developmental, physical, and psychosocial changes that occur with aging contribute to the late-onset abuse of alcohol and other drugs by older adults. The older adult may have difficulty coping with losses that occur with increasing age, such as retirement, death of family and friends, relocation, social isolation, and poor health. When risks are identified, these individuals can be taught coping skills and introduced to support services. Home visits by a nurse provide a good source of assessment of the problems and also provide valuable support. When the nurse suspects an alcohol or substance dependence in the older patient, the nurse should refer the patient for treatment. It is a mistaken belief that older persons have little to gain from alcohol and drug dependence treatment. The rewards of treatment can lead to greater quality and quantity of life for older adults.

CRITICAL THINKING EXERCISE

CASE STUDY

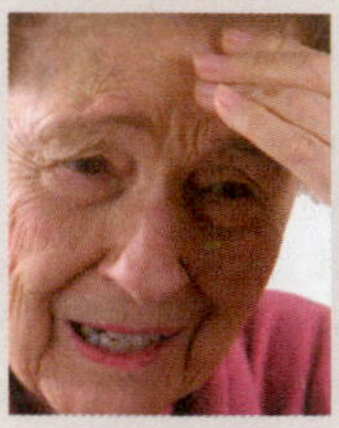

Case Study photo ©iStockphoto.com/ Lisa Kyle Young.

Substance Misuse and Abuse

Patient Profile. Mrs. Carla Miller, a 78-year-old white woman, is admitted to the emergency department after falling and injuring her right shoulder and arm. She has been widowed for 4 years and lives alone. Recently her best friend died. Her only family is a daughter who lives out of town. When the nurse contacts the daughter by phone, she tells the nurse that her mother has appeared to be more disoriented and confused over the past year when she has talked to her on the phone.

Subjective Data

- Is complaining of severe pain in her right shoulder and upper arm
- Admits she had some wine in the late afternoon to stimulate her appetite
- Has experienced several falls in the past 2 months
- Reports that she fell after taking her sleeping pill prescribed by her physician because she does not sleep well
- Speech is hesitant and slurred
- Says she smokes about one-half pack of cigarettes a day

Objective Data

Physical Examination

- Oriented to person and place, but not time
- Blood pressure 162/94, pulse 92, respirations 24
- Bruising and edema of right upper arm
- Tremors of hands

Diagnostic Tests

- X-ray reveals comminuted fracture of the proximal humerus requiring surgical repair
- Blood alcohol concentration (BAC) 120 mg/dl (0.12 mg%)
- Complete blood count: hemoglobin 10.6 g/dl, hematocrit 38%

Critical Thinking Questions

1. What other information is needed to assess Mrs. Miller's condition?
2. How should questions regarding these areas be addressed?
3. What factors may contribute to Mrs. Miller's use of psychoactive substances?
4. What nursing interventions are appropriate during Mrs. Miller's preoperative period?
5. What possible complications and other health problems may become apparent during Mrs. Miller's postoperative recovery?
6. What nursing interventions are appropriate following Mrs. Miller's surgery?
7. Based on the assessment data presented, write one or more nursing diagnoses. Are there any collaborative problems?

NCLEX EXAMINATION REVIEW QUESTIONS

The number of the question corresponds to the same-numbered objective at the beginning of the chapter.

1. A person who injects heroin to experience the euphoria it causes is demonstrating
   a. abuse.
   b. addiction.
   c. tolerance.
   d. addictive behavior.
2. The effects of long-term addictive substances on the brain lead to
   a. increased availability of dopamine.
   b. destruction of the mesolimbic system.
   c. loss of pleasure from experiences that previously resulted in enjoyment.
   d. potentiation of effects of similar drugs taken when the individual is drug free.
3. A major public health problem related to the behaviors of substance abuse is the prevalence of
   a. hepatitis C.
   b. malnutrition.
   c. infective endocarditis.
   d. respiratory depression and arrest.
4. The nurse would suspect cocaine overdose in the patient who is experiencing
   a. craving, restlessness, and irritability.
   b. agitation, cardiac dysrhythmia, and seizures.
   c. diarrhea, nausea and vomiting, and confusion.
   d. slow, shallow respirations, hyporeflexia, and blurred vision.
5. The most appropriate nursing intervention for a patient who is seen at the clinic for increasing shortness of breath but who is not interested in quitting smoking is to
   a. accept the patient's decision and not intervene until the patient expresses a desire to quit.
   b. realize that some smokers will never quit, and trying to assist them only increases the patient's and the nurse's frustration.
   c. increase the patient's motivation to quit by explaining that continued smoking will only increase the breathing problems.
   d. ask the patient at every clinic visit to identify the relevance, risks, and benefits of quitting and what barriers to quitting are present.
6. While caring for a patient who is experiencing alcohol withdrawal the nurse should
   a. provide a quiet, nonstimulating, dimly lit environment.
   b. orient the patient to the environment and personnel with each contact.
   c. assist the patient to ambulate frequently to increase the metabolism of alcohol.
   d. provide stimulant beverages such as coffee or tea to counteract the effects of alcohol.
7. A patient who is dependent on intravenous barbiturates is scheduled for surgery following an automobile accident. The nurse recognizes that this patient
   a. may need less pain medication during the postoperative period.
   b. should be provided with tapering doses of barbiturates following surgery.
   c. may have an immediate onset of withdrawal symptoms when given anesthetic and analgesic agents.
   d. has a low risk for physical withdrawal symptoms but is likely to experience craving and drug-seeking behavior during the postoperative period.
8. When caring for a patient following surgery for a fractured femur who is dependent on opioids, the nurse should
   a. avoid giving narcotics.
   b. provide patient-controlled analgesia.
   c. insist that the patient stop all drugs of abuse.
   d. treat the patient's report of pain with opioids.
9. During motivational interviewing with a patient, the nurse should
   a. insist that the patient maintain abstinence while undergoing therapy.
   b. relate motivational techniques to the patient's stage of behavior change.

c. use any method of communication that will make the patient change behavior.
d. ask a prescribed set of questions to increase the patient's awareness of addiction behaviors.

10. Substance abuse problems in older adults are most commonly related to
    a. use of drugs and alcohol as a social activity.
    b. misuse of prescribed and over-the-counter drugs and alcohol.
    c. continuing the use of illegal drugs initiated during middle age.
    d. a pattern of binge drinking for weeks or months with periods of sobriety.

REFERENCES

1. Office of Applied Studies: *Overview of findings from the 2003 national survey on drug use and health*, DHHS Publication No. SMA 04-3963, Rockville, Md, 2004, Substance Abuse and Mental Health Services Administration (SAMHSA), US Department of Health and Human Services.
2. American Psychiatric Association: *The diagnostic and statistical manual of mental disorders DMS-IV-TR,* ed 4, Washington, DC, 2000, American Psychiatric Association.
3. Goulding PM: *Drugs of abuse*, Lakeway, Tex, 2003, National Center of Continuing Education, Inc.
4. Johnson BA: The biologic basis of alcohol dependence, *Advanced Studies in Nursing* 2(2):48, 2004.
5. Zickler P: Genetic variation may increase nicotine craving and smoking relapse, *NIDA Notes* 18:3, 2003.
6. Hanson GR: In drug abuse, gender matters, *NIDA Notes* 17:2, 2002.
7. Lehne RA: *Pharmacology for nursing care*, ed 5, St Louis, 2004, Saunders.
8. Zickler P: Nicotine's multiple effects on the brain's reward system drive addiction, *NIDA Notes* 17:6, 2003.
9. National Institute on Drug Abuse: *NIDA infofacts: cigarettes and other nicotine products*, Bethesda, MD, 2005, NIDA. Available at *www.drugabuse.gov/infofacts/tobacco.html* (accessed June 20, 2005).
10. Sarna L, Bialous SA: Why tobacco is a women's health issue, *Nurs Clin North Am* 39:165, 2004.
11. Asplund K: Smokeless tobacco and cardiovascular disease, *Prog Cardiovasc Dis* 45(5):383, 2003.
12. Zickler P: Early nicotine initiation increases severity of addiction, vulnerability to some effects of cocaine, *NIDA Notes* 19:2, 2004.
13. Anthonisen NR, Skeans MA, Wise RA, et al: The effects of a smoking cesstion intervention on 14.5-year mortality: a randomized clinical trial, *Ann Intern Med* 142(4):233, 2005.
14. FDA News: FDA approves novel medication for smoking cessation, 2006, Food and Drug Administration. Available at *www.fda.gov/bbs/topics/NEWS/2006/NEW01370.html* (accessed May 17, 2006).
15. Bialous SA, Sarna L: Sparing a few minutes for tobacco cessation, *Am J Nurs* 104(12):54, 2004.
16. US Department of Health and Human Services: *Healthy people 2010*, Washington, DC, 2004, US Department of Health and Human Services. Available at *www.healthypeople.gov* (accessed May 12, 2006).
17. US Department of Health and Human Services: *Clinical practice guideline: treating tobacco use and dependence,* Washington, DC, 2000, US Public Health Service.
18. National Institute on Drug Abuse: *NIDA infofacts: methamphetamines*, Bethesda, Md, 2005, NIDA. Available at *www.nida.nih.gov/infofacts/methamphetamine.html* (accessed May 12, 2006).
19. Reid TR: Caffeine, *National Geographic* 204(1):2, 2005.
20. Bridle L, Remick J, Duffy E: Is caffeine excess part of your differential diagnosis? *Nurse Pract* 29(4):39, 2004.
21. Yost DA: Acute care for alcohol intoxication, *Postgrad Med* 112(6):14, 2002.
22. Mayo-Smith MF, Beecher LH, Fischer TL, et al: Management of alcohol withdrawal delirium. An evidence-based practice guideline, *Arch Intern Med* 164(18):1405, 2004.
23. FDA talk paper: FDA approves new drug for treatment of alcoholism, 2004, Food and Drug Administration. Available at *www.fda.gov/bbs/topics/ANSWERS/2004/ANS01302.html* (accessed June 20, 2005).
24. National Institute on Drug Abuse: *NIDA research report series: heroin abuse and addiction*, NIH Publication No. 05-4165, 2005, NIDA. Available at *www.nida.nih/gov/ResearchReports/Heroin/heroin4.html* (accessed May 12, 2006).
25. Substance Abuse and Mental Health Services Administration: Buprenorphine, 2003, SAMHSA. Available at *http://buprenorphine.samhsa.gov/about.html* (accessed May 12, 2006).
26. Kelly AE, Saucier J: Is your patient suffering from alcohol withdrawal? *RN* 67(2):27, 2004.
27. Smith-Alnimer M, Watford MF: Alcohol withdrawal and delirium tremens, *Am J Nurs* 104(5):72A, 2004.
28. Nichols R: Pain management in patients with addictive disease, *Am J Nurs* 103(3):87, 2003.
29. Miller WR: Enhancing motivation for change in substance abuse treatment: treatment improvement protocol (TIP) series 35, DHHS Publication No. (SMA) 99-3354, Rockville, Md, 1999, US Department of Health and Human Services. Available at *http://hstat.nlm.nih.gov/hp/Hquest/db/local.tip.tip35/screen/TocDisplay/da/1/s/36610/action/Toc* (accessed May 12, 2006).
30. Miller RW, Rollnick S: Preparing people to change addictive behavior, New York, 1991, Guilford Press.
31. Prochaska JO, DiClemente CC: *The transtheoretical approach: crossing traditional boundaries of therapy,* Homewood, Ill, 1984, Dow Jones–Irwin.
32. Lange N, Tigges BB: Influence positive change with motivational interviewing, *Nurse Pract* 30(3):44, 2005.
33. Office of Applied Studies: *The NSDUH report: substance use among older adults: 2002 and 2003 update,* Rockville, Md, 2005, Substance Abuse and Mental Health Services Administration (SAMHSA), US Department of Health and Human Services.
34. Lantz MS: Prescription drug and alcohol abuse in an older woman, *Clin Geriatr* 13(1):39, 2005.
35. O'Connell H, Chin AV, Hamilton F, et al: A systematic review of the utility of self-report alcohol screening instruments in the elderly, *Int J Geriatr Psychiatry* 19(11):1074, 2004.
36. Lantz MS: Smoking cessation: don't give up on older adults, *Clin Geriatr* 12(8):11, 2004.

RESOURCES

Alcoholics Anonymous
212-870-3400
www.alcoholics-anonymous.org

American Lung Association
212-315-8700
www.lungusa.org

American Psychiatric Nurses Association
703-243-2443
Email: info@apna.org
www.apna.org

American Society of Addiction Medicine
301-656-3920
Email: Email@asam.org
www.asam.org

International Nurses Society on Addictions
919-821-1292
www.intnsa.org

Narcotics Anonymous
818-773-9999
www.na.org

National Clearinghouse for Alcohol and Drug Information
301-468-2600
800-729-6686
Email: info@health.org
www.health.org/about

National Council on Alcoholism and Drug Dependence, Inc.
212-269-7797
Hope Line: 800-NCA-CALL
Email: national@ncadd.org
www.ncadd.org

National Institute on Drug Abuse
301-443-1124
www.nida.nih.gov

Tobacco Information and Prevention Source (TIPS)
404-488-5705
Email: tobaccoinfo@cdc.gov
www.cdc.gov/tobacco

For additional Internet resources, see the website for this book at *http://evolve.elsevier.com/Lewis/medsurg.*

Section

2

Pathophysiologic Mechanisms of Disease

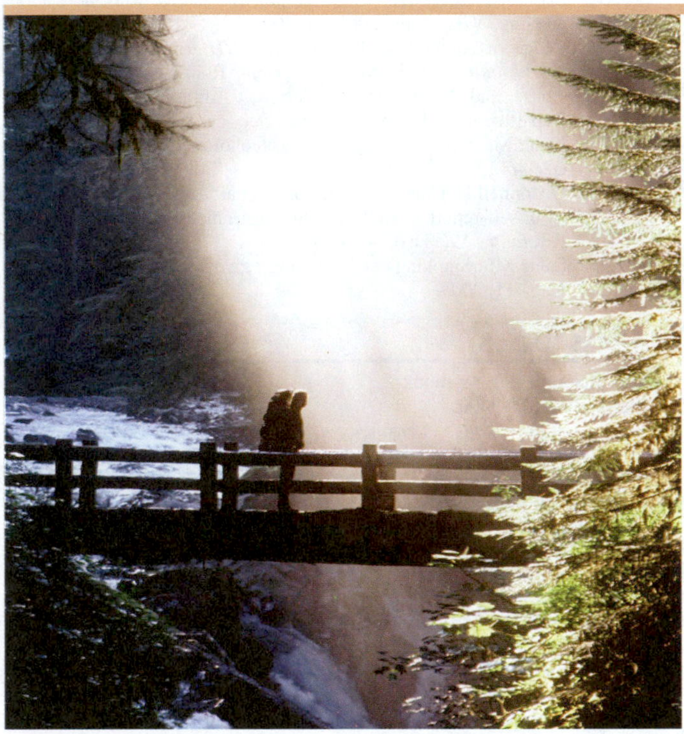

Section Outline

How wonderful it is that nobody need wait a single moment before starting to improve the world.
Anne Frank

Inflammation and Wound Healing

13

Sharon L. Lewis

LEARNING OBJECTIVES

1. Describe the inflammatory response, including vascular and cellular responses and exudate formation.
2. Explain local and systemic manifestations of inflammation and their physiologic bases.
3. Differentiate among healing by primary, secondary, and tertiary intention.
4. Describe the factors that delay wound healing and common complications of wound healing.
5. Describe the drug therapy, nutrition therapy, and nursing management of inflammation.
6. Describe the nursing and collaborative management of wound healing.
7. Describe a patient risk assessment for pressure ulcers and measures to prevent the development of pressure ulcers.
8. Explain the etiology and clinical manifestations of pressure ulcers.
9. Discuss nursing and collaborative management of a patient with pressure ulcers.

KEY TERMS

adhesions, p. 201
dehiscence, p. 201
evisceration, p. 201
fibroblasts, p. 198
hypertrophic scar, p. 201
inflammatory response, p. 193
pressure ulcer, p. 206
regeneration, p. 197
repair, p. 198
shearing force, p. 206

Electronic Resources

Supplemental content related to Chapter 13 can be found . . .

Companion CD

- Stress-Busting Kit for Nursing Students
- Interactive Case Study: Pressure Ulcers
- NCLEX Examination Review Questions
- Comprehensive Glossary

Evolve Website evolve

http://evolve.elsevier.com/Lewis/medsurg

- Content Updates
- Key Points (Printable and CD/MP3 Download)
- Concept Map Creator
- Expanded Audio Glossary
- Key Term Flash Cards
- Customizable Nursing Care Plans:
  - Fever
  - Pressure Ulcer
- Electronic Calculators
- WebLinks

This chapter focuses on inflammation and wound healing. Assessment of pressure ulcer risk factors, and interventions to prevent and treat pressure ulcers are also described.

INFLAMMATORY RESPONSE

The **inflammatory response** is a sequential reaction to cell injury. It neutralizes and dilutes the inflammatory agent, removes necrotic materials, and establishes an environment suitable for healing and repair. The term *inflammation* is often but incorrectly used as a synonym for the term *infection.* Inflammation is always present with infection, but infection is not always present with inflammation. However, a person who is neutropenic may not be able to mount an inflammatory response. An infection involves invasion of tissues or cells by microorganisms such as bacteria, fungi, and viruses. In contrast, inflammation can also be caused by nonliving agents such as heat, radiation, trauma, and allergens. If infection is present with inflammation, it is from a superimposed invasion of microorganisms.

The mechanism of inflammation is basically the same regardless of the injuring agent. The intensity of the response depends on the extent and severity of injury and on the reactive capacity of the injured person. The inflammatory response can be divided into a vascular response, a cellular response, formation of exudate, and healing.

Vascular Response

After cell injury, arterioles in the area briefly undergo transient vasoconstriction. After release of histamine and other chemicals by the injured cells, the vessels dilate. This vasodilation results in *hyperemia* (increased blood flow in the area), which raises fil-

Reviewed by Robert B. Babiak, RN, BSN, CWOCN, Wound, Ostomy, Continent Nurse, St. Luke's Baptist Hospital, San Antonio, Tex.; and Sandra Hoffman, APRN-BC, MSN, Clinical Assistant Professor, School of Nursing, University of North Carolina at Chapel Hill, Chapel Hill, N. C.

tration pressure. Vasodilation and chemical mediators cause endothelial cell retraction, which increases capillary permeability. Movement of fluid from capillaries into tissue spaces is facilitated by both of these responses. Initially composed of serous fluid, this inflammatory exudate later contains plasma proteins, primarily albumin, because of increased permeability of blood vessels. The proteins exert oncotic pressure that further draws fluid from blood vessels. The tissue becomes edematous. This response is illustrated in Fig. 13-1.

As the plasma protein fibrinogen leaves the blood, it is activated to fibrin by the products of the injured cells. Fibrin strengthens a blood clot formed by platelets. In tissue the clot functions to trap bacteria, to prevent their spread, and to serve as a framework for the healing process.

Cellular Response

The cellular response to injury is illustrated in Fig. 13-2. The blood flow through capillaries in the area slows as fluid is lost and viscosity increases. Neutrophils and monocytes move to the inner surface of the capillaries *(margination)* and then, in ameboid fashion, through the capillary wall *(diapedesis)* to the site of injury (Fig. 13-3).

Chemotaxis is the directional migration of white blood cells (WBCs) along a concentration gradient of chemotactic factors, which are substances that attract leukocytes to the site of inflammation. Chemotaxis is the mechanism for ensuring accumulation of neutrophils and monocytes at the focus of injury.

Neutrophils. Neutrophils are the first leukocytes to arrive (usually within 6 to 12 hours). They phagocytize (engulf) bacteria, other foreign material, and damaged cells. With their short life span (24 to 48 hours), dead neutrophils soon accumulate. In time a mixture of dead neutrophils, digested bacteria, and other cell debris accumulates as a creamy substance termed *pus.*

To keep up with the demand for neutrophils, the bone marrow releases more neutrophils into circulation. This results in an elevated WBC count, especially the neutrophil count. Sometimes the demand for neutrophils increases to the extent that the bone marrow releases immature forms of neutrophils *(bands)* into circulation. (Mature neutrophils are called segmented neutrophils.) The finding of increased numbers of band neutrophils in circulation is called a *shift to the left,* which is commonly found in patients with acute bacterial infections. (See Chapter 30 for a discussion on neutrophils.)

Monocytes. Monocytes are the second type of phagocytic cells that migrate from circulating blood. They are attracted to the site by chemotactic factors and usually arrive at the site within 3 to 7 days after the onset of inflammation. On entering the tissue spaces, monocytes transform into macrophages. Together with the tissue macrophages, these newly arrived macrophages assist in phagocytosis of the inflammatory debris. The macrophage role is important in cleaning the area before healing can occur. Macrophages have a long life span; they can multiply and may stay in the

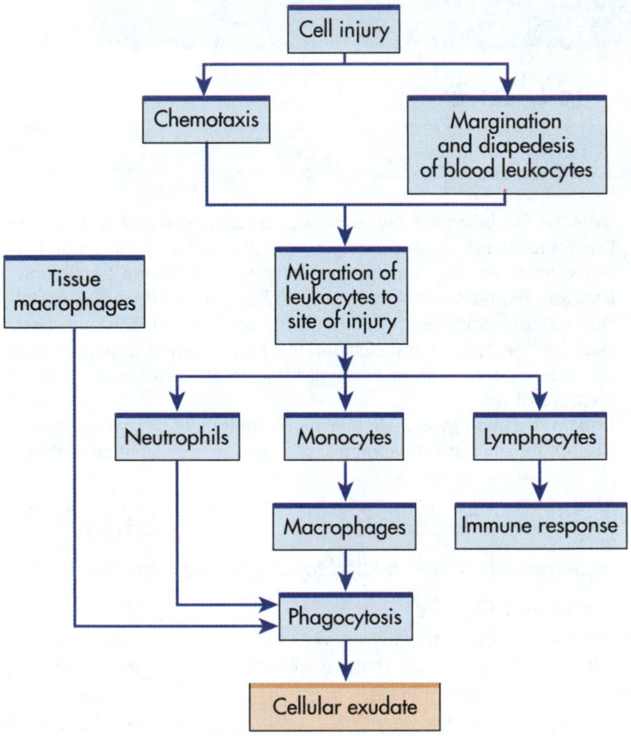

FIG. 13-2 Cellular response in inflammation.

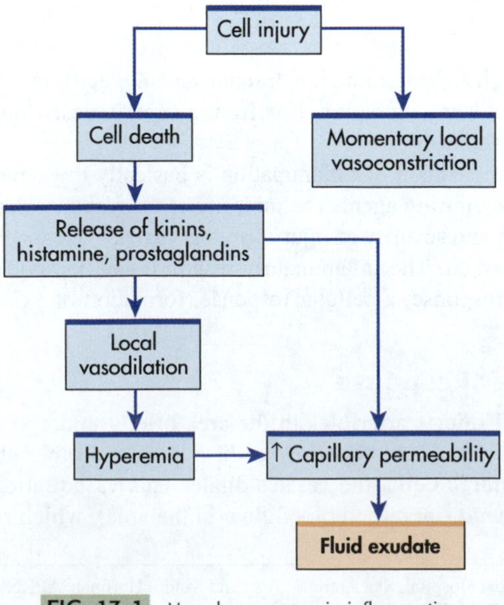

FIG. 13-1 Vascular response in inflammation.

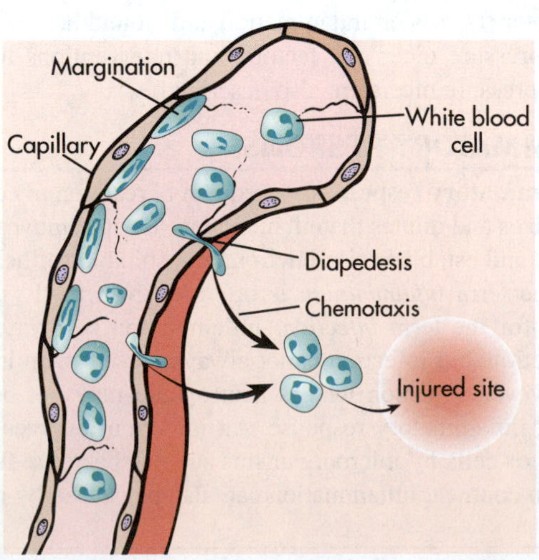

FIG. 13-3 Margination, diapedesis, and chemotaxis of white blood cells.

damaged tissues for weeks. These long-lived cells are important in orchestrating the healing process.

In some cases, macrophages perform tasks other than phagocytosis. They may accumulate and fuse to form a *multinucleated giant cell.* The giant cell attempts to phagocytize particles too large for macrophages. The giant cell is then encapsulated by collagen, leading to the formation of a granuloma. A classic example of this process occurs with the tubercle bacillus in the lung. While the bacillus is walled off, a chronic state of inflammation exists. The granuloma formed is a cavity of necrotic tissue.

Lymphocytes. Lymphocytes arrive later at the site of injury. Their primary role is related to humoral and cell-mediated immunity (see Chapter 14).

Eosinophils and Basophils. Eosinophils and basophils have a more selective role in inflammation. Eosinophils are released in large quantities during an allergic reaction. They release chemicals that act to control the effects of histamine and serotonin. They are also involved in phagocytosis of the allergen-antibody complex. Eosinophils also contain highly caustic chemicals that are capable of destroying a parasite's cell surfaces. The histamine and heparin that basophils carry in their granules are released during inflammation.

Chemical Mediators

Mediators of the inflammatory response are presented in Table 13-1.

Complement System. The complement system is a major mediator of the inflammatory response. Major functions of the complement system are enhanced phagocytosis, increased vascular permeability, chemotaxis, and cellular lysis. All of these activities are important in the inflammatory response.

When activated, the components occur in the sequential order of C1, C4, C2, C3, C5, C6, C7, C8, and C9 (Fig. 13-4). The numbering reflects the order of their discovery. Some components have subparts designated by lowercase letters, such as C3a, C3b, and C5a. The primary pathway for activation of the complement system is through fixation of component C1 to an antigen-antibody complex. The immunoglobulins IgG and IgM are responsible for fixing complement. Each activated complex can act on the next component, thus creating a cascade effect.

An alternative pathway exists in which C3 is activated without prior antigen-antibody fixation. Bacterial products, lipopolysaccharides, and neutrophil proteases can stimulate the complement sequence at the C3 level with activation of C5 through C9.

Complement activation increases phagocytosis through opsonization and chemotaxis. *Opsonization* occurs when the antigen, in combination with complement factor C3b and immunoglobulin, sticks to the surface of phagocytic cells. This leads to more rapid phagocytosis. In addition, complement component C5a promotes chemotaxis.

Complement activation is also involved in the anaphylactoid reaction. The components C3a, C5a, and C4a are termed *anaphylatoxins* and bind to receptors on mast cells and basophils, thus triggering histamine release. Histamine causes smooth muscle contraction, vasodilation, and an increase in vascular permeability.

The entire complement sequence of C1 to C9 must be activated for cell lysis to occur. The final components (C8, C9) act on the cell surface, causing rupture of the cell membrane and lysis. Bacteria, red blood cells (RBCs), and nucleated cells are susceptible to the lysis.

Prostaglandins and Leukotrienes. Prostaglandins (PGs) are substances that can be synthesized from the phospholipids of cell membranes of most body tissues, including blood cells. On stimulation by chemotactic factors or phagocytosis or after cell injury, phospholipids can be converted to arachidonic acid (a 20-carbon polyunsaturated fatty acid), which is then oxidized by two different pathways (Fig. 13-5).

The *cyclooxygenase metabolic pathway* leads to the production of PGs of the D, E, F, and I series and thromboxanes (formed on activation of platelets). PGs of the E and I series are potent vasodilators and inhibit platelet and neutrophil aggregation. PGE_2 can also sensitize pain receptors to arousal by stimuli that would normally be painless. PGE_2 is also a potent pyrogen, acting on the temperature-regulating area of the hypothalamus. Thromboxane A_2 is a powerful vasoconstrictor and platelet-aggregating agent. PGs are generally considered proinflammatory, contributing to increased blood flow, edema, and pain. Metabolism of arachidonic acid by the *lipoxygenase pathway* leads to the production of leukotrienes (LTs). LTB_4 is a potent chemotactic factor. LTC_4, LTD_4, and LTE_4 form the slow-reacting substance of anaphylaxis (SRS-A), which constricts smooth muscles of bronchi and increases capillary permeability.

Drugs that inhibit PG synthesis are useful clinically. Nonsteroidal antiinflammatory drugs (NSAIDs), one type of these drugs, are a prototype drug treatment for many acute and chronic inflammatory

TABLE 13-1 Mediators of Inflammation

Mediator	Source	Mechanisms of Action
Histamine	Stored in granules of basophils, mast cells, platelets	Causes vasodilation and increased vascular permeability by stimulating contraction of endothelial cells and creating widened gaps between cells
Serotonin	Stored in platelets, mast cells, enterochromaffin cells of GI tract	Same as above; stimulates smooth muscle contraction
Kinins (e.g., bradykinin)	Produced from precursor factor kininogen as a result of activation of Hageman factor (XII) of clotting system	Cause contraction of smooth muscle and dilation of blood vessels; result in stimulation of pain
Complement components (C3a, C4a, C5a)	Anaphylatoxic agents generated from complement pathway activation	Stimulate histamine release; stimulate chemotaxis
Prostaglandins and leukotrienes	Produced from arachidonic acid (see Fig. 13-5)	PGE_1 and PGE_2 cause vasodilation; LTB_4 stimulates chemotaxis
Cytokines	For information on cytokines, see Table 14-5	

GI, Gastrointestinal; *LT,* leukotriene; *PG,* prostaglandin.

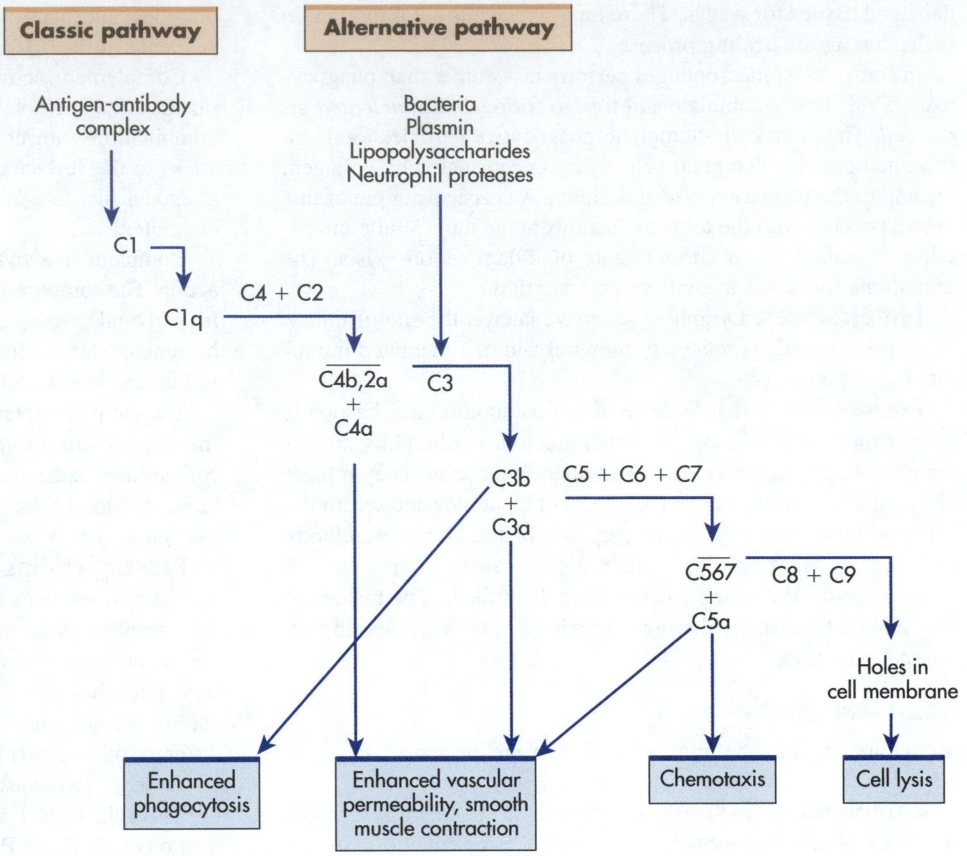

FIG. 13-4 Sequential activation and biologic effects of the complement system.

conditions. Acetylsalicylic acid (ASA; aspirin) blocks platelet aggregation; it also has antiinflammatory action. Prostacyclin (PGI_2) has been used to prevent platelet deposition in extracorporeal systems, such as hemodialysis and heart-lung bypass oxygenators.

Another group of drugs that inhibit PGs are corticosteroids. They are valuable in the treatment of asthma because they inhibit leukotriene production and thus prevent bronchoconstriction. (Other mediators of the inflammatory response are described in Table 13-1.)

Exudate Formation

Exudate consists of fluid and leukocytes that move from the circulation to the site of injury. The nature and quantity of exudate depend on the type and severity of the injury and the tissues involved (Table 13-2).

Clinical Manifestations

The local response to inflammation includes the manifestations of redness, heat, pain, swelling, and loss of function (Table 13-3). Systemic manifestations of inflammation include an increased WBC count with a shift to the left, malaise, nausea and anorexia, increased pulse and respiratory rate, and fever.

Leukocytosis results from the increased release of leukocytes from the bone marrow. An increase in the circulating number of one or more types of leukocytes may be found. Inflammatory reactions are accompanied by the vaguely defined constitutional symptoms of malaise, nausea, anorexia, and fatigue. The causes of these systemic changes are poorly understood, but the changes are probably due to complement activation and the release of cytokines (soluble factors secreted by WBCs and other types of cells that act as intercellular messengers). Some of these cytokines (e.g., interleukin-1 [IL-1], interleukin-6 [IL-6], tumor necrosis factor [TNF]) are important in causing the systemic manifestations of inflammation, as well as inducing the production of fever. An increase in pulse and respiration follows the rise in metabolism as a result of an increase in body temperature. (Cytokines are discussed in Chapter 14.)

Fever. The onset of fever is triggered by the release of cytokines. The most potent of these cytokines are IL-1, IL-6, and TNF (released from mononuclear phagocyte cells). α-Interferon (α-IFN), β-interferon (β-IFN), and γ-interferon (γ-IFN) are also cytokines that can stimulate the responses to cause a fever. These cytokines cause fever by their ability to initiate metabolic changes in the temperature-regulating center (Fig. 13-6). The synthesis of prostaglandin E_2 (PGE_2) is the most critical metabolic change. PGE_2 acts directly to increase the thermostatic set point. The hypothalamus then activates the autonomic nervous system to stimulate increased muscle tone and shivering and decreased perspiration and blood flow to the periphery. Epinephrine released from the adrenal medulla increases the metabolic rate. The net result is fever.

With the physiologic thermostat fixed at a higher-than-normal temperature, the rate of heat production is increased until the body temperature reaches the new set point. As the set point is raised, the hypothalamus signals an increase in heat production and conservation to raise the body temperature to the new level. At this point the individual feels chilled and shivers. The shivering response is the body's method of raising the body's temperature until the new set point is attained. This seeming paradox is dramatic: the body is hot, yet an individual piles on blankets and may go to bed

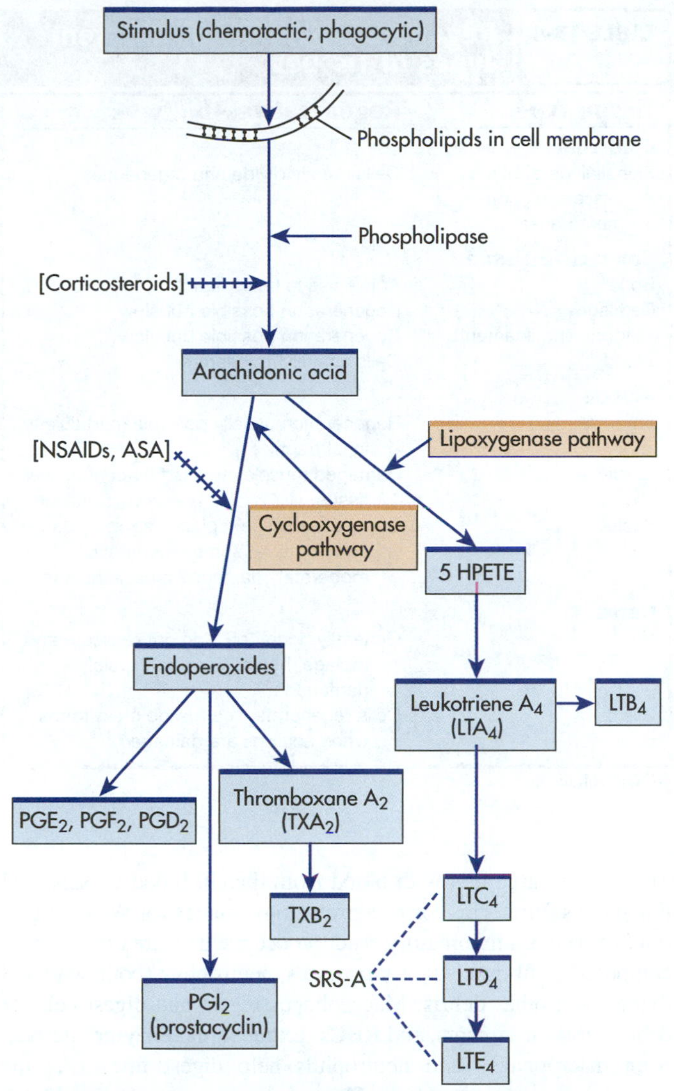

FIG. 13-5 Pathway of arachidonic acid oxygenation and generation of prostaglandins and leukotrienes. Corticosteroids, nonsteroidal antiinflammatory drugs (NSAIDs), and acetylsalicylic acid (ASA) act to inhibit various steps in this pathway. LTC_4, LTD_4, and LTE_4 form the slow-reacting substance of anaphylaxis (SRS-A), an important mediator of allergic responses, by causing bronchoconstriction and increased vascular permeability. *5-HPETE,* 5-hydroperoxyeicosatetraenoic acid; *PG,* prostaglandins.

to get warm. When the circulating body temperature reaches the set point of the core body temperature, the chills and warmth-seeking behavior cease.

The released cytokines and the fever they trigger activate the body's defense mechanisms. Beneficial aspects of fever include increased killing of microorganisms, increased phagocytosis by neutrophils, and increased proliferation of T cells. Higher body temperatures may also enhance the activity of interferon, the body's natural virus-fighting substance[1] (see Chapter 14).

Types of Inflammation

The basic types of inflammation are acute, subacute, and chronic. In *acute inflammation,* the healing occurs in 2 to 3 weeks and usually leaves no residual damage. Neutrophils are the predominant cell type at the site of inflammation. A *subacute inflammation* has the features of the acute process but lasts longer. For example, infective endocarditis is a smoldering infection with acute inflammation, but it persists for weeks or months (see Chapter 37).

Chronic inflammation lasts for weeks, months, or even years. The injurious agent persists or repeatedly injures tissue. The predominant cell types present at the site of inflammation are lymphocytes and macrophages. Examples of chronic inflammation include rheumatoid arthritis and tuberculosis. Tuberculosis is a type of chronic granulomatous inflammation. A chronic inflammatory process is debilitating and can be devastating. The prolongation and chronicity of any inflammation may be the result of an alteration in the immune response (e.g., autoimmune disease).

TABLE 13-2 Types of Inflammatory Exudate

Type	Description	Examples
Serous	Results from outpouring of fluid that has low cell and protein content; seen in early stages of inflammation or when injury is mild.	Skin blisters, pleural effusion
Catarrhal	Found in tissues where cells produce mucus. Mucus production is accelerated by inflammatory response.	Runny nose associated with upper respiratory tract infection
Fibrinous	Occurs with increasing vascular permeability and fibrinogen leakage into interstitial spaces. Excessive amounts of fibrin coating tissue surfaces may cause them to adhere.	Adhesions
Purulent (pus)	Consists of WBCs, microorganisms (dead and alive), liquefied dead cells, and other debris.	Furuncle (boil), abscess, cellulitis (diffuse inflammation in connective tissue)
Hemorrhagic	Results from rupture or necrosis of blood vessel walls; it consists of RBCs that escape into tissue.	Hematoma

RBCs, Red blood cells; *WBCs,* white blood cells.

TABLE 13-3 Local Manifestations of Inflammation

Manifestations	Cause
Redness (rubor)	Hyperemia from vasodilation
Heat (calor)	Increased metabolism at inflammatory site
Pain (dolor)	Change in pH; change in local ionic concentration; nerve stimulation by chemicals (e.g., histamine, prostaglandins); pressure from fluid exudate
Swelling (tumor)	Fluid shift to interstitial spaces; fluid exudate accumulation
Loss of function (functio laesa)	Swelling and pain

HEALING PROCESS

The final phase of the inflammatory response is healing. Healing includes the two major components of regeneration and repair. **Regeneration** is the replacement of lost cells and tissues with cells

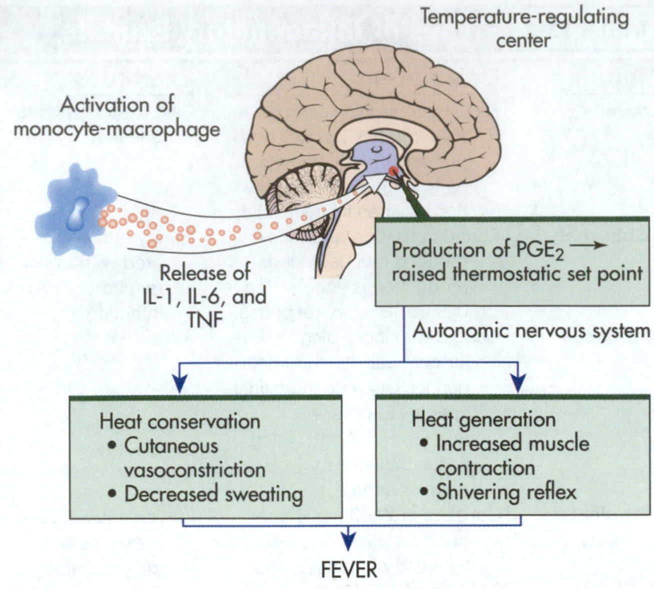

FIG. 13-6 Production of fever. When monocytes-macrophages are activated, they secrete cytokines such as interleukin-1 *(IL-1)*, interleukin-6 *(IL-6)*, and tumor necrosis factor *(TNF)*, which reach the hypothalamic temperature-regulating center. These cytokines promote the synthesis and secretion of prostaglandin E_2 *(PGE_2)* in the anterior hypothalamus. PGE_2 increases the thermostatic set point, and the autonomic nervous system is stimulated, resulting in shivering, muscle contraction, and peripheral vasoconstriction.

TABLE 13-4 Regenerative Ability of Different Types of Tissues

Tissue Type	Regenerative Ability
Epithelial	
Skin, linings of blood vessels, mucous membranes	Cells readily divide and regenerate
Connective Tissue	
Bone	Active tissue heals rapidly
Cartilage	Regeneration possible but slow
Tendons and ligaments	Regeneration possible but slow
Blood	Cells actively regenerate
Muscle	
Smooth	Regeneration usually possible (particularly in GI tract)
Cardiac	Damaged muscle replaced by connective tissue
Skeletal	Connective tissue replaces severely damaged muscle; some regeneration in moderately damaged muscle occurs
Nerve	
Neuron	Generally nonmitotic; do not replicate and replace themselves if irreversibly damaged
Glial	Cells regenerate; scar tissue often forms when neurons are damaged

GI, Gastrointestinal.

of the same type. **Repair** is healing as a result of lost cells being replaced by connective tissue. Repair is the more common type of healing and usually results in scar formation.

Regeneration

The ability of cells to regenerate depends on the cell type (Table 13-4). Labile cells divide constantly. Examples include cells of the skin, lymphoid organs, bone marrow, and mucous membranes of the gastrointestinal (GI), urinary, and reproductive tracts. Injury to these organs is followed by rapid regeneration.

Stable cells retain their ability to regenerate but do so only if the organ is injured. Examples of stable cells are liver, pancreas, kidney, and bone cells.

Permanent cells have left the cell cycle and do not divide. Examples of these cells are neurons of the central nervous system (CNS), and skeletal and cardiac muscle cells. Damage to CNS neurons or heart or skeletal muscle can lead to permanent loss. If neurons in the CNS are destroyed, the tissue is generally replaced by glial cells. However, recent research demonstrates that neurogenesis may occur from stem cells (see Chapter 56.) Healing of skeletal and cardiac muscle will occur by repair with scar tissue.

Repair

Repair is a more complex process than regeneration. Most injuries heal by connective tissue repair. Repair healing occurs by primary, secondary, or tertiary intention[2] (Fig. 13-7).

Primary Intention. *Primary intention* healing takes place when wound margins are neatly approximated, such as in a surgical incision or a paper cut. A continuum of processes is associated with primary healing (Table 13-5). These processes include three phases.

Initial Phase. The initial phase lasts for 3 to 5 days. The edges of the incision are first aligned and sutured (or stapled) in place. The incision area fills with blood from the cut blood vessels, and blood clots form. This forms a provisional matrix for WBC migration. An acute inflammatory reaction occurs. The area of injury is composed of fibrin clots, erythrocytes, neutrophils (both dead and dying), and other debris. Macrophages ingest and digest cellular debris, fibrin fragments, and RBCs. Extracellular enzymes derived from macrophages and neutrophils help digest fibrin. As the wound debris is removed, the fibrin clot serves as a meshwork for future capillary growth and migration of epithelial cells.

Granulation Phase. The *granulation (fibroblastic, proliferative, reconstructive)* phase is the second step and lasts from 5 days to 3 weeks. The components of granulation tissue include proliferating fibroblasts; proliferating capillary sprouts (angioblasts); various types of WBCs; exudate; and loose, semifluid, ground substance.

Fibroblasts are immature connective tissue cells that migrate into the healing site and secrete collagen. In time the collagen is organized and restructured to strengthen the healing site. At this stage it is termed *fibrous* or *scar tissue*.

During the granulation phase, the wound is pink and vascular. Numerous red granules (young budding capillaries) are present. At this point the wound is friable, at risk for dehiscence, and resistant to infection.

Surface epithelium at the wound edges begins to regenerate. In a few days, a thin layer of epithelium migrates across the wound surface. The epithelium thickens and begins to mature, and the wound now closely resembles the adjacent skin. In a superficial wound, reepithelialization may take 3 to 5 days.

Maturation Phase and Scar Contraction. The maturation phase, during which scar contraction occurs, overlaps with the granulation phase. It may begin 7 days after the injury and continue for several months or years. Collagen fibers are further orga-

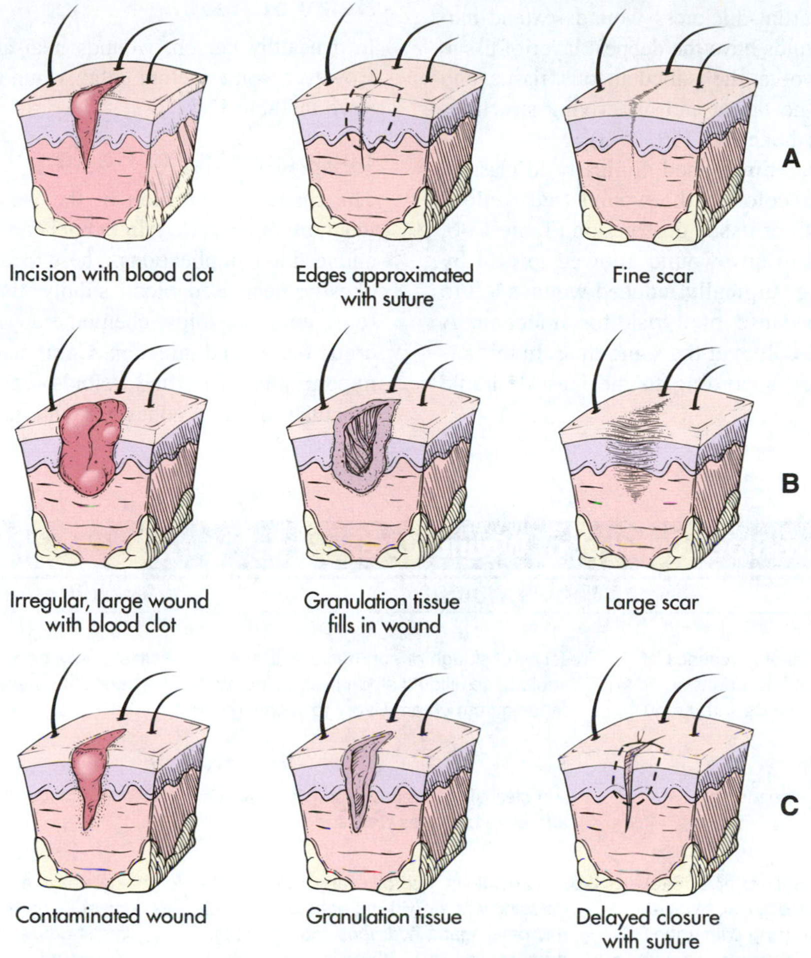

FIG. 13-7 Types of wound healing. **A,** Primary intention. **B,** Secondary intention. **C,** Tertiary intention.

TABLE 13-5 Phases in Primary Intention Healing

Phase	Activity
Initial (3 to 5 days)	Approximation of incision edges; migration of epithelial cells; clot serving as meshwork for starting capillary growth
Granulation (5 days to 4 weeks)	Migration of fibroblasts; secretion of collagen; abundance of capillary buds; fragility of wound
Scar contracture (7 days to several months)	Remodeling of collagen; strengthening of scar

nized, and the remodeling process occurs. Fibroblasts disappear as the wound becomes stronger. The active movement of the myofibroblasts causes contraction of the healing area, helping to close the defect and bring the skin edges closer together. A mature scar is then formed. In contrast to granulation tissue, a mature scar is virtually avascular and pale. The scar may be more painful at this phase than in the granulation phase.

Secondary Intention. Wounds that occur from trauma, ulceration, and infection have large amounts of exudate and wide, irregular wound margins with extensive tissue loss. These wounds may have edges that can be approximated. The inflammatory reaction may be greater than in primary healing. This results in more debris, cells, and exudate. The debris may have to be cleaned away *(debrided)* before healing can take place.

In some instances a primary incision may become infected, creating additional inflammation. The wound may reopen, and healing by *secondary intention* takes place.

The process of healing by secondary intention is essentially the same as healing by primary intention. The major differences are the greater defect and the gaping wound edges. Healing and granulation take place from the edges inward and from the bottom of the wound upward until the defect is filled. There is more granulation tissue, and the result is a much larger scar.

Tertiary Intention. *Tertiary intention* (delayed primary intention) healing occurs with delayed suturing of a wound in which two layers of granulation tissue are sutured together. This occurs when a contaminated wound is left open and sutured closed after the infection is controlled. It also occurs when a primary wound becomes infected, is opened, is allowed to granulate, and is then sutured. Tertiary intention usually results in a larger and deeper scar than primary or secondary intention.

Wound Classification

Identifying the etiology of a wound is essential to classifying the wound properly. Wounds can be classified by their cause (surgical or nonsurgical; acute or chronic) or depth of tissue affected (superficial, partial thickness, or full thickness). A superficial wound involves only the epidermis. Partial-thickness wounds extend into the dermis. Full-thickness wounds have the deepest layer of tissue destruction because they involve the subcutaneous tissue and sometimes even extend into the fascia and underlying structures such as the muscle, tendon, or bone (see Fig. 25-3).

Another system that is sometimes used clinically to classify open wounds is based on the color of the wound (red, yellow, black) rather than on the depth of tissue destruction (Table 13-6, Fig. 13-8). It can be applied to any wound allowed to heal by secondary intention, including surgically induced wounds left to heal without skin closure because of a risk for infection. A wound may have two or three colors at the same time. In this situation the wound is classified according to the least-desirable color present.

Delay of Healing

In a healthy person, wounds heal at a normal, predictable rate. However, some factors delay wound healing. These are summarized in Table 13-7.

Complications of Healing

The shape and location of the wound determine how well the wound will heal. Certain factors can interfere with wound healing and lead to complications. These factors may include malnutrition, obesity, decreased blood supply, tissue trauma, smoking, drugs (e.g., corticosteroids, chemotherapy), wound debris such as necrotic tissue, and infection. Complications that may result include hypertrophic scars and keloids, contracture, dehiscence, excess granulation tissue, adhesions, and major organ dysfunction.

TABLE 13-6 Red-Yellow-Black Concept of Wound Care

	Red Wound	Yellow Wound	Black Wound
Characteristics	Traumatic or surgical wound, possible presence of serosanguineous drainage, pink to bright or dark red healing or chronic wounds with granulating tissue	Presence of slough or soft necrotic tissue; liquid to semiliquid slough with exudate ranging from creamy ivory to yellow-green	Black, gray, or brown adherent necrotic tissue; possible presence of purulent drainage
Purpose of Treatment	Protection and gentle atraumatic cleansing	Wound cleansing to remove nonviable tissue and absorb excess drainage	Debridement of eschar and nonviable tissue
Dressings and Therapy	Transparent film dressing (e.g., Tegaderm, OpSite), hydrocolloid dressing (e.g., DuoDerm), hydrogels (e.g., Tegagel), gauze dressing with antimicrobial ointment or solution, Telfa dressing with antibiotic ointment	Wound irrigations, hydrotherapy, moist gauze dressing with or without antibiotic or antimicrobial agent, hydrocolloidal dressing, hydrogel covered with gauze, absorptive dressing	Topical enzyme debridement, surgical debridement, hydrotherapy, chemical debridement, moist gauze dressing, hydrogel covered with gauze, absorptive dressing covered with gauze

A B

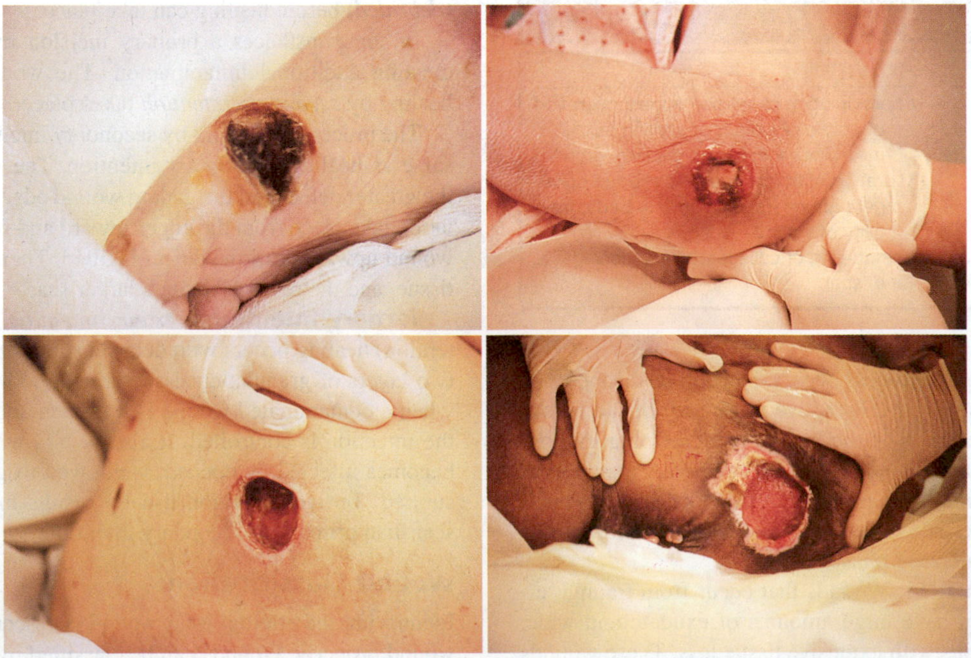

C D

FIG. 13-8 Wounds classified by color assessment. **A,** Black wound. **B,** Yellow wound. **C,** Red wound. **D,** Mixed-color wound.

TABLE 13-7 Factors Delaying Wound Healing

Factor	Effect on Wound Healing
Nutritional deficiencies	
Vitamin C	Delays formation of collagen fibers and capillary development
Protein	Decreases supply of amino acids for tissue repair
Zinc	Impairs epithelialization
Inadequate blood supply	Decreases supply of nutrients to injured area, decreases removal of exudative debris, inhibits inflammatory response
Corticosteroid drugs	Impair phagocytosis by WBCs, inhibit fibroblast proliferation and function, depress formation of granulation tissue, inhibit wound contraction
Infection	Increases inflammatory response and tissue destruction
Smoking	Nicotine is a potent vasoconstrictor and impedes blood flow to healing areas
Mechanical friction on wound	Destroys granulation tissue, prevents apposition of wound edges
Advanced age	Slows collagen synthesis by fibroblasts, impairs circulation, requires longer time for epithelialization of skin, alters phagocytic and immune responses
Obesity	Decreases blood supply in fatty tissue
Diabetes mellitus	Decreases collagen synthesis, retards early capillary growth, impairs phagocytosis (result of hyperglycemia), reduces supply of O_2 and nutrients secondary to vascular disease
Poor general health	Causes generalized absence of factors necessary to promote wound healing
Anemia	Supplies less oxygen at tissue level

WBCs, White blood cells.

Hypertrophic Scars and Keloid Formation. Hypertrophic scars and keloid formation occur when the body produces excess collagen tissue. A **hypertrophic scar** is inappropriately large, red, raised, and hard. However, it remains confined to the wound edges and regresses in time. In contrast, a *keloid* is an even greater protrusion of scar tissue that extends beyond the wound edges and may form tumorlike masses (Fig. 13-9). In addition, keloids are permanent, without any tendency to subside. The patient with keloids often complains of tenderness, pain, and hyperesthesia, particularly in the early stages of development. A predisposition to keloid formation is thought to be hereditary and occurs more often in dark-skinned people, particularly African Americans. Neither complication is life threatening, but both can have serious cosmetic implications.

Contracture. Wound contraction is necessary for healing. This process may become abnormal when there is excessive contraction resulting in deformity or contracture. A shortening of muscle or scar tissue results from excessive fibrous tissue formation, especially if the wound is near a joint (see Fig. 25-13). Contracture frequently occurs in an area that has been burned.

Dehiscence. **Dehiscence** is the separation and disruption of previously joined wound edges. It usually occurs when a primary healing site bursts open. There are three possible contributing causes of dehiscence. First, an infection may cause an inflammatory process. Second, the granulation tissue may not be strong enough to withstand the forces imposed on the wound. For example, during the granulation phase of wound healing, the patient is at risk for wound dehiscence. Third, obese individuals are at a high risk for dehiscence because adipose tissue interferes with healing. **Evisceration** occurs when wound edges separate to the extent that intestines protrude through the wound.

Excess Granulation Tissue. Excess granulation tissue ("proud flesh") may protrude above the surface of the healing wound. If the granulation tissue is cauterized or cut off, healing continues in a normal manner. Fig. 13-10 shows an example of poor-quality granulation tissue.

Adhesions. **Adhesions** are bands of scar tissue between or around organs. Adhesions may occur in the abdominal cavity or between the lungs and pleura. Adhesions in the abdomen may cause an intestinal obstruction. Adhesions between the lungs and

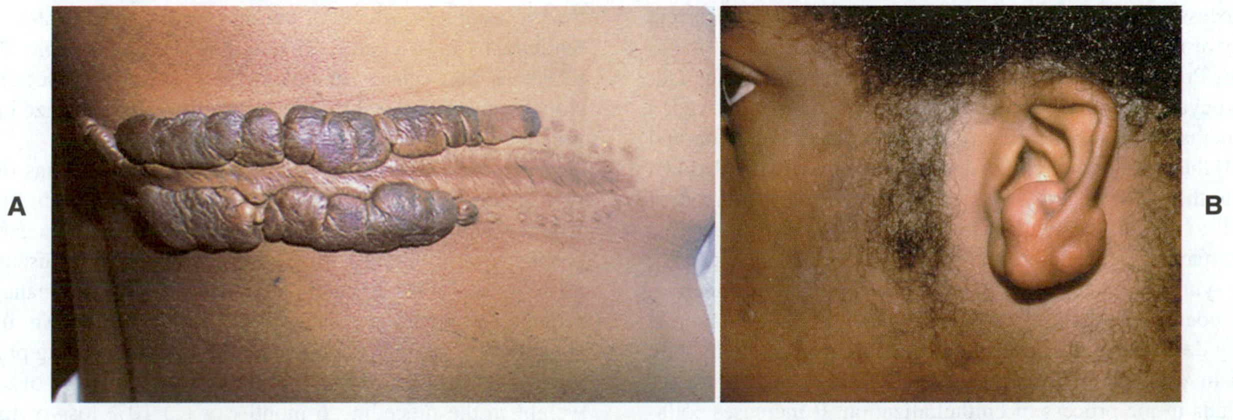

FIG. 13-9 **A,** Keloid formation resulting from suture mark. **B,** Large keloid scar in African American male.

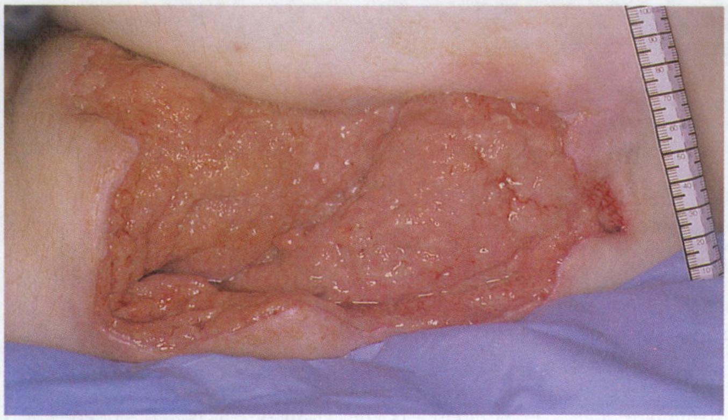

FIG. 13-10 Poor-quality granulation tissue.

pleura require decortication, or stripping of pleura, to permit normal ventilation.

Collaborative Care

Collaborative care for the patient with an inflammatory problem is highly variable. It depends on the causative agent, the degree of injury, and the patient's condition. Superficial skin injuries may only need cleansing. Adhesive strips may be used instead of sutures. The treatment plan can include covering these wounds with a film dressing to provide a moist healing environment and wound protection from trauma. Deeper skin wounds can be closed by suturing the edges together. If the wound is contaminated, it must be converted into a clean wound before healing can occur normally. Debridement of a wound that has multiple fragments or devitalized tissue may be necessary. If the source of inflammation is an internal organ (e.g., appendix, ruptured spleen), surgical removal of the organ is the treatment of choice.

Drug Therapy. Drugs are used to decrease the inflammatory response (Table 13-8). Antihistamine drugs may also be used to inhibit the action of histamine. (Antihistamines are discussed in Chapters 14 and 27.)

Nutritional Therapy. There are special nutritional measures to consider to facilitate wound healing. A high fluid intake is needed to replace fluid loss from perspiration and exudate formation. An increased metabolic rate intensifies water loss. There is a 7% increase in metabolism for every 1° F increase in temperature above 100° F (37.8° C), or a 13% increase for every 1° C increase.

Undernutrition puts a person at the risk for poor healing.[3] A diet high in protein, carbohydrate, and vitamins with moderate fat intake is necessary to promote healing. Protein is needed to correct the negative nitrogen balance resulting from the increased metabolic rate. Protein is also necessary for synthesis of immune factors, leukocytes, fibroblasts, and collagen. Carbohydrate is needed for the increased metabolic energy required in inflammation and healing. If there is a carbohydrate deficit, the body will break down protein for the needed energy. Fats are also a necessary component in the diet to help in the synthesis of fatty acids and triglycerides, which are part of the cellular membrane. Vitamin C is needed for capillary synthesis and collagen. The B-complex vitamins are necessary as coenzymes for many metabolic reactions. If a vitamin B deficiency develops, a disruption of protein, fat, and carbohydrate metabolism will occur. Vitamin A is also needed in healing because it aids in the process of epithelialization. It increases collagen synthesis and tensile strength of the healing wound.

TABLE 13-8 DRUG THERAPY
Inflammation and Healing

Drug	Mechanisms of Action
Antipyretic Drugs	
Salicylates (aspirin)	Lower temperature by action on heat-regulating center in hypothalamus, resulting in peripheral dilation and heat loss; interfere with formation and release of PGs; selectively depress CNS
acetaminophen (Tylenol)	Lowers temperature by action on heat-regulating center in hypothalamus
NSAIDs (e.g., ibuprofen [Motrin, Advil])	Inhibit synthesis of PGs
Antiinflammatory Drugs	
Salicylates	Inhibit synthesis of PGs, reduce capillary permeability
Corticosteroids	Interfere with tissue granulation, induce immunosuppressive effects (decreased synthesis of lymphocytes), prevent liberation of lysosomes
NSAIDs (e.g., ibuprofen [Motrin], piroxicam [Feldene])	Inhibit synthesis of PGs (see Fig. 13-5)
Vitamins	
Vitamin A	Accelerates epithelialization
Vitamin B complex	Acts as coenzymes
Vitamin C	Assists in synthesis of collagen and new capillaries
Vitamin D	Facilitates calcium absorption

CNS, Central nervous system; *NSAIDs,* nonsteroidal antiinflammatory drugs; *PGs,* prostaglandins.

If the patient is unable to eat, enteral feedings and supplements should be the first choice if the GI tract is functional. Parenteral nutrition is indicated when enteral feedings are contraindicated or not tolerated. (Enteral and parenteral nutrition are discussed in Chapter 40.)

NURSING MANAGEMENT INFLAMMATION

■ Nursing Implementation

Health Promotion. The best management of inflammation is the prevention of infection, trauma, surgery, and contact with potentially harmful agents. This is not always possible. A simple mosquito bite causes an inflammatory response. Because occasional injury is inevitable, concerted efforts to minimize inflammation and infection are needed.

Adequate nutrition is essential so that the body has the necessary factors to promote healing when injury occurs. Individuals at risk for wound-healing problems are those with malabsorption problems (e.g., Crohn's disease, GI surgery, liver disease), deficient intake or high energy demands (e.g., malignancy, major trauma or surgery, sepsis, fever), and diabetes. An individual should always be considered at risk for wound-healing problems if the following have occurred: (1) loss of 20% or more of total body weight in the preceding 6 months or (2) 10% loss of total body weight in the preceding 2 months.[4]

Early recognition of the manifestations of inflammation is necessary so that appropriate treatment can begin. This may be rest, drug therapy, or specific treatment of the injured site. Immediate treatment may prevent the extension and complications of inflammation.

Acute Intervention

Observation and Vital Signs. The ability to recognize the clinical manifestations of inflammation is important. In the individual who is immunosuppressed (e.g., taking corticosteroids or receiving chemotherapy), the classic manifestations of inflammation may be masked. In this individual, early symptoms of inflammation may be malaise or "just not feeling well."

Vital signs are important to note with any inflammation, especially when an infectious process is present. When infection is present, temperature may rise, and pulse and respiration rates may increase. If a wound infection develops in a postoperative patient, vital signs will show a change within 3 to 5 days after surgery.

Fever. The most important aspect of fever management should be determining its cause. Although fever is usually regarded as harmful, an increase in body temperature is an important host defense mechanism. In the seventeenth century, Thomas Sydenham noted that "fever is a mighty engine which nature brings into the world for the conquest of her enemies."[5] Steps are frequently taken to lower body temperature to relieve the anxiety of the patient and medical personnel. Because mild to moderate fever usually does little harm, imposes no great discomfort, and may benefit host defense mechanisms, antipyretic drugs are rarely essential to patient welfare. Moderate fevers (up to 103° F [39.5° C]) usually produce few problems in most patients. However, if the patient is very young or very old, is extremely uncomfortable, or has a significant medical problem (e.g., severe cardiopulmonary disease, brain injury), the use of antipyretics should be considered. Fever in the immunosuppressed patient should be treated rapidly and antibiotic therapy begun because infections can rapidly progress to septicemia.

Fever (especially if greater than 104° F [40° C]) can be damaging to body cells, and delirium and seizures can occur. At temperatures greater than 105.8° F (41° C), regulation by the hypothalamic temperature control center becomes impaired, and damage can occur to many cells, including those in the brain.

Older adults have a blunted febrile response to infection. The body temperature may not rise to the level expected for a younger adult or may be delayed in its onset. The blunted response can delay diagnosis and treatment. By the time fever (as defined for younger adults) is present, the illness may be more severe.

Several drugs are commonly used to lower the body temperature set point in the hypothalamus. Aspirin specifically blocks prostaglandin (PG) synthesis in the hypothalamus and elsewhere in the body. Acetaminophen acts on the heat-regulating center in the hypothalamus. Some NSAIDs (e.g., ibuprofen [Motrin, Advil]) have antipyretic effects (see Fig. 13-5). Corticosteroids are antipyretic through the dual mechanisms of inhibiting IL-1 production and preventing PG synthesis. The action of these drugs results in dilation of superficial blood vessels, increased skin temperature, and sweating.

Antipyretics should be given around the clock to prevent acute swings in temperature. Chills may be evoked or perpetuated by the intermittent administration of antipyretics. These agents cause a sharp decrease in temperature. When the antipyretic wears off, the body may initiate a compensatory involuntary muscular contraction (i.e., chill) to raise the body temperature back up to its previous level. This unpleasant side effect of antipyretic drugs can be prevented by administering these agents regularly and frequently at 2- to 4-hour intervals. Although sponge baths increase evaporative heat loss, there is no evidence that they decrease the body temperature unless antipyretic drugs have been given to lower the set point; otherwise, the body will initiate compensatory mechanisms (e.g., shivering) to restore body heat. The same principle applies to the use of cooling blankets; they are most effective in lowering body temperature when the set point has also been lowered. A nursing care plan for the patient with a fever is available on the Evolve website *(http://evolve.elsevier.com/Lewis/medsurg)*.

RICE. Rest, ice, compression, and elevation (RICE) is a key concept in treating soft tissue injuries.

Rest. Rest helps the body better use its nutrients and oxygen for the healing process. The repair process is facilitated by allowing fibrin and collagen to form across the wound edges with little disruption.

Cold and Heat. Cold application is usually appropriate at the time of the initial trauma to cause vasoconstriction and decrease swelling, pain, and congestion from increased metabolism in the area of inflammation. Heat may be used later (e.g., after 24 to 48 hours) to promote healing by increasing the circulation to the inflamed site and subsequent removal of debris. Heat is also used to localize the inflammatory agents. Warm, moist heat may help debride the wound site if necrotic material is present.

Compression and Immobilization. Compression and immobilization of the inflamed area promote healing by decreasing the inflammatory process, assisting in the repair process, and decreasing metabolic needs. Immobilization with a cast, splint, or bandage lessens wound debris and the possibility of hemorrhage.

Elevation. Elevating the injured extremity will reduce the edema at the inflammatory site and increase venous return. Elevation helps reduce pain and improve the circulation of blood, which provides the oxygen and nutrients needed for healing.

NURSING *and* COLLABORATIVE MANAGEMENT WOUND HEALING

■ *Nursing Assessment*

Observation and recording of wound characteristics are essential.[6,7] The wound should be measured. One method for measuring wounds is presented in Fig. 13-11. The consistency, color, and odor of any drainage should be recorded and reported if abnormal for the situation. *Staphylococcus* and *Pseudomonas* species are common organisms that cause purulent, draining wounds.

■ *Nursing Implementation*

The type of wound management and dressings required depend on the type, extent, and characteristics of the wound. The purposes of wound management include (1) cleaning a wound to remove any dirt and debris from the wound bed, (2) treating infection to prepare the wound for healing, and (3) protecting a clean wound from trauma so it can heal normally.

Sutures and fibrin sealant are used to facilitate wound closure and create an optimal setting for wound healing. Most commonly sutures are used to close wounds because suture material provides the mechanical support necessary to sustain closure. A wide variety of suturing materials are available. In contrast, fibrin sealant is a biologic tissue adhesive that can function as a useful adjunct to

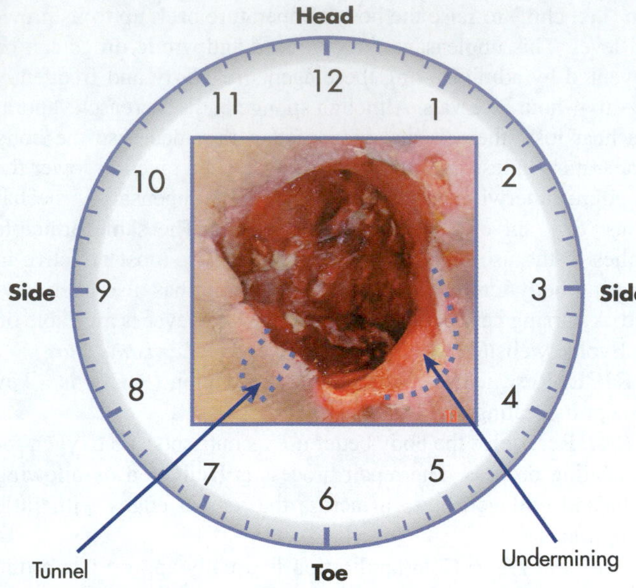

FIG. 13-11 Wound measurements are made in centimeters. The first measurement is oriented from head to toe, the second is from side to side, and the third is the depth (if any). If there is any tunneling (when cotton-tipped applicator is placed in wound, there is movement) or undermining (when cotton-tipped applicator placed in wound, there is a "lip") around the wound, this is charted in respect to a clock with 12 o'clock being toward the patient's head. This wound would be charted as a full-thickness, red wound, 7 cm × 5 cm × 3 cm, with a 3-cm tunnel at 7 o'clock and 2-cm undermining from 3 o'clock to 5 o'clock.

sutures. Fibrin sealant can be used in conjunction with sutures or tape to promote optimal wound integrity. It can be used independently to seal wound sites where sutures cannot control bleeding or would aggravate bleeding. This adhesive can effectively seal tissue and eliminate potential spaces. The use of fibrin sealant has resulted in a low rate of infection and has promoted healing.[8]

For wounds that heal by primary intention, it is common to cover the incision with a dry, sterile dressing that is removed as soon as the drainage stops or in 2 to 3 days. Medicated sprays that form a transparent film on the skin may be used for dressings on a clean incision or injury. Transparent film dressings are also commonly used (Fig. 13-12). Sometimes a surgeon will leave a surgical wound uncovered.

Wound healing management by secondary intention depends on the wound etiology and type of tissue in the wound. This type of management can be described as the red-yellow-black concept of

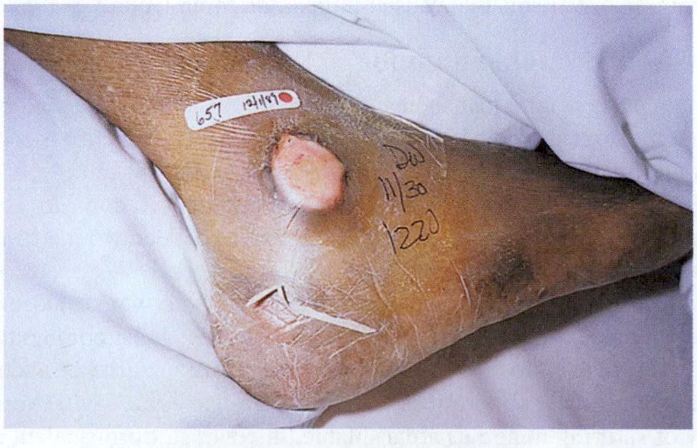

FIG. 13-12 Transparent film dressing.

wound care (see Table 13-6 and Fig. 13-8). Examples of types of wound dressings are presented in Table 13-9.[9]

Red Wound. A *red wound* can be a superficial or deep wound if it is clean and pink in appearance. Examples include skin tears, pressure ulcers (stage II), partial-thickness or second-degree burns, and wounds created surgically that are allowed to heal by secondary intention. The purpose of treatment is protection of the wound and gentle cleansing (if indicated). Clean wounds that are granulating and reepithelializing should be kept slightly moist and protected from further trauma until they heal naturally. A dressing material that keeps the wound surface clean and slightly moist is optimal to promote epithelialization. Transparent film or adhesive semipermeable dressings (e.g., OpSite, Tegaderm) are occlusive dressings that are permeable to oxygen. The wound is then usually covered with a sterile dressing. Unnecessary manipulation during dressing changes may destroy new granulation tissue and break down fibrin formation.[10]

Yellow Wound. A *yellow wound* has nonviable necrotic tissue, which creates an ideal situation for bacterial growth and therefore must be removed. The purpose of treatment is continual cleansing to remove nonviable tissue and to absorb excessive drainage. A type of dressing used in yellow wounds is an absorption dressing (e.g., calcium alginate, foam, hydrogel), which absorbs exudate and cleanses the wound surface. Absorption dressings work by drawing excess drainage from the wound surface. After these preparations are saturated with exudate, they should be removed by washing with sterile saline or water. The amount of wound secretions determines the number of dressing changes.

Hydrocolloid dressings such as DuoDerm are also used to treat yellow wounds. The inner part of these dressings interacts with the exudate, forming a hydrated gel over the wound. When the dressing is removed, the gel separates and stays over the wound. The wound must be cleansed gently to prevent damage to newly formed tissue. These types of dressings are designed to be left in place for up to 7 days or until leakage occurs around the dressing.

Black Wound. A *black wound* is covered with thick, dry, black necrotic tissue called *eschar*. Examples of black wounds include full-thickness or third-degree burns, pressure ulcers (stages III and IV) (described later in this chapter), and gangrenous ulcers. The risk of wound infection increases in proportion to the amount of necrotic tissue present. The immediate treatment is debridement of the nonviable, eschar tissue. The debridement method used depends on the amount of debris and the condition of the wound tissue. There are several approaches to debridement: [11]

1. *Surgical debridement.* This quickest method of debridement is indicated when large amounts of nonviable tissue are present and the patient is septic.
2. *Mechanical debridement.* This method is used when minimal debris is present. A common form of mechanical debridement is wet-to-dry dressings in which open-mesh gauze is moistened with normal saline, packed on or into the wound surface, and allowed to dry. Wound debris adheres to the dressing. When the dressing is removed, the coarse debris is entrapped in the gauze. One disadvantage to this method is that it is nonselective and will also debride some healthy tissue. This method of mechanical debridement is painful, and the patient should receive appropriate pain management before the removal of a wet-to-dry dressing.

Topical antimicrobials and antibactericidals (e.g., povidone-iodine [Betadine], Dakin's solution [sodium hy-

TABLE 13-9 Types of Wound Dressings

Type	Description	Examples
Gauzes and nonwovens	Provides absorption of exudates. Supports debridement if applied and kept moist. Can be used to maintain moist wound surface. Can be used for cleansing, packing, and covering a variety of wounds.	Numerous products available (e.g., Curity, Kling, Kerlix)
Nonadherent dressings	Woven or nonwoven dressings; may be impregnated with saline, petrolatum, or antimicrobials. Are minimally absorbent. Used mainly on minor wounds or as a second dressing.	Adaptic, Vaseline gauze, Xeroform
Transparent films	Semipermeable membrane that permits gaseous exchange between wound and environment. Transparency allows visualization of the wound. Minimally absorbent so fluid environment is created in presence of exudate. Used for dry noninfected wounds or wounds with minimal drainage.	Bioclusive, BlisterFilm, CarraFilm, Omniderm, OpSite, Polyskin, Suresite, Tegaderm, Transeal
Hydrocolloids	Wafers, powders, or pastes composed of gelatin, pectin, or carboxymethylcellulose. Occlusive dressing does not allow O_2 to diffuse from atmosphere to wound. Occlusion does not interfere with wound healing. Supports debridement and prevents secondary infections. Used for superficial and partial-thickness wounds with light to moderate drainage.	Comfeel, DuoDerm, Exuderm, Hydrocol, NU-DERM, RepliCare, Restore, Ultec
Foams	Sheets and other shapes of foamed polymer solutions (most commonly polyurethane) with small, open cells capable of holding fluids. Moderate to heavy amounts of exudates can be absorbed. The area in contact with the wound surface is nonadhesive for easy removal. Used for partial- or full-thickness wounds or infected wounds.	Allevyn, Curafoam, Flexzan, Hydrasorb, Lyofoam, Mepilex, Polyderm
Absorptive dressings	Large volumes of exudates can be absorbed. Maintain moist wound surface. Placed into wounds and can obliterate dead space. For partial- or full-thickness wounds or infected wounds.	ABD Combine Pads, Covaderm, Curity Abdominal Pads, Multipad
Hydrogel	Available as sheet, gel, and gauze designed to donate moisture to a dry wound and to maintain a moist healing environment. High moisture content serves to rehydrate wound tissue. Debridement because of moisturizing effects. Provides limited absorption of exudates. Most types require a secondary dressing. Used for partial- or full-thickness wounds, deep wounds with minimal drainage, and necrotic wounds.	AquaSite, Carrasyn Gel, Curasol Gel, Hypergel, Geliperm, IntraSite, Saf-Gel, SoloSite, Tegagel, Woun'Dres
Alginates	Nonwoven, nonadhesive pads and ribbons composed of natural polysaccharide fibers or xerogel derived from seaweed. On contact with exudate, form a moist gel. Easy to use over irregular-shaped wounds. Indicated for wounds with moderate to heavy exudates (e.g., pressure ulcers, infected wounds). Generally require a secondary dressing.	AlgiCELL, AlgiSite, CarraSorb, Kalginate, Maxorb, SeaSorb, Sorbalgon
Antimicrobials	Wound covers that deliver agents such as silver and polyhexamethylene biguanide (PHMB), which have antibacterial properties. Indicated in partial- and full-thickness wounds, over skin line sites and surgical incisions, or around tracheostomies. Available as sponges, impregnated woven gauzes, film dressings, absorptive products, island dressings, nylon fabric, nonadherent barriers, or a combination of materials.	Acticoat, BIOPATCH, Curity AMD, Island Wound Dressing with Microban, SilverDerm, SilverIon

For more information, see *http://search.woundsource.com.*

pochlorite], hydrogen peroxide [H_2O_2], and chlorhexidine [Hibiclens]) should be used with caution in wound care because they can damage the new epithelium of healing tissue. Therefore they should never be used in a clean granulating wound.

Another method of mechanical debridement is wound irrigation. It is important to make sure that bacteria are not accidentally driven into the wound. Whirlpool is another method of mechanical debridement. Mechanical debridement should not be used in a clean granulating wound.

3. *Autolytic debridement.* Semiocclusive or occlusive dressings (see Table 13-9) may be used to promote softening of dry eschar by autolysis. These types of dressings are used in open wounds with necrotic debris and no infection. The area around the wound must be assessed for maceration when these dressings are used.
4. *Enzymatic debridement.* This method uses drugs that are applied topically to the necrotic tissue in the wound and then covered with moist dressing such as saline-moistened gauze. Examples of these drugs include collagenase and papain-urea (e.g., Panafil, Gladase). These drugs dissolve necrotic tissue. The manufacturer's directions must be followed because these products are different in terms of the pH range of use, frequency of application, and type of cleaning solutions to avoid.

Negative-Pressure Wound Therapy. Negative-pressure wound therapy *(vacuum-assisted wound closure)* is a type of therapy that uses suction to remove drainage and speed wound healing.[12] In this therapy the wound is cleaned, and a special dressing consisting of sponges packed with tubing and a transparent adhesive dressing is used. Sponges are placed into the wound to absorb drainage. Tubing from the wound is then attached to a pump, which creates a negative pressure in the wound bed. Wound types suitable for this therapy include acute or traumatic wounds, surgical wounds that have dehisced, pressure ulcers, and chronic ulcers.[13]

Hyperbaric Oxygen Therapy. Hyperbaric O_2 therapy is the delivery of O_2 at increased atmospheric pressures.[14] It can be given systemically with the patient placed in an enclosed chamber where 100% O_2 is administered at 1.5 to 3 times the normal atmospheric pressure. An alternative approach is to topically administer hyperbaric O_2 by creating a chamber around the injured limb. Most systemic treatments last from 90 to 120 minutes, and the number of treatments may vary from 10 to 60 minutes depending on the condition being treated. The topical treatments can last 20 minutes twice daily or 4 to 6 hours daily. The number of treatments is highly variable. Hyperbaric O_2 therapy accelerates granulation tissue formation and wound healing.

Infection Prevention and Control. The nurse and the patient must scrupulously follow aseptic procedures for keeping the wound free from infection. The patient should not be allowed to touch a recently injured area. The patient's environment should be as free as possible from contamination from items introduced by roommates and visitors. Antibiotics may be administered prophylactically to some patients. If an infection develops, a culture and sensitivity test should be done to determine the organism and the most effective antibiotic for that specific organism. The culture should be taken before the first dose of antibiotic is given.

Psychologic Implications. The patient may be distressed at the thought or sight of an incision or wound because of fear of scarring or disfigurement. Drainage from a wound often causes increased alarm. The patient needs to understand the healing process and the normal changes that occur as the wound heals. When a nurse is changing a dressing, inappropriate facial expressions can alert the patient to problems with the wound or the nurse's ability to care for it. Wrinkling of the nose by the nurse may convey disgust to the patient. A nurse should also be careful not to focus on the wound to the extent that the patient is not treated as a total person.

Patient Teaching. Because patients are being discharged earlier after surgery and many have surgery as outpatients, it is important that the patient, the family, or both know how to care for the wound and perform dressing changes. Wound healing may not be complete for 4 to 6 weeks or longer. Adequate rest and good nutrition should be continued throughout this time. Physical and emotional stress should be minimal. Observing the wound for complications such as contractures, adhesions, and secondary infection is important. The patient should understand the signs and symptoms of infection. The patient should note changes in wound color and the amount of drainage. The health care provider should be notified of any signs of abnormal wound healing.

Drugs will often be taken for a period of time after recovery from the acute infection. Drug-specific side effects and adverse effects should be reviewed with the patient; the patient should be instructed to contact the health care provider if any of these effects occur. Awareness of the necessity to continue the drugs for the specified time is an important point to teach the patient. For example, a patient who is instructed to take an antibiotic for 10 days may stop taking the drug after 5 days because of decreased or absent symptoms. However, the organism may not be entirely eliminated, and it may also become resistant to the antibiotic if the drug is not continued (see Table 15-7).

PRESSURE ULCERS

Etiology and Pathophysiology

A **pressure ulcer** is a localized area (usually over a bony prominence) of tissue necrosis caused by unrelieved pressure that occludes blood flow to the tissues. Pressure ulcers generally fall under the category of healing by secondary intention. The most common site for pressure ulcers is the sacrum, with heels being second. Factors that influence the development of pressure ulcers include the amount of pressure (intensity), the length of time the pressure is exerted on the skin (duration), and the ability of the patient's tissue to tolerate the externally applied pressure. Besides pressure, **shearing force** (pressure exerted on the skin when it adheres to the bed and the skin layers slide in the direction of body movement), *friction* (two surfaces rubbing against each other), and *excessive moisture* contribute to pressure ulcer formation.

TABLE 13-10 Risk Factors for Pressure Ulcers

• Advanced age	• Low diastolic blood pressure (<60 mm Hg)
• Anemia	• Mental deterioration
• Contractures	• Neurologic disorders
• Diabetes mellitus	• Obesity
• Elevated body temperature	• Pain
• Immobility	• Prolonged surgery
• Impaired circulation	• Vascular disease
• Incontinence	

Factors that put a patient at risk for the development of pressure ulcers are presented in Table 13-10. Individuals at risk include those who are elderly, incontinent, bed- or wheelchair-bound, or recovering from spinal cord injuries.

The incidence of pressure ulcers is estimated to be about 23% among residents of long-term care facilities. The prevalence is between 5% and 10% of hospitalized patients and about 15% of residents of long-term care facilities.[15]

Clinical Manifestations

The clinical manifestations of pressure ulcers depend on the extent of the tissue that is involved. Pressure ulcers are graded or staged according to their deepest level of tissue damage or "wounding." Table 13-11 illustrates the four pressure ulcer stages based on the National Pressure Ulcer Advisory Panel (NPUAP) guidelines.[16-18]

A pressure ulcer may be unstageable. The actual depth of tissue loss is obscured by slough (yellow, tan, gray, green, or brown) and/or eschar (tan, brown, or black) in the wound bed. A pressure ulcer may also present as a blood-filled blister. Until enough slough and/or eschar is removed to expose the base of the wound, the true depth, and therefore stage, cannot be determined. Stable (dry, adherent, intact) eschar on the heels serves as "the body's natural (biological) cover" and should not be removed.[19]

If the pressure ulcer becomes infected, the patient may display signs of infection, such as leukocytosis and fever. In addition, the pressure ulcer may increase in size, odor, and drainage; have necrotic tissue; and be indurated, warm, and painful. Untreated ulcers may lead to cellulitis, chronic infection, or osteomyelitis. The most common complication of a pressure ulcer is recurrence. Therefore, it is important to note the location of previously healed pressure ulcers on an initial admission assessment of a patient.

NURSING *and* COLLABORATIVE MANAGEMENT
PRESSURE ULCERS

Care of a patient with a pressure ulcer requires local care of the wound and support measures of the whole person, such as adequate nutrition, pain management, control of other medical conditions, and pressure relief. The current trend is to keep a pressure ulcer slightly moist, rather than dry, to enhance reepithelialization. In addition to the nurse, other members of the health team, such as the plastic surgeon, the dietitian, the physical therapist, and the occupational therapist, can provide valuable input into the com-

TABLE 13-11 Staging of Pressure Ulcers

Definition/Description	Diagram	Clinical Presentation
Stage I A stage I pressure ulcer is an observable pressure-related change of intact skin whose indicators, as compared to an adjacent or opposite area on the body, may include changes in one or more of the following: Skin temperature (warmth or coolness) Tissue consistency (firm or boggy feel) Sensation (pain, itching) The ulcer appears as a defined area of persistent redness in lightly pigmented skin, whereas in darker skin tones, the ulcer may appear with persistent red, blue, or purple hues.	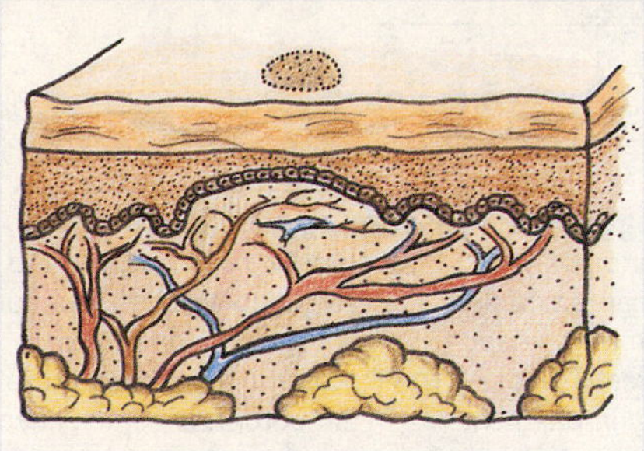	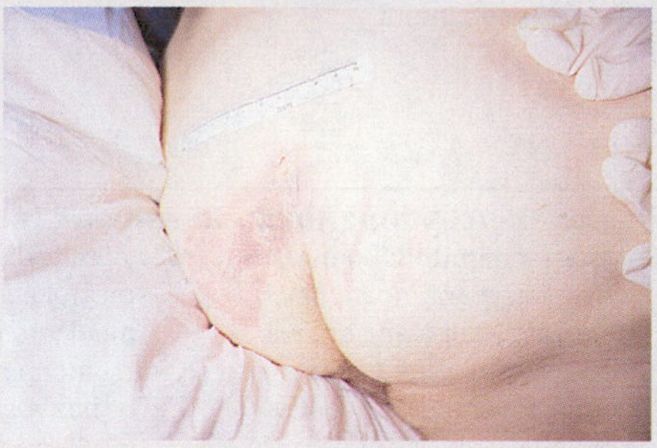
Stage II Partial-thickness skin loss involving epidermis, dermis, or both. The ulcer is superficial and presents clinically as an abrasion, blister, or shallow crater.	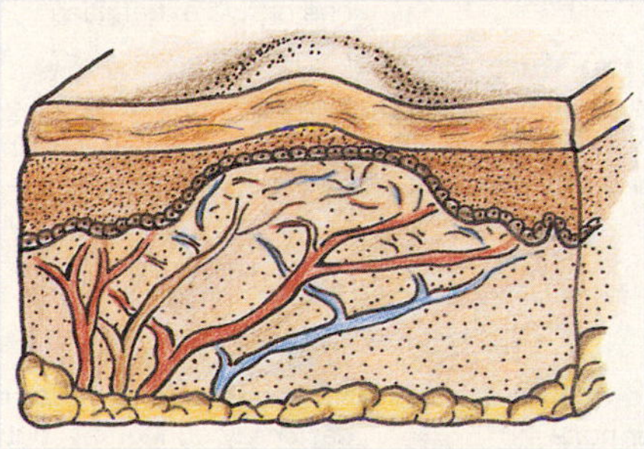	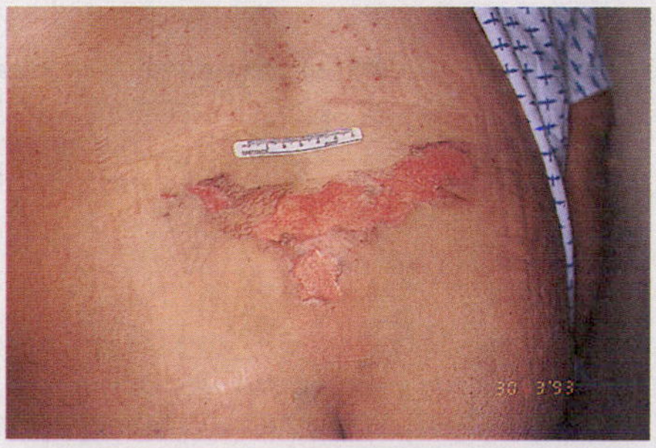
Stage III Full-thickness skin loss involving damage to, or necrosis of, subcutaneous tissue that may extend down to, but not through, underlying fascia. The ulcer presents clinically as a deep crater with or without undermining of adjacent tissue.	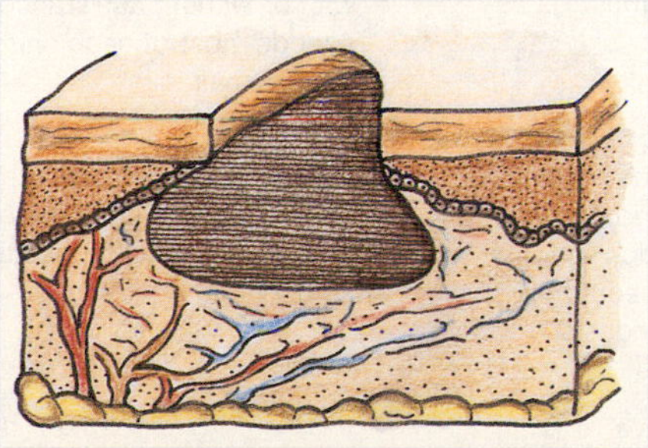	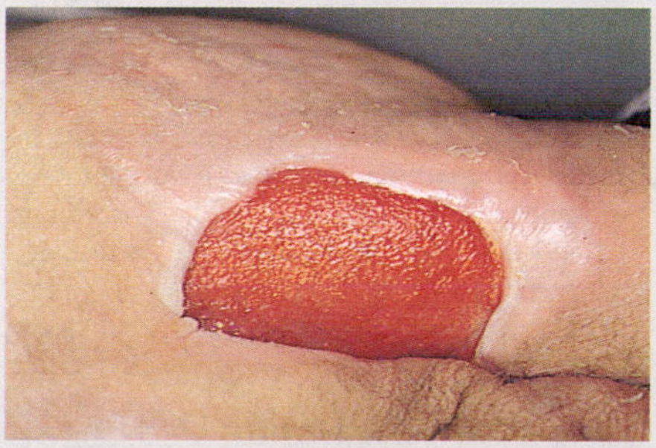
Stage IV Full-thickness skin loss with extensive destruction, tissue necrosis, or damage to muscle, bone, or supporting structures (e.g., tendon, joint capsule). Undermining and sinus tracts may also be associated with stage IV pressure ulcers.	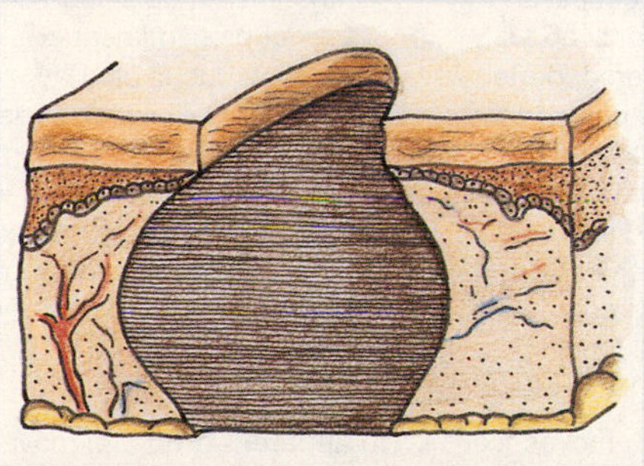	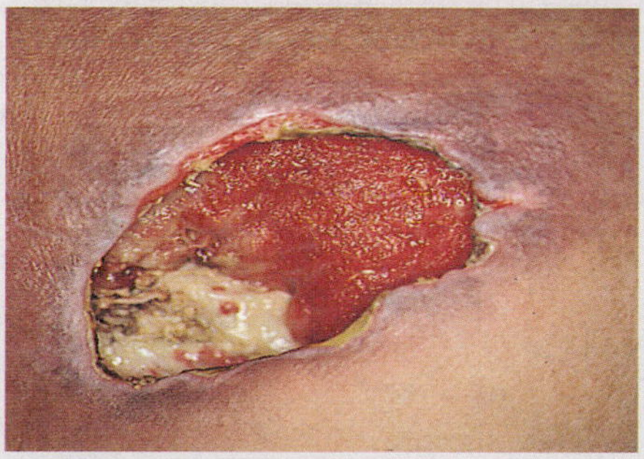

Source: National Pressure Ulcer Advisory Board. Staging criteria were undergoing final revisions at publication. Check website for National Pressure Ulcer Advisory Panel Board at *www.npuap.org*.

plex treatment necessary to prevent and treat pressure ulcers. Both conservative and surgical strategies are used in the treatment of pressure ulcers, depending on the stage and condition of the ulcer. Therapeutic and nursing management are discussed together because the activities are interrelated.

Nursing Assessment

Patients should be assessed for pressure ulcer risk initially on admission and at periodic intervals based on the patient's condition and care setting. For example, in acute care a patient should be reassessed every 48 hours; in long-term care, a resident should be reassessed weekly for the first 4 weeks after admission and then minimally monthly or quarterly; in home care, a person should be reassessed at every nurse visit.

Risk assessment should be done using a validated assessment tool such as the Braden scale[20] (Table 13-12). To obtain a patient's pressure ulcer risk assessment score on the Braden scale, add the numeric scores for the factors in each of the six subscales (sensory perception, moisture, activity, mobility, nutrition, and friction and shear) to obtain the total score. Scores can range from 6 to 23. The lower the numeric score on the Braden scale, the higher the patient's predicted risk of developing a pressure ulcer. Incremental

TABLE 13-12 Braden Scale for Predicting Pressure Sore Risk

Patient Name ______________________ Evaluator's Name ______________________

Date of Assessment ______________________

	Point Value				
	1	2	3	4	Score
Sensory Perception: Ability to respond meaningfully to pressure-related discomfort	**Completely limited:** unresponsive (does not moan, flinch, or grasp) to painful stimuli, due to diminished level of consciousness or sedation or limited ability to feel pain over most of body	**Very limited:** responds only to painful stimuli; cannot communicate discomfort except by moaning or restlessness or has a sensory impairment that limits the ability to feel pain or discomfort over half of body	**Slightly limited:** responds to verbal commands, but cannot always communicate discomfort or the need to be turned or has some sensory impairment that limits ability to feel pain or discomfort in one or two extremities	**No impairment:** responds to verbal commands; has no sensory deficit that would limit ability to feel or to voice pain or discomfort	
Moisture: Degree to which skin is exposed to moisture	**Constantly moist:** skin is kept moist almost constantly by perspiration, urine, etc.; dampness is detected every time patient is moved or turned	**Very moist:** skin is often, but not always, moist; linen must be changed at least once per shift	**Occasionally moist:** skin is occasionally moist, requiring an extra linen change approximately once per day	**Rarely moist:** skin is usually dry, linen only requires changing at routine intervals	
Activity: Degree of physical activity	**Bedfast:** confined to bed	**Chairfast:** ability to walk severely limited or nonexistent; cannot bear own weight and/or must be assisted into chair or wheelchair	**Walks occasionally:** walks occasionally during day, but for very short distances, with or without assistance; spends most of each shift in bed or chair	**Walks frequently:** walks outside room at least twice per day and inside room at least once every 2 hours during waking hours	
Mobility: Ability to change and control body position	**Completely immobile:** does not make even slight changes in body or extremity position without assistance	**Very limited:** makes occasional slight changes in body or extremity position but unable to make frequent or significant changes independently	**Slightly limited:** makes frequent though slight changes in body or extremity position independently	**No limitation:** makes major and frequent changes in position without assistance	
Nutrition: Usual food intake pattern	**Very poor:** never eats a complete meal; rarely eats more than ½ of any food offered; eats two servings or less of protein (meat or dairy products) per day; takes fluids poorly; does not take a liquid dietary supplement or is NPO and/or maintained on clear liquids or IVs for more than 5 days	**Probably inadequate:** rarely eats a complete meal and generally eats only about ½ of any food offered; protein intake includes only three servings of meat or dairy products per day; occasionally will take a dietary supplement or receives less than optimum amount of liquid diet or tube feeding	**Adequate:** eats over half of most meals; eats four servings of protein (meat or dairy products) per day; occasionally will refuse a meal, but will usually take a supplement when offered or is on a tube feeding or parenteral nutrition regimen that probably meets most of nutritional needs	**Excellent:** eats most of every meal; never refuses a meal; eats four or more servings of protein (meat or dairy products); occasionally eats between meals; does not require supplementation	
Friction and Shear	**Problem:** requires moderate to maximum assistance in moving; complete lifting without sliding against sheets is impossible; frequently slides down in bed or chair, requiring frequent repositioning with maximum assistance; spasticity, contractures, or agitation lead to almost constant friction	**Potential problem:** moves feebly or requires minimum assistance; during a move skin probably slides to some extent against sheets, chair, restraints, or other devices; maintains relatively good position in chair or bed most of the time but occasionally slides down	**No apparent problem:** moves in bed and in chair independently and has sufficient muscle strength to lift up completely during move; maintains good position in bed or chair		

From Braden B, Bergstrom N: Predictive validity of the Braden scale for pressure sore risk in a nursing home population, *Res Nurs Health* 17:459, 1994.
Available at no charge at *www.bradenscale.com/bradenscale.htm.*

changes in the score indicate the level of risk: no risk (19 to 23), at risk (15 to 18), moderate risk (13 to 14), high risk (10 to 12), and very high risk (9 or below). Knowing the level of risk can determine how aggressive preventive measures should be.

Identification of stage I pressure ulcers may be difficult in patients with dark skin. Table 13-13 presents techniques to help assess darker skin. Subjective and objective data that should be obtained from a person with a pressure ulcer are presented in Table 13-14.

Nursing Diagnoses

Nursing diagnoses for the patient with a pressure ulcer may include, but are not limited to, those presented in NCP 13-1.

TABLE 13-13 Assessing Patients with Dark Skin

- Look for changes in skin color, such as skin that is darker (purplish, brownish, bluish) than surrounding skin.
- Use natural or halogen light source to accurately assess the skin color. Fluorescent light casts blue color, which can make skin assessment difficult.
- Assess the area for the skin temperature using your hand. The area may feel initially warm, then cooler.
- Touch the skin to feel its consistency. Boggy or edematous feel may indicate a stage I pressure ulcer.
- Ask the patient if he or she has any pain or itchy sensation.

TABLE 13-14 *NURSING ASSESSMENT* Pressure Ulcers

Subjective Data

Important Health Information

Past health history: Stroke, spinal cord injury; prolonged bed rest or immobility; circulatory impairment; poor nutrition; altered level of consciousness; prior history of pressure ulcer; immunologic abnormalities; advanced age; diabetes; anemia; trauma

Medications: Use of opioids, hypnotics, systemic corticosteroids

Surgery or other treatments: Recent surgery

Functional Health Patterns

Nutritional-metabolic: Obesity, emaciation; decreased fluid, calorie, or protein intake; vitamin or mineral deficiencies; clinically significant malnutrition as indicated by low serum albumin, decreased total lymphocyte count, and decreased body weight (15% less than ideal body weight)

Elimination: Incontinence of urine, feces, or both

Activity-exercise: Weakness, debilitation, inability to turn and position body; contractures

Cognitive-perceptual: Pain or altered cutaneous sensation in pressure ulcer area; decreased awareness of pressure on body areas; capacity to follow treatment plan

Objective Data

General

Fever

Integumentary

Diaphoresis, edema, and discoloration, especially over bony areas such as sacrum, hips, elbows, heels, knees, ankles, shoulders, and ear rims, progressing to increased tissue damage characteristic of ulcer stages*

Possible Findings

Leukocytosis, positive cultures for microorganisms from pressure ulcer

*See Table 13-11.

Planning

The overall goals are that the patient with a pressure ulcer will (1) have no deterioration of the ulcer stage, (2) reduce or eliminate the factors that lead to pressure ulcers, (3) not develop an infection in the pressure ulcer, (4) have healing of pressure ulcers, and (5) have no recurrence.

Nursing Implementation

Health Promotion. A primary nursing responsibility is the identification of patients at risk for the development of pressure ulcers (see Tables 13-12 and 13-14) and implementing pressure ulcer prevention strategies for those identified as being at risk. Prevention remains the best treatment for pressure ulcers. Devices such as alternating pressure mattresses, foam mattresses with adequate stiffness and thickness, wheelchair cushions, padded commode seats, boots (foam, air), and lift sheets are useful in reducing pressure and shearing force. However, they are not adequate substitutes for frequent repositioning. Once a person has been identified as being at risk for pressure ulcer development, prevention strategies should be implemented[21] (Table 13-15).

Acute Intervention. Once a pressure ulcer has developed, the nurse should initiate interventions based on the ulcer characteristics (e.g., stage, size, location, amount of exudate, type of wound, presence of infection or pain) and the patient's general status (e.g., nutritional state, age, cardiovascular status, level of mobility). Careful documentation should be made of the size of the pressure ulcer. A wound-measuring card or tape can be used to note the ulcer's maximum length and width in centimeters. To find the depth of the ulcer, gently place a sterile cotton-tipped applicator into the deepest part of the ulcer. The length of the portion of the applicator that probed the ulcer can then be measured. Documentation of the healing wound can be done by using several available pressure ulcer healing tools such as the NPUAP Pressure Ulcer Scale of Healing (PUSH) tool.[22] Some agencies require that pictures of the pressure ulcer be taken initially and at regular intervals during the course of treatment.

Local care of the pressure ulcer may involve debridement, wound cleaning, application of a dressing, and relief of pressure. It is important to select the appropriate pressure-relieving technique (e.g., pad, overlay, mattress, specialty bed) to relieve pressure and keep the patient off of the pressure ulcer. A pressure ulcer that has necrotic tissue or eschar (except for dry, stable necrotic feet or heels) must have the tissue removed by either surgical, mechanical, enzymatic, or autolytic debridement methods. Once the pressure ulcer has been successfully debrided and has a clean granulating base, the goal is to provide an appropriate wound environment that supports moist wound healing and prevents disruption of the newly formed granulation tissue. Reconstruction of the pressure ulcer site by operative repair, including skin grafting, skin flaps, musculocutaneous flaps, or free flaps, may be necessary.

Pressure ulcers should be cleaned with noncytotoxic solutions that do not kill or damage cells, especially fibroblasts. Solutions such as Dakin's solution (sodium hypochlorite solution), acetic acid, povidone-iodine, and hydrogen peroxide (H_2O_2) are cytotoxic and therefore should not be used to clean pressure ulcers. It is also important to use enough irrigation pressure to adequately clean the pressure ulcer (4 to 15 psi) without causing trauma or damage to the wound. To obtain this pressure, a 30-ml syringe and a 19-gauge needle can be used.

NURSING CARE PLAN 13-1

Patient with a Pressure Ulcer

NURSING DIAGNOSIS **Impaired skin integrity** *related to* pressure and inadequate circulation *as evidenced by* presence of pressure ulcer

PATIENT GOALS
1. Maintains intact skin with no further pressure ulcers
2. Experiences healing of pressure ulcer

OUTCOMES (NOC)

Tissue Integrity: Skin and Mucous Membranes

- Skin temperature ____
- Sensation ____
- Tissue perfusion ____
- Skin intactness ____

Measurement Scale

1 = Severely compromised
2 = Substantially compromised
3 = Moderately compromised
4 = Mildly compromised
5 = Not compromised

- Erythema ____
- Blanching ____
- Necrosis ____

Measurement Scale

1 = Severe
2 = Substantial
3 = Moderate
4 = Mild
5 = None

Wound Healing: Secondary Intention

- Purulent drainage ____
- Serous drainage ____
- Serosanguineous drainage ____
- Necrosis ____
- Sloughing ____
- Tunneling ____

Measurement Scale

1 = Extensive
2 = Substantial
3 = Moderate
4 = Limited
5 = None

INTERVENTIONS (NIC) and *RATIONALES*

Pressure Ulcer Prevention

- Use an established risk assessment tool to monitor individual's risk factors (e.g., Braden scale) *to reduce or eliminate factors that contribute to development or progression of the pressure ulcer*
- Remove excessive moisture on the skin resulting from perspiration, wound drainage, and fecal or urinary incontinence *to prevent maceration*
- Avoid massaging over bony prominences *to prevent further tissue damage*
- Turn every 1 to 2 hours *to avoid prolonged pressure in one area*
- Turn with care (e.g., avoid shearing) *to prevent injury to fragile skin*
- Position with pillows *to elevate pressure points off the bed*
- Utilize specialty beds and mattresses *as needed to provide pressure relief*
- Use devices on the bed (e.g., sheepskin) that protect the individual from pressure
- Apply elbow and heel protectors as appropriate *to avoid pressure*
- Assist individual in maintaining a healthy weight *as the risk for pressure ulcers is increased in people who are obese or very thin*

Pressure Ulcer Care

- Describe characteristics of the ulcer at regular intervals, including size (length × width × depth), stage (I–IV), location, exudate, granulation or necrotic tissue, and epithelialization *to provide baseline and ongoing data for monitoring pressure ulcer*
- Keep the ulcer moist *to aid in healing*
- Cleanse the ulcer with the appropriate nontoxic solution, working in a circular motion from the center
- Debride ulcer, as needed, *to promote new tissue growth*
- Apply a permeable adhesive membrane, saline soaks, ointments, and/or dressings, as appropriate, *to promote healing*
- Verify adequate caloric and high-quality protein intake *to provide nutrients necessary for tissue repair*
- Teach individual or family member(s) wound care procedures *to enhance self-care*
- Instruct family member/caregiver about signs of skin breakdown *to prevent recurrence*
- Initiate consultation services of the enterostomal therapy nurse, as needed, *for specialized direction of ulcer care*

TABLE 13-15 *PATIENT AND FAMILY TEACHING GUIDE*
Pressure Ulcer

1. Identify and explain risk factors and etiology of pressure ulcers to patient and family.
2. Assess all at-risk patients at time of first hospital and/or home visit or whenever the patient's condition changes.
   Thereafter assess at regular intervals based on care setting (every 48 hours for acute care or every visit in home care).
3. Teach family care techniques for incontinence. If incontinence occurs, cleanse skin at time of soiling and use pads or briefs that are absorbent.
4. Demonstrate correct positioning to decrease risk of skin breakdown. Instruct family to reposition bed-bound patient at least every 2 hours, chair-bound patient every hour. NEVER position the patient directly on the pressure ulcer.
5. Assess resources (i.e., adequacy of caregiver availability and skill, finances, and equipment) of patients requiring pressure ulcer care at home. When selecting ulcer care dressing, consider cost and amount of caregiver time.
6. Teach patient and/or caregiver to place clean dressings over sterile dressings using "no touch" technique when changing dressings. Instruct family on disposal of contaminated dressings.
7. Teach patient and family to inspect skin daily. Assess and document pressure ulcer status at least weekly; may require help from patient and family.
8. Teach patient and family the importance of good nutrition to enhance ulcer healing.
9. Evaluate program effectiveness.

After the pressure ulcer has been cleansed, it should be covered with an appropriate dressing. Some factors to consider when selecting a dressing are maintenance of a moist environment, prevention of wound desiccation (drying out), ability to absorb the wound drainage, location of the wound, amount of caregiver time, cost of the dressing, presence of infection, clean versus sterile dressings, and care delivery setting. A wet-to-dry dressing should never be used on a clean granulating pressure ulcer; this type of dressing should be used only for mechanical debridement of the wound. (Dressings are discussed in Table 13-9.)

Stages II through IV pressure ulcers are considered to be contaminated or colonized with bacteria. It is important to remember that, in persons who have chronic wounds or who are immunocompromised, the clinical signs of infection (purulent exudate, odor, erythema, warmth, tenderness, edema, pain, fever, and elevated WBC count) may not be present even though the pressure ulcer is infected.

The maintenance of adequate nutrition is an important nursing responsibility for the patient with a pressure ulcer. Often, the patient is debilitated and has a poor appetite secondary to inactivity. Clinically significant malnutrition occurs when the serum albumin is less than 3.0 g/dl, total lymphocyte count is less than 1800/μl, or body weight decreases by more than 15%. Oral feedings must be adequate in calories, proteins, fluids, vitamins, and minerals to meet the patient's nutritional requirements. The caloric intake needed to correct and maintain nutritional balance may be 30 to 35 calories/kg/day and 1.25 to 1.50 g of protein/kg/day. Nasogastric or gastrostomy feedings can be used to supplement the oral feedings. If necessary, parenteral nutrition consisting of amino acid and glucose solutions is used when oral and nasogastric feedings are inadequate. (Parenteral and enteral nutrition are discussed in Chapter 40.) NCP 13-1 outlines the care for the patient with a pressure ulcer.

Ambulatory and Home Care. Pressure ulcers affect the quality of life of patients and their caregivers. Because the recurrence of pressure ulcers is common, the education of both the patient and the care provider in prevention techniques is extremely important (see Table 13-15). (A sixth-grade level version of the patient guide to pressure ulcer prevention is available on the NPUAP website for use in patient teaching.) The care provider needs to know the etiology of pressure ulcers, prevention techniques, early signs, nutritional support, and care techniques for actual pressure ulcers. Because the patient with a pressure ulcer often requires extensive care for other health problems, it is important that the nurse support the caregiver through the added responsibility of pressure ulcer treatment.

■ Evaluation

Expected outcomes for the patient with a pressure ulcer are presented in NCP 13-1.

CRITICAL THINKING EXERCISE

CASE STUDY

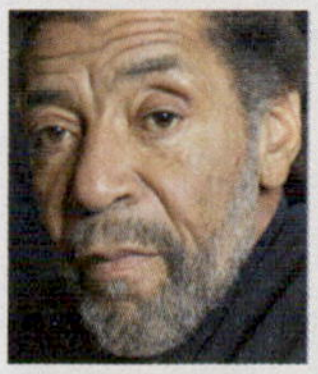

Case Study photo ©iStockphoto.com/ Gisele's Gaze.

Inflammation and Infection

Patient Profile. George, a 58-year-old African American man, was admitted to the hospital emergency department with partial-thickness burns that involved his face, neck, and upper trunk. He also had a lacerated right leg. His injuries occurred about 36 hours earlier when he fell out of a tree onto his gas grill (which was lit) while trying to get his cat.

Subjective Data

- Complains of slightly hoarse voice and irritated throat
- States that he tried to treat himself because he does not have health insurance
- Has been coughing up sooty sputum
- Complains of severe pain in left hip

Objective Data

Physical Examination

- Leg wound is gaping and has drainage: temperature 101.1° F (38.4° C)
- X-rays reveal a fractured right tibia and fractured left hip

Laboratory Studies

- WBC count 26,400/μl (26.4 × 10^9/L) with 80% neutrophils (10% bands)

Collaborative Care

- Surgery is performed to repair the left hip

Critical Thinking Questions

1. What clinical manifestations of inflammation did George exhibit, and what are their pathophysiologic mechanisms?
2. What type of exudate formation did he develop?
3. What is the basis for the development of the temperature?
4. What is the significance of his WBC count and differential?
5. Because his wound was deep, primary tissue healing was not possible. How would you expect healing to take place? What complications could he develop?
6. What risk factors does George have to develop a pressure ulcer?
7. Based on the assessment data provided, write one or more appropriate nursing diagnoses. Are there any collaborative problems?

NCLEX EXAMINATION REVIEW QUESTIONS

The number of the question corresponds to the same-numbered objective at the beginning of the chapter.

1. The role of the complement system in opsonization affects which response of the inflammatory process?
   a. Healing
   b. Cellular
   c. Vascular
   d. Formation of exudate
2. Fever that accompanies inflammation is most likely caused by
   a. activation of the complement system.
   b. release of IL-1, IL-6, and TNF from monocytes.
   c. increased production and activity of neutrophils.
   d. massive vasodilation during the vascular response.
3. A patient has an open, infected surgical wound that is treated with irrigations and moist gauze dressings. The nurse expects that this wound
   a. is classified as a black wound.
   b. has to heal by tertiary intention.
   c. heals by regeneration of epithelial cells.
   d. heals by the same processes as an uninfected deep wound.
4. Contractures frequently occur after burn healing because of
   a. secondary infection.
   b. lack of adequate blood supply.
   c. weakness of connective tissue.
   d. excess fibrous tissue formation.

5. Rest and immobilization are important measures of acute care for wound healing because they
   a. decrease the inflammatory response.
   b. increase the circulation to the affected area.
   c. increase the body's production of corticosteroids.
   d. are known mechanisms to increase cytokine production.
6. Which one of the following orders should a nurse question as part of the plan of care for a patient with a stage III pressure ulcer?
   a. Pack the ulcer with foam dressing.
   b. Turn and position the patient every 2 hours.
   c. Clean the ulcer every shift with Dakin's solution.
   d. Assess for pain and medicate before dressing change.
7. An 85-year-old patient is assessed to have a score of 15 on the Braden scale. This means that the patient
   a. has an existing stage I pressure ulcer.
   b. is at risk for developing a pressure ulcer.
   c. is in need of a weekly pressure ulcer risk assessment.
   d. is not at risk for developing a pressure ulcer at this time.
8. A 65-year-old stroke patient who is confined to bed is assessed to be at risk for the development of a pressure ulcer. Based on this information, the nurse should
   a. implement a q2hr turning schedule.
   b. have the patient maintain a high-fat diet.
   c. keep head of bed elevated to 90 degrees at all times.
   d. vigorously massage reddened bony prominences daily.
9. An 82-year-old man is being cared for at home by his family. A pressure ulcer on his right buttock measures 1 cm × 2 cm × 0.8 cm in depth, and pink tissue is completely visible on the wound bed. This pressure ulcer should be documented as
   a. stage I.
   b. stage II.
   c. stage III.
   d. stage IV.

REFERENCES

1. Thompson HJ: Fever: a concept analysis, *J Adv Nursing Sci* 51:484, 2005.
2. Ayello E, Schultz G, Sibbald G, et al: Time heals all wounds, *Nursing* 34:36, 2004.
3. MacKay D, Miller AL: Nutritional support for wound healing, *Altern Med Res* 8:359, 2003.
4. Zulkowski K: How nutrition and aging affect wound healing, *Nursing* 33:70, 2003.
5. Atkins E: Fever: its history, cause, and function, *Yale J Biol Med* 55:283, 1982.
6. Baranoski S: Using a wound assessment form, *Nursing* 35:14, 2005.
7. Langemo D: Sizing up wounds accurately, *Nursing* 35:70, 2005.
8. Baranoski S, Ayello EA: *Wound care essentials*, Philadelphia, 2004, Lippincott Williams & Wilkins.
9. Worley C: So, what do I put on this wound? Making sense of the wound dressing puzzle: part II, *Dermatol Nurs* 17:204, 2005.
10. Rijswijk L: Bridging the gap between research and practice, *AJN* 104:28, 2004.
11. Morison MJ, Ovington LG, Wilkie K: *Chronic wound care: a problem-based learning approach*, London, 2004, Mosby.
12. Mendez-Eastman S: Using negative-pressure for positive results, *Nursing* 35:48, 2005.
13. Malli S: Keep a close eye on vacuum-assisted wound closure, *Nursing* 35:25, 2005.
14. Anderson D: Using hyperbaric oxygen therapy to heal radiation wounds, *Nursing* 33:50, 2003.
15. Horn SD, Bender MS, Ferguson ML, et al: The National Pressure Ulcers Long-Term Care Study: pressure ulcer development in long-term care residents, *J Am Geriatric Soc* 52:359, 2004.
16. National Pressure Ulcer Advisory Panel (NPUAP), Cuddigan J, Ayello EA, Sussman C, editors: *Pressure ulcers in America: prevalence, incidence, and implications for the future,* Reston, Va., 2001, NPUAP.
17. AHCPR Panel for the Prediction and Prevention of Pressure Ulcers in Adults: *Pressure ulcers in adults: prediction and prevention. Clinical practice guideline, number 3* (AHCPR Publication No. 92-0047), Rockville, Md., 1992, Agency for Health Care Policy and Research.
18. National Pressure Ulcer Advisory Panel Board of Directors, Cuddigan J, Berlowitz DR, Ayello EA, editors: Pressure ulcers in America: prevalence, incidence, and implications for the future—an executive summary of the National Pressure Ulcer Advisory Panel monograph, *Adv Skin Wound Care* 14:208, 2001.
19. National Pressure Ulcer Advisory Board. *www.npuap.org* (accessed April 28, 2006).
20. Braden B, Maklebust J: Preventing pressure ulcers with the Braden scale, *AJN* 105:70, 2005.
21. Eaton-Bancroft I: Teaming up for wound care, *Nursing* 35:32, 2005.
22. National Pressure Ulcer Advisory Panel: PUSH tool information and registration form. Available at *www.npuap.org.*

RESOURCES

Advances in Skin and Wound Care
www.woundcarenet.com

Agency for Healthcare Research and Quality
301-427-1364
www.ahcpr.gov

American Academy of Wound Management
202-521-0368
www.aawm.org

American Society for Microbiology
202-737-3600
www.asmusa.org

Association for Professionals in Infection Control and Epidemiology, Inc.
202-789-1890
www.apic.org

Braden Risk Assessment Scale
www.bradenscale.com/bradenscale.htm

The European Wound Management Association
457-020-0305
www.ewma.org

Infectious Disease Society of America (IDSA)
703-299-0200
www.IDSociety.org

Johns Hopkins Healthcare Epidemiology and Infection Control
410-502-4003
www.hopkinsmedicine.org

National Center for Infectious Diseases, Antimicrobial Resistance
404-639-3311
www.cdc.gov/drugresistance

National Foundation for Infectious Diseases
301-656-0003
www.NFID.org

National Pressure Ulcer Advisory Panel
202-521-6789
www.npuap.org

Wound Ostomy and Continence Nurses Certification Board
888-496-2622
www.wocncb.org

Wound Ostomy and Continence Nurses Society
888-224-9626
www.wocn.org

For additional Internet resources, see the website for this book at *http://evolve.elsevier.com/Lewis/medsurg*.

Always remember that you are absolutely unique. Just like everybody else.

Margaret Mead

Genetics, Altered Immune Responses, and Transplantation

14

Sharon L. Lewis and Cory A. Shaw

LEARNING OBJECTIVES

1. Define com mon terms related to genetics and genetic disorders: Autosome, carrier, heterozygous, homozygous, mutation, recessive, and sex-linked.
2. Compare and contrast the most common classifications of genetic disorders.
3. Describe the functions and components of the immune system.
4. Compare and contrast humoral and cell-mediated immunity regarding lymphocytes involved, types of reactions, and effects on antigens.
5. Identify the five types of immunoglobulins and their characteristics.
6. Differentiate among the four types of hypersensitivity reactions in terms of immunologic mechanisms and resulting alterations.
7. Identify the clinical manifestations and emergency management of a systemic anaphylactic reaction.
8. Describe the assessment and collaborative care of a patient with chronic allergies.
9. Explain the relationship between the human leukocyte antigen system and certain diseases.
10. Describe the etiologic factors, clinical manifestations, and treatment modalities of autoimmune diseases.
11. Describe the etiologic factors and categories of immunodeficiency disorders.
12. Describe the various kinds of organ transplants and the types of rejections following transplantation.
13. Identify the types and side effects of immunosuppressive therapy.

KEY TERMS

anergy, p. 224
antigen, p. 219
autoimmunity, p. 234
cell-mediated immunity, p. 224
cytokines, p. 223
human leukocyte antigen, p. 233
humoral immunity, p. 223
hypersensitivity reaction, p. 224
immunocompetence, p. 224
immunodeficiency, p. 235
immunosuppressive therapy, p. 238
monoclonal antibodies, p. 240

Electronic Resources

Supplemental content related to Chapter 14 can be found . . .

Companion CD

- Stress-Busting Kit for Nursing Students
- NCLEX Examination Review Questions
- Comprehensive Glossary
- Animations
  - Function of B Cells
  - Function of T Cytotoxic Cells

Evolve Website evolve

http://evolve.elsevier.com/Lewis/medsurg

- Content Updates
- Key Points (Printable and CD/MP3 Download)
- Concept Map Creator
- Expanded Audio Glossary
- Key Term Flash Cards
- Electronic Calculators
- WebLinks

GENETICS

Genetics has a profound impact on health and disease. The study of genetics has become increasingly important for health care professionals. More than 4000 diseases are thought to be related to mutated genes. Common disorders such as heart disease and most cancers arise from a complex interplay among multiple genes and between genes and factors in the environment.[1,2]

The identification of a genetic basis for many diseases has affected the study of genetics and its relevance to nurses. This has directly influenced the care of patients at risk for or diagnosed with a disease that has a genetic basis. Nurses need to know the basic principles of genetics, be familiar with the impact that genetics has on health and disease, and be prepared to assist the patient and family in dealing with genetic issues.

Basic Principles of Genetics

In the 1860s, a monk named Gregor Mendel discovered how traits are transmitted from parents to offspring while experimenting with

Reviewed by Karen E. Greco, RN, MN, PhD, ANP, Instructor, School of Nursing, Oregon Health and Science University, Portland, Ore.; and Shelia Grossman, PhD, APRN-BC, Professor, School of Nursing, Fairfield University, Fairfield, Conn.

pea plants. This discovery led to the study of *genetics,* also known as the study of inheritance. (Common terms used in the study of genetics are listed and defined in Table 14-1.)

Genes. *Genes* are the basic units of heredity. There are approximately 20,000 to 25,000 genes in each person's genetic makeup, or *genome.* The Human Genome Project was an effort to map all of the human genome (see Genetics in Clinical Practice box). Any change in gene structure leads to a *mutation* that may alter the type and amount of protein produced.

Genes are arranged in a specific linear formation along a chromosome. Each gene has a specific location on a chromosome, termed a *locus.* An *allele* is one of two or more alternative forms of a gene that occupy corresponding loci on homologous chromosomes. Each allele codes for a specific inherited characteristic. When two gene pairs are different alleles, the allele that is fully expressed is the *dominant allele.* The other allele that lacks the ability to express itself in the presence of a dominant allele is the *recessive allele.* Physical traits expressed by a person are termed the *phenotype,* and the actual genetic makeup of the person is termed the *genotype.*

Chromosomes. *Chromosomes* are contained in the nucleus of a cell and occur in pairs. There are 23 pairs of chromosomes; 22 of the 23 pairs of chromosomes are said to be *homologous* and are termed *autosomes.* Autosomes are the same in both males and females. The sex chromosomes make up the twenty-third pair of chromosomes. A female has two X chromosomes, and a male has one X and one Y chromosome. One chromosome of each pair is inherited from the mother and one from the father. One half of each child's chromosomes (and therefore the genetic makeup) comes from his or her father and one half from his or her mother.

DNA. Genes are made up of a nucleic acid called *deoxyribonucleic acid* (DNA). DNA stores genetic information and encodes the instructions for synthesizing specific proteins needed to maintain life. DNA also dictates the rate at which proteins will be made. The DNA molecule is double stranded and is identified as a double helix. Each DNA molecule is made up of many smaller molecules, including sugar, nitrogenous bases, and phosphate units. The four nitrogenous bases making up DNA are adenine, thymine, guanine, and cytosine.

RNA. *Ribonucleic acid* (RNA) is very similar to DNA. Although they are very similar, there are some significant differences. Like DNA, RNA contains the nitrogenous bases adenine, guanine, and cytosine. However, RNA lacks the nitrogenous base thymine and instead contains uracil. RNA is single stranded and contains ribose instead of deoxyribose sugar. RNA transfers the genetic information obtained from DNA to the proper location for protein synthesis and plays a critical role during the synthesis of proteins (Fig. 14-1).

Protein Synthesis. *Protein synthesis,* or the making of proteins, occurs in two steps: *transcription* and *translation* (see Fig. 14-1). Transcription is the process by which messenger RNA (mRNA) is synthesized from single-stranded DNA. The mRNA becomes attached to a ribosome, where translation occurs. At this point another specialized type of RNA, transfer RNA (tRNA), arranges the amino acids in the correct sequence to assemble the protein. Once the protein is made, it is released from the ribosome and is able to perform its specific function.

TABLE 14-1 Glossary of Genetic Terms

Term	Definition
Allele	One of two or more alternative forms of a gene that can occupy a particular chromosomal locus
Autosome	Any chromosome that is not a sex chromosome
Carrier	Individual who carries a copy of a mutated gene for a recessive disorder
Chromosome	Gene-carrying structure in the nucleus of all human cells consisting of DNA and protein
Codominance	Two dominant versions of a trait that are both expressed in the same individual
Congenital	Condition present at birth
Dominant allele	Gene that is expressed in the phenotype of a heterozygous individual
Gene	Unit of hereditary information located on a specific part of a chromosome
Genetics	Study of inheritance; study of individual genes and their impact on relatively rare single gene disorders
Genome	Complete genetic information of an organism
Hereditary	Transmission of a disease or condition from parent to offspring
Heterozygous	Having two different alleles for one given gene
Homozygous	Having two identical alleles for one given gene
Locus	Position of a gene on a chromosome
Mutation	Change in the DNA sequence of a gene affecting the original expression of the gene
Oncogene	Gene that is able to initiate and contribute to the conversion of normal cells to cancer cells
Pedigree	Family tree that contains the genetic characteristics and disorders of that particular family
Phenotype	Clinically expressed traits of an individual
Protooncogene	Normal cellular genes that are important regulators of normal cellular processes; mutations can activate them to become oncogenes
Recessive allele	Allele that has no noticeable effect on the phenotype in a heterozygous individual
Sex-linked gene	Gene located on a sex chromosome
Trait	Physical characteristic that one inherits, such as hair and eye color

GENETICS IN CLINICAL PRACTICE
Human Genome Project

The Human Genome Project (HGP), which was initiated in 1990 and completed in 2003, was an international effort to map all 20,000 to 25,000 human genes (the human genome) and determine the complete sequence of more than 3 billion DNA bases. It involved more than 2000 scientists from 20 institutions in 6 countries. The legal, social, and ethical issues that may arise from the project are still being addressed. The U.S. HGP was sponsored by the Department of Energy (DOE) and the National Institutes of Health (NIH).

Although mapping of the human genome is complete, analysis of the data will continue for many years to come. It is believed that the knowledge gained through the HGP will help improve the diagnosis of diseases, allow for earlier detection of genetic predisposition to diseases, and play a critical role in determining risk assessment for genetic-related diseases. In addition, the results of the HGP will assist in matching organ donors with recipients in transplant programs.

Websites covering the topic of the HGP include *Human Genome Project Information* at *www.ornl.gov/hgmis* and *NIH National Human Genome Research Institute* at *www.nhgri.nih.gov.*

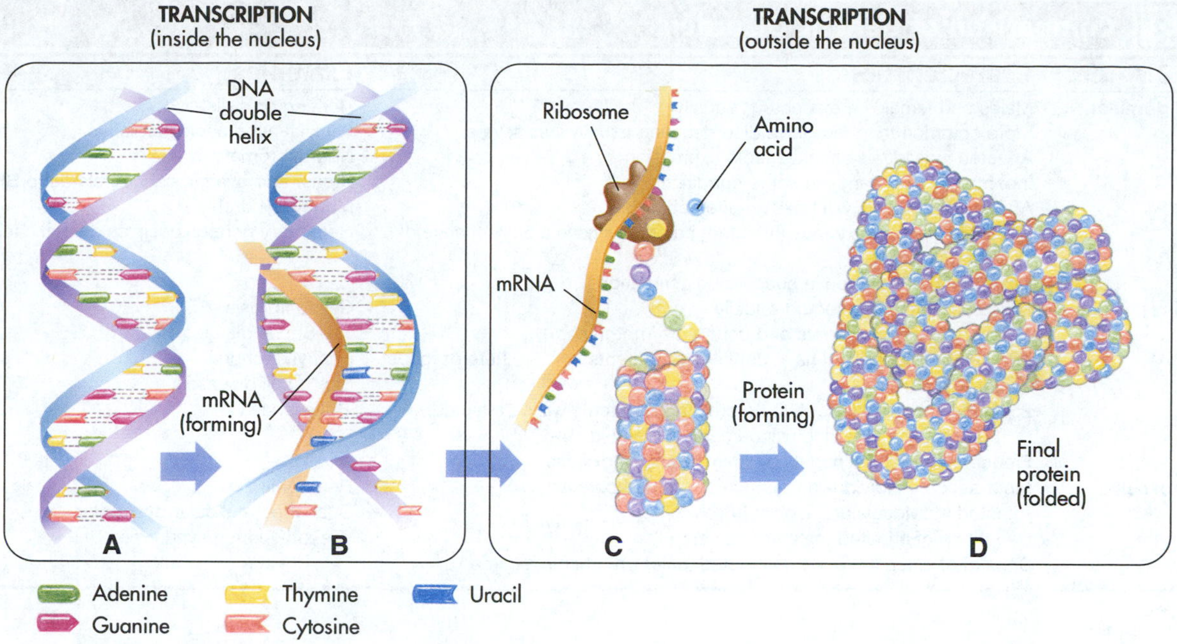

FIG. 14-1 **A,** The DNA molecule contains a sequence of genes. **B,** During transcription, the DNA code is transcribed as messenger RNA (mRNA). **C,** During translation, the mRNA code is translated at the ribosome and the proper sequence of amino acids is assembled. The amino acid strand coils or folds as it is formed. **D,** The coiled amino acid strand folds again to form a protein molecule with a specific, complex shape.

Mitosis. *Mitosis* is a type of cell division that results in the formation of genetically identical daughter cells. The chromosomes of each cell duplicate. As a result of the division, two cells (daughter cells) form. These daughter cells contain identical sets of chromosomes, which are also identical to the cell that divided, or the parent cell.

Meiosis. *Meiosis* occurs only in sexual reproductive cells. In meiosis, the number of chromosomes is reduced, resulting in half of the usual number of chromosomes. Therefore oocytes and sperm contain only a single copy of each chromosome, whereas all other body cells contain duplicates of each chromosome.

In meiosis, a process known as crossing over may occur. *Crossing over* is when genetic material is exchanged between the two chromosomes in the cell. Because one chromosome is from the mother and the other from the father, the recombination from the process of crossing over creates a greater amount of diversity in the genetic makeup of the oocytes and sperm. During meiosis, a pair of chromosomes normally separates. However, sometimes this does not completely occur. *Nondisjunction,* the failure of the two chromosomes to separate during meiosis, causes an abnormal number of chromosomes. The result is that an oocyte or sperm may have two copies of the same chromosome, or a chromosome may be missing. Examples of disorders caused by chromosome abnormalities include Down syndrome and Turner syndrome. These disorders are characterized by physical and/or mental defects.

Inheritance Patterns

Genetic disorders can be categorized into autosomal dominant, autosomal recessive, or sex-linked (X-linked) recessive disorders (Table 14-2). If the mutant gene is located on an autosome, the genetic disorder is called *autosomal.* If the mutant gene is on the X chromosome, the genetic disorder is called *X-linked.*

Autosomal dominant disorders are caused by a mutation of a single gene pair (heterozygous) on a chromosome. A dominant allele prevails over a normal allele. Autosomal dominant disorders show variable expression. *Variable expression* means that the symptoms expressed by the individuals with the mutated gene vary from person to person even though they have the same mutated gene. Although autosomal dominant disorders have a high probability of occurring in families, sometimes these disorders cause a new mutation or skip a generation. This is termed *incomplete penetrance.*

Autosomal recessive disorders are caused by mutations of two gene pairs (homozygous) on a chromosome. Fig. 14-2 shows a family pedigree with an autosomal recessive disorder. A person who inherits one copy of the recessive allele does not develop the disease because the normal allele predominates. However, such a person is a *carrier.*

X-linked recessive disorders are caused by a mutation on the X chromosome. Usually only men are affected by this disorder because women who carry the mutated gene on one X chromosome have another X chromosome to compensate for the mutation. However, women who carry the mutated gene can transmit the mutated gene to their offspring.

Multifactorial inherited conditions are caused by a combination of genetic and environmental factors. These disorders run in families but do not show the same inherited characteristics as the single-gene mutation conditions. Multifactorial conditions are poorly understood but include diabetes mellitus, obesity, hypertension, cancer, and coronary artery disease.[2]

Genetic Testing

Genetic testing includes any procedure done to analyze chromosomes, genes, or any gene product that can determine a mutation or a predisposition to a condition. Genetic tests include direct testing,

TABLE 14-2 Comparison of Genetic Disorders

Genetic Disorder	Characteristics	Examples
Autosomal dominant	Males and females are affected* equally More common than recessive disorders and usually less severe Affected individuals show variable expression Incomplete penetrance in some conditions Affected individuals will have an affected parent Children of a heterozygous (affected) parent will have a 50% chance of being affected Individuals are affected in successive generations	Huntington's disease Familial hypercholesterolemia Neurofibromatosis Breast and ovarian cancer related to BRCA genes Marfan syndrome Hereditary nonpolyposis colorectal cancer
Autosomal recessive	Males and females affected equally Heterozygotes are carriers and usually asymptomatic Affected individuals will have unaffected† parents who are heterozygous for trait 25% chance offspring of two heterozygous parents will be affected; 50% chance offspring will be carriers (see Fig. 14-2) Frequently there is a negative family history of disease	Cystic fibrosis Tay-Sachs disease Phenylketonuria Sickle cell disease Thalassemia
X-linked recessive	Most affected individuals will have unaffected parents Affected individuals are usually males Daughters of affected male are carriers Sons of affected male are unaffected (unless mother is a carrier)	Hemophilia Duchenne muscular dystrophy Wiskott-Aldrich syndrome

*Have the disease.
†Do not have the disease.

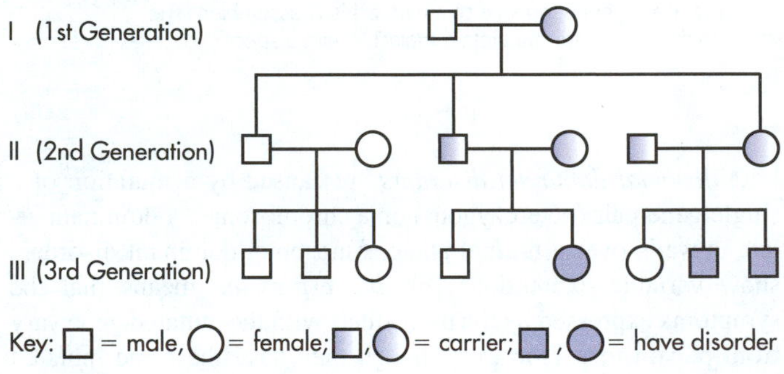

FIG. 14-2 Example of family pedigree in autosomal recessive disorder. Possible conditions represented by this family pedigree are cystic fibrosis, sickle cell anemia, thalassemia, and phenylketonuria.

linkage testing, biochemical testing, and karyotyping. Direct testing examines the DNA for any mutations. Linkage testing looks for gene markers that cause disease in family members from at least two generations. Biochemical testing includes analyzing gene products such as enzymes and proteins. *Karyotyping* investigates the number, form, size, and arrangement of the chromosomes.

A blood sample or buccal smear (skin or hair can also be used) is frequently used to obtain samples for genetic testing. Individual genetic testing may be used to confirm findings when a patient's signs and symptoms suggest a genetic disorder. Also, genetic testing can provide assessment of the risk for a presymptomatic diagnosis and assist in assessing the risk of genetic adverse outcomes of a child by testing both members of a couple for mutations.[3]

For example, genetic testing for BRCA-1 and BRCA-2 mutations can be done in women believed to be at risk for developing breast cancer. A genetic mutation in these genes has been found in 5% to 10% of all breast cancer patients. Therefore women can be tested if they develop breast cancer at a young age or have a first-degree relative with breast or ovarian cancer or a known BRCA-1 or BRCA-2 mutation. Presymptomatic testing allows physicians to take prophylactic steps, such as performing a mastectomy or oophorectomy, to avoid the development of cancer.

GENETICS IN CLINICAL PRACTICE

Genetics in Clinical Practice Boxes

Genetic Disorder	Location of Genetics Box: Chapter	Page
α_1-Antitrypsin deficiency	29	632
Alzheimer's disease	60	1565
Ankylosing spondylitis	65	1712
Breast cancer	52	1349
Cystic fibrosis	29	656
Duchenne muscular dystrophy	64	1675
Familial adenomatous polyposis (FAP)	43	1063
Familial hypercholesterolemia	34	788
Hemochromatosis	31	699
Hemophilia A and B	31	707
Hereditary nonpolyposis colorectal cancer (HNPCC)	43	1064
Human Genome Project	14	214
Huntington's disease	59	1559
Ovarian cancer	54	1402
Polycystic kidney disease	46	1176
Sickle cell disease	31	696
Types 1 and 2 diabetes mellitus	49	1256

Genetic testing of individuals opens the door for ethical and social issues. People making decisions about genetic testing should be aware that, when test results are placed in their medical records, the results might not be kept private. If an individual is tested, it may uncover information about a family member who was not tested, and these individuals are frequently not a part of the decision to undergo testing. Similarly, if a whole family is tested, the results may indicate that the biologic relationship is not what the family believed it to be.[4] Some tests are used to help guide physicians' choices about treatment. Other tests allow families to avoid having children with devastating diseases or identify people at high risk for conditions that may be prevented by monitoring or having surgery.

Widespread genetic testing has limitations. For example, many people who test positive for apolipoprotein E-4 (Apo E-4) will never develop Alzheimer's disease (see Chapter 60).

Populations of people may be tested for multiple reasons. It may be a public health matter that propels the testing, such as the practice of testing newborn children, or it may be community-based testing (i.e., screening for Tay-Sachs disease among the Ashkenazi Jewish population). All states currently test every newborn for phenylketonuria and congenital hypothyroidism. Most states also test for other genetic disorders. Also, population testing may be performed as a matter of practice, such as the testing offered to all prenatal women. These group testings identify a treatable disease before the onset of symptoms, which can be especially helpful in diseases in which early identification improves the outcome.[5]

Prenatal genetic testing can involve an amniocentesis or chorionic villus sampling (CVS) to obtain fetal cells. In an amniocentesis, a small amount of amniotic fluid is removed. CVS involves the removal of a small amount of tissue from the placenta. The tissue has the same genetic makeup as the fetus.

Genetic testing is also available on fertilized embryos prior to implantation. This is called preimplantation genetic diagnosis (PGD). This allows embryos free of particular disorders to be placed into the uterus. Embryos that test positive for genetic disorders can be destroyed. This may be a consideration for a couple at high risk for a certain genetic disorder.

Currently, over 900 genetic tests are available from testing laboratories. For more information about genetic testing, see the GeneTests website *www.genetests.org.*

Gene Therapy

Gene therapy is an experimental technique that is used to replace or repair defective or missing genes with normal genes. A normal gene can be inserted into a human chromosome to counteract the effects of a missing or abnormal gene. Although gene therapy is a promising treatment option for a number of diseases (including inherited disorders, some types of cancer, and certain viral infections), the technique remains risky and is still under study to make sure that it will be safe and effective. Gene therapy is currently only being tested for the treatment of diseases that have no other cures.[6]

The first approved gene therapy trials involved children with severe combined immunodeficiency disease caused by adenosine deaminase deficiency. T lymphocytes from these children were obtained, and the missing gene was inserted into these T cells (Fig. 14-3). The new T cells were then reinjected into the children's bloodstreams. The gene signaled the cells to produce the missing enzyme, and these children were capable of developing a functioning immune system.

Gene therapy has promise for treating a wide array of problems that do not respond to conventional methods of intervention. Although no gene therapy is used in clinical practice, the treatment strategies closest to being incorporated into mainstream therapies include those that address immunodeficiency disease, hemophilia, and ischemic vascular disease. Before gene therapy may become a practical approach to treating disease, scientists must find improved methods of delivering the genes to directly target the affected cells and must ensure that the new genes can be controlled by the body.[7]

Methods of Gene Delivery. One of the major hurdles in gene therapy is finding a way to insert the gene into the body. Genes that are inserted directly into a cell usually do not function.

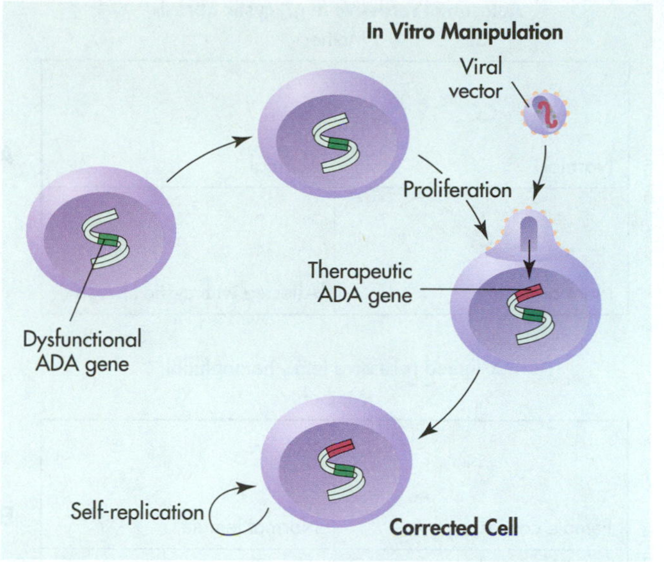

FIG. 14-3 Gene therapy for adenosine deaminase (ADA) deficiency attempts to correct this immunodeficiency state. The viral vector containing the therapeutic ADA gene is inserted into the patient's lymphocytes. These cells can then make the ADA enzyme.

Instead, a carrier, called a *vector,* is used to deliver the gene. The most common vectors are attenuated or modified versions of viruses. The viruses are modified so they cannot cause disease when used in humans.[6]

Some types of viruses, such as retroviruses, integrate their genetic material (including the new gene) into a chromosome in the human cell. Other viruses, such as adenoviruses, introduce their DNA into the nucleus of the cell, but the DNA is not integrated into a chromosome.

The vector can be injected or given intravenously (IV) directly into a specific tissue in the body, where it is taken up by the individual cells. Alternatively, a sample of the patient's cells can be removed and exposed to the vector in a laboratory setting. The cells containing the vector are returned to the patient. If the treatment is successful, the new gene delivered by the vector will make a functioning protein.

NURSING MANAGEMENT GENETICS

Nurses must be knowledgeable about the fundamentals of genetics. By understanding the profound influence that genetics has on health and disease, the nurse can assist the patient and family in making critical decisions related to genetic issues, such as genetic testing. The nurse also needs to collaborate with the team or physician to involve a genetics counselor.[8] The nurse should be able to give patients and their families accurate information pertaining to genetics, genetic diseases, and probabilities of genetic disorders. Inheritance patterns can be assessed by the nurse and explained to the patient and family through the use of Punnett squares (Fig. 14-4) and/or family pedigrees (Fig. 14-2). Maintaining patient confidentiality and respecting the patient's values and beliefs are critical since the information from the counselor may have major implications for many persons who are involved.[9]

Genetic testing may raise many psychologic issues. Knowledge of carrier status of a genetic disorder may influence a person's ca-

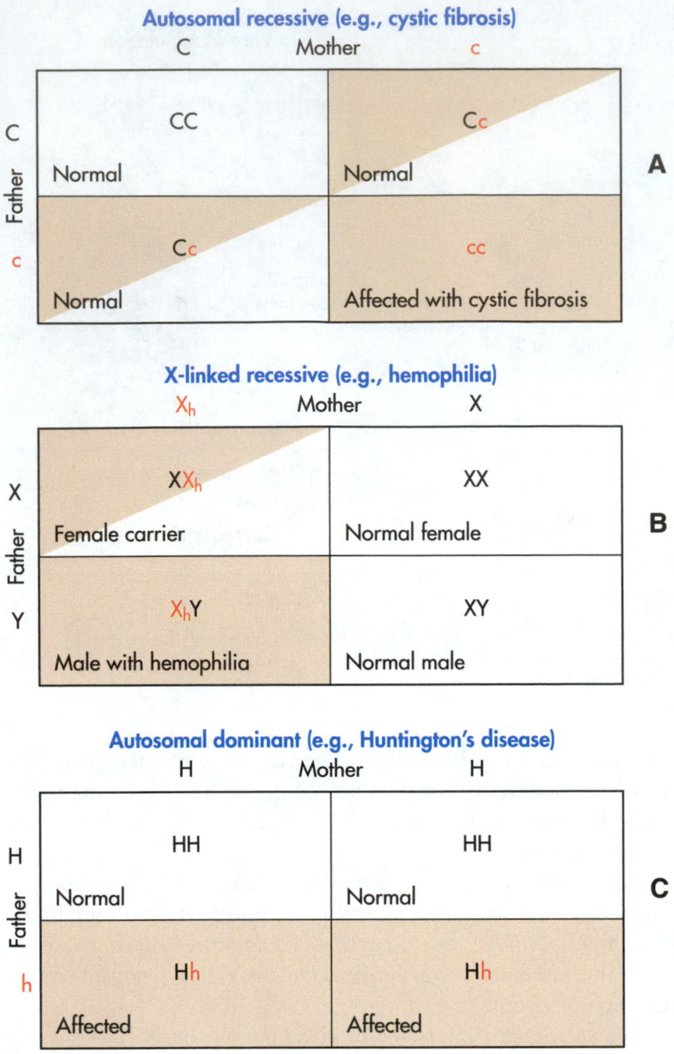

FIG. 14-4 Punnett squares can be used to determine inheritance possibilities. **A,** If the mother and father are both carriers for cystic fibrosis, there is a 25% chance that offspring will have cystic fibrosis. **B,** If the mother is a carrier for the hemophilia gene and the father has a normal genotype, there is a 50% chance that any male offspring will have hemophilia. There is a 50% chance that any female offspring will be a carrier. **C,** If the mother has a normal genotype and the father has Huntington's disease, there is a 50% chance that offspring will have the disease.

reer plans and decisions for marriage and childbearing. It may also affect significant others in grappling with serious life and health care issues. Furthermore, there are ethical concerns.[5] Who should know the results of a genetic test? How should society or the government protect individuals' privacy of test results and prevent individuals from encountering discrimination? Genetic information should not be misused to stigmatize individuals or particular ethnic groups. Attention must be paid to better understand psychosocial needs of individuals and societal responses and health care policy related to genetic testing.[10] (Genetics resources for nurses are listed at the end of the chapter.)

STEM CELLS

Stem cells are the subject of much discussion because it is believed that they may offer treatment for many chronic illnesses. The use of stem cells may allow for the regeneration of lost tissue and restoration of function in diseases such as Parkinson's disease, Alzheimer's disease, heart disease, diabetes mellitus, and spinal cord injuries.

Stem cells are cells in the body that have the ability to differentiate into other cells. Stem cells can be divided into two types: embryonic and adult.

Embryonic stem cells have the ability to become any one of the hundreds of types of cells in the human body. They are derived from human embryo cells that are 4 to 5 days old. These stem cells are pluripotent and can differentiate into any cell type that they are stimulated to become. Because of their versatility, embryonic stem cells are preferred for use in medical research.

Similar to embryonic stem cells, donor eggs can be used with existing adult tissue to produce new tissue. In a process known as nuclear transfer or therapeutic cloning, the nucleus is removed from the egg and replaced with the nucleus of the desired tissue. Then, as the egg divides, a 200-cell blastocyst of the desired tissue is created.

Adult stem cells are undifferentiated cells that are found in small numbers in most adult tissues. They are also found in children and can be extracted from umbilical cord blood. The primary roles of adult stem cells in the body are to maintain and repair tissues in which they are found. They are usually thought of as multipotent cells, giving rise to a closely related family of cells within the tissue. For example, hematopoietic stem cells form all the various cells in blood. Skin stem cells produce new skin cells. Adult stem cells have been discovered in the skin, gastrointestinal tract,

ETHICAL DILEMMAS

Genetic Testing

Situation

A 30-year-old woman informs you that she is 3 months pregnant. She has 2 children with her current husband. This pregnancy was unplanned, and her youngest child has cystic fibrosis (CF). She expresses concern regarding the possibility of having another child with CF. She mentions that she would like to have genetic testing on her fetus. Her husband asks you if they will have another child with CF.

Important Points for Consideration

- With complete and accurate information, the woman and her husband can make a decision on their own without coercion from others.
- With genetic testing, the patient and her family can find out whether or not their child will have CF.
- Genetic counseling is recommended prior to and after obtaining genetic testing because of the complexity of the information and the emotional issues involved.
- The nurse, knowing that CF is an autosomal recessive condition, can use Punnett squares (see Fig. 14-4) or a family pedigree (see Fig. 14-2) to show the woman and her husband the probability of having another child with CF.

Critical Thinking Questions

1. What information would you give the patient regarding genetic testing in order for her and her husband to make an informed decision?
2. What options are available for this couple?
3. How would you assist this couple in making a decision about possibly terminating the pregnancy if the results of the genetic testing show that the fetus tested positive for the CF gene?

and bone marrow. Scientists hope that adult stem cells can be coaxed into providing tissue for unrelated organs.

Stem cells found within the bone marrow are the body's site of hematopoiesis. The cells are prolific by design and are already being donated in the treatment of certain diseases, such as leukemia. Cells similar to the stem cells found in bone marrow can be found in the umbilical cord and blood from the placenta. These cells are used in situations similar to those of bone marrow. Studies are being conducted to find future uses that will allow the cells to become other tissues in the body.[11]

NORMAL IMMUNE RESPONSE

Immunity is a state of responsiveness to foreign substances such as microorganisms and tumor proteins.[12] Immune responses serve three functions:

1. *Defense.* The body protects against invasions by microorganisms and prevents the development of infection by attacking foreign antigens and pathogens.
2. *Homeostasis.* Damaged cellular substances are digested and removed. Through this mechanism, the body's different cell types remain uniform and unchanged.
3. *Surveillance.* Mutations continually arise in the body but are normally recognized as foreign cells and destroyed.

Types of Immunity

Immunity is classified as innate (natural) or acquired. *Innate immunity* exists in a person without prior contact with an antigen. This type of immunity involves a nonspecific response, and neutrophils and monocytes are the primary white blood cells (WBCs) involved. One type of innate immunity present at birth is species specificity of infectious agents. Humans are naturally immune to some of the infectious agents that cause illnesses in other species. *Acquired immunity* is the development of immunity, either actively or passively[13] (Table 14-3).

Active Acquired Immunity. *Active acquired immunity* results from the invasion of the body by foreign substances such as microorganisms and subsequent development of antibodies and sensitized lymphocytes. With each reinvasion of the microorganisms, the body responds more rapidly and vigorously to fight off the invader. Active acquired immunity may result naturally from a disease or artificially through inoculation of a less virulent antigen (e.g., immunizations). Because antibodies are synthesized, immunity takes time to develop but is long lasting.

Passive Acquired Immunity. *Passive acquired immunity* implies that the host receives antibodies to an antigen rather than synthesizing them. This may take place naturally through the transfer of immunoglobulins across the placental membrane from mother to fetus. Artificial passive acquired immunity occurs through injection with gamma globulin (serum antibodies). The benefit of this immunity is its immediate effect. Unfortunately, passive immunity is short lived, because the host did not synthesize the antibodies and consequently does not retain memory cells for the antigen.

TABLE 14-3 Types of Acquired Specific Immunity

Active

Natural

Natural contact with antigen through clinical infection (e.g., recovery from chickenpox, measles, mumps)

Artificial

Immunization with antigen (e.g., immunization with live or killed vaccines)

Passive

Natural

Transplacental and colostrum transfer from mother to child (e.g., maternal immunoglobulins in neonate)

Artificial

Injection of serum from immune human (e.g., injection of human gamma globulin)

HEALTHY PEOPLE

Health Impact of Immunization

- Can help control the spread of infections within communities
- Can prevent disability and death from infectious disease for individuals
- Reduces and can possibly eliminate polio, measles, and other diseases with widespread use

Note: Recommended immunizations for adults 65 years and older include a yearly immunization against influenza and a one-time immunization against pneumococcal disease.

Antigens

An **antigen** is a substance that elicits an immune response. Most antigens are composed of protein. However, other substances such as large-size polysaccharides, lipoproteins, and nucleic acids can act as antigens. All of the body's cells have antigens on their surface that are unique to that person and enable the body to recognize itself. The immune system becomes "tolerant" to the body's own molecules and therefore is nonresponsive to "self" antigens.

Lymphoid Organs

The lymphoid system is composed of central (or primary) and peripheral lymphoid organs. The *central lymphoid organs* are the thymus gland and bone marrow. The *peripheral lymphoid organs* are the tonsils; gut-, genital-, bronchial-, and skin-associated lymphoid tissues; lymph nodes; and spleen (Fig. 14-5).

Lymphocytes are produced in the bone marrow and eventually migrate to the peripheral organs. The thymus is important in the differentiation and maturation of T lymphocytes and is therefore essential for a cell-mediated immune response. During childhood the gland is large. The gland shrinks with age and is a collection of reticular fibers, lymphocytes, and connective tissue in older persons.

Lymphoid tissue is found in the submucosa of the respiratory (bronchial-associated), genitourinary (genital-associated), and gastrointestinal (gut-associated) tracts. This tissue protects the body surface from external microorganisms. The tonsils are a typical example of lymphoid tissue.

The skin-associated lymph tissue primarily consists of lymphocytes and Langerhans cells (a type of dendritic cell) found in the epidermis of skin. When Langerhans cells are depleted, the skin can neither initiate an immune response nor support a skin-localized delayed hypersensitivity response.

When antigens are introduced into the body, they may be carried by the bloodstream or lymph channels to regional lymph nodes. The antigens interact with B and T lymphocytes and mac-

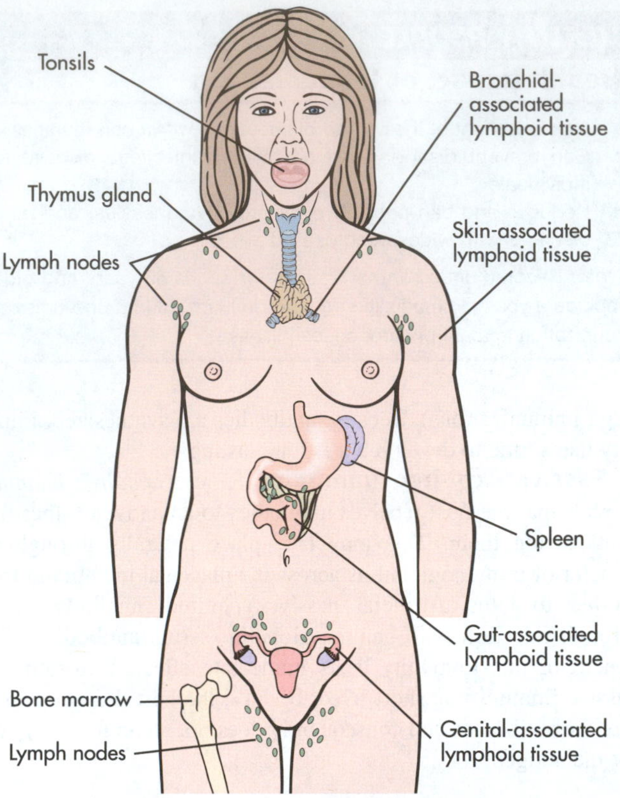

FIG. 14-5 Organs of the immune system.

rophages in the lymph nodes. The two important functions of lymph nodes are (1) filtration of foreign material brought to the site and (2) circulation of lymphocytes.

The spleen is important as the primary site for filtering foreign substances from the blood. It consists of two kinds of tissue: white pulp containing B and T lymphocytes and red pulp containing erythrocytes. Macrophages line the pulp and sinuses of the spleen. The spleen is the major site of immune responses to blood-borne antigens.

Cells Involved in Immune Response

Mononuclear Phagocytes. The *mononuclear phagocyte system* includes monocytes in the blood and macrophages found throughout the body. Mononuclear phagocytes have a critical role in the immune system. They are responsible for capturing, processing, and presenting the antigen to the lymphocytes. This stimulates a humoral or cell-mediated immune response. Capturing is accomplished through phagocytosis. The macrophage-bound antigen, which is highly immunogenic, is presented to circulating T or B lymphocytes and thus triggers an immune response (Fig. 14-6).

Lymphocytes. Lymphocytes are produced in the bone marrow (Fig. 14-7). Lymphocytes differentiate into B and T lymphocytes.

B Lymphocytes. In the early research on *B lymphocytes* (bursa-equivalent lymphocytes) in birds, it was discovered that they mature under the influence of the bursa of Fabricius. Hence the name of B-cells. However, this lymphoid organ does not exist in humans. The bursa-equivalent tissue in humans is the bone marrow. B cells differentiate into *plasma cells* when activated. Plasma cells produce antibodies (immunoglobulins) (Table 14-4).

T Lymphocytes. Cells that migrate from the bone marrow to the thymus differentiate into *T lymphocytes* (thymus-dependent cells). The thymus secretes hormones, including thymosin, that stimulate the maturation and differentiation of T lymphocytes. T cells compose 70% to 80% of the circulating lymphocytes and are primarily responsible for immunity to intracellular viruses, tumor cells, and fungi. T cells live from a few months to the life span of an individual and account for long-term immunity.

T lymphocytes can be categorized into T cytotoxic and T helper cells. Antigenic characteristics of WBCs have now been classified using monoclonal antibodies. These antigens are classified as *clusters of differentiation* or *CD antigens.* Many types of WBCs, especially lymphocytes, are referred to by their CD designations. All mature T cells have the CD3 antigen.

T Cytotoxic Cells. T cytotoxic (or cytolytic) (CD8) cells are involved in attacking antigens on the cell membrane of foreign pathogens and releasing cytolytic substances that destroy the pathogen. These cells have antigen specificity and are sensitized by exposure to the antigen. Similar to B lymphocytes, some sensitized T cells do not attack the antigen but remain as memory T cells. As in the humoral immune response, a second exposure to the antigen will result in a more intense and rapid cell-mediated immune response.

T Helper Cells. T helper (CD4) cells are involved in the regulation of cell-mediated immunity and the humoral antibody response. T helper cells differentiate into subsets of cells that produce distinct types of cytokines (discussed in a later section). These subsets are called T_H1 cells and T_H2 cells. T_H1 cells stimulate phagocyte-mediated ingestion and killing of microbes, the key component of cell-mediated immunity. T_H2 cells stimulate phagocyte independent, eosinophil-mediated immunity, which is effective against parasites. They are also involved in allergic responses.

TABLE 14-4 Characteristics of Immunoglobulins

Class	Relative Serum Concentration (%)	Location	Characteristics
IgG	76	Plasma, interstitial fluid	Is only immunoglobulin that crosses placenta Is responsible for secondary immune response
IgA	15	Body secretions, including tears, saliva, breast milk, colostrum	Lines mucous membranes and protects body surfaces
IgM	8	Plasma	Is responsible for primary immune response Forms antibodies to ABO blood antigens
IgD	1	Plasma	Is present on lymphocyte surface Assists in the differentiation of B lymphocytes
IgE	0.002	Plasma, interstitial fluids	Causes symptoms of allergic reactions Fixes to mast cells and basophils Assists in defense against parasitic infections

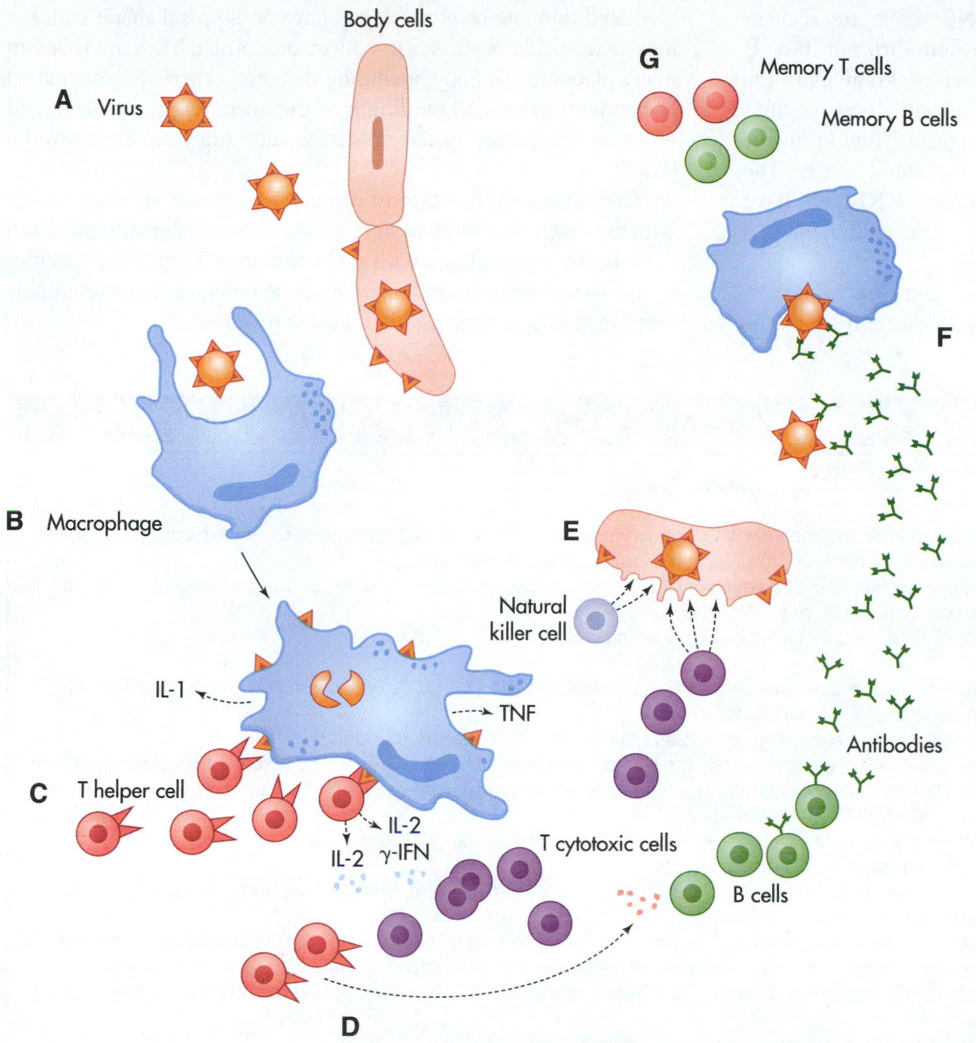

FIG. 14-6 The immune response to a virus. **A,** A virus invades the body through a break in the skin or another portal of entry. The virus must make its way inside a cell in order to replicate itself. **B,** A macrophage recognizes the antigens on the surface of the virus. The macrophage digests the virus and displays pieces of the virus (antigens) on its surface. **C,** A T helper cell recognizes the antigen displayed and binds to the macrophage. This binding stimulates the production of cytokines (interleukin-1 [IL-1] and tumor necrosis factor [TNF]) by the macrophage and interleukin-2 (IL-2) and γ-interferon (γ-IFN) by the T cell. These cytokines are intracellular messengers that provide communication among the cells. **D,** IL-2 instructs other T helper cells and T cytotoxic cells to proliferate (multiply). T helper cells release cytokines, causing B cells to multiply and produce antibodies. **E,** T cytotoxic cells and natural killer cells destroy infected body cells. **F,** The antibodies bind to the virus and mark it for macrophage destruction. **G,** Memory B and T cells remain behind to respond quickly if the same virus attacks again.

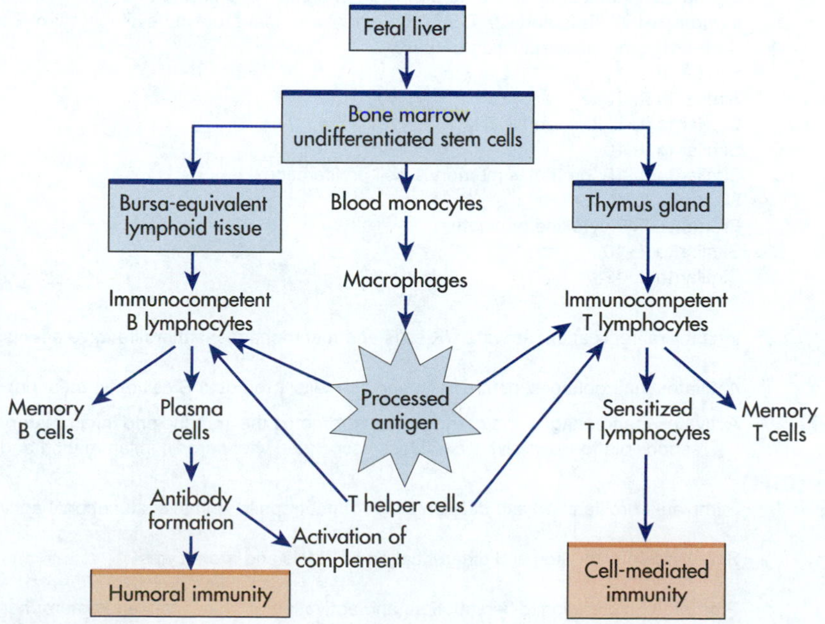

FIG. 14-7 Relationships and functions of macrophages, B lymphocytes, and T lymphocytes in an immune response.

Natural Killer Cells. Natural killer (NK) cells are also involved in cell-mediated immunity. These cells are not T or B cells, but are large lymphocytes with numerous granules in the cytoplasm. NK cells do not require prior sensitization for their generation. These cells are involved in recognition and killing of virus-infected cells, tumor cells, and transplanted grafts. The mechanism of recognition is not fully understood. NK cells have a significant role in immune surveillance for malignant cell changes.

Dendritic Cells. *Dendritic cells* make up a system of cells that are important to the immune system, especially the cell-mediated immune response. They have an atypical shape with extensive dendritic processes that form and retract. They are found in many places in the body, including the skin (where they are called Langerhans cells) and the lining of the nose, lungs, stomach, and intestine. Especially in the immature state, they are found in the blood.

They primarily function to capture antigens at sites of contact with the external environment (e.g., skin, mucous membranes) and then transport an antigen until it encounters a T cell with specificity for the antigen. In this role, dendritic cells can have an important function in activating the immune response.

TABLE 14-5 Types and Functions of Cytokines

Type	Primary Functions
Interleukins (ILs)	
IL-1	Augments the immune response; inflammatory mediator; promotes maturation and clonal expansion of B cells; enhances activity of NK cells; activates T cells, activates macrophages
IL-2	Induces proliferation and differentiation of T cells; activation of T cells, NK cells, and macrophages; stimulates release of other cytokines (α-IFN, TNF, IL-1, IL-6)
IL-3 (multicolony colony-stimulating factor)	Hematopoietic growth factor for hematopoietic precursor cells
IL-4	B-cell growth factor; stimulates proliferation and differentiation of B cells; induces differentiation into T_H2 cells; stimulates growth of mast cells
IL-5	B cell growth and differentiation; promotes growth and differentiation of eosinophils
IL-6	T- and B-cell growth factor; enhances the inflammatory response; promotes differentiation of B cells into plasma cells; stimulates antibody secretion; induces fever; synergistic effects with IL-1 and TNF
IL-7	Promotes growth of T and B cells
IL-8	Chemotaxis of neutrophils and T cells; stimulates superoxide and granule release
IL-9	Enhances T-cell survival; mast cell activation
IL-10	Inhibits cytokine production by T and NK cells; promotes B-cell proliferation and antibody responses; potent suppressor of macrophage function
IL-11	Synergistic action with IL-3 and IL-4 in hematopoiesis; is a multifunctional regulator of hematopoiesis and lymphopoiesis; osteoclast formation; elevates platelet count; inhibits proinflammatory cytokine production
IL-12	Promotes α-IFN production; induction of T helper cells; activates NK cells; stimulates proliferation of activated T and NK cells
IL-13	B cell growth and differentiation; inhibits proinflammatory cytokine production
IL-14	Stimulates proliferation of activated B cells
IL-15	Mimics IL-2 effects; stimulates proliferation of T cells and NK cells
IL-16	Proinflammatory cytokine; chemoattractant of T cells, eosinophils, and monocytes
IL-17	Promotes release of IL-6, IL-8, and G-CSF; enhances expression of adhesion molecules
IL-18	Induces α-IFN, IL-2, and GM-CSF production; important role in development of T helper cells; enhances NK activity; inhibits production of IL-10
IL-19	Similar to IL-10
IL-20	Similar to IL-10
IL-21	Similar to IL-2, IL-4, and IL-5
IL-22	Similar to IL-10
IL-23	Similar to IL-12; promotes memory T cell proliferation
IL-24	Similar to IL-10
IL-25	Promotes T_H2 cytokine production
IL-26	Similar to IL-10
IL-27	Similar to IL-12
Interferons (IFNs)	
α-Interferon (α-IFN)	Inhibit viral replication; activate NK cells and macrophages; antiproliferative effects on tumor cells
β-Interferon (β-IFN)	
γ-Interferon (γ-IFN)	Activates macrophages, neutrophils, and NK cells; promotes B cell differentiation; inhibits viral replication
Tumor Necrosis Factor (TNF)	Activates macrophages and granulocytes; promotes the immune and inflammatory responses; kills tumor cells; is responsible for extensive weight loss associated with chronic inflammation and cancer
Colony-Stimulating Factors (CSFs)	
Granulocyte colony-stimulating factor (G-CSF)	Stimulates proliferation and differentiation of neutrophils; enhances functional activity of mature PMNs
Granulocyte-macrophage colony-stimulating factor (GM-CSF)	Stimulates proliferation and differentiation of PMNs and monocytes
Macrophage colony-stimulating factor (M-CSF)	Promotes proliferation, differentiation, and activation of monocytes and macrophages
Erythropoietin	Stimulates erythroid progenitor cells in bone marrow to produce red blood cells

NK, Natural killer; *PMN,* polymorphonuclear neutrophil.

Cytokines

The immune response involves complex interactions of T cells, B cells, monocytes, and neutrophils. These interactions depend on **cytokines** (soluble factors secreted by WBCs and a variety of other cells in the body) that act as messengers between the cell types. Cytokines instruct cells to alter their proliferation, differentiation, secretion, or activity. There are currently at least 100 different cytokines, and they can be classified into distinct categories. Some of these cytokines are listed in Table 14-5. In general, the interleukins act as immunomodulatory factors, colony-stimulating factors act as growth-regulating factors for hematopoietic cells, and interferons are antiviral and immunomodulatory.

Cytokines have a beneficial role in hematopoiesis and immune function. They can also have detrimental effects such as those seen in chronic inflammation, autoimmune diseases, and sepsis. Cytokines such as erythropoietin (see Chapter 47), colony-stimulating factors (see Table 16-18), interferons (see Table 16-17), and interleukin-2 (see Table 16-17) are used clinically to (1) stimulate hematopoiesis, (2) stimulate the bone marrow to make WBCs, and (3) treat various malignancies. In addition, inhibitors of cytokines such as soluble tumor necrosis factor receptor antagonist and interleukin-1 are being used in clinical trials as antiinflammatory agents. (Clinical uses of cytokines are listed in Table 14-6.)

Interferon helps the body's natural defenses attack tumors and viruses. Three types of interferon have now been identified (see Table 14-5). In addition to their direct antiviral properties, interferons have immunoregulatory functions. These include enhancement of NK cell production and activation, and inhibition of tumor cell growth.

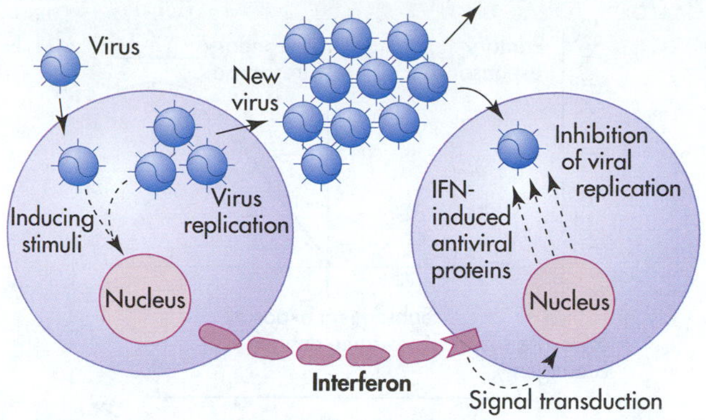

FIG. 14-8 Mechanism of action of interferon. When a virus attacks a cell, the cell begins to synthesize viral DNA and interferon. Interferon serves as an intercellular messenger. Interferon induces the production of antiviral proteins. Then the virus is not able to replicate in the cell.

Interferon is not directly antiviral but produces an antiviral effect in cells by reacting with them and inducing the formation of a second protein termed *antiviral protein* (Fig. 14-8). This protein mediates the antiviral action of interferon by altering the cell's protein synthesis and preventing new viruses from becoming assembled.[13,14]

TABLE 14-6 Clinical Uses of Cytokines

Cytokine	Clinical Uses
α-Interferon (Roferon-A, Intron A)	Hairy-cell leukemia, chronic myelogenous leukemia, malignant melanoma, renal cell carcinoma, non-Hodgkin's lymphoma, ovarian cancer, multiple myeloma, Kaposi sarcoma
β-Interferon (Betaseron, Avonex, Rebif)	Multiple sclerosis
Colony-Stimulating Factors	
G-CSF	
filgrastim (Neupogen), pegfilgrastim (Neulasta)	Chemotherapy-induced neutropenia
GM-CSF	
sargramostim (Leukine)	Neutropenia, myeloid recovery after bone marrow transplantation
Soluble TNF Receptor	
etanercept (Enbrel)	Rheumatoid arthritis
Interleukin-2	
aldesleukin (Proleukin)	Metastatic renal cell carcinoma, metastatic melanoma
Interleukin 11 (platelet growth factor)	
oprelvekin (Neumega)	Prevention of thrombocytopenia following chemotherapy
Erythropoetin	
epoetin alfa (Epogen, Procrit), darbepoetin alfa (Aranesp)	Anemia of chronic cancer, anemia related to chemotherapy
IL-1 Receptor Antagonist	
anakinra (Kineret)	Rheumatoid arthritis

G-CSF, Granulocyte colony-stimulating factor; *GM-CSF,* granulocyte-macrophage colony-stimulating factor; *IL,* interleukin; *TNF,* tumor necrosis factor.

Comparison of Humoral and Cell-Mediated Immunity

Humans need both humoral and cell-mediated immunity to remain healthy. Each type of immunity has unique properties and different methods of action; each reacts against particular antigens. Table 14-7 compares humoral and cell-mediated immunity.[12]

Humoral Immunity. **Humoral immunity** consists of antibody-mediated immunity. The term *humoral* comes from the Greek word *humor,* which means body fluid. Antibodies are produced by plasma cells (differentiated B cells) and found in plasma; therefore the term *humoral immunity* is used. Production of antibodies is an essential component in a humoral immune response. Each

TABLE 14-7 Comparison of Humoral Immunity and Cell-Mediated Immunity

Characteristics	Humoral Immunity	Cell-Mediated Immunity
Cells involved	B lymphocytes	T lymphocytes, macrophages
Products	Antibodies	Sensitized T cells, cytokines
Memory cells	Present	Present
Protection	Bacteria Viruses (extracellular) Respiratory and gastrointestinal pathogens	Fungus Viruses (intracellular) Chronic infectious agents Tumor cells
Examples	Anaphylactic shock Atopic diseases Transfusion reaction Bacterial infections	Tuberculosis Fungal infections Contact dermatitis Graft rejection Destruction of cancer cells

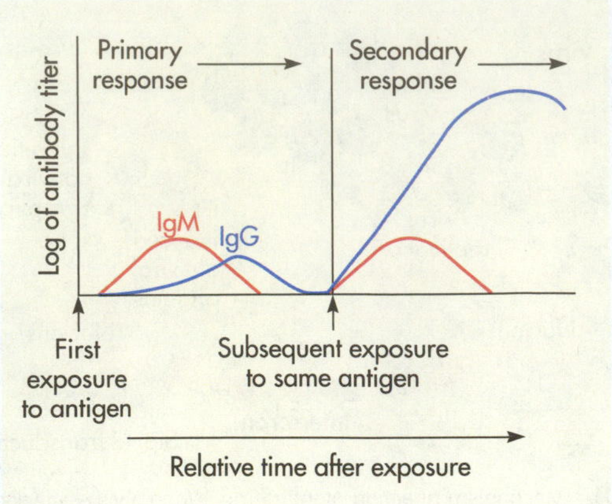

FIG. 14-9 Primary and secondary immune responses. The introduction of antigen induces a response dominated by two classes of immunoglobulins, IgM and IgG. IgM predominates in the primary response, with some IgG appearing later. After the host's immune system is primed, another challenge with the same antigen induces the secondary response, in which some IgM and large amounts of IgG are produced.

of the five classes of immunoglobulins (Igs), which are IgG, IgA, IgM, IgD, and IgE, has specific characteristics (see Table 14-4).

When a pathogen (especially bacteria) enters the body, it may encounter a B lymphocyte that is specific for antigens located on that bacterial cell wall. In addition, a monocyte or macrophage may phagocytize the bacteria and present its antigens to a B lymphocyte. The B lymphocyte recognizes the antigen because it has receptors on its cell surface specific for that antigen. When the antigen comes in contact with the cell surface receptor, the B cell becomes activated, and most B cells will differentiate into plasma cells (see Fig. 14-7). The mature plasma cell secretes immunoglobulins. Some stimulated B lymphocytes remain as memory cells.

The primary immune response is evident 4 to 8 days after the initial exposure to the antigen (Fig. 14-9). IgM is the first type of antibody formed. Because of the large size of the IgM molecule, this immunoglobulin is confined to the intravascular space. As the immune response progresses, IgG is produced and can move from intravascular to extravascular spaces.

When the individual is exposed to the antigen the second time, a secondary antibody response occurs. This response occurs faster (1 to 3 days), is stronger, and lasts for a longer time than a primary response. Memory cells account for the memory of the first exposure to the antigen and the more rapid production of antibodies. IgG is the primary antibody found in a secondary immune response.

IgG crosses the placental membrane and provides the newborn with passive acquired immunity for at least 3 months. Infants may also get some passive immunity from IgA in breast milk and colostrum.

Cell-Mediated Immunity. Immune responses that are initiated through specific antigen recognition by T cells are termed **cell-mediated immunity.** Although these reactions were initially considered to be solely mediated by T cells, several cell types and factors are involved in cell-mediated immunity. The cell types involved include T lymphocytes, macrophages, and NK cells. Cell-mediated immunity is of primary importance in (1) immunity against pathogens that survive inside of cells, including viruses and some bacteria (e.g., *Mycobacterium*); (2) fungal infections; (3) rejection of transplanted tissues; (4) contact hypersensitivity reactions; and (5) tumor immunity.[15]

TABLE 14-8 GERONTOLOGIC DIFFERENCES IN ASSESSMENT
Effects of Aging on the Immune System

- Thymic involution
- ↓ Cell-mediated immunity
- ↓ Delayed hypersensitivity reaction
- ↓ IL-1 and IL-2 synthesis
- ↓ Expression of IL-2 receptors
- ↓ Proliferative response of T and B cells
- ↓ Primary and secondary antibody responses
- ↓ Autoantibodies

IL, Interleukin.

GERONTOLOGIC CONSIDERATIONS
EFFECTS OF AGING ON THE IMMUNE SYSTEM

With advancing age, there is a decline in the immune system[16] (Table 14-8). The primary clinical evidence for this *immunosenescence* is the high incidence of tumors in older adults. A greater susceptibility also occurs to infections (e.g., influenza, pneumonia) from pathogens that an older person had been relatively immunocompetent against earlier in life.

Aging does not affect all aspects of the immune system. The bone marrow is relatively unaffected by increasing age. However, aging has a pronounced effect on the thymus, which decreases in size and activity with aging. These changes in the thymus are probably a primary cause of immunosenescence. Both T and B cells show deficiencies in activation, transit time through the cell cycle, and subsequent differentiation. However, the most significant alterations involve T cells. As thymic output of T cells diminishes, the differentiation of T cells increases. Consequently, there is an accumulation of memory cells rather than new precursor cells responsive to previously unencountered antigens.

The delayed hypersensitivity reaction, as determined by skin testing with injected antigens, is frequently decreased or absent in older adults. This altered response reflects **anergy** (an immunodeficient condition characterized by lack of or diminished reaction to an antigen or a group of antigens). The clinical consequences of a decline in cell-mediated immunity are evident.

ALTERED IMMUNE RESPONSE

Immunocompetence exists when the body's immune system can identify and inactivate or destroy foreign substances. When the immune system is incompetent or underresponsive, severe infections, immunodeficiency diseases, and malignancies may occur. When the immune system overreacts, hypersensitivity disorders such as allergies and autoimmune diseases may occur.

Hypersensitivity Reactions

Sometimes the immune response is overreactive against foreign antigens or fails to maintain self-tolerance, and this results in tissue damage. This is termed a **hypersensitivity reaction.** A type of hypersensitivity response occurs when the body fails to recognize self-proteins and reacts against its own protein. The diseases that occur as a result of immune responses against self-antigens are termed *autoimmune diseases.*

Classification of hypersensitivity reactions may be done according to the source of the antigen, the time sequence (immediate or delayed), or the basic immunologic mechanisms causing the in-

TABLE 14-9 Types of Hypersensitivity Reactions

	Type I: IgE-Mediated	Type II: Cytotoxic Reactions	Type III: Immune-Complex Reactions	Type IV: Delayed Hypersensitivity Reactions
Antigen	Exogenous pollen, food, drugs, dust	Cell surface of RBCs Basement membrane	Extracellular fungal, viral, bacterial	Intracellular or extracellular
Antibody involved	IgE	IgG IgM	IgG IgM	None
Complement involved	No	Frequently	Yes	No
Mediators of injury	Histamine Mast cells Leukotrienes Prostaglandins	Complement lysis Macrophages in tissues	Neutrophils Complement lysis	Cytokines T cytotoxic cells Monocytes/macrophages Lysosomal enzymes
Examples	Allergic rhinitis Asthma	Transfusion reaction Goodpasture syndrome Autoimmune thrombocytopenic purpura Graves' disease	Systemic lupus erythematosus Rheumatoid arthritis	Contact dermatitis to poison ivy
Skin test	Wheal and flare	None	Erythema and edema in 3-8 hr	Erythema and edema in 24-48 hr (e.g., TB test)

RBCs, Red blood cells; *TB,* tuberculosis.

jury. Basically, four types of hypersensitivity reactions exist. Types I, II, and III are immediate and are examples of humoral immunity. Type IV is a delayed hypersensitivity reaction and is related to cell-mediated immunity. Table 14-9 presents a summary of the four types of hypersensitivity reactions.

Type I: IgE-Mediated Reactions. *Anaphylactic reactions* are type I reactions that occur only in susceptible persons who are highly sensitized to specific allergens. IgE antibodies, produced in response to the allergen, have a characteristic property of attaching to mast cells and basophils (see Fig. 14-10 and Fig. 29-2). Within these cells are granules containing potent chemical mediators (histamine, serotonin, leukotrienes, eosinophil chemotactic factor of anaphylaxis [ECF-A], kinins, and bradykinin). (Chemical mediators of inflammation are discussed in Chapter 13 and Fig. 13-5.) On the first exposure to the allergen, IgE antibodies are produced and bind to mast cells and basophils. On any subsequent exposures, the allergen links with the IgE bound to mast cells or basophils and triggers degranulation of the cells and the release of chemical mediators from the granules. In this process, the mediators that are released attack target organs, causing clinical allergy symptoms. These effects include smooth muscle contraction, increased vascular permeability, vasodilation, hypotension, increased secretion of mucus, and itching. Fortunately, the mediators are short acting and their effects are reversible. (The mediators and their effects are summarized in Table 14-10.)

A genetic predisposition to the development of allergic diseases exists. The capacity to become sensitized to an allergen appears to be the inherited trait, rather than the specific allergic disorder. For example, a father with asthma may have a son who has allergic rhinitis.

The clinical manifestations of an anaphylactic reaction depend on whether the mediators remain local or become systemic or whether they affect particular organs. When the mediators remain localized, a cutaneous response termed the *wheal-and-flare reaction* occurs. This reaction is characterized by a pale wheal containing edematous fluid surrounded by a red flare from the hyperemia. The reaction occurs in minutes or hours and is usually not danger-

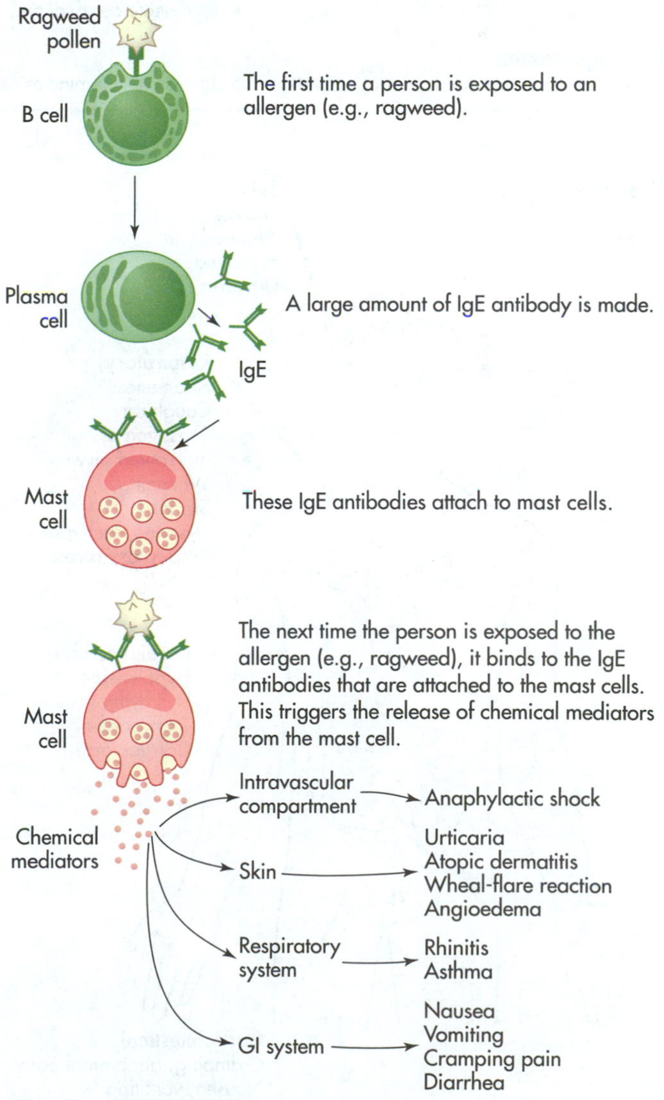

FIG. 14-10 Steps in a type I allergic reaction.

TABLE 14-10 Mediators of Allergic Response

Type and Source	Biologic Activity	Clinical Outcomes
Histamine Mast cell and basophil granules	Increases vascular permeability; constricts smooth muscle; stimulates irritant receptors	Edema of airways and larynx; bronchial constriction; urticaria, angioedema, pruritus; nausea, vomiting, diarrhea; shock
Leukotrienes Metabolites of arachidonic acid by lipoxygenase pathway*	Constrict bronchial smooth muscle; increase vascular permeability	Bronchial constriction; enhanced effect of histamine on smooth muscle
Prostaglandins Metabolites of arachidonic acid by cyclooxygenase pathway*	Stimulate vasodilation; constrict smooth muscle	Wheal-and-flare reaction on skin; hypotension; bronchospasm
Platelet-Activating Factor Mast cell	Aggregates platelets; stimulates vasodilation	Increase in pulmonary artery pressure; systemic hypotension
Kinins Kininogen	Stimulate slow, sustained smooth muscle contraction; increase vascular permeability; stimulate secretion of mucus; stimulate pain receptors	Angioedema with painful swelling; bronchial constriction
Serotonin Platelets	Increases vascular permeability; stimulates smooth muscle contraction	Mucosal edema; bronchial constriction
Anaphylatoxins C3a, C4a, C5a from complement activation	Stimulate histamine release	Same as for histamine

*See Chapter 13, Fig. 13-5.

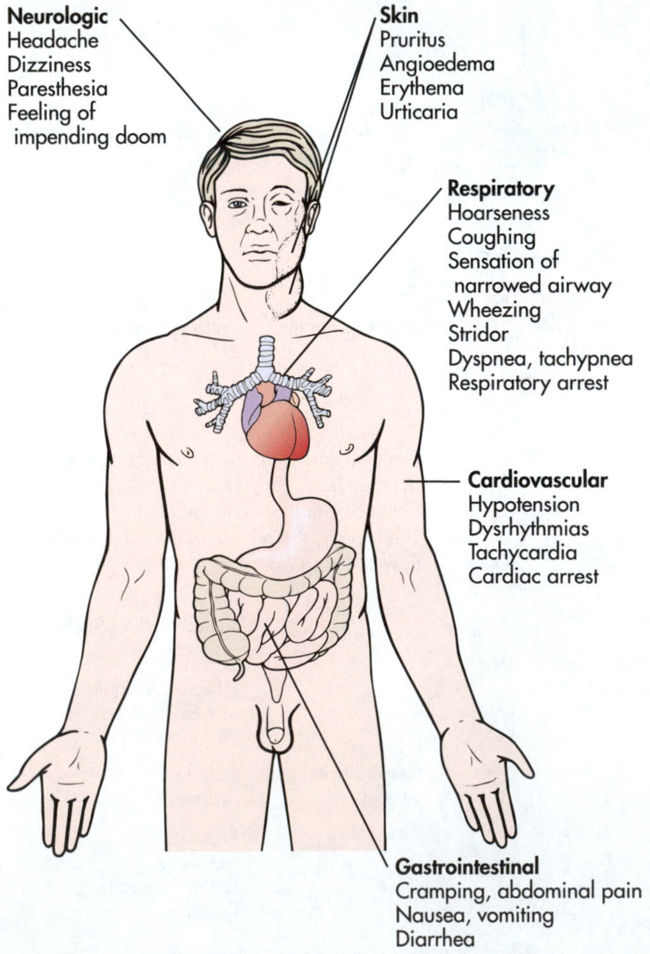

FIG. 14-11 Clinical manifestations of a systemic anaphylactic reaction.

ous. A classic example of a wheal-and-flare reaction is the mosquito bite. The wheal-and-flare reaction serves a diagnostic purpose as a means of demonstrating allergic reactions to specific allergens during skin tests.

Common allergic reactions include anaphylaxis and atopic reactions.

Anaphylaxis. *Anaphylaxis* can occur when mediators are released systemically (e.g., after injection of a drug, after an insect sting). The reaction occurs within minutes and can be life threatening because of bronchial constriction and subsequent airway obstruction and vascular collapse. The target organs affected are seen in Fig. 14-11. Initial symptoms include edema and itching at the site of the exposure to the allergen. Shock can occur rapidly and is manifested by rapid, weak pulse; hypotension; dilated pupils; dyspnea; and possibly cyanosis. This is compounded by bronchial edema and angioedema. Death will occur if emergency treatment is not initiated. Some of the important allergens leading to anaphylactic shock in hypersensitive persons are listed in Table 14-11.

Atopic Reactions. An estimated 20% of the population is *atopic,* having an inherited tendency to become sensitive to environmental allergens. The atopic diseases that can result are allergic rhinitis, asthma, atopic dermatitis, urticaria, and angioedema.

Allergic rhinitis, or hay fever, is the most common type I hypersensitivity reaction. It may occur year-round (perennial allergic rhinitis), or it may be seasonal (seasonal allergic rhinitis). Airborne substances such as pollens, dust, and molds are the primary cause of allergic rhinitis. Perennial allergic rhinitis may be caused by dust, molds, and animal dander. Seasonal allergic rhinitis is commonly caused by pollens from trees, weeds, or grasses. The target areas affected are the conjunctiva of the eyes and the mucosa of the upper respiratory tract. Symptoms include nasal discharge, sneezing, lacrimation, mucosal swelling with airway obstruction, and

TABLE 14-11 Allergens Causing Anaphylactic Shock

Drugs
Penicillins
Sulfonamides
Insulins
Aspirin
Tetracycline
Local anesthetics
Chemotherapeutic agents
Cephalosporins
Nonsteroidal antiinflammatory drugs
Insect Venoms
Wasps, hornets, yellow jackets, bumblebees, ants
Foods
Eggs
Milk
Nuts
Peanuts
Shellfish
Fish
Chocolate
Strawberries
Animal Sera
Tetanus antitoxin
Rabies antitoxin
Diphtheria antitoxin
Snake venom antitoxin
Treatment Measures
Blood products (whole blood and components)
Iodine-contrast media for IVP or angiogram test
Allergenic extracts in hyposensitization therapy

IVP, Intravenous pyelogram.

pruritus around the eyes, nose, throat, and mouth.[17] (Treatment of allergic rhinitis is discussed in Chapter 27.)

Many patients with *asthma* have an allergic component to their disease. These patients frequently have a history of atopic disorders (e.g., infantile eczema, allergic rhinitis, food intolerances). Inflammatory mediators produce bronchial smooth muscle constriction, excessive secretion of viscoid mucus, edema of the mucous membranes of the bronchi, and decreased lung compliance. Because of these physiologic alterations, patients manifest dyspnea, wheezing, coughing, tightness in the chest, and thick sputum. (Pathophysiology and management of asthma are discussed in Chapter 29.)

Atopic dermatitis is a chronic, inherited skin disorder characterized by exacerbations and remissions. It is caused by several environmental allergens that are difficult to identify. Although patients with atopic dermatitis have elevated IgE levels and positive skin tests, the histopathologic features do not represent the typical, localized wheal-and-flare type I reactions. The skin lesions are more generalized and involve vasodilation of blood vessels, resulting in interstitial edema with vesicle formation (Fig. 14-12). (Dermatitis is discussed in Chapter 24.)

Urticaria (hives) is a cutaneous reaction against systemic allergens occurring in atopic persons. It is characterized by transient wheals (pink, raised, edematous, pruritic areas) that vary in size and shape and may occur throughout the body. Urticaria develops rapidly after exposure to an allergen and may last minutes or hours. Histamine causes localized vasodilation (erythema), transudation of fluid (wheal), and flaring. Flaring is due to blood vessels on the edge of the wheal dilating in response to a reaction augmented by the sympathetic nervous system. Histamine is responsible for the pruritus associated with the lesions. (Urticaria is discussed in Chapter 24.)

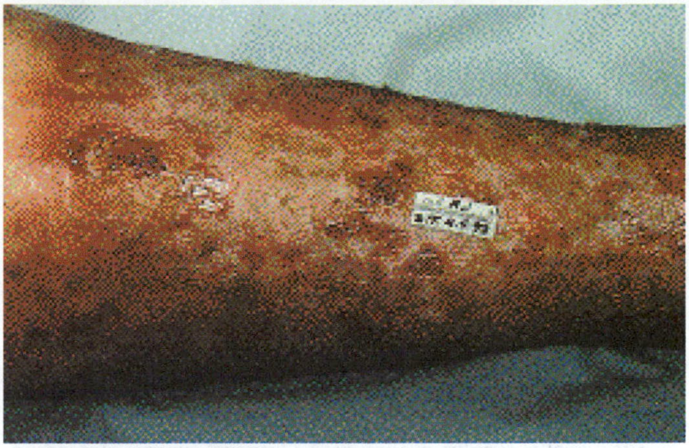

FIG. 14-12 Eczema of the lower leg.

Angioedema is a localized cutaneous lesion similar to urticaria but involving deeper layers of the skin and the submucosa. The principal areas of involvement include the eyelids, lips, tongue, larynx, hands, feet, gastrointestinal (GI) tract, and genitalia. Swelling usually begins in the face and then progresses to the airways and other parts of the body. Dilation and engorgement of the capillaries secondary to release of histamine cause the diffuse swelling. Welts are not apparent as in urticaria; the outer skin appears normal or has a reddish hue. The lesions may burn, sting, or itch and can cause acute abdominal pain if in the GI tract. The swelling may occur suddenly or over several hours and usually lasts for 24 hours.

Type II: Cytotoxic and Cytolytic Reactions. Cytotoxic and cytolytic reactions are type II hypersensitivity reactions involving the direct binding of IgG or IgM antibodies to an antigen on the cell surface. Antigen-antibody complexes activate the complement system, which mediates the reaction. Cellular tissue is destroyed in one of two ways: (1) activation of the complement cascade resulting in cytolysis or (2) enhanced phagocytosis.

Target cells frequently destroyed in type II reactions are erythrocytes, platelets, and leukocytes. Some of the antigens involved are the ABO blood group, Rh factor, and drugs. Pathophysiologic disorders characteristic of type II reactions include ABO incompatibility transfusion reaction, Rh incompatibility transfusion reaction, autoimmune and drug-related hemolytic anemias, leukopenias, thrombocytopenias, erythroblastosis fetalis (hemolytic disease of the newborn), and Goodpasture syndrome. The tissue damage usually occurs rapidly.

Hemolytic Transfusion Reactions. A classic type II reaction occurs when a recipient receives ABO-incompatible blood from a donor. Naturally acquired antibodies to antigens of the ABO blood group are in the recipient's serum but are not present on the erythrocyte membranes (see Chapter 30, Table 30-10). For example, a person with type A blood has anti-B antibodies, a person with type B blood has anti-A antibodies, a person with type AB blood has no antibodies, and a person with type O blood has both anti-A and anti-B antibodies.

If the recipient is transfused with incompatible blood, antibodies immediately coat the foreign erythrocytes, causing *agglutination* (clumping). The clumping of cells blocks small blood vessels in the body, uses existing clotting factors, and depletes them, leading to bleeding. Within hours, neutrophils and macrophages phagocytize the agglutinated cells. As complement is fixed to the antigen, cytolysis occurs. Cellular lysis causes the release of hemoglobin into the urine and plasma. In addition, a cytotoxic reaction causes vascular spasms in the kidney that further block the renal tubules. Acute renal failure can result from the hemoglobinuria. (Blood transfusions are discussed in Chapter 31.)

Goodpasture Syndrome. *Goodpasture syndrome* is a disorder involving the lungs and kidneys. An antibody-mediated autoimmune reaction occurs involving the glomerular and alveolar basement membranes. The circulating antibodies combine with tissue antigen to activate complement, which causes deposits of IgG to form along the basement membranes of the lungs or kidneys. This reaction may result in pulmonary hemorrhage and glomerulonephritis. The disease is usually rapidly progressive. Corticosteroids, immunosuppressive drugs (e.g., cyclophosphamide [Cytoxan]), and plasmapheresis have been used effectively to slow the progression of the disease. (Goodpasture syndrome is discussed in Chapter 46.)

Type III: Immune-Complex Reactions. Tissue damage in immune-complex reactions, which are type III reactions, occurs secondary to antigen-antibody complexes. Soluble antigens combine with immunoglobulins of the IgG and IgM classes to form complexes that are too small to be effectively removed by the mononuclear phagocyte system. Therefore the complexes deposit in tissue or small blood vessels. They cause the fixation of complement and the release of chemotactic factors that lead to inflammation and destruction of the involved tissue.

Type III reactions may be local or systemic and immediate or delayed. The clinical manifestations depend on the number of complexes and the location in the body. Common sites for deposit are the kidneys, skin, joints, blood vessels, and lungs. Severe type III reactions are associated with autoimmune disorders such as systemic lupus erythematosus (SLE), acute glomerulonephritis, and rheumatoid arthritis (RA). (SLE and RA are discussed in Chapter 65, and acute glomerulonephritis is discussed in Chapter 46.)

Type IV: Delayed Hypersensitivity Reactions. A *delayed hypersensitivity reaction*—a type IV reaction—is also termed a *cell-mediated immune response.* Although cell-mediated responses are usually protective mechanisms, tissue damage occurs in delayed hypersensitivity reactions.

The tissue damage in a type IV reaction does not occur in the presence of antibodies or complement. Rather, sensitized T lymphocytes attack antigens or release cytokines. Some of these cytokines attract macrophages into the area. The macrophages and enzymes released by them are responsible for most of the tissue destruction. In the delayed hypersensitivity reaction, it takes 24 to 48 hours for a response to occur.

Clinical examples of a delayed hypersensitivity reaction include contact dermatitis (Fig. 14-13); hypersensitivity reactions to bacterial, fungal, and viral infections; and transplant rejections. Some drug sensitivity reactions also fit this category.

Contact Dermatitis. *Allergic contact dermatitis* is an example of a delayed hypersensitivity reaction involving the skin. The reaction occurs when the skin is exposed to substances that easily penetrate the skin to combine with epidermal proteins. The substance then becomes antigenic. Over a period of 7 to 14 days, memory cells form to the antigen. On subsequent exposure to the substance, a sensitized person develops eczematous skin lesions within 48 hours. The most common potentially antigenic substances encountered are metal compounds (e.g., those containing nickel or mercury); rubber compounds; catechols present in poison ivy, poison oak, and poison sumac; cosmetics; and some dyes.

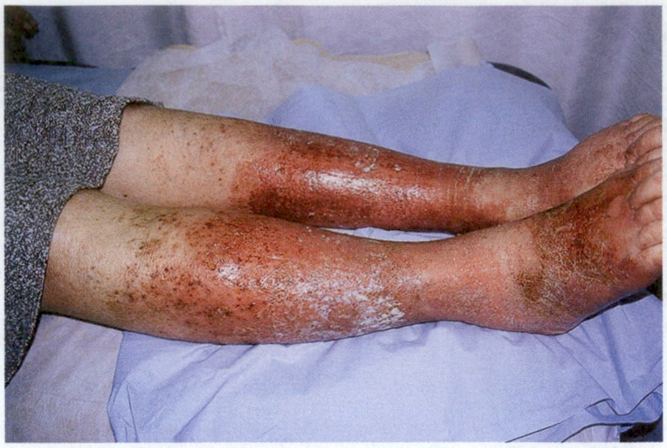

FIG. 14-13 Contact dermatitis to rubber.

In acute contact dermatitis, the skin lesions appear erythematous and edematous and are covered with papules, vesicles, and bullae. The involved area is very pruritic but may also burn or sting. When contact dermatitis becomes chronic, the lesions resemble atopic dermatitis because they are thickened, scaly, and lichenified. The main difference between contact dermatitis and atopic dermatitis is that contact dermatitis is localized and restricted to the area exposed to the allergens, whereas atopic dermatitis is usually widespread.

Microbial Hypersensitivity Reactions. The classic example of a microbial cell-mediated immune reaction is the body's defense against the tubercle bacillus. Tuberculosis results from invasion of lung tissue by the highly resistant tubercle bacillus. The organism itself does not directly damage the lung tissue. However, antigenic material released from the tubercle bacilli reacts with T lymphocytes, initiating a cell-mediated immune response. The resulting response causes extensive caseous necrosis of the lung.

After the initial cell-mediated reaction, memory cells persist, so subsequent contact with the tubercle bacillus or an extract of purified protein from the organism causes a delayed hypersensitivity reaction. This is the basis for the purified protein derivative (PPD) tuberculosis skin test, which is read 48 to 72 hours after the injection. (Tuberculosis is discussed in Chapter 28.)

ALLERGIC DISORDERS

Although an alteration of the immune system may be manifested in many ways, allergies or type I hypersensitivity reactions are seen most frequently.

Assessment

For a thorough assessment of a patient with allergies, a complete database must be obtained. This consists of a comprehensive patient history, physical examination, diagnostic workup, and skin testing for allergens.

Health History. A comprehensive history that covers family allergies, past and present allergies, and social and environmental factors is essential. The information may be obtained from the patient or the patient's caregiver.

Family history, including information about atopic reactions in relatives, is especially important in identifying at-risk patients. The specific disorder, clinical manifestations, and treatments prescribed should be assessed.

Past and present allergies must be noted. Identifying the allergens that may have triggered a reaction is essential to control allergic reactions. Determination of the time of year that an allergic reaction occurs can be a clue to a seasonal allergen. Information should also be obtained about any over-the-counter or prescription medications used to treat the allergies.

In addition to identification of the allergen, information about the clinical manifestations and course of allergic reaction should be obtained. If the patient is a woman, assessment of symptoms during pregnancy, menstruation, or menopause may be important. Social and environmental factors, especially the physical environment, are important. Questions about pets, trees, and plants on the property; pollutants in the air; and floor coverings, houseplants, and cooling and heating systems in the home and workplace can provide valuable information about allergens. In addition, a daily or weekly food diary with a description of any untoward reactions is important. Of particular interest is a screening for any reaction to medication. Finally, questions about the patient's lifestyle and stress level should be reviewed in connection with the appearance of allergic symptoms.[17]

Physical Examination. A comprehensive head-to-toe physical examination should be given to a patient with allergies, with particular attention focused on the site of the allergic manifestations. A comprehensive assessment that includes subjective and objective data should be obtained from the patient (Table 14-12).

TABLE 14-12 *NURSING ASSESSMENT* Allergies

Subjective Data

Important Health Information

Past health history: Recurrent respiratory problems, seasonal exacerbations; unusual reactions to insect bites or stings; past and present allergies

Medications: Unusual reactions to any medications; use of over-the-counter drugs, use of medications for allergies

Functional Health Patterns

Health perception–health management: Family history of allergies; malaise

Nutritional-metabolic: Food intolerances; vomiting

Elimination: Abdominal cramps, diarrhea

Activity-exercise: Fatigue; hoarseness, cough, dyspnea

Cognitive-perceptual: Itching, burning, stinging of eyes, nose, throat, or skin; chest tightness

Role-relationship: Altered home and work environment, presence of pets

Objective Data

Integumentary

Rashes, including urticaria, wheal and flare, papules, vesicles, bullae; dryness, scaliness, scratches, irritation

Eyes, Ears, Nose, and Throat

Eyes: Conjunctivitis; lacrimation; rubbing or excessive blinking; dark circles under the eyes ("allergic shiner")

Ears: Diminished hearing; immobile or scarred tympanic membranes; recurrent ear infections

Nose: Nasal polyps; nasal voice; nose twitching; itchy nose; rhinitis; pale, boggy mucous membranes; sniffling; repeated sneezing; swollen nasal passages; recurrent, unexplained nosebleeds; crease across the bridge of nose ("allergic salute")

Throat: Continual throat clearing; swollen lips or tongue; red throat; palpable neck lymph nodes

Respiratory

Wheezing, stridor; thick sputum

Possible Findings

Eosinophilia of serum, sputum, or nasal and bronchial secretions; ↑ serum IgE levels; positive skin tests; abnormal chest and sinus x-rays

Diagnostic Studies

Many specialized immunologic techniques can be performed to detect abnormalities of lymphocytes, eosinophils, and immunoglobulins. A complete blood count (CBC) and serology tests are commonly done.

A CBC with WBC differential is required, with an absolute lymphocyte count and eosinophil count. Cellular immunodeficiency is diagnosed if the lymphocyte count is below 1200/μl (1.2×10^9/L). T cell and B cell quantification is used to diagnose specific immunodeficiency syndromes. The eosinophil count is elevated with type I hypersensitivity reactions involving IgE immunoglobulins. Serum IgE level is also generally elevated in type I hypersensitivity reactions and serves as a diagnostic indicator of atopic diseases.

The radioallergosorbent test (RAST) is an in vitro diagnostic test for IgE antibodies to specific allergens. Although expensive, it is safe but less sensitive and takes longer than skin tests for detecting allergens. RAST is helpful in confirming reactivity to various foods or drugs in individuals with a history of severe anaphylactic reactions.

Sputum, nasal, and bronchial secretions also may be tested for the presence of eosinophils. If asthma is suspected, pulmonary function tests for vital capacity, forced expiratory volume, and maximum midexpiratory flow rates are helpful.[18]

Skin Tests. Skin testing is generally used to confirm specific sensitivity in patients with atopic disease after the history has suggested possible allergens for testing. With empiric allergy medications as the treatment of choice for most allergic rhinitis, it has become common practice to omit skin testing for specific allergens in these patients. However, diagnosing an allergy to a specific antigen enables the patient to avoid an allergen and makes him or her a candidate for immunotherapy. Unfortunately, skin testing cannot be performed on patients who cannot be removed from medications that suppress the histamine response or patients with food allergies.

Procedure. Skin testing may be done by one of two methods: (1) a cutaneous scratch or prick or (2) an intracutaneous injection. The areas of the body usually used in testing are the arms and back. Allergen extracts are applied to the skin in rows with a corresponding control site opposite the test site. Saline or another diluent is applied to the control site. In the scratch test, the epidermal skin layer is scratched with a lancet and the allergen extract is applied at the site. The prick test involves placing a drop of allergen extract on the skin and then piercing the underlying epidermis with a needle. In the intracutaneous method, the allergen extract is injected intradermally in rows. Because the allergic reaction is more severe with this method, the test is used only for persons who did not react to cutaneous methods.

Results. If the person is hypersensitive to the allergen, a positive reaction will occur within minutes after insertion in the skin and may last for 8 to 12 hours. A positive reaction is manifested by a local wheal-and-flare response. The size of the positive reaction does not always correlate with the severity of allergy symptoms. False-positive and false-negative results may occur. Negative results from skin testing do not necessarily mean the person does not have an allergic disorder, and positive results do not necessarily mean that the allergen was causing the clinical manifestations. Positive results imply that the person is sensitized to that allergen.

Therefore, correlating skin test results with the patient's history is important.[18]

Precautions. A highly sensitive person is always at risk for developing an anaphylactic reaction to skin tests. Therefore a patient should never be left alone during the testing period. Sometimes skin testing is completely contraindicated and the RAST test is used. If a severe reaction does occur with a cutaneous test, the extract is immediately removed and antiinflammatory topical cream is applied to the site. For intracutaneous testing, the arm is used so that a tourniquet can be applied during a severe reaction. A subcutaneous injection of epinephrine may also be necessary.

Collaborative Care

After an allergic disorder is diagnosed, the therapeutic treatment is aimed at reducing exposure to the offending allergen, treating the symptoms, and, if necessary, desensitizing the person through immunotherapy. All health care workers must be prepared for the rare but life-threatening anaphylactic reaction, which requires immediate medical and nursing interventions. It is extremely important that all of a patient's allergies be listed on the chart, the nursing care plan, and the medication record.

Anaphylaxis. Anaphylactic reactions occur suddenly in hypersensitive patients after exposure to the offending allergen. They may occur following parenteral injection of drugs (especially antibiotics) or blood products, and following insect stings. The cardinal principle in therapeutic management is speed in (1) recognition of signs and symptoms of an anaphylactic reaction, (2) maintenance of a patent airway, (3) prevention of spread of the allergen by using a tourniquet, (4) administration of drugs, and (5) treatment for shock. Table 14-13 summarizes the emergency treatment of anaphylactic shock.

Mild symptoms such as pruritus and urticaria can be controlled by administration of 0.2 to 0.5 ml of epinephrine, diluted 1:1000, given subcutaneously or intramuscularly every 10 to 15 minutes according to the health care provider's orders or a hospital emergency drug protocol. An IV infusion should be initiated to provide a route for administration of 0.5 ml of epinephrine, diluted 1:10,000, at 5- to 10-minute intervals; volume expanders; and vasopressor agents such as dopamine (Intropin) if intractable hypotension occurs.[19]

Oxygen via a non-rebreather mask should be administered. Endotracheal intubation or a tracheostomy is mandatory for O_2 delivery if progressive hypoxia exists. Other second-line agents are used, including an antihistamine such as diphenhydramine (Benadryl) IV or intramuscularly for urticaria and angioedema.

In more severe cases of anaphylaxis, hypovolemic shock may occur because of the loss of intravascular fluid into interstitial spaces that occurs secondary to increased capillary permeability. Peripheral vasoconstriction and stimulation of the sympathetic nervous system occur to compensate for the fluid shift. However, unless shock is treated early, the body will no longer be able to compensate, and irreversible tissue damage will occur, leading to death. (Hypovolemic shock is discussed in Chapter 67.)

Chronic Allergies. Most allergic reactions are chronic and are characterized by remissions and exacerbations of symptoms. Treatment focuses on identification and control of allergens, relief of symptoms through drug therapy, and hyposensitization of a patient to an offending allergen.

Allergen Recognition and Control. The nurse plays an important role in helping the patient make lifestyle adjustments so that there is minimal exposure to offending allergens. The nurse must reinforce that, even with drug therapy and immunotherapy, the patient will never be desensitized or completely symptom free. The nurse can initiate various preventive measures that will help control the allergic symptoms.

Of primary importance is the need to identify the offending allergen. Sometimes this is done through skin testing. In the case of food allergies, an elimination diet is sometimes valuable. If an allergic reaction occurs, all foods eaten shortly before the reaction should be eliminated and gradually reintroduced one at a time until the offending food is detected.

Many allergic reactions, especially asthma and urticaria, may be aggravated by fatigue and emotional stress. The nurse can be instrumental in initiating a stress management program with the

TABLE 14-13 *EMERGENCY MANAGEMENT* Anaphylactic Shock

Etiology	Assessment Findings	Interventions
• Injection of, inhalation of, ingestion of, or topical exposure to substance that produces profound allergic response • See Table 14-11 for more complete listing	See Fig. 14-11	**Initial** • Ensure patent airway. • Remove insect stinger if present. • Epinephrine 1:1000, 0.2-0.5 ml subcutaneously for mild symptoms; repeat at 10- to 15-minute intervals. • Epinephrine 1:10,000, 0.5 ml IV at 5- to 10-minute intervals for severe reaction. • Administer high-flow oxygen via non-rebreather mask. • Place recumbent and elevate legs. • Keep warm. • Administer diphenhydramine (Benadryl) IM or IV. • Administer histamine H_2 blockers such as cimetidine (Tagamet). • Maintain blood pressure with fluids, volume expanders, vasopressors (e.g., dopamine [Intropin], norepinephrine bitartrate [Levophed]). **Ongoing Monitoring** • Monitor vital signs, respiratory effort, oxygen saturation, level of consciousness, and cardiac rhythm. • Anticipate intubation with severe respiratory distress. • Anticipate cricothyrotomy or tracheostomy with severe laryngeal edema.

IM, Intramuscular; *IV*, intravenous.

patient. Relaxation techniques can be practiced when the patient comes for frequent immunotherapy treatments.

Sometimes control of allergic symptoms requires environmental control, including changing an occupation, moving to a different climate, or giving up a favorite pet. In the case of airborne allergens, sleeping in an air-conditioned room, damp dusting daily, covering mattresses and pillows with hypoallergenic covers, and wearing a mask outdoors may be helpful.

If the allergen is a drug, the patient should be instructed to avoid the drug. The patient also has the responsibility to make the drug intolerance well known to all health care providers. The patient should wear a Medic Alert bracelet listing the particular drug allergy and have the offending drug listed on all medical and dental records.

For a patient allergic to insect stings, commercial bee-sting kits containing preinjectable epinephrine and a tourniquet are available. The nurse has the responsibility to instruct the patient about the technique of applying the tourniquet and self-injecting the subcutaneous epinephrine. This patient also should wear a Medic Alert bracelet and carry a bee-sting kit whenever going outdoors.

Drug Therapy. The major categories of drugs used for symptomatic relief of chronic allergic disorders include antihistamines, sympathomimetic/decongestant drugs, corticosteroids, antipruritic drugs, and mast cell–stabilizing drugs. Many of these drugs may be obtained over the counter and are often misused by patients.

Antihistamines. Antihistamines are the best drugs for treatment of allergic rhinitis and urticaria (see Chapter 27, Table 27-2). They are less effective for severe allergic reactions. They act by competing with histamine for H_1-receptor sites and thus blocking the effect of histamine. Best results are achieved if they are taken as soon as allergy signs and symptoms appear. Antihistamines can be used effectively to treat edema and pruritus but are relatively ineffective in preventing bronchoconstriction. With seasonal rhinitis, antihistamines should be taken during peak pollen seasons. (Antihistamines are discussed in Chapter 27.)

Sympathomimetic/Decongestant Drugs. The major sympathomimetic drug is epinephrine (Adrenalin), which is the drug of choice to treat an anaphylactic reaction. Epinephrine is a hormone produced by the adrenal medulla that stimulates α- and β-adrenergic receptors. Stimulation of the α-adrenergic receptors causes vasoconstriction of peripheral blood vessels. β-Receptor stimulation relaxes bronchial smooth muscles. Epinephrine also acts directly on mast cells to stabilize them against further degranulation. The action of epinephrine lasts only a few minutes. For the treatment of anaphylaxis, the drug must be given parenterally (usually subcutaneously).

Several specific, minor sympathomimetic drugs differ from epinephrine because they can be taken orally or nasally and last for several hours. Included in this category are phenylephrine (Neo-Synephrine) and pseudoephedrine (Sudafed). The minor sympathomimetic drugs are used primarily to treat allergic rhinitis.

Corticosteroids. Nasal corticosteroid sprays are very effective in relieving the symptoms of allergic rhinitis (see Chapter 27 and Table 27-2). Occasionally patients have such severe manifestations of allergies that they are truly incapacitated. In these situations, a brief course of oral corticosteroids can be used.

Antipruritic Drugs. Topically applied antipruritic drugs are most effective when the skin is not broken. These drugs protect the skin and provide relief from itching. Common over-the-counter drugs include calamine lotion, coal tar solutions, and camphor. Menthol and phenol may be added to other lotions to produce an antipruritic effect. Some more potent drugs that require a prescription include methdilazine (Tacaryl) and trimeprazine (Temaril). These drugs should be used with great caution because of the associated risk of agranulocytosis.

Mast Cell–Stabilizing Drugs. Cromolyn (Intal, Nasalcrom, Rynacrom) and nedocromil (Tilade) are mast cell–stabilizing agents that inhibit the release of histamines, leukotrienes, and other agents from the mast cell after antigen-IgE interaction. They are available as an inhalant nebulizer solution or a nasal spray. They are used in the management of asthma (see Chapter 29) and in the treatment of allergic rhinitis (see Chapter 27). An important feature of these drugs is a very low incidence of side effects.

Leukotriene Receptor Antagonists. Leukotriene receptor antagonists (LTRAs) block leukotriene, one of the major mediators of the allergic inflammatory process. These medications can be taken orally. They may be used in the treatment of allergic rhinitis and asthma. For more information, refer to Chapters 27 and 29.

Immunotherapy. Immunotherapy is the recommended treatment for control of allergic symptoms when the allergen cannot be avoided and drug therapy is not effective. Relatively few patients with allergies have symptoms so intolerable that they require allergy immunotherapy. Immunotherapy is absolutely indicated only in individuals with anaphylactic reactions to insect venom. It involves administration of small titers of an allergen extract in increasing strengths until hyposensitivity to the specific allergen is achieved. For best results, the patient should continue to avoid the offending allergen whenever possible because complete desensitization is impossible. Unfortunately, not all allergy-related conditions respond to immunotherapy. Food allergies cannot be safely treated with this therapy, and eczema may worsen with immunotherapy.

Mechanism of Action. IgE immunoglobulin level is elevated in atopic individuals. When IgE combines with an allergen in a hypersensitive person, a reaction occurs, releasing histamine in various body tissues. Allergens more readily combine with IgG immunoglobulin than with other immunoglobulins. Therefore immunotherapy involves injecting allergen extracts that will stimulate increased IgG levels. The binding of IgG to allergen-reactive sites interferes with allergen binding to mast cell–bound IgE, preventing mast cell degranulation, and thus reduces the number of reactions that cause tissue damage. The goal of long-term immunotherapy is to keep "blocking" IgG levels high. In addition, allergen-specific T suppressor cells develop in individuals receiving immunotherapy.[20]

Method of Administration. The allergens included in immunotherapy are chosen on the basis of the results of skin testing with a panel of allergens found in the local geographic area. Immunotherapy involves the subcutaneous injection of titrated amounts of allergen extracts biweekly or weekly. The dose is small at first and is increased slowly until a maintenance dosage is reached. Generally it takes 1 to 2 years of immunotherapy to reach the maximal therapeutic effect. Therapy may be continued for about 5 years. After that, consideration is given to discontinuing therapy. In many patients, a decrease in symptoms is sustained after the treatment is discontinued. For patients with severe allergies or sensitivity to insect stings, maintenance therapy is continued indefinitely. Best results are achieved when immunotherapy is administered throughout the year.[21]

Sublingual immunotherapy has been developed and investigated for years, but is now gaining support through many European studies. Taken under the tongue, this method of immunotherapy has a lower risk of severe adverse reaction than the traditional subcutaneous administration. Although available in commercial preparations in Europe, sublingual immunotherapy is not yet available in the United States.[22]

NURSING MANAGEMENT IMMUNOTHERAPY

The nurse is often primarily responsible for giving immunotherapy. Adverse reactions should always be anticipated, especially when using a new-strength dose, after a previous reaction, or after a missed dose. Early signs and symptoms indicative of a systemic reaction include pruritus, urticaria, sneezing, laryngeal edema, and hypotension. Emergency measures for anaphylactic shock should be initiated immediately. A local reaction should be described according to the degree of redness and swelling at the injection site. If the area is greater than the size of a quarter in an adult, the reaction should be reported to the health care provider so that the allergen dosage may be decreased.

Immunotherapy always carries the risk of a severe anaphylactic reaction. Therefore a health care provider, emergency equipment, and essential drugs should be available whenever injections are given.

Record keeping must be accurate and can be invaluable in preventing an adverse reaction to the allergen extract. Before giving an injection, the nurse should check the patient's name with the name on the vial. Next, the vial strength, amount of last dose, date of last dose, and any reaction information should be screened.

The nurse should always administer the allergen extract in an extremity away from a joint so that a tourniquet can be applied for a severe reaction. The site should be rotated for each injection. The nurse must aspirate for blood before giving an injection to ensure that the allergen extract is not injected into a blood vessel. An injection directly into the bloodstream can potentiate an anaphylactic reaction. After the injection is given, the patient should be carefully observed for 20 minutes because systemic reactions are most likely to occur immediately. However, the patient should be warned that a delayed reaction can occur as long as 24 hours later.[21]

Latex Allergies

Allergies to latex products have become a problem of increasing proportion, affecting both patients and health care professionals. The increase in allergic reactions has coincided with the sharp increase in glove use.[23] It is estimated that 5% to 18% of health care workers regularly exposed to latex are sensitized. The more frequent and prolonged the exposure to latex, the greater the likelihood of developing a latex allergy.[24] In addition to gloves, many latex-containing products are used in health care, such as blood pressure cuffs, stethoscopes, tourniquets, IV tubing, syringes, electrode pads, O_2 masks, tracheal tubes, colostomy and ileostomy pouches, urinary catheters, anesthetic masks, and adhesive tape. Latex proteins can become aerosolized through powder on gloves and can result in serious reactions when inhaled by sensitized individuals. It is recommended that all health care facilities use powder-free gloves to avoid respiratory exposure to latex proteins. Because some proteins in rubber are similar to food proteins, some foods may cause an allergic reaction in people who are allergic to latex. The most common of these foods are banana, avocado, chestnut, kiwi fruit, tomato, water chestnuts, guava, hazelnuts, potatoes, peaches, grapes, and apricots.

Types of Latex Allergies. Two types of latex allergies that can occur are type IV allergic contact dermatitis and type I allergic reactions. Type IV contact dermatitis is caused by the chemicals used in the manufacturing process of latex gloves. It is a delayed reaction that occurs within 6 to 48 hours. Typically the person first has dryness, pruritus, fissuring, and cracking of the skin, followed by redness, swelling, and crusting at 24 to 48 hours. Chronic exposure can lead to lichenification, scaling, and hyperpigmentation. The dermatitis may extend beyond the area of physical contact with the allergen.

A type I allergic reaction is a response to the natural rubber latex proteins and occurs within minutes of contact with the proteins. These types of allergic reactions can manifest as various reactions ranging from skin redness, urticaria, rhinitis, conjunctivitis, or asthma to full-blown anaphylactic shock. Systemic reactions to latex may result from exposure to latex protein via various routes, including the skin, mucous membranes, inhalation, and blood.[24]

NURSING *and* COLLABORATIVE MANAGEMENT LATEX ALLERGIES

The identification of patients and health care workers sensitive to latex is crucial in the prevention of adverse reactions. A thorough health history and history of any allergies should be collected, especially on patients with any complaints of latex contact symptoms. Not all latex-sensitive individuals can be identified, even with a careful and thorough history. The greatest risk factor is long-term multiple exposures to latex products (e.g., health care personnel, individuals who have had multiple surgeries, rubber industry workers). Additional risk factors include a patient history of hay fever, asthma, and allergies to certain foods (see earlier).[25]

Latex precaution protocols should be used for those patients identified as having a positive latex allergy test or a history of signs and symptoms related to latex exposure. Many health care facilities have created latex-free product carts that can be used for patients with latex allergies. The National Institute for Occupational Safety and Health (NIOSH) has published recommendations for preventing allergic reactions to latex in the workplace (Table 14-14).

TABLE 14-14 Guidelines for Preventing Allergic Latex Reactions

- Use nonlatex gloves for activities that are not likely to involve contact with infectious materials (e.g., food preparation, housekeeping).
- Use powder-free gloves with reduced protein content.
- Do not use oil-based hand creams or lotions when wearing gloves.
- After removing gloves, wash hands with mild soap and dry thoroughly.
- Frequently clean work areas that are contaminated with latex-containing dust.
- Know the symptoms of latex allergy, including skin rash; hives; flushing; itching; nasal, eye, or sinus symptoms; asthma; and shock.
- If symptoms of latex allergy develop, avoid direct contact with latex gloves and products.
- Wear a medical alert bracelet and carry an epinephrine pen.

Source: The National Institute for Occupational Safety and Health (NIOSH) (*www.cdc.gov/niosh*).

Multiple Chemical Sensitivities

Multiple chemical sensitivities (MCS) is an acquired disorder in which certain people exposed to various foods and chemicals in the environment have many symptoms related to multiple body systems. These symptoms are usually subjective and are not found during physical examination. The patient experiences wide-ranging symptoms, but evidence of pathology or physiologic dysfunction is lacking.

Primarily, MCS is found in women. Symptoms include fatigue, headache, nausea, pain, irritable bowel symptoms, dizziness, mouth irritation, disorientation, and cough. Almost any chemical can initiate the symptoms of MCS.[26] Odor seems to be the principal trigger. Gas exhaust, perfumes, cigarette smoke, plastics, pesticides, and industrial solvents are some of the most common odors associated with MCS. Also, food additives, drugs, and naturally occurring foods, including drinking water, often cause sensitivity. The uniqueness of MCS is that symptoms occur at levels below the established guidelines of toxic levels and concentrations.

The causes of MCS are thought to be immunologic, psychologic, toxicologic, and sociologic factors. Diagnosis is usually made based on a patient's health history. There is no established test used to diagnose MCS. Diagnostic tests that are used include provocation-neutralization and immunologic testing (e.g., CBC, lymphocyte subsets, antibody titers). Immunologic testing, however, has not been widely accepted as a diagnostic test. The provocation-neutralization test is done by exposing the patient to certain environmental substances to produce symptoms and then repeating the exposure at higher and lower doses to initiate the disappearance of symptoms.

The most effective treatment for MCS is to avoid the chemicals that may trigger the symptoms and create a chemical-free home/workplace. However, this can be difficult in a chemical-dependent society. Other commonly recommended treatments include regular exercise, physical therapy, massage, prayer, and meditation.[27]

HUMAN LEUKOCYTE ANTIGEN SYSTEM

The **human leukocyte antigen** (HLA) system consists of a series of linked genes that occur together on the sixth chromosome in humans.[28] The products of these genes include the cell membrane antigens of the HLA series. Because of its importance in the study of tissue matching, the chromosomal region incorporating the HLA genes is termed the *major histocompatibility complex.* The genes determining the products recognized as the HLA-A, HLA-B, HLA-C, HLA-D, and HLA-DR antigens are clustered together (Fig. 14-14). HLAs are present on all nucleated cells and platelets.

An important characteristic of HLA genes is that they are highly polymorphic. Each HLA locus can have many different possible alleles. The specific allele is identified by a number. For example, a person could be A6, B7, C8, D1, DR7. With many alleles possible at each HLA locus, many combinations exist. Each person has two antigens for each locus, one inherited from each parent. Both antigens of a locus are expressed independently (i.e., they are codominant). The entire set of A, B, C, D, and DR antigens located on one chromosome is termed a *haplotype.* A complete set of antigens located on a chromosome is inherited as a unit (haplotype). One haplotype is inherited from each parent (see Fig. 14-14).

Because of the polymorphic nature of the HLA system, it is an ideal marker for genetic studies. This characteristic also makes it a useful tool in settling paternity disputes. The frequencies of HLAs vary considerably among different races. For example, HLA-B8 is relatively high in American whites, but it is very low in Native American and Japanese persons.

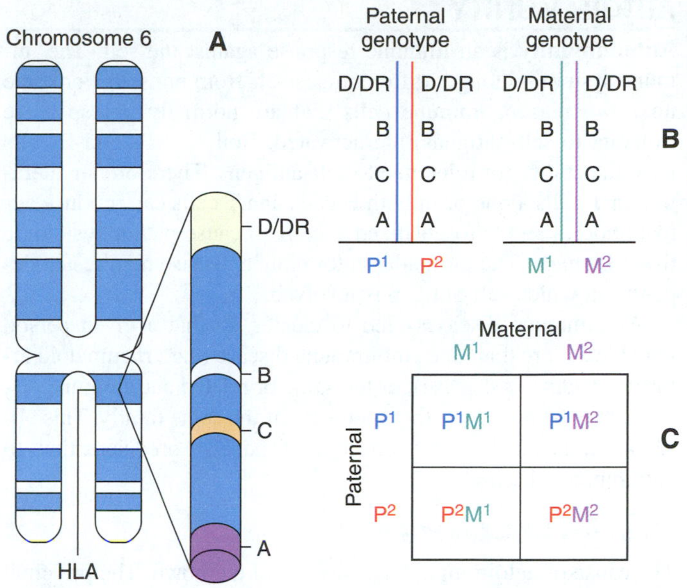

FIG. 14-14 Patterns of human leukocyte antigen (HLA) inheritance. **A,** HLA genes are located on chromosome 6. **B,** The two haplotypes of the father are labeled P^1 and P^2 and the haplotypes of the mother are labeled M^1 and M^2. Each child inherits two haplotypes, one from each parent. **C,** Therefore only four combinations—P^1M^1, P^1M^2, P^2M^1, and P^2M^2—are possible, and 25% of the offspring will have identical HLA haplotypes.

Human Leukocyte Antigen and Disease Associations

The early interest in HLAs was stimulated by its potential role in matching donors and recipients of organ transplants. During the last few years, interest in the association between HLAs and disease has grown. Strong associations between HLA type and susceptibility to certain diseases have been demonstrated.[29] HLA disease associations mean that the frequency of a defined HLA allele is significantly increased in patients with a certain disease when compared with ethnically matched controls. Most of the HLA-associated diseases are classified as autoimmune disorders. Examples of HLA types and disease associations include (1) HLA-B27 and ankylosing spondylitis, (2) HLA-DR2 and HLA-DR3 and SLE, and (3) HLA-DR3 and HLA-DR4 and diabetes mellitus.

The discovery of HLA associations with certain diseases is a major breakthrough in understanding the genetic bases of these diseases. It is now known that at least part of the genetic bases of HLA-associated diseases lies in the HLA region, but the actual mechanism or mechanisms involved in these associations are still unknown. However, most individuals who inherit an HLA type associated with a disease will never develop the disease.

The association between HLAs and certain diseases is presently of little practical clinical importance. Nevertheless, there is promise for the development of clinical applications in the future. For example, with certain autoimmune diseases, it may be possible to identify members of a family at greatest risk for developing the same or a related autoimmune disease. These persons would need close medical supervision, implementation of preventive measures (if possible), and institution of early diagnosis and treatment to prevent chronic complications.

AUTOIMMUNITY

Autoimmunity is an immune response against the self. The immune system no longer differentiates self from nonself. For some unknown reason, immune cells that are normally unresponsive (tolerant to self-antigens) are activated. Both T cells and B cells have the ability for tolerance to self-antigens. Therefore an alteration in T cells alone or in both B cells and T cells can produce autoantibodies and autosensitized T cells to cause pathophysiologic tissue damage. The particular autoimmune disease manifested depends on which self-antigen is involved.[30]

Autoimmune diseases tend to cluster, so that a given person may have more than one autoimmune disease (e.g., rheumatoid arthritis, Addison's disease), or the same or related autoimmune diseases may be found in other members of the same family. This observation has led to the concept of genetic predisposition to autoimmune disease.

Theories of Causation

The cause of autoimmune diseases is still unknown. The principal factors in the development of autoimmunity are (1) the inheritance of susceptibility genes, which may contribute to the failure of self-tolerance and (2) initiation of autoreactivity by triggers, such as infections, which may activate self-reactive lymphocytes. Age is thought to play some role, because the number of circulating autoantibodies increases in persons over age 50.

Genetic Susceptibility. Most autoimmune diseases have a genetic basis. Most of the research work in this area correlates certain HLA types with an autoimmune condition.[31] (HLAs and disease association were discussed earlier in this chapter.)

Initiation of Autoreactivity. Even in a genetically predisposed person, some trigger is required for the initiation of autoreactivity. This may include infectious agents such as a virus.[30] Viral infections can cause an alteration of cells or tissues that are not normally antigenic. The virally induced changes can make the cells or tissues antigenic. There is some evidence that viruses may be involved in the development of multiple sclerosis and type 1 diabetes mellitus. Rheumatic fever and rheumatic heart disease are autoimmune responses triggered by streptococcal infection and mediated by antibodies against group A β-hemolytic streptococci that cross-react with heart muscles and valves and synovial membranes.

Drugs can also be precipitating factors in autoimmune disease. Hemolytic anemia can result from methyldopa (Aldomet) administration. Procainamide (Pronestyl) can induce the formation of antinuclear antibodies and cause a lupus-like syndrome.

Hormones also have a role in autoimmune disease. More women than men have autoimmune disease. During pregnancy, many autoimmune diseases get better. Following delivery, the woman with an autoimmune disease frequently has an exacerbation.

Autoimmune Diseases

Generally, autoimmune diseases are grouped according to organ-specific and systemic diseases. (Table 14-15 presents examples of autoimmune diseases.) Systemic lupus erythematosus (SLE) is a classic example of a systemic autoimmune disease characterized by damage to multiple organs. It occurs most frequently in women ages 20 to 40 years. The etiology is unknown, but there appears to be a loss of self-tolerance for the body's own DNA antigens.

TABLE 14-15 Examples of Autoimmune Diseases*

Systemic Diseases	***Endocrine System***
Systemic lupus erythematosus	Addison's disease
Rheumatoid arthritis	Thyroiditis
Progressive systemic sclerosis (scleroderma)	Hypothyroidism
Mixed connective tissue disease	Type 1 diabetes mellitus
Organ-Specific Diseases	***Gastrointestinal System***
Blood	Pernicious anemia
Autoimmune hemolytic anemia	Ulcerative colitis
Immune thrombocytopenic purpura	***Kidney***
Central Nervous System	Goodpasture syndrome
Multiple sclerosis	Glomerulonephritis
Guillain-Barré syndrome	***Liver***
Muscle	Primary biliary cirrhosis
Myasthenia gravis	Autoimmune hepatitis
Heart	***Eye***
Rheumatic fever	Uveitis

*These diseases are discussed in various chapters throughout the book.

In SLE, tissue injury appears to be the result of the formation of antinuclear antibodies. For some reason (possibly a viral infection), the cell membrane is damaged and DNA is released into the systemic circulation, where it is viewed as nonself. This DNA is normally sequestered inside the nucleus of cells. On release into the circulation, the DNA antigen reacts with an antibody. Some antibodies are involved in immune complex formation, and others may cause damage directly. Once the complexes are deposited, complement is activated and further damages the tissue, especially the renal glomerulus. (Systemic lupus erythematosus is discussed in Chapter 65.)

Apheresis

Apheresis has been effectively used to treat autoimmune diseases and other diseases and disorders. *Apheresis* is the use of a procedure to separate components of the blood followed by the removal of one or more of these components. Compound words are often used to describe any particular apheresis procedure, depending on the blood components being collected. *Cytapheresis* is a general term for cell separation and removal. *Plateletpheresis* is the removal of platelets, usually for collection from normal individuals to infuse into patients with low platelet counts (e.g., patients taking chemotherapy who develop thrombocytopenia). *Leukocytapheresis* is a general term indicating the removal of WBCs and is used in chronic myelogenous leukemia to remove high numbers of leukemic cells. *Lymphocytapheresis* is used to decrease high lymphocyte counts, such as in individuals with chronic lymphocytic leukemia.

Plasmapheresis. *Plasmapheresis* is the removal of plasma containing components causing or thought to cause disease. When plasma is removed, it is replaced by substitute fluids such as saline or albumin. Therefore, the term *plasma exchange* more accurately describes this procedure.

Plasmapheresis has been used to treat autoimmune diseases such SLE, glomerulonephritis, Goodpasture syndrome, myasthenia gravis, thrombocytopenic purpura, rheumatoid arthritis, and Guillain-Barré syndrome. Apheresis procedures are also done on healthy donors to obtain plasma and selected blood components to administer to patients as replacement therapy.

TABLE 14-16 Primary Immunodeficiency Disorders

Disorder	Affected Cells	Genetic Basis
Chronic granulomatous disease	PMNs, monocytes	Sex-linked
Job syndrome	PMNs, monocytes	
Bruton's X-linked agammaglobulinemia	B	Sex-linked
Common variable hypogammaglobulinemia	B	
Selective IgA, IgM, or IgG deficiency	B	Some sex-linked
DiGeorge syndrome (thymic hypoplasia)	T	
Severe combined immunodeficiency disease	Stem, B, T	Sex-linked or autosomal recessive
Ataxia-telangiectasia	B, T	Autosomal recessive
Wiskott-Aldrich syndrome	B, T	Sex-linked
Graft-versus-host disease	B, T	

PMNs, Polymorphonuclear neutrophils.

The rationale for performing therapeutic plasmapheresis in autoimmune disorders is to remove pathologic substances present in plasma. Many disorders for which plasmapheresis is being used are characterized by circulating autoantibodies (usually of the IgG class) and antigen-antibody complexes. Immunosuppressive therapy has been used to prevent recovery of IgG production, and plasmapheresis has been used to prevent antibody rebound.

In addition to removing antibodies and antigen-antibody complexes, plasmapheresis may also remove inflammatory mediators (e.g., complement) that are responsible for tissue damage. In the treatment of SLE, plasmapheresis is usually reserved for the patient having an acute attack who is unresponsive to conventional therapy.

Plasmapheresis involves the removal of whole blood through a needle inserted in one arm and circulation of the blood through a cell separator. Inside the separator, the blood is divided into plasma and its cellular components by centrifugation or membrane filtration. A needle is inserted into the opposite arm for return of the blood to the patient. Plasma, platelets, WBCs, or red blood cells can be separated selectively. The undesirable component is removed, and the remainder is returned to the patient. The plasma is generally replaced with normal saline, lactated Ringer's solution, fresh frozen plasma, plasma protein fractions, or albumin. When blood is manually removed, only 500 ml may be taken at one time. However, with the use of apheresis procedures, over 4 L of plasma can be pheresed in 2 to 3 hours.

As with administration of other blood products, nurses must be aware of side effects associated with plasmapheresis. The most common complications are hypotension and citrate toxicity. Hypotension is usually the result of vasovagal reaction or transient volume changes. Citrate is used as an anticoagulant and may cause hypocalcemia, which may manifest as headache, paresthesias, and dizziness.

IMMUNODEFICIENCY DISORDERS

When the immune system does not adequately protect the body, **immunodeficiency** exists. Immunodeficiency disorders involve an impairment of one or more immune mechanisms, which include (1) phagocytosis, (2) humoral response, (3) cell-mediated response, (4) complement, and (5) a combined humoral and cell-mediated deficiency. Immunodeficiency disorders are *primary* if the immune cells are improperly developed or absent and *secondary* if the deficiency is caused by illnesses or treatment. Primary immunodeficiency disorders are rare and often serious, whereas secondary disorders are more common and less severe.

Primary Immunodeficiency Disorders

The basic categories of primary immunodeficiency disorders are (1) phagocytic defects, (2) B-cell deficiency, (3) T-cell deficiency, and (4) a combined B-cell and T-cell deficiency (Table 14-16).

Secondary Immunodeficiency Disorders

Some of the important factors that may cause secondary immunodeficiency disorders are listed in Table 14-17. Drug-induced immunosuppression is the most common. Immunosuppressive therapy is prescribed for patients to treat autoimmune disorders and to prevent transplant rejection. In addition, immunosuppression is a serious side effect of drugs used in cancer chemotherapy. Generalized leukopenia often results, leading to a decreased humoral and cell-mediated response. Therefore secondary infections are common in immunosuppressed patients.

TABLE 14-17 Causes of Secondary Immunodeficiency

Drug-Induced Immunodeficiency
- Chemotherapy drugs
- Corticosteroids

Age
- Infants
- Older adults

Malnutrition
- Dietary deficiency
- Cachexia

Diseases/Disorders
- Acquired immunodeficiency syndrome (AIDS)
- Cirrhosis
- Chronic kidney disease
- Diabetes mellitus
- Malignancies
- Systemic lupus erythematosus
- Burns
- Trauma
- Severe infection

Therapies
- Radiation
- Surgery
- Anesthesia

Stress
- Chronic stress
- Emotional trauma

Stress may alter the immune response. This response involves interrelationships among the nervous, endocrine, and immune systems (see Chapter 9).

A hypofunctional state of the immune system exists in young children and older adults. Laboratory studies have demonstrated that immunoglobulin levels decrease with age and therefore lead to a suppressed humoral immune response in older adults. Thymic involution occurs with aging along with decreased numbers of T cells. The incidence of malignancies and autoimmune diseases increases with aging and may be related to immunologic alterations.

Malnutrition alters cell-mediated immune responses. When protein is deficient over a prolonged period, atrophy of the thymus gland occurs and lymphoid tissue decreases. In addition, an increased susceptibility to infections always exists.

Radiation destroys lymphocytes either directly or through depletion of stem cells. As the radiation dose is increased, more bone marrow atrophies, leading to severe pancytopenia and suppression of immune function.

Surgical removal of lymph nodes, thymus, or spleen can suppress the immune response. Splenectomy in children is especially dangerous and may lead to septicemia from simple respiratory infections.

Hodgkin's lymphoma greatly impairs the cell-mediated immune response, and patients may die from severe viral or fungal infections. (Hodgkin's lymphoma is discussed in Chapter 31.) Viruses, especially rubella, may cause immunodeficiency by direct cytotoxic damage to lymphoid cells. Systemic infections can place such a demand on the immune system that resistance to a secondary or subsequent infection is impaired.

Graft-versus-Host Disease

Graft-versus-host (GVH) disease occurs when an immunoincompetent (immunodeficient) patient is transfused or transplanted with immunocompetent cells. A GVH response may result from the infusion of any blood product containing viable lymphocytes, such as in therapeutic blood transfusions, and from the transplantation of fetal thymus, fetal liver, or bone marrow. In most transplantation situations, the biggest concern is the host's rejection of the graft. However, in GVH disease, the graft rejects the host or recipient tissue.

The GVH response may have its onset 7 to 30 days after transplantation. Once the reaction is started, little can be done to modify its course. The exact mechanism involved in this reaction is not completely understood. However, it involves donor T cells attacking and destroying vulnerable host cells.

The target organs for the GVH phenomenon are the skin, GI tract, and liver. The skin disease may be a maculopapular rash, which may be pruritic or painful. It initially involves the palms and soles of the feet but can progress to a generalized erythema with bullous formation and desquamation. The liver disease may range from mild jaundice with elevated liver enzymes to hepatic coma. The intestinal disease may be manifested by mild to severe diarrhea, severe abdominal pain, GI bleeding, and malabsorption. The biggest problem with GVH disease is infection, with different types of infections seen in different periods. Bacterial and fungal infections predominate immediately after transplantation when granulocytopenia exists. The development of interstitial pneumonitis is the predominant later problem.

There is no adequate treatment of GVH disease once it is established. Although corticosteroids are often used, they enhance the susceptibility to infection. The use of immunosuppressive agents (e.g., methotrexate, cyclosporine) has been most effective as a preventive rather than a treatment measure. Radiation of blood products before they are administered is another measure to prevent T-cell replication.

ORGAN TRANSPLANTATION

During the 1960s, organ and tissue transplantation was considered to be experimental and reserved for patients who had no other medical options. Overall, transplantation success improved in the 1980s with advances in surgical technique and more effective immunosuppressants (e.g., cyclosporine). Now, most organs and tissues are transplanted successfully with good survival rates.

Common transplants include corneas, kidneys, skin, bone marrow, heart valves, bone, and connective tissues (Fig. 14-15). Corneas are often transplanted to prevent or correct blindness. Skin grafts are used to assist in managing burn patients. Bone marrow is donated to help patients with leukemias and other malignancies.

Transplanted organs currently come from many different body systems. These organs include the heart, lung, liver, kidney, pancreas, and intestine. Certain organs can be transplanted together, such as kidney and pancreas. For example, many patients who receive a pancreas transplant also receive a kidney transplant because a patient with diabetes may not only have lost his or her

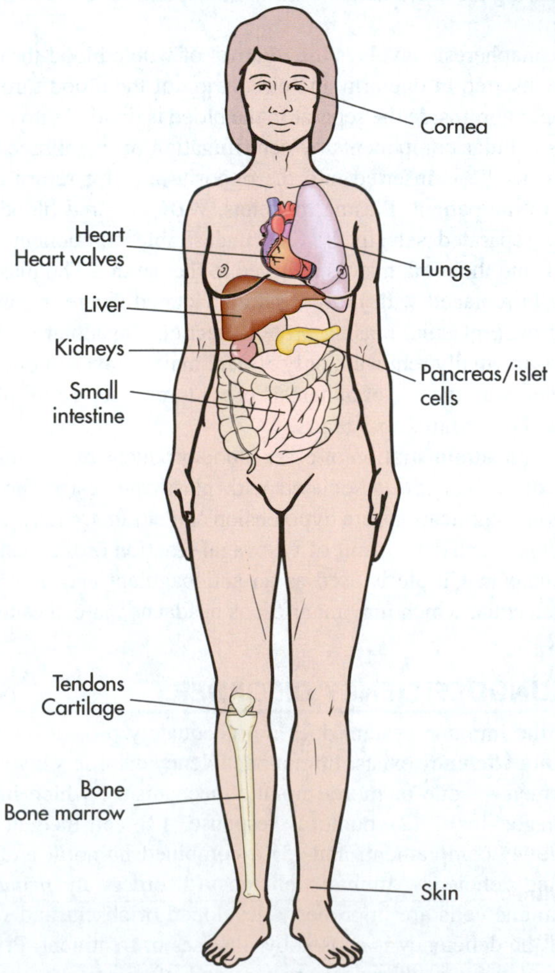

FIG. 14-15 Tissues and organs that can be transplanted.

pancreatic ability to produce insulin but may also have renal failure.

Some organs can be transplanted in parts or segments instead of transplanting an entire organ. Liver and lung lobes (rather than the whole organ) may be transplanted, or an intestine may be used in segments, thus allowing for one person's organ donation to benefit many recipients. This technique also enables living donors to donate part of an organ while maintaining the functional organ themselves.

Organ donations are taken from two sources, deceased (cadaveric) and living donors. Most organs used currently originate from deceased donors. Although there are nonrelated living donors, the majority of living donors are typically a family member of the recipient.

In order to become an organ and tissue donor, an individual notifies the state of his or her decision when receiving a new driver's license. At that time, he or she should receive an organ/tissue donor card (Fig. 14-16). An organ donor should also notify his or her family of the decision because the family members are ultimately the people who give the medical community the approval to enroll a deceased individual as an organ donor.

Currently there are 90,645 people on the Organ Procurement and Transplantation Network's national waiting list to receive organ donations, and there are only 10,932 donors. Each day, around 74 people receive an organ transplant, but another 17 people die waiting for a transplant. The organs with the highest demand are kidneys, hearts, and livers; these are also the most commonly transplanted organs.[32] Organ and tissue donations are all regulated by the Uniform Anatomical Gift Act in order to allow for fair and consistent transplantation laws among all states. Patients are matched to available donors based on a number of factors: ABO blood and human leukocyte antigen (HLA) typing, medical urgency, time on the waiting list, and geographic location.

Histocompatibility Studies

The purpose of histocompatibility testing is to identify the HLAs for both donors and potential recipients. A serologic or polymerase chain reaction (PCR) test is used to type for the antigens at all five loci (A, B, C, D, and DR). (PCR is explained later in the chapter.) Lymphocytes are isolated from peripheral blood and then combined with serum that contains antibodies to HLAs. Currently only the A, B, and DR antigens are thought to be clinically significant for transplantation. Because there are two antigens at each locus, a total of six antigens are identified. In deceased donor transplantation, an attempt is made to match as many antigens as possible between the HLA-A, HLA-B, and HLA-DR loci. Antigen matches of five and six antigens and certain four-antigen matches have been found to have better clinical outcomes (i.e., the patient is less likely to reject the transplanted organ), especially in kidney and bone marrow transplants.

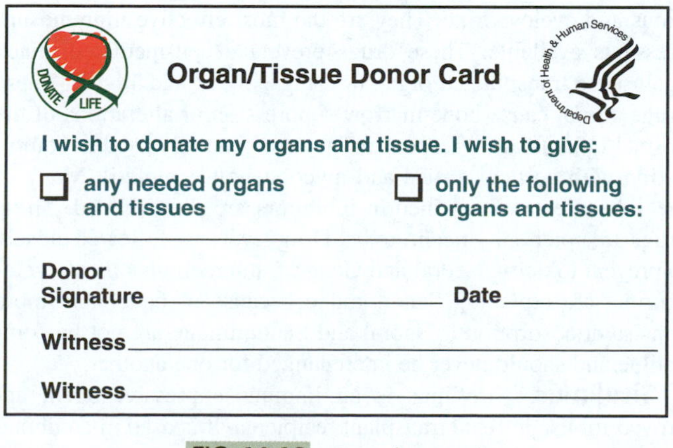

DONATE LIFE
Organ/Tissue Donor Card
Department of Health & Human Services
I wish to donate my organs and tissue. I wish to give:
any needed organs and tissues
only the following organs and tissues:
Donor Signature
Date
Witness
Witness

FIG. 14-16 Organ donor card.

Another test done is called a *crossmatch.* This is done at the time a living donor is being evaluated and just before surgery for deceased donors. A crossmatch uses serum from the recipient mixed with donor lymphocytes to test for any preformed cytotoxic (anti-HLA) antibodies to the potential donor organ. A positive crossmatch indicates that the recipient has cytotoxic antibodies to the donor and is an absolute contraindication to transplantation. The potential recipient may have been exposed to antigens similar to those of the donor by means of previous blood transfusions, pregnancy, or a previous organ transplant. If transplanted, the organ would undergo hyperacute rejection. A negative crossmatch indicates that no preformed antibodies are present and it is safe to proceed with transplantation.

Crossmatching is also performed to detect preformed cytotoxic antibodies in the recipient serum to HLAs on lymphocytes from random donors. In this situation, rather than using specific donor lymphocytes, the recipient serum is mixed with a randomly selected panel of donor lymphocytes to determine reactivity. This is called the panel of reactive antibodies (PRA) and indicates the recipient's sensitivity to various HLAs. The results are calculated in percentages. A high PRA indicates that the person has a large number of cytotoxic antibodies, which means that there is a poor chance of finding a crossmatch-negative donor. In patients awaiting transplantation, a PRA panel is usually done on a regular basis.

Clinical Significance of HLA Matching. The degree of HLA matching required or deemed suitable for successful solid organ transplantation is dependent on the type of organ and the transplant center at which the transplantation is being performed. Certain organ and tissue transplants require a closer histocompatibility match than other organs. For example, a cornea transplant can be accepted by nearly any individual because the corneas are avascular and therefore no antibodies reach the cornea to cause rejection.

HLA matching is not used extensively for liver, lung, and heart transplants. For liver transplants, HLA mismatches have shown little impact on graft survival. For heart and lung transplants, minimizing HLA mismatches significantly improves survivals. However, another major consideration is the time and distance that a HLA-compatible organ has to be transported. This can result in damage to the donor organ. In addition, there are fewer donors available for these organs and it is difficult to get good HLA matches.

In kidney and bone marrow transplantation, HLA matching is important. Whenever possible, especially with deceased donors, kidneys are usually only exchanged when there are no HLA-A, -B, and -DR mismatches between the donor and the recipient.[33]

Transplant Rejection

Rejection is one of the major problems following organ transplantation. Rejection of organs occurs if the donor organ does not perfectly match the recipient's HLAs. The rejection can be prevented by closely matching ABO, Rh, and HLAs between donor and recipient. Unfortunately, many different HLAs exist, and a perfect match is nearly impossible unless the tissue is from oneself or an identical twin. Rejection can be hyperacute, acute, or chronic. Prevention, early diagnosis, and treatment of rejection are essential for long-term graft function.

Hyperacute Rejection. *Hyperacute (antibody-mediated, humoral) rejection* occurs minutes to hours after transplantation. There is no treatment for hyperacute rejection, and the transplanted organ is removed. Hyperacute rejection is a rare event because the final crossmatch will usually identify if the recipient is sensitized to any of the donor HLAs. On occasion, for unclear reasons, the final crossmatch does not detect these preformed antibodies, and hyperacute rejection occurs.

Acute Rejection. *Acute rejection* most commonly occurs days to months after transplantation. This type of rejection is mediated by the recipient's T cytotoxic lymphocytes, which attack the foreign organ (Fig. 14-17). It is not uncommon to have at least one rejection episode, especially with organs from deceased donors. These episodes are usually reversible with additional immunosuppressive therapy that may include increased corticosteroid doses or polyclonal or monoclonal antibodies. Unfortunately, immunosuppressants do increase the risk for infection. In order to combat acute rejection, certain organ transplants, such as pancreas transplants, require long-term use of immunosuppressants, putting those patients at a high risk for infection for a longer period of time.

Chronic Rejection. *Chronic rejection* is a process that occurs over months or years and is irreversible. The transplanted organ is infiltrated with large numbers of T and B cells characteristic of an ongoing, low-grade, immune-mediated injury. Chronic rejection is more common in some organ transplants than others. Lung chronic rejection is the form of organ chronic rejection seen most often and is commonly due to bronchiolitis obliterans. Liver chronic rejection is rare and typically a result of repeated bouts of acute rejection.[34]

There is no definitive therapy for this type of rejection. Changing immunosuppressive therapy to include tacrolimus (Prograf) or mycophenolate mofetil (CellCept) has brought some improvement for some patients who were not previously taking these drugs. Treatment is mainly supportive. This type of rejection is difficult to manage and is not associated with the optimistic prognosis of acute rejection. Patients with chronic rejection should be put on the transplant list in the hope that they can be retransplanted.

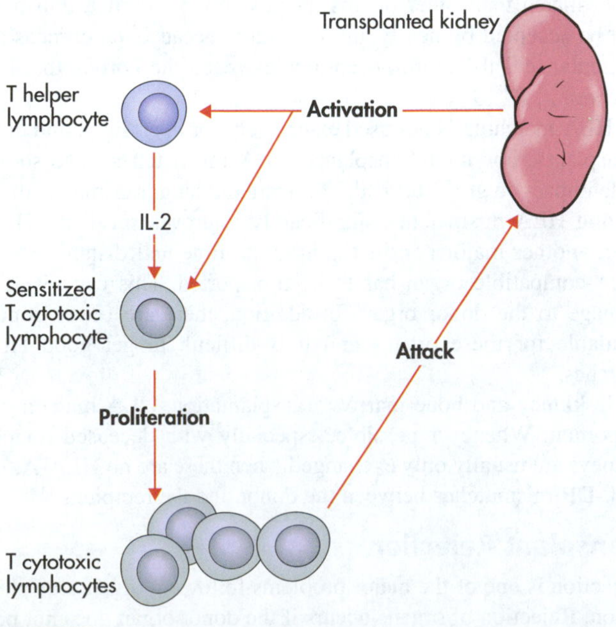

FIG. 14-17 Mechanism of action of T cytotoxic lymphocyte activation and attack of transplanted tissue. The transplanted organ (e.g., kidney) is recognized as foreign and activates the immune system. T helper cells are activated to produce interleukin-2 (IL-2), and T cytotoxic lymphocytes are sensitized. After the T cytotoxic cells proliferate, they attack the transplanted organ.

Immunosuppressive Therapy

The goal of **immunosuppressive therapy** is to adequately suppress the immune response to prevent rejection of the transplanted organ while maintaining sufficient immunity to prevent overwhelming infection. Many of the medications used to achieve immunosuppression have significant side effects. Two are of particular concern: (1) increased risk of infection and (2) increased risk of malignancies. Furthermore, because transplant recipients must take immunosuppressants for life, the risk of toxicity continues for the rest of their lives.

Immunosuppressant drugs are presented in Table 14-18 and Fig. 14-18. By using a combination of medications that work in different phases of the immune response (see Fig. 14-18), lower doses of each drug produce effective immunosuppression while minimizing side effects.[35]

The major immunosuppressive agents are (1) calcineurin inhibitors, including cyclosporine (Sandimmune, Neoral, Gengraf) and tacrolimus (Prograf, FK506); (2) corticosteroids (prednisone, methylprednisolone [Solu-Medrol] IV); (3) mycophenolate mofetil (CellCept); and (4) sirolimus (Rapamune). Azathioprine (Imuran) and cyclophosphamide (Cytoxan) have been used in the past, but are not commonly used now because they have been replaced with safer, more effective drugs. Antilymphocyte globulin (ALG) and muromonab-CD3 are IV medications used for short periods to prevent early rejection or reverse acute rejection.

***Drug Alert** - Cyclosporine*
- *Compound present in grapefruit juice prevents metabolism of drug.*
- *Consuming grapefruit juice while using drug could increase its toxicity.*

Immunosuppressive protocols are highly variable among transplant centers, with different combinations of medications being used. Most patients are initially on triple therapy. The standard triple therapy usually includes a calcineurin inhibitor, a corticosteroid, and mycophenolate mofetil (CellCept). Doses of some immunosupressant drugs may be decreased over time. Some patients may be weaned off corticosteroids (prednisone) after a few years.

Calcineurin Inhibitors. This group of drugs includes tacrolimus and cyclosporine. They are the most effective immunosuppressants available. These drugs prevent a cell-mediated attack against the transplanted organ (see Figs. 14-17 and 14-18). These drugs do not cause bone marrow suppression or alterations of the normal inflammatory response. They are generally used in combination with corticosteroids and mycophenolate mofetil. Many of the side effects of calcineurin inhibitors are dose related. These drugs are potentially nephrotoxic. Drug levels are followed closely to prevent toxicity. Neoral and Gengraf, microemulsions of cyclosporine, are replacing Sandimmune because of better and more consistent absorption.[36] Neoral and Sandimmune are not biocompatible and should never be interchanged for one another.

Sirolimus. Sirolimus is an immunosuppressive agent approved for use in renal transplant recipients. It is used in combination with corticosteroids and cyclosporine.[36] It is also used in combination with tacrolimus.

TABLE 14-18 DRUG THERAPY
Immunosuppressive Therapy

Agent	Route	Mechanism of Action	Side Effects
Corticosteroids			
prednisone, methylprednisolone (Solu-Medrol)	PO, IV	Suppress inflammatory response; inhibit cytokine production and T-cell activation and proliferation	Peptic ulcers, hypertension, osteoporosis, Na^+ and H_2O retention, muscle weakness, easy bruising, delayed healing, hyperglycemia, ↑ risk for infection
Calcineurin Inhibitors			
cyclosporine (Sandimmune,* Neoral,* Gengraf*) (Neoral and Gengraf are microemulsions with better absorption than Sandimmune)	PO, IV	Acts on T helper cells to prevent production and release of IL-2 and γ-interferon; inhibits production of T cytotoxic lymphocytes and B cells	Nephrotoxicity, ↑ risk for infection, hepatotoxicity, lymphoma, hypertension, tremors, hirsutism, leukopenia, gingival hyperplasia
tacrolimus (Prograf, FK506)	PO, IV	Same as cyclosporine but more effective	Same as cyclosporine but more toxic
Cytotoxic Drugs			
mycophenolate mofetil (CellCept)	PO, IV	Inhibits purine synthesis; suppresses proliferation of T and B cells	Diarrhea, nausea and vomiting, severe neutropenia, thrombocytopenia, ↑ risk for infection, ↑ incidence of malignancies
cyclophosphamide (Cytoxan, Neosar)	PO	Cross-links DNA, leading to cell injury and death. Results in decrease in number and activity of T and B cells	Neutropenia, hemorrhagic cystitis
azathioprine (Imuran)	PO, IV	Suppresses cell-mediated and humoral immune responses by inhibiting proliferation of T and B cells	Neutropenia, thrombocytopenia
sirolimus (Rapamune)	PO	Suppresses T-cell activation and proliferation	↑ Risk for infection, hyperlipidemia, hypercholesterolemia, arthralgias, diarrhea, thrombocytopenia, ↑ incidence of malignancies. Not used in liver or lung transplantation
Monoclonal Antibodies			
muromonab-CD3 (Orthoclone OKT3)	IV push	Monoclonal antibody that binds to CD3 receptors on T cells, causing cell lysis; inhibits function of cytotoxic T cells	Fever, chills, dyspnea, chest pain, nausea and vomiting. Anaphylactic reactions include pulmonary edema, cardiac or respiratory arrest
daclizumab (Zenapax)	IV	Monoclonal antibody that acts as IL-2 receptor antagonist by inhibiting the binding of IL-2; inhibits T-cell activation and proliferation	Generally no side effects. Rarely causes acute hypersensitivity reaction, including anaphylaxis
basiliximab (Simulect)	IV	Same as daclizumab	Same as daclizumab
Polyclonal Antibody			
Lymphocyte immune globulin (Atgam)	IV	Prepared by immunizing horse with human T cells. Polyclonal antibodies directed against T cells, thus depleting them	Serum sickness (fever, chills, muscle and joint pain), tachycardia, back pain, shortness of breath, hypotension, anaphylaxis, leukopenia, thrombocytopenia, rash, ↑ risk for infection

IL, Interleukin.
*Not bioequivalent and cannot be interchanged.

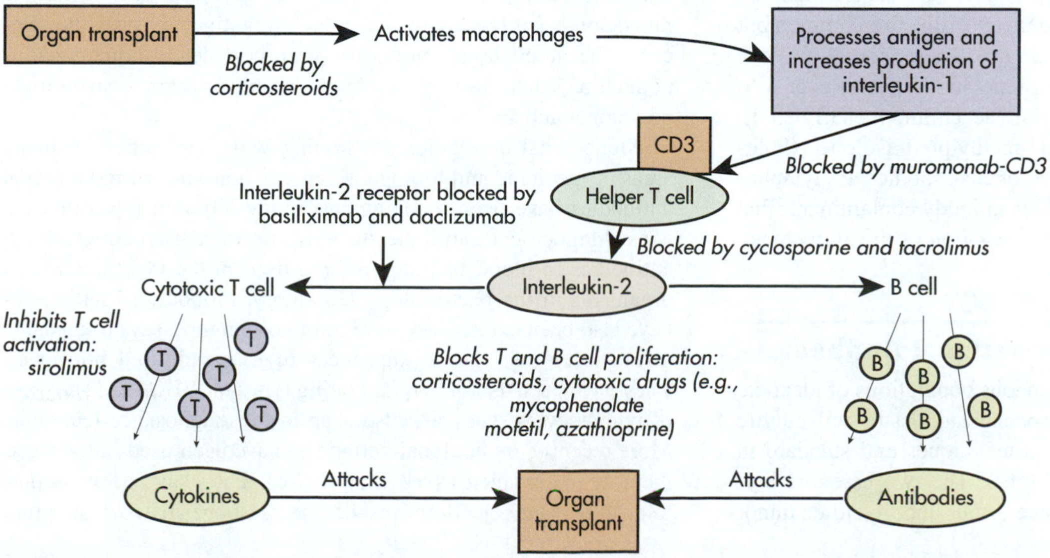

FIG. 14-18 Sites of action for immunosuppressive agents.

Mycophenolate Mofetil. Mycophenolate mofetil (CellCept) is a lymphocyte-specific inhibitor of purine synthesis with suppressive effects on both T and B lymphocytes. This drug appears to be most effective when used in combination with tacrolimus or cyclosporine. Its effects are additive because it acts later in the lymphocyte activation pathway by a different mechanism. It is used in place of azathioprine at many transplant centers because of its lymphocyte-specific effects. It has also been shown to decrease the incidence of late graft loss. The major limitation of this drug is its GI toxicities, including nausea, vomiting, and diarrhea. In many cases the side effects can be diminished by lowering the dose or giving smaller doses more frequently.

Monoclonal Antibodies. Monoclonal antibodies are used for preventing and treating acute rejection episodes. (Monoclonal antibodies are discussed later in this chapter.) Muromonab-CD3 was the first of these monoclonal antibodies to be used in clinical transplantation. It is a mouse monoclonal antibody that binds with the CD3 antigen found on the surface of human thymocytes and mature T cells. It is an anti–antigen receptor antibody that interferes with the function of the T lymphocyte, the pivotal cell in the response to graft rejection. It is administered via IV push daily for 7 to 14 days. All T cells are affected rather than just the subset active in graft rejection. Within minutes after the initial infusion of muromonab-CD3, the number of circulating T cells decreases significantly.

A flu-like syndrome occurs during the first few days of treatment due to cytokine release. Side effects include fever, rigors, headache, myalgias, and various GI disturbances. To reduce the expected side effects of muromonab-CD3, patients should receive acetaminophen, diphenhydramine, and IV corticosteroids before administering the dose.

Newer generation monoclonal antibodies include daclizumab (Zenapax) and basiliximab (Simulect). These monoclonal antibodies are a hybrid of mouse and human antibodies and have fewer side effects than muromonab-CD3 because they have been humanized by replacing large parts of the molecule with human IgG.

Polyclonal Antibody. Lymphocyte immune globulin (Atgam) is used as induction therapy or to treat acute rejection. The purpose of induction therapy is to severely immunosuppress an individual immediately after transplantation to prevent early rejection. It is made by immunizing horses with human lymphocytes. The antibody made against the human lymphocytes is then purified and administered IV.

Allergic reactions to the foreign proteins from the host animal, manifested by fever, arthralgias, and tachycardia, are common but usually not severe enough to preclude use. These side effects can be attenuated by administering the preparation slowly, over 4 to 6 hours, and premedicating patients with acetaminophen (Tylenol), diphenhydramine (Benadryl), and methylprednisolone (Solu-Medrol). The main toxicities of polyclonal antibodies are lymphopenia and thrombocytopenia caused by antibody contaminants that are not completely removed during preparation of the antibodies.

TECHNOLOGIES IN IMMUNOLOGY

Hybridoma Technology: Monoclonal Antibodies

Monoclonal antibodies are homogeneous populations of identical antibody molecules produced by specialized tissue cell culture lines. The procedure uses cell fusion techniques and standard in vitro tissue culture systems (Fig. 14-19). The two essential biologic components are immunized mice or rats and myeloma tumor cell lines, which are of lymphoid origin. Single antibody-forming cells (lymphocytes) from rodents previously immunized with antigen are fused with myeloma cells to create hybrid cells with properties of both parent cell types. The hybrids have an unlimited capacity to grow, similar to that of the myeloma parent cell. The hybrids produce the single type of antibody molecule that they inherited from the normal, antibody-forming parent cell. Hybrid cells derived in this way can produce unlimited quantities of specific antibodies. With appropriate selection techniques, producing monoclonal antibodies to virtually any antigen is possible. Because the monoclonal antibodies are a completely homogeneous population, their use incurs fewer problems than conventional polyclonal antisera.

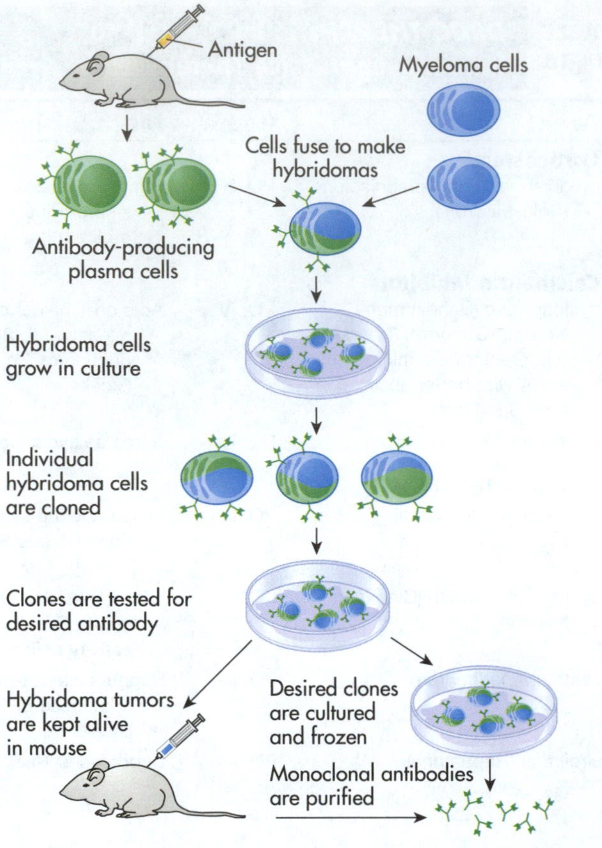

FIG. 14-19 Monoclonal antibodies are identical antibodies made by clones of a single antibody-producing cell. The target antigen is injected into a mouse. Plasma cells are harvested from the spleen of the mouse and fused with myeloma cells. The fused cells, or hybridomas, are then cloned. A clone can secrete monoclonal antibodies over a long period of time.

Monoclonal antibodies are finding wide application in many areas of medicine and biologic science. Thousands of monoclonal antibodies have been made against many different types of antigens. Monoclonal antibodies have begun to replace conventional antibodies in blood banking and are used in the identification of organisms in the bacteriology laboratory. Monoclonal antibodies have also been extensively used in radioimmunoassays to measure serum levels of various substances (e.g., parathyroid hormone). They have been useful in quantitating types of WBCs and subtypes of lymphocytes. They are also used in the diagnosis of leukemia. More recently, monoclonal antibodies have been used in the treatment of malignancies (see Chapter 16). They have been used to treat transplant rejection episodes, purge bone marrow of tumor cells in bone marrow transplants, and remove mature T cells that cause GVH disease in bone marrow transplant patients.

A major limitation of monoclonal antibodies used for humans is that they are mouse antibodies and therefore can elicit an antibody response by the host against the foreign agent. Recently, human hybridomas have been produced using human myelomas. These hybrids synthesize human monoclonals and are therefore advantageous for in vivo use in diagnosis and therapy.

Recombinant DNA Technology

Recombinant DNA technology, a form of genetic engineering, involves taking segments of DNA from one type of organism and combining them with genes from a second organism (Fig. 14-20). When the cell divides, the DNA is transcribed and a specific protein coded by the DNA is made. In this way, relatively simple organisms such as *Escherichia coli,* yeast, or mammalian tissue culture cells can be used to make large quantities of human proteins. This process is used to make human insulin and cytokines (e.g., α-interferon, interleukin-2), as well as many other substances.

Polymerase Chain Reaction

When rapid genetic diagnosis is necessary, *polymerase chain reaction* (PCR) can provide a way to make many copies of a DNA or RNA sequence in only a few hours. PCR involves the artificial replication of a DNA or RNA sequence. The DNA or RNA strands can be separated to form new templates that are used for replication. PCR requires only small amounts of sample (e.g., blood, buccal swabs, secretions), in contrast to other laboratory assays. PCR is used extensively in forensic medicine to identify DNA of criminal suspects by using samples from blood, hair, and semen. PCR can also be used as a confirmatory test in human immunodeficiency virus (HIV) testing. This is especially important when an infant of a mother who is HIV-antibody positive also tests HIV positive. In this situation, it is not known whether the antibodies from the infant's blood are from the baby or the mother. PCR techniques can be used on the baby's lymphocytes to determine whether the baby is infected with HIV.

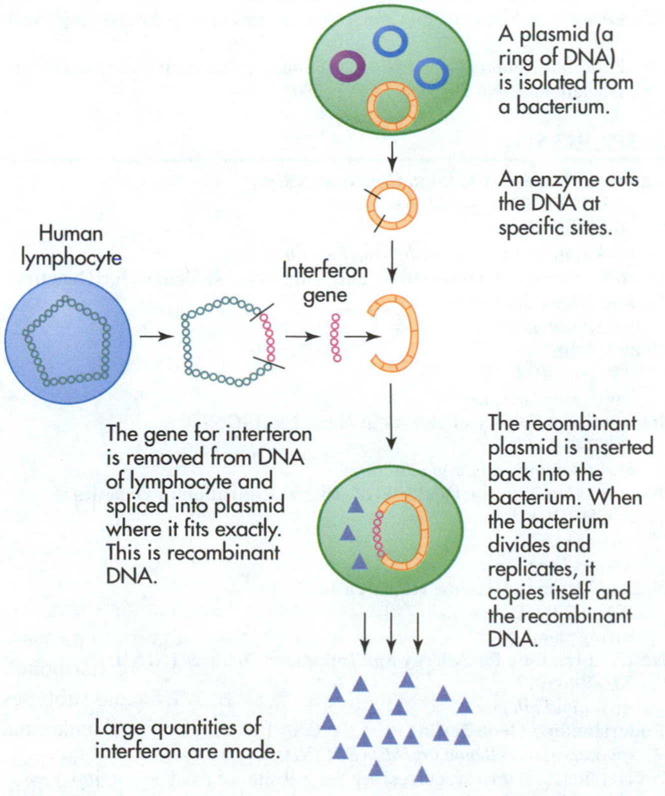
A plasmid (a ring of DNA) is isolated from a bacterium.
An enzyme cuts the DNA at specific sites.
Human lymphocyte
Interferon gene
The gene for interferon is removed from DNA of lymphocyte and spliced into plasmid where it fits exactly. This is recombinant DNA.
The recombinant plasmid is inserted back into the bacterium. When the bacterium divides and replicates, it copies itself and the recombinant DNA.
Large quantities of interferon are made.

FIG. 14-20 Mass production of interferon by recombinant gene technology.

NCLEX EXAMINATION REVIEW QUESTIONS

The number of the question corresponds to the same-numbered objective at the beginning of the chapter.

1. If a person is heterozygous for a given gene, it means that the person
   a. is a carrier for a genetic disorder.
   b. is affected by the genetic disorder.
   c. has two identical alleles for the gene.
   d. has two different alleles for the gene.
2. A father who has a sex-linked recessive disorder and a wife with a normal genotype will
   a. pass the carrier state to his male children.
   b. pass the carrier state to all of his children.
   c. pass the carrier state to his female children.
   d. not pass on the genetic mutation to any of his children.
3. The function of monocytes in immunity is related to their ability to
   a. stimulate the production of T and B lymphocytes.
   b. produce antibodies on exposure to foreign substances.
   c. bind antigens and stimulate natural killer cell activation.
   d. capture antigens by phagocytosis and present them to lymphocytes.
4. One function of cell-mediated immunity is
   a. formation of antibodies.
   b. activation of the complement system.
   c. surveillance for malignant cell changes.
   d. opsonization of antigens to allow phagocytosis by neutrophils.
5. The reason newborns are protected for the first 6 months of life from bacterial infections is because of the maternal transmission of
   a. IgG.
   b. IgA.
   c. IgM.
   d. IgE.
6. In a type I hypersensitivity reaction, the primary immunologic disorder appears to be
   a. binding of IgG to an antigen on a cell surface.
   b. deposit of antigen-antibody complexes in small vessels.
   c. release of cytokines to interact with specific antigens.
   d. release of chemical mediators from IgE-bound mast cells and basophils.
7. The nurse is alerted to possible anaphylactic shock immediately after a patient has received intramuscular penicillin by the development of
   a. edema and itching at the injection site.
   b. sneezing and itching of the nose and eyes.
   c. a wheal-and-flare reaction at the injection site.
   d. chest tightness and production of thick sputum.
8. The nurse advises a friend who asks him to administer his allergy shots that
   a. it is illegal for nurses to administer injections outside of a medical setting.
   b. he is qualified to do it if the friend has epinephrine in an injectible syringe provided with his extract.
   c. avoiding the allergens is a more effective way of controlling allergies, and allergy shots are not usually effective.
   d. immunotherapy should only be administered in a setting where emergency equipment and drugs are available.

9. Association between HLA antigens and diseases is most commonly found in what disease conditions?
   a. Malignancies
   b. Infectious diseases
   c. Neurologic diseases
   d. Autoimmune disorders
10. A patient is undergoing plasmapheresis for treatment of systemic lupus erythematosus. The nurse explains that plasmapheresis is used in her treatment to
    a. remove T lymphocytes in her blood that are producing antinuclear antibodies.
    b. remove normal particles in her blood that are being damaged by autoantibodies.
    c. exchange her plasma that contains antinuclear antibodies with a substitute fluid.
    d. replace viral-damaged cellular components of her blood with replacement whole blood.
11. The most common cause of secondary immunodeficiencies is
    a. drugs.
    b. stress.
    c. malnutrition.
    d. human immunodeficiency virus.
12. Which of the following accurately describes rejection following transplantation?
    a. Hyperacute rejection can be treated with OKT3.
    b. Acute rejection can be treated with sirolimus or tacrolimus.
    c. Chronic rejection can be treated with tacrolimus or cyclosporine.
    d. Hyperacute reaction can usually be avoided if crossmatching is done prior to the transplantation.
13. If a person is having an acute rejection of a transplanted organ, which of the following drugs would most likely be used?
    a. Tacrolimus
    b. Daclizumab
    c. Cyclosporine
    d. Mycophenolate mofetil

REFERENCES

1. Beery TA, Hern MJ: Genetic practice, education, and research: an overview for advanced practice nurses, *Clin Nurse Specialist* 18:126, 2004.
2. Lashley FR: *Clinical genetics in nursing practice*, ed 3, New York, 2005, Springer.
3. Gaff C: Identifying clients who might benefit from genetic services and information, *Nurs Standard* 20:49, 2005.
4. Skirton H, Barnes C: Obtaining and communicating information about genetics, *Nurs Standard* 20:50, 2005.
5. Bradley AN: Utility and limitations of genetic testing and information, *Nurs Standard* 20:52, 2005.
6. National Library of Medicine: Handbook: gene therapy, experimental techniques, safety, ethics, and availability, May 7, 2006. Available at *http://ghr.nlm.nih.gov/handbook/therapy.*
7. National Library of Medicine: Genetics Home Reference home page. Available at *http://ghr.nlm.nih.gov/.*
8. Benjamin CM, Gamet K: Recognizing the limitations of your genetic expertise, *Nurs Standard* 20:49, 2005.
9. Haydon J: Genetics: uphold the rights of all clients to informed decision-making and voluntary action, *Nurs Standard* 20:48, 2005.
10. Jenkins JF, Lea DH: *Nursing care in the genomic era: a case-based approach,* Boston, 2005, Jones & Bartlett.
11. National Institutes of Health: Stem cell Information home page. Available at *http://stemcells.nih.gov/.*
12. Abbas AK, Lichtman AH: *Basic immunology: functions and disorders of the immune system,* ed 2, Philadelphia, 2006, Saunders.
13. Rabson A, Roitt IM, Delves PJ: *Really essential medical immunology,* ed 2, Malden, Mass., 2005, Blackwell.
14. Doan T, Melvold R, Waltenbaugh C: *Concise medical immunology,* Philadelphia, 2005, Lippincott Williams & Wilkins.
15. Nairn R, Helbert M: *Immunology for medical students,* Edinburgh, 2002, Elsevier Mosby.
16. Birrin JE: *Encyclopedia of gerontology,* ed 2, St Louis, 2007, Academic Press (in press).
17. Hayden ML: Allergic rhinitis: proper management benefits concomitant diseases, *Nurse Practitioner* 29:26, 2004.
18. Gendo K, Larson EB: Evidence-based diagnosis strategies for evaluating suspected allergic rhinitis, *Ann Intern Med* 140:278, 2004.
19. Anchor J, Settipane RA: Appropriate use of epinephrine in anaphylaxis, *Am J Emerg Med* 22:488, 2004.
20. Schmidt-Weber CB, Blaser K: New insights into the mechanisms of allergen-specific immunotherapy, *Curr Opin Allergy Clin Immunol* 5:525, 2005.
21. Norman PS: Immunotherapy: 1999–2004, *J Allergy Clin Immunol* 113:1013, 2004.
22. Wilson DR, Lima MT, Durham SR: Sublingual immunotherapy for allergic rhinitis: systemic review and meta-analysis, *Allergy* 60:4, 2005.
23. Rolland JM, Drew AC, O'Hehir RE: Advances in development of hypoallergenic latex immunotherapy, *Curr Opin Allergy Clin Immunol* 5:544, 2005.
24. Amr S, Bollinger ME: Latex allergy and occupational asthma in health care workers: adverse outcomes, *Environ Health Perspect* 112:378, 2004.
25. National Institute for Occupational Safety and Health: Preventing allergic reactions to natural rubber latex in the workplace (Publication No. 97-135), Atlanta, 1997, Centers for Disease Control and Prevention. Available at *www.cdc.gov/niosh.*
26. Richardson RD, Engel CC: Evaluation and management of medically unexplained physical symptoms, *Neurologist* 10:18, 2004.
27. Glinton GJ: Multiple-chemical sensitivity, *MEDSURG Nurs* 14:365, 2005.
28. Janeway CA, Travers P, Walport M, Shlomchik MJ: *Immunobiology,* New York, 2005, Garland Science.
29. Turner D: The human leucocyte antigen (HLA) system, *Vox Sang* 87(Suppl 1):87, 2004.
30. Christen U, von Herrath MG: Initiation of autoimmunity, *Curr Opin Immunol* 16:759, 2004.
31. Rioux JD, Abbas AK: Paths to understanding the genetic basis of autoimmune disease, *Nature* 435:584, 2005.
32. Organ Procurement and Transplant Network home page. Available at *www.optn.org.*
33. Dyer PA, Langton A, Liggett H, et al: Testing for histocompatibility. In Forsythe JLR, editor: *Transplantation: a companion to specialist surgical practice,* ed 3, pp 84–98, Amsterdam, 2005, Elsevier Saunders.
34. Forsythe JLR: *Transplantation: a companion to specialist surgical practice,* ed 3, Amsterdam, 2005, Elsevier Saunders.
35. Lehne RA: *Pharmacology for nursing care,* ed. 6, St Louis, 2007, Saunders.
36. Zand MS: Immunosuppression and immune monitoring after renal transplantation, *Semin Dialysis* 18:511, 2005.

RESOURCES

American Society of Human Genetics (ASHG)
866-HUMGENE (486-4363)
301-634-7300
www.ashg.org/genetics/ashg/ashgmenu.htm

Essential Nursing Competencies and Curricula Guidelines for Genetics and Genomics
www.genome.gov/17517146

Gene Clinics
206-606-4033
www.geneclinics.org

International Society of Nurses in Genetics (ISONG)
412-344-1414
http://nursing.creighton.edu/isong

National Coalition for Health Professional Education in Genetics (NCHPEG)
410-583-0600
www.nchpeg.org

National Human Genome Research Institute
301-402-0911
www.genome.gov

National Institute for Allergy and Infectious Diseases (NIAID)
301-496-5717
www.niaid.nih.gov

Understanding Gene Testing
www.accessexcellence.org/AE/AEPC/NIH

For additional Internet resources, see the website for this book at *http://evolve.elsevier.com/Lewis/medsurg.*

Learning without thought is labor lost; thought without learning is perilous.

Confucius

Infection and Human Immunodeficiency Virus Infection

15

Lucy Bradley-Springer, Cory A. Shaw, and Sharon L. Lewis*

LEARNING OBJECTIVES

1. Discuss the impact of emerging and reemerging infections on health care.
2. List ways that nurses can decrease the development of resistance to antibiotics.
3. List the ways human immunodeficiency virus (HIV) is transmitted and the factors that affect transmission.
4. Describe the pathophysiology of HIV infection.
5. Outline HIV disease progression in the spectrum of untreated infection.
6. Identify the diagnostic criteria for acquired immunodeficiency syndrome (AIDS).
7. Explain methods of testing for HIV infection.
8. Discuss the collaborative management of HIV infection.
9. Summarize the characteristics of opportunistic diseases associated with AIDS.
10. Describe the long-term consequences of HIV infection and/or treatment of HIV infection.
11. Compare and contrast the methods of HIV prevention that eliminate risk and those that decrease risk.
12. Describe the nursing management of HIV-infected patients and HIV-at-risk patients.

KEY TERMS

acquired immunodeficiency syndrome (AIDS), p. 252
emerging infection, p. 245
human immunodeficiency virus (HIV), p. 250
opportunistic diseases, p. 252
oral hairy leukoplakia, p. 252
retroviruses, p. 250
reverse transcriptase, p. 251
seroconversion, p. 252
viral load, p. 249
viremia, p. 251
window period, p. 253

Electronic Resources

Supplemental content related to Chapter 15 can be found . . .

Companion CD

- Stress-Busting Kit for Nursing Students
- Interactive Case Study: Human Immunodeficiency Virus (HIV) Infection and Acquired Immunodeficiency Syndrome (AIDS)
- NCLEX Examination Review Questions
- Comprehensive Glossary

Evolve Website evolve

http://evolve.elsevier.com/Lewis/medsurg

- Content Updates
- Key Points (Printable and CD/MP3 Download)
- Concept Map Creator
- Expanded Audio Glossary
- Key Term Flash Cards
- Patient and Family Instruction Guides in English and Spanish:
  - The Proper Use of Drug Using Equipment
  - Signs and Symptoms that HIV-Infected Patients Need to Report
  - Use of Antiretroviral Drugs
  - The Right Way to Use Antibiotics
- Electronic Calculators
- WebLinks

Infections

An infection is an invasion of the body by a *pathogen* (any microorganism that causes disease) and the resulting signs and symptoms that develop in response to the invasion. Infections can be divided into two categories: localized and systemic. A localized infection is limited to a small area. Systemic infections are widespread throughout the body and are often spread via the blood.

CAUSES OF INFECTIONS

A number of microorganisms can cause infections. The most common are bacteria, viruses, fungi, and protozoa. **Bacteria** were first

Reviewed by Suzanne L. Jed, APRN-BC, MSN, FNP, Instructor, School of Medicine, Division of Infectious Diseases, University of Colorado at Denver and Health Sciences Center, Denver, Colo.

*Contributor for content on HIV.

observed by Anton Van Leeuwenhoek, who named them "animalcules." A number of bacteria are considered to be normal flora. They live harmoniously in or on the human body without causing disease under normal circumstances. These normal flora act protectively and prevent the overgrowth of other microorganisms. *Escherichia coli,* for example, are bacteria that are normal flora in the large intestine.[1]

Bacteria cause disease in two ways. They can enter the body and grow inside human cells (e.g., tuberculosis [TB]) or they can secrete toxins that damage cells. Bacteria are divided into categories based on the shape of their cells. Cocci are round cells that include streptococci and staphylococci. Bacilli are rod shaped and include tetanus and TB. Curved rods include *Vibrio* bacteria, one of which causes cholera. Table 15-1 lists common pathogenic bacteria and the diseases that they cause.[1,2]

Viruses can also cause infections. The word "virus" comes from the Latin term meaning poison. Unlike bacteria, viruses are not cells. They consist of either ribonucleic acid (RNA) or deoxyribonucleic acid (DNA) and a protein envelope. Viruses can only reproduce in the cells of a living organism and are therefore obligate parasites. Examples of diseases caused by viruses are presented in Table 15-2.[1]

Fungi are organisms similar to plants, but they lack chlorophyll. Mycosis is any disease caused by a fungus. Pathogenic fungi cause infections that are usually localized to a small area, but can become disseminated in an immunocompromised person. Athlete's foot and ringworm are two common mycotic infections. Some fungi are normal flora in various places in the body, but when overgrowth occurs, disease can result. Overgrowth of *Candida albicans,* for example, causes oral candidiasis (thrush), esophageal candidiasis, intestinal symptoms, and vaginitis, depending on the affected site.[1] Other fungi and their respective mycotic infections can be found in Table 15-3. Fungal infections of the lungs are presented in Table 28-12 and fungal infections of the skin in Table 24-6.

TABLE 15-1 Common Disease-Causing Bacteria

Type	Diseases Caused
Clostridia	
• *C. botulinum*	Food poisoning with progressive muscle paralysis
• *C. tetani*	Tetanus (lockjaw)
Corynebacterium diphtheriae	Diphtheria
Escherichia coli	Urinary tract infections, peritonitis
Haemophilus organisms	
• *H. influenzae*	Nasopharyngitis, meningitis, pneumonia
• *H. pertussis*	Whooping cough
Helicobacter pylori	Peptic ulcers, gastritis
Klebsiella-Enterobacter organisms	Urinary tract infections, peritonitis, pneumonia
Legionella pneumophila	Pneumonia (Legionnaires' disease)
Mycobacteria	
• *M. leprae*	Hansen's disease (leprosy)
• *M. tuberculosis*	Tuberculosis
Neisseriae	
• *N. gonorrhoeae*	Gonorrhea, pelvic inflammatory disease
• *N. meningitidis*	Meningococcemia, meningitis
Proteus species	Urinary tract infections, peritonitis
Pseudomonas aeruginosa	Urinary tract infections, meningitis
Salmonella species	
• *S. typhi*	Typhoid fever
• Other *Salmonella* organisms	Food poisoning, gastroenteritis
Shigella species	Shigellosis, diarrhea with abdominal pain and fever (dysentery)
Staphylococcus aureus	Skin infections, pneumonia, urinary tract infections, acute osteomyelitis, toxic shock syndrome
Streptococci	
• *S. faecalis*	Genitourinary infection, infection of surgical wounds
• *S. pneumoniae*	Pneumococcal pneumonia
• *S. pyogenes* (group A β-hemolytic streptococci)	Pharyngitis, scarlet fever, rheumatic fever, acute glomerulonephritis, erysipelas, pneumonia
• *S. pyogenes* (group B β-hemolytic streptococci)	Urinary tract infections
• *S. viridans*	Bacterial endocarditis
Treponema pallidum	Syphilis

TABLE 15-2 Common Disease-Causing Viruses

Type	Diseases Caused
Adenoviruses	Upper respiratory tract infection, pneumonia
Arbovirus	Syndrome of fever, malaise, headache, myalgia; aseptic meningitis; encephalitis
Coronavirus	Upper respiratory tract infection
Coxsackieviruses A and B	Upper respiratory tract infection, gastroenteritis, acute myocarditis, aseptic meningitis
Echoviruses	Upper respiratory tract infection, gastroenteritis, aseptic meningitis
Hepatitis	
• A	Viral hepatitis
• B	Viral hepatitis
• C	Viral hepatitis
Herpesviruses	
• Cytomegalovirus (CMV)	Gastroenteritis; pneumonia and retinal damages in immunosuppressed individuals, infectious mononucleosis–like syndrome
• Epstein-Barr	Mononucleosis, Burkitt's lymphoma (possibly)
• Herpes simplex, type 1	Herpes labialis ("fever blisters"), genital herpes infection
• Herpes simplex, type 2	Genital herpes infection
• Varicella-zoster	Chickenpox; shingles
Human immunodeficiency virus (HIV)	HIV infection, acquired immunodeficiency syndrome (AIDS)
Influenza A and B	Upper respiratory tract infection
Mumps	Parotitis, orchitis in postpubertal males
Papovavirus	Warts
Parainfluenza 1-4	Upper respiratory tract infection
Parvovirus	Gastroenteritis
Poliovirus	Poliomyelitis
Pox viruses	Smallpox
Reoviruses 1, 2, 3	Upper respiratory tract infection
Respiratory syncytial virus	Gastroenteritis, respiratory tract infection
Rhabdovirus	Rabies
Rhinovirus	Upper respiratory tract infection, pneumonia
Rotaviruses	Gastroenteritis
Rubella	German measles
Rubeola	Measles
West Nile virus	Flu-like symptoms, meningitis, encephalitis

TABLE 15-3 Common Disease-Causing Fungi

Organism	Diseases Caused	Organs Affected
Aspergillus fumigatus	Aspergillosis	Lungs*
	Otomycosis	Ears
Blastomyces dermatitidis	Blastomycosis	Lungs, various organs
Candida albicans	Candidiasis	Intestines
	Vaginitis	Vagina
	Thrush	Skin,† mouth
Coccidioides immitis	Coccidioidomycosis	Lungs*
Pneumocystis jiroveci	*Pneumocystis* pneumonia	Lungs*
Sporothrix schenckii	Sporotrichosis	Skin, lymph vessels
Trichophyton species	Tinea pedis	Skin†
Microsporum species	Tinea capitis	
Epidermophyton species	Tinea corporis	

*See Table 28-12: Fungal Infections of the Lung.
†See Table 24-6: Common Fungal Infections of the Skin.

Protozoa are single-cell, animal-like microorganisms. Protozoa can be divided into four categories: amebas, ciliates, flagellates, and sporozoa. Protozoa normally live in soil and bodies of water. When introduced into the human body, infection can result. Amebic dysentery and giardiasis are caused by protozoan parasites. Malaria is caused by a sporozoa called *Plasmodium malariae.*[1,2]

EMERGING INFECTIONS

An **emerging infection** is an infectious disease whose incidence has increased in the past 20 years or threatens to increase in the immediate future. Examples of emerging infections are described in Table 15-4. Emerging infectious diseases can originate from unknown sources, from contact with animals, changes in known diseases, or even biologic warfare. For example, severe acute respiratory syndrome (SARS) and the West Nile virus come from animal sources, whereas others, such as *Staphylococcus aureus*, have emerged as a result of a previously treatable organism developing resistance to antibiotics. The battle against infectious disease is an age-old problem. However, modern technologies have changed the rules of the game. Global travel, population density, encroachment into new environments, and misused antibiotics have all increased the risk for widespread new or untreatable infectious diseases.[3]

TABLE 15-4 Examples of Emerging Infections

Microbe	Related Disease
Bacteria	
Borrelia burgdorferi	Lyme disease
Campylobacter jejuni	Diarrhea
Escherichia coli 0157:H7	Hemorrhagic colitis, hemolytic uremic syndrome
Helicobacter pylori	Peptic ulcer disease
Legionella pneumophila	Legionnaires' disease
Vibrio cholerae 0139	New strain associated with epidemic cholera
Virus	
Ebola virus	Ebola hemorrhagic fever
Hantavirus	Hemorrhagic fever associated with severe pulmonary syndrome
Hepatitis C	Parenterally transmitted hepatits
Hepatitis E	Enterically transmitted hepatits
Human immunodeficiency virus (HIV)	HIV disease and AIDS
Human herpesvirus 6 (HHV-6)	Roseola subitum
Human herpesvirus 8 (HHV-8)	Associated with Kaposi's sarcoma in immunosuppressed patients, AIDS patients
West Nile virus	West Nile fever
Parasite	
Cryptosporidium parvum	Acute and chronic diarrhea

AIDS, Acquired immunodeficiency syndrome.

It is interesting that only a generation ago many believed that science had conquered infectious disease. Unfortunately, infections remain the third leading killer of Americans and the leading cause of death worldwide. More than 30 newly recognized infectious diseases have emerged in the last two decades, including human immunodeficiency virus (HIV), Lyme disease, hepatitis C, SARS, and Ebola virus, and some diseases once thought to be under control, including TB and drug-resistant strains of other bacteria, have reemerged.[4]

Studies in zoonosis (the science of transmission of diseases from animals to humans) indicate that many known infectious diseases come from animals and insects (vectors). The SARS outbreak in China in 2003, for instance, was linked to the civet cat, a small carnivorous mammal found throughout much of Asia and Africa. (SARS is discussed in Chapter 68.) Animal-borne infections are difficult to predict and prevent.

West Nile virus is transmitted by a virus carried by mosquitoes. Mosquitoes acquire the virus as they draw blood from infected animals and people. The virus does not cause illness in the mosquito, but can be transferred to uninfected animals and humans as the mosquito continues to feed. Bird deaths are an indicator of the spread of the West Nile virus and can serve as an early warning sign of an outbreak that can spread quickly if action is not taken in a timely manner.[5] (West Nile virus is discussed in Chapter 57.)

Sometimes an organism alters its normal path of transmission. In the past, influenza A viruses were typically spread from birds to pigs to humans. Recently, in cases such as the avian flu outbreak, the virus has been spread directly from chickens to humans. This was first demonstrated in Hong Kong in 1997 and also in the Netherlands in 2003. Infected people generally suffer from conjunctivitis or mild influenza-like symptoms. However, 130 deaths related to avian flu have occurred.[6] Upon discovery of an outbreak, all chickens in the area are typically slaughtered to remove the source of the infection.

The Ebola virus is an emerging disease that has presented an ongoing challenge to public health since it was first seen in 1976. Ebola virus causes a severe hemorrhagic fever and is usually lethal. Therapeutic and preventive measures are extremely limited. The natural reservoir and path of transmission of the virus are unknown, which makes it impossible to effectively combat the disease.[6]

Reemerging Infections

Vaccines and proper medications have led to the near eradication of some infections. However, infective agents can always reemerge if conditions are right. Table 15-5 illustrates some diseases that have reemerged in recent decades.

For example, the incidence of TB was steadily decreasing beginning in the mid-1950s. However, in 1984 the trend changed and TB cases began to rise, with the total U.S. cases peaking in 1992.

TABLE 15-5 Examples of Reemerging Infections

Microbe	Description
Bacteria	
Diphtheria	Localized infection of mucous membranes or skin
Escherichia coli O157:H7	Acute infection causing abdominal cramping, inflammatory colitis, profuse diarrhea, and hemolytic uremic syndrome
Pertussis	Acute, highly contagious respiratory disease that is characterized by loud whooping inspiration; also known as whooping cough
Tuberculosis	Chronic infection caused by *Mycobacterium tuberculosis;* transmitted by inhalation of infected droplets (see Chapter 28)
Virus	
Dengue fever	Acute infection transmitted by mosquitoes and occurring mainly in tropical and subtropical regions
Parasite	
Giardiasis	Diarrheal illness that usually originates in fecal-contaminated water; also known as traveler's diarrhea

TABLE 15-6 Common Antibiotic-Resistant Organisms and Treatment

Bacteria	Resistant to	Preferred Treatment
Staphylococcus aureus	Methicillin	Vancomycin
Staphylococcus epidermidis	Methicillin	Vancomycin
Enterococcus faecalis	Vancomycin (Vancocin), streptomycin, gentamicin (Garamycin)	Penicillin G or ampicillin
Enterococcus faecium	Vancomycin, streptomycin, gentamicin	Penicillin G or ampicillin
Streptococcus pneumoniae	Penicillin G	Ceftriaxone (Rocephin), cefotaxime (Claforan)
Klebsiella pneumoniae	Third-generation cephalosporins (e.g., ceftazidime [Ceptaz, Fortaz])	Imipenem/cilastatin (Primaxin), meropenem (Merrem IV)

Local and federal governments responded and measures were taken to curb the increase. As a result, the incidence of TB declined to an all-time low in 2003.[7] One factor that led to the increase in TB cases was the increase in people with HIV, whose depressed immune systems allow diseases such as TB to cause infection. Other factors leading to the rise included major cutbacks in public health funds and the development of multidrug-resistant forms of TB (MDR-TB).[7]

International travel creates a new dilemma for the local eradication of diseases. Measles, for instance, is no longer considered endemic in the United States, but it remains a leading cause of morbidity in developing countries. Some measles cases in the United States have been found in people with recent travel to these measles-endemic countries.[8]

Antibiotic-Resistant Organisms

Resistance occurs when pathologic organisms change in ways that decrease the ability of a drug (or a family of drugs) to treat disease. Microorganisms can become resistant to classical (e.g., penicillin) as well as newer antibiotic and antiviral agents. Methicillin-resistant *Staphylococcus aureus* (MRSA), vancomycin-resistant enterococci (VRE), and penicillin-resistant *Streptococcus pneumoniae* are three of the most troublesome resistant bacteria currently causing problems in North America. Table 15-6 describes the most common antibiotic-resistant bacteria.

Bacteria are highly adaptable organisms that have evolved genetic and biochemical means of resisting antimicrobial actions. Genetic mechanisms include mutation and acquisition of new DNA. Biochemically, bacteria resist antibiotics by producing enzymes that destroy or inactivate the drugs. Drug target sites are then altered so that the antibiotic cannot bind to or enter the bacteria. If the drug cannot enter the cell, it cannot kill the bacteria.[5]

MRSA can be acquired in a hospital setting as well as in the community. Health care workers exposed to MRSA can become infected and spread the infection to other health care workers and patients. The organism can remain viable for days on environmental surfaces and clothing. Hospital patients most at risk include those who are immunosuppressed (e.g., receiving chemotherapy), have invasive devices (e.g., indwelling catheters), or have breaks in the skin barrier (e.g., surgical wound). VRE are hardier than MRSA and can remain viable on environmental surfaces for weeks. An antiseptic soap such as chlorhexidine is needed to kill these bacteria.[9] The Centers for Disease Control and Prevention (CDC) recommend that infection control for antibiotic-resistant organisms consist of Standard Precautions (see Tables 15-8 and 15-9 on pp. 248 to 249), which should be used for all patient care.

Certain gram-negative bacteria have developed the ability to produce β-lactamase, an enzyme that makes them resistant to third-generation cephalosporins (e.g., ceftriaxone [Rocephin], cefixime [Suprax]). Infections caused by these bacteria present with signs and symptoms similar to nonresistant strains but require different antibiotics to be effectively treated. Culture specimens should be tested to determine if the bacteria is β-lactamase producing and that the organism is sensitive to the antibiotic selected for treatment.[10]

Drug resistance is a particularly difficult problem when dealing with infectious diseases. Health care providers can contribute to the development of drug-resistant organisms. They can do this by (1) administering antibiotics for viral infections, (2) succumbing to pressures from patients to prescribe unnecessary antibiotic therapy, (3) using inadequate drug regimens to treat infections, or (4) using broad-spectrum or combination agents for infections that should be treated with first-line medications. Patients who miss doses or do not take antibiotics for the full duration of the prescribed therapy also contribute to the development of resistance. In addition, limited resources and/or access to medications make it difficult for some patients to get adequate treatment for infections. Patients and their families should be taught that the proper use of antibiotics (Table 15-7) is crucial to treatment success and prevention of drug-resistant pathogens.

NOSOCOMIAL INFECTIONS

Nosocomial infections are infections that are acquired as a result of exposure to a microorganism in a hospital setting. These infections typically occur within 72 hours of hospitalization. Approximately 2 million nosocomial infections occur in the United States each

TABLE 15-7 ***PATIENT AND FAMILY TEACHING GUIDE***
Decrease Risk for Antibiotic-Resistant Infection

1. Do Not Take Antibiotics to Prevent Illness.
Doing this increases your risk for developing resistant infection.
Exceptions include taking antibiotics before certain surgeries and taking antibiotics before dental work if you have a heart valve disorder.

2. Wash Your Hands Frequently.
Handwashing is the single most important thing you can do to prevent an infection.

3. Follow Directions.
Not taking your antibiotic as prescribed or skipping doses can encourage the development of antibiotic-resistant bacteria.

4. Finish Your Antibiotic.
Do not stop taking your antibiotic when you feel better. If you stop taking your antibiotic early, the hardiest bacteria survive and multiply. Eventually you could develop an infection resistant to many antibiotics. You should never have leftover antibiotics.

5. Do Not Request an Antibiotic for Flu or Colds.
If your health care provider says that you do not need an antibiotic, chances are you do not. Antibiotics are effective against bacterial infections but not viruses, which cause colds and flus.

6. Do Not Take Leftover Antibiotics.
People often save unfinished antibiotics for later use or borrow leftover drugs from family or friends. This is dangerous because (1) the leftover antibiotic may not be appropriate for you, (2) your illness may not be a bacterial infection, (3) old antibiotics can lose their effectiveness and in some cases can even be fatal, and (4) there will not be enough doses in a leftover bottle to allow for a full treatment.

year, and 50% are caused by antibiotic-resistant organisms.[3] According to the Centers for Disease Control and Prevention (CDC), up to 10% of hospital patients will acquire a nosocomial infection, and surgical patients are at even greater risk. In addition, some bacteria that are not normally pathologic can cause infections in patients who are immunocompromised as a result of illness or treatment of illness. Nosocomial infections can be caused by any organism, but certain bacteria, including *Escherichia coli, Staphylococcus aureus, Enterobacter aerogenes,* and various types of streptococci, are the more common culprits.[3]

Approximately one third of nosocomial infections are preventable. Nosocomial infections are often transmitted from patient to patient through direct contact by health care providers. Hand washing (or using an alcohol-based hand sanitizer) between patients and procedures as well as appropriate use of protective equipment such as gloves remain the first lines of defense in preventing the spread of nosocomial infections. Isolated infections can be caused when bacteria that are normally present in one area of the body are introduced into another area. Therefore care must be taken to change gloves and wash hands when moving from one task to another, even when working with one patient.[11]

GERONTOLOGIC CONSIDERATIONS
INFECTION IN OLDER ADULTS

For older adult patients, the rate of nosocomial infection is 2 to 3 times higher than for younger patients. Individuals in long-term care facilities have a greater incidence of illness and are at special risk. Age-related changes of decreased immunocompetence, the presence of comorbidities, and an increase in disability all contribute to higher infection rates.[12]

Infections common in older adults include pneumonia, urinary tract infections, skin infections, and TB.[12] Urinary tract infections are the most common nosocomial infections in older adults residing in long-term care facilities. They are often found in patients who have indwelling catheters. Infections in older adults often have atypical presentations showing cognitive and behavioral changes before alterations occur in laboratory values.[13] Suspicion of disease should typically begin when changes in ability to perform daily activities or in cognitive function occur. Fever should not be relied upon to indicate infection in older adults because many have lower core body temperatures and decreased immune responses. In addition, underlying diseases, increased frequency of drug reactions, and institutionalization can all complicate the management of the older adult with infection.

INFECTION PREVENTION AND CONTROL

Occupational Safety and Health Administration Guidelines

The Occupational Safety and Health Administration (OSHA) is a federal agency that protects workers from injury and illness in their places of employment. It has a standard that mandates that any employer whose employees are potentially exposed to blood from needles and other sharps must implement sharps safety devices wherever feasible. In addition, employees at risk need to be provided appropriate personal protective equipment (PPE). The nurse needs to minimize or eliminate exposure to infectious material. When that is not possible, appropriate PPE must be selected. These include gloves, clothing, and facial protection (Table 15-8). Appropriate PPE will vary depending on the situation.

Infection Precautions

If the patient develops an infection that is considered a risk to others, infection precautions may be needed. The purpose of these precautions is to prevent the transmission of organisms from patients to health care providers, from health care providers to patients, and from one patient to another.

The CDC developed guidelines that contain two levels of precautions (Table 15-9): (1) *standard precautions,* which are designed for the care of all patients in hospitals and health care facilities regardless of diagnosis or presumed infection status, and (2) *transmission-based precautions,* which are used for patients known to be or suspected of being infected with epidemiologically important pathogens that can be transmitted by airborne or droplet transmission or by contact with dry skin or contaminated surfaces.

The standard precautions system applies to (1) blood; (2) all body fluids, secretions, and excretions regardless of whether they contain visible blood; (3) nonintact skin; and (4) mucous membranes. Standard precautions are designed to reduce the risk of transmission of microorganisms from both recognized and unrecognized sources of infection in hospitals. Standard precautions should be applied to all patients regardless of diagnosis or infection status. The CDC's standard precautions incorporate all requirements of OSHA's blood-borne pathogens standard.

Transmission-based precautions are designed for patients suspected of or documented with highly transmissible or epidemiologically important pathogens for which additional precautions

TABLE 15-8 Occupational Safety and Health Administration (OSHA) Requirements for Personal Protective Equipment to Minimize Exposure to Blood-Borne Pathogens*

Equipment	Indications for Use
Gloves	Must be used when it can be reasonably anticipated that the employee may have contact with blood or other potentially infectious materials, when performing vascular access procedures,* and when handling or touching contaminated items or surfaces. Gloves must be replaced if torn, punctured, or contaminated or their ability to function as a barrier is compromised.
Clothing (gowns, aprons, caps, boots)	Needs to be used when occupational exposure is anticipated. The type and characteristics will depend on the task and degree of exposure anticipated.
Facial protection (mask with glasses with solid side shields or a chin-length face shield)	Must be used when splashes, sprays, spatters, or droplets of blood or other potentially infectious materials pose a hazard to the eyes, nose, or mouth.

Source: OSHA website, *www.osha.gov/SLTC/bloodbornepathogens/.*

NOTE: Employers must provide, make accessible, and require the use of personal protective equipment (PPE) at no cost to the employee. PPE also must be provided in appropriate sizes. Hypoallergenic gloves or other similar alternatives must be made available to employees who have an allergic sensitivity to gloves.

*Some exceptions are made for voluntary blood donation centers.

TABLE 15-9 CDC Recommendations for Isolation Precautions in Health Care Facilities

Standard Precautions	Transmission-Based Precautions: Airborne	Transmission-Based Precautions: Droplet	Transmission-Based Precautions: Contact
When to Use			
All patients	Use in addition to standard precautions for patients known to be or suspected of being infected with microorganisms transmitted by airborne droplet (e.g., measles, varicella, tuberculosis).	Use in addition to standard precautions for patients known to be or suspected of being infected with microorganisms transmitted by droplets (e.g., *Haemophilus influenzae, Neisseria meningitidis, Streptococcus pneumoniae, Mycoplasma pneumoniae*).	Use in addition to standard precautions for specified patients known to be or suspected of being infected with epidemiologically important microorganisms that can be transmitted by direct contact with patient (e.g., enteric pathogens, multidrug-resistant bacteria, *Staphylococcus aureus, Clostridium difficile*, herpes simplex) or by direct contact with environmental surface or patient care items in the patient's environment.
Handwashing			
Wash hands after touching blood, body fluids, secretions, excretions, and contaminated items, regardless of whether gloves are worn; wash hands immediately after gloves are removed, between patient contacts, and to prevent transfer of microorganisms to other patients or environments.	Same as standard precautions.	Same as standard precautions.	Same as standard precautions.
Gloves			
Wear nonsterile gloves when touching blood, body fluids, secretions, excretions, and contaminated items; put on clean gloves just before touching mucous membranes and nonintact skin; remove gloves promptly after use, before touching noncontaminated items, or environmental surfaces, or going to another patient.	Same as standard precautions.	Same as standard precautions.	In addition to glove use as described in standard precautions, wear gloves when entering the room whenever providing direct patient care or having hand contact with potentially contaminated surfaces or items in patient's environment.
Mask, Eye Protection, Face Shield			
Wear mask and eye protection or face shield to protect mucous membranes of eyes, nose, and mouth during procedures and patient care activities likely to generate splashes or sprays of blood, body fluids, secretions, and excretions.	In addition to standard precautions, wear respiratory protection when entering room of patient known to have or suspected of having tuberculosis.	In addition to standard precautions, wear a mask when working within 3 ft of patient.	Same as standard precautions.

Source: CDC website, *www.cdc.gov/ncidod/dhqp/gl_isolation.html.*

CDC, Centers for Disease Control and Prevention.

TABLE 15-9 CDC Recommendations for Isolation Precautions in Health Care Facilities—cont'd

Standard Precautions	Transmission-Based Precautions: Airborne	Droplet	Contact
Gown			
Wear clean, nonsterile gown to protect skin and prevent soiling of clothing during procedures and patient care activities likely to generate splashes or sprays of blood, body fluids, secretions, or excretions or likely to cause soiling of clothing; remove gown promptly when tasks are completed; wash hands.	Same as standard precautions.	Same as standard precautions.	Wear clean, nonsterile gown if substantial contact is anticipated with patient, surfaces, or items in environment; wear gown if patient is incontinent or has diarrhea, an ileostomy, a colostomy, or uncontained wound drainage; remove gown carefully when tasks are completed; wash hands.
Linen			
Handle, transport, and process used linen in manner that prevents skin and mucous membrane exposure, contamination of clothing, and environmental soiling.	Same as standard precautions.	Same as standard precautions.	Same as standard precautions.
Patient Transport			
	Limit movement and transport of patient from room to essential purposes only; if transport or movement is necessary, minimize patient dispersal of droplet nuclei by placing surgical mask on patient, if possible.	Limit movement and transport of patient from room to essential purposes only; if transport or movement is necessary, minimize patient dispersal of droplet nuclei by masking patient, if possible.	Limit movement and transport of patient from room to essential purposes only; if transport is necessary, ensure that precautions are maintained to minimize contamination of environmental surfaces or equipment.

beyond standard precautions are needed to interrupt transmission in hospitals. The three types of transmission-based precautions are *airborne precautions, droplet precautions,* and *contact precautions.* They may be combined for diseases that have multiple routes of transmission. Whether used by themselves or in combination, these precautions are employed in addition to standard precautions.

Human Immunodeficiency Virus Infection

The history of the human immunodeficiency virus (HIV) epidemic in the United States and Canada has unfolded since the mid-1970s. Although HIV obviously had been present prior to 1981, it was not until that year that public health officials documented the presence of a new disease that would become known as the acquired immunodeficiency syndrome (AIDS). By 1985 the causative agent, HIV, had been identified, and AIDS was determined to be an advanced stage of chronic HIV infection. In addition, an antibody test was developed and routes of transmission were determined. Drug therapy to treat the infection became available in 1987 with the release of zidovudine (ZDV, AZT, Retrovir) and has since expanded dramatically. Since 1994 several important advances have been made, including the development of laboratory tests to assess the number of HIV particles in the plasma **(viral load),** the production of new drugs, the use of combination drug therapy, the ability to test for antiretroviral drug resistance, and treatment to decrease the risk of transmission from mother to baby.[14] In developed countries, the result has been decreases in the number of HIV-related deaths, improved quality of life, and a significant decrease in children born with HIV.[15,16] Unfortunately, these advances are not available to all who need them. Although great progress has been made, the epidemic is not over; North American and global numbers continue to increase, and leveling off, typical of a waning epidemic, has not yet started.[17] Nursing care for patients with HIV infection continues to be a critical need that will evolve as advances in prevention and care emerge.

Significance of the Problem

One million people were living with HIV in North America at the end of 2004, with an estimated 44,000 new infections and 16,000 HIV-related deaths that year. Of those living with the infection, 260,000 (25%) were adolescent and adult women and 11,000 were children under the age of 15. The number of new cases each year in the United States has remained consistent at 40,000 for several years, but the epidemic is growing at faster rates among women, people of color, people who live in poverty, and adolescents. In addition, treatment has provided major advances in the ability to keep HIV-infected people healthy for longer periods of time, and the death rate has fallen dramatically.[18]

Globally, HIV has been devastating. Since the beginning of the *pandemic,* more than 60 million people have been infected and more than 20 million of those have died.[19] At the end of 2004, an estimated 39.4 million people, including 2.2 million children under age 15, were living with HIV. During that year, 4.9 million people were newly infected with HIV and over 3 million died of HIV-related causes.[18]

The burden of HIV is not evenly distributed. Since the beginning of the epidemic, sub-Saharan Africa has been the most devastated, but the Caribbean, Asia, Eastern Europe, Central America, and South America also have growing epidemics. In developing countries, the major route of transmission is heterosexual sex, and women and children bear a large part of the burden of illness. Industrialized countries have fared better, but have not eliminated the infection or provided appropriate care to all HIV-infected individuals. For the most part, HIV remains a disease of marginalized individuals: those who are disenfranchised by virtue of gender, race, sexual orientation, poverty, drug use, or lack of access to health care.[19-22]

Transmission of HIV

HIV is a fragile virus. It can only be transmitted under specific conditions that allow contact with infected body fluids, including blood, semen, vaginal secretions, and breast milk. Transmission of HIV occurs through sexual intercourse with an infected partner, exposure to HIV-infected blood or blood products, and perinatal transmission during pregnancy, at the time of delivery, or through breastfeeding.[23]

HIV-infected individuals can transmit HIV to others within a few days after becoming infected. After that, the ability to transmit HIV is lifelong. Transmission of HIV is subject to the same requirements as other microorganisms (i.e., a large enough amount of the virus must enter the body of a susceptible host). Duration and frequency of contact, volume of fluid, virulence and concentration of the organism, and host immune status all affect whether infection is established after an exposure. The viral load (or the number of viruses) in the blood, semen, vaginal secretions, or breast milk of the "donor" is an important variable. Large amounts of HIV can be found in the blood during the first 6 months of infection and again during the late stages of the disease (Fig. 15-1). Unprotected sexual or blood exposure to an infected individual is more risky during these periods, although HIV can be transmitted during all phases of the disease.[24-26]

HIV is not spread casually. The virus cannot be transmitted through hugging, dry kissing, shaking hands, sharing eating utensils, using toilet seats, or attending school or working with an HIV-infected person. It is not transmitted through tears, saliva, urine, emesis, sputum, feces, or sweat. Repeated studies have failed to demonstrate transmission of the virus by respiratory droplets, enteric routes, or casual encounters in any setting. Health care workers have a very low risk of acquiring HIV at work, even after a needle-stick injury.[24-26]

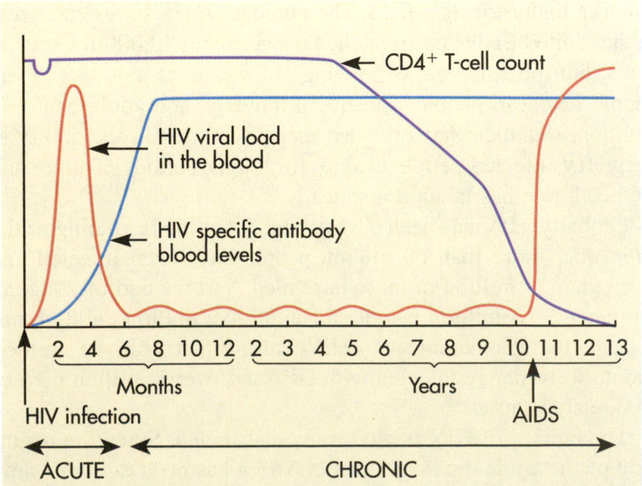

FIG. 15-1 Viral load in the blood and CD4+ T-cell counts over the spectrum of untreated human immunodeficiency virus (HIV) infection.

Sexual Transmission. Unprotected sexual contact with an HIV-infected partner is the most common mode of transmission. Sexual activity provides an opportunity for contact with semen, vaginal secretions, and/or blood, all of which have lymphocytes that may contain HIV.

Although *men who have sex with men* (MSM) still account for most cases of HIV in the United States and Canada, heterosexual transmission has become more prevalent and is now the most common method of infection for women.[15] The riskiest sexual activity is unprotected anal intercourse. During any form of sexual intercourse (anal, vaginal, or oral), the risk of infection is greater for the partner who receives the semen, although infection can also be transmitted to an inserting partner. This occurs because the receiver has prolonged contact with infected fluids, and helps explain why women are more easily infected than men during heterosexual intercourse. Sexual activities that involve blood, such as during menstruation or as a result of trauma to local tissues, also increase the risk of transmission. In addition, the presence of genital lesions caused by other sexually transmitted diseases (e.g., herpes, syphilis) significantly increases the likelihood of infection.[25]

Contact with Blood and Blood Products. HIV can be transmitted during exposure to blood through drug-using equipment. Used equipment may be contaminated with HIV and other blood-borne organisms, and sharing that equipment can result in disease transmission.[24,26]

In North America, transfusion of infected blood and blood products has caused only 1% of adult AIDS cases.[15,16] In 1985, routine screening of blood donors to identify at-risk individuals and testing donated blood for the presence of HIV were implemented, thereby improving the safety of the blood supply. HIV infection as a result of blood transfusions is now unlikely, but still possible because blood donated during the first few months of infection may not test positive for HIV antibodies[27] (see Fig. 15-1). Clotting factors used by people with hemophilia are now treated with heat or chemicals that kill HIV and other blood-borne viruses, thus eliminating that risk.[28]

Puncture wounds are the most common means of work-related transmission. The risk of infection after a needle-stick exposure to HIV-infected blood is 0.3% to 0.4% (or 3 to 4 out of 1000). The risk is higher if the exposure involves blood from a patient with a high viral load, a deep puncture wound, a needle with a hollow bore and visible blood, a device used for venous or arterial access, or a patient who dies within 60 days. Splash exposures of blood on skin with an open lesion present some risk, but it is much lower than from a puncture wound.[26]

Perinatal Transmission. Perinatal transmission is the most common route of infection for children. Transmission from an HIV-infected mother to her infant can occur during pregnancy, at the time of delivery, or after birth through breastfeeding. On average, 25% of infants born to untreated HIV-infected women will be born with HIV. This means that 75% of these infants would not have been infected even without treatment.[29]

Pathophysiology

The **human immunodeficiency virus (HIV),** a ribonucleic acid (RNA) virus, was discovered in 1983. RNA viruses are called **retroviruses** because they replicate in a "backward" manner (going from RNA to deoxyribonucleic acid [DNA]). Like all viruses, HIV cannot replicate unless it is inside a living cell. HIV can enter a cell when the gp120 "knobs" (Fig. 15-2) on the viral envelope bind to

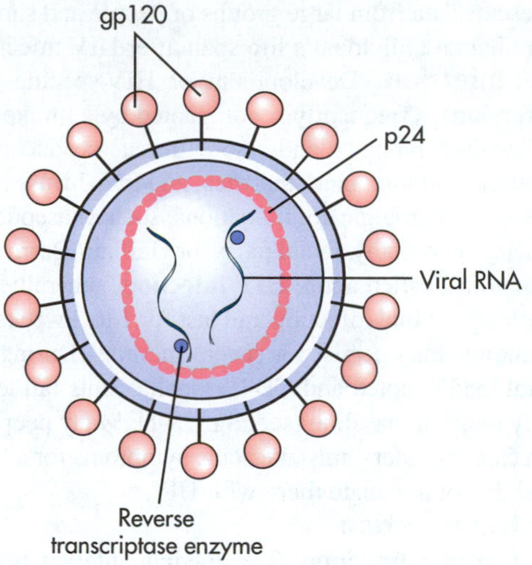

FIG. 15-2 HIV is surrounded by an envelope made up of proteins (including gp120) and contains a core of viral RNA and proteins.

specific CD4 and chemokine receptor sites on the cell's surface **(fusion)** (Fig. 15-3). Chemokine receptors are proteins normally found in cell membranes that respond to chemokines outside the cell to trigger a response inside the cell. HIV uses the chemokine receptors CXCR4 and CCR5 as co-receptors (CD4 being the main receptor) to make binding and entry into the $CD4^+$ T cells possible.

Once bound, viral RNA enters the cell, where it is transcribed into a single strand of viral DNA with the assistance of **reverse transcriptase,** an enzyme made by retroviruses. This strand copies itself, becoming double-stranded viral DNA, which then enters the cell's nucleus and, using another enzyme called **integrase,** splices itself into the genome, becoming a permanent part of the cell's genetic structure. There are two consequences of this action: (1) because all genetic material is replicated during cell division, all daughter cells will also be infected; and (2) viral DNA in the genome will direct the cell to make new HIV. HIV production in the cell starts with long strands of HIV RNA. These are cut into appropriate lengths in the presence of the enzyme **protease** during the budding sequence.[30]

Initial infection with HIV results in **viremia** (large amounts of virus in the blood). This is followed within a few weeks by a prolonged period in which HIV levels in the blood remain low even without treatment (see Fig. 15-1). During this time, which may last for 10 to 12 years, there are few clinical symptoms. Even without symptoms, however, HIV replication occurs at a rapid and constant rate in the blood and lymph tissues. A steady-state viral load can be maintained in the body of infected individuals for many years. To do this, 10^8 to 10^9 new viruses are produced each day. A major consequence of rapid replication is that copy errors can occur, causing mutations that contribute to difficulties in treatment and vaccine development.[23,31]

In a normal immune response, foreign antigens interact with B cells and T cells. In the initial stages of HIV infection, these cells

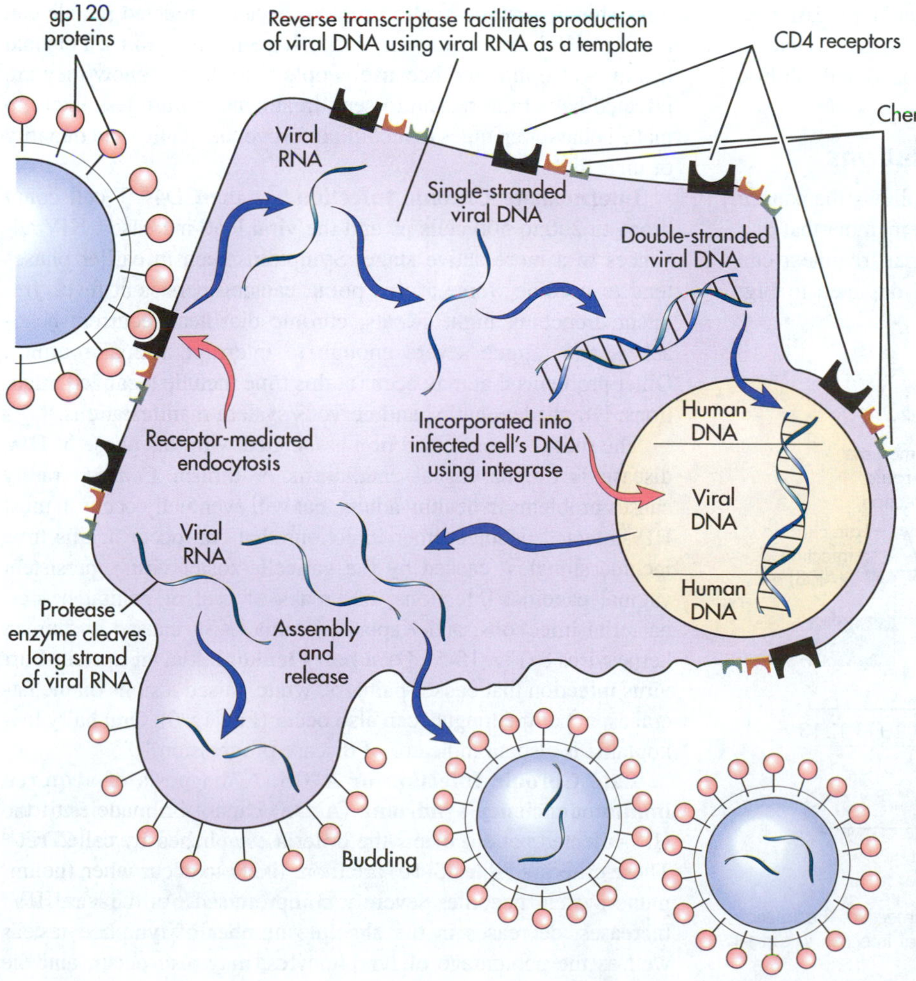

FIG. 15-3 HIV has gp120 glycoproteins that attach to CD4 and chemokine CXCR4 and CCR5 receptors on the surface of $CD4^+$ T cells. Viral RNA then enters the cell, produces viral DNA in the presence of reverse transcriptase, and incorporates itself into the cellular genome in the presence of integrase, causing permanent cellular infection and the production of new virions. New viral RNA develops initially in long strands that are cut in the presence of protease and leave the cell through a budding process that ultimately contributes to cellular destruction.

respond and function normally. B cells make HIV-specific antibodies that are effective in reducing viral loads in the blood, and activated T cells mount a cellular immune response to viruses trapped in the lymph nodes.[31]

HIV infects human cells with CD4 receptors on their surfaces. These include lymphocytes, monocytes/macrophages, astrocytes, and oligodendrocytes. Immune dysfunction in HIV disease is caused predominantly by damage to and destruction of $CD4^+$ T cells (also known as T helper cells or $CD4^+$ T lymphocytes). These cells are targeted because they have more CD4 receptors on their surfaces than other CD4 receptor–bearing cells. This is unfortunate because $CD4^+$ T cells play a key role in the ability of the immune system to recognize and defend against pathogens. Adults normally have 800 to 1200 $CD4^+$ T cells per microliter (μl) of blood. The normal life span of a $CD4^+$ T cell is about 100 days, but HIV-infected $CD4^+$ T cells will die after an average of only 2 days.[31]

Viral activity destroys about 1 billion $CD4^+$ T cells every day. Fortunately, the bone marrow and thymus are able to produce enough new $CD4^+$ T cells to replace the destroyed cells for many years. Eventually, however, the ability of HIV to destroy $CD4^+$ T cells exceeds the body's ability to replace the cells. The result is a decline in the $CD4^+$ T cell count and impaired immune function. Generally the immune system will remain healthy with more than 500 $CD4^+$ T cells/μl. Immune problems start to occur when the count drops below 500 $CD4^+$ T cells/μl, and severe problems develop below 200 $CD4^+$ T cells/μl. In HIV infection, a point is eventually reached where so many $CD4^+$ T cells have been destroyed that not enough remain to regulate immune responses (see Fig. 15-1). The major concern related to immune suppression is the development of **opportunistic diseases** (infections and cancers that occur in immunosuppressed patients that can lead to disability, disease, and death).[32,33]

Clinical Manifestations and Complications

The typical course of untreated HIV infection follows the pattern shown in Fig. 15-4. However, it is important to remember that disease progression is highly individualized and that treatment can significantly alter this pattern. The information depicted in Fig. 15-4 represents data from large groups of people and should not be used to predict an individual's life span after HIV infection.

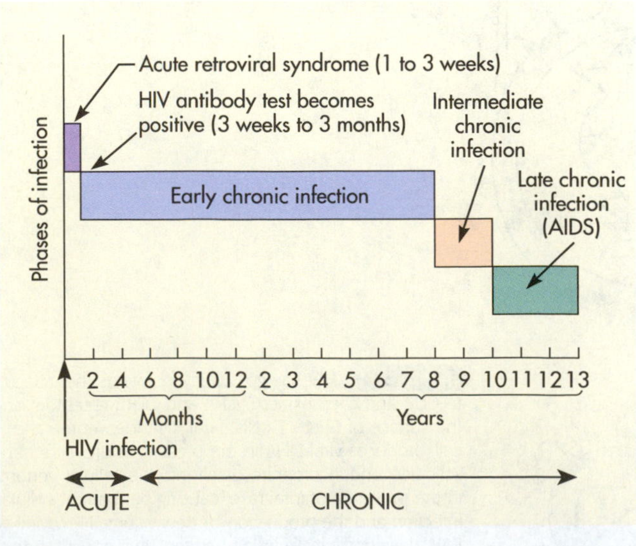

FIG. 15-4 Timeline for the spectrum of untreated HIV infection. The timeline represents the course of untreated illness from the time of infection to clinical manifestations of disease.

Acute Infection.

Development of HIV-specific antibodies (**seroconversion**) is frequently accompanied by a flulike syndrome of fever, swollen lymph glands, sore throat, headache, malaise, nausea, muscle and joint pain, diarrhea, and/or a diffuse rash. Some people develop neurologic complications, such as aseptic meningitis, peripheral neuropathy, facial palsy, or Guillain-Barré syndrome. These symptoms, called **acute HIV infection,** generally occur 1 to 3 weeks after the initial infection and last for 1 to 2 weeks, although some symptoms may persist for several months. During this time, a high viral load is noted and $CD4^+$ T cell counts fall temporarily but quickly return to baseline (see Fig. 15-1). Many people, including health care providers, mistake acute symptoms for a bad case of the flu and do not associate them with HIV.[34]

Chronic HIV Infection

Early Chronic Infection. The median interval between untreated HIV infection and a diagnosis of AIDS is about 11 years. During this time, $CD4^+$ T-lymphocyte counts remain above 500 cells/μl (normal or slightly decreased) and the viral load in the blood will be low. This phase has been referred to as *asymptomatic disease,* although fatigue, headache, low-grade fever, night sweats, *persistent generalized lymphadenopathy* (PGL), and other symptoms often occur.[34]

Because most of the symptoms during early infection are vague and nonspecific for HIV, people may not be aware that they are infected. During this time, infected people continue their usual activities, which may include high-risk sexual and drug-using behaviors. This is a public health problem because infected people can transmit HIV to others even if they have no symptoms. Personal health is also affected because people who do not know they are infected have little reason to seek treatment and are less likely to make behavior changes that could improve the quality and quantity of their lives.[35]

Intermediate Chronic Infection. As the $CD4^+$ T cell count drops to 200 to 500 cells/μl and the viral load increases, HIV advances to a more active stage. Symptoms seen in earlier phases tend to become worse at this point, causing persistent fever, frequent drenching night sweats, chronic diarrhea, recurrent headaches, and fatigue severe enough to interrupt normal routines. Other problems that may occur at this time include localized infections, lymphadenopathy, and nervous system manifestations.[34]

The most common infection associated with this phase of HIV disease is oropharyngeal candidiasis or thrush. *Candida* rarely causes problems in healthy adults, but will eventually occur in most HIV-infected people. Other infections that can occur at this time include shingles (caused by the varicella-zoster virus), persistent vaginal candidal infections, outbreaks of oral or genital herpes, bacterial infections, and Kaposi sarcoma (KS), caused by human herpesvirus 8 (Fig. 15-5). **Oral hairy leukoplakia,** an Epstein-Barr virus infection that causes painless, white, raised lesions on the lateral aspect of the tongue, can also occur (Fig. 15-6). Oral hairy leukoplakia is also an indicator of disease progression.[36]

Late Chronic Infection or AIDS. A diagnosis of **acquired immunodeficiency syndrome (AIDS)** cannot be made until the HIV-infected patient meets the criteria established by the CDC.[36] These criteria (Table 15-10) are more likely to occur when the immune system becomes severely compromised. As the viral load increases, decreases in the absolute number of lymphocytes, as well as the percentage of lymphocytes, may also occur, and the

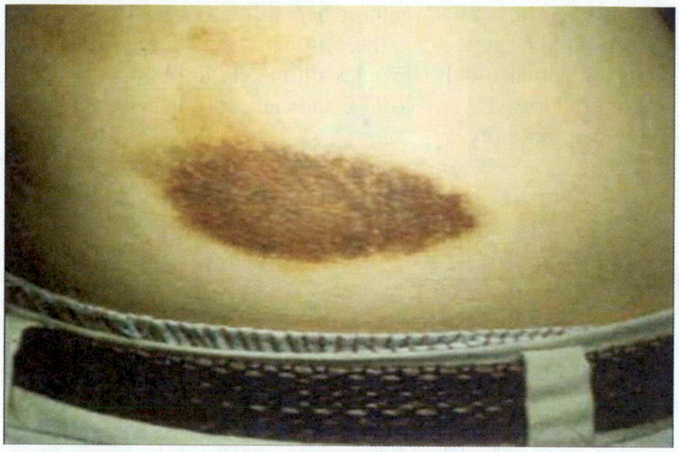

FIG. 15-5 Kaposi sarcoma (KS). Malignant vascular lesion on the torso. KS lesions can appear anywhere on the skin surface or on internal organs. Lesions vary in size from pinpoint to very large and may appear in a variety of shades.

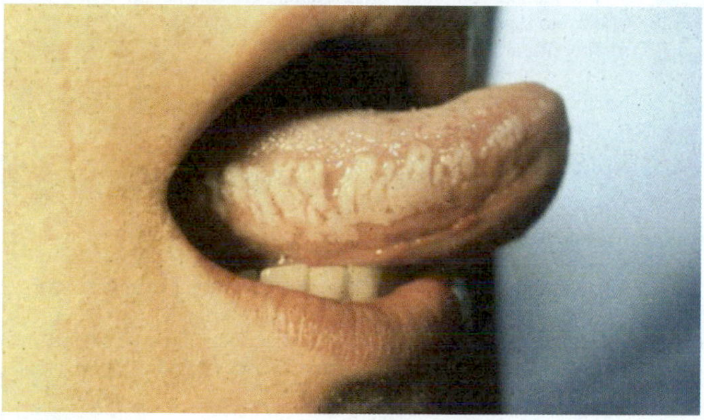

FIG. 15-6 Oral hairy leukoplakia on the lateral aspect of the tongue.

risk of developing one or more of the opportunistic diseases that contribute to disability and death increases.[31]

Opportunistic diseases, often a reactivation of a prior infection, generally do not occur in the presence of a functioning immune system. Numerous infections, a variety of malignancies, wasting, and dementia can result from HIV-related immune impairment (Table 15-11). Organisms that do not usually cause disease in people with functioning immune systems can cause severe, debilitating, disseminated, and life-threatening infections during this stage. Several opportunistic diseases are likely to occur at the same time, further compounding the difficulties of diagnosis and treatment. Advances in HIV treatment have led to significant decreases in opportunistic diseases because successful treatment helps maintain a functioning immune system.[32,33]

Diagnostic Studies

Diagnosis of HIV Infection. The most useful screening tests for HIV are those that detect HIV-specific antibodies. The major problem with these tests is that there is a median delay of 2 months after infection before antibodies can be detected (see Fig. 15-1). This creates a **window period** during which an infected individual may not test HIV-antibody positive. HIV-antibody screening is generally done in the sequence shown in Table 15-12. This process produces highly accurate results.[37] New "rapid" HIV-antibody tests provide results in 20 minutes and are strongly recommended by the CDC.[35] Rapid testing is highly reliable and provides immediate feedback to patients who can then be counseled about treatment and prevention. Positive rapid tests must be confirmed as described in Table 15-12, but results can be given to the patient as soon as they are available.[38] This is an important advantage because many people do not return to get their test results when other tests are used.

TABLE 15-10 Diagnostic Criteria for AIDS

AIDS is diagnosed when an individual with HIV develops at least one of these conditions:

1. $CD4^+$ T cell count drops below 200 cells/μl.
2. Development of one of the following opportunistic infections (OIs):
   - *Fungal*: candidiasis of bronchi, trachea, lungs, or esophagus; *Pneumocystis jiroveci* pneumonia (PCP); disseminated or extrapulmonary coccidioidomycosis; disseminated or extrapulmonary histoplasmosis
   - *Viral*: cytomegalovirus (CMV) disease other than liver, spleen, or nodes; CMV retinitis (with loss of vision); herpes simplex with chronic ulcer(s) or bronchitis, pneumonitis, or esophagitis; progressive multifocal leukoencephalopathy (PML); extrapulmonary cryptococcosis
   - *Protozoal*: toxoplasmosis of the brain, chronic intestinal isosporiasis; chronic intestinal cryptosporidiosis
   - *Bacterial*: *Mycobacterium tuberculosis* (any site); any disseminated or extrapulmonary *Mycobacterium,* including *M. avium* complex (MAC) or *M. kansasii;* recurrent pneumonia; recurrent *Salmonella* septicemia
3. Development of one of the following opportunistic cancers:
   - Invasive cervical cancer, Kaposi's sarcoma (KS), Burkitt's lymphoma, immunoblastic lymphoma, or primary lymphoma of the brain
4. Wasting syndrome occurs. *Wasting* is defined as a loss of 10% or more of ideal body mass.
5. AIDS dementia complex (ADC) develops.

Modified from Centers for Disease Control and Prevention (CDC): 1993 Revised classification system for HIV infection and expanded surveillance case definition for AIDS among adolescents and adults, 1993. Available at *www.cdc.gov/hiv/surveillance.htm#Tools* (accessed April 22, 2006).
CMV, Cytomegalovirus.

Laboratory Studies in HIV Infection. The progression of HIV infection is monitored by two important laboratory assessments: $CD4^+$ T cell counts and viral load. $CD4^+$ T cell counts provide a marker for immune function. As the disease progresses, there is usually a decrease in the number of $CD4^+$ T cells (see Fig. 15-1). Although labs vary, the $CD4^+$ counts of 800 to 1200 cells/μl are generally considered normal. Laboratory tests that measure viral activity provide an assessment of disease progression. The lower the viral load, the less active the disease. In HIV, viral loads are reported as real numbers (i.e., 1260 copies/μl) or as undetectable. "Undetectable" indicates the viral load is lower than the test is able to report; "undetectable" does ***not*** mean that the virus has been eliminated from the body or that the individual can no longer transmit HIV to others. The combination of these tests provides information that helps determine when to initiate therapy, the efficacy of therapy, and whether clinical goals are being met.[34]

A variety of abnormal blood tests are common in HIV infection and may be caused by HIV, opportunistic diseases, or complications of therapy. A decreased white blood cell (WBC) count, especially low neutrophil counts (neutropenia), is often seen; low platelet counts (thrombocytopenia) may be caused by HIV, antiplatelet antibodies, or drug therapy; and anemia is associated with the chronic disease process as well as with adverse effects of some antiretroviral agents. Altered liver function tests, caused by HIV disease, drug therapy, or co-infection with a hepatitis virus, are also common. Early identification of co-infection with hepatitis B virus (HBV) and/or hepatitis C virus (HCV) is extremely important because these infections have a more serious course in patients with HIV, may ultimately limit options for antiretroviral drug therapy (ART), and can cause liver-related morbidity and mortality.[32,33]

TABLE 15-11 Manifestations and Treatment of Common Opportunistic Diseases Associated with HIV Infection

Organism/Disease	Clinical Manifestations	Prophylaxis* and Treatment†
Candida albicans	Thrush, esophagitis, vaginitis; whitish yellow patches in mouth, esophagus, GI tract, vagina	Treatment: fluconazole (Diflucan), clotrimazole (Lotrimin), nystatin (Mycostatin), itraconazole (Sporanox); if fluconazole refractory: amphotericin B (Fungizone) 2° Prophylaxis: only if subsequent episodes are frequent or severe recurrences: fluconazole (Diflucan), itraconazole (Sporanox)
Coccidioides immitis	Pneumonia/fever, weight loss, cough	Treatment: amphotericin B (Fungizone), fluconazole (Diflucan), itraconazole (Sporanox) 2° Prophylaxis: to prevent recurrence of documented disease: fluconazole (Diflucan), amphotericin B (Fungizone), itraconazole (Sporanox)
CNS lymphoma	Cognitive dysfunction, motor impairment, aphasia, seizures, personality changes, headache	Treatment: radiation, chemotherapy
Cryptococcosus neoformans	Meningitis, cognitive impairment, motor dysfunction, fever, seizures, headache	Treatment: amphotericin B (Fungizone), fluconazole (Diflucan), itraconazole (Sporanox) 2° Prophylaxis: to prevent recurrence of documented disease: fluconazole (Diflucan), amphotericin B (Fungizone), itraconazole (Sporanox)
Cryptosporidium muris	Gastroenteritis, watery diarrhea, abdominal pain, weight loss	Treatment: antidiarrheals, nitazoxanide (Alinia), paromomycin (Humatin)
Cytomegalovirus (CMV)	Retinitis—retinal lesions, blurred vision, loss of vision Esophagitis/stomatitis—difficulty swallowing; colitis/gastritis—bloody diarrhea, pain, weight loss Pneumonitis—respiratory symptoms Neurologic disease—CNS manifestations	Treatment: ganciclovir (Cytovene), foscarnet (Foscavir), cidofovir (Vistide), valganciclovir (Valcyte) 2° Prophylaxis: to prevent recurrence of documented disease: ganciclovir (Cytovene), foscarnet (Foscavir), cidofovir (Vistide), valganciclovir (Valcyte)
Hepatitis B virus (HBV)	Jaundice, fatigue, abdominal pain, loss of appetite, nausea, vomiting, joint pain; 30% may have no signs or symptoms	1° Prevention: Hepatitis B vaccine series; screen and vaccinate those with no evidence of previous HBV infection; encourage for IDU, sexually active MSM, sexual partners or household contacts of HBV-infected individuals, and those with hepatitis C virus; hepatitis A vaccine series should be given to prevent additive effects and advanced liver damage; screen and vaccinate those without evidence of previous HAV infection Treatment: adefovir dipivoxil (Hepsera), α-interferon, lamivudine (Epivir), entecavir (Baraclude)
Hepatitis C virus (HCV)	Jaundice, fatigue, abdominal pain, loss of appetite, nausea, vomiting, dark urine; 80% may have no signs or symptoms	Prophylaxis: None for HCV. Hepatitis A and B vaccine series should be given to prevent additive affects and advanced liver damage; screen and vaccinate those without evidence of previous HAV/HBV infection Treatment: α-interferon, ribavirin (Virazole)
Herpes simplex	HSV1 (type 1): orolabial and mucocutaneous vesicular and ulcerative lesions; keratitis—visual disturbances; encephalitis—CNS manifestations HSV2 (type 2): genital and perianal vesicular and ulcerative lesions	Treatment: acyclovir (Zovirax), famciclovir (Famvir), valacyclovir (Valtrex), foscarnet (Foscavir), cidofovir (Vistide) 2° Prophylaxis: only if subsequent episodes are frequent or severe: acyclovir (Zovirax), famciclovir (Famvir), valacyclovir (Valtrex)
Histoplasma capsulatum	Pneumonia—fever, cough, weight loss Meningitis—CNS manifestations; disseminated disease	Treatment: amphotericin B (Fungizone), itraconazole (Sporanox), fluconazole (Diflucan) 2° Prophylaxis: to prevent recurrence of documented disease: itraconazole (Sporanox), amphotericin B (Fungizone)
Influenza virus	Fever (usually high), headache, extreme tiredness, dry cough, sore throat, runny or stuffy nose, muscle aches; nausea, vomiting, and diarrhea can occur	1° Prevention: Inactivated trivalent influenza virus vaccine; provide annually, before influenza virus season; revaccinate if initial vaccine was given when CD4+ T cell count was $<200/\mu l$ Treatment: supportive therapy

Sources: Centers for Disease Control and Prevention (CDC): Treating opportunistic infections among HIV-infected adults and adolescents, 2004; and USPHS/IDSA guidelines for the prevention of opportunistic infections in persons with human immunodeficiency virus, 2001. Available at *http://aidsinfo.nih.gov* (accessed July 18, 2005).
CNS, Central nervous system; *GI,* gastrointestinal; *IDU,* injection drug use; *IgG,* immunoglobulin G; *MSM,* men who have sex with men; *1°,* primary; *2°,* secondary.
*If available. In most cases, effective antiretroviral therapy is the best prevention for all opportunistic diseases.
†In most cases, adequate antiretroviral therapy is the best treatment for all opportunistic diseases.

TABLE 15-11 **Manifestations and Treatment of Common Opportunistic Diseases Associated with HIV Infection—cont'd**

Organism/Disease	Clinical Manifestations	Prophylaxis* and Treatment†
JC papovavirus	Progressive multifocal leukoencephalopathy (PML), CNS manifestations, mental and motor declines	Treatment: supportive therapy
Kaposi's sarcoma (KS) caused by human herpesvirus 8 (HHV8)	Vascular lesions on the skin, mucous membranes, and viscera with wide range of presentation: firm, flat, raised, or nodular; pinpoint to several cm in size; hyperpigmented, multicentric; can cause lymphedema and disfigurement, particularly when confluent; not usually serious unless it occurs in the respiratory or gastrointestinal systems	Treatment: dependent on severity of lesions: cancer chemotherapy, α-interferon, local radiation; cryotherapy for skin lesions
***Mycobacterium avium* complex** (MAC)	Gastroenteritis, watery diarrhea, weight loss	1° Prophylaxis: Initiate when $CD4^+$ T cells <50/μl; rule out disseminated disease or tuberculosis: clarithromycin (Biaxin) or azithromycin (Zithromax), rifabutin (Mycobutin). Prophylaxis may be stopped when $CD4^+$ T cell count of >100/μl is documented for 6-12 mo; restart if $CD4^+$ T-cell count falls to <50/μl Treatment: clarithromycin (Biaxin), ethambutol (Myambutol), rifabutin (Mycobutin), azithromycin (Zithromax), ciprofloxacin (Cipro), levofloxacin (Levaquin), amikacin (Amikin)
Mycobacterium tuberculosis	Respiratory and disseminated disease; productive cough, fever, night sweats, weight loss	1° Prophylaxis: Initiate if TB testing is ≥0.5 mm reactive, after high-risk exposure, or if prior positive TB testing without treatment: isoniazid (INH) + pyridoxine for 9 mo; consider directly observed therapy. Rule out active disease, extrapulmonary disease, or drug-resistant strain, all of which require multidrug therapy Treatment: isoniazid (INH), rifampin (Rifadin), rifabutin (Mycobutin), pyrazinamide, ethambutol (Myambutol)
***Pneumocystis jiroveci* pneumonia** (PCP)	Pneumonia, nonproductive cough, hypoxemia, progressive shortness of breath, fever, night sweats, fatigue	1° Prophylaxis: Initiate when $CD4^+$ T cells <200/μl: trimethoprim/sulfamethoxazole (TMP/SMX), dapsone, dapsone with pyrimethamine + folinic acid, aerosolized pentamidine, atovaquone. Side effects of TMP/SMX and dapsone (especially rash, fever, and anemia) are common and may limit use Treatment: trimethoprim/sulfamethoxazole (Bactrim), pentamidine (NebuPent), dapsone + trimethoprim, clindamycin (Cleocin) + primaquine, atovaquone (Mepron); with hypoxia, use corticosteroids
Toxoplasma gondii	Encephalitis, cognitive dysfunction, motor impairment, fever, altered mental status, headache, seizures, sensory abnormalities	1° Prophylaxis: Initiate with positive toxoplasmosis IgG titer when $CD4^+$ T cells <100/μl: trimethoprim/sulfamethoxazole (TMP/SMX) or dapsone with pyrimethamine + folinic acid or atovaquone ± pyrimethamine + folinic acid Treatment: pyrimethamine + folinic acid + sulfadiazine, clindamycin (Cleocin), azithromycin (Zithromax), atovaquone (Mepron)
Varicella-zoster virus (VZV)	Shingles: erythematous maculopapular rash along dermatomal planes, pain, pruritis Ocular: progressive outer retinal necrosis (PORN)	1° Prophylaxis: varicella-zoster immune globulin (VZIG) administered only after significant exposure to chickenpox or shingles for patients with no history of disease or negative VZV antibody test Treatment: acyclovir (Zovirax), famciclovir (Famvir), valacyclovir (Valtrex)

It is now possible to test for resistance to antiretroviral drugs in people being treated for HIV infection. Two types of resistance assays are used: genotype and phenotype. The *genotype assay* detects drug-resistant viral mutations that are present in reverse transcriptase and protease genes. The *phenotype assay* measures the growth of the virus in various concentrations of antiretroviral drugs (much like bacteria-antibiotic sensitivity tests). These assays are especially useful in making decisions about new drug combinations in patients who do not respond to therapy.[34,39]

Collaborative Care

Collaborative management of the HIV-infected patient focuses on monitoring HIV disease progression and immune function, initiating and monitoring antiretroviral therapy (ART), preventing the development of opportunistic diseases, detecting and treating opportunistic diseases, managing symptoms, preventing or decreasing the complications of treatment, and preventing further transmission of HIV. Ongoing assessment, clinician–patient interactions, and patient education and support are required to accomplish these objectives.[34,35]

The initial visit provides an opportunity to gather baseline data and to start establishing rapport. A complete history and physical examination, including an immunization history and psychosocial and dietary evaluations, should be conducted. Findings from the history, assessment, and laboratory tests help determine patient needs. This is a good time to initiate patient education related to the spectrum of HIV disease, treatment, preventing transmission to others, improving health, and family planning. Patient input should

TABLE 15-12 HIV-Antibody Test Screening Process

All HIV testing should be accompanied by pretest and posttest counseling. The following additional steps are used in the process of testing blood for antibodies to HIV:

1. A highly sensitive enzyme immunoassay (EIA) is done to detect serum antibodies that bind to HIV antigens on test plates. Blood samples that are negative on this test are reported as negative.
   - Posttest counseling should include an assessment of risk behaviors, especially looking for recent risks.
   - If recent risks are found, encourage retesting at 3 weeks, 6 weeks, and 3 months.
2. If the blood is EIA-antibody positive, the test is repeated.
3. If the blood is repeatedly EIA-antibody positive, a more specific confirming test, such as the Western blot (WB) or immunofluorescence assay (IFA), is done.
   - WB testing uses purified HIV antigens electrophoresed on gels. These are incubated with serum samples. If antibody in the serum is present, it can be detected.
   - IFA is used to identify HIV in infected cells. Blood is treated with a fluorescent antibody against p17 or p24 antigen and then examined using a fluorescent microscope.
4. Blood that is reactive in all of the first three steps is reported as HIV-antibody positive.
5. If the results are indeterminate, the following steps are taken:
   - If in-depth risk assessment reveals that the individual does not have a history of high-risk activities, reassure the patient that she or he is extremely unlikely to be infected with HIV and suggest retesting in 3 months.
   - If in-depth risk assessment reveals that the individual does have a history of high-risk activities, repeat antibody test at 1, 2, and 6 months; discuss risk reduction measures to protect partners from infection; consider tests for HIV-antigen detection.

Special Considerations for Rapid HIV-Antibody Testing

1. Rapid testing is strongly recommended by the CDC. Results are highly accurate, can be done in a variety of settings, and can be reported within 20 minutes. A major advantage of rapid tests is that patients do not have to return to the testing site to get their results.
2. Rapid tests also test for antibodies and not for antigen (the virus itself).
3. Negative tests should be followed by the risk assessment discussed above. Positive tests can also be disclosed to the patient, but need to be confirmed with the more specific WB or IFA (as above). This step will necessitate a blood draw and a return appointment to get results.
4. Rapid test kits are more expensive than established testing methods and have a relatively short shelf life. In addition, false-positive results are more likely to occur in low-incidence populations. For these reasons, some rural areas have opted not to start using rapid tests.

be used to develop a plan of care, and necessary referrals can be made. It is important to remember that a newly diagnosed patient may be in a state of shock or denial and unable to retain or understand information. The nurse should be prepared to repeat and clarify information over the course of several months. This is also a good time to assure that case reports required by the state health department have been completed.[40]

Drug Therapy for HIV Infection. The goals of drug therapy in HIV infection are to (1) decrease the viral load, (2) maintain or raise $CD4^+$ T cell counts, and (3) delay the development of HIV-related symptoms and opportunistic diseases. Guidelines on the use of antiretroviral agents are updated regularly.[34]

HIV treatment guidelines incorporate the use of the following principles: (1) Treatment decisions should be individualized by risk for disease progression indicated by higher viral loads and lower $CD4^+$ T-cell counts and by a patient's desires for therapy. (2) Combination ART suppresses HIV replication and limits the potential for antiretroviral resistance, which is the major factor limiting treatment effect. The most effective means to suppress HIV replication is simultaneous initiation of at least three effective antiretroviral drugs from at least two different drug classes used in optimum schedules and full dosages. (3) Women should receive optimal ART regardless of pregnancy status. (4) HIV-infected persons, even those with viral loads below detectable limits and those on effective ART, should be considered infectious and should avoid behaviors associated with transmission of HIV and other infectious pathogens.[34,35] There is evidence, however, that the risk of HIV transmission decreases with lower viral loads. Recommendations for starting therapy in the chronically infected patient are summarized in Table 15-13.

No drug or combination of drugs can cure HIV, but therapy can decrease viral replication and delay progression of disease in most patients. Drugs used to treat HIV work at various points in the HIV replication cycle (Table 15-14). The major advantage of using antiretroviral drugs from different drug groups is that combination

ETHICAL DILEMMAS

Individual vs. Public Health Protection

Situation

A nurse in a community clinic was having a follow-up visit with Virginia, a 38-year-old woman who tested positive for HIV during her annual exam 2 weeks ago. While obtaining her history and physical examination, Virginia disclosed that she has been verbally and physically abused by her partner. During the discussion, Virginia indicated that she had not yet told her partner about her positive HIV test because she is afraid that he will hurt her. She has not used any protection during sex with him since she learned of her test results and she says, "He probably already has it and infected me!"

Important Points for Consideration

- Since the nurse's primary obligation is to the patient, patient teaching and support are paramount.
- A conflict exists for the nurse between preventing further harm to Virginia (possible increase in intimate partner violence) and protecting public health (potential spread of HIV infection to her partner).
- HIV is a reportable communicable disease in most, but not all, states. Reporting should have been done when the test came back positive. The nurse needs to determine if this was explained to Virginia, and if Virginia provided her partner's name and contact information to the reporting individual.
- If she did disclose his name and contact information, Virginia's partner will be notified by public health officials of an intimate partner testing positive for HIV. He will then be encouraged to be tested for HIV. While her name should not be used in this communication, he may be able to guess that she has HIV.

Critical Thinking Questions

1. Within the parameters of your state's requirements for reportable conditions, how can the nurse protect the patient's confidentiality to prevent further intimate partner violence?
2. Since it is unclear whether Virginia acquired the HIV infection from her partner, how can the nurse protect the partner from possible infection while also attempting to protect Virginia from further violence?
3. How can the nurse address the issues of intimate partner violence? What resources would Virginia have in your community?

TABLE 15-13 DRUG THERAPY
Indications for Initiation of Antiretroviral Therapy in the Chronically HIV-Infected Patient

Clinical Category	$CD4^+$ T cell Count	Plasma HIV RNA	Recommendation
Symptomatic (AIDS-defining illness or severe symptoms)	Any value	Any value	Treat
Asymptomatic*	<200/μl	Any value	Treat
Asymptomatic	200/μl-350/μl	Any value	Treatment should be offered following full discussion of pros and cons of treatment
Asymptomatic	>350/μl	>100,000	Most clinicians recommend deferring therapy, but some clinicians will treat
Asymptomatic	>350/μl	<100,000	Defer therapy

Revised from Centers for Disease Control and Prevention (CDC): Guidelines for the use of antiretroviral agents in HIV-infected adults and adolescents, 2005. Available at *http://aidsinfo.nih.gov/* (accessed July 10, 2005).

*Clinical benefit has been demonstrated in controlled trials only for patients with $CD4^+$ T cells <200/μl. However, the majority of clinicians would offer therapy at a $CD4^+$ T cell threshold <350/μl. A collaborative analysis of data from 13 cohort studies from Europe and North America found that lower CD4 count, higher HIV viral load, injection drug use, and age over 50 were all predictors of progression to AIDS or death in antiretroviral-naive patients beginning combination antiretroviral therapy (ART). These data indicate that the prognosis is better for patients who initiate therapy at >200 cells/μl, but risk after initiation of therapy does not vary considerably at >200 cells/μl.

TABLE 15-14 DRUG THERAPY
Mechanisms of Action of Drugs Used to Treat HIV Infection

Drug Classification	Mechanism of Action
Nonnucleoside reverse transcriptase inhibitors (NNRTIs)	Combine with reverse transcriptase enzyme to block the process needed to convert HIV RNA into HIV DNA
Nucleoside reverse transcriptase inhibitors (NRTIs)	Insert a piece of DNA into the developing HIV DNA chain, blocking further development of the chain and leaving the production of the new strand of HIV DNA incomplete
Nucleotide reverse transcriptase inhibitors (NtRTI)	Inhibit the action of reverse transcriptase
Protease inhibitors (PIs)	Prevent the protease enzyme from cutting HIV proteins into the proper lengths needed to allow viable virions to assemble and bud out from the cell membrane
Entry inhibitors	Prevent binding of HIV to cells, thus preventing entry of HIV into cells where replication would occur

therapy can attack viral replication in several different ways, making it more difficult for the virus to recover and decreasing the likelihood of drug resistance. An additional advantage is that alternatives exist for those patients who do not (or who no longer) respond to a specific drug regimen.[34,39]

Currently approved drugs include three groups that inhibit the ability of HIV to make a DNA copy early in replication, one group that inhibits the ability of the virus to reproduce in the late stages of replication, and one group that prevents entry of HIV into the cell (Table 15-15). *Nucleoside reverse transcriptase inhibitors* (NRTIs), *nonnucleoside reverse transcriptase inhibitors* (NNRTIs), and *nucleotide reverse transcriptase inhibitors* (NtRTIs) work by inhibiting the activity of reverse transcriptase. *Protease inhibitors* (PIs) work by interfering with the activity of the enzyme protease. *Entry inhibitors* interfere with HIV CD4 receptor site binding and entry into the cell. A major problem with most drugs used in ART is that resistance develops rapidly when they are used alone *(monotherapy)* or taken in inadequate doses. For that reason, combinations of three or more antiretroviral drugs, prescribed at full strength, should be used. Many antiretroviral drugs can cause dangerous and potentially lethal interactions with other commonly used drugs, including over-the-counter drugs and herbal therapies.[34,41] For example, St. John's wort, commonly used to alleviate depression, can interfere with ART.[42] In fact, all herbal products should be used with caution by people with HIV infection.[43]

Drug Alert - *Enfuvirtide (Fuzeon)*
- *Do not shake vial during reconstitution—roll vial gently between palms to dissolve powder and prevent foam from forming.*
- *Decrease the occurrence of local injection site reactions by rotating injection sites and using warm compresses after injection.*

Drug Alert - *Efavirenz (Sustiva)*
- *Do not use in pregnancy as large doses could cause fetal anomalies.*
- *Once-a-day dose should be taken before bed (at least initially) to help patient cope with side effects of dizziness and confusion.*

Treatment protocols can reduce viral loads by 90% to 99% in most cases, but side effects and other problems are common.[34] Some patients will not be able to use combination therapies because of the expense, side effects, or inability to adhere to required schedules. Combination ART is more cost effective than the cost of advancing disease, but the drugs are not universally available.[44]

Drug Therapy for Opportunistic Diseases. Management of HIV is complicated by the many opportunistic diseases that can develop as the immune system deteriorates (see Table 15-11). A preferred approach to opportunistic diseases is to prevent their occurrence. A number of opportunistic diseases associated with HIV can be delayed or prevented through the use of adequate ART, vaccines (including hepatitis B, influenza, and pneumococcal), and disease-specific prevention measures. Prophylaxis, used according to established criteria, contributes significantly to preventing morbidity and mortality. Although it is usually not possible to eradicate opportunistic diseases once they occur, treatments that can control them are available. Advances in the prevention, diagnosis, and treatment of opportunistic diseases have contributed significantly to increased life expectancy.[32,33] Table 15-11 lists prophylaxis and treatments for some common HIV-related opportunistic diseases.

Vaccination. Despite considerable research, a vaccine for HIV still eludes scientists. The problems that impede HIV vaccine development are numerous.[45] HIV lives inside cells, where it can "hide" from circulating immune factors. HIV also mutates rapidly, so that infected individuals develop HIV variants that may not all respond to a simple vaccine. In addition, two strains of HIV (HIV-1 and HIV-2) cause AIDS and at least nine *clades* (subtypes) of HIV-1 exist around the world. Development of an effective vaccine for clade B (the predominant group in the Americas and Western Europe) may not be effective in developing countries, where the need is even greater.[46]

There are also social, ethical, and economic issues related to vaccination. Vaccine efficacy will eventually have to be established

TABLE 15-15 *DRUG THERAPY* Antiretroviral Agents Used in HIV Infection*†

Drug	Adverse Effects
Nucleoside Reverse Transcriptase Inhibitors (NRTIs)	Adverse effects common to NRTIs: lactic acidosis with hepatic steatosis is a rare but potentially life-threatening problem; lipodystrophy, especially fat atrophy and mitochondrial toxicity
zidovudine (AZT, ZDV, Retrovir)	Nausea, vomiting, anemia, leukopenia, fatigue, headache, insomnia, pancreatitis
didanosine (ddI, Videx, Videx-EC [time-released])	Nausea, diarrhea, peripheral neuropathy (dose related and reversible), pancreatitis
stavudine (d4T, Zerit)	Peripheral neuropathy, nausea, pancreatitis
lamivudine (3TC, Epivir)	Minimal toxicities, nausea, nasal congestion
abacavir (Ziagen)	Nausea; hypersensitivity reaction, including fever, nausea, vomiting, diarrhea, lethargy, malaise, sore throat, shortness of breath, cough, rash; may produce life-threatening event if hypersensitivity is rechallenged
emtricitabine (FTC, Emtriva)	Headache, diarrhea, nausea, rash, skin discoloration
Combivir (lamivudine and zidovudine combination)	Combines side effects of lamivudine and zidovudine
Trizivir (lamivudine, zidovudine, and abacavir combination)	Combines side effects of lamivudine, zidovudine, and abacavir
Epizicom (lamivudine and abacavir combination)	Combines side effects of lamivudine and abacavir
Nucleotide Reverse Transcriptase Inhibitor (NtRTI)	
tenofovir DF (Viread)	Nausea, vomiting, diarrhea
Truvada (tenofovir and emtricitabine combination)	Combines side effects of tenofovir and emtricitabine
Nonnucleoside Reverse Transcriptase Inhibitors (NNRTIs)	Adverse effects common to NNRTIs: Rash, erythema multiforme, increased liver enzymes, hepatotoxicity
nevirapine (Viramune)	GI upset, headache
delavirdine (Rescriptor)	Headache, fatigue, GI upset, neutropenia, pruritis
efavirenz (Sustiva)	Dizziness, trouble concentrating, unusual dreams, confusion, anxiety, depression, diarrhea, encephalopathy; false-positive cannabinoid test
Protease Inhibitors (PIs)	Adverse effects common to PIs: hyperglycemia, hyperlipidemia, lipodystrophy
saquinavir (Fortovase, Invirase)	Diarrhea, nausea, headache
indinavir (Crixivan)	Nausea, diarrhea, asymptomatic hyperbilirubinemia, interstitial nephritis, kidney stones (patient should drink 2–4 L of fluid a day)
ritonavir (Norvir)—most often used in low doses with other PIs to boost effect	Nausea, diarrhea, vomiting, taste perversion, circumoral and perioral paresthesia, hepatitis
nelfinavir (Viracept)	Diarrhea, flatulence, nausea, rash
amprenavir (Agenerase)	Nausea, vomiting, headache, taste perversion, perioral paresthesia, severe skin rashes, diarrhea, periorbital paresthesia
Kaletra (lopinavir and ritonavir combination)	Nausea, diarrhea, taste perversion, perioral and circumoral paresthesia, hepatitis
atazanavir (Reyataz)	Nausea, diarrhea, hyperbilirubinemia
fosamprenavir (Lexiva)	Diarrhea, nausea, vomiting, headache
tipranavir (Aptivus)	Nausea, diarrhea, headache, clinical hepatitis, increased transaminases, hepatic decompensation, symptoms of sulfa allergy, rash, or photosensitivity
darunavir (Prezista)	Diarrhea, nausea, headache
Entry Inhibitor	
enfuvirtide (Fuzeon)	Injection site reactions (ISRs), fatigue, nausea, diarrhea, insomnia, peripheral neuropathy, hypersensitivity reaction, pneumonia
Combination Therapy	
Atripla (tenovir, emtricitabine, and efavirenz combination)	Combined side effects of tenovir, emtricitabine, and efavirenz

Sources: Centers for Disease Control and Prevention (CDC): Guidelines for the use of antiretroviral agents in HIV-infected adults and adolescents, 2005. Available at *http://aidsinfo.nih.gov* (accessed April 22, 2006); Wolbach J, Jed SL, Johnson SC, et al: *A pharmacist's guide to antiretroviral medications for HIV-infected adults and adolescents,* Mountain Plains AIDS Education and Training Center, Denver, Colo., 2005. Available at *www.mpaetc.org* (accessed July 18, 2005).

GI, gastrointestinal.

*Current recommendations for therapy require combinations of three or more of these drugs. Treatment with only one drug is rarely acceptable.

†Many of these drugs cause serious and potentially fatal interactions when used in combination with other commonly used drugs, some of which are available over the counter.

in human testing: How will volunteers be recruited? How will true protection be determined? Will volunteers be exposed to HIV after immunization to test immunity? Because HIV is a global problem, with developing countries bearing the brunt of the epidemic, there is also concern about developing a vaccine that can be widely distributed in a short amount of time at an acceptable cost. Will vaccines, once developed, be accepted?[47] Despite the overwhelming nature of these issues, considerable research is in progress. Vaccines in various stages of development are being tested. The development of a successful vaccine would be extremely helpful in controlling the epidemic, but would not replace current prevention methods because no vaccine is likely to be 100% effective.[46]

NURSING MANAGEMENT HIV INFECTION

Nursing Assessment

Nursing assessment for individuals not known to be infected with HIV should focus on behaviors that could put the person at risk for HIV infection and other sexually transmitted and blood-borne diseases. All patients should be assessed for risky behaviors on a regular basis. The assumption should not be made that someone is without risk because he is too old or too young or because she is married or sings in the church choir. Nurses can help individuals assess risk by asking four basic questions: (1) Have you ever had a blood transfusion or used clotting factors? If so, was it before 1985? (2) Have you ever shared drug-using equipment with another person? (3) Have you ever had a sexual experience in which your penis, vagina, rectum, or mouth came into contact with another person's penis, vagina, rectum, or mouth? and (4) Have you ever had a sexually transmitted disease (STD)? These questions provide the minimum data needed to initiate a risk assessment. A positive response to any of these questions requires an in-depth exploration of issues related to the identified risk.[48,49]

Specific assessments are needed when an individual has been diagnosed with HIV infection. Subjective and objective data that should be obtained are presented in Table 15-16. Repeated nursing assessments over time are essential because people's circumstances change. Early recognition and treatment of problems can decrease the progression of HIV infection and prevent new infections. A complete history and thorough systems review can help the nurse identify and address problems in a timely manner.

TABLE 15-16 *NURSING ASSESSMENT* HIV-Infected Patient

Subjective Data

Important Health Information

Past health history: Route of infection; hepatitis; other STDs; tuberculosis; frequent viral, fungal, and/or bacterial infections

Medications: Use of immunosuppressive drugs

Functional Health Patterns

Health perception–health management: Perception of illness; alcohol and drug use; malaise

Nutritional-metabolic: Weight loss, anorexia, nausea, vomiting; lesions, bleeding, or ulcerations of lips, mouth, gums, tongue, or throat; sensitivity to acidic, salty, or spicy foods; difficulty swallowing; abdominal cramping; skin rashes, lesions, or color changes; nonhealing wounds

Elimination: Persistent diarrhea, change in character of stools; painful urination, low back pain

Activity-exercise: Chronic fatigue, muscle weakness, difficulty walking; cough, shortness of breath

Sleep-rest: Insomnia; night sweats, fatigue

Cognitive-perceptual: Headaches, stiff neck, chest pain, rectal pain, retrosternal pain; blurred vision, photophobia, diplopia, loss of vision; hearing impairment; confusion, forgetfulness, attention deficit, changes in mental status, memory loss, personality changes; paresthesias, hypersensitivity in feet, pruritus

Role-relationship: Support system(s), financial resources

Sexuality-reproductive: Lesions on genitalia (internal or external), pruritus or burning in vagina, penis, or anus; painful sexual intercourse, rectal pain or bleeding, changes in menstruation, vaginal or penile discharge; use of birth control measures, pregnancies, desire for future children

Coping–stress tolerance: Stress levels, previous losses, coping patterns, self-concept

Objective Data

General

Lethargy, persistent fever, lymphadenopathy, peripheral wasting, fat deposits in truncal areas and upper back; social withdrawal

Integumentary

Decreased skin turgor, dry skin, or diaphoresis; pallor, cyanosis; lesions, eruptions, discolorations, or bruises of skin or mucous membranes; vaginal or perianal excoriation; alopecia, delayed wound healing

Eyes

Presence of exudate; retinal lesions or hemorrhage; papilledema

Respiratory

Tachypnea, dyspnea, intercostal retractions; crackles, wheezing, productive or nonproductive cough

Cardiovascular

Pericardial friction rub, murmur, bradycardia, tachycardia

Gastrointestinal

Mouth lesions, including blisters (HSV), white-gray patches *(Candida),* painless white lesions on lateral aspect of the tongue (hairy leukoplakia), discolorations (KS); gingivitis, tooth decay or loosening; redness or white patchy lesions of throat; vomiting, diarrhea, incontinence; rectal lesions; hyperactive bowel sounds, abdominal masses, hepatosplenomegaly

Musculoskeletal

Muscle wasting

Neurologic

Ataxia, tremors, lack of coordination; sensory loss; slurred speech, aphasia; memory loss, peripheral neuropathy, apathy, agitation, depression, inappropriate behavior; decreasing levels of consciousness, seizures, paralysis, coma

Reproductive

Genital lesions or discharge, abdominal tenderness secondary to pelvic inflammatory disease (PID)

Possible Findings

Positive HIV antibody assay (EIA or ELISA, confirmed by WB or IFA); detectable viral load levels by bDNA or PCR; ↓ $CD4^+$ lymphocytes, ↓ WBC count, lymphopenia, anemia, thrombocytopenia; electrolyte imbalances; abnormal liver function tests; ↑ cholesterol, triglycerides, and blood glucose

bDNA, Branched chain DNA; *EIA,* enzyme immunoassay; *ELISA,* enzyme-linked immunosorbent assay; *HSV,* herpes simplex virus; *IFA,* immunofluorescence assay; *KS,* Kaposi's sarcoma; *PCR,* polymerase chain reaction; *STDs,* sexually transmitted diseases; *WB,* Western blot; *WBC,* white blood cell.

Nursing Diagnoses

Nursing diagnoses related to HIV infection are dictated by several variables: the stage (e.g., Is prevention of HIV infection the issue? Are there concerns related to ongoing infection? Is the patient dying?); the presence of specific etiologic problems (e.g., respiratory distress, depression, pain); and psychosocial factors (e.g., issues related to self-esteem, sexuality, family interactions, finances). Because HIV infection is a complex and individually experienced disease, a broad spectrum of nursing diagnoses may include, but are not limited to, those presented in Table 15-17.

Planning

Prevention of HIV infection presents a number of challenges for the patient, many of which are related to the difficulties of behavior change. Nurses can be instrumental in this process. Nursing interventions to prevent disease transmission depend on assessment of the patient's individual risk behaviors, knowledge, and skills. Nursing orders based on these assessments can encourage the patient to adopt safer, healthier, and less risky behaviors.[35]

Infection with HIV affects the entire range of a person's life from physical health to social, emotional, economic, and spiritual well-being. Once infected, no known treatment can eliminate HIV from the body. Therefore the overriding goals of therapy are to keep the viral load as low as possible for as long as possible, maintain or restore a functioning immune system, improve the patient's quality of life, prevent opportunistic disease, reduce HIV-related disability and death, and prevent new infections. Nursing interventions can assist the patient to (1) adhere to drug regimens; (2) promote a healthy lifestyle that includes avoiding exposure to additional sexual and blood-borne diseases; (3) protect others from HIV; (4) maintain or develop healthy and supportive relationships; (5) maintain activities and productivity; (6) explore spiritual issues; (7) come to terms with issues related to disease, disability, and death; and (8) cope with the frequent symptoms caused by HIV and its treatments.[32,34,49,50] Goals are individualized and change as new treatment protocols develop and/or as HIV disease progresses.

Nursing Implementation

The complexity of HIV disease is related to its chronic nature. As with most chronic and infectious diseases, primary prevention and health promotion are the most effective health care strategies. When prevention fails, disease results. HIV has no cure, continues for life, causes increasing physical disability, contributes to impaired health, and ultimately leads to death.

Nursing interventions at every stage of HIV disease can be instrumental in improving the quality and quantity of the patient's life. Nurses who emphasize a holistic and individualized approach to care are well suited to provide optimal care to these patients. Table 15-18 presents a synopsis of nursing goals, assessments, and interventions at each stage of HIV infection.

Health Promotion. A major goal of health promotion is to prevent disease. Even with recent successes in the treatment of HIV, prevention is crucial for control of the epidemic. In addition, health promotion encourages early detection of disease so that, if primary prevention has failed, early intervention can be implemented.[34,35,49]

Prevention of HIV Infection. HIV infection is preventable. Avoiding and/or modifying risky behaviors are the most effective prevention tools. All patients should be provided with education and behavior change counseling that is specific to the patient's need, culturally sensitive, language appropriate, and age specific. Nurses are excellent resources for this type of education, but they must be comfortable with and know how to talk about sensitive topics such as sexuality and drug use.[49,51]

Prevention behaviors have been known and recommended since the mid-1980s. It is important to remember that a range of activities can reduce the risk of HIV infection and that individuals will choose methods that best fit their life circumstances. The goal is for the person to develop safer, healthier, and less risky behaviors. These techniques can be divided into *safe activities* (those that eliminate risk) and *risk-reducing activities* (those that decrease risk, but do not eliminate it). The more consistently and correctly

TABLE 15-17 NURSING DIAGNOSES
HIV Infection

- Acute pain
- Anxiety
- Caregiver role strain
- Chronic low self-esteem
- Decisional conflict
- Diarrhea
- Disturbed body image
- Disturbed thought processes
- Fatigue
- Fear
- Grieving
- Hyperthermia
- Imbalanced nutrition: less than body requirements
- Impaired oral mucous membrane
- Ineffective coping
- Ineffective denial
- Ineffective therapeutic regimen management
- Insomnia
- Interrupted family processes
- Noncompliance
- Powerlessness
- Relocation stress syndrome
- Risk for disuse syndrome
- Self-care deficit
- Situational low self-esteem
- Social isolation
- Spiritual distress

HEALTHY PEOPLE
Prevention and Early Detection of HIV

- Increase safe sexual practices, including condom use
- Decrease equipment sharing among intravenous drug users
- Increase clinician skills to assess for risk factors for HIV infection, to recommend HIV testing, and to provide counseling for behavior change
- Make voluntary HIV testing a routine part of health care
- Increase access to HIV testing facilities in traditional health care settings as well as in alternate sites such as drug and alcohol treatment facilities and community-based organizations
- Increase access to new HIV testing technologies, especially rapid testing
- Increase risk assessment and individualized behavior change messages to people with HIV to prevent new infections
- Further decrease perinatal HIV infection by including voluntary HIV testing as a part of routine prenatal care and providing counseling and appropriate HIV therapy to those found to be infected

TABLE 15-18 Nursing Interventions in HIV Disease

Levels of Nursing Care/Goals	Assess	Interventions
Health Promotion 1. Prevent HIV infection 2. Detect HIV infection early	*Risk factors:* What behaviors or social, physical, emotional, pathologic, and immune factors place the patient at risk? Does the patient need to be tested for HIV?	• Education, including knowledge, attitudes, and behaviors, with an emphasis on risk reduction to: • *General population:* cover general information • *Pregnant women:* general information and information specific to HIV infection and pregnancy • *Individual patient:* specific to assessed need • Empower patients to take control of prevention measures. • Provide HIV antibody testing with pretest and posttest counseling.
Acute Intervention 1. Promote health and limit disability 2. Manage problems caused by HIV infection	*Physical health:* Is patient experiencing problems? *Mental health status:* How is the patient coping? *Resources:* Does the patient have family/social support? Is patient accessing community services? Is money/ insurance a problem? Does the patient have access to spiritual support?	• Provide case management. • Educate regarding HIV, the spectrum of infection, options for care, signs and symptoms to report, treatment options, immune enhancement, risk reduction, and ways to adhere to treatment regimens. • Refer to needed resources. • Establish long-term, trusting relationship with patient, family, and significant others. • Provide emotional and spiritual support. • Provide care during acute exacerbations: recognition of life-threatening developments, life support, rapid intervention with treatments and drugs, patient and family emotional support during crisis, comfort, and hygiene needs. • Develop resources for legal needs: discrimination prevention, wills and powers of attorney, child care wishes. • Empower patient to identify needs, direct care, seek services.
Ambulatory and Home Care 1. Maximize quality of life 2. Resolve life and death issues	*Physical health:* Are new symptoms developing? Is the patient experiencing drug side effects or interactions? *Mental health:* How is the patient coping? What adjustments have been made? *Finances:* Can the patient maintain health care and basic standards of living? *Family/social/community supports:* Are these available? Is the patient using supports in an effective manner? Do family/significant others need education, encouragement, or stress relief? *Spirituality issues:* Does the patient desire support from a religious organization? Are spirituality issues private and personal? What assistance does the patient need?	• Continue case management. • Educate about changing treatment options and continued adherence. • Empower patient to continue to direct care and to make desires known to family members and significant others. • Continue physical care for chronic disease process: treatments, drugs, comfort, and hygiene needs. • Support patient and family/significant others in a trusting relationship. • Refer to resources that will assist in meeting identified needs. • Encourage health promotion measures (as above). • Assist with end-of-life issues: resuscitation orders, comfort measures, funeral plans, estate planning, child care continuation, etc.

prevention methods are used, the more effective they are in preventing HIV infection.

Research shows that the majority of new HIV infections were transmitted by individuals who were not aware that they were infected. An estimated 25% to 30% of HIV-infected people in the United States and Canada do not know that they are infected.[16,35] These facts helped the Centers for Disease Control and Prevention (CDC) develop four strategies in the *Advancing HIV Prevention* (AHP) initiative: (1) HIV testing should be a part of routine health care based on risk assessment and clinical need; (2) rapid HIV testing should also be used to diagnose HIV outside of traditional care settings (e.g., in community-based organizations and at health fairs), (3) providers should work with HIV-infected patients and their partners to change risky behaviors and decrease the risks of HIV transmission, and (4) perinatal transmission should be further reduced by universally offering HIV tests to pregnant women and appropriate treatment to those found to be infected.[35,52]

Decreasing Risks Related to Sexual Intercourse. Safe sexual activities eliminate the risk of exposure to HIV in semen and vaginal secretions. Abstaining from all sexual activity is the most effective way to accomplish this goal, but there are safe options for those who cannot or do not wish to abstain. Limiting sexual behavior to activities in which the mouth, penis, vagina, or rectum does not come into contact with a partner's mouth, penis, vagina, or rectum is safe because there is no contact with blood, semen, or vaginal secretions. Safe activities include massage, masturbation, mutual masturbation ("hand job"), telephone sex, and other activities that meet the "no contact" requirements. *Insertive sex* between partners who are not infected with HIV or not at risk of becoming infected with HIV is also considered to be safe.

Risk-reducing sexual activities decrease the risk of contact with HIV through the use of barriers. Barriers should be used when engaging in insertive sexual activity (oral, vaginal, or anal) with a partner whose HIV status is not known or with a partner who is known to have HIV. The most commonly used barrier is the male condom (Fig. 15-7). The *efficacy* (protection provided under ideal circumstances) of male condoms is essentially 100%; their *effectiveness* (protection provided in actual or "real life" circumstances) is 80% to 90%. Correct use of male condoms, as discussed in Table 15-19, increases effectiveness. Female condoms provide an excellent alternative to male condoms (Fig. 15-8). Female condom efficacy is also close to 100% and effectiveness is 94% to 97% against HIV and STD transmission. Use can be complicated, so careful instruction and practice are required[53] (Table 15-20). In addition, squares of latex (known as dental dams) or plastic food wrap can be used to cover the external female genitalia during oral sexual activity.

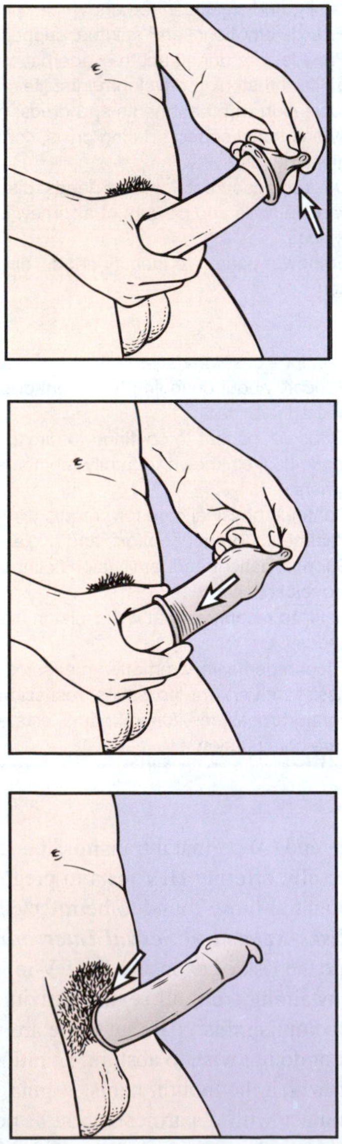

FIG. 15-7 Proper placement of the male condom. **A,** The condom is placed over the glans of the erect penis, being careful to squeeze air out of the reservoir (tip). **B** and **C,** The condom is then rolled down the shaft of the penis to the hairline.

Decreasing Risks Related to Drug Use. Drug use, including alcohol, is harmful. It can cause immune suppression and malnutrition, as well as a host of psychosocial problems. However, drug use in and of itself does not cause HIV infection. The major risk for HIV infection is related to sharing equipment and/or having unsafe sexual experiences while under the influence of drugs. Basic risk reduction rules are: (1) do not use drugs; (2) if you use drugs, do not share equipment; and (3) do not have sexual intercourse when under the influence of any drug (including alcohol) that impairs decision-making ability.[22]

The safest mechanism is to abstain from drugs. Although this is the best option for those who do not currently use drugs, it may not be a viable option for users who are not prepared to quit or for those who have no access to drug treatment services. The risk of HIV for these individuals can be eliminated if they do not share equipment. Injecting equipment ("works") includes needles, syringes, cookers (spoons or bottle caps used to mix the drug), cotton, and rinse water. Equipment used to snort (straws) or smoke (pipes) drugs can also be contaminated with blood. None of this equipment should be shared. Access to sterile equipment is an important risk elimination tactic. Some communities have needle and syringe exchange programs (NSEPs) that provide sterile equipment to users in exchange for used equipment. Opposition to these programs is supported by the fear that ready access to injecting supplies will increase drug use. However, studies have shown that, in communities where exchange programs have been established, drug use does not increase, rates of HIV and other blood-borne infections are controlled, and an overall cost benefit results.[54] Cleaning equipment before use is a risk-reducing activity. It decreases the risk for those who share equipment (Table 15-21), but cleaning requires equipment, takes time, and may be difficult for a person in drug withdrawal.

Decreasing Risks of Perinatal Transmission. The best way to prevent HIV infection in infants is to prevent HIV infection in women. Women who are already infected with HIV should be

TABLE 15-19 PATIENT TEACHING GUIDE
Proper Use of the Male Condom

1. Use only condoms that are made with latex or polyurethane. "Natural skin" condoms have pores that are large enough for HIV to penetrate.
2. Store condoms in a cool, dry place and protect them from trauma. The friction caused by carrying them in a back pocket, for instance, can damage the latex.
3. Do not use a condom if the expiration date has passed or if the package looks worn or punctured.
4. Lubricants used in conjunction with condoms must be water soluble. Oil-based lubricants can weaken latex and increase the risk of tearing or breaking.
5. Nonlubricated, flavored, or unflavored condoms can provide protection during oral intercourse.
6. The condom must be placed on the erect penis before any contact is made with the partner's mouth, vagina, or rectum to prevent exposure to preejaculatory secretions that may contain HIV.
7. See Fig. 15-7 for proper steps in male condom placement.
8. Remove the penis and condom from the partner's body immediately after ejaculation and before the erection is lost. Hold the condom at the base of the penis and remove both from the partner's body at the same time. This keeps semen from leaking around the condom as the penis becomes flaccid.
9. Remove the condom after use, wrap in tissue, and discard. Do not dispose in the toilet, as this can cause plumbing problems.
10. Condoms are not reusable! A new condom must be used for every act of intercourse.

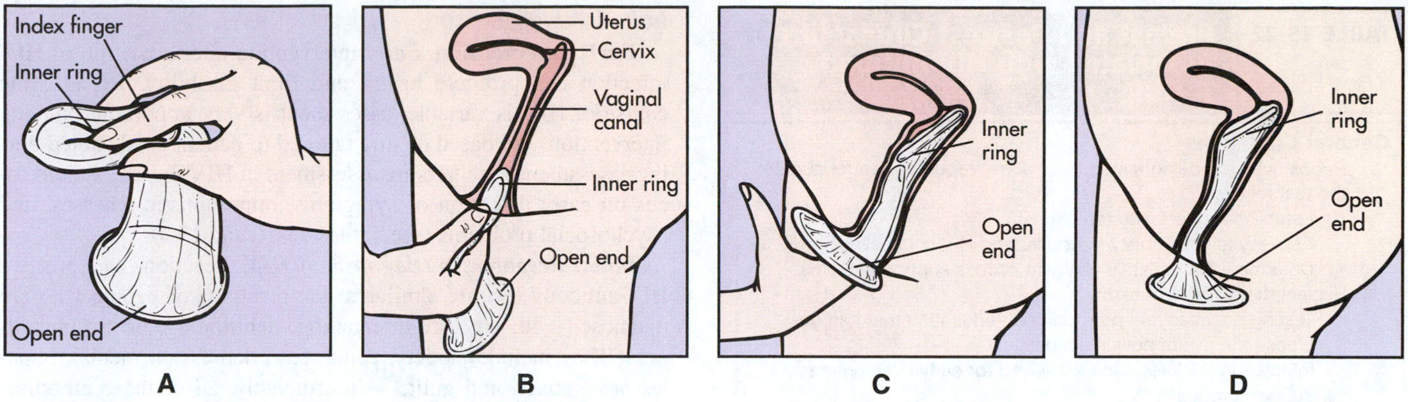

FIG. 15-8 Proper placement of the female condom. **A,** Inner ring is squeezed for insertion. **B,** Sheath is inserted similarly to a diaphragm. **C,** Inner ring is pushed up as far as it can go with the index finger. **D,** Proper placement of female condom.

TABLE 15-20 ***PATIENT TEACHING GUIDE*** **Proper Use of the Female Condom**

1. Female condoms consist of a polyurethane sheath with two spring-form rings.
   - The smaller ring is inserted into the vagina and holds the condom in place internally. This ring can be removed if the condom is to be used for anal intercourse. It should not be removed if the condom is to be used for vaginal intercourse.
   - The larger ring surrounds the opening to the condom. It functions to keep the condom in place while protecting the external genitalia.
2. Use only water-soluble lubricants with female condoms.
   - Female condoms come prelubricated and with a tube of additional lubricant.
   - Lubrication is needed to protect the condom from tearing during sexual intercourse and can also decrease noise that results from friction of the penis against the condom.
3. Some men have reported that the female condom feels better than the male condom. Other men like male condoms better. The only way to find out which type of condom works best is to try them both.
4. Practice inserting the female condom. The steps for proper insertion are shown in Fig. 15-8. Lubrication makes the condom slippery, but do not get discouraged, just keep trying.
5. During sexual intercourse, ensure that the penis is inserted into the female condom through the outer ring. It is possible for the penis to miss the opening, thus making contact with the vaginal or rectal mucosa, and defeating the purpose of the condom.
6. Do not use a male condom at the same time as a female condom as this is unnecessary and could result in less adherence to consistent condom use.
7. After intercourse, remove the condom before standing up.
8. Twist the outer ring to keep the semen inside, gently pull the condom out of the vagina or rectum, and discard.
9. Do not dispose in the toilet, as this can cause plumbing problems.
10. Do not reuse a female condom.

asked about their reproductive desires. Those who choose not to have children need to have family planning methods discussed in detail. Should they become pregnant, abortion may be desired and should be discussed in conjunction with other options.[29]

If HIV-infected pregnant women are appropriately treated during pregnancy, the rate of perinatal transmission can be decreased from 25% to less than 2%. The current standard of care is that all women who are pregnant or contemplating pregnancy should be counseled about HIV infection, informed of their choices, routinely offered access to voluntary HIV-antibody testing, and, if infected, offered optimal ART.[29,35]

TABLE 15-21 ***PATIENT AND FAMILY TEACHING GUIDE*** **Proper Use of Drug-Using Equipment**

1. When injecting drugs, it is always preferable to use new, sterile syringes, needles, cookers, and cotton (works). When snorting or smoking drugs, it is important to use clean pipes and straws.
2. Find out if there is a needle and syringe exchange program in your community. If there is, take used equipment in and you will be provided with new works.
3. In many states, sterile equipment can be purchased without a prescription.
4. Reusing your own equipment is acceptable. Just ensure that no one else uses your equipment.
5. If you must share injecting equipment, it is very important to clean the works thoroughly before use.
   - First, rinse the used needle and syringe twice with tap water.
   - Next, fill the syringe with full-strength household bleach, shake for 30 seconds, and squirt the bleach out.
   - Repeat the bleaching process a second time, being sure to shake the bleach-filled syringe for 30 seconds.
   - Finally, rinse equipment twice with tap water.
   - Do not share your bleach or rinse water.
   - Do not share your cooker. If you must share your cooker, clean it with bleach and water before using it again.
6. If you must share pipes or straws, it is very important to clean them thoroughly before use. Soak in bleach and rinse with water.

Decreasing Risks at Work. The risk of infection from occupational exposure to HIV is small but real. The Occupational Safety and Health Administration (OSHA) requires employers to protect workers from exposure to blood and other potentially infectious materials. Precautions and safety devices decrease the risk of direct contact with blood and body fluids (see Chapter 13). Should exposure to HIV-infected fluids occur, **postexposure prophylaxis (PEP)** with combination ART based on the type of exposure, the volume of the exposure, and the status of the source patient can significantly decrease the risk of infection. The possibility of treatment makes reporting of all blood exposures even more critical.[26]

HIV Testing and Counseling. Testing is the only sure way to determine if a person has HIV infection. Any individual who is at risk for HIV should be encouraged to be tested. When negative, testing can relieve anxieties about past behaviors and provide opportunities for prevention education. When positive, testing provides the needed impetus to seek treatment and to protect sexual and drug-using partners. HIV testing should be accompanied by pretest and posttest counseling[35,37] (Table 15-22).

TABLE 15-22 Pretest and Posttest Counseling Associated with HIV-Antibody Testing

General Guidelines

1. People who are being tested for HIV are frequently fearful about the test results.
   - Establish rapport with the patient.
   - Assess patient's ability to understand HIV counseling.
   - Determine the patient's ability to access support systems.
2. Explain the benefits of testing.
   - Testing provides an opportunity for education that can decrease the risk of new infections.
   - Infected individuals can be referred for early intervention and support programs.
3. Discuss negative aspects of testing.
   - Confidentiality issues: breaches of confidentiality have led to discrimination.
   - A positive test affects all aspects of the patient's life (personal, social, economic, etc.) and can raise difficult emotions (anger, anxiety, guilt, and thoughts of suicide).

Pretest Counseling

1. Determine the patient's risk factors and when the last risk occurred. Counseling should be individualized according to these parameters.
2. Provide education to decrease future risk of exposure.
3. Provide education that will help the patient protect sexual and drug-sharing partners.
4. Discuss problems related to the delay between infection and an accurate test. Testing will need to be repeated at intervals for up to 6 months after each possible exposure. Discuss the need to use measures to decrease the risks to the patient and the patient's partners during that interval.
5. Discuss the possibility of false-negative tests, which are most likely to occur during the window period.
6. Assess support systems. Provide telephone numbers and resources as needed.
7. Discuss patient's personally anticipated responses to test results (positive and negative).
8. Outline assistance that will be offered if the test is positive.

Posttest Counseling

1. If the test is negative, reinforce pretest counseling and prevention education. Remind patient that test needs to be repeated at intervals for up to 6 months after the most recent exposure risk.
2. If the test is positive, understand that the patient may be in shock and not hear much of what you say.
3. Provide resources for medical and emotional support and help the patient get immediate assistance.
   - Evaluate suicide risk and follow-up as needed.
   - Determine need to test others who have had risky contact with the patient.
   - Discuss retesting to verify results. This tactic supports hope for the patient, but more importantly, it keeps the patient in the system. While waiting for the second test result, the patient has time to think about and adjust to the possibility of being HIV infected.
   - Encourage optimism.
4. Remind patient that effective treatments are available; HIV is not a death sentence.
5. Review health habits that can improve the immune system.
6. Arrange for patient to speak to HIV-infected people who are willing to share with and assist newly diagnosed patients during the transition period.
7. Reinforce that a positive HIV test means that the patient is infected, but does not necessarily mean that the patient has progressed to AIDS.
8. Educate to prevent new infections. HIV-infected people should be instructed to avoid donating blood, organs, or semen; to avoid sharing razors, toothbrushes, or other household items that may contain blood or other body fluids; and to protect sexual and needle-sharing partners from blood, semen, and vaginal secretions.

Acute Intervention

Early Intervention. Early intervention after detection of HIV infection can promote health and limit disability. Because the course of HIV is variable, assessment is very important. Nursing interventions are based on and tailored to patient needs noted during assessment. The nursing assessment in HIV disease should focus on early detection of symptoms, opportunistic diseases, and psychosocial problems (see Tables 15-16 and 15-18).

Initial Response to Diagnosis of HIV. Reactions to a positive HIV-antibody test are similar to the reactions of people who are diagnosed with any life-threatening, debilitating, or chronic illness. They include anxiety, panic, fear, depression, denial, hopelessness, anger, and guilt.[37] Unfortunately, all of these emotions are overlaid with the stigma and discrimination that continue to pervade social reactions to HIV.[55] Many of these reactions are also seen in the patient's family members, friends, and caregivers. As time passes, patients and their loved ones must confront common issues associated with any life-threatening illness. These include complex treatment decisions; feelings of loss, anger, powerlessness, depression, and grief; social isolation imposed by self or others; altered concepts of the physical, social, emotional, and creative self; thoughts of suicide; and the possibility of death.

Antiretroviral Therapy. Multidrug-therapy protocols have been shown to significantly reduce viral loads and reverse clinical progression of HIV.[34] However, nurses must be aware that the protocols can be complex, the drugs have side effects and potential interactions with other medications, and ART does not work for everyone. All of these factors contribute to problems with adherence to treatment, a dangerous situation because of the risk of developing drug resistance. Frequently, nurses are the clinicians who work most closely with patients who are trying to cope with these issues. Interventions include education about (1) the advantages and disadvantages of new treatments, (2) the dangers of nonadherence to therapeutic regimens, (3) how and when to take each drug, (4) drug interactions to avoid, and (5) side effects that must be reported to the health care provider.[50] Table 15-23 provides guidance for patient teaching in these areas.

When to Start Antiretroviral Therapy. ART has evolved continuously since the first antiretroviral drug was released in 1987. When new drugs were developed, clinicians had the ability to combine and substitute medications. For a while, the preferred treatment strategy was known as "hit it early, hit it hard." This was thought to be appropriate because decreasing the viral load provides for better health outcomes. However, side effects and treatment "burnout" often led to nonadherence, which increased the risk of developing resistance to medications. For this reason, federal guidelines now suggest that treatment can be delayed until greater immune suppression is observed[34] (see Table 15-13). The most important consideration for initiating therapy is patient readiness. Nurses can provide in-depth education and counseling for patients as they struggle to make this decision.

Adherence. Adherence is the accurate and consistent fidelity to a treatment regimen. Adherence to drug regimens is a critical component of drug therapy for people with HIV infection and an area where nurses are uniquely well prepared to provide assistance. Taking drugs as ordered (right dose and time) every day is important for all drug therapy. The difference with HIV is that missing even a few doses can lead to viral mutations that allow HIV to become resistant to the drug.[34-36]

The difficulty of adhering consistently is probably clear to anyone who has tried to take a 10-day course of antibiotics. Patients with HIV infection have to take anywhere from 2 to 20 pills a day, at precise times during the day. This process must be repeated every day for the rest of their lives even though they often suffer uncomfortable side effects. Nurses have learned that helping people adhere to difficult treatment regimens requires a number of things. The most important is to remember that each patient is a unique individual with unique ways of dealing with therapy. Patients may be helped with technologies such as electronic reminders, beepers, or timers on pillboxes. Group support and individual counseling can also help, but the best approach is to learn about the patient's life and assist with problem solving within the confines of that life.[56-58] Table 15-24 lists strategies proven to assist with adherence.

Health Promotion. HIV disease progression may be delayed by promoting a healthy immune system whether the patient chooses to use ART or not. Useful interventions for HIV-infected patients include (1) nutritional support to maintain lean body mass and ensure appropriate levels of vitamins and micronutrients; (2) moderation or elimination of alcohol, tobacco, and drug use; (3) keeping recommended vaccines up to date; (4) adequate rest, exercise, and stress reduction; (5) avoiding exposure to new infectious agents; (6) mental health counseling; and (7) getting involved in support groups and community activities.

Patients should be taught to recognize symptoms that may indicate disease progression and/or drug side effects so that prompt medical care can be initiated. Table 15-25 provides an overview of symptoms that patients should report. In general, patients should have as much information as needed to make the informed decisions that guide appropriate nursing intervention.

Acute Exacerbations. Chronic diseases are characterized by acute exacerbations of recurring problems. This is especially true in HIV disease where infections, cancers, debility, and psychosocial/economic issues may interact to overwhelm the patient's ability to cope. Nursing care becomes more complex as the patient's immune system deteriorates and new problems arise to compound existing difficulties. When opportunistic diseases or difficult side effects of treatment develop, symptom management, education, and emotional support are necessary.[50]

Nursing care assumes primary importance in helping patients prevent the many opportunistic diseases associated with HIV infection. The best prevention of opportunistic disease is adequate treatment of the underlying HIV infection. In addition to assisting the patient with the medications prescribed for these diseases, the nurse will need to provide appropriate supportive care. If the patient has *Pneumocystis jiroveci* pneumonia (PCP), for example, nursing interventions will be required to assure adequate oxygenation (Fig. 15-9); if the patient has cryptococcal meningitis, an important nursing concern will be to maintain a safe environment for a confused patient.[50]

Ambulatory and Home Care

Ongoing Care. HIV-infected patients share problems experienced by all individuals with chronic diseases, but these problems are exacerbated by negative social constructs surrounding HIV. In HIV, the stigma of illness is compounded by several factors. HIV-infected people may be seen as lacking control over urges to have sex or use drugs. It is then easy to jump to the conclusion that they brought the disease on themselves and therefore deserve to be sick. Behaviors associated with HIV infection may be viewed as immoral (e.g., homosexuality, having many sexual partners) and are sometimes illegal (e.g., using drugs, sex work). The fact that infected individuals can transmit HIV to others increases stigma, and stigma leads to discrimination in all facets of life. In the United

TABLE 15-23 PATIENT AND FAMILY TEACHING GUIDE — Use of Antiretroviral Drugs

Resistance to antiretroviral drugs is a major problem in treating HIV infection. To decrease the risk of developing resistance:

1. Take at least three different antiretroviral drugs from at least two different drug classes; discuss options with your health care provider to find the best regimen for you.
2. Know what you are taking and how to take them (some have to be taken with food, some must be taken on an empty stomach, some cannot be taken together). If you do not understand, ask. Get your nurse to write the instructions clearly for you.
3. Take the full dose prescribed and take it on schedule. If you cannot take the drug because of side effects or other problems, report it to your health care provider immediately.
4. Take all of the drugs as prescribed. Do not quit taking one drug while continuing the others. If you cannot tolerate one of your drugs, talk to your health care provider, who will recommend a new set of drugs.
5. Many of the antiretroviral drugs interact with other drugs, including a number of common drugs you can buy without a prescription. Be sure your health care provider and pharmacist know all of the drugs that you are taking, and do not take any new drugs without checking for possible interactions.
6. The goal of antiretroviral therapy is to decrease the amount of virus in your blood. This is called your *viral load.* The best result is to get your viral load below detectable levels. Most health care providers will check your blood for your viral load on a regular basis whether you are taking antiretroviral agents or not.
7. Two to 4 weeks after you start on drug therapy (or change your therapy), your health care provider will test your viral load to find out if the drugs are working. These results are reported in absolute numbers or in logarithms (a mathematical concept). All you need to know is that you want to see the viral load drop. If reports are in logarithms, you want to see a drop of at least 1 unit, which means that 90% of your viral load has been eliminated. If your viral load drops by 2 units, your viral load will have decreased by 95%. If your viral load drops by 3 units, your viral load will have decreased by 99%.
8. An undetectable viral load means that the amount of virus is extremely low and viruses cannot be found in the blood using the current technology. It does *not* mean that the virus is gone because much of the virus will be in lymph nodes and organs that the tests cannot detect. It also does *not* mean that you are no longer able to transmit HIV to others; you will need to continue protecting all of your sexual and drug-using partners from HIV.

TABLE 15-24 Strategies to Improve Adherence to Antiretroviral Therapy

- Establish the patient's readiness to start therapy
- Provide education on dosing of medication
- Review potential side effects of drugs
- Anticipate and treat side effects
- Use educational aids, including pictures, pillboxes, and calendars
- Engage family and friends in the education process
- Simplify regimens, dosing, and food requirements
- Use team approach with nurses, pharmacists, and peer counselors
- Provide accessible and trusting health care team
- Integrate medication doses into patient's life and work schedules

Revised from Centers for Disease Control and Prevention (CDC): Guidelines for the use of antiretroviral agents in HIV-infected adults and adolescents, 2005. Available at *http://aidsinfo.nih.gov/* (accessed April 22, 2006).

TABLE 15-25 ***PATIENT AND FAMILY TEACHING GUIDE***
Signs and Symptoms That HIV-Infected Patients Need to Report

Report the Following Signs and Symptoms Immediately to Health Care Provider

- Any change in level of consciousness: lethargy, hard to arouse, unable to arouse, unresponsive, unconscious
- Headache accompanied by nausea and vomiting, changes in vision, changes in ability to perform coordinated activities, or after any head trauma
- Vision changes: blurry or black areas in vision field, new floaters, double vision
- Persistent shortness of breath related to activity and not relieved by a short rest period
- Nausea and vomiting accompanied by abdominal pain
- Vomiting blood
- Dehydration: unable to eat or drink because of nausea, diarrhea, or mouth lesions; severe diarrhea or vomiting; dizziness when standing
- Yellow discoloration of the skin
- Any bleeding from the rectum that is not related to hemorrhoids or trauma (from anal sexual intercourse)
- Pain in the flank with fever and unable to urinate for more than 6 hours
- Blood in the urine
- New onset of weakness in any part of the body, new onset of numbness that is not obviously related to pressure, new onset of difficulty speaking
- Chest pain not obviously related to cough
- Seizures
- New rash accompanied by fever
- New oral lesions accompanied by fever
- Severe depression, anxiety, hallucinations, delusions, or thoughts of causing danger to self or others

Report the Following Signs and Symptoms within 24 Hours

- New or different headache; constant headache not relieved by aspirin or acetaminophen
- Headache accompanied by fever, nasal congestion, or cough
- Burning, itching, or discharge from the eyes
- New or productive cough
- Vomiting 2-3 times a day
- Vomiting accompanied by fever
- New, significant, or watery diarrhea (more than 6 times a day)
- Painful urination, bloody urine, urethral discharge
- New, significant rash (widespread, painful, itchy, or following a path down the leg or arm, around the chest, or on the face)
- Difficulty eating or drinking because of mouth lesions
- Vaginal discharge, pain, or itching

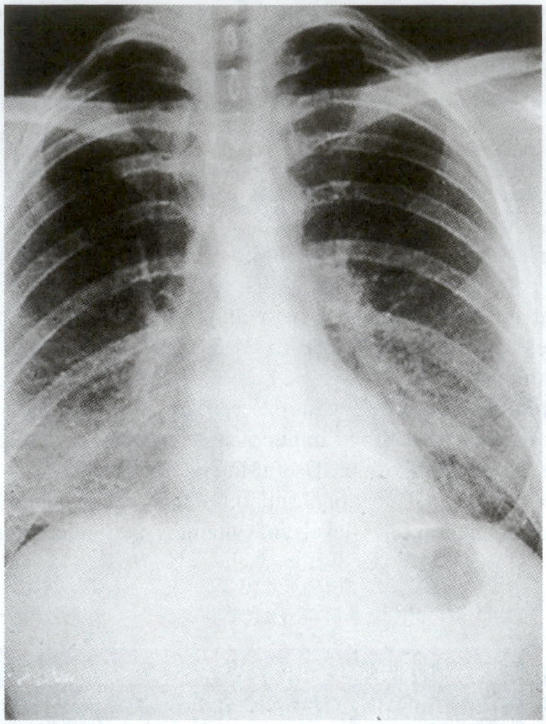

FIG. 15-9 Chest x-ray showing interstitial infiltrates as the result of *Pneumocystis jiroveci* pneumonia.

States, for example, HIV-infected people have lost jobs, homes, and insurance, even though these forms of discrimination are illegal according to the Americans with Disabilities Act (ADA).[14,59] Unfortunately, this problem occurs all over the world and is often more severe for women.[20,21,55]

Discrimination related to HIV infection can lead to social isolation, dependence, frustration, lowered self-image, loss of control, and economic pressures. It is of interest that all of these variables may have contributed to the patient's infection in the first place. Low self-esteem, searching for social contact, frustration, and economic difficulties can all contribute to drug use and risky sexual behaviors.

Disease and Drug Side Effects. Physical problems related to HIV and/or the treatment of HIV can interrupt the patient's ability to maintain a desired lifestyle. HIV-infected patients frequently experience anxiety, fear, depression, diarrhea, peripheral neuropathy, pain, nausea, vomiting, and fatigue. These are symptoms that nurses deal with routinely. Interventions for these symptoms do not change significantly based on the primary diagnosis. Individual considerations will, of course, influence the way that the nurse approaches each patient. Nursing management of diarrhea, for instance, still includes helping patients collect specimens, recommending dietary changes, encouraging fluid and electrolyte replacement, instructing the patient about skin care, and managing skin breakdown around the perianal area. Nursing approaches for fatigue in HIV include teaching patients to assess fatigue patterns, determine contributing factors, set activity priorities, conserve energy, schedule rest periods, exercise, and avoid substances such as caffeine, nicotine, alcohol, and other drugs that may disturb sleep.[50]

Some HIV-infected patients, especially those who have been infected for a long time and who have been on ART, develop a set of metabolic disorders that include changes in body shape (fat deposits in the abdomen, upper back, and breasts along with fat loss in the arms, legs, and face) due to lipodystrophy (Fig. 15-10), hyperlipidemia (elevated triglycerides and decreases in high-density lipoproteins), insulin resistance and hyperglycemia, bone disease (osteoporosis, osteopenia, avascular necrosis), lactic acidosis, and cardiovascular disease. It is still not clear why these disorders develop, but it is probably a combination of factors such as long-term infection with HIV, side effects of ART, genetic predisposition, and chronic stress.[60,61]

Management of metabolic disorders currently focuses on detecting problems early, dealing with the symptoms, and helping the patient cope with new problems and changes to treatment regimens. It is important to recognize and treat these problems early, especially since cardiovascular disease and lactic acidosis are potentially fatal complications. A frequent first intervention is to change ART medications because some drugs are more often associated with these

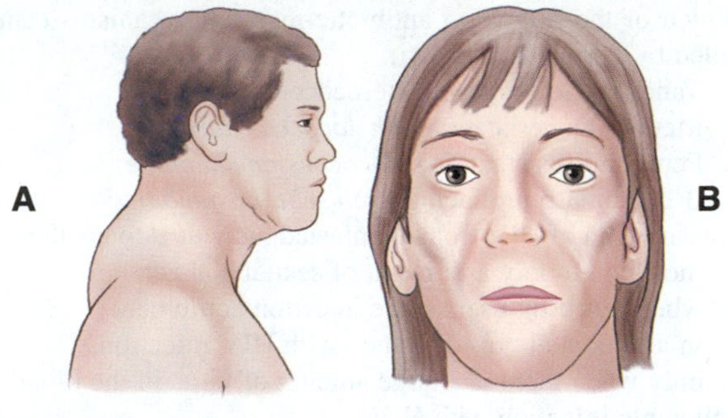

FIG. 15-10 Lipodystrophy manifestations: **A,** Buffalo hump (hypertrophy). **B,** Facial wasting.

problems (see Table 15-15). Lipid abnormalities are generally treated with lipid-lowering drugs (see Table 34-6), dietary changes, and exercise. Insulin resistance is treated with hypoglycemic drugs and weight loss. Bone disease may be improved with exercise, dietary changes, and calcium and vitamin D supplements.[50]

Body changes that combine fat accumulation and wasting are major problems for patients with this syndrome. There is little evidence that exercise or dietary changes make any difference. Human growth hormone, testosterone, and anabolic steroids have been used to help resolve these changes, but they frequently are not effective or even available. Some patients have had plastic surgery to reduce areas of fat and to build up sunken areas of the face, but access to these procedures is limited. Nursing interventions can focus on helping the patient to make treatment decisions and cope with negative changes in body image.[50]

Terminal Care. Despite exciting new developments in the treatment of HIV infection, many patients eventually experience disease progression, disability, and death. Sometimes these occur because treatments do not work for the patient. Sometimes the patient's HIV becomes resistant to all available drug therapies. In other cases, a patient may make a calculated decision to forego further treatment, allowing the disease to progress toward death. Nursing care during the terminal phase of any disease needs to focus on keeping the patient comfortable, facilitating emotional and spiritual acceptance of the finite nature of life, helping the patient's significant others deal with grief and loss, and maintaining a safe environment. Nurses become pivotal care providers during the terminal phase of illness, especially when patients and families choose terminal care at home. (End-of-life care is discussed in Chapter 11.)

Evaluation

The expected outcomes are that the patient at risk for HIV infection will

- analyze personal risk factors
- develop and implement a flexible and progressive personal plan to decrease risks
- get tested for HIV

The expected outcomes are that the patient with HIV infection will

- describe basic aspects of the effects of HIV on the immune system
- compare and contrast various treatment options for HIV disease
- work with a team of health care providers to achieve optimal health
- prevent transmission of HIV to others

CRITICAL THINKING EXERCISES

CASE STUDY

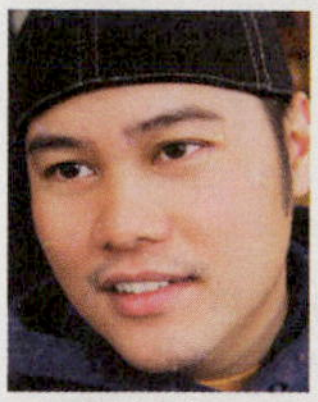

Case Study photo ©iStockphoto.com/ Roberta Osborne.

At Risk for HIV Disease

Patient Profile. Emilio, a 20-year-old Hispanic male college student, comes to the student health center with pain on urination.

Subjective Data

- Describes pain as, "Just like it felt when I had the clap last year"
- Provides a history of sexual activity since age 15, reports lifetime sexual partners as six women and two men; states he is always the "top" (inserting partner)
- Denies injected drug, tobacco, or steroid use
- Uses alcohol (mainly beer) at weekend parties and has smoked marijuana, but not recently
- Sexual activity in the past month has been with one woman and two men and includes vaginal and anal intercourse

Objective Data

Physical Examination

- 5 feet 11 inches tall, 168 pounds, temperature 100.4° F (38° C), purulent urethral discharge noted

Laboratory Studies

- Urine test for *Neisseria gonorrhoeae* is positive

Collaborative Care

- IM injection with 250 mg ceftriaxone (Rocephin)
- Doxycycline 100 mg PO bid for 7 days

Critical Thinking Questions

1. Why should Emilio be encouraged to be tested for HIV?
2. How will you counsel Emilio about the testing process? How can you help him prepare for the test and the test results?
3. Ask a classmate to be "Emilio" and role-play HIV risk assessment, risk reduction counseling, and pretest and posttest counseling.
4. What are the main considerations to cover when teaching about barrier methods of protection? Are there components of the Hispanic culture that may affect your approach to teaching about condoms?
5. Emilio has at least one STD. How will you discuss the issue of partner notification with him? If he is positive for HIV, will that change the partner notification process?
6. If Emilio's HIV test is positive, what nursing diagnoses apply? If his HIV test is negative, what nursing diagnoses apply?

CASE STUDY

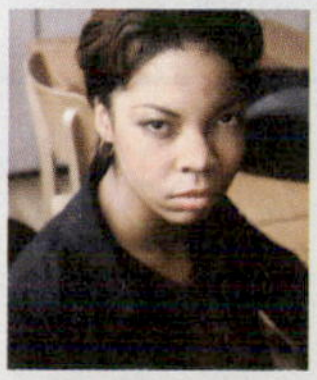

Case Study photo ©iStockphoto.com/ Mike Manzano.

Symptomatic HIV Disease

Patient Profile. Janelle, a 35-year-old African American single mother, was admitted to the hospital with AIDS and cytomegalovirus (CMV) retinitis that were both diagnosed 2 days ago.

Subjective Data

- Seen by a doctor 6 years ago for pain behind the sternum and difficulty swallowing, diagnosed as esophageal candidiasis; positive HIV-antibody test at that time
- Has consistently refused ART because "We can't afford it"

CASE STUDY—cont'd

- Married to Jim, a former IV drug user, for 15 years until his recent death from AIDS-related complications
- Has two children, ages 10 and 13, who are both HIV-antibody negative
- Experiences fatigue and frequent oral and vaginal candidiasis outbreaks
- Expresses concern about the welfare of her children, who are at home with her sister, and says, "Maybe I should take better care of myself for them"

Objective Data

Physical Examination

- 5 feet 6 inches tall, 100 pounds, temperature 99.8° F (37.7° C)

Laboratory Studies

- $CD4^+$ T cell count 185/μl
- Viral load 25,328 copies/μl
- Hematocrit 30%

Collaborative Care

- Insertion of central venous catheter to be used for CMV treatment
- Trimethoprim/sulfamethoxazole
- Triple antiretroviral therapy: zidovudine with lamivudine (Combivir) and efavirenz (Sustiva)

Critical Thinking Questions

1. Why was Janelle's initial medical problem (esophageal candidiasis) unusual?
2. Why was trimethoprim/sulfamethoxazole ordered and what are its common side effects?
3. What diagnostic criteria for AIDS are present in Janelle's history?
4. Is there a potential advantage to Janelle's refusal to take antiretroviral drugs in the past? If so, why?
5. Women often put their children's welfare first. What barriers could this cause for Janelle's treatment? How can these problems be resolved?
6. What teaching needs to be done before Janelle is allowed to return home after this hospitalization? What referrals need to be made?
7. How can Janelle be helped to adhere to her medications?
8. What nursing interventions are immediately appropriate? What plans need to be made for continued nursing care after discharge?
9. Based on the assessment data presented, choose at least three appropriate nursing diagnoses. Are there any collaborative problems?

NCLEX EXAMINATION REVIEW QUESTIONS

The number of the question corresponds to the same-numbered objective at the beginning of the chapter.

1. Sources of emerging infections include all of the following except
   a. plants.
   b. animals.
   c. biologic warfare.
   d. antibiotic resistance.
2. Which of the following antibiotic-resistant organisms cannot be killed by normal hand soap?
   a. Vancomycin-resistant enterococci
   b. Methicillin-resistant *Staphylococcus aureus*
   c. Penicillin-resistant *Streptococcus pneumoniae*
   d. β-Lactamase producing *Klebisella pneumoniae*
3. Transmission of HIV from an infected individual to another occurs
   a. most commonly as a result of sexual contact.
   b. whenever drug users share injection equipment.
   c. in all infants born to women with HIV infection.
   d. only when there is a large amount of virus in the blood.
4. Following infection with HIV
   a. the virus replicates mainly in B lymphocytes before spreading to $CD4^+$ T cells.
   b. infection of monocytes may occur, but these cells are quickly destroyed by antibodies.
   c. the immune system is impaired predominantly by the eventual widespread destruction of $CD4^+$ T cells.
   d. a long period of dormancy develops during which HIV cannot be found in the blood and there is little viral replication.
5. Which of the following statements is false?
   a. Infection with HIV results in a chronic disease with acute exacerbations.
   b. Late-stage infection is called acquired immunodeficiency syndrome (AIDS).
   c. Untreated HIV infection can remain in the early chronic stage for a decade or more.
   d. Opportunistic diseases occur more often when the $CD4^+$ T cell count is high and the viral load is low.
6. A diagnosis of AIDS is made when an HIV-infected patient has
   a. a $CD4^+$ T cell count below 200/μl.
   b. an increasing amount of HIV in the blood.
   c. lipodystrophy with metabolic abnormalities.
   d. oral hairy leukoplakia, an infection caused by Epstein-Barr virus.
7. Screening for HIV infection generally involves
   a. laboratory analysis of blood to detect HIV antigen.
   b. electrophoretic analysis for HIV antigen in plasma.
   c. laboratory analysis of blood to detect HIV antibodies.
   d. analysis of lymph tissues for the presence of HIV RNA.
8. Antiretroviral drugs are used to
   a. cure acute HIV infection.
   b. decrease viral RNA levels.
   c. treat opportunistic diseases.
   d. decrease pain and symptoms in terminal disease.
9. Opportunistic diseases in HIV infection
   a. are usually benign.
   b. are generally slow to develop and progress.
   c. occur in the presence of immunosuppression.
   d. are curable with appropriate pharmacologic intervention.
10. Which of the following statements about metabolic side effects of ART is false?
    a. These are an annoying set of symptoms that are ultimately harmless.
    b. Changes in body shape and size are often difficult for patients to accept.
    c. Lipid abnormalities include increases of triglycerides and decreases in high-density cholesterol.
    d. Insulin resistance and hyperlipidemia can be treated with drugs to control glucose and cholesterol.
11. Which of the following eliminates the risk of transmission of HIV?
    a. Using sterile equipment to inject drugs
    b. Cleaning equipment used to inject drugs

c. Taking zidovudine (AZT, ZDV, Retrovir) during pregnancy
d. Using latex or polyurethane barriers to cover genitals during sexual contact

12. Of the following, which is the most appropriate nursing intervention to help an HIV-infected patient adhere to a treatment regimen?
a. "Set up" a drug pillbox for the patient every week.
b. Give the patient a videotape and a brochure to view and read at home.
c. Tell the patient that the side effects of the drugs are bad but that they go away after awhile.
d. Assess the patient's routines and find adherence cues that fit into the patient's life circumstances.

REFERENCES

1. Herlihy B, Maebius NK: *The human body in health and illness*, St Louis, 2003, Elsevier.
2. Pommerville JC: *Alcamo's fundamentals of microbiology*, Boston, 2004, Jones & Bartlett.
3. Emerging Infectious Diseases. Available at *www.cdc.gov/ncidod/diseases/eid/index.htm.*
4. Madoff LC, Kasper DL: Introduction to infectious diseases: host-pathogen interaction. In Kasper DL, Braunwald E, Fauci AS, et al, editors: *Harrison's principles of internal medicine,* New York, 2005, McGraw-Hill.
5. Goldrick BA: 21st century emerging and reemerging infections, *Am J Nurs* 104:67, 2004.
6. *www.who.int/csr/disease/avian_influenza/country/cases_table_2006_06_20/en/index.htm.*
7. Schneider E, Castro KG: Tuberculosis trends in the United States, *Tuberculosis* 83:21, 2003.
8. Krilov LR: Emerging infectious diseases in international adoptions: severe acute respiratory syndrome, avian influenza and measles, *Curr Opin Infect Dis* 17:391, 2004.
9. Sheff B: Multi-drug resistant microorganisms: still making waves, *Nursing* 33:59, 2003.
10. Kjonegaard R, Myers FE: Arresting drug-resistant organisms, *Nursing* 35:48, 2005.
11. Bock-Avalos S, Campbell V: Knocking out nosocomial infections, *Nursing* 34:24, 2004.
12. Furman CD, Rayner AV, Tobin EP: Pneumonia in older residents of long-term care facilities, *Am Fam Physician* 15:1495, 2004.
13. Thrupp L, Bradley S, Smith P, et al for the SHEA Long-Term-Care Committee: Tuberculosis prevention and control in long-term care facilities for older adults, *Infect Control Hospital Epidemiol* 25:1097, 2004.
14. Ungvarski P: The past 20 years of AIDS through the eyes of one nurse, *Am J Nurs* 101:26, 2001.
15. Centers for Disease Control and Prevention (CDC): Cases of HIV infection and AIDS in the United States, 2003. Available at *www.cdc.gov/hiv/surveillance.htm* (accessed April 22, 2006).
16. Public Health Agency of Canada: HIV/AIDS epi updates, 2005. Available at *www.hc-sc.gc.ca/* (accessed July 18, 2005).
17. World Health Organization (WHO): Access to HIV treatment continues to accelerate in developing countries, but bottlenecks persist says WHO/UNAIDS report, press release, June 29, 2005. Available at *www.who.int/3by5/progressreportJune2005/en/* (accessed April 22, 2006).
18. Facts at a glance: Regional/global HIV/AIDS statistics, 2004. Available at *www.globalhealthreporting.org* (accessed July 18, 2005).
19. Overview: Regional/global HIV/AIDS statistics, 2004. Available at *www.globalhealthreporting.org* (accessed April 22, 2006).
20. American Foundation for AIDS Research (amfAR): Gender-based violence and HIV among women: assessing the evidence, *Issue Brief* 1:3, 2005. Available at *www.amfar.org/cgi-bin/iowa/programs/publicp/index.html* (accessed July 18, 2005).
*21. Carr RL, Gramling LF: Stigma: a health barrier for women with HIV/AIDS, *J Assoc Nurses AIDS Care* 15:30, 2004.
22. Drug use and HIV: Fact Sheet 154, New Mexico AIDS InfoNet, 2005. Available at *www.aidsinfonet.org* (accessed April 22, 2006).
23. National Institute of Allergy and Infectious Diseases (NIAID): HIV Infection and AIDS: an overview, 2005. Available at *www.niaid.nih.gov/factsheets/hivinf.htm* (accessed July 18, 2005).
24. Centers for Disease Control and Prevention (CDC): HIV and its transmission, 2003. Available at *www.cdc.gov/hiv/pubs/facts/transmission.htm* (accessed April 22, 2006).
25. Cohen MS, Pilcher CD: Amplified HIV transmission and new approaches to HIV prevention, *J Infect Dis* 191:1391, 2005.
26. Centers for Disease Control and Prevention (CDC): Updated U.S. Public Health Service guidelines for the management of occupational exposures to HBV, HCV, and HIV and recommendations for postexposure prophylaxis, 2001. Available at *http://aidsinfo.nih.gov* (accessed July 18, 2005).
27. Centers for Disease Control and Prevention (CDC): How safe is the blood supply in the United States? 2003. Available at *www.cdc.gov/hiv/pubs/faq/faq15.htm* (accessed April 22, 2006).
28. Centers for Disease Control and Prevention (CDC): How is HIV passed from one person to another? 2003. Available at *www.cdc.gov/hiv/pubs/faq/faq16.htm* (accessed July 18, 2005).
29. Centers for Disease Control and Prevention (CDC): Public Health Service Task Force recommendations for use of antiretroviral drugs in pregnant HIV-1-infected women for maternal health and interventions to reduce perinatal HIV-1 transmission in the United States—February 24, 2005. Available at *http://aidsinfo.nih.gov* (accessed April 22, 2006).
30. AIDSinfo: The HIV life cycle, 2005. Available at *http://aidsinfo.nih.gov/other/factsheet.asp* (accessed July 18, 2005).
31. Paranjape RS: Immunopathogenesis of HIV infection, *Indian J Med Res* 121:240, 2005. Available at *www/icmr.nic.in/ijmr/2005/April/0405.pdf* (accessed April 22, 2006).
32. Centers for Disease Control and Prevention (CDC): USPHS/IDSA guidelines for the prevention of opportunistic infections in persons with human immunodeficiency virus, 2001. Available at *http://aidsinfo.nih.gov* (accessed July 18, 2005).
33. Centers for Disease Control and Prevention (CDC): Treating opportunistic infections among HIV-infected adults and adolescents, 2004. Available at *http://aidsinfo.nih.gov* (accessed April 22, 2006).
34. Centers for Disease Control and Prevention (CDC): Guidelines for the use of antiretroviral agents in HIV-infected adults and adolescents, 2005. Available at *http://aidsinfo.nih.gov* (accessed July 18, 2005).
35. Centers for Disease Control and Prevention (CDC): Advancing HIV prevention: new strategies for a changing epidemic—United States, 2003. Available at *www.cdc.gov/mmwr/preview/mmwrhtml/mm5215a1.htm* (accessed April 22, 2006).
36. Centers for Disease Control and Prevention (CDC): 1993 revised classification system for HIV infection and expanded surveillance case definition for AIDS among adolescents and adults, 1993. Available at *www.cdc.gov/hiv/surveillance.htm#Tools* (accessed July 18, 2005).
37. Centers for Disease Control and Prevention (CDC): Revised guidelines for HIV counseling, testing, and referral, 2001. Available at *http://aidsinfo.nih.gov* (accessed April 22, 2006).
38. Armington K: Integrating rapid HIV testing into fast-paced private practice settings, *PRN Notebook* 10:7, 2005.
39. O'Brien WA: Genotyping vs. phenotyping: Which test when? In *Resistance testing in HIV: An in-depth series, Clinical Care Options for HIV*, Northwestern University, Chicago, 2004.
40. Brown B: *First visit basics: initiating care for the HIV-infected patient*, Mountain Plains AIDS Education and Training Center, Denver, Colo, 2004.
41. Wolbach J, Jed SL, Johnson SC, et al: *A pharmacist's guide to antiretroviral medications for HIV-infected adults and adolescents,* Mountain Plains AIDS Education and Training Center, Denver, Colo, 2005. Available at *www.mpaetc.org* (accessed July 18, 2005).
42. St. John's Wort (hypericin): Fact Sheet 729, New Mexico AIDS InfoNet, 2004. Available at *www.aidsinfonet.org* (accessed April 22, 2006).
43. Alternative and complementary therapies: Fact Sheet 700, New Mexico AIDS InfoNet, 2005. Available at *www.aidsinfonet.org* (accessed July 18, 2005).
44. Bozzette SA: The economics of HIV in the HAART era, *Clinical Care Options for HIV*, Northwestern University, Chicago, 2004.
45. Smith KA: The continuing HIV vaccine saga: naked emperors alongside fairy godmothers, *Med Immunol* 4:6, 2005.
46. Brown BK, Darden JM, Tovanabutra S, et al: Biologic and genetic characterization of a panel of 60 human immunodeficiency virus type 1 iso-

*Nursing research–based reference.

lates, representing clades A, B, C, D, CRF01_AE, and CRF02_AG, for the development and assessment of candidate vaccines, *J Virol* 79:6089, 2005.

47. Rudy ET, Newman, PA, Duan N, et al: HIV vaccine acceptability among women at risk: perceived barriers and facilitators to future HIV vaccine uptake, *AIDS Educ Prevent* 17:253, 2005.
48. *STD/HIV risk assessment: A quick reference guide,* Mountain Plains AIDS Education and Training Center, Denver, Colo, n.d. Available at *www.mpaetc.org* (accessed April 22, 2006).
49. Centers for Disease Control and Prevention (CDC): Incorporating HIV prevention into the medical care of persons living with HIV, 2003. Available at *http://aidsinfo.nih.gov* (accessed July 18, 2005).
50. Bradley-Springer L, editor: *HIV symptom management*, Association of Nurses in AIDS Care (ANAC), Akron, Ohio, 2005.

*51. Whyte J, Standing T, Madigan E: The relationship between HIV-related knowledge and safe sexual behavior in African American women dwelling in the rural southeast, *J Assoc Nurses AIDS Care* 15:51, 2004.

52. U.S. Preventive Services Task Force: Screening for HIV: recommendation statement, *Ann Intern Med* 143:32, 2005.
53. American Foundation for AIDS Research (amfAR): The effectiveness of condoms in preventing HIV transmission, *Issue Brief,* 1:1, 2005. Available at *www.amfar.org/cgi-bin/iowa/programs/publicp/index.html* (accessed April 22, 2006).
54. Downing M, Riess TH, Vernon K, et al: What's community got to do with it? Implementation models or syringe exchange programs, *AIDS Ed and Prevention* 17:68, 2005.

*55. Duffy L: Suffering, shame, and silence: the stigma of HIV/AIDS, *J Assoc Nurses AIDS Care* 16:13, 2005.

56. Centers for Disease Control and Prevention (CDC): Adherence to potent antiretroviral therapy, 2004. Available at *http://aidsinfo.nih.gov* (accessed July 18, 2005).

*57. Russell J, Krantz S, Neville S: The patient-provider relationship and adherence to highly active antiretroviral therapy, *J Assoc Nurses AIDS Care* 15:40, 2004.

*58. Williams AB, Burgess JD, Danvers K, et al: Kitchen table wisdom: a Freirian approach to medication adherence, *J Assoc Nurses AIDS Care* 16:3, 2005.

59. The Americans with Disability Act, 42 U.S.C. § 1201 et seq. (1992 and 1994).
60. Norris A, Dreher HM: Lipodystrophy syndrome: the morphologic and metabolic effects of antiretroviral therapy in HIV infection, *J Assoc Nurses AIDS Care* 15:46, 2004.
61. Robinson FP: HIV lipodystrophy syndrome: a primer, *J Assoc Nurses AIDS Care* 15:15, 2004.

*Nursing research–based reference.

RESOURCES

Advancing HIV Prevention
Centers for Disease Control and Prevention
1-800-CDC-INFO
www.cdc.gov/hiv/partners/ahp.htm

AIDS Action
202-530-8030
www.aidsaction.org

AIDS Info
800-HIV-0440
http://aidsinfo.nih.gov

Association of Nurses in AIDS Care (ANAC)
800-260-6780
www.anacnet.org

CDC National Prevention Information Network (NPIN)
800-458-5231
www.cdcnpin.org

International AIDS Society–USA (IAS-USA)
415-544-9401
www.iasusa.org

Journal of the Association of Nurses in AIDS Care
800-462-6198
www.janacnet.org

National Association of People with AIDS (NAPWA)
240-247-0880
www.napwa.org

National HIV/AIDS Clinical Consultation Center
800-933-3413
www.ucsf.edu/hivcntr

National Minority AIDS Council (NMAC)
202-234-5120
www.nmac.org

National Native American AIDS Prevention Center (NNAAPC)
510-494-2051
www.nnaapc.org

For additional Internet resources, see the website for this book at *http://evolve.elsevier.com/Lewis/medsurg.*

The scientific mind does not so much provide the right answers as ask the right questions.

Claude Levi-Strauss

Cancer 16

Connie Engelking and Jormain Cady

LEARNING OBJECTIVES

1. Describe the prevalence, incidence, survival, and mortality rates of cancer in the United States.
2. Describe the processes involved in the biology of cancer.
3. Differentiate the three phases of cancer development.
4. Describe the role of the immune system related to cancer.
5. Describe the use of the classification systems for cancer.
6. Explain the role of the nurse in the prevention and detection of cancer.
7. Explain the use of surgery, chemotherapy, radiation therapy, and biologic and targeted therapy in the treatment of cancer.
8. Identify the classifications of chemotherapeutic agents and methods of administration.
9. Differentiate between teletherapy (external beam radiation) and brachytherapy.
10. Describe the effects of radiation therapy and chemotherapy on normal tissues.
11. Identify the types and effects of biologic and targeted therapy agents.
12. Describe the nursing management of patients receiving chemotherapy, radiation therapy, and biologic and targeted therapy.
13. Describe the nutritional therapy for patients with cancer.
14. Describe the complications associated with advanced cancer.
15. Describe the psychologic support interventions for cancer patients, cancer survivors, and family members.

KEY TERMS

benign neoplasms, p. 274
biologic therapy, p. 302
brachytherapy, p. 293
cancer, p. 271
carcinogens, p. 275
carcinomas, p. 279
chemotherapy, p. 285
hematopoietic stem cell transplantation, p. 304
malignant neoplasms, p. 274
metastasis, p. 276
oncogenes, p. 274
protooncogenes, p. 274
radiation, p. 292
sarcomas, p. 279
staging, p. 280
targeted therapy, p. 302
teletherapy, p. 293
vesicants, p. 286

Electronic Resources

Supplemental content related to Chapter 16 can be found . . .

Companion CD

- Stress-Busting Kit for Nursing Students
- NCLEX Examination Review Questions
- Comprehensive Glossary

Evolve Website

http://evolve.elsevier.com/Lewis/medsurg

- Content Updates
- Key Points (Printable and CD/MP3 Download)
- Concept Map Creator
- Expanded Audio Glossary
- Key Term Flash Cards
- Tables:
  - Neutropenic Diet
  - Precautions to Minimize Risks from Neutropenia
- Electronic Calculators
- WebLinks

Cancer is a group of more than 200 diseases characterized by uncontrolled and unregulated growth of cells. It is a major health problem that occurs in people of all ethnicities. Although cancer is often considered a disease of aging, with the majority of cases (76%) diagnosed in those over the age of 55 years, it occurs in people of all ages. An estimated 1,399,790 persons were diagnosed in 2006 (excluding basal and squamous cell skin cancers and carcinoma in situ except of the urinary bladder).[1] More than 1 million cases of basal and squamous cell skin cancers are diagnosed annually.[1] Overall cancer incidence rates have been relatively stable since 1992. The incidence of some cancers, such as colorectal, lung, and oral and pharyngeal cancers, have declined (largely as a

Reviewed by Barbara Owens, RN, PhD, OCN, Clinical Assistant Professor, University of Texas Health Science Center, San Antonio, Tex.; and Karen K. Swenson, RN, PhD (c), AOCN, Oncology Research Manager, Park Nicollet Institute, St. Louis Park, Minn.

result of preventive efforts). However, the incidence of other types of cancers, such as non-Hodgkin's lymphoma and skin cancers, is on the rise. Notably, the incidence of melanoma is rising faster than any other malignancy in the United States, which is a combined result of genetic predisposition and sun exposure.

Cancer incidence overall is higher in men than women. Gender differences in incidence and in death rates for specific cancers are presented in Tables 16-1 and 16-2 and the Gender Differences box. Although mortality rates from all cancers combined are on the decline, cancer is still the second most common cause of death in the United States (heart disease is the most common). However, in people less than 85 years of age, cancer is the leading cause of death. In 2006, an estimated 564,830 Americans died as a result of cancer, which is more than 1500 people per day.[1]

Both cancer incidence and death rates are disproportionately higher in African Americans than in whites and other minority groups (see Cultural and Ethnic Health Disparities box). These rates are especially high among male African Americans, who have a 25% higher incidence rate and 43% higher death rate than whites.[2] Differences in survival from cancer are attributed primarily to a combination of several factors, including poverty, difficult access to and poorer quality of health care, more comorbid conditions, and differences in tumor biology. In addition, African Americans are more likely to present with later stage disease than whites.[3]

Considerable progress has been made in controlling cancer for long periods of time. More than 10 million Americans are alive today who have a history of cancer. The 5-year survival rate is now 65% (an 11% gain over the past 20 years). This statistic represents Americans living with cancer, including those who are disease free, in remission, or undergoing treatment. (Cancer survivors are discussed at the end of this chapter.)

Statistics are helpful in describing the scope of cancer as a public health problem, but they cannot describe the combined physiologic, psychologic, and social impact of cancer on individual patients and their families. There is considerable apprehension associated with a cancer diagnosis, proportionally more so than with other chronic diseases such as heart disease. Despite advances in treatment and care, there continues to be a great deal of anxiety and fear associated with a diagnosis of cancer. Education of health care professionals and the public is essential to promote realistic attitudes about cancer and cancer treatment.

Nurses are in a strategic position to lead efforts at changing attitudes and behaviors about cancer. Furthermore, it is clearly an important nursing goal to implement educational interventions that will assist individuals to (1) understand, reduce, or eliminate their risk of cancer development; (2) comply with cancer management regimens; and (3) cope with the effects of cancer and related treatment. The nurse needs to be knowledgeable about specific types of cancer, treatment options, protocols for the management of side effects of therapy, and supportive therapies for individuals who are diagnosed with cancer. Understanding the principles of palliative and end-of-life care can position the nurse to help those patients whose cancers do not respond to treatment to experience a "good death."

BIOLOGY OF CANCER

Cancer encompasses a broad range of diseases of multiple causes that can arise in any cell of the body capable of evading regulatory controls over proliferation and differentiation. Two major dysfunc-

TABLE 16-1 Cancer Incidence by Site and Gender*

Male		Female	
Type	**%**	**Type**	**%**
Prostate	33	Breast	31
Lung	13	Lung	12
Colon/rectum	10	Colon/rectum	11
Urinary bladder	6	Uterus	6
Melanoma (skin)	5	Non-Hodgkin's lymphoma	4
Non-Hodgkin's lymphoma	4	Melanoma (skin)	4

Source: *Cancer facts and figures,* Atlanta, 2006, American Cancer Society.
*Numbers are estimates based on 2006 statistics excluding basal and squamous cell skin cancers and carcinoma in situ.

TABLE 16-2 Cancer Deaths by Site and Gender*

Male		Female	
Type	**%**	**Type**	**%**
Lung and bronchus	31	Lung and bronchus	26
Prostate	10	Breast	15
Colon/rectum	9	Colon/rectum	10
Pancreas	6	Pancreas	6
Leukemia	4	Ovary	6
Liver	4	Leukemia	4
Esophagus	4	Non-Hodgkin's lymphoma	3
Non-Hodgkin's lymphoma	3	Uterus	3

Source: *Cancer facts and figures,* Atlanta, 2006, American Cancer Society.
*Numbers are estimates based on 2006 statistics.

GENDER DIFFERENCES

Cancer

Men

- Mortality from lung cancer is higher in men than women
- More men than women die from cancer-related deaths each year
- Esophageal cancer is more prevalent in men than in women
- Cancer with the highest incidence among men is prostate cancer
- Men are more likely to develop liver cancer than women
- Head and neck cancer occurs more frequently in men than women
- Bladder cancer is at least three times as common in men as in women

Women

- Cancer with the highest death rate among women is lung cancer
- Nonsmoking women are at a greater risk than men of developing lung cancer
- Thyroid cancer is more prevalent in women than men
- Cancer with the highest incidence among women is breast cancer
- Women are less likely to have colon cancer screenings than men

CULTURAL AND ETHNIC HEALTH DISPARITIES

Cancer

- African Americans have the highest average annual death rate from all cancers compared to all other ethnicities. Whites have the second highest.
- Cancer incidence and death rates for men are highest among African Americans, followed by whites, Hispanics, and Asian/Pacific Islanders.
- Cancer incidence rates for women are highest among whites, followed by African Americans, Hispanics, and Asian/Pacific Islanders.
- However, cancer death rates for women are highest among African Americans, followed by whites, Hispanics, and Asian/Pacific Islanders.
- Prostate cancer incidence rates are about 3.5 times higher among African American men than among Asian/Pacific Islander men, and prostate cancer death rates are almost 6 times higher among African American men than among Asian/Pacific Islander men.
- Breast cancer incidence rates are about 2 times higher among white women than among Asian/Pacific Islander women, and breast cancer death rates are about 2.7 times higher among African American women than among Asian/Pacific Islander women.
- Overall, Asian women have low cervical cancer incidence rates, yet Vietnamese women have a high rate of cervical cancer.
- African American men have more cancers of the lung, prostate, colon, and rectum than do men of other ethnicities.
- Asian/Pacific Islander men and Hispanic men have the lowest mortality rates from lung cancer, while African American men have the highest rate.
- For women, African American women and white women have the highest rates of dying from lung cancer.

Source: Centers for Disease Control, 2005.

tions present in the process of cancer are defective cellular proliferation (growth) and defective cellular differentiation.

Defect in Cellular Proliferation

Normally, most tissues of the human adult contain a population of predetermined, undifferentiated cells known as stem cells. *Predetermined* means that the stem cells of a particular tissue will ultimately differentiate and become mature, functioning cells of that tissue and only that tissue.

Cell proliferation originates in the stem cell and begins when the stem cell enters the cell cycle (Fig. 16-1). The time from when a cell enters the cell cycle to when the cell divides into two identical cells is called the *generation time of the cell.* A mature cell continues to function until it degenerates and dies.

All cells of the body are controlled by an intracellular mechanism that determines when cellular proliferation is necessary. Under normal conditions, a state of dynamic equilibrium is constantly maintained (i.e., cellular proliferation equals cellular degeneration or death). Normally the process of cellular division and proliferation is activated only in the presence of cellular degeneration or death. Cellular proliferation will also occur if the body has a physiologic need for more cells. For example, a normal increase in white blood cell (WBC) count occurs in the presence of infection.

Another explanation for the phenomenon of proliferation control in normal cells is *contact inhibition.* Normal cells respect the boundaries and territory of the cells surrounding them. They will not invade a territory that is not their own. The neighboring cells are thought to inhibit cellular growth through the physical contact of the surrounding cell membranes. Cancer cells grown in tissue culture are characterized by loss of contact inhibition. These cells have no regard for cellular boundaries and will grow on top of one another and also on top of or between normal cells.

The rate of normal cellular proliferation (from the time of cellular birth to the time of cellular death) differs in each body tissue.

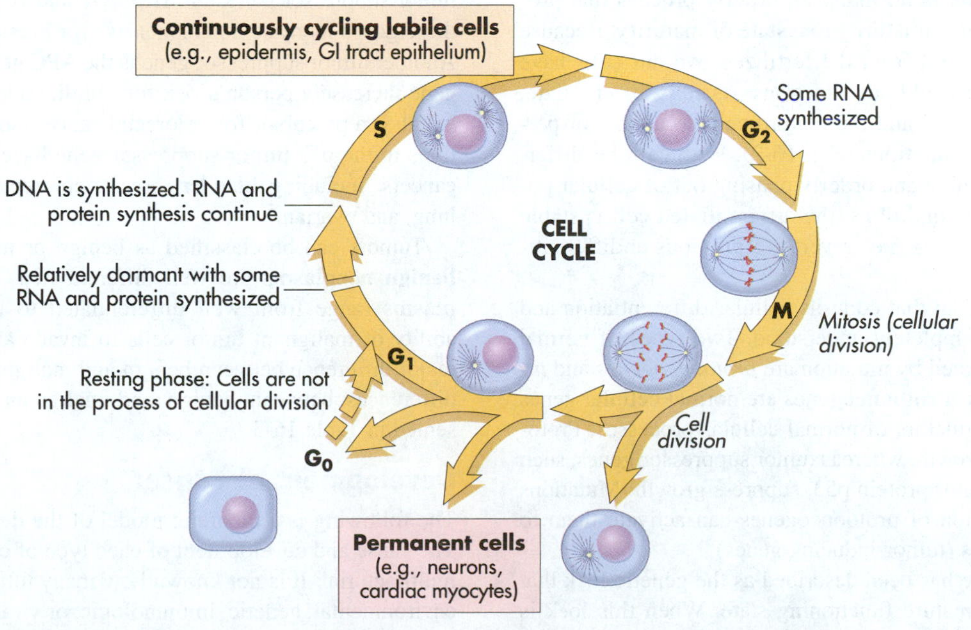

FIG. 16-1 Cell life cycle and metabolic activity. Generation time is the period from *M* phase to *M* phase. Cells not in the cycle but capable of division are in the resting phase (G_0).

In some tissues, such as bone marrow, hair follicles, and epithelial lining of the gastrointestinal (GI) tract, the rate of cellular proliferation is rapid. In other tissues, such as myocardium and cartilage, cellular proliferation does not occur or is slow.

Cancer cells usually proliferate at the same rate as the normal cells of the tissue from which they arise. However, cancer cells respond differently than normal cells to the intracellular signals that regulate the state of dynamic equilibrium. Cancer cells divide indiscriminately and haphazardly. Sometimes they produce more than two cells at the time of mitosis.

The stem cell theory proposes that the loss of intracellular control of proliferation results from a mutation of the stem cells. The stem cells are viewed as the target or the origin of cancer development. The deoxyribonucleic acid (DNA) of the stem cell is substituted or permanently rearranged. When this happens, the stem cell is mutated. Once the cell has mutated, one of three things can occur: (1) the cell can die, either from the damage resulting from the mutation or by initiating a programmed cellular suicide called *apoptosis;* (2) the cell can recognize the damage and repair itself; or (3) the mutated cell can survive and pass along the damage to its daughter cells. Mutated cells that survive have the potential to become malignant (i.e., cells with invasive and metastatic potential). The stem cell theory of cancer development is not complete because malignant stem cells can differentiate to form normal tissue cells.[4]

A common misconception regarding the characteristics of cancer cells is that the rate of proliferation is more rapid than that of any normal body cell. In most situations, cancer cells proliferate at the same rate as the normal cells of the tissue from which they originate. The difference is that proliferation of the cancer cells is indiscriminate and continuous. In this way, with each cell division creating two or more offspring cells, there is continuous growth of a tumor mass: $1 \rightarrow 2 \rightarrow 4 \rightarrow 8 \rightarrow 16$ and so on. This is termed the *pyramid effect.* The time required for a tumor mass to double in size is known as its *doubling time.*

Defect in Cellular Differentiation

Cellular differentiation is normally an orderly process that progresses from a state of immaturity to a state of maturity. Because all body cells are derived from the fertilized ova, all cells have the potential to perform all body functions. As cells differentiate, this potential is repressed and the mature cell is capable of performing only specific functions (Fig. 16-2). With cellular differentiation, there is a stable and orderly phasing out of cellular potential. Under normal conditions, the differentiated cell is stable and will not *dedifferentiate* (i.e., revert to a previous undifferentiated state).

The exact mechanism that controls cellular differentiation and proliferation is not completely understood. Two types of normal genes that can be affected by mutation are *protooncogenes* and *tumor suppressor genes.* **Protooncogenes** are normal cellular genes that are important regulators of normal cellular processes. Protooncogenes promote growth, whereas tumor suppressor genes, such as the gene for the tumor protein p53, suppress growth. Mutations that alter the expression of protooncogenes can activate them to function as **oncogenes** (tumor-inducing genes).

The protooncogene has been described as the genetic lock that keeps the cell in its mature functioning state. When this lock is "unlocked," as may occur through exposure to *carcinogens* (agents

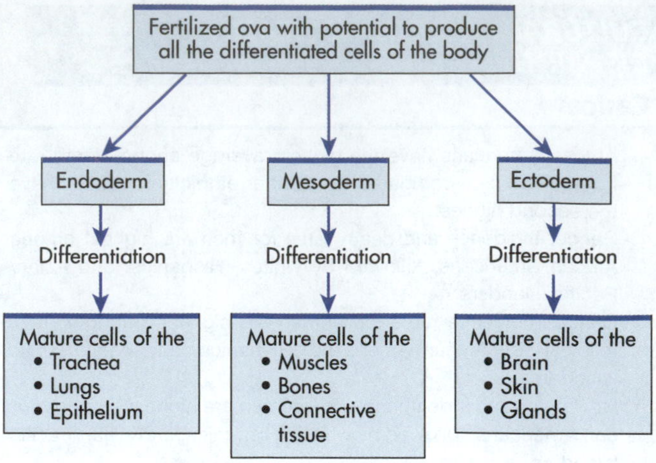

FIG. 16-2 Normal cellular differentiation.

that cause cancer) or oncogenic viruses, genetic alterations and mutations occur. The abilities and properties that the cell had in fetal development are again expressed. Oncogenes interfere with normal cell expression under some conditions, causing the cell to become malignant. This cell regains a fetal appearance and function. For example, some cancer cells produce new proteins, such as those characteristic of the embryonic and fetal periods of life. These proteins, located on the cell membrane, include carcinoembryonic antigen (CEA) and α-fetoprotein (FP). They can be detected in human blood by laboratory studies (see Role of the Immune System later in this chapter). Other cancer cells, such as small cell carcinoma of the lung, produce hormones (see Complications Resulting from Cancer, later in this chapter) that are ordinarily produced by cells arising from the same embryonic cells as the tumor cells.

Tumor suppressor genes function to regulate cell growth. Mutations that alter tumor suppressor genes render them inactive, resulting in a loss of their tumor-suppressing action. Examples of tumor suppressor genes are BRCA-1 and BRCA-2. Alterations in these genes increase a person's risk for breast and ovarian cancer. Another tumor suppressor gene is the APC gene. Alterations in this gene increase a person's risk for familial adenomatous polyposis, which is a precursor for colorectal cancer (see Chapter 43). Mutations in the p53 tumor suppressor gene have been found in many cancers, including bladder, breast, colorectal, esophageal, liver, lung, and ovarian.[5]

Tumors can be classified as benign or malignant. In general, **benign neoplasms** are well differentiated, and **malignant neoplasms** range from well differentiated to undifferentiated. The ability of malignant tumor cells to invade and metastasize is the major difference between benign and malignant neoplasms. Other differences between benign and malignant neoplasms are presented in Table 16-3.

Development of Cancer

The following is a theoretic model of the development of cancer. The cause and development of each type of cancer are likely to be multifactorial. It is not known how many tumors have a chemical, environmental, genetic, immunologic, or viral origin. Cancers may arise spontaneously from causes that are thus far unexplained.

TABLE 16-3 Comparison of Benign and Malignant Neoplasms

Characteristic	Benign	Malignant
Encapsulated	Usually	Rarely
Differentiated	Normally	Poorly
Metastasis	Absent	Capable
Recurrence	Rare	Possible
Vascularity	Slight	Moderate to marked
Mode of growth	Expansive	Infiltrative and expansive
Cell characteristics	Fairly normal; similar to parent cells	Cells abnormal, become more unlike parent cells

It is a common belief that the development of cancer is a rapid, haphazard event. However, the natural history of cancer is an orderly process comprising several stages and occurring over a period of time. These stages include initiation, promotion, and progression (Fig. 16-3).

Initiation. The first stage, *initiation,* is a mutation in the cell's genetic structure resulting from an inherited mutation (an error that occurs during DNA replication), or following exposure to a chemical, radiation, or viral agent. This altered cell has the potential for developing into a *clone* (group of identical cells) of neoplastic cells.

Initiation is irreversible, but not all altered cells go on to establish a tumor because many undergo apoptosis. An initiated cell is not yet a tumor cell because it has not established the ability to self-replicate and grow. The DNA alteration may remain undetected throughout the lifetime of an individual unless further events stimulate development of a tumor.

Many **carcinogens** (cancer-causing agents capable of producing cellular alterations) are detoxified by protective enzymes and are harmlessly excreted. If this protective mechanism fails, carcinogens can enter the cell's nucleus and alter DNA. The cell may die or repair itself. However, if cell death or repair does not occur before cell division, the cell will replicate into daughter cells, each with the same genetic alteration.[4]

Carcinogens may be chemical, radiation, or viral in nature. In addition, some genetic anomalies increase the susceptibility of individuals to certain cancers. Common characteristics of carcinogens are that their effects in the stage of initiation are usually irreversible and additive.

Chemical Carcinogens. Chemicals were identified as cancer-causing agents in the latter part of the eighteenth century when Percival Pott noted that chimney sweeps had a higher incidence of cancer of the scrotum associated with exposure to soot residues in chimneys. As the years passed, more chemical agents were identified as actual and potential carcinogens. Evidence indicated that persons exposed to certain chemicals over a period of time had a greater incidence of certain cancers than others. The long latency period from the time of exposure to the development of cancer makes it difficult to identify cancer-causing chemicals. Also, those chemicals that cause cancer in animals may or may not cause the same specific cancer in humans. Some chemicals are cancer causative in their environmental form, but others must first undergo certain changes to become carcinogenic.

Certain drugs have also been identified as carcinogens. Drugs that are capable of interacting with DNA (e.g., alkylating agents) and immunosuppressive agents have the potential to cause neoplasms in humans. The use of alkylating agents (e.g., cyclophosphamide [Cytoxan] and nitrogen mustard), either alone or in combination with radiation therapy, has been associated with an increased incidence of acute myelogenous leukemia in persons treated for Hodgkin's lymphoma, non-Hodgkin's lymphomas, and multiple myeloma. These *secondary leukemias* are relatively refractory to induction of remission with combination chemotherapy. Secondary leukemia has also been observed in persons who have undergone transplant surgery and who have taken immunosuppressive drugs.

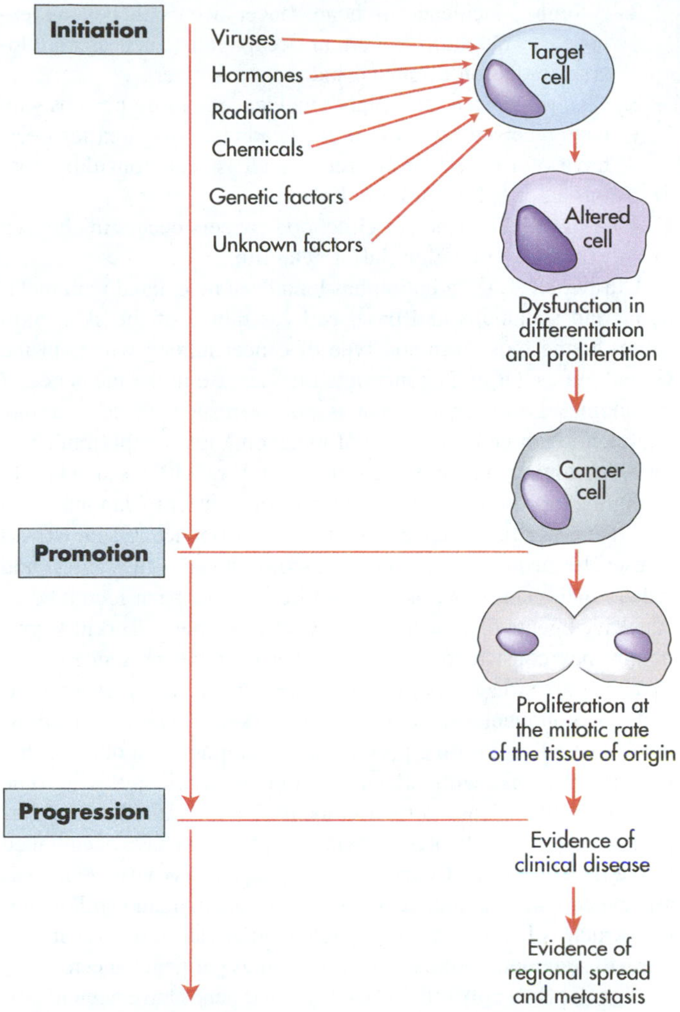

FIG. 16-3 Process of cancer development.

Radiation. Since the beginning of the twentieth century, it has been known that ionizing radiation can cause cancer in almost any human body tissue. Presently, the dose of radiation that causes cancer is not known, and there is considerable debate surrounding the effect of exposure to low-dose radiation over a period of time. When cells are exposed to a source of radiation, damage occurs to one or both strands of DNA. Certain malignancies have been correlated with radiation as a carcinogenic agent:

1. Leukemia, lymphoma, thyroid cancer, and other cancers increased in incidence in the general population of Hiroshima and Nagasaki after the atomic bomb explosions.

2. A higher incidence of bone cancer occurs in persons exposed to radiation in certain occupations, such as radiologists, radiation chemists, and uranium miners.
3. Thyroid cancer has a higher incidence in those persons who have received radiation to the head and neck area for treatment of a variety of disorders, such as acne, tonsillitis, sore throat, or enlarged thyroid gland.
4. A higher incidence of childhood cancers occurs in children exposed to radiation during fetal life.

Ultraviolet (UV) radiation has long been associated with melanoma and squamous and basal cell carcinoma of the skin. Skin cancer is the most common type of cancer among whites in the United States. Of great concern is the increase in the incidence of melanoma, a skin cancer that is poorly responsive to systemic treatment. Although the cause of melanoma is probably multifactorial, mounting evidence suggests that UV radiation secondary to sunlight exposure is linked to the development of melanoma.

Viral Carcinogens. Certain DNA and ribonucleic acid (RNA) viruses, termed *oncogenic,* can transform the cells they infect and induce malignant transformation. Viruses have been identified as causative agents of cancer in animals and humans. Burkitt's lymphoma has consistently shown evidence of the presence of the Epstein-Barr virus (EBV) in vitro. This virus is also present in infectious mononucleosis, but the explanation of why an infectious disease develops in some persons and a lymphoma in others is not known. Persons with acquired immunodeficiency syndrome (AIDS), which is caused by a virus, have a high incidence of Kaposi sarcoma (see Chapter 15). Other viruses that have been linked to the development of cancer include hepatitis B virus, which is associated with hepatocellular carcinoma, and human papillomavirus, which is believed to be capable of inducing lesions that progress to squamous cell carcinomas, such as cervical cancers.

Genetic Susceptibility. Cancer-related genes have been identified that increase an individual's susceptibility to development of certain cancers. For example, a woman who carries the genes BRCA1 or BRCA2 has a 40% to 80% risk of developing breast cancer in her lifetime. However, in reality, 95% of women who develop breast cancer do not possess these genes. Based on current knowledge, it is believed that only 10% of cancers have a strong genetic link.[4]

Promotion. A single alteration of the genetic structure of the cell is not sufficient to result in cancer. However, the odds of cancer development are increased with the presence of promoting agents. *Promotion,* the second stage in the development of cancer, is characterized by the reversible proliferation of the altered cells. Consequently, with an increase in the altered cell population, the likelihood of additional mutations is increased.

An important distinction between initiation and promotion is that the activity of promoters is reversible. This is a key concept in cancer prevention. Promoting factors include such agents as dietary fat, obesity, cigarette smoking, and alcohol consumption. Changing a person's lifestyle to modify these risk factors can reduce the chance of cancer development. Approximately half of cancer-related deaths in the United States are related to tobacco use, unhealthy diet, physical inactivity, and obesity.[1]

Several promoting agents exert activity against specific types of body tissues or organs. Therefore these agents tend to promote specific kinds of cancer. For example, cigarette smoke is a promoting agent in bronchogenic carcinoma and, in conjunction with alcohol intake, promotes esophageal and bladder cancers. Some carcinogens (complete carcinogens) are capable of both initiating and promoting the development of cancer. Cigarette smoke is an example of a complete carcinogen capable of initiating and promoting cancer.

A period of time, ranging from 1 to 40 years, elapses between the initial genetic alteration and the actual clinical evidence of cancer. This period, called the *latent* period, is now theorized to comprise both the initiation and the promotion stages in the natural history of cancer. The variation in the length of time that elapses before the cancer becomes clinically evident is associated with the mitotic rate of the tissue of origin and environmental factors. In most cancers, the process of developing cancer is years or even decades in length.

For the disease process to become clinically evident, the cells must reach a critical mass. A 1-cm tumor (the size usually detectable by palpation) contains 1 billion cancer cells. A 0.5-cm tumor is the smallest that can be detected by current diagnostic measures, such as magnetic resonance imaging (MRI).

Progression. *Progression* is the final stage in the natural history of a cancer. This stage is characterized by increased growth rate of the tumor, increased invasiveness, and spread of the cancer to a distant site **(metastasis).** Certain cancers seem to have an affinity for a particular tissue or organ as a site of metastasis (e.g., colon cancer spreads to the liver). Other cancers are unpredictable in their pattern of metastasis (e.g., melanoma). The most frequent sites of metastasis are the lungs, brain, bone, liver, and adrenal glands (Fig. 16-4).

Metastasis is a multistep process beginning with the rapid growth of the primary tumor (Fig. 16-5). As the tumor increases in size, development of its own blood supply is critical to its survival and growth. The process of the formation of blood vessels within the tumor itself is termed **tumor angiogenesis** and is facilitated by tumor angiogenesis factors produced by the cancer cells. As the tumor grows, it can begin to mechanically invade surrounding tissues, growing into areas of least resistance.

Certain subpopulations (segments) of tumor cells are able to detach from the primary tumor, invade the tissue surrounding the tumor, and penetrate the walls of lymph or vascular vessels for metastasis to a distant site. Unique capabilities of some tumor cells facilitate this process. First, rapid proliferation of malignant cells causes mechanical pressure leading to penetration of surrounding tissues. Second, certain malignant cells have decreased cell-to-cell adhesion in comparison with normal cells. This property equips these cancer cells with the mobility needed to move to the exterior of the primary tumor and to move within other vascular and organ structures. Some cancer cells produce metalloproteinase enzymes, a family of enzymes that are capable of destroying the basement membrane (a tough barrier surrounding tissues and blood vessels) not only of the tumor itself, but also of lymph and blood vessels, muscles, nerves, and most epithelial boundaries. Once free from the primary tumor, metastatic tumor cells frequently travel to distant organ sites via lymphatic and hematogenous routes. These two routes of metastasis are interconnected. Thus it is theorized that tumor cells metastasize via both routes.

Hematogenous metastasis involves several steps beginning with the penetration of blood vessels by primary tumor cells via the release of metalloproteinase enzymes (described previously). These tumor cells then enter the circulation, travel through the

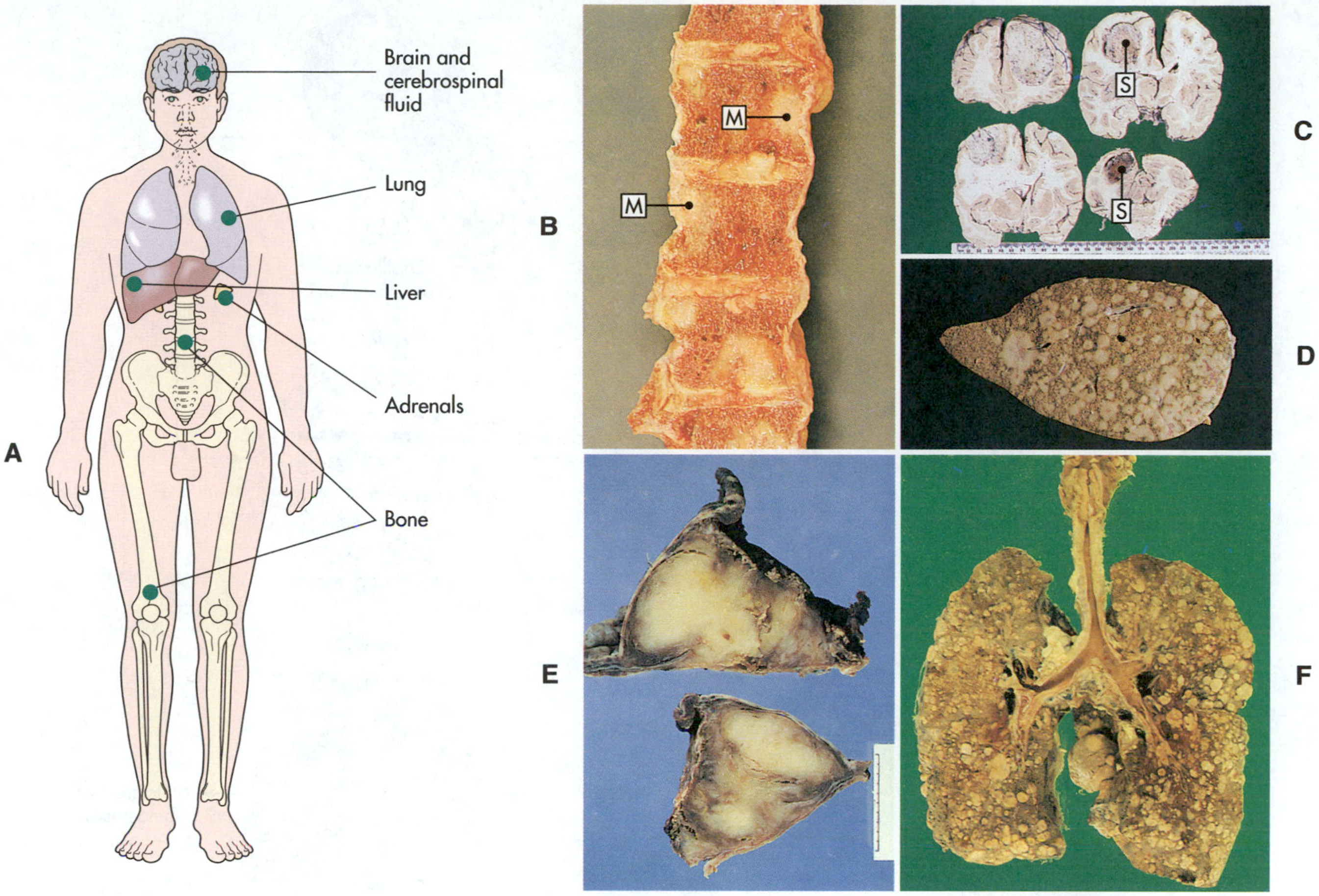

FIG. 16-4 Main sites of blood-borne metastasis. **A,** Sites of hematogenous metastasis. **B,** Metastasis in bone. **C,** Metastasis in brain. **D,** Metastasis in liver. **E,** Metastasis in adrenals. **F,** Metastasis in lungs. *M,* Lesions in vertebrae; *S,* metastasis from neoplasm of the stomach. (From Stevens A, Lowe J: *Pathology: an illustrated review in color,* ed 2, London, 2000, Mosby.)

body, and adhere to small blood vessels of distant organs. Tumor cells are then able to penetrate the blood vessels of these distant organs by releasing the same types of enzymes. Most tumor cells do not survive this process and are destroyed by mechanical mechanisms (e.g., turbulence of blood flow) and cells of the immune system. However, the formation of a combination of tumor cells, platelets, and fibrin deposits may protect some tumor cells from destruction in blood vessels.

In the lymphatic system, tumor cells may be "trapped" in the first lymph node confronted or they may bypass regional lymph nodes and travel to more distant lymph nodes, a phenomenon termed *skip metastasis.* This phenomenon is exhibited in malignancies such as esophageal cancers and is the basis for questions about the effectiveness of dissection of regional lymph nodes for the prevention of some distant metastases.[6] Tumor cells that do survive the process of metastasis must create an environment in the distant organ site that is conducive to their growth and development. This growth and development is facilitated by the ability of tumor cells to evade cells of the immune system and to produce a vascular supply within the metastatic site similar to that developed in the primary tumor site. Vascularization is critical to the supply of nutrients to the metastatic tumor and to the removal of waste products. Vascularization of the metastatic site is also facilitated by tumor angiogenesis factors produced by the cancer cells.

Role of the Immune System

This section is limited to a discussion of the role of the immune system in the recognition and destruction of tumor cells. (For a detailed discussion of immune system function, see Chapter 14.)

The immune system has the potential to distinguish cells that are normal (self) from abnormal (nonself) cells. For example, cells of transplanted organs can be recognized by the immune system as *nonself* and thus elicit an immune response. This response can ultimately result in the rejection of the organ. Similarly, cancer cells can be perceived as nonself and elicit an immune response resulting in their rejection and destruction. However, unlike transplanted cells, cancer cells arise from normal human cells and, although they are mutated and thus different, the immune response that is mounted against cancer cells may be inadequate to effectively eradicate them.

Cancer cells may display altered cell surface antigens as a result of malignant transformation. These antigens are termed **tumor-associated antigens** (TAAs) (Fig. 16-6). It is believed that one of the functions of the immune system is to respond to TAAs. The response of the immune system to antigens of the malignant cells is termed **immunologic surveillance.** Lymphocytes continually check cell surface antigens and detect and destroy cells with abnormal or altered antigenic determinants. It has been proposed that malignant transformation occurs continuously and that the

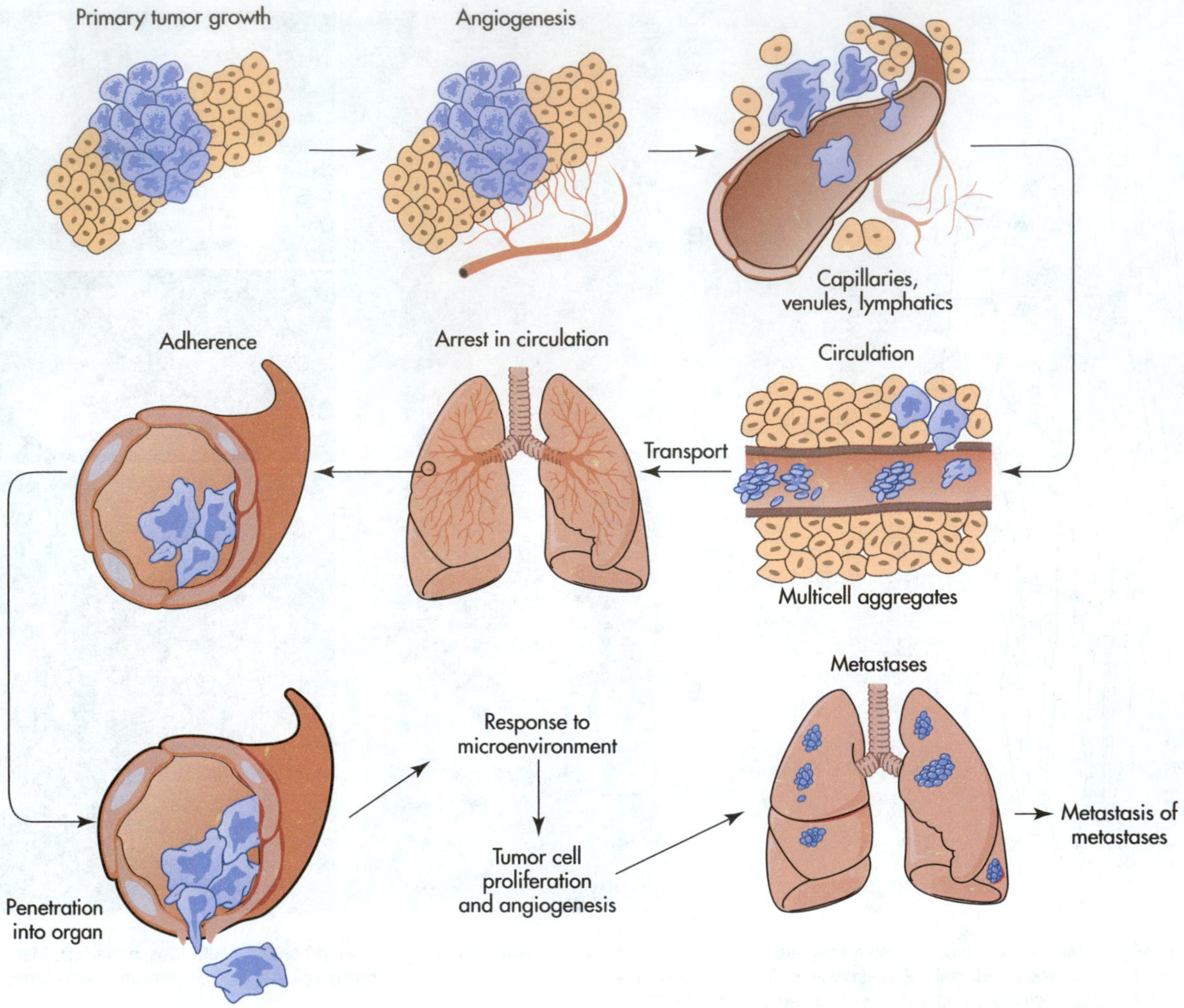

FIG. 16-5 The pathogenesis of cancer metastasis. To produce metastases, tumor cells must detach from the primary tumor and enter the circulation, survive in the circulation to arrest in the capillary bed, adhere to capillary basement membrane, gain entrance into the organ parenchyma, respond to growth factors, proliferate and induce angiogenesis, and evade host defenses.

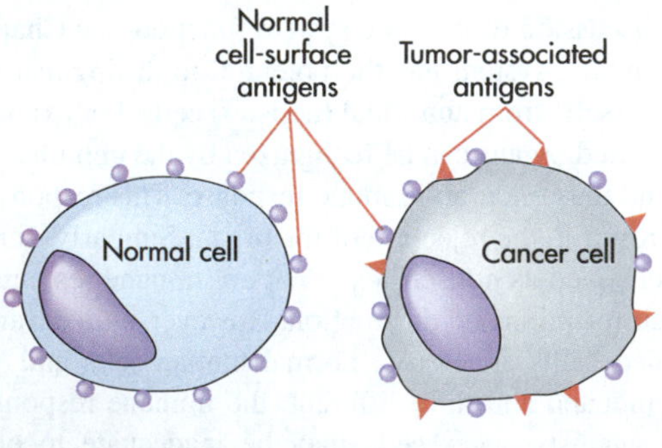

FIG. 16-6 Tumor-associated antigens appear on the cell surface of malignant cells.

malignant cells are destroyed by the immune response. Under most circumstances, immune surveillance will prevent these transformed cells from developing into clinically detectable tumors.

Virtually every cell type involved in normal immune responses and every function used to inactivate or remove antigens has been demonstrated in immune responses to tumors. These immune responses involve cytotoxic T cells, natural killer cells, macrophages, and B lymphocytes.

Cytotoxic T cells are thought to play a dominant role in resisting tumor growth. These cells are capable of killing tumor cells. T cells are also important in the production of cytokines (e.g., interleukin-2 [IL-2] and γ-interferon), which stimulate T cells, natural killer cells, B cells, and macrophages.

Natural killer (NK) cells are able to directly lyse tumor cells spontaneously without any prior sensitization. These cells are stimulated by γ-interferon and IL-2 (released from T cells), resulting in increased cytotoxic activity. Monocytes and macrophages have several important roles in tumor immunity (Fig. 16-7). Macrophages can be activated by γ-interferon (produced by T cells) to become nonspecifically lytic for tumor cells. Macrophages also secrete cytokines, including interleukin-1 (IL-1), tumor necrosis factor (TNF), and colony-stimulating factors. The release of IL-1, coupled with the presentation of the processed antigen, stimulates T lymphocyte activation and production. α-Interferon augments the killing ability of NK cells. TNF causes hemorrhagic necrosis of tumors and exerts cytocidal or cytostatic actions against tumor cells. Colony-stimulating factors regulate the production of various blood cells in the bone marrow and stimulate the function of various WBCs.

B lymphocytes can produce specific antibodies that bind to tumor cells and can kill these cells by complement fixation and lysis

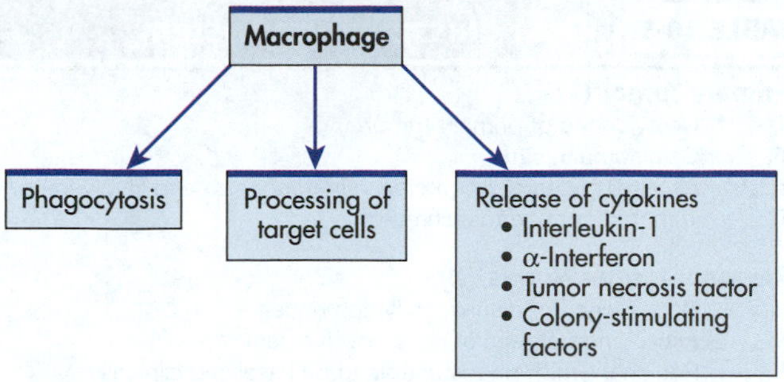

FIG. 16-7 Macrophage functioning in response to malignant target cells.

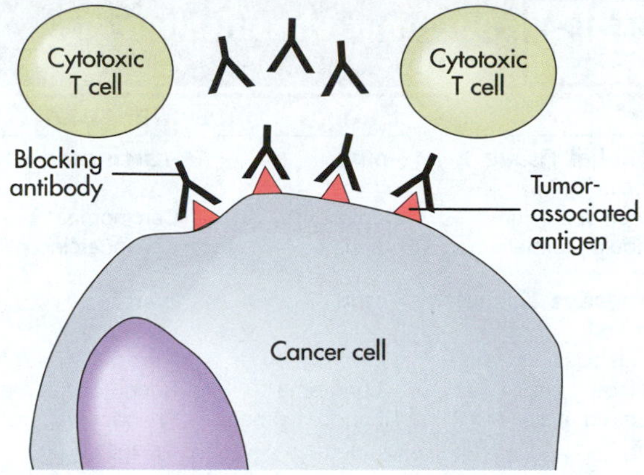

FIG. 16-8 Blocking antibodies prevent T cells from interacting with tumor-associated antigens and from destroying the malignant cell.

(see Chapter 13). These antibodies are often detectable in the serum and saliva of the patient. In some persons, antibodies that are specific for both the person's own tumor and a similar tumor in other persons have been found.

Escape Mechanisms from Immunologic Surveillance. The process by which cancer cells evade the immune system is termed *immunologic escape.* Theorized mechanisms by which cancer cells can escape immunologic surveillance include (1) suppression of factors that stimulate T cells to react to cancer cells, (2) weak surface antigens allowing cancer cells to "sneak through" immunologic surveillance, (3) the development of tolerance of the immune system to some tumor antigens, (4) suppression of the immune response by products secreted by cancer cells, (5) the induction of suppressor T cells by the tumor, and (6) blocking antibodies that bind TAAs, thus preventing their recognition by T cells (Fig. 16-8).

Oncofetal Antigens. *Oncofetal antigens* are a type of tumor antigen. They are found on both the surfaces and the inside of cancer cells, as well as fetal cells. These antigens are an expression of the shift of cancerous cells to a more immature metabolic pathway, an expression usually associated with embryonic or fetal periods of life. The reappearance of fetal antigens in malignant disease is not well understood, but it is believed to occur as a result of the cell regaining its embryonic capability to differentiate into many different cell types.

Examples of oncofetal antigens are carcinoembryonic antigen (CEA) and α-fetoprotein (AFP). CEA is found on the surfaces of cancer cells derived from the GI tract and from normal cells from the fetal gut, liver, and pancreas. Normally, it disappears during the last 3 months of fetal life. CEA was originally isolated from colorectal cancer cells. However, elevated CEA levels have also been found in nonmalignant conditions (e.g., cirrhosis of the liver, ulcerative colitis, and heavy smoking). Presently, the major value of CEA is its use as an indicator of the success of cancer treatment. For example, the persistence of elevated preoperative CEA titers after surgery indicates that the tumor is not completely removed. A rise in CEA levels after chemotherapy or radiation therapy may indicate recurrence or spread of the cancer.

AFP is produced by malignant liver cells, as well as fetal liver cells. AFP levels have also been found to be elevated in some cases of testicular carcinoma, viral hepatitis, and nonmalignant liver disorders. AFP has diagnostic value in primary cancer of the liver (hepatocellular cancer), but it is also produced when metastatic liver growth occurs. The detection of AFP is of value in tumor detection and determination of tumor progression.

Other examples of oncofetal antigens currently being studied are CA-125, found in ovarian carcinoma; CA-19-9, found in pancreatic and gallbladder cancer; and prostate-specific antigen (PSA), found in prostate cancer.

CLASSIFICATION OF CANCER

Tumors can be classified according to anatomic site, histology (grading), and extent of disease (staging). Tumor classification systems are intended to provide a standardized way to (1) communicate the status of the cancer to all members of the health care team, (2) assist in determining the most effective treatment plan, (3) evaluate the treatment plan, (4) serve as a factor in determining the prognosis, and (5) compare like groups for statistical purposes.

Anatomic Site Classification

In the *anatomic classification* of tumors, the tumor is identified by the tissue of origin, the anatomic site, and the behavior of the tumor (i.e., benign or malignant) (Table 16-4). **Carcinomas** originate from embryonal *ectoderm* (skin and glands) and *endoderm* (mucous membrane linings of the respiratory tract, gastrointestinal tract, and genitourinary [GU] tract). **Sarcomas** originate from embryonal *mesoderm* (connective tissue, muscle, bone, and fat). Lymphomas and leukemias originate from the hematopoietic system.

Histologic Classification

In **histologic grading** of tumors, the appearance of cells and the degree of differentiation are evaluated pathologically. For many tumor types, four grades are used to evaluate abnormal cells based on the degree to which the cells resemble the tissue of origin. Tumors that are poorly differentiated (undifferentiated) have a worse prognosis than those that are closer in appearance to the normal tissue of origin:

Grade I: Cells differ slightly from normal cells (mild dysplasia) and are well differentiated.

Grade II: Cells are more abnormal (moderate dysplasia) and moderately differentiated.

Grade III: Cells are very abnormal (severe dysplasia) and poorly differentiated.

Grade IV: Cells are immature and primitive *(anaplasia)* and undifferentiated; cell of origin is difficult to determine.

Cancer

TABLE 16-4 Anatomic Classification of Tumors

Site	Benign	Malignant
Epithelial Tissue Tumors*	**-oma**	**-carcinoma**
Surface epithelium	Papilloma	Carcinoma
Glandular epithelium	Adenoma	Adenocarcinoma
Connective Tissue Tumors†	**-oma**	**-sarcoma**
Fibrous tissue	Fibroma	Fibrosarcoma
Cartilage	Chondroma	Chondrosarcoma
Striated muscle	Rhabdomyoma	Rhabdomyosarcoma
Bone	Osteoma	Osteosarcoma
Nervous Tissue Tumors	**-oma**	**-oma**
Meninges	Meningioma	Meningeal sarcoma
Nerve cells	Ganglioneuroma	Neuroblastoma
Hematopoietic Tissue Tumors		
Lymphoid tissue		Hodgkin's lymphoma, non-Hodgkin's lymphoma
Plasma cells		Multiple myeloma
Bone marrow		Lymphocytic and myelogenous leukemia

*Body surfaces, lining of body cavities, and glandular structures.
†Supporting tissue, fibrotic tissue, and blood vessels.

Extent of Disease Classification

Classifying the extent and spread of disease is termed **staging.** This classification system is based on a description of the extent of the disease rather than on cell appearance. Although there are similarities in the staging of cancers, there are many differences based on a thorough knowledge of the natural history of each specific type of cancer.

Clinical Staging. The clinical staging classification system determines the anatomic extent of the malignant disease process by stages:

Stage 0: cancer in situ
Stage I: tumor limited to the tissue of origin; localized tumor growth
Stage II: limited local spread
Stage III: extensive local and regional spread
Stage IV: metastasis

Stage grouping is based on American Joint Committee on Cancer (AJCC) tumor site–specific rules. This classification system has been used as a basis for staging a variety of tumor types, including cancer of the cervix (see Chapter 54, Table 54-11) and Hodgkin's lymphoma (see Chapter 31, Fig. 31-15). Other malignant diseases (e.g., leukemia) do not use this staging approach. Clinical staging assignment is completed after the diagnostic workup but before treatment begins.

TNM Classification System. The *TNM classification system* represents the AJCC modification of the clinical staging of cancer originally developed by the International Union Against Cancer (UICC). The modification was made to achieve consistency with American medical practice. This classification system (Table 16-5) is used to determine the anatomic extent of the disease involvement according to three parameters: tumor size and invasiveness (T), presence or absence of regional spread to the lymph nodes (N), and metastasis to distant organ sites (M). (Examples of the TNM classification system can be found in Tables 28-16 and 52-6.) TNM staging cannot be applied to all malignancies. For example, the leukemias are not solid tumors and therefore cannot be staged using these guidelines. *Carcinoma in situ* has its own designation in the system (T_{is}) since it has all the histologic characteristics of cancer except invasion—a primary feature of the TNM staging system.

TABLE 16-5 TNM Classification System

Primary Tumor (T)	
T_0	No evidence of primary tumor
T_{is}	Carcinoma in situ
T_{1-4}	Ascending degrees of increase in tumor size and involvement
T_x	Tumor cannot be measured or found
Regional Lymph Nodes (N)	
N_0	No evidence of disease in lymph nodes
N_{1-4}	Ascending degrees of nodal involvement
N_x	Regional lymph nodes unable to be assessed clinically
Distant Metastases (M)	
M_0	No evidence of distant metastases
M_{1-4}	Ascending degrees of metastatic involvement of the host, including distant nodes
M_x	Cannot be determined

Note: For examples of TNM classification system applied to diseases, see Fig. 31-15, Table 28-16, and Table 52-6.

Staging of the disease can be performed initially and at several evaluation points. Clinical diagnostic staging is done at the completion of the diagnostic workup to determine the most effective treatment plan. Examples of diagnostic studies that may be performed to assess for extent of disease include radiologic studies, such as bone and liver scans; ultrasonography; computed tomography (CT); and MRI.

Surgical staging refers to the extent of the disease as determined by surgical excision, exploration, and/or lymph node sampling. For example, a laparotomy and a splenectomy may be performed in staging of Hodgkin's lymphoma. During a staging laparotomy, lymph node biopsies may be done and margins of any masses may be marked with metal clips. These clips are used as markers when radiotherapy is used as a treatment modality. Exploratory surgical staging, however, is being used less frequently as noninvasive diagnostic technology becomes increasingly sophisticated.

After the extent of the disease is determined, the stage classification is not changed. The original description of the extent of the tumor remains part of the original record. If additional treatment is needed, or if treatment fails, retreatment staging is done to determine the extent of the disease process prior to retreatment. "Restaging" classification (rTNM) is differentiated from stage at diagnosis as the clinical significance may be quite different.

In addition to tumor classification systems, other rating scales can be used to describe and document the status of patients with cancer at the time of diagnosis, treatment, and retreatment and at each follow-up examination. For example, the Karnofsky Functional Performance Scale describes patient performance in terms of functionality on a percentage basis (Table 16-6).

TABLE 16-6 Karnofsky Functional Performance Scale

Definitions	Percentage	Criteria
Able to carry on normal activity and to work; no special care needed	100	Normal; no complaints; no evidence of disease
	90	Ability to carry on normal activity; minor signs or symptoms of disease
	80	Normal activity with effort; some signs or symptoms of disease
Unable to work; able to live at home and care for most personal needs; varying amount of assistance needed	70	Ability to care for self; inability to carry on normal activity or do active work
	60	Occasional assistance necessary but ability to care for most needs
	50	Considerable assistance and frequent medical care necessary
Unable to care for self; requires equivalent of institutional or hospital care; disease may be progressing rapidly	40	Disabled; special care and assistance necessary
	30	Severely disabled; indication for hospitalization although death not imminent
	20	Very sick; hospitalization necessary; active supportive treatment necessary
	10	Moribund; fatal processes progressing rapidly
	0	Dead

PREVENTION AND DETECTION OF CANCER

The nurse plays a prominent role in the prevention and detection of cancer. Elimination of predisposing risk factors reduces the incidence of cancer and increases the survival of patients who have cancer. For example, following reduction in smoking rates, there was a decrease in lung cancer. Early detection and prompt treatment are directly responsible for increased survival rates in patients with cancer.[7] One important aspect is to educate the public to do the following:

1. Reduce or avoid exposure to known or suspected carcinogens and cancer-promoting agents, including cigarette smoke and sun exposure.
2. Eat a balanced diet that includes vegetables and fresh fruits (see Fig. 40-1 and Table 40-1), whole grains, and adequate amounts of fiber, and reduce the amount of fat and preservatives, including smoked and salt-cured meats containing high nitrite concentrations.
3. Participate in a regular exercise regimen (i.e., ≥30 minutes moderate physical activity 5 times weekly).
4. Obtain adequate, consistent periods of rest (at least 6 to 8 hours per night).
5. Have a health examination on a regular basis that includes a health history, a physical examination, and specific diagnostic tests for common cancers in accordance with the guidelines published by the American Cancer Society *(www.cancer.org)* (Table 16-7).
6. Eliminate, reduce, or change the perceptions of stressors and enhance the ability to effectively cope with stressors (see Chapter 9).
7. Know the seven warning signs of cancer (Table 16-8). (These actually detect fairly advanced disease.)
8. Learn and practice recommended cancer screenings on a timely basis (e.g., colonoscopy in average-risk people beginning at 50 years and every 10 years thereafter).
9. Learn and practice self-examination (e.g., testicular self-examination).
10. Seek immediate medical care if you notice a change in what is normal for you and if cancer is suspected. Early detection of cancer has a positive impact on prognosis.

When the public is educated about cancer, care should be taken to minimize the fear that surrounds the diagnosis. Teaching approaches that minimize anxiety and address the special needs of the learner or group are preferable. For example, older adults may have visual and hearing acuity deficits or difficulty processing information. For some, English may be a second language. Reinforcement with large-type print materials that include graphics and repetition of key concepts will increase the success of educational efforts for these groups. The goal of public education is to motivate learners to change their negative health behavior patterns to achieve and maintain an optimal state of health. Nurses play a significant role in meeting this goal. Although the general public can benefit from education, those at increased risk of cancer are the target population for educational cancer control efforts[8] (see Table 16-7). Nurses can have a definite impact in persuading people that a change in lifestyle patterns can have a positive influence on their health. To achieve the desired effect, nurses must recognize the challenge and proactively develop strategies to effectively teach cancer prevention and early detection principles.

Diagnosis of Cancer

When a patient has a possible diagnosis of cancer, it is a stressful time for the patient and the family. Patients may undergo several days to weeks of diagnostic studies. During this time fear of the unknown may be more stressful than the actual diagnosis of cancer.

While the patient is waiting for the results of the diagnostic studies, the nurse should be available to actively listen to the patient's concerns and skilled in techniques that will engage the patient and the family members or significant others in discussion about their cancer-related fears. It is important to recognize that their anxiety may arise from myths and misconceptions about cancer (e.g., cancer is a "death sentence," cancer treatment is worse than the illness). Correcting those misconceptions can help to minimize their anxiety. Nurses should also learn to recognize their own discomfort when faced with discussions about cancer. Therefore to protect themselves, they often use communication patterns that close off the interaction. It is important to avoid false reassurance that everything will be all right (e.g., "It's probably nothing"), redirecting the discussion (e.g., "Let's discuss that later"), and generalizing (e.g., "Everyone feels this way") as these are closed communication patterns that may shut off further communication with the patient.[9]

During this time of high anxiety, the patient may need repeated explanations regarding the diagnostic workup. Explanations should include as much information as needed by the patient and the family. The information should be given in clear, understandable terms and should be reinforced as necessary. Written information is helpful for reinforcement of verbal information.

TABLE 16-7 Screening Guidelines for Early Detection of Cancer in Asymptomatic People*

Site	Recommendation
Breast	Women 40 and older should have an annual mammogram and annual clinical breast examination (CBE) by a health care provider. Women ages 20–39 should have a CBE by a health care provider every 3 years. A monthly breast self-examination (BSE) is an option for women starting in their 20s. Women at increased risk (e.g., family history, genetic tendency) should talk with their doctors about the benefits and limitations of starting mammography screening earlier, having additional tests (i.e., breast ultrasound and MRI), or having more frequent exams.
Colon and rectum	Beginning at age 50, men and women should follow *one* of the examination schedules below: • Yearly fecal occult blood test (FOBT)† or fecal immunochemical test (FIT) • Flexible sigmoidoscopy every 5 years • Yearly FOBT† or FIT plus flexible sigmoidoscopy every 5 years‡ • Double-contrast barium enema every 5 years • Colonoscopy every 10 years
Prostate	Both the prostate-specific antigen (PSA) blood test and digital rectal examination (DRE) should be offered annually, beginning at age 50, to men who have at least a 10-year life expectancy. Men at high risk (African American men and men with a strong family history of one or more first-degree relatives [father, brothers] diagnosed at an early age) should begin testing at age 45. For both men at average risk and those at high risk, information should be provided about what is known and what is uncertain about the benefits and limitations of early detection and treatment of prostate cancer so that they can make an informed decision about testing.
Uterus	*Cervix:* Screening should begin 3 years after having vaginal intercourse but no later than 21 years of age. Conventional Pap test should be performed annually or every 2 years using liquid-based tests. Beginning at age 30, women who have had three normal Pap test results in a row may get screened every 2–3 years with either the conventional or liquid-based Pap test. Alternatively, cervical cancer screening with human papillomavirus (HPV) DNA testing and conventional or liquid-based cytology could be performed every 3 years. Women 70 years of age or older who have had three or more normal Pap tests in a row and no abnormal Pap test results in the last 10 years may choose to stop having cervical cancer screening. Women who have had a total hysterectomy may also choose to stop having cervical cancer screening, unless the surgery was done as a treatment for cervical cancer. *Endometrium:* At the time of menopause, all should be informed about the risks and symptoms of endometrial cancer, and strongly encouraged to report any unexpected bleeding or spotting to their health care providers. For women with or at high risk for hereditary nonpolyposis colon cancer (HNPCC), annual screening should be offered for endometrial cancer with endometrial biopsy beginning at age 35.
Cancer-related checkup	For individuals undergoing periodic health examinations, a cancer-related checkup should include health counseling and, depending on a person's age and gender, might include examinations for cancers of the thyroid, oral cavity, skin, lymph nodes, testes, and ovaries, as well as some nonmalignant diseases.

Source: *Cancer facts and figures,* Atlanta, 2006, American Cancer Society.
*These recommendations are for people at average risk for cancer. People at increased risk may need to follow a different screening schedule, such as starting at an earlier age or being screened more often.
†For FOBT, the take-home multiple sample method should be used.
‡The combination of yearly FOBT or FIT plus flexible sigmoidoscopy every 5 years is preferred over either of these options alone.

TABLE 16-8 Seven Warning Signs of Cancer

C hange in bowel or bladder habits
A sore that does not heal
U nusual bleeding or discharge from any body orifice
T hickening or a lump in the breast or elsewhere
I ndigestion or difficulty in swallowing
O bvious change in a wart or mole
N agging cough or hoarseness

A diagnostic plan for the person in whom cancer is suspected includes health history, identification of risk factors, physical examination, and specific diagnostic studies. (The specifics of the health history and the screening physical examination are presented in Chapter 4.)

The health history includes particular emphasis on risk factors, such as family or personal history of cancer, exposure to or use of known carcinogens (e.g., cigarette smoking, exposure to occupational pollutants or chemicals), diseases characterized by chronic inflammation (e.g., ulcerative colitis), and drug ingestion (e.g., hormone therapy, previous anticancer therapies). Other important information relates to dietary habits, ingestion of alcohol, lifestyle, and patterns and degree of coping with perceived stressors.

HEALTHY PEOPLE

Prevention and Early Detection of Cancer

- Limit alcohol use
- Get regular physical activity
- Maintain a normal body weight
- Obtain regular colorectal screening
- Avoid cigarette smoking and other tobacco use
- Get regular mammography screening and Pap tests
- Use sunscreen with a sun protection factor of 15 or higher
- Practice healthy dietary habits, such as reduced fat consumption and increased fruit and vegetable consumption

The physical examination should be thorough, and particular attention should be given to the respiratory system, the GI system (including the colon, rectum, and liver), the lymphatic system (including the spleen), the breasts, the skin, the reproductive system (testes and prostate gland in men; cervix, uterus, and ovaries in women), and the musculoskeletal and neurologic systems.

Diagnostic studies to be performed will depend on the suspected primary or metastatic site(s) of the cancer. (Specific procedures as they relate to each body system are discussed in the respective assessment chapters.) Examples of studies or procedures that may be included in the process of diagnosing cancer include the following:

1. Cytology studies (e.g., Papanicolaou [Pap] test, bronchial washings)
2. Tissue biopsy
3. Chest x-ray
4. Complete blood count, chemistry profile
5. Sigmoidoscopy or colonoscopy examination (including guaiac test for occult blood)
6. Liver function studies (e.g., aspartate aminotransferase [AST])
7. Radiologic studies (e.g., mammography, ultrasound)
8. Radioisotope scans (e.g., bone, lung, liver, brain)
9. CT scan (e.g., spiral)
10. Positron emission tomography (PET) scan[10]
11. Presence of tumor markers (e.g., CEA, AFP, PSA, CA-125) or genetic markers (e.g., BRCA-1, BRCA-2)
12. Bone marrow examination (if a hematolymphoid malignancy is suspected or to document metastatic disease)

Biopsy. The *biopsy* procedure is the only definitive means of diagnosing cancer and, as such, is essential in planning a treatment regimen for the patient. It involves the surgical acquisition of tissue from the suspicious area for histologic examination by a pathologist. A biopsy will determine whether the tissue is benign or malignant, the anatomic tissue from which the tumor arises, and the degree of cellular differentiation (i.e., how closely the cells resemble the normal cellular structure) of the cancer cells present in the tumor.

The procedure may be a needle or aspiration biopsy, an incisional biopsy, or an excisional biopsy. A *needle* biopsy is used to obtain cells and tissue fragments through a large-bore needle that is guided into the tissue in question (e.g., bone marrow aspiration; core biopsy of prostate gland, breast, liver, and kidney tissues). Cytologic analysis is then performed to determine the presence of tumor. *Incisional biopsy,* performed with a scalpel or dermal punch, is a common technique used for obtaining a tissue sample for making a diagnosis of cancer. The premise that incisional biopsy may contribute to the spread of cancer has not been proven.

Excisional biopsy involves removal of the entire tumor. It is usually used for small tumors (smaller than 2 cm), skin lesions, intestinal polyps, and breast masses. This procedure can be considered therapeutic as well as diagnostic. When a tumor is not easily accessible, a major surgical procedure (laparotomy, thoracotomy, craniotomy) is often necessary to obtain a piece of the tumor tissue. Biopsy specimens of the GI, respiratory, and GU systems can usually be obtained by endoscopic procedures.

COLLABORATIVE CARE

Goals and Modalities

The goal of cancer treatment is cure, control, or palliation (Fig. 16-9). Factors that determine the therapeutic approach are tumor cell type, location, and size and the systemic extent of disease. Other important considerations in determining the treatment plan are the patient's physiologic status (e.g., presence of comorbid illnesses), psychologic status, and personal desires (e.g., active treatment versus palliation of symptoms). These factors influence

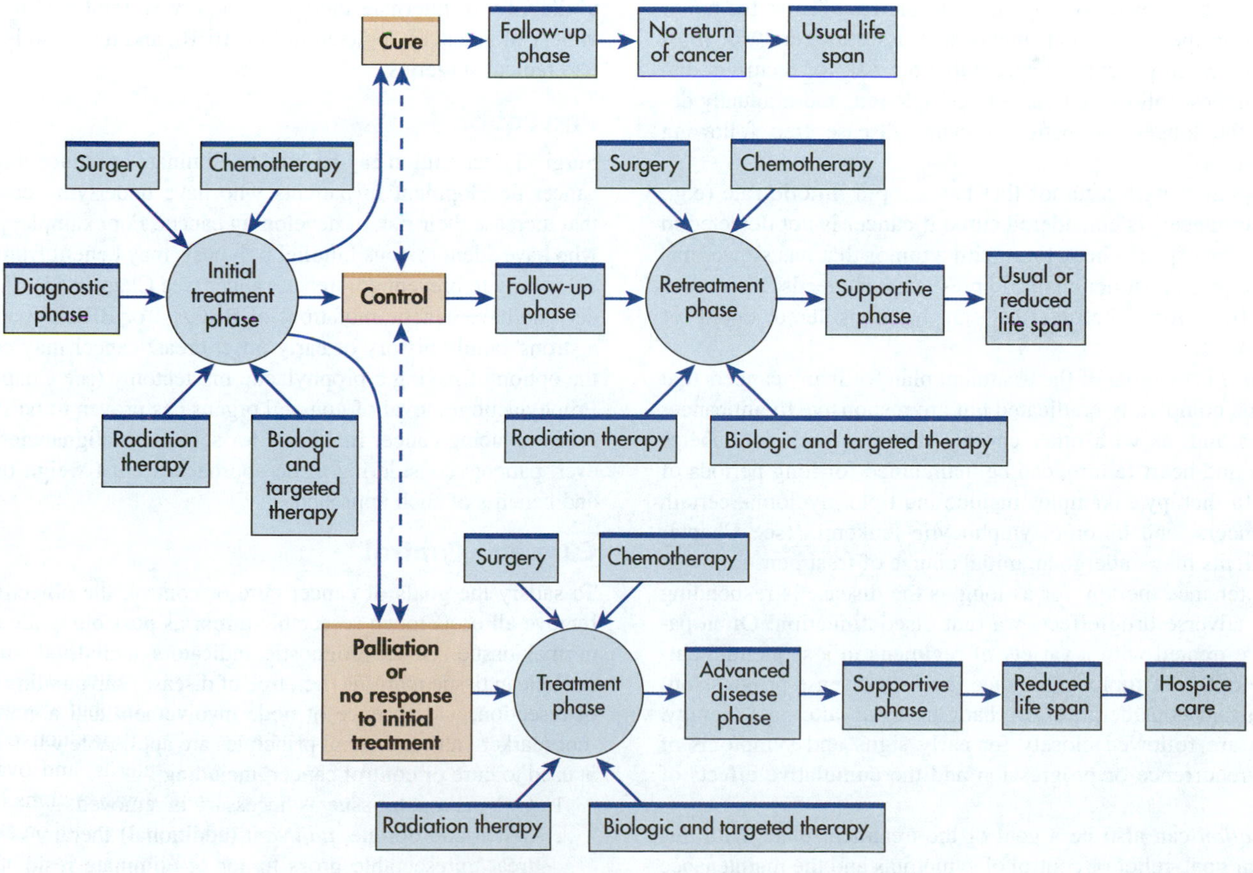

FIG. 16-9 Goals of cancer treatment.

the modalities chosen for treatment (i.e., surgery, radiation therapy, chemotherapy), how therapies are sequenced, and the length of time the treatment is prescribed. A variety of evidence-based cancer treatment guidelines have been developed to guide the formulation of appropriate treatment recommendations for individual patients. Some examples include guidelines of the American Society of Clinical Oncologists (ASCO) and the National Comprehensive Cancer Network (NCCN). These guidelines have been developed for both clinicians and consumers. They provide valuable patient education and treatment decision-making resources and are readily available online at *www.asco.org* and *www.nccn.org*.

When caring for the patient with cancer, the nurse should know the goals of the treatment plan to appropriately communicate with, educate, and support the patient. When *cure* is the goal, treatment is offered that is expected to have the greatest chance of disease eradication. Curative cancer therapy differs according to the particular cancer being treated and may involve local therapies (i.e., surgery or radiation) alone or in combination, with or without periods of adjunctive systemic therapy (i.e., chemotherapy). For example, basal cell carcinoma of the skin is usually cured by surgical removal of the lesion or by several weeks of radiation therapy. Acute promyelocytic leukemia in adults also has curative potential. The treatment plan for acute leukemias involves administration of several chemotherapy drugs on a scheduled basis over a period of 6 months to several years in sequential phases known as remission induction, remission consolidation, and maintenance therapy. Head and neck cancers can be cured with a combination of surgery and pre- or postoperative radiation, with or without chemotherapy.

Risk of recurrence over time may differ according to the tumor type. While there is no benchmark that assures "cure" for most malignancies, in general it appears that the risk for recurrent disease is highest following treatment completion, and gradually decreases the longer the patient remains disease free following treatment.

The patient with a tumor that has a rapid mitotic rate (e.g., testicular cancer) is considered cured if cancer is not detected in a 2-year time span. The patient with a tumor that has slower mitotic rate (e.g., postmenopausal breast cancer) needs 20 or more disease-free years before she can be considered cured of cancer.

Control is the goal of the treatment plan for many cancers that cannot be completely eradicated but are responsive to anticancer therapies and, as with other chronic illnesses such as diabetes mellitus and heart failure, can be maintained for long periods of time with therapy. Examples include multiple myeloma, certain lung cancers, and chronic lymphocytic leukemia (see Chapter 31). Patients may undergo an initial course of treatment followed by maintenance therapy for as long as the disease is responding or until adverse drug effects warrant discontinuation. Often patients are treated with a variety of regimens in a sequential pattern. Evidence of tumor resistance (such as disease progression) may warrant consideration of changing to an alternate therapy. Patients are followed closely for early signs and symptoms of disease recurrence or progression and the cumulative effects of therapy.

Palliation can also be a goal of the treatment plan. With this treatment goal, relief or control of symptoms and the maintenance of a satisfactory quality of life are the primary goals rather than cure or control of the disease process. It should be noted that palliation and disease control are not mutually exclusive. Radiation therapy or chemotherapy given to reduce tumor size and relieve subsequent symptoms such as the pain of bone metastasis or discomforts associated with lymphedema are examples of treatment in which palliation is the primary goal. Palliative care goals may be in effect for months to years.

The goals of cure, control, and palliation are achieved through the use of four treatment modalities for cancer: surgery, radiation therapy, chemotherapy, and biologic and targeted therapy. Each can be used alone or in any combination during initial treatment or as maintenance therapy as well as in retreatment if the disease does not respond or recurs after remission. For many cancers, two or more of the treatment modalities (known as "multimodality therapy" or "combined modality therapy") are used to achieve the goal of cure or control for a long period of time. Multimodality therapy has the benefit of being more effective (given it takes advantage of more than one mechanism of action), but often at the expense of some increased toxicity.

SURGICAL THERAPY

Surgery is the oldest form of local cancer treatment, and in the early days it was the only effective method of cancer diagnosis and treatment. The treatment of choice for many years was to remove the cancer and as much of the surrounding normal tissue as possible. What this approach did not fully consider was the ability of malignant cells to travel from the original tumor site to other locations, making surgical cure possible only when the tumor was localized and relatively small. Today, with improved surgical techniques, expanded knowledge of tumor metastasis patterns, and the availability of alternate therapies, surgery is employed to meet a variety of goals, as depicted in Fig. 16-10, and the trend is toward less radical surgeries.

Prevention

Surgical intervention can be used to eliminate or reduce the risk of cancer development in patients who have underlying conditions that increase their risk of developing cancer. For example, patients who have adenomatous familial polyposis may benefit from a total colostomy to prevent colorectal cancer (see Chapter 43). Individuals who have genetic mutations of BRCA-1 or BRCA-2 and have a strong family history of early-onset breast cancer may consider the option of having a prophylactic mastectomy (see Chapter 52). Prophylactic removal of nonvital organs has proven to be successful in reducing cancer incidence for selected malignancies. However, patients considering these approaches must weigh the risks and benefits of such approaches.

Cure and Control

To satisfy the goals of cancer cure or control, the objective is to remove all or as much resectable tumor as possible while sparing normal tissue. Good prognostic indicators include small tumor size, clean tissue margins (i.e., free of disease) surrounding the site of resection, and absence of node involvement and abnormal tumor marker values. Several principles are applicable when surgery is used to cure or control cancer, including

1. Only as much tissue as necessary is removed.
2. When appropriate, *adjuvant* (additional) therapy is used to treat unresectable gross tumor or eliminate residual undetectable micrometastases. The risk for metastatic disease is

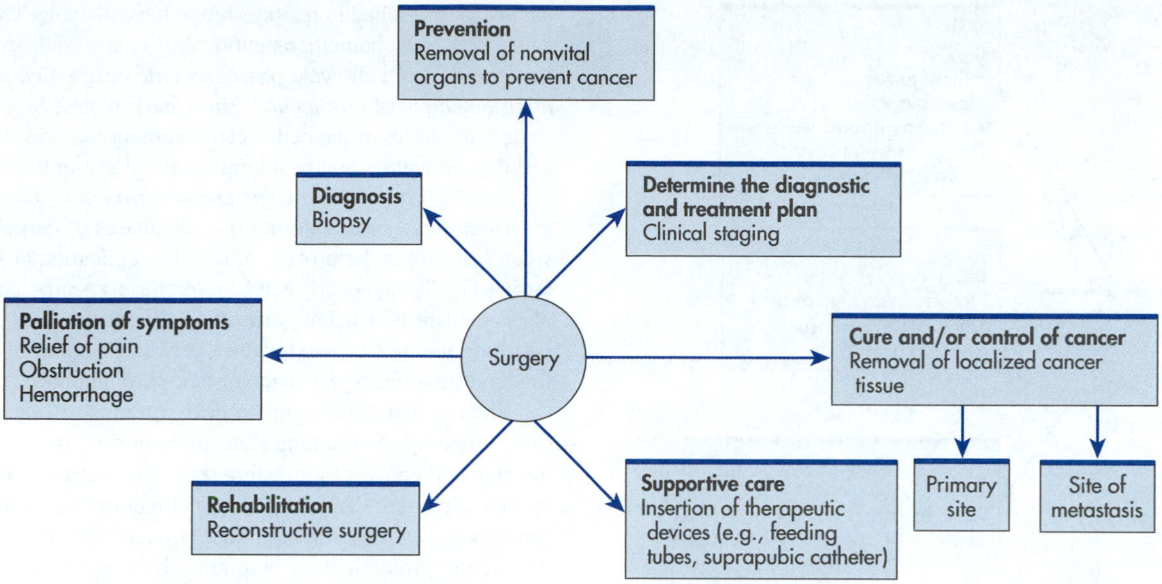

FIG. 16-10 Role of surgery in the treatment of cancer.

tumor dependent. The decision regarding adjuvant therapy is customized to the patient's tumor type, stage, level of risk for residual or metastatic disease, comorbidities, and patient preferences.

3. Preventive measures are used to reduce the surgical seeding of cancer cells.
4. The usual sites of regional spread may be surgically removed to evaluate presence of microscopic disease or to minimize the risk of recurrence.

Examples of surgical procedures used for cure or control of cancer include radical neck dissection, lumpectomy, mastectomy, pneumonectomy, orchiectomy, thyroidectomy, nephrectomy, hysterectomy and oophorectomy, and bowel resection.

A *debulking* or *cytoreductive procedure* may be used if the tumor cannot be completely removed (e.g., a tumor attached to a vital organ). When this occurs, as much tumor as possible is removed and the patient is given chemotherapy and/or radiation therapy. This type of surgical procedure can make chemotherapy or radiation therapy more effective since the tumor mass is reduced prior to the initiation of treatment.

Supportive and Palliative Care

When cure or control of cancer is no longer possible, the focus shifts to preservation of quality of life at the highest possible level for the longest possible period of time. Supportive care and palliation of symptoms are the primary goals.

Surgical procedures may be used to provide supportive care that maximizes bodily function or facilitates cancer treatment. Examples of supportive surgical procedures include the following:

1. Insertion of gastric feeding tube to maintain nutrition during head and neck cancer treatment
2. Creation of a colostomy to allow healing of rectal abscess
3. Suprapubic cystostomy for the patient with advanced prostatic cancer
4. Placement of venous access devices to deliver chemotherapy, pain medication, parenteral nutrition, blood products, and other supplements

Quality of life is also affected by distressing symptoms (e.g., pain). Examples of surgical procedures performed for palliation of symptoms associated with cancer include

1. Debulking of tumor or radiation therapy to relieve pain or pressure
2. Colostomy for the relief of a bowel obstruction (see Chapter 43)
3. Laminectomy for the relief of a spinal cord compression (see Chapter 61)

Rehabilitative Care

Cancer surgery can produce a change in body image and function. It is often difficult for the patient to cope with these changes in conjunction with a diagnosis of cancer while attempting to maintain usual lifestyle patterns. As the treatment for certain cancers becomes more effective, the length of time the patient must live with an alteration created by surgery will be increased. If quality of life is to be maintained, patients must be able to accept and cope with their altered body image and functional ability on a daily basis. Increasingly greater emphasis is being placed on the rehabilitative role of surgery in cancer care to increase the quality of life. Examples of rehabilitative surgical procedures include creation of a bladder reservoir at the time of cystectomy and breast reconstruction after a mastectomy. The insertion of appliances to facilitate functionality (e.g., spinal or joint stabilizing rods) and the creation of ostomies are other major contributions to rehabilitative management.

CHEMOTHERAPY

Chemotherapy (the use of chemicals as a systemic therapy for cancer) has been evolving over the past six decades. In the 1940s chemotherapy was in its infancy. Nitrogen mustard, a chemical warfare agent used in World Wars I and II, was used in the treatment of lymphoma and acute leukemia, and a folic acid antimetabolite (5-FU) was found to have antitumor activity. In the 1970s chemotherapy was established as an effective treatment modality for cancer. Chemotherapy is now a mainstay of cancer therapy used in the treatment of most solid tumors and hematologic malignancies (e.g., leukemias,

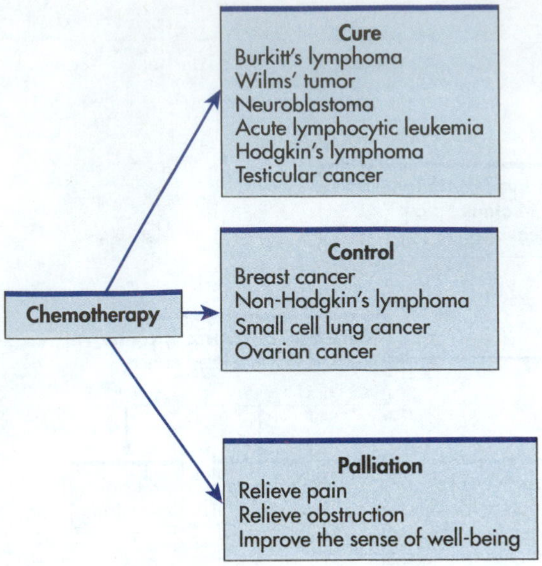

FIG. 16-11 Goals of chemotherapy.

lymphomas, myeloma, and myelodysplastic syndromes). Chemotherapy has evolved to become a therapeutic option that can offer cure for certain cancers, control other cancers for long periods of time, and in some instances offer palliative relief of symptoms when cure or control no longer is possible (Fig. 16-11).

The goal of chemotherapy is to eliminate or reduce the number of malignant cells present in the primary tumor and metastatic tumor site(s).[11] Several factors determine the response of cancer cells to chemotherapy:

1. *Mitotic rate of the tissue from which the tumor arises.* The more rapid the mitotic rate, the greater the potential for response. Examples of tumors with rapid proliferative rates include acute leukemia and small cell lung cancer.
2. *Size of the tumor.* The lower the tumor burden (i.e., smaller the number of cancer cells), the greater the potential for response.
3. *Age of the tumor.* The younger the tumor, the greater the response to chemotherapy. Newly developing tumors tend to have a greater percentage of proliferating cells.
4. *Location of the tumor.* Certain anatomic sites provide a protected environment from the effects of chemotherapy. For example, only a few drugs (nitrosoureas, bleomycin, temozolomide) cross the blood-brain barrier. New agents and techniques are being developed to more effectively cross this barrier.
5. *Presence of resistant tumor cells.* Mutation of cancer cells within the tumor mass can result in variant cells that are resistant to chemotherapy. Resistance can also occur because of the biochemical inability of some cancer cells to convert the drug to its active form. Malignant cells unresponsive to chemotherapy are essentially selected for during treatment, and pass this resistance on to daughter cells, diminishing response to further treatment over time.

Effect on Cells

The effect of chemotherapy is at the cellular level. All cells (cancer cells and normal cells) enter the cell cycle for replication and proliferation (see Fig. 16-1). The effects of the chemotherapeutic agents are described in relationship to the cell cycle. The two major categories of chemotherapeutic drugs are cell cycle phase–nonspecific and cell cycle phase–specific drugs. *Cell cycle phase–nonspecific chemotherapeutic drugs* have their effect on the cells during all phases of the cell cycle, including those in the process of cellular replication and proliferation and those in the resting phase (G_0). *Cell cycle phase–specific chemotherapeutic drugs* exert their most significant effects during specific phases of the cell cycle (i.e., when cells are in the process of cellular replication or proliferation during G_1, S_1, G_2, or M). Cell cycle phase–specific and cell cycle phase–nonspecific agents are often administered in combination with one another to maximize effectiveness by using agents that function by differing mechanisms and throughout the cell cycle.

When cancer first begins to develop, most of the cells are actively dividing. As the tumor increases in size, more cells become inactive and convert to a resting state (G_0). Because most chemotherapeutic agents are most effective against dividing cells, cells can escape death by staying in the G_0 phase. A major challenge in developing protocols is overcoming the effect of resistant resting and noncycling cells.

Classification of Chemotherapeutic Drugs

Chemotherapeutic drugs are classified in general groups according to their molecular structure and mechanisms of action (Table 16-9). Each drug in a particular classification has many similarities. However, there are major differences in how the drugs work and unique side effects associated with drugs in each class.

Preparation and Administration of Chemotherapy

It is very important to know the specific guidelines for administration of chemotherapeutic drugs. In addition, it is important to understand that drugs may pose an occupational hazard to health care professionals who do not follow safe handling guidelines. A person preparing, transporting, or administering chemotherapy may absorb the drug through inhalation of particles when reconstituting a powder in an open ampule and through skin contact if there is droplet exposure. There may also be some risk in handling the body fluids and excretions of persons receiving chemotherapy. Guidelines for the safe handling of chemotherapeutic agents have been developed by the Occupational Safety and Health Administration (OSHA) and the Oncology Nursing Society.[12,13] Only those personnel specifically trained in chemotherapy handling techniques should be involved with the preparation and administration of antineoplastic agents.

Methods of Administration

Chemotherapy can be administered by multiple routes (Table 16-10). The intravenous (IV) route is most common. Advances in drug formulation techniques are driving the reemergence of oral antineoplastic agents. Major concerns associated with the IV administration of antineoplastic drugs include venous access difficulties, device- or catheter-related infection, and *extravasation* (infiltration of drugs into tissues surrounding the infusion site) causing local tissue damage (Fig. 16-12).

Many chemotherapeutic drugs may be either irritants or **vesicants**. Irritants will damage the intima of the vein, casing phlebitis and sclerosis and limiting future peripheral venous access, but will not cause tissue damage if infiltrated. Vesicants, however, if inadvertently infiltrated into the skin, may cause severe local tissue

TABLE 16-9 ***DRUG THERAPY*** **Classification of Chemotherapy Drugs**

Mechanisms of Action	Examples
Alkylating Agents ***Cell Cycle Phase–Nonspecific Agents*** Damage DNA by causing breaks in the double-stranded helix; if repair does not occur, cells will die immediately (cytocidal) or when they attempt to divide (cytostatic)	nitrogen mustards: mechlorethamine (Mustargen), cyclophosphamide (Cytoxan, Neosar), chlorambucil (Leukeran), ifosfamide (Ifex), melphalan (Alkeran); busulfan (Myleran), dacarbazine (DTIC-Dome), temozolomide (Temodar), thiotepa (Thioplex)
Nitrosoureas ***Cell Cycle Phase–Nonspecific Agents*** Like alkylating agents, break DNA helix, interfering with DNA replication; cross blood-brain barrier	carmustine (BiCNU, Gliadel), lomustine (CeeNu), streptozocin (Zanosar)
Platinum Drugs ***Cell Cycle Phase–Nonspecific Agents*** Bind to DNA and RNA, miscoding information and/or inhibiting DNA replication, and cells die	oxaliplatin (Eloxatin), cisplatin (Platinol-AQ), carboplatin (Paraplatin)
Antimetabolites ***Cell Cycle Phase–Specific Agents*** Mimic naturally occurring substances, thus interfering with enzyme function or DNA synthesis. Primarily act during S phase. Purine and pyrimidine are building blocks of nucleic acids needed for DNA and RNA synthesis.	
• Interfere with purine metabolism	mercaptopurine (Purinethol), thioguanine, fludarabine (Fludara), pentostatin (Nipent), cladribine (Leustatin)
• Interfere with pyrimidine metabolism	capecitabine (Xeloda); cytarabine (Ara-C [Cytosar-U, DepoCyt]), fluorouracil (5-FU [Adrucil]), floxuridine (FUDR), gemcitabine (Gemzar)
• Interfere with folic acid metabolism	methotrexate (Rheumatrex, Trexall), pemetrexed (Alimta)
• Interferes with DNA synthesis	hydroxyurea (Hydrea, Droxia)
Antitumor Antibiotics ***Cell Cycle Phase–Nonspecific Agents*** Bind directly to DNA, thus inhibiting the synthesis of DNA and interfering with transcription of RNA	doxorubicin (Adriamycin, Rubex, Doxil), bleomycin (Blenoxane), mitomycin (Mutamycin), daunorubicin (Cerubidine, DaunoXome), dactinomycin (Cosmegen), idarubicin (Idamycin), plicamycin (Mithracin), epirubicin (Ellence), mitoxantrone (Novantrone), valrubicin (Valstar)
Mitotic Inhibitors ***Cell Cycle Phase–Specific Agents*** *Taxanes* Antimicrotubule agents that interfere with mitosis. Act during the late G_2 phase and mitosis to stabilize microtubules, thus inhibiting cell division.	paclitaxel (Taxol), docetaxel (Taxotere), paclitaxel albumin-bound particles (Abraxane)
Vinca Alkaloids Act in M phase to inhibit mitosis	vinblastine (Velban), vincristine (Oncovin), vinorelbine (Navelbine)
Topoisomerase Inhibitors ***Cell Cycle Phase–Specific Agents*** Inhibit the normal enzymes (topoisomerases) that function to make reversible breaks and repairs in DNA that allow for flexibility of DNA in replication	irinotecan (Camptosar), topotecan (Hycamtin), etoposide (VePesid), teniposide (Vumon)
Corticosteroids ***Cell Cycle Phase–Nonspecific Agents*** Disrupt the cell membrane and inhibit synthesis of protein; decrease circulating lymphocytes; inhibit mitosis; depress immune system; increase sense of well-being	cortisone (Cortone), hydrocortisone (Cortef), methylprednisolone (Medrol), prednisone, dexamethasone (Decadron)

Note: Many of these drugs are irritants or vesicants that require special attention during administration to avoid extravasation. It is important to know this information about a drug before administering it.

Continued

TABLE 16-9 DRUG THERAPY
Classification of Chemotherapy Drugs—cont'd

Mechanisms of Action	Examples
Hormone Therapy	
Cell Cycle Phase–Nonspecific Agents	
Antiestrogens	
Selectively attach to estrogen receptors, causing down-regulation of them and inhibiting tumor growth; also known as SERMs (selective estrogen receptor modulators)	tamoxifen (Nolvadex), fulvestrant (Faslodex), raloxifene (Evista), toremifene (Fareston)
Estrogens	
Interfere with hormone receptors and proteins	diethylstilbestrol (DES [Stilphostrol]), estramustine (Emcyt), estrogen (Menest), estradiol (Estrace)
Aromatase Inhibitors	
Inhibit aromatase, an enzyme that converts adrenal androgen to estrogen	anastrozole (Arimidex), letrozole (Femara), exemestane (Aromasin)
Miscellaneous	
Inhibits protein synthesis; enzyme derived from the yeast *Erwinia* used to deplete the supply of asparagines for leukemic cells that are dependent on an exogenous source of this amino acid	L-asparaginase (Elspar), *Erwinia* asparaginase
Causes changes in DNA in leukemia cells and degrades the fusion protein PML-RAR-α	arsenic trioxide (Trisenox)
Suppresses mitosis at interphase; appears to alter preformed DNA, RNA, and protein	procarbazine (Matulane, Natulan)

TABLE 16-10 DRUG THERAPY
Methods of Chemotherapy Administration

Method	Examples
Oral	cyclophosphamide (Cytoxan), capecitabine (Xeloda), temozolomide (Temodar)
Intramuscular	bleomycin (Blenoxane)
Intravenous	doxorubicin (Adriamycin), vincristine (Oncovin), cisplatin (Platinol), 5-FU, paclitaxel (Taxol)
Intracavitary (pleural, peritoneal)	radioisotopes, alkylating agents, methotrexate
Intrathecal	methotrexate, cytarabine
Intraarterial	DTIC, 5-FU, methotrexate
Perfusion	alkylating agents
Continuous infusion	5-FU, methotrexate, cytarabine
Subcutaneous	cytarabine
Topical	5-FU cream

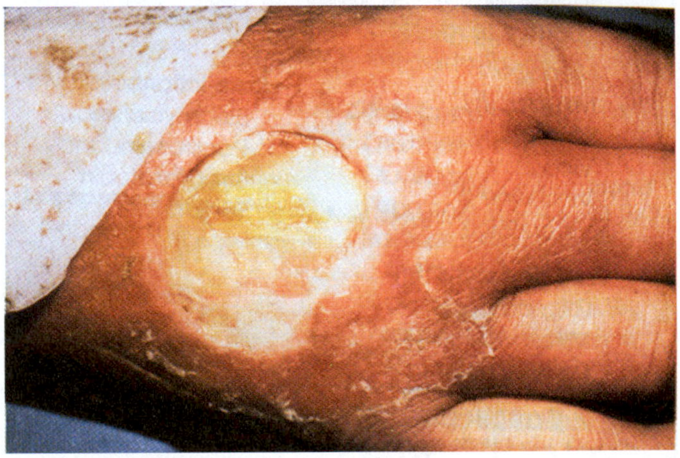

FIG. 16-12 Extravasation injury from infiltration of chemotherapy drug.

breakdown and necrosis. It is extremely important to monitor for and promptly recognize symptoms associated with extravasation of a vesicant and to take immediate action if it occurs. The infusion should be immediately turned off, and protocols for drug-specific extravasation procedures should be followed to minimize further tissue damage.[14]

Although pain is the cardinal symptom of extravasation, it has been known to occur without causing pain. Swelling, redness, and the presence of vesicles on the skin are other signs of extravasation. After a few days, the tissue may begin to ulcerate and necrose. The process has the potential to progress to a deep, wide crater that often warrants closure with skin grafts.[12]

To minimize the associated physical discomforts, emotional distress, and risks of infection and infiltration, IV chemotherapy can be administered by means of a *central vascular access device* (CVAD). CVADs are placed in large blood vessels and permit frequent, continuous, or intermittent administration of chemotherapy, biologic and targeted therapy, and other products, thus avoiding multiple venipunctures for vascular access. These devices are indicated in instances of limited vascular access, intensive chemotherapy, repetitive or continuous infusion of vesicant agents, and projected long-term need for vascular access. In addition to their usefulness in administration of chemotherapeutic agents, CVADs can also be used to administer additional fluids and electrolytes, blood products, parenteral nutrition, or other medications (e.g., antiemetics) and for venous blood sampling.

Advantages of CVADs include reduced need for venipuncture, decreased risk of extravasation injury, and facilitation of supportive therapies. The major disadvantage is risk of systemic infection,

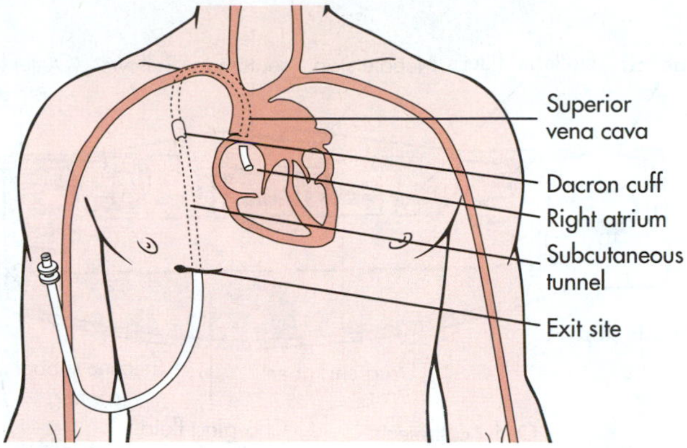

FIG. 16-13 Tunneled catheter placement. Note tip of the catheter in the right atrium.

particularly if the patient becomes immunosuppressed during therapy.[15] While the incidence is decreased, extravasation can still occur if there is displacement of or damage to the particular device being used for central venous access. Three major types of vascular access devices used in oncology patients are tunneled catheters, peripherally inserted central catheters (PICCs), and implanted infusion ports.

Tunneled Catheters

Tunneled catheters are single-, double-, or triple-lumen catheters approximately 90 cm in length with internal diameters ranging from 1 to 2 mm (Fig. 16-13). These catheters are inserted with the aid of local or general anesthesia through a central vein with the tip resting in the distal end of the superior vena cava or the right atrium of the heart. The other end of the catheter is tunneled through subcutaneous tissue and exits through a separate incision on the chest or abdominal wall. A Dacron cuff on the catheter serves to stabilize the catheter and may decrease the incidence of infection by impeding bacteria migration along the catheter beyond the cuff. Accurate placement must be verified by chest x-ray before the catheter can be used. Care requirements include cap change, cleansing, heparin flush, and dressing change. The exact frequency and procedures for these requirements vary from institution to institution. Complications with these catheters include occlusion, sepsis, bleeding, venous thrombosis, technical problems, and local infection at the exit site.

The Groshong catheter is a special type of tunneled central venous catheter device. The catheter is unique in that it is closed ended with a slit valve (or pressure-activated valve) on the side of the catheter near the distal end. This valve opens with infusion, flushing, or aspirating blood. When not being used, the valve is at rest and closed, preventing the backflow of blood or the entry of air. This precludes the need for heparin flushing or clamping.

Peripherally Inserted Central Venous Catheters. Venous PICCs are single- or double-lumen, nontunneled, polymer catheters that are primarily used in cancer care for immediate central venous access or when the need for infusion therapy is beyond the capacity of the patient's existing, long-term venous access device (Fig. 16-14). These catheters are used for short-term IV therapy, frequent administration of blood products, blood drawing, and intermittent or continuous drug infusions. A physician or a specially trained nurse places these catheters.

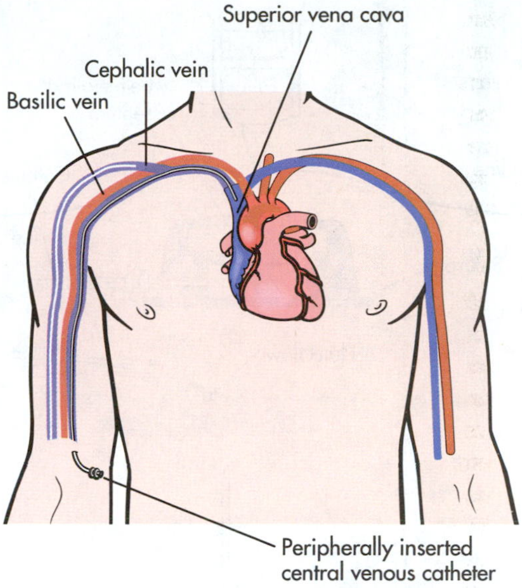

FIG. 16-14 Placement of peripherally inserted central venous catheter (PICC).

PICC lines are inserted at or just above the antecubital fossa and advanced to a position with the tip ending in the distal one third of the superior vena cava. These lines are up to 60 cm in length with gauges ranging from 24 to 16. They can be in place for up to 6 months. The technique for placement of a PICC line involves insertion of the catheter through a needle with the use of a guidewire or forceps to advance the line.

Complications of PICC lines include catheter occlusion and phlebitis. A thrombolytic agent can be used to lyse obstructions. If phlebitis occurs, it usually appears within 7 to 10 days following insertion. Signs of phlebitis include redness, edema, and tenderness along the track of the catheter line. The catheter should be removed, and the tip of the catheter must be cultured. The arm in which a PICC is in place should not be used for blood pressures or blood drawing.

Implanted Infusion Ports. Implanted infusion ports consist of a central venous catheter connected to an implanted, single or double subcutaneous injection port (Fig. 16-15). The catheter is placed into the desired vein and the other end is connected to a port that is sutured to the chest wall muscle and surgically implanted in a subcutaneous pocket on the chest wall. The port consists of a metal sheath with a self-sealing silicone septum. It is accessed via the septum by means of a special Huber-point needle that has a deflected tip to prevent coring of the septum. Huber-point needles are also available with the tip at a 90-degree angle for longer infusions. Care requirements include regular flushing. Complications attributed to implanted infusion ports include clotting, catheter migration, infection, bleeding, thrombosis, air embolism, and infection at the exit site or in the pocket. Formation of "sludge" (accumulation of clotted blood and drug precipitate) may also occur within the port septum.

Infusion Pumps. Infusion pumps are used primarily for the continuous infusion of chemotherapy by IV, subcutaneous, intraarterial, and epidural routes. Infusion pumps can be worn externally or implanted surgically. The various types of external infusion pumps differ in terms of their mechanisms of action, components, and capabilities.

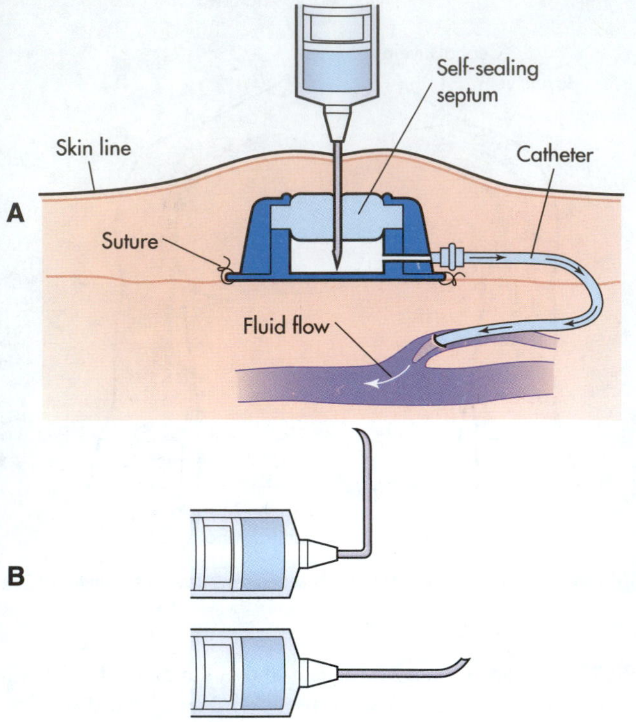

FIG. 16-15 **A,** Cross section of implantable port displaying access of the port with the Huber-point needle. Note the deflected point of the Huber-point needle, which prevents coring of the port's septum. **B,** Two Huber-point needles used to enter the implanted port. The 90-degree needle is used for top-entry ports for continuous infusion.

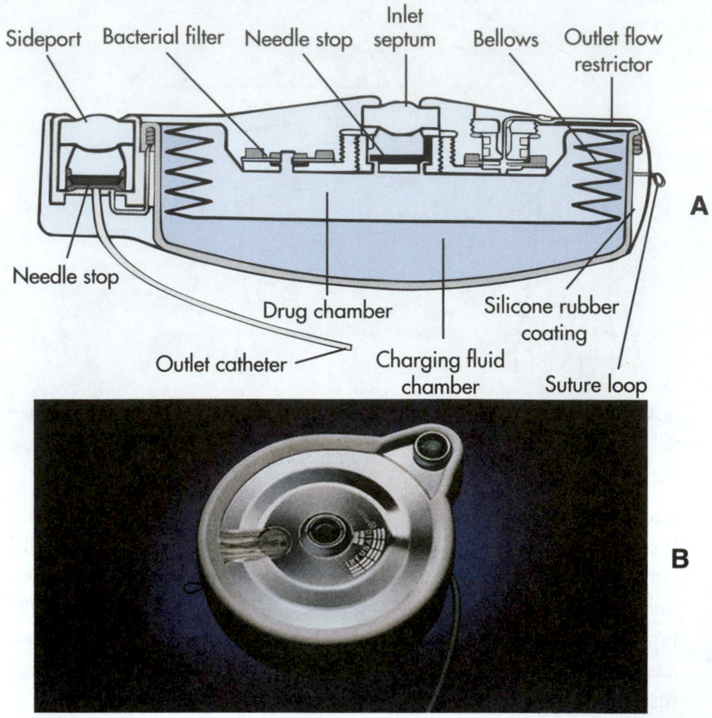

FIG. 16-16 **A,** Cross section of the implantable pump displaying its two chambers: the drug chamber (inner) and the charging fluid chamber (outer). As the drug chamber is filled, the bellows expand, compressing the charging fluid in the outer chamber. The resulting increased pressure in the outer chamber forces the drug through a membrane filter and preset flow restrictor, thus ensuring a nearly constant flow. **B,** Infusaid pump.

Implanted infusion pumps are used primarily for intraarterial administration of chemotherapy (Fig. 16-16). This approach permits continuous infusion of the chemotherapeutic agent directly to the area of the tumor while sparing the patient the systemic effects of the drug. Some implanted pumps have two silicone septa. The second septum can be used for bolus medication administration. The most common use of this method of chemotherapy administration has been hepatic artery infusion in the treatment of liver metastasis, usually from primary colorectal cancer.

Implanted pumps also consist of a catheter that is threaded into the designated artery. The catheter is attached to a pump apparatus that consists of two chambers: an inner chamber that serves as the drug reservoir and an outer chamber that contains vapor pressure providing a source of power for the pump. The pump is implanted surgically in a subcutaneous pocket. Access to the pump is via a silicone septum with a Huber-point needle. Flow rate of the pump can be affected by drug concentration, the length and diameter of the Silastic catheter, and the patient's body temperature. Thus dose alterations may be required if the patient experiences a change in temperature or travels to higher altitudes. Complications that have been associated with implanted infusion pumps include infection, thrombosis, clotting of the catheter, and pump malfunction.

Other access devices used in the treatment of the person with cancer include the Tenckhoff catheter used in the administration of intraperitoneal chemotherapy and the Ommaya reservoir, which delivers agents directly to the central nervous system (CNS).

Regional Chemotherapy Administration

Regional treatment with chemotherapy involves the delivery of the drug directly to the tumor site. The advantage of administering chemotherapy by this method is that higher concentrations of the drug can be delivered to the tumor with reduced systemic toxicity. Several regional delivery methods have been developed, including intraarterial, intraperitoneal, intrathecal or intraventricular, and intravesical bladder chemotherapy.

Intraarterial Chemotherapy. Intraarterial chemotherapy delivers the drug to the tumor via the arterial vessel supplying the tumor. This method has been used for the treatment of osteogenic sarcoma; cancers of the head and neck, bladder, brain, and cervix; melanoma; primary liver cancer; and metastatic liver disease. One method of intraarterial drug delivery involves the surgical placement of a catheter that is subsequently connected to an external infusion pump or an implanted infusion pump for infusion of the chemotherapeutic agent. Generally, intraarterial chemotherapy results in reduced systemic toxicity. The type of toxicity experienced by the patient depends on the site of the tumor being treated.

Intraperitoneal Chemotherapy. Intraperitoneal chemotherapy involves the delivery of chemotherapy to the peritoneal cavity for treatment of peritoneal metastases from primary colorectal and ovarian cancers and malignant ascites. Temporary Silastic catheters (Tenckhoff, Hickman, and Groshong) are percutaneously or surgically placed into the peritoneal cavity for short-term administration of chemotherapy. Alternatively, an implanted port can be used to administer chemotherapy intraperitoneally. Chemotherapy is generally infused into the peritoneum in 1 to 2 L of fluid and allowed to "dwell" in the peritoneum for a period of 1 to 4 hours. Following the "dwell time," the fluid is usually drained from the peritoneum. Complications of peritoneal chemotherapy include abdominal pain; catheter occlusion, dislodgement, and migration; and infection.

Intrathecal or Intraventricular Chemotherapy. Cancers that metastasize to the CNS—most commonly breast, lung, and GI tumors, leukemia, and lymphoma—are difficult to treat because the blood-brain barrier often prevents distribution of chemotherapy to this area. One method used to treat metastasis to the CNS is intrathecal chemotherapy. This method involves a lumbar puncture and injection of chemotherapy into the subarachnoid space. However, this method has resulted in incomplete distribution of the drug in the CNS, particularly to the cisternal and ventricular areas.

To ensure more uniform distribution of chemotherapy to the cisternal and ventricular areas, an Ommaya reservoir is often inserted. An Ommaya reservoir is a Silastic, dome-shaped disk with an extension catheter that is surgically implanted through the cranium into a lateral ventricle. In addition to more consistent drug distribution, the Ommaya reservoir precludes the use of repeated, painful lumbar punctures. Complications of intrathecal or intraventricular chemotherapy include headache, nausea, vomiting, fever, and nuchal rigidity.

Intravesical Bladder Chemotherapy. The patient with superficial transitional cell cancer of the bladder often has recurrent disease following traditional surgical therapy. Instillation of chemotherapy into the bladder promotes destruction of cancer cells and reduces the incidence of recurrent disease. Additional benefits of this therapy include reduced urinary and sexual dysfunction. The chemotherapeutic agent is instilled into the bladder via a urinary catheter and retained for 1 to 3 hours. Complications of this therapy include dysuria, urinary frequency, hematuria, and bladder spasms.

TABLE 16-11 Cells with Rapid Rate of Proliferation

Cells and Generation Time	Effect of Cell Destruction
Bone marrow stem cell, 6–24 hr	Myelosuppression; infection, bleeding, anemia
Neutrophils, 12 hr	Leukopenia, infection
Epithelial cells lining the gastrointestinal tract, 12–24 hr	Anorexia, mucositis (including stomatitis, esophagitis), nausea and vomiting, diarrhea
Cells of the hair follicle, 24 hr	Alopecia
Ova or testes, 24–36 hr	Reproductive dysfunction

Effects of Chemotherapy on Normal Tissues

Chemotherapeutic agents cannot selectively distinguish between normal cells and cancer cells. Chemotherapy-induced side effects are the result of the destruction of normal cells, especially those that are rapidly proliferating such as those in the bone marrow, the lining of the gastrointestinal system, and the integumentary system (skin, hair, and nails) (Table 16-11). Effects of chemotherapy are caused by general cytotoxicity and organ-specific drug toxicities. Response of the body to the products of cellular destruction in circulation may cause fatigue, anorexia, and taste alterations.

The general and drug-specific adverse effects of these drugs are classified as acute, delayed, or chronic. *Acute toxicity* occurs during and immediately after drug administration and includes anaphylactic and hypersensitivity reactions, extravasation or a flare reaction, anticipatory nausea and vomiting, and cardiac dysrhythmias. *Delayed effects* are numerous and include delayed nausea and vomiting, mucositis, alopecia, skin rashes, bone marrow suppression, altered bowel function (diarrhea or constipation), and a variety of cumulative neurotoxicities depending on the affected component of the nervous system (i.e., central or peripheral nervous system or cranial nerves). *Chronic toxicities* involve damage to organs such as the heart, liver, kidneys, and lungs. Some side effects fall into more than one category. For example, nausea and vomiting can be both acute and delayed.

Treatment Plan

While single-drug chemotherapy can be and sometimes is prescribed, combining agents in multidrug regimens has proven to be more effective in managing most cancers. Choosing agents with different mechanisms of action and varying toxicity profiles avoids tumor cell resistance and minimizes the occurrence and severity of side effects. Drug regimens are selected based on evidence supporting their use in specific cancers, and are sometimes customized to meet the needs of an individual patient. Chemotherapy is most effective when tumor burden is low, therapy is not interrupted, and the patient receives the intended dose. The dose of each drug is carefully calculated according to the patient's body surface area (i.e., calculation of the drug is based on body weight and height). An example of a FOLFOX treatment regimen is provided in Table 16-12.

TABLE 16-12 *DRUG THERAPY* Example of Chemotherapeutic Drug Schedule

Schedule: FOLFOX + bevacizumab (Avastin) is given to treat advanced colon cancer. FOLFOX* includes 5-FU (**FOL**) given IV as a continuous infusion over 46 hours on days 1 and 2; leucovorin (folinic acid) (**F**) given IV over 2 hours on days 1 and 2; and oxaliplatin (Eloxatin) (**OX**) given IV over 2 hours on day 1. Bevacizumab (Avastin) is given IV over 2 hours on day 1. This is repeated every 2 weeks. The number of cycles depends on a patient's situation.

Weeks	1			3			5			7		
Days	1	2	3	1	2	3	1	2	3	1	2	3
Drug												
5-FU	↔	↔		↔	↔		↔	↔		↔	↔	
leucovorin (folinic acid)	↔	↔		↔	↔		↔	↔		↔	↔	
oxaliplatin (Eloxatin)	↔			↔			↔			↔		
bevacizumab (Avastin)	↔			↔			↔			↔		

*There are slightly different versions of the FOLFOX regimen.

RADIATION THERAPY

Radiation therapy is a local treatment modality for cancer. Along with surgery, it is one of the oldest methods of cancer treatment. Historically, workers exposed to radiation were noted to have a higher incidence of skin desquamation and developed carcinomas of the fingers related to the handling of radioactive substances and primitive x-ray equipment. In fact, Marie and Pierre Curie (scientists of the late nineteenth century credited with advancing our understanding of radioactivity) both developed leukemia related to radiation exposure.

The observation that radiation exposure caused tissue damage led scientists in the early twentieth century to explore the use of radiation to treat tumors. The hypothesized association was that, if radiation resulted in the destruction of the highly mitotic skin cells of workers, it could be used in a controlled way to prevent the continued growth of highly mitotic cancer cells. It was not until the 1960s that sophisticated equipment and treatment planning facilitated the delivery of adequate radiation doses to tumors and tolerable doses to normal tissues. It is estimated in current practice that up to 60% of all persons with cancer will receive radiation therapy at some point in the treatment of their disease.

Effects of Radiation

Radiation is the emission and distribution of energy through space or a material medium. Delivery of high-energy beams, when absorbed into tissue, produces ionization of atomic particles. The local energy in ionizing radiation and resultant generation of free radicals act to break the chemical bonds in DNA. Damage to cellular DNA may be either lethal or sublethal. Lethal damage causes sufficient chromosomal disruption that the cell is unable to replicate, or may also impair protein synthesis functions necessary for survival. When sublethal DNA damage occurs, there is potential for repair in between radiation doses, or potential for accumulated damage to occur with repetitive doses, which ultimately leads to cell death. Cancer cells are more likely to be permanently damaged by cumulative doses of radiation because they are less capable of repairing sublethal DNA damage than healthy cells.

Different types of ionizing radiation are used to treat cancer, including electromagnetic radiation (i.e., x-rays, gamma rays) and particulate radiation (alpha particles, electrons, neutrons, protons). The primary difference between x-rays and gamma rays is that gamma rays are emitted from a radioactive source through the process of constant decay. High-energy x-rays (photons) are generated by an electric machine such as a linear accelerator. The main problem with emitted radiation (such as historic cobalt technology introduced in the 1960s) is that over time the source deteriorates, thus emitting less energy and requiring periodic replacement. Safety issues relating to housing the radioactive source are also a consideration. Technologic advances have expanded and refined the sources and methods of delivering radiation therapy, thus offering more accurate and less invasive radiation treatment options.[16] Most radiation centers in the United States currently use linear accelerator technology, and larger radiation facilities may offer a combination of treatment machines that permit expanded treatment options for patients at one treatment site.

Principles of Radiobiology. As the radiation beam passes through the treatment field, energy deposited is determined by the properties of the energy used and the absorptive properties of the matter through which the beams pass. *Low-energy beams* (such as electrons) expend energy quickly upon impact with matter. Therefore they penetrate only a short distance. (They are clinically useful in treating superficial skin lesions). *High-energy beams* (such as photons) have greater depth of penetration, not attaining full intensity until they reach a certain depth. Therefore they are suitable for delivering optimal doses to internal targets while sparing the skin.

The radiation dose is determined based on tumor volume, type of tumor, and treatment setting. Technically, all cancer cells could be eradicated with radiation given in high enough doses. However, to avoid serious toxicity and long-term complications of treatment, radiation to surrounding healthy tissue must be limited to the *maximal tolerated dose* for that specific tissue. Improvements in planning and in delivery technology (such as *intensity-modulated radiotherapy [IMRT]*) have greatly improved the ability to deliver maximal doses to the target volume while sparing critical structures such as the spinal cord, small bowel, carotid arteries, parotid glands, optic chiasm, and other important structures as much as possible.

Historically, the radiation dose was expressed in units called rads (radiation absorbed doses). Current nomenclature is *gray* (Gy) or centigray (cGy). A *centigray* is equivalent to 1 rad, and 100 centigray equals 1 gray (Table 16-13).

Once the total dose to be delivered is determined, that dose is divided into daily "fractions" (generally between 180 and 200 cGy). Treatment is typically delivered once a day Monday through Friday for a period of 2 to 8 weeks (depending on the desired total dose). Other treatment schedules may be prescribed based on principles of radiobiologic effect. High daily doses of radiation may be given with fewer fractions *(hypofractionated),* lower daily doses may be given over a longer period of time *(hyperfractionated),* or doses may be delivered twice daily *(accelerated fractionation).*

The amount of time that is required for the manifestations of radiation damage is determined by the mitotic rate of the tissue, with rapidly proliferating tissues being more sensitive. Sufficient cells within the tissue must be killed to establish a noticeable effect. This is true in both normal and cancer cells. Rapidly dividing cells in the GI tract, oral mucosa, and bone marrow will die quickly and exhibit early acute responses to radiation. Tissues with slowly proliferating cells, such as cartilage, bone, and kidneys, manifest later responses to radiation. This differential rate of cellular death explains the timing of clinical manifestations related to radiation therapy. Certain cancers are more susceptible to the effects of radiation than others. Table 16-14 describes the relative radiosensitivity of a variety of tumors. In responsive tumors (such as lymphomas), even a large tumor burden will be affected by therapy. In less responsive tumors, a large tumor burden may result

TABLE 16-13 Measurement of Radiation

Unit	Definition
Curie (Ci)	A measure of the number of atoms of a particular radioisotope that disintegrate in 1 sec
Roentgen (R)	A measure of the radiation required to produce a standard number of ions in air; a unit of exposure to radiation
Rad	Measurement of radiation dosage absorbed by the tissues
Rem	Measurement of the biologic effectiveness of various forms of radiation on the human cell (1 rem = 1 rad)
Gray (Gy)	1 Gy = 100 rads; 1 centigray (cGy) = 1 rad

TABLE 16-14 Tumor Radiosensitivity

High Radiosensitivity	Moderate Radiosensitivity	Mild Radiosensitivity	Poor Radiosensitivity
Ovarian dysgerminoma	Oropharyngeal carcinoma	Soft tissue sarcomas (e.g., chondrosarcoma)	Osteosarcoma
Testicular seminoma	Esophageal carcinoma	Gastric adenocarcinoma	Malignant melanoma
Hodgkin's lymphoma	Breast adenocarcinoma	Renal adenocarcinoma	Malignant gliomas
Non-Hodgkin's lymphoma	Uterine and cervical carcinoma	Colon adenocarcinoma	Testicular nonseminoma
Wilms' tumor	Prostate carcinoma		
Neuroblastoma	Bladder carcinoma		

in a slower and perhaps incomplete response. Localized prostate cancer responds very slowly to radiation (over a period of several months). For some benign diseases (such as meningiomas), arrested growth (rather than disease regression) may be considered successful.

Simulation

Simulation is a part of radiation treatment planning used to determine the optimal treatment method by focusing on the geometric aspects of treatment (i.e., orientation and size of radiation beams, location of field-shaping blocks, and outlining the field on the patient's skin). Simulation is the process used to define and aim the radiation beams to meet the goals of the prescribed plan. The patient lies on a table in a position that permits maximal treatment of tumor while minimizing exposure of normal tissue. Immobilization devices (e.g., casts, bite blocks, thermoplastic face masks) are typically used to help the patient maintain a stable position (Fig. 16-17). The target is defined using a variety of possible imaging techniques (e.g., x-rays, CT, MRI, PET scans), physical examination, and surgical reports.[17] Under fluoroscopy, the critical normal structures that will be included in the treatment field (or portal) are identified so they can be protected. A film is taken to verify the field, and marks are placed on the skin to delineate the "treatment port"; small tattoos may be placed to ensure the patient position is precisely reproduced on a daily basis. Computerized dosimetry using CT scanning (or fused CT/MRI) is used to produce a treatment plan that delivers the maximum amount of radiation to the tumor within the acceptable dose to normal tissue.

Treatment

Radiation is used to treat a carefully defined area of the body to achieve local control of disease. As radiation only has an affect on tissues within the treatment field, it is not appropriate as an independent modality for patients with systemic disease. However, radiation may be used, independently or in combination with chemotherapy, to treat primary tumors or for palliative control of metastatic lesions. Radiation can be delivered externally *(teletherapy)* or internally *(brachytherapy).* As with other cancer therapies, the goals of radiation therapy are cure, control, or palliation. There are multiple settings in which radiation may be used, including

- *Definitive or primary therapy:* used as an independent treatment modality with curative intent (e.g., for cancers of the lung, prostate, bladder, and head/neck; Hodgkin's lymphoma)
- *Neoadjuvant therapy:* given (with or without chemotherapy) preoperatively to minimize tumor burden and improve the likelihood of complete surgical resection, making a previously inoperable tumor (such as one adjacent to a critical structure) operable (e.g., lung, esophageal, or colorectal cancers)

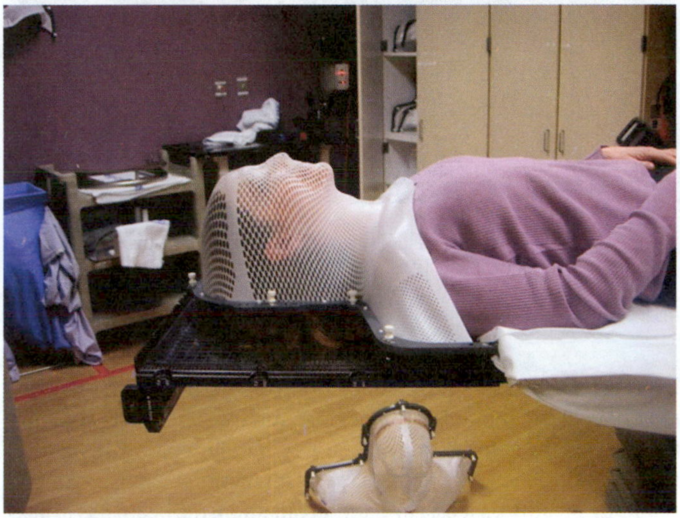

FIG. 16-17 Immobilization device. Use of a head holder and immobilization mask may be used to ensure accurate positioning for daily treatment of head and neck cancer.

- *Adjuvant therapy:* administered following surgery or chemotherapy to improve local control of disease and reduce risk of local disease recurrence (e.g., glioblastoma, head and neck cancers, cancers of the breast, lung, rectum, pancreas)
- *Prophylaxis:* administered to high risk areas to prevent future cancer development (such as prophylactic cranial irradiation to prevent brain metastasis secondary to small cell lung cancer)
- *Disease control:* limiting tumor growth to extend the symptom-free period as much as possible
- *Palliation:* given to prevent or relieve distressing symptoms such as pain (bone metastasis) or shortness of breath (obstructing bronchial tumor), and for preservation of neurologic function (brain metastasis or spinal cord compression)

External Radiation. **Teletherapy** *(external beam radiation)* is the most common form of radiation treatment delivery. With this technique, the patient is exposed to radiation from a megavoltage treatment machine. Machines that are used to deliver treatment may include the cobalt-60 machine, which emits gamma rays from a radioactive source (the original technology, still in limited use in the United States); a cyclotron, which produces neutrons or protons; and a linear accelerator, which generates ionizing radiation from electricity and can have multiple energies (Fig. 16-18).

Internal Radiation. Radiation can also be delivered as **brachytherapy,** which means "close" or internal radiation treat-

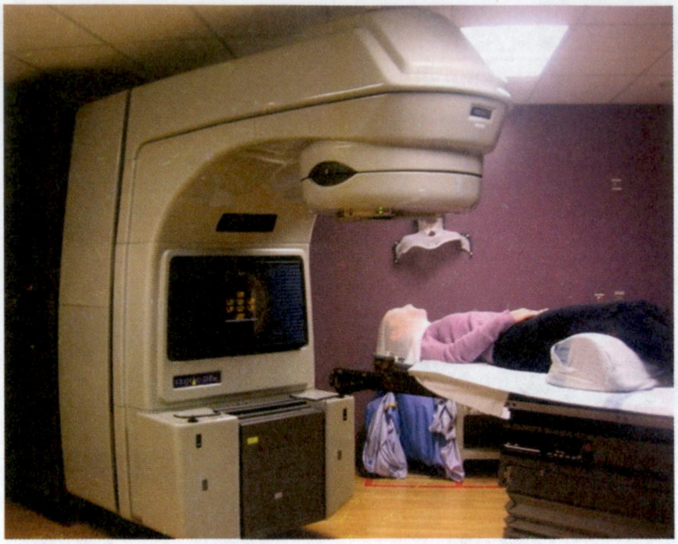

FIG. 16-18 Linear accelerator. Varian Clinac EX linear accelerator with multiple photon and electron energies available for use according to the treatment plan. Patient is positioned on radiation treatment table for treatment of head and neck cancer.

ment. It consists of the implantation or insertion of radioactive materials directly into the tumor (interstitial) or in close proximity adjacent to the tumor (intracavitary or intraluminal). This allows for direct dose delivery to the target with minimal exposure to surrounding healthy tissues. (In external radiation, the beam has to pass through external tissues to reach the internal source). Brachytherapy is commonly used in combination with external radiation as a supplemental "boost" treatment.

Sources of radiation for brachytherapy include temporary sealed sources such as iridium-192 and cesium-137 and permanent sealed sources such as iodine-125, gold-198, and palladium-103. These are supplied in the form of seeds or ribbons. With a temporary implant, the source may be placed into a special catheter or metal tube that has been inserted into the tumor area. It is left in place until the prescribed dose of radiation has been reached in the calculated number of hours. This method is commonly used for tumors of the head and neck, and lung and gynecologic malignancies.

Brachytherapy is delivered as high-dose-rate (HDR) treatment (i.e., several doses administered at varying intervals over a few minutes each time) or low-dose-rate (LDR) treatment (i.e., continuous treatment over several hours or days). A remote "afterloading" technique (i.e., the source is inserted after the applicator is in place) is designed to enhance physician and patient safety and is used for HDR brachytherapy with iridium-192. Permanent implants, such as for prostate brachytherapy, involve the insertion of radioactive seeds directly into the tumor tissue, where they remain permanently. As interstitial seeds used for treatment emit low energies with limited tissue penetration, patients are not considered radioactive. However, some initial radiation precautions may be recommended as there is a small risk of seed dislodgement. Over time, the isotopes that are used decay and are no longer radioactive. The time frame for side effects induced by treatment can be predicted based on the rate of decay for the specific isotope used.

Radiopharmaceutical therapy employs unsealed liquid radioactive sources that are administered orally as a drink, such as iodine-131 for thyroid cancer, or intravenously as with yttrium-90 administered for refractory lymphomas or samarium-153 used to treat bone metastases.[17]

Caring for the person undergoing brachytherapy or receiving radiopharmaceuticals requires that the nurse be aware that the patient is emitting radioactivity. Patients with temporary implants are radioactive only during the time the source is in place. In patients with permanent implants, because the sources have fairly short half-lives and are weak emitters, the radioactive exposure to the outside and to others is low. These patients may be discharged with precautions.

The principles of *ALARA (as low as reasonably achievable)* and *time, distance,* and *shielding* are vital to health care professional safety when caring for the person with a source of internal radiation. Care should be organized to limit the amount of time spent in direct contact with the patient. To minimize anxiety and confusion, the patient should be made aware of the reason for time and distance limitations before the procedure. The radiation safety officer will indicate how much time at a specific distance can be spent with the patient. This is determined by the dose delivered by the implant. Because the source is nonpenetrating, small differences in distance are critical. Only care that must be delivered near the source, such as checking placement of the implant, is performed in close proximity. Shielding, if available, should be used, and no care should be delivered without wearing a film badge. This badge will indicate cumulative radiation exposure. The film badge should not be shared, should not be worn other than at work, and should be returned according to the agency's protocol.

NURSING MANAGEMENT
PATIENTS UNDERGOING CHEMOTHERAPY AND RADIATION THERAPY

The nurse plays an important role in identifying, reporting, and helping patients deal with the side effects of radiation and chemotherapy. Educating patients about their treatment regimen, supportive care options (e.g., antiemetics, antidiarrheals), and what to expect during the course of treatment is important to help decrease fear and anxiety, encourage adherence, and guide at-home self-management. Before initiating education, however, the patient's ability and desire to process information should be assessed. Teaching should then be customized to meet the patient's and family's learning needs.

Common side effects of chemotherapy and radiation are presented in Table 16-15. Bone marrow suppression, fatigue, GI disturbances, integumentary and mucosal reactions, and pulmonary and reproductive effects are discussed in this section.

▪ *Nursing Implementation*

Bone Marrow Suppression. Myelosuppression is one of the most common effects of chemotherapy and, to a lesser extent, it can also occur with radiation. Since bone marrow is responsible for producing critically important blood cells (red blood cells, white blood cells, and platelets), treatment-induced reductions in blood cell production can result in life-threatening and distressing effects including infection, hemorrhage, and overwhelming fatigue. The major difference in manifestations between radiation and chemotherapy is that with radiation (a local therapy) only bone marrow within the treatment field will be affected, whereas chemotherapy (a systemic therapy) affects bone marrow function

TABLE 16-15 Nursing Management of Problems Caused by Chemotherapy and Radiation Therapy

Problem	Etiology	Nursing Management
Gastrointestinal System		
Stomatitis, mucositis, esophagitis	• Epithelial cells are destroyed by chemotherapy or radiation treatment when located in field (e.g., head and neck, stomach, esophagus) • Inflammation and ulceration occur due to rapid cell destruction	• Assess oral mucosa daily and teach patient to do this • Be aware that eating, swallowing, and talking may be difficult (may require analgesics) • Encourage patient to use artificial saliva to manage dryness (radiation) • Discourage use of irritants such as tobacco and alcohol • Apply topical anesthetics (e.g., viscous lidocaine, oxethazine)
Nausea and vomiting	• Release of intracellular breakdown products stimulates vomiting center in brain • Drugs also stimulate vomiting center in brain (see Fig. 42-1) • GI lining destroyed with radiation and chemotherapy	• Teach patient to eat and drink when not nauseated • Administer antiemetics prophylactically prior to chemotherapy and also on as-needed basis • Use diversional activities (if appropriate)
Anorexia	• Release of TNF and IL-1 from macrophages has appetite-suppressant effect • Therapy-induced GI effects (mucositis, nausea, and vomiting, bowel disturbances) and anxiety that reduce appetite	• Monitor weight • Encourage patient to eat small, frequent meals of high-protein, high-calorie foods • Gently encourage patient to eat, but avoid nagging • Serve food in pleasant environment
Diarrhea	• Denuding of epithelial lining of intestines • Side effect of chemotherapy • Radiation to abdomen, pelvis, lumbosacral areas	• Give antidiarrheal agents as needed • Encourage low-fiber, low-residue diet • Encourage fluid intake of at least 3 L

Constipation	• Decreased intestinal motility related to autonomic nervous system dysfunction
	• Caused by neurotoxic effects of plant alkaloids (vincristine, vinblastine)
		• Instruct patients to
		  • Take stool softeners as needed
		  • Eat high-fiber foods
		  • Increase fluid intake

Hepatotoxicity	• Toxic effects from chemotherapy drugs (usually transient and resolves when drug is stopped)	• Monitor liver function tests
Hematologic System		
Anemia	• Bone marrow depressed secondary to therapy • Malignant infiltration of bone marrow by cancer	• Monitor hemoglobin and hematocrit levels • Administer iron supplements and erythropoietin • Encourage intake of foods that promote RBC production (see Table 31-5)
Leukopenia	• Depression of bone marrow secondary to chemotherapy or radiation therapy • Infection most frequent cause of morbidity and death in cancer patients • Respiratory and genitourinary system usual sites of infection	• Monitor WBC count, especially neutrophils • Teach patient to report temperature elevation and any other manifestations of infection • Teach patient to avoid large crowds and people with infections • Administer WBC growth factors (see Table 16-18) • For patient teaching, see Table 31-23
Thrombocytopenia	• Bone marrow depressed secondary to chemotherapy • Malignant infiltration of bone marrow that crowds out normal marrow • Spontaneous bleeding can occur with platelet counts ≤20,000/μl	• Observe for signs of bleeding (e.g., petechiae, ecchymosis) • Monitor platelet counts • For patient teaching, see Table 31-15
Integumentary System		
Alopecia	• Destruction of hair follicles by chemotherapy or radiation to scalp • Hair loss usually temporary with chemotherapy; usually permanent in response to radiation	• Suggest ways to cope with hair loss (e.g., hair pieces, scarves, wigs) • Cut long hair before therapy • Avoid excessive shampooing, brushing, and combing of hair • Avoid use of electric hair dryers, curlers, and curling rods • Discuss impact of hair loss on self-image
Radiation skin changes (dry to moist desquamation)	• Radiation damage to skin	• Keep treatment field protected; do not apply any lotions, creams, cosmetics, or other products unless prescribed by physician • See Table 16-16 for additional patient management details

BUN, Blood urea nitrogen; *ECG,* electrocardiogram; *GI,* gastrointestinal; *IL-1,* interleukin-1; *RBC,* red blood cell; *TNF,* tumor necrosis factor; *WBC,* white blood cell.

Continued

Cancer

TABLE 16-15 Nursing Management of Problems Caused by Chemotherapy and Radiation Therapy—cont'd

Problem	Etiology	Nursing Management
Integumentary System—cont'd		
Chemotherapy-induced skin changes	• Hyperpigmentation • Telangiectasis • Photosensitivity • Acneiform eruptions • Acral erythema	• Alert patient to potential skin changes • Encourage patient to avoid sun exposure • Implement symptomatic management as needed depending on specific skin effect (e.g., application of lotions, benzoyl peroxide for acne, corticosteroid creams)
Genitourinary Tract		
Hemorrhagic cystitis	• Cells lining bladder destroyed from chemotherapy (e.g., cyclophosphamide, ifosfamide) • Side effect of radiation when located in treatment field	• Monitor manifestations such as urgency, frequency, and hematuria • Administer cytoprotectant agent (mesna [Mesnex]) and hydration • Administer supportive care agents to manage symptoms (e.g., Urimax, flavozate)
Reproductive dysfunction	• Cells of testes or ova are damaged from therapy	• Discuss possibility with patients prior to treatment initiation • Offer opportunity for sperm and ova banking prior to treatment for patients of childbearing age
Nephrotoxicity	• Direct renal cell damage due to exposure to nephrotoxic agents (cisplatin and high-dose methotrexate) • Precipitation of metabolites of cellular breakdown (tumor lysis syndrome [TLS])	• Monitor BUN and serum creatinine levels • Avoid potentiating drugs • Alkalinize the urine with sodium bicarbonate and administer allopurinol or rasburicase for TLS prevention
Nervous System		
Increased intracranial pressure	• May result from radiation edema in central nervous system	• Monitor neurologic status • May be controlled with corticosteroids
Peripheral neuropathy	• Paresthesias, areflexia, skeletal muscle weakness, and smooth muscle dysfunction can occur as a side effect of plant alkaloids and cisplatin	• Monitor for these manifestations in patients on these drugs
Respiratory System		
Pneumonitis	• Radiation pneumonitis develops 2-3 mo after start of treatment • After 6-12 mo, fibrosis occurs and is evident on x-ray • Side effect of some chemotherapy drugs	• Monitor for dry, hacking cough, fever, and exertional dyspnea
Cardiovascular System		
Pericarditis and myocarditis	• Inflammation secondary to radiation injury • Complication when chest wall is irradiated; may occur up to 1 yr after treatment • Side effect of some chemotherapy drugs	• Monitor for clinical manifestations of these disorders
Cardiotoxicity	• Some chemotherapy drugs (e.g., anthracyclines, taxanes) can cause ECG changes and rapidly progressive heart failure	• Monitor heart with ECG and cardiac ejection fractions • Drug therapy may need to be modified for symptoms or deteriorating cardiac function studies
Biochemical		
Hyperuricemia	• Increased uric acid levels due to chemotherapy-induced cell destruction • Can cause secondary gout and obstructive uropathy	• Monitor uric acid levels • Allopurinol (Zyloprim) may be given as a prophylactic measure • Encourage high fluid intake
Psychoemotional		
Fatigue	• Anabolic processes resulting in accumulation of metabolites from cell breakdown	• Tell patient that fatigue is an expected side effect of therapy • Encourage patient to rest when fatigued, to maintain usual lifestyle patterns as closely as possible, and to pace activities in accordance with energy level

throughout the body. Therefore effects are more profound with chemotherapy and when the two therapies are combined.

In general, the onset of bone marrow suppression is related to the lifespan of the type of blood cell. WBCs (especially neutrophils) are affected most acutely—within 1 to 2 weeks—platelets in 2 to 3 weeks, and red blood cells (RBCs), with a longer life span of 120 days, at a later time. The severity of myelosuppression is dependent on the chemotherapy drugs used, dosages of drugs, and the specific radiation treatment field. Radiation to large marrow-containing regions of the body produces the most clinically significant myelosuppression. In the adult, about 40% of active marrow is in the pelvis and 25% is in the thoracic and lumbar vertebrae.[17] Certain chemotherapy agents are more myelosuppressive than others, and some drug regimens that include multiple myelosuppressive agents can result in significant effects.

Monitoring the complete blood count is critical in patients receiving radiation and/or chemotherapy, particularly the neutrophil, platelet, and RBC counts. It is typical for patients to experience the lowest blood cell counts (called the **nadir**) between 7 and 10 days after initiation of therapy. However, the exact onset depends on the particular drug regimen and host factors.

Neutropenia is most common in patients receiving chemotherapy and can place them at significant risk for serious infection or sepsis. Neutropenia at certain levels is a trigger to delay or otherwise modify treatment (i.e., lower dosages). Every possible measure must be taken to prevent infections in these patients. (See nursing care plan on neutropenia [NCP 31-3].) WBC growth factors (i.e., filgrastim [Neupogen], pegfilgrastim [Neulasta]) are routinely used to reduce the duration of chemotherapy-induced neutropenia, and as a prophylactic measure to prevent neutropenia when highly myelosuppressive chemotherapy drugs are used.[18] (Neutropenia is discussed in Chapter 31, where a patient teaching guide is also available [see Table 31-23].) Precautions to minimize risks from neutropenia and a neutropenia diet are available on the website for this chapter.

Thrombocytopenia can result in spontaneous bleeding or major hemorrhage. (See the nursing care plan on thrombocytopenia [NCP 31-2].) Risk of serious bleeding is generally not apparent until the platelet count falls below 50,000/μl. Platelet transfusions may be necessary and are usually administered when platelet counts fall below 20,000/μl.

Anemia is common in patients undergoing either radiation or chemotherapy and generally has a later onset (about 3 to 4 months after treatment initiation). For patients with low hemoglobin levels (i.e., below 11 g/dl), red blood cell growth factors (i.e., darbepoetin [Aranesp], epoetin [Procrit]) are initiated and administered until the hemoglobin is between 11 and 13 g/dl. In extreme circumstances (i.e., symptomatic anemia), RBC transfusions may also be indicated. In general, efforts are increasingly being made to avoid RBC transfusion. (Hematopoietic growth factors are discussed later in this chapter and presented in Table 16-18.)

Fatigue. Fatigue is a nearly universal symptom affecting 70% to 100% of patients with cancer.[19] It is commonly reported by patients undergoing active treatment as the most distressful of treatment-related side effects. It is defined as the persistent subjective sense of tiredness associated with cancer and its treatment that interferes with usual day-to-day functioning. The pathophysiologic mechanisms of fatigue are unclear. One theory is that the accumulation of muscle metabolites such as lactate, hydrogen ions, and other end products from the destruction of cells results in decreased muscle strength. Other explanations include cytokine production, changes in neuromuscular function, serotonin dysregulation, and an indirect association with anorexia, fever, and infection typical in patients undergoing treatment. Finally, fatigue is an associated effect of treatment-induced anemia. Fatigue associated with radiation therapy generally begins during the third to fourth week of treatment, persists after treatment ends, and then gradually subsides. Factors such as weight loss, depression, nausea, and other symptoms can exacerbate the sensation of fatigue. For many patients, fatigue continues after the completion of treatment.

The nurse can help patients recognize that fatigue is a common side effect of therapy rather than a sign that treatment is not effective or that their cancer is progressing. A patient may report more energy on some days than on others. Encouraging the individual to identify days or times during the day when he or she typically is feeling better may allow the patient to remain more active. Resting before activity and having others assist with work or home management may be necessary. Ignoring the fatigue or overstressing the body when fatigue is tolerable may lead to an increase in symptoms. Maintaining good nutritional and hydration status and managing other symptoms also helps reduce fatigue. Walking programs are a way for most patients to keep active without overtaxing them. The ability to remain active helps to improve mood and avoid the debilitating cycle of fatigue-depression-fatigue that can occur in patients with cancer.

Gastrointestinal Effects. The cells of the mucosal lining of the GI tract are highly proliferative, with surface cells replaced every 2 to 6 days. The intestinal mucosa is one of the most sensitive tissues to radiation and chemotherapy. The etiology of GI reactions is related to a variety of mechanisms, including (1) the release of serotonin from the GI tract, which then stimulates the chemoreceptor trigger zone (CTZ) and the vomiting center in the brain; and (2) cellular death and resulting damage to mucosal tissues and underlying structures in the GI lining responsible for digestion, secretion, and absorption. Additionally, radiation to treatment fields that contain GI structures (i.e., abdominopelvic, lumbosacral, and lower thoracic areas) and selected chemotherapy agents produce direct injury to GI epithelial cells. These effects result in a variety of GI effects—nausea and vomiting, diarrhea, mucositis, and anorexia—all of which can significantly effect the patient's hydration and nutritional status and sense of well-being.

Nausea and Vomiting. Nausea and vomiting are common sequelae of chemotherapy, and in some instances radiation therapy. Vomiting may occur within 1 hour of chemotherapy administration or a few hours after radiation therapy to the chest or abdomen and may persist for 24 hours or more. Several antiemetic drugs are available (see Chapter 42 and Table 42-1). Metoclopramide (Reglan); serotonin receptor antagonists (ondansetron [Zofran], granisetron [(Kytril], dolasetron [Anzemet], and palonosetron [Aloxi]); and dexamethasone (Decadron) have been used to decrease nausea and vomiting caused by chemotherapy. Aprepitant (Emend) is the first agent in a class of antiemetics known as neurokinin 1 receptor antagonists, and is effective in preventing nausea and vomiting on the day of chemotherapy as well as for delayed symptoms. The 3-drug combination of a serotonin receptor antagonist, dexamethasone, and aprepitant is recommended before chemotherapy of high emetic risk (e.g., cyclophosphamide, anthracyclines).[20]

Patients may also develop *anticipatory nausea and vomiting* if they experience poorly controlled nausea and vomiting following chemotherapy administration. In this phenomenon, encountering the cues even without receiving treatment may precipitate nausea and vomiting. Aggressive emesis control, including the use of prophylactic administration of antiemetic and antianxiety medication 1 hour before treatment, is recommended. The patient may find that eating a light meal of nonirritating food before treatment is also helpful.

Delayed nausea and vomiting can develop 24 hours and up to a week following treatment. Patients experiencing nausea and vomiting must be assessed for signs and symptoms of dehydration and metabolic alkalosis. Fluid intake is recorded to ensure that an adequate volume is being consumed and retained. Nausea and vomiting can be successfully managed with antiemetic regimens, dietary modification, and other nonpharmacologic interventions.

Diarrhea. Diarrhea is a reaction of the bowel mucosa to radiation and to certain antineoplastic agents. It is characterized by an increase in frequency of liquidity of stool. Pathophysiology of treatment-induced diarrhea is multifaceted. The most common mechanisms are osmotic, secretory, hypermotility, and exudative. The small bowel is extremely sensitive and does not tolerate significant radiation doses. With radiation, treating patients with a full bladder may be done to move the small bowel out of the treatment field. Both radiation and chemotherapy-induced diarrhea are best managed with antidiarrheals, antimotility agents, and antispasmodics (see Table 43-3).

A diet low in fiber and residue should be recommended prior to treatment with chemotherapy known to cause diarrhea. This includes limiting foods that are high in roughage (e.g., fresh fruits, vegetables, seeds, nuts) (see Table 43-9). To prevent diarrhea, other foods that may be avoided include fried or highly seasoned foods, or other foods that are gas producing. Depending on severity, hydration and electrolyte supplementation are also recommended. Lukewarm sitz baths may alleviate discomfort and cleanse the rectal area if significant rectal irritation has developed. The rectal area must be kept clean and dry to maintain skin integrity. The nurse should visually inspect the perianal area for evidence of skin breakdown. Systemic analgesia may be warranted for the painful skin irritations that may develop. The number, volume, consistency, and character of stools per day should be noted. Patients can be taught to maintain a diary or log to record episodes, and aggravating and alleviating factors.[21]

Mucositis. Oral mucositis (irritation, inflammation, and/or ulceration of the mucosa) is a common complication in almost all patients receiving radiation to the head and neck and in a significant number of patients receiving certain antineoplastic agents, especially 5-fluorouracil (5-FU). Similar to the bowel mucosa, the mucosal linings of the oral cavity, oropharynx, and esophagus are extremely sensitive to the effects of radiation and chemotherapy. Oral mucositis (or stomatitis) is a complex problem involving not only the epithelial lining but also other mucosal components, including the endothelial, extracellular matrix, and connective tissues. Greater understanding of mucositis pathophysiology is opening doors to the development of new interventions, including cytoprotectant and keratinocyte growth factors.[22]

Certain factors can compound the problem. For example, patients undergoing head and neck radiation may face the additional challenge of radiation-induced parotid gland dysfunction. This may result in decreased salivary flow, causing acute and/or chronic *xerostomia* (dry mouth). Dryness or thick saliva compromises the protective salivary functions of assisting with cleansing teeth, moistening food and swallowing. Meticulous oral care during and after treatment reduces the risk of radiation caries, which develop as a result of diminished saliva. Saliva substitutes are available and may be offered to patients with xerostomia, although many patients find that drinking small amounts of water frequently has an equivalent effect. Amifostine (a cytoprotectant) is often used during radiation treatment.

Taste loss may develop during therapy, and by the end of treatment patients often report that all food has lost its flavor. Ultimately nutritional status may be compromised. *Dysphagia* (difficulty swallowing), which characterizes esophageal involvement, further impedes eating. Patients may report feeling that they have a "lump" as they swallow and that "foods get stuck."

Oral assessment and meticulous intervention to keep the oral cavity moist, clean, and free of debris are essential to prevent infection and to facilitate nutritional intake. The patient should be taught to self-examine the oral cavity. The mucous membranes, characteristics of saliva, and ability to swallow must be assessed. Oral care includes pretreatment evaluation by a dentist to perform all necessary dental work before the initiation of treatment. The patient should also be taught how to perform oral care (proper toothbrushing, flossing, and use of fluoride trays to prevent caries). Oral care should be performed at least before and after each meal and at bedtime. A saline solution of 1 teaspoon of salt in 1 L of water is an effective cleansing agent. One teaspoon of sodium bicarbonate may be added to the oral care solution to decrease odor, alleviate pain, and dissolve mucin. Toothbrushing and flossing are critical unless contraindicated by decreased platelet counts.

Alleviation of mucositis or pain in the throat can be achieved by systemic and/or topical analgesics and, if infection is documented, antibiotics. The past practices of creating combination regimens of antacids, diphenhydramine (Benadryl), and viscous lidocaine (Xylocaine) and the use of antiinfective rinses such as chlorhexidine are no longer supported. Current evidence reveals that there are no benefits, and that use of these cocktails produces thick secretions and they could serve as a medium for infection, particularly with *Candida albicans.* Instead, frequent cleansing with saline and water and topical application of anesthetic gels directly to the lesions are standard care.[23]

Palifermin (Kepivance), a synthetic version of keratinocyte growth factor, is available to prevent and shorten the duration of mucositis if it develops. It is given IV and stimulates cells on the surface layer of the mouth to grow. This is thought to lead to faster replacement of these cells when killed by cancer treatment and is believed to speed up the healing process of mouth ulcers. Palifermin has not been shown to be safe and effective in patients being treated for forms of cancer other than leukemia or lymphoma. The safety and efficacy of palifermin have not been established in patients with nonhematologic malignancies.

Feedings of soft, nonirritating high-protein and high-calorie foods should be offered frequently throughout the day. Extremes of temperature, as well as tobacco and alcohol, should be avoided. Nutritional supplements (e.g., Ensure) as an adjunct to meals and fluid intake must be encouraged. The patient should be weighed at least twice each week to monitor for weight loss. Families are an integral part of the health care team. As symptom severity increases, the family's role in assisting the patient to eat becomes increasingly critical. If family members are not available, alternative support such as volunteers and home aides is indicated.

Anorexia. Anorexia may develop as a general reaction to treatment. The mechanisms for anorexia are unclear, but several theories exist. Macrophages release tumor necrosis factor (TNF) and interleukin-1 (IL-1) in an attempt to fight the cancer. Both TNF and IL-1 have an appetite-suppressing *(anorectic)* effect. As tumors are destroyed by therapy, it is proposed that increased levels of these factors may be released into the system and cross the blood-brain barrier, exerting an influence on the satiety center. Large tumors produce more of these factors, thus resulting in the cachexia seen in advanced cancer. Other treatment-induced GI side effects can also interfere with appetite. Patients experiencing nausea and vomiting, bowel disturbances, mucositis, and taste alterations typically have little desire and actual mechanical difficulty with eating and drinking. Although it is highly individual, anorexia seems to peak at about 4 weeks of treatment and seems to resolve more quickly than fatigue when treatment ends. The patient with anorexia will need to be monitored carefully during treatment to ensure that weight loss does not become excessive. Body weight should be measured at least twice weekly. Small, frequent meals of high-protein, high-calorie foods are better tolerated than large meals. Nutritional supplements can be helpful as well. Parenteral nutrition may be indicated if the patient is severely malnourished or expected to have symptoms that interfere with nutrition for a protracted period or when the bowel is being rested.

Skin Reactions. Like the bone marrow and the GI lining, the skin contains rapidly proliferating cells and therefore is affected by radiation and chemotherapy. With radiation, skin effects are local, occurring only in the treatment field. In contrast, there are a range of chemotherapy-related skin effects that occur throughout the integumentary system—hair, skin, and nails. Combination chemotherapy can increase the severity of skin reactions experienced, especially with selected agents. Some examples are photosensitivity reactions with methotrexate and the "radiation recall" phenomenon with anthracyclines.

Radiation-induced skin changes can be acute or chronic depending on the area irradiated, dosage, and technique. The skin-sparing ability of modern radiation equipment limits the severity of these reactions. Although skin reactions can begin as early as the first treatment, this is initially transitory.[24] Erythema may develop 1 to 24 hours after a single treatment. Erythema is an acute response followed by dry desquamation (Fig. 16-19). If the rate of cellular sloughing is faster than the ability of the new epidermal cells to replace dead cells, a wet desquamation occurs with exposure of the dermis and weeping of serous fluid (Fig. 16-20). Skin reactions are particularly evident in areas of skinfolds or where skin is subjected to pressure, such as behind the ear and in gluteal folds, perineum, breast, collar line, and bony prominences.

Although skin care protocols vary among institutions, all are founded on basic skin care principles. Prevention of infection and facilitation of wound healing are the therapeutic goals. Irradiated skin should be protected from temperature extremes. Heating pads, ice packs, and hot water bottles cannot be used in the treatment field. Constricting garments, rubbing, harsh chemicals, and deodorants may also traumatize the skin and should be avoided. Dry reactions are uncomfortable and result in pruritus. Dry skin should be lubricated with a nonirritating lotion emollient (such as aloe vera) that contains no metal, alcohol, perfume, or additives that can be irritating to the skin. Wet desquamation of tissues generally produces pain, drainage, and increased infection risk. Skin care to manage most desquamation includes keeping tissues clean with normal saline compresses or modified Burow's solution soaks and protected from further damage with moisture vapor–permeable dressings or Vaseline petrolatum gauze. The use of corticosteroids and hydrogen peroxide remains controversial because of their interference with wound healing. Because protocols vary widely, the guidelines presented in Table 16-16 should be clarified with the department of radiotherapy before being instituted.

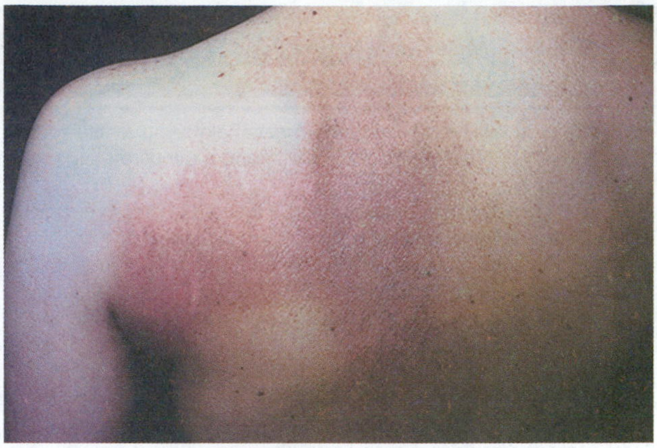

FIG. 16-19 Dry desquamation.

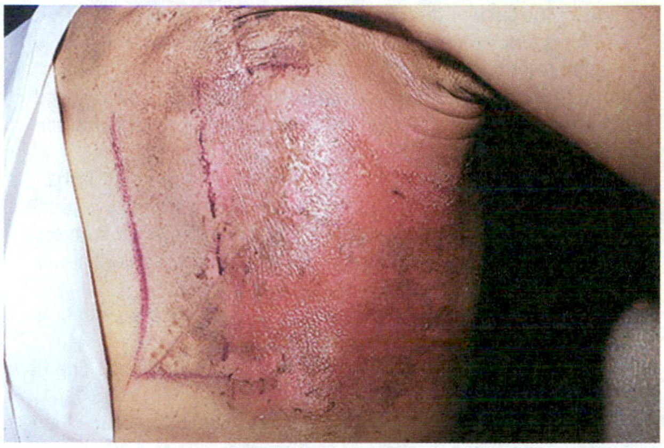

FIG. 16-20 Wet desquamation.

Chemotherapy produces a wide array of cutaneous toxicities ranging from mild erythema and hyperpigmentation to more distressing effects such as acral erythema and palmar-plantar erythrodyesthesia (PPE), or hand-foot syndrome, common with some of the targeted therapies. PPE can cause mild symptoms of redness and tingling of the palms of the hands and soles of the feet. PPE may also cause severe symptoms of painful moist desquamation, ulceration, blistering, and pain. If severe symptoms occur, the chemotherapy drug should be withheld for 1 to 2 weeks to allow the skin to regenerate. (Consult the Oncology Nursing Society's Chemotherapy and Biotherapy Guidelines for more detailed descriptions of specific reactions and recommendations for management.[12])

Cancer

TABLE 16-16 PATIENT AND FAMILY TEACHING GUIDE
Radiation Skin Reactions

1. Gently cleanse the skin in the treatment field using a mild soap (Ivory, Dove), tepid water, a soft cloth, and a gentle patting motion. Rinse thoroughly and pat dry.
2. Apply nonmedicated, nonperfumed, moisturizing lotion or creams, such as aloe gel aquaphor or biafine cream to alleviate dry skin. This substance must be gently cleansed from the treatment field before each treatment and reapplied. (NOTE: Care differs from institution to institution.) Over-the-counter hydrocortisone cream 1% may reduce itching.
3. Rinse the area with saline solution. Expose the area to air as often as possible. If copious drainage is present, use of astringent compresses (such as Domeboro solution) and nonadhesive absorbent dressings are warranted (they must be changed as soon as they become wet). Observe the area daily for signs of infection.
4. Instruct the patient to avoid wearing tight-fitting clothing such as brassieres, girdles, and belts over the treatment field.
5. Instruct the patient to avoid wearing harsh fabrics, such as wool and corduroy. A lightweight cotton garment is best. If possible, expose the treatment field to air.
6. Instruct the patient to use gentle detergents such as Dreft and Ivory Snow to wash clothing that will come in contact with the treatment field.
7. Instruct the patient to avoid direct exposure to the sun. If the treatment field is in an area that is exposed to the sun, protective clothing such as a wide-brimmed hat should be worn during exposure to the sun. Encourage use of appropriate sunscreen application.
8. Avoid all sources of excessive heat (hot water bottles, heating pads, and sunlamps) on the treatment field.
9. Avoid exposing the treatment field to cold temperatures (ice bags or cold weather).
10. Instruct the patient to avoid swimming in salt water or in chlorinated pools during the time of treatment.
11. Instruct the patient to avoid the use of all medications, deodorants, perfumes, powders, or cosmetics on the skin in the treatment field. Tape, dressings, and adhesive bandages should also be avoided unless permitted by the radiation therapist. Avoid shaving the hair in the treatment field.
12. Sensitive skin must continue to be protected after the treatment is completed. Teach the patient to do the following:
    a. Avoid direct exposure to the sun. A sunscreen agent and protective clothing must be worn if the potential of exposure to the sun is present.
    b. Use an electric razor if shaving is necessary in the treatment field.

Alopecia (hair loss) is an easily recognizable effect of cancer therapy. It is frequently associated with varying degrees of emotional distress. Hair loss associated with radiation is local, whereas chemotherapy affects hair throughout the body. The degree and duration of hair loss experienced by patients undergoing radiation and chemotherapy depend on the type and dose of the chemotherapeutic agent, and the location of the radiation field and radiation dosage. Alopecia caused by the administration of chemotherapeutic agents is usually reversible, while radiation produces temporary and partial hair loss at 30 Gy and permanent hair loss at 55 Gy. Sometimes the hair grows back while the patient is still receiving chemotherapeutic agents, but generally the hair does not grow back until 3 to 4 weeks after the drugs are discontinued. Often the new hair has a different color and texture than the hair that was lost. Patients experience a range of emotions at the prospect of losing their hair and when hair loss actually occurs. These include anger, grief, embarrassment, and fear. Hair loss is a constant reminder of their cancer and the challenges of treatment. For some persons, the loss of hair is one of the most stressful events experienced during the course of treatment. The American Cancer Society's "Look Good, Feel Better" program is an excellent support and resource for people experiencing not just hair loss but body image changes in general.

Pulmonary Effects. Both chemotherapy and radiation have the potential to produce pulmonary toxicity and tissue damage that is irreversible and progressive. Distinguishing between the complications of treatment and those related to disease is challenging since the manifestations of therapy-induced toxicity to the lungs can mimic a broad array of problems. The type and severity of therapy-induced pulmonary effects is related to the actual radiation field (i.e., thoracic field) and volume treated, specific chemotherapeutic agents, dosages, past treatment, and comorbid conditions. The effects of radiation on the lung include both acute and late reactions. Radiation doses in the lung are magnified because there is no reduction of the dose through tissue. Pneumonitis can be an acute inflammatory reaction related to radiation. This reaction is often asymptomatic, although an increase in cough, fever, and night sweats may occur. Treatment with bronchodilators, expectorants, bed rest, and oxygen is preferable to treatment with corticosteroids. The pulmonary effects of radiation are frightening to the patient because they may involve an exacerbation of the symptoms that precipitated the cancer diagnosis. Cough and dyspnea may increase. The cough becomes more productive as alveoli that had been blocked are opened as the tumor responds to treatment. As treatment continues, the cough can become dry as the mucosa begins to be altered by the radiation. Cough suppressants may be indicated at night. Oxygen, if prescribed for symptomatic pneumonitis, must be used judiciously if the patient has chronic obstructive pulmonary disease (see Chapter 29). The patient may mistakenly believe that increasing oxygen flow is an appropriate response to treat increasing dyspnea. If the patient experiences dyspnea, anxiety may be pronounced. Lying flat on the radiation treatment table and being alone in the room may potentiate anxiety.

The most common pulmonary toxicities associated with chemotherapy include pulmonary edema (noncardiogenic) related to capillary leak syndrome or fluid retention, hypersensitivity pneumonitis, interstitial fibrosis, and pneumonitis produced by an inflammatory reaction or destruction of alveolar-capillary endothelium. Though other agents are implicated, the highest risk for chemotherapy-induced pulmonary toxicity is associated with bleomycin, busulfan, carmustine, cyclophosphamide, cytosine arabinoside, gemcitabine, high-dose methotrexate, mitomycin, and some targeted therapy agents (e.g., gefitinib). Patients are managed according to the offending agent and the manifestations of toxicity.

Cardiovascular Effects. Radiation to the thorax can damage the pericardium, myocardium, valves, and coronary blood vessels. The pericardium is the most commonly involved, with pericardial effusion or pericarditis the key problems.[25] The incidence of radiation-induced heart disease is higher in patients given high doses of radiation or radiation therapy concurrent with doxorubicin. Patients with preexisting coronary artery disease are especially vulnerable.[26]

Anthracyclines (e.g., doxorubicin, daunorubicin) are the best studied of the anticancer drugs that cause cardiotoxicity. Acute cardiotoxicities may cause electrocardiographic (ECG) abnormalities, and late effects are left ventricular dysfunction and heart failure. Anthracycline toxicity can be decreased by changing administration from a rapid infusion to a continuous infusion.

5-FU can cause cardiac ischemic syndrome. Monoclonal antibodies, when infused, commonly cause hypotension because of a massive release of cytokines. One type of monoclonal antibody, trastuzumab (Herceptin), which is used in the treatment of breast cancer, is cardiotoxic and may result in ventricular dysfunction and heart failure. Trastuzumab-related cardiomyopathy is managed with angiotensin-converting enzyme inhibitors and β-adrenergic blockers.

Reproductive Effects. Reproductive dysfunction secondary to radiation and chemotherapy varies according to the radiation treatment field and dosage and the particular chemotherapy agent and dose as well as host factors (e.g., age). Treatment can cause temporary or permanent gonadal failure. Reproductive effects occur most often when reproductive organs are included in the radiation treatment field and with alkylating agents. The testes are highly sensitive to radiation, and protection of the testicles with a testicular shield should be done whenever possible. Radiation doses of 15 to 30 cGy temporarily decrease the sperm count, with temporary aspermia developing at 35 to 230 cGy. The patient receiving 200 to 300 cGy may recover sperm production by 3 years following treatment. In some cases, 200 to 300 cGy may result in permanent aspermia. The patient receiving 400 to 600 cGy either recovers in 2 to 5 years or not at all. Greater than 600 cGy exposure is associated with permanent sterility. Pretreatment status may be a significant factor because a low sperm count and loss of motility are seen in individuals with testicular cancer and Hodgkin's lymphoma before any therapy. Combined modality treatment or prior chemotherapy with alkylating agents enhances and prolongs the effects of radiation on the testes. When radiation is used alone with conventional doses and appropriate shielding, testicular recovery often occurs. Compromise of reproductive function in men may also result from erectile dysfunction following pelvic radiation due to related vascular and neurologic effects.

The radiation dose necessary to induce ovarian failure changes with age. Permanent cessation of menses occurs at 500 to 1000 cGy in 95% of women less than 40 years of age and at 375 cGy in women more than 40 years of age. Unlike the testes, there is no avenue for repair of ovarian function. The ovaries are shielded whenever possible. Other factors that influence reproductive or sexual functioning in women include reactions in the cervix and endometrium. These tissues withstand a high radiation dose with minimal sequelae, accounting for the ability to treat endometrial and cervical cancer with high external and brachytherapy doses. Acute reactions such as tenderness, irritation, and loss of lubrication compromise sexual activity. Late effects of combined internal and external therapy include vaginal shortening related to fibrosis and loss of elasticity and lubrication.

The patient and her or his partner require information about the expected effects of treatment relative to reproductive and sexual issues. Potential infertility can be a significant consequence for the individual, and counseling may be indicated. However, in no case should the patient think that conception is not possible during treatment. Pretreatment harvesting of sperm or ova may be considered. Specific suggestions to manage side effects that have an impact on sexual functioning include using a water-soluble vaginal lubricant and a vaginal dilator after pelvic irradiation. The nurse needs to encourage discussion of issues related to sexuality, offer specific suggestions, and make referrals for ongoing counseling when indicated.

Coping with Therapy. Nurses play a key role in assisting patients to cope with the psychoemotional issues associated with receiving cancer treatment. Anxiety is common among patients receiving anticancer therapy—anxieties about various aspects of treatment administration (i.e., repeated venipuncture), dependency on others, ability to pay, potential side effects, and poor outcomes. Repetitive office visits or hospitalizations, as well as continuing medications and laboratory testing, force the individual to confront the cancer on a daily basis. Treatment-related uncertainties and fears are often most evident at the beginning of therapy. For those patients completing curative therapy, anxiety may surface again when therapy comes to an end (i.e., fear of recurrence, less available support). Telling patients that they will be followed and that support is ongoing can be reassuring. Providing information and support can help to minimize the negative impact of anticancer therapy on quality of life. Patient teaching, symptom management, and interventions designed to help patients self-manage their illness and normalize their experience (e.g., adjusting treatment schedules to permit patients to work when possible, referral to support groups) facilitate personal coping during and after cancer therapy and optimizing lifestyle patterns that comprise quality of life. Arranging for patients to meet with individuals who have successfully completed therapy can offer hopefulness and confidence. In addition, nurses can make regular supportive telephone contacts between office visits and assist with planning for transportation, nutrition, and emotional support with available resources such as the American Cancer Society, churches, and other community resources.

LATE EFFECTS OF RADIATION AND CHEMOTHERAPY

Cancer survivors are achieving long-term remission and survival rates with advancements in treatment modalities. However, these forms of therapy (especially radiation and chemotherapy) may produce long-term sequelae termed *physiologic late effects* that occur months to years after cessation of therapy. Every body system can be affected to some extent by chemotherapy and radiation therapy. The effects of radiation on the body's tissues are caused by cellular hypoplasia of stem cells and alterations in the fine vasculature and fibroconnective tissues. In addition to the acute toxicities, chemotherapy can have long-term effects related to the loss of cells' proliferative reserve capacity. The additive effects of multiagent chemotherapy before, during, or after a course of radiotherapy can significantly increase the resulting physiologic late effects.

The cancer survivor may also be at risk for leukemias and other secondary malignancies resulting from therapy for the primary cancer. However, the potential risk for developing a second malignancy does not contraindicate the use of cancer treatment. The overall risk of developing neoplastic complications is low, and the latency period may be long.

The cancer treatments most frequently implicated in causing secondary malignancy are the alkylating chemotherapeutic agents and high-dose radiation, which can induce cancers at the exposure site. The exact mechanism of oncogenesis secondary to radiation and chemotherapy remains unclear. It could be related to interactions between immunosuppressive factors, direct cellular damage, and carcinogenic effects along with other environmental carcinogens.

Acute leukemias occurring as secondary malignancies have been most widely reported after treatment for Hodgkin's lymphoma, but they also occur in survivors of ovarian, lung, and breast cancers. Secondary malignancies other than leukemias include multiple myeloma after radiation therapy for breast cancer; non-Hodgkin's lymphoma after treatment for Hodgkin's lymphoma; and cancers of the bladder, kidney, and ureters after the use of cyclophosphamide. Radiation therapy for breast, lung, ovarian, uterine, and thyroid cancers, non-Hodgkin's lymphoma, and Hodgkin's lymphoma has been linked to secondary osteosarcoma of the rib, scapula, clavicle, humerus, sternum, ilium, and pelvis. Fibrosarcomas have been reported several years after radiation therapy for astrocytoma, glioblastoma, and pituitary adenoma. Unfortunately, secondary malignancies are usually resistant to therapy.

BIOLOGIC AND TARGETED THERAPY

Biologic and targeted therapy is the fourth type of cancer treatment modality. Biologic and targeted therapy can be effective alone or in combination with surgery, radiation therapy, and chemotherapy. **Biologic therapy,** or *biologic response modifier* therapy, consists of agents that modify the relationship between the host and the tumor by altering the biologic response of the host to the tumor cells. Biologic agents may affect host-tumor response in three ways: (1) they have direct antitumor effects; (2) they restore, augment, or modulate host immune system mechanisms; and (3) they have other biologic effects, such as interfering with the cancer cells' ability to metastasize or differentiate (Table 16-17).

Targeted therapy interferes with cancer growth by targeting specific cellular receptors and pathways that are important in tumor growth (see Table 16-17 and Fig. 16-21). The targeted therapies are more selective for specific molecular targets than cytotoxic anticancer drugs. Thus they are able to kill cancer cells without damaging normal cells. Targeted therapies include various tyrosine kinase inhibitors, monoclonal antibodies (MoAb), antiangiogenic agents known as vascular endothelial growth factor (VEGF) receptor inhibitors, and proteasome inhibitors. Tyrosine kinase is an important enzyme that activates the signaling pathways that regulate cell proliferation and survival. Monoclonal antibodies are capable of binding to specific target cells, including tumor cells. They function by being directed at specific binding sites, thus inhibiting the internalization of receptor-antibody complexes and signaling pathways. They may also stimulate an immunologic response in the patient.[27] (Hybridoma technology for the production of MoAbs is described in Chapter 14.)

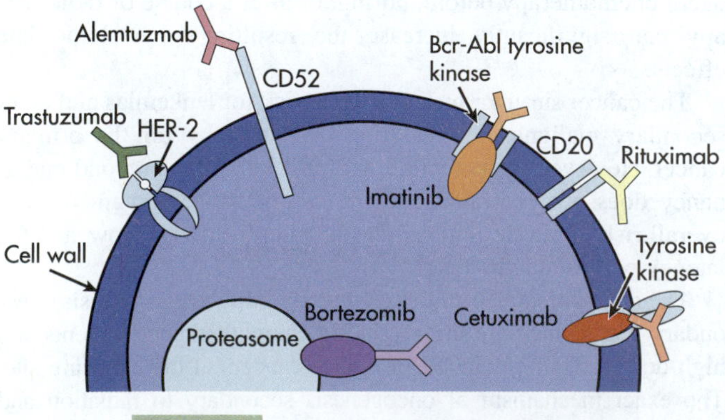

FIG. 16-21 Sites of action of targeted therapy.

Human epidermal growth factor receptor 2 (HER-2) is overexpressed in certain cancers (especially breast cancers) and is associated with more aggressive disease and decreased survival. Trastuzumab (Herceptin) is a MoAb that binds to HER-2 and inhibits the growth of breast cancer cells that overexpress the HER-2 protein. Trastuzumab is used in the treatment of metastatic breast cancers that overexpress HER-2.

Angiogenesis inhibitors work by preventing the mechanisms and pathways necessary for vascularization of tumors. Bevacizumab (Avastin), a recombinant human MoAb, is indicated in combination with chemotherapy (e.g., 5-FU) for the management of metastatic colorectal cancer.

Proteasomes are intracellular multienzyme complexes that degrade proteins. Proteasome inhibitors can cause these proteins to accumulate, thus leading to altered cell function. Normal cells are capable of recovering from proteasome inhibition, but cancer cells undergo death when proteasomes are inhibited.

Side Effects of Biologic and Targeted Therapy

The administration of one biologic agent usually induces the endogenous release of other biologic agents. The release and action of these biologic agents results in systemic immune and inflammatory responses. The toxicities and side effects of biologic agents are related to dose and schedule. Table 16-17 summarizes the potential side effects associated with specific biologic and targeted therapies.

Common side effects include constitutional flu-like symptoms, including headache, fever, chills, myalgias, fatigue, malaise, weakness, photosensitivity, anorexia, and nausea. With interferon therapy, these flu-like symptoms almost invariably appear. However, the severity of the flu-like syndrome associated with interferon therapy generally decreases over time. Acetaminophen administered every 4 hours, as prescribed, often reduces the severity of the flu-like syndrome. The patient is commonly premedicated with acetaminophen in an attempt to prevent or decrease the intensity of these symptoms. In addition, large amounts of fluids help decrease the symptoms.

Tachycardia and orthostatic hypotension are also commonly reported. IL-2 and monoclonal antibodies can cause capillary leak syndrome, which can result in pulmonary edema. Other toxic and side effects may involve the CNS, renal and hepatic systems, and cardiovascular system. These effects are found particularly with interferons and IL-2.

A wide range of neurologic deficits has been observed with interferon and IL-2 therapy. The nature and extent of these problems are not yet completely understood. However, these problems are understandably frightening to the patient and the family, who must be taught to observe for neurologic problems (e.g., confusion, memory loss, difficulty making decisions, insomnia), report their occurrence, and institute appropriate safety and support measures.

MoAbs are administered by the infusion method. Patients may experience infusion-related symptoms, which can include fever, chills, urticaria, mucosal congestion, nausea, diarrhea, and myalgias. There is also a risk, although rare, of anaphylaxis associated with the administration of MoAbs. This potential exists because most MoAbs are produced by mouse lymphocytes and thus represent a foreign protein to the human body. Onset of anaphylaxis can occur within 5 minutes of administration and can be a life-

TABLE 16-17 DRUG THERAPY
Biologic and Targeted Therapy

Drug	Mechanism of Action	Indications	Side Effects
α-interferon (Roferon-A, Intron A)	Inhibits DNA and protein synthesis Suppresses cell proliferation Increases cytotoxic effects of natural killer (NK) cells	Hairy cell leukemia, chronic myelogenous leukemia, malignant melanoma, renal cell carcinoma, non-Hodgkin's lymphoma, ovarian cancer, multiple myeloma, Kaposi sarcoma, pancreatic carcinoma	Flu-like syndrome (fever, chills, myalgia, headache), cognitive changes, fatigue, nausea, vomiting, anorexia, weight loss
interleukin-2 (aldesleukin [Proleukin])	Stimulates proliferation of T and B cells Activates NK cells	Metastatic renal cell cancer, metastatic melanoma	Same as above; capillary leak syndrome resulting in hypotension; bone marrow suppression
levamisole (Ergamisol)	Potentiates monocytes and macrophage function	Duke's stage C colon cancer (given in combination with 5-FU)	Diarrhea, metallic taste, nausea, fever, chills, mouth sores, headache
BCG vaccine (TheraCys)	Induces an immune response that prevents angiogenesis of tumor	In situ bladder cancer	Flu-like syndrome, nausea, vomiting, rash, cough
Tyrosine Kinase Inhibitors			
cetuximab (Erbitux)	Inhibits epidermal growth factor receptor, which is coupled with tyrosine kinase	Colorectal cancer, in combination with radiotherapy for head and neck carcinoma	Rash, dry skin, infusion reactions, interstitial lung disease, fatigue, fever
erlotinib (Tarceva)	Same as above	Non–small cell lung cancer	Rash, diarrhea, interstitial lung disease
gefitinib (Iressa)	Same as above	Non–small cell lung cancer	Rash, diarrhea, interstitial lung disease
imatinib (Gleevec)	Inhibits Bcr-Abl tyrosine kinase	Chronic myeloid leukemia	Nausea, diarrhea, myalgia, fuid retention
sorafenib (Nexavar)	Inhibits several tyrosine kinases, some of which are involved in angiogenesis	Advanced renal cell carcinoma	Rash, diarrhea, hypertension; redness, pain, swelling, or blisters on hands/feet
Monoclonal Antibody to CD20			
rituximab (Rituxan)	Binds CD20 antigen, causing cytotoxicity	Non-Hodgkin's lymphoma (B cell)	Fever, chills, nausea, headache, angioedema
ibritumomab tiuxetan/yttrium-90 (Zevalin)	Binds CD20 antigen, causing cytotoxicity and radiation injury	Non-Hodgkin's lymphoma (B cell)	Bone marrow suppression, fatigue, nausea, chills
tositumomab/tositumomab-^{131}I (Bexxar)	Binds CD20 antigen, causing immune attack and radiation injury	Non-Hodgkin's lymphoma (B cell)	Bone marrow suppression, fever, chills, nausea, headache
Angiogenesis Inhibitor			
bevacizumab (Avastin)	Binds vascular endothelial growth factor, thereby inhibiting angiogenesis	Colorectal cancer	Hypertension, colon bleeding and perforation, impaired wound healing, thromboembolism, diarrhea
Proteasome Inhibitor			
bortezomib (Velcade)	Inhibits proteasome activity, which functions to regulate cell growth	Multiple myeloma	Bone marrow suppression, nausea, vomiting, diarrhea, peripheral neuropathy, fatigue
Monoclonal Antibodies			
gemtuzumab ozogamicin (Mylotarg)	Binds CD33 antigen (expressed on leukemic cells) to deliver cytotoxic drug into the DNA	Acute myeloid leukemia	Bone marrow suppression, fever, chills, nausea
alemtuzumab (Campath)	Binds CD52 antigen (found on T and B cells, monocytes, NK cells, neutrophils)	Chronic lymphocytic leukemia (B cell)	Bone marrow suppression, chills, fever, vomiting, diarrhea, fatigue
trastuzumab (Herceptin)	Binds human epidermal growth factor receptor 2 (HER-2)	Breast cancer (HER-2 positive)	Cardiotoxicity

threatening event. If this occurs, administration of the MoAb should be stopped immediately, emergency assistance obtained, and resuscitation measures implemented. (See Chapter 14 for a discussion of nursing management of anaphylaxis.)

Skin rashes are common in patients receiving epidermal growth factor receptor (EGFR) inhibitors and manifest generally as erythema and acneiform rashes that can cover up to 50% of the upper body. Antiangiogenics can produce life-threatening problems of arterial thrombi, hemorrhage, hypertension, and proteinuria.[27] Other toxicities of MoAbs can include capillary leak syndrome, hepatotoxicity, bone marrow depression, and central nervous system effects. Patients who receive traztuzumab may also experience cardiac dysfunction, especially when it is administered in higher doses or in combination with anthracycline antibiotics such as doxorubicin (Adriamycin).

NURSING MANAGEMENT
BIOLOGIC AND TARGETED THERAPY

Some problems experienced by the patient receiving biologic and targeted therapy are different from those observed with more traditional forms of cancer therapy. These effects occur more acutely and are dose limited (i.e., effects resolve when the agent is discontinued). Capillary leak syndrome and pulmonary edema are problems that require critical care nursing. Bone marrow depression occurring with biologic therapy administration is generally more transient and less severe than that observed with chemotherapy. Fatigue associated with biologic therapy can be so severe that it can constitute a dose-limiting toxicity. As these agents are increasingly combined with cytotoxic therapies, the spectrum of therapy-related effects expands.

Nursing interventions for flu-like syndrome include the administration of acetaminophen before treatment and every 4 hours after treatment. IV meperidine (Demerol) has been used to control the severe chills associated with some biologic agents. Other nursing measures include monitoring of vital signs and temperature, planning for periods of rest for the patient, assisting with activities of daily living (ADLs), and monitoring for adequate oral intake.

HEMATOPOIETIC GROWTH FACTORS

Hematopoietic growth factors are used to support cancer patients through the treatment of the disease (Table 16-18). Colony-stimulating factors (CSFs) are a family of glycoproteins produced by various cells. CSFs stimulate production, maturation, regulation, and activation of cells of the hematologic system. The name of the CSF is based on the specific cell line it affects (see Table 16-18). Erythropoietin stimulates erythroid precursor cells in the kidneys to make red blood cells (see Chapter 45).

HEMATOPOIETIC STEM CELL TRANSPLANTATION

Bone marrow transplantation (BMT) and **peripheral stem cell transplantation** (PSCT) are effective, lifesaving procedures for a number of malignant and nonmalignant diseases (Table 16-19). BMT and PSCT allow for the safe use of very high doses of chemotherapy and/or radiation therapy in patients whose tumors have developed resistance or failed to respond to standard doses of chemotherapy and radiation.

This therapeutic approach was typically referred in prior years to as BMT because the bone marrow was the original source of stem cells when the procedure was first developed. However, advances in harvesting and cryopreservation technologies have opened new pathways to the collection of stem cells from the peripheral blood. Consequently, the terminology is changing and it is now typical to refer to these procedures in general as **hematopoietic stem cell transplantation** (HSCT).[28] Whether the diagnosis is a malignant or nonmalignant disease, the goal of HSCT is cure. Overall cure rates are still low, but are steadily increasing. Even when cure is not achieved, transplantation can result in a period of remission.

The approach is to eradicate tumor cells and/or clear the marrow of its components to make way for engraftment of the transplanted stem cells. This is accomplished by administering higher than usual dosages of chemotherapy with or without radiation therapy, which can produce life-threatening consequences associated with pancytopenia and other adverse effects. Infusing healthy stem cells after therapy has been completed "rescues" the damaged bone marrow through the engraftment and subsequent normal proliferation and differentiation of the donated stem cells in the recipient. HSCT is an intensive procedure with many risks, and some patients die from treatment-related complications or from relapse of the original disease. Because it is a highly toxic therapy, the patient must weigh the significant risks of treatment-related death or treatment failure (relapse) against the hope of cure.

Types of Hematopoietic Stem Cell Transplants

HSCTs are categorized as allogeneic, syngeneic, or autologous. The sources of stem cells include the bone marrow, peripheral circulating blood, and umbilical cord blood. In *allogeneic transplantation,* stem

TABLE 16-18 *DRUG THERAPY*
Hematopoietic Growth Factors Used in Cancer Treatment

Growth Factor	Drug Name	Indications	Side Effects
Granulocyte-macrophage colony-stimulating factor (GM-CSF)	sargramostin (Leukine)	Myeloid cell recovery after bone marrow transplantation	Nausea, vomiting, diarrhea, fever, chills, myalgia, headache, fatigue
Granulocyte colony-stimulating factor (G-CSF)	filgrastim (Neupogen) pegfilgrastim (Neulasta)	Chemotherapy-induced neutropenia	Bone pain, nausea, vomiting
Erythropoietin	epoetin (Epogen, Procrit) darbepoetin (Aranesp)	Anemia of chronic cancer Anemia related to chemotherapy	Hypertension, thrombosis, headache
Interleukin-11 (platelet growth factor)	oprelvekin (Neumega)	Thrombocytopenia related to chemotherapy	Fluid retention, peripheral edema, dyspnea, tachycardia, nausea, mouth sores

TABLE 16-19 Indications for Hematopoietic Stem Cell Transplantation

Malignant Diseases	Nonmalignant Diseases
Acute and chronic myelogenous leukemia	Hematologic diseases
Acute lymphocytic leukemia	Aplastic anemia
Hodgkin's lymphoma	Chronic granulomatous disease
Multiple myeloma	Fanconi's anemia
Myelodysplastic syndrome	Sickle cell disease (severe)
Neuroblastoma	Thalassemia
Non-Hodgkin's lymphoma	Immunodeficiency diseases
Ovarian cancer	Severe combined immunodeficiency disease (SCID)
Sarcoma	Wiskott-Aldrich syndrome
Testicular cancer	

cells are acquired from a donor who, through human leukocyte antigen (HLA) tissue typing, has been determined to be HLA matched to the recipient. HLA typing involves testing WBCs to identify genetically inherited antigens common to both donor and recipient that are important in compatibility of transplanted tissue. (HLA tissue typing is discussed in Chapter 14.) Often this is a family member but may be an unrelated donor found through a national or international bone marrow registry (i.e., National Marrow Donor Program). While there may be more risks and toxicities associated with an unrelated allogeneic transplant, an added benefit of this type of transplant is not only eradication of the tumor cells with high-dose therapy, but also the potential stimulation of the graft-versus-tumor effect in which donor WBCs identify and attack malignant cells in the recipient. Common indications for allogeneic transplant are certain leukemias, multiple myeloma, and lymphoma.

Syngeneic transplantation is a type of allogeneic transplant that involves obtaining stem cells from one identical twin and infusing them into the other. Identical twins have identical HLA types and are a perfect match. Therefore neither the graft-versus-host nor the graft-versus-tumor effect occurs.

In *autologous transplantation,* patients receive their own stem cells back following *myeloablative* (destroying bone marrow) chemotherapy (Fig. 16-22). The aim of this approach is purely "rescue." It enables patients to receive intensive chemotherapy and/or radiation by supporting them with their previously harvested stem cells until their marrow is generating blood cells again on its own. Restoration usually takes 4 to 6 weeks depending on the particular conditioning regimen administered. Autologous transplants are typically used to treat hematologic malignancies if there is no suitable donor or the patient cannot undergo allogeneic transplantation. HSCT continues to be investigated in the management of some solid tumors refractory to treatment.[28]

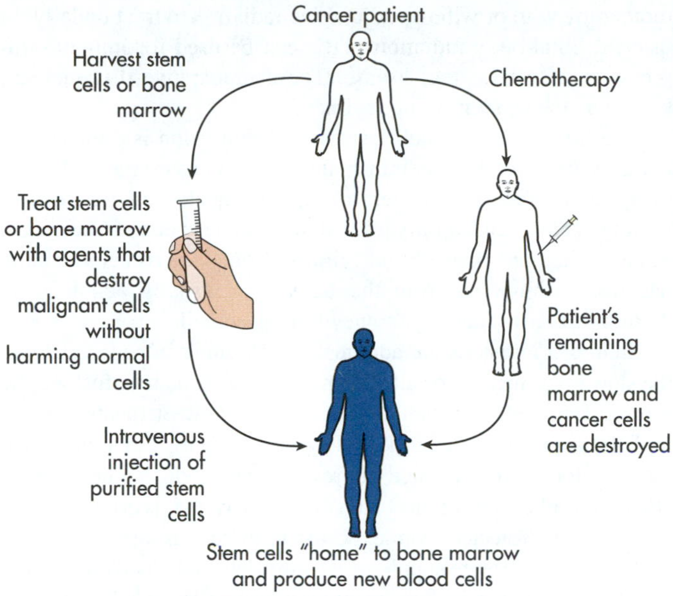

FIG. 16-22 Autologous stem cell transplant.

Procedures

Harvest Procedures. Hematopoetic stem cells are "harvested" from a unique donor (for allogeneic transplantation) or from the recipient (for autologous transplantation) via two different methods. In one type of procedure, used for harvesting of stem cells residing in bone marrow (as the process was originally developed), the procedure is performed in the operating room using general or spinal anesthesia. Multiple bone marrow aspirations (usually from the iliac crest, but sometimes from the sternum) are carried out to obtain a specific quantity of stem cells (i.e., the number needed to ensure engraftment). The entire bone marrow harvest procedure takes about 1 to 2 hours, and the patient can be discharged following recovery. Postharvest, the donor may experience pain at the collection site, which can be treated with mild analgesics. The donor's body will replenish the bone marrow removed in a few weeks.

In the other type of procedure, peripheral stem cell transplants are obtained from the peripheral blood in an outpatient procedure. It is done using cell separator equipment that automatically separates the stem cells from the blood circulating through the machine and returns the remaining blood components to the donor. The process averages about 2 to 4 hours but can sometimes be longer depending on donor factors and the quality of the venous access. Often it takes more than one procedure to obtain enough stem cells. Because there are fewer stem cells in the blood than in the bone marrow, "mobilization" of stem cells from the bone marrow into the peripheral blood can be accomplished using chemotherapy and/or hematopoietic growth factors. Common growth factors that are used are GM-CSF and G-CSF (see Table 16-18), but chemotherapeutic agents, typically cyclophosphamide (Cytoxan), can also be used if there is a need to reduce tumor burden.

Harvested marrow is processed to strain out bone fragments (this is not necessary with peripheral collections). The marrow or peripherally collected stem cells are then bagged with preservative for cryopreservation and storage until they are needed or used for more immediate administration. Since it is coming from the patient, autologous stem cells are sometimes treated (purged) to remove undetected cancer cells. Many different pharmacologic, immunologic, physical, and chemical agents have been used for this purpose.

Umbilical cord blood is also rich in hematopoietic stem cells, and successful allogeneic transplants have been performed using this source. Cord blood can be HLA-typed and cryopreserved. A disadvantage of cord blood is the possibility of insufficient numbers of stem cells to permit transplant to adults. Considerable research is currently ongoing to define the optimal application of this technology.[29]

Preparative Regimens and Stem Cell Infusions. In malignant diseases, patients receive myeloablative dosages of chemotherapy with or without adjunctive radiation to treat underlying disease. Total-body radiation (TBI) can be used for immunosuppression or to treat the disease. These preparative therapies are known as the "conditioning regimen."

The timing of stem cell harvest and reinfusion is critical, particularly with autologous transplantation. To ensure the collection of optimally functioning stem cells in adequate numbers, conditioning is commenced only after stem cells have already been harvested. They are thawed and reinfused only after chemotherapy has been eliminated from the body (i.e., usually about 24 to 48 hours) to avoid damage to newly infused cells.

Stem cell infusions are administered IV, and can be injected via the slow bolus method or infused much like a blood transfusion. The infused stem cells reconstitute the bone marrow elements, "rescuing" the recipient's hematopoietic system. Usually 2 to 4 weeks are required for the transplanted marrow to start producing hematopoietic blood cells. During this pancytopenic period, it is critical for the patient to be protected from exposure to infectious agents and supported with electrolyte supplements, nutrition, and blood component transfusions (as needed) to maintain adequate levels of circulating RBCs and platelets.

Complications. Bacterial, viral, and fungal infections are common following HSCT. Prophylactic antibiotic therapy may reduce their incidence. A potentially serious complication of allogeneic transplant is graft-versus-host disease. This occurs when the T lymphocytes from the donated marrow (graft) recognize the recipient (host) as foreign and begin to attack certain organs such as the skin, liver, and GI tract. (Graft-versus-host disease is discussed in Chapter 14.) The occurrence and severity of posttransplant complications are also dependent on the drugs comprising the patient's particular conditioning regimen (some are more toxic than others) and the stem cell source. Because stem cells in the peripheral blood are more mature than those harvested from the marrow, the hematologic recovery period in PSCT is shorter, and fewer, less severe complications are seen.[30]

GENE THERAPY

Gene therapy is an experimental therapy that involves introducing genetic material into a person's cells to fight disease. Researchers are studying several ways to treat cancer using gene therapy. Some approaches target healthy cells to enhance their ability to fight cancer. Other approaches target cancer cell to destroy them or prevent their growth. In one approach, researchers replace missing or altered genes with healthy genes. Because some missing or altered genes (e.g., *p53*) may lead to cancer, substituting "working" copies of these genes may keep cancer from developing. Researchers are also studying ways to improve a patient's immune response to cancer. In this approach, gene therapy is used to stimulate the body's natural ability to attack cancer cells. Other research is focused on the use of gene therapy to prevent cancer cells from developing new blood vessels (angiogenesis). At this time, the use of gene therapy is investigational. Additional information can be found on the National Cancer Institute's website at *www.nci.gov.* (Gene therapy is discussed in Chapter 14.)

COMPLICATIONS RESULTING FROM CANCER

The patient may develop complications related to the continual growth of the malignancy into normal tissue or to the side effects of treatment.

Nutritional Problems

Malnutrition. The patient with cancer often experiences protein and calorie malnutrition characterized by fat and muscle depletion. (Assessment of the degree of malnutrition is discussed in Chapter 40.) Foods suggested for increasing the protein intake to facilitate repair and regeneration of cells are presented in Table 16-20. High-calorie foods that provide energy and minimize weight loss are presented in Table 16-21. (A sample high-calorie, high-protein diet is presented in Table 40-14.)

The nurse should suggest the need for a nutritional supplement to the health care provider as soon as a 5% weight loss is noted or if the patient has the potential for protein and calorie malnutrition. Albumin and prealbumin levels should be monitored. Once a 10-lb (4.5-kg) weight loss occurs, it is difficult to maintain the nutritional status. The patient can be taught to use nutritional supple-

TABLE 16-20 *NUTRITIONAL THERAPY* Protein Foods with High Biologic Value

Milk

Whole milk (1 cup) = 9 g protein

Double-strength milk—1 quart of whole milk plus 1 cup of dried skim milk blended and chilled: 1 cup = 14 g protein

Milk shake—1 cup of ice cream plus 1 cup of milk = 15 g protein, 416 calories

Use evaporated milk, double-strength milk, or half-and-half to make casseroles, hot cereals, sauces, gravies, puddings, milkshakes, and soups.

Yogurt (regular and frozen)—check labels and purchase brand with highest protein content: 1 cup = 10 g protein

Eggs

Egg = 6 g protein

Eggnog (1 cup) = 15.5 g protein

Add eggs to salads, casseroles, and sauces. Deviled eggs are especially well tolerated.

Desserts that contain eggs include angel food cake, sponge cake, custard, and cheesecake.

Cheese

Cottage	½ cup	15 g protein
American	1 slice	3 g protein
Cheddar	1 slice	6 g protein
Cream	1 tbs	1 g protein

Use cheese in a sandwich or as a snack.

Add cheese to salads, casseroles, sauces, and baked potatoes.

Cheese spread with crackers is a wholesome snack that can be made and stored in the refrigerator for easy accessibility.

Meat, Poultry, Fish

Beef	3 oz	approx. 21 g protein
Pork	3 oz	approx. 19 g protein
Chicken	½ breast	approx. 26 g protein
Fish	3 oz	approx. 30 g protein
Tuna fish	6½ oz	approx. 44.5 g protein

Add meat, poultry, and fish to salads, casseroles, and sandwiches.

Add strained and junior baby meats to soups and casseroles.

Cocktail weiners or deviled ham on crackers are wholesome snacks. These snacks can be made and stored in the refrigerator for easy accessibility.

TABLE 16-21 NUTRITIONAL THERAPY High-Calorie Foods

Mayonnaise	1 tbs	=	101 cal
Butter or margarine	1 tsp	=	35 cal
Sour cream	1 tbs	=	72 cal
Peanut butter	1 tbs	=	94 cal
Whipped cream	1 tbs	=	53 cal
Corn oil	1 tbs	=	119 cal
Jelly	1 tbs	=	49 cal
Ice cream	1 cup	=	256 cal
Honey	1 tbs	=	64 cal

ments in place of milk when cooking or baking. Foods to which nutritional supplements can be easily added include scrambled eggs, pudding, custard, mashed potatoes, cereal, and cream sauces. Packages of instant breakfast can be used as indicated or sprinkled on cereals, desserts, and casseroles.

If the malnutrition cannot be treated with dietary intake, it may be necessary to use enteral or parenteral nutrition as an adjunct nutritional measure. (Enteral and parenteral nutrition are discussed in Chapter 40.)

Altered Taste Sensation. It is theorized that cancer cells release substances that resemble amino acids and stimulate the bitter taste buds. The patient may also experience an alteration in the sweet taste sensation, as well as in the sour and salty taste sensations. Meat may also taste bitter to the patient. At this time, the physiologic basis of these varied taste alterations is unknown. The patient with an altered taste problem should be instructed to avoid foods that are disliked. Frequently the patient may feel compelled to eat certain foods because those foods are believed to be beneficial. The patient can be taught to experiment with spices and other seasoning agents in an attempt to mask the taste alterations that are occurring. Lemon juice, onion, mint, basil, and fruit juice marinades may improve the taste of certain meats and fish. Bacon bits, onion, and pieces of ham may enhance the taste of vegetables. An additional amount of a spice or seasoning agent is usually not an effective way to enhance the taste.

Infection

Infection is a primary cause of death in the patient with cancer. The usual sites of infection include the lungs, GU system, mouth, rectum, peritoneal cavity, and blood (septicemia). Infection occurs as a result of the ulceration and necrosis caused by the tumor, compression of vital organs by the tumor, and neutropenia caused by the disease process or the treatment of cancer. Outpatients with risk for neutropenia should be instructed to call with a temperature of 100.5° F (38° C) or greater. Assessment most often includes signs and symptoms of fever, determination of possible etiology, and complete blood count.

Many patients are neutropenic when an infection develops. In these individuals, infection may cause significant morbidity and may be rapidly fatal if not treated promptly. The classic manifestations of infection are not often present in a patient with neutropenia and a depressed immune system. (Neutropenia is discussed in Chapter 31.)

Oncologic Emergencies

Oncologic emergencies are life-threatening emergencies that can occur as a result of cancer or cancer treatment. These emergencies can be obstructive, metabolic, or infiltrative.

Obstructive Emergencies. Obstructive emergencies are primarily caused by tumor obstruction of an organ or blood vessel. Obstructive emergencies include superior vena cava syndrome, spinal cord compression syndrome, third space syndrome, and intestinal obstruction.

Superior Vena Cava Syndrome. *Superior vena cava syndrome* results from obstruction of the superior vena cava by a tumor or thrombosis. The clinical manifestations include facial edema, periorbital edema, distention of veins of the head, neck, and chest (Fig. 16-23), headache, and seizures. A mediastinal mass is often visible on chest x-ray. The most common causes are lung cancer, non-Hodgkin's lymphoma, and metastatic breast cancer. Superior vena cava syndrome is considered a serious medical problem. Management usually involves radiation therapy to the site of obstruction. However, chemotherapy may be administered for tumors more sensitive to this form of therapy.

Spinal Cord Compression. Spinal cord compression is a neurologic emergency caused by the presence of a malignant tumor in the epidural space of the spinal cord. The most common primary tumors that produce this problem are breast, lung, prostate, GI, and renal tumors and melanoma.[31] Lymphomas also pose a risk if diseased lymph tissue invades the epidural space. The manifestations are back pain that is intense, localized, and persistent, accompanied by vertebral tenderness and aggravated by the Valsalva maneuver; motor weakness and dysfunction; sensory paresthesia and loss; and autonomic dysfunction. One of the clinical symptoms that reflects autonomic dysfunction is a reported change in bowel or bladder function. Radiation therapy in conjunction with prompt initiation of corticosteroids is generally associated with some initial improvement. Surgical decompressive laminectomy is used less commonly. It may be considered for patients with tumors that are relatively radioresistant or when the tumor is in a previously irradiated area. Activity limitations and pain management are important nursing interventions.

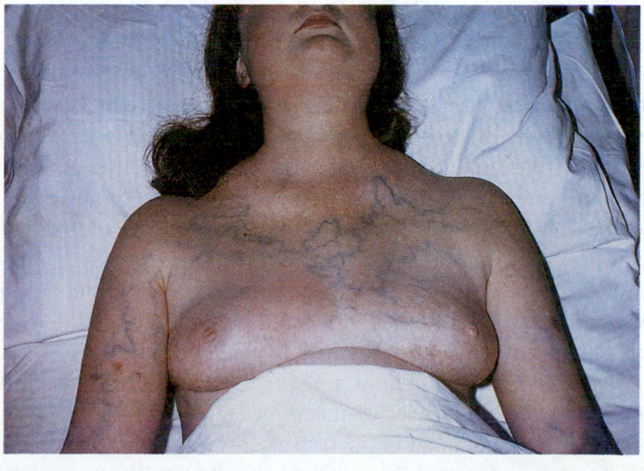

FIG. 16-23 Superior vena caval obstruction in bronchial carcinoma. Note the swelling of the face and neck and the development of collateral circulation in the veins.

Third Space Syndrome. Third space syndrome involves a shifting of fluid from the vascular space to the interstitial space that primarily occurs secondary to extensive surgical procedures, biologic therapy, or septic shock. Initially patients exhibit signs of hypovolemia, including hypotension, tachycardia, low central venous pressure, and decreased urine output. Treatment includes fluid, electrolyte, and plasma protein replacement. During recovery hypervolemia can occur, resulting in hypertension, elevated central venous pressure, weight gain, and shortness of breath. Treatment generally involves reduction in fluid administration and fluid balance monitoring.

Intestinal Obstruction. Chapter 43 presents a complete discussion of intestinal obstruction.

Metabolic Emergencies. Metabolic emergencies are caused by the production of ectopic hormones directly from the tumor or are secondary to metabolic alterations caused by the presence of the tumor or cancer treatment. Ectopic hormones arise from tissues that do not normally produce these hormones. Cancer cells return to a more embryologic form, thus allowing the stored potential of the cells to become evident. Metabolic emergencies include syndrome of inappropriate antidiuretic hormone secretion, hypercalcemia, tumor lysis syndrome, septic shock, and disseminated intravascular coagulation.

Syndrome of Inappropriate Antidiuretic Hormone Secretion. Syndrome of inappropriate antidiuretic hormone secretion (SIADH) results from abnormal or sustained production of antidiuretic hormone (ADH) with resultant H_2O retention and hyponatremia (see Chapter 50). SIADH occurs most frequently in carcinoma of the lung (especially small cell lung cancer) but can also occur in cancer of the pancreas, duodenum, brain, esophagus, colon, ovary, prostate, bronchus, and nasopharynx; leukemia; mesothelioma; reticulum cell sarcoma; Hodgkin's lymphoma; and thymoma. Cancer cells in these tumors are actually able to manufacture, store, and release ADH. The chemotherapeutic agents vincristine and cyclophosphamide (Cytoxan) also stimulate the release of ADH from the pituitary or tumor cells. Symptoms of SIADH include weight gain, weakness, anorexia, nausea, vomiting, personality changes, seizures, and coma. Treatment of SIADH includes treating the underlying malignancy and measures to correct the sodium-water imbalance, including fluid restriction and, in severe cases, IV administration of 3% sodium chloride solution.

Hypercalcemia. Hypercalcemia can occur in the presence of cancer that involves metastatic disease of the bone or multiple myeloma, or when a parathyroid hormone–like substance is secreted by cancer cells in the absence of bony metastasis. Hypercalcemia resulting from malignancies that have metastasized occurs most frequently in patients with lung, breast, kidney, colon, ovarian, or thyroid cancer. Hypercalcemia resulting from secretion of parathyroid hormone–like substance occurs most frequently in squamous cell carcinoma of the lung; head and neck, cervical, and esophageal cancer; lymphomas; and leukemia. Immobility and dehydration can contribute to or exacerbate hypercalcemia.

The primary manifestations of hypercalcemia include apathy, depression, fatigue, muscle weakness, electrocardiogram changes, polyuria and nocturia, anorexia, nausea, and vomiting. Serum levels of calcium in excess of 12 mg/dl (3 mmol/L) will often produce symptoms, and significant calcium elevations can be life threatening. Chronic hypercalcemia can result in nephrocalcinosis and irreversible renal failure. The long-term treatment of hypercalcemia is aimed at the primary disease. Acute hypercalcemia is treated by hydration (3 L/day), diuretic (particularly loop diuretics) administration, and a bisphosphonate, a drug that inhibits the action of osteoclasts. Infusion of the bisphosphonate zoledronate (Zometa) or pamidronate (Aredia) is the treatment of choice. These drugs are also used to prevent bone complications in patients with bone metastasis.

Tumor Lysis Syndrome. Acute *tumor lysis syndrome* (TLS) is a metabolic complication characterized by rapid release of intracellular components in response to chemotherapy. It occurs less commonly with radiation therapy. TLS is often associated with tumors that have high growth rates and are sensitive to the effects of chemotherapy. Massive cellular destruction, associated with aggressive chemotherapy for rapidly growing tumors, releases a host of intracellular components into the bloodstream, including potassium, phosphate, and DNA and RNA components (which are metabolized to uric acid by the liver). Rise in serum phosphate drives serum calcium levels down, with resultant hypocalcemia. Metabolic abnormalities and concentrated uric acid (which crystallizes in the distal tubules of the kidneys) lead quickly to acute renal failure if not identified and treated early.

The four hallmark signs of TLS are hyperuricemia, hyperphosphatemia, hyperkalemia, and hypocalcemia. TLS usually occurs within the first 24 to 48 hours after the initiation of chemotherapy and may persist for approximately 5 to 7 days. The primary goal of TLS management is preventing renal failure and severe electrolyte imbalances. The primary treatment includes increasing urine production using hydration therapy and decreasing uric acid concentrations using allopurinol.[32]

Septic Shock and Disseminated Intravascular Coagulation. Septic shock is discussed in Chapter 67, and disseminated intravascular coagulation is discussed in Chapter 31.

Infiltrative Emergencies. Infiltrative emergencies occur when malignant tumors infiltrate major organs or secondary to cancer therapy. The most common infiltrative emergencies are cardiac tamponade and carotid artery rupture.

Cardiac Tamponade. Cardiac tamponade results from fluid accumulation in the pericardial sac, constriction of the pericardium by tumor, or pericarditis secondary to radiation therapy to the chest. Manifestations include a heavy feeling over the chest, shortness of breath, tachycardia, cough, dysphagia, hiccups, hoarseness, nausea, vomiting, excessive perspiration, decreased level of consciousness, pulsus paradoxus, distant or muted heart sounds, and extreme anxiety. Emergency management is aimed at reduction of fluid around the heart and includes surgical establishment of a pericardial window or an indwelling pericardial catheter. Supportive therapy includes administration of oxygen therapy, intravenous hydration, and vasopressor therapy.

Carotid Artery Rupture. Rupture of the carotid artery occurs most frequently in patients with cancer of the head and neck secondary to invasion of the arterial wall by tumor or to erosion following surgery or radiation therapy. Bleeding can manifest as minor oozing or spurting of blood in the case of a "blowout" of the artery. In the presence of a blowout, pressure should be applied to the site with a finger. Intravenous fluid and blood products are administered in an attempt to stabilize the patient for surgery. Surgical management involves ligation of the carotid artery above and below the rupture site and reduction of local tumor.

MANAGEMENT OF CANCER PAIN

Moderate to severe pain occurs in approximately 50% of patients who are receiving active treatment for their cancer and in 80% to 90% of patients with advanced cancer. What is not considered is that these statistics have not changed in the past 30 years. Undertreatment of cancer pain is common and causes needless suffering, hampers quality of life, and increases the burden on family caregivers.[33]

The American Pain Society has released a new clinical practice guideline that describes the management of cancer pain.[34] Inadequate pain assessment is the single greatest barrier to effective pain management. Data such as vital signs and patient behaviors are not reliable indicators of pain, especially long-standing, chronic pain. It is important to distinguish between persistent and breakthrough pain. Therefore it is essential that a comprehensive pain assessment include a detailed history to determine the presence of persistent pain and breakthrough pain. Pain management plans need to be developed to address both components of pain if they are present.

As part of the plan, patients should be taught how to keep a pain management diary. Ongoing assessment of cancer pain is needed to determine the effectiveness of the treatment plan. Data need to be obtained and documented initially and at regular intervals on the location and intensity of the pain, what it feels like, and how it is relieved. Patterns of change also should be assessed. The patient report should always be believed and accepted as the primary source of assessment data. Table 16-22 presents assessment questions that may facilitate this data collection.

Drug therapy, including nonsteroidal antiinflammatory drugs, opioids, and adjuvant pain medications, should be used. Opioids normally are prescribed for the treatment of moderate to severe cancer pain. Analgesic medications (e.g., morphine, fentanyl) should be given on a regular schedule (around the clock) with additional doses available as needed for breakthrough pain. In general, oral administration of the medication is preferred, but other routes (e.g., transdermal) are also available. It is important to remember that, with opioid drugs such as morphine, the appropriate dose is whatever is necessary to control the pain with the least side effects. Fear of addiction is not warranted but must be addressed as part of patient teaching relevant to pain control, since it is a significant barrier for both the patient and the nurse to appropriate pain management.

Patient education should clarify myths and misconceptions and reassure patients and family caregivers that cancer pain can be effectively relieved. Furthermore, addiction and tolerance are not problems associated with effective cancer pain management.[34] Nonpharmacologic interventions, including relaxation therapy and imagery, can be effectively used to manage pain (see Chapter 9). Additional strategies to relieve pain are discussed in Chapter 10.

TABLE 16-22 Pain Assessment in Cancer Patients

Location	• Where is the pain? • Is there more than one place? Is there a new location of pain? • Does location of pain correlate with known diagnosis?
Intensity	• How bad is the pain? • Rate the pain on a scale of 0–10. (See Chapter 10 for rating scales.)
Quality	• What does the pain feel like? • Sharp, dull, burning, shooting, aching, or others? (See Chapter 10 for descriptors.)
Pattern	• Has the pain changed? • Is the pain getting better, worse, or unchanged? • What makes the pain better or worse?
Relief measures	• What do you do to control your pain? • Are medications used? • Do the relief measures help much? How much?

PSYCHOLOGIC SUPPORT

Psychologic support of the patient is an important aspect of cancer care. A positive attitude of patient, family, and health care providers toward cancer and cancer treatment can have an effect on the patient's quality of life. A positive attitude may also influence the prognosis of the patient, although there is no scientific evidence to support that concept.

ETHICAL DILEMMAS
Medical Futility

Situation

A 65-year-old Jewish woman has breast cancer with metastasis to the liver and bone. The family asks the nurse why their mother is not receiving chemotherapy. In addition, they want to make certain that she will be resuscitated should her heart stop. They are aware of her diagnosis and that she may have less than 1 month to live. The nurse was told in morning rounds that the woman does not want any treatment that would prolong her life.

Important Points for Consideration

- If the patient is competent, the patient is legally and ethically the decision maker regarding his or her own care in consultation with the family and the health care team as desired.
- Members of the health care team have no obligation to provide care that is medically futile, that is, care that will not support a person to be able to pursue his or her life goals. Care that is futile may be inappropriate, prolong dying, or provide little or no physical benefit to the patient.
- Palliative care is health care that would provide comfort, control pain, reduce symptoms, or improve the quality of her remaining life as defined by the patient.
- Patients or families do not have a right to demand treatment that offers no clear benefit to the patient.
- In the Jewish faith, withdrawing care is usually acceptable when the patient is terminally ill and suffering.
- The nurse should work in collaboration with other members of the health care team to have discussions with the family, ease the acceptance of their mother's diagnosis, incorporate their mother's goals into the plan of care, discuss a Do Not Resuscitate order and a referral to hospice, and plan for her eventual death.

Critical Thinking Questions

1. How can the nurse assist the patient to communicate her wishes to her family?
2. How can the nurse and the health care team assist the family to plan end-of-life care that incorporates the wishes of their mother?
3. What are the cultural issues in this case?

The diagnosis of cancer is viewed as a crisis. Common fears experienced by the patient with cancer include disfigurement, dependency, disruption of relationships, pain, emaciation, financial depletion, abandonment, and death.

To cope with these fears, the patient with cancer may use and experience different behavioral patterns: shock, anger, denial, bargaining, depression, helplessness, hopelessness, rationalization, acceptance, and intellectualization. These behavioral patterns may occur at any time during the process of cancer. However, some patterns appear to occur more frequently or at a greater intensity at certain specific stages of the disease process. The following factors may influence how the patient will cope with the diagnosis of cancer:

1. *Ability to cope with stressful events in the past* (e.g., loss of job, major disappointment). By simply asking how the patient has coped with previous stressful events, the nurse can gain an understanding of the patient's coping patterns, the effectiveness of the usual coping patterns, and the usual coping time frame.
2. *Availability of significant others.* The patient who has effective support systems tends to cope more effectively than the patient who does not have a meaningful, available support system.
3. *Ability to express feelings and concerns.* The patient who is able to express feelings and needs and who seeks and asks for help appears to cope more effectively than the patient who internalizes feelings and needs.
4. *Age at the time of diagnosis.* Age determines the coping strategies to a great degree. For example, a young mother with cancer may have concerns that differ from those of a 70-year-old woman with cancer.
5. *Extent of disease.* Cure or control of the disease process is usually easier to cope with than the reality of terminal illness.
6. *Disruption of body image.* Disruption of the body image (e.g., radical neck dissection, alopecia, mastectomy) may intensify the psychologic impact of cancer.
7. *Presence of symptoms.* Symptoms such as fatigue, nausea, diarrhea, and pain may intensify the psychologic impact of cancer.
8. *Past experience with cancer.* Negative experiences with cancer (personal or in others) are likely to influence perceptions about current situation.
9. *Attitude associated with the cancer.* A patient who feels in control and has a positive attitude about cancer and cancer treatment is better able to cope with the diagnosis and treatment of cancer than the patient who feels hopeless, helpless, and out of control.

To facilitate the development of a hopeful attitude about cancer and to support the patient and the family during the various stages of the process of cancer, the nurse should do the following:

1. Be available and continue to be available, especially during difficult times.
2. Exhibit a caring attitude.
3. Listen actively to fears and concerns.
4. Provide relief from distressing symptoms.
5. Provide essential information regarding cancer and cancer care.
6. Maintain a relationship based on trust and confidence; be open, honest, and caring in the approach.
7. Use touch to exhibit caring. A squeeze of the hand or a hug may at times be more effective than words.
8. Assist the patient in setting realistic, reachable short-term and long-term goals.
9. Assist the patient in maintaining usual lifestyle patterns.
10. Maintain hope, which is the key to effective cancer care. Hope varies, depending on the status of the patient—hope that the symptoms are not serious, hope that the treatment is curative, hope for independence, hope for relief of pain, hope for a longer life, or hope for a peaceful death. Hope provides control over what is occurring and is the basis of a positive attitude toward cancer and cancer care.

Organizations and journals available as resources for the nurse are listed in the Resources section at the end of this chapter. In many cities, local units of the American Cancer Society provide a wide variety of services.

GERONTOLOGIC CONSIDERATIONS
CANCER

Cancer is a disease of aging. Most cancers occur in people over age 65. Cancer is the leading cause of death in people 65 to 74 years of age. Cancer mortality is exceedingly high in the elderly, with 70% of all deaths due to malignancies occurring in those over the age of 65. This is especially important since life span is lengthening and the elderly population (>65 years) is expected to double from 35 to 70 million by 2050.[35]

Clinical manifestations of cancer in older adults may be mistakenly attributed to age-related changes and ignored by the person.[36] Older adults are particularly vulnerable to the complications of both cancer and cancer therapy. This is due to their decline in physiologic functioning, social and emotional resources, and cognitive function. The functional status of an older adult should be taken into consideration when selecting a treatment plan. Age alone is not a good predictor of tolerance or response to treatment. Advances in the treatment of cancer are making cancer therapies beneficial to an increasing number of older adults, including patients with suboptimal health. Some important questions to consider when an older person is diagnosed with cancer include the following: Will the treatment provide more benefits than harm? Will he or she be able to tolerate the treatment safely? What is the patient's choice of therapy?

CANCER SURVIVORSHIP

Because of the effectiveness of cancer treatment, many patients with cancer are cured or their disease is controlled for long periods. Survival rates from cancer have steadily increased over the past 30 years. There are almost 10 million survivors of cancer in the United States, and the number is expected to rise. Because of this trend, emphasis must be placed on maintaining an optimal quality of life after the diagnosis of cancer. Many long-term and late effects of cancer and cancer therapies can be seen in cancer survivors.[37] These effects may include secondary cancer, cognitive changes, cardiovascular dysfunction, sexual dysfunction, and psychosocial effects. In addition, there can be changes in interpersonal relationships and financial status.[38]

TABLE 16-23 Resources for Cancer Survivors

Resource	Website
National Coalition for Cancer Survivorship (NCCS)	*www.canceradvocacy.org*
Office of Cancer Survivorship	*www.cancercontrol.cancer.gov/ocs/*
Lance Armstrong Foundation, Live Strong Survivor Care	*www.livestrong.org*
Life after Cancer Care, The University of Texas M.D. Anderson Cancer Center, Houston	*www.mdanderson.org/Departments/LACC*
The Long-Term Follow-Up Program, Memorial Sloan-Kettering Cancer Center, New York City	*www.mskcc.org/mskcc/html/2936.cfm*
The Lance Armstrong Foundation Adult Survivorship Clinic, Dana Farber Cancer Center, Boston	*www.dana-farber.org/pat/surviving*

The psychosocial effects experienced after cancer treatment can play a profound role in a patient's life after cancer. Fear of cancer recurrence often dominates the minds of the cancer survivor and the family members. Depression and anxiety are also challenges that are commonly faced by cancer survivors. Individuals who continue to experience late effects or develop other medical problems experience greater depression and posttraumatic stress characteristics.

While some survivors continue to worry about the possibility of a cancer recurrence or fear of a secondary cancer, others recognize the positive changes that the illness has made on their lives, such as feelings of personal growth and resilience. Long-term cancer survivors have the opportunity to reflect upon their cancer experience and find meaning from it. It is common for this reflection to result in the creation of a new identity or social role.

Understanding the meaning of the cancer experience for each individual is essential for nurses to better assist survivors. Some patients may wish to return to their normal lives as soon as possible. Such behavior could potentially result in patients not attending scheduled follow-up appointments. Other survivors may become cancer advocates or become active members of a cancer support group. Still others may allow their lives to revolve around the cancer and may even become resistant to giving up the illness role. Resources for survivors are listed in Table 16-23.

Nurses can help cancer survivors by

1. Educating health care providers about the needs of cancer survivors, including long-term effects of cancer and cancer treatments.
2. Teaching cancer survivors to look for and report late effects of radiation therapy and chemotherapy.
3. Promoting healthy behaviors such as making sure to get health screenings (e.g., breast and colon screening), good nutrition, exercise, and maintaining proper weight.
4. Encouraging cancer survivors to have regular follow-up examinations.
5. Assessing for psychoemotional problems related to cancer and assisting patients in getting appropriate help if necessary.

NCLEX EXAMINATION REVIEW QUESTIONS

The number of the question corresponds to the same-numbered objective at the beginning of the chapter.

1. Trends in the incidence and death rates of cancer include the fact that
   a. lung cancer is the most common type of cancer in men.
   b. a higher percentage of women than men have lung cancer.
   c. breast cancer is the leading cause of cancer deaths in women.
   d. African Americans have a higher death rate from cancer than whites.
2. Cancer is a name for a large group of diseases, all of which are characterized by
   a. increasing differentiation of cells.
   b. production of toxins that alter cells.
   c. rapid, explosive proliferation of cells.
   d. cell growth that escapes normal control.
3. A characteristic of the stage of progression in the development of cancer is
   a. oncogenic viral transformation of target cells.
   b. a reversible steady growth facilitated by carcinogens.
   c. a period of latency before clinical detection of cancer.
   d. proliferation of cancer cells in spite of host control mechanisms.
4. The primary protective role of the immune system related to malignant cells is
   a. surveillance for cells with tumor-associated antigens.
   b. binding with free antigen released by malignant cells.
   c. production of blocking factors that immobilize cancer cells.
   d. responding to a new set of antigenic determinants on cancer cells.
5. The primary difference between benign and malignant neoplasms is the
   a. rate of cell proliferation.
   b. site of malignant tumor.
   c. requirements for cellular nutrients.
   d. characteristic of tissue invasiveness.
6. Important nursing roles related to prevention and detection of cancer include
   a. instructing people to eat low-fiber, refined-carbohydrate diets.
   b. instructing persons on ways to increase capacity to cope with stress.
   c. teaching people to have annual screening tests for all detectable cancer sites.
   d. using people's natural fear of cancer to motivate changes in unhealthy lifestyles.
7. The goals of cancer treatment are based on the principle that
   a. surgery is the single most effective treatment for cancer.
   b. initial treatment is always directed toward cure of the cancer.
   c. a combination of treatment modalities is effective for controlling many cancers.
   d. although cancer cure is rare, quality of life can be increased with treatment modalities.
8. The most effective method of administering a chemotherapeutic agent that is a vesicant is to
   a. give it orally.
   b. give it intraarterially.
   c. use an Ommaya reservoir.
   d. use a central venous access device.
9. The nurse explains to a patient undergoing brachytherapy of the cervix that she
   a. must undergo simulation to locate the treatment area.
   b. requires the use of radioactive precautions during nursing care.

c. may experience desquamation of the skin on the abdomen and upper legs.
d. requires shielding of the ovaries during treatment to prevent ovarian damage.

10. Stomatitis, a common side effect of chemotherapeutic agents, occurs because the
 a. site of the malignancy is near the oral cavity.
 b. general health of the patient with cancer is poor.
 c. chemotherapeutic drugs have an external, local, and irritating effect.
 d. rapidly dividing cells of the mucous membranes of the mouth are being destroyed.
11. The nurse teaches the patient receiving IL-2 about the drug based on the knowledge that this agent is administered primarily for the purpose of
 a. stimulating the immune system.
 b. inhibiting DNA and protein synthesis in tumor cells.
 c. decreasing the antigenic expression of antigens on tumor cell surfaces.
 d. preventing bone marrow suppression associated with chemotherapy administration.
12. The nurse counsels the patient receiving radiation therapy or chemotherapy that
 a. effective birth control methods should be used for the rest of the patient's life.
 b. if nausea and vomiting occur during treatment, the treatment plan will be modified.
 c. following successful treatment, a return to the person's previous functional level can be expected.
 d. the cycle of fatigue-depression-fatigue that may occur during treatment can be reduced by restricting activity.
13. An inappropriate nursing intervention to promote nutrition in the patient with cancer is
 a. providing bland, pureed food because the person's taste sensation is altered.
 b. providing increased protein for normal cell recovery and immune system function.
 c. encouraging the patient to eat a high-calorie, high-protein snack every few hours to prevent weight loss.
 d. alerting the physician that nutritional supplements may be needed when the patient has a 10-lb weight loss.
14. Syndrome of inappropriate ADH secretion (SIADH) that occurs in certain types of cancer is primarily due to
 a. autoimmune reaction.
 b. gram-negative septicemia.
 c. invasiveness of cancer cells.
 d. ectopic hormonal production.
15. A patient has recently been diagnosed with early stages of breast cancer. Which of the following is most appropriate for the nurse to focus on?
 a. Maintaining patient's hope
 b. Preparing a will and advance directives
 c. Discussing replacement child care for patient's children
 d. Discussing the patient's past experiences with her grandmother's cancer

REFERENCES

1. *Cancer facts and figures,* Atlanta, 2006, American Cancer Society.
2. National Cancer Institute: *Cancer trends progress report update, 2005,* Bethesda, MD, 2005, National Institutes of Health. Available at *http://progressreport.cancer.gov.*
3. American Cancer Society: *Cancer facts and figures for African Americans, 2005–2006,* Atlanta, 2005, American Cancer Society.
4. Tannock IF, Hill RP, Bristow RG, et al: *The basic science of oncology,* ed 4, New York, 2005, McGraw-Hill.
5. Ewart-Toland A, Balmain A: The genetics of cancer susceptibility: from mouse to man, *Toxicol Pathol* 32(Suppl 1):26, 2004.
6. Abeloff MD: *Clinical oncology,* London, 2005, Churchill Livingstone.
7. Stewart B, Coates A: Cancer prevention: a global perspective, *J Clin Oncol* 23:392, 2005.
8. Kemp C, Potyk D: Cancer screening: principles and controversies, *Nurse Practitioner* 30:47, 2005.
9. Engelking C: Communication in cancer care: making every word count. In Gates RA, Fink RM, editors: *Oncology nursing secrets,* ed 2, Philadelphia, 2001, Hanley & Belfus.
10. Juweid ME, Cheson BD: Positron-emission tomography and assessment of cancer therapy, *N Engl J Med* 354:496, 2006.
11. Otto SE: *Oncology nursing: clinical reference,* St Louis, 2004, Mosby.
12. Polovitch M, White J, Kelleher L, editors: *Chemotherapy and biotherapy guidelines and recommendations for practice,* ed 2, Pittsburgh, 2005, Oncology Nursing Society. Available at *www.ons.org.*
13. *http://www.osha.gov/dts/osta/otm/otm_vi/otm_vi_2.html#3.*
14. Hadaway L: Preventing and managing peripheral extravasation, *Nursing* 34:66, 2004.
15. Camp-Sorrell D: *Access device guidelines: recommendations for nursing practice and education,* Pittsburgh, 2005, Oncology Nursing Society.
16. Moran J, Elshikh M, Lawrence T: Radiotherapy: what can be achieved by technical improvements in dose delivery? *Lancet Oncol* 6:51, 2005.
17. Bruner DW, Haas ML, Gosselin-Acomb TK: *Radiation oncology nursing practice and education,* ed 3, Pittsburgh, 2005, Oncology Nursing Society.
18. National Comprehensive Cancer Network: NCCN Clinical Practice Guidelines—Myeloid Growth Factors. Available at *www.nccn.org.*
19. Ahlberg K, Ekman T, Gaston-Johansson F: The experience of fatigue, other symptoms and global quality of life during radiotherapy for uterine cancer, *Int J Nurs Studies* 42:377, 2005.
20. Kris MG, Hesketh PJ, Somerfield MR, et al: American Society of Clinical Oncology Guideline for Antiemetics in Oncology: Update 2006, *Journal of Clinical Oncology* 24:2932-2947, 2006.
21. Benson AB, Ajani J, Catalano R, et al: Recommended guidelines for the treatment of cancer treatment-induced diarrhea, *J Clin Oncol* 22:2918, 2004.
22. Sonis ST: Oral mucositis in cancer therapy, *J Supportive Oncol* 2(Suppl 3):3, 2004.
23. Rubenstein EB, Peterson DE, Schubert M, et al: Clinical practice guidelines for the prevention and treatment of cancer therapy-induced oral and gastrointestinal mucositis, *Cancer* 100(9 Suppl):2026, 2004.
24. D'Haese S, Bate T, Claeus S, et al: Management of skin reactions during radiotherapy: a study of nursing practice, *Eur J Cancer Care* 14:28, 2005.
25. Yeh E, Tong AT, Lenihan D, et al: Cardiovascular complications of cancer therapy: diagnosis, pathogenesis, and management, *Circulation* 109:3122, 2004.
26. Lee PJ, Mallik R: Cardiovascular effects of radiation therapy: practical approach to radiation therapy-induced heart disease, *Cardiol Rev* 13:80, 2005.
27. Viele C: Keys to unlock cancer: targeted therapy, *Oncol Nurs Forum* 32:935, 2005.
28. Neiss D, Duffy KM: Basic concepts of transplantation. In Ezzone S, editor: *Hematopoietic stem cell transplantation: a manual for nursing practice,* Pittsburgh, 2004, Oncology Nursing Society.
29. Schmit-Pokorny K: Stem cell collection. In Ezzone S, editor: *Hematopoietic stem cell transplantation: a manual for nursing practice,* Pittsburgh, 2004, Oncology Nursing Society.
30. McAdams FW, Burgunder MR: Transplant course. In Ezzone S, editor: *Hematopoietic stem cell transplantation: a manual for nursing practice,* Pittsburgh, 2004, Oncology Nursing Society.
31. Held-Warmkessel J: Managing critical cancer, *Nursing* 35:58, 2005.
32. Del Toro G, Morris E, Cairo MS: Tumor lysis syndrome: pathophysiology, definition, and alternative treatment approaches, *Clinical Advances in Hematology & Oncology* 3(1):54, 2005.
33. Miaskowski C: The next step to improving cancer pain management, *Pain Management Nurs* 6:1, 2005.
34. Miaskowski C, Clearly J, Burney R, et al: *Guideline for the management of cancer pain in adults and children,* APS Clinical Practice Guidelines Series, No 3, Glenview, Ill., 2005, American Pain Society.
35. Erschler WB: Cancer: a disease of the elderly, *J Supportive Oncol* 4(Suppl 2):5, 2003.
36. Coleman E, Hutchins L, Goodwin J: An overview of cancer in the older adult, *Medsurg Nurs* 13:75, 2005.

37. Dow KH, Loerzel VW: Cancer survivorship: a critical aspect of care. In Yarbo CH, Frogge MH, Goodman M, editors: *Cancer nursing: principles and practice*, ed 6, Boston, 2005, Jones & Bartlett.
38. Curtis CP, Haylock PJ, Hawkins R: Improving the care of cancer survivors, *AJN* 106:48, 2006.

RESOURCES

American Association for Cancer Education (AACE)
www.aaceonline.com

American Cancer Society
800-ACS-2345 or 404-320-3333
www.cancer.org

American Institute for Cancer Research
800-843-8114 or 202-328-7744
www.aicr.org

American Society of Clinical Oncology (ASCO)
703-299-0150
www.asco.org

Association of Community Cancer Centers (ACCC)
301-984-9496
www.accc-cancer.org

Canadian Cancer Society
416-961-7223

Cancer Care, Inc.
800-813-HOPE or 212-712-8080
www.cancercare.org

Cancer Federation, Inc.
909-849-4325
www.cancerfed.com

Cancer Guide
http://cancerguide.org

Cancer Hotline
800-525-3777
800-638-6070 (Alaska)
800-636-5700 (District of Columbia)
808-524-1234 (Hawaii; call collect)

Cancer Information Service
888-939-3333
www.cancer.ca

Cancer Information Service (CIS), a program of the National Cancer Institute (NCI)
800-4-CANCER
http://cis.nci.nih.gov

Cancer News on the Net
www.cancernews.com

International Society of Nurses in Cancer Care (ISNCC)
44 (0) 1625-428-192
www.isncc.org

International Union Against Cancer (UICC)
41-22-809-18-11
www.uicc.ch

Memorial Sloan-Kettering Cancer Center (MSKCC)
212-639-2000
www.mskcc.org

National Cancer Institute (NCI)
NCI Public Inquiries Office
800-4-CANCER or 301-496-4907
www.nci.nih.gov

National Coalition for Cancer Survivorship (NCCS)
877-NCCS-YES or 301-650-9127
www.canceradvocacy.org

National Foundation for Cancer Research
800-321-CURE or 301-654-1250
www.researchforacure.com

OncoLink (cancer information site)
www.oncolink.upenn.edu

Oncology Nursing Society (ONS)
412-859-6100
www.ons.org

Society of Gynecologic Oncologists (SGO)
312-644-6610
www.sgo.org

For additional Internet resources, see the website for this book at *http://evolve.elsevier.com/Lewis/medsurg*.

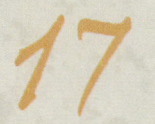

There are many trails up the mountain, but in time they all reach the top.

Anya Seton

17 Fluid, Electrolyte, and Acid-Base Imbalances

Audrey J. Bopp

LEARNING OBJECTIVES

1. Describe the composition of the major body fluid compartments.
2. Define the following processes involved in the regulation of movement of water and electrolytes between the body fluid compartments: Diffusion, osmosis, filtration, hydrostatic pressure, oncotic pressure, and osmotic pressure.
3. Describe the etiology, laboratory diagnostic findings, clinical manifestations, and nursing and collaborative management of the following disorders:
   a. Extracellular fluid volume imbalances: Fluid volume deficit and fluid volume excess
   b. Sodium imbalances: Hypernatremia and hyponatremia
   c. Potassium imbalances: Hyperkalemia and hypokalemia
   d. Magnesium imbalances: Hypermagnesemia and hypomagnesemia
   e. Calcium imbalances: Hypercalcemia and hypocalcemia
   f. Phosphate imbalances: Hyperphosphatemia and hypophosphatemia
4. Identify the processes to maintain acid-base balance.
5. Discuss the etiology, laboratory diagnostic findings, clinical manifestations, and nursing and collaborative management of the following acid-base imbalances: Metabolic acidosis, metabolic alkalosis, respiratory acidosis, and respiratory alkalosis.
6. Describe the composition and indications of common intravenous fluid solutions.

KEY TERMS

acidosis, p. 333
active transport, p. 317
alkalosis, p. 333
anions, p. 315
buffers, p. 334
diffusion, p. 316
electrolytes, p. 315
fluid spacing, p. 319
hydrostatic pressure, p. 318
hypertonic, p. 318
hypotonic, p. 318
isotonic, p. 318
oncotic pressure, p. 318
osmolality, p. 317
osmolarity, p. 317
osmosis, p. 317
osmotic pressure, p. 317

Electronic Resources

Supplemental content related to Chapter 17 can be found . . .

Companion CD

- Stress-Busting Kit for Nursing Students
- Interactive Case Study: Hyponatremia/Fluid Volume Imbalance
- NCLEX Examination Review Questions
- Comprehensive Glossary

Evolve Website evolve

http://evolve.elsevier.com/Lewis/medsurg

- Content Updates
- Key Points (Printable and CD/MP3 Download)
- Concept Map Creator
- Expanded Audio Glossary
- Key Term Flash Cards
- Fluid and Electrolyte Tutorial
- Electronic Calculators
- WebLinks

HOMEOSTASIS

Body fluids and electrolytes play an important role in homeostasis. **Homeostasis** is the state of equilibrium in the internal environment of the body, naturally maintained by adaptive responses that promote healthy survival.[1] Maintenance of the composition and volume of body fluids within narrow limits of normal is necessary to maintain homeostasis.[2] During normal metabolism, the body produces many acids. These acids alter the internal environment of the body, including fluid and electrolyte balances, and must also be regulated to maintain homeostasis. Many diseases and their treatments have the ability to affect fluid and electrolyte balance. For example, a patient with metastatic breast or lung cancer may develop hypercalcemia as a result of bone destruction from tumor invasion. Chemotherapy prescribed to treat the cancer may result in nausea and vomiting and, subsequently, dehydration and acid-base imbalances. Correction of the dehydration with intravenous (IV) fluids must be monitored closely to prevent fluid overload.

Reviewed by Cheryl Swallow, RN, MSN, Associate Professor, St Louis Community College–Forest Park, St Louis, Mo.

It is important for the nurse to anticipate the potential for alterations in fluid and electrolyte balance associated with certain disorders and medical therapies, to recognize the signs and symptoms of imbalances, and to intervene with the appropriate action. This chapter describes the normal control of fluids, electrolytes, and acid-base balance; etiologies that disrupt homeostasis and resultant manifestations; and actions that the health care provider can take to prevent or restore fluid, electrolyte, and acid-base balance.

WATER CONTENT OF THE BODY

Water is the primary component of the body, accounting for approximately 60% of the body weight in the adult. Water is the solvent in which body salts, nutrients, and wastes are dissolved and transported. The water content varies with gender, body mass, and age (Fig. 17-1). The percentage of body weight that is composed of water is generally greater in men than in women because men tend to have more lean body mass than women. Fat cells contain less water than an equivalent volume of lean tissue.[3] In the older adult, body water content averages 45% to 55% of body weight. In the infant, water content is 70% to 80% of the body weight. Thus infants and the elderly are at a higher risk for fluid-related problems than young adults.

Body Fluid Compartments

The two major fluid compartments in the body are intracellular and extracellular (Fig. 17-2). Approximately two thirds of the body water is located within cells and is termed *intracellular fluid* (ICF); the ICF constitutes approximately 40% of body weight. The body of a 70-kg man would contain approximately 42 L of water, of which 30 L would be located within cells. *Extracellular fluid* (ECF) consists of *interstitial fluid,* composed of the fluid in the interstitium (the space between cells) and lymph; the fluid in blood (plasma); and a very small amount of fluid contained within specialized cavities of the body (cerebrospinal fluid, fluid in the gastrointestinal [GI] tract, and pleural, synovial, and peritoneal fluid). The fluid in the specialized cavities is sometimes referred to as *transcellular fluid.* The ECF consists of one third of the body water, or about 20% of the total weight; this would amount to about 11 L in a 70-kg man. About one third of the ECF is in the plasma space (3 L in a 70-kg man), and two thirds is in the interstitial space (8 L in a 70-kg man). The fluid in the specialized cavities totals about 1 L at any given time, but because 3 to 6 L of fluid is secreted into and reabsorbed from the GI tract every day, loss of this fluid from vomiting or diarrhea can produce serious fluid and electrolyte imbalances.

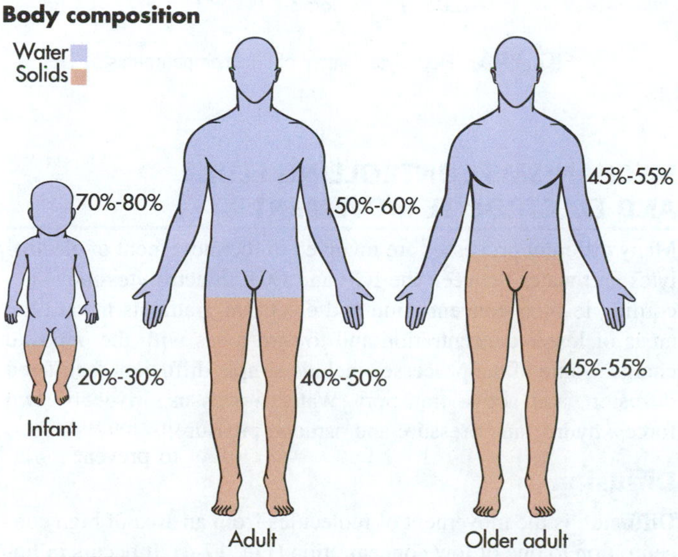

FIG. 17-1 Changes in body water content with age.

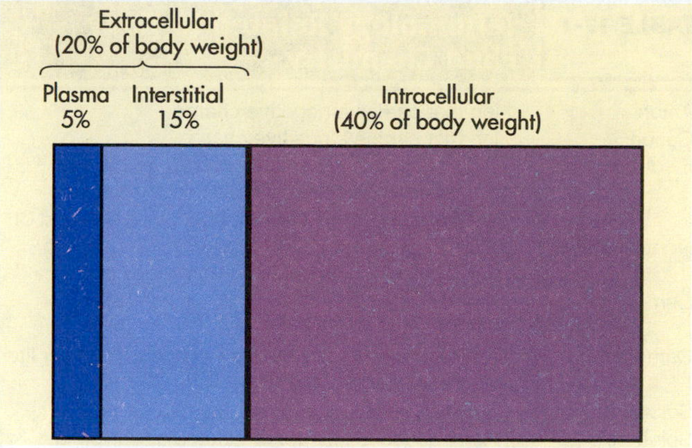

FIG. 17-2 Fluid compartments in the body.

Functions of Body Water

Body fluids are in constant motion transporting nutrients, electrolytes, and oxygen to cells and carrying waste products away from cells. Water is necessary in the regulation of body temperature. In addition, it lubricates joints and membranes and is a medium for food digestion.[3]

Calculation of Fluid Gain or Loss

One liter of water weighs 2.2 lb (1 kg). Body weight change, especially sudden change, is an excellent indicator of overall fluid volume loss or gain. For example, if a patient drinks 240 ml (8 oz) of fluid, weight gain will be 0.5 lb (0.24 kg). A patient receiving diuretic therapy who loses 4.4 lb (2 kg) in 24 hours has experienced a fluid loss of approximately 2 L. An adult patient who is fasting might lose approximately 1 to 2 lb per day. A weight loss exceeding this is likely due to loss of body fluid.

ELECTROLYTES

Electrolytes are substances whose molecules dissociate, or split into ions, when placed in water. **Ions** are electrically charged particles. **Cations** are positively charged ions. Examples include sodium (Na^+), potassium (K^+), calcium (Ca^{2+}), and magnesium (Mg^{2+}) ions. **Anions** are negatively charged ions. Examples include bicarbonate (HCO_3^-), chloride (Cl^-), and phosphate (PO_4^{3-}) ions. Most proteins bear a negative charge and are thus anions. The electrical charge of an ion is termed its **valence.** Cations and anions combine according to their valences. (Definitions of terminology related to body fluid chemistry is presented in Table 17-1.)

Measurement of Electrolytes

The measurement of electrolytes is important to the nurse in evaluating electrolyte balance, as well as determining the composition of electrolyte preparations. The concentration of electrolytes can be expressed in milligrams per deciliter (mg/dl), millimoles per liter (mmol/L), or milliequivalents per liter (mEq/L). The interna-

TABLE 17-1 Terminology Related to Body Fluid Chemistry

Anion	Ion that carries a negative charge
Cation	Ion that carries a positive charge
Electrolyte	Substance that dissociates in solution into ions (charged particles); a molecule of sodium chloride (NaCl) in solution becomes Na^+ and Cl^-
Nonelectrolyte	Substance that does not dissociate into ions in solution; examples include glucose and urea
Osmolality	A measure of the total solute concentration per kilogram of solvent
Osmolarity	A measure of the total solute concentration per liter of solution
Solute	Substance that is dissolved in a solvent
Solution	Homogeneous mixture of solutes dissolved in a solvent
Solvent	Substance that is capable of dissolving a solute (liquid or gas)
Valence	The degree of combining power of an ion

tional standard for measuring electrolytes is mmol/L. One mole (mol) of a substance is the molecular (or atomic) weight of that substance in grams; hence a millimole (mmol) of a substance is the atomic weight in milligrams. Sodium's atomic weight is 23 mg; therefore 23 mg of sodium is 1 mmol of sodium. Sodium and chloride are monovalent elements that carry one electron and will match one to one. One mmol of sodium combines with one mmol of chloride. An element with two electrons, such as calcium, will require two monovalent partners.

The milliequivalent is the commonly used unit of measure for electrolytes in the United States. The following formula is used to convert millimoles to milliequivalents:

$$\text{mEq} = \text{mmol/L} \times \text{valence}$$

Electrolytes in body fluids are active chemicals that unite in varying combinations. Thus it is more practical to express their concentration as a measure of chemical activity (or milliequivalents) rather than as a measure of weight. Ions combine milliequivalent for milliequivalent. For example, 1 mEq (1 mmol) of sodium combines with 1 mEq (1 mmol) of chloride, and 1 mEq (0.5 mmol) of calcium combines with 1 mEq (1 mmol) of chloride. This combining power of electrolytes is important to maintain the balance of positively charged (cation) and negatively charged (anion) ions within body fluids.

Electrolyte Composition of Fluid Compartments

Electrolyte composition varies between the ECF and ICF. The overall concentration of the electrolytes is approximately the same in the two compartments. However, concentrations of specific ions differ greatly (Fig. 17-3). In the ICF, the most prevalent cation is potassium with small amounts of magnesium and sodium. The prevalent ICF anion is phosphate with some protein and a small amount of bicarbonate.

In the ECF, the main cation is sodium with small amounts of potassium, calcium, and magnesium. The primary ECF anion is chloride with small amounts of bicarbonate, sulfate, and phosphate anions. The plasma has substantial amounts of protein. However, the amount of protein in the plasma is less than in the ICF. There is a very small amount of protein in the interstitium.

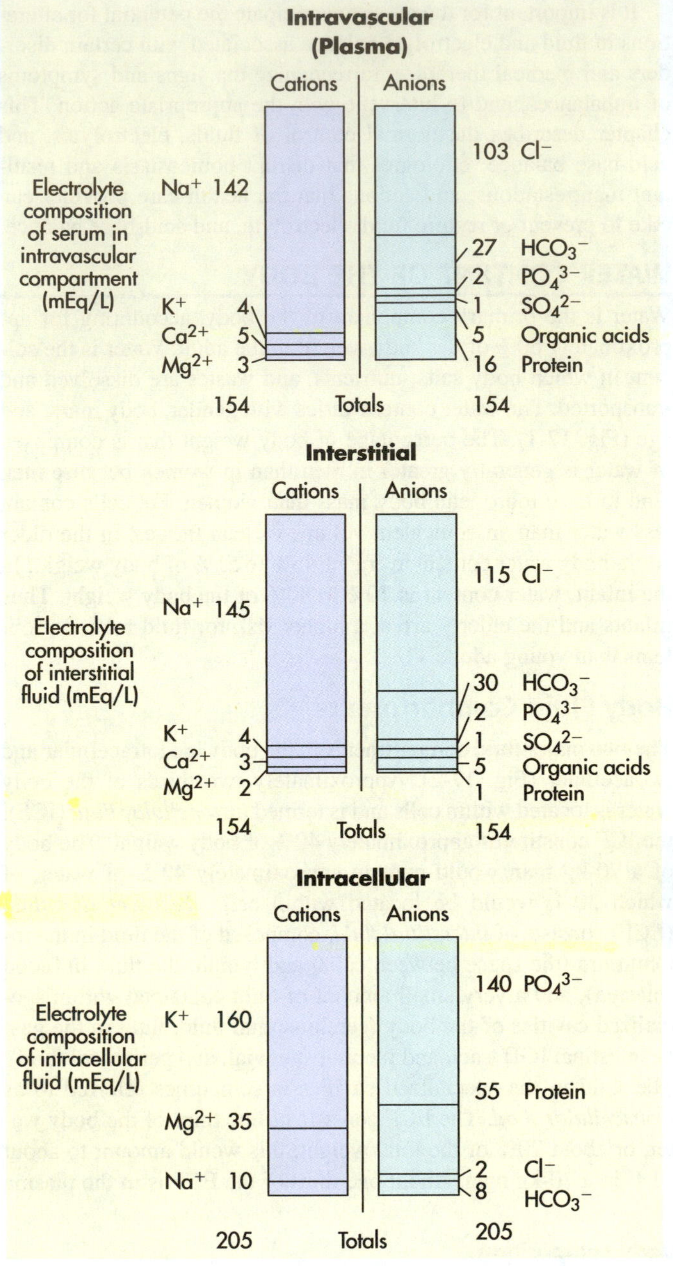

FIG. 17-3 Electrolyte content of fluid compartments.

MECHANISMS CONTROLLING FLUID AND ELECTROLYTE MOVEMENT

Many different processes are involved in the movement of electrolytes and water between the ICF and ECF. Electrolytes move according to their concentration and electrical gradients toward the areas of lower concentration and toward areas with the opposite charge. Some of the processes include simple diffusion, facilitated diffusion, and active transport. Water moves as driven by two forces: hydrostatic pressure and osmotic pressure.

Diffusion

Diffusion is the movement of molecules from an area of high concentration to one of low concentration (Fig. 17-4). It occurs in liquids, gases, and solids. Net movement of molecules stops when the

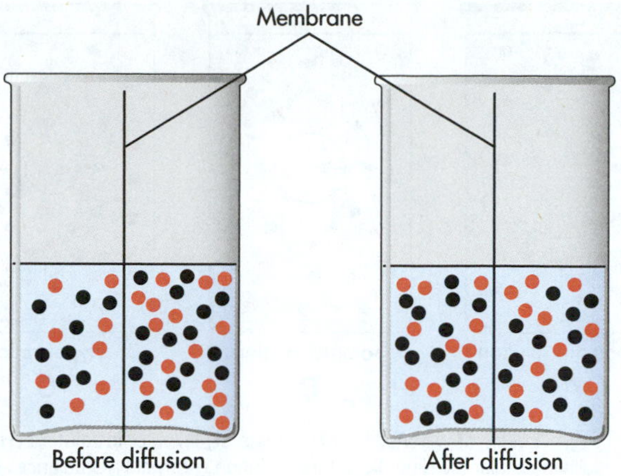

FIG. 17-4 Diffusion is the movement of molecules from an area of high concentration to an area of low concentration.

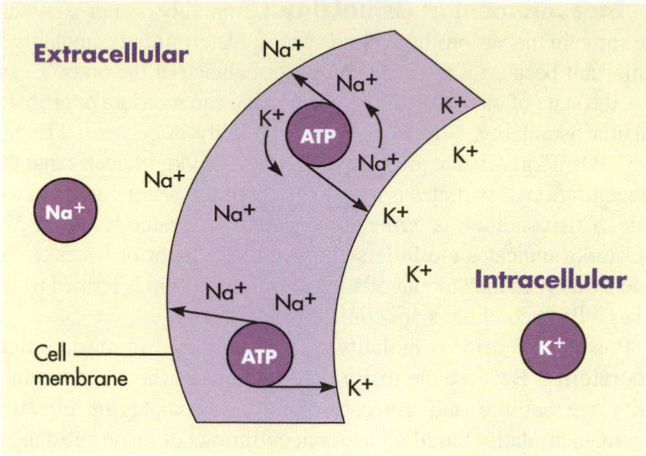

FIG. 17-5 Sodium-potassium pump. As sodium (Na^+) diffuses into the cell and potassium (K^+) diffuses out of the cell, an active transport system supplied with energy delivers Na^+ back to the extracellular compartment and K^+ to the intracellular compartment. *ATP,* Adenosine triphosphate.

concentrations are equal in both areas. The membrane separating the two areas must be permeable to the diffusing substance for the process to occur. Simple diffusion requires no external energy. Gases (e.g., oxygen, nitrogen, carbon dioxide) and other substances (e.g., urea) can permeate through cell membranes and are distributed throughout the body.

Facilitated Diffusion

Because of the composition of cellular membranes, some molecules diffuse slowly into the cell. However, when they are combined with a specific carrier molecule, the rate of diffusion accelerates. Like simple diffusion, **facilitated diffusion** moves molecules from an area of high concentration to one of low concentration. Facilitated diffusion is passive and requires no energy other than that of the concentration gradient. Glucose transport into the cell is an example of facilitated diffusion. There is a carrier molecule on most cells that increases or facilitates the rate of diffusion of glucose into these cells.

Active Transport

Active transport is a process in which molecules move against the concentration gradient. External energy is required for this process. The concentrations of sodium and potassium differ greatly intracellularly and extracellularly (see Fig. 17-3). By active transport, sodium moves out of the cell and potassium moves into the cell to maintain this concentration difference (Fig. 17-5). This active transport mechanism is referred to as the sodium-potassium pump. The energy source for this mechanism is adenosine triphosphate (ATP), which is produced in the cell's mitochondria.

Osmosis

Osmosis is the movement of water between two compartments separated by a semipermeable membrane (a membrane permeable to water but not to a solute). Water moves through the membrane from an area of low solute concentration to an area of high solute concentration (Fig. 17-6); that is, water moves from the more dilute compartment (has more water) to the side that is more concentrated (has less water). Osmosis requires no outside energy sources and stops when the concentration differences disappear or when hydrostatic pressure builds and is sufficient to oppose any further movement of water. Diffusion and osmosis are important in maintaining the fluid volume of body cells and the concentration of the solute.

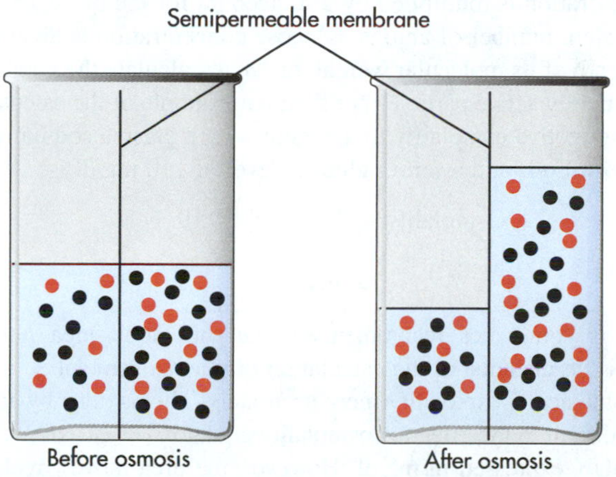

FIG. 17-6 Osmosis is the process of water movement through a semipermeable membrane from an area of low solute concentration to an area of high solute concentration.

Osmotic pressure is the amount of pressure required to stop the osmotic flow of water. Osmotic pressure can be understood in terms of imagining a chamber in which two compartments are separated by a semipermeable membrane (see Fig. 17-6). Water will move from the less concentrated side to the more concentrated side of the chamber. At some point the pressure generated by the height of the higher column of water will oppose the further movement of water.

Osmotic pressure is determined by the concentration of solutes in solution. It is measured in milliosmoles (mOsm) and may be expressed as either fluid osmolarity or fluid osmolality. **Osmolality** measures the osmotic force of solute per unit of weight of solvent (mOsm/kg or mmol/kg). **Osmolarity** measures the total milliosmoles of solute per unit of total volume of solution (mOsm/L). Although osmolality and osmolarity are often used interchangeably, osmolality is used to describe fluids inside the body and osmolarity pertains to fluids outside the body.[4] Osmolality is the test typically performed to evaluate the concentration of plasma and urine.

Measurement of Osmolality. Osmolality is approximately the same in the various body fluid spaces. Determining osmolality is important because it indicates the water balance of the body. To assess the state of the body water balance, one can measure or estimate plasma osmolality. Normal plasma osmolality is between 275 and 295 mOsm/kg. A value greater than 295 mOsm/kg indicates that the concentration of particles is too great or that the water content is too little. This condition is termed *water deficit.* A value less than 275 mOsm/kg indicates too little solute for the amount of water or too much water for the amount of solute. This condition is termed *water excess.* Both conditions are clinically significant.

Plasma and urine osmolality can be measured in most clinical laboratories. Because the major determinants of the plasma osmolality are sodium and glucose, one can calculate the effective plasma osmolality based on the concentrations of those substances by using the following equation:

$$\text{Effective osmolality} = (2 \times [\text{Na}^+]\text{p}) + ([\text{glucose}]/18)$$

where $[\text{Na}^+]$p and [glucose] are the plasma concentrations of sodium and glucose in mEq/L and mg/dl, respectively. The sodium concentration is multiplied by 2 to account for the presence of an equivalent number of anions. Glucose concentration is divided by one tenth of its molecular weight, or 18, to calculate the number of osmotically active particles per liter. An example of the calculation of an effective osmolality in a patient with a plasma sodium value of 139 mEq/L and a serum glucose level of 110 mg/dl is:

$$\begin{aligned}\text{Osmolality} &= 2 \times 139 + 110 \div 18 \\ &= 278 + 6.11 \\ &= 284.11\end{aligned}$$

It is sometimes recommended that the blood urea nitrogen (BUN) be included in the calculation of plasma osmolality to estimate the actual osmolality more accurately. This is done by adding a third term to the effective osmolality equation (+ BUN/2.8), with the BUN expressed in mg/dl. However, the urea moves freely between body fluid compartments; it has no lasting effect on water movement across cell membranes and is sometimes dubbed an "ineffective osmole." As a result, the measure of the effective plasma osmolality without consideration of the BUN term is the more physiologically meaningful estimate. Osmolality of urine can range from 100 to 1300 mOsm/kg, depending on the amount of antidiuretic hormone (ADH) in circulation and the renal response to it.

Osmotic Movement of Fluids. Cells are affected by the osmolality of the fluid that surrounds them. Fluids with the same osmolality as the cell interior are termed **isotonic.** Solutions in which the solutes are less concentrated than the cells are termed **hypotonic** (hypoosmolar). Those with solutes more concentrated than cells are termed **hypertonic** (hyperosmolar).

Normally, the ECF and ICF are isotonic to one another; hence no net movement of water occurs. In the metabolically active cell, there is a constant exchange of substances between the cell and the interstitium, but no net gain or loss of water occurs.

If a cell is surrounded by hypotonic fluid, water moves into the cell, causing it to swell and possibly to burst. If a cell is surrounded by hypertonic fluid, water leaves the cell to dilute the ECF; the cell shrinks and may eventually die (Fig. 17-7).

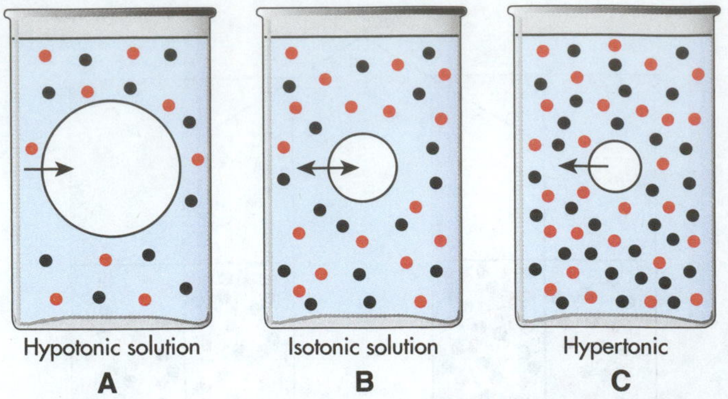

FIG. 17-7 Effects of water status on cell size. **A,** Hypotonic solution (H_2O excess) results in cellular swelling. **B,** Isotonic solution (normal H_2O balance) results in no change. **C,** Hypertonic solution (H_2O deficit) results in cellular shrinking.

Hydrostatic Pressure

Hydrostatic pressure is the force within a fluid compartment. In the blood vessels, hydrostatic pressure is the blood pressure generated by the contraction of the heart.[2] Hydrostatic pressure in the vascular system gradually decreases as the blood moves through the arteries until it is about 40 mm Hg at the arterial end of a capillary. Because of the size of the capillary bed and fluid movement into the interstitium, the pressure decreases to about 10 mm Hg at the venous end of the capillary. Hydrostatic pressure is the major force that pushes water out of the vascular system at the capillary level.

Oncotic Pressure

Oncotic pressure (colloidal osmotic pressure) is osmotic pressure exerted by colloids in solution. The major colloid in the vascular system contributing to the total osmotic pressure is protein. Protein molecules attract water, pulling fluid from the tissue space to the vascular space.[4] Unlike electrolytes, the large molecular size prevents proteins from leaving the vascular space through pores in capillary walls. Under normal conditions, plasma oncotic pressure is approximately 25 mm Hg. Some proteins are found in the interstitial space; they exert an oncotic pressure of approximately 1 mm Hg.

FLUID MOVEMENT IN CAPILLARIES

There is normal movement of fluid between the capillary and the interstitium. The amount and direction of movement are determined by the interaction of (1) capillary hydrostatic pressure, (2) plasma oncotic pressure, (3) interstitial hydrostatic pressure, and (4) interstitial oncotic pressure.

Capillary hydrostatic pressure and interstitial oncotic pressure cause the movement of water out of the capillaries. Plasma oncotic pressure and interstitial hydrostatic pressure cause the movement of fluid into the capillary. At the arterial end of the capillary (Fig. 17-8), capillary hydrostatic pressure exceeds plasma oncotic pressure, and fluid is moved into the interstitium. At the venous end of the capillary, the capillary hydrostatic pressure is lower than plasma oncotic pressure, and fluid is drawn back into the capillary by the oncotic pressure created by plasma proteins.

Fluid Shifts

If capillary or interstitial pressures are altered, fluid may abnormally shift from one compartment to another, resulting in edema or dehydration.

Shifts of Plasma to Interstitial Fluid. Accumulation of fluid in the interstitium *(edema)* occurs if venous hydrostatic pressure rises, plasma oncotic pressure decreases, or interstitial oncotic pressure rises. Edema may also develop if there is an obstruction of lymphatic outflow that causes decreased removal of interstitial fluid.

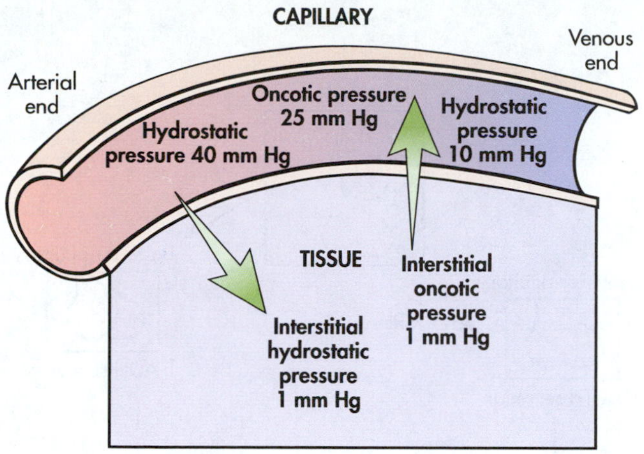

FIG. 17-8 Dynamics of fluid exchange between the capillary and the tissue. An equilibrium exists between forces filtering fluid out of the capillary and forces absorbing fluid back into the capillary. Note that the hydrostatic pressure is greater at the arterial end of the capillary than the venous end. The net effect of pressures at the arterial end of the capillary causes a movement of fluid into the tissue. At the venous end of the capillary, there is net movement of fluid back into the capillary.

Elevation of Venous Hydrostatic Pressure. Increasing the pressure at the venous end of the capillary inhibits fluid movement back into the capillary. Causes of increased venous pressure include fluid overload, heart failure, liver failure, obstruction of venous return to the heart (e.g., tourniquets, restrictive clothing, venous thrombosis), and venous insufficiency (e.g., varicose veins).

Decrease in Plasma Oncotic Pressure. Fluid remains in the interstitium if the plasma oncotic pressure is too low to draw fluid back into the capillary. Decreased oncotic pressure is seen when the plasma protein content is low. This can result from excessive protein loss (renal disorders), deficient protein synthesis (liver disease), and deficient protein intake (malnutrition).

Elevation of Interstitial Oncotic Pressure. Trauma, burns, and inflammation can damage capillary walls and allow plasma proteins to accumulate in the interstitium. The resultant increased interstitial oncotic pressure draws fluid into the interstitium and holds it there.

Shifts of Interstitial Fluid to Plasma. Fluid is drawn into the plasma space whenever there is an increase in the plasma osmotic or oncotic pressure. This could happen with administration of colloids, dextran, mannitol, or hypertonic solutions. Fluid is drawn from the interstitium. In turn, water is drawn from cells via osmosis, equilibrating the osmolality between ICF and ECF.

Increasing the tissue hydrostatic pressure is another way of causing a shift of fluid into plasma. The wearing of elastic compression gradient stockings or hose to decrease peripheral edema is a therapeutic application of this effect.

FLUID MOVEMENT BETWEEN EXTRACELLULAR FLUID AND INTRACELLULAR FLUID

Changes in the osmolality of the ECF alter the volume of cells. Increased ECF osmolality *(water deficit)* pulls water out of cells until the two compartments have a similar osmolality. Water deficit is associated with symptoms that result from cell shrinkage as water is pulled into the vascular system. For example, neurologic symptoms are caused by altered central nervous system (CNS) function as brain cells shrink. Decreased ECF osmolality *(water excess)* develops as the result of gain or retention of excess water. In this case, cells swell. Again, the primary symptoms are neurologic as a result of brain cell swelling as water shifts into the cells.

FLUID SPACING

Fluid spacing is a term sometimes used to describe the distribution of body water. *First spacing* describes the normal distribution of fluid in the ICF and ECF compartments. *Second spacing* refers to an abnormal accumulation of interstitial fluid (i.e., edema). *Third spacing* occurs when fluid accumulates in a portion of the body from which it is not easily exchanged with the rest of the ECF. Third-spaced fluid is trapped and essentially unavailable for functional use. Examples of third spacing are ascites, sequestration of fluid in the abdominal cavity with peritonitis, and edema associated with burns.

REGULATION OF WATER BALANCE

Hypothalamic Regulation

Water balance is maintained via the finely tuned balance of water intake and excretion. A body fluid deficit or increase in plasma osmolality is sensed by osmoreceptors in the hypothalamus, which in turn stimulates thirst and antidiuretic hormone (ADH) release. Thirst causes the patient to drink water. ADH, which is synthesized in the hypothalamus and stored in the posterior pituitary, acts in the renal distal and collecting tubules causing water reabsorption. Together these factors result in increased free water in the body and decreased plasma osmolality. If the plasma osmolality is diminished or there is water excess, secretion of ADH is suppressed, resulting in urinary excretion of water.

An intact thirst mechanism is critical because it is the primary protection against the development of hyperosmolality. The patient who cannot recognize or act on the sensation of thirst is at risk for fluid deficit and hyperosmolality. The sensitivity of the thirst mechanism decreases in older adults.

The desire to consume fluids is also affected by social and psychologic factors not related to fluid balance. A dry mouth will cause the patient to drink, even when there is no measurable body water deficit. Water ingestion will equal water loss in the individual who has free access to water, a normal thirst and ADH mechanism, and normally functioning kidneys.

Pituitary Regulation

Under hypothalamic control, the posterior pituitary releases ADH, which regulates water retention by the kidneys. The distal tubules and collecting ducts in the kidneys respond to ADH by becoming more permeable to water so that water is reabsorbed from the tubular filtrate into the blood and not excreted in urine. An increase in plasma osmolality or a decrease in circulating blood volume will stimulate ADH secretion. Other factors that stimulate ADH release include stress, nausea, nicotine, and morphine. These factors usually result in shifts of osmolality within the range of normal values. It is common for the postoperative patient to have a lower serum osmolality after surgery, possibly because of the stress of surgery and narcotic analgesia.

A pathologic condition seen occasionally is *syndrome of inappropriate antidiuretic hormone secretion* (SIADH) (see Chapter 50). Causes of SIADH include abnormal ADH production in CNS disorders (e.g., brain tumors, brain injury) and certain malignancies (e.g., small cell lung cancer). The inappropriate ADH causes water retention, which produces a decrease in plasma osmolality below the normal value and a relative increase in urine osmolality with a decrease in urine volume.

Reduction in the release or action of ADH produces diabetes insipidus (see Chapter 50). A copious amount of dilute urine is excreted because the renal tubules and collecting ducts do not appropriately reabsorb water. The patient with diabetes insipidus exhibits extreme polyuria and, if the patient is alert, *polydipsia* (excessive thirst). Symptoms of dehydration and hypernatremia develop if the water losses are not adequately replaced.

Adrenal Cortical Regulation

While ADH affects only water reabsorption, glucocorticoids and mineralocorticoids secreted by the adrenal cortex help regulate both water and electrolytes. The glucocorticoids (e.g., cortisol) primarily have an antiinflammatory effect and increase serum glucose levels, whereas the mineralocorticoids (e.g., aldosterone) enhance sodium retention and potassium excretion (Fig. 17-9). When sodium is reabsorbed, water follows as a result of osmotic changes.

Cortisol is the most abundant glucocorticoid. In large doses, cortisol has both glucocorticoid (glucose-elevating and antiinflammatory) and mineralocorticoid (sodium-retention) effects. Cortisol is normally secreted in a diurnal, or circadian, pattern and also in response to increased physical and psychologic stress. Many body functions, including fluid and electrolyte balance, are affected by stress (Fig. 17-10).

Aldosterone is a mineralocorticoid with potent sodium-retaining and potassium-excreting capability. The secretion of aldosterone may be stimulated by decreased renal perfusion or decreased sodium delivery to the distal portion of the renal tubule. The kidneys respond by secreting renin into the plasma. Angiotensinogen, produced in the liver and normally found in blood, is acted on by the renin to form angiotensin I, which converts to angiotensin II, which stimulates the adrenal cortex to secrete aldosterone. In addition to the renin-angiotensin mechanism, increased plasma potassium, decreased plasma sodium, and adrenocorticotropic hormone (ACTH) from the anterior pituitary all act directly on the adrenal cortex to stimulate the secretion of aldosterone (see Fig. 17-9).

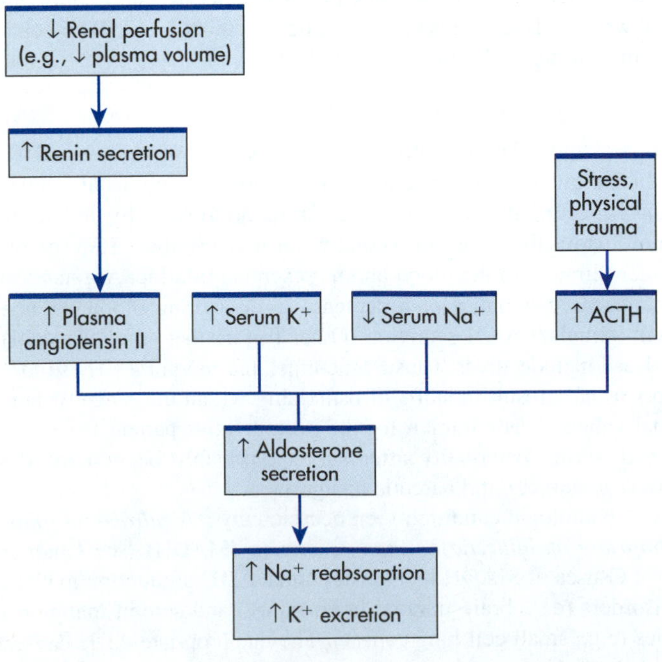

FIG. 17-9 Factors affecting aldosterone secretion. *ACTH,* Adrenocorticotropic hormone.

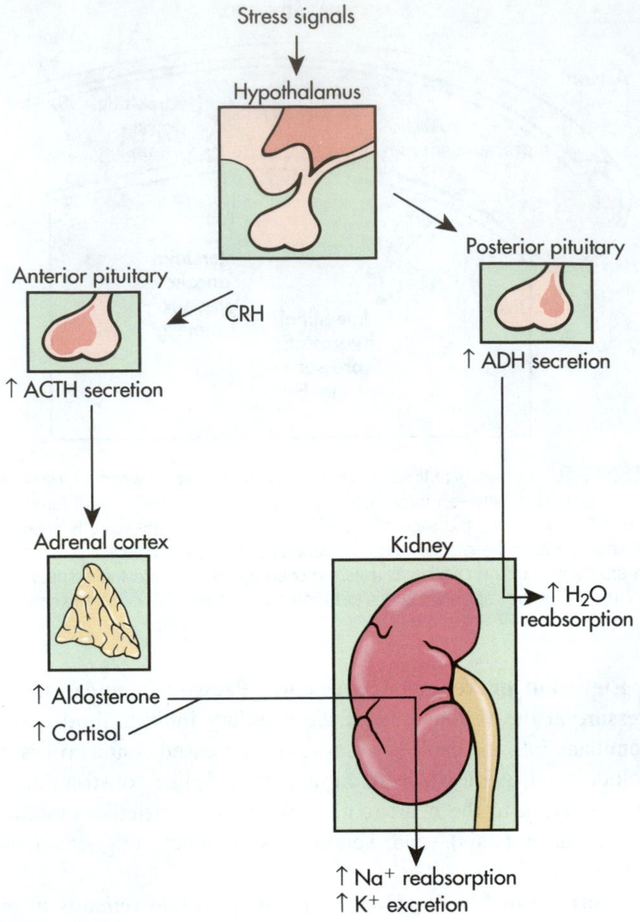

FIG. 17-10 Effects of stress on fluid and electrolyte balance. *ACTH,* Adrenocorticotropic hormone; *ADH,* antidiuretic hormone; *CRH,* corticotropin-releasing hormone.

Renal Regulation

The primary organs for regulating fluid and electrolyte balance are the kidneys (see Chapter 45). The kidneys regulate water balance through adjustments in urine volume. Similarly, urinary excretion of most electrolytes is adjusted so that a balance is maintained between overall intake and output. The total plasma volume is filtered by the kidneys many times each day. In the average adult, the kidney reabsorbs 99% of this filtrate, producing approximately 1.5 L of urine per day. As the filtrate moves through the renal tubules, selective reabsorption of water and electrolytes and secretion of electrolytes result in the production of urine that is greatly different in composition and concentration than the plasma. This process helps maintain normal plasma osmolality, electrolyte balance, blood volume, and acid-base balance. The renal tubules are the site for the actions of ADH and aldosterone.

With severely impaired renal function, the kidneys cannot maintain fluid and electrolyte balance. This condition results in edema, potassium and phosphorus retention, acidosis, and other electrolyte imbalances (see Chapter 47).

Cardiac Regulation

Natriuretic peptides, including atrial natriuretic peptide (ANP) and b-type natriuretic peptide (BNP), are hormones produced by cardiomyocytes. They are natural antagonists to the renin-angiotensin-aldosterone system (RAAS). They are produced in response to in-

TABLE 17-2 Normal Fluid Balance in the Adult

Intake	
Fluids	1200 ml
Solid food	1000 ml
Water from oxidation	300 ml
	2500 ml
Output	
Insensible loss (skin and lungs)	900 ml
In feces	100 ml
Urine	1500 ml
	2500 ml

TABLE 17-3 Normal Serum Electrolyte Values

Anions	Normal Value
Bicarbonate (HCO_3^-)	22-26 mEq/L (22-26 mmol/L)
Chloride (Cl^-)	96-106 mEq/L (96-106 mmol/L)
Phosphate (PO_4^{3-})	2.8-4.5 mg/dl (0.90-1.45 mmol/L)
Cations	**Normal Value**
Potassium (K^+)	3.5-5.0 mEq/L (3.5-5.0 mmol/L)
Magnesium (Mg^{2+})	1.5-2.5 mEq/L (0.75-1.25 mmol/L)
Sodium (Na^+)	135-145 mEq/L (135-145 mmol/L)
Calcium (Ca^{2+}) (total)	9-11 mg/dl (2.25-2.75 mmol/L) 4.5-5.5 mEq/L
Calcium (ionized)	4.5-5.5 mg/dl (1.13-1.38 mmol/L) 2.25-2.75 mEq/L

creased atrial pressure (increased volume) and high serum sodium levels. They suppress secretion of aldosterone, renin, and ADH, and the action of angiotensin II.[2] They act on the renal tubules to promote excretion of sodium and water, resulting in a decrease in blood volume and blood pressure.

Gastrointestinal Regulation

Daily water intake and output are normally between 2000 and 3000 ml (Table 17-2). Oral intake of fluids accounts for most of the water intake. Water intake also includes water from food metabolism and water present in solid foods. Lean meat is approximately 70% water, whereas the water content of many fruits and vegetables approaches 100%.

In addition to oral intake, the GI tract normally secretes approximately 8000 ml of digestive fluids each day that are reabsorbed. A small amount of the fluid in the GI tract is normally eliminated in feces, but diarrhea and vomiting that prevent GI absorption of secretions and fluids can lead to significant fluid and electrolyte loss.

Insensible Water Loss

Insensible water loss, which is invisible vaporization from the lungs and skin, assists in regulating body temperature. Normally, about 600 to 900 ml/day is lost. The amount of water loss is increased by accelerated body metabolism, which occurs with increased body temperature and exercise.

Water loss through the skin should not be confused with the vaporization of water excreted by sweat glands. Only water is lost by insensible perspiration. Excessive sweating *(sensible perspiration)* caused by fever or high environmental temperatures may lead to large losses of water and electrolytes.

GERONTOLOGIC CONSIDERATIONS
FLUID AND ELECTROLYTES

The older adult experiences normal physiologic changes that increase susceptibility to fluid and electrolyte imbalances. Structural changes to the kidney and a decrease in the renal blood flow lead to a decrease in the glomerular filtration rate, decreased creatinine clearance, the loss of the ability to concentrate urine and conserve water, and narrowed limits for the excretion of water, sodium, potassium, and hydrogen ions. Hormonal changes include a decrease in renin and aldosterone and an increase in ADH and ANP.[5,6] Loss of subcutaneous tissue and thinning of the dermis lead to increased loss of moisture through the skin and an inability to respond to heat or cold quickly. Older adults experience a decrease in the thirst mechanism resulting in decreased fluid intake despite increases in osmolality and serum sodium level. The frail elderly, especially if ill, are at increased risk of free-water loss and subsequent development of hypernatremia secondary to impairment of the thirst mechanism and barriers to accessible fluids.[7]

Healthy older adults usually consume adequate fluids to remain well hydrated. However, functional changes may occur that affect the individual's ability to independently obtain fluids. Musculoskeletal changes, such as stiffness of the hands and fingers, can lead to a decreased ability to hold a glass or cup. Mental status changes, such as confusion or disorientation, or changes in ambulation status may lead to a decreased ability to obtain fluids. As a result of incontinent episodes, the older adult may intentionally restrict fluid intake.[6]

To best serve the older adult patient, the health care provider must understand the homeostatic changes that occur in the elderly. It is important to avoid the pitfalls of ageism, wherein elderly patients' fluid and electrolyte problems may be inappropriately attributed to the natural processes of aging.[8] The nurse must adjust assessment and nursing implementation to account for these physiologic and functional changes. Suggestions for alterations in nursing care for the older adult are presented throughout this chapter and in Chapter 6.

Fluid and Electrolyte Imbalances

Fluid and electrolyte imbalances occur to some degree in most patients with a major illness or injury because illness disrupts the normal homeostatic mechanism. Some fluid and electrolyte imbalances are directly caused by illness or disease (e.g., burns, heart failure). At other times, therapeutic measures (e.g., IV fluid replacement, diuretics) cause or contribute to fluid and electrolyte imbalances.

The imbalances are commonly classified as *deficits* or *excesses.* Each imbalance is discussed separately. (For normal values, see Table 17-3.) In actual clinical situations, more than one imbalance occurring in the same patient is common. For example, a patient with prolonged nasogastric suction will lose Na^+, K^+, H^+, and Cl^-. These imbalances may result in a deficiency of both Na^+ and K^+, a fluid volume deficit, and a metabolic alkalosis due to loss of HCl.

EXTRACELLULAR FLUID VOLUME IMBALANCES

ECF volume deficit (hypovolemia) and ECF volume excess (hypervolemia) are commonly occurring clinical conditions. ECF volume imbalances are typically accompanied by one or more electrolyte imbalances, particularly changes in the serum sodium level.

FLUID VOLUME DEFICIT

Fluid volume deficit can occur with abnormal loss of body fluids (e.g., diarrhea, fistula drainage, hemorrhage, polyuria), inadequate intake, or a plasma-to–interstitial fluid shift. The term *fluid volume deficit* should not be used interchangeably with the term *dehydration*. **Dehydration** refers to loss of pure water alone without corresponding loss of sodium. The clinical manifestations of fluid volume deficit are listed in Table 17-4.

Collaborative Care

The goal of treatment for fluid volume deficit is to correct the underlying cause and to replace both water and any needed electrolytes. Balanced IV solutions, such as lactated Ringer's solution, are usually given. Isotonic (0.9%) sodium chloride is used when rapid volume replacement is indicated. Blood is administered when volume loss is due to blood loss.

FLUID VOLUME EXCESS

Fluid volume excess may result from excessive intake of fluids, abnormal retention of fluids (e.g., heart failure, renal failure), or interstitial-to–plasma fluid shift. Although shifts in fluid between the plasma and interstitium do not alter the overall volume of the ECF, these shifts do result in changes in the intravascular volume. The clinical manifestations of fluid volume excess are listed in Table 17-4.

Collaborative Care

The goal of treatment for fluid volume excess is removal of fluid without producing abnormal changes in the electrolyte composition or osmolality of ECF. The primary cause must be identified and treated. Diuretics and fluid restriction are the primary forms of therapy. Restriction of sodium intake may also be indicated. If the fluid excess leads to ascites or pleural effusion, an abdominal paracentesis or thoracentesis may be necessary.

NURSING MANAGEMENT
EXTRACELLULAR FLUID VOLUME IMBALANCES

Nursing Diagnoses

Nursing diagnoses and collaborative problems for the patient with fluid imbalances include, but are not limited to, the following:

Extracellular fluid volume deficit:
- Deficient fluid volume *related to* excessive ECF losses or decreased fluid intake
- Decreased cardiac output *related to* excessive ECF losses or decreased fluid intake
- Potential complication: hypovolemic shock

Extracellular fluid volume excess:
- Excess fluid volume *related to* increased water and/or sodium retention
- Impaired gas exchange *related to* water retention leading to pulmonary edema
- Risk for impaired skin integrity *related to* edema
- Disturbed body image *related to* altered body appearance secondary to edema
- Potential complications: pulmonary edema, ascites

Nursing Implementation

Intake and Output. The use of 24-hour intake and output records gives valuable information regarding fluid and electrolyte problems. Sources of excessive intake or fluid losses can be identified on an accurately recorded intake-and-output flowsheet. Intake should include oral, IV, and tube feedings and retained irrigants. Output includes urine, excess perspiration, wound or tube drainage, vomitus, and diarrhea. Fluid loss from wounds and perspiration should be estimated. Urine specific gravity measurements can be done. Readings of greater than 1.025 indicate concentrated urine, whereas those of less than 1.010 indicate dilute urine.

Cardiovascular Changes. Monitoring the patient for cardiovascular changes is necessary to prevent or detect complications from

TABLE 17-4 Extracellular Fluid Imbalances: Causes and Clinical Manifestations

ECF Volume Deficit	ECF Volume Excess
Causes	
↑ Insensible water loss or perspiration (high fever, heatstroke)	Excessive isotonic or hypotonic IV fluids
Diabetes insipidus	Heart failure
Osmotic diuresis	Renal failure
Hemorrhage	Primary polydipsia
GI losses—vomiting, NG suction, diarrhea, fistula drainage	SIADH
Overuse of diuretics	Cushing syndrome
Inadequate fluid intake	Long-term use of corticosteroids
Third-space fluid shifts—burns, intestinal obstruction	
Clinical Manifestations	
Restlessness, drowsiness, lethargy, confusion	Headache, confusion, lethargy
Thirst, dry mouth	Peripheral edema
Decreased skin turgor, ↓ capillary refill	Distended neck veins
Postural hypotension, ↑ pulse, ↓ CVP	Bounding pulse, ↑ BP, ↑ CVP
↓ Urine output, concentrated urine	Polyuria (with normal renal function)
↑ Respiratory rate	Dyspnea, crackles (rales), pulmonary edema
Weakness, dizziness	Muscle spasms
Weight loss	Weight gain
Seizures, coma	Seizures, coma

BP, Blood pressure; *CVP,* central venous pressure; *GI,* gastrointestinal; *IV,* intravenous; *NG,* nasogastric; *SIADH,* syndrome of inappropriate antidiuretic hormone.

fluid and electrolyte imbalances. Signs and symptoms of ECF volume excess and deficit are reflected in changes in blood pressure, pulse force, and jugular venous distention. In fluid volume excess, the pulse is full and bounding. Because of the expanded intravascular volume, the pulse is not easily obliterated. Increased volume causes distended neck veins (jugular venous distention) and increased blood pressure.

In mild to moderate fluid volume deficit, compensatory mechanisms include sympathetic nervous system stimulation of the heart and peripheral vasoconstriction. Stimulation of the heart increases heart rate and, combined with vasoconstriction, maintains blood pressure within normal limits. A change in position from lying to sitting or standing may elicit a further increase in heart rate or a decrease in blood pressure (orthostatic hypotension). If vasoconstriction and tachycardia provide inadequate compensation, hypotension occurs when the patient is recumbent. Severe fluid volume deficit can cause a weak, thready pulse that is easily obliterated and flattened neck veins. Severe, untreated fluid deficit will result in shock.

Respiratory Changes. Both fluid excess and fluid deficit affect respiratory status. ECF excess results in pulmonary congestion and pulmonary edema as increased hydrostatic pressure in the pulmonary vessels forces fluid into the alveoli. The patient will experience shortness of breath, irritative cough, and moist crackles on auscultation.[3] The patient with ECF deficit will demonstrate an increased respiratory rate due to decreased tissue perfusion and resultant hypoxia.

Neurologic Changes. Changes in neurologic function may occur with fluid volume excesses or deficits. ECF excess may result in cerebral edema as a result of increased hydrostatic pressure in cerebral vessels. Alternatively, profound volume depletion may cause an alteration in sensorium secondary to reduced cerebral tissue perfusion.

Assessment of neurologic function includes evaluation of (1) the level of consciousness, which includes responses to verbal and painful stimuli and the determination of a person's orientation to time, place, and person; (2) pupillary response to light and equality of pupil size; and (3) voluntary movement of the extremities, degree of muscle strength, and reflexes. Nursing care focuses on maintaining patient safety.

Daily Weights. Accurate daily weights provide the easiest measurement of volume status. An increase of 1 kg (2.2 lb) is equal to 1000 ml (1 L) of fluid retention (provided the person has maintained usual dietary intake or has not been on nothing-by-mouth [NPO] status). However, weight changes must be obtained under standardized conditions. An accurate weight requires the patient to be weighed at the same time every day, wearing the same garments, and on the same carefully calibrated scale. Excess bedding should be removed and all drainage bags should be emptied before the weighing. If bulky dressings or tubes are present, which may not necessarily be used every day, a notation regarding these variables should be recorded on the flowsheet or nursing notes.

Skin Assessment and Care. Clues to ECF volume deficit and excess can be detected by inspection of the skin. Skin should be examined for turgor and mobility. Normally a fold of skin, when pinched, will readily move and, on release, will rapidly return to its former position. Skin areas over the sternum, abdomen, and anterior forearm are the usual sites for evaluation of tissue turgor (Fig. 17-11). The preferred areas to assess for tissue turgor in the older person are areas where decreases in skin elasticity is less significant, such as the forehead or over the sternum.[6]

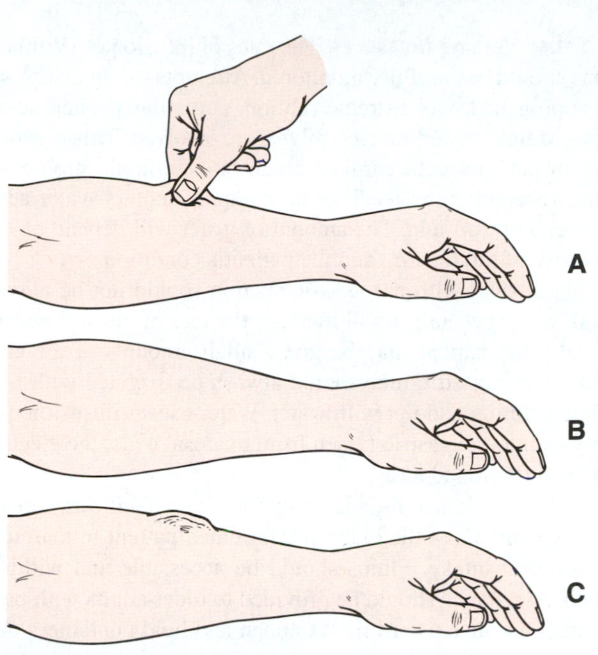

FIG. 17-11 Assessment of skin turgor. **A** and **B,** When normal skin is pinched, it resumes shape in seconds. **C,** If the skin remains wrinkled for 20 to 30 seconds, the patient has poor skin turgor.

In ECF volume deficit, skin turgor is diminished; there is a lag in the pinched skinfold's return to its original state (referred to as *tenting*). The skin may be cool and moist if there is vasoconstriction to compensate for the decreased fluid volume. Mild hypovolemia usually does not stimulate this compensatory response; consequently, the skin will be warm and dry. Volume deficit may also cause the skin to appear dry and wrinkled. These signs may be difficult to evaluate in the older adult because the patient's skin may be normally dry, wrinkled, and nonelastic. Oral mucous membranes will be dry, the tongue may be furrowed, and the individual often complains of thirst. Routine oral care is critical to the comfort of the dehydrated patient and the patient who is fluid restricted for management of fluid volume excess.

Skin that is edematous may feel cool because of fluid accumulation and a decrease in blood flow secondary to the pressure of the fluid. The fluid can also stretch the skin, causing it to feel taut and hard. Edema is assessed by pressing with a thumb or forefinger over the edematous area. A grading scale is used to standardize the description if an indentation (ranging from 1+ [slight edema; 2-mm indentation] to 4+ [pitting edema; 8-mm indentation]) remains when pressure is released. The areas to be evaluated for edema are those where soft tissues overlie a bone. Skin areas over the tibia, fibula, and sacrum are the preferred sites.

Good skin care for the person with ECF volume excess or deficit is important. Edematous tissues must be protected from extremes of heat and cold, prolonged pressure, and trauma. Frequent skin care and changes in position will protect the patient from skin breakdown. Elevation of edematous extremities helps promote venous return and fluid reabsorption. Dehydrated skin needs frequent care without the use of soap. The application of moisturizing creams or oils will increase moisture retention and stimulate circulation.

Other Nursing Measures. The rates of infusion of IV fluid solutions should be carefully monitored. Attempts to "catch up" should be approached with extreme caution, particularly when large volumes of fluid or certain electrolytes are involved. This is especially true in patients with cardiac, renal, or neurologic problems. Patients receiving tube feedings need supplementary water added to their enteral formula. The amount of water will depend on the osmolarity of the feeding and the patient's condition.

The patient with nasogastric suction should not be allowed to drink water because it will increase the loss of electrolytes. Occasionally the patient may be given small amounts of ice chips to suck. A nasogastric tube should always be irrigated with isotonic saline solution and not with water. Water causes diffusion of electrolytes into the gastric lumen from mucosal cells; the electrolytes are then suctioned away.

Nurses in hospitals and long-term care facilities should encourage and assist the older or debilitated patient to maintain adequate oral intake. Fluids should be accessible and within easy reach. Assistance should be provided to older adults with physical limitations, such as arthritis, to open and hold containers. A variety of types of fluids should be available, and individual preferences should be assessed. Room-temperature drinks often lack appeal; therefore fluids should be served at a temperature that is preferred by the patient. Seventy percent to 80% of the daily intake of fluids should be with meals, with the addition of fluid supplements between meals. Older adults may choose to decrease or eliminate fluids 2 hours before bedtime to decrease nocturia or incontinence. The unconscious or cognitively impaired patient is at increased risk because of an inability to express thirst and act on it. Therefore fluid intake and losses must be accurately documented. Careful evaluation of adequacy of intake must occur, and appropriate fluid intake must be administered.[6,7,9]

SODIUM IMBALANCES

Sodium is the main cation of the ECF and plays a major role in maintaining the concentration and volume of the ECF. Therefore sodium is the primary determinant of ECF osmolality. Sodium imbalances are typically associated with parallel changes in osmolality. Because of its impact on osmolality, sodium affects the water distribution between the ECF and the ICF. Sodium is also important in the generation and transmission of nerve impulses and the regulation of acid-base balance. Serum sodium is measured in milliequivalents per liter (mEq/L) or millimoles per liter (mmol/L).

The GI tract absorbs sodium from foods. Typically, daily intake of sodium far exceeds the body's daily requirements. Sodium leaves the body through urine, sweat, and feces. The kidneys are the primary regulator of sodium balance. The kidneys regulate the ECF concentration of sodium by excreting or retaining water under the influence of ADH. Aldosterone also plays a role in sodium regulation by promoting sodium reabsorption from the renal tubules. The serum sodium level reflects the ratio of sodium to water, not necessarily the loss or gain of sodium. Thus changes in the serum sodium level may reflect a primary water imbalance, a primary sodium imbalance, or a combination of the two. Sodium imbalances are typically associated with imbalances in ECF volume (Figs. 17-12 and 17-13).

HYPERNATREMIA

Common causes of hypernatremia are listed in Table 17-5. An elevated serum sodium may occur with water loss or sodium gain. Because sodium is the major determinant of the ECF osmolality, hypernatremia causes hyperosmolality. In turn, ECF hyperosmolality causes a shift of water out of the cells, which leads to cellular dehydration.

As discussed earlier, the primary protection against the development of hyperosmolality is thirst. As the plasma osmolality increases, the thirst center in the hypothalamus is stimulated, and the individual seeks fluids. Hypernatremia is not a problem in an alert person who has access to water, can sense thirst, and is able to swallow. Hypernatremia secondary to water deficiency is often the result of an impaired level of consciousness or an inability to obtain fluids.

Several clinical states can produce water loss and hypernatremia. A deficiency in the synthesis or release of ADH from the posterior pituitary gland (central diabetes insipidus) or a decrease in kidney responsiveness to ADH (nephrogenic diabetes insipidus) can result in profound diuresis resulting in a water deficit and hypernatremia. Hyperosmolality can result from administration of

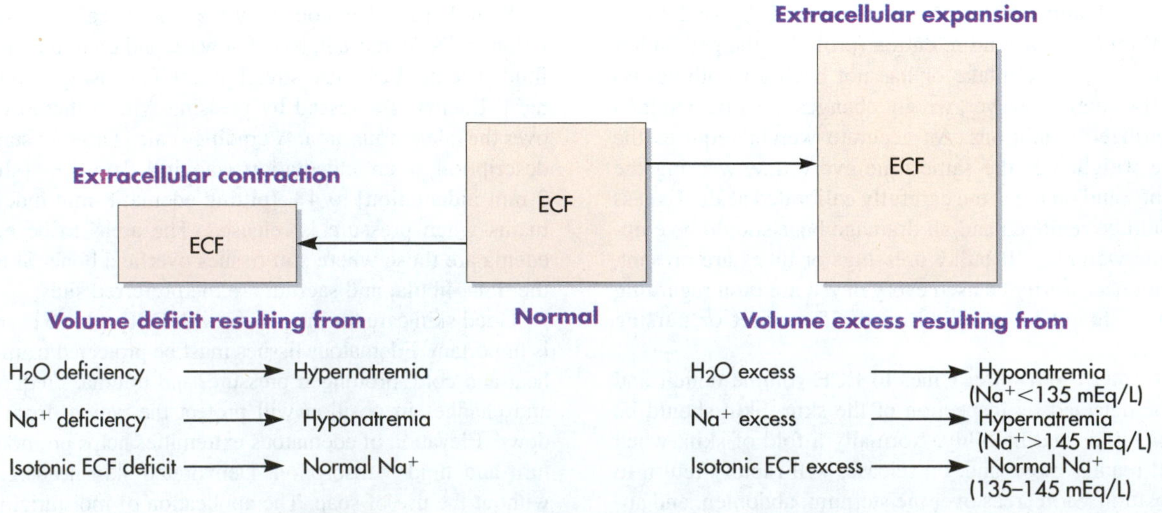

FIG. 17-12 Differential assessment of extracellular fluid (ECF) volume.

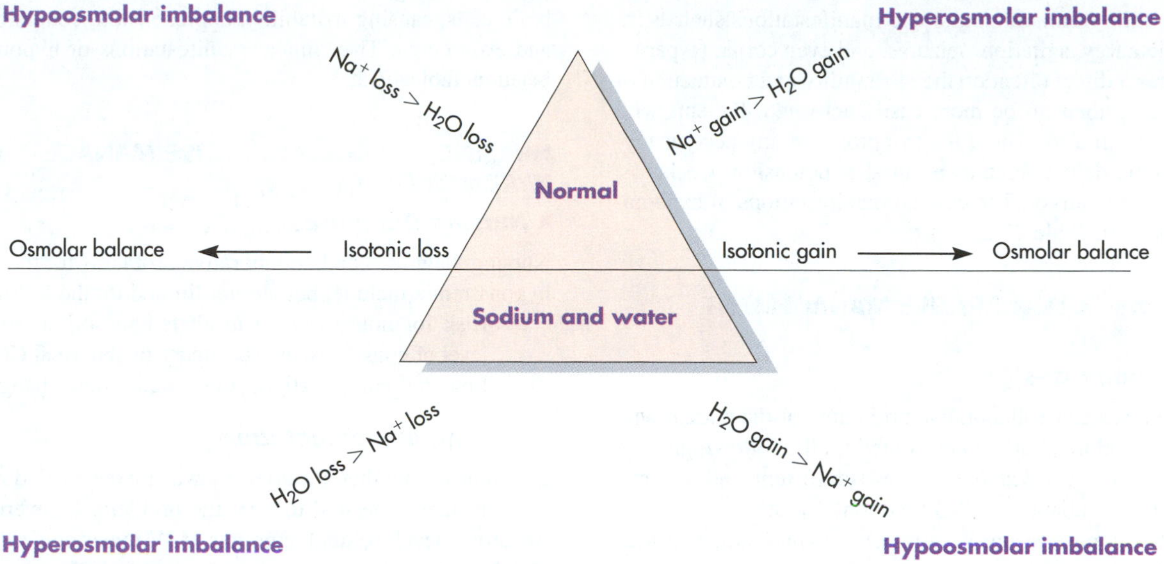

FIG. 17-13 Isotonic gains and losses affect mainly the extracellular fluid (ECF) compartment with little or no water movement into the cells. Hypertonic imbalances cause water to move from inside the cell into the ECF to dilute the concentrated sodium, causing cell shrinkage. Hypotonic imbalances cause water to move into the cell, causing cell swelling.

concentrated hyperosmolar tube feedings and osmotic diuretics (mannitol), as well as hyperglycemia associated with uncontrolled diabetes mellitus. These situations result in osmotic diuresis. Dilute urine is lost, leaving behind a high solute load. Other causes of hypernatremia include excessive sweating and increased sensible losses from high fever.

Excessive sodium intake with inadequate water intake can also lead to hypernatremia. Examples of sodium gain include intravenous administration of hypertonic saline or sodium bicarbonate, use of sodium-containing drugs, concentrated enteral tube feedings, excessive oral intake of sodium (ingestion of seawater), and *primary aldosteronism* (hypersecretion of aldosterone) caused by a tumor of the adrenal glands.

Clinical Manifestations. Symptomatic hypernatremia is rare except in cases in which individuals do not have access to water or have an altered thirst mechanism. When symptoms do occur, they are primarily the result of water shifting out of cells into the ECF with resultant dehydration and shrinkage of cells. Dehydra-

TABLE 17-5 Sodium Imbalances: Causes and Clinical Manifestations

Hyponatremia (Na^+ <135 mEq/L [mmol/L])	Hypernatremia (Na^+ >145 mEq/L [mmol/L])
Causes	
Excessive sodium loss: GI losses: diarrhea, vomiting, fistulas, NG suction Renal losses: diuretics, adrenal insufficiency, Na^+ wasting renal disease Skin losses: burns, wound drainage Inadequate sodium intake: fasting diets Excessive water gain (↓ sodium concentration): excessive hypotonic IV fluids, primary polydipsia Disease states: SIADH, heart failure, primary hypoaldosteronism	Excessive sodium intake: IV fluids: hypertonic NaCl, excessive isotonic NaCl, IV sodium bicarbonate Hypertonic tube feedings without water supplements Near-drowning in salt water Inadequate water intake: unconscious or cognitively impaired individuals Excessive water loss (↑ sodium concentration): ↑ insensible water loss (high fever, heatstroke, prolonged hyperventilation), osmotic diuretic therapy, diarrhea Disease states: diabetes insipidus, primary hyperaldosteronism, Cushing syndrome, uncontrolled diabetes mellitus
Clinical Manifestations	
Hyponatremia with Decreased ECF Volume	***Hypernatremia with Decreased ECF Volume***
Irritability, apprehension, confusion, dizziness, personality changes, tremors, seizures, coma Dry mucous membranes Postural hypotension, ↓ CVP, ↓ jugular venous filling, tachycardia, thready pulse Cold and clammy skin	Restlessness, agitation, twitching, seizures, coma Intense thirst; dry, swollen tongue, sticky mucous membranes Postural hypotension, ↓ CVP, weight loss Weakness, lethargy
Hyponatremia with Normal/Increased ECF Volume	***Hypernatremia with Normal/Increased ECF Volume***
Headache, apathy, confusion, muscle spasms, seizures, coma Nausea, vomiting, diarrhea, abdominal cramps Weight gain, ↑ BP, ↑ CVP	Restlessness, agitation, twitching, seizures, coma Intense thirst, flushed skin Weight gain, peripheral and pulmonary edema, ↑ BP, ↑ CVP

BP, Blood pressure; *CVP*, central venous pressure; *ECF*, extracellular fluid; *GI*, gastrointestinal; *IV*, intravenous; *NG*, nasogastric; *SIADH*, syndrome of inappropriate antidiuretic hormone.

tion of brain cells results in neurologic manifestations such as intense thirst, lethargy, agitation, seizures, and even coma. Hypernatremia also has a direct effect on the excitability and conduction of neurons, causing them to be more easily activated. Patients with hypernatremia will also exhibit the symptoms of any accompanying ECF volume deficit, such as postural hypotension, weakness, and decreased skin turgor. The clinical manifestations of hypernatremia are listed in Table 17-5.

NURSING *and* COLLABORATIVE MANAGEMENT HYPERNATREMIA

■ *Nursing Diagnoses*

Nursing diagnoses and collaborative problems for the patient with hypernatremia include, but are not limited to, the following:

- Risk for injury *related to* altered sensorium and seizures secondary to abnormal CNS function
- Potential complication: seizures and coma leading to irreversible brain damage

■ *Nursing Implementation*

The goal of treatment in hypernatremia is to treat the underlying cause. In primary water deficit, the continued water loss must be prevented and water replacement must be provided. If oral fluids cannot be ingested, intravenous solutions of 5% dextrose in water or hypotonic saline may be given initially. Serum sodium levels must be reduced gradually to prevent too rapid a shift of water back into the cells. Overly rapid correction of hypernatremia can result in cerebral edema. The risk is greatest in the patient who has developed hypernatremia over several days or longer.

The goal of treatment for sodium excess is to dilute the sodium concentration with sodium-free IV fluids, such as 5% dextrose in water, and to promote excretion of the excess sodium by administering diuretics. Dietary sodium intake will also be restricted. (See Chapter 50 for specific treatment of diabetes insipidus.)

HYPONATREMIA

Hyponatremia may result from loss of sodium-containing fluids, from water excess (dilutional hyponatremia), or a combination of both. Hyponatremia causes hypoosmolality with a shift of water into the cells.

Common causes of hyponatremia caused by water excess are inappropriate use of sodium-free or hypotonic IV fluids. This may occur in patients after surgery or major trauma, during administration of fluids in patients with renal failure, or in patients with psychiatric disorders associated with excessive water intake. SIADH will result in dilutional hyponatremia caused by abnormal retention of water. (See Chapter 50 for a discussion of the causes of SIADH.)

Losses of sodium-rich body fluids from the GI tract, kidney, or skin indirectly result in hyponatremia. Because these fluids are either isotonic or hypotonic, sodium is lost with an equal or greater proportion of water. However, hyponatremia develops as the body responds to the fluid volume deficit with activation of the thirst mechanism and by releasing ADH. The resultant retention of water lowers the sodium concentration.[3]

Clinical Manifestations. Symptoms of hyponatremia are related to cellular swelling and are first manifested in the CNS.[3] The excess water lowers plasma osmolality, shifting fluid into brain cells, causing irritability, apprehension, confusion, seizures, and even coma. The clinical manifestations of hyponatremia are listed in Table 17-5.

NURSING *and* COLLABORATIVE MANAGEMENT HYPONATREMIA

■ *Nursing Diagnoses*

Nursing diagnoses and collaborative problems for the patient with hyponatremia include, but are not limited to, the following:

- Risk for injury *related to* altered sensorium and decreased level of consciousness secondary to abnormal CNS function
- Potential complication: severe neurologic changes

■ *Nursing Implementation*

In hyponatremia that is caused by water excess, fluid restriction is often all that is needed to treat the problem. If severe symptoms (seizures) develop, small amounts of IV hypertonic saline solution (3% NaCl) are given to restore the serum sodium level while the body is returning to a normal water balance. Treatment of hyponatremia associated with abnormal fluid loss includes fluid replacement with sodium-containing solutions.

POTASSIUM IMBALANCES

Potassium is the major ICF cation, with 98% of the body potassium being intracellular. For example, potassium concentration within muscle cells is approximately 140 mEq/L; potassium concentration in the ECF is 3.5 to 5.0 mEq/L. The sodium-potassium pump in cell membranes maintains this concentration difference by pumping potassium into the cell and sodium out, a process fueled by the breakdown of ATP. Adequate intracellular magnesium is necessary for normal function of the pump. Because the ratio of ECF potassium to ICF potassium is the major factor in the resting membrane potential of nerve and muscle cells, neuromuscular and cardiac function are commonly affected by potassium imbalances.[2]

Potassium is critical for many cellular and metabolic functions. In addition to its role in neuromuscular and cardiac function, potassium regulates intracellular osmolality and promotes cellular growth. Potassium moves into cells during the formation of new tissues and leaves the cell during tissue breakdown.[3] Potassium also plays a role in acid-base balance that is discussed in acid-base regulation later in this chapter.

Diet is the source of potassium. The typical Western diet contains approximately 50 to 100 mEq of potassium daily, mainly from fruits, dried fruits, and vegetables. Many salt substitutes used in low-sodium diets contain substantial potassium. Patients may receive potassium from parenteral sources, including IV fluids; transfusions of stored, hemolyzed blood; and medications (e.g., potassium-penicillin).

The kidneys are the primary route for potassium loss. About 90% of the daily potassium intake is eliminated by the kidneys; the remainder is lost in the stool and sweat. If kidney function is significantly impaired, toxic levels of potassium may be retained. There is an inverse relationship between sodium and potassium reabsorption in the kidneys. Factors that cause sodium retention (e.g., low blood volume, increased aldosterone level) cause potassium loss in the urine. Large urine volumes can be associated with excess loss of potassium in the urine. The ability of the kidneys to conserve potassium is weak even when body stores are depleted.[2,10]

Disruptions in the dynamic equilibrium between ICF and ECF potassium often cause clinical problems. Among the factors causing potassium to move from the ECF to the ICF are the following:

- Insulin
- Alkalosis
- β-Adrenergic stimulation (catecholamine release in stress, coronary ischemia, delirium tremens, or administration of β-adrenergic agonist drugs)
- Rapid cell building (administration of folic acid or cobalamin [vitamin B_{12}] to patients with megaloblastic anemia resulting in marked production of red blood cells)

Factors that cause potassium to move from the ICF to the ECF include acidosis, trauma to cells (as in massive soft tissue damage or in tumor lysis), and exercise. Both digoxin-like drugs and β-adrenergic blocking drugs (e.g., propranolol [Inderal]) can impair entry of potassium into cells, resulting in a higher ECF potassium concentration. Causes of potassium imbalance are summarized in Table 17-6.

HYPERKALEMIA

Hyperkalemia (high serum potassium) may be caused by a massive intake of potassium, impaired renal excretion, shift of potassium from the ICF to the ECF, or a combination of these factors. The most common cause of hyperkalemia is renal failure. Hyperkalemia is also common in patients with massive cell destruction (e.g., burn or crush injury, tumor lysis); rapid transfusion of stored, hemolyzed blood; and catabolic states (e.g., severe infections). Metabolic acidosis is associated with a shift of potassium ions from the ICF to the ECF as hydrogen ions move into the cell. Adrenal insufficiency with a subsequent aldosterone deficiency leads to retention of K^+. Certain drugs, such as potassium-sparing diuretics (e.g., spironolactone [Aldactone], triamterene [Dyrenium]) and angiotensin-converting enzyme (ACE) inhibitors (e.g., enalapril [Vasotec], lisinopril [Prinivil]), may contribute to the development of hyperkalemia. Both of these types of drugs reduce the kidney's ability to excrete potassium (see Table 17-6).

Clinical Manifestations. Hyperkalemia increases the concentration of potassium outside of the cell, altering the normal ECF and ICF ratio, resulting in increased cellular excitability. Initially the patient may experience cramping leg pain, followed by weakness or paralysis of skeletal muscles. Leg muscles are affected initially; respiratory muscles are spared. Disturbances in cardiac conduction occur as the potassium level rises.[3] Cardiac depolarization is decreased, leading to flattening of the P wave and widening of the QRS complex. Repolarization occurs more rapidly, resulting in shortening of the QT in-

TABLE 17-6 Potassium Imbalances: Causes and Clinical Manifestations

Hypokalemia (K^+ <3.5 mEq/L [mmol/L])	Hyperkalemia (K^+ >5.0 mEq/L [mmol/L])
Causes	
Potassium Loss	***Excess Potassium Intake***
GI losses: diarrhea, vomiting, fistulas, NG suction	Excessive or rapid parenteral administration
Renal losses: diuretics, hyperaldosteronism, magnesium depletion	Potassium-containing drugs (e.g., potassium-penicillin)
Skin losses: diaphoresis	Potassium-containing salt substitute
Dialysis	
Shift of Potassium Into Cells	***Shift of Potassium Out of Cells***
Increased insulin (e.g., IV dextrose load)	Acidosis
Alkalosis	Tissue catabolism (e.g., fever, sepsis, burns)
Tissue repair	Crush injury
↑ Epinephrine (e.g., stress)	Tumor lysis syndrome
Lack of Potassium Intake	***Failure to Eliminate Potassium***
Starvation	Renal disease
Diet low in potassium	Potassium-sparing diuretics
Failure to include potassium in parenteral fluids if NPO	Adrenal insufficiency
	ACE inhibitors
Clinical Manifestations	
Fatigue	Irritability
Muscle weakness, leg cramps	Anxiety
Nausea, vomiting, paralytic ileus	Abdominal cramping, diarrhea
Soft, flabby muscles	Weakness of lower extremities
Paresthesias, decreased reflexes	Paresthesias
Weak, irregular pulse	Irregular pulse
Polyuria	Cardiac arrest if hyperkalemia sudden or severe
Hyperglycemia	
Electrocardiogram Changes	***Electrocardiogram Changes***
ST segment depression	Tall, peaked T wave
Flattened T wave	Prolonged PR interval
Presence of U wave	ST segment depression
Ventricular dysrhythmias (e.g., PVCs)	Loss of P wave
Bradycardia	Widening QRS
Enhanced digitalis effect	Ventricular fibrillation
	Ventricular standstill

ACE, Angiotensin-converting enzyme; *GI,* gastrointestinal; *NG,* nasogastric; *NPO,* nothing by mouth; *PVC,* premature ventricular contraction.

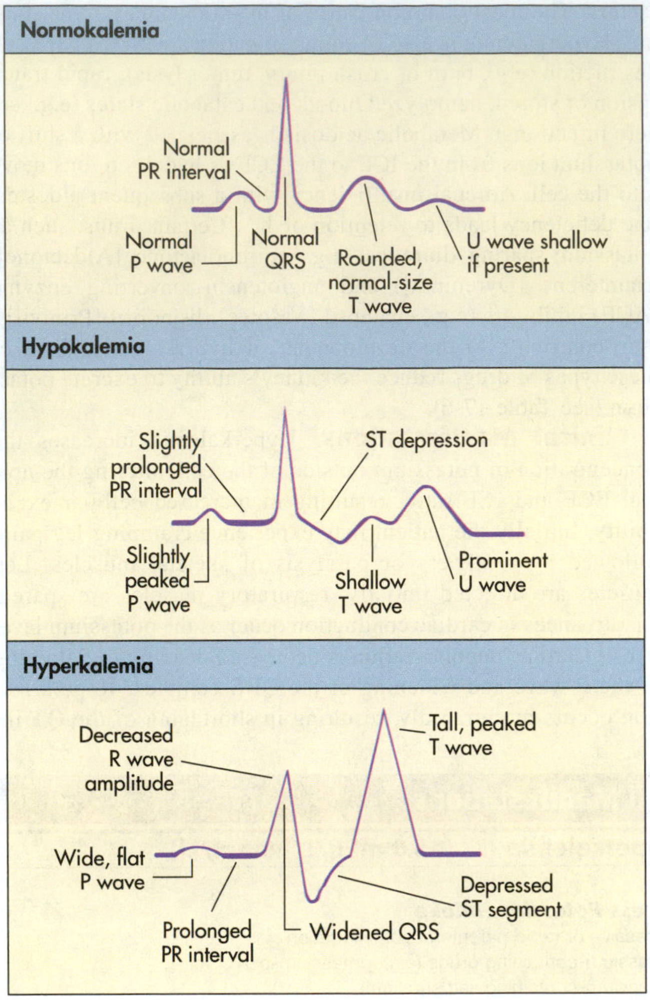

FIG. 17-14 Electrocardiographic changes associated with alterations in potassium status.

terval and causing the T wave to be narrower and more peaked. Ventricular fibrillation or cardiac standstill may occur. Fig. 17-14 illustrates the electrocardiographic (ECG) effects of hyperkalemia. Abdominal cramping and diarrhea occur from hyperactivity of smooth muscles. Other clinical manifestations are listed in Table 17-6.

NURSING *and* COLLABORATIVE MANAGEMENT HYPERKALEMIA

■ *Nursing Diagnoses*

Nursing diagnoses and collaborative problems for the patient with hyperkalemia include, but are not limited to, the following:

- Risk for injury *related to* lower extremity muscle weakness and seizures
- Potential complication: dysrhythmias

■ *Nursing Implementation*

Treatment of hyperkalemia consists of the following:

1. Eliminate oral and parenteral potassium intake (see Table 47-9).
2. Increase elimination of potassium. This is accomplished via diuretics, dialysis, and use of ion-exchange resins such as sodium polystyrene sulfonate (Kayexalate). Increased fluid intake can enhance renal potassium elimination.
3. Force potassium from the ECF to the ICF. This is accomplished by administration of intravenous insulin (along with glucose so the patient does not become hypoglycemic) or via administration of IV sodium bicarbonate in the correction of acidosis. Rarely, a β-adrenergic agonist (e.g., epinephrine) is administered.
4. Reverse the membrane potential effects of the elevated ECF potassium by administering calcium gluconate IV. Calcium ion can immediately reverse the membrane excitability.

In cases in which the elevation of potassium is mild and the kidneys are functioning, it may be sufficient to withhold potassium from the diet and IV sources and increase renal elimination by administering fluids and possibly diuretics. Kayexalate, which is administered via the GI tract, binds potassium in exchange for sodium, and the resin is excreted in feces (see Chapter 47). All patients with clinically significant hyperkalemia should be monitored electrocardiographically to detect dysrhythmias and to monitor the effects of therapy. Patients with moderate hyperkalemia should additionally receive one of the treatments to force potassium into cells, usually IV insulin and glucose. The patient experiencing dangerous cardiac dysrhythmias should receive IV calcium gluconate immediately while the potassium is being eliminated and forced into cells. Hemodialysis is an effective means of removing potassium from the body in the patient with renal failure.

HYPOKALEMIA

Hypokalemia (low serum potassium) can result from abnormal losses of potassium from a shift of potassium from ECF to ICF, or rarely from deficient dietary potassium intake. The most common causes of hypokalemia are abnormal losses, via either the kidneys or the GI tract. Abnormal losses occur when the patient is diuresing, particularly in the patient with an elevated aldosterone level. Aldosterone is released when the circulating blood volume is low; it causes sodium retention in the kidneys but loss of potassium in the urine. Magnesium deficiency may contribute to the development of potassium depletion. Low plasma magnesium stimulates renin release and subsequent increased aldosterone levels, which results in potassium excretion.[2] GI tract losses of potassium secondary to diarrhea, laxative abuse, vomiting, and ileostomy drainage can cause hypokalemia.

Metabolic alkalosis can cause a shift of potassium into cells in exchange for hydrogen, thus lowering the potassium in the ECF and causing symptomatic hypokalemia. Hypokalemia is sometimes associated with the treatment of diabetic ketoacidosis because of a combination of factors, including an increased urinary potassium loss and a shift of potassium into cells with the administration of insulin and correction of metabolic acidosis. A less common cause of hypokalemia is the sudden initiation of cell formation; for example, the formation of red blood cells (RBCs) as in treatment of anemia with cobalamin (vitamin B_{12}), folic acid, or erythropoietin.

Clinical Manifestations. Hypokalemia alters the resting membrane potential. It most commonly is associated with hyperpolarization, or increased negative charge within the cell. This causes reduced excitability of cells. The most serious clinical problems are cardiac. Cardiac changes include impaired repolarization, resulting in a flattening of the T wave and eventually in emergence of a U wave. The P wave amplitude may increase and may become peaked (see Fig. 17-14). The incidence of potentially lethal ventricular dysrhythmias is increased in hypokalemia. Patients at risk for hypokalemia and those who are critically ill should have cardiac monitoring to detect cardiac changes related to potassium imbalances. Patients taking digoxin experience increased digoxin toxicity if their serum potassium level is low. Skeletal muscle weakness and paralysis may occur with hypokalemia. As with hyperkalemia, symptoms are often observed initially in the legs. Severe hypokalemia can cause weakness or paralysis of respiratory muscles, leading to shallow respirations and respiratory arrest.

Smooth muscle function is also altered by hypokalemia. The patient may experience decreased GI motility (e.g., paralytic ileus), decreased airway responsiveness, and impaired regulation of arteriolar blood flow, possibly contributing to smooth muscle cell breakdown. Finally, hypokalemia can impair function in nonmuscle tissue. Release of insulin is impaired, leading to hyperglycemia. With prolonged hypokalemia, the kidneys are unable to concentrate urine and diuresis occurs.[9] Clinical manifestations of hypokalemia are presented in Table 17-6.

NURSING *and* COLLABORATIVE MANAGEMENT HYPOKALEMIA

Nursing Diagnoses

Nursing diagnoses and collaborative problems for the patient with hypokalemia include, but are not limited to, the following:

- Risk for injury *related to* muscle weakness and hyporeflexia
- Potential complication: dysrhythmias

Nursing Implementation

Hypokalemia is treated by giving potassium chloride supplements and increasing dietary intake of potassium. Potassium chloride (KCl) supplements can be given orally or IV. Except in severe deficiencies, KCl is never given unless there is urine output of at least 0.5 ml/kg of body weight per hour. KCl supplements added to IV solutions should never exceed 60 mEq/L. The preferred level is 40 mEq/L. The rate of IV administration of KCl should not exceed 10 to 20 mEq per hour to prevent hyperkalemia and cardiac arrest. When given IV, potassium may cause pain in the area of the vein where it is entering. Central IV lines should be used when rapid correction of hypokalemia is necessary. Patients should be taught methods to prevent hypokalemia depending on their individual situations. Patients at risk should obtain regular serum potassium levels to monitor for hypokalemia. A teaching guide for prevention of hypokalemia is found in Table 17-7, and foods high in potassium are identified in Table 47-9.

TABLE 17-7 PATIENT AND FAMILY TEACHING GUIDE Prevention of Hypokalemia

1. Teach the patient and family the signs and symptoms of hypokalemia (see Table 17-6) and to report them to the health care provider.
2. For patient taking diuretics:
   - Explain the importance of increasing dietary potassium intake, especially if on a thiazide or loop diuretic (see Chapter 33, Table 33-8).
   - Teach patient which foods are high in potassium (see Chapter 47, Table 47-9).
   - Explain that salt substitutes contain approximately 50 to 60 mEq of potassium per teaspoon and help raise potassium if taking a potassium-losing diuretic. Salt substitutes should be avoided if taking a potassium-sparing diuretic (see Chapter 33, Table 33-8).
3. For patient taking oral potassium supplements:
   - Instruct the patient to take the medication as prescribed to prevent overdosage and to take the supplement with a full glass of water to help it dissolve in the GI tract.
4. For patient taking digitalis preparations and others at risk for hypokalemia:
   - Explain the importance of having serum potassium levels regularly monitored because low potassium enhances the action of digitalis.

CALCIUM IMBALANCES

Calcium is obtained from ingested foods. However, only about 30% of the calcium from foods is absorbed in the GI tract. More than 99% of the body's calcium is combined with phosphorus and concentrated in the skeletal system. Bones serve as a readily available store of calcium. Thus wide variations in serum calcium levels are avoided by regulating the movement of calcium into or out of the bone. Usually the amount of calcium and phosphorus found in the serum has an inverse relationship; that is, as one increases, the other decreases.[11] The functions of calcium include transmission of nerve impulses, myocardial contractions, blood clotting, formation of teeth and bone, and muscle contractions.

Calcium is present in the serum in three forms: free or ionized; bound to protein (primarily albumin); and complexed with phosphate, citrate, or carbonate. The ionized form is the biologically active form. Approximately one half of the total serum calcium is ionized.

Calcium is measured in milligrams per deciliter (mg/dl) and milliequivalents per liter (mEq/L). As usually reported, serum calcium levels reflect the total calcium level (all three forms), although ionized calcium levels may be reported separately. The levels listed in Table 17-8 reflect total calcium levels. Changes in serum pH will alter the level of ionized calcium without altering the total calcium level. A decreased plasma pH (acidosis) decreases calcium binding to albumin, leading to more ionized calcium. An increased plasma pH (alkalosis) increases calcium binding, leading to decreased ionized calcium. Alterations in serum albumin levels affect the interpretation of total calcium levels. Low albumin levels result in a drop in the total calcium level, although the level of ionized calcium is not affected.

Calcium balance is controlled by parathyroid hormone (PTH), calcitonin, and vitamin D.[11,12] PTH is produced by the parathyroid gland. Its production and release are stimulated by low serum calcium levels. PTH increases bone resorption (movement of calcium out of bones), increases GI absorption of calcium, and increases renal tubule reabsorption of calcium.

Calcitonin is produced by the thyroid gland and is stimulated by high serum calcium levels. It opposes the action of PTH and thus lowers the serum calcium level by decreasing GI absorption, increasing calcium deposition into bone, and promoting renal excretion.

Vitamin D is formed through the action of ultraviolet (UV) rays on a precursor found in the skin or is ingested in the diet. Vitamin D is important for absorption of calcium from the GI tract. Causes of calcium imbalances are listed in Table 17-8.

HYPERCALCEMIA

About two thirds of hypercalcemia cases are caused by hyperparathyroidism and one third are caused by malignancy, especially from breast cancer, lung cancer, and multiple myeloma.[11] Malignancies lead to hypercalcemia through bone destruction from tumor invasion or through tumor secretion of a parathyroid-related

TABLE 17-8 Calcium Imbalances: Causes and Clinical Manifestations

Hypocalcemia (Ca^{2+} <9 mg/dl; 4.5 mEq/L [2.25 mmol/L])	Hypercalcemia (Ca^{2+} >11 mg/dl; 5.5 mEq/L [2.75 mmol/L])
Causes	
Decreased Total Calcium	***Increased Total Calcium***
Chronic renal failure	Multiple myeloma
Elevated phosphorus	Malignancies with bone metastasis
Primary hypoparathyroidism	Prolonged immobilization
Vitamin D deficiency	Hyperparathyroidism
Magnesium deficiency	Vitamin D overdose
Acute pancreatitis	Thiazide diuretics
Loop diuretics (e.g., furosemide [Lasix])	Milk-alkali syndrome
Chronic alcoholism	
Diarrhea	
↓ Serum albumin (patient is usually asymptomatic due to normal ionized calcium level)	
Decreased Ionized Calcium	***Increased Ionized Calcium***
Alkalosis	Acidosis
Excess administration of citrated blood	
Clinical Manifestations	
Easy fatigability	Lethargy, weakness
Depression, anxiety, confusion	Depressed reflexes
Numbness and tingling in extremities and region around mouth	Decreased memory
Hyperreflexia, muscle cramps	Confusion, personality changes, psychosis
Chvostek's sign	Anorexia, nausea, vomiting
Trousseau's sign	Bone pain, fractures
Laryngeal spasm	Polyuria, dehydration
Tetany, seizures	Nephrolithiasis
	Stupor, coma
Electrocardiogram Changes	***Electrocardiogram Changes***
Elongation of ST segment	Shortened ST segment
Prolonged QT interval	Shortened QT interval
Ventricular tachycardia	Ventricular dysrhythmias
	Increased digitalis effect

protein, which stimulates calcium release from bones. Hypercalcemia is also associated with vitamin D overdose. Prolonged immobilization results in bone mineral loss and increased plasma calcium concentration. Hypercalcemia rarely occurs from increased calcium intake (e.g., ingestion of antacids containing calcium, excessive administration during cardiac arrest).

Excess calcium leads to reduced excitability of both muscles and nerves. Manifestations of hypercalcemia include decreased memory, confusion, disorientation, fatigue, muscle weakness, constipation, cardiac dysrhythmias, and renal calculi (see Table 17-8).

NURSING *and* COLLABORATIVE MANAGEMENT HYPERCALCEMIA

▪ *Nursing Diagnoses*

Nursing diagnoses and collaborative problems for the patient with hypercalcemia include, but are not limited to, the following:

- Risk for injury *related to* neuromuscular and sensorium changes
- Potential complication: dysrhythmias

▪ *Nursing Implementation*

The basic treatment of hypercalcemia is promotion of excretion of calcium in urine by administration of a loop diuretic (e.g., furosemide [Lasix]), and hydration of the patient with isotonic saline infusions. In hypercalcemia, the patient must drink 3000 to 4000 ml of fluid daily to promote the renal excretion of calcium and to decrease the possibility of kidney stone formation.

Synthetic calcitonin can also be administered to lower serum calcium levels. A diet low in calcium may be prescribed. Mobilization with weight-bearing activity is encouraged to enhance bone mineralization. Plicamycin (Mithracin), a cytotoxic antibiotic, inhibits bone resorption and thus lowers the serum calcium level. In hypercalcemia associated with malignancy, the drug of choice is pamidronate (Aredia), which inhibits the activity of osteoclasts (cells that break down bone and result in calcium release). Pamidronate is preferred over plicamycin because it does not have cytotoxic side effects and it inhibits bone resorption without inhibiting bone formation and mineralization.

HYPOCALCEMIA

Any condition that causes a decrease in the production of PTH may result in the development of hypocalcemia. This may occur with surgical removal of a portion of or injury to the parathyroid glands during thyroid or neck surgery. Acute pancreatitis is another potential cause of hypocalcemia. Lipolysis, a consequence of pancreatitis, produces fatty acids that combine with calcium ions, decreasing serum calcium levels.[13] The patient who receives multiple blood transfusions can become hypocalcemic because the citrate used to anticoagulate the blood binds with the calcium. Sudden alkalosis may also result in symptomatic hypocalcemia despite a normal total serum calcium level. The high pH increases calcium binding to protein, decreasing the amount of ionized calcium. Hypocalcemia can occur if the diet is low in calcium or if there is increased loss of calcium due to laxative abuse and malabsorption syndromes. (See Table 17-8 for the clinical manifestations and etiologies of hypocalcemia.)

Low calcium levels allow sodium to move into excitable cells, decreasing the threshold of action potentials with subsequent depolarization of the cells. This results in increased nerve excitability and sustained muscle contraction that is referred to as **tetany.** Clinical signs of tetany include Trousseau's sign and Chvostek's sign. *Trousseau's sign* refers to carpal spasms induced by inflating a blood pressure cuff on the arm (Fig. 17-15, *B* and *C*). The blood pressure cuff is inflated above the systolic pressure. Carpal spasms become evident within 3 minutes if hypocalcemia is present. *Chvostek's sign* is contraction of facial muscles in response to a tap over the facial nerve in front of the ear (see Fig. 17-15, *A*), and it also indicates hypocalcemia with latent tetany. Other manifestations of tetany are laryngeal stridor, dysphagia, and numbness and tingling around the mouth or in the extremities.

Cardiac effects of hypocalcemia include decreased cardiac contractility and ECG changes. A prolonged QT interval may develop into a ventricular tachycardia. Clinical manifestations of hypocalcemia are listed in Table 17-8.

NURSING *and* COLLABORATIVE MANAGEMENT HYPOCALCEMIA

■ *Nursing Diagnoses*

Nursing diagnoses and collaborative problems for the patient with hypocalcemia include, but are not limited to, the following:

- Risk for injury *related to* tetany and seizures
- Potential complications: fracture, respiratory arrest

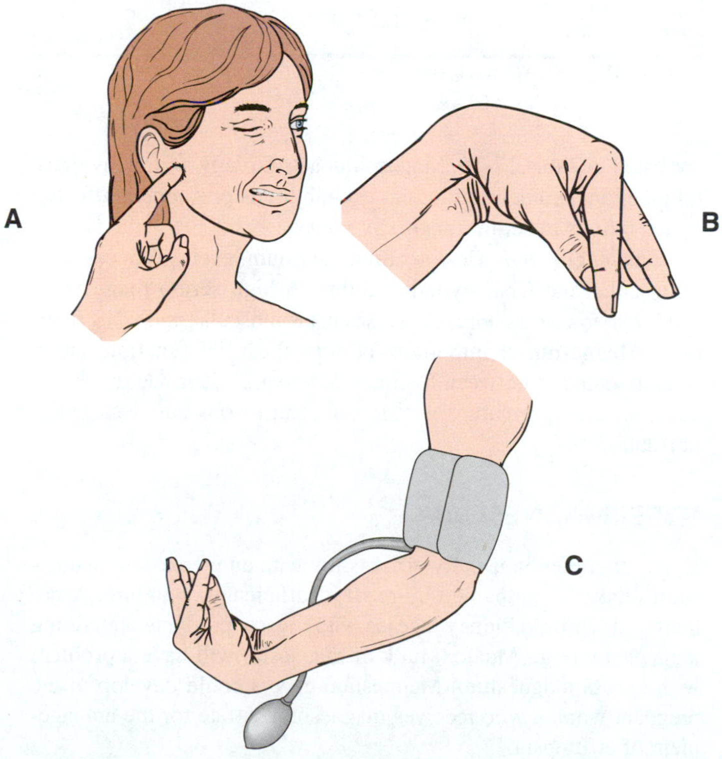

FIG. 17-15 Tests for hypocalcemia. **A,** Chvostek's sign is contraction of facial muscles in response to a light tap over the facial nerve in front of the ear. **B,** Trousseau's sign is a carpal spasm induced by **C,** inflating a blood pressure cuff above the systolic pressure for a few minutes.

■ *Nursing Implementation*

The primary goal in treatment of hypocalcemia is aimed at treating the cause. Hypocalcemia can be treated with oral or IV calcium supplements. Calcium is not given intramuscularly (IM) because it may cause severe local reactions, such as burning, necrosis, and tissue sloughing. Intravenous preparations of calcium, such as calcium gluconate, are administered when severe symptoms of hypocalcemia are impending or present. A diet high in calcium-rich foods is usually ordered along with vitamin D supplements for the patient with hypocalcemia. Oral calcium supplements, such as calcium carbonate, may be used when patients are unable to consume enough calcium in the diet, such as those who do not tolerate dairy products. Pain and anxiety must be adequately treated in the patient with suspected hypocalcemia because hyperventilation-induced respiratory alkalosis can precipitate hypocalcemic symptoms. Any patient who has had thyroid or neck surgery must be observed closely in the immediate postoperative period for manifestations of hypocalcemia because of the proximity of the surgery to the parathyroid glands.

PHOSPHATE IMBALANCES

Phosphorus is a primary anion in the ICF and is essential to the function of muscle, RBCs, and the nervous system. It is deposited with calcium for bone and tooth structure. It is also involved in the acid-base buffering system, the mitochondrial energy production of ATP, cellular uptake and use of glucose, and the metabolism of carbohydrates, proteins, and fats.

Maintenance of normal phosphate balance requires adequate renal functioning because the kidneys are the major route of phosphate excretion. A small amount is lost in the feces. A reciprocal relationship exists between phosphorus and calcium in that a high serum phosphate level tends to cause a low calcium concentration in the serum.

HYPERPHOSPHATEMIA

The major condition that can lead to hyperphosphatemia is acute or chronic renal failure that results in an altered ability of the kidneys to excrete phosphate. Other causes include chemotherapy for certain malignancies (lymphomas), excessive ingestion of milk or phosphate-containing laxatives, and large intakes of vitamin D that increase GI absorption of phosphorus (Table 17-9).

Clinical manifestations of hyperphosphatemia (Table 17-9) primarily relate to metastatic calcium-phosphate precipitates. Ordinarily, calcium and phosphate are deposited only in bone. However, an increased serum phosphate concentration along with calcium precipitates readily, and calcified deposits can occur in soft tissue such as joints, arteries, skin, kidneys, and corneas (see Chapter 47). Other manifestations of hyperphosphatemia are neuromuscular irritability and tetany, which are related to the low serum calcium levels often associated with high serum phosphate levels.

Management of hyperphosphatemia is aimed at identifying and treating the underlying cause. Ingestion of foods and fluids high in phosphorus (e.g., dairy products) should be restricted. Adequate hydration and correction of hypocalcemic conditions can enhance the renal excretion of phosphate through the action of PTH. As the serum calcium level increases, it causes the renal excretion of phosphorus. For the patient with renal failure, measures to reduce serum phosphate levels include calcium supplements, phosphate-binding agents or gels, and dietary phosphate restrictions (see Chapter 47).

TABLE 17-9 Phosphate Imbalances: Causes and Clinical Manifestations

	Hypophosphatemia (PO_4^{3-} <2.8 mg/dl [0.9 mmol/L])	Hyperphosphatemia (PO_4^{3-} >4.5 mg/dl [1.45 mmol/L])
Causes	Malabsorption syndrome Nutritional recovery syndrome (reversal or treatment of starvation) Glucose administration Parenteral nutrition Alcohol withdrawal Phosphate-binding antacids Recovery from diabetic ketoacidosis Respiratory alkalosis	Renal failure Chemotherapeutic agents Enemas containing phosphorus (e.g., Fleet Enema) Excessive ingestion (e.g., milk, phosphate-containing laxatives) Large vitamin D intake Hypoparathyroidism
Clinical Manifestations	Central nervous system dysfunction (confusion, coma) Muscle weakness, including respiratory muscle weakness and difficulty weaning from ventilator Renal tubular wasting of Mg^{2+}, Ca^{2+}, HCO_3^- Cardiac problems (dysrhythmias, decreased stroke volume) Osteomalacia Rhabdomyolysis	Hypocalcemia Muscle problems; tetany Deposition of calcium-phosphate precipitates in skin, soft tissue, corneas, viscera, blood vessels

HYPOPHOSPHATEMIA

Hypophosphatemia (low serum phosphate) is seen in the patient who is malnourished or has a malabsorption syndrome. Other causes include alcohol withdrawal and use of phosphate-binding antacids. Hypophosphatemia may also occur during parenteral nutrition with inadequate phosphorus replacement. Table 17-9 lists causes of phosphorus imbalances.

Most clinical manifestations of hypophosphatemia (see Table 17-9) relate to a deficiency of cellular ATP or 2,3-diphosphoglycerate (2,3-DPG), an enzyme in RBCs that facilitates oxygen delivery to the tissues. Because phosphorus is needed for formation of ATP and 2,3-DPG, its deficit results in impaired cellular energy and oxygen delivery. Mild to moderate hypophosphatemia is often asymptomatic. Severe hypophosphatemia may be fatal because of decreased cellular function. Acute symptoms include CNS depression, confusion, and other mental changes. Other manifestations include muscle weakness and pain, dysrhythmias, and cardiomyopathy.

Management of a mild phosphorus deficiency may involve oral supplementation (e.g., Neutra-Phos) and ingestion of foods high in phosphorus (e.g., dairy products). Severe hypophosphatemia can be serious and may require IV administration of sodium phosphate or potassium phosphate. Frequent monitoring of serum phosphate levels is necessary to guide IV therapy. Sudden symptomatic hypocalcemia, secondary to increased calcium phosphorus binding, is a potential complication of IV phosphorus administration.

MAGNESIUM IMBALANCES

Magnesium is the second most abundant intracellular cation. Approximately 50% to 60% of the body's magnesium is contained in bone. Magnesium functions as a coenzyme in the metabolism of carbohydrates and protein. It is also involved in metabolism of cellular nucleic acids and proteins. Magnesium is regulated by GI absorption and renal excretion.[3] The kidneys are able to conserve magnesium in times of need and excrete excesses. Factors that regulate calcium balance (e.g., PTH) appear to similarly influence magnesium balance. Manifestations of magnesium imbalance are often mistaken for calcium imbalances. Because magnesium balance is related to calcium and potassium balance, all three cations should be assessed together.[10] Causes of magnesium imbalances are listed in Table 17-10. Magnesium acts directly on the myoneural junction, and neuromuscular excitability is profoundly affected by alterations in serum magnesium levels.

TABLE 17-10 Causes of Magnesium Imbalances

Hypomagnesemia	Hypermagnesemia
Diarrhea Vomiting Chronic alcoholism Impaired GI absorption Malabsorption syndrome Prolonged malnutrition Large urine output NG suction Poorly controlled diabetes mellitus Hyperaldosteronism	Renal failure (especially if patient is given magnesium products) Excessive administration of magnesium for treatment of eclampsia Adrenal insufficiency

GI, Gastrointestinal; *NG*, nasogastric.

Hypomagnesemia (low serum magnesium level) produces neuromuscular and CNS hyperirritability. A high serum magnesium level *(hypermagnesemia)* depresses neuromuscular and CNS functions. Magnesium is important for normal cardiac function. There is an association between hypomagnesemia and cardiac dysrhythmias, such as premature ventricular contractions and ventricular fibrillation.

HYPERMAGNESEMIA

Hypermagnesemia usually occurs only with an increase in magnesium intake accompanied by renal insufficiency or failure. A patient with chronic kidney disease who ingests products containing magnesium (e.g., Maalox, milk of magnesia) will have a problem with excess magnesium. Magnesium excess could develop in the pregnant woman who receives magnesium sulfate for the management of eclampsia.

Initial clinical manifestations of a mildly elevated serum magnesium concentration include lethargy, drowsiness, and nausea and vomiting. As the levels of serum magnesium increase, deep tendon reflexes are lost, followed by somnolence, and then respiratory and, ultimately, cardiac arrest can occur.

Management of hypermagnesemia should focus on prevention. Persons with chronic kidney disease should not take magnesium-containing drugs and must be cautioned to review all over-the-counter drug labels for magnesium content. The emergency treatment of hypermagnesemia is IV administration of calcium chloride or calcium gluconate to physiologically oppose the effects of the magnesium on cardiac muscle. Promoting urinary excretion with fluid will decrease serum magnesium levels. The patient with impaired renal function will require dialysis because the kidneys are the major route of excretion for magnesium.

HYPOMAGNESEMIA

A major cause of magnesium deficiency is prolonged fasting or starvation. Chronic alcoholism commonly causes hypomagnesemia as a result of insufficient food intake. Fluid loss from the GI tract interferes with magnesium absorption. Another potential cause of hypomagnesemia is prolonged parenteral nutrition without magnesium supplementation. Many diuretics increase the risk of magnesium loss through renal excretion.[3] In addition, osmotic diuresis caused by high glucose levels in uncontrolled diabetes mellitus increases renal excretion of magnesium. The significant clinical manifestations include confusion, hyperactive deep tendon reflexes, tremors, and seizures. Magnesium deficiency also predisposes to cardiac dysrhythmias. Clinically, hypomagnesemia resembles hypocalcemia and may contribute to the development of hypocalcemia as a result of the decreased action of PTH. Hypomagnesemia may also be associated with hypokalemia that does not respond well to potassium replacement. This occurs because intracellular magnesium is critical to normal function of the sodium-potassium pump.

Mild magnesium deficiencies can be treated with oral supplements and increased dietary intake of foods high in magnesium (e.g., green vegetables, nuts, bananas, oranges, peanut butter, chocolate). If the condition is severe, parenteral IV or IM magnesium (e.g., magnesium sulfate) should be administered. Too rapid administration of magnesium can lead to cardiac or respiratory arrest.

ACID-BASE IMBALANCES

The body normally maintains a steady balance between acids produced during metabolism and bases that neutralize and promote the excretion of the acids. Many health problems may lead to acid-base imbalances in addition to fluid and electrolyte imbalances. Patients with diabetes mellitus, chronic obstructive pulmonary disease, and kidney disease frequently develop acid-base imbalances. Vomiting and diarrhea may cause loss of acids and bases in addition to fluids and electrolytes. The kidneys are an essential buffer system for acids, and in the older adult, the kidneys are less able to compensate for an acid load. The older adult also has decreased respiratory function, leading to impaired compensation for acid-base imbalances. In addition, tissue hypoxia from any cause may alter acid-base balance. The nurse must always consider the possibility of acid-base imbalance in patients with serious illnesses.

pH and Hydrogen Ion Concentration

The acidity or alkalinity of a solution depends on its hydrogen ion (H^+) concentration. An increase in H^+ concentration leads to acidity; a decrease leads to alkalinity. (Definitions of terminology related to acid-base balance are presented in Table 17-11.)

TABLE 17-11 Terminology Related to Acid-Base Physiology

Acid	Donor of hydrogen ion (H^+); separation of an acid into H^+ and its accompanying anion in solution
Acidemia	Signifying an arterial blood pH of less than 7.35
Acidosis	Process that adds acid or eliminates base from body fluids
Alkalemia	Signifying an arterial blood pH of more than 7.45
Alkalosis	Process that adds base or eliminates acid from body fluids
Anion gap	Reflection of normally unmeasured anions in the plasma; helpful in differential diagnosis of acidosis
Base	Acceptor of hydrogen ions; bicarbonate (HCO_3^-) most abundant base in body fluids; chemical combining of acid and base when hydrogen ions are added to a solution containing a base
Buffer	Substance that reacts with an acid or base to prevent a large change in pH
pH	Negative logarithm of the H^+ concentration

Despite the fact that acids are produced by the body daily, the H^+ concentration of body fluids is small (0.0004 mEq/L). This tiny amount is maintained within a narrow range to ensure optimal cellular function. Hydrogen ion concentration is usually expressed as a negative logarithm (symbolized as **pH**) rather than in milliequivalents. The use of the negative logarithm means that the lower the pH, the higher the H^+ concentration. In contrast to a pH of 7, a pH of 8 represents a 10-fold decrease in H^+ concentration.

The pH of a chemical solution may range from 1 to 14. A solution with a pH of 7 is considered neutral. An acid solution has a pH less than 7, and an alkaline solution has a pH greater than 7. Blood is slightly alkaline (pH 7.35 to 7.45); yet if it drops below 7.35, the person has **acidosis,** even though the blood may never become truly acidic. If the blood pH is greater than 7.45, the person has **alkalosis** (Fig. 17-16).

Acid-Base Regulation

The body's metabolic processes constantly produce acids. These acids must be neutralized and excreted to maintain acid-base balance. Normally the body has three mechanisms by which it regu-

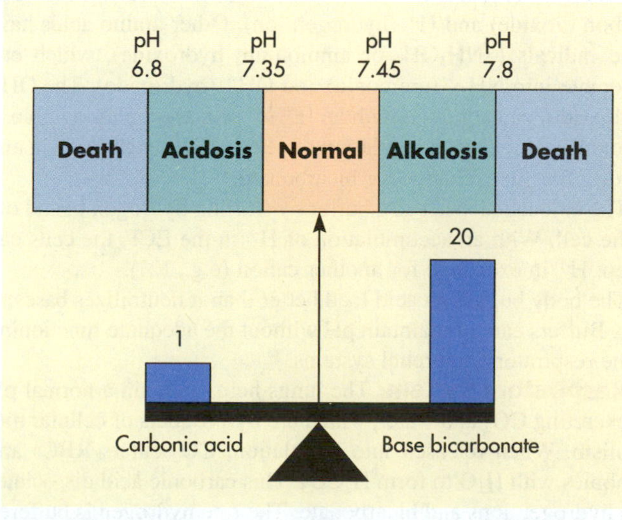

FIG. 17-16 The normal range of plasma pH is 7.35 to 7.45. A normal pH is maintained by a ratio of 1 part carbonic acid to 20 parts bicarbonate.

lates acid-base balance to maintain the arterial pH between 7.35 and 7.45. These mechanisms are the buffer systems, the respiratory system, and the renal system.

The regulatory mechanisms react at different speeds. Buffers react immediately; the respiratory system responds in minutes and reaches maximum effectiveness in hours; the renal response takes 2 to 3 days to respond maximally, but the kidneys can maintain balance indefinitely in chronic imbalances.

Buffer System. The buffer system is the fastest acting system and the primary regulator of acid-base balance. **Buffers** act chemically to change strong acids into weaker acids or to bind acids to neutralize their effect. The buffers in the body include carbonic acid–bicarbonate, monohydrogen-dihydrogen phosphate, intracellular and plasma protein, and hemoglobin buffers.

A buffer consists of a weakly ionized acid or a base and its salt. Buffers function to minimize the effect of acids on blood pH until they can be excreted from the body. The carbonic acid (H_2CO_3)–bicarbonate (HCO_3^-) buffer system neutralizes hydrochloric acid (HCl) in the following manner:

HCl	+	NaH_2CO_3	→	NaCl	+	H_2CO_3
strong acid		strong base		salt		weak acid

In this way, an acid is prevented from making a large change in the blood's pH, and more H_2CO_3 is formed. The carbonic acid, in turn, is broken down to H_2O and CO_2. The CO_2 is excreted by the lungs, either combined with insensible H_2O as carbonic acid, or alone as CO_2. In this process the buffer system maintains the 20:1 ratio between bicarbonate and carbonic acid and the normal pH.

The phosphate buffer system is composed of sodium and other cations in combination with monohydrogen phosphate (HPO_4^{2-}) or dihydrogen phosphate ($H_2PO_4^-$). This intracellular buffer system acts in the same manner as the bicarbonate system. Strong acids are neutralized to form sodium chloride (NaCl) and sodium biphosphate (NaH_2PO_4), a weak acid that can be excreted in the urine. When a strong base such as sodium hydroxide (NaOH) is added to the system, it can be neutralized by sodium dihydrogen phosphate (NaH_2PO_4) to a weak base (Na_2HPO_4) and H_2O.

Intracellular and extracellular proteins are an effective buffering system throughout the body. The protein buffering system acts like the bicarbonate system. Some of the amino acids of proteins contain free acid radicals (–COOH), which can dissociate into CO_2 (carbon dioxide) and H^+ (hydrogen ion). Other amino acids have basic radicals (–NH_3OH, or ammonium hydroxide), which can dissociate into NH_3^+ (ammonia) and OH^- (hydroxide). The OH^- (hydroxide) can combine with an H^+ to form H_2O. Hemoglobin is a protein that assists in regulation of pH by shifting chloride in and out of RBCs in exchange for bicarbonate.

The cell can also act as a buffer by shifting hydrogen in and out of the cell. With an accumulation of H^+ in the ECF, the cells can accept H^+ in exchange for another cation (e.g., K^+).

The body buffers an acid load better than it neutralizes base excess. Buffers cannot maintain pH without the adequate functioning of the respiratory and renal systems.

Respiratory System. The lungs help maintain a normal pH by excreting CO_2 and water, which are by-products of cellular metabolism. When released into circulation, CO_2 enters RBCs and combines with H_2O to form H_2CO_3. This carbonic acid dissociates into hydrogen ions and bicarbonate. The free hydrogen is buffered by hemoglobin molecules, and the bicarbonate diffuses into the plasma. In the pulmonary capillaries, this process is reversed, and CO_2 is formed and excreted by the lungs. The overall reversible reaction is expressed as the following:

$$CO_2 + H_2O \rightleftarrows H_2CO_3 \rightleftarrows H^+ + HCO_3^-$$

The amount of CO_2 in the blood directly relates to carbonic acid concentration and subsequently to H^+ concentration. With increased respirations, more CO_2 is expelled and less remains in the blood. This leads to less carbonic acid and less H^+. With decreased respirations, more CO_2 remains in the blood. This leads to increased carbonic acid and more H^+.

The rate of excretion of CO_2 is controlled by the respiratory center in the medulla in the brainstem. If increased amounts of CO_2 or H^+ are present, the respiratory center stimulates an increased rate and depth of breathing. Respirations are inhibited if the center senses low H^+ or CO_2 levels.

As a compensatory mechanism, the respiratory system acts on the $CO_2 + H_2O$ side of the reaction by altering the rate and depth of breathing to "blow off" (through hyperventilation) or "retain" (through hypoventilation) CO_2. If a respiratory problem is the cause of an acid-base imbalance (e.g., respiratory failure), the respiratory system loses its ability to correct a pH alteration.

Renal System. Under normal conditions, the kidneys reabsorb and conserve all of the bicarbonate they filter. The kidneys can generate additional bicarbonate and eliminate excess H^+ as compensation for acidosis. The three mechanisms of acid elimination are (1) secretion of small amounts of free hydrogen into the renal tubule, (2) combination of H^+ with ammonia (NH_3) to form ammonium (NH_4^+), and (3) excretion of weak acids.

The body depends on the kidneys to excrete a portion of the acid produced by cellular metabolism. Thus the kidneys normally excrete acidic urine (average pH equals 6). As a compensatory mechanism, the pH of the urine can decrease to 4 and increase to 8. If the renal system is the cause of an acid-base imbalance (e.g., renal failure), it loses its ability to correct a pH alteration.

Alterations in Acid-Base Balance

An acid-base imbalance is produced when the ratio of 1:20 between acid and base content is altered (Table 17-12). A primary disease or process may alter one side of the ratio (e.g., CO_2 retention in pulmonary disease). The compensatory process attempts to maintain the other side of the ratio (e.g., increased renal bicarbonate reabsorption). When the compensatory mechanism fails, an acid-base imbalance results. The compensatory process may be inadequate because either the pathophysiologic process is overwhelming or there is insufficient time for the compensatory process to function.

Acid-base imbalances are classified as respiratory or metabolic. *Respiratory imbalances* affect carbonic acid concentrations; *metabolic imbalances* affect the base bicarbonate. Therefore acidosis can be caused by an increase in carbonic acid (respiratory acidosis) or a decrease in bicarbonate (metabolic acidosis). Alkalosis can be caused by a decrease in carbonic acid (respiratory alkalosis) or an increase in bicarbonate (metabolic alkalosis). Imbalances may be further classified as acute or chronic. Chronic imbalances allow greater time for compensatory changes.

Respiratory Acidosis. *Respiratory acidosis* (carbonic acid excess) occurs whenever there is hypoventilation (see Table 17-12). Hypoventilation results in a buildup of CO_2; subsequently, carbonic acid accumulates in the blood. Carbonic acid dissociates, liberating H^+, and there is a decrease in pH. If CO_2 is not eliminated from the blood, acidosis results from the accumulation of carbonic acid (Fig. 17-17, *A*).

To compensate, the kidneys conserve bicarbonate and secrete increased concentrations of hydrogen ion into the urine. In acute respiratory acidosis, the renal compensatory mechanisms begin to operate within 24 hours. Until the renal mechanisms have an effect, the serum bicarbonate level will usually be normal.

Respiratory Alkalosis. *Respiratory alkalosis* (carbonic acid deficit) occurs with hyperventilation (see Table 17-12). The primary cause of respiratory alkalosis is hypoxemia from acute pulmonary disorders. Anxiety, CNS disorders, and mechanical overventilation also increase ventilation rate and decrease the partial pressure of arterial carbon dioxide ($PaCO_2$) level. This leads to decreased carbonic acid and alkalosis (see Fig. 17-17, *A*).

Compensated respiratory alkalosis is rare. In acute respiratory alkalosis, aggressive treatment of the causes of hypoxemia is essential and usually does not allow time for compensation to occur. However, buffering of acute respiratory alkalosis may occur with shifting of bicarbonate (HCO_3^-) into cells in exchange for Cl^-. In chronic respiratory alkalosis that occurs with pulmonary fibrosis or CNS disorders, compensation may include renal excretion of bicarbonate.

Metabolic Acidosis. *Metabolic acidosis* (base bicarbonate deficit) occurs when an acid other than carbonic acid accumulates in the body or when bicarbonate is lost from body fluids (see Table 17-12 and Fig. 17-17, *B*). In both cases a bicarbonate deficit results. Ketoacid accumulation in diabetic ketoacidosis and lactic acid accumulation with shock are examples of accumulation of acids. Severe diarrhea results in loss of bicarbonate. In renal disease, the kidneys lose their ability to reabsorb bicarbonate and secrete hydrogen ions.

The compensatory response to metabolic acidosis is to increase CO_2 excretion by the lungs. The patient often develops *Kussmaul respiration* (deep, rapid breathing). In addition, the kidneys attempt to excrete additional acid.

Metabolic Alkalosis. *Metabolic alkalosis* (base bicarbonate excess) occurs when a loss of acid (prolonged vomiting or gastric suction) or a gain in bicarbonate (ingestion of baking soda) occurs (see Table 17-12 and Fig. 17-17, *B*). The compensatory mechanism is a decreased respiratory rate to increase plasma CO_2. Renal excretion of bicarbonate also occurs in response to metabolic alkalosis.

Mixed Acid-Base Disorders. A mixed acid-base disorder occurs when two or more disorders are present at the same time. The pH will depend on the type, severity, and acuity of each of the disorders involved and any compensation mechanisms at work. Respiratory acidosis combined with metabolic alkalosis (e.g., a patient with chronic obstructive lung disease also treated with a thiazide diuretic) may result in a near-normal pH, while respiratory acidosis combined with metabolic acidosis will cause a greater decrease in pH than either disorder alone. An example of a mixed acidosis appears in a patient in cardiopulmonary arrest. Hypoven-

TABLE 17-12 Acid-Base Imbalances

Common Causes	Pathophysiology	Laboratory Findings
Respiratory Acidosis		
Chronic obstructive pulmonary disease Barbiturate or sedative overdose Chest wall abnormality (e.g., obesity) Severe pneumonia Atelectasis Respiratory muscle weakness (e.g., Guillain-Barré syndrome) Mechanical hypoventilation	CO_2 retention from hypoventilation Compensatory response to HCO_3^- retention by kidney	Plasma pH ↓ $PaCO_2$ ↑ HCO_3^- normal (uncompensated) HCO_3^- ↑ (compensated) Urine pH <6 (compensated)
Respiratory Alkalosis		
Hyperventilation (caused by hypoxia, pulmonary emboli, anxiety, fear, pain, exercise, fever) Stimulated respiratory center caused by septicemia, encephalitis, brain injury, salicylate poisoning Mechanical hyperventilation	Increased CO_2 excretion from hyperventilation Compensatory response of HCO_3^- excretion by kidney	Plasma pH ↑ $PaCO_2$ ↓ HCO_3^- normal (uncompensated) HCO_3^- ↓ (compensated) Urine pH >6 (compensated)
Metabolic Acidosis		
Diabetic ketoacidosis Lactic acidosis Starvation Severe diarrhea Renal tubular acidosis Renal failure Gastrointestinal fistulas Shock	Gain of fixed acid, inability to excrete acid or loss of base Compensatory response of CO_2 excretion by lungs	Plasma pH ↓ $PaCO_2$ normal (uncompensated) $PaCO_2$ ↓ (compensated) HCO_3^- ↓ Urine pH <6 (compensated)
Metabolic Alkalosis		
Severe vomiting Excess gastric suctioning Diuretic therapy Potassium deficit Excess $NaHCO_3$ intake Excessive mineralocorticoids	Loss of strong acid or gain of base Compensatory response of CO_2 retention by lungs	Plasma pH ↑ $PaCO_2$ normal (uncompensated) $PaCO_2$ ↑ (compensated) HCO_3^- ↑ Urine pH >6 (compensated)

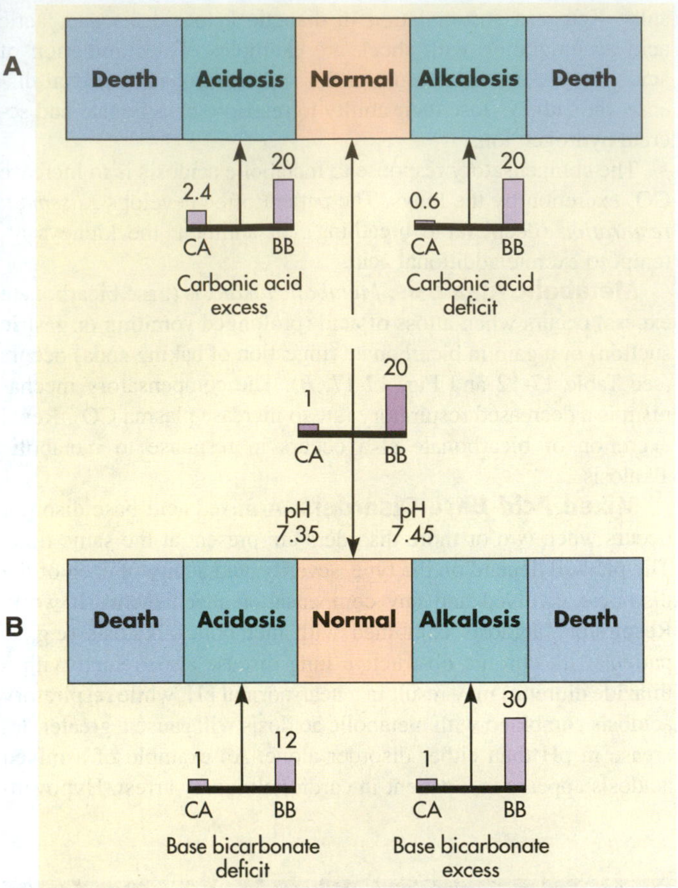

FIG. 17-17 Kinds of acid-base imbalances. **A,** Respiratory imbalances caused by carbonic acid *(CA)* excess and carbonic acid deficit. **B,** Metabolic imbalances caused by base bicarbonate *(BB)* deficit and base bicarbonate excess.

TABLE 17-13 Clinical Manifestations of Acidosis

Respiratory (↑ $PaCO_2$)	Metabolic (↓ HCO_3^-)
Neurologic	
Drowsiness	Drowsiness
Disorientation	Confusion
Dizziness	Headache
Headache	Coma
Coma	
Cardiovascular	
↓ Blood pressure	↓ Blood pressure
Ventricular fibrillation (related to hyperkalemia from compensation)	Dysrhythmias (related to hyperkalemia from compensation)
Warm, flushed skin (related to peripheral vasodilation)	Warm, flushed skin (related to peripheral vasodilation)
Gastrointestinal	
No significant findings	Nausea, vomiting, diarrhea, abdominal pain
Neuromuscular	
Seizures	No significant findings
Respiratory	
Hypoventilation with hypoxia (lungs are unable to compensate when there is a respiratory problem)	Deep, rapid respirations (compensatory action by the lungs)

tilation elevates the CO_2 level, and anaerobic metabolism due to decreased perfusion produces lactic acid accumulation. An example of a mixed alkalosis is the case of a patient who is hyperventilating because of postoperative pain and is also losing acid secondary to nasogastric suctioning.

Clinical Manifestations

Clinical manifestations of acidosis and alkalosis are summarized in Tables 17-13 and 17-14. Because a normal pH is vital to all cellular reactions, the clinical manifestations of acid-base imbalances are generalized and nonspecific. The compensatory mechanisms also produce some clinical manifestations. For example, the deep, rapid respirations of a patient with metabolic acidosis are an example of respiratory compensation. In alkalosis, hypocalcemia occurs due to increased calcium binding with albumin, lowering the amount of ionized, biologically active calcium. The hypocalcemia accounts for many of the clinical manifestations of alkalosis.

Blood Gas Values. Arterial blood gas (ABG) values provide valuable information about a patient's acid-base status, the underlying cause of the imbalance, the body's ability to regulate pH, and the patient's overall oxygen status.[14] Diagnosis of acid-base disturbances and identification of compensatory processes are done by performing the following six steps:

1. Determine whether the pH is acidotic or alkalotic. Use 7.4 as the starting point. Label values less than 7.4 as acidotic and values greater than 7.4 as alkalotic.
2. Analyze the $PaCO_2$ to determine if the patient has respiratory acidosis or alkalosis. $PaCO_2$ is controlled by the lungs and is thus considered the respiratory component of the

TABLE 17-14 Clinical Manifestations of Alkalosis

Respiratory (↓ $PaCO_2$)	Metabolic (↑ HCO_3^-)
Neurologic	
Lethargy	Dizziness
Light-headedness	Irritability
Confusion	Nervousness, confusion
Cardiovascular	
Tachycardia	Tachycardia
Dysrhythmias (related to hypokalemia from compensation)	Dysrhythmias (related to hypokalemia from compensation)
Gastrointestinal	
Nausea	Nausea
Vomiting	Vomiting
Epigastric pain	Anorexia
Neuromuscular*	
Tetany	Tetany
Numbness	Tremors
Tingling of extremities	Tingling of fingers and toes
Hyperreflexia	Muscle cramps, hypertonic muscles
Seizures	Seizures
Respiratory	
Hyperventilation (lungs are unable to compensate when there is a respiratory problem)	Hypoventilation (compensatory action by the lungs)

*Alkalosis increases calcium binding to protein, leading to decreased ionized calcium.

ABG. Because CO_2 forms carbonic acid when dissolved in blood, high CO_2 levels indicate acidosis and low CO_2 levels indicate alkalosis.

3. Analyze the HCO_3^- to determine if the patient has metabolic acidosis or alkalosis. HCO_3^-, the metabolic component of the ABG, is controlled primarily by the kidneys. Because HCO_3^- is a base, high levels of HCO_3^- result in alkalosis and low levels result in acidosis.
4. At this point, if the CO_2 and the HCO_3^- are within normal limits, the ABGs are normal if the pH is between 7.35 and 7.45.
5. Determine if the CO_2 or the HCO_3^- matches the acid or base alteration of the pH. For example, if the pH is acidotic and the CO_2 is high (respiratory acidosis), but the HCO_3^- is high (metabolic alkalosis), the CO_2 is the parameter that matches the pH alteration. The patient's acid-base imbalance would be diagnosed as respiratory acidosis.
6. Decide if the body is attempting to compensate for the pH change. If the parameter that does not match the pH is moving in the opposite direction, the body is attempting to compensate. In the example in step 5, the HCO_3^- level is alkalotic; this is in the opposite direction of respiratory acidosis and considered compensation. If compensatory mechanisms are functioning, the pH will return toward 7.40. When the pH is back to normal, the patient has *full compensation.* The body will not overcompensate for pH changes.

Table 17-15 lists normal blood gas values and Table 17-16 provides a sample ABG with interpretation. (Refer to the laboratory findings section of Table 17-12 for the ABG findings of the four major acid-base disturbances.) Knowledge of the patient's clinical situation and the physiologic extent of renal and respiratory compensation enables the nurse to identify mixed acid-base disorders as well as the patient's ability to compensate.

Blood gas analysis will also show the partial pressure of arterial oxygen (PaO_2) and oxygen saturation. These values are used to identify hypoxemia. The values of blood gases differ slightly between arterial and venous samples (see Table 17-15). (Blood gases are discussed further in Chapter 26.)

TABLE 17-15 Normal Arterial and Venous Blood Gas Values

Parameter	Arterial	Venous
pH	7.35-7.45	7.35-7.45
$PaCO_2$	35-45 mm Hg	40-45 mm Hg
Bicarbonate (HCO_3^-)	22-26 mEq/L (mmol/L)	22-26 mEq/L (mmol/L)
PaO_2*	80-100 mm Hg	40-50 mm Hg
Oxygen saturation	96%-100%	60%-85%
Base excess	±2.0 mEq/L	±2.0 mEq/L

*Decreases above sea level and with increasing age.

TABLE 17-16 Arterial Blood Gas (ABG) Analysis

ABG Values	Analysis
pH 7.30	1. pH <7.4 indicates acidosis.
$PaCO_2$ 25 mm Hg	2. $PaCO_2$ is low, indicating respiratory alkalosis.
HCO_3^- 16 mEq/L	3. HCO_3^- is low, indicating metabolic acidosis.
	4. Metabolic acidosis matches the pH.
	5. The CO_2 does not match, but is moving in the opposite direction, which indicates the lungs are attempting to compensate for the metabolic acidosis.

Interpretation

This ABG is interpreted as metabolic acidosis with partial compensation. If the pH returns to the normal range, the patient is said to have full compensation.

ASSESSMENT OF FLUID, ELECTROLYTE, AND ACID-BASE IMBALANCES

Clinical manifestations for specific fluid, electrolyte, and acid-base imbalances have been presented earlier in this chapter. In addition to assessing for those clinical manifestations, subjective and objective data that should be obtained from any patient with suspected fluid, electrolyte, or acid-base imbalances are outlined below.

Subjective Data

Important Health Information

Past Health History. The patient should be questioned about any past history of problems involving the kidneys, heart, GI system, or lungs that could affect the present fluid, electrolyte, and acid-base balance. Information about specific diseases such as diabetes mellitus, diabetes insipidus, chronic obstructive pulmonary disease, renal failure, ulcerative colitis, and Crohn's disease should be obtained from the patient. The patient should also be questioned about the incidence of prior fluid, electrolyte, or acid-base disorders.

Medications. An assessment of the patient's current and past use of medications is important. The ingredients in many drugs, especially over-the-counter drugs, are often overlooked as sources of sodium, potassium, calcium, magnesium, and other electrolytes. Many prescription drugs, including diuretics, corticosteroids, and electrolyte supplements, can cause fluid and electrolyte imbalances.

Surgery or Other Treatments. The patient should be asked about past or present renal dialysis, kidney surgery, or bowel surgery resulting in a temporary or permanent external collecting system such as a colostomy or nephrostomy.

Functional Health Patterns

Health Perception–Health Management Pattern. If the patient is currently experiencing a problem related to fluid, electrolyte, and acid-base balance, a careful description of the illness, including onset, course, and treatment, should be obtained. The patient should be questioned about any recent changes in body weight.

Nutritional-Metabolic Pattern. The patient should be questioned regarding diet, and any special dietary practices should be noted. Weight reduction diets, fad diets, or any eating disorders, such as anorexia or bulimia, can lead to fluid and electrolyte problems. If the patient is on a special diet, such as low sodium or high potassium, the ability to comply with the dietary prescription should be assessed.

Elimination Pattern. Note should be made of the patient's usual bowel and bladder habits. Any deviations from the expected elimination pattern, such as diarrhea, oliguria, nocturia, polyuria, or incontinence, should be carefully documented.

Activity-Exercise Pattern. The patient's exercise pattern is important to determine because excessive perspiration secondary to exercise could result in a fluid and electrolyte problem. Also, the patient's exposure to extremely high temperatures as a result of leisure or work activity should be determined. The patient should be asked what practices are followed to replace fluid and electrolytes lost through excessive perspiration. An assessment of the patient's activity level should be done to determine any functional problems that could lead to lack of ability to obtain food or fluids.

Cognitive-Perceptual Pattern. The patient should be asked about any changes in sensations, such as numbness, tingling, *fasciculations* (uncoordinated twitching of a single muscle group), or muscle weakness, that could indicate a fluid and electrolyte problem. Additionally, both the patient and the family should be asked if any changes in mentation or alertness have been noted, such as confusion, memory impairment, or lethargy.

Objective Data

Physical Examination. There is no specific physical examination to assess fluid, electrolyte, and acid-base balance. Common abnormal assessment findings of major body systems offer clues to possible imbalances (Table 17-17).

Laboratory Values. Assessment of serum electrolyte values is a good starting point for identifying fluid and electrolyte imbalance (see Table 17-3). However, serum electrolyte values often provide only limited information. They reflect the concentration of that electrolyte in the ECF but do not necessarily provide information concerning the concentration of the electrolyte in the ICF. For example, the majority of the potassium in the body is found intracellularly. Changes in serum potassium values may be the result of a true deficit or excess of potassium or may reflect the movement of potassium into or out of the cell during acid-base imbalances.

An abnormal serum sodium level may reflect a sodium problem or, more likely, a water problem. A reduced hematocrit value could indicate anemia, or it could be caused by fluid volume excess.

Other laboratory tests that are helpful in evaluating the presence of or risk for fluid, electrolyte, and acid-base imbalances include serum and urine osmolality, serum glucose, BUN, serum creatinine, urine specific gravity, and urine electrolytes.

In addition to arterial and venous blood gases, serum electrolytes can provide important information concerning a patient's acid-base balance. Changes in the serum bicarbonate (often reported as total CO_2 or CO_2 content on an electrolyte panel) will indicate the presence of metabolic acidosis (low bicarbonate level) or alkalosis (high bicarbonate level). Calculation of the *anion gap* (serum sodium level minus the sum of the chloride and bicarbonate levels) can help to determine the source of metabolic acidosis. The anion gap is increased in metabolic acidosis associated with acid gain (e.g., lactic acidosis, diabetic ketoacidosis) but remains normal (10 to 14 mmol/L) in metabolic acidosis caused by bicarbonate loss (e.g., diarrhea).

ORAL FLUID AND ELECTROLYTE REPLACEMENT

In all cases of fluid, electrolyte, and acid-base imbalances, the treatment is directed toward correction of the underlying cause. The specific diseases or disorders that cause these imbalances are discussed in various chapters throughout this text. Mild fluid and electrolyte deficits can be corrected using oral rehydration solutions containing water, electrolytes, and glucose. Glucose not only provides calories but also promotes sodium absorption in the small intestine. Commercial oral rehydration solutions are now available for home use.

TABLE 17-17 COMMON ASSESSMENT ABNORMALITIES Fluid and Electrolyte Imbalances

Finding	Possible Cause
Skin	
Poor skin turgor	Fluid volume deficit
Cold, clammy skin	Na^+ deficit, shift of plasma to interstitial fluid
Pitting edema	Fluid volume excess
Flushed, dry skin	Na^+ excess
Pulse	
Bounding pulse	Fluid volume excess, shift of interstitial fluid to plasma
Rapid, weak, thready pulse	Shift of plasma to interstitial fluid, Na^+ deficit, fluid volume deficit
Weak, irregular, rapid pulse	Severe K^+ deficit
Weak, irregular, slow pulse	Severe K^+ excess
Blood Pressure	
Hypotension	Fluid volume deficit, shift of plasma to interstitial fluid, Na^+ deficit
Hypertension	Fluid volume excess, shift of interstitial fluid to plasma
Respirations	
Deep, rapid breathing	Compensation for metabolic acidosis
Shallow, slow, irregular breathing	Compensation for metabolic alkalosis
Shortness of breath	Fluid volume excess
Moist crackles	Fluid volume excess, shift of interstitial fluid to plasma
Restricted airway	Ca^{2+} deficit
Skeletal Muscles	
Cramping of exercised muscle	Ca^{2+} deficit, Mg^+ deficit, alkalosis
Carpal spasm (Trousseau's sign)	Ca^{2+} deficit, Mg^+ deficit, alkalosis
Flabby muscles	K^+ deficit
Positive Chvostek's sign	Ca^{2+} deficit, Mg^+ deficit, alkalosis
Behavior or Mental State	
Picking at bedclothes	K^+ deficit, Mg^+ deficit
Indifference	Fluid volume deficit, Na^+ deficit
Apprehension	Shift of plasma to interstitial fluid
Extreme restlessness	K^+ excess, Na^+ excess, fluid volume deficit
Confusion and irritability	K^+ deficit, fluid volume excess, Ca^{2+} excess, Mg^+ excess, H_2O excess, Na^+ deficit
Decreased level of consciousness	Na^+ deficit, H_2O excess

INTRAVENOUS FLUID AND ELECTROLYTE REPLACEMENT

Intravenous fluid and electrolyte therapy are commonly used to treat many different fluid and electrolyte imbalances. Many patients need maintenance IV fluid therapy only while they cannot take oral fluids (e.g., during and after surgery). Other patients need corrective or replacement therapy for losses that have already oc-

TABLE 17-18 Composition and Use of Commonly Prescribed Crystalloid Solutions

Solution	Tonicity	mOsm/kg	Glucose (g/L)	Indications and Considerations
Dextrose in Water				
5%	Isotonic, but physiologically hypotonic	278	50	• Provides free water necessary for renal excretion of solutes • Used to replace water losses and treat hypernatremia • Provides 170 calories/L • Does not provide any electrolytes
10%	Hypertonic	556	100	• Provides free water only, no electrolytes • Provides 340 calories/L
Saline				
0.45%	Hypotonic	154	0	• Provides free water in addition to Na^+ and Cl^- • Used to replace hypotonic fluid losses • Used as maintenance solution, although it does not replace daily losses of other electrolytes • Provides no calories
0.9%	Isotonic	308	0	• Used to expand intravascular volume and replace extracellular fluid losses • Only solution that may be administered with blood products • Contains Na^+ and Cl^- in excess of plasma levels • Does not provide free water, calories, other electrolytes • May cause intravascular overload or hyperchloremic acidosis
3.0%	Hypertonic	1026	0	• Used to treat symptomatic hyponatremia • Must be administered slowly and with extreme caution because it may cause dangerous intravascular volume overload and pulmonary edema
Dextrose in Saline				
5% in 0.225%	Isotonic	355	50	• Provides Na^+, Cl^-, and free water • Used to replace hypotonic losses and treat hypernatremia • Provides 170 calories/L
5% in 0.45%	Hypertonic	432	50	• Same as 0.45% NaCl except provides 170 calories/L
5% in 0.9%	Hypertonic	586	50	• Same as 0.9% NaCl except provides 170 calories/L
Multiple Electrolyte Solutions				
Ringer's solution	Isotonic	309	0	• Similar in composition to plasma except that it has excess Cl^-, no Mg^{2+}, and no HCO_3^- • Does not provide free water or calories • Used to expand the intravascular volume and replace extracellular fluid losses
Lactated Ringer's (Hartmann's) solution	Isotonic	274	0	• Similar in composition to normal plasma except does not contain Mg^{2+} • Used to treat losses from burns and lower GI • May be used to treat mild metabolic acidosis but should not be used to treat lactic acidosis • Does not provide free water or calories

Modified from Heitz UE, Horne MM: *Pocket guide to fluid, electrolyte, and acid-base balance,* ed 5, St Louis, 2005, Mosby.

curred. The amount and type of solution are determined by the normal daily maintenance requirements and by imbalances identified by laboratory results. Table 17-18 provides a list of commonly prescribed IV solutions.

Solutions

Hypotonic. A hypotonic solution provides more water than electrolytes, diluting the ECF. Osmosis then produces a movement of water from the ECF to the ICF. After osmotic equilibrium has been achieved, the ICF and the ECF have the same osmolality, and both compartments have been expanded. Examples of hypotonic fluids are given in Table 17-18. Maintenance fluids are usually hypotonic solutions (e.g., 0.45% NaCl) because normal daily losses are hypotonic. Additional electrolytes (e.g., KCl) may be added to maintain normal levels. Hypotonic solutions have the potential to cause cellular swelling, and patients should be monitored for changes in mentation that may indicate cerebral edema.[4,15]

Although 5% dextrose in water is considered an isotonic solution, the dextrose is quickly metabolized, and the net result is the administration of free water (hypotonic) with proportionately equal expansion of the ECF and ICF. One liter of a 5% dextrose solution provides 50 g of dextrose, or 170 calories. Although this amount of dextrose is not enough to meet caloric requirements, it helps prevent ketosis associated with starvation. Pure water cannot be administered IV because it would cause hemolysis of RBCs.

Isotonic. Administration of an isotonic solution expands only the ECF. There is no net loss or gain from the ICF. An isotonic solution is the ideal fluid replacement for a patient with an ECF volume deficit. Examples of isotonic solutions include lactated Ringer's solution and 0.9% NaCl. Lactated Ringer's solution contains sodium, potassium, chloride, calcium, and lactate (the precursor of bicarbonate) in about the same concentrations as those of the ECF. It is contraindicated in the presence of lactic acidosis because of the body's decreased ability to convert lactate to bicarbonate.

Isotonic saline (0.9% NaCl) has a sodium concentration (154 mEq/L) somewhat higher than plasma (135 to 145 mEq/L) and a chloride concentration (154 mEq/L) significantly higher than the plasma chloride level (96 to 106 mEq/L). Thus excessive administration of isotonic NaCl can result in elevated sodium and chloride levels. Isotonic saline may be used when a patient has experienced both fluid and sodium losses or as vascular fluid replacement in hypovolemic shock.

Hypertonic. A hypertonic solution initially raises the osmolality of ECF and expands it. It is useful in the treatment of hypovolemia and hyponatremia. Examples are listed in Table 17-18. In addition, the higher osmotic pressure draws water out of the cells into the ECF. Hypertonic solutions (e.g., 3% NaCl) require frequent monitoring of blood pressure, lung sounds, and serum sodium levels and should be used with caution because of the risk for intravascular fluid volume excess.[15]

Although concentrated dextrose and water solutions (10% dextrose or greater) are hypertonic solutions, once the dextrose is metabolized, the net result is the administration of water. The free water provided by these solutions will ultimately expand both the ECF and ICF. The primary use of these solutions is in the provision of calories. Concentrated dextrose solutions may be combined with amino acid solutions, electrolytes, vitamins, and trace elements to provide parenteral nutrition (see Chapter 40). Solutions containing 10% dextrose or less may be administered through a peripheral IV line. Solutions with concentrations greater than 10% must be administered through a central line so that there is adequate dilution to prevent shrinkage of RBCs.

Intravenous Additives. In addition to the basic solutions that provide water and a minimum amount of calories and electrolytes, there are additives to replace specific losses. These additives were mentioned previously during the discussion of the particular electrolyte deficiencies. KCl, CaCl, $MgSO_4$, and HCO_3^- are common additives to the basic IV solutions.

Plasma Expanders. Plasma expanders stay in the vascular space and increase the osmotic pressure. Plasma expanders include colloids, dextran, and hetastarch. Colloids are protein solutions such as plasma, albumin, and commercial plasmas (e.g., Plasmanate). Albumin is available in 5% and 25% solutions. The 5% solution has an albumin concentration similar to plasma and will expand the intravascular fluid milliliter for milliliter. In contrast, the 25% albumin solution is hypertonic and will draw additional fluid from the interstitium. Dextran is a complex synthetic sugar. Because dextran is metabolized slowly, it remains in the vascular system for a prolonged period but not as long as the colloids. It pulls additional fluid into the intravascular space. Hetastarch (Hespan) is a synthetic colloid that works similarly to dextran to expand plasma volume. (Indications for plasma volume expanders are discussed in Chapter 67.)

If the patient has lost blood, whole blood or packed RBCs are necessary. Packed RBCs have the advantage of giving the patient primarily RBCs; the blood bank can use the plasma for blood components. Whole blood, with its additional fluid volume, may cause circulatory overload. Although packed RBCs have a decreased plasma volume, they will increase the oncotic pressure and pull fluid into the intravascular space. Loop diuretics may be administered with blood to prevent symptoms of fluid volume excess in anemic patients who are not volume depleted. (Administration of blood and blood products is discussed in Chapter 31.)

CRITICAL THINKING EXERCISE

CASE STUDY

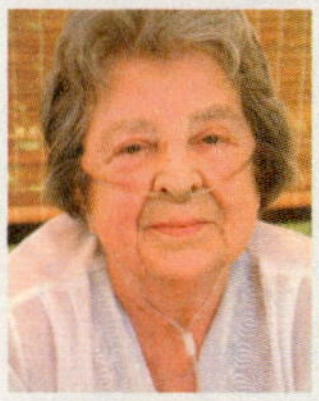

Case Study photo ©iStockphoto.com/ Jessica Jones Photography.

Fluid and Electrolyte Imbalance

Patient Profile. Sarah Smith, a 73-year-old white female with lung cancer, has been receiving chemotherapy on an outpatient basis. She completed her third treatment 5 days ago and has been experiencing nausea and vomiting for 2 days even though she has been using ondansetron (Zofran) orally as directed. Ms. Smith's daughter brings her to the hospital, where she is admitted to the medical unit. The admitting nurse performs a thorough assessment.

Subjective Data

- Complains of lethargy, weakness, dizziness, and a dry mouth
- States she has been too nauseated to eat or drink anything for 2 days

Objective Data

- Heart rate 110 beats/min, pulse thready
- Blood pressure 100/65
- Weight loss of 5 pounds since she received her chemotherapy treatment 5 days ago
- Dry oral mucous membranes

Critical Thinking Questions

1. Based on her clinical manifestations, what fluid imbalance does Ms. Smith have?
2. What additional assessment data should the nurse obtain?
3. What are the patient's risk factors for fluid and electrolyte imbalances?
4. The nurse draws blood for a serum chemistry evaluation. What electrolyte imbalances are likely and why?
5. The physician orders dextrose 5% in 0.45% saline to infuse at 100 ml/hr. What type of solution is this and how will it help Ms. Smith's fluid imbalance?
6. What are the priority nursing interventions for Ms. Smith?
7. Because of the nature of her disease process, Ms. Smith is at risk for the development of SIADH. How would the nurse recognize this complication and what is the anticipated treatment?
8. Based on the assessment data presented, write one or more appropriate nursing diagnoses. Are there any collaborative problems?

NCLEX EXAMINATION REVIEW QUESTIONS

The number of the question corresponds to the same-numbered objective at the beginning of the chapter.

1. During the postoperative care of a 76-year-old patient, the nurse monitors the patient's intake and output carefully, knowing that the patient is at risk for fluid and electrolyte imbalances primarily because
   a. older adults have an impaired thirst mechanism and need reminding to drink fluids.
   b. water accounts for a greater percentage of body weight in the older adult than in younger adults.
   c. older adults are more likely than younger adults to lose extracellular fluid during surgical procedures.
   d. small losses of fluid are more significant because body fluids account for only about 50% of body weight in older adults.
2. If the blood plasma has a higher osmolality than the fluid within a red blood cell, the mechanism involved in equalizing the fluid concentration is
   a. osmosis.
   b. diffusion.
   c. active transport.
   d. facilitated diffusion.

3a. An elderly woman was admitted to the medical unit with dehydration. A clinical indication of this problem is
   a. weight loss.
   b. full bounding pulse.
   c. engorged neck veins.
   d. Kussmaul respiration.

3b. Implementation of nursing care for the patient with hyponatremia includes
   a. fluid restriction.
   b. administration of hypotonic IV fluids.
   c. administration of a cation-exchange resin.
   d. increased water intake for patients on nasogastric suction.

3c. A patient is receiving a loop diuretic. The nurse should be alert for which symptoms?
   a. Restlessness and agitation
   b. Paresthesias and irritability
   c. Weak, irregular pulse, and poor muscle tone
   d. Increased blood pressure and muscle spasms

3d. Which patient would be at greatest risk for the potential development of hypermagnesemia?
   a. 83-year-old man with lung cancer and hypertension
   b. 65-year-old woman with hypertension taking β-adrenergic blockers
   c. 42-year-old woman with systemic lupus erythematosus and renal failure
   d. 50-year-old man with benign prostatic hyperplasia and a urinary tract infection

3e. It is especially important for the nurse to assess for which clinical manifestation(s) in a patient who has just undergone a total thyroidectomy?
   a. Weight gain
   b. Depressed reflexes
   c. Positive Chvostek sign
   d. Confusion and personality changes

3f. The nurse anticipates that the patient with hyperphosphatemia secondary to renal failure will require
   a. calcium supplements.
   b. potassium supplements.
   c. magnesium supplements.
   d. fluid replacement therapy.

4. The lungs act as an acid-base buffer by
   a. increasing respiratory rate and depth when CO_2 levels in the blood are high, reducing acid load.
   b. increasing respiratory rate and depth when CO_2 levels in the blood are low, reducing base load.
   c. decreasing respiratory rate and depth when CO_2 levels in the blood are high, reducing acid load.
   d. decreasing respiratory rate and depth when CO_2 levels in the blood are low, increasing acid load.
5. A patient has the following arterial blood gas results: pH 7.52; $PaCO_2$ 30 mm Hg; HCO_3^- 24 mEq/L. The nurse determines that these results indicate
   a. metabolic acidosis.
   b. metabolic alkalosis.
   c. respiratory acidosis.
   d. respiratory alkalosis.
6. The typical fluid replacement for the patient with an ICF fluid volume deficit is
   a. isotonic.
   b. hypotonic.
   c. hypertonic.
   d. a plasma expander.

REFERENCES

1. Anderson DM: *Mosby's medical, nursing, and allied health dictionary,* ed 6, St Louis, 2005, Mosby.
2. Huether SE, McCance K: *Understanding pathophysiology,* ed 3, St Louis, 2004, Mosby.
3. Kee JL, Paulanka BJ, Purnell LD: *Handbook of fluids, electrolytes and acid-base imbalances,* ed 2, Clifton Park, NY, 2004, Thompson/Delmar.
4. Porth CM: *Pathophysiology: concepts of altered health states,* ed 7, Philadelphia, 2004, Lippincott.
5. Ebersole P, Hess P, Luggen AS: *Toward healthy aging,* ed 6, St Louis, 2004, Mosby.
6. Larson K: Fluid balance in the elderly, *Geriatr Nurs* 24:5, 2003.
7. Amella EJ: Feeding and hydration issues for older adults with dementia, *Nurs Clin North Am* 39:3, 2004.
8. Luckey AE: Fluid and electrolytes in the aged, *Arch Surg* 138:10, 2003.
9. Woodrow P: Assessing fluid balance in older people, *Nurs Older People* 14:10, 2003.
10. Burger C: Hypokalemia, *AJN* 104:11, 2004.
11. Singh S, Frances S: Management of hypercalcaemia, *Geriatr Med* 34:5, 2004.
12. Shuey KM: Hypercalcemia of malignancy: part I, *Clin J Oncol Nurs* 8:2, 2004.
13. Price SA, Wilson LM: *Pathophysiology: clinical concepts of disease processes,* ed 6, St Louis, 2003, Mosby.
14. Pruitt WC: Interpreting arterial blood gases: easy as ABC, *Nursing* 38:8, 2004.
15. Phillips LD: *Manual of IV therapeutics,* ed 4, Philadelphia, 2005, FA Davis.

RESOURCE

Infusion Nurses Society
781-440-9408
Fax: 781-440-9409
www.ins1.org

For additional Internet resources, see the website for this book at *http://evolve.elsevier.com/Lewis/medsurg.*

Section 3

Perioperative Care

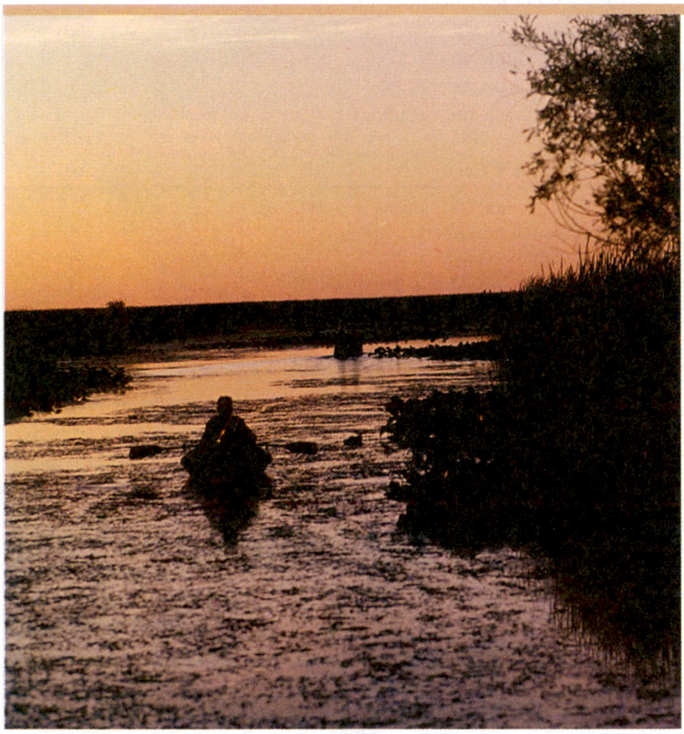

Section Outline

The wisest mind has something yet to learn.

George Santayana

Nursing Management Preoperative Care

18

Janice A. Neil

LEARNING OBJECTIVES

1. Identify the common purposes and settings of surgery.
2. Describe the purpose and components of a preoperative nursing assessment.
3. Interpret the significance of data related to the preoperative patient's health status and operative risk.
4. Explain the components and purpose of informed consent for surgery.
5. Describe the nursing role in the physical, psychologic, and educational preparation of the surgical patient.
6. Discuss the day-of-surgery preparation for the surgical patient.
7. Identify the purposes and types of preoperative medications.
8. Identify the special considerations of preoperative preparation for the older adult surgical patient.

KEY TERMS

ambulatory surgery, p. 344
elective surgery, p. 343
emergency surgery, p. 343
informed consent, p. 352
same-day admission, p. 344
surgery, p. 343

Electronic Resources

Supplemental content related to Chapter 18 can be found . . .

Companion CD

- Stress-Busting Kit for Nursing Students
- NCLEX Examination Review Questions
- Comprehensive Glossary

Evolve Website evolve

http://evolve.elsevier.com/Lewis/medsurg

- Content Updates
- Key Points (Printable and CD/MP3 Download)
- Concept Map Creator
- Expanded Audio Glossary
- Key Term Flash Cards
- Electronic Calculators
- WebLinks

Surgery can be defined as the art and science of treating diseases, injuries, and deformities by operation and instrumentation. The surgical procedure involves the interaction of the patient, surgeon, anesthesia care provider (ACP), and nurse. Surgery may be performed for any of the following purposes:

1. *Diagnosis:* determination of the presence and/or extent of pathology (e.g., lymph node biopsy or bronchoscopy)
2. *Cure:* elimination or repair of pathology (e.g., removal of a ruptured appendix or benign ovarian cyst)
3. *Palliation:* alleviation of symptoms without cure (e.g., cutting a nerve root [rhizotomy] to remove symptoms of pain, or creating a colostomy to bypass an inoperable bowel obstruction)
4. *Prevention:* examples include removal of a mole before it becomes malignant or removal of the colon in a patient with familial polyposis to prevent cancer
5. *Exploration:* surgical examination to determine the nature or extent of a disease (e.g., laparotomy)
6. *Cosmetic improvement:* examples include repairing a burn scar or changing breast shape

Specific suffixes are commonly used in combination with identifying a body part or organ in naming surgical procedures (Table 18-1).

SURGICAL SETTINGS

Surgery may be a carefully planned event **(elective surgery)** or may arise with unexpected urgency **(emergency surgery).** Both elective and emergency surgery may be performed in a variety of settings. The setting in which a surgical procedure may be safely and effectively performed is influenced by the complexity of the surgery, the potential complications, and the general health status of the patient.

Reviewed by Mary Ann Wehmer, RN, MSN, CNOR, Nursing Instructor, University of Southern Indiana, Evansville, Ind.

TABLE 18-1 Suffixes Describing Surgical Procedures

Suffix	Meaning	Example
-ectomy	Excision or removal of	Appendectomy
-lysis	Destruction of	Electrolysis
-orrhaphy	Repair or suture of	Herniorrhaphy
-oscopy	Looking into	Endoscopy
-ostomy	Creation of opening into	Colostomy
-otomy	Cutting into or incision of	Tracheotomy
-plasty	Repair or reconstruction of	Mammoplasty

For inpatient surgery, patients who are going to be admitted to the hospital are usually admitted on the day of surgery **(same-day admission).** Patients who are in the hospital before surgery are usually there because of their medical conditions.

Many types of surgical procedures are being performed as **ambulatory surgery** (also called *same-day* or *outpatient surgery*). Many of these surgeries involve the use of endoscopic techniques and are described in chapters throughout the text that discuss surgical intervention for specific medical problems. Ambulatory surgery is conducted in emergency departments, endoscopy clinics, doctors' offices, freestanding surgical clinics, and outpatient surgery units in hospitals. These procedures can be performed with the use of a general, regional, or local anesthetic; usually take less than 2 hours; require less than a 3- to 4-hour stay in the postanesthesia care unit (PACU); and do not require an overnight hospital stay. In some cases, the patient will stay in the hospital overnight after surgery, but for less than 24 hours. This is known as a "23-hour" stay.

Ambulatory surgery is generally preferred by patients, physicians, and third-party payers. Patients like the convenience of recovering at home, physicians prefer the flexibility in scheduling and availability of operating rooms, and the cost is usually less for both the patient and the insurer. Ambulatory surgery generally involves fewer laboratory tests, fewer preoperative and postoperative medications, less psychologic stress (especially for older adults), and less susceptibility to hospital-acquired infections. In some cases it is mandated by third-party payers, such as private insurance companies, government insurers (Medicare and Medicaid), and health maintenance organizations (HMOs).

Regardless of where the surgery is performed, the nurse is vital in preparing the patient for surgery, caring for the patient during surgery, and facilitating the patient's recovery following surgery. To perform these functions effectively, the nurse must have certain basic information. First, the nurse must have knowledge of the nature of the disorder requiring surgery and any coexisting disease processes. Second, the nurse must identify the individual patient's response to the stress of surgery. Third, the nurse must assess the results of appropriate preoperative diagnostic tests. Finally, the nurse must consider the bodily alterations and potential risks and complications associated with the surgical procedure and any coexisting medical problems. The nurse caring for the patient preoperatively is likely to be different from the nurse in the operating room (OR), PACU, surgical intensive care unit (SICU), or surgical unit. Thus communication and documentation of important preoperative assessment findings are essential to the continuity of care.

The preoperative nursing measures included in this chapter are those that apply to the preparation of any surgical patient. Preparation measures for specific surgical procedures (e.g., abdominal, thoracic, or orthopedic surgery) are covered in appropriate chapters of this text.

PATIENT INTERVIEW

The patient may be seen multiple times by multiple health care team members before surgery. To prevent the patient from having to repeat the same information over and over, the nurse should check the documentation for information before asking common questions. Regardless of the source of information, one of the most important nursing actions is the preoperative interview. The interview may be done by the nurse who works in the physician's office, a preoperative admission clinic, the ambulatory surgery center, or the hospital preoperative area. The site of the interview and the time before surgery will dictate the depth and completeness of the interview. Important findings must be documented and communicated to others so that continuity of care will be maintained.

The preoperative interview may occur in advance or on the patient's day of surgery. The primary purposes of the patient interview are to (1) obtain the patient's health information, (2) determine the patient's expectations about surgery and anesthesia, (3) provide and clarify information about the surgical experience, and (4) assess the patient's emotional state and readiness for surgery. The nurse may also ensure that the patient's consent form for surgery has been signed and witnessed.

The interview also provides the patient and family an opportunity to ask questions about surgery, anesthesia, and postoperative care. Often patients will ask about taking their routine medications, such as insulin or heart medications, or if they will experience pain. The nurse who is aware of a patient's and family's needs and perception of stressors can provide or arrange for the support needed during the perioperative period.

NURSING ASSESSMENT OF THE PREOPERATIVE PATIENT

The overall goal of the preoperative assessment is to gather data in order to identify risk factors and plan care to ensure patient safety throughout the surgical experience. Goals of the assessment are to:

1. Determine the psychologic status of the patient in order to reinforce the use of coping strategies during the surgical experience.
2. Determine physiologic factors that are directly or indirectly related to the surgical procedure that may contribute to operative risk factors.
3. Establish baseline data for comparison in the intraoperative and postoperative period.
4. Identify and document the surgical site and/or side on which the surgical procedure will be performed.
5. Identify prescription medications and over-the-counter drugs and herbs that have been taken by the patient that may affect the surgical outcome.
6. Confirm that the results of all preoperative laboratory and diagnostic tests are documented in the patient's record and communicated to appropriate personnel.
7. Identify cultural and ethnic factors that may affect the surgical experience.
8. Determine if the patient has received adequate information from the surgeon to make an informed decision to have surgery and that the consent form is signed and witnessed.

Subjective Data

Psychosocial Assessment. Surgery is a frightening event, even when the procedure is considered relatively minor. The psychologic and physiologic reactions to the surgical procedure and anesthesia elicit the stress response.[1] The stress response enables the body to prepare to meet the demands in the perioperative period. If stressors or the response to the stressors are excessive, the stress response can be magnified and recovery can be affected. Many factors influence the patient's susceptibility to stress, including age, past experiences with stress, current health, and socioeconomic status. The nurse who is aware of a patient's perceived or actual stressors can provide support and the needed information during the preoperative period so that stress will not become distress. (See Chapter 9 for a discussion of stress.)

The nurse must use common language and avoid medical jargon. Words and language that are familiar to the patient should be used to increase the patient's understanding of surgical consent and the surgical experience. Familiar language will also help reduce preoperative anxiety.

The nurse's role in psychologically preparing the patient for surgery is to assess the patient for potential stressors that could negatively affect surgery (Table 18-2). The nurse should communicate all concerns to the appropriate surgical team member, especially if the concern requires intervention later in the surgical experience. Because the patient may be admitted directly into the preoperative area from the community or home, the nurse must be skilled in assessing vital psychologic factors in a very short time. The most common psychologic factors are anxiety, fear, and hope.

Anxiety. Everyone is anxious when facing surgery because of the unknown. This is normal and is an inherent survival mechanism. However, if the anxiety level is extremely high, cognition, decision making, and coping abilities are diminished. Anxiety can arise from lack of knowledge, which may range from not knowing what to expect during the surgical experience to uncertainty about the outcome of surgery. The potential outcome often contributes to anxiety when the surgery is for diagnostic purposes. The patient may have totally unrealistic expectations of what surgery will be like, or what it will accomplish. This may be a result of past experiences or the vicarious experiences provided by friends' stories and the mass media, especially television. The nurse can decrease some anxiety for the patient by providing information about what can be expected.[2] The surgeon should be informed if the patient requires any additional information or if anxiety seems excessive.

The patient may experience anxiety when surgical interventions are in conflict with his or her religious and cultural beliefs. In particular, the nurse should identify the patient's religious and cultural beliefs about the possibility of blood transfusions.[1] The need for blood replacement should have been discussed with the physician before admission, but may not have been communicated to all of the perioperative staff.

Common Fears. There are many reasons patients fear surgery. The most prevalent is the potential for death or permanent disability resulting from surgery. Sometimes the fear arises after hearing or reading about the risks during the informed consent process. Other fears can be pain, change in body image, or results of a diagnostic procedure.

Fear of death can be extremely detrimental. The nurse should notify the physician if the patient has a strong fear of death. A patient's strong fear of impending death may prompt the physician to postpone the surgery until this situation improves because attitude and emotional state influence the stress response, and thus the surgical outcome.

Fear of pain and discomfort during and after surgery is universal. If the fear appears extreme, the nurse should notify the anesthesia care provider (ACP) so that an appropriate preoperative medication can be given. The nurse can encourage the patient to talk with the ACP for clarification. The patient should be reassured that drugs are available for both anesthesia and analgesia during surgery. The nurse should stress that the patient should ask for medications following surgery if pain is present, and that taking these medications will not contribute to an addiction.

TABLE 18-2 Psychosocial Assessment of the Preoperative Patient

Situational Changes
- Determine support systems, including family, significant others, group and institutional structure, and religious and spiritual orientation.
- Define current degree of personal control, decision making, and independence.
- Consider the impact of surgery and hospitalization and the possible effects on lifestyle.
- Identify the presence of hope and anticipation of positive results.

Concerns with the Unknown
- Identify specific areas and depth of anxiety and fears.
- Identify expectations of surgery, changes in current health status, and effects on daily living.

Concerns with Body Image
- Identify current roles or relationships and view of self.
- Determine perceived or potential changes in role or relationships and their impact on body image.

Past Experiences
- Review previous surgical experiences, hospitalizations, and treatments.
- Determine responses to those experiences (positive and negative).
- Identify current perceptions of surgical procedure in relation to the above and information from others (e.g., a neighbor's view of a personal surgical experience).

Knowledge Deficit
- Identify the amount and type of preoperative information the patient requires.
- Assess understanding of the surgical procedure, including preparation, care, interventions, preoperative activities, restrictions, and expected outcomes.
- Identify the accuracy of information the patient has received from others, including health care team, family, friends, and the media.

Drugs may also be given that provide an amnesic effect so that the patient will not remember what occurs during the surgical episode. The patient should be told preoperatively that these medications are expected to cause temporary cognitive deficits after surgery to prevent anxiety related to memory lapses.

Fear of mutilation or alteration in body image can occur whether the surgery is radical, such as amputation, or minor, such as a bunion repair. The presence of even a small scar on the body can be repulsive to some, and others fear keloid development (overgrowth of a scar). The nurse must listen to and assess the patient's concern about this aspect of surgery with an open, nonjudgmental attitude.

Fear of anesthesia may arise from the unknown, from personal past experience, and/or from tales of others' unpleasant experiences. These concerns can result from a prior induction of anesthesia or information about hazards or complications (e.g., brain damage, paralysis). Many patients also fear losing control while under the influence of anesthesia. If these fears are identified, the nurse should inform the ACP immediately so that he or she can talk further with the patient. The patient should also be reassured that a nurse and the ACP will be present at all times during surgery.

Fear of disruption of life functioning or patterns may be present in varying degrees. It can range from fear of permanent disability and loss of life to concern about not being able to engage in leisure activities for a few weeks. Concerns about separation from family and about how spouse or children are managing may be exhibited. Financial concerns may be related either to an anticipated loss of income or to the costs of surgery.

If the nurse identifies any of these fears, consultation with a social worker, a spiritual or cultural advisor, a psychologist, or family members may prove valuable in providing assistance to the patient. Financial advisors at the hospital may be able to provide information about financial support for the uninsured, such as Medicaid.

Hope. Most psychologic factors related to surgery seem to be negative, but hope stands out as a positive attribute.[2] Hope may be the patient's strongest method of coping. To deny or minimize hope may negate the positive mental attitude necessary for a quick and full recovery. Some surgeries are hopefully anticipated. These can be the surgeries that repair (e.g., plastic surgery for burn scars), rebuild (e.g., total joint replacement to minimize pain and improve function), or save and extend life (e.g., repair of aneurysm, coronary artery bypass surgery). The nurse should assess and support the presence of hope and anticipation of positive results that the patient is expecting.

Past Health History. The nurse should ask the patient about medical conditions diagnosed in the past, as well as current health problems. A guideline for preoperative review of the patient's past health history and other subjective data will assist in asking the patient about specific problems. Initially the nurse should determine if the patient understands the reason for surgery. For example, the patient scheduled for a total knee replacement may indicate that increasing pain and immobility are the reasons for the surgery.

The reason for past hospitalizations should be documented. Any previous surgeries and dates of the surgeries should also be documented. Any problems with previous surgeries should be identified. For example, the patient may have experienced a wound infection or a reaction to an analgesic.

Women should be asked about their menstrual and obstetric history. This includes obtaining the date of the patient's last menstrual period and the number of pregnancies. The surgeon should be informed immediately if the patient states that she might be pregnant because maternal and subsequent fetal exposure to anesthetics during the first trimester can be avoided. Questions regarding reproductive function may be embarrassing for a teenager in the presence of parents or guardians. The nurse may elect to ask these questions with parents or guardians out of the room.

Inherited traits may contribute to the surgical outcome and need to be considered when obtaining family history information. Possible inherited conditions may be identified by asking both the patient and family members about the family health history. A family history of cardiac and endocrine disease should be recorded. For example, if a patient reports a mother or father with hypertension, sudden cardiac death, myocardial infarction, or coronary artery disease, the nurse should be alerted to the possibility that the patient may also have a similar predisposition or condition. A family history of diabetes should also be investigated because of the familial predisposition to both type 1 and type 2 diabetes mellitus. Tendencies toward these conditions may be exacerbated during surgery and affect physiologic function during and after surgery.

Information should also be obtained about the patient's family history of adverse reactions to or problems with anesthesia. Anesthesia care providers first became aware of a condition, later to be known as malignant hyperthermia, when a young man in Australia reported that 10 of his family members had died while undergoing anesthesia. The genetic predisposition for malignant hyperthermia is now well documented, and measures to minimize complications associated with this condition can be taken. (For further information on malignant hyperthermia, see Chapter 19.)

Medications. Current routine and intermittent medication use, including the use of over-the-counter drugs and herbal products, should be documented. In many ambulatory surgery centers, the patients are asked to bring their bottles of medications with them when reporting for surgery to facilitate accurate assessment and documentation of both the name and dosage of home medication. Information regarding the patient's compliance with the medication regimen should also be assessed and evaluated to identify other concerns.

Drugs and herbal products may interact with anesthetics. The interaction of the patient's home medication and anesthesia agents can increase or decrease the desired physiologic effect. It is also important to consider the effects of opioids and prescribed medications for heart disease, hypertension, immunosuppression, seizure control, anticoagulation, and endocrine replacement. For example, tranquilizers potentiate the effect of opioids and barbiturates, which are agents that can be used for anesthesia. Antihypertensive drugs may predispose the patient to shock from the combined effect of the drug and the vasodilator effect of some anesthetic agents. Insulin or oral hypoglycemic agents may require dose or agent adjustments during the perioperative period because of increased body metabolism, decreased caloric intake, stress, and anesthesia. Aspirin and nonsteroidal antiinflammatory drugs (NSAIDs) may inhibit platelet aggregation and may contribute to postoperative bleeding complications. Surgeons often require that patients not take any aspirin or NSAIDs for 1 to 2 weeks before surgery.

The nurse must specifically ask about the use of herbs and dietary supplements because their use is so prevalent. Many patients do not think to include herbal products in their list of medications. Many patients believe that herbal products are "natural" and therefore do not pose a surgical risk.[3] (See Complementary and Alternative Therapy box in Chapter 4 on p. 44 on how to assess for the use of herbal products.) Excessive use of vitamins and herbs can cause detrimental effects in patients undergoing surgery, such as changes in blood pressure, cardiac effects, electrolyte alterations, delayed awakening from anesthesia, and inhibition of platelet aggregation.[3,4] In patients taking anticoagulants or drugs that inhibit platelet aggregation, the additional use of herbal products can produce excessive postoperative bleeding that may necessitate a return to the operating room.[4] The effects of specific herbs that are of concern during the perioperative period are listed in the Complementary and Alternative Therapies box on p. 347.

The nurse must also ask the patient about possible recreational drug use, abuse, and addiction. The substances most likely to be abused include tobacco, alcohol, opioids, marijuana, and cocaine. Questions about the use of these substances should be asked matter-of-factly. The nurse should stress that recreational drug use may affect the type and amount of anesthesia that will be needed. When patients become aware of the potential interactions of these substances with anesthetics, most patients will respond honestly about their using them. Chronic alcohol use will place the surgical patient at risk because of lung, gastrointestinal, or liver damage. When liver function is decreased, metabolism of anesthetic agents is prolonged, nutritional status is altered, and the potential for postoperative complications is increased. Alcohol withdrawal can also occur during lengthy surgery or in the postoperative period. This can be a life-threatening

COMPLEMENTARY AND ALTERNATIVE THERAPIES

Herbs and Supplements: Effects during the Perioperative Period

Herb or Supplement	Perioperative Considerations
Echinacea	May cause inflammation of the liver if used with certain medications
Feverfew	May inhibit platelet activity and increase bleeding
Garlic	May increase bleeding, especially in patients taking anticoagulants
Ginger	May increase bleeding, especially in patients taking anticoagulants
Ginkgo biloba	May increase bleeding, especially in patients taking anticoagulants
Ginseng	May increase bleeding, especially in patients taking anticoagulants; may cause increased heart rate or elevated BP
Goldenseal	May cause increased BP; may increase swelling
Kava	May prolong the effects of certain anesthetics or antiseizure medications; may cause liver injury
Licorice	Certain preparations may cause elevated BP, swelling, or electrolyte imbalance
Saw palmetto	May have additive effects with other hormone therapies
St. John's wort	May prolong the effects of anesthetic agents
Valerian	May prolong the effects of certain anesthetics or antiseizure medications; may cause liver injury
Vitamin E	May increase bleeding, especially in patients taking anticoagulants; may affect thyroid gland function; in high doses may cause increased BP in patients who already have high BP

Source: American Society of Anesthesiologists (2005). What you should know about herbal and dietary supplement use and anesthesia. Available at *www.asahq.org/patientEducation.htm*.

event, but it can be avoided with appropriate planning and management (see Chapter 12).

While assessing the patient's home medications, the nurse must also question the patient about drug intolerance and drug allergies. Drug intolerance usually results in side effects that are uncomfortable or unpleasant for the patient but are not life threatening. These effects can include nausea, constipation, diarrhea, or *idiosyncratic* (opposite than expected) reactions. A true drug allergy produces hives and/or an anaphylactic reaction, causing cardiopulmonary compromise, including hypotension, tachycardia, bronchospasm, and possibly pulmonary edema. By being aware of drug intolerance and drug allergies, it will be possible to maintain patient comfort, safety, and stability. For example, some anesthetic agents contain sulfur, so the ACP should be notified if a history of allergy to sulfur is given. If a drug intolerance or drug allergy is noted, it must be documented, and an allergy wristband should be put on the patient on the day of surgery.

All findings of the medication history should be documented and communicated to the intraoperative and postoperative personnel. Although the ACP will determine the appropriate schedule and dose of the patient's routine medications before and after surgery, the nurse must ensure that all of the patient's medications are identified, implement the alterations in medication administration, and monitor the patient for potential interactions and complications.

Allergies. The nurse should inquire about nondrug allergies, including allergies to foods, chemicals, and pollen. The patient with a history of any allergic responsiveness has a greater potential for demonstrating hypersensitivity reactions to drugs administered during anesthesia.

Patients should also be screened for possible latex allergies.[5] The American College of Allergy, Asthma, and Immunology (ACAAI) recommends that patients be screened in the following five areas:

1. Risk factors
2. Contact dermatitis
3. Contact urticaria (e.g., hives)
4. Aerosol reactions
5. History of reactions that suggest an allergy to latex

Risk factors include long-term, multiple exposures to latex products, such as those experienced by health care personnel and rubber industry workers. Additional risk factors include a history of hay fever, asthma, and allergies to certain foods, such as avocados, kiwi, bananas, chestnuts, potatoes, peaches, and apricots.[6] (Latex allergies are discussed in Chapter 14.)

Review of Systems. The last component of the patient history is the body systems review. Specific questions should be asked to confirm the presence or absence of any diseases. Past medical problems can alert the nurse to areas that should be more closely examined in the preoperative physical examination. When the nurse evaluates the patient before the day of surgery and combines the review of systems with the patient history data, the need for specific preoperative laboratory tests can be assessed and implemented.

Cardiovascular System. Cardiovascular (CV) function is evaluated to determine the presence of preexisting disease or existing problems (e.g., mitral valve prolapse, valve replacements) so that the patient's CV status can be monitored during the surgical and recovery periods. In reviewing the CV system, the nurse may find that there is a history of cardiac problems, including hypertension, angina, dysrhythmias, heart failure, and/or myocardial infarction. The nurse should also inquire about the patient's treatment for the CV condition and the level of maintenance and functioning. The patient and family should be questioned if the patient has seen or is seeing a cardiologist, correct identification of the cardiologist, and the use of CV medication or treatment. If the patient has had a recent myocardial infarction or has a pacemaker, a cardiologist should be consulted before surgery.

The patient's heart will be monitored continuously during surgery and, if indicated, postoperatively. The vital signs recorded preoperatively will be the baseline for the perioperative period. If pertinent, clotting and bleeding times should be present on the chart before surgery, as well as other laboratory reports. For example, the patient who receives digitalis therapy will have serum potassium levels drawn preoperatively and results should be available. If the patient has a history of hypertension, the ACP may administer vasoactive drugs to maintain adequate blood pressure during the surgery. If the patient has a history of congenital, rheumatic, or valvular heart disease, antibiotic prophylaxis may be given before surgery to decrease the risk of bacterial endocarditis (see Chapter 37).

Respiratory System. The patient should be asked about any recent or chronic upper respiratory infections. The presence of an upper airway infection may result in the cancellation or postponement of elective surgery because the existing infection will place the patient at an increased risk of bronchospasm, laryngospasm, decreased oxygen saturation, and problems with respiratory secretions. The nurse should also report a patient's history of dyspnea at rest or with exertion (e.g., breathing hard when carrying groceries), coughing (dry or productive), or hemoptysis (coughing blood) to the ACP and surgeon.

If a patient has a history of asthma, the nurse should inquire about the patient's use of inhaled or oral corticosteroids and bronchodilators, as well as the frequency and triggers of asthma attacks. The patient with a history of chronic obstructive pulmonary disease (COPD) and asthma is at high risk for postoperative pulmonary complications, which include hypoxemia and atelectasis.

The patient who smokes should be encouraged to stop at least 6 weeks preoperatively to decrease the risk of intraoperative and postoperative respiratory complications, but may find this difficult during such a stressful time. The greater the patient's pack-years of smoking (packs smoked per day times years), the greater the patient's potential for pulmonary complications during or after surgery. Conditions likely to influence or compromise respiratory function such as obesity and spinal, chest, and airway deformities should also be noted and reported. Depending on the patient's history and physical examination, baseline pulmonary function tests and arterial blood gases (ABGs) may be ordered preoperatively.

Nervous System. Preoperative evaluation of neurologic functioning includes assessing the patient's ability to respond to questions, follow commands, and maintain orderly thought patterns. Alterations in the patient's hearing and vision may affect responses and ability to follow directions throughout the perioperative assessment and evaluation. The patient's ability to pay attention, concentrate, and respond appropriately in the preoperative phase must be documented to establish an accurate baseline for postoperative comparison.

Cognitive function is particularly important for the patient who is expected to prepare for surgery and to complete preoperative preparation on an outpatient basis. If deficits are noted, careful assessment should determine the extent of the problems and if the problems can be corrected before surgery. If the problems cannot be corrected, it is important that a guardian or a person with durable power of attorney for health care be involved to assist the patient and provide informed consent for surgery.

The preoperative assessment of the older person's baseline cognitive function is especially crucial for intraoperative and postoperative evaluation.[7] The older adult may have intact mental abilities preoperatively, but is more prone to be adversely affected than younger adults by the additional stressors of the surgical procedure, dehydration, hypothermia, and anesthesia and adjunctive medications. These factors may contribute to the development of postoperative delirium, a condition that may be falsely labeled as senility or dementia. Thus preoperative findings are extremely important for postoperative comparison.

In the review of the nervous system it is also important for the nurse to inquire about any presence of strokes, transient ischemic attacks, or spinal cord injury. The nurse should ask about diseases of the nervous system, such as myasthenia gravis, Parkinson's disease, and multiple sclerosis and any treatments used.

Urinary System. The preoperative patient should be assessed for a history of renal or urinary diseases, such as glomerulonephritis, chronic kidney disease, or repeated urinary tract infections. The present disease state and treatment used to control the disease should be noted and documented. Renal dysfunction is associated with a number of alterations, including fluid and electrolyte imbalances, coagulopathies, increased risk for infection, and impaired wound healing. Another important consideration is the recognition that many drugs are metabolized and excreted by the kidneys. A decrease in renal function may contribute to an altered response to drugs and unpredictable drug elimination. Renal function tests, such as serum creatinine and blood urea nitrogen, are commonly ordered preoperatively, and results should be available on the chart before the patient goes to surgery.

The nurse should document and report to the perioperative team if the patient has problems voiding. Male patients may have physical alterations, such as an enlarged prostate, which can interfere with the insertion of a urinary catheter during surgery or impair voiding in the postoperative period.

Hepatic System. The liver is involved in glucose homeostasis, fat metabolism, protein synthesis, drug and hormone metabolism, and bilirubin formation and excretion. The liver detoxifies many anesthetics and adjunctive drugs. The patient with hepatic dysfunction may have an increased perioperative risk for clotting abnormalities and adverse responses to medications. The nurse should consider the presence of liver disease if there is a history of jaundice, hepatitis, or alcohol abuse.

Integumentary System. The nurse should inquire about a history of skin problems. The current status of the skin, especially at the incision site, should be assessed for rashes, boils, ulcers, or other dermatologic conditions. A patient with a history of pressure ulcers may require extra padding during surgery. Skin problems may affect postoperative healing.

Musculoskeletal System. Musculoskeletal and mobility problems, especially in the older adult, should be noted. If the patient has arthritis, all affected joints should be identified. Mobility restrictions may influence intraoperative and postoperative positioning and ambulation. Spinal anesthesia may be difficult if the patient cannot flex his or her lumbar spine adequately to allow easy needle insertion. If the neck is affected, intubation and airway management may be difficult. Any mobility aids such as a cane, a walker, or crutches should be brought with the patient on the day of surgery. Frequently, postoperative pain is due to chronic musculoskeletal pain and positioning during surgery, rather than the acute pain of the surgical procedure.

Endocrine System. The patient with diabetes mellitus is especially at risk for adverse effects of anesthesia and surgery. Hypoglycemia, hyperglycemia, ketosis, cardiovascular alterations, delayed wound healing, and infection are common complications of diabetes during the perioperative period. Serum glucose tests should be completed the morning of surgery to determine baseline levels. It is important to clarify with the patient's surgeon or ACP whether the patient should take the usual dose of insulin or oral hypoglycemic agents on the day of surgery. ACP practitioners may vary the usual insulin dose based on the patient's current status and history of glucose control. Regardless of the preoperative insulin orders, the patient's serum glucose will be determined periodically and managed, if necessary, with regular (short-acting, rapid-onset) insulin.

It should also be determined if the patient has a history of thyroid dysfunction. Either hyperthyroidism or hypothyroidism can place the patient at surgical risk because of alterations in metabolic rate. If the patient takes a thyroid replacement drug, the nurse should check with the ACP about administration of the drug the day of surgery. If the patient has a history of thyroid dysfunction, laboratory tests may be ordered to determine current levels of thyroid function.

The patient with Addison's disease also requires special consideration during surgery. Addisonian crisis or shock can occur if a patient abruptly stops taking replacement corticosteroids, and the stress of surgery may require additional intravenous (IV) corticosteroid therapy.[8]

Immune System. If the patient has a history of a compromised immune system or takes immunosuppressive drugs, it must be documented. Corticosteroids used in immunosuppressive doses may be tapered before surgery. Impairment of the immune system can lead to delayed wound healing and increased risk for postoperative infections. If the patient has an acute infection (e.g., acute upper respiratory tract infection, acute sinusitis, influenza), elective surgery is frequently cancelled. Patients with active chronic infections such as hepatitis B or C, acquired immunodeficiency syndrome (AIDS), and tuberculosis may have surgery if treatment for the infections is continued. When preparing the patient for surgery, it should be remembered that infection control precautions must be taken with every patient. (Infection control guidelines are discussed in Chapter 15 and Tables 15-8 and 15-9.)

Fluid and Electrolyte Status. The patient should be questioned about the recent presence of conditions that increase the risk for fluid and electrolyte imbalances, such as vomiting, diarrhea, or difficulty swallowing. For example, surgery may be planned for a patient with cholecystitis who has been vomiting for several days. Drugs that the patient takes that alter fluid and electrolyte status, such as diuretics, should also be identified. Serum electrolyte levels are often evaluated before surgery. Some patients may have restricted fluids for some time before surgery, and if the surgery is delayed, they could develop dehydration. A patient with or at risk for dehydration may require additional fluids and electrolytes before or during surgery. Although a preoperative fluid balance history should be completed for all patients, it is especially critical for the older adult because the reduced adaptive capacity leaves a narrow margin of safety between overhydration and underhydration.

Nutritional Status. Nutritional deficits include overnutrition and undernutrition, both of which require considerable time to correct. However, knowing that a patient exhibits either undernutrition or overnutrition can help the team provide more individualized care. For example, timely notification that the patient is very obese allows the perioperative nurse time to obtain a large operating bed on which surgery can be performed and the patient does not have to be moved. Longer instruments can also be prepared, especially for abdominal surgery.

Obesity stresses both the cardiac and pulmonary systems and makes access to the surgical site and anesthesia administration more difficult.[3] It predisposes the patient to wound dehiscence, wound infection, and incisional herniation postoperatively. Adipose tissue is less vascular than other types of tissue.[3] In addition, the patient may be slower to recovery from anesthesia because the inhalation anesthetic is absorbed and stored by adipose tissue, thus leaving the body more slowly.

Nutritional deficiencies of protein and vitamins A, C, and B complex are particularly significant because these substances are essential for wound healing.[9] Supplemental IV and oral nutrients can be administered during the perioperative period to promote adequate healing ability if the patient is malnourished. The older adult is often at risk for malnutrition and fluid volume deficits.[10] If the patient is very thin, the perioperative team should be notified in order to provide more padding than usual (pressure points on all patients are protected routinely) on the operating bed. This is necessary to prevent pressure ulcers, especially during a lengthy procedure. Nutritional deficiencies impair the ability to recover from surgery. It is important to remember that the obese patient can also be protein and vitamin deficient. If the nutritional problem is severe, the surgery may be postponed until the patient loses or gains weight and nutritional deficiencies are corrected.

Dietary habits may affect postoperative recovery and should be identified if the patient will remain in the hospital postoperatively. For example, patients who consume large quantities of coffee or soft drinks containing high caffeine levels should be identified. In many cases, the withholding of caffeinated beverages preoperatively, as well as for a considerable length of time postoperatively, can lead to severe withdrawal headaches.[11] Caffeine withdrawal headaches could be confused with spinal headaches if the preoperative data are not documented. Caffeinated beverages given postoperatively to the patient, when possible, will prevent caffeine withdrawal headaches.

Functional Health Patterns. The review of each functional health pattern of the patient provides valuable subjective data about the patient's physical and psychologic status, as well as cultural values and beliefs related to his or her health care. Questions to ask a preoperative patient are listed in Table 18-3.

Objective Data

Physical Examination. The Joint Commission on Accreditation of Healthcare Organizations (JCAHO)[12] requires that all patients admitted to the operating room have a documented physical examination (PE) in the chart. This examination may be done in advance of surgery or on the day of surgery. The PE may be performed by any number of qualified people, including nurses, nurse practitioners, physicians, physician assistants, or ACPs.

Findings from the patient's history and PE will enable the ACP to assign the patient a physical status rating for anesthesia administration (Table 18-4). This rating is an indicator of the patient's perioperative risk and may influence perioperative decisions.

Many physiologic stressors may put the patient at risk for surgical complications. A physiologic assessment of the preoperative patient is presented in Table 18-5. A focused physical examination should be completed immediately before surgery. The nurse should review the documentation already present on the patient's chart, including the review of systems and the physician's PE report, to better proceed with the examination. All findings must be documented, with any relevant findings immediately communicated to the surgeon or ACP.

Laboratory and Diagnostic Testing. The nurse should obtain and evaluate the results of laboratory and diagnostic tests ordered preoperatively. For example, if the patient is taking an anticoagulant (including aspirin), a coagulation profile may be ordered; if a patient is on diuretic therapy, a potassium level may need to be assessed; or if a patient is taking medications for dysrhythmias, a preoperative electrocardiogram (ECG) will probably be performed. Blood glucose monitoring should be done for patients with diabetes. Commonly ordered preoperative laboratory tests can be found in Table 18-6.

Ideally, preoperative laboratory tests are ordered on the basis of the individual patient history and physical examination. However, many facilities and/or third-party reimbursement agencies have a written protocol or standards for preoperative laboratory tests,

TABLE 18-3 HEALTH HISTORY Preoperative Patient

Health Perception–Health Management Pattern
- What has the doctor explained to you about your surgery?
- Have you had surgery before?*
- Have you or any family members ever experienced any problems with anesthesia?*
- Do you smoke?* If yes, how many packs daily? For how many years?
- Do you have any chronic illnesses?*
- Are you taking any medications?* Are you allergic to any foods or medications?*
- What is your usual use of alcohol?

Nutritional-Metabolic Pattern
- What is your usual or present height and weight?
- Have you had a recent weight gain or loss?*
- Do you have any food preferences or dislikes?*
- Do you have any difficulty chewing or swallowing?*
- Do you take vitamins?* Supplements?*
- Do you have any problems healing?*
- Do you have a history of liver problems?*

Elimination Pattern
- Do you experience any problems with constipation?*
- Do you experience any problems with urinary elimination?*

Activity-Exercise Pattern
- Do you have a history of high blood pressure or cardiac disease?*
- Do you have any history of dyspnea, coughing, hemoptysis, COPD, or asthma?*
- Do you presently have an upper respiratory infection?*
- Do you have any musculoskeletal problems that might affect positioning during surgery or activity level after surgery?*
- Do you have any limitation in mobility of your neck?*
- Do you require any special equipment for ambulation?*

Sleep-Rest Pattern
- Describe any problems you have with sleeping.
- Do you use sleeping pills?*
- Do you snore?

Cognitive-Perceptual Pattern
- Do you wear glasses, contact lenses, or a hearing aid?*
- How would you describe your pain tolerance?
- What methods have you found effective for pain relief?

Self-Perception–Self-Concept Pattern
- How do you feel about having this surgery?
- Have you experienced any changes in the way you feel about yourself or your body?*

Role-Relationship Pattern
- Will this surgery create any problems in your usual roles or relationships?*
- Will you have the support you feel you need following discharge?

Sexuality-Reproductive Pattern
- Do you expect this surgery to have any impact on your usual sexual activity?*

Coping–Stress Tolerance Pattern
- How do you feel about this surgery?

Value-Belief Pattern
- Do you have a conflict between your planned surgery and your value or belief system?*

COPD, Chronic obstructive pulmonary disease.
*If yes, describe.

which may or may not include all the identified needed areas. In addition, offices and preadmission clinics may do the preoperative tests days before surgery at sites some distance from the surgical facility. Thus the nurse must ensure that all laboratory reports have arrived at the place of surgery at the right time and are on the chart.

TABLE 18-4 American Society of Anesthesiologists Physical Classification System

Rating	Definition
P1	A normal healthy person
P2	A patient with mild systemic disease
P3	A patient with severe systemic disease
P4	A patient with severe systemic disease that is a constant threat to life
P5	A moribund patient who is not expected to survive without surgery
P6	A declared brain-dead patient whose organs are being removed for donor purposes

Source: American Society of Anesthesiologists (2005). Available at *www.asahq.org/clinical/physicalstatus.htm.*

Lack of required diagnostic reports may result in a delay or cancellation of the surgery.

NURSING MANAGEMENT PREOPERATIVE PATIENT

Preoperative nursing interventions are derived from the nursing assessment and must reflect each individual patient's specific needs. Physical preparations will be determined by the pending surgery and the routines of the surgery setting. Preoperative teaching may be minimal or extensive. General information for surgery should be given.

Preoperative Teaching

The patient has a right to know what to expect and how to participate effectively during the surgical experience. Preoperative teaching increases patient satisfaction and may reduce postoperative fear, anxiety, and stress.[3] Teaching may also decrease complications, the duration of hospitalization, and the recovery time following discharge.

In most surgical settings, patients often arrive only a short time before surgery is scheduled. This includes patients arriving for ambulatory surgery and patients who will be hospitalized postoperatively. Preoperative teaching for these patients is generally done in the surgeon's office or preadmission surgical clinic and reinforced on the day of surgery. After ambulatory surgery, the patient usually goes home several hours after recovery depending on the patient's progress and procedure-specific needs. If ambulatory patients have not had preoperative teaching in an outpatient setting before surgery, teaching before they are discharged is necessary. In this case, patient teaching must address needs of the highest priority and include information that focuses on the safety of the patient. Written materials must be provided for patients to use for review and reinforcement at home.

When providing preoperative teaching for a patient several days before surgery, the nurse must provide a balance between telling so little that the patient is unprepared and explaining so much that the patient is overwhelmed. The nurse who observes carefully and listens sensitively to the patient can usually determine how much information is enough in each instance, remembering that anxiety and fear may decrease learning ability. The nurse must also assess what the patient wants to know right away and give priority to his or her concerns.

TABLE 18-5 Physiologic Assessment of the Preoperative Patient*

Cardiovascular System
- Identify acute or chronic problems; focus on presence of angina, hypertension, heart failure, recent history of myocardial infarction.
- Auscultate and palpate baseline pulses: apical, radial, and pedal for rate and characteristics (compare one side to the other).
- Inspect and palpate for presence of edema (including dependent areas), noting location and severity.
- Inspect and palpate neck veins for distention.
- Take baseline blood pressure in both arms.
- Identify any drug or herbal product that may affect coagulation (e.g., aspirin, ginkgo, ginger).
- Review laboratory and diagnostic tests for cardiovascular function.
- Identify patients with pacemakers and/or implantable defibrillators.

Respiratory System
- Identify acute or chronic problems; note the presence of infection or chronic obstructive pulmonary disease (COPD), asthma.
- Assess history of smoking, including the time interval since the last cigarette and the number of pack-years. (Remember that although smoking should be discouraged preoperatively, it may be difficult for patients to stop during this time of anxiety.)
- Auscultate lungs for normal and adventitious breath sounds.
- Determine baseline respiratory rate and rhythm, and regularity of pattern.
- Observe for cough, dyspnea, and use of accessory muscles of respiration.

Neurologic System
- Determine orientation to time, place, and person.
- Identify presence of confusion, disorderly thinking, or inability to follow commands.
- Identify past history of strokes, transient ischemic attacks or nervous system diseases (e.g., Parkinson's disease, multiple sclerosis).

Urinary System
- Identify any preexisting disease.
- Determine ability to void. Prostate enlargement may affect catheterization during surgery and ability to void postoperatively.
- If necessary, note color, amount, and characteristics of urine.
- Review laboratory and diagnostic tests for renal function.

Hepatic System
- Inspect skin color and sclera of eyes for any signs of jaundice.
- Review past history of substance abuse, especially alcohol and IV drug use.
- Review laboratory and diagnostic tests for liver function.

Integumentary System
- Assess mucous membranes for dryness and intactness.
- Determine skin status; note drying, bruising, or breaks in surface.
- Inspect skin for rashes, boils, or infection, especially around the planned surgical site.
- Assess skin moisture and temperature.
- Inspect the mucous membranes and skin turgor for dehydration.

Musculoskeletal System
- Examine skin/bone pressure points.
- Assess for presence of any pressure ulcers.
- Assess for limitations in joint range of motion and muscle weakness.
- Assess mobility, gait, and balance.
- Assess for presence of joint pain.

Gastrointestinal System
- Determine food and fluid intake patterns and any recent weight loss.
- Weigh and measure patient.
- Assess for the presence of dentures and bridges (loose dentures or teeth may be dislodged during intubation).

Immune System
- Identify any immunodeficiency or autoimmune disorders.
- Assess for use of corticosteroids or other immunosuppressant drugs.

*See related body system chapters for more specific assessments and related laboratory studies.

TABLE 18-6 Common Preoperative Diagnostic Tests

Test	Assessment
Urinalysis	Renal status, hydration, urinary tract infection and disease
Chest x-ray	Pulmonary disorders, cardiac enlargement
Blood studies: RBC, Hb, Hct, WBC, WBC differential	Anemia, immune status, infection
Electrolytes	Metabolic status, renal function, diuretic side effects
ABGs, oximetry	Pulmonary and metabolic function
PT, PTT, INR, platelet count	Bleeding tendencies
Blood glucose	Metabolic status, diabetes mellitus
Creatinine	Renal function
Blood urea nitrogen	Renal function
Serum albumin	Nutritional status
Electrocardiogram	Cardiac disease, electrolyte abnormalities
Pulmonary function studies	Pulmonary status
Liver function tests	Liver function
Type and crossmatch	Blood availability for replacement (elective surgery patients may have own blood available)
hCG	Pregnancy

ABGs, Arterial blood gases; *Hb,* hemoglobin; *hCG,* human chorionic gonadotropin; *Hct,* hematocrit; *INR,* international normalized ratio; *PT,* prothrombin time, *PTT;* partial thromboplastin time; *RBC,* red blood cells; *WBC,* white blood cells.

Generally, preoperative teaching concerns three types of information: sensory, process, and procedural. Different patients, with varying cultures, backgrounds, and experience, may want different types of information. With *sensory information,* patients want to know what they will see, hear, smell, and feel during the surgery. For example, the nurse may tell them that the OR will be cold, but they can ask the OR nurse for a warm blanket; the lights in the OR are very bright; or there will be lots of sounds that are unfamiliar and there may be specific smells present. Patients wanting *process information* may not want specific details but desire the general flow of what is going to happen. This information would include the patients' transfer to the holding area, visits by the nurse and ACP before transfer to the OR, and waking up in the PACU. Patients may also be informed that as soon as they are awake, their family may come in to visit them. With *procedural information,* desired details are more specific. For example, this information would include that an IV line will be started while patients are in the holding area and the surgeon may mark the operative site with an indelible marker to verify site and side. Other procedural information includes that when patients are transferred to the OR, they will be asked to move onto the narrow bed and a safety strap will be put over their thighs.[13]

Preoperative teaching provided to the patient must be communicated to the nurses providing postoperative care so that learning can be evaluated and duplication of teaching can be prevented. Because the nurse has limited time for teaching, the team approach is usually used. Nurses in offices, homes, or clinics may initiate the teaching. The perioperative nurses continue teaching and evaluate the patient's understanding of the content. The discharge nurse provides written instructions and additional information for reinforcement. Community nurses may also be involved if the patient has continuing learning needs that these nurses can address during home visits after patients are discharged.

TABLE 18-7 PATIENT AND FAMILY TEACHING GUIDE
Preoperative Preparation

Sensory Information
- Holding area may be noisy.
- Drugs and cleaning solutions may be smelled.
- Operating room (OR) can be cold; warm blankets are available.
- Talking may be heard in the OR but may be distorted because of masks. Questions should be asked if something is not understood.
- OR bed will be narrow. A safety strap will be applied over the knees.
- Lights in the OR may be very bright.
- Monitoring machines (ticking and pinging noises) may be heard when awake. Their purpose is to monitor and ensure safety.

Procedural Information
- What to bring and what type of clothing to wear to the ambulatory surgery center.
- Any changes in time of surgery.
- Fluid and food restrictions.
- Physical preparation required (e.g., bowel or skin preparation).
- Purpose of frequent vital signs assessment.
- Pain control and other comfort measures.
- Why turning, coughing, and deep breathing postoperatively is important; practice sessions need to be done preoperatively.
- Insertion of intravenous lines.
- Procedure for anesthesia administration.
- Expect surgical site and/or side to be marked with indelible ink or marker.

Process Information
Information About General Flow of Surgery
- Admission area.
- Preoperative holding area, OR, and recovery area.
- Families can usually stay in holding area until surgery.
- Families may be able to enter recovery area as soon as patient is awake.
- Identification of any technology that may be present on awakening, such as monitors and central lines.

Where Families Can Wait during Surgery
- Patient and family members need to be encouraged to verbalize concerns.
- OR staff will notify family when surgery is completed.
- Surgeon will usually talk with family following surgery.

All teaching should be documented in the patient's medical record. A patient and family teaching guide for preoperative preparation is presented in Table 18-7. Additional information related to patient teaching may be found in Chapter 5.

General Surgery Information. All patients should receive instruction about deep breathing, coughing, and moving postoperatively. This is essential because patients may not want to do these activities postoperatively unless they are taught the rationale for them and practice them preoperatively. Patients and families should be told if there will be tubes, drains, monitoring devices, or special equipment after surgery, and that these devices enable the nurse to safely care for the patient.

Examples of individualized teaching may include how to use incentive spirometers or postoperative patient-controlled analgesia pumps. The patient should also receive accurate surgery-specific information, such as a patient having an immobilizer following a total joint replacement, a patient having an epidural catheter for postoperative pain control, or the patient being told about waking up in the intensive care unit following extensive surgery.

Ambulatory Surgery Information. The ambulatory surgery patient or the patient admitted to the hospital the day of surgery will need to receive information before admission. Some ambulatory surgical centers have the staff telephone the patients the evening before surgery to answer last-minute questions and to reinforce teaching. Each surgical center has policies and procedures that direct and enable this communication in a timely manner.

The patient will need basic information such as the time to arrive at the surgery center and the time of surgery. Arrival time is usually 1 to 2 hours before the scheduled time of surgery to allow for the completion of the preoperative assessment and paperwork preparation. Information can also include the day-of-surgery events such as patient registration, parking, what to wear, what to bring, and the need to have a responsible adult present for transportation home after surgery.

To provide for general hygiene and preparation of surgical areas the surgeon may order a preoperative shower, an enema, and food and fluid restrictions. Historically, patients having elective surgery were usually instructed by the ACP to have nothing by mouth (NPO) starting at midnight on the night before surgery. Current guidelines published by the American Society of Anesthesiologists are much less stringent (Table 18-8). Protocols may vary if the patient is having local anesthesia or the surgery is scheduled for late in the day. The NPO protocol of each surgical facility should be followed because varying NPO protocols exist. Providing the patient with the rationale for adhering to NPO orders can significantly increase the patient's perception of their importance.[14] Restriction of fluids and food is designed to minimize the potential risk of aspiration and to decrease the risk of postoperative nausea and vomiting. The patient who has not followed this instruction may have surgery delayed or cancelled, so it is critical that the surgical patient understands and adheres to these restrictions.

TABLE 18-8 Preoperative Fasting Recommendations*

Liquid and Food Intake	Minimum Fasting Period (hr)
Clear liquids (e.g., water, clear tea, black coffee, carbonated beverages, and fruit juice without pulp)	2
Breast milk	4
Nonhuman milk, including infant formula	6
Light meal (e.g., toast and clear liquids)	6
Regular or heavy meal (may include fried or fatty food, meat)	8

Source: Practice guidelines for preoperative fasting and the use of pharmacologic agents to reduce the risk of pulmonary aspiration: application to healthy patients undergoing elective procedures: a report by the American Society of Anesthesiologists. Available at *www.asahq.org/publicationsAndServices/NPO.pdf*.
*For healthy patients of all ages undergoing elective surgery (excluding women in labor).

Legal Preparation for Surgery

Legal preparation for surgery consists of checking that all required forms have been correctly signed and are present on the chart, and that the patient and family clearly understand what is going to happen. Standard consent forms include those for the surgical procedure and blood transfusions. Other forms may include those that have been completed for advance directives and power of attorney (see Chapter 11).

Consent for Surgery. Before nonemergency surgery can be legally performed, the patient must voluntarily sign an informed consent form in the presence of a witness. **Informed consent** is an active, shared decision-making process between the provider and the recipient of care. Three conditions must be met for consent to be valid. First, there must be *adequate disclosure* of the diagnosis; the nature and purpose of the proposed treatment; the risks and consequences of the proposed treatment; the probability of a successful outcome; the availability, benefits, and risks of alternative treatments; and the prognosis if treatment is not instituted. Second, the patient must demonstrate clear *understanding* and *comprehension* of the information being provided before receiving sedating preoperative medications. Third, the recipient of care must *give consent voluntarily.* The patient must not be persuaded or coerced in any way by anyone to undergo the procedure.[15]

Although the physician is ultimately responsible for obtaining the patient's consent for surgical treatment, the nurse may be responsible for witnessing the patient's signature on the consent form. At this time the nurse can be a patient advocate, verifying that the patient (or family member) understands the information presented in the consent form, the implications of consent, and that consent for surgery is truly voluntary. If the patient is unclear about operative plans, the nurse should contact the surgeon about the patient's need for additional information. The patient also should be aware that consent, even when signed, can be withdrawn at any time if the desire to give permission for the procedure changes.

If the patient is a minor, is unconscious, or is mentally incompetent to sign the permit, the written permission may be given by a legally appointed representative or responsible family member.[16] Procedures for obtaining consent, especially from minors and patients who are mentally incompetent, vary among states and institutions. Therefore the nurse should follow specifics required by the state's nurse practice act and the institutional or agency policies that apply to an individual situation.

A true medical emergency may override the need to obtain consent. When immediate medical treatment is needed to preserve life or to prevent serious impairment to life and the individual patient is incapable of giving consent, the next of kin may give consent. If reaching the next of kin is not possible, the physician may institute treatment without written consent. A note is written in the chart documenting the medical necessity of the procedure. In the case of

EVIDENCE-BASED PRACTICE

How Long Should Patients Have Fluids Withheld Before Elective Surgery?

Clinical Question

Do adult patients undergoing elective surgery with general anesthetic (P) receiving clear liquids up to 2 hours before surgery (I) versus remaining NPO after midnight (C) experience higher rates of regurgitation/aspiration (O)?

Best Available Evidence

- Systematic review of randomized controlled trials (RCTs)
- NPO guidelines published by American Society of Anesthesiologists, 1999
- NPO guidelines published by Canadian Anesthesiologists' Society, 2004

Critical Appraisal and Synthesis of Evidence

- Two RCTs ($n = 2270$) adult participants not at risk for aspiration (*at risk* defined as pregnant, obese, elderly, stomach disorders).
- Parameters assessed: duration of fast, type and volume of intake permitted, rate of regurgitation/aspiration.
- Measures included volume, pH, and marker dye concentrations of postoperative gastric contents.
- No evidence of increased rates or risk of regurgitation or aspiration as measured by actual occurrence in patients given fluids up to 2 hours before surgery.

Conclusions

- In patients not considered to be at risk, clear fluids up to 2 hours before surgery may be appropriate.
- Patients reported less thirst and mouth dryness with no increase in nausea or vomiting.
- Pulmonary aspiration is a rare complication with modern anesthesia.

Implications for Nursing Practice

- The former order of NPO after midnight for all food or fluids is no longer appropriate for all patients.
- NPO orders need to be individualized for each patient.
- Clear liquids up to 2 hours before surgery for patients not at risk for regurgitation/aspiration may be given.
- Risk of regurgitation/aspiration (i.e., those who are pregnant, obese, elderly, history of stomach disorders) should be included in the preoperative assessment.
- Conduct studies examining safety of NPO guidelines in patients identified in the higher risk categories.

References for Evidence

American Society of Anesthesiologists: Practice guidelines for preoperative fasting and the use of pharmacologic agents to reduce the risk of pulmonary aspiration: application to healthy patients undergoing elective procedure, *Anesthesiology* 90:896, 1999.

Brady M, Kinn S, Stuart P: Preoperative fasting for adults to prevent perioperative complications. Cochrane Wounds Group, *Cochrane Database of Systematic Reviews* 4, 2005.

Canadian Anesthesiologists' Society: *Guidelines to the practice of anesthesia. Revised edition,* 2004. Available at *www.cas.ca* (accessed May 20, 2006).

Critical appraisal of Brady systematic review, *Evidence Based Nursing Journal* 7(2):44. PMID: 15106594, 2004.

PICO: P, Patient population of interest; *I,* intervention or area of interest; *C,* comparison of interest or comparison group; *O,* outcome(s) of interest (see p. 6).

ETHICAL DILEMMAS

Informed Consent

Situation

The nurse discusses a patient's impending surgery in the preoperative holding area. It becomes obvious that this competent adult patient was not fully informed of the alternatives to this surgery. She has signed the consent form but clearly was not fully informed about her treatment options.

Important Points for Consideration

- Informed consent requires that patients have complete information about the proposed treatment and its possible consequences, as well as alternative treatments and possible consequences.
- Risks and benefits of each treatment option must also be explained in order for patients to weigh treatment options.
- An opportunity to have questions answered about the various treatment options and their possible outcomes is also an important element of informed consent.
- Informed consent is an ongoing process that needs periodic assessment and discussion, not an event where a person signs a document.
- Paternalism results when health care providers do not provide complete information for patients to make fully informed decisions or when they decide what is best for patients.

Critical Thinking Questions

1. What should the nurse do?
2. What is the nurse's role as patient advocate in the informed consent process?

emergency where consent cannot be obtained, the intraoperative nurse will usually need to complete an incident report because it is an occurrence that is inconsistent with routine facility operations.[17]

Day-of-Surgery Preparation

Nursing Role. Day-of-surgery preparation will vary a great deal depending on whether the patient is an inpatient or an outpatient. The nursing responsibilities immediately before surgery include final preoperative teaching, assessment and communication of pertinent findings, ensuring that all preoperative preparation orders have been completed, and ensuring that records and reports are present and complete to accompany the patient to the OR (Fig. 18-1). It is especially important to verify the presence of a signed operative consent, laboratory data, a history and physical examination report, a record of any consultations, baseline vital signs, and nurses' notes complete to that point. In addition, the site and side of the anticipated surgery may be marked with an indelible marker and documented to indicate agreement with the patient.[13]

If the patient is an inpatient, the hospital nurse is responsible to ensure that the patient is ready and appropriately prepared for surgery. If the patient is an outpatient, the patient or family member will share the responsibility for preoperative preparation.

Hospitals may require that a patient wear a hospital gown with no underclothes, whereas surgery centers may allow the patient to wear underwear, depending on the surgical procedure to be performed. The patient should not wear cosmetics because observation of skin color will be important. Nail polish and artificial nails should be removed so that capillary refill and pulse oximetry can be assessed. An identification band is put on the patient and, if applicable, an allergy band. All patient valuables are returned to a family member or secured according to institutional protocol. If the patient prefers not to remove a wedding ring, the ring can be taped securely to the finger to prevent loss. All prostheses, including dentures, contact lenses, and glasses, are generally removed to prevent loss or damage to them. Hearing aids may be left in place to allow the patient to better follow instructions. Glasses and hearing aids must be returned to the patient as soon as possible following surgery.

The patient should be encouraged to void before preoperative medications are administered if the medications will interfere with maintaining balance and increase the risk for a fall when ambulating to the bathroom. The patient should also have an empty bladder on transfer to the OR to prevent involuntary elimination under anesthesia and reduce the possibility of urinary retention during early postoperative recovery. The use of a preoperative checklist (Table 18-9) ensures that all preoperative preparations have been completed before the patient is given any sedating medications.

Preoperative Medications. Preoperative medications are used for a variety of reasons. A patient may receive a single drug or a combination of drugs. Benzodiazepines and barbiturates are used for their sedative and amnesic properties. Anticholinergics are given to reduce secretions. Opioids may be given to decrease intraoperative anesthetic requirements and to decrease pain. Antiemetics may be given to decrease nausea and vomiting. Table 18-10 identifies common preoperative medications and the purposes of their use preoperatively.

Other medications that may be administered preoperatively include antibiotics, eyedrops, and routine prescription drugs. Antibiotics may be administered throughout the perioperative period for a patient with a history of congenital or valvular heart disease to prevent the development of infective endocarditis. Antibiotics may also be ordered for the patient undergoing surgery where wound contamination is either a potential risk (e.g., gastrointestinal surgery) or where wound infection could have serious postoperative consequences (e.g., cardiac and joint replacement surgery). Antibiotics are most commonly administered intravenously (IV) and may be started either preoperatively or in the OR.

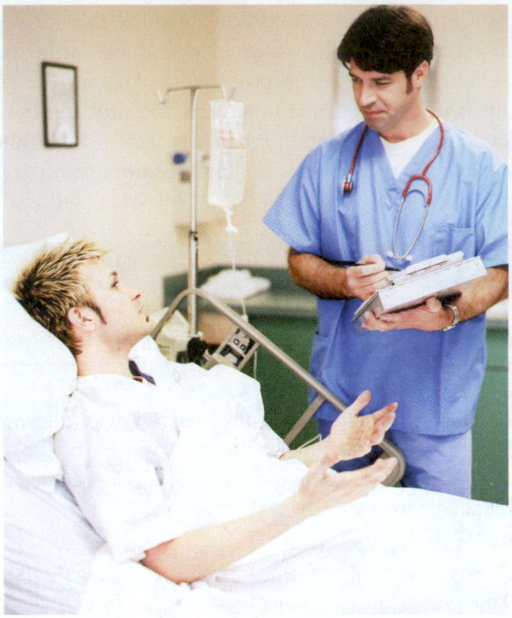

FIG. 18-1 The nurse makes final preoperative preparations with the patient before he goes to surgery.

Eyedrops are commonly ordered and administered preoperatively for the patient undergoing cataract and other eye surgery. Many times the patient will require multiple sets of eyedrops administered at 5-minute intervals. It is important to administer these drugs as ordered and on time to adequately prepare the eye for surgery.

Medications that patients routinely use for health maintenance or disease management may or may not be used on the day of surgery. To facilitate patient teaching and eliminate confusion about which medications should be taken, the nurse should carefully check written preoperative orders and clarify the orders with the surgeon and/or ACP if there is any question.

Premedications may be administered orally (PO), IV, subcutaneously (SC), or intramuscularly (IM). Oral medications are given 60 to 90 minutes before the patient goes to the OR unless otherwise ordered. Because patients are fluid restricted before surgery, the patient should swallow these medications with a minimal amount of water. IM and SC injections are usually to be given 30 to 60 minutes before arrival at the OR (minimally 20 minutes). Intravenous medications are usually administered to the patient after arrival in the preoperative holding area or operating room. The patient should be informed about the expected effects of the medications, such as relaxation, drowsiness, and dryness of the mouth.

Transportation to the Operating Room

If the patient is an inpatient, the OR staff sends transport personnel to the patient's room with a cart to transport the patient to surgery. The nurse assists the patient in transferring from the hospital bed to the OR cart, and the side rails of the cart are raised and secured. The nurse should ensure that the completed chart goes with the

TABLE 18-9 Preoperative Checklist

Preoperative Requirements	Initials	Day of Surgery	Initials
Height _____ Weight _____		Surgical site marked Y N NA	
Isolation? _____ Type _____		ID band on patient	
Allergies noted on chart		Allergy band on patient Y NA	
Vital signs (Initial) T ____ P ____ R ____ BP ____		Vital signs Time _____ T ____ P ____ R ____ BP ____	
Chart Review		**Procedures**	
H&P on chart		NPO since _____	
H&P within 30 days? Y N		Capillary blood glucose Y NA	
Signed and witnessed informed consent form on chart		Preoperative skin prep Y NA	
		Shower Scrub Shave	
Signed consent for blood administration Y NA		Makeup, nail polish, false fingernails, and false eyelashes removed Y NA	
Blood type and cross match Y NA		Hospital gown applied Y NA	
Name plate on chart		**Valuables** Y or N	
Old chart requested and sent Y NA		Dentures _____	
Diagnostic Results		Wig or hairpiece _____	
Hb/ Hct ____/____ NA		Eyeglasses _____	
PT/INR/PTT ____/____/____ NA		Contact lenses _____	
CXR _____ NA		Hearing aid _____	
ECG _____ NA		Prosthesis _____	
Other labs		Jewelry _____	
		Clothing _____	
Final chart review:		Disposition of valuables:	
New forms added		Family Rings taped Safe	
Signed off		Voided/catheter Time: _____	
		Preoperative medications given	
		Time _____ NA	
		Preoperative antibiotics given	
		Time _____ NA	

Time to OR _____ Date _____
Transported to OR by _____
Final Check by _____ RN

CXR, Chest x-ray; *ECG*, electrocardiogram; *H&P*, history and physical examination; *Hb*, hemoglobin; *Hct*, hematocrit; *INR*, international normalized ratio; *NPO*, nothing by mouth; *PT*, prothrombin time, *PTT*, partial thromboplastin time.

TABLE 18-10 *DRUG THERAPY* Commonly Used Preoperative Medications

Class	Drug	Purpose and Effects
Benzodiazepines	midazolam (Versed) diazepam (Valium) lorazepam (Ativan)	Reduce anxiety, amnesic effects Induce sedation Induce amnesia
Opioids	morphine meperidine (Demerol) fentanyl (Sublimaze)	Relieve discomfort during preoperative procedures
Histamine (H_2)-receptor antagonists	cimetidine (Tagamet) famotidine (Pepcid) ranitidine (Zantac)	Decrease HCl acid secretion Increase gastric pH Decrease gastric volume
Antiemetics	metoclopramide (Reglan) droperidol (Inapsine) ondansetron (Zofran)	Increase gastric emptying Decrease nausea and vomiting Prevent nausea and vomiting
Anticholinergics	atropine glycopyrrolate (Robinul) scopolamine	Decrease oral and respiratory secretions Prevent bradycardia

patient, as well as any ordered preoperative equipment, such as antiembolism devices or the patient's inhaler. In many institutions the family may accompany the patient to the holding area.

In an ambulatory surgical center, the patient may be transported to the OR by cart or wheelchair, or, if no sedatives have been administered, the patient may even walk accompanied to the OR. In all cases it is important for the nurse to ensure patient safety during transport. The method of transportation and the person who transported the patient should be documented by the nurse responsible for the transfer.

The family should be instructed where to wait for the patient during surgery. Many hospitals have a surgical waiting room where OR personnel communicate the status of the patient to the family. It is in this waiting room that the surgeon can locate the family after surgery and where families can be notified that the surgery is complete. Some hospitals provide pagers to waiting family members so that they may eat or do errands during the surgery.

While the patient is in surgery the inpatient nurse should have the patient's room prepared for the postoperative arrival. Any additional necessary equipment, including IV poles, oxygen, suction, and additional pillows for positioning, should also be placed in the room. The room also is organized to facilitate entry of the transport cart.

CULTURALLY COMPETENT CARE
PREOPERATIVE PATIENT

The nurse should include cultural and ethnic considerations when assessing and implementing care for the preoperative needs of a patient. For example, culture might determine one's expression of pain coping strategies, family expectations, and ability to verbally express needs. Cultural considerations may require that the family be included in any decision making. For example, many older Hispanic women may defer to their family for the decision to have or not to have surgery. These decisions must be respected and valued. If the patient and family do not speak English, it is essential that the services of a competent translator are obtained. Hospitals are now required to provide translators for common languages other than English. (Culturally competent care is discussed in Chapter 3.)

GERONTOLOGIC CONSIDERATIONS
PREOPERATIVE PATIENT

Many surgical procedures are performed on patients older than 65 years of age. Surgery can even be safely performed on patients in their nineties. Surgery on the elderly requires careful evaluation. Frequently performed procedures in the older adult are cataract extraction, coronary and vascular procedures, prostate surgery, herniorrhaphy, cholecystectomy, and hip repair.

The nurse must be particularly alert when assessing and caring for the older adult surgical patient. An event that has little effect on a younger patient may be overwhelming to the older patient. Emotional reactions to impending surgery and hospitalization often intensify in the older adult. To the older patient, hospitalization may represent a physical decline and loss of health, mobility, and/or independence. The older adult may view the hospital as a place to die or as a stepping-stone to nursing home placement. The nurse can be instrumental in decreasing anxieties and fears, as well as maintaining and restoring the self-esteem of the older adult during the surgical experience.

The risks associated with anesthesia and surgery increase in the older patient.[3] In general, the older the patient, the greater the risk of complications after surgery. It is important to consider the physiologic status or condition of the patient in planning care and not simply the chronologic age. The surgical risk in the older adult relates to normal physiologic aging and changes that compromise organ function, reduce reserve capacity, and limit the body's ability to adapt to stress. This decreased ability to cope with stress, frequently compounded by the additional burden of one or more chronic illnesses, and the surgery itself increases the risk of complications.

When preparing the older adult for surgery, it is important to obtain a detailed history and complete physical examination. Preoperative laboratory tests, an ECG, and a chest x-ray can be important in planning the choice and technique of anesthesia. The patient's primary physician is usually not the surgeon, and frequently several physicians are involved in the patient's care. It is important for the nurse to help coordinate the care and the physicians' orders for the patient.

Consideration of family support is important with the older adult. With the increase in outpatient surgical procedures and shorter postoperative hospitalization, family support is an important consideration in the continuity of care for the older patient.

The nurse must remember that many older adults have sensory deficits. Vision and hearing may be diminished, and bright lights may bother those with eye problems. Thought processes and cognitive abilities may be slowed or impaired. Sensory function and cognition must be assessed and documented. Physical reactions are often slowed as a result of mobility and balance problems. All of these changes may require more time for the older adult to complete preoperative testing and understand preoperative instructions. These changes also require attention to promote patient safety and prevent injury.

When older adults live in some type of long-term care facility, transportation from these agencies must be coordinated so that timely arrival allows for surgery preparation. A legal representative of the patient must be present to provide consent for surgery if the patient cannot sign for himself or herself.

Following surgery the patient may experience additional stress from the changes and losses (perceived or real) because of the surgical procedure. The threat to independence, lifestyle, and self-esteem may result in ineffective coping. The nurse must be particularly supportive and help the older adult cope with the surgical experience.

CRITICAL THINKING EXERCISE
CASE STUDY

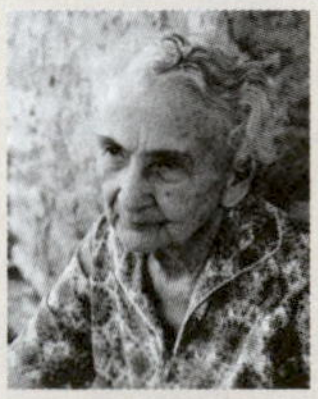

Case Study photo ©iStockphoto.com/ bbear.

Preoperative Patient

Patient Profile. Mrs. Frances Delarosa, an 82-year-old Hispanic retired librarian, is admitted to the hospital with compromised circulation of the right lower leg and a necrotic right foot. She is a diabetic and takes insulin to maintain appropriate blood glucose levels. She has not had anything to eat since last night at 8:00 PM. It is now 1:00 PM in the afternoon of the next day (surgery day).

Subjective Data
- History of type 2 diabetes mellitus for 40 years
- History of renal problems
- History of vision problems
- Surgical history that includes a cesarean section at age 30 and a cholecystectomy at age 65; did not heal well following the last surgery
- Blood glucose has not been well controlled
- Social security checks barely cover the cost of living and medications
- Lives alone but has family who want her to move in with them following surgery
- Uses herbs to control blood glucose levels and frequently refuses to take insulin

Objective Data

Physical Examination
- Alert, cognitively intact, anxious, thin, elderly woman with complaints of numbness and lack of feeling in right leg
- Weight 110 lb, height 5 ft 3 in
- Wears glasses for close work and reading
- Has macular degeneration in right eye

Diagnostic Studies
- Admission laboratory blood glucose level was 537 mg/dl (29.8 mmol/L)
- Morning finger-stick blood glucose level was 97 mg/dl (5.39 mmol/L)
- Doppler pulses for lower leg very weak; absent in right foot
- Doppler pulses in left leg present, weak in left foot
- Serum creatinine 2.5 mg/dl (221 mmol/L)

Collaborative Care
- Scheduled for a below-the-knee amputation of the right leg as the last case of the day.

Critical Thinking Questions

1. What factors may influence Mrs. Delarosa's response to hospitalization and surgery?
2. Given Mrs. Delarosa's history, what preoperative nursing assessments would you want to complete and why?
3. What potential perioperative complications might you expect for Mrs. Delarosa?
4. What topics would you include in Mrs. Delarosa's preoperative teaching plan?
5. What is the priority nursing intervention for Mrs. Delarosa?
6. Based on the assessment data presented, identify one or more appropriate nursing diagnoses. What would be your plans and interventions for those diagnoses? Are there any collaborative problems?

NCLEX EXAMINATION REVIEW QUESTIONS

The number of the question corresponds to the same-numbered objective at the beginning of the chapter.

1. Which of the following surgical procedures involves removal of a body organ?
   a. Colostomy
   b. Laparotomy
   c. Mammoplasty
   d. Cholecystectomy
2. One of the most important goals of the preoperative assessment by the nurse is to
   a. determine if the patient's psychologic stress is too high to undergo surgery.
   b. identify what information the patient needs to give voluntary, informed consent for surgery.
   c. establish baseline data for comparison of the patient's status in the intraoperative and postoperative period.
   d. determine whether the patient's surgery should be done as an inpatient, an outpatient, or a same-day admission.
3. A patient who is scheduled for a hysterectomy reports using ginkgo biloba to improve her memory. Which of the following questions is the most important for the perioperative nurse to ask the patient?
   a. "How long have you used ginkgo biloba?"
   b. "How have you been able to tell if this herb is effective?"
   c. "Have you been taking this herb during the last several weeks?"
   d. "Have you experienced any side effects of taking this herbal product?"
4. The nurse's role in informed consent for surgery may include
   a. obtaining the patient's signature on the consent form.
   b. asking the patient for consent for the planned procedure.
   c. explaining the risks and consequences of the proposed surgery.
   d. informing the patient of the prognosis if the surgical procedure is refused.
5. A nursing intervention to assist a preoperative patient in coping with fear of pain would be to
   a. describe the degree of pain expected.
   b. explain the availability of pain medication.
   c. divert the patient when talking about pain.
   d. inform the patient of the frequency of pain medication.
6. The nursing measure that should be performed last on the morning of surgery is to
   a. ask patient to void in the bathroom.
   b. check chart for signed consent form.
   c. administer preanesthetic medications.
   d. lock up the patient's jewelry and money.
7. The nurse administering preoperative medications recognizes that
   a. preoperative medications may help reduce anesthetic requirements.
   b. intravenous medications can be administered only by an anesthesiologist on the day of surgery.
   c. a preoperative diazepam (Valium) tablet should be administered within 15 minutes of scheduled surgery.
   d. an intramuscular injection of secobarbital (Seconal) should be administered 2 hours before the scheduled surgery.
8. A primary consideration in the instruction of the older preoperative patient is
   a. using large-print material.
   b. teaching early in the morning.
   c. standing very close to aid communication.
   d. recognizing that cognitive function may be decreased.

REFERENCES

1. Nash MJ, Cohen H: Management of Jehovah's Witness patients with hematological problems, *Blood Reviews* 18:21, 2004.
2. Snyder CR, et al: Hope theory: updating a common process for psychological change. In Snyder CR, Ingram RE, editors: *Handbook of psychological change: psychotherapy processes and practices for the 21st century,* New York, 2000, Wiley.
3. Steele SM, Nielsen KC, Klein SM: *Ambulatory anesthesia and perioperative analgesia*, New York, 2005, McGraw-Hill.
4. American Society of Anesthesiologists: What you should know about your patients' use of herbal medicines and other dietary supplements. Available at *www.asahq.org/clinical/physicalstatus.htm* (accessed May 20, 2006).

5. Latex allergy, protect yourself, protect your patients, *Nursing World: Workplace Issues.* Available at *www.nursingworld.org/dlwa/osh/wp7.htm#1* (accessed May 20, 2006).
6. Patients and consumers: tips to remember: latex allergy, *American Academy of Allergy and Immunology,* 2003. Available at *www.aaaai.org/patients/publicedmat/tips/latexallergy.stm* (accessed August 1, 2005).
7. Saufl NM: Preparing the older adult for surgery and anesthesia, *J Perianesth Nurs* 19(6):372, 2004.
8. Yalamarthi S: Perioperative steroids in surgical patients, *Royal College of Surgeons at Edinburgh. Surgical Knowledge and Skills.* Available at *www.edu.rcsed.ac.uk/lectures/lt4.htm* (accessed May 20, 2006).
9. MacKay D, Miller AL: Nutritional support for wound healing, *Alternative Medicine Review* 8:359, 2003.
10. Harris CL, Frasier C: Malnutrition in the institutionalized elderly: the effects on wound healing, *Ostomy Wound Management* 50:54, 2004.
11. Sjaastad O, Bakketeig LS: Caffeine-withdrawal headache: the Vaga study of headache epidemiology, *Cephalalgia* 24:241, 2004.
12. Joint Commission on Accreditation of Healthcare Organizations: *Comprehensive accreditation manual for hospitals: the official handbook,* Oakbrook Terrace, Ill, 2005, The Joint Commission.
13. AORN position statement on correct site surgery. *AORN Online*, 2003. Available at *www.aorn.org/about/positions/correctsite.htm* (accessed May 20, 2006).
*14. Kramer FM: Patient perceptions of the importance of maintaining preoperative NPO status, *AANA J* 68:321, 2000.
15. Giving your informed consent. Public information from the American College of Surgeons. Available at *www.facs.org/public_info/operation/consent.html* (accessed August 1, 2005).
16. Yeh EL, Freas G: Consent. eMedicine: instant access to medicine, 2005. Available at *www.emedicine.com/emerg/topic740.htm* (accessed May 20, 2006).
17. Dunn D: Incident reports—their purpose and scope, *AORN J* 78:49, 2003.

RESOURCES

Resources for this chapter are listed in Chapter 20 on p. 396.

For additional Internet resources, see the website for this book at *http://evolve.elsevier.com/Lewis/medsurg.*

*Nursing research–based reference.

It is not how much we do—it is how much love we put into the doing.

Mother Teresa

Nursing Management
Intraoperative Care

19

Anita J. Shoup, Maureen Reilly, and Jack R. Kless**

LEARNING OBJECTIVES

1. Describe the three different areas of the surgery department and the proper attire for each area.
2. Describe the physical environment of the operating room and the holding area.
3. Describe the functions of the members of the surgical team.
4. Identify needs experienced by the patient undergoing surgical procedures.
5. Discuss the role of the perioperative nurse when managing the care of the patient undergoing surgery.
6. Describe basic principles of aseptic technique used in the operating room.
7. Discuss the importance of safety in the positioning of patients.
8. Differentiate between general and regional or local anesthesia, including advantages, disadvantages, and rationale for choice of the anesthetic technique.
9. Identify the basic techniques used to induce and maintain general anesthesia.
10. Discuss techniques for administering local and regional anesthesia.

KEY TERMS

anesthesia care provider, p. 362
anesthesiology, p. 362
conscious sedation, p. 367
epidural block, p. 372
general anesthesia, p. 367
holding area, p. 360
local anesthesia, p. 367
malignant hyperthermia, p. 373
nurse anesthetist, p. 363
regional anesthesia, p. 367
spinal anesthesia, p. 371

Electronic Resources

Supplemental content related to Chapter 19 can be found . . .

Companion CD
- Stress-Busting Kit for Nursing Students
- NCLEX Examination Review Questions
- Comprehensive Glossary

Evolve Website
http://evolve.elsevier.com/Lewis/medsurg
- Content Updates
- Key Points (Printable and CD/MP3 Download)
- Concept Map Creator
- Expanded Audio Glossary
- Key Term Flash Cards
- Electronic Calculators
- WebLinks

Nursing care of the surgical patient requires an understanding of surgery and surgical interventions. This knowledge allows the nurse to monitor the patient's response to the stressors related to the surgical experience. Use of the nursing process during the operative phase of care is necessary as a framework for the delivery of care. The needs of the patient determine the type of nursing care delivered. These needs are based on the current health status of the patient and the type of surgical intervention anticipated.

Historically, surgical interventions have taken place in the traditional environment of the hospital operating room (OR) suite. Advancements in surgical technology, improvements in the administration of anesthesia, and changes in the health care environment have altered where and how surgery is performed. The trend in surgical settings is a decrease of in-hospital surgical procedures and an increase in outpatient procedures in hospitals, surgery centers, and physician offices. Although all surgical specialties are represented in the ambulatory surgery setting, ophthalmology, gynecology, plastic surgery, otorhinolaryngology, orthopedic surgery, and general surgery are the specialties with the highest patient loads. In addition, the demand for some types of surgeries, such as cataracts, may increase by as much as 47% in the next 20 years.[1]

The perioperative nurse must remember that the surgical procedure has the same seriousness and potential for complications regardless of where it is performed. The patient and family members still have the same needs and fears. The nurse must still maintain asepsis in the surgical environment, keep current on new technologies, and continue to be a strong advocate for safe patient care.

Reviewed by Virginia E. Printz-Feddersen, RN, MSN, CNS, Clinical Nurse Specialist, Anesthesia/OR, Lovelace Medical Center, Albuquerque, N.Mex.; and Kathleen R. Wren, CRNA, PhD, Program Director, Louisiana State University Health Science Center School of Nursing, New Orleans, La.
*Contributed section on anesthesia content.

Differences in the ambulatory surgery setting as compared with the traditional in-hospital surgery setting include healthier patient populations, shorter procedures, quicker patient turnovers, and less time available for perioperative teaching of the patient and family.

PHYSICAL ENVIRONMENT OF OPERATING ROOM

Department Layout

The **surgical suite** is a controlled environment designed to minimize the spread of infectious organisms and allow a smooth flow of patients, personnel, and the instruments and equipment needed to provide safe patient care. The suite is divided into three distinct areas: the unrestricted, semirestricted, and restricted areas. The *unrestricted area* is where personnel in street clothes can interact with those in scrub clothing. These areas typically include the points of entry for patients (e.g., holding area), staff (e.g., locker rooms), and information (e.g., nursing station or control desk). The *semirestricted area* includes the peripheral support areas and corridors. Only authorized personnel are allowed access to the semirestricted areas. All personnel in the semirestricted area must wear surgical attire and cover all head and facial hair. In the *restricted area* masks are required to supplement surgical attire. The restricted area can include the ORs, scrub sink areas, and clean core.

In addition, the physical layout is designed to reduce cross-contamination. The flow of clean and sterile supplies and equipment should be separated from contaminated supplies, equipment, and waste by space, time, and traffic patterns.[2] Personnel move supplies from clean areas, such as the clean core, through the OR for surgery, and on to peripheral areas, such as the instrument decontamination area.[2]

Holding Area

The **holding area,** frequently called the preoperative holding area, is a special waiting area inside or adjacent to the surgical suite. The size varies according to hospital design and can range from a centralized area to accommodate numerous patients to a small designated area immediately outside the actual room scheduled for the surgical procedure. In the holding area the perioperative nurse makes the final identification and assessment before the patient is transferred into the OR for surgery. Many minor procedures can also be performed in the holding area, such as inserting intravenous (IV) catheters and arterial lines, removing casts, and drug administration.

In some settings another area for holding is identified as the admission, observation, and discharge (AOD) area. This area is designed to allow early-morning admissions for outpatient surgery, same-day admission, and inpatient holding before surgery. In this holding area the nurse can assess the patient for preoperative data, observe the patient both before and after surgery, and allow recovery for a sufficient length of time before discharge to either the home or an inpatient room. The AOD area significantly affects the patient's stay throughout outpatient surgery and prevents unnecessary overnight stays in the inpatient setting.

Separation from loved ones just before surgery can produce anxiety. This anxiety can be reduced when institutions permit the family or a friend to wait with the patient in the holding area until the patient is transferred to the OR.

Operating Room

The traditional surgical environment, or **operating room (OR),** is a unique acute care setting removed from other hospital clinical units. It is controlled geographically, environmentally, and bacteriologically, and it is restricted in terms of the inflow and outflow of personnel (Fig. 19-1). It is preferable to have the physical location of the OR adjacent to the postanesthesia care unit (PACU) and the surgical intensive care unit for quick transportation of the surgical postoperative patient and close proximity to anesthesia personnel if complications arise. This allows for close collaboration for postanesthesia recovery and intensive care follow-up. Careful consideration of the design, location, and control of the physical environment assists with the prevention of infection and provides physical safety and comfort for the patient.

Several methods are used to prevent the transmission of infection. Filters and controlled airflow in the ventilating systems provide dust control. Positive air pressure in the rooms prevents air from entering the OR from the halls and corridors. Dust-collecting surfaces such as open shelves and tables are omitted. Materials that are resistant to the corroding effects of strong disinfectants are used. The functional design facilitates the practice of aseptic technique by the OR team.

Physical safety and comfort are aided by the use of OR furniture that is adjustable, easy to clean, and easy to move. All equipment is checked frequently to ensure electrical safety. The lighting is designed to provide a low- to high-intensity range for a precise view of the surgical site. A communication system provides a means for the delivery of routine and emergency messages.[3,4]

The privacy of the patient is achieved by restricting the influx of hospital personnel and visitors. The complexity of operative procedures does not allow for the presence of extraneous personnel and visitors (Fig. 19-2).

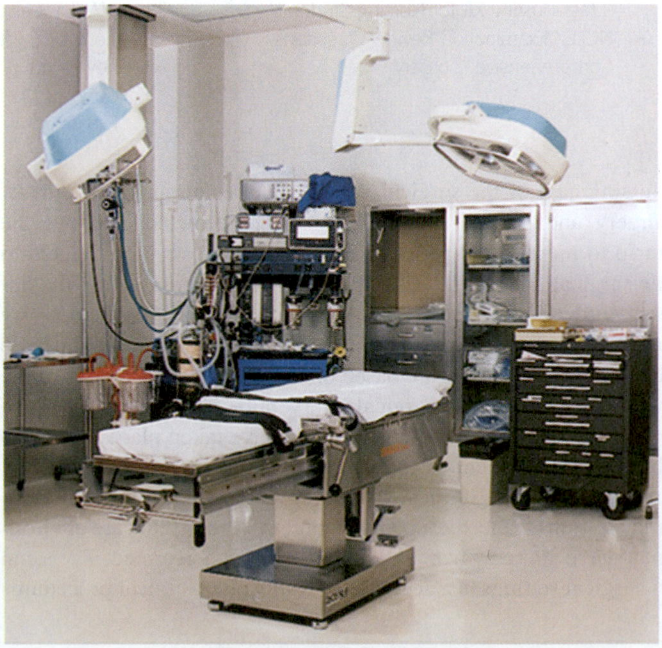

FIG. 19-1 Traditional operating room.

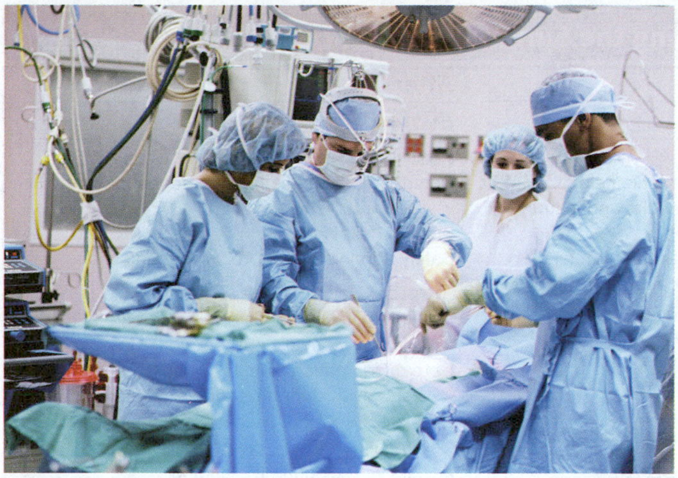

FIG. 19-2 The complexity of the operative procedure does not allow for the influx of extra personnel or visitors.

SURGICAL TEAM

Registered Nurse

The **perioperative nurse** is a registered nurse who implements patient care during the perioperative period based on the nursing process. Before the patient's arrival in the OR, the nurse, through close collaboration with the other members of the surgical team, prepares the OR for the patient. When the patient arrives from home or is transported from the acute care inpatient area to the holding area, the nurse is usually the first member of the surgical team encountered. The nurse is the patient's advocate throughout the intraoperative experience. This encompasses protecting the patient, communicating with the patient, doing things for the patient, and comforting and caring for the patient.[5] The nurse assesses the patient to determine any additional needs or tasks to complete before surgery to meet the patient's individual plan of care. The nurse provides preoperative education regarding the upcoming experience and physical comfort measures. In addition, the nurse works with the patient's family and/or significant others, keeping them informed and answering questions. This is particularly important in day surgery areas where families may have less contact with staff members and must assume greater responsibility for preoperative and postoperative care.[6]

The perioperative nurse may assume functions that involve either sterile or unsterile activities. If the nurse is not scrubbed, gowned, and gloved and remains in the unsterile field, the **function of circulating** is implemented. If the nurse follows the designated scrub procedure, is gowned and gloved in sterile attire, and remains in the sterile field, the **function of scrubbing** is implemented. Some specific intraoperative activities of each function are outlined in Table 19-1.

The perioperative nurse is not limited to task-oriented duties and actively implements nursing care throughout the patient's surgical experience. The majority of behaviors of perioperative nurses reflect critical thinking regarding safe patient care.[7] The nurse must anticipate the needs of not only the patient, but other members of the team as well. Ongoing assessment of the patient is essential because the patient's condition may change quickly. The perioperative nurse responds to these changes and revises the plan of care as needed. Examples of nursing activities that characterize each phase surrounding the surgical experience are presented in Table 19-2.

TABLE 19-1 Intraoperative Activities of the Perioperative Nurse

Circulating/Nonsterile Activities

- Reviews anatomy, physiology, and the surgical procedure.
- Assists with preparing the room.
- Practices aseptic technique in all required activities.
- Monitors practices of aseptic technique in self and others.
- Ensures that needed items are available and sterile (if required).
- Checks mechanical and electrical equipment and environmental factors.
- Identifies and admits the patient to the OR suite.
- Assesses the patient's physical and emotional status.
- Plans and coordinates the intraoperative nursing care.
- Checks the chart and relates pertinent data.
- Admits the patient to the operating room suite.
- Assists with transferring the patient to the operating room bed.
- Ensures patient safety in transferring and positioning the patient.
- Participates in insertion and application of monitoring devices.
- Assists with the induction of anesthesia.
- Monitors the draping procedure.
- Documents intraoperative care.
- Records, labels, and sends to proper locations tissue specimens and cultures.
- Measures blood and fluid loss.
- Records amount of drugs used during local anesthesia.
- Coordinates all activities in the room with team members and other health-related personnel and departments.
- Counts sponges, needles, and instruments.
- Accompanies the patient to the postanesthesia recovery area.
- Reports information relevant to the care of the patient to the recovery area nurses.

Scrubbed/Sterile Activities

- Reviews anatomy, physiology, and the surgical procedure.
- Assists with preparation of the room.
- Scrubs, gowns, and gloves self and other members of the surgical team.
- Prepares the instrument table and organizes sterile equipment for functional use.
- Assists with the draping procedure.
- Passes instruments to the surgeon and assistants by anticipating their needs.
- Counts sponges, needles, and instruments.
- Monitors practices of aseptic technique in self and others.
- Keeps track of irrigation solutions used for calculation of blood loss.
- Reports amounts of local anesthesia and epinephrine solutions used by ACP and/or surgeon.

ACP, Anesthesia care provider.

The nurse in the circulating role documents the nursing care of the patient. Documentation may be written or electronic. Documentation of the assessment and identification of clinical problems, diagnoses, and intervention differentiates the perioperative nurse's role from other members of the surgical team.

The perioperative nurse has the opportunity to become certified in the specialty. Certification reflects expertise and leadership within the surgical and health care communities. The credential is a personal commitment to higher standards that inspires credibility and confidence with patients and peers in the workplace.[8]

TABLE 19-2 Examples of Nursing Activities Surrounding the Surgical Experience

Before	During	After
Assessment	***Implementation***	***Evaluation***
Home/Clinic/Holding Area	**Maintenance of Safety**	**Postanesthesia/Discharge Area**
Initiates preoperative assessment Plans teaching methods appropriate to patient's needs Involves family in interview	Ensures the integrity of the sterile field Ensures that the sponge, needle, and instrument counts are correct Positions the patient to ensure correct alignment, exposure of surgical site, and prevention of injury Prevents chemical injury from prepping solutions, pharmaceuticals, etc. Ensures safe use of electrical equipment, lasers, and radiation Safely administers appropriate medications	Determines patient's immediate response to surgical intervention Monitors vital signs Safely administers appropriate medications
Surgical Unit	**Monitoring of Physical Status**	**Surgical Unit**
Completes preoperative assessment Coordinates patient teaching with other nursing staff Develops a plan of care	Monitors and reports changes in patient's vital signs Monitors blood loss Monitors urine output as applicable	Evaluates effectiveness of nursing care in the OR using patient outcome criteria Determines patient's level of satisfaction with care given during perioperative period Evaluates products used on patient in the OR Determines patient's psychologic status Assists with discharge planning
Surgical Suite	**Monitoring of Psychologic Status**	**Home/Clinic**
Identifies patient Verifies surgical site Assesses patient's level of consciousness, skin integrity, mobility, emotional status, and functional limitations Reviews chart	Provides emotional support to patient Stands near or touches patient during procedures and induction Ensures the patient's right to privacy is maintained Communicates patient's emotional status to other appropriate members of the health care team	Seeks patient's perception of surgery in terms of the effects of anesthetic agents, impact on body image, immobilization Determines family's perceptions of surgery
Planning		
Determines a plan of care that incorporates and respects the patient's value system, lifestyle, ethnicity, and culture; care plan reflects the patient's level of function and ability during the perioperative period Ensures all supplies and equipment needed for surgery are available, functioning properly, and sterile, if appropriate		

OR, Operating room.

Licensed Practical Nurse and Surgical Technologist

In many institutions a surgical technologist or a licensed practical nurse performs the scrubbed function. Surgical technologists may have attended an associate degree program, a vocational training program, or a hospital or military training program. The Association of Surgical Technologists (AST) is a national organization that sets standards for education and provides continuing education opportunities to advance knowledge and skill. Certification as a surgical technologist is available when specific criteria are met.[9]

The person in the scrubbed function assists the surgeon by passing instruments and implementing other technical functions during the surgical procedure. This role is supervised by and can also be assumed by a registered nurse.

Surgeon and Assistant

The *surgeon* is the physician who performs the surgical procedure. The surgeon is primarily responsible for the following:

1. Preoperative medical history and physical assessment, including need for surgical intervention, choice of surgical procedure, management of preoperative workup, and discussion of the risks of and alternatives to surgical intervention
2. Patient safety and management in the OR
3. Postoperative management of the patient

The surgeon's assistant can be a physician who functions in an assisting role during the surgical procedure. The assistant usually holds retractors to expose surgical areas and assists with hemostasis and suturing. In some instances, especially in educational settings, the assistant may perform some portions of the operative procedure under the direct supervision of the surgeon.

In some institutions the surgeon's assistant is a registered nurse or a nonphysician who functions in the role of the assistant under the direct supervision of the physician. Hospital policies define this role and physician responsibility when a nonphysician fills the assistant's position.

Registered Nurse First Assistant

Nursing roles in the perioperative setting change and evolve as technology and health care change. One of these changes is the use of the *registered nurse first assistant* (RNFA). The RNFA works in collaboration with the surgeon to produce an optimal surgical outcome for the patient. The Association of periOperative Registered Nurses (AORN) position statement on RNFAs states that this perioperative nurse must have formal education for this role and works collaboratively with the surgeon, patient, and surgical team by handling tissue, using instruments, providing exposure to the surgical site, assisting with hemostasis, and suturing.[4,10] The RNFA can also obtain certification.

Anesthesia Care Provider

The **anesthesia care provider** (ACP) is one who administers anesthesia and can be an anesthesiologist or a nurse anesthetist. **Anesthesiology** is a discipline within the practice of medicine specializing in the following:

1. Medical management of patients who are rendered unconscious and/or insensible to pain and emotional stress during surgical, obstetric, and certain other medical procedures

2. Protection of life functions and vital organs under the stress of anesthetic, surgical, or other medical procedures
3. Management of problems in pain relief
4. Management of cardiopulmonary resuscitation
5. Management of problems in pulmonary care
6. Management of critically ill patients in special care units

The anesthesiologist is responsible for on-site medical direction of any nonphysician who participates in the delivery of anesthesia care to the patient.[11]

A **nurse anesthetist** is a registered nurse who has graduated from an accredited nurse anesthesia program (minimally a master's degree program) and successfully completed a national certification examination to become a certified registered nurse anesthetist (CRNA). The CRNA scope of practice includes, but is not limited to, the following:

1. Performing and documenting a preanesthetic assessment and evaluation
2. Developing and implementing an anesthetic plan
3. Selecting and initiating the planned anesthetic technique
4. Selecting, obtaining, and administering the anesthesia, adjuvant drugs, accessory drugs, and fluids
5. Selecting, applying, and inserting appropriate noninvasive and invasive monitoring devices
6. Managing a patient's airway and pulmonary status
7. Managing emergence and recovery from anesthesia
8. Releasing or discharging patients from a postanesthesia care area
9. Ordering, initiating, or modifying pain relief therapy
10. Responding to emergency situations by providing airway management, administering emergency fluids, and/or emergency drugs
11. Additional responsibilities within the expertise of the individual[12]

In preparation for and carrying out the surgical procedure, all members of the surgical team (circulating nurse, scrub assistant, surgeon[s], surgeon's assistant, and ACP) collaborate to ensure that the patient receives optimum care.

NURSING MANAGEMENT PATIENT BEFORE SURGERY

The preoperative assessment of the surgical patient establishes baseline data for intraoperative and postanesthesia care. Assessment data provided by the patient and family in the holding area and data from the inpatient nursing units are verified and used to develop a plan of care for the patient.

Psychosocial Assessment

The perioperative nurse who cares for the patient in the OR is knowledgeable about the activities that occur when a patient is transferred into the surgical suite. This knowledge allows for informative and reassuring explanations, especially to the anxious patient. General questions regarding surgery or anesthesia can usually be answered by the perioperative nurse. Examples of these questions include, "When will I go to sleep?" "Who will be in the room?" "When will my doctor arrive?" "How much of my body will be exposed and to whom?" "Will I be cold?" "When will I wake up?" Specific questions relating to details of the surgical procedure and anesthesia may be referred to the surgeon or ACP.

Cultural assessment is essential to understanding the patient's response to the surgical experience (see Chapter 3 for cultural assessment and considerations). For example, members of the Jehovah's Witness community may refuse blood transfusions.[13] For Muslims, the left hand is considered unclean, so the nurse should use the right hand to administer forms, drugs, and treatments.[14] Some Native American patients may request that surgically removed body tissue be preserved so that it may be ritually buried. Some body piercings may also have cultural meaning.[15] An interpreter may be necessary if the patient does not speak English. Spiritual considerations, attitudes, and expression regarding pain and health beliefs and practices should individualize the plan of care.

Physical Assessment

A thorough physical assessment should be made during the preoperative preparation of the patient (see Chapter 18). Physical assessment data that are specifically important to intraoperative nursing care include baseline data such as vital signs, height, weight, and age; allergic reactions to food, drugs, and latex; condition and cleanliness of skin; skeletal and muscle impairments; perceptual difficulties; level of consciousness; nothing-by-mouth (NPO) status; and any sources of pain or discomfort. Vital signs are important as baseline data to evaluate the effects of intraoperative medications and body positioning. Height and weight of the patient guide the nurse regarding the width and length of the OR bed. The need for extra warmth is indicated by the patient's age, metabolic problems, and planned surgical procedures.

Some allergic reactions may be avoided with such simple measures as a change in "prepping" solutions or the type of tape used with dressings.[16] Catastrophic reactions can possibly be avoided if latex sensitivity is determined before the procedure begins. (See the discussion of latex allergies in Chapter 14.) The condition and cleanliness of the skin determine the amount and type of intraoperative skin preparation solutions, and will alert the team to the potential for infection as a result of open or closed skin lesions. Knowledge of skeletal and muscle impairments helps prevent injury during positioning. Knowledge of the presence of piercings will allow jewelry to be removed to prevent site burns when using electrosurgery.[15] Perceptual difficulty, such as a vision or hearing impairment, will guide the nurse in adapting communication techniques to individual needs. An altered level of consciousness necessitates increased safety and protection techniques. Communicating identified sources of pain to other health team members prevents subjecting the patient to unnecessary discomfort.

The increased use of herbs and dietary supplements has increased the risk of complications for patients undergoing surgery. Herbs can potentially inhibit coagulation, alter blood pressure, cause sedation, have cardiac effects, or alter electrolyte levels.[4,17,18] (See the Complementary and Alternative Therapies box in Chapter 18, p. 347.)

Chart Review

Required chart data vary with hospital policy, patient condition, and specific surgical procedures. Because ambulatory surgery facilities tend to have a healthier population, fewer tests may be required. Examples of data that are obtained during the preoperative assessment include the following:

1. History and physical examination
2. Allergies

3. Urinalysis
4. Complete blood cell count
5. Serum electrolyte values
6. Chest x-ray
7. Electrocardiogram (ECG)
8. Other diagnostic tests (e.g., computed tomography [CT] scan, magnetic resonance imaging [MRI])
9. Pregnancy testing (if applicable)
10. Surgical and blood transfusion consent
11. Blood type and crossmatch (if applicable)

This information contributes to an understanding of past and present history, cardiopulmonary status, and potential for infection and other complications.

Admitting the Patient

Hospital policy designates the protocol to be followed when admitting the patient to the holding area and OR suite. A general routine includes initial greeting, extension of human contact and warmth, and proper identification. The identification process includes asking the patient to state her or his name, the surgeon's name, and the operative procedure and location. In addition, the hospital identification numbers are compared with the patient's own identification band and chart. The patient may be further identified by the surgeon before anesthesia induction. In some institutions, identification takes place in the holding area; in others, it takes place in the OR itself.

Complementary and alternative therapies such as therapeutic touch, aromatherapy, music therapy, guided imagery, humor, and even movies are some of the therapies that are being used for surgical patients. (See the Complementary and Alternative Therapies box at right and Scripps Center for Integrative Medicine in Chapter 8, p. 108.) These therapies may decrease anxiety, promote relaxation, reduce pain, and accelerate the healing process.[4,19-23] In some facilities these are initiated before the patient's admission to the OR. In others, such as ambulatory settings, they may be started after the patient's arrival in the holding area.

The admitting procedure is continued with reassessment of the patient and with time allowed for last-minute questions. The nurse completes the review of the chart for the previously mentioned data and notes any abnormalities or changes. The patient is questioned concerning valuables, prostheses, and last intake of food and fluid. Validation is made that the correct preoperative medication was given, if ordered. A warm blanket, pillow, or position adjustment is provided if the patient is uncomfortable. Most hospitals require the patient's hair to be covered just before transfer to the OR suite to reduce potential shedding.

COMPLEMENTARY AND ALTERNATIVE THERAPIES

Music Therapy

Clinical Uses

Music can be used to (1) decrease stress, anxiety, and pain; (2) improve cognitive functioning; (3) alter mood states; (4) promote relaxation and sleep; and (5) enhance alertness. Music can be used in many different clinical settings, including occupational and physical therapy, elder care facilities, operating or procedure rooms, and hospices. Playing music in the background while a person is seemingly unaware of the music itself can reduce stress.

Preoperatively, music can be used to decrease anxiety. Before and during surgery, music can be used to distract attention of patients from their discomfort and the sounds of the equipment and staff. Surgical patients exposed to music have diminished analgesic and hypnotic requirements during conscious sedation. Postoperatively, music can decrease pain and the need for analgesics.

Effects

Music can have many different physiologic effects. Listening to calming music can result in slower, deeper breathing and a decrease in heart rate and blood pressure. Both of these indicate relaxation. Music with a faster pace can energize a person and promote mental alertness.

Nursing Implications

To be effective, music selection needs to be appropriate for the situation. No single type of music is good for everyone. People have different tastes. It is important that the person likes the music being played. There are no known side effects of this low-cost intervention. It is also well suited as a self-care technique. Combining music with relaxation therapy is more effective than doing relaxation therapy alone. Additional information can be found at *www.musictherapy.org*.

NURSING MANAGEMENT PATIENT DURING SURGERY

Room Preparation

Before transferring the patient into the scheduled OR, the nurse spends significant time preparing the room to ensure privacy, safety, and prevention of infection. Surgical attire (pants and shirts, masks, protective eyewear, and caps or hoods) is worn by all persons entering the OR suite (Fig. 19-3). All electrical and mechanical equipment is checked for proper functioning. Aseptic technique is practiced as each surgical item is opened and placed systematically on the instrument table.[24] Sponges, needles, and instruments are counted to ensure accurate retrieval at the close of the procedure.[25]

During room preparation and during the procedure the functions of the team members are delineated. The scrub person will scrub hands and arms, don sterile gown and gloves, and touch only those items in the sterile field. The circulating nurse remains in the unsterile field and implements those activities that permit touching all unsterile items and the patient. Every person on the surgical team must share the responsibility for monitoring aseptic practice and initiating corrective action when a sterile field is compromised.[4]

Transferring the Patient

Once the patient has been properly identified and the OR has been adequately prepared, the patient is transported into the room for the surgery. Each time a patient is transferred from one bed to another, the wheels of the stretcher should be locked, and a sufficient number of personnel should be available to lift, guide, and prevent accidental falling. Once the patient is on the OR bed, safety straps should be snugly placed across the patient's thighs. At this time the monitor leads (e.g., ECG leads), blood pressure cuff, and pulse oximeter are usually applied and an IV catheter is inserted if it was not in place when the patient arrived from the holding area.

Scrubbing, Gowning, and Gloving

Surgical hand antisepsis is required of all sterile members of the surgical team (scrub assistant, surgeon, and assistant). This is done to eliminate dirt, skin oil, and transient microorganisms; to decrease the

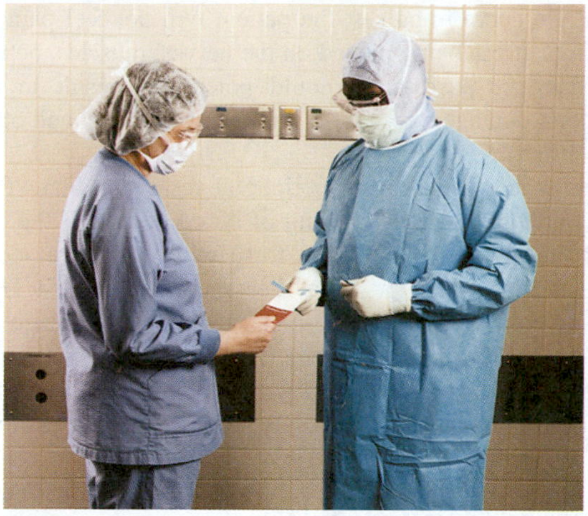

FIG. 19-3 Surgical attire is worn by all persons entering the operating room suite.

microbial count as much as possible; and to inhibit rapid rebound growth of microorganisms.[26,27] The agent used for antisepsis should be an effective antimicrobial agent. It should significantly reduce microorganisms on the skin; contain a nonirritating, antimicrobial preparation; be broad spectrum and fast acting; and have a persistent effect.[26,27] The procedure should be standardized for all personnel. When the procedure of scrubbing is the chosen method for surgical hand antisepsis, the team members' fingers and hands should be scrubbed first with progression to the forearms and elbows. The hands should be held away from surgical attire and higher than the elbows at all times to prevent contamination from clothing or detergent suds and water from draining from the unclean area above the elbows to the clean and previously scrubbed areas of the hands and fingers.[4,26] Waterless, alcohol-based agents are replacing traditional soap and water in many facilities. When a waterless hand rub product is chosen, the team member should first wash and dry hands and forearms with soap and water.[26,27]

Once surgical hand antisepsis is completed, the team members enter the OR to put on the surgical gowns and gloves. Because the gowns and gloves are sterile, it is permissible for the scrubbed people to manipulate and organize all sterile items for use during the procedure.

Basic Aseptic Technique

To prevent infections, aseptic technique is practiced in the OR. This is implemented through the creation and maintenance of a sterile field (Fig. 19-4). The center of the sterile field is the site of the surgical incision. Inanimate items in the sterile field include surgical items and equipment that have been sterilized by appropriate sterilization methods.

There are specific principles that the team members should understand to practice aseptic technique. Unless these principles are followed, the safety of the patient is compromised, and the potential for postoperative infection is increased. Table 19-3 presents basic principles of aseptic technique.[4,24]

In addition to following the principles of aseptic technique, the surgical team is responsible for following the guidelines established by the U.S. Occupational Safety and Health Administration (OSHA) and AORN to protect the patient and the team from exposure to blood-borne pathogens.[28] These guidelines emphasize standard and transmission-based precautions (see Table 15-9); engineering and work practice controls; and the use of personal protective equipment such as gloves, gowns, aprons, caps, face shields, masks, and protective eyewear (see Table 15-8). This is especially important in the OR environment because of the high potential for exposure to blood-borne pathogens.

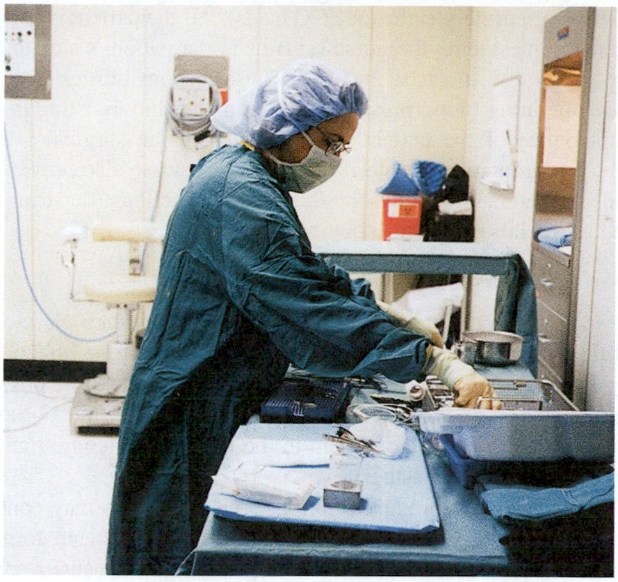

FIG. 19-4 A sterile field is created before surgery.

TABLE 19-3 Principles of Basic Aseptic Technique in the Operating Room

1. All materials that enter the sterile field must be sterile.
2. If a sterile item comes in contact with an unsterile item, it is contaminated.
3. Contaminated items should be removed immediately from the sterile field.
4. Sterile team members must wear only sterile gowns and gloves; once dressed for the procedure, they should recognize that the only parts of the gown considered sterile are the front from chest to table level and the sleeves to 2 inches above the elbow.
5. A wide margin of safety must be maintained between the sterile and unsterile fields.
6. Tables are considered sterile only at tabletop level; items extending beneath this level are considered contaminated.
7. The edges of a sterile package are considered contaminated once the package has been opened.
8. Bacteria travel on airborne particles and will enter the sterile field with excessive air movements and currents.
9. Bacteria travel by capillary action through moist fabrics and contamination occurs.
10. Bacteria harbor on the patient's and the team members' hair, skin, and respiratory tracts and must be confined by appropriate attire.

Assisting the Anesthesia Care Provider

While the perioperative nurse checks the OR to complete its preparation, the anesthesia care provider (ACP) prepares the patient for the administration of the anesthetic. The nurse must understand the mechanism of anesthetic administration and the pharmacologic effects of the agents. The nurse should know the location of all emergency drugs and equipment in the OR area.

The circulating nonsterile perioperative nurse may be involved in placing monitoring devices to be used during the surgical procedure (e.g., urinary catheter, ECG leads).[29] If the patient is to have a general anesthetic, the nurse remains at the patient's side to ensure safety and to assist the ACP. These responsibilities may include obtaining blood pressure measurements and assisting in the maintenance of the patient's airway. During the surgical procedure, the circulating nonsterile perioperative nurse also provides a vital communication link for the ACP to ancillary departments such as the laboratory or blood bank.

Safety Considerations

All surgical procedures, regardless of where they take place, can put the patient at risk for injury. These injuries can be infections, physical trauma from positioning or equipment used, or physiologic effects of surgery itself. The perioperative nurse must be alert to all safety issues as the patient in the OR is often compromised from the effects of anesthesia.

Smoke particles produced during laser procedures may contain trace hydrocarbons, including acetone, isopropanol, toluene, formaldehyde, and cyanide. These airborne contaminates can cause respiratory irritation and have mutagenic and carcinogenic potential. Smoke evacuators may be used to minimize this exposure. Care must be taken with correct placement of the grounding pad and all aspects of the electrosurgical equipment to prevent injury from burns or fire.[30]

The Joint Commission on Accreditation of Healthcare Organizations (JCAHO) developed the first National Patient Safety Goals. These goals are intended to assist accredited health care institutions address patient safety concerns. Preventing wrong site, wrong procedure, and wrong surgery has become known as the *Universal Protocol*.[31] AORN has developed a position statement regarding correct site surgery and guidelines for implementing the Universal Protocol.[32] All members of the surgical team stop what they are doing during a *surgical time-out* just before the procedure is started to verify patient identification, surgical procedure, and surgical site.

Positioning the Patient

Positioning the patient is a critical part of every procedure and usually follows administration of the anesthetic. The ACP will indicate when to begin the positioning. The position of the patient should allow for accessibility to the operative site, administration and monitoring of anesthetic agents, and maintenance of the patient's airway. When positioning for the surgical procedure, care must be used to (1) provide correct skeletal alignment; (2) prevent undue pressure on nerves, skin over bony prominences, and eyes; (3) provide for adequate thoracic excursion; (4) prevent occlusion of arteries and veins; (5) provide modesty in exposure; and (6) recognize and respect individual needs such as previously assessed aches, pains, or deformities. It is a nursing responsibility to secure the extremities, provide adequate padding and support, and obtain sufficient physical or mechanical help to avoid unnecessary straining of self or patient.[33]

Various positions in which the patient may be placed include supine, prone, Trendelenburg, lateral, kidney, lithotomy, jackknife, and sitting. The supine is the most common position used. It is suited for surgery involving the abdomen, heart, and breast. The prone position allows easy access for back surgeries (e.g., laminectomies). The lithotomy position is used for some types of pelvic organ surgery (e.g., vaginal hysterectomy).

Whatever position is required for the procedure, great care is taken to prevent injury to the patient. Because anesthesia has blocked the nerve impulses, the patient will not feel pain or discomfort, or stress being placed on the nerves, muscles, bones, and skin. Improper positioning could potentially result in muscle strain, joint damage, pressure ulcers, nerve damage, and other untoward effects.

General anesthesia causes peripheral vessels to dilate. Position changes affect where the pooling of blood occurs. If the head of the OR bed is raised, the lower torso will have increased blood volume and the upper torso may become compromised. Hypovolemia and cardiovascular disease can further compromise the patient's status. Consequently the perioperative nurse, working with the entire surgical team, carefully plans and implements the patient's positioning, and then closely monitors the patient throughout the surgical procedure.[4]

Preparing the Surgical Site

The purpose of skin preparation, or "prepping," is to reduce the number of organisms available to migrate to the surgical wound. The task of prepping is usually the responsibility of the circulating nurse.

The skin is prepared by mechanically scrubbing or cleansing around the surgical site with antimicrobial agents identified as being nonallergenic to the patient. Hair that will interfere with the surgical procedure is removed. The area is then scrubbed in a circular motion. The principle of scrubbing from the clean area (site of the incision) to the dirty area (periphery) is observed at all times. A liberal area is cleansed to allow for added protection and unexpected occurrences during the procedure.[34]

After preparation of the skin, the sterile members of the surgical team drape the area. Only the site to be incised is left exposed.

Patient After Surgery

Through constant observation of the surgical progress, the ACP anticipates the end of the surgical procedure and uses appropriate types and doses of anesthetic agents so that their effects will be minimal at the end of the surgical procedure. This also allows greater physiologic control of the patient during the transfer to the postanesthesia care unit (PACU).

The patient's response to nursing care is evaluated by the OR nurse based on outcome criteria established during the development of the patient's plan of care. These outcome criteria are published as the *Perioperative Nursing Data Set (PNDS)* by AORN. The PNDS reflects standards and recommended practices related to the delivery of nursing care in any perioperative setting.[4,35,36]

The ACP and the perioperative nurse or another member of the surgical team accompany the patient to the PACU. A report of the patient's status and the procedure is communicated to the nurse receiving the patient in the PACU to promote safe, continuing care.

Anesthesia

The art and science of anesthesia has dramatically changed in the last 20 years. Agents and equipment have become more plentiful, and monitoring systems have become more sophisticated in the information that they provide. These changes have led to a number of new techniques and modes of delivery of anesthetic agents. To provide effective care for the patient during surgery, it is important that the perioperative nurse have an understanding of the types of anesthetics and the role of the perioperative nurse in their delivery.

The anesthetic technique and agents are selected by the ACP in collaboration with the surgeon and the patient. However, the ultimate responsibility for the choice of anesthetic remains the responsibility of the ACP. Factors contributing to the decision include the patient's current health status and history, emotional stability, and factors relating to the operative procedure (e.g., length, position, site). An absolute contraindication of any anesthetic technique is patient refusal. The ACP validates this information during the preoperative assessment, obtains anesthesia consent, writes orders for the preoperative medication, and assigns the patient an anesthesia classification. The American Society of Anesthesiologists' (ASAs') physical status classification, an independent guideline for the ACP, is based on the physiologic status of the patient with no regard to the surgical procedure to be performed. A scale of 1 to 6 is used, with 1 assigned to a healthy patient, 5 assigned to a patient not expected to survive the operation because of multiorgan dysfunction, and 6 assigned to a brain-dead patient who has been designated as an organ donor (see Chapter 18, Table 18-4). An intraoperative complication is more likely to develop with a higher classification number. In addition to the numerical scale, an "E" is added for an emergent procedure that is considered necessary to save life or limb. These physical status classes are dynamic and represent the status of the patient as he or she is immediately before the operative procedure. For example, a healthy 21-year-old man who is in an automobile accident may be classified as a P5E because of severe injuries that require emergent surgery.

CLASSIFICATION OF ANESTHESIA

Anesthesia can be classified according to the effect that it has on the patient's sensorium and pain perception. Four levels of sedation and anesthesia have been defined: (1) At *minimal sedation* the patient responds normally; (2) at *moderate sedation/analgesia (conscious sedation)* airway and cardiovascular function are maintained; (3) at *deep sedation/analgesia* the patient is not easily aroused; and (4) at *anesthesia* level the patient requires assisted ventilation.[37,38]

Moderate sedation/analgesia **(conscious sedation)** is a drug-induced depression of consciousness that retains the patient's ability to maintain her or his own airway and respond appropriately to verbal commands, yet the patient achieves a level of emotional and physical acceptance of a painful procedure (e.g., colonoscopy). Often a combination of anxiolytic (e.g., midazolam [Versed]) and opioid (e.g., fentanyl) drugs is used to provide analgesia, relieve anxiety, and/or provide amnesia.[39] Conscious sedation is also widely used for diagnostic and minor surgical procedures outside of the OR and may be administered by personnel other than anesthesiologists (e.g., nurses) under the direct orders of a physician. Although managing the care of patients receiving conscious sedation falls within the professional nurse's scope of practice, the risks of conscious sedation for the patient are considerable. Complications include airway obstruction, respiratory depression, hypoxia, and hypotension that can develop into clinical emergencies. Only those nurses specially trained in the techniques of conscious sedation should carry out these procedures. Guidelines for sedation by the non-ACP are available from the American Association of Nurse Anesthetists, the American Society of Anesthesiologists, and AORN.[40-42] Nurses providing conscious sedation should comply with these guidelines, the protocols of the employing institution, and the scope of nursing practice identified in applicable state nurse practice acts.

Anesthesia can be classified into general, local, and regional anesthesia. **General anesthesia** is the loss of sensation with loss of consciousness; skeletal muscle relaxation; possible impaired ventilatory and cardiovascular function; and elimination of the somatic, autonomic, and endocrine responses, including coughing, gagging, vomiting, and sympathetic nervous system responsiveness. **Local anesthesia** is the loss of sensation without loss of consciousness. Local anesthesia may be induced topically or via infiltration intracutaneously or subcutaneously. **Regional anesthesia** is the loss of sensation to a region of the body without loss of consciousness when a specific nerve or group of nerves is blocked with the administration of a local anesthetic (e.g., spinal, epidural, or peripheral nerve block).

General Anesthesia

Traditionally, general anesthesia was induced primarily though the use of inhalation agents that provided a complete anesthetic. Today the ACP has the choice of a variety of anesthetic agents and techniques to meet the predominant goal of anesthesia (i.e., to facilitate a faster return to baseline function and thereby decrease the risk of anesthesia).[43] To this end, the IV and inhalation agents used today have a faster onset with a shortened duration of action to facilitate earlier discharge from both the PACU and outpatient surgery facilities.

General anesthesia is usually the technique of choice for patients who (1) are having surgical procedures that require significant skeletal muscle relaxation, last for long periods of time, require awkward positions because of the location of the incision site, or require control of respiration; (2) are extremely anxious; (3) refuse or have contraindications for local or regional anesthetic techniques; and (4) are uncooperative because of their emotional status, lack of maturity, intoxication, head injury, or pathophysiologic processes that do not permit them to remain immobile for any length of time. Phases of general anesthesia are presented in Table 19-4.

General anesthesia may be administered intravenously, by inhalation, or rectally. A balanced technique (use of drugs from different classes) is the most common method used for general anesthesia. Table 19-5 presents common anesthetic drugs with advantages, disadvantages, and nursing interventions that are indicated for patients receiving these agents.

Intravenous Agents. Virtually all routine general anesthetics begin with an IV induction agent. When used during the initial period of anesthesia, these agents induce a pleasant sleep with a rapid onset of action that patients find desirable. A single dose lasts only a few minutes, which is long enough for an endotracheal tube to be placed and an inhalation agent to be started.

Recent advances in IV anesthetics have created a new type of general anesthesia named *total IV anesthesia* (TIVA). All medications are delivered intravenously in TIVA, thus eliminating the need for inhalation agents. However, the patient may still require advanced airway management such as endotracheal intubation and will receive oxygen/air mixtures via the endotracheal tube.

Inhalation Agents. Inhalation agents are the foundation of general anesthesia. The inhalation agents used for general anesthesia may be volatile liquids (liquid at room temperature) or gases (gas at room temperature). Volatile liquids are administered through a specially designed vaporizer after being mixed with oxygen as a carrier gas. This gas mixture is then delivered to the patient via the anesthesia circuit/apparatus.

TABLE 19-4 Phases of General Anesthesia

	Phases			
	Preinduction	**Induction**	**Maintenance**	**Emergence**
Description	Time period starting with preoperative medication, initiation of appropriate IV/arterial access, application of monitors	Initiation of sequence of medications that render the patient unconscious, securing the airway	Time period during which the surgical procedure is performed; patient remains in an unconscious state with appropriate measures to ensure safety of the airway	Time period during which the surgical procedure is completed; patient is prepared for return to consciousness and removal of airway assist devices
ACP role	Preanesthetic assessment • Determination of final anesthetic care plan • Application and monitoring of IV/arterial access	• Administration of appropriate drugs • Securing the airway	• Monitor physiologic status of patient • Administer incremental medications as appropriate	• Reversal of residual neuromuscular blocking agents • Assessment for return of adequate respiratory reflexes and function • Removal of airway assist devices
Role of perioperative nurse related to anesthesia	• Completion of preoperative assessment • Check and confirm operative permits • Complete the "time-out" for patient identification and confirmation of correct procedure and site • Administration of aspiration prophylaxis	• Assist with application of monitors (noninvasive and invasive) • Assist with airway management	• Adjust patient position as necessary • Monitor patient safety	• Assist in placement of dressing • Prepare the patient for movement to PACU
Anticipated classes of drugs to be used	Benzodiazepines Antibiotics Aspiration prophylaxis: • Nonparticulate antacids • H_2-receptor blockers (e.g., cimetidine [Tagamet], famotidine [Pepcid]) • Gastric motility agents (e.g., metoclopramide [Reglan])	Benzodiazepines Opioids Hypnotics Volatile gases	Benzodiazepines Opioids Hypnotics Volatile gases	Reversal agents: • Anticholinergics • Sympathomimetics • Opioid antagonists (prn) • Benzodiazepine antagonists Supplemental narcotics (prn) Antiemetics

ACP, Anesthesia care provider; *IV,* intravenous; *PACU,* postanesthesia care unit.

Inhalation agents enter the body through the alveoli in the lungs. The apparatus used for administration may be a mask, an endotracheal tube, a laryngeal mask airway, or a tracheostomy. Ease of administration and rapid excretion by ventilation make them desirable agents. One undesirable characteristic is the irritating effect of inhalation agents on the respiratory tract. Each agent has its own specific characteristics, which include to what degree irritation of the respiratory tract will occur. Complications that may arise are coughing, laryngospasm (muscular constriction of the larynx), bronchospasm, increased secretions, and respiratory depression.[44] The newer, less soluble agents provide for faster induction and emergence from general anesthesia.

Inhalation agents are most commonly administered via an endotracheal tube placed into the trachea once the patient has been induced with an IV agent. The endotracheal tube permits control of ventilation and airway protection, both for patency and to prevent aspiration. Complications of endotracheal intubation include those primarily associated with its insertion and removal. These include failure to intubate, damage to teeth and lips, laryngospasm, laryngeal edema, postoperative sore throat, and hoarseness caused by injury or irritation of the vocal cords or surrounding tissues.

Adjuncts to General Anesthesia. The administration of general anesthesia is rarely limited to one agent. Drugs added to an inhalation anesthetic (other than an IV induction agent) are termed *adjuncts*. These agents are added to the anesthetic regimen specifically to achieve unconsciousness, analgesia, amnesia, muscle relaxation, or autonomic nervous system control. Adjuncts include opioids, benzodiazepines, neuromuscular blocking agents (muscle relaxants), and antiemetics. It is important for the nurse to know that these agents are often given in combination and may have synergistic or additive effects. In this case, the PACU nurse may observe deeper levels of sedation than would be expected when an agent is given alone. See Table 19-6 for commonly used adjunct agents, their uses during anesthesia, adverse effects, and nursing interventions.

Opioids. Opioids are used preoperatively for sedation and analgesia, intraoperatively for induction and maintenance of anesthesia and analgesia, and postoperatively for pain management. Opioids alter the perception of pain and the response to painful stimuli. When administered before the end of a surgical procedure, the residual analgesia often carries over into the PACU, allowing the patient to awaken relatively pain free.

All opioids produce dose-related respiratory depression.[45] Respiratory depression may be difficult to detect in the OR and

TABLE 19-5 DRUG THERAPY
General Anesthesia

Drugs	Advantages	Disadvantages	Nursing Interventions
Intravenous Agents			
Barbiturates			
thiopental (Pentothal) methohexital (Brevital)	Rapid induction, duration of action less than 5 min	Adverse cardiac effects, hypotension, tachycardia, respiratory depression	Usually have minimal postoperative effects because of extremely short effects Repeated doses may lead to "hangover effect"
Nonbarbiturate Hypnotics			
etomidate (Amidate)	Produces little change in cardiovascular dynamics; useful for hemodynamically unstable patients	Associated with adverse effects of myoclonia, nausea and vomiting, hiccups, and adrenocortical inhibition	Observe for transient skeletal muscle movements (myoclonia), nausea and vomiting, hiccups, hypotension, and hypoglycemia
propofol (Diprivan)	Ideal for short outpatient procedures because of rapid onset of action, rapid distribution, and high metabolic clearance; may be used for maintenance of anesthesia, as well as induction	May cause bradycardia and other dysrhythmias, hypotension; apnea, phlebitis, nausea and vomiting, hiccups May cause hypertriglyceridemia	Short action leads to minimal postoperative effects; monitor injection site for phlebitis; cardiac monitoring if unstable Monitor serum triglycerides every 24 hr for sedation >24 hr
Inhalation Agents			
Volatile Liquids			
halothane (Fluothane) enflurane (Ethrane) isoflurane (Forane) desflurane (Suprane) sevoflurane (Ultane)	All volatile liquids: muscle relaxation, low incidence of nausea and vomiting Halothane: bronchodilation Isoflurane: less cardiac depression, devoid of toxicity to body organs Desflurane: rapid induction and emergence, widely used volatile agent Sevoflurane: predictable effects on cardiovascular and respiratory systems, rapid acting, nonirritating to respiratory system	All volatile liquids: myocardial depression, early onset of pain because of rapid elimination Halothane: hypotension and possible hepatotoxicity Enflurane: increased intracranial pressure, seizures, unpredictable duration of action Sevoflurane: may be associated with emergence delirium	Assess and treat pain during early anesthesia recovery; assess for adverse reactions such as cardiopulmonary depression with hypotension and prolonged respiratory depression; monitor for nausea and vomiting
Gaseous Agents			
nitrous oxide	Potentiates volatile agents, allowing a reduction in their dosage and their negative side effects, and increases the rate of induction; has high analgesic potency	Weak anesthetic, rarely used alone; must be administered with oxygen to prevent hypoxemia; nausea and vomiting more common than with other inhaled anesthetics	Produces little or no toxicity at therapeutic concentrations; monitor for effects of volatile liquids when nitrous oxide used as an adjunct
Dissociative Anesthetic			
ketamine (Ketalar)	Can be administered IV or IM; potent analgesic and amnesic	May cause hallucinations and nightmares, increased intracranial and intraocular pressure, increased heart rate, hypertension	Anticipate administration of a benzodiazepine if agitation and hallucinations occur; calm, quiet environment is essential in postoperative care

therefore requires close observation and pulse oximetry monitoring. Decreased SaO_2 recorded by pulse oximetry is a late sign of respiratory depression. Assessment of respiratory rate and depth is critical in the management of the patient who has received opioids. Opioid-induced respiratory depression can be reversed with naloxone (Narcan). However, its use is often associated with a reversal of the analgesic effects of the opioids as well.

Benzodiazepines. Sedative-hypnotic benzodiazepines are widely used for premedication before surgery for their amnesic effects, as agents for the induction and maintenance of anesthesia, for conscious sedation, as supplemental IV sedation during local and regional anesthesia, and for postoperative anxiety and agitation. Because of its excellent amnesic property, shorter duration of action, and absence of pain on injection, midazolam (Versed) is presently the most frequently used benzodiazepine. The other agents in this drug class are limited in their usefulness because of their long duration of action. In both ambulatory surgery settings and in conscious sedation, midazolam is the most common anesthesia adjunct used. It is commonly administered intravenously or intramuscularly. Flumazenil (Romazicon) is a specific benzodiazepine antagonist that may be used to reverse marked benzodiazepine-induced respiratory depression.[46] However, the use of a reversal agent may also cause unwanted or untoward side effects.

TABLE 19-6 DRUG THERAPY
Adjuncts to General Anesthesia

Agents	Uses during Anesthesia	Adverse Effects	Nursing Interventions
Opioids			
fentanyl (Sublimaze) sufentanil (Sufenta) morphine sulfate meperidine (Demerol) alfentanil (Alfenta) remifentanil (Ultiva) methadone (Dolophine)	Induce and maintain anesthesia, reduce stimuli from sensory nerve endings, provide analgesia during surgery and anesthetic recovery	Respiratory depression, stimulation of vomiting center, possible bradycardia and peripheral vasodilation (when combined with anesthetics), high incidence of pruritus in both regional and IV administration	Assess respiratory status, monitor pulse oximetry findings, protect airway in anticipation of vomiting, use standing orders for antipruritics such as diphenhydramine
Benzodiazepines			
midazolam (Versed) diazepam (Valium) lorazepam (Ativan)	Induce and maintain anesthesia	Potentiation of the effects of opioids, increasing the potential for respiratory depression; hypotension and tachycardia	Monitor cardiopulmonary status, level of consciousness
Neuromuscular Blocking Agents			
Depolarizing agents: succinylcholine (Anectine) Nondepolarizing agents: vecuronium (Norcuron) atracurium (Tracrium) pancuronium (Pavulon) tubocurarine (Tubarine) pipecuronium (Arduan) doxacurium (Nuromax) rocuronium (Zemuron) mivacurium (Mivacron)	Facilitate endotracheal intubation, promote skeletal muscle relaxation (paralysis) to enhance access to surgical sites; effects of nondepolarizing agents are usually reversed toward the end of surgery by the administration of anticholinesterase agents (e.g., neostigmine, pyridostigmine, edrophonium)	Apnea related to paralysis of respiratory muscles, prolonged muscle relaxation because of longer action of nondepolarizing agents than reversal agents, cardiac alterations; recurrence of muscle weakness with correction of hypothermia	Monitor respiratory rate and pattern until patient able to cough and return to previous levels of muscle strength; maintain patent airway; ensure availability of nondepolarizing reversal agents and respiratory support equipment, monitor temperature and levels of muscle strength with temperature changes
Antiemetics			
droperidol (Inapsine) ondansetron (Zofran) dolansetron (Anzemet) metoclopramide (Reglan) prochlorperazine (Compazine) promethazine (Phenergan)	Prevention of vomiting with aspiration during surgery, counteract the emetic effects of inhalation agents and opioids; droperidol often used during surgery; others more often used postoperatively	Droperidol: dysrhythmias, laryngospasm, bronchospasm, tachycardia, hypotension, central nervous system alterations, extrapyramidal reactions, contraindicated in patients with Parkinson's disease or hypomagnesemia Other antiemetics: headache, dizziness, sedation, malaise, fatigue, musculoskeletal pain, shivers, diarrhea, acute dystonic reactions, cardiovascular alterations, contraindicated in patients with hypomagnesemia	Monitor cardiopulmonary status, level of consciousness, and ability to move limbs Droperidol: administer with caution in patients with heart disease

Neuromuscular Blocking Agents. Neuromuscular blocking agents (muscle relaxants) are used as adjuncts to general anesthesia to facilitate endotracheal intubation and to optimize surgical working conditions by providing relaxation (paralysis) of skeletal muscles. Neuromuscular blocking agents interrupt the transmission of nerve impulses at the neuromuscular junction. Succinylcholine (Anectine), the only depolarizing muscle relaxant, works on the nerve side of the neuromuscular junction, whereas all other muscle relaxants (nondepolarizing) act on the muscle side of the junction. The site and mode of action determine whether or not the effects of the drugs can be chemically reversed. Succinylcholine cannot be reversed. The effects of nondepolarizing muscle relaxants are frequently reversed toward the end of the surgery by the administration of anticholinesterase agents (e.g., neostigmine [Prostigmin], pyridostigmine [Mestinon], edrophonium [Tensilon]).[4,47]

Disadvantages of the use of muscle relaxants are of special concern to the ACP and postanesthesia nurse. The duration of their action may be longer than the surgical procedure, or reversal agents may not be effective in completely eliminating the residual effects. Confusion and nausea are known side effects of these drugs because of their central nervous system (CNS) activity. The patient should be carefully observed for airway patency and adequacy of respiratory muscle movement. Change of patient temperature can greatly alter the metabolism and effectiveness of neuromuscular blocking agents. Therefore temperature should be closely monitored. For example, a patient who arrives in the PACU with a temperature of 95.7° F (35.4° C) is strong and easily managing his or her airway. As the patient is warmed to a temperature of 98° F (36.7° C), weakness induced by the action of the neuromuscular blocking drugs may reoccur. Lack of movement or poor return of reflexes and strength may indicate the need for an artificial airway and ventilator. If the patient is intubated, the endotracheal tube should not be removed without careful assessment of return of muscular strength, level of consciousness, and the minute ventilation (respiratory rate times tidal volume [amount of air inhaled and exhaled during a normal ventilation]).

Antiemetics. Antiemetics are used preoperatively, intraoperatively, and postoperatively to prevent and treat nausea and vomiting associated with the administration of anesthesia. Antiemetics are used prophylactically in patients who are most at risk for nausea and vomiting. Risk factors include gender, age, smoking history, history of motion sickness, and history of prior postoperative nausea. At highest risk is the female nonsmoker with a history of motion sickness. An additional risk factor is the surgical procedure. High-risk procedures include abdominal or gynecologic laparoscopic procedures, facial cosmetic procedures, and a variety of ear, nose, and throat (ENT) procedures. Treatment includes the use of medications from more than one drug class along with appropriate hydration. Antiemetics listed in Table 19-7 are most frequently used preoperatively or postoperatively.

Dissociative Anesthesia. Dissociative anesthesia interrupts associative brain pathways while blocking sensory pathways. The patient appears catatonic, is amnesic, and experiences profound analgesia that lasts into the postoperative period. Ketamine (Ketalar) is a commonly administered dissociative anesthetic. Ketamine is particularly advantageous because it can be administered intravenously or intramuscularly; it is a potent analgesic and amnesic. It is used in asthmatic patients undergoing surgery because it promotes bronchodilation and in trauma patients requiring surgery because it increases heart rate and helps maintain cardiac output. Because ketamine is a phencyclidine (PCP) derivative, the drug may cause hallucinations and nightmares, particularly in adult patients, greatly limiting its usefulness.[48]

Local Anesthesia

Local anesthetics block the initiation and transmission of electrical impulses along nerve fibers. With progressive increases in local anesthetic concentration, the transmission of autonomic, then somatic sensory, and finally somatic motor impulses is blocked. This produces autonomic nervous system blockade, anesthesia, and skeletal muscle paralysis in the area of the affected nerve.

Local anesthesia allows an operative procedure to be performed on a particular part of the body without loss of consciousness or sedation. Because there is little systemic absorption of the drug, recovery is rapid with little residual drug "hangover." The duration of action of the local anesthetic frequently carries over into the postoperative period, providing continued analgesia.[49] In addition, the use of a local anesthetic in a regional technique provides an alternative to a general anesthetic in a physiologically compromised patient.

The disadvantages of local anesthetics include the technical difficulty and discomfort that may be associated with injections, inadvertent IV administration producing hypotension and potential seizures, and the inability to precisely match the duration of action of the agents administered to the duration of the surgical procedure.

In ambulatory or outpatient procedures, the nurse may assist a physician in the administration of a peripheral or "field" anesthesia block. Consequently, the nurse must be familiar with the drugs, the methods of administration, and adverse and toxic effects of the drugs. Initial assessment of the patient should include detailed questioning of the patient's history with local anesthetics and any adverse events associated with the use of local anesthetics experienced by the patient or blood relatives.

Many patients report "allergies" to local anesthetics. Although true allergies to local anesthetics occur, they are rare. Allergies are most likely to be a result of additives or preservatives in the preparation. There are two classes of local anesthetics: esters and amides. It is highly unlikely that an individual is allergic to both. Therefore it is important to carefully question the patient concerning the agent and the symptoms experienced so that an agent in the proper class may be selected for the procedure.

Methods of Administration. There are a variety of methods for administering local anesthetics (Table 19-7). Topical application is application of the agent directly to the skin, mucous membranes, or open surface. Eutectic mixture of local anesthetics (EMLA cream), a combination of lidocaine and prilocaine, can be applied to the skin to produce localized dermal anesthesia. EMLA should be applied to the site 30 to 60 minutes before painful procedures. Local infiltration is the injection of the agent into the tissues through which the surgical incision will pass.

Regional (peripheral) nerve block is achieved by the injection of a local anesthetic into or around a specific nerve or group of nerves. Nerve blocks may be used to provide intraoperative anesthesia and postoperative analgesia and for the diagnosis and treatment of chronic pain. Whenever a patient is prepared for regional anesthesia, airway equipment, emergency drugs, and monitors should be immediately available to induce a general endotracheal anesthesia if necessary.

Examples of common regional nerve blocks include brachial plexus, intercostal, and retrobulbar blocks. Intravenous regional nerve block (Bier block) is the IV injection of a local anesthetic into an extremity following mechanical exsanguination using a compression bandage and a tourniquet. A fully functioning tourniquet is a necessity. Function and status of the tourniquet should be checked and documented immediately before use. This type of block provides not only analgesia, but also the ability to work in a bloodless field.

Spinal and Epidural Anesthesia. Spinal and epidural anesthesia are also types of regional anesthesia (Fig. 19-5). **Spinal anesthesia** involves the injection of a local anesthetic into the cerebrospinal fluid found in the subarachnoid space, usually below the level of L2. The local anesthetic mixes with cerebrospinal fluid, and, depending on the extent of its spread, various levels of anes-

TABLE 19-7 Methods for Administering Local Anesthesia

- Topical application
  - Aerosolized
  - Nebulized
- Local infiltration
- Regional injection
  - Peripheral nerve block
  - Intravenous regional block (Bier block)
  - Spinal anesthesia (block)
  - Epidural anesthesia (block)

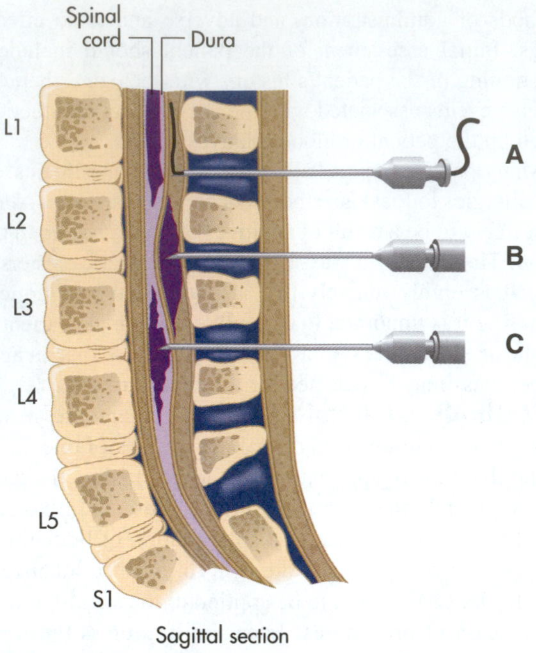

FIG. 19-5 Location of needle point and injected anesthetic relative to dura. *A*, Epidural catheter. *B*, Single-injection epidural. *C*, Spinal anesthesia. (Interspaces most commonly used are L4-5, L3-4, and L2-3.)

thesia are achieved. Because the local anesthetic is administered directly into the cerebrospinal fluid, a spinal anesthetic produces an autonomic, sensory, and motor blockade. Patients experience vasodilation and may become hypotensive as a result of the autonomic block, feel no pain as a result of the sensory block, and are unable to move as a result of the motor block. The duration of action of the spinal anesthetic depends on the agent selected and the dose administered. A spinal anesthetic may be used for procedures involving the lower abdomen, groin, perineum, or lower extremity.[49]

An **epidural block** involves injection of a local anesthetic into the epidural (extradural) space via either a thoracic or lumbar approach. The anesthetic agent does not enter the cerebrospinal fluid, but works by binding to nerve roots as they enter and exit the spinal cord. By using a low concentration of local anesthetic, sensory pathways are blocked, but motor fibers remain intact. In higher doses, both sensory and motor fibers are blocked. Epidural anesthesia may be used as the sole anesthetic for a surgical procedure, or a catheter may be placed to allow for intraoperative use with continued use into the postoperative period to provide analgesia. This method of postoperative analgesia uses lower doses of epidurally administered local anesthetic, usually in combination with an opioid.[49] Epidural anesthesia is commonly used for obstetrics, vascular procedures involving the lower extremities, and hip and knee replacement surgeries.

During the surgical procedure when spinal or epidural anesthesia is used, the patient can remain fully conscious or IV sedation can be achieved. The onset of spinal anesthesia is faster than that seen with an epidural, but the end results with either approach are usually similar. The patient must be closely observed for signs of autonomic nervous system blockade, including hypotension, bradycardia, nausea, and vomiting. There is less autonomic nervous system blockade with epidural anesthesia than with spinal anesthesia. Should "too high" a block be achieved, the patient may experience inadequate breathing and apnea.[49]

One advantage of epidural (extradural) injection over spinal (subarachnoid) injection is a decreased incidence of headache. A headache may be experienced after spinal anesthesia if leakage of spinal fluid occurs at the site of injection. The incidence of headache is decreasing with the common use of smaller-gauge (25 to 27) needles and the use of noncutting, "pencil-point" spinal needles.

Additional Anesthetic Considerations

Controlled hypotension is a technique used to decrease the amount of expected blood loss by lowering the blood pressure during the administration of anesthesia. *Hypothermia* is the deliberate lowering of body temperature to decrease metabolism, thus reducing both the demand for oxygen and anesthetic requirements. *Cryoanesthesia* involves cooling or freezing a localized area to block pain impulses. Acupuncture is also used to produce decreased sensation[50] (see Chapter 8).

GERONTOLOGIC CONSIDERATIONS
PATIENT DURING SURGERY

Although anesthetic agents have become safer and more predictable, the onset, peak, and duration of medications administered by any route are greatly altered in the older adult. Because of this, anesthetic drugs should be carefully titrated when given to older adults. Physiologic changes in aging may alter the patient's response not only to the anesthetic, but also to blood and fluid loss and replacement, hypothermia, pain, and the tolerance of the surgical procedure and positioning. The older adult's response to all anesthetic agents must be carefully monitored and the postoperative recovery assessed before the patient is left without close supervision (e.g., transferred from the PACU to a surgical unit).

Many older adults experience a decrease in their ability to communicate and follow directions as a result of alterations in vision or hearing. These factors pose a special need for clear and concise communication in the OR, especially when preoperative sedation is superimposed on the existing sensory deficit. Because of decreased ability to perceive discomfort or pressure on vulnerable areas and a loss of skin elasticity, the skin of the older adult is at risk for injury from tape, electrodes, warming and cooling blankets, and certain types of dressing. In addition, pooling of solutions used to prepare the skin in dependent areas can quickly create skin burns or abrasions.

The care and vigilance of the entire surgical team is needed in preparing and positioning the older patient. The older adult often has osteoporosis and osteoarthritis. Bad positioning of arthritic joints that may be desensitized by administration of an anesthetic may create long-term injury and disability. Older adults are also at a greater risk of perioperative hypothermia. The use of a variety of warming devices should be considered and carefully monitored if used.

CATASTROPHIC EVENTS IN THE OPERATING ROOM

Unanticipated intraoperative events occasionally occur. Although some might be anticipated (e.g., cardiac arrest in an unstable patient, massive blood loss during trauma surgery), others may occur without warning, demanding immediate intervention by all members of the OR team. Two such events are anaphylactic reactions and malignant hyperthermia.

Anaphylactic Reactions

Anaphylaxis is the most severe form of an allergic reaction, manifesting with life-threatening pulmonary and circulatory complications. The initial clinical manifestations of anaphylaxis may be masked by anesthesia. ACPs administer an array of drugs to patients, such as anesthetics, antibiotics, blood products, and plasma expanders. Because any parenterally administered material can theoretically produce an allergic response, vigilance and rapid intervention are essential. An anaphylactic reaction causes hypotension, tachycardia, bronchospasm, and possibly pulmonary edema. Antibiotics and latex are responsible for many perioperative allergic reactions. (Anaphylaxis is discussed in Chapter 14.)

Latex allergy has become a particular concern in the perioperative setting, given the use of gloves, catheters, and many other devices containing natural rubber latex (NRL). Reactions to NRL have ranged from urticaria to anaphylaxis with symptoms appearing immediately or at some time during the surgical procedure. Latex allergy protocols should be set up in each institution so that a latex-safe environment can be provided in susceptible individuals.[51] (Latex allergies are discussed in Chapter 14.)

Malignant Hyperthermia

Malignant hyperthermia (MH) is a rare metabolic disease characterized by hyperthermia with rigidity of skeletal muscles that can result in death. It occurs in affected people exposed to certain anesthetic agents. Succinylcholine (Anectine), especially in conjunction with the volatile inhalation agents, appears to be the primary trigger of the disorder, although other factors, such as stress, trauma, and heat, have been implicated. When it does occur, it is usually during general anesthesia, but it may manifest in the recovery period as well. It is autosomal dominant in inheritance but is variable in its genetic penetrance, so predictions based on family history are important but inconsistent. (Autosomal dominant disorders are discussed in Chapter 14.) The fundamental defect is hypermetabolism of skeletal muscle resulting from altered control of intracellular calcium, leading to muscle contracture, hyperthermia, hypoxemia, lactic acidosis, and hemodynamic and cardiac alterations.

Tachycardia, tachypnea, hypercarbia, and ventricular dysrhythmias are generally seen but are nonspecific to MH. MH is generally diagnosed after all other causes of the hypermetabolism are ruled out. The rise in body temperature is not an early sign of MH. Unless promptly detected with rapid initiation of appropriate intervention, MH can result in cardiac arrest and death. The definitive treatment of MH is prompt administration of dantrolene (Dantrium), which slows metabolism, along with symptomatic support to correct hemodynamic instability, acidosis, hypoxemia, and elevated temperature. A treatment protocol is available from the Malignant Hyperthermia Association of the United States (available at *www.mhaus.org*) and is usually displayed in the OR.

To prevent MH, it is important for the nurse to obtain a careful family history and be alert to its development perioperatively. The patient known or suspected to be at risk for this disorder can be anesthetized with minimal risks if appropriate precautions are taken. Patients with MH should be informed of the condition so that family members may be genetically tested.[52]

NEW AND FUTURE CONSIDERATIONS

Changes in technology and new developments in science provide new and better treatment modalities for the patient undergoing surgery. Historically, patients having surgery were instructed to be NPO starting at midnight the night before their surgery. The American Society of Anesthesiologists (ASA) published new practice guidelines that are much less stringent (see Table 18-8 and Evidence-Based Practice box in Chapter 18, p. 353). Investigators have determined that ingestion of water, apple juice, black tea and coffee, pulp-free orange juice, and carbonated beverages 2 to 3 hours before surgery has no detrimental effect on the risk factors of gastric aspiration in healthy nonobese adults.[53]

"Bloodless surgery" is becoming more of a reality. Various techniques can minimize blood loss during and after surgery, and allow the surgical team to manage blood loss without the need for a blood transfusion. These include drug therapy and techniques for managing low hematocrit, hemostatic agents to enhance clotting and control bleeding, surgical devices and techniques to locate and stop internal bleeding, and surgical and anesthetic techniques to limit blood loss. There are also new alternatives to blood transfusions such as erythropoietin.[54] Research is also continuing on the development of a synthetic, oxygen-carrying blood alternative.

After years of development and implementation in other fields, robotics is now a technology in the OR as robots are being used to assist in surgery. The use of robots for surgery is expected to grow over the next 5 years. Although the first surgical systems were passive robotic aides, today most robotic aides have active mechanisms with a degree of autonomy. The number of different procedures that can be performed using robotics is growing. For example, laparoscopic procedures using robotics include cholecystectomy, common bile duct injury repair, small bowel operation, tubal reanastomosis, Nissen fundoplication, and internal mammary artery harvesting.[55] Surgical intervention using robotics, combined with advances in computer technology and communication systems, will vastly change and broaden the scope of practice for the perioperative nurse.

Technologic developments have also made telesurgery a reality. The first transatlantic operation was performed in September 2001 with the patient in Strasbourg, France, and the surgeon in New York City.[56] Many other telesurgeries have occurred since then.

Telesurgery will reduce the need for seriously ill patients to travel long distances for care. Surgeons can perform procedures in locations in which their expertise is not readily available. In addition, surgeons can perform procedures on patients in hazardous environments such as battlefields.

NCLEX EXAMINATION REVIEW QUESTIONS

The number of the question corresponds to the same-numbered objective at the beginning of the chapter.

1. Proper attire for the semirestricted area of the surgery department is
   a. street clothing.
   b. surgical attire and head cover.
   c. surgical attire, head cover, and mask.
   d. street clothing with the addition of shoe covers.

2. The characteristic of the operating room environment that facilitates the prevention of infection in the surgical patient is
   a. adjustable lighting.
   b. conductive furniture.
   c. filters in the ventilating system.
   d. explosion-proof electrical plugs.
3. An activity that is carried out by nurses performing both sterile and nonsterile activities in the operating room is
   a. checking electrical equipment.
   b. passing instruments to the surgeon and assistants.
   c. coordinating activities occurring in the operating room.
   d. assisting the ACP with monitoring of patient during surgery.
4. Assessment of a patient with a musculoskeletal impairment on arrival to the operating room enables the nurse to meet the patient's needs during
   a. preparation of the skin.
   b. induction of anesthesia.
   c. positioning on the operating room bed.
   d. explanations about the surgical activities.
5. The perioperative nurse's primary responsibility for the care of the patient undergoing surgery is
   a. developing an individualized plan of nursing care for the patient.
   b. carrying out specific tasks related to surgical policies and procedures.
   c. ensuring that the patient has been assessed for safe administration of anesthesia.
   d. performing a preoperative history and physical assessment to identify patient needs.
6. When scrubbing at the scrub sink, the surgical team members should
   a. scrub from elbows to hands.
   b. scrub without mechanical friction.
   c. scrub for a minimum of 10 minutes.
   d. hold the hands higher than the elbows
7. When positioning a patient in preparation for surgery, the perioperative nurse understands that injury to the patient is most likely to occur as a result of
   a. incorrect skeletal alignment.
   b. loss of perception of pain or pressure.
   c. pooling of blood in peripheral vessels.
   d. disregarding the patient's need for modesty.
8. A patient being prepared for surgery tells the nurse that the anesthesia care provider told her that she would receive "laughing gas" in addition to some other inhaled drug for her anesthesia. The nurse recognizes that an advantage of this anesthetic agent is that it
   a. is safer than other inhaled anesthetic agents.
   b. has a strong analgesic effect during surgery.
   c. is easier to administer than other anesthetic agents.
   d. has strong anesthetic properties, allowing a decreased dose of other anesthetics.
9. Intravenous induction for general anesthesia is the method of choice for most patients because
   a. the patient is not intubated.
   b. the agents are nonexplosive.
   c. induction is rapid and pleasant.
   d. the odor of the agent is not offensive.
10. The injection of the local anesthetic into the tissues through which the surgical incision will pass is the technique of
   a. nerve block.
   b. local infiltration.
   c. topical application.
   d. regional application.

REFERENCES

1. Liu JH, Etzioni DA, O'Connell JB, et al: The increasing workload of general surgery, *Arch Surg* 139(4):423, 2004.
2. Association of periOperative Registered Nurses: Recommended practice for traffic patterns in the perioperative practice setting. In *Standards, recommended practices and guidelines*, Denver, 2005, Association of periOperative Registered Nurses.
3. Phillips N: *Berry and Kohn's operating room technique*, ed 10, St Louis, 2004, Mosby.
4. Rothrock JC: *Alexander's care of the patient in surgery*, ed 12, St Louis, 2003, Mosby.

*5. Boyle HJ: Patient advocacy in the perioperative setting, *AORN J* 82:2, 2005.

*6. Majasaari H, Sarajarvi A, Koskinen H, et al: Patients' perceptions of emotional support and information provided to family members, *AORN J* 81:5, 2005.

*7. Reavis CW, Sandidge J, Bauer K: Critical thinking's role in perioperative patient safety outcomes, *AORN J* 68:5, 1998.

8. Competency and Credentialing Institute. Available at *www.cc-institute.org* (accessed May 25, 2006).
9. Association of Surgical Technologists: Enhancing the profession to ensure quality patient care. Available at *www.ast.org* (accessed May 23, 2006).
10. Association of periOperative Registered Nurses: *AORN official statement on RN first assistants,* Denver, 2005, Association of periOperative Registered Nurses.
11. American Society of Anesthesiologists: Standards, guidelines, and statements. Available at *www.asahq.org/publications* (accessed May 23, 2006).
12. American Association of Nurse Anesthetists: Qualifications and capabilities of the certified registered nurse anesthetist. Available at *www.aana.com/crna/qualifications.asp* (accessed May 23, 2006).
13. Jehovah's Witnesses oppositions to blood transfusions. Available at *www.religioustolerance.org/witness5.htm* (accessed May 25, 2006).
14. 30 days of prayer for the Muslim world: about Islam. Available at *www.30-days.net/islam/customs.htm* (accessed May 25, 2006).
15. Larkin BG: The ins and outs of body piercings, *AORN J* 79:2, 2004.

*16. Hammarsten R, Hammarsten J, Jemsby P: Preoperative skin testing of materials used in surgical procedures, *AORN J* 77:4, 2003.

17. Haynes LC, Martin JH, Endres D: Use of non-traditional therapies: implications for older adults, *AORN J* 77:5, 2003.
18. MacKichan C, Ruthman J: Herbal product use and perioperative patients, *AORN J* 79:5, 2004.
19. Ellison DJ: A guideline for incorporating holistic nursing interventions into perianesthesia nursing, *J Perianesth Nurs* 20:1, 2005.

*20. Mok E, Wong KY: Effects of music on patient anxiety, *AORN J* 77:2, 2003.

*21. McRee LD, Noble S, Pasvogel A: Using massage and music therapy to improve postoperative outcomes, *AORN J* 78:3, 2003.

*22. Anderson LA, Gross JB: Aromatherapy with peppermint, isopropyl alcohol, or placebo is equally effective in relieving postoperative nausea, *J Perianesth Nurs* 19:1, 2004.

23. Favorite movie helps patients get through surgery, *OR Manager* 20:12, 2004.
24. Association of periOperative Registered Nurses: Recommended practice for sterile field—maintaining. In *Standards, recommended practices and guidelines*, Denver, 2005, Association of periOperative Registered Nurses.
25. Association of periOperative Registered Nurses: Recommended practice for counts—sponge, sharp and instrument. In *Standards, recommended practices and guidelines*, Denver, 2005, Association of periOperative Registered Nurses.
26. Association of periOperative Registered Nurses: Recommended practice for hand antisepsis—surgical. In *Standards, recommended practices and guidelines*, Denver, 2005, Association of periOperative Registered Nurses.
27. Centers for Disease Control and Prevention: Guideline for hand hygiene in health-care settings, *MMWR* 51:RR-16, 2002.
28. Association of periOperative Registered Nurses: Recommended practice for standard and transmission-based precautions. In *Standards, recommended practices and guidelines*, Denver, 2005, Association of periOperative Registered Nurses.

*Nursing research–based reference.

29. Keller J: Top ten safety issues with medical devices, *OR Manager* 19:4, 2002.
30. Association of periOperative Registered Nurses: Recommended practice for electrosurgery. In *Standards, recommended practices and guidelines*, Denver, 2005, Association of periOperative Registered Nurses.
31. Joint Commission on Accreditation of Healthcare Organizations: Universal protocol for preventing wrong site, wrong procedure, wrong person surgery. Available at *www.jcaho.org/accredited +organizations/patient+safety/universal+protocol/universal+protocol.pdf* (accessed May 23, 2006).
32. Association of periOperative Registered Nurses: AORN correct site surgery position statement. Available at *www.aorn.org/about/positions/pdf/Final%20PS%20on%20Correct%20Site%20Surgery.pdf* (accessed May 23, 2006).
33. Association of periOperative Registered Nurses: Recommended practice for positioning the patient in the perioperative practice setting. In *Standards, recommended practices and guidelines*, Denver, 2001, Association of periOperative Registered Nurses.
34. Association of periOperative Registered Nurses: Recommended practice for skin preparation of patients. In *Standards, recommended practices and guidelines*, Denver, 2005, Association of periOperative Registered Nurses.
35. Association of periOperative Registered Nurses: Patient outcomes: standards of perioperative care. In *Standards, recommended practices and guidelines*, Denver, 2001, Association of periOperative Registered Nurses.
*36. Association of periOperative Registered Nurses: *Perioperative nursing data set: the perioperative nursing vocabulary*, Denver, 2000, Association of periOperative Registered Nurses.
37. Joint Commission on Accreditation of Healthcare Organizations: *Hospital accreditation standards*, Oakbrook Terrace, Ill, 2005, The Commission.
38. American Society of Anesthesiologists: Continuum of depth of sedation: definition of general anesthesia and levels of sedation/analgesia, 2004. Available at *www.asahq.org/publicationsAndServices/standards/20.pdf* (accessed February 8, 2006).
39. Kost M: Moderate sedation/analgesia. In Defazio DM, Schick L, editors: *Perianesthesia nursing core curriculum*, St Louis, 2004, Saunders.
40. American Association of Nurse Anesthetists: Considerations for policy guidelines for registered nurses engaged in the administration of sedation and analgesia, 2003. Available at *www.aana.com/practice/conscious.asp* (accessed May 25, 2006).
41. American Society of Anesthesiologists: Practice guidelines for sedation and analgesia by non-anesthesiologists: a report by the American Society of Anesthesiologists task force on sedation and analgesia by non-anesthesiologists, *Anesthesiology* 84(2):459, 1996.
42. Association of periOperative Registered Nurses: Recommended practice for conscious sedation/analgesia: managing the patient. In *Standards, recommended practices and guidelines*, Denver, 2005, Association of periOperative Registered Nurses.
43. Hassan ZU: Anesthetic choices in surgery, *Surg Clin North Am* 85:1075, 2005.
44. Kossick MA: Inhalation anesthetics. In Naglehout JJ, Zaglaniczny KL, editors: *Nurse anesthesia*, ed 3, St Louis, 2005, Saunders.
45. Wilson WO: Opioid agonists and antagonists. In Naglehout JJ, Zaglaniczny KL, editors: *Nurse anesthesia*, ed 3, St Louis, 2005, Saunders.
46. Reves JG et al: Intravenous nonopioid anesthetics. In Miller RD, editor: *Miller's anesthesia*, ed 6, Philadelphia, 2005, Elsevier Churchill Livingstone.
47. Hass RE, Darsey A, Powell D: Neuromuscular blocking agents, reversal agents and their monitoring. In Naglehout JJ, Zaglaniczny KL, editors: *Nurse anesthesia*, ed 3, St Louis, 2005, Saunders.
48. Fallacaro NA, Fallacaro MD: Intravenous induction agents. In Naglehout JJ, Zaglaniczny KL, editors: *Nurse anesthesia*, ed 3, St Louis, 2005, Saunders.
49. Burkard J, Olson RL, Vacchiano CA: Regional anesthesia. In Naglehout JJ, Zaglaniczny KL, editors: *Nurse anesthesia*, ed 3, St Louis, 2005, Saunders.
50. Ang-Lee M, Yuan C, Moss J: Complementary and alternative therapies. In Miller RD, editor: *Miller's anesthesia*, ed 6, Philadelphia, 2005, Elsevier Churchill Livingstone.
51. Association of periOperative Registered Nurses: Latex guideline. In *Standards, recommended practices and guidelines*, Denver, 2005, Association of periOperative Registered Nurses.
52. Rosenberg H: Malignant hyperthermia slide show. Available at *www.mhaus.org* (accessed May 25, 2006).
53. American Society of Anesthesiologists: Practice guidelines for preoperative fasting and use of pharmacologic agents to reduce the risk of pulmonary aspiration: application to healthy patients undergoing elective procedures, *Anesthesiology* 90:3, 1999.
54. Karkouti K, McCluskey SA, Evans L, et al: Erythropoietin is an effective clinical modality for reducing RBC transfusion in joint surgery, *Can J Anesth* 52:4, 2005.
55. Reger TB, Janhke ME: Robotic cardiac surgery, *AORN J* 77:1, 2003.
56. Larkin M: Transatlantic, robotic-assisted telesurgery deemed a success, *Lancet* 358(9287):1074, 2001.

RESOURCES

Resources for this chapter are listed in Chapter 20 on p. 396. For additional Internet resources, see the website for this book at *http://evolve.elsevier.com/Lewis/medsurg.*

When love and skill work together, expect a masterpiece.

John Ruskin

20 Nursing Management
Postoperative Care

Debra J. Smith

LEARNING OBJECTIVES

1. Identify the components of an initial postanesthesia assessment.
2. Identify the nursing responsibilities in admitting patients to the postanesthesia care unit (PACU).
3. Explain the etiology and the nursing assessment and management of potential problems of patients in the PACU.
4. Describe the initial nursing assessment and management after transfer from the PACU to the general care unit.
5. Explain the etiology and the nursing assessment and management of potential problems during the postoperative period.
6. Identify the information needed by the postoperative patient in preparation for discharge.

KEY TERMS

airway obstruction, p. 378
atelectasis, p. 378
bronchospasm, p. 378
delayed emergence, p. 387
emergence delirium, p. 387
epidural analgesia, p. 389
hypothermia, p. 389
hypoventilation, p. 380
hypoxemia, p. 378

Electronic Resources

Supplemental content related to Chapter 20 can be found . . .

Companion CD

- Stress-Busting Kit for Nursing Students
- Interactive Case Study: Surgery
- NCLEX Examination Review Questions
- Comprehensive Glossary

Evolve Website

http://evolve.elsevier.com/Lewis/medsurg

- Content Updates
- Key Points (Printable and CD/MP3 Download)
- Concept Map Creator
- Expanded Audio Glossary
- Key Term Flash Cards
- Customizable Nursing Care Plan: Postoperative Patient
- Electronic Calculators
- WebLinks

The postoperative period begins immediately after surgery and continues until the patient is discharged from medical care. This chapter focuses on the common features of postoperative nursing care for the patient undergoing surgery. Much of postoperative nursing care involves (1) protecting the patient, who has been placed at physiologic risk during surgery, and (2) preventing complications while the body repairs itself during the recovery process. Many of the effects and potential complications of surgery identified in this chapter are discussed as clinical problems in other chapters. In addition, the problems and nursing care related to specific surgical procedures are discussed in the appropriate chapters of this text.

POSTOPERATIVE CARE OF THE SURGICAL PATIENT

The patient's immediate recovery period is supervised by a postanesthesia care nurse, a nurse specialist working in a *postanesthesia care unit* (PACU). The PACU is located adjacent to the operating room (OR) to minimize transportation of the patient immediately after surgery and to provide ready access to anesthesia and surgical personnel. Three phases of postanesthesia care provide different levels of care depending on the needs of individual patients. These different phases of postanesthesia care have been identified because the current variety of types of surgery, levels of anesthesia, and ambulatory surgeries results in patients with wide variation in postoperative care needs.

Reviewed by Nancy H. Wright, RN, BS, CNOR, Director, Surgical Technology, Virginia College, Birmingham, Ala.

TABLE 20-1 Phases of Postanesthesia Care

Phase I
- ECG and more intense monitoring
- Providing care during the immediate postanesthesia period
- **Goal:** Preparing patient for transfer to Phase II or inpatient unit

Phase II
- Ambulatory surgery patients
- **Goal:** Preparing patient for transfer to Phase III, home, or extended care facility

Phase III
- Extended care/observation unit
- **Goal:** Preparing patient for self-care

Source: Quinn DMD, Schick L: *PeriAnesthesia nursing core curriculum: preoperative, phase I and phase II PACU nursing,* Philadelphia, 2004, Saunders.
ECG, Electrocardiogram.

Phase I postanesthesia care involves providing intensive monitoring and care of the patient in the immediate postoperative period. Patients move from Phase I care either to Phase II care in the PACU or to an inpatient unit. *Phase II postanesthesia care* provides less intensive care to surgery patients who will then be transferred to Phase III care, to home, or to an extended care facility. *Phase III postanesthesia care* is provided when patients are being prepared for self-care and discharge from the surgical facility (Table 20-1).[1]

Postanesthesia Care Unit Admission

The initial admission of the patient to the PACU is a joint effort between the anesthesia care provider (ACP) and the PACU nurse. This collaborative effort fosters a smooth transfer of care to the PACU and helps determine the phase to which the patient is assigned.

PACU Progression. How patients move through the phases of care in the PACU is determined by their condition. If a patient assigned to Phase I care on admission to the PACU is stable and recovering well, the patient may rapidly progress through Phase I to discharge to either Phase II care or an inpatient unit. This accelerated progress can occur with either inpatients or outpatients, and is termed **rapid postanesthesia care unit progression (RPP).** Another accelerated system of care is **fast-tracking,** which involves admitting ambulatory surgery patients who have received general, regional, or local anesthesia directly to Phase II care.[1] One study that evaluated the effects of fast-tracking on patient recovery time and nursing workload and costs found that this system significantly reduced the overall recovery time without compromising patient satisfaction. However, the overall nursing workload and the associated cost were not significantly affected.[2] Although both RPP and fast-tracking can potentially result in time and cost savings, the patient's safety should be the primary determining factor of where or at what level postoperative care is provided.

Phase I Initial Assessment. On admission of the patient to the PACU, the ACP gives a verbal report to the admitting PACU nurse. Table 20-2 summarizes the components of a complete anesthesia report. While the patient is in the PACU, priority care includes monitoring and management of respiratory and circulatory function, pain, temperature, and the surgical site.[1] Table 20-3 identifies key components of a PACU assessment.

Assessment should begin with an evaluation of the airway, breathing, and circulation (ABC) status of the patient. During the initial assessment, signs of inadequate oxygenation and ventilation should be identified (Table 20-4). Any evidence of respiratory compromise requires prompt intervention.

Pulse oximetry monitoring is initiated because it provides a noninvasive means of assessing the adequacy of oxygenation. (Pulse oximetry is discussed in Chapter 26.) The greatest value of pulse oximetry is to provide an early warning of hypoxemia and significant reduction of arterial blood gases. However, it has not been shown to affect the outcome of anesthesia recovery.[3]

TABLE 20-2 Postanesthesia Admission Report

General Information
- Patient name
- Age
- Anesthesia care provider
- Surgeon
- Surgical procedure

Patient History
- Indication for surgery
- Medical history, medications, allergies

Intraoperative Management
- Anesthetic medications
- Other medications received preoperatively or intraoperatively
- Blood loss
- Fluid replacement totals, including blood transfusions
- Urine output

Intraoperative Course
- Unexpected anesthetic events or reactions
- Unexpected surgical events
- Vital signs and monitoring trends
- Results of intraoperative laboratory tests

TABLE 20-3 Initial Postanesthesia Care Unit Assessment

Airway
- Patency
- Oral or nasal airway
- Endotracheal tube

Breathing
- Respiratory rate and quality
- Auscultated breath sounds
- Pulse oximetry
- Supplemental oxygen

Circulation
- ECG monitoring—rate and rhythm
- Blood pressure
- Temperature and color of skin
- Peripheral pulses

Neurologic
- Level of consciousness
- Orientation
- Sensory and motor status

Genitourinary
- Intake (fluids, irrigations)
- Output (urine, drains)

Surgical Site
- Dressings/drainage

Pain
- Incision
- Other

ECG, Electrocardiogram.

TABLE 20-4 Clinical Manifestations of Inadequate Oxygenation

Central Nervous System
- Restlessness
- Agitation
- Muscle twitching
- Seizures
- Coma

Cardiovascular System
- Hypertension
- Hypotension
- Tachycardia
- Bradycardia
- Dysrhythmias

Integumentary System
- Cyanosis
- Prolonged capillary refill
- Flushed and moist skin

Respiratory System
- Increased to absent respiratory effort
- Use of accessory muscles
- Abnormal breath sounds
- Abnormal arterial blood gases

Renal System
- Urine output <0.5 ml/kg/hr

Electrocardiographic (ECG) monitoring is initiated to determine cardiac rate and rhythm. Deviations from preoperative findings should be noted and evaluated. Blood pressure (BP) should be measured and compared with baseline readings. Invasive monitoring (e.g., arterial monitoring) can be initiated if needed. Body temperature and skin color and condition should also be assessed. Any evidence of inadequate circulatory status requires prompt intervention.

The initial neurologic assessment focuses on level of consciousness, orientation, sensory and motor status, and size, equality, and reactivity of the pupils. The patient may be awake, drowsy but arousable, or asleep. Because hearing is the first sense to return in the unconscious patient, the nurse should explain all activities to the patient from the moment of his or her admission to the PACU. If the patient has had a regional anesthetic (e.g., spinal or epidural), sensory and motor blockade may still be present.

The assessment of the urinary system focuses on intake and output as well as fluid balance. Intraoperative fluid totals are communicated as part of the anesthesia report. The PACU nurse should note the presence of all intravenous (IV) lines, all irrigation solutions and infusions, and all output devices, including catheters and wound drains. Intravenous infusions are regulated according to postoperative orders.

The PACU nurse should also assess the surgical site, noting the condition of any dressings and the type and amount of any drainage. Postoperative orders related to site care are instituted. All data obtained in the admission assessment are documented on a PACU record, a form specific to postanesthesia and postsurgical care.

After the initial assessment is completed, the PACU nurse continues to apply the skills of ongoing assessment, diagnosis, and intervention. The patient's response to intervention is also noted. The goal of PACU care is to identify actual and potential patient problems that may occur as a result of anesthetic administration and surgical intervention and to intervene appropriately. The most recent core curriculum (2004) of the American Society of periAnesthesia Nurses (ASPAN) helps to guide the practice of preoperative, Phase I, and Phase II PACU nursing.[1]

Potential problems in the postoperative period are identified in Fig. 20-1. Nursing management of these problems is discussed in the following pages and can be applied to patients in both the PACU and the clinical unit.

POTENTIAL RESPIRATORY PROBLEMS

Etiology

PACU. In the immediate postanesthetic period, the most common causes of airway compromise include obstruction, hypoxemia, and hypoventilation (Table 20-5). Patients at risk include those who have had general anesthesia, are older, smoke heavily, have lung disease, are obese, or have undergone airway, thoracic, or abdominal surgery. However, respiratory problems may occur with any patient who has been anesthetized.

Airway obstruction is most commonly caused by blockage of the airway by the patient's tongue (Fig. 20-2). The base of the tongue falls backward against the soft palate and occludes the pharynx. It is most pronounced in the supine position and in the patient who is extremely sleepy after surgery. Less common causes of airway obstruction include laryngospasm, retained secretions, and laryngeal edema.

Hypoxemia, specifically a partial pressure of arterial oxygen (PaO_2) of less than 60 mm Hg, is characterized by a variety of nonspecific clinical signs and symptoms, ranging from agitation to somnolence, hypertension to hypotension, and tachycardia to bradycardia. Pulse oximetry will indicate a low oxygen saturation (less than 90% to 92%). Arterial blood gas analysis should be used to confirm hypoxemia if the pulse oximetry indicates a low oxygen saturation.

The most common cause of postoperative hypoxemia is atelectasis. **Atelectasis** (alveolar collapse) may be the result of bronchial obstruction caused by retained secretions or decreased respiratory excursion. Atelectasis occurs when mucus blocks bronchioles or when the amount of alveolar surfactant (the substance that holds the alveoli open) is reduced (Fig. 20-3). As air becomes trapped beyond the plug and is eventually absorbed, the alveoli collapse. Atelectasis may affect a portion or an entire lobe of the lungs. Hypotension and low cardiac output states can also contribute to the development of atelectasis.

Other causes of hypoxemia that may occur in the PACU include pulmonary edema, aspiration, and bronchospasm. *Pulmonary edema* is caused by an accumulation of fluid in the alveoli and may be the result of fluid overload; left ventricular failure; or prolonged airway obstruction, sepsis, or aspiration. Pulmonary edema is characterized by hypoxemia, crackles on auscultation, decreased pulmonary compliance, and the presence of infiltrates on chest x-ray.

Aspiration of gastric contents into the lungs is a potentially serious airway emergency. Symptoms include bronchospasm, hypoxemia, atelectasis, interstitial edema, alveolar hemorrhage, and respiratory failure. Gastric aspiration may also cause laryngospasm, infection, and pulmonary edema. Because of the serious consequences of gastric aspiration, prevention, as opposed to treatment, is the goal.

Bronchospasm is the result of an increase in bronchial smooth muscle tone with resultant closure of small airways. Airway edema develops, causing secretions to build up in the airway. The patient

TABLE 20-5 Common Immediate Postoperative Respiratory Complications

Complications and Causes	Mechanisms	Manifestations	Interventions
Airway Obstruction			
Tongue falling back	Muscular flaccidity associated with ↓ consciousness and muscle relaxants	Use of accessory muscles Snoring respirations ↓ Air movement	Patient stimulation Jaw thrust Chin lift Artificial airway
Retained thick secretions	Secretion stimulation by anesthetic agents Dehydration of secretions	Noisy respirations Coarse crackles	Suctioning Deep breathing and coughing IV hydration Chest physical therapy
Laryngospasm	Irritation from endotracheal tube or anesthetic gases Most likely to occur after removal of endotracheal tube	Inspiratory stridor (crowing respiration) Sternal retraction Acute respiratory distress	O_2 Positive pressure ventilation IV muscle relaxant Lidocaine Corticosteroids
Laryngeal edema	Allergic drug reaction Mechanical irritation from intubation Fluid overload	Similar to laryngospasm	O_2 Antihistamines Corticosteroids Sedatives Possible intubation
Hypoxemia			
Atelectasis	Bronchial obstruction caused by secretions or ↓ lung volumes	↓ Breath sounds ↓ O_2 saturation	Humidified O_2 Deep breathing Incentive spirometry Early mobilization
Pulmonary edema	↑ Hydrostatic pressure ↓ Interstitial pressure ↑ Capillary permeability	Crackles Infiltrates on chest x-ray Fluid overload ↓ O_2 saturation	O_2 therapy Diuretics Fluid restriction
Pulmonary embolism	Thrombus dislodged from peripheral venous system; lodged in pulmonary arterial system	Acute tachypnea Dyspnea Tachycardia Hypotension ↓ O_2 saturation	O_2 therapy Cardiopulmonary support Anticoagulant therapy
Aspiration	Inhalation of gastric contents	Bronchospasm Atelectasis Crackles Respiratory distress ↓ O_2 saturation	O_2 therapy Cardiac support Antibiotics
Bronchospasm	↑ Smooth muscle tone with closure of small airways	Wheezing Dyspnea Tachypnea ↓ O_2 saturation	O_2 therapy Bronchodilators
Hypoventilation			
Depression of central respiratory drive	Medullary depression from anesthetics/opioids/sedatives	Shallow respirations ↓ Respiratory rate/apnea ↓ PaO_2 ↑ $PaCO_2$	Stimulation Reversal of opioids/benzodiazepines Mechanical ventilation
Poor respiratory muscle tone	Neuromuscular blockade Neuromuscular disease	As above	Reversal of paralysis Mechanical ventilation
Mechanical restriction	Tight casts, dressings, positioning, and obesity preventing lung expansion	As above	Elevate head of bed Repositioning Loosen dressings
Pain	Shallow breathing to prevent incisional pain	As above Complaints of pain Guarding behavior	Opioid analgesic therapy in reduced dose

$PaCO_2$, Partial pressure of arterial carbon dioxide; *PaO_2*, partial pressure of arterial oxygen.

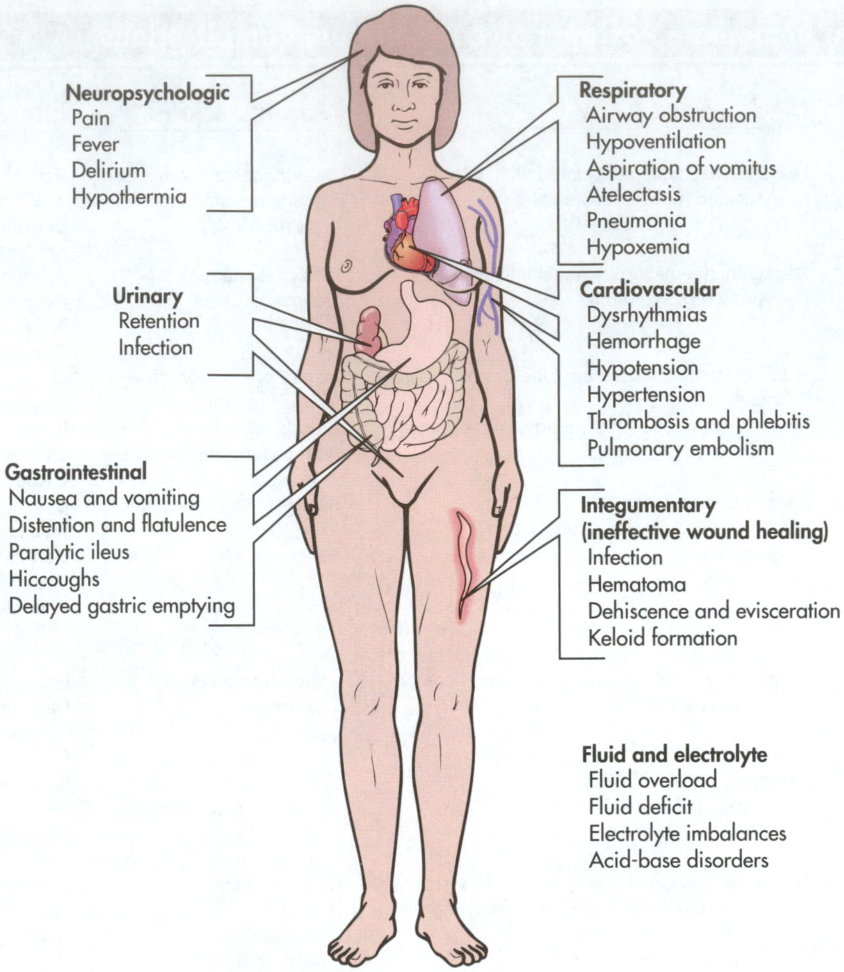

FIG. 20-1 Potential problems in the postoperative period.

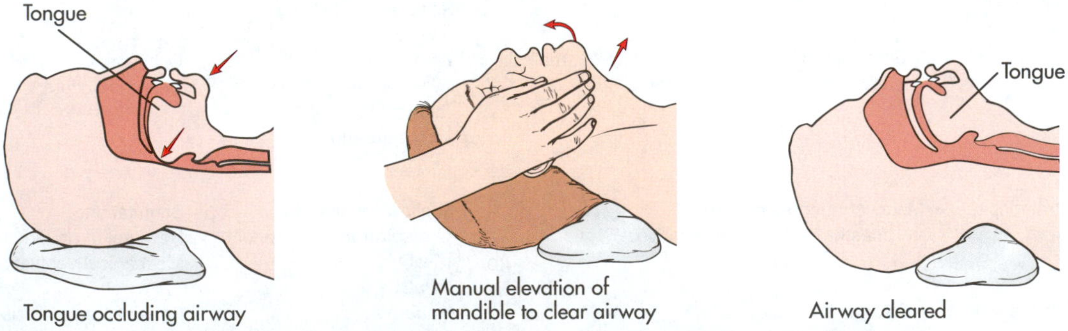

FIG. 20-2 Etiology and relief of airway obstruction caused by patient's tongue.

will have wheezing, dyspnea, use of accessory muscles, hypoxemia, and tachypnea. Bronchospasm may be due to aspiration, endotracheal intubation, suctioning, or chemical mediator release as a result of an allergic response. (Allergic responses are discussed in Chapter 14.) Bronchospasm is seen more frequently in patients with asthma and chronic obstructive pulmonary disease (COPD).

Hypoventilation, a common complication in the PACU, is characterized by a decreased respiratory rate or effort, hypoxemia, and an increasing partial pressure of arterial carbon dioxide ($PaCO_2$), also known as hypercapnia. Hypoventilation may occur as a result of depression of the central respiratory drive (secondary to anesthesia or pain medication), poor respiratory muscle tone (secondary to neuromuscular blockade or disease), or a combination of both.

Clinical Unit. Common causes of respiratory problems for postoperative patients in the clinical unit are atelectasis and pneumonia, especially after abdominal and thoracic surgery. The postoperative development of mucous plugs and decreased surfactant production are directly related to hypoventilation, constant recumbent position, ineffective coughing, and history of smoking. Increased bronchial secretions occur when the respiratory passages have been irritated by heavy smoking, acute or chronic pulmonary infection or disease, and the drying of mucous membranes that occurs with intubation, inhalation anesthesia, and dehydration. Without intervention,

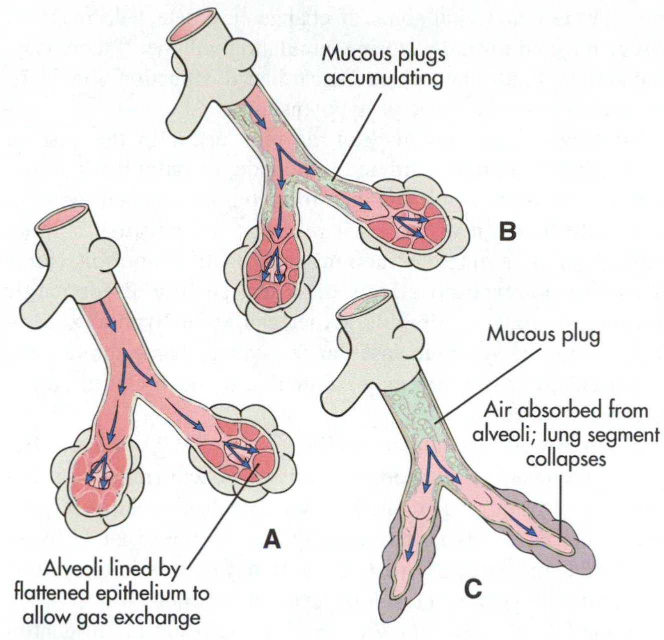

FIG. 20-3 Postoperative atelectasis. **A,** Normal bronchiole and alveoli. **B,** Mucous plug in bronchiole. **C,** Collapse of alveoli due to atelectasis following absorption of air.

atelectasis can progress to pneumonia when microorganisms grow in the stagnant mucus and an infection develops.

NURSING MANAGEMENT RESPIRATORY PROBLEMS

■ Nursing Assessment

For an adequate respiratory assessment, the nurse must evaluate airway patency; chest symmetry; and the depth, rate, and character of respirations. The chest wall should be observed for symmetry of movement with a hand placed lightly over the xiphoid process. Impaired ventilation may initially be detected by the observation of slowed breathing or diminished chest and abdominal movement during the respiratory cycle. It should also be determined whether abdominal or accessory muscles are being used for breathing. Observable use of these muscles may indicate respiratory distress. Breath sounds should be auscultated anteriorly, laterally, and posteriorly. Decreased or absent breath sounds will be detected when airflow is diminished or obstructed.

Regular monitoring of vital signs and use of pulse oximetry in conjunction with thorough respiratory assessment permit the nurse to recognize early signs of respiratory problems. The presence of hypoxemia from any cause may be reflected by rapid breathing, gasping, apprehension, restlessness, and a rapid or thready pulse.

The characteristics of sputum or mucus should be noted and recorded. Mucus from the trachea and throat is normally colorless and thin in consistency. Sputum from the lungs and bronchi is normally thick with a slight yellow tinge.

■ Nursing Diagnoses

Nursing diagnoses and collaborative problems related to potential respiratory problems for the postoperative patient include, but are not limited to, the following:

- Ineffective airway clearance
- Ineffective breathing pattern
- Impaired gas exchange

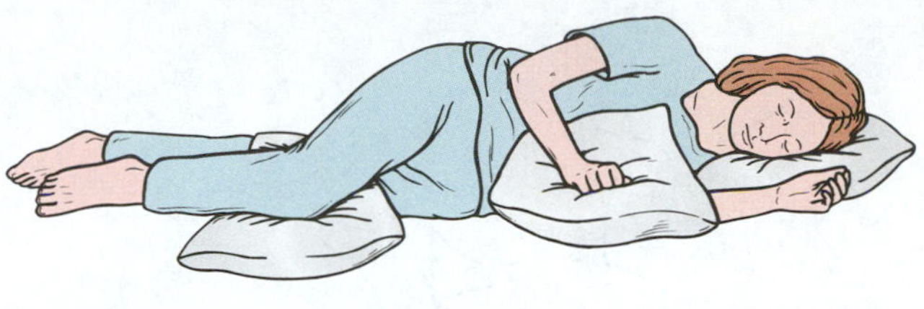

FIG. 20-4 Position of patient during recovery from general anesthesia.

- Risk for aspiration
- Potential complication: hypoxemia
- Potential complication: pneumonia
- Potential complication: atelectasis

■ Nursing Implementation

In the PACU, nursing interventions are designed to both prevent and treat respiratory problems. Proper positioning of the patient to facilitate respirations and protect the airway is essential. Unless contraindicated by the surgical procedure, the unconscious patient is positioned in a lateral "recovery" position (Fig. 20-4). This recovery position keeps the airway open and reduces the risk of aspiration if vomiting occurs. Once conscious, the patient is usually returned to a supine position with the head of the bed elevated. This position maximizes expansion of the thorax by decreasing the pressure of the abdominal contents on the diaphragm.

Oxygen therapy will be used if the patient has had general anesthesia and/or the ACP orders it. Oxygen therapy is given via nasal cannula or face mask. The use of oxygen aids in the elimination of anesthetic gases and helps meet the increased demand for oxygen resulting from decreased blood volume or increased cellular metabolism. If the patient requires postoperative breathing assistance, a mechanical ventilator will be provided.

Deep breathing is encouraged to facilitate gas exchange and to promote the return to consciousness. Once the patient is more awake, deep-breathing and coughing techniques help the patient prevent alveolar collapse and move respiratory secretions to larger airway passages for expectoration. The patient should be encouraged to breathe deeply 10 times every hour while awake. The use of an incentive spirometer is helpful in providing visual feedback of respiratory effort. Diaphragmatic or abdominal breathing is accomplished by inhaling slowly and deeply through the nose, holding the breath for a few seconds, and then exhaling slowly and completely through the mouth. The patient's hands should be placed lightly over the lower ribs and upper abdomen. This allows the patient to feel the abdomen rise during inspiration and fall during expiration.

Effective coughing is essential in mobilizing secretions (see Chapter 29). If secretions are present in the respiratory passages, deep breathing often will move them up to stimulate the cough reflex without any voluntary effort by the patient, and then they can be expectorated. Splinting an abdominal incision with a pillow or a rolled blanket provides support to the incision and aids in coughing and expectoration of secretions (Fig. 20-5).

The patient's position should be changed every 1 to 2 hours to allow full chest expansion and to increase perfusion of both lungs. Ambulation, not just sitting in a chair, should be aggressively carried out as soon as physician approval is given. Adequate and regular analgesic medication should be provided because incisional pain often is the greatest deterrent to patient participation in effective ventilation and ambulation. The patient should also be reas-

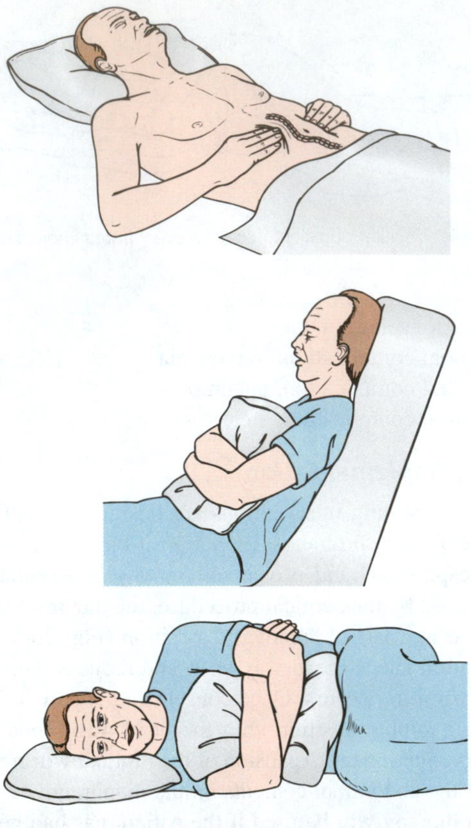

FIG. 20-5 Techniques for splinting wound when coughing.

sured that these activities will not cause the incision to separate. Adequate hydration, either parenteral or oral, is essential to maintain the integrity of mucous membranes and to keep secretions thin and loose for easy expectoration.

Other nursing interventions appropriate for specific respiratory problems are detailed in Table 20-5. Nursing care for the postoperative patient is presented in NCP 20-1.

POTENTIAL CARDIOVASCULAR PROBLEMS

Etiology

PACU. In the immediate postanesthetic period, the most common cardiovascular problems include hypotension, hypertension, and dysrhythmias. Patients at greatest risk for alterations in cardiovascular function include those with alterations in respiratory function, those with a history of cardiovascular disease, the elderly, the debilitated, and the critically ill.

Hypotension is evidenced by signs of hypoperfusion to the vital organs, especially the brain, heart, and kidneys. Clinical signs of disorientation, loss of consciousness, chest pain, oliguria, and anuria reflect hypoxemia and the loss of physiologic compensation. Intervention must be timely to prevent the devastating complications of cardiac ischemia or infarction, cerebral ischemia, renal ischemia, and bowel infarction.

The most common cause of hypotension in the PACU is unreplaced fluid and blood loss, which may lead to hypovolemic shock. Hemorrhage is always a risk of surgery, and marked blood loss is possible when cauterization or ligatures fail. Hemorrhage most often occurs internally, requiring assessment for changes in level of consciousness and vital signs. If changes are detected, treatment will be directed toward restoring circulating volume. If there is no response to fluid administration, cardiac dysfunction should be considered to be the cause of hypotension.

Primary cardiac dysfunction, as may occur in the case of myocardial infarction, cardiac tamponade, or pulmonary embolism, results in an acute fall in cardiac output. Secondary myocardial dysfunction occurs as a result of the negative chronotropic (rate of cardiac contraction) and negative inotropic (force of cardiac contraction) effects of drugs, such as β-adrenergic blockers, digoxin, or opioids. Other causes of hypotension include decreased systemic vascular resistance, dysrhythmias, and measurement errors that may occur if a blood pressure cuff is incorrectly sized.

Hypertension, a common finding in the PACU, is most frequently the result of sympathetic nervous system stimulation that may be the result of pain, anxiety, bladder distention, or respiratory compromise. Hypertension may also be the result of hypothermia and preexisting hypertension. It may be seen after vascular and cardiac surgery as a result of revascularization.

In the PACU, *dysrhythmias* are often the result of an identifiable cause other than myocardial injury. The leading causes include hypokalemia, hypoxemia, hypercarbia, alterations in acid-base status, circulatory instability, and preexisting heart disease. Hypothermia, pain, surgical stress, and many anesthetic agents are also capable of causing dysrhythmias.

Clinical Unit. In the clinical unit, postoperative fluid and electrolyte imbalances are contributing factors to cardiovascular problems. Such imbalances may develop as a result of a combination of the body's normal response to the stress of surgery, excessive fluid losses, and improper IV fluid replacement. The body's fluid status directly affects cardiac output. Fluid retention during the first 2 to 5 postoperative days can be the result of the stress response. This response serves to maintain both blood volume and blood pressure. Fluid retention results from the secretion and release of two hormones by the pituitary—antidiuretic hormone (ADH) and adrenocorticotropic hormone (ACTH)—and activation of the renin-angiotensin-aldosterone system. ADH release leads to increased water reabsorption and decreased urinary output, increasing blood volume. ACTH stimulates the adrenal cortex to secrete cortisol and, to a lesser degree, aldosterone. Fluid losses resulting from surgery decrease kidney perfusion, stimulating the renin-angiotensin-aldosterone system and causing marked release of aldosterone (see Chapter 17). Both of the mechanisms that increase aldosterone lead to significant sodium and fluid retention, increasing blood volume.

Fluid overload may occur during this period of fluid retention when IV fluids are administered too rapidly, when chronic (e.g., cardiac, renal) disease exists, or when the patient is an older adult. Conversely, fluid deficit may be related to slow or inadequate fluid replacement, which leads to decreases in cardiac output and tissue perfusion. Untreated preoperative dehydration or intraoperative or postoperative losses from vomiting, bleeding, wound drainage, or suctioning may be contributing factors to fluid deficits.

Hypokalemia can be a consequence of urinary and gastrointestinal (GI) tract losses, and it results when potassium is not replaced in IV fluids. Low serum potassium levels directly affect the contractility of the heart and thus may also contribute to decreases in cardiac output and in overall body tissue perfusion. Adequate re-

NURSING CARE PLAN 20-1

Postoperative Patient

NURSING DIAGNOSIS **Ineffective breathing pattern** *related to* respiratory irritation, increased secretions, and airway obstruction *as evidenced by* dyspnea, crowing, shallow chest excursion, or low oxygen saturation

PATIENT GOAL Maintains a breathing pattern that meets oxygen needs of the body

OUTCOMES (NOC)

Respiratory Status: Airway Patency

- Ease of breathing ___
- Respiratory rate ___
- Respiratory rhythm ___

Measurement Scale

1 = Severely compromised
2 = Substantially compromised
3 = Moderately compromised
4 = Mildly compromised
5 = Not compromised

INTERVENTIONS (NIC) and *RATIONALES*

Respiratory Monitoring

- Monitor rate, rhythm, depth, and effort of respirations *to determine need for additional respiratory support.*
- Monitor pulse oximetry *to assess oxygen status.*
- Auscultate breath sounds noting *whether there are areas of decreased/absent ventilation and presence of adventitious sounds.*
- Place the patient on side *to prevent aspiration.*

NURSING DIAGNOSIS **Acute pain** *related to* surgical incision and reflex muscle spasm *as evidenced by* complaints of pain, tense and guarded body posture, facial grimacing, restlessness, irritability, moaning, diaphoresis, tachycardia

PATIENT GOALS
1. Reports satisfaction with pain relief
2. Uses pain relief techniques effectively

OUTCOMES (NOC)

Pain Control

- Uses analgesics appropriately ___
- Uses nonanalgesic relief ___
- Reports changes in pain symptoms or site to health care professional ___
- Reports pain controlled ___

Measurement Scale

1 = Never demonstrated
2 = Rarely demonstrated
3 = Sometimes demonstrated
4 = Often demonstrated
5 = Consistently demonstrated

INTERVENTIONS (NIC) and *RATIONALES*

Pain Management

- Perform a comprehensive assessment of pain to include location, characteristics, onset/duration, frequency, quality, intensity or severity of pain, and precipitating factors *to plan appropriate interventions.*
- Provide the person optimal pain relief with prescribed analgesics *to relieve acute pain.*
- Implement the use of patient-controlled analgesia (PCA) *to permit patient control of analgesic dosing.*
- Teach the use of nonpharmacologic techniques (e.g., relaxation, guided imagery, music therapy, distraction, massage) before, after, and, if possible, during painful activities; before pain occurs or increases; and along with other pain relief measures *for patient to use in lieu of or in conjunction with analgesics to obtain pain relief.*
- Use pain control measures before pain becomes severe *to prevent breakthrough pain that is difficult to control.*
- Institute and modify pain control measures on the basis of the patient's response.

NURSING DIAGNOSIS **Nausea** *related to* effects of anesthetic agents and gastrointestinal distention *as evidenced by* complaints of nausea, refusal to take fluids or solids, observed or reported vomiting

PATIENT GOAL Experiences reduced or no episodes of nausea and vomiting

OUTCOMES (NOC)

Nausea and Vomiting Control

- Uses antiemetic medications ___
- Reports nausea, retching, and vomiting controlled ___

Measurement Scale

1 = Never demonstrated
2 = Rarely demonstrated
3 = Sometimes demonstrated
4 = Often demonstrated
5 = Consistently demonstrated

INTERVENTIONS (NIC) and *RATIONALES*

Nausea Management

- Provide information about the nausea, such as causes of the nausea and how long it will last, *to prevent negative anticipation of the nausea.*
- Ensure that effective antiemetic drugs are given *to prevent nausea.*
- Identify factors (e.g., medications, procedures) that may cause or contribute to nausea.
- Reduce or eliminate factors that precipitate or increase nausea (anxiety, fear, fatigue, and lack of knowledge).

Vomiting Management

- Assess emesis for color, consistency, blood, timing, and extent to which it is forceful.
- Position to prevent aspiration.
- Provide comfort (such as cool cloths to forehead, sponging face, or clean dry clothes) during/after the vomiting episode.
- Use oral hygiene to clean mouth and nose.

This is a general nursing care plan for the postoperative patient. It should be used in conjunction with a nursing care plan specific to the type of surgery performed.

Continued

NURSING CARE PLAN 20-1

Postoperative Patient—cont'd

NURSING DIAGNOSIS **Risk for imbalanced fluid volume** *related to* stress response to surgery and abnormal fluid loss and gain

PATIENT GOALS
1. Maintains fluid and electrolyte balance required for metabolic needs
2. Demonstrates no signs of hypo- or hypervolemia

OUTCOMES (NOC)

Fluid Balance

- Blood pressure ___
- Radial pulse rate ___
- Peripheral pulses ___
- Serum electrolytes ___
- 24-hour intake and output balance ___

Measurement Scale

1 = Severely compromised
2 = Substantially compromised
3 = Moderately compromised
4 = Mildly compromised
5 = Not compromised

INTERVENTIONS (NIC) and *RATIONALES*

Fluid/Electrolyte Management

- Monitor for abnormal serum electrolyte levels *to determine need for supplements.*
- Obtain laboratory specimens for monitoring of altered fluid or electrolyte levels (e.g., hematocrit; blood urea nitrogen; protein, sodium, and potassium levels) *to determine presence of fluid imbalance.*
- Monitor vital signs *to detect fluid imbalances and plan appropriate interventions.*
- Maintain intravenous solution containing electrolyte(s) at constant flow rate *to prevent fluid and electrolyte overload.*
- Keep an accurate record of intake and output.
- Administer prescribed supplemental electrolytes *to maintain electrolyte balance.*
- Consult physician if signs and symptoms of fluid and/or electrolyte imbalance persist or worsen.

NURSING DIAGNOSIS **Risk for infection** *related to* altered skin integrity, inadequate nutrition and fluid intake, presence of environmental pathogens, invasive instrumentation, and immobility

PATIENT GOAL Experiences no evidence of infection

OUTCOMES (NOC)

Infection Severity

- Fever ___
- White blood cell count elevation ___
- Purulent sputum ___
- Urine culture colonization ___
- Wound site culture colonization ___

Measurement Scale

1 = Severe
2 = Substantial
3 = Moderate
4 = Mild
5 = None

Wound Healing: Primary Intention

- Purulent drainage ___
- Serosanguineous drainage ___
- Surrounding skin erythema ___
- Periwound edema ___
- Skin temperature elevation___
- Foul wound odor ___

Measurement Scale

1 = Extensive
2 = Substantial
3 = Moderate
4 = Limited
5 = None

INTERVENTIONS (NIC) and *RATIONALES*

Airway Management

- Position patient to maximize ventilation potential.
- Remove secretions by encouraging coughing or by suctioning *to prevent colonization of respiratory secretions.*
- Encourage slow, deep breathing as well as turning and coughing *to remove secretions and prevent atelectasis.*
- Assist with incentive spirometer

Tube Care

- Administer skin care at the tube insertion site *to avoid infection.*
- Inspect the area around the tube insertion site for redness and skin breakdown *to identify infection.*
- Monitor amount, color, and consistency of drainage from tube *to detect infection.*

Incision Site Care

- Inspect the incision site for redness, swelling, or signs of dehiscence or evisceration *to detect infection.*
- Note characteristics of drainage *to detect infection.*
- Cleanse the area around the incision with an appropriate cleaning solution *to reduce local pathogens.*
- Cleanse the area around any drain site or drainage tube last *to prevent wound contamination.*
- Change the dressing at appropriate intervals *to reduce microbial colonization.*

Nutrition Management

- Determine, in collaboration with dietitian, number of calories and type of nutrients needed to meet nutrition requirements.
- Encourage calorie intake appropriate for body type and lifestyle.

placement of potassium is usually 40 mEq/day. However, potassium should not be given until adequate renal function has been established. A urine output of at least 0.5 ml/kg/hr is generally considered indicative of adequate renal function.

Cardiovascular status is also affected by the state of tissue perfusion or blood flow. The stress response contributes to an increase in clotting tendencies in the postoperative patient by increasing platelet production. Deep vein thrombosis (DVT) may form in leg veins as a result of inactivity, body position, and pressure, all of which lead to venous stasis and decreased perfusion. DVT, especially common in the older adult, obese individual, and immobilized patient, is a potentially life-threatening compli-

NURSING CARE PLAN 20-1

Postoperative Patient—cont'd

NURSING DIAGNOSIS **Effective therapeutic regimen management** *as evidenced by* verbalized desire to manage postoperative care and intent to reduce risk factors for complications

PATIENT GOALS
1. Describes home management of surgical wound and pain
2. Identifies signs and symptoms that must be reported to a health care professional

OUTCOMES (NOC)

Compliance Behavior

- Discusses prescribed treatment regimen with health care professional ___
- Performs treatment regimen as prescribed ___
- Reports changes in symptoms to health care professional ___
- Monitors treatment response ___

Measurement Scale

1 = Never demonstrated
2 = Rarely demonstrated
3 = Sometimes demonstrated
4 = Often demonstrated
5 = Consistently demonstrated

INTERVENTIONS (NIC) and *RATIONALES*

Incision Site Care

- Instruct the patient on how to care for the incision during bathing or showering *to avoid infection.*
- Teach the patient and/or the family how to care for the incision, including signs and symptoms of infection, *to enhance the patient's management of care.*

Infection Control

- Teach patient and family about signs and symptoms of infection and when to report them to the health care provider *to enhance the patient's management of care.*

Teaching: Individual

- Appraise the patient's current level of knowledge and understanding of content *to identify learning needs.*
- Tailor the content to the patient's cognitive, psychomotor, and/or affective abilities/ disabilities *to promote learning.*
- Provide time for the patient to ask questions and discuss concerns.

COLLABORATIVE PROBLEMS

NURSING GOALS

Potential Complication

- Monitor operative site for signs of hemorrhage
- Report deviations from acceptable parameters
- Carry out appropriate medical and nursing interventions

NURSING INTERVENTIONS and *RATIONALES*

Hemorrhage *related to* ineffective vascular closure or alterations in coagulation

- Observe surgical site and dressings regularly, including dependent sites (qhr for 4 hr, then q4hr) *to detect signs of bleeding.*
- Monitor vital signs regularly from q15min to q2-4hr as indicated *to detect signs of hypovolemia.*
- Report abnormalities such as decreasing blood pressure; rapid pulse and respirations; cool, clammy skin; pallor; and bright red blood on dressing.
- Monitor for changes in mental status, such as restlessness and sense of impending doom, *as indicators of inadequate cerebral perfusion.*
- Monitor hematocrit and hemoglobin levels *because decreases may indicate hemorrhage.*
- Monitor platelet levels and coagulation function tests *because alterations indicate bleeding tendencies.*

Potential Complication

- Monitor for signs of thromboembolism
- Report deviations from acceptable parameters
- Carry out appropriate medical and nursing interventions

Thromboembolism *related to* dehydration, immobility, vascular manipulation, or injury

- Assess for signs of thromboembolism, such as redness, swelling, and pain; increased warmth along path of vein; edema or pain in extremity; chest pain; hemoptysis; tachypnea; dyspnea; and restlessness.
- Administer anticoagulants (e.g., heparin, enoxaparin [Lovenox]) as ordered *to decrease clot formation.*
- Teach or perform range-of-motion exercises for lower extremities and encourage early ambulation *to maintain muscle contractions and adequate vascular flow.*
- Avoid pressure under knees from bed or pillows *to avoid pressure on veins, constriction of circulation, or pooling and stasis of blood.*
- Apply antiembolism stockings and sequential compression device, if ordered. Remove for 1 hr every 8-10 hr *to allow for skin assessment.*

Continued

cation because it may lead to pulmonary embolism. Patients with a history of DVT have a greater risk for pulmonary embolism. Pulmonary embolism should be suspected in any patient complaining of tachypnea, dyspnea, and tachycardia, particularly when the patient is already receiving oxygen therapy. Other manifestations may include chest pain, hypotension, hemoptysis, dysrhythmias, and heart failure. Superficial thrombophlebitis is an uncomfortable but less ominous complication that may develop in a leg vein as a result of venous stasis or in the arm veins as a result of irritation from IV catheters or solutions. If a piece of a clot becomes dislodged and travels to the lung, it can cause a pulmonary infarction of a size proportionate to the vessel in

NURSING CARE PLAN 20-1
Postoperative Patient—cont'd

COLLABORATIVE PROBLEMS—cont'd

NURSING GOALS	NURSING INTERVENTIONS and *RATIONALES*
Potential Complication • Monitor for signs of urinary retention • Report deviation from acceptable parameters • Carry out appropriate medical and nursing interventions	**Urinary retention** *related to* horizontal positioning, pain, fear, analgesic and anesthetic medications, or surgical procedure • Assess for bladder pain and distention, or decreased or absent urinary output *to determine if a problem is present.* • Percuss bladder routinely for 48 hr postoperatively *to assess for distention.* • Notify physician if patient does not urinate within 6 hr after surgery *to prevent bladder distention and discomfort.* • Position patient in as normal a position as possible for voiding. • Use appropriate pain measures and provide privacy to reduce anxiety *so voiding will be easier.*
Potential Complication • Monitor for signs of paralytic ileus • Report deviation from acceptable parameters • Carry out appropriate medical and nursing interventions	**Paralytic ileus** *related to* bowel manipulation, immobility, pain medication, and anesthetics • Assess for abdominal distention, presence of flatus or stool, bowel sounds, or nausea and vomiting *to determine if paralytic ileus is present.* • Maintain nothing-by-mouth (NPO) status until peristalsis returns and ensure patency of nasogastric tube *to prevent vomiting and abdominal distention.*

which it lodges. (DVT and pulmonary embolism are discussed in Chapters 38 and 28, respectively.)

Syncope (fainting) is another factor that reflects the cardiovascular status. It may indicate decreased cardiac output, fluid deficits, or defects in cerebral perfusion. Syncope frequently occurs as a result of postural hypotension when the patient ambulates. It is more common in the older adult or in the patient who has been immobile for long periods of time. Normally when the patient quickly moves to a standing position, the arterial pressoreceptors respond to the accompanying fall in blood pressure with sympathetic nervous system stimulation, which produces vasoconstriction and thereby maintains blood pressure. These sympathetic and vasomotor functions may be diminished in the older adult and the immobile or postanesthetic patient.

NURSING MANAGEMENT
CARDIOVASCULAR PROBLEMS

■ *Nursing Assessment*

The most important aspect of the cardiovascular assessment is frequent monitoring of vital signs. They are usually monitored every 15 minutes in Phase I, or more often until stabilized, and then at less frequent intervals. Postoperative vital signs should be compared with preoperative and intraoperative readings to determine when the signs are stabilizing at a level that is normal for the patient's condition. The ACP or surgeon should be notified if the following occur:

1. Systolic BP is less than 90 mm Hg or greater than 160 mm Hg.
2. Pulse rate is less than 60 beats per minute or greater than 120 beats per minute.
3. Pulse pressure (difference between systolic and diastolic pressures) narrows.
4. BP gradually decreases during several consecutive readings.
5. There is a change in cardiac rhythm.
6. There is a significant variation from preoperative readings.

Cardiac monitoring is recommended for patients who have a history of cardiac disease and for all older adult patients who have undergone major surgery, regardless of whether they have cardiac problems. The apical-radial pulse should be assessed carefully, and any irregularities should be reported.

Assessment of skin color, temperature, and moisture provides valuable information in detecting cardiovascular problems. Hypotension accompanied by a normal pulse and warm, dry, pink skin usually represents the residual vasodilating effects of anesthesia and suggests only a need for continued observation. Hypotension accompanied by a rapid pulse and cold, clammy, pale skin may be caused by impending hypovolemic shock and requires immediate treatment.

■ *Nursing Diagnoses*

Nursing diagnoses and collaborative problems related to potential cardiovascular problems for the postoperative patient include, but are not limited to, the following:

- Decreased cardiac output
- Deficient fluid volume
- Excess fluid volume
- Ineffective tissue perfusion
- Activity intolerance
- Potential complication: hypovolemic shock
- Potential complication: thromboembolism

■ *Nursing Implementation*

PACU. Nursing interventions in the PACU are designed to prevent and treat cardiovascular problems. Treatment of hypotension should always begin with oxygen therapy to promote oxygenation of hypoperfused organs. Volume status should be assessed as described, and errors of BP measurement should be ruled out. Because the most common cause of hypotension is fluid loss, IV fluid boluses will be given to normalize BP. Primary cardiac dysfunction may require drug intervention. Peripheral vasodilation and hypotension may require vasoconstrictive agents to normalize systemic vascular resistance.

Treatment of hypertension will center on addressing the cause of sympathetic nervous system stimulation and eliminating the precipitating cause. Treatment may include the use of analgesics, assistance in voiding, and correction of respiratory problems. Rewarming will correct hypothermia-induced hypertension. If the patient has preexisting hypertension or has undergone cardiac or vascular surgery, drug therapy designed to reduce BP will usually be required.

Because the majority of dysrhythmias seen in the PACU have identifiable causes, treatment is directed toward eliminating the cause. Correction of these physiologic alterations will, in most instances, correct the dysrhythmias. In the event of life-threatening dysrhythmias (e.g., ventricular tachycardia), protocols for cardiac life support will be applied.

Clinical Unit. An accurate intake and output record should be kept during the postoperative period, and laboratory findings (e.g., electrolytes, hematocrit) should be monitored. Nursing responsibilities relating to IV management are critical during this period. In particular, the nurse should be alert for symptoms of too slow or too rapid a rate of fluid replacement. Assessment should also be made of the hazards associated with the IV administration of potassium, such as cardiac dysrhythmias and pain at the infusion site.

Leg exercises (Fig. 20-6) should be encouraged 10 to 12 times every 1 to 2 hours while awake. The muscular contraction produced by these exercises and by ambulation facilitates venous return from the lower extremities. When confined to bed, the patient should alternately flex and extend the legs. When the patient is sitting in a chair or lying in bed, there should be no pressure to impede venous flow through the popliteal space. Crossed legs, pillows behind the knees, and extreme elevation of the knee gatch of the bed must be avoided.

Early ambulation is the most significant general nursing measure to prevent postoperative complications. The exercise associated with walking (1) increases muscle tone; (2) improves GI and urinary tract function; (3) stimulates circulation, which prevents venous stasis and speeds wound healing; and (4) increases vital capacity and maintains normal respiratory function.

Currently the most effective means of preventing DVT and pulmonary emboli in surgical patients is use of subcutaneous heparin (or low-molecular-weight heparin [LMWH]) in combination with antiembolism stockings.[4,5] One recent study indicated that the combination of LMWH and thigh-length stockings was the best method to decrease the risk for developing a DVT.[4]

The nurse may prevent syncope by making changes slowly in the patient's position. Progression to ambulation can be achieved by first raising the head of the patient's bed for 1 to 2 minutes and then by assisting the patient to sit on the side of the bed while monitoring the radial pulse for rate and quality. If no changes or complaints are noted, ambulation can be started. If faintness occurs, the nurse can help the patient sit on the edge of the bed while continuing to monitor the pulse. If changes occur or if the patient complains of feeling faint during ambulation, the nurse should provide assistance to a nearby chair or ease the patient to the floor. The patient should remain in either location until recovery is evidenced by BP stability, and then be helped back to the bed. If faintness occurs, it is often frightening for the patient and for the unprepared nurse, but syncope poses no real physiologic danger, although injury can result from a fall.

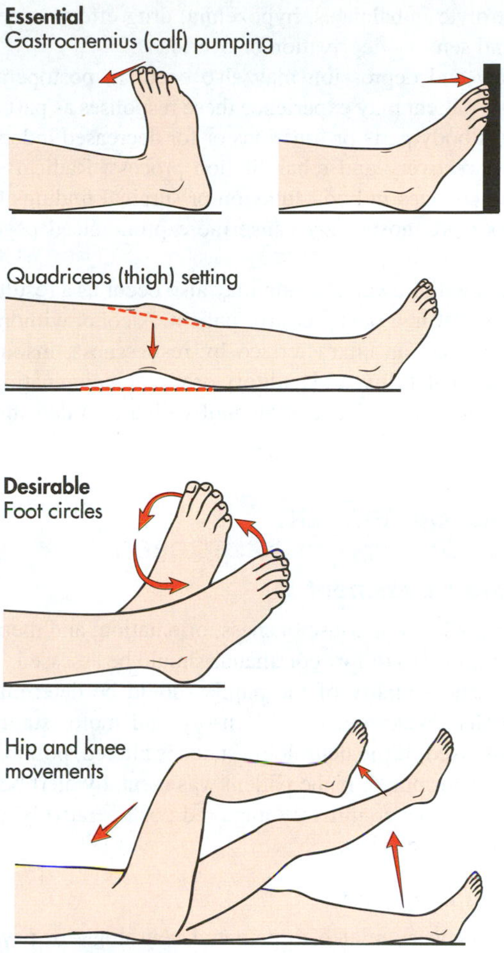

FIG. 20-6 Postoperative leg exercises.

POTENTIAL NEUROLOGIC/PSYCHOLOGIC PROBLEMS

Etiology

PACU. Postoperatively, emergence delirium is the neurologic alteration that causes the most concern. **Emergence delirium,** or *waking up wild,* can include behaviors such as restlessness, agitation, disorientation, thrashing, and shouting. This condition may be caused by anesthetic agents, hypoxia, bladder distention, pain, electrolyte abnormalities, or the patient's state of anxiety preoperatively. Hypoxia should be suspected first.[1]

Delayed emergence may also be a problem postoperatively. Fortunately, the most common cause of delayed emergence is prolonged drug action, particularly of opioids, sedatives, and inhalational anesthetics, as opposed to neurologic injury. Normal awakening can be predicted by the ACP based on the drugs used in surgery.

Clinical Unit. Two types of postoperative cognitive impairment are seen in surgical patients: delirium and postoperative cognitive dysfunction (POCD).[6] POCD is almost exclusively seen in the older surgical patient. While postoperative confusion and delirium are also more commonly seen in the older patient, they may occur in patients of any age. Confusion or delirium may arise from a variety of psychologic and physiologic sources, including fluid and electrolyte imbalances, hypoxemia, drug effects, sleep deprivation, and sensory deprivation or overload.

Anxiety and depression may also occur in postoperative patients. Any patient may experience these responses as part of grieving for lost body parts or functions or for decreased independence during the recovery and rehabilitation process. Radical surgeries leading to changes in body function or surgical findings that suggest a poor prognosis may cause more pronounced psychologic reactions.

Alcohol withdrawal delirium may also occur as a result of alcohol withdrawal in a postoperative patient. Alcohol withdrawal delirium is a reaction characterized by restlessness, insomnia and nightmares, irritability, and auditory or visual hallucinations. Identification and management of alcohol withdrawal delirium is discussed in Chapter 12.

NURSING MANAGEMENT NEUROLOGIC/PSYCHOLOGIC PROBLEMS

■ *Nursing Assessment*

The patient's level of consciousness, orientation, and memory and his or her ability to follow commands should be assessed. The size, reactivity, and equality of the pupils should be determined. The patient's sleep/wake cycle and sensory and motor status should also be assessed. If the neurologic status is altered, possible causes should be determined. If the patient was mentally alert before surgery and becomes cognitively impaired postoperatively, the nurse should suspect delirium.

■ *Nursing Diagnoses*

Nursing diagnoses related to potential neurologic or psychologic problems for the postoperative patient include, but are not limited to, the following:

- Disturbed sensory perception
- Risk for injury
- Disturbed thought processes
- Impaired verbal communication
- Anxiety
- Ineffective coping
- Disturbed body image
- Fear

■ *Nursing Implementation*

PACU. The most common cause of postoperative agitation in the PACU is hypoxemia. As a result, attention must focus on evaluating respiratory function. Once hypoxemia has been ruled out as the cause of postoperative delirium and all potentially known causes have been addressed, sedation may prove beneficial in controlling the agitation and providing for patient and staff safety. Emergence delirium is usually time limited and will resolve before the patient is discharged from the PACU. Because the most common cause of delayed emergence is prolonged drug action, delays in awakening usually spontaneously resolve with time. If necessary, benzodiazepines and opioids may be pharmacologically reversed with antagonists.

Until the patient is awake and able to communicate effectively, it is the responsibility of the PACU nurse to act as a patient advocate and to maintain patient safety at all times. This includes having the side rails up, securing IV lines and artificial airways, verifying the presence of identification and allergy bands, and monitoring physiologic status.

Clinical Unit. To prevent or manage postoperative delirium, the nurse should address factors that are known to contribute to the condition. Maintenance of normal physiologic function is important and includes fluid and electrolyte balance, adequate nutrition, pain management, proper bowel and bladder function, and early mobilization. The nurse can also use environmental aids, such as clocks, calendars, and photographs, to help orient the patient.

The nurse should attempt to prevent psychologic problems in the postoperative period by providing adequate support for the patient. Supportive measures include taking time to listen to and talk with the patient, offering explanations and genuine reassurance, and encouraging the presence and assistance of significant others. The nurse must observe and evaluate the patient's behavior to distinguish a normal reaction to the stress situation from one that is becoming abnormal or excessive.

The nurse should discuss the patient's expectations regarding activity and assistance needed following discharge. The patient must be included in discharge planning and should be provided with the information and support to make informed decisions about continuing care.

The recognition of alcohol withdrawal delirium in a patient not previously known to be an alcoholic presents a particular challenge. Any unusual or disturbed behavior should be reported immediately so that diagnosis and treatment may be instituted.

PAIN AND DISCOMFORT

Etiology

Despite the availability of analgesic drugs and pain-relieving techniques, pain remains a common problem and a significant fear for the patient in the PACU and during the postoperative period. Postoperative pain is caused by the interaction of a number of physiologic and psychologic factors. The skin and underlying tissues have been traumatized by the incision and retraction during surgery. In addition, there may be reflex muscle spasms around the incision. Anxiety and fear, sometimes related to the anticipation of pain, create tension and further increase muscle tone and spasm. Positioning during surgery or the use of internal devices such as an endotracheal tube or catheters may also result in pain. The effort and movement associated with deep breathing, coughing, and ambulating may aggravate pain by creating tension on the incision area.

Pain can contribute to complications such as dysfunction of the immune system and blood clotting, and delayed return of normal gastric and bowel function.[7] It also increases the risk of atelectasis and impaired respiratory function.[8]

When the internal viscera are cut, no pain is felt. However, pressure in the internal viscera elicits pain. Therefore deep visceral pain may signal the presence of a complication such as intestinal distention, bleeding, or abscess formation.

NURSING MANAGEMENT PAIN

■ *Nursing Assessment*

The patient's self-report is the single most reliable indicator of pain.[7] Since this is not always possible in the PACU, the patient should also be observed for other indications of pain (e.g., restlessness, increased heart rate, diaphoresis). Identifying the location of the pain is important. Incisional pain is to be expected, but other causes of pain, such as a full bladder, may be present. The Joint Commission on Accreditation of Healthcare Organizations (JCAHO) has published monographs listing numerous clinical practice guidelines from a variety of sources to aid in the assessment and treatment of pain.[9,10] ASPAN also has published the "Pain and Comfort Clinical Guideline," which is directed at caring for patients throughout their perioperative experience.[11]

Nursing Diagnoses

Nursing diagnoses for the patient experiencing pain and discomfort include, but are not limited to, the following:

- Acute pain
- Anxiety

Nursing Implementation

The most effective interventions for postoperative pain management include using a variety of analgesics.[12] Intravenous opioids provide the most rapid relief. Drugs are administered slowly and titrated to allow for optimal pain management with minimal to no adverse drug side effects. More sustained relief may be obtained through the use of epidural catheters, patient-controlled analgesia, or regional anesthetic blockade.

Postoperative pain relief is a nursing responsibility because the surgeon's orders for analgesic medication and other comfort measures are usually written on an as-needed basis. During the first 48 hours or longer, opioid analgesics (e.g., morphine) are required to relieve moderate to severe pain. After that time, nonopioid analgesics, such as nonsteroidal antiinflammatory agents, may be sufficient as pain intensity decreases.

Analgesic administration should be timed to ensure that it is in effect during activities that may be painful for the patient, such as ambulating. Although opioid analgesics are often essential for the postoperative patient's comfort, there are undesirable side effects. Side effects such as constipation, nausea and vomiting, respiratory and cough depression, and hypotension are most common with the opioids. Before administering any analgesic, the nurse should first assess the nature of the patient's pain, including location, quality, and intensity. If it is incisional pain, analgesic administration is appropriate. If it is chest or leg pain, medication may simply mask a complication that must be reported and documented. If it is gas pain, opioids can aggravate it. The nurse should notify the physician and request a change in the order if the analgesic either fails to relieve the pain or makes the patient excessively lethargic or somnolent.

Patient-controlled analgesia (PCA) and epidural analgesia are two alternative approaches for pain control. The goals of PCA are to provide immediate analgesia and to maintain a constant, steady blood level of the analgesic agent. PCA involves self-administration of predetermined doses of analgesia by the patient. The route of delivery may be IV, oral, or epidural. (PCA is discussed in Chapter 10.) Some advantages of PCA are early ambulation, improved wound healing, and earlier hospital discharge.[8]

Epidural analgesia is the infusion of opioid analgesics through a catheter placed into the epidural space surrounding the spinal cord. The goal of epidural analgesia is delivery of medication directly to opiate receptors in the spinal cord. Administration methods include intermittent bolus dosing, continuous infusion, and patient-controlled epidural analgesia (PCEA). The overall effectiveness and the technique of administration result in a constant circulating level and a reduced total dose of medication. The use of epidural analgesia for postoperative pain is increasing based on research that has demonstrated superior pain relief and improved functional outcomes after major surgery in patients who receive epidural analgesia compared with patients receiving IV PCA.[13]

The acute pain of surgery almost always requires the use of analgesics. However, nonpharmacologic approaches such as repositioning, massage, distraction, relaxation, and deep breathing can enhance pain management. Music and educational interventions have also been shown to be effective adjuncts to pain medication.[14]

EVIDENCE-BASED PRACTICE

Which Postoperative Analgesia Is the Most Effective for Pain Control?

Clinical Question

In postoperative patients (P), does epidural analgesia (I) or IV patient-controlled analgesia (C) provide better pain control (O)?

Best Available Evidence

Systematic review of randomized controlled trials (RCTs)

Critical Appraisal and Synthesis of Evidence

- Meta-analysis of 50 RCTs (n = 3208).
- Epidural analgesia was administered continuously or self-administered while IV analgesia was only self-administered.
- Surgical sites included abdominal, thoracic, pelvic, lower extremity, and others.
- Epidural analgesia (with one exception), regardless of analgesic agent, was superior to self-administered IV analgesia.
- Continuous epidural infusion provided better pain control than patient-administered epidural analgesia. However, patient-controlled epidural analgesia resulted in a lower incidence of nausea/vomiting and motor block.

Conclusions

- Epidural analgesia is a better choice for postoperative pain than IV patient-administered analgesia.
- Continuous epidural infusion gives superior pain relief when compared to patient-administered epidural analgesia.

Implications for Nursing Practice

Provide information and allow patients to actively participate in determining which analgesia option is the best for them.

Reference for Evidence

Wu CL, Cohen BS, Richman J et al: Efficacy of postoperative patient-controlled and continuous infusion epidural analgesia versus intravenous patient-controlled analgesia with opioids, *Anesthesiology* 103:1079, 2005.

PICO: P, Patient population of interest; *I*, intervention or area of interest; *C*, comparison of interest or comparison group; *O*, outcome(s) of interest (see p. 6).

POTENTIAL ALTERATIONS IN TEMPERATURE

Etiology

Hypothermia, a core temperature of less than 96.8° F (36° C), occurs when heat loss exceeds heat production. In addition to the usual heat loss mechanisms of radiation, convection, conduction, and evaporation, heat loss may occur in the perioperative setting because of infusion of cool IV fluids and ventilation with dry gases.[1]

Although all patients are at risk for hypothermia, the older, debilitated, or intoxicated patient is at an increased risk. Long surgical procedures and prolonged anesthetic administration lead to re-

TABLE 20-6 Significance of Postoperative Temperature Changes

Time After Surgery	Temperature	Possible Causes
Up to 12 hr	Hypothermia to 96.8° F (36° C)	Effects of anesthesia Body heat loss during surgical exposure
First 24-48 hr	Elevation to 100.4° F (38° C)	Inflammatory response to surgical stress
	Above 100.4° F (38° C)	Lung congestion, atelectasis
Third day and later	Elevation above 100° F (37.7° C)	Wound infection Urinary infection Respiratory infection Phlebitis

distribution of body heat from the core to the periphery. This places the patient at increased risk for hypothermia. Complications from hypothermia may include compromised immune function, postoperative pain, bleeding, myocardial ischemia, impaired wound healing, and delayed drug metabolism.[1]

Another complication of hypothermia is shivering. Shivering can increase oxygen consumption, carbon dioxide production, and cardiac output, as well as significantly affect the patient's comfort level.[15]

Temperature variation in the postoperative period provides valuable information about the patient's status. Fever may occur at any time during the postoperative period (Table 20-6). A mild elevation (up to 100.4° F [38° C]) during the first 48 hours usually reflects the surgical stress response. A moderate elevation (higher than 100.4° F [38° C]) is caused more frequently by respiratory congestion or atelectasis and less frequently by dehydration. After the first 48 hours, a moderate to marked elevation (higher than 99.9° F [37.7° C]) is usually caused by infection.

Wound infection, particularly from aerobic organisms, is often accompanied by a fever that spikes in the afternoon or evening and returns to near-normal levels in the morning. The respiratory tract may be infected secondary to stasis of secretions in areas of atelectasis. The urinary tract may be infected secondary to catheterization. Superficial thrombophlebitis may occur at the IV site or in the leg veins. Thrombophlebitis in the leg veins may produce a temperature elevation between 7 and 10 days after surgery.

Nosocomial infectious diarrhea caused by *Clostridium difficile* may be signaled by fever, diarrhea, and abdominal pain. Surgical patients who receive antibiotics for a period of time are at risk.

Intermittent high fever accompanied by shaking chills and diaphoresis suggests septicemia. This may occur at any time during the postoperative period because microorganisms may have been introduced into the bloodstream during surgery, especially in GI or genitourinary (GU) procedures, or picked up later from the site of a wound or from a urinary tract or vein infection.

NURSING MANAGEMENT
ALTERED TEMPERATURE

▪ *Nursing Assessment*

Frequent assessment of the patient's temperature is important to detect patterns of hypothermia and/or fever that may be present in the postoperative period. Temperature may be taken orally, or via the tympanic membrane or axilla. The color and temperature of the skin should also be assessed. The nurse should observe the patient for early signs of inflammation and infection that may precede a fever so that any complications that arise may be treated in a timely manner.

▪ *Nursing Diagnoses*

Nursing diagnoses for the patient with an altered temperature include, but are not limited to, the following:

- Hyperthermia
- Hypothermia
- Risk for imbalanced body temperature

▪ *Nursing Implementation*

Passive rewarming in a patient with hypothermia (i.e., shivering) raises basal body metabolism. *Active rewarming* requires the application of external warming devices, including warm blankets, heated aerosols, radiant warmers, forced air warmers, and heated water mattresses. When using any external warming device, body temperature should be monitored at 15-minute intervals, and care should be taken to prevent skin injuries. In addition, oxygen therapy via nasal prongs or mask is used to treat the increased demand for oxygen accompanying the increase in body temperature. Shivering is usually quickly suppressed by opioids.[15] (See Chapter 69 for additional management of hypothermia.)

The nurse's role with respect to postoperative fever may be preventive, diagnostic, and therapeutic. The patient's temperature is usually measured every 4 hours for the first 48 hours postoperatively and then less frequently if no problems develop. Meticulous asepsis is maintained with regard to the wound and the IV site, and airway clearance is encouraged. If fever develops, chest x-rays may be taken, and, depending on the suspected cause, cultures of the wound, urine, or blood are obtained. If infection is the source of the fever, antibiotics are started as soon as cultures have been obtained. If the fever rises above 103° F (39.4° C), antipyretic drugs and body-cooling measures may be employed.

POTENTIAL GASTROINTESTINAL PROBLEMS

Etiology

Postoperative nausea and vomiting occur in 20% to 30% of adult patients. These problems are responsible for unanticipated hospital admission of day-surgery patients, increased patient discomfort, delays in discharge, and patient dissatisfaction with the surgical experience. Numerous factors have been identified as contributing to the development of nausea and vomiting, including gender (female), history of motion sickness or previous postoperative nausea and vomiting, and action of anesthetics or opioids, as well as duration and type of surgery.[16] Delayed gastric emptying and slowed peristalsis that result from handling of the bowel during abdominal surgery also contribute to nausea and vomiting, as does the resumption of oral intake too soon after surgery.

Abdominal distention is another common problem caused by decreased peristalsis as a result of handling of the intestine during surgery and limited dietary intake before and after surgery. Following abdominal surgery, motility in the large intestine may be reduced for 3 to 5 days, although motility in the small intestine resumes within 24 hours. Swallowed air and GI secretions may accumulate in the colon, producing distention and gas pains.

Hiccups *(singultus)* are intermittent spasms of the diaphragm caused by irritation of the phrenic nerve, which innervates the diaphragm. Postoperative sources of direct irritation of the phrenic nerve may be gastric distention, intestinal obstruction, intraabdominal bleeding, and a subphrenic abscess. Indirect irritation of the phrenic nerve may be produced by acid-base and electrolyte imbalances. Reflex irritation may come from drinking hot or cold liquids or from the presence of a nasogastric tube. Hiccups usually last a short time and subside spontaneously; occasionally they may be persistent, but they are rarely debilitating.

NURSING MANAGEMENT GASTROINTESTINAL PROBLEMS

Nursing Assessment

The patient should be questioned about feelings of nausea. If vomiting occurs, it is important to determine the quantity, characteristics, and color of the vomitus. The abdomen should be assessed for distention and the presence of bowel sounds. Because bowel sounds are frequently absent or diminished in the immediate postoperative period, all four quadrants should be auscultated to determine the presence, frequency, and characteristics of the sounds. The return of normal bowel motility is usually accompanied by the passage of flatus in addition to normal bowel sounds and the absence of distention.

Nursing Diagnoses

Nursing diagnoses for the patient experiencing GI problems include, but are not limited to, the following:

- Nausea
- Risk for aspiration
- Risk for deficient fluid volume
- Imbalanced nutrition: less than body requirements
- Potential complication: fluid and electrolyte imbalance
- Potential complication: hiccups

Nursing Implementation

Postoperative nausea and vomiting are treated with the use of antiemetic or prokinetic drugs (see Chapter 42, Table 42-1). Other methods of decreasing nausea and vomiting are being tested, such as giving carbohydrate-rich fluid to patients before laparoscopic cholecystectomy.[16] In the PACU, oral fluids should be given only as indicated and tolerated. Intravenous fluids will provide hydration until the patient is able to tolerate oral fluids. Care should also be taken to prevent aspiration if the patient vomits while still sleepy from anesthesia. Having suction equipment readily available at the bedside and turning the patient's head to the side will help protect the patient from aspiration. Other nonpharmacologic nursing interventions that may be effective include biofeedback, hypnosis, relaxation, guided imagery, music therapy, distraction, and acupressure.[17]

Depending on the nature of the surgery, the patient may resume oral intake as soon as the gag reflex returns. The patient who had abdominal surgery is usually allowed nothing by mouth (NPO) until the presence of bowel sounds indicates the return of peristalsis. When the patient is NPO, IV infusions are given to maintain fluid and electrolyte balance. A nasogastric tube may be used to decompress the stomach to prevent nausea, vomiting, and abdominal distention. Regular mouth care is essential for comfort and stimulation of salivary glands when the patient is NPO or has a nasogastric tube. When oral intake is allowed, clear liquids are offered first and the IV infusion is continued, usually at a reduced rate. If oral intake is well tolerated by the patient, the IV infusion is discontinued, and the diet is advanced until a regular diet is tolerated.

Abdominal distention may be prevented or minimized by early and frequent ambulation, which stimulates intestinal motility. The nurse should assess the patient regularly to detect the resumption of normal intestinal peristalsis as evidenced by the return of bowel sounds and the passage of flatus. The nasogastric tube must be clamped or the suction turned off when the abdomen is auscultated. Resumption of a normal diet after bowel sounds have returned will also enhance the return of normal peristalsis.

The patient may need to be encouraged to expel flatus and assured that expulsion is necessary and desirable. Gas pains, which tend to become pronounced on the second or third postoperative day, may be relieved by ambulation and frequent repositioning. Positioning the patient on the right side permits gas to rise along the transverse colon and facilitates its release. Bisacodyl (Dulcolax) suppositories may be ordered to stimulate colonic peristalsis and expulsion of flatus and feces.

POTENTIAL URINARY PROBLEMS

Etiology

Low urine output (800 to 1500 ml) in the first 24 hours after surgery may be expected, regardless of fluid intake. This low output is caused by increased aldosterone and ADH secretion resulting from the stress of surgery, fluid restriction before surgery, and fluid loss through surgery, drainage, and diaphoresis. By the second or third day, the patient will begin to have increasing urinary output after fluid has been mobilized and the immediate stress reaction subsides.

Acute urinary retention can occur in the postoperative period for a variety of reasons. Anesthesia depresses the nervous system, including the micturition reflex arc and the higher centers that influence it. This allows the bladder to fill more completely than normal before the urge to void is felt. Anesthesia also impedes voluntary micturition. Anticholinergic and opioid drugs may also interfere with the ability to initiate voiding or to empty the bladder completely.

Retention is more likely to occur after lower abdominal or pelvic surgery because spasms or guarding of the abdominal and pelvic muscles interferes with their normal function in micturition. Pain may alter perception and interfere with the patient's awareness of bladder filling. Voiding ability is probably impaired to the greatest extent by immobility and the recumbent position in bed. The supine position reduces the ability to relax the perineal muscles and external sphincter.

Oliguria (the diminished output of urine) can be a manifestation of renal failure and is a less common, although more serious, problem after surgery. It may result from renal ischemia caused by inadequate renal perfusion or altered cardiovascular function.

NURSING MANAGEMENT URINARY PROBLEMS

Nursing Assessment

The urine of the postoperative patient should be examined for both quantity and quality. The color, amount, consistency, and odor of the urine should be noted. Indwelling catheters should be assessed for patency, and urine output should be at least 0.5 ml/kg/hr. Most patients urinate within 6 to 8 hours after surgery. If no voiding occurs, the abdominal contour should be inspected and the bladder assessed for distention.

▪ Nursing Diagnoses

Nursing diagnoses and collaborative problems related to potential urinary problems for the postoperative patient include, but are not limited to, the following:

- Impaired urinary elimination
- Potential complication: acute urinary retention

▪ Nursing Implementation

The nurse may facilitate voiding by normal positioning of the patient—sitting for women and standing for men. Providing reassurance to the patient regarding the ability to void and the use of techniques such as providing privacy, running water, having the patient drink water, or pouring warm water over the perineum may also be of assistance. Ambulation, preferably to the bathroom, and the use of a bedside commode are additional helpful measures to assist in voiding.

The surgeon often leaves an order to catheterize the patient in 6 to 8 hours if voiding has not occurred. Because of the possibility of infection associated with catheterization, the nurse should first try other measures to induce voiding and validate that the bladder is actually full. In assessing the need for catheterization, the nurse should consider fluid intake during and after surgery and determine bladder fullness (e.g., palpable fullness above the symphysis pubis, discomfort when pressure is applied over the bladder, or the presence of the urge to void). Straight catheterization is preferred because of the possibility of infection associated with an indwelling catheter.

POTENTIAL INTEGUMENTARY PROBLEMS

Etiology

Surgery generally involves an incision through the skin and underlying tissues. An incision disrupts the protective skin barrier. Therefore, wound healing is one of the major concerns during the postoperative period.

An adequate nutritional state is essential for wound healing. Amino acids are readily available for the healing process because of the catabolic effects of the stress-related hormones (e.g., cortisol). The patient who was well nourished preoperatively can tolerate the postoperative delay in nutritional intake for several days. However, the patient with preexisting nutritional deficits that occur with chronic diseases (e.g., diabetes, ulcerative colitis, alcoholism) is more prone to problems of wound healing. Abdominal wound healing is affected by obesity. Wound healing is also a concern for the older adult. The patient who is unable to meet nutritional needs postoperatively may be provided with enteral nutrition or parenteral nutrition to promote healing.

Wound infection may result from contamination of the wound from three major sources: (1) exogenous flora present in the environment and on the skin, (2) oral flora, and (3) intestinal flora. The incidence of wound sepsis is higher in patients who are malnourished, immunosuppressed, or older, or who have had a prolonged hospital stay or a lengthy surgical procedure (lasting more than 3 hours). Patients undergoing bowel surgery, particularly following a traumatic injury, are at particularly high risk. Infection may involve the entire incision and may extend downward through the deeper tissue layers. An abscess may form locally, or the infection may spread throughout entire body cavities, as in peritonitis. Evidence of wound infection usually does not become apparent before the third to the fifth postoperative day. Local manifestations include redness, swelling, and increasing pain and tenderness at the site. Systemic manifestations are fever and leukocytosis.

An accumulation of fluid in a wound may create pressure, impair circulation and wound healing, and predispose to infection. For these reasons, the surgeon may place a drain in the incision or make a stab wound adjacent to the incision to allow for drainage. These drains may be made of soft rubber and drain into a dressing, or they may be firm catheters attached to a Hemovac or other source of gentle suction.

NURSING MANAGEMENT
SURGICAL WOUNDS

▪ Nursing Assessment

Nursing assessment of the wound and dressing requires knowledge of the type of wound, the drains inserted, and expected drainage related to the specific type of surgery. A small amount of serous drainage is common from any type of wound. If a drain is in place, a moderate to large amount of drainage may be expected. For example, an abdominal incision with an accompanying drain is expected to have a moderate amount of serosanguineous drainage in the first 24 hours. In contrast, an inguinal herniorrhaphy should have only minimal serous drainage during the postoperative period.

In general, drainage is expected to change from sanguineous (red) to serosanguineous (pink) to serous (clear yellow). The drainage output should decrease over hours or days, depending on the type of surgery. Wound infection may be accompanied by purulent drainage. **Wound dehiscence** (separation and disruption of previously joined wound edges) may be preceded by a sudden discharge of brown, pink, or clear drainage.

▪ Nursing Diagnoses

Nursing diagnoses related to surgical wounds of the postoperative patient include, but are not limited to, the following:

- Risk for infection
- Potential complication: impaired wound healing

▪ Nursing Implementation

When drainage occurs on the dressing, the type, amount, color, consistency, and odor of drainage should be noted and recorded. Expected drainage from tubes is outlined in Table 20-7. The effect of position changes on drainage should also be assessed. The surgeon should be notified of any excessive or abnormal drainage and significant changes in vital signs.

The incision may be covered with a dressing immediately after surgery. If there is no drainage after 24 to 48 hours, the dressing may be removed and the incision left open to the air. If the initial operative dressing is saturated, institutional policy determines whether the nurse may change the dressing or simply reinforce it.

When a dressing is changed, the number and type of drains present should be noted. Care should be taken to avoid dislodging drains during dressing removal. When the dressing is changed, the incision site should be examined carefully. The area around the sutures may be slightly reddened and swollen, which is an expected inflammatory response. However, the skin around the incision should be of

TABLE 20-7 Expected Drainage from Tubes and Catheters

Substance	Daily Amount	Color	Odor	Consistency
Indwelling Catheter				
Urine	500-700 ml for 1-2 days postoperative; 1500-2500 ml thereafter	Clear, yellow	Ammonia	Watery
Nasogastric Tube/Gastrostomy Tube				
Gastric contents	Up to 1500 ml/day	Pale, yellow-green Bloody following gastrointestinal surgery	Sour	Watery
Hemovac				
Wound drainage	Variable with procedure	Variable with procedure Usually serosanguineous	Same as wound dressing	Variable
T-Tube				
Bile	500 ml	Bright yellow to dark green	Acid	Thick

normal color and temperature. Clinical manifestations of infection include redness, swelling, pain, fever, and increased white blood cell count. If healing is by primary intention, little or no drainage is present, and no drains are in place, a single-layer dressing or no dressing is sufficient. When drains are in place, when moderate to heavy drainage is occurring, or when healing occurs other than by primary intention, a multiple-layer dressing is needed. Wound healing and care are discussed in Chapter 13.

DISCHARGE FROM THE PACU

The choice of discharge site is based on patient acuity, access to follow-up care, and the potential for postoperative complications. The decision to discharge the patient from the PACU is based on written discharge criteria. Examples of discharge criteria are provided in Table 20-8.

Discharge to the Clinical Unit

Before discharging the patient from the PACU to the clinical unit, the PACU nurse provides a verbal report about the patient to the receiving nurse. The report summarizes the operative and postanesthetic period.

TABLE 20-8 Postanesthesia and Ambulatory Surgery Discharge Criteria

Postanesthesia Discharge Criteria (Phase I)
- Patient awake (or baseline)
- Vital signs stable
- No excess bleeding or drainage
- No respiratory depression
- Oxygen saturation >90%
- Report given

Ambulatory Surgery Discharge Criteria (Phase II/III)
- All PACU discharge criteria met
- No IV opioid drugs for last 30 min
- Minimal nausea and vomiting
- Voided (if appropriate to surgical procedure/orders)
- Able to ambulate if age appropriate and not contraindicated
- Responsible adult present to accompany patient
- Discharge instructions given and understood

PACU, Postanesthesia care unit.

The nurse who receives the patient on the clinical unit assists PACU transport personnel in transferring the patient from the PACU cart onto the bed. Care must be taken to protect IV lines, wound drains, dressings, and traction devices. The use of a draw sheet or transfer board and sufficient personnel facilitates transfer of the patient.

Vital signs should be obtained, and patient status should be compared with the report provided by the PACU. Documentation of the transfer is then completed, followed by a more in-depth assessment (Table 20-9). Postoperative orders and appropriate nursing care are then initiated.

TABLE 20-9 Nursing Assessment and Care of Patient on Admission to Clinical Unit

1. Record time of patient's return to unit
2. Take baseline vital signs
3. Assess pain and discomfort
   - Note last dose and type of pain control
   - Note current pain intensity
4. Assess airway and breath sounds
5. Assess neurologic status, including level of consciousness and movement of extremities
6. Assess wound, dressing, and drainage tubes:
   - Type and amount of drainage
   - Connect tubing to gravity or suction drainage (per orders)
7. Assess color and appearance of skin
8. Assess urinary status:
   - Time of voiding
   - Presence of catheter, patency, and total output
   - Bladder distention or urge to void
9. Position for airway maintenance, comfort, and safety (bed in low position, side rails up)
10. Check IV infusion:
    - Type of solution
    - Amount of fluid remaining
    - Flow rate
    - Integrity of insertion site and size of catheter
11. Attach call light within reach, and orient patient to use of call light
12. Ensure that emesis basin and tissues are available
13. Determine emotional condition and support
14. Check for presence of family member or significant other:
    - Orient patient and family to immediate environment
15. Check and carry out postoperative orders

AMBULATORY SURGERY: PHASE II AND III POSTOPERATIVE CARE

Ambulatory surgery has many advantages, including greater convenience, lower rates of hospital-acquired infections, and reduced costs.[18] Seventy percent of all surgical procedures in North America are considered ambulatory surgery.[19] Ambulatory surgery patients include those patients receiving Phase II and III postoperative care (see Table 20-1).

Pain following ambulatory surgery is a significant problem that can lead to increased symptoms of nausea, anxiety, and delirium; prolonged PACU stay; delayed discharge; readmission; and delayed resumption of normal activities at home.[20,21]

Ambulatory Surgery Discharge

The patient leaving an ambulatory surgery setting must be mobile and alert to provide a degree of self-care when discharged to home. Postoperative pain and nausea and vomiting must be controlled. Overall, the patient must be stable and near the level of preoperative functioning for discharge from the unit. At discharge, instructions specific to the type of anesthesia received and the surgery are given to the patient verbally and reinforced with written directions. The patient may not drive and must be accompanied by a responsible adult at the time of discharge. A follow-up evaluation of the patient's status is made by telephone, and any specific questions and concerns are addressed.

The nurse must carefully determine not only readiness for discharge, but home care needs of the individual. It is important to determine availability of assistive personnel (e.g., family, friends), access to a pharmacy for prescriptions, access to a phone in the event of an emergency, and access to follow-up care.

Planning for Discharge and Follow-up Care

Preparation for the patient's discharge should be an ongoing process throughout the surgical experience that begins during the preoperative period. The informed patient is prepared as events unfold and gradually assumes greater responsibility for self-care during the postoperative period. As the time of discharge approaches, the nurse should be certain that the patient and any caregivers have the following information:

1. Care of wound site and any dressings, including bathing recommendations
2. Action and possible side effects of any drugs; when and how to take them
3. Activities allowed and prohibited; when various physical activities can be resumed safely (e.g., driving a car, returning to work, sexual intercourse, leisure activities)
4. Dietary restrictions or modifications
5. Symptoms to be reported (e.g., development of incisional tenderness or increased drainage, discomfort in other parts of the body)
6. Where and when to return for follow-up care
7. Answers to any individual questions or concerns

Common reasons patients seek help after discharge include pain, need for advice about medications, and wound oozing and bleeding.[22] Attention to complete discharge instructions may prevent needless distress for the patient. Written instructions are important for reinforcing verbal information. The nurse should specifically document in the record the discharge instructions provided to the patient and family. For the patient, the postoperative phase of care continues and extends into the recuperative period. Assessment and evaluation of the patient after discharge may be accomplished by a follow-up call or by a visit from a nurse (e.g., home health nurse). The Joint Commission on Accreditation of Healthcare Organizations has developed patient education standards that give guidelines for content, materials used, and evaluation.[1]

Increasingly, patients are being discharged from the hospital with many care needs. They may be transferred to transitional care facilities, long-term care facilities, or directly to their homes (see Chapter 7). When discharged directly to home, it is expected that the patient, with assistance from family, friends, or home health care, will continue self-care in the home. This may include dressing changes, wound care, catheter or drain care, home antibiotics, or continued physical therapy. Working with the discharge planner for the hospital unit, or the case manager, the nurse can facilitate the transition of care from hospital-based to community-based and home care, without jeopardizing the quality of care.

GERONTOLOGIC CONSIDERATIONS
POSTOPERATIVE PATIENT

The older postoperative patient deserves special consideration. The older adult has decreased respiratory function, including decreased ability to cough, decreased thoracic compliance, and decreased lung tissue. These alterations in pulmonary status lead to an increase in the work of ventilation and a decreased ability to readily eliminate pharmacologic agents. Reactions to anesthetic agents must be carefully monitored and their postoperative elimination assessed before the patient is left without close supervision. Pneumonia is a common postoperative complication in the elderly.

Vascular function in the older adult is altered because of atherosclerosis and decreased elasticity in the blood vessels. Cardiac function is often compromised, and compensatory responses to changes in blood pressure and volume are limited. Circulating blood volume is decreased, and hypertension is common. Cardiovascular parameters must be closely monitored throughout surgery and the postoperative period.

Drug toxicity is a potential problem in the older adult. Renal perfusion in the older adult normally decreases, with a reduction in the ability to eliminate drugs that are excreted by the kidney. Decreased liver function in the older adult also leads to decreased drug metabolism and increased drug activity. Renal and liver function must be carefully assessed in the postoperative phase of the patient's care to prevent drug overdosage and toxicity.[23]

Observing for changes in mental status is an important part of postoperative care in older adults. Postoperative delirium is common (up to 60%) in the elderly in the postoperative period.[24] Factors such as age, alcohol abuse, low baseline cognition, severe metabolic derangement, hypoxia, hypotension, and type of surgery appear to contribute to postoperative delirium. Despite knowledge of risk factors, postoperative delirium in the elderly is poorly understood. Anesthetics, notably anticholinergic drugs and benzodiazepines, increase the risk for delirium. Delirium is an acute disorder of cognition and primarily affects attention and concentration. In contrast, the onset of dementia is usually slow.[24] (Dementia and delirium are discussed in Chapter 60.)

Pain control in the older adult patient is challenging because of possible preexisting cognitive impairment, impaired communication, and physiologic changes that affect how drugs are metabolized.[25] Older patients may be hesitant to request pain medication. They may believe that pain is an inevitable consequence of surgery that needs to be tolerated. Nurses may not appropriately assess pain in patients who do not report their pain. Some older patients are hesitant to learn how to use PCA machines. The nurse should encourage the use of analgesics, explaining to the patient and family that untreated pain could have a negative effect on recovery.

A comprehensive, multidisciplinary approach to caring for all of the health needs of the older adult patient is recommended by health professionals working with this population. When the older adult must undergo surgery, the same approach to care of the patient during the perioperative period can improve the outcome and decrease the risk for these patients.

CRITICAL THINKING EXERCISE

CASE STUDY

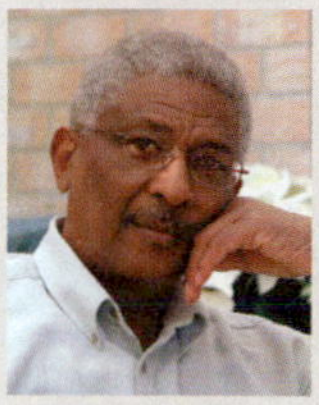

Case Study photo ©iStockphoto.com/ Malcolm Romain.

Postoperative Patient

Patient Profile. Edward Gray, a 74-year-old African American retired college professor, has just undergone surgery for a fractured hip. He fell off of a ladder while painting his house. The surgery, performed while the patient was under general anesthesia, lasted 4 hours.

Subjective Data

- Was in good health before his fall
- Played tennis three times each week
- Has smoked 1 pack of cigarettes per day × 58 years
- Always had problems sleeping
- Difficulty hearing, wears hearing aid
- Upset with injury and its impact on activity
- Has no relatives or friends to assist with care

Objective Data

- Admitted to PACU with abduction pillow between his legs, two peripheral IV catheters, a self-suction drain from the hip dressing, an indwelling urinary catheter, and a 40% face mask

Collaborative Care

Postoperative Orders

- Vital signs per PACU routine
- Dextrose 5% in 0.45 normal saline at 100 ml/hr
- Morphine via patient-controlled analgesia 1 mg q6min (30 mg max in 4 hr) for pain
- Advance diet as tolerated
- Incentive spirometry qhr × 10 while awake
- O_2 to keep oxygen saturation >90%

Critical Thinking Questions

1. What are the potential postanesthetic problems that the nurse might expect with Mr. Gray?
2. What nursing interventions would be appropriate to prevent these complications from occurring?
3. What factors may predispose Mr. Gray to the following problems: atelectasis, infection, pulmonary embolism, nausea and vomiting?
4. How should it be determined when Mr. Gray is sufficiently recovered from general anesthesia to be discharged to the clinical unit?
5. What potential postoperative problems might the nurse on the clinical unit expect?
6. What are risk factors for this patient developing postoperative delirium? What are the signs and symptoms?
7. Why is drug toxicity a potential problem for this patient?
8. Based on the assessment data presented, write one or more appropriate nursing diagnoses. Are there any collaborative problems?

NCLEX EXAMINATION REVIEW QUESTIONS

The number of the question corresponds to the same-numbered objective at the beginning of the chapter.

1. The components of an initial postanesthesia assessment that should be considered by the PACU nurse include
   a. the indication for the surgery.
   b. the status of the surgical incision.
   c. the results of intraoperative laboratory tests.
   d. the amount of fluid and blood replaced during surgery.
2. During the patient's admission to the PACU, the priority responsibility of the nurse is assessment of
   a. urinary output.
   b. airway patency.
   c. ECG monitoring.
   d. level of consciousness.
3. The nurse determines that the postoperative patient needs additional information before discharge when the patient tells the nurse
   a. "I don't have an appointment for a check-up with the surgeon."
   b. "The doctor told me I should not drive or return to work for 6 weeks."
   c. "I have a prescription for some pills that I can take until the pain gets better."
   d. "I should call the doctor if I have increased drainage or pain at the incision site."
4. Following admission of the postoperative patient to the clinical unit, which of the following assessment data requires the most immediate attention?
   a. Oxygen saturation of 85%
   b. Respiratory rate of 13/min
   c. Temperature of 100.4° F (38° C)
   d. Blood pressure of 90/60 mm Hg
5. A urine output averaging 20 ml/hr for the first postoperative day in a 154-pound patient
   a. is a normal, expected finding.
   b. requires a return to the operating room.
   c. requires an evaluation of the patient's fluid status.
   d. is normal if the patient had genitourinary surgery.
6. Discharge criteria for the Phase II patient include all of the following except
   a. ability to drive self home.
   b. no respiratory depression.
   c. minimal nausea and vomiting.
   d. written discharge instructions.

REFERENCES

1. Quinn DMD, Schick L: *PeriAnesthesia nursing core curriculum: preoperative, phase I and phase II PACU nursing,* Philadelphia, 2004, Saunders.

*2. Song D, Chung F, Ronayne M, et al: Fast-tracking (bypassing the PACU) does not reduce nursing workload after ambulatory surgery, *Br J Anaesth* 93:768, 2004.

*Nursing research–based reference.

*3. Pedersen T, Dyrlund Pedersen B, Moller AM: Pulse oximetry for perioperative monitoring, *The Cochrane Database of Systematic Reviews 2003*, Issue 2, Art. No. CD002013. (DOI: 10.1002/14651858.CD002013.)
*4. Howard A, Zaccagnini D, Ellis M, et al: Randomized clinical trial of low molecular weight heparin with thigh-length or knee-length antiembolism stockings for patients undergoing surgery, *Br J Surg* 91:842, 2004.
*5. Wells PS, Anderson DR, Rodger MA, et al: A randomized trial comparing 2 low-molecular-weight heparins for the outpatient treatment of deep vein thrombosis and pulmonary embolism, *Arch Intern Med* 165:733, 2005.
6. Souders JE, Rooke GA: Perioperative care for geriatric patients, *Ann Long-Term Care* 13(6):17, 2005.
7. Ang P, Knight H, Matadial C, et al: Managing acute postoperative pain: is 3 hours too long? *J PeriAnesth Nurs* 19:312, 2004.
*8. Chang AM, Ip WY, Cheung TH: Patient-controlled analgesia versus conventional intramuscular injection: a cost effectiveness analysis, *J Adv Nurs* 46:531, 2004.
9. National Pharmaceutical Council, Inc. and Joint Commission on Accreditation of Healthcare Organizations: *Pain: current understanding of assessment, management, and treatments* [monograph], Chicago, 2001, Joint Commission.
10. Joint Commission on Accreditation of Healthcare Organizations and National Pharmaceutical Council, Inc: *Improving the quality of pain management through measurement and action* [monograph], Chicago, 2003, Joint Commission.
11. American Society of PeriAnesthesia Nurses: ASPAN pain and comfort clinical guideline, *J PeriAnesth Nurs* 18:232, 2003.
12. Windle PE: The challenges of pain management: adverse effects of analgesics, *J PeriAnesth Nurs* 19:212, 2004.
13. Pasero C: Epidural analgesia for postoperative pain, *Am J Nurs* 103(10):62, 2003.
*14. Sherwood GD, McNeill JA, Starck PL, et al: Changing acute pain management outcomes in surgical patients, *AORN J* 77:374, 2003.
*15. Kiekkas P, Poulopoulou M, Papahatzi A, et al: Effects of hypothermia and shivering on standard PACU monitoring of patients, *AANA J* 73:47, 2005.
*16. Hausel J, Mygren J, Thorell A, et al: Randomized clinical trial of the effects of oral preoperative carbohydrates on postoperative nausea and vomiting after laparoscopic cholecystectomy, *Br J Surg* 92:415, 2005.
17. Dochterman JM, Bulechek GM: *Nursing interventions classification,* ed 4, St Louis, 2004, Mosby.
*18. Horvath, KJ: Postoperative recovery at home after ambulatory gynecologic laparoscopic surgery, *J PeriAnesth Nurs* 18:324, 2003.
19. Kamming D, et al: Pain management in ambulatory surgery, *J PeriAnesth Nurs* 19:174, 2004.
*20. Watt-Watson J, Chung F, Chan VWS, et al: Pain management following discharge after ambulatory same-day surgery, *J Nurs Management* 12:153, 2004.
*21. Pavlin DJ, Chen C, Penaloza DA, et al: Pain as a factor complicating recovery and discharge after ambulatory surgery, *Anesth Analg* 95:627, 2002.
*22. Kamming D, et al: Postoperative pain following discharge after ambulatory surgery, *Can J Anaesth* 50:A20, 2003.
23. Kuchta A, Golembiewski J: Medication use in the elderly patient: focus on the perioperative/perianesthesia setting, *J PeriAnesth Nurs* 19:415, 2004.
24. Dibert C: Delirium and the older adult after surgery, *Perspectives* 28:10, 2004.
25. Paynter D, Mamaril ME: Perianesthesia challenges in geriatric pain management, *J PeriAnesth Nurs* 19:385, 2004.

*Nursing research–based reference.

RESOURCES

American Association of Nurse Anesthetists (AANA)
847-692-7050
www.aana.com

American College of Surgeons
312-202-5000
800-621-4111
www.facs.org

American Pain Society
847-375-4715
www.ampainsoc.org

American Society of Anesthesiologists
847-825-5586
www.asahq.org

American Society of PeriAnesthesia Nurses (ASPAN)
877-737-9696
www.aspan.org

Association of periOperative Registered Nurses (AORN)
303-755-6300
800-755-2676
www.aorn.org

Association of Surgical Technologists
303-694-9130
800-637-7433
www.ast.org

Canadian Anesthesiologists Society
416-480-0602
www.cas.ca

Centers for Disease Control and Prevention, Division of Healthcare Quality Promotion
404-639-3311
www.cdc.gov/ncidod/hip

Malignant Hyperthermia Association of the United States
607-674-7901
www.mhaus.org

National Latex Allergy Network: Latex Allergy Links
http://latexallergylinks.tripod.com

Operating Room Nurses Association of Canada
www.ornac.ca

For additional Internet resources, see the website for this book at *http://evolve.elsevier.com/Lewis/medsurg*.

Section
4

Problems Related to Altered Sensory Input

Section Outline

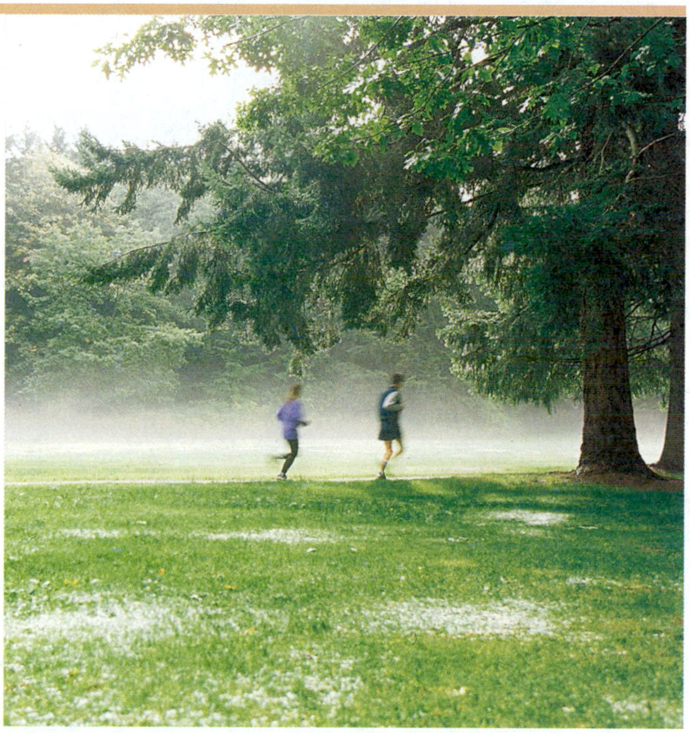

Everything has its beauty but not everyone sees it.

Confucius

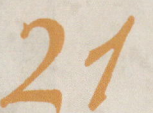

21 Nursing Assessment
Visual and Auditory Systems

Sarah C. Smith and Sherry Neely

LEARNING OBJECTIVES

1. Describe the structures and functions of the visual and auditory systems.
2. Describe the physiologic processes involved in normal vision and hearing.
3. Identify the significant subjective and objective assessment data related to the visual and auditory systems that should be obtained from the patient.
4. Describe the appropriate techniques used in the physical assessment of the visual and auditory systems.
5. Differentiate normal from common abnormal findings of a physical assessment of the visual and auditory systems.
6. Describe age-related changes in the visual and auditory systems and differences in assessment findings.
7. Describe the purpose, significance of results, and nursing responsibilities related to diagnostic studies of the visual and auditory systems.

KEY TERMS

aqueous humor, p. 399
astigmatism, p. 400
conjunctiva, p. 400
hyperopia, p. 400
lens, p. 401
nystagmus, p. 409
retina, p. 401
sclera, p. 400
tinnitus, p. 409
vertigo, p. 409

Electronic Resources

Supplemental content related to Chapter 21 can be found . . .

Companion CD

- Stress-Busting Kit for Nursing Students
- NCLEX Examination Review Questions
- Comprehensive Glossary
- Animation: Ears: Weber Test
- Video Clips:
  - Evaluation: Central Vision and Visual Acuity
  - Evaluation: Pupil Responses, Direct and Consensual
  - Inspection and Palpation: External Ear
  - Inspection and Palpation: External Eye
  - Inspection: Ear Canal

Evolve Website

http://evolve.elsevier.com/Lewis/medsurg

- Content Updates
- Key Points (Printable and CD/MP3 Download)
- Concept Map Creator
- Expanded Audio Glossary
- Key Term Flash Cards
- Electronic Calculators
- Physical Examination Videos:
  - Eyes
  - Ears
- WebLinks

STRUCTURES AND FUNCTIONS OF THE VISUAL SYSTEM

The visual system consists of the external tissues and structures surrounding the eye, the external and internal structures of the eye, the refractive media, and the visual pathway. The external structures are the eyebrows, eyelids, eyelashes, lacrimal system, conjunctiva, cornea, sclera, and extraocular muscles. The internal structures are the iris, lens, ciliary body, choroid, and retina. The entire visual system is important for visual function. Light reflected from an object in the field of vision passes through the transparent structures of the eye and, in doing so, is *refracted* (bent) so that a clear image can fall on the retina. From the retina, the visual stimuli travel through the visual pathway to the occipital cortex, where they are perceived as an image.

Structures and Functions of Vision

Eyeball. The eyeball, or globe, is composed of three layers (Fig. 21-1). The tough outer layer is composed of the sclera and the transparent cornea. The middle layer consists of the uveal tract (iris, choroid, and ciliary body), and the innermost layer is the retina. The an-

Reviewed by Beth Hurley, BSN, CRNO, COE, President, Ophthalmic Surgery Resources Inc., Phoenix, Ariz.; and Susan E. Sitter, RN, MSN, Research Assistant, Edinboro University of Pennsylvania, Edinboro, Pa.

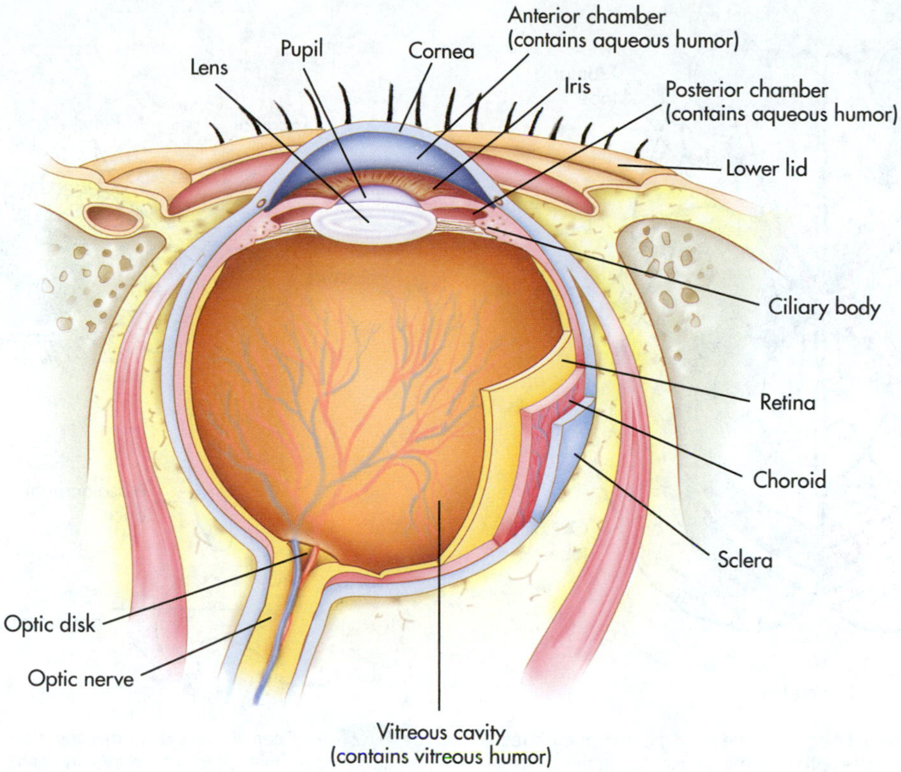

FIG. 21-1 The human eye.

terior chamber lies between the iris and the posterior surface of the cornea, whereas the posterior chamber lies between the anterior surface of the lens and the posterior surface of the iris. These chambers are filled with aqueous humor secreted by the ciliary body (Fig. 21-2). The anatomic space *(vitreous cavity)* between the posterior lens and the retina is filled with a gel substance *(vitreous humor).*

Refractive Media. For light to reach the retina, it must pass through a number of structures: the cornea, aqueous humor, lens, and vitreous. All of these structures must remain clear for light to reach the retina and stimulate the photoreceptor cells. The transparent cornea is the first structure through which light passes. It is responsible for the majority of light refraction necessary for clear vision.[1]

Aqueous humor, a clear watery fluid, fills the anterior and posterior chambers of the anterior cavity of the eye. Aqueous humor is produced by the ciliary process (see Fig. 21-2). It drains through the trabecular meshwork located in the angle. This circular canal conveys fluid into scleral veins, which enter the circulation of the body. The aqueous humor bathes and nourishes the lens and the endothelium of the cornea. Excess production or decreased outflow can elevate intraocular pressure above the normal 10 to 21 mm Hg, a condition termed *glaucoma.*

The lens is a biconvex structure located behind the iris and supported in place by small fibers called *zonules.* The primary function of the lens is to bend light rays, allowing the rays to fall onto the retina. The lens shape is modified by action of the ciliary zonules as part of *accommodation,* a process that allows the patient to focus on near objects, such as in reading. Anything altering the clarity of the lens affects light transmission.

Vitreous humor is located in the vitreous cavity, the large area behind the lens and in front of the retina (see Fig. 21-1). Light passing through the vitreous may be blocked by any nontransparent substance within the vitreous. The effect on vision varies, depending on the amount, type, and location of the substance blocking the light. The vitreous becomes more liquid with aging.[1]

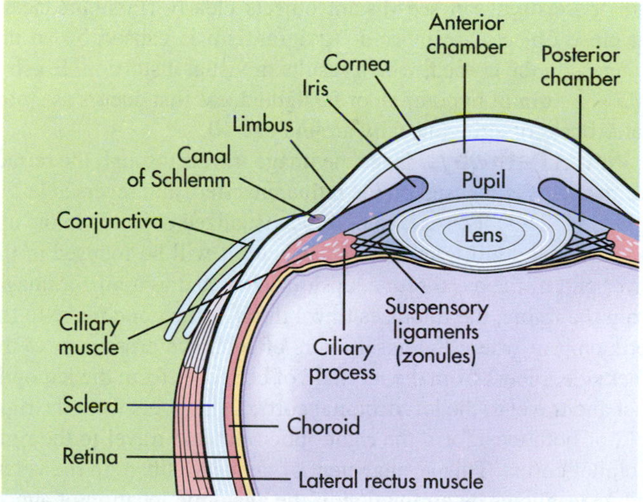

FIG. 21-2 Close-up view of ciliary body, zonules, lens, and anterior and posterior chambers. The aqueous humor flows from the ciliary process, over the anterior lens, and into the anterior chamber through the pupil, where it drains through the canal of Schlemm.

Refractive Errors. Refraction is the ability of the eye to bend light rays so that they fall on the retina. In the normal eye, parallel light rays are focused through the lens into a sharp image on the retina. This condition is termed *emmetropia* and means that light is focused exactly on the retina, not in front of it or behind it. When the light does not focus properly, it is called a *refractive error.*

The individual with **myopia** can see near objects clearly (nearsightedness), but objects in the distance are blurred. The individual

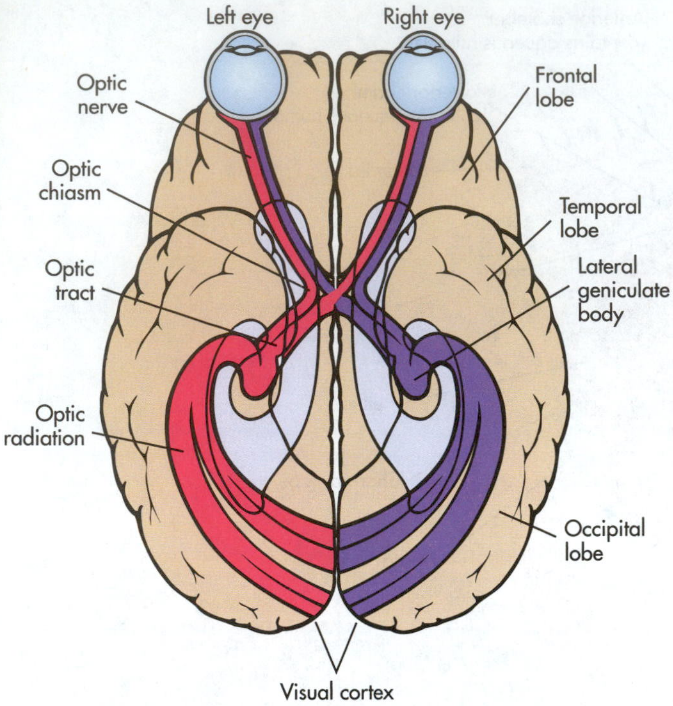

FIG. 21-3 The visual pathway. Fibers from the nasal portion of each retina cross over to the opposite side of the optic chiasma, terminating in the lateral geniculate body of the opposite side. Location of a lesion in the visual pathway determines the resulting visual defect.

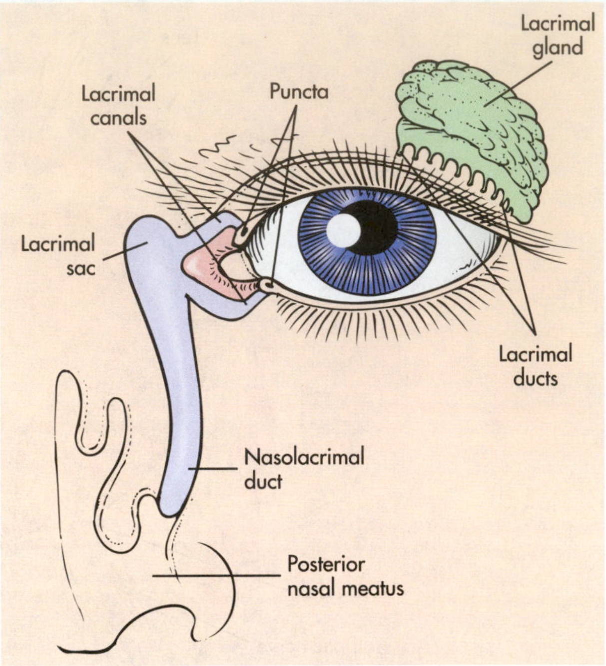

FIG. 21-4 External eye and lacrimal apparatus. Tears produced in the lacrimal gland pass over the surface of the eye and enter the lacrimal canal. From there the tears are carried through the nasolacrimal duct to the nasal cavity.

with **hyperopia** can see distant objects clearly (farsightedness), but close objects are blurred. **Astigmatism** is caused by an unevenness in the cornea, which results in visual distortion. **Presbyopia** is a form of hyperopia, or farsightedness that occurs as a normal process of aging, usually around age 40.

Visual Pathways. Once the image travels through the refractive media, it is focused on the retina, inverted, and reversed left to right (Fig. 21-3). For example, if the visualized object is in the upper part of the left temporal visual field, it will be focused in the lower part of the nasal retina, upside down, and as a mirror image. From the retina, the impulses travel through the optic nerve to the optic chiasm where the nasal fibers of each eye cross over to the other side. Fibers from the left field of both eyes form the left optic tract and travel to the left occipital cortex. The fibers from the right field of both eyes form the right optic tract and travel to the right occipital cortex. This arrangement of the nerve fibers in the visual pathways allows determination of the anatomic location of abnormalities in those nerve fibers by interpretation of the specific visual field defect (see Fig. 21-3).

External Structures and Functions

Eyebrows, Eyelids, and Eyelashes. The eyebrows, eyelids, and eyelashes serve an important role in protecting the eye. They provide a physical barrier to dust and foreign particles (Fig. 21-4). The eye is further protected by the surrounding bony orbit and by fat pads located below and behind the globe, or eyeball.

The upper and lower eyelids join at the medial and lateral canthi. The upper eyelid blinks spontaneously approximately 15 times a minute. Blinking distributes tears over the anterior surface of the eyeball and helps control the amount of light entering the visual pathway.

The eyelids open and close through the action of muscles innervated by cranial nerve (CN) VII, which is the facial nerve. Muscular action also helps hold the eyelids against the eyeball.

Conjunctiva. The **conjunctiva** is a transparent mucous membrane that covers the inner surfaces of the eyelids (the palpebral conjunctiva) and also extends over the sclera (bulbar conjunctiva), forming a "pocket" under each eyelid. Glands in the conjunctiva secrete mucus and tears.

Sclera. The **sclera** is composed of collagen fibers meshed together to form an opaque structure commonly referred to as the "white" of the eye. The sclera forms a tough shell that helps protect the intraocular structures.

Cornea. The transparent and avascular cornea allows light to enter the eye (see Fig. 21-1). The curved cornea refracts (bends) incoming light rays to help focus them on the retina. The cornea consists of five layers: the epithelium, Bowman's layer, the stroma, Descemet's membrane, and the endothelium. The epithelium consists of a layer of cells that helps protect the eye. Epithelial cells regenerate when damaged. The stroma consists of collagen fibrils.

Lacrimal Apparatus. The lacrimal system consists of the lacrimal gland and ducts, lacrimal canals and puncta, lacrimal sac, and nasolacrimal duct. In addition to the lacrimal gland, other glands provide secretions to make up the mucous, aqueous, and lipid layers of the tear film. The tear film moistens the eye and provides oxygen to the cornea.

Extraocular Muscles. Each eye is moved by three pairs of extraocular muscles: (1) superior and inferior rectus muscles, (2) medial and lateral rectus muscles, and (3) superior and inferior oblique muscles. Neuromuscular coordination produces simultaneous movement of the eyes in the same direction *(conjugate movement).*

Internal Structures and Functions

Iris. The iris provides the color of the eye. This structure has a small round opening in its center, the *pupil,* which allows light to enter the eye. The pupil constricts via action of the iris sphincter muscle (innervated by CN III [oculomotor nerve]) and dilates via action of the iris dilator muscle (innervated by CN V [trigeminal nerve]) to control the amount of light that enters the eye.

Lens. The **lens** is a biconvex, avascular, transparent structure located behind the iris. It is supported by the anterior and posterior ciliary zonules. The primary function of the lens is to bend light rays so that they fall onto the retina. Accommodation occurs when the eye focuses on a near object and is facilitated by contraction of the ciliary body, which changes the shape of the lens.

Ciliary Body. The ciliary body consists of the ciliary muscles, which surround the lens and lie parallel to the sclera; the ciliary zonules, which attach to the lens capsule; and the ciliary processes, which constitute the terminal portion of the ciliary body. The ciliary processes lie behind the peripheral part of the iris and secrete aqueous humor.

Choroid. The *choroid* is a highly vascular structure that serves to nourish the ciliary body, the iris, and the outer portion of the retina. It lies inside and parallel to the sclera and extends from the area where the optic nerve enters the eye to the ciliary body (see Fig. 21-1).

Retina. The **retina** is the innermost layer of the eye that extends and forms the optic nerve. Neurons make up the major portion of the retina. Therefore retinal cells are unable to regenerate if destroyed.

TABLE 21-1 GERONTOLOGIC DIFFERENCES IN ASSESSMENT Visual System

Changes	Differences in Assessment Findings
Eyebrows and Eyelashes	
Loss of pigment in the hair	Graying of eyebrows, eyelashes
Eyelids	
Loss of orbital fat, decreased muscle tone	Entropion, ectropion, mild ptosis
Tissue atrophy, prolapse of fat into eyelid tissue	Blepharodermachalasis (excessive upper lid skin)
Conjunctiva	
Tissue damage related to chronic exposure to ultraviolet light or to other chronic environmental exposure	Pinguecula (small yellowish spot usually on the medial aspect of the conjunctiva)
Sclera	
Lipid deposition	Scleral color yellowish as opposed to bluish
Cornea	
Cholesterol deposits in peripheral cornea	Arcus senilis (milky or yellow ring encircling periphery of cornea)
Tissue damage related to chronic exposure	Pterygium (thickened, triangular bit of pale tissue that extends from the inner canthus of eye to the nasal border of the cornea)
Decrease in water content, atrophy of nerve fibers	Decreased corneal sensitivity and corneal reflex
Epithelial changes	Loss of corneal luster
Accumulation of lipid deposits	Blurring of vision
Lacrimal Apparatus	
Decreased tear secretion	Dryness
Malposition of the eyelid resulting in tears overflowing the lid margins instead of draining through the puncta	Tearing, irritated eyes
Iris	
Increased rigidity of iris	Decreased pupil size
Dilator muscle atrophy or weakness	Slower recovery of pupil size after light stimulation
Loss of pigment	Change of iris color
Ciliary muscle becomes smaller, stiffer	Decrease in near vision and accommodation
Lens	
Biochemical changes in lens proteins, oxidative damage, chronic exposure to ultraviolet light	Cataracts
Increased rigidity of lens	Presbyopia
Opacities in the lens (may also be related to opacities in the cornea and vitreous)	Complaints of glare, night vision impaired
Accumulation of yellow substances	Yellow color of lens
Retina	
Retinal vascular changes related to atherosclerosis and hypertension	Narrowed, pale, straighter arterioles; acute branching
Decrease in cones	Changes in color perception, especially blue and violet
Loss of photoreceptor cells, retinal pigment, epithelial cells, and melanin	Decreased visual acuity
Age-related macular degeneration as a result of vascular changes	Loss of central vision
Vitreous	
Liquefaction and detachment of the vitreous	Increased complaints of "floaters"

The retina lines the inside of the eyeball, extending from the area of optic nerve to the ciliary body (see Fig. 21-1). It is responsible for converting images into a form that the brain can understand and process as vision. The retina is composed of two types of photoreceptor cells: rods and cones. Rods are stimulated in dim or darkened environments, and cones are receptive to colors in bright environments.[2] The center of the retina is the *fovea centralis,* a pinpoint depression composed only of densely packed cones. This area of the retina provides the sharpest visual acuity. Surrounding the fovea is the *macula,* an area less than 1 square millimeter, which has a high concentration of cones and is relatively free of blood vessels.

GERONTOLOGIC CONSIDERATIONS
EFFECTS OF AGING ON THE VISUAL SYSTEM

Every structure of the visual system is subject to changes as the individual ages. Whereas many of these changes are relatively benign, others may result in severely compromised visual acuity in the older adult. The psychosocial impact of poor vision or blindness can be highly significant. Age-related changes in the visual system and differences in assessment findings are presented in Table 21-1 on p. 401.

ASSESSMENT OF THE VISUAL SYSTEM

Assessment of the visual system may be as simple as determining a patient's visual acuity or as complex as collecting complete subjective and objective data pertinent to the visual system. To do an appropriate ophthalmic evaluation, the nurse must determine which parts of the data collection are important for each patient.

Subjective Data

Important Health Information

Past Health History. Information about the patient's past health history should include both ocular and nonocular history. The nurse should ask the patient specifically about systemic diseases, such as diabetes, hypertension, cancer, rheumatoid arthritis, syphilis and other sexually transmitted diseases (STDs), acquired immunodeficiency syndrome (AIDS), muscular dystrophy, myasthenia gravis, multiple sclerosis, inflammatory bowel disease, and hypothyroidism or hyperthyroidism, because many of these diseases have ocular manifestations. It is particularly important to determine if the patient has any history of cardiac or pulmonary disease because β-adrenergic blockers are often used to treat glaucoma. These medications can slow heart rate, decrease blood pressure, and exacerbate asthma or emphysema.[3]

A history of tests for visual acuity should be obtained, including the date of the last examination and change in glasses or contact lenses. The nurse should specifically ask about a history of strabismus, amblyopia, cataracts, retinal detachment, refractive surgery, or glaucoma. Any trauma to the eye, its treatment, and sequelae should be noted.

The patient's nonocular history can be significant in assessing or treating the ophthalmic condition. Specifically, the nurse should ask the patient about previous surgeries or treatments related to the head, as well as about previous trauma to the head.

Medications. If the patient takes medication, the nurse should obtain a complete list, including over-the-counter (OTC) medicines, eyedrops, and herbal therapies or dietary supplements. Many patients do not think OTC drugs, eyedrops, or herbal therapies are "real" drugs and may not mention their use unless specifically questioned. However, many of these drugs have ocular effects. For example, many cold preparations contain a form of epinephrine (e.g., pseudoephedrine) that can dilate the pupil. The nurse should also note the use of any antihistamines or decongestants, because these drugs can cause ocular dryness. The nurse should specifically ask whether the patient uses any prescription drugs such as corticosteroids, thyroid medications, or agents such as oral hypoglycemics and insulin to lower blood glucose levels. Long-term use of corticosteroid preparations can contribute to the development of glaucoma or cataracts. It is especially important to indicate whether the patient is taking any β-adrenergic blockers, because these can be potentiated by the β-adrenergic blockers used to treat glaucoma.

Each drug that the patient uses should correspond with a disease or disorder described in the patient's history. If a medication cannot be correlated with a disease or disorder, the nurse should ask the patient to explain why the drug is used. Finally, the nurse should determine whether the patient has allergies to medications or other substances.

Surgery or Other Treatments. Surgical procedures related to the eye or brain should be noted. Brain surgery and the subsequent swelling can cause pressure on the optic nerve or tract, resulting in visual alterations. Any laser procedures to the eye should also be documented. The effect of any eye surgery or laser treatment on visual acuity is important information for the nurse to obtain.

Functional Health Patterns. The ophthalmic patient may seek health care for a specific problem or for regular ophthalmic care. When the patient needs routine ophthalmic care, the nurse will focus the assessment of functional patterns on issues related to health promotion. When the patient has a recognized problem, the nurse will direct the assessment to identify those issues related to the patient's specific problem.

Ocular problems do not always affect the patient's visual acuity. For example, patients with blepharitis or diabetic retinopathy may not have any visual deficit. The nurse should be aware that many conditions can cause vision loss. The focus of the functional health pattern assessment depends on the presence or absence of vision loss and whether the loss is permanent or temporary. Table 21-2 lists suggested health history questions to obtain data relating to the functional health patterns.

Health Perception–Health Management Pattern. The patient's age is pertinent in considering cataracts, macular problems, glaucoma, and other ophthalmic conditions. Men are more likely than women to have color blindness. African Americans and older individuals are at higher risk of damage to the optic nerve from glaucoma.[4]

The ophthalmic patient in a clinic or office setting is often seeking routine eye care or a change in the prescription of eyewear. However, there can be some underlying concern that the patient may not mention or even recognize. The nurse should ask the patient, "Why are you here today?"

The patient's visual health can affect activities at home or at work. It is important to know how the patient perceives the current health problem. As outlined in Table 21-2, the nurse can guide the patient in defining the current problem and how it affects the patient's normal activities. The nurse should also assess the patient's ability to accomplish all necessary self-care, especially any eye care related to the patient's ophthalmic problem.

The nurse should assess the patient's ocular health care activities. The patient may not recognize the importance of eye-safety

TABLE 21-2 HEALTH HISTORY
Visual System

Health Perception–Health Management Pattern
- Describe the change in your vision. Describe how this affects your daily life.
- Do you wear protective eyewear (sunglasses, safety goggles, or hats)?*
- Do you wear contact lenses? If so, how do you take care of them?
- If you use eyedrops, how do you instill them?
- Do you have any allergies that cause eye symptoms?
- Do you have a family history of cataracts, glaucoma, or macular degeneration?

Nutritional-Metabolic Pattern
- Do you take any nutritional supplements?
- Does your visual problem affect your ability to obtain and prepare food?*

Elimination Pattern
- Do you have to strain to void or defecate?*

Activity-Exercise Pattern
- Are your activities limited in any way by your eye problem?*
- Do you participate in any leisure activities that have the potential for eye injury?*

Sleep-Rest Pattern
- Is your vision affected by the amount of sleep you get?*

Cognitive-Perceptual Pattern
- Does your eye problem affect your ability to read?*
- Do you have any eye pain?* Do you have any eye itching, burning, or foreign body sensation?*

Self-Perception–Self-Concept Pattern
- How does your eye problem make you feel about yourself?

Role-Relationship Pattern
- Do you have any problems at work or home because of your eyes?*
- Have you made any changes in your social activities because of your eyes?

Sexuality-Reproductive Pattern
- Has your eye problem caused a change in your sex life?*
- For women: Are you pregnant? Do you use birth control pills?*

Coping–Stress Tolerance Pattern
- Do you feel able to cope with your eye problem?*
- Are you able to acknowledge the effects of your eye problem on your life?*

Value-Belief Pattern
- Do you have any conflicts about the treatment of your eye problem?*

*If yes, describe.

practices such as wearing protective eyewear during potentially hazardous activities or avoiding noxious fumes and other eye irritants. Information about the use of sunglasses in bright light should be obtained. Prolonged exposure to ultraviolet (UV) light can affect the retina. Night driving habits and any problems encountered should be noted. Today, millions of people wear contact lenses, but many do not care for them properly.[5] The type of contact lenses used and the patient's wearing and care habits may provide information for teaching.

Information about allergies should be obtained. Allergies often cause eye symptoms such as itching, burning, watering, drainage, and blurred vision.

Many hereditary systemic diseases (e.g., sickle cell anemia) can significantly affect ocular health. In addition, many refractive errors and other eye problems are hereditary. For these reasons the nurse should obtain a careful family history of both ocular and nonocular diseases. Specifically, the nurse should ask if the patient has a family history of diseases such as atherosclerosis, diabetes, thyroid disease, hypertension, arthritis, or cancer. The nurse should also determine whether the patient has a family history of ocular problems such as cataracts, tumors, glaucoma, refractive errors (especially myopia and hyperopia), or retinal degenerative conditions (e.g., macular degeneration, retinal detachment, retinitis pigmentosa).

Nutritional-Metabolic Pattern. The patient's intake of antioxidants (vitamins C and E) and trace minerals can be important to ocular health.[6] Adequate intake of vitamins C and E may be beneficial in preventing or delaying retinal damage, and zinc deficiency is linked to erythematous scales in the periorbital area.

Elimination Pattern. Straining to defecate (Valsalva maneuver) can raise the intraocular pressure. Although there is some evidence that elevating the intraocular pressure by normal activities is not detrimental to the surgical incision made during eye surgery, many surgeons do not want the patient to strain. The nurse should assess the patient's usual pattern of elimination and determine whether there is the potential for constipation in the patient who has had ophthalmic surgical procedures.

Activity-Exercise Pattern. The patient's usual level of activity or exercise may be affected by reduced vision, by symptoms accompanying an ocular problem, or by activity restrictions following a surgical procedure. For example, a patient with *hyphema* (intraocular bleeding) may be on bed rest or have severely restricted activity. The diabetic patient with lower limb prostheses will have additional ambulation difficulties if diabetic retinopathy with vision loss is present.

The nurse should also inquire about leisure activities during which the patient may incur an ocular injury. For example, gardening, woodworking, and other craft activities can result in corneal or conjunctival foreign bodies or even penetrating injuries of the globe. Injuries to the globe or bony orbit can also occur after blows to the head or eye during sports activities such as racquetball, baseball, and tennis. Cross-country skiers may develop corneal fungal ulcers after an abrasion caused by low-hanging tree limbs. Other leisure activities such as needlepoint, fly tying, or bird watching may have high-level visual demands and produce eye strain.

Sleep-Rest Pattern. In the otherwise healthy person, lack of sleep may cause ocular irritation, especially in the patient who wears contact lenses. Normal sleep patterns may be disrupted in the patient with painful eye problems such as corneal abrasions. The patient with alkali burns of the eye requires continuous irrigation of the ocular surface.[7] Normal sleep will be disrupted during this time.

Cognitive-Perceptual Pattern. The entire assessment of the ophthalmic patient focuses on the sense of sight, but it is important not to overlook other cognitive or perceptual problems. For example, the functional ability of a patient with a visual deficit will be further compromised if the patient also has hearing problems. The patient who cannot see to read has increased difficulty in following postoperative instructions if there is also trouble hearing or remembering verbal instructions. The patient who does not understand or read English may require written or verbal instructions and information in the native language.

Eye pain is always an important symptom to assess. Corneal abrasions, iritis, and acute glaucoma manifest with pain and are serious eye problems. Infections and foreign bodies can also cause less severe eye discomfort and are also potentially serious. If eye pain is present, the patient should be questioned about treatment and response.

Self-Perception–Self-Concept Pattern. The loss of independence that can follow a partial or complete loss of vision, even if the condition is temporary, can have devastating effects on the patient's self-concept. The nurse should carefully evaluate the potential effect of vision loss on the patient's self-image. For instance, disabling glare from a cataract may prevent nighttime driving or even limit daytime driving, resulting in a diminished self-image. In today's highly mobile society, loss of ability to drive can represent a significant loss of independence and self-esteem. The patient with severe ptosis or other disfiguring ophthalmic conditions may be embarrassed by her or his appearance and suffer from a poor self-image.

Role-Relationship Pattern. The patient's ability to maintain the necessary or desired roles and responsibilities in the home, work, and social environments can be negatively affected by ocular problems. For example, macular degeneration may decrease the patient's visual acuity to a level inadequate to function at work. Many occupations place workers in conditions in which eye injury may occur. For example, factory workers may be at risk from flying metal debris. Information should be obtained about eye-safety practices, such as the use of goggles or safety glasses. Workers can also be exposed to eyestrain in the office from video display terminals, poor lighting, and glare. An ergonomic consultation may be beneficial.

The patient with diabetes may not be able to see well enough to self-administer insulin. This patient may resent the dependence on a family member who takes over this function. The patient with *exophthalmos* (marked protrusion of eyeballs) may be embarrassed by his or her appearance and avoid usual social activities. The nurse should sensitively inquire if the patient's preferred roles and responsibilities have been affected by the ocular problem.

Sexuality-Reproductive Pattern. The inactivity that may be associated with low vision, blindness, and certain eye problems and surgeries can negatively affect a patient's sexuality. The patient with severe vision loss may develop such a poor self-image that the ability to be sexually intimate is lost. The nurse can assure the patient that low vision or blindness does not affect a person's ability to be sexually expressive. For many sexually expressive acts, touch is more important than vision.

If a patient with low vision or blindness has a family, assistance with child-rearing tasks may be necessary. The nurse should determine the need and availability of help if this situation is present.

Coping–Stress Tolerance Pattern. The patient with temporary or permanent visual problems will experience emotional stress. The nurse should assess the patient's coping level, coping mechanisms, and availability of social and personal support systems.

The patient with permanent visual loss experiences the usual stages of grief after the loss. The nurse should assess the potential need for psychosocial counseling and eventual vocational rehabilitation.

Value-Belief Pattern. The nurse must be sensitive to the individual values and spiritual beliefs of each patient, because the patient makes decisions regarding ophthalmic care based on those values and beliefs. It can be difficult to understand why a patient refuses treatment that has potential benefit or wants treatment that may have limited potential benefit. The nurse should assess the patient's value-belief pattern that serves as the basis for making those decisions.

Objective Data

Physical Examination. Physical examination of the visual system includes inspecting the ocular structures and determining the status of their respective functions. Physiologic functional assessment includes determining the patient's visual acuity, determining the patient's ability to judge closeness and distance, assessing extraocular muscle function, evaluating the visual fields, observing pupil function, and measuring the intraocular pressure. Assessment of ocular structures should include examining the ocular adnexa, external eye, and internal structures. Some structures, such as the retina and blood vessels, must be visualized with the aid of ophthalmic observation equipment, such as the ophthalmoscope.

Assessment of the visual system may include all of the following components, or it may be as brief as measuring the patient's visual acuity. The nurse will assess what is appropriate and necessary for the specific patient. All of the following assessments are in the nurse's scope of practice, but some require special training. Normal physical assessment of the visual system is outlined in Table 21-3. Age-related visual changes and differences in assessment findings are listed in Table 21-1. Assessment techniques related to vision are summarized in Table 21-4, and common assessment abnormalities are listed in Table 21-5 on p. 406.

Initial Observation. The initial observation of the patient can provide information that will help the nurse focus the assessment. When first encountering the patient, the nurse may observe that the patient is dressed in clothing with unusual color combinations. This may indicate a color-vision deficit. The nurse may also note an unusual head position. The patient with diplopia may hold the head in a skewed position in an attempt to see a single image. The patient with a corneal abrasion or photophobia will cover the eyes with the hands to try to block out room light. The nurse can make a crude estimate of depth perception by extending a hand for the patient to shake.

During the initial observation, the nurse should also observe the overall facial and ophthalmic appearance of the patient. The eyes should be symmetric and normally placed on the face. The globes should not have a bulging or sunken appearance.

Assessing Functional Status

Visual Acuity. The nurse should always record the patient's visual acuity for medical and legal reasons. The nurse must document the patient's visual acuity before the patient receives any care.

The patient sits or stands 20 feet (6 meters) from the Snellen chart with the usual correction (glasses or contact lenses) left in place unless they are used solely for reading. The nurse asks the

TABLE 21-3 Normal Physical Assessment of the Visual System

- Visual acuity 20/20 OU; no diplopia
- External eye structures symmetric and without lesions or deformities
- Lacrimal apparatus nontender and without drainage
- Conjunctiva clear; sclera white
- PERRLA
- Lens clear
- EOMI
- Disc margins sharp
- Retinal vessels normal, with no hemorrhages or spots

EOMI, Extraocular movements intact; *OU,* both eyes; *PERRLA,* pupils equal, round, reactive to light and accommodation.

TABLE 21-4 Assessment Techniques
Visual System

Technique	Description	Purpose
Visual acuity testing	Patient reads from Snellen chart at 20 ft (distance vision test) or Jaeger's chart at 14 in (near vision test); examiner notes smallest print patient can read on each chart.	To determine patient's distance and near visual acuity
Confrontation visual field test	Patient faces examiner, covers one eye, fixates on examiner's face, and counts number of fingers that the examiner brings into patient's field of vision.	To determine if patient has a full field of vision, without obvious scotomas
Pupil function testing	Examiner shines light into patient's pupil and observes pupillary response; each pupil is examined independently; examiner also checks for consensual and accommodative response.	To determine if patient has normal pupillary response
Tono-pen tonometry	Covered end of probe is gently touched several times to the anesthetized corneal surface; examiner records several readings to obtain a mean intraocular pressure (see Fig. 21-6).	To measure intraocular pressure (normal pressure is 10-22 mm Hg)
Ophthalmoscopy	Examiner holds ophthalmoscope close to patient's eye, shining light into back of eye and looking through aperture on ophthalmoscope; examiner adjusts dial to select one of the lenses in ophthalmoscope that produces the desired amount of magnification to inspect ocular fundus.	To provide magnified view of retina and optic nerve head
Color vision testing	Patient identifies numbers or paths formed by pattern of dots in series of color plates.	To determine patient's ability to distinguish colors
Keratometry	Examiner aligns the projection and notes the readings of corneal curvature.	To measure the corneal curvature; often done before fitting contact lenses, before doing refractive surgery, or after corneal transplantation

patient to cover the left eye and read the smallest line that the patient can read comfortably. If the patient reads that line with 50% or fewer errors, the examiner instructs the patient to read the next lower line. The nurse notes the smallest line the patient can read with 50% or fewer errors, and records the standard of 20 feet (6 meters) and then the distance in feet on the line of the Snellen chart the patient read successfully. The nurse records the visual acuities using the ophthalmic abbreviations for right eye (*oculus dexter* [OD]), left eye (*oculus sinister* [OS]), and both eyes (*oculus uterque* [OU]). For example, for the patient who reads to the 30-foot (9-meter) line with the right eye, the nurse records the acuity as 20/30 OD. *Legal blindness* is defined as the best-corrected vision in the better eye of 20/200 or less. The nurse then asks the patient to cover the right eye, and the process is repeated.

To evaluate visual acuity when the patient is unable to see the 20/400 letter, the nurse holds up a number of fingers 3 to 5 feet (0.9 to 1.5 meters) in front of the patient and asks the patient to count them.[8] If the patient is unable to count the fingers, the nurse holds up a different number of fingers at successively closer distances up to 1 foot and again asks the patient to count them. The examiner tests the opposite eye in the same manner and records the acuities of each eye. If the patient can count the number of fingers at 2 feet (0.6 meters), the nurse records the acuity as FC or CF ("finger counting" or "counts fingers") at 2 feet (0.6 meters). If the patient cannot count fingers, the nurse asks the patient to indicate if moving the hand is seen in front of the face. This level of visual acuity is HM ("hand motion").

If the patient has a complaint of visual problems with near vision, and for all patients 40 years of age or older, the nurse tests the near visual acuity. The patient is instructed to hold a Jaeger chart 14 inches (35.6 cm) from the eyes. The nurse covers the patient's left eye with the occluder, asks the patient to read successively smaller lines of print from the chart, and records the visual acuity that corresponds to the smallest line of print the patient can read comfortably. The procedure is repeated while covering the right eye. A near acuity of $Jaeger_1$ (J_1) indicates that the patient can read 4-point type at 14 inches (35.6 cm) and is considered normal. A near acuity of J_{10} indicates that the smallest print the patient can read at 14 inches (35.6 cm) is 14-point type and is moderately impaired.

If the nurse must assess visual acuity without access to an eye chart, an accurate assessment is still possible. Examples of other stimuli acceptable for use include newsprint or the label on a container. The examiner records the acuity as "reads newspaper headline at _X_ inches."

Extraocular Muscle Functions. The nurse observes the corneal light reflex to evaluate for weakness or imbalance of the extraocular muscles. In a darkened room, the nurse asks the patient to look straight ahead while a penlight is shone directly on the cornea. The light reflection should be located in the center of both corneas as the patient faces the light source.

To assess eye movement the nurse should hold a finger or an object within 10 to 12 inches from the patient's nose. Ask the patient to follow with eyes only the movement of the object or finger in the six cardinal positions of gaze (Fig. 21-5). This test can indicate weakness or paralysis in the extraocular muscles and cranial nerves (oculomotor nerve [CN III], trochlear nerve [CN IV], and abducens nerve [CN VI]).

Pupil Function. Pupil function is determined by inspecting the pupils and their reactions to light. The pupils should be equal in size, round, and react briskly to light. In a small percentage of the population the pupils are unequal in size (anisocoria). The pupils should react to light directly (the pupil constricts when a light shines into the same eye) and consensually (the pupil constricts when a light shines into the opposite eye).

Intraocular Pressure. Intraocular pressure can be measured by a variety of methods, including the Tono-pen (Fig. 21-6). The Tono-pen is commonly used because it is simple to use and very accurate. The surface of the anesthetized cornea is touched lightly several times with the covered end of the probe. The instrument records several readings and provides a mean measurement on a

TABLE 21-5 COMMON ASSESSMENT ABNORMALITIES
Visual System

Finding	Description	Possible Etiology and Significance
Subjective Data		
Pain	Foreign body sensation	Superficial corneal erosion or abrasion; can result from contact lens wear or trauma; conjunctival or corneal foreign body
	Severe, deep, throbbing	Anterior uveitis, acute glaucoma, infection; acute glaucoma also associated with nausea, vomiting
Photophobia	Persistent abnormal intolerance to light	Inflammation or infection of cornea or anterior uveal tract (iris and ciliary body)
Blurred vision	Gradual or sudden inability to see clearly	Refractive errors, corneal opacities, cataracts, migraine aura, retinal changes (detachment, macular degeneration)
Spots, floaters	Patient describes seeing spots, "spider webs," "curtain," or floaters within the field of vision	Most common cause is vitreous liquefaction (benign phenomenon); other possible causes include hemorrhage into the vitreous humor, retinal holes or tears
Dryness	Discomfort, sandy, gritty, irritation, or burning	Decreased tear formation or changes in tear composition because of aging or various systemic diseases
Diplopia	Double vision	Abnormalities of extraocular muscle action related to muscle or cranial nerve pathology
Objective Data		
Eyelids		
Allergic reactions	Redness, excessive tearing, and itching of lid margins	Many possible allergens; associated eye trauma can occur from rubbing itchy eyelids
Hordeolum (sty)	Small, superficial white nodule along lid margin	Infection of a sebaceous gland of eyelid; causative organism is usually bacterial (most commonly *Staphylococcus aureus*)
Blepharitis	Redness, swelling, and crusting along lid margins	Bacterial invasion of lid margins; often chronic
Ptosis	Dropping of upper lid margin, unilateral or bilateral	Mechanical causes as a result of eyelid tumors or excess skin; myogenic causes such as myasthenia gravis
Entropion	Inward turning of upper or lower lid margin, unilateral or bilateral	Congenital causes resulting in development abnormalities
Ectropion	Outward turning of lower lid margin	Mechanical causes as a result of eyelid tumors, herniated orbital fat, or extravasation of fluid
Conjunctiva		
Conjunctivitis	Redness, swelling of conjunctiva; may be itchy	Bacterial or viral infection; may be allergic response or inflammatory response to chemical exposure
Subconjunctival hemorrhage	Appearance of blood spot on sclera; may be small or can affect entire sclera	Conjunctival blood vessels rupture, leaking blood into the subconjunctival space
Cornea		
Corneal abrasion	Localized painful disruption of the epithelial layer of cornea, can be visualized with fluorescein dye	Trauma; overwear or improper fit of contact lenses
Globe		
Exophthalmos	Protrusion of globe beyond its normal position within bony orbit; sclera often visible above iris when eyelids are open	Intraocular or periorbital tumors; hyperthyroidism
Pupil		
Anisocoria	Pupils are unequal (constricted)	Central nervous system disorders; slight difference in pupil size is normal in a small percentage of the population
Abnormal response to light or accommodation	Pupils respond asymmetrically or abnormally to light stimulus or accommodation	Central nervous system disorders, general anesthesia
Iris		
Extraocular Muscles		
Strabismus	Deviation of eye position in one or more directions	Overaction or underaction of one or more extraocular muscles
Visual Field Defect		
Peripheral	Partial or complete loss of peripheral vision	Glaucoma; interruption of visual pathway (e.g., tumor); migraine headache
Central	Loss of central vision	Macular disease
Lens		
Cataract	Opacification of lens, pupil can appear cloudy or white when opacity is visible behind pupil opening	Aging, trauma, diabetes, long-term systemic corticosteroid therapy

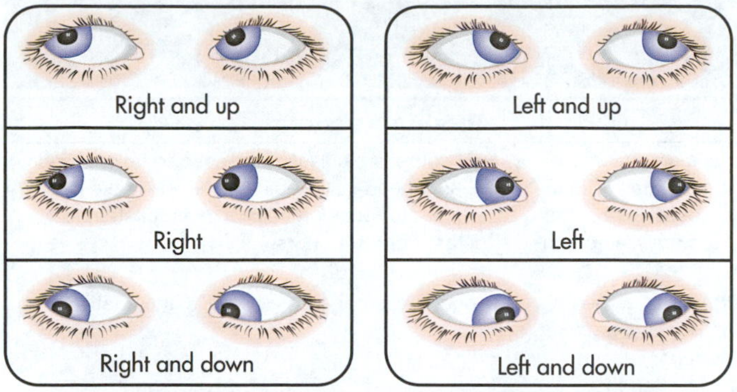

FIG. 21-5 Six cardinal positions of gaze.

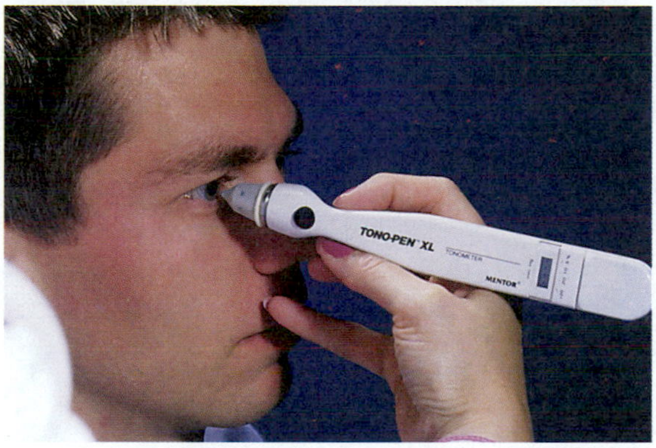

FIG. 21-6 Tono-pen tonometry.

digital light-emitting diode (LED) screen located on the front surface. Normal intraocular pressure ranges from 10 to 22 mm Hg.

Assessing Structures. The structures that constitute the visual system are assessed primarily by inspection. The visual system is unique because the nurse can directly inspect not only the external structures but also many of the internal structures. The iris, lens, vitreous, retina, and optic nerve can all be visualized directly through the clear cornea and pupil opening.

This direct inspection requires the examiner to use special observation equipment such as the slit lamp microscope and the ophthalmoscope. This equipment permits examination of the conjunctiva, sclera, cornea, anterior chamber, iris, lens, vitreous, and retina under magnification. The *ophthalmoscope* is a handheld instrument with a light source and magnifying lenses that is held close to the patient's eye to visualize the posterior part of the eye. Little pain or discomfort is associated with these examinations.

Eyebrows, Eyelashes, and Eyelids. All structures should be present and symmetric, and without deformities, redness, or swelling. Eyelashes extend outward from the lid margins. In normal closing, the upper and lower eyelid margins just touch. The lacrimal puncta should be open and positioned properly against the globe.

Conjunctiva and Sclera. The nurse can easily examine the conjunctiva and sclera at the same time. The examiner evaluates the color, smoothness, and presence of lesions or foreign bodies. The conjunctiva covering the sclera is normally clear, with fine blood vessels visible. These blood vessels are more common in the periphery.

The sclera is normally white, but it may take on a yellowish hue in the older individual because of lipid deposition. A pale blue cast caused by scleral thinning can also be normal in the older adult and in the infant (who have naturally thinner sclerae). A slight yellow cast may also be found in some dark-skinned persons, such as African Americans and Native Americans.

Cornea. The cornea should be clear, transparent, and shiny. The iris should appear flat and not bulging toward the cornea. The area between the cornea and the iris should be clear, with no blood or purulent material visible in the anterior chamber.

Iris. Both irides should be of similar color and shape. However, a color difference between the irides occurs normally in a small portion of the population.

Retina and Optic Nerve. To assess these structures, the nurse uses an ophthalmoscope to magnify the ocular structures and bring them into crisp focus. The ability to directly view arteries, veins, and the optic nerve in this manner is unique.

The optic nerve or disc is examined for size, color, and abnormalities. The optic disc is creamy yellow with distinct margins. A slight blurring of the nasal margin is common.

A central depression in the disc, called the *physiologic cup,* may be seen. This area is the exit site for the optic nerve. The cup should be less than one half the diameter of the disc. Normally, no hemorrhages or exudates are present in the fundus (retinal background). Careful inspection of the fundus can reveal the presence of retinal holes, tears, detachments, or lesions. Small hemorrhages can be associated with diabetes or hypertension and can appear in various shapes, such as dots or flames. Finally, the nurse examines the macula for shape and appearance. This area of high reflectivity is devoid of any blood vessels.

The nurse can obtain important information about the vascular system and the central nervous system (CNS) through direct visualization with an ophthalmoscope. Skilled use of this instrument requires practice.

Special Assessment Techniques

Color Vision. Testing the patient's ability to distinguish colors can be an important part of the overall assessment because some occupations may require accurate color discrimination. The Ishihara color test determines the patient's ability to distinguish a pattern of color in a series of color plates. Older adults have a loss of color discrimination at the blue end of the color spectrum and loss of sensitivity throughout the entire spectrum, especially when cataracts are present.

Stereopsis. *Stereoscopic vision* allows a patient to see objects in three dimensions. Any event that causes a patient to have monocular vision (e.g., enucleation, patching) results in the loss of stereoscopic vision. When stereopsis is not present, the individual's ability to judge distances is impaired. This disability can have serious consequences if the patient trips over a step when walking or follows too closely behind another vehicle when driving.

DIAGNOSTIC STUDIES OF THE VISUAL SYSTEM

Diagnostic studies provide important information to the nurse in monitoring the patient's condition and planning appropriate interventions. These studies are considered objective data. Table 21-6 presents the most common basic diagnostic studies of the visual system.

STRUCTURES AND FUNCTIONS OF THE AUDITORY SYSTEM

The auditory system is composed of the peripheral auditory system and the central auditory system. The peripheral system includes the structures of the ear itself: the external, middle, and inner ear (Fig. 21-7). This system is concerned with the reception and perception of sound. The inner ear functions in hearing and balance. The central system (the brain and its pathways) integrates and as-

TABLE 21-6 ***DIAGNOSTIC STUDIES***
Visual System

Study	Description and Purpose	Nursing Responsibility*
Refractometry	Subjective measure of refractive error; multiple lenses are mounted on rotating wheels; patient sits looking through apertures at Snellen acuity chart, lenses are changed; patient chooses lenses that make acuity sharpest; cycloplegic drugs used to paralyze accommodation during refraction process.	Procedure is painless, may need to help patient hold head still. Pupil dilation will make it difficult to focus on near objects; dilation may last from 3-4 hours.
Ultrasonography	A-scan probe is applanated against patient's anesthetized cornea; used primarily for axial length measurement for calculating power of intraocular lens implanted after cataract extraction; B-scan probe is applied to patient's closed lid; used more often than A-scan for diagnosis of ocular pathology such as intraocular foreign bodies or tumors, vitreous opacities, retinal detachments.	Procedure is painless (cornea is anesthetized).
Fluorescein angiography	Fluorescein (a nonradioactive, noniodine dye) is intravenously injected into antecubital or other peripheral vein, followed by serial photographs (over 10-minute period) of the retina through dilated pupils; provides diagnostic information about flow of blood through pigment epithelial and retinal vessels; often used in diabetic patients to accurately locate areas of diabetic retinopathy before laser destruction of neovascularization.	If extravasation occurs, fluorescein is toxic to tissue; systemic allergic reactions are rare, but nurse should be familiar with emergency equipment and procedures; tell patient that dye can sometimes cause transient nausea or vomiting; yellow discoloration of urine and skin is normal and transient.
Amsler grid test	Test is self-administered using a handheld card printed with a grid of lines (similar to graph paper); patient fixates on center dot and records any abnormalities of the grid lines, such as wavy, missing, or distorted areas; used to monitor macular problems.	Regular testing is necessary to identify any changes in macular function.

*Patient education regarding the purpose and method of testing is a nursing responsibility for all diagnostic procedures.

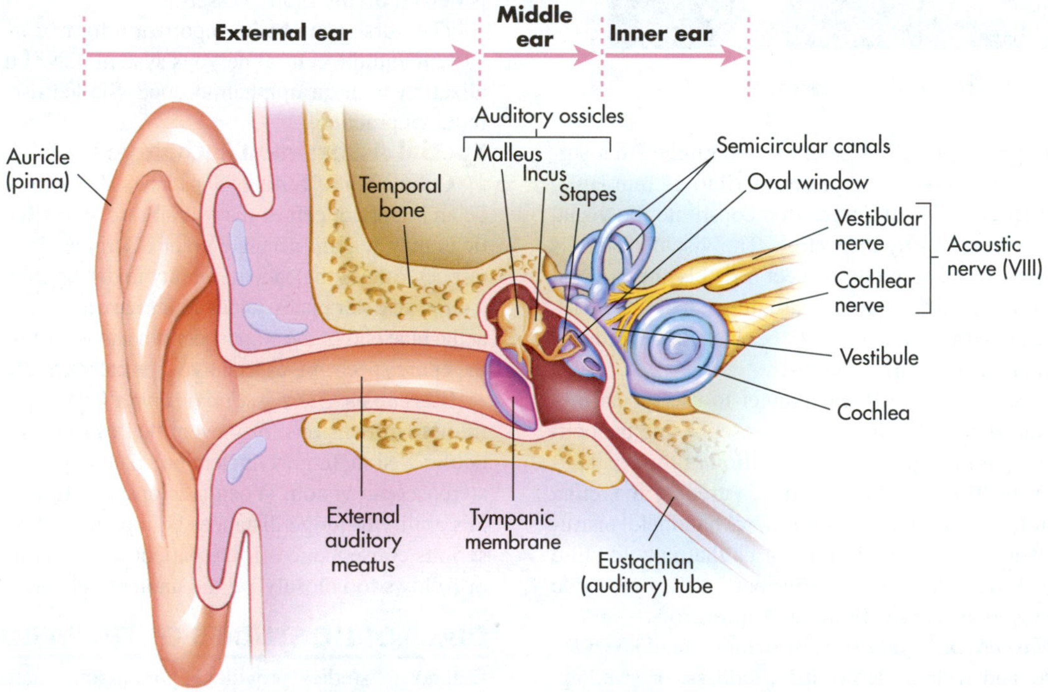

FIG. 21-7 External, middle, and inner ear.

signs meaning to what is heard. The external and middle portions of the ear function to conduct and amplify sound waves from the environment. This portion of sound conduction is termed *air conduction.* Problems in these two parts of the ear may cause *conductive hearing loss,* resulting in an alteration in the patient's perception of or sensitivity to sounds.

The inner ear functions in hearing and balance. Pathology of the inner ear or along the nerve pathway from the inner ear to the brain can result in *sensorineural hearing loss.* This may result in an alteration of the patient's perception of or sensitivity to specific tones. Impairment within the central auditory system causes *central hearing loss.* This type of hearing loss causes difficulty in understanding the meaning of words that are heard. (Types of hearing loss are discussed in Chapter 22.)

External Ear

The external ear consists of the *auricle,* or pinna, and the external auditory canal. The auricle is composed of cartilage and connective tissue covered with epithelium, which also lines the external auditory canal (see Fig. 21-7). The external auditory canal is a slightly S-shaped tube about 1 inch (2.5 cm) in length in the adult. The skin that lines the canal contains fine hairs and sebaceous (oil) glands and ceruminous (wax) glands. The oil and wax lubricate the ear canal and keep it free from debris and kill bacteria.[9]

Hair is present in the outer half of the canal. The inner half of the ear canal is highly sensitive. The function of the external ear and canal is to collect and transmit sound waves to the *tympanic membrane* (eardrum). This shiny, translucent, pearl-gray membrane is composed of epithelial cells, connective tissue, and mucous membrane. It serves as a partition and an instrument of sound transmission between the external auditory canal and the middle ear.

Middle Ear

The middle ear cavity is an air space located in the temporal bone. Mucous membrane lines the middle ear and is continuous from the nasal pharynx via the eustachian (auditory) tube. The eustachian tube functions to equalize atmospheric air pressure between the middle ear and the throat and allows the tympanic membrane to move freely. It opens during yawning and swallowing. Blockage of this tube can occur with allergies, nasopharyngeal infections, or enlarged adenoids. The middle ear contains three tiny bones: *malleus, incus,* and *stapes* (ossicles). Vibrations of the tympanic membrane cause the ossicles to move and transmit sound waves to the oval window. This oval window vibration causes the fluid in the inner ear to move and stimulate the receptors of hearing. The round window covered with mucous membrane also opens into the inner ear to help maintain fluid balance in the inner ear. The superior part of the middle ear is called the *epitympanum,* or the attic. It also communicates with air cells within the mastoid bone. The facial nerve (CN VII) traverses above the oval window of the middle ear. The thin, bony covering of the facial nerve can become damaged by chronic ear infection, skull fracture, or trauma during ear surgery. Problems may occur related to voluntary facial movements, eyelid closure, and taste discrimination. Permanent damage to the facial nerve can also result.

Inner Ear

The inner ear is composed of a bony labyrinth (maze) surrounding a membrane. This complex contains the functional organs for hearing and balance. The receptor organ for hearing is the *cochlea,* a coiled structure. It contains the *organ of Corti,* whose tiny hair cells respond to stimulation of selected portions of the basilar membrane according to pitch. This stimulus is converted into an electrochemical impulse and then transmitted by the acoustic portion of the vestibulocochlear nerve (CN VIII) to the temporal lobe of the brain to process and interpret the sound.

Three semicircular canals and the vestibule make up the organ of balance. These structures make up the membranous labyrinth, which is housed in the bony labyrinth. The membranous labyrinth is filled with endolymphatic fluid, and the bony labyrinth is filled with perilymphatic fluid. The fluid cushions these two sensitive organs and communicates with the brain and the subarachnoid spaces of the brain. The nervous stimuli are communicated by the vestibular portion of CN VIII.[10] Debris or excessive pressure within the lymphatic fluid can cause disorders such as vertigo.

Transmission of Sound. Sound waves are conducted by air (air conduction) and picked up by the auricles and auditory canal. The tympanic membrane is struck by the sound waves, causing it to vibrate. The central area of the tympanic membrane is connected to the malleus, which also starts to vibrate, transmitting the vibration to the incus and then the stapes. As the stapes moves back and forth, it pushes the membrane of the oval window in and out. Movement of the oval window produces waves in the perilymph.

Once sound has been transmitted to the liquid medium of the inner ear, the vibration is picked up by the tiny sensory hair cells of the cochlea, which initiate nerve impulses. These impulses are carried by nerve fibers to the main branch of the acoustic portion of CN VIII and then to the brain.[10]

The bones of the skull can also transmit sound directly to the inner ear (bone conduction). This can be demonstrated by placing the stem of a vibrating tuning fork on the skull.

GERONTOLOGIC CONSIDERATIONS
EFFECTS OF AGING ON THE AUDITORY SYSTEM

Age-related changes of the auditory system can result in impaired hearing. **Presbycusis,** or hearing loss due to aging, can result from aging or insults from a variety of sources. Noise exposure, vascular or systemic diseases, poor or inadequate nutrition, ototoxic drugs, and pollution during the life span can damage the delicate hair cells of the organ of Corti or atrophy lymph-producing cells. Sound transmission is diminished by calcification of the ossicles. Dry cerumen in the external canal can also interfere with the transmission of sound. **Tinnitus,** or ringing in the ears, may accompany the hearing loss that results from the aging process.

Hearing loss, especially in the older adult, can have serious implications for the quality of life, including progressive physical and psychosocial dysfunction.[11] As the average life span increases, the number of people with hearing loss will also increase. Early identification of problems will ensure a more active and healthy patient population in their seventh and eighth decades.

Age-related changes in the auditory system and differences in assessment findings are presented in Table 21-7.

ASSESSMENT OF THE AUDITORY SYSTEM

Assessment of the auditory system includes assessment of the *vestibular* (balance) system because the auditory and vestibular systems are so closely related. It is often difficult to separate symptoms from the two systems. The nurse needs to help the patient describe symptoms and problems in order to differentiate the source of the problems. Health history questions to ask a patient with an auditory problem are listed in Table 21-8.

Problems with balance may manifest as nystagmus or vertigo. **Nystagmus** is abnormal eye movements that may be observed by others as twitching of the eyeball or described by the patient as a blurring of vision with head or eye movement. **Vertigo** is a sense that the person or objects around the person are moving or spinning and is usually stimulated by movement of the head. Dizziness is a sensation of being off-balance that occurs when standing or walking. It does not occur when lying down.

Initially the nurse should try to categorize symptoms related to balance and separate them from symptoms related to hearing loss or tinnitus. The symptoms can be combined later in the assessment to help make the diagnosis and plan for the patient.

Subjective Data

Important Health Information

Past Health History. Many problems related to the ear are sequelae of childhood illnesses or result from problems of adjacent organs. Consequently, a careful assessment of past health problems is important.

The patient should be questioned about previous problems regarding the ears, especially problems experienced during childhood. The frequency of acute middle ear infections (otitis media), surgical procedures (e.g., myringotomy), perforations of the eardrum, drainage, and history of mumps, measles, or scarlet fever should be recorded. Congenital hearing loss can result from infectious diseases (e.g., rubella, influenza, or syphilis), teratogenic medications, or hypoxia in the first trimester of pregnancy. Head injury should be documented because it may result in hearing loss. Information about food and environmental allergies is important

TABLE 21-7 GERONTOLOGIC DIFFERENCES IN ASSESSMENT
Auditory System

Changes	Differences in Assessment Findings
External Ear	
Increased production of and drier cerumen	Impacted cerumen; potential hearing loss
Increased hair growth	Visible hair, especially in men
Loss of elasticity in cartilage	Collapsed ear canal
Middle Ear	
Atrophic changes of tympanic membrane	Conductive hearing loss
Inner Ear	
Hair cell degeneration, neuron degeneration in auditory nerve and central pathways, reduced blood supply to cochlea, calcification of ossicles	Presbycusis, diminished sensitivity to high-pitched sounds, impaired speech reception, tinnitus
Less effective vestibular apparatus in semicircular canals	Alterations in balance and body orientation

TABLE 21-8 HEALTH HISTORY
Auditory System

Health Perception–Health Management Pattern

Hearing
- Have you had a change in your hearing?*
- If yes, how does this change affect your daily life?
- Do you use any devices to improve your hearing (e.g., hearing aid, special volume control, headphones for television or stereo)?*
- How do you protect your hearing?
- Do you have any allergies that result in ear problems?*

Balance
- When did the dizziness first occur?
- Is your walking affected by dizziness or vertigo?*
- Have you ever fallen because of the dizziness?
- Does movement cause nausea or vomiting?
- Can you drive or walk alone? If no, elaborate.
- Are there any times of the day when your symptoms are worse?*
- In women, is your dizziness connected with your menstrual cycle?*

Tinnitus
- How long have you experienced ringing in your ears? Has it changed?
- When does it bother you the most?
- What things have you tried that help?

Nutritional-Metabolic Pattern
- Do you have any food allergies that affect your ears?*
- Do you notice any differences in symptoms with changes in diet?*

Elimination Pattern
- Does straining during a bowel movement cause you ear pain?*
- Does your ear problem cause nausea that interferes with your food intake?*
- Does chewing or swallowing cause you any ear discomfort?

Activity-Exercise Pattern
- Does your ear problem result in any change in your usual activity or exercise?*
- Do you need help with certain activities (e.g., lifting, bending, climbing stairs, driving, speaking) because of symptoms?*
- Do you have any limitations in activities of daily living because of your symptoms?*

Sleep-Rest Pattern
- Is your sleep disturbed by symptoms of tinnitus or dizziness?*

Cognitive-Perceptual Pattern
- Do you experience pain associated with your hearing or balance problem?* What relieves the pain? What makes it worse?
- Is your ability to communicate and understand affected by your symptoms?*

Self-Perception–Self-Concept Pattern
- Have changes in your hearing affected your self-esteem or feeling of independence?*

Role-Relationship Pattern
- What effect has your ear problem had on your work, family, or social life?
- Are you able to recognize the effects of your ear problems on your life?*
- Do you consider your ear problem a stressor?*

Sexuality-Reproductive Pattern
- Has your ear problem caused a change in your sex life?*

Coping–Stress Tolerance Pattern
- What coping mechanisms do you use during times of exacerbation of symptoms?
- Do you feel able to cope with your hearing or balance problem? If no, describe.

Value-Belief Pattern
- Do you have a conflict between your planned treatment and your value-belief system?*

*If yes, describe.

because they can cause the eustachian tube to become edematous and prevent aeration of the middle ear.

Symptoms such as dizziness, tinnitus, and hearing loss are recorded in the patient's words. It may be difficult for the patient to describe the dizziness. However, it is important that the patient describe the dizziness in detail using her or his own words. This careful description could help differentiate the cause.

Information regarding family members with hearing loss and type of hearing loss is important. Some congenital hearing loss is hereditary. The age of onset of presbycusis also follows a familial pattern.

Medications. Information about present or past medications that are *ototoxic* (cause damage to CN VIII) and can produce hearing loss, tinnitus, and vertigo should be obtained. The amount and frequency of aspirin use are important because tinnitus can result from high aspirin intake. Aminoglycosides, any other antibiotics, salicylates, antimalarial agents, chemotherapeutic drugs, diuretics, and nonsteroidal antiinflammatory drugs (NSAIDs) are groups of drugs that are potentially ototoxic.[12] Careful monitoring for hearing and balance problems is essential. Many drugs produce hearing loss that may be reversible if treatment is stopped.

Surgery or Other Treatments. Information regarding previous hospitalizations for ear surgery (e.g., myringotomy, tympanoplasty), as well as for tonsillectomy and adenoidectomy, should be obtained. Use of and satisfaction with a hearing aid should be documented. Problems with impacted cerumen should also be noted.

Functional Health Patterns. Hearing and balance problems can affect all aspects of a person's life. To assess the impact of hearing loss, health history questions can be asked based on a functional health pattern approach (see Table 21-8).

Health Perception–Health Management Pattern. The nurse should note the onset of hearing loss, whether sudden or gradual. It should be recorded who noted the onset, whether it be the patient, family, or significant others. Gradual hearing losses are most often noted by those who communicate with the patient. Sudden losses and those exacerbated by some other condition are most often reported by the patient.

The patient should be questioned about personal practices used to preserve hearing. The use of protective ear covers or earplugs is good practice for persons in high-noise environments. If the patient is a swimmer, the frequency and duration of swimming and use of ear protection should be documented. It is also important to note the type of water (pool, lake, or ocean) in which the swimming takes place to help identify contact with contaminated water. Placement of any item in the ear, including hearing aids, that can cause trauma to the skin increases risk of infection.

Nutritional-Metabolic Pattern. Both alcohol and sodium affect the amount of endolymph in the inner ear system. Patients with Ménière's disease generally notice some improvement in their symptoms with alcohol restriction and a low-sodium diet. Improvements and exacerbations associated with food intake should be noted. The patient should also be questioned about any ear pain or discomfort associated with chewing or swallowing that might decrease nutritional intake. This situation is often associated with a problem in the middle ear.

Assessment of clenching or grinding of the teeth helps differentiate problems of the ear from referred pain of the temporomandibular joint (TMJ). Ask about dental problems and dentures. There is a higher incidence of hearing loss in individuals who wear dentures.[13]

Elimination Pattern. Elimination patterns and their association with ear problems are mainly of interest in the patient with perilymph fistula or the patient who is immediately postoperative. If the patient experiences frequent constipation or straining with bowel or bladder elimination, this may interfere with healing of a perilymph fistula or its repair. The post-stapedectomy patient especially needs to prevent the increased intracranial (and consequent inner ear) pressure associated with straining during bowel movements. Stool softeners may be ordered postoperatively for the patient who reports chronic problems with constipation.

Activity-Exercise Pattern. Activity-exercise review is most important when assessing the patient with vestibular problems. The patient should be questioned specifically about activities that relieve or exacerbate symptoms of dizziness or cause nausea or vomiting. If vertigo is a problem, the patient should be questioned about the onset, duration, and frequency of this symptom. Patients with Ménière's disease demonstrate increasing inability to compensate for environmental input as the day progresses. Symptoms are experienced particularly in the evening. In contrast, the patient with chronic vertigo syndrome (benign paroxysmal positional vertigo [BPPV]) notes that the symptoms improve throughout the day as adjustment to the visual and positional input from the environment occurs. The nurse and the patient should identify a list of activities and exercises that aggravate and relieve dizziness and vertigo. Frequent repetition of an activity that causes symptoms (habituation) may help the body adjust so that the activity is no longer a problem.

Sleep-Rest Pattern. The patient with chronic tinnitus should be questioned about sleep problems. Tinnitus can disturb sleep and activities conducted in a quiet environment. The patient should be asked if any masking devices or techniques are used or have been tried to drown out the tinnitus. The nurse should also assess for snoring because it can be caused by swelling or hypertrophy of tissue in the nasopharynx. This excessive tissue can impair the functioning of the eustachian tube and cause the sensation of ear fullness or pain.

Cognitive-Perceptual Pattern. Pain is associated with some ear problems, particularly those involving the middle ear. If pain is present, the patient should be asked to describe the pain and the treatments used for relief. The effect on the pain level when the auricle is moved or the tragus is palpated should be noted.

Difficulties relating to attending and following directions might be an indication of early hearing loss. A gradual hearing loss may not be recognized by the patient. Gradual hearing losses are most often noted by those who communicate with the patient. Ask significant others if they have noted any change in the patient's hearing. When hearing loss is present, the nurse should note the onset and whether onset was sudden or gradual.

Self-Perception–Self-Concept Pattern. The patient should be asked to describe how the ear problem has affected his or her personal life and feelings about himself or herself. Hearing loss and chronic vertigo are particularly distressing for the patient. Hearing loss can result in embarrassing social situations that cause the patient to have a diminished self-concept. The nurse should sensitively question the patient about the occurrence of such situations.

The patient with chronic vertigo may at times be accused of alcohol intoxication. The patient should be asked if this has happened and how the situation was handled.

Role-Relationship Pattern. The patient should be questioned about the effect the ear problem has had on family life, work responsibilities, and social relationships. Hearing loss can result in strained family relations and misunderstandings. Failure to acknowledge hearing loss and failure to seek treatment can further hinder family relationships.

The patient should be questioned regarding employment or contact with environments that have excessive noise levels, such as work with jet engines and machinery, contact with the firing of firearms, and electronically amplified music. The use of preventive devices worn in noisy environments is important to document.

Many jobs rely on the ability to hear accurately and respond appropriately. If a hearing loss is present, the nurse should gather detailed information of the effect this has on the patient's job. The patient should be assisted to realistically evaluate the job situation.

Hearing loss often leaves the patient feeling isolated from valued social relationships. The nurse should gather information about social activities such as playing cards, going to movies, and attending church from before and since the hearing loss occurred. Comparison of the frequency and enjoyment of the events can indicate if a problem is present.

The unpredictability of vertigo attacks can have devastating effects on all aspects of a patient's life. Ordinary activities such as driving, child care, housework, climbing stairs, and cooking all have an element of danger. The patient should be asked to describe the effect of the vertigo on the many roles and responsibilities of life. Compensatory practices to avoid the development of dangerous situations should also be noted.

Sexuality-Reproductive Pattern. It should be determined if hearing loss or deafness has interfered with the establishment of a satisfactory sex life. Although intimacy does not depend on the ability to hear, it could interfere with establishing or maintaining a relationship.

Coping–Stress Tolerance Pattern. The patient should be asked to report the usual coping style, tolerance for stress, stress-reducing behaviors, and available support. This information enables the nurse to determine if the patient's resources are adequate to meet the demands imposed by the ear problem. If the nurse concludes that the patient seems unable to manage the situation, outside intervention may be required. Denial is a common response to a hearing problem and should be assessed.

Value-Belief Pattern. The patient should be questioned about any conflicts produced by the problem or treatment related to values or beliefs. Every effort should be made to resolve the problem so the patient does not experience additional stress. Ask about the use of home remedies such as hot oil in the ear.

Objective Data

Physical Examination. The nurse can collect valuable objective data regarding the patient's ability to hear during the health-history interview. Clues such as posturing of the head and appropriateness of responses should be noted. Does the patient ask to have certain words repeated? Does the patient intently watch the examiner but miss comments when not looking at the examiner? Such observations are significant and should be recorded. This is also important because the patient is often unaware of hearing loss or does not admit to changes in hearing until moderate losses have occurred. A normal assessment of the ear is listed in Table 21-9. Age-related changes of the auditory system and differences in assessment findings are listed in Table 21-7.

TABLE 21-9 Normal Physical Assessment of the Auditory System

- Ears symmetric in location and shape
- Auricles and tragus nontender, without lesions
- Canal clear, tympanic membrane intact, landmarks and light reflex intact
- Able to hear low whisper at 30 cm; Rinne test results AC > BC; Weber's test results, no lateralization

AC, Air conduction; *BC,* bone conduction.

External Ear. The external ear is inspected and palpated before examination of the external canal and tympanum. The auricle, preauricular area, and mastoid area are observed for symmetry of both ears, color of skin, nodules, swelling, redness, and lesions. The auricle and mastoid areas are then palpated for tenderness and nodules. Grasping the auricle may elicit pain, especially if inflammation of the external ear or canal is present.

External Auditory Canal and Tympanum. Before inserting an otoscope, the nurse should inspect the canal opening for patency, palpate the tragus, and gently move the auricle to check for discomfort. Key factors in proper use of the otoscope are adequate illumination, absence or clearing of cerumen, and tight seal of the speculum in the ear canal.[14] A speculum slightly smaller than the size of the ear canal is selected. The patient's head is tipped to the opposite shoulder. The top of the auricle is grasped and gently pulled up and backward in adults and slightly down and backward in children to straighten the canal. The otoscope, held in the examiner's hand and stabilized on the patient's head by the fingers, is inserted slowly (Fig. 21-8). The canal is observed for size and shape and the color, amount, and type of cerumen. The tympanic membrane (TM) separates the external ear from the middle ear. If a large amount of cerumen is present, the TM may not be visible. The TM is observed for color, landmarks, contour, and intactness (Fig. 21-9). It is pearl gray, white, or pink; shiny; and translucent. The handle *(manubrium)* of the malleus and the end *(umbo)* are formed from the short process of the malleus and should be visible through the membrane. The somewhat anterior position and concave shape of the TM causes the light from the otoscope to reflect back as a cone of light with crisp edges. If the TM is bulging or retracted, the edges of the light reflex will lose their cone shape, spread out or move, and have irregular edges (diffuse). The circumference of the tympanum is thickened into a dense, whitish, fibrous ring, or *annulus,* except in the superior area. The tympanum within the annulus is taut and is called the *pars tensa.* Above the short process of the malleus is the *pars flaccida,* the flaccid part of the tympanum. The malleolar folds are anterior and posterior to the short process of the malleus. The middle and inner ear cannot be examined with the otoscope because of the TM. Table 21-10 summarizes common assessment abnormalities of the auditory system.

DIAGNOSTIC STUDIES OF THE AUDITORY SYSTEM

Table 21-11 (p. 414) describes diagnostic studies commonly used to assess the auditory system.

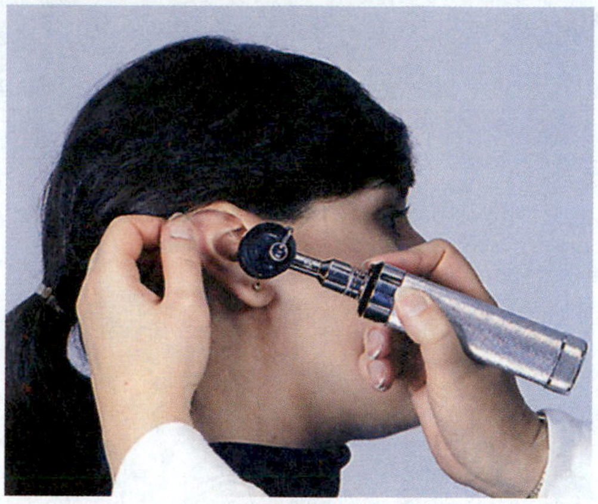

FIG. 21-8 Otoscopic examination of the adult ear. Auricle is pulled up and back. The hand holding the otoscope is braced against the face for stabilization.

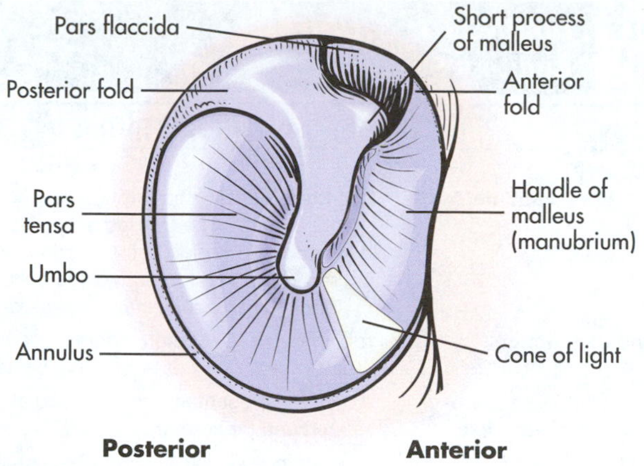

FIG. 21-9 Normal landmarks of the right tympanic membrane as seen through an otoscope.

TABLE 21-10 ***COMMON ASSESSMENT ABNORMALITIES*** **Auditory System**

Finding	Description	Possible Etiology and Significance
External Ear and Canal		
Sebaceous cyst behind ear	Usually within skin, possible presence of black dot (opening to sebaceous gland)	Removal or incision and drainage if painful
Tophi	Hard nodules in the helix or antihelix consisting of uric acid crystals	Associated with gout, metabolic disorder; further diagnosis needed
Impacted cerumen	Wax that has not normally been excreted from the ear; no visualization of eardrum	Decreased hearing possible, sensation of fullness in auditory canal, removal necessary before otoscopic examination
Discharge in canal	Infection of external ear, usually painful	Swimmer's ear, infection of external ear; possibly caused by ruptured eardrum and otitis media
Swelling of pinna, pain	Infection of glands of skin, hematoma caused by trauma	Aspiration (for hematoma)
Scaling or lesions	Change in usual appearance of skin	Seborrheic dermatitis, squamous cell carcinoma, atrophic dermatitis
Exostosis	Bony growth extending into canal causing narrowing of canal	Possible interference with visualization of tympanum, usually asymptomatic
Tympanum		
Retracted eardrum	Appearance of shorter, more horizontal malleus; absent or bent cone of light	Vacuum in middle ear, blockage of eustachian tube, negative pressure in middle ear
Hairline fluid level, yellow-amber bubbles above fluid level	Caused by transudate of blood and serum, meniscus of fluid producing hairline appearance	Serous otitis media
Bulging red or blue eardrum, lack of landmarks	Fluid-filled middle ear, pus, blood	Acute otitis media, perforation possible
Perforation of eardrum (central or marginal)	Previous perforations of the eardrum that have failed to heal; thin, transparent layer of epithelium surrounding eardrum	Chronic otitis media, mastoiditis
Recruitment	Disproportionate loudness of sound from malfunction of inner ear	Hearing aid difficult to use

Tests for Hearing Acuity

Tests involving the whispered and spoken voice can provide gross screening information about the patient's ability to hear. Audiometric testing provides more detailed information that can be used for diagnosis and treatment.

In the whispered test the examiner stands 12 to 24 inches (30 to 61 cm) to the side of the patient and, after exhaling, speaks using a low whisper. A louder whisper is used if the patient does not respond correctly. Spoken voice, increasing in loudness, is similarly used. The patient is asked to repeat numbers or words or answer questions. Each ear is tested. The ear not being tested is masked with the patient occluding the ear or with the examiner moving a finger rapidly, close to the ear canal.

Tuning-Fork Tests. Tuning-fork tests aid in differentiating between conductive and sensorineural hearing loss. Tuning forks of 512 Hz are generally used for this examination. Both skill and expe-

TABLE 21-11 DIAGNOSTIC STUDIES
Auditory System

Study	Description and Purpose	Nursing Responsibility
Auditory		
Pure-tone audiometry	Sounds are presented through earphones in soundproof room. Patient responds nonverbally when sound is heard. Response is recorded on an audiogram. Purpose is to determine hearing range of patient in terms of decibels (dB) and Hertz (Hz) for diagnosing conductive and sensorineural hearing loss. Tinnitus can cause inconsistent results.	Nurse does not usually participate in examination.
Bone conduction	Tuning fork is placed on mastoid process, and hearing by bone conduction is recorded. Diagnoses conductive hearing loss.	
One-syllable and two-syllable word lists	Words are presented and recorded at comfortable level of hearing to determine percentage correct and word understanding.	
Auditory evoked potential (AEP)	Procedure is similar to electroencephalogram (see Chapter 56 and Table 56-9). Electrodes are attached to patient in a darkened room. Electrodes are placed typically at the vertex, mastoid process, or earlobes and forehead. A computer is used to isolate the auditory from other electrical activity of the brain.	Explain procedure to patient. Do not leave patient alone in the darkened room.
Electrocochleography	Test is useful for uncooperative patient or patient who cannot volunteer useful information. Test records electrical activity in the cochlea and auditory nerve.	Nurse does not usually participate in examination.
Auditory brainstem response (ABR)	Study measures electrical peaks along auditory pathway of inner ear to brain and provides diagnostic information related to acoustical neuromas, brainstem problems, and stroke.	Nurse does not usually participate in examination.
Tympanometry (impedance audiometry)	Useful in diagnosis of middle ear effusions. A probe is placed snugly in the external ear canal and positive and negative pressures are then applied. Compliance of the middle ear is then noted in response to the pressures.	
Vestibular		
Caloric test stimulus	Endolymph of the semicircular canals is stimulated by irrigation of cold (68° F [20° C]) or warm (97° F [36° C]) solution into ear. Patient is seated or in supine position. Observation of type of nystagmus, nausea and vomiting, falling, or vertigo is helpful in diagnosing disease of labyrinth. Decreased function is indicated by decreased response and indicates disease of vestibular system. Other ear is tested similarly and results are compared.	Instruct patient to eat light meal before the test to avoid nausea. Observe patient for vomiting; assist if necessary. Ensure patient safety.
Electronystagmography (ENG)	Electrodes are placed near patient's eyes and movement of eyes (nystagmus) is recorded on graph during specific eye movements and when ear is irrigated. Study diagnoses diseases of vestibular system.	
Posturography	Balance test that can isolate one semicircular canal from others to determine site of lesion.	Inform patient that test is time consuming and uncomfortable; test can be discontinued at any time at patient's request.
Rotary chair testing	The patient is seated in a chair driven by a motor under computer control. Evaluates peripheral vestibular system.	

rience are required to ensure accurate results. If a problem is suspected, further evaluation by pure-tone audiometry is essential. The most common tuning-fork tests are the Rinne test and Weber's test.

For the Rinne test the base of an activated tuning fork is held first against the mastoid bone and then in front of the ear canal (0.5 to 2 inches). The patient reports whether the sound is louder behind the ear (on the mastoid bone) or next to the ear canal. When the sound is no longer perceived behind the ear, the fork is moved next to the ear canal until the patient indicates that the sound is no longer heard. The Rinne test is positive when the patient reports that air conduction (AC) is heard longer than bone conduction (BC). This can indicate normal hearing or a sensorineural loss. If the patient hears the tuning fork better by bone conduction, the Rinne test is negative and indicates that a conductive hearing loss is present.

For Weber's test an activated tuning fork is placed on the midline of the skull, the forehead, or the teeth. The patient is asked to indicate where the sound is heard best. In normal auditory function the patient perceives a midline tone. If a patient has a conductive hearing loss in one ear, sound is heard louder (lateralizes) in that ear. If a sensorineural loss is present, sound is louder (lateralizes) in the unaffected ear.

Results of tuning fork tests are subjective. The patient with inconsistent test results or questionable results should be referred for more objective audiometric evaluation.

Audiometry. *Audiometry* is beneficial as a screening test for hearing acuity and as a diagnostic test for determining the degree and type of hearing loss. The audiometer produces pure tones at varying intensities to which the patient can respond. Sound is characterized by the number of vibrations or cycles that occur each second. *Hertz* (Hz) is the unit of measurement used to classify the frequency of a tone; the higher the frequency, the higher the pitch. Hearing loss can affect certain sound frequencies. The specific pattern produced on the audiogram by these losses can assist in the diagnosis of the type of hearing loss. The intensity or strength of a sound wave is expressed in terms of decibels (dB), ranging from 0 to 110 dB. The intensity of a sound required to make any frequency barely audible to the average normal ear is 0 dB. *Threshold* refers to the signal level at which pure tones are detected (pure tone thresholds) or the signal level at which the patient correctly hears 50% of the signals (speech detection thresholds).

Normal speech is approximately 40 to 65 dB; a soft whisper is 20 dB. Normally, a child and a young adult can hear frequencies from about 16 to 20,000 Hz, but hearing is most sensitive between 500 and 4000 Hz. This is similar to the frequencies contained in speech. A 40- to 45-dB loss in these frequencies causes moderate difficulty in hearing normal speech. A hearing aid may be helpful because it makes sound information louder but not clearer. A hearing aid may not be helpful to the patient who has problems with discrimination of sounds or sound information because the consonants are still not heard enough to make speech understandable.

Screening Audiometry. Screening audiometry is the testing of large numbers of persons with a fast, simple test to detect possible hearing problems. A pass-fail criterion is used to screen persons who will or will not be given additional diagnostic testing. Persons who fail the screening should be referred to an audiologist for pure-tone (threshold) audiometry.

Pure-Tone Audiometry. A pure-tone audiometer produces pure tones at varied frequencies and intensities and is performed by an audiologist. The purpose is to determine the hearing range of the patient in terms of decibels and Hertz. Tinnitus can cause inconsistent results.

Specialized Tests

The more specialized tests of the auditory system are most often performed in an outpatient setting by an audiologist. An audiologist can perform many additional tests with the use of audiometers and computers that record electrical activity from the middle ear, inner ear, and brain (see Table 21-11). The most common test performed by the audiologist is pure-tone audiometry. The audiologist can also test air conduction and bone conduction to aid in differentiating sensorineural from conductive hearing losses.[15] The nursing responsibilities include (1) explaining the examination in general terms, (2) informing the patient if there are any dietary restrictions such as caffeine or other stimulants, and (3) advising the patient if sedation will be used.

More sophisticated tests are available to determine the origin of certain hearing losses. These include evoked potential studies (also called auditory brainstem response) and electrocochleography. Computed tomography (CT) and magnetic resonance imaging (MRI) scans are used to diagnose the site of a lesion, such as a tumor of the auditory nerve.

Test for Vestibular Function

Table 21-11 describes diagnostic studies commonly used to assess vestibular function. Results of these tests can be altered by use of caffeine, other stimulants, sedatives, and antivertigo agents.

NCLEX EXAMINATION REVIEW QUESTIONS

The number of the question corresponds to the same-numbered objective at the beginning of the chapter.

1. In a patient who has a hemorrhage in the vitreous cavity of the eye, the nurse knows that blood is accumulating
   a. in the aqueous humor.
   b. between the lens and the retina.
   c. between the cornea and the lens.
   d. in the space between the iris and the lens.
2. Increased intraocular pressure may occur as a result of
   a. edema of the corneal stroma.
   b. dilation of the retinal arterioles.
   c. blockage of the lacrimal canals and ducts.
   d. increased production of aqueous humor by the ciliary process.
3. The nurse should specifically question patients using eyedrops to treat glaucoma about
   a. use of corrective lenses.
   b. their usual sleep pattern.
   c. a history of heart or lung disease.
   d. sensitivity to opioids or depressants.
4. The nurse should always assess the patient with an ophthalmic problem for
   a. visual acuity.
   b. pupillary reactions.
   c. intraocular pressure.
   d. confrontation visual fields.
5. During assessment of hearing, the nurse would expect to find
   a. absent cone of light.
   b. pearl-gray tympanic membrane.
   c. lateralization with Weber's test.
   d. bone conduction (BC) greater than air conduction (AC).
6. Arcus senilis is due to
   a. tissue atrophy.
   b. decreased pupil size.
   c. opacities in the lens.
   d. cholesterol deposits in the cornea.
7. Before injecting fluorescein for angiography, it is important to
   a. obtain an emesis basin.
   b. ask if the patient is fatigued.
   c. administer topical anesthesia.
   d. determine whether the patient has a peripheral scotoma.

REFERENCES

1. Kanski JJ: *Clinical ophthalmology: a systematic approach*, ed 5, New York, 2003, Butterworth/Heinemann.
2. Horton J: Disorders of the eye. In Kasper D, et al, editors: *Harrison's principles of internal medicine*, ed 16, New York, 2005, McGraw-Hill.
3. Hodgson B, Kizior R: *Saunders nursing drug handbook*, St Louis, 2005, Elsevier Saunders.
4. Jarvis C: *Physical examination and health assessment,* ed 4, Philadelphia, 2004, Saunders.
5. Nammis JM, Zadnik K, Carol-Ghanem C, et al.: *Contact lenses in ophthalmic practice*, New York, 2004, Springer.
6. Johns Hopkins Medical Letter: *Health After 50,* 15:4, 2004.
7. Riordan-Eva P: Eye. In Tierney L, McPhee S, Papakadis M, editors: *Current medical diagnosis and treatment 2005,* ed 44, New York, 2005, McGraw-Hill.
8. Gillett P, Goldblum K: Opthalmic patient assessment, *INSIGHT—J Am Soc Ophth RNs* 39:23, 2004.
9. Herlihy B, Maebius N: *Human body in health and illness*, ed 3, St Louis, 2007, Elsevier Saunders.

*10. Finegold LS, et al: The effect of noise on public health: International Congress explores global impact, *American Speech-Language-Hearing Association (ASHI) Leader* 9:15, 2004.

11. Seidel H, et al: *Mosby's guide to physical examination,* ed 6, St Louis, 2006, Mosby.
12. Mosby: *Mosby's drug consult 2004*, St Louis, 2004, Mosby.
13. Peeters J: A potential link between oral status and hearing impairment: preliminary observations, *J Oral Rehabilitation* 31:306, 2004.
14. Holcomb SS: New guidelines improve treatment of otitis media, *Nurse Pract* 29:6, 2004.
15. Chernecky C, Berger B: *Laboratory tests and diagnostic procedures*, Philadelphia, 2004, Elsevier Saunders.

RESOURCES

Resources for this chapter are listed after Chapter 22 on page 448.
For additional resources, see the website for this book at *http://evolve.elsevier.com/Lewis/medsurg*.

*Nursing research–based reference.

The years teach much the days never knew.

Ralph Waldo Emerson

22 Nursing Management Visual and Auditory Problems

Sarah C. Smith and Sherry Neely

LEARNING OBJECTIVES

1. Describe the types of refractive errors and appropriate corrections.
2. Describe the etiology and collaborative care of extraocular disorders.
3. Explain the pathophysiology, clinical manifestations, and nursing management and collaborative care of the patient with selected intraocular disorders.
4. Describe the nursing measures that promote the health of the eyes and ears.
5. Explain the general preoperative and postoperative care of the patient undergoing surgery of the eye or ear.
6. Describe the action and uses of drug therapy for treating problems of the eyes and ears.
7. Explain the pathophysiology, clinical manifestations, and nursing management and collaborative care of common ear problems.
8. Compare the causes, management, and rehabilitative potential of conductive and sensorineural hearing loss.
9. Explain the use, care, and patient teaching related to assistive devices for eye and ear problems.
10. Describe the common causes and assistive measures for uncorrectable visual impairment and deafness.
11. Describe the measures used to assist the patient in adapting psychologically to decreased vision and hearing.

KEY TERMS

Electronic Resources

Supplemental content related to Chapter 22 can be found . . .

Companion CD

- Stress-Busting Kit for Nursing Students
- Interactive Case Study: Cataract Surgery
- NCLEX Examination Review Questions
- Comprehensive Glossary

Evolve Website evolve

http://evolve.elsevier.com/Lewis/medsurg

- Content Updates
- Key Points (Printable and CD/MP3 Download)
- Concept Map Creator
- Expanded Audio Glossary
- Key Term Flash Cards
- Customizable Nursing Care Plan: Patient After Eye Surgery
- Electronic Calculators
- WebLinks
- Figure: Refractive Errors

Visual Problems

CORRECTABLE REFRACTIVE ERRORS

The most common visual problem is **refractive error.**[1] This defect prevents light rays from converging into a single focus on the retina. Defects are a result of irregularities of the corneal curvature, the focusing power of the lens, or the length of the eye. The major symptom is blurred vision. In some cases the patient may also complain of ocular discomfort, eyestrain, or headaches. *Myopia* (nearsightedness) is the most common refractive error, with approximately 25% of Americans exhibiting this disorder. The prevalence of *hyperopia* (farsightedness) and *presbyopia* (farsightedness resulting from a decrease in the accommodative ability of the eye as a result of aging) is less common. The principal refractive errors

Reviewed by Beth Hurley, BSN, CRNO, COE, President, Ophthalmic Surgery Resources Inc., Phoenix, Ariz.; and Susan E. Sitter, RN, MSN, Research Assistant, Edinboro University of Pennsylvania, Edinboro, Pa.

of the eye can be corrected by the use of lenses in the form of eyeglasses or contact lenses, refractive surgery, or surgical implantation of an artificial lens. Refractive errors in young children should be corrected because children may develop **amblyopia** (reduced vision in the affected eye) if their refractive error is uncorrected.[2] Contrary to popular belief, uncorrected refractive errors do not worsen the error, nor do they cause further pathology after age 6.

Myopia

Myopia (nearsightedness) causes light rays to be focused in front of the retina. Myopia may occur because of excessive light refraction by the cornea or lens or because of an abnormally long eye. There is an inability to accommodate for objects at a distance. (Refractive error figure available at http://evolve.elsevier.com/Lewis/medsurg.)

Hyperopia

Hyperopia (farsightedness) causes the light rays to focus behind the retina and requires the patient to use accommodation to focus the light rays on the retina for near and far objects. This type of refractive error occurs when the cornea or lens does not have adequate focusing power or when the eyeball is too short.

Presbyopia

Presbyopia is the loss of accommodation associated with age. This condition generally appears at about age 45 years. As the eye ages, the lens becomes larger, firmer, and less elastic. These changes, which progress with aging, decrease the eye's accommodative ability. There is an inability to accommodate for near objects.

Astigmatism

Astigmatism is caused by an irregular corneal curvature. This irregularity causes the incoming light rays to be bent unequally. Consequently, the light rays do not come to a single point of focus on the retina. Astigmatism can occur in conjunction with any of the other refractive errors.

Aphakia

Aphakia is defined as the absence of the lens. The lens may be absent congenitally, or it may be removed during cataract surgery. A lens that is traumatically dislocated results in functional aphakia, although the lens remains in the eye. The lens accounts for approximately 30% of ocular refractive power. The absence of the lens results in a significant refractive error.[3] Without the focusing ability of the lens, images are projected behind the retina.

CULTURAL AND ETHNIC HEALTH DISPARITIES

Visual and Auditory Problems

- Whites have a higher incidence of hearing impairment than African Americans or Asian Americans.
- Incidence and severity of glaucoma are greater among African Americans than among whites.
- Hispanic Americans have an increased incidence of diabetic retinopathy.
- Native Americans have an increased incidence of otitis media when compared with whites.
- Whites have a higher incidence of macular degeneration than Hispanics, African Americans, and Asian Americans.

Nonsurgical Corrections

Corrective Glasses. Myopia, hyperopia, presbyopia, astigmatism, and aphakia can be modified by using the appropriate corrective lens. Myopia requires a minus corrective lens *(concave),* whereas hyperopia, presbyopia, and aphakia all require a plus corrective lens *(convex).* Glasses for presbyopia are often called "reading glasses" because they are usually worn for close work only. The presbyopic correction may also be combined with a correction for another refractive error, such as myopia or astigmatism. In these combined glasses the presbyopic correction is in the lower portion of bifocal or trifocal glasses. A newer type of correction for presbyopia, the "no-line" bifocal, is actually a multifocal lens that allows the patient to see clearly at any distance.

Aphakic glasses are very thick, making them heavy and unattractive to wear. The high degree of correction also causes images to be magnified about 25%. With the modern surgical procedures prevalent today, patients seldom wear aphakic glasses for correction because of the associated visual problems.

Contact Lenses. Contact lenses are another way to correct refractive errors. Table 22-1 describes the various contact lenses and the advantages and disadvantages of each type. Contact lenses generally provide better vision than glasses because the patient has more normal peripheral vision without the distortion and obstruction of glasses and their frames. This is especially true with high refractive errors. Contact lenses are made from various plastic and silicone substances, which are very permeable to oxygen and have a high water content, which allows increased wearing time with greater comfort. If the oxygen supply to the cornea is decreased, it becomes swollen, visual acuity decreases, and the patient experiences severe discomfort.

Altered or decreased tear formation can make wearing contact lenses difficult. Tear production can be decreased by medications such as antihistamines, decongestants, diuretics, birth control pills, and the hormones produced during pregnancy. Environmental factors such as wind, fans, and dust may also decrease the tear film. Allergic conjunctivitis with itching, tearing, and redness can also affect contact lens wear.

In general, the nurse must know whether the patient wears contact lenses, the pattern of wear (daily versus extended), and care practices. Shining a light obliquely on the eyeball can help the nurse visualize a contact lens. The patient should know the signs and symptoms of contact lens problems that must be managed by the eye care professional. The patient may remember these symptoms better if the nurse uses the mnemonic device RSVP:

Redness
Sensitivity
Vision problems
Pain

The nurse must stress the importance of removing contact lenses immediately if any of these problems occur.

Corneal Molding. *Corneal molding,* also called orthokeratology, is the use of specially designed, rigid, gas-permeable contact lenses to alter the shape of the cornea. It reduces or corrects myopia and moderate degrees of astigmatism. The cornea is molded by fitting progressively flatter rigid contact lenses and requires regular wearing of "retainer" contact lenses to maintain corneal shape.

TABLE 22-1 Types of Contact Lenses

Type	Description	Advantages	Disadvantages	Wearing Schedule
Rigid Lenses				
Standard	Rigid plastic; smaller than cornea	Can be tinted for easier visibility out of the eye; longer lasting, least expensive to purchase; corrects all types of refractive errors	Requires separate care solutions for cleaning, storing, wetting; new patients (or those resuming wear after a period of nonwear) must gradually increase wearing time; initially uncomfortable; requires adaptation to obtain adequate comfort level	Daily wear; sleeping in lenses (either inadvertently or purposely) can cause corneal edema or severe pain from lack of oxygen to cornea
Gas permeable	Similar to standard rigid lenses, but plastic allows oxygen to pass through to cornea	Longer lasting than soft lenses; corrects all types of refractive errors; more comfortable initially than standard hard lenses; less adaptation time and fewer problems with corneal edema than standard hard lenses; flexible wearing schedule	Requires separate care solutions for cleaning, storing, wetting; more expensive to purchase than rigid standard contact lens	Daily wear
Soft Lenses				
Standard	Soft, flexible plastic; covers entire cornea and a small rim of sclera	Fits snugly on eye, allowing less invasion of foreign particles under the lens; initially more comfortable and less adaptation time than rigid lenses; can be worn intermittently	Less durable and more expensive than rigid lenses (cost may be similar to gas-permeable rigid lenses); more susceptible to surface protein deposition that causes discomfort and vision problems; requires cleaning, sterilizing, and enzymatic removal of protein deposition, cannot correct for higher degrees of astigmatism	Daily wear only; sleeping in these lenses causes similar problems as sleeping in standard rigid lenses
High water content	Similar to standard soft lenses, but with a higher water content	Similar to standard soft lenses; allows more oxygen through lens so lens can be worn up to a week at a time without removal	Similar to standard soft lenses (with the exception that these can be extended wear); greater risk of complications related to contact lens wear than with standard soft lenses	Daily wear or extended wear
Toric	Similar to other standard soft lenses; special design to correct astigmatism	Similar to other soft lenses; can be custom ordered to correct patient's individual type of astigmatism	Similar to other soft lenses; more expensive than other types of lenses; can be more difficult to fit than nontoric soft lenses	Daily wear or extended wear
Disposable	Similar to other soft lenses but thinner	Similar to other soft lenses; frequent replacement decreases risk of complications related to contact lens wear	Similar to other soft lenses; cost may be greater (can be similar, depending on prevalent charges for replacement lenses)	Daily wear or extended wear; each lens can be worn as long as 2 weeks before disposal
Daily disposable	Similar to disposable	Similar to other soft lenses; daily disposal decreases risk of complications; no cleaning or disinfection necessary; commonly dispensed for new users, teenagers, and frequent travelers	Greater expense	Daily wear only; each lens is worn for 1 day and then discarded

Surgical Therapy

Surgical procedures are designed to eliminate or reduce the need for eyeglasses or contact lenses and correct refractive errors by changing the focus of the eye. Surgical management for refractive errors includes laser surgery, intraocular lens (IOL) implantation, and thermal procedures.

Laser. *Laser-assisted in-situ keratomileusis* (LASIK) may be considered for patients with low to moderately high amounts of myopia, hyperopia, and astigmatism. The procedure first involves using a laser or surgical blade to create a thin flap in the cornea. Using new technology called "wave-front," the laser is then programmed to use a map of the patient's cornea to sculpt the cornea and correct the refractive error. The flap is then repositioned and adheres on its own without sutures in a few minutes.[4,5]

Photorefractive keratectomy (PRK) is indicated for low to moderate amounts of myopia, hyperopia, and astigmatism and is a good option for a patient with insufficient corneal thickness for a LASIK flap. In PRK only the epithelium is removed and the laser sculpts the cornea to correct the refractive error. *Laser-assisted epithelial keratomileusis* (LASEK) is similar to PRK except that the epithelium is replaced after surgery.

Implant. *Intracorneal ring segments* (ICRs) are two semicircular pieces of plastic that are implanted between the layers of the cornea to treat mild forms of myopia. They are designed to change the shape of the cornea by adjusting the focusing power. ICRs can be removed and the cornea will usually return to its original shape within a few weeks.

Refractive intraocular lens (refractive IOL) implantation is an option for patients with a high degree of myopia or hyperopia. Like cataract surgery, it involves the removal of the patient's natural lens and implantation of an IOL, which is a small plastic lens to correct a patient's refractive error. Since this requires entering the eye, the risk of complications is higher. New accommodating IOLs will correct both myopia and presbyopia.

Phakic intraocular lenses (phakic IOLs) are sometimes referred to as an implantable contact lens. They are implanted into the eye without removing the eye's natural lens. They are used for patients with high degrees of myopia and hyperopia. Unlike refractive IOLs, the phakic IOL is placed in front of the eye's natural lens. Leaving the natural lens in the eye preserves the ability of the eye to focus for reading vision. Artisan is one type of phakic IOL used for moderate to severe myopia. For more information, see *www.fda.gov/cdrh/phakic*.

Thermal Procedures. *Laser thermal keratoplasty* (LTK) and *conductive keratoplasty* (CK) are procedures for patients with hyperopia or presbyopia. Using laser or high radio frequency, heat is applied to the peripheral area of the cornea to tighten it like a belt and make the central cornea steeper. Only the less dominant eye is treated, and the desired effect is monovision. Monovision enables one eye to focus at close proximity; the other eye is left untreated or, if needed, is treated to focus at a distance. A preoperative trial with contact lenses is a useful test to see if a patient will adapt to the intended refractive outcome.

UNCORRECTABLE VISUAL IMPAIRMENT

Approximately 4.8 million people in the United States have *severe visual impairment,* which is defined as the inability to read newsprint even with glasses. Of those individuals, only 9% have no useful vision, and the remaining 91% are considered partially sighted. The partially sighted individual may have significant visual abilities. It is important in working with the visually impaired patient to understand that a person classified as blind may have useful vision. Appropriate responses and interventions depend on the nurse's understanding of each patient's visual abilities.

Levels of Visual Impairment

The patient may be categorized by the level of visual loss.[6] *Total blindness* is defined as no light perception and no usable vision. *Functional blindness* is present when the patient has some light perception but no usable vision. The patient with either total or functional blindness is considered legally blind and may use vision substitutes such as guide dogs and canes for ambulation. Vision enhancement techniques are not helpful.

Almost all blindness in the United States is the result of common eye diseases. Less than 4% is the result of injuries. There are 1 million people who are blind in the United States. The most common causes of blindness are cataracts, glaucoma, age-related macular degeneration, diabetic retinopathy, and corneal diseases (e.g., herpes eye infection).

The *legally blind individual* meets the criteria developed by the federal government to determine eligibility for federal and state assistance and income tax benefits (Table 22-2). A legally blind individual may have some usable vision. The *partially sighted individual* who is not legally blind has a corrected visual acuity greater than 20/200 in the better eye and greater than 20 degrees of visual field, but the visual acuity is 20/50 or worse in the better eye. The patient who is partially sighted or legally blind can benefit greatly from vision enhancement techniques.

TABLE 22-2 Definition of Legal Blindness in the United States

- Central visual acuity for distance of 20/200 or worse in the better eye (with correction)
- Visual field no greater than 20 degrees in its widest diameter or in the better eye

NURSING MANAGEMENT
VISUAL IMPAIRMENT

Nursing Assessment

It is important to determine how long the patient has had a visual impairment because recent loss of vision has different implications for nursing care. The nurse should determine how the patient's visual impairment affects normal functioning. This may be done by questioning the patient about the level of difficulty encountered when doing certain tasks. For example, the nurse may ask how much difficulty the patient has when reading a newspaper, writing a check, moving from one room to the next, or viewing television. Other questions can help the nurse determine the personal meaning that the patient attaches to the visual impairment. The nurse can ask how the vision loss has affected specific aspects of the patient's life, whether the patient has lost a job, or what activities the patient does not engage in because of the visual impairment. The patient may attach many negative meanings to the impairment because of societal views of blindness. For example, the patient may view the impairment as punishment or view himself or herself as useless and burdensome. It is also important to determine the patient's primary coping strategies, the patient's emotional reactions, and the availability and strength of the patient's support systems.

Nursing Diagnoses

Nursing diagnoses depend on the degree of visual impairment and how long it has been present. Nursing diagnoses for the visually impaired patient include, but are not limited to, the following:

- Disturbed sensory perception *related to* visual deficit
- Risk for injury *related to* visual impairment and inability to see potential dangers
- Self-care deficits *related to* visual impairment
- Fear *related to* inability to see potential danger or accurately interpret environment
- Grieving *related to* loss of functional vision

Planning

The overall goals are that the patient with recently impaired vision or the patient with impaired adjustment to long-standing visual impairment will (1) make a successful adjustment to the impairment, (2) verbalize feelings related to the loss, (3) identify personal strengths and external support systems, and (4) use appropriate coping strategies. If the patient has been functioning at an appropriate or acceptable level, the goal is to maintain the current level of function.

HEALTHY PEOPLE
Health Impact of Responsible Eye Care

- Regular hand washing prevents the spread of disease from one eye to the other
- Seeking appropriate health care can lead to early detection of disease and prevent patients with certain types of partial vision loss from undergoing further loss of vision
- Wearing sunglasses and practicing proper nutrition may contribute toward the prevention of cataract development and age-related macular degeneration
- Wearing eye protection during potentially hazardous work, hobby, and sport activities reduces the risk of eye injuries

Nursing Implementation

Health Promotion. The nurse should encourage the partially sighted patient with preventable causes for further visual impairment to seek appropriate health care. For example, the patient with vision loss from glaucoma may prevent further visual impairment by complying with prescribed therapies and suggested ophthalmic evaluations.

Acute Intervention. The nurse provides emotional support and direct care to the patient with recent visual impairment. Active listening and facilitating are important components of nursing care for the recently visually impaired patient. The nurse should allow the patient to express anger and grief and should help the patient to identify fears and successful coping strategies. The family is intimately involved in the experiences that follow vision loss. With the patient's knowledge and permission, the nurse should include family members in discussions and encourage members to express their concerns.

Many people are uncomfortable around a blind or partially sighted individual because they are not sure what behaviors are appropriate. Sensitivity to the patient's feelings without being overly solicitous or stifling the patient's independence is vital in creating a therapeutic nursing presence. The nurse should always communicate in a normal conversational tone and manner with the patient, and the nurse should address the patient, not a family member or friend that may be with the patient. Common courtesy dictates introducing oneself and any other persons who approach the blind or partially sighted patient and saying good-bye on leaving. Making eye contact with the partially sighted patient accomplishes several objectives. It ensures that the nurse speaks while facing the patient so the patient has no difficulty hearing the nurse. The nurse's head position validates that the nurse is attentive to the patient. Also, establishing eye contact ensures that the nurse can observe the patient's facial expressions and reactions.

Orientation to the environment lessens the patient's anxiety or discomfort and facilitates independence. In orienting the partially sighted or blind patient to a new area, the nurse should identify one object as the focal point and describe the location of other objects in relation to it. For example, the nurse may say, "The bed is straight ahead, approximately 10 steps. The chair is to the left, and the nightstand is to the right, near the head of the bed. The bathroom is to the left of the foot of the bed." The nurse should explain any activities or noises occurring in the patient's immediate surroundings.

The nurse should assist the patient to each major object in the area, using the sighted-guide technique. When using this technique, the nurse stands slightly in front and to one side of the patient and offers an elbow for the patient to hold. The nurse serves as the sighted guide, walking slightly ahead of the patient with the patient holding the back of the nurse's arm (Fig. 22-1). When using this technique in any situation, the nurse should describe the environment to help orient the patient. For example, the nurse may say, "We're going through an open doorway and approaching two steps down. There is an obstacle on the left." To assist the patient to sit, place one of his or her hands on the back of the chair.

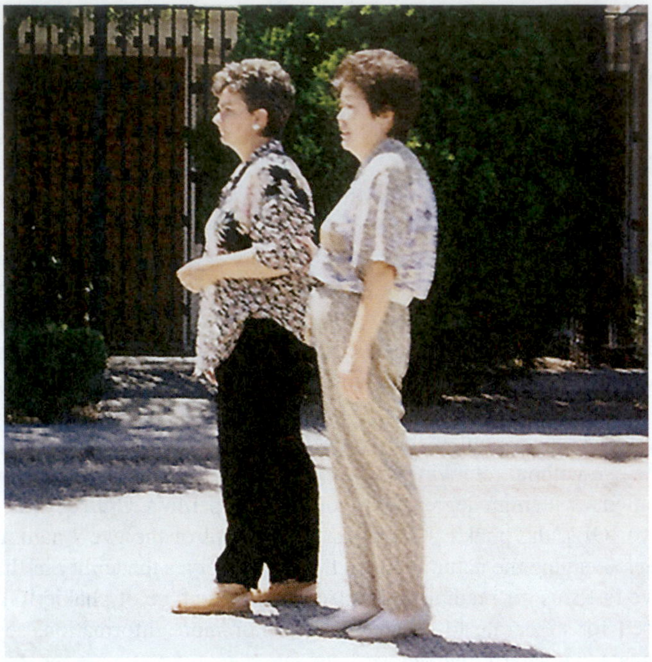

FIG. 22-1 Sighted-guide technique. The nurse serves as the sighted guide, walking slightly ahead of the patient with the patient holding the back of the nurse's arm.

Ambulatory and Home Care. Rehabilitation after partial or total loss of vision can foster independence, self-esteem, and productivity. The nurse should know what services and devices are available for the partially sighted or blind patient and should be prepared to make appropriate referrals for those services and devices. For the legally blind patient, the primary resource for services is the state agency for rehabilitation of the blind.[7] A list of agencies that serve the partially sighted or blind patient is available from the American Foundation for the Blind *(www.afb.org)*. Many of these agencies are listed in the resources section at the end of the chapter.

Braille or audio books for reading and a cane or guide dog for ambulation are examples of vision substitution techniques. These are usually most appropriate for the patient with no functional vision. For most patients who have some remaining vision, vision enhancement techniques can provide enough help for many patients to learn to ambulate, read printed material, and accomplish activities of daily living (ADLs).

Optical Devices for Vision Enhancement. Telescopic lenses for near or far vision and magnifiers of various types can often enhance the patient's remaining vision enough to allow the performance of many previously impossible tasks and activities. Most of these devices require some training and practice for successful use. Closed circuit television can provide magnification up to 60 times, allowing some patients to read, write, use computers, and do crafts. Although these systems are expensive and have limited portability, they are available in some public or university libraries.

Nonoptical Methods for Vision Enhancement. *Approach magnification* is a simple but sometimes overlooked technique for enhancing the patient's residual vision. The nurse can recommend that the patient sit closer to the television or hold books closer to the eyes, which the patient may be reluctant to do unless encouraged. Contrast enhancement techniques include watching television in black and white, placing dark objects against a light background (e.g., a white plate on a black place mat), using a black felt-tip marker, and using contrasting colors (e.g., a red stripe at the edge of steps or curbs). Increased lighting can be provided by halogen lamps, direct sunlight, or gooseneck lamps that can be aimed directly at the reading material or other near objects. Large type is often helpful, especially in conjunction with other optical or nonoptical vision enhancements.

Evaluation

The overall expected outcomes are that the patient with severe visual impairment will

- have no further progressive loss of vision
- be able to express adaptive coping strategies
- not experience a decrease in self-esteem or social interactions
- function safely within her or his own environment

GERONTOLOGIC CONSIDERATIONS
VISUAL IMPAIRMENT

The elderly patient is at an increased risk for vision loss because of cataracts, glaucoma, diabetic retinopathy, and macular degeneration. The older patient may have other deficits, such as cognitive impairment or limited mobility, that further affect the ability to function in usual ways. Societal devaluation of the elderly may compound the self-esteem or isolation issues associated with the older patient's visual impairment. Financial resources may meet normal needs but can be inadequate in meeting increased demands of vision services or devices.

The older patient may become confused or disoriented when visually compromised. The combination of decreased vision and confusion increases the risk of falls, which have potentially serious consequences for the older adult. Decreased vision may compromise the older patient's ability to function, causing concerns about maintaining independence and causing a decreased self-image. Decreased manual dexterity may make the instillation of prescribed eyedrops difficult for some older adults.

EYE TRAUMA

Although the eyes are well protected by the bony orbit and by fat pads, everyday activities can result in ocular trauma. Ocular injuries can involve the ocular adnexa, the superficial structures, or the deeper ocular structures. In the United States an estimated 1.3 million eye injuries occur each year. Of these injuries, 40,000 result in permanent visual impairment. Table 22-3 outlines emergency

TABLE 22-3 *EMERGENCY MANAGEMENT* Eye Injury

Etiology

Blunt Injury
Fist
Other blunt objects

Penetrating Injury
Fragments such as glass, metal, wood
Knife, stick, or other large object

Chemical Injury
Alkaline
Acid

Thermal Injury
Direct burn from curling iron or other hot surface
Indirect burn from UV light (e.g., welding torch, sun lamp)

Foreign Bodies
Glass
Metal
Wood
Plastic

Trauma
Blunt
Penetrating/perforating

Burns
Chemical
Thermal

Assessment Findings

- Pain
- Photophobia
- Redness—diffuse or localized
- Swelling
- Ecchymosis
- Tearing
- Blood in the anterior chamber
- Absent eye movements
- Fluid drainage from eye (e.g., blood, CSF, aqueous humor)
- Abnormal or decreased vision
- Visible foreign body
- Prolapsed globe
- Abnormal intraocular pressure
- Visual field defect

Interventions

Initial

- Determine mechanism of injury.
- Ensure airway, breathing, circulation.
- Assess for other injuries.
- Assess for chemical exposure.
- Begin ocular irrigation *immediately* in case of chemical exposure; do not stop until emergency personnel arrive to continue irrigation; sterile, pH-balanced, physiologic solution is best; if unavailable, use any nontoxic liquid. Use sterile saline or water if saline is unavailable.
- Assess visual acuity.
- Do not put pressure on the eye.
- Instruct patient not to blow nose.
- Do not attempt to treat the injury (except as noted above for chemical exposure).
- Stabilize foreign objects.
- Cover the eye(s) with dry, sterile patches and a protective shield.
- Do not give the patient food or fluids.
- Elevate head of bed 45 degrees.
- Do not put medication or solutions in the eye unless ordered by physician.
- Administer analgesia as appropriate.

Ongoing Monitoring

- Reassure the patient.
- Monitor pain.
- Anticipate surgical repair for penetrating injury, globe rupture, or globe avulsion.

CSF, Cerebrospinal fluid; *UV*, ultraviolet.

management of the patient with an eye injury. Types of ocular trauma include blunt injuries, penetrating injuries, and chemical exposure injuries. Causes of ocular injuries include automobile accidents, falls, sports and leisure activity injuries, assaults, and work-related situations. Trauma is often a preventable cause of visual impairment. Almost 90% of all sports-related eye injuries could be prevented by wearing protective eyewear during potentially hazardous work, hobbies, or sports activities. The nurse's role in individual and community education is extremely important in reducing the incidence of ocular trauma.[8]

Extraocular Disorders

INFLAMMATION AND INFECTION

One of the most common conditions encountered by the ophthalmologist is inflammation or infection of the external eye. Many external irritants or microorganisms affect the lids and conjunctiva and can involve the avascular cornea. It is a nursing responsibility to teach the patient appropriate interventions related to the specific disorder.

Hordeolum

An external **hordeolum** (commonly called a *sty*) is an infection of the sebaceous glands in the lid margin (Fig. 22-2). The most common bacterial infective agent is *Staphylococcus aureus.* A red, swollen, circumscribed, and acutely tender area develops rapidly. The nurse should instruct the patient to apply warm, moist compresses at least four times a day until it improves. This may be the only treatment necessary. If there is a tendency for recurrence, the patient should be taught to perform lid scrubs daily. In addition, appropriate antibiotic ointments or drops may be indicated.

Chalazion

A **chalazion** is a chronic inflammatory granuloma of the meibomian (sebaceous) glands in the lid. It may evolve from a hordeolum. It may also occur as a response to the material released into the lid when a blocked gland ruptures. The chalazion usually appears on the upper lid as a swollen, tender, reddened area that may be painful. Initial treatment is similar to that for a hordeolum. If warm, moist compresses are ineffective in causing spontaneous drainage, the ophthalmologist may surgically remove the lesion (this is normally an office procedure), or the ophthalmologist may inject the lesion with corticosteroids.

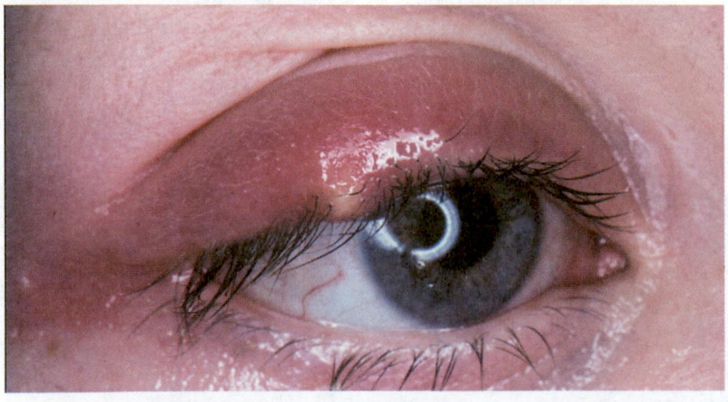

FIG. 22-2 External hordeolum (sty) on the upper eyelid caused by staphylococcal infection.

Blepharitis

Blepharitis is a common chronic bilateral inflammation of the lid margins. The lids are red rimmed with many scales or crusts on the lid margins and lashes. The patient may primarily complain of itching but may also experience burning, irritation, and photophobia. Conjunctivitis may occur simultaneously.

If the blepharitis is caused by a staphylococcal infection, collaborative care includes the use of an appropriate ophthalmic antibiotic ointment.[9] Seborrheic blepharitis, related to seborrhea of the scalp and eyebrows, is treated with an antiseborrheic shampoo for the scalp and eyebrows. Often blepharitis is caused by both staphylococcal and seborrheal microorganisms, and the treatment must be more vigorous to avoid hordeolum, *keratitis* (inflammation of the cornea), and other eye infections. Conscientious hygienic practices involving skin and scalp must be emphasized. Gentle cleansing of the lid margins with baby shampoo can effectively soften and remove crusting.

Conjunctivitis

Conjunctivitis is an infection or inflammation of the conjunctiva. Conjunctival infections may be caused by bacterial or viral microorganisms. Conjunctival inflammation may result from exposure to allergens or chemical irritants (including cigarette smoke). The tarsal conjunctiva (lining the interior surface of the lids) may become inflamed as a result of a chronic foreign body in the eye, such as a contact lens or an ocular prosthesis. Careful hand washing and using individual or disposable towels helps prevent spreading the condition.

Bacterial Infections. Acute bacterial conjunctivitis (pinkeye) is a common infection. Although it occurs in every age-group, epidemics commonly occur in children because of their poor hygienic habits. In adults and children the most common causative microorganism is *S. aureus. Streptococcus pneumoniae* and *Haemophilus influenzae* are other common causative agents, but they are seen more often in children than adults. The patient with bacterial conjunctivitis may complain of irritation, tearing, redness, and a mucopurulent drainage. Although this typically occurs initially in one eye, it spreads rapidly to the unaffected eye.[10] It is usually self-limiting, but treatment with antibiotic drops shortens the course of the disorder.

Viral Infections. Conjunctival infections may be caused by many different viruses. The patient with viral conjunctivitis may complain of tearing, foreign body sensation, redness, and mild photophobia. This condition is usually mild and self-limiting. However, it can be severe, with increased discomfort and subconjunctival hemorrhaging. Adenovirus conjunctivitis may be contracted in contaminated swimming pools and through direct contact with an infected patient. Treatment is usually palliative. If the patient is severely symptomatic, topical corticosteroids provide temporary relief but have no benefit in the final outcome. Antiviral drops are ineffective and therefore not indicated.

Chlamydial Infections. Trachoma is a chronic conjunctivitis caused by *Chlamydia trachomatis* (serotypes A through C). It is a major cause of blindness worldwide, with the incidence estimated at 146 million.[11] This preventable eye disease is transmitted mainly by the hands and by flies. Adult inclusion conjunctivitis (AIC) is caused by *C. trachomatis* (serotypes D through K). AIC is becoming more prevalent in the United States because of the increase in sexually transmitted chlamydial disease. Manifestations for both trachoma and AIC are mucopurulent ocular discharge, irritation, redness, and lid swelling. For unknown reasons, AIC does not carry the long-term consequences of trachoma. AIC also differs from trachoma in that it is common in economically developed countries, whereas trachoma is most commonly seen in underdeveloped countries. Antibiotic therapy is usually effective for trachoma and AIC.

Although antibiotic treatment may be successful in the adult with AIC, these patients have a high risk of concurrent chlamydial genital infection, as well as other sexually transmitted diseases. The nurse's responsibility with the patient with AIC includes education about the ocular condition, as well as the sexual implications of the condition.

Allergic Conjunctivitis. Conjunctivitis caused by exposure to some allergen can be mild and transitory, or it can be severe enough to cause significant swelling, sometimes ballooning the conjunctiva beyond the eyelids. The defining symptom of allergic conjunctivitis is itching.[12] The patient may also complain of burning, redness, and tearing. Acutely, the patient may also have white or clear exudate. If the condition is chronic, the exudate is thicker and becomes mucopurulent. In addition to pollens, the patient may develop allergic conjunctivitis in response to animal dander, ocular solutions and medications, or even contact lenses. The nurse should instruct the patient to avoid the allergen if it is known. Artificial tears can be effective in diluting the allergen and washing it from the eye. Effective topical medications include antihistamines and corticosteroids.

Keratitis

Keratitis is an inflammation or infection of the cornea that can be caused by a variety of microorganisms or by other factors. The condition may involve the conjunctiva and/or the cornea. When it involves both, the disorder is termed *keratoconjunctivitis.*

Bacterial Infections. The intact cornea provides an effective defense against infection. When the epithelial layer is disrupted, the cornea can become infected by a variety of bacteria. Topical antibiotics are generally effective, but eradicating the infection may require subconjunctival antibiotic injection or, in severe cases, intravenous (IV) antibiotics. Risk factors include mechanical or chemical corneal epithelial damage, contact lens wear, debilitation, nutritional deficiencies, immunosuppressed states, and contaminated products (e.g., lens care solutions and cases, topical medications, cosmetics).

Viral Infections. Herpes simplex virus (HSV) keratitis is the most frequently occurring infectious cause of corneal blindness in the Western hemisphere. It is a growing problem, especially with immunosuppressed patients. It may be caused by HSV-1 or HSV-2 (genital herpes), although HSV-2 ocular infection is much less common. The resulting corneal ulcer has a characteristic dendritic (tree-branching) appearance, and it is often, although not always, preceded by infection of the conjunctiva or eyelids. Pain and photophobia are common. Up to 40% of patients with herpetic keratitis heal spontaneously. The spontaneous healing rate increases to 70% if the cornea is debrided to remove infected cells. Collaborative therapy includes corneal debridement followed by topical therapy with vidarabine (Vira-A) or trifluridine (Viroptic) used for 2 to 3 weeks. Topical corticosteroids are usually contraindicated because they contribute to a longer course and possible deeper ulceration of the cornea. Drug therapy may also include oral acyclovir (Zovirax).

The varicella-zoster virus (VZV) causes both chickenpox and herpes zoster ophthalmicus (HZO). HZO may occur by reactivation of an endogenous infection that has persisted in latent form after an earlier attack of varicella or by direct or indirect contact with a patient with chickenpox or herpes zoster. It occurs most frequently in the older adult and in the immunosuppressed patient. Collaborative care of the patient with acute HZO may include opioid or nonopioid analgesics for the pain, topical corticosteroids to reduce inflammation, antiviral agents such as acyclovir (Zovirax) to reduce viral replication, mydriatic agents to dilate the pupil and relieve pain, and topical antibiotics to combat secondary infection. The patient may apply warm compresses and povidone-iodine gel to the affected skin (gel should not be applied near the eye).

Epidemic keratoconjunctivitis (EKC) is the most serious ocular adenoviral disease. EKC is spread by direct contact, including sexual activity. In the medical setting, contaminated hands and instruments can be the source of spread. The patient may complain of tearing, redness, photophobia, and foreign body sensation. In most patients, the disease involves only one eye. Treatment is primarily palliative and includes ice packs and dark glasses. In severe cases, therapy can include mild topical corticosteroids to temporarily relieve symptoms and topical antibiotic ointment. The nurse's most important role is to teach the patient and family members regarding good hygienic practices to avoid spreading the disease.

Other Causes of Keratitis. Keratitis may also be caused by fungi (most commonly *Aspergillus, Candida,* and *Fusarium* species), especially in the case of ocular trauma in an outdoor setting where fungi are prevalent in the soil and moist organic matter. *Acanthamoeba* keratitis is caused by a parasite that is associated with contact lens wear, probably as a result of contaminated lens care solutions or cases (Fig. 22-3). Homemade saline solution is particularly susceptible to *Acanthamoeba* contamination. The nurse should instruct the patient who wears contact lenses about good lens care practices. Medical treatment of fungal and *Acanthamoeba* keratitis is difficult. The *Acanthamoeba* organism is resistant to most drugs. Only one antifungal eyedrop (natamycin [Natacyn]) is approved by the Food and Drug Administration (FDA). If antimicrobial therapy fails, the patient may require a corneal transplant.

Exposure keratitis occurs when the patient cannot adequately close the eyelids. The patient with exophthalmos (protruding eyeball) from thyroid eye disease or masses posterior to the globe is susceptible to exposure keratitis.

Corneal Ulcer. Tissue loss caused by infection of the cornea produces a *corneal ulcer* (infectious keratitis). The infection can be due to bacteria, viruses, or fungi. Corneal ulcers are often very painful, and patients may feel as if there is a foreign body in their eye. Other symptoms can include tearing, purulent or watery discharge, redness, and photophobia. Treatment is generally aggressive to avoid permanent loss of vision. Antibiotic, antiviral, or an-

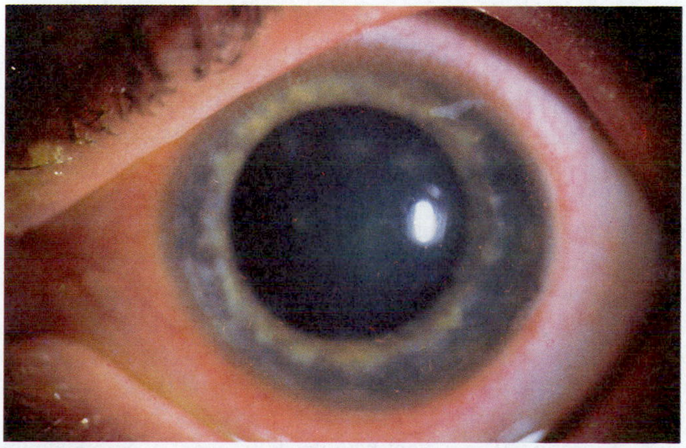

FIG. 22-3 *Acanthamoeba* keratitis. Corneal infection associated with contact lens wear.

tifungal eyedrops may be prescribed as frequently as every hour night and day for the first 24 hours. An untreated corneal ulcer can result in corneal scarring and perforation (hole in the cornea). A corneal transplant may be indicated.

NURSING MANAGEMENT INFLAMMATION AND INFECTION

■ Nursing Assessment

The nurse should assess ocular changes, such as edema, redness, decreasing visual acuity, feeling as if a foreign body is present, or discomfort, and document the findings in the patient's record. The nurse's assessment should also consider the psychosocial aspects of the patient's condition, especially when the patient has visual impairment associated with the condition.

■ Nursing Diagnoses

Nursing diagnoses for the patient with inflammation or infection of the external eye include, but are not limited to, the following:

- Acute pain *related to* irritation or infection of the external eye
- Anxiety *related to* uncertainty of cause of disease and outcome of treatment
- Disturbed sensory perception (visual) *related to* diminished or absent vision

■ Planning

The overall goals are that the patient with inflammation or infection of the external eye will (1) avoid spread of infection, (2) maintain an acceptable level of comfort and functioning during the course of the specific ocular problem, (3) maintain or improve visual acuity, (4) comply with the prescribed therapy, and (5) promote appropriate health-seeking behaviors.

■ Nursing Implementation

Health Promotion. Careful asepsis and frequent, thorough hand washing are essential to prevent spreading organisms from one eye to the other, to other patients, to family members, and to the nurse. The nurse should dispose of any contaminated dressings in a proper waste container. The patient and family need information about avoiding sources of ocular irritation or infection and responding appropriately if an ocular problem occurs. The patient with infective disorders that may have a sexual mode of transmission or an associated sexually transmitted disease (STD) needs specific information about those disorders. The patient needs information about appropriate use and care of lenses and lens care products. The nurse should encourage the patient to follow the recommended regimens.

Acute Intervention. The nurse may apply warm or cool compresses if indicated for the patient's condition. Darkening the room and providing an appropriate analgesic are other comfort measures. If the patient's visual acuity is decreased, the nurse may need to modify the patient's environment or activities for safety.

The patient may require eyedrops as frequently as every hour. If the patient receives two or more different drops, the nurse should stagger the eyedrops to promote maximum absorption. For example, if two different eyedrops are ordered hourly, the nurse should administer one drop on the hour and one drop on the half hour unless otherwise prescribed. This staggered schedule promotes maximum absorption. The patient who needs frequent eyedrop administration may experience sleep deprivation.

Ambulatory and Home Care. The patient's primary need in the home environment is for information about required care and how to accomplish that care. The patient and family also need information about proper techniques for medication administration. If the patient's vision is compromised, the nurse should provide suggestions for alternative ways to accomplish necessary daily activities and self-care. The patient who wears contact lenses and develops infections should discard all opened or used lens care products and cosmetics to decrease the risk of reinfection from contaminated products (a common problem and a probable source of infection for many patients).

■ Evaluation

The overall expected outcomes are that the patient with inflammation or infection of the external eye will

- cooperate with the treatment plan
- experience relief of ocular discomfort
- effectively cope with functional changes if decreased visual acuity is present
- obtain specific information to prevent recurrent disease

DRY EYE DISORDERS

Keratoconjunctivitis sicca (dry eyes) is a common complaint, particularly of the elderly and individuals with certain systemic diseases such as scleroderma and systemic lupus erythematosus.[13] Patients with dry eyes complain of irritation or "sand in my eye" and that the sensation typically worsens through the day. This condition is caused by a decrease in the quality or quantity of the tear film, and treatment is directed at the underlying cause. Dry eyes caused by lacrimal duct dysfunction may respond to hot compresses and lid massage. With decreased tear secretion, the patient may use artificial tears or ointments. In severe cases, closure of the lacrimal puncta may be necessary. Patients with dry eyes associated with dry mouth may have Sjögren's syndrome (see Chapter 65).

STRABISMUS

Strabismus is a condition in which the patient cannot consistently focus two eyes simultaneously on the same object. One eye may deviate in *(esotropia),* out *(exotropia),* up *(hypertropia),* or down *(hypotropia).* Strabismus in the adult may be caused by thyroid disease, neuromuscular problems of the eye muscles, entrapment of the extraocular muscles in orbital floor fractures, retinal detachment repair, or cerebral lesions. In the adult, the primary complaint with strabismus is double vision.

CORNEAL DISORDERS

Corneal Scars and Opacities

The cornea is an optically transparent tissue that allows light rays to enter the eye and focus on the retina, thus producing a visual image. Any wound causes the cornea to become abnormally hydrated and decreases the normal transparency. A rigid contact lens can be effective in correcting the irregular astigmatism that results from corneal scars. In other situations the treatment for corneal scars or opacities is *penetrating keratoplasty* (corneal transplant). In penetrating keratoplasty the ophthalmic surgeon removes the full thickness of the patient's cornea and replaces it with a donor cornea or "button" that is sutured into place. Although corneal problems leading to blindness are uncommon, a corneal transplant can restore vision that otherwise would be lost. Approximately 40,000 corneal transplants are performed in the United States each year.

The time between the donor's death and the removal of the tissue should be as short as possible. Most surgeons prefer this interval to be 4 hours or less. The eye banks test donors for human immunodeficiency virus (HIV) and hepatitis B and C. The tissue is preserved in a special nutritive solution, and it can be kept for up to 5 days in the storage medium, if used for transplantation. Improved methods of tissue procurement and preservation, refined surgical techniques, postoperative topical corticosteroids, and careful follow-up have decreased graft rejection.

Keratoconus

Keratoconus is a noninflammatory, usually bilateral disease that is familial but has no exclusive inheritance pattern. It can be associated with Down syndrome, atopic dermatitis, Marfan syndrome, aniridia (congenital absence of the iris), and retinitis pigmentosa (hereditary disease characterized by bilateral primary degeneration of the retina beginning in childhood and progressing to blindness by middle age).

The anterior cornea thins and protrudes forward, taking on a cone shape. Keratoconus usually appears during adolescence and slowly progresses between ages 20 and 60 years. The only symptom is blurred vision caused by the variable astigmatism associated with the altered corneal shape. The astigmatism may be corrected with glasses or rigid contact lenses. INTACS inserts are two clear plastic lenses surgically inserted on the cornea perimeter to reduce astigmatism and myopia. INTACS are generally used to delay the need for a corneal transplant when contact lenses or glasses no longer help a patient achieve adequate vision. The cornea can perforate as central corneal thinning progresses. In advanced cases, a penetrating keratoplasty is indicated before perforation.

Intraocular Disorders

CATARACT

A **cataract** is an opacity within the lens. The patient may have a cataract in one or both eyes. If present in both eyes, one cataract may affect the patient's vision more than the other. Cataracts are the third leading cause of preventable blindness and the most common cause of self-declared visual disability in the United States. Approximately 50% of Americans between ages 65 and 74 years have some degree of cataract formation, and for those older than 75 years, the incidence increases to approximately 70%. Cataract removal is the most common surgical procedure for Americans older than 65 years. Congenital cataracts are relatively common, occurring in 1 of every 250 newborns (0.4%).[14]

Etiology and Pathophysiology

Although most cataracts are age related *(senile cataracts),* they can be associated with other factors. These include blunt or penetrating trauma, congenital factors such as maternal rubella, radiation or ultraviolet (UV) light exposure, certain drugs such as systemic corticosteroids or long-term topical corticosteroids, and ocular inflammation.[15] The patient with diabetes mellitus tends to develop cataracts at a younger age than does the patient without diabetes.

Cataract development is mediated by a number of factors. In senile cataract formation, it appears that altered metabolic processes within the lens cause an accumulation of water and alterations in the lens fiber structure. These changes affect lens transparency, causing vision changes.[15]

COMPLEMENTARY AND ALTERNATIVE THERAPIES

Bilberry

Clinical Uses

- Cataracts, retinopathy, peripheral vascular disease, varicose veins, diabetes mellitus*
- Night blindness†

Effects

Has been evaluated for its effect as an antioxidant, antiinflammatory, mucostimulant, and vasoprotective. At this time there is not sufficient evidence in support of or against the use of bilberry for most indications.

Nursing Implications

May lower blood glucose. Caution is advised when using drugs, herbs, or supplements that lower blood glucose. May lower BP. Caution is advised when using drugs, herbs, and supplements that lower BP. May increase risk of bleeding when taken with drugs, herbs, or supplements that increase the risk of bleeding. Unclear evidence related to safety during pregnancy or lactation. Should not be used in large doses over extended periods of time.

Ulbricht CE, Basch EM: *Natural standard herb and supplement reference: evidence-based clinical reviews,* St Louis, 2005, Mosby. Available at *www.naturalstandard.com.*
*Unclear scientific evidence for use.
†Fair scientific evidence against its use.

Clinical Manifestations

The patient with cataracts may complain of a decrease in vision, abnormal color perception, and glare. Glare is due to light scatter caused by the lens opacities, and it may be significantly worse at night when the pupil dilates. The visual decline is gradual, but the rate of cataract development varies from patient to patient. Secondary glaucoma can also occur if the enlarging lens causes increased intraocular pressure (IOP).

Diagnostic Studies

Diagnosis is based on decreased visual acuity or other complaints of visual dysfunction. The opacity is directly observable by ophthalmoscopic or slit lamp microscopic examination. As noted earlier, a totally opaque lens creates the appearance of a white pupil. Table 22-4 outlines other diagnostic studies that may be helpful in evaluating the visual impact of a cataract.

Collaborative Care

The presence of a cataract does not necessarily indicate a need for surgery. For many patients the diagnosis is made long before they actually decide to have surgery. Nonsurgical therapy may postpone the need for surgery. Collaborative care for cataracts is presented in Table 22-4.

Nonsurgical Therapy. Currently, there is no available treatment to "cure" cataracts other than surgical removal. If the cataract is not removed, the patient's vision will continue to deteriorate. However, palliative measures alone may help the patient. Often, changing the patient's eyewear prescription can improve the level of visual acuity, at least temporarily. Other visual aids, such as

TABLE 22-4 COLLABORATIVE CARE
Cataract

Diagnostic
History and physical examination
Visual acuity measurement
Ophthalmoscopy (direct and indirect)
Slit lamp microscopy
Glare testing, potential acuity testing in selected patients
Keratometry and A-scan ultrasound (if surgery is planned)
Other tests (e.g., visual field perimetry) may be indicated to differentiate visual loss of cataract from visual loss of other causes

Collaborative Therapy
Nonsurgical
Change prescription of glasses
Strong reading glasses or magnifiers
Increased lighting
Lifestyle adjustment
Reassurance

Acute Care: Surgical Therapy
Preoperative
Mydriatic, cycloplegic agents
Nonsteroidal antiinflammatory drugs
Topical antibiotics
Antianxiety medications
Surgery
Removal of lens
- Phacoemulsification
- Extracapsular extraction

Correction of surgical aphakia
Intraocular lens implantation (most frequent type of correction)
Contact lens
Postoperative
Topical antibiotic
Topical corticosteroid or other antiinflammatory agent
Mild analgesia if necessary
Eye shield and activity as preferred by patient's surgeon

strong reading glasses or magnifiers of some type, may help the patient with close vision. Increasing the amount of light to read or accomplish other near-vision tasks is another useful measure. The patient may be willing to adjust his or her lifestyle to accommodate for visual decline. For example, if glare makes it difficult to drive at night, a patient may elect to drive only during daylight hours or to have a family member drive at night. Sometimes informing and reassuring the patient about the disease process makes the patient comfortable about choosing nonsurgical measures, at least temporarily.

Surgical Therapy. When palliative measures no longer provide an acceptable level of visual function, the patient is an appropriate candidate for surgery. The patient's occupational needs and lifestyle changes are also factors affecting the decision to have surgery. In some instances, factors other than the patient's visual needs may influence the need for surgery. Lens-induced problems such as increased IOP may require lens removal. Opacities may prevent the ophthalmologist from obtaining a clear view of the retina in the patient with diabetic retinopathy or other sight-threatening pathology. In those cases the cataract may be removed to allow visualization of the retina and adequate management of the problem.

Preoperative Phase. The patient's preoperative preparation should include an appropriate history and physical examination. Because almost all patients have local anesthesia, many physicians and surgical facilities do not require an extensive preoperative physical assessment. However, most cataract patients are older adults and may have several medical problems that should be evaluated and controlled before surgery. The surgeon may order preoperative antibiotic eyedrops. The patient should not have food or fluids for approximately 6 to 8 hours before surgery. Almost all patients with cataracts are admitted to a surgical facility on an outpatient basis. The patient is normally admitted several hours before surgery to allow adequate time for necessary preoperative procedures.

The nurse will instill dilating drops and a nonsteroidal antiinflammatory eyedrop to reduce inflammation and to help maintain pupil dilation. One type of drug used for dilation is a *mydriatic,* an α-adrenergic agonist that produces pupillary dilation by contraction of the iris dilator muscle. Another type of drug is a *cycloplegic,* an anticholinergic agent that produces paralysis of accommodation (cycloplegia) by blocking the effect of acetylcholine on the ciliary body muscles. Cycloplegics produce pupillary dilation (mydriasis) by blocking the effect of acetylcholine on the iris sphincter muscle. Examples of mydriatics and cycloplegics are listed in Table 22-5, and nursing considerations are discussed on p. 428. The patient often receives preoperative antianxiety medication before the local anesthesia injection.

***Drug Alert** - Anticholinergic Agents*
Cycloplegics and Mydriatics
- *Instruct patient to wear dark glasses to minimize photophobia.*
- *Monitor for signs of systemic toxicity (e.g., tachycardia, central nervous system effects).*

Intraoperative Phase. Cataract extraction is an intraocular procedure. Rarely, intracapsular extraction is performed, in which the entire lens is removed with the capsule intact (this procedure may be necessary in instances of trauma). More commonly, extracapsular extraction is done, in which the anterior capsule is opened and the lens nucleus and cortex are removed, leaving the remaining capsular bag intact. In extracapsular extraction, the surgeon can remove the lens nucleus by "scooping" it out with a lens loop, or by *phacoemulsification,* in which the nucleus is fragmented by ultrasonic vibration and aspirated from inside the capsular bag[16] (Fig. 22-4). In either case, the remaining cortex is aspirated with an irrigation and aspiration instrument. The placement and type of incision vary among surgeons. Corneoscleral incisions require closure with sutures, whereas scleral tunnel incisions are self-sealing and require no closing suture. The incision required for phacoemulsification is considerably smaller than that required with intracapsular or standard extracapsular surgery.

Almost all patients now have an intraocular lens implanted at the time of cataract extraction surgery. Because most patients have an extracapsular procedure, the lens of choice is a posterior chamber lens that is implanted in the capsular bag behind the iris. At the end of the procedure, the patient receives injections of corticosteroid and antibiotic medications. Then an antibiotic and corticosteroid ointment is applied. Depending on the type of anesthesia, the patient's eye is covered with a patch and protective shield. If used, a patch is usually worn overnight and removed during the first postoperative visit.

TABLE 22-5 *DRUG THERAPY*
Topical Medications for Pupil Dilation

Examples	Onset	Duration	Comments
Mydriatics			
phenylephrine HCl acid (Neo-Synephrine, Mydfrin)	45-60 min	4-6 hr	May cause tachycardia and elevated blood pressure, especially in elderly patient; can cause a reflexive decrease in heart rate when blood pressure rises; use punctal occlusion to limit systemic absorption
Cycloplegics			
tropicamide (Mydriacyl, Tropicacyl)	20-40 min	4-6 hr	1% solution used in cycloplegic refraction; 0.5% solution used in fundus examination
cyclopentolate HCl acid (AK-Pentolate, Cyclogyl, Ocu-Pentolate, Pentolair)	30-75 min	6-24 hr	Has been associated with psychotic reactions and behavioral disturbances; used in cycloplegic refraction, fundus examination, and uveitis
homatropine hydrobromide (AK-Homatropine, Isopto Homatropine)	30-60 min	1-3 days	Used in cycloplegic refraction, uveitis; may be used for pupil dilation to allow patient to see around a central lens opacity
scopolamine (Isopto Hyoscine)	20-60 min	3-7 days	Used in cycloplegic refraction, uveitis
atropine (Atropisol, Atropair, Bufopto, Atropine, Isopto Atropine, Ocu-Tropine)	30-180 min	6-12 days	Used in cycloplegic refraction, uveitis

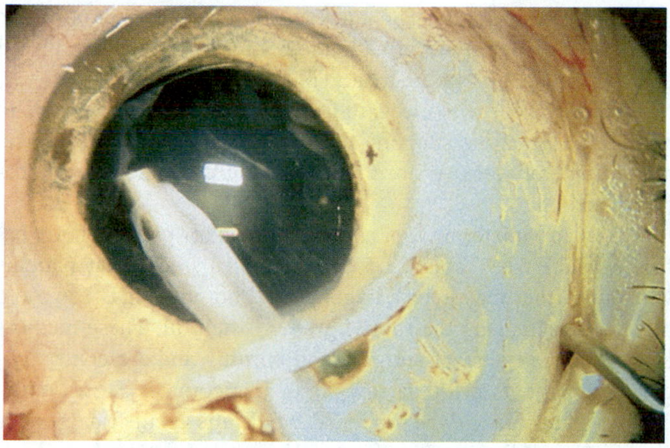

FIG. 22-4 Phacoemulsification of a cataractous lens through a self-sealing, scleral-tunnel incision. Note the circular opening in the anterior lens capsule.

Postoperative Phase. Unless complications occur, the patient is usually ready to go home as soon as the effects of sedative agents have worn off. Postoperative medications usually include antibiotic drops to prevent infection and corticosteroid drops to decrease the postoperative inflammatory response. There is some evidence that postoperative activity restrictions and nighttime eye shielding are unnecessary. However, many ophthalmologists still prefer that the patient avoid activities that increase the IOP, such as bending or stooping, coughing, or lifting. Ophthalmologists may also recommend using an eye shield over the operative eye at night for protection.

The ophthalmologist will usually see the patient four to five times at increasing intervals throughout the 6 to 8 weeks following surgery. During each postoperative examination the surgeon will measure the patient's visual acuity, check anterior chamber depth, assess corneal clarity, and measure IOP. A flat anterior chamber may cause adhesions of the iris and cornea. The cornea may become hazy or cloudy from intraoperative trauma to the endothelium. Even on the operative day the patient's uncorrected visual acuity in the operative eye may be good. However, it is not unusual or indicative of any problem if the patient's visual acuity is reduced immediately after surgery. The postoperative eyedrops will be gradually reduced in frequency and finally discontinued when the eye has healed. When the eye is fully recovered, the patient will receive a final prescription for glasses. Although the majority of the postoperative refractive error is corrected with the intraocular lens, the patient will still need corrective eyewear for near vision and for any residual refractive error.[17] This is prescribed when healing is complete, approximately 6 to 8 weeks postoperatively.

NURSING MANAGEMENT
CATARACTS

■ *Nursing Assessment*

The nurse should assess the patient's distance and near visual acuity. If the patient is going to have surgery, the nurse should especially note the visual acuity in the patient's unoperated eye. With this information the nurse can determine how visually compromised the patient may be while the operative eye is healing. In addition, the nurse should assess the psychosocial impact of the patient's visual disability and the patient's level of knowledge regarding the disease process and therapeutic options. Postoperatively it is important to assess the patient's level of comfort and ability to follow the postoperative regimen.

■ *Nursing Diagnoses*

Nursing diagnoses for the patient with a cataract include, but are not limited to, the following:

- Self-care deficits *related to* visual deficit
- Anxiety *related to* lack of knowledge about the surgical and postoperative experience

EVIDENCE-BASED PRACTICE

What Surgical Location Has Better Outcomes for Cataract Surgery?

Clinical Question

In adults with cataracts (P), does day surgery (I) or inpatient surgery (C) result in better visual acuity 4 months postoperatively, and which surgical location is safer and more cost-effective (O)?

Best Available Evidence

Systematic review of randomized controlled trials (RCTs)

Critical Appraisal and Synthesis of Evidence

- Meta-analysis of two RCTs ($n = 1284$). Only one study with 1034 subjects was methodologically sound, and evidence is based primarily on this study.
- No significant differences in visual acuity as measured by the Snellen chart at 4 months postoperatively.
- Significantly more early complications (e.g., increased intraocular pressure) were reported in the day-surgery patients with no relevance to vision acuity at 4 months.
- Costs for inpatient surgery were 20% higher than day surgery.
- Quality-of-life scores, patient satisfaction, and cataract symptom scores were similar for both patient groups.

Conclusions

- Day surgery is safe and subjectively preferred by patients.
- Day surgery provides the same visual outcome as inpatient surgery.

Implications for Nursing Practice

- Provide information that day-surgery outcomes for cataract surgery are comparable to inpatient surgery and less costly.
- Quality of life may be improved if day surgery allows the patient to begin home recuperation sooner.

Reference for Evidence

Fedorowicz Z, Lawrence D, Gutierrez P: Day care versus in-patient surgery for age-related cataract, Cochrane Eyes and Vision Group, *Cochrane Database of Systematic Reviews* 4, 2005.

PICO: P, Patient population of interest; *I*, intervention or area of interest; *C*, comparison of interest or comparison group; *O*, outcome(s) of interest (see p. 6).

▪ Planning

Preoperatively the overall goals are that the patient with a cataract will (1) make informed decisions regarding therapeutic options and (2) experience minimal anxiety. Postoperatively the overall goals are that the patient with a cataract will (1) understand and comply with postoperative therapy, (2) maintain an acceptable level of physical and emotional comfort, and (3) remain free of infection and other complications.

▪ Nursing Implementation

Health Promotion. There are no proven measures to prevent cataract development. However, it is probably wise (and certainly does no harm) to suggest that the patient wear sunglasses, avoid extraneous or unnecessary radiation, and maintain appropriate intake of antioxidant vitamins (e.g., vitamins C and E) and good nutrition. The nurse can also provide information about vision enhancement techniques for the patient who chooses not to have surgery.

Acute Intervention. Preoperatively the patient with cataracts needs accurate information about the disease process and the treatment options, especially because cataract surgery is considered an elective procedure. For the patient who wants or needs to see better without surgical interventions, cataract surgery may not seem elective. Although cataracts are not a life-threatening condition, the patient needs to know that without surgery there will be some degree of visual disability. The nurse should be available to give the patient and the family information to help them make an informed decision about appropriate treatment.

For the patient who elects to have surgery, the nurse is able to provide information, support, and reassurance about the surgical and postoperative experience that can reduce or alleviate the patient's anxiety.

When administering topical medications for pupil dilation before surgery (see Table 22-5 for examples), note that patients with dark irides may need a larger dose. Photophobia is common; therefore decreasing the room lighting is helpful. These medications produce transient stinging and burning and are contraindicated in patients with narrow-angle glaucoma because angle-closure glaucoma may be produced. Mydriatic agents can produce significant cardiovascular effects. When administering mydriatics, use punctal occlusion, especially in older and susceptible patients.

Table 22-6 outlines patient and family teaching following eye surgery. The nurse should inform patients with a patch that they will not have depth perception until their patch is removed (usually within 24 hours). This necessitates special considerations to avoid possible falls or other injuries. The patient with significant visual impairment in the unoperated eye requires more assistance while the operative eye is patched. Once the patch is removed (usually within 24 hours), most patients with visual impairment in the unoperated eye will have adequate vision for necessary activities because the implanted IOL provides immediate visual rehabilitation in the operated eye. Occasionally the patient may require 1 or 2 weeks for the visual acuity in the operated eye to reach an adequate level for most visual needs. This patient will also need some special assistance until the vision improves.

The postoperative cataract patient usually experiences little or no pain. There may be some scratchiness in the operative eye. Mild analgesics are usually sufficient to relieve any pain. If the pain is intense, the patient should notify the surgeon because this may indicate hemorrhage, infection, or increased IOP. The nurse should also

TABLE 22-6 PATIENT AND FAMILY TEACHING GUIDE: After Eye Surgery

Teach patient or patient and family the following:

1. Proper hygiene and eye care techniques to ensure that medications, dressings, and/or surgical wound are not contaminated during necessary eye care.
2. Signs and symptoms of infection and when and how to report those to allow early recognition and treatment of possible infection.
3. Importance of complying with postoperative restrictions on head positioning, bending, coughing, and Valsalva maneuver to optimize visual outcomes and prevent increased intraocular pressure.
4. How to instill eye medications using aseptic techniques and to comply with prescribed eye medication routine to prevent infection.
5. How to monitor pain and take prescribed medication for pain as directed and to report pain not relieved by prescribed medications.
6. Importance of continued follow-up as recommended to maximize potential visual outcomes.

Source: American Society of Ophthalmic Registered Nurses: *Core curriculum for ophthalmic nursing,* ed 2, Dubuque, Iowa, 2004, Kendall/Hunt Publishing.

instruct the patient to notify the surgeon if there is increased or purulent drainage, increased redness, or any decrease in visual acuity. A nursing care plan for the patient after eye surgery is available on the Evolve website at *http://evolve.elsevier.com/Lewis/medsurg*.

Ambulatory and Home Care. For the patient with cataracts who has not had surgery, the nurse can suggest ways in which the patient may modify activities or lifestyle to accommodate the visual deficit caused by the cataract. The nurse should also provide the patient with accurate information about appropriate long-term eye care.

Patients with cataracts who have surgery remain in the surgical facility for only a few hours. The patient and the family are responsible for almost all postoperative care. It is essential that the nurse give them written and verbal instructions before discharge. These teachings should include information about postoperative eye care, activity restrictions, medications, follow-up visit schedule, and signs and symptoms of possible complications. The patient's family should be included in the instruction because some patients may have difficulty with self-care activities, especially if the vision in the unoperated eye is poor. The nurse should provide an opportunity for the patient and family to perform return demonstrations of any necessary self-care activities.

Most patients experience little visual impairment following surgery. IOL implants provide immediate visual rehabilitation, and many patients achieve a usable level of visual acuity within a few days following surgery. Also, the patient's eye may remain patched for only 24 hours, and many patients have good vision in their unoperated eye. A few patients may experience significant visual impairment postoperatively. These include patients who do not have an IOL implanted at the time of surgery, those who require several weeks to achieve a usable level of visual acuity following surgery, or those with poor vision in their unoperated eye. For those patients the time between surgery and receiving aphakic glasses or contacts can be a period of significant visual disability. The nurse can suggest ways in which the patient and the family can modify activities and the environment to maintain an adequate level of safe functioning. Suggestions may include getting assistance with steps, removing area rugs and other potential obstacles, preparing meals for freezing before surgery, or obtaining audio books for diversion until visual acuity improves.

▪ *Evaluation*

The overall expected outcomes are that the patient following cataract surgery will

- have improved vision
- be better able to take care of self
- have minimal to no pain
- be optimistic about expected outcomes

GERONTOLOGIC CONSIDERATIONS
CATARACTS

Most patients with cataracts are elderly. When the older patient is visually impaired, even temporarily, the patient may experience a loss of independence, lack of control over her or his life, and a significant change in self-perception. Societal devaluation of the older individual complicates these experiences. The older patient often needs emotional support and encouragement, as well as specific suggestions to allow a maximum level of independent function. The nurse can assure the older patient that cataract surgery can be accomplished safely and comfortably with minimal sedation. The use of outpatient surgery for cataract surgery is particularly beneficial for the older patient who may become confused or disoriented during hospitalization.

RETINOPATHY

Retinopathy is a process of microvascular damage to the retina. It can develop slowly or rapidly and lead to blurred vision and progressive vision loss. Retinopathy is most often associated in adults with diabetes mellitus and hypertension.

Diabetic retinopathy is the leading cause of visual disability and blindness in persons with long-standing uncontrolled diabetes. (Diabetes is discussed in Chapter 49.) *Nonproliferative retinopathy* is the most common form of diabetic retinopathy and is characterized by capillary microaneuryms, retinal swelling, and hard exudates. Macular edema represents a worsening of the retinopathy as plasma leaks from macular blood vessels. This can lead to a severe loss in central vision.[18] As the disease advances, *proliferative retinopathy* may occur where new blood vessels grow. However, these blood vessels are abnormal, fragile, and predisposed to leak, thus causing severe vision loss. Fluorescein angiography is used to detect diabetic macular edema, which may be treated with laser photocoagulation.

Hypertensive retinopathy is caused by high blood pressure creating blockages in retinal blood vessels. (Hypertension is discussed in Chapter 33.) These changes may not initially affect a person's vision. On a routine eye examination, retinal hemorrhages and macula swelling can be noted. Sustained, severe hypertension can cause sudden visual loss from swelling of the optic disc and nerve *(papilledema)*. Treatment, which may be an emergency, focuses on lowering the blood pressure. Signs of retinal damage may persist for weeks to months after the pressure has been reduced.[19]

RETINAL DETACHMENT

A **retinal detachment** is a separation of the sensory retina and the underlying pigment epithelium, with fluid accumulation between the two layers. The incidence of nontraumatic retinal detachment is approximately 1 out of every 10,000 individuals each year. This number increases when aphakic individuals are included because retinal detachment is more likely to occur in aphakic patients. If traumatic retinal detachments are included, the incidence is only slightly increased. In the patient with no other risk factors who has had a retinal detachment in one eye, the risk of detachment in the second eye is 2% to 25%. Almost all patients with an untreated, symptomatic retinal detachment become blind in the involved eye.

Etiology and Pathophysiology

There are many causes of retinal detachment. The most common cause is a retinal break. *Retinal breaks* are an interruption in the full thickness of the retinal tissue, and they can be classified as tears or holes. *Retinal holes* are atrophic retinal breaks that occur spontaneously. *Retinal tears* can occur as the vitreous humor shrinks during aging and pulls on the retina. The retina tears when the traction force exceeds the strength of the retina. Once there is a break in the retina, liquid vitreous can enter the subretinal space between the sensory layer and the retinal pigment epithelium layer, causing a *rhegmatogenous* retinal detachment.[20] Less frequently, retinal detachment can occur when abnormal membranes mechanically pull on the retina. These are called *tractional* detachments. A third type of retinal detachment is the *secondary* or *exudative* detachment that

TABLE 22-7 Risk Factors for Retinal Detachment

- Increasing age
- Severe myopia
- Eye trauma
- Retinopathy (diabetic)
- Cataract or glaucoma surgery
- Family or personal history

Source: Johns Hopkins Medical Letter: *Health After 50,* 17:8, 2005. Available at *www.hopkinsafter50.com.*

occurs with conditions that allow fluid to accumulate in the subretinal space (e.g., choroidal tumors, intraocular inflammation). Risk factors for retinal detachment are listed in Table 22-7.

Clinical Manifestations

Patients with a detaching retina describe symptoms that include *photopsia* (light flashes), floaters, and a "cobweb," "hairnet," or ring in the field of vision. Once the retina has detached, the patient describes a painless loss of peripheral or central vision, "like a curtain" coming across the field of vision. The area of visual loss corresponds to the area of detachment. If the detachment is in the superior nasal retina, the visual field loss will be in the inferior temporal area. If the detachment is small or develops slowly in the periphery, the patient may not be aware of a visual problem.

Diagnostic Studies

Visual acuity measurements should be the first diagnostic procedure with any complaint of vision loss (Table 22-8). The retinal detachment can be directly visualized using direct and indirect ophthalmoscopy or slit lamp microscopy in conjunction with a special lens to view the far periphery of the retina. Ultrasound may be useful to identify a retinal detachment if the retina cannot be directly visualized (e.g., when the cornea, lens, or vitreous is hazy or opaque).

TABLE 22-8 COLLABORATIVE CARE Retinal Detachment

Diagnostic
History and physical examination
Visual acuity measurement
Ophthalmoscopy (direct and indirect)
Slit lamp microscopy
Ultrasound if cornea, lens, or vitreous is hazy or opaque

Collaborative Therapy
Preoperative
Mydriatic, cycloplegic
Photocoagulation of retinal break that has not progressed to detachment

Surgery to Seal Retinal Breaks and Relieve Traction on Retina
Laser photocoagulation
Cryoretinopexy
Scleral buckling procedure
Draining of subretinal fluid
Vitrectomy
Intravitreal bubble

Postoperative
Topical antibiotic
Topical corticosteroid
Analgesia
Mydriatics
Positioning and activity as preferred by patient's surgeon

Collaborative Care

The ophthalmologist will carefully evaluate the patient with retinal breaks to determine if prophylactic laser photocoagulation or cryopexy is necessary to avoid possible retinal detachment. Some retinal breaks are not likely to progress to detachment, and the ophthalmologist will simply watch the patient, giving precise information about the warning signs and symptoms of impending detachment and instructing the patient to seek immediate evaluation if any of those signs or symptoms are recognized. The general ophthalmologist will usually refer the patient with retinal detachments to a retinal specialist. Treatment of retinal detachment has two objectives. The first is to seal any retinal breaks, and the second is to relieve inward traction on the retina. Several techniques are used to accomplish these objectives.

Surgical Therapy

Laser Photocoagulation and Cryopexy. These techniques seal retinal breaks by creating an inflammatory reaction that causes a chorioretinal adhesion or scar. *Laser photocoagulation* involves using an intense, precisely focused light beam, such as the argon laser, to create an inflammatory reaction. The light is directed at the area of the retinal break. This produces a scar that seals the edges of the hole or tear, and prevents fluid from collecting in the subretinal space and causing a detachment. The retinal specialist may use photocoagulation alone if there is a single small tear with little or no detachment in the periphery and minimal subretinal fluid. For retinal breaks accompanied by significant detachment, the retinal specialist may use photocoagulation intraoperatively in conjunction with scleral buckling. Tears or holes without accompanying retinal detachment may be treated prophylactically with laser photocoagulation if the retinal specialist judges them to be at high risk of progressing to retinal detachment.[21] When used alone, laser therapy is an outpatient procedure that usually requires only topical anesthesia, and the patient usually experiences minimal adverse symptoms during or following the procedure.

An alternative method used to seal retinal breaks is *cryopexy.* This procedure involves using extreme cold to create the inflammatory reaction that produces the sealing scar. The ophthalmologist applies the cryoprobe instrument to the external globe in the area over the tear. This is usually done on an outpatient basis and under local anesthesia. As with photocoagulation, cryotherapy may be used alone or during scleral buckling surgery. The patient may experience significant discomfort and eye pain following cryopexy. The nurse should encourage the patient to take the prescribed pain medication following the procedure.

Scleral Buckling. *Scleral buckling* is an extraocular surgical procedure that involves indenting the globe so that the pigment epithelium, choroid, and sclera move toward the detached retina. This not only helps seal retinal breaks, but also helps relieve inward traction on the retina. The retinal surgeon sutures a silicone implant against the sclera, causing the sclera to buckle inward. The surgeon may place an encircling band over the implant if there are multiple retinal breaks, if the surgeon cannot locate suspected breaks, or if there is widespread inward traction on the retina (Fig. 22-5). If present, subretinal fluid may be drained by inserting a small-gauge needle to facilitate contact between the retina and the buckled sclera. Scleral buckling is usually accomplished under local anesthesia, and the patient may be discharged on the first postoperative day. Scleral buckling surgery is often performed as an outpatient procedure.

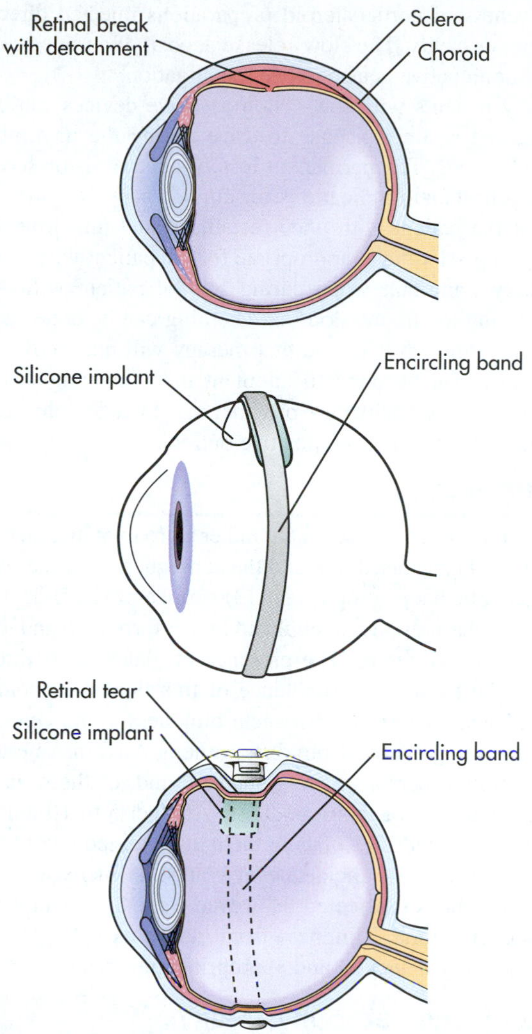

FIG. 22-5 Retinal break with detachment: surgical repair by scleral buckling technique.

Intraocular Procedures. In addition to the extraocular procedures described, retinal surgeons may use one or more intraocular procedures in treating some retinal detachments. *Pneumatic retinopexy* is the intravitreal injection of a gas to form a temporary bubble in the vitreous that closes retinal breaks and provides apposition of the separated retinal layers. Because the intravitreal bubble is temporary, this technique is combined with laser photocoagulation or cryotherapy. The patient with an intravitreal bubble must position the head so that the bubble is in contact with the retinal break. It may be necessary for the patient to maintain this position as much as possible for up to several weeks.

Vitrectomy (surgical removal of the vitreous) may be used to relieve traction on the retina, especially when the traction results from proliferative diabetic retinopathy. Vitrectomy may be combined with scleral buckling to provide a dual effect in relieving traction. In *proliferative vitreoretinopathy* (PVR), membranes develop in the vitreous cavity and on the retinal surface, exerting traction that causes folds in the retina. Vitrectomy may be combined with membrane peeling to relieve traction in those cases.

Postoperative Considerations in Scleral Buckling and Intraocular Procedures. Reattachment is successful in 90% of retinal detachments. Visual prognosis varies, depending on the extent, length, and area of detachment. Postoperatively, the patient may be on bed rest and may require special positioning to maintain proper position of an intravitreal bubble. The patient may need multiple topical medications, including antibiotics, antiinflammatory agents, or dilating agents. Activity recommendations vary according to physician preference, extent of the detachment, and the particular repair procedure.

The nurse should teach the patient at risk for retinal detachment the signs and symptoms of retinal detachment. The nurse can also promote use of proper protective eyewear to help avoid retinal detachments related to trauma.

In most cases retinal detachment is an urgent situation, and the patient is confronted suddenly with the need for surgery. The patient needs emotional support, especially during the immediate preoperative period when preparations for surgery can lead to additional anxiety. When the patient experiences postoperative pain, the nurse should administer prescribed pain medications and teach the patient to take the medication as necessary after being discharged. The patient may go home within a few hours of surgery or may remain in the hospital for several days, depending on the surgeon and the type of repair.

Discharge planning and teaching is important, and the nurse should begin this process as early as possible because the patient does not remain hospitalized long. Patient and family teaching following eye surgery is discussed in Table 22-6. The patient is at risk for retinal detachment in the other eye. Therefore the nurse should teach the patient the signs and symptoms of retinal detachment.

The level of activity restriction following retinal detachment surgeries varies greatly. The nurse should verify the prescribed level of activity with each patient's surgeon and help the patient plan for any necessary assistance related to activity restrictions.

AGE-RELATED MACULAR DEGENERATION

Age-related macular degeneration (AMD) is the most common cause of irreversible central vision loss in persons over age 60. AMD is divided into two forms: dry (nonexudative) and wet (exudative). People with dry AMD, which is the more common form (90% of all cases), may often notice close vision tasks becoming more difficult. In this form the macular cells start to atrophy, leading to a slowly progressive and painless vision loss.

Wet AMD is the more severe form. Untreated, the majority of patients with eyes affected with wet AMD become functionally blind. Wet AMD accounts for 90% of the cases of AMD-related blindness. Wet AMD has a more rapid onset and is noted by the development of abnormal blood vessels in or near the macula. Only 10% to 15% of patients with dry AMD go on to develop the wet form.

Etiology and Pathophysiology

AMD is related to retinal aging. Genetic factors also appear to play a major role as family history is a major risk factor for AMD. A gene responsible for some cases of AMD has been recently identified. Long-term exposure to UV light, hyperopia, cigarette smoking, and light-colored eyes may be additional risk factors.[22] Nutritional factors may play a role in the progression of AMD. A dietary supplement of vitamin C, vitamin E, beta-carotene, and zinc was shown in the Age-Related Eye Disease Study (AREDS) to lower the development of advancing AMD but appeared to have no effect on persons with minimal AMD or those with no evidence of AMD.[23] Additional studies *(www.nei.hih.gov/amd)* indicate that eating lots of dark green, leafy vegetables containing lutein (i.e., kale and spinach) may help reduce the risk of AMD.

The dry form of AMD starts with the abnormal accumulation of yellowish colored extracellular deposits called *drusen* in the retinal pigment epithelium. The atrophy and degeneration of macular cells then results. Wet AMD is characterized by the growth of new blood vessels from their normal location in the choroids to an abnormal location in the retinal epithelium. As the new blood vessels leak, scar tissue gradually forms. Acute vision loss may occur in some cases with bleeding from subretinal neovascular membranes.

Clinical Manifestations

The patient may complain of blurred and darkened vision, the presence of *scotomas* (blind spots in the visual field), and *metamorphopsia* (distortion of vision). Many people may not notice unilateral early changes in their vision if the other eye is not affected.

Diagnostic Studies

In addition to visual acuity measurement, the primary diagnostic procedure is ophthalmoscopy. The examiner looks for drusen and other fundus changes associated with AMD. The Amsler grid test may help define the involved area, and it provides a baseline for future comparison. Fundus photography and IV angiography with fluorescein and/or indocyanine green dyes may be helpful in further defining the extent and type of AMD.

Collaborative Care

Until recently, laser macular photocoagulation of the abnormal blood vessels when visual acuity is already compromised extensively has been the therapy of choice. The destruction of blood vessels prevents additional central vision loss. However, the laser beam also destroys the retinal pigment epithelium and photoreceptor cells where it is applied, leaving a blind spot due to the scarred area in the retina.

A new therapy available for patients with wet AMD called *photodynamic therapy* (PDT) uses verteporfin (Visudyne) intravenously and a "cold" laser to excite the dye. This procedure destroys the abnormal blood vessels without permanent damage to the retinal pigment epithelium and photoreceptor cells. Current criteria for its use are very specific, and only about 10% of patients with wet AMD are eligible at this time. Verteporfin is a photosensitizing drug that becomes active when exposed to the low-level laser light wave. Until the drug is completely excreted by the body, it can be activated by exposure to sunlight or other high-intensity light such as halogen. Therefore patients are cautioned to avoid direct exposure to sunlight and other intense forms of light for 5 days after treatment. After receiving therapy, patients must be completely covered because any exposure to skin by sunlight could activate the drug in that area, resulting in a thermal burn.

Pegaptanib (Macugen), an intravitreous injectable drug, is a selective inhibitor of endothelial growth factor, which helps to slow vision loss in wet AMD. Side effects of the drug include blurred vision, eye irritation, eye pain, and photosensitivity. Rare side effects can include retinal detachment, infection, and traumatic cataract.

Ranibizumab (Lucentis), a new type of biologic therapy, can assist in preserving the vision of patients with wet AMD. Ranibizumab is an injectable monthly treatment that blocks new blood vessel growth and leakiness. Side effects include conjunctival hemorrhage, eye pain and inflammation, and floaters.

People at risk for developing advanced AMD (in consultation with their health care provider) should consider supplements of vitamins and minerals.[23] Current clinical trials aimed at reducing the progression and slowing vision loss of AMD are examining the effectiveness of corticosteroid preparations injected directly into the vitreous cavity. The slow-release deposit of corticosteroids under the conjunctiva is also under investigation.

Many patients with low-vision assistive devices can continue reading and retain a license to drive during the daytime and at lowered speeds. The permanent loss of central vision has significant psychosocial implications for nursing care. Nursing management of the patient with uncorrectable visual impairment is discussed on p. 419 and is appropriate for the patient with AMD. It is especially important when caring for the patient with AMD to avoid giving the impression that "nothing can be done" about the problem. Although it is true that therapy will not recover lost vision, much can be done to augment the remaining vision. Just knowing that the health care provider has not abandoned them can give these patients a more positive outlook.

GLAUCOMA

Glaucoma is not one disease but rather a group of disorders characterized by (1) increased IOP and the consequences of elevated pressure, (2) optic nerve atrophy, and (3) peripheral visual field loss.

Intraocular pressure is regulated by the formation and reabsorption of aqueous humor. The presence of glaucoma is directly related to the balance or imbalance of this fluid. Glaucoma is the second leading cause of permanent blindness in the United States and the leading cause of blindness among African Americans. At least 2 million persons have glaucoma, and, of these, more than 50% are unaware of their condition. Another 5 to 10 million persons have elevated IOP, placing them at increased risk of developing the disease. The incidence of glaucoma increases with age. One in 50 whites is affected. However, 1 in 10 African Americans develops glaucoma. Blindness from glaucoma is largely preventable with early detection and appropriate treatment.

Etiology and Pathophysiology

The etiology of glaucoma is related to the consequences of elevated IOP. A proper balance between the rate of aqueous production (referred to as inflow) and the rate of aqueous reabsorption (referred to as outflow) is essential to maintain the IOP within normal limits. When the rate of inflow is greater than the rate of outflow, IOP can rise above the normal limits. If IOP remains elevated, permanent vision loss may occur.

Primary open-angle glaucoma (POAG) represents 90% of the cases of primary glaucoma. In POAG, the outflow of aqueous humor is decreased in the trabecular meshwork. In essence, the drainage channels become clogged, like a clogged kitchen sink.

Primary angle-closure glaucoma (PACG) represents approximately 10% of the total number of glaucoma cases in the United States. As the name implies, the mechanism reducing the outflow of aqueous is angle closure. Usually, this is caused from the lens bulging forward as a result of an age-related process. Angle closure may also occur as a result of pupil dilation in the patient with anatomically narrow angles. Dilation causes peripheral iris bulging with the same outcome of covering the trabecular meshwork and blocking the outflow channels. An acute attack may be precipitated by situations during which the pupil remains in a partially dilated state long enough to cause an acute and significant rise in the IOP. This may occur because of drug-induced mydriasis, emotional excitement, or darkness. Drug-induced mydriasis may occur not only from topical ophthalmic preparations but also from many systemic medications (both prescription drugs and over-the-counter [OTC] drugs). The nurse should check drug records and documentation before administering medications to the patient with angle-closure glaucoma and should instruct the patient not to take any mydriatic-producing medications.

In *secondary glaucoma,* increased IOP results from other ocular or systemic conditions that may block the outflow channels in some way. Secondary glaucoma may be associated with inflammatory processes that block the outflow channels such as trauma and ocular neoplasms.

Clinical Manifestations

POAG develops slowly and without symptoms. The patient with POAG reports no symptoms of pain or pressure. The patient usually does not notice the gradual visual field loss until peripheral vision has been severely compromised. Eventually the patient with untreated glaucoma has "tunnel vision" in which only a small center field can be seen, and all peripheral vision is absent.

Acute angle-closure glaucoma causes definite symptoms, including sudden, excruciating pain in or around the eye. This is often accompanied by nausea and vomiting. Visual symptoms include seeing colored halos around lights, blurred vision, and ocular redness. The acute rise in IOP may also cause corneal edema, giving the cornea a frosted appearance.

Manifestations of subacute or chronic angle-closure glaucoma appear more gradually. The patient who has had a previous, unrecognized episode of subacute angle-closure glaucoma may report a history of blurred vision, seeing colored halos around lights, ocular redness, or eye or brow pain.

Diagnostic Studies

IOP is usually elevated in glaucoma. Normal IOP is 10 to 21 mm Hg. In the patient with elevated pressures, the ophthalmologist will usually repeat the measurements over a period of time to verify the elevation. In open-angle glaucoma, IOP is usually between 22 and 32 mm Hg. In acute angle-closure glaucoma, IOP may be 50 mm Hg or higher.

In open-angle glaucoma, slit lamp microscopy reveals a normal angle. In angle-closure glaucoma, the examiner may note a markedly narrow or flat anterior chamber angle, an edematous cornea, a fixed and moderately dilated pupil, and ciliary injection. Gonioscopy allows better visualization of the anterior chamber angle.

Measures of peripheral and central vision provide other diagnostic information. Whereas central acuity may remain 20/20 even in the presence of severe peripheral visual field loss, visual field perimetry may reveal subtle changes in the peripheral retina early in the disease process, long before actual scotomas develop. When visual field defects begin to appear, the initial scotoma is a small, football-shaped defect that gradually progresses to a nasal and superior field defect in chronic open-angle glaucoma. In acute angle-closure glaucoma, central visual acuity will be reduced if the patient has corneal edema, and the visual fields may be markedly decreased.

As glaucoma progresses, *optic disc cupping* occurs. This is visible with direct or indirect ophthalmoscopy (Fig. 22-6). The optic disc becomes wider, deeper, and paler (light gray or white). Optic disc cupping may be one of the first signs of chronic open-angle glaucoma. Optic disc photographs are useful for comparison over time to demonstrate an increase in the cup-to-disc ratio and progressive blanching.

Collaborative Care

The primary focus of glaucoma therapy is to keep the IOP low enough to prevent the patient from developing optic nerve damage. This damage is manifested by increasing visual field loss and progressive optic disc cupping. Specific therapies vary with the type of glaucoma. The diagnostic and collaborative care of glaucoma is summarized in Table 22-9.

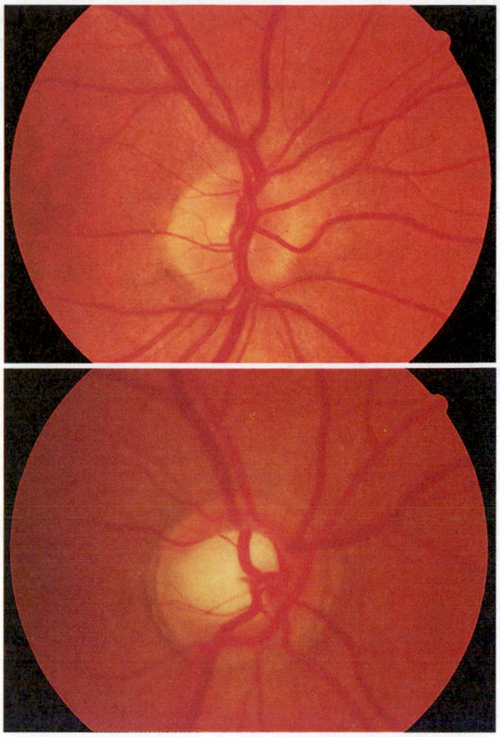

FIG. 22-6 **A,** In the normal eye, the optic cup is pink with little cupping. **B,** In the glaucomatous eye, the optic disc is bleached and optic cupping is present. (Note the appearance of the retinal vessels, which travel over the edge of the optic cup and appear to dip into it.)

Chronic Open-Angle Glaucoma. Initial treatment in chronic open-angle glaucoma is with drugs (Table 22-10). With all drug therapy, the patient must understand that continued treatment and supervision are necessary because the drugs control, but do not cure, the disease.

Argon laser trabeculoplasty (ALT) is a therapeutic option to lower IOP when medications are not successful or when the patient either cannot or will not use the drug therapy as recommended. ALT is an outpatient procedure that requires only topical anesthetic. The topical drops anesthetize the cornea before the gonioscopy lens is applied, allowing visualization of the treatment area. Approximately 50 laser "spots" are evenly spaced around the superior or inferior 180 degrees of the trabecular meshwork. The laser stimulates scarring and contraction of the trabecular meshwork, opening the outflow channels. ALT reduces IOP approximately 75% of the time. A second 180-degree area may be treated in a subsequent procedure. The patient uses topical corticosteroids for approximately 3 to 5 days following the procedure. The most common complication is an acute postoperative IOP rise. Because the decrease in pressure is gradual, the patient continues taking the preoperative glaucoma medication. The ophthalmologist examines the patient 1 week after the procedure and again 4 to 6 weeks following surgery.

A *filtering procedure,* such as trabeculectomy, may be indicated if medical management and laser therapy are not successful. In this procedure the surgeon makes conjunctival and scleral flaps, removes part of the iris and trabecular meshwork, and closes the scleral flap loosely. Aqueous humor may now "percolate" out through the area of missing iris where it is trapped under the repaired conjunctiva and absorbed into the systemic circulation. The

TABLE 22-9 COLLABORATIVE CARE Glaucoma

Diagnostic
History and physical examination
Visual acuity measurement
Tonometry
Ophthalmoscopy (direct and indirect)
Slit lamp microscopy
Gonioscopy
Visual field perimetry
Fundus photography
Collaborative Therapy
Ambulatory/Home Care for Open-Angle Glaucoma
Drug therapy
β-adrenergic blockers
α-adrenergic agonists
Cholinergic agents (miotics)
Carbonic anhydrase inhibitors
Surgical therapy
Argon laser trabeculoplasty (ALT)
Trabeculectomy with or without filtering implant
Acute Care Angle-Closure Glaucoma
Topical cholinergic agent
Hyperosmotic agent
Laser peripheral iridotomy
Surgical iridectomy

success rate of this filtering surgery is 75% to 85%. The subconjunctival application of mitomycin (Mutamycin) or 5-fluorouracil (5-FU) may increase the success rate by preventing scarring and subsequent closure of the opening created during surgery.

An implant is another surgical option, usually reserved for the patient in whom filtration surgery has failed. It involves surgical placement of a small tube and reservoir to shunt aqueous humor from the anterior chamber to the implanted reservoir.

Acute Angle-Closure Glaucoma. Acute angle-closure glaucoma is an ocular emergency that requires immediate intervention. Miotics and oral or IV hyperosmotic agents are usually successful in immediately lowering the IOP (see Table 22-9). A laser peripheral iridotomy or surgical iridectomy is necessary for long-term treatment and prevention of subsequent episodes. These procedures allow the aqueous humor to flow through a newly created opening in the iris and into normal outflow channels. One of these procedures may also be performed on the other eye as a precaution because many patients often experience an acute attack in the other eye.

***Drug Alert** - Miotics*

- *Warn patients about decreased visual acuity, especially in dim light.*

Secondary Glaucoma. Secondary glaucoma is managed by treating the underlying problem and by using antiglaucoma drugs. If treatment fails, glaucoma can progress to absolute glaucoma, resulting in a hard, sightless, and usually painful eye requiring enucleation (surgical removal of the eye).

TABLE 22-10 DRUG THERAPY Acute and Chronic Glaucoma

Drug	Action	Side Effects	Nursing Considerations
β-Adrenergic Blockers			
betaxolol (Betoptic)	β_1 cardioselective blocker; probably decreases aqueous humor production	Transient discomfort; systemic reactions rarely reported but include bradycardia, heart block, pulmonary distress, headache, depression	Topical drugs; minimal effect on pulmonary and cardiovascular parameters; contraindicated in patient with bradycardia, cardiogenic shock, or overt cardiac failure; systemic absorption can have additive effect with systemic β_1-blocking agents
carteolol (Ocupress) levobunolol (Betagan) metipranolol (OptiPranolol) timolol maleate (Timoptic, Istalol)	β_1 and β_2 noncardioselective blockers; probably decrease aqueous humor production	Transient ocular discomfort, blurred vision, photophobia, blepharoconjunctivitis, bradycardia, decreased BP, bronchospasm, headache, depression	Topical drops; same as betaxolol; these noncardioselective β_2-blockers are also contraindicated in patients with asthma or severe COPD
α-Adrenergic Agonists			
dipivefrin (Propine)	α- and β-adrenergic agonist; converted to epinephrine inside the eye; decreases aqueous humor production, enhances outflow facility	Ocular discomfort and redness, tachycardia, hypertension	Topical drops; contraindicated in patient with narrow-angle glaucoma; teach punctal occlusion to patient at risk of systemic reactions
epinephrine (Epifrin, Eppy, Gaucon, Epitrate, Epinal, Eppy/N)	Same as dipivefrin	Same as dipivefrin, but can be more pronounced	Topical drops; same as dipivefrin
apraclonidine (Lopidine) brimonidine (Alphagan)	α-adrenergic agonists; probably decrease aqueous humor production	Ocular redness; irregular heart rate	Topical drops; used to control or prevent acute postlaser IOP rise (used before and immediately after ALT and iridotomy, Nd:YAG laser capsulotomy); teach patient at risk of systemic reactions to occlude puncta

ALT, Argon laser trabeculoplasty; *BP,* blood pressure; *COPD,* chronic obstructive pulmonary disease; *GI,* gastrointestinal; *HP,* heart failure; *IOP,* intraocular pressure; *IV,* intravenous.

NURSING MANAGEMENT
GLAUCOMA

Nursing Assessment

Because glaucoma is a chronic condition requiring long-term management, the nurse must carefully assess the patient's ability to understand and comply with the rationale and regimen of the prescribed therapy. In addition, the nurse should assess the patient's psychologic reaction to the diagnosis of a potentially sight-threatening chronic disorder. The nurse must include the patient's family in the assessment process because the chronic nature of this disorder affects the family in many ways. Some families may become the primary providers of necessary care, such as eyedrop administration, if the patient is unwilling or unable to accomplish these self-care activities. The nurse also assesses visual acuity, visual fields, IOP, and fundus changes when appropriate.

TABLE 22-10 DRUG THERAPY
Acute and Chronic Glaucoma—cont'd

Drug	Action	Side Effects	Nursing Considerations
α-Adrenergic Agonists—cont'd			
latanoprost (Xalatan)	Prostaglandin F analog	Increased brown iris pigmentation, ocular discomfort and redness, dryness, itching, and foreign body sensation	Topical drops; teach patient to not exceed 1 drop per evening; have patient remove contact lens 15 min before instilling
Cholinergic Agents (Miotics)			
carbachol (Isopto Carbachol)	Parasympathomimetic; stimulates iris sphincter contraction, causing miosis and opening of trabecular meshwork, facilitating aqueous outflow; also partially inhibits cholinesterase	Transient ocular discomfort, headache, browache, blurred vision, decreased dark adaptation, syncope, salivation, dysrhythmias, vomiting, diarrhea, hypotension, retinal detachment in susceptible individual (rare)	Topical drops; caution patient about decreased visual acuity caused by miosis, particularly in dim light
pilocarpine (Akarpine; Isopto Carpine, Pilocar, Pilopine, Piloptic, Pilostat)	Parasympathomimetic; stimulates iris sphincter contraction, causing miosis and opening of trabecular meshwork, facilitating aqueous humor outflow	Same as carbachol	Topical drops; same as carbachol
Carbonic Anhydrase Inhibitors			
Systemic			
acetazolamide (Diamox) dichlorphenamide (Daranide) methazolamide (Neptazane)	Decreases aqueous humor production	Paresthesias, especially "tingling" in extremities; hearing dysfunction or tinnitus; loss of appetite; taste alteration; GI disturbances; drowsiness; confusion	Oral nonbacteriostatic sulfonamides; anaphylaxis and other sulfa-type allergic reactions may occur in patient allergic to sulfa; diuretic effect can lower electrolyte levels; ask patient about aspirin use; drug should not be given to patient on high-dose aspirin therapy
Topical			
brinzolamide (Azopt) dorzolamide (Trusopt)		Transient stinging, blurred vision, redness	Same as above
Combination Therapy			
timolol maleate and dorzolamide (Cosopt)	Combination of two drugs	See individual drugs for side effects	
Hyperosmolar Agents			
glycerin liquid (Ophthalgan, Osmoglyn Oral)	Increases extracellular osmolarity so intracellular water moves to the extracellular and vascular spaces, reducing IOP	Nausea, vomiting, headache, confusion, disorientation, dysrhythmia, severe dehydration	Oral liquid; used in acute glaucoma attacks or preoperatively when decreased IOP is desired; assess patient for susceptibility to pulmonary edema and HF before administering hyperosmolar agents
isosorbide solution (Ismotic)	Same as glycerin	Nausea, vomiting, headache, confusion, disorientation, syncope, lethargy, irritability	Oral liquid; same as glycerin
mannitol solution (Osmitrol)	Same as glycerin	Nausea, vomiting, diarrhea, thrombophlebitis, hypertension, hypotension, tachycardia	IV solution; same as glycerin

Nursing Diagnoses

Nursing diagnoses for the patient with glaucoma include, but are not limited to, the following:

- Risk for injury *related to* visual acuity deficits
- Self-care deficits *related to* visual acuity deficits
- Acute pain *related to* pathophysiologic process and surgical correction
- Noncompliance *related to* the inconvenience and side effects of glaucoma medications

Planning

The overall goals are that the patient with glaucoma will (1) have no progression of visual impairment, (2) understand the disease process and rationale for therapy, (3) comply with all aspects of therapy (including medication administration and follow-up care), and (4) have no postoperative complications.

Nursing Implementation

Health Promotion. Loss of vision due to glaucoma is a preventable problem.[24] The nurse has an important role in teaching the patient and family about the risk of glaucoma. The nurse should stress the importance of early detection and treatment in preventing visual impairment. This knowledge should encourage the patient to seek appropriate ophthalmic health care. The patient should know that the incidence of glaucoma increases with age and that a comprehensive ophthalmic examination is invaluable in identifying persons with glaucoma or those at risk of developing glaucoma. The current recommendation is for an ophthalmologic examination every 2 to 4 years for persons between ages 40 and 64 years, and every 1 to 2 years for persons age 65 years or older. African Americans in every age category should have examinations more often because of the increased incidence and more aggressive course of glaucoma in these individuals.

Acute Intervention. Acute nursing interventions are directed primarily toward the patient with acute angle-closure glaucoma and the surgical patient. The patient with acute angle-closure glaucoma requires immediate medication to lower the IOP, which the nurse must administer in a timely and appropriate manner according to the ophthalmologist's prescription. This patient may also be uncomfortable, and appropriate nursing comfort interventions may include darkening the environment, applying cool compresses to the patient's forehead, and providing a quiet and private space for the patient. Most surgical procedures for glaucoma are outpatient procedures. Acutely, the patient needs postoperative instructions and may require nursing comfort measures to relieve discomfort related to the procedure. Patient and family teaching after eye surgery is discussed in Table 22-6.

Ambulatory and Home Care. Because of the chronic nature of glaucoma, the patient needs encouragement to follow the therapeutic regimen and follow-up recommendations prescribed by the ophthalmologist. The patient needs accurate information about the disease process and treatment options, including the rationale underlying each option. In addition, the patient needs information about the purpose, frequency, and technique for administration of prescribed antiglaucoma agents. In addition to verbal instructions, all patients should receive written instructions that contain the same information. This should be sufficiently detailed to provide all the necessary information without being so extensive that the patient becomes overwhelmed. The patient may be encouraged to comply with the medication regimen if the nurse promotes consideration of the sight-saving nature of the drops. The nurse can further encourage compliance by helping the patient identify the most convenient and appropriate times for medication administration or advocating a change in therapy if the patient reports unacceptable side effects.

Evaluation

The overall expected outcomes are that the patient with glaucoma will

- have no further loss of vision
- comply with recommended therapy
- safely function within own environment
- obtain relief from pain associated with the disease and surgery

GERONTOLOGIC CONSIDERATIONS
GLAUCOMA

Many older patients with glaucoma have systemic illnesses or take systemic medications that may affect their therapy. In particular, the patient using a β-adrenergic blocking glaucoma agent may experience an additive effect if a systemic β-adrenergic blocking drug is also being taken. All β-adrenergic blocking glaucoma agents are contraindicated in the patient with bradycardia, greater than first-degree heart block, cardiogenic shock, and overt cardiac failure. The noncardioselective β-adrenergic blocker glaucoma agents are also contraindicated in the patient with severe chronic obstructive pulmonary disease (COPD) or asthma. The hyperosmolar agents may precipitate heart failure or pulmonary edema in the susceptible patient. The older patient on high-dose aspirin therapy for rheumatoid arthritis should not take carbonic anhydrase inhibitors. The α-adrenergic agonists can cause tachycardia or hypertension, which may have serious consequences in the older patient. The nurse should teach the older patient to occlude the puncta to limit the systemic absorption of glaucoma medications.

INTRAOCULAR INFLAMMATION AND INFECTION

The term *uveitis* is used to describe inflammation of the uveal tract, the retina, the vitreous body, or the optic nerve. This inflammation may be caused by bacteria, viruses, fungi, or parasites. *Cytomegalovirus retinitis* (CMV retinitis) is an opportunistic infection that occurs in patients with acquired immunodeficiency syndrome (AIDS) and in other immunosuppressed patients. The etiology of sterile intraocular inflammation includes autoimmune disorders, AIDS, malignancies, or those associated with systemic diseases such as juvenile rheumatoid arthritis and inflammatory bowel disease. Pain and photophobia are common symptoms.

Endophthalmitis is an extensive intraocular inflammation of the vitreous cavity. Bacteria, viruses, fungi, or parasites can all induce this serious inflammatory response. The mechanism of infection may be endogenous, in which the infecting agent arrives at the eye through the bloodstream, or exogenous, in which the infecting agent is introduced through a surgical wound or a penetrating injury. Although rare, most cases of endophthalmitis are a devastating complication of intraocular surgery or penetrating ocular injury and can lead to irreversible blindness within hours or days. Manifestations include ocular pain, photophobia, decreased visual acuity, headaches, upper lid edema, reddened and swollen conjunctiva, and corneal edema.

When all the layers of the eye (vitreous, retina, choroid, and sclera) are involved in the inflammatory response, the patient has *panophthalmitis.* In the final stages of extensive cases, the scleral coat may undergo bacterial or inflammatory dissolution. Subsequent rupture of the globe spreads the infection into the orbit or eyelids.

Treatment of intraocular inflammation depends on the underlying cause. Intraocular infections require antimicrobial agents, which may be delivered topically, subconjunctivally, intravitreally, systemically, or in some combination. Sterile inflammatory responses require antiinflammatory agents such as corticosteroids. The site and the severity of the sterile inflammatory response determine whether topical, subconjunctival, or systemic corticosteroids are necessary.

The patient with intraocular inflammation is usually uncomfortable and may be noticeably anxious and frightened. The patient may fear sudden and total loss of vision. In some cases this fear is realistic, and the nurse should provide accurate information and emotional support to the patient and the family. In severe cases enucleation may be necessary. When the patient has lost visual function or even the entire eye, the patient will grieve the loss. The nurse's role includes helping the patient through the grieving process.

ENUCLEATION

Enucleation is the removal of the eye. The primary indication for enucleation is a blind, painful eye. This may result from absolute glaucoma, infection, or trauma. Enucleation may also be indicated in ocular malignancies, although many malignancies can be managed with cryotherapy, radiation, and chemotherapy. An extremely rare indication is *sympathetic ophthalmia,* in which the untraumatized eye develops an inflammatory response following the primary eye trauma. In this situation the traumatized eye is enucleated. The surgical procedure includes severing the extraocular muscles close to their insertion on the globe, inserting an implant to maintain the intraorbital anatomy, and suturing the ends of the extraocular muscles over the implant. The conjunctiva covers the joined muscles, and a clear conformer is placed over the conjunctiva until the permanent prosthesis is fitted. A pressure dressing helps prevent postoperative bleeding.

Postoperatively the nurse observes the patient for signs of complications, including excessive bleeding or swelling, increased pain, displacement of the implant, or temperature elevation. Patient teaching should include the instillation of topical ointments or drops and wound cleansing. The nurse should also instruct the patient in the method of inserting the conformer into the socket in case it falls out. The patient is often devastated by the loss of an eye, even when enucleation occurs following a lengthy period of painful blindness. The nurse should recognize and validate the patient's emotional response and provide support to the patient and the family.

Approximately 6 weeks following surgery, the wound is sufficiently healed for the permanent prosthesis. The prosthesis is fitted by an ocularist and designed to match the remaining eye. The patient should learn how to remove, cleanse, and insert the prosthesis. Special polishing is required periodically to remove dried protein secretions.

OCULAR MANIFESTATIONS OF SYSTEMIC DISEASES

Many systemic diseases have significant ocular manifestations. Although it is not the purpose of this discussion to provide a full description of these disorders, it is important for the nurse to recognize that many systemic diseases have ocular symptoms. Conversely, ocular signs and symptoms may be the first finding or complaint in the patient with a systemic disease. One example is the patient with undiagnosed diabetes who seeks ophthalmic care for blurred vision. A careful history and examination of the patient can reveal that the underlying cause of the blurred vision is lens swelling caused by hyperglycemia. Another example is the patient who seeks care for a conjunctival lesion. The ophthalmologist may be the first health care professional to make the diagnosis of AIDS based on the presence of a conjunctival Kaposi sarcoma (KS). Table 22-11 lists some systemic diseases and disorders and the associated ophthalmic manifestations.

TABLE 22-11 Ocular Manifestations of Systemic Diseases or Disorders

Systemic Entity	Ocular Manifestations
AIDS	Herpes zoster ophthalmicus, keratitis (bacterial and viral), CMV retinitis, endophthalmitis (bacterial and fungal), cotton-wool spots and microvasculopathy of the retina, KS of eyelids or conjunctiva
Albinism	Decreased visual acuity, photophobia, nystagmus, strabismus
Diabetes mellitus	Fluctuating refractive errors, diabetic retinopathy, macular edema, premature cataract development, increased incidence of glaucoma
Down syndrome	Myopia, cataracts, nystagmus, strabismus, keratoconus, upward and outward slant of palpebral fissures
Hypertension	Cotton-wool spots and hemorrhage of the retina, retinal lipid deposits
Systemic lupus erythematosus	Dry eye, retinal changes, uveitis, scleritis
Marfan syndrome	Lens dislocation, severe myopia, keratoconus, retinal detachment
Rheumatoid arthritis	Dry eye, keratitis, scleritis
Infections	
Botulism	Blurred vision, ptosis, diplopia, fixed, dilated pupil
Endocarditis	Subconjunctival or retinal petechiae
Tuberculosis	Conjunctivitis, keratitis, uveitis
Leprosy	Conjunctivitis, keratitis, uveitis, ptosis
Herpes	Herpes simplex keratitis
CMV infection	CMV retinitis
Measles	Conjunctivitis, keratitis, retinopathy
Congenital rubella	Cataracts, glaucoma
Histoplasmosis	Chorioretinal lesions, subretinal neovascularization
Toxoplasmosis	Necrotic retinal lesions, vitreal inflammation, retinochoroiditis
Lyme disease	Conjunctivitis, keratitis, episcleritis, panophthalmitis, retinal detachment, diplopia
Syphilis	Conjunctivitis, keratitis, uveitis, retinal detachment, macular edema, lens dislocation, glaucoma (congenital syphilis)
Temporal arteritis	Vision loss; palsies of CNs III, IV, and VI; nystagmus; ptosis
Thyroid disease	Lid retraction, lid lag, exophthalmos, abnormal eye movement, increased IOP
Vitamin deficiencies	
A	Night blindness, corneal ulceration
B	Optic neuropathy, corneal changes, retinal hemorrhage, nystagmus
C	Hemorrhage in anterior chamber, retina, conjunctiva
D	Exophthalmos

AIDS, Acquired immunodeficiency syndrome; *CMV,* cytomegalovirus; *CN,* cranial nerve; *IOP,* intraocular pressure; *KS,* Kaposi sarcoma.

Auditory Problems External Ear and Canal

TRAUMA

Trauma to the external ear can cause injury to the subcutaneous tissue that may result in a hematoma. If the hematoma is not aspirated, inflammation of the membranes of the ear cartilage (perichondritis) can result. Antibiotics are given to prevent infection. Blows to the ear can also cause a conductive hearing loss if there is damage to the ossicles in the middle ear or if a perforation of the tympanic membrane results. Head trauma that injures the temporal lobe of the cerebral cortex can impair the ability to understand the meaning of sounds.

EXTERNAL OTITIS

The skin of the external ear and canal is subject to the same problems as skin anywhere on the body. **External otitis** involves inflammation or infection of the epithelium of the auricle and ear canal. Frequent swimming may alter the flora of the external canal, resulting in an infection often referred to as "swimmer's ear." Trauma caused by picking the ear or the use of sharp objects, such as hairpins, frequently causes the initial break in the skin. Piercing of cartilage in the upper part of the auricle is at higher risk for infection than earlobe piercing.[25]

Etiology

Infections, dermatitis, or both may cause external otitis. Bacteria or fungi may be the cause. The bacteria most commonly cultured are *Pseudomonas aeruginosa* followed by *Klebsiella, Proteus, Escherichia coli,* and *S. aureus.* The most common fungi are *Candida albicans* and *Aspergillus* organisms.[26] Fungi are often the causative agents of external otitis, especially in warm, moist climates. The warm, dark environment of the ear canal provides a good medium for the growth of microorganisms.

Malignant external otitis is an infection caused by *P. aeruginosa.* The infection occurs mainly in elderly patients with diabetes. It can spread from the external ear to the parotid gland and temporal bone.

Clinical Manifestations and Complications

Pain *(otalgia)* is one of the first signs of external otitis. Even in mild cases, the patient may experience pain that is disproportionate to the infection. The swelling of the bony ear canal as a result of the inflammatory process causes pain. Pain is especially noted on movement of the auricle or on application of pressure to the tragus (directly in front of the ear). Drainage from the ear may be serosanguineous or purulent. If it is the result of an infection caused by *Pseudomonas,* the drainage will be green and have a musty smell. Temperature elevations occur when there is extensive involvement of the tissue. The swelling of the ear canal can block hearing and cause dizziness. Facial nerve paralysis may occur with malignant external otitis.

NURSING MANAGEMENT EXTERNAL OTITIS

Diagnosis of external otitis is made by observation with the otoscope light using the largest speculum that the ear will accommodate without causing the patient unnecessary discomfort. The eardrum may be normal if it can be seen. Culture and sensitivity studies of the drainage may be done. Mild analgesics will usually control the pain. After the ear canal is cleansed, a wick of cotton is placed in the canal to help deliver the antibiotic eardrops. Cotton wicks should be used with caution in young patients and confused or psychotic patients, who may push them farther into the ear. Topical antibiotics include polymyxin B and neomycin (Neosporin) and chloramphenicol (Chloromycetin). Nystatin (Mycostatin) is used for fungal infections. Corticosteroids may also be used to decrease inflammation unless the infection is fungal, in which case they are contraindicated. If the surrounding tissue is involved, systemic antibiotics are prescribed. Warm, moist compresses or heat may be applied. Improvement should occur in 48 hours, but 7 to 14 days are required for complete resolution.

Careful handling and disposal of material saturated with drainage are important. Hands should be washed before and after administration of otic drops (eardrops). The drops should be administered at room temperature because cold drops can cause dizziness in the patient, due to stimulation of the semicircular canals. The tip of the dropper should not touch the ear during administration to prevent contamination of the entire bottle of drops. The ear is positioned so that the drops can run down the canal. This position should be maintained for 2 minutes after eardrop administration to allow dispersion of drops. Collaborative care of external otitis is shown in Table 22-12.

TABLE 22-12 COLLABORATIVE CARE External Otitis

Diagnostic
History and physical examination
Otoscopic examination
Culture and sensitivity
Collaborative Therapy
Analgesics (depending on severity)
Warm compresses
Cleansing of canal
Ear wick
Antibiotic otic drops
Systemic antibiotics

CERUMEN AND FOREIGN BODIES IN THE EXTERNAL EAR CANAL

Impacted cerumen (earwax) can cause discomfort and decreased hearing. In the older person, the earwax becomes dense and drier. Hair becomes thicker and coarser, entrapping the hard dry cerumen in the canal. Water that enters the canal during a shower or swimming may cause swelling of the cerumen, resulting in complete blockage of the canal. Symptoms of cerumen impaction are outlined in Table 22-13. Management involves irrigation of the canal with body-temperature solutions. Special syringes can be used and vary from the simple bulb syringe to special irrigating equipment used in the health care provider's office or clinic. The patient is placed in a sitting position with an emesis basin under the ear. The auricle is pulled up and back, and the flow of solution is directed above or below the impaction. It is important that the ear canal not be completely occluded with the syringe tip. If irrigation does not remove the wax, mild lubricant drops may be used to soften the earwax. Irrigation may then be effective in removing the impacted cerumen. It may need to be removed by a physician using an operating microscope, suction, and microsurgical instruments.

The list of foreign objects removed from the ear is extensive and includes animate, inanimate, vegetable, and mineral objects.

TABLE 22-13 Manifestations of Cerumen Impaction

- Hearing loss
- Otalgia
- Tinnitus
- Vertigo
- Cough
- Cardiac depression (vagal stimulation)

Attempts to remove the object occasionally result in pushing it further into the canal. An otolaryngologist should remove the object. Vegetable matter tends to swell and may create a secondary inflammation, making removal more difficult.

Animate objects must be immobilized before removal. Mineral oil or lidocaine can be used to drown an insect. The organism can then be removed with microscope guidance. The use of general anesthesia or conscious sedation may be necessary depending on the level of patient cooperation. Rarely, it may be necessary to make a canal incision to remove the foreign body.

The patient should be instructed to keep objects out of the ear. Ears should be cleaned only with a washcloth and finger. Hairpins and cotton-tipped applicators should especially be avoided. Penetration of the middle ear by a cotton-tipped applicator can cause serious injury to the tympanic membrane and ossicles and may result in facial paralysis as a result of nerve damage. The use of cotton-tipped applicators can also impact cerumen against the tympanic membrane and impair hearing.

MALIGNANCY OF THE EXTERNAL EAR

Malignancies of the external ear (other than skin cancers) and canal are uncommon. Because of long-term sun exposure, the superior border of the auricle is at risk for the development of skin cancer. The most common malignant neoplasms of the auricle are basal cell and squamous cell cancers. These skin cancers can be excised surgically. Auricular skin cancers are usually not life threatening, and the cure rate after resection is greater than 90% in most cases. Melanoma occurs rarely on the external ear. Cancer of the ear often results in cosmetic deformities that are difficult to reconstruct. An important nursing role is teaching about the danger of sun exposure. Hats and sunscreen should be used regularly.

Middle Ear and Mastoid

ACUTE OTITIS MEDIA

The most common problem of the middle ear is *acute otitis media,* usually a childhood disease associated with colds, allergies, sore throats, and blockage of the eustachian tube. The earlier the first episode, the greater the risk of subsequent episodes occurring. Infection can be due to viruses or bacteria. Pain, fever, malaise, headache, and reduced hearing are signs and symptoms of acute otitis media.

Collaborative care involves the use of antibiotics to eradicate the causative organism. Amoxicillin is the current therapy of choice in the United States. Surgical intervention is generally reserved for the patient who does not respond to medical treatment.[27] A *myringotomy* involves an incision in the tympanum to release the increased pressure and exudate from the middle ear. A tympanostomy tube may be placed for short- or long-term use. Prompt treatment of an episode of acute otitis media generally prevents spontaneous perforation of the tympanic membrane. In the adult patient for whom allergy may be a causative factor, antihistamines may also be prescribed.

CHRONIC OTITIS MEDIA AND MASTOIDITIS

Etiology and Pathophysiology

Untreated or repeated attacks of acute otitis media may lead to a chronic condition. Chronic infection of the middle ear is more common in persons who experience episodes of acute otitis media in early childhood. Organisms involved in chronic otitis media include *S. aureus*, *Proteus mirabilis*, and *P. aeruginosa*. Because the mucous membrane is continuous, both the middle ear and the air cells of the mastoid can be involved in the chronic infectious process.

Clinical Manifestations

Chronic otitis media is characterized by a purulent exudate and inflammation that can involve the ossicles, eustachian tube, and mastoid bone. It is often painless. Nausea and episodes of dizziness can occur. The patient may complain of hearing loss that may be a result of destruction of the ossicles, a tympanic membrane perforation, or the accumulation of fluid in the middle ear space. Occasionally a facial palsy or an attack of vertigo may alert the patient to this condition.

Complications

Untreated conditions can result in perforation of the tympanic membrane and the formation of a **cholesteatoma** (a mass of epithelial cells and cholesterol in the middle ear). Its enlarging tumorlike behavior may destroy the adjacent bones, including the ossicles. Unless removed surgically, a cholesteatoma can cause extensive damage to the structures of the middle ear, can erode the bony protection of the facial nerve, may create a labyrinthine fistula, or can even invade the dura, threatening the brain.

Diagnostic Studies

Otoscopic examination may reveal color changes, decreased tympanic membrane mobility, and a marginal or central perforation of the tympanic membrane (Fig. 22-7). Culture and sensitivity tests are necessary to identify the organisms involved so that the appropriate antibiotic therapy can be prescribed. The audiogram may demonstrate no loss in hearing or a loss as great as 50 to 60 dB if the ossicles have been partially destroyed or separated. Sinus x-rays, magnetic resonance imaging (MRI), or a computed tomography (CT) scan of the temporal bone may demonstrate bone destruction, absence of ossicles, or the presence of a mass.

Collaborative Care

The aims of treatment are to clear the middle ear of infection, repair the perforation, and preserve hearing (Table 22-14). Systemic antibiotic therapy is initiated based on the culture and sensitivity results. In addition, the patient may need to undergo frequent evacuation of drainage and debris in an outpatient setting. Otic and oral antibiotics are used to reduce infection. In many cases of chronic otitis media, antibiotic resistance is present.

Surgical Therapy. Often chronic tympanic membrane perforations will not heal with conservative treatment, and surgery is necessary. Surgery involving reconstruction of the tympanic mem-

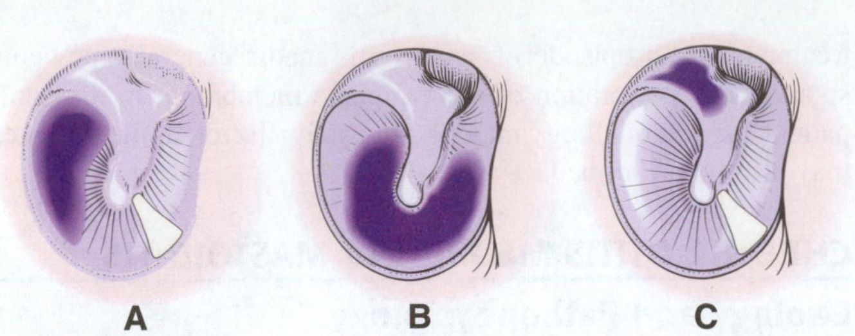

FIG. 22-7 Three common tympanic perforations. **A,** Small central perforation (hearing is usually good). **B,** Large central perforation around the handle of the malleus (hearing is usually poor). **C,** Marginal perforation of Shrapnell's membrane (hearing is usually good). Cholesteatomas commonly occur in patients with a marginal perforation and are always present with attic perforation.

TABLE 22-14 COLLABORATIVE CARE
Chronic Otitis Media

Diagnostic
History and physical examination
Otoscopic examination
Culture and sensitivity of middle ear drainage
Mastoid x-ray

Collaborative Therapy
Ear irrigations
Otic, oral, or parenteral antibiotics
Analgesics
Antiemetics
Surgery
  Tympanoplasty*
  Mastoidectomy

*See Table 22-15.

brane and/or the ossicular chain is called a *tympanoplasty.* A *mastoidectomy* is often performed with a tympanoplasty to remove diseased tissue and the source of infection. Removal of tissue stops at the middle ear structures that appear capable of functioning in the conduction of sound. A *myringoplasty* is surgical reconstruction limited to repair of a tympanic membrane perforation.

NURSING MANAGEMENT CHRONIC OTITIS MEDIA

■ Following Tympanoplasty

Routine preoperative care is provided before tympanoplasty and includes teaching postoperative expectations (Table 22-15). Postoperative concerns are the avoidance of complications such as disruption of the repair during the healing phase, and facial nerve paralysis.

After surgery the patient will be positioned flat and side-lying with the operative side up. It is normal to have impaired hearing during the postoperative period if there is packing in the ear. A cotton ball dressing is used for an endaural incision. The patient should be instructed to change the cotton packing and dressing daily. If a postauricular incision is used and a drain is in place, a mastoid dressing is used. A small gauze pad is cut to fit behind the ear, and fluffs are applied over the ear to prevent the outer circular head dressing from placing pressure on the auricle. It is necessary to monitor the tightness of the dressing to prevent tissue necrosis and the amount and type of drainage postoperatively.

TABLE 22-15 PATIENT AND FAMILY TEACHING GUIDE
After Ear Surgery

1. Avoid sudden head movements.
2. Do not try to get out of bed without assistance.
3. Take antivertigo agents if prescribed.
4. Change positions slowly.
5. Avoid getting the head wet (including showering) until directed by surgeon.
6. Report fever, pain, an increase in hearing loss, or drainage from the ear.
7. Do not cough or blow the nose because this causes increased pressure in the eustachian tube and middle ear cavity and disrupts healing.
8. If need to cough or sneeze, leave the mouth open to help reduce the pressure.
9. Avoid crowds where respiratory infections may be contracted.
10. Avoid situations where pressure or popping in the ears is normally experienced, such as high elevations or airplane travel.

OTITIS MEDIA WITH EFFUSION

Otitis media with effusion is an inflammation of the middle ear in which a collection of fluid is present in the middle ear space. The fluid may be thin, mucoid, or purulent. This condition is commonly called *serous otitis media,* "glue ear," or *secretory otitis media.* The fluid usually collects because of a malfunction of the eustachian tube, which commonly follows upper respiratory and/or chronic sinus infections, barotrauma (caused by pressure change), or otitis media. If the eustachian tube does not open and allow equalization of atmospheric pressure, negative pressure within the middle ear causes fluid to seep from the tissues.

Complaints include a feeling of fullness of the ear, "plugged" feeling or popping, and decreased hearing. The patient does not experience pain, fever, or discharge from the ear. Pneumatic otoscopy is a critical assessment tool in differentiating otitis media with effusion from acute otitis media.[28] It is normal to have otitis media with effusion for weeks to months after an episode of acute otitis media. It usually resolves in 75% to 90% of cases without treatment but may recur.

OTOSCLEROSIS

Otosclerosis, an autosomal dominant disease, is the fixation of the footplate of the stapes in the oval window. Spongy bone develops from the bony labyrinth, causing immobilization of the footplate of the stapes, which reduces the transmission of vibrations to the inner ear fluids. It is a common cause of conductive hearing loss in young adults, especially women, and may accelerate during pregnancy. Otosclerosis is bilateral in about 80% of patients. Although hearing loss is typically bilateral, one ear may show faster hearing loss progression. The patient is often unaware of the problem until the loss becomes so severe that communication is difficult.

Otoscopic examination may reveal a reddish blush of the tympanum (Schwartz's sign) caused by the vascular and bony changes within the middle ear. Tuning fork tests help identify the conductive component of the hearing loss. On the Rinne test, sound will be heard longer when the stem of the tuning fork is touching the mastoid bone (bone conduction) than when placed next to the ear (air conduction). In Weber's test, the sound is heard better through the skull bone in the ear with the greater conductive hearing loss than through air. An audiogram demonstrates good hearing by bone conduction, but air conduction demonstrates poor hearing (air-bone gap). Usually at least a difference of 20 to 25 dB between air and bone conduction levels of hearing is seen in otosclerosis.

Collaborative Care

The hearing loss associated with otosclerosis may be stabilized by the use of sodium fluoride with vitamin D and calcium carbonate to retard bone resorption and encourage calcification of bony lesions. Amplification of sound by a hearing aid can be effective because the inner ear function is normal. Surgical treatment involves partial removal of the stapes *(stapedectomy)* or complete removal with prosthesis insertion *(fenestration)*. Collaborative care of otosclerosis is shown in Table 22-16.

Surgery is usually performed under local anesthesia with sedation. The ear with poorer hearing is repaired first, and the other ear may be operated on 6 months to 1 year later. An endaural incision is made using the operating microscope for visualization. Gelfoam is used on the incision flap to limit bleeding. A cotton ball is placed in the ear canal and a small dressing is used to cover the ear.

During surgery the patient will often report an immediate improvement in hearing in the operative ear. Because of the accumulation of blood and fluid in the middle ear, the hearing level decreases postoperatively but will improve with healing. After stapedectomy, 90% of patients experience an improvement in hearing, in many instances to near normal.

NURSING MANAGEMENT
OTOSCLEROSIS

Nursing management of the patient undergoing a stapedectomy or fenestration is similar to that for the patient who has undergone a tympanoplasty. Postoperatively, the patient may experience dizziness, nausea, and vomiting as a result of stimulation of the labyrinth intraoperatively. Some patients demonstrate nystagmus because of disturbance of the perilymph fluid. Care should be taken to decrease sudden movements by the patient that may bring on or exacerbate dizziness. Actions such as coughing, sneezing, lifting, bending, and straining during bowel movements should also be minimized.

TABLE 22-16 *COLLABORATIVE CARE* Otosclerosis

Diagnostic
History and physical examination
Otoscopic examination
Rinne test
Weber's test
Audiometry
Tympanometry
Collaborative Therapy
Hearing aid
Surgery (stapedectomy or fenestration)
Drug therapy
Sodium fluoride
Vitamin D
Calcium carbonate

Inner Ear Problems

Three symptoms that indicate disease of the inner ear are vertigo, sensorineural hearing loss, and tinnitus. Symptoms of vertigo arise from the vestibular labyrinth, whereas hearing loss and tinnitus arise from the auditory labyrinth. There is an overlap between manifestations of inner ear problems and central nervous system (CNS) disorders.

MÉNIÈRE'S DISEASE

Ménière's disease (endolymphatic hydrops) is characterized by symptoms caused by inner ear disease, including episodic vertigo, tinnitus, fluctuating sensorineural hearing loss, and aural fullness. This disease causes significant disability for the patient because of sudden, severe attacks of vertigo with nausea and vomiting. Symptoms usually begin between 30 and 60 years of age.

The cause of the disease is unknown, but it results in an excessive accumulation of endolymph in the membranous labyrinth. The volume of endolymph increases until the membranous labyrinth ruptures, mixing high-potassium endolymph with low-potassium perilymph. Attacks may be preceded by a sense of fullness in the ear, increasing tinnitus, and a decrease in hearing acuity. The patient may experience the feeling of being pulled to the ground ("drop attacks"). Some patients report that they feel as if they are whirling in space. The duration of attacks may be hours or days, and attacks may occur several times a year. Autonomic symptoms include pallor, sweating, nausea, and vomiting.

The clinical course of the disease is highly variable. Low-pitched tinnitus may be present continuously in the affected ear or it may be intensified during an attack. It is often described as a "roar," or "like the ocean." Hearing loss fluctuates, and with continued attacks, hearing recovery is often less complete with each episode, eventually leading to progressive permanent hearing loss.

NURSING *and* COLLABORATIVE MANAGEMENT
MÉNIÈRE'S DISEASE

Collaborative care of Ménière's disease (Table 22-17) includes diagnostic tests to rule out CNS disease. The audiogram demonstrates a mild, low-frequency sensorineural hearing loss. Vestibular tests indicate decreased function.

A glycerol test may aid in the diagnosis of Ménière's disease. An oral dose of glycerol is given, followed by serial audiograms over 3 hours. Improvement in hearing or speech discrimination supports a diagnosis of Ménière's disease. The improvement is attributed to the osmotic effect of glycerol that pulls fluid from the inner ear. Although a positive test is diagnostic of Ménière's disease, a negative test does not rule out the condition.

During the acute attack, antihistamines, anticholinergics, and benzodiazepines can be used to decrease the abnormal sensation and lessen symptoms such as nausea and vomiting. Acute vertigo is treated symptomatically with bed rest, sedation, and antiemetics or antivertigo drugs for motion sickness administered orally, rectally, or intravenously. The patient requires reassurance and counseling that the condition is not life threatening. Management between attacks may include diuretics, antihistamines, and a low-sodium diet. Diazepam (Valium), meclizine (Antivert [Bonamine plus nicotinic acid]), and fentanyl with droperidol (Innovar) may be used to reduce the vertigo. Over a period of time, most pa-

TABLE 22-17 COLLABORATIVE CARE
Ménière's Disease

Diagnostic
History and physical examination
Audiometric studies, including speech discrimination, tone decay
Vestibular tests, including caloric test, positional test
Electronystagmography
Neurologic examination
Glycerol test
Collaborative Therapy
Acute Care (one or more)
Sedative (diazepam [Valium])
Anticholinergic (atropine)
Vasodilators
Antihistamine (diphenhydramine [Benadryl])
Surgical Therapy
Conservative Surgical Intervention
Endolymphatic shunt
Vestibular nerve section
Destructive Surgical Intervention
Labyrinthotomy
Labyrinthectomy
Ambulatory/Home Care (one or more)
Diuretics
Antihistamines
Vasodilators
Antiseizure drugs
Vitamins
diazepam (Valium)
Low-salt diet
Restriction of caffeine, nicotine, and alcohol intake

tients respond to the prescribed medications but must learn to live with the unpredictability of the attacks. The remainder of patients may, in time, require surgical intervention.

Frequent and incapacitating attacks, reduced quality of life, and threatened unemployment are indications for surgical intervention. Surgical decompression of the endolymphatic sac is performed to reduce the pressure on the cochlear hair cells and to prevent further damage and hearing loss.[29] If relief is not achieved with endolymphatic shunt surgery and hearing remains good, vestibular nerve resection may be performed to alleviate vertigo and preserve hearing. When involvement is unilateral, surgical ablation of the labyrinth, resulting in loss of the vestibular and hearing cochlear function, is performed. Careful management can decrease the possibility of progressive sensorineural loss in many patients.

Nursing interventions are planned to minimize vertigo and provide for patient safety. During an acute attack the patient is kept in a quiet, darkened room in a comfortable position. The patient needs to be taught to avoid sudden head movements or position changes. Fluorescent or flickering lights or watching television may exacerbate symptoms and should be avoided. An emesis basin should be available because vomiting is common. To minimize the risk of falling, the nurse should keep the side rails up and the bed low in position when the patient is in bed. The patient should be instructed to call for assistance when getting out of bed. Medications and fluids are administered parenterally, and intake and output are monitored. When the attack subsides, the patient should be assisted with ambulation because unsteadiness may remain. Similar nursing care is provided after surgical ablation of the labyrinth. The patient will have severe tinnitus and vertigo, which decrease during a period of days or weeks as the brain adjusts to loss of vestibular input and postural stability is regained.

LABYRINTHITIS

Labyrinthitis is an inflammation of the inner ear affecting the cochlear and/or vestibular portion of the labyrinth. Infection can enter from the meninges, the middle ear, or the bloodstream. Symptoms include vertigo, tinnitus, and sensorineural hearing loss on the affected side. This condition is rare since the advent of antibiotics. *Nystagmus*, an abnormal rhythmic, jerking movement of the eyes, accompanies the vertigo and has a horizontal beat.

Suppurative labyrinthitis from infection causes severe vertigo with nausea and vomiting similar to that of an attack of Ménière's disease. Complete destruction of the cochlea and labyrinth may occur, causing permanent deafness. Loss of vestibular input causes extreme unsteadiness in the patient. The patient requires physical therapy to recondition the brain to interpret vestibular input.

The most common complication of labyrinthitis is meningitis. It is important for the nurse to assess for changes in level of consciousness, headache, and nuchal rigidity (stiff neck). The patient may become very lethargic or easily agitated. These changes should be reported immediately to the health care provider. It is important for the nurse to document these assessments even if they are normal. (Meningitis is discussed in Chapter 57.)

ACOUSTIC NEUROMA

An **acoustic neuroma** (or *vestibular schwannoma*) is a benign tumor that occurs where the acoustic nerve (CN VIII) enters the internal auditory canal or the temporal bone from the brain. It is important that an early diagnosis be made because the tumor can compress the facial nerve and arteries within the internal auditory canal. Once the tumor has expanded and become an intracranial neoplasm, more extensive surgery is necessary, reducing the chances of preserving hearing and normal facial nerve function.

Early symptoms are associated with CN VIII compression and destruction. They include unilateral, progressive, sensorineural hearing loss; unilateral tinnitus; and mild, intermittent vertigo. One of the earliest symptoms of an acoustic neuroma is reduced touch sensation in the posterior ear canal. Diagnostic tests include neurologic, audiometric, and vestibular tests and CT scans and MRI with gadolinium enhancement.

Surgery to remove small tumors is performed through the middle cranial fossa or retrolabyrinthine approach, which preserves hearing and vestibular function. A translabyrinthine approach is usually used for medium-sized tumors and when hearing is minimal. Although hearing is destroyed by this approach, advantages include good access to the tumor and preservation of the facial nerve. Retrosigmoid (suboccipital) or transotic approaches are used for large tumors (larger than 3 cm). It is almost impossible to preserve hearing when the tumor is larger than 2 cm. Stereotactic radiosurgery may slow tumor growth and preserve the facial nerve.[30]

HEARING LOSS AND DEAFNESS

Hearing disorders are the primary handicapping disability in the United States. The majority of persons lose their hearing as adults. Hearing impairment is common among older adults. Nearly half of the persons who need assistance with hearing disorders are 65 years of age or older. With the aging of the population, hearing

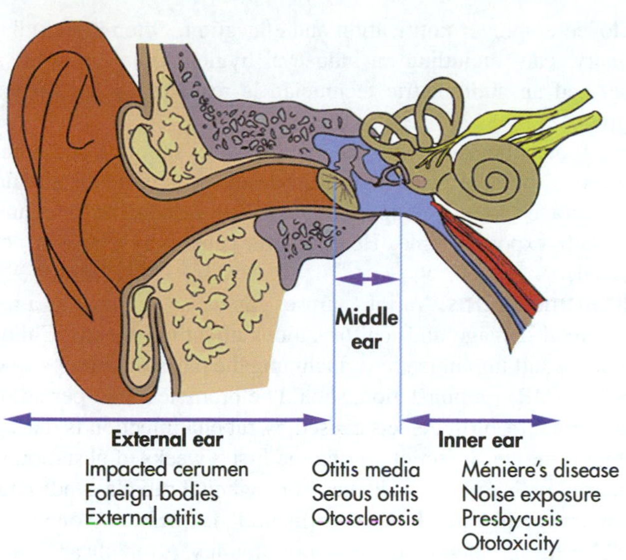

FIG. 22-8 Causes of hearing loss.

loss is increasing. At age 50, one of every eight persons is hearing impaired. Causes of hearing loss are shown in Fig. 22-8.

Types of Hearing Loss

Conductive Hearing Loss. *Conductive hearing loss* occurs in the outer and middle ear and impairs the sound being conducted from the outer to the inner ear.[31] It is caused by conditions interfering with air conduction, such as impacted cerumen and foreign bodies, middle ear disease, otosclerosis, and stenosis of the external auditory canal. The most common cause is otitis media with effusion. The audiogram demonstrates an air-bone gap of at least 15 dB.

An air-bone gap occurs when hearing sensitivity by bone conduction is better than by air conduction. The patient may speak softly because he or she hears his or her voice, which is conducted by bone, as being loud. This patient hears better in a noisy environment. A hearing aid is helpful for a patient with a 40- to 50-dB loss or more if correction of the cause is not possible.

Sensorineural Hearing Loss. *Sensorineural hearing loss* is caused by impairment of function of the inner ear or the vestibulocochlear nerve (CN VIII). Congenital and hereditary factors, noise trauma during a period of time, aging (presbycusis), Ménière's disease, and ototoxicity can cause sensorineural hearing loss. Systemic diseases, such as tuberculosis, syphilis, Lyme disease, cytomegalovirus, HIV, and Paget's disease of the bone, can also cause sensorineural deafness. Immune diseases, diabetes mellitus, bacterial meningitis, and trauma are also causes of this type of hearing loss.

The two main problems associated with sensorineural loss are the ability to hear sound but not to understand speech, and the lack of understanding of the problem by others. The ability to hear high-pitched sounds diminishes with a sensorineural hearing loss. Consonants are high-pitched sounds that give intelligibility to speech. Words become difficult to distinguish, and sound becomes muffled. An audiogram demonstrates a loss in dB levels of the 4000-Hz range, which can progress to the 2000-Hz range. A hearing aid may help the patient who has a 30-dB loss or more by reducing the strain of trying to hear, but the sounds will still be muffled.

Mixed Hearing Loss. Mixed hearing loss is caused by a combination of conductive and sensorineural losses. Careful evaluation is needed before corrective surgery for conductive loss is planned because the sensorineural component of the hearing loss will still remain.

Central and Functional Hearing Loss. Central hearing loss is caused by a problem along the pathway from the inner ear to the auditory region of the brain or in the brain itself. The patient is unable to understand or to put meaning to the incoming sound. A careful history is helpful because there is usually a reference to deafness within the family. Referral to qualified hearing and speech services is indicated.

Functional hearing loss may be caused by an emotional or a psychologic factor. The patient does not seem to hear or respond to pure-tone subjective hearing tests, but no organic cause can be identified. Psychologic counseling may help.

Classification of Hearing Loss. Hearing loss can also be classified by the decibel (dB) level or loss as recorded on the audiogram. Normal hearing is in the 0- to 15-dB range. Slight hearing loss is in the 16- to 25-dB range. A mild impairment is present at the 26- to 40-dB hearing level. A moderate impairment is in the 41- to 55-dB range. A moderately severe impairment is in the 56- to 70-dB range. The severely impaired have a loss in the 71- to 90-dB range. The profoundly deaf have a loss greater than 91 dB. Many persons in this last group are congenitally deaf.

Clinical Manifestations

Manifestations that indicate hearing loss include asking others to speak up, answering questions inappropriately, not responding when not looking at the speaker, straining to hear, cupping hand around ear, showing irritability with others who do not speak up, and increasing sensitivity to slight increases in noise level. Often the patient is unaware of minimal hearing loss or may compensate by using these mannerisms. Family and friends who get tired of repeating or talking loudly are often first to notice hearing loss. Pressure exerted by significant others is a significant factor in whether the patient seeks help for hearing impairement.[32]

Deafness is often called the "unseen handicap" because it is not until conversation is initiated with a deaf adult that the difficulty in communication is realized. It is important that the health professional be aware of the need for thorough validation of the deaf person's understanding of health teaching. Descriptive visual aids can be helpful.

Interference in communication and interaction with others can be the source of many problems for the patient and family. Often the patient refuses to admit or may be unaware of impaired hearing. Irritability is common because of the concentration with which the patient must listen to understand speech. The loss of clarity of speech in the patient with sensorineural hearing loss is most frustrating. The patient may hear what is said but not understand it. Withdrawal, suspicion, loss of self-esteem, and insecurity are commonly associated with advancing hearing loss.

NURSING *and* COLLABORATIVE MANAGEMENT
HEARING LOSS AND DEAFNESS

■ *Health Promotion*

Environmental Noise Control. Hearing loss can be caused by acute loud noise (acoustic trauma) or by the chronic exposure to loud noise (noise-induced hearing loss). Acoustic trauma causes hearing loss from mechanical destruction of parts of the organ of Corti. Some recovery of function may occur in the first weeks after injury, but the remaining loss is permanent. Noise-induced hearing loss is probably caused by high-intensity stimulation of the cochlea resulting in mechanical damage of the hair cells and basal membrane in the organ of Corti.

Sensorineural hearing loss as a result of increased and prolonged environmental noise, such as amplified sound, is occurring in young adults at an increasing rate. Health teaching regarding avoidance of continued exposure to noise levels greater than 85 to 95 dB is essential. Table 22-18 describes the range of sounds audible to humans.

In work environments known to have high noise levels (greater than 85 dB), ear protection should be worn. Occupational Safety and Health Administration (OSHA) standards require ear protection for workers in environments where the noise levels exceed 85 dB consistently. A variety of protectors are available that are worn over the ears or in the ears to prevent hearing loss. Periodic audiometric screening should be part of the health maintenance policies of industry. This provides baseline data on hearing to measure subsequent hearing loss.

The nurse should participate in hearing conservation programs in work environments. A hearing conservation program should include noise exposure analysis, provision for control of noise exposure (hearing protectors), measurements of hearing, and employee-employer notification and education. Often a multidisciplinary team including an industrial hygienist, an engineer, a nurse, and an audiometric technician is responsible for such a program.

Ear protection should be worn during skeet shooting and other recreational pursuits with high noise levels. Young adults should be encouraged to keep amplified music at a reasonable level and limit their exposure time. Hearing loss caused by noise is not reversible.

Immunizations. Various viruses can cause deafness as a result of fetal damage and malformations affecting the ear. Childhood and adult immunizations, including the measles, mumps, and rubella (MMR) immunization, should be promoted. The period of greatest risk for birth defects caused by rubella infection is during the first trimester. Infection during the first 8 weeks of gestation is associated with an 85% incidence of congenital rubella syndrome, which commonly involves sensorineural deafness.[33] Women of childbearing age should be tested for immunity. A rubella antibody titer of 1:8 or greater shows that the individual has immunity to rubella. If the titer is less, immunization with live vaccine should be given. The woman should avoid pregnancy for at least 3 months after being immunized. Immunization must be delayed if the woman is pregnant. Women who are susceptible to rubella can be vaccinated safely during the postpartum period.

Ototoxic Substances. Ototoxic drugs and chemicals used in industry (e.g., toluene, carbon disulfide, mercury) may damage the inner ear.[34] Drugs commonly associated with ototoxicity include salicylates, diuretics, antineoplastic drugs, and antibiotics. The patient who is receiving ototoxic drugs or is exposed to ototoxic chemicals should be monitored for signs and symptoms associated with ototoxicity. The most common symptoms of ototoxicity are tinnitus, sensorineural hearing loss, and vestibular dysfunction. If these symptoms develop, immediate withdrawal of the drug may prevent further damage and may cause the symptoms to disappear.

TABLE 22-18 Range of Sounds Audible to Human Ear

Typical Decibel	Example
0	Faintest sound audible to the human ear.
30	Quiet library, soft whisper.
40	Living room, quiet office, bedroom away from traffic.
50	Light traffic at a distance, refrigerator, gentle breeze.
60	Air conditioner at 20 ft, conversation, sewing machine.
70	Busy traffic, noisy restaurant. At this decibel level, noise may begin to affect hearing if exposure is constant.
Hazardous Zone for Hearing Loss	
80	Subway, heavy city traffic, alarm clock at 2 ft, factory noise. These noises are dangerous if exposure to them lasts for more than 8 hr.
90	Truck traffic, noisy home appliances, shop tools, lawn mower. As loudness increases, the "safe" time exposure decreases; damage can occur in less than 8 hr.
100	Chain saw, snowmobile, pneumatic drill. Even 2 hr of exposure can be dangerous at this decibel level; with each 5-dB increase, the safe time is cut in half.
120	Loud rock concert, sandblasting, auto horn. The danger is immediate; exposure of 120 dB can injure ears.
140	Gunshot blast, jet plane. Any length of exposure time is dangerous; noise at this level may cause actual pain in the ear. Maximum allowed noise without ear protectors.
180	Rocket launching pad. Without ear protection, noise at this level causes irreversible damage; hearing loss is inevitable.

Adapted from American Academy of Otolaryngology, 2005. Available at *www.entnet.org* (accessed May 17, 2005).

Assistive Devices and Techniques

Hearing Aids. It is important that the patient with a suspected hearing loss have a hearing assessment by a qualified audiologist, including examination and audiometric testing. If a hearing aid is indicated, it should be fitted by an audiologist or a speech and hearing specialist. Many types of hearing aids are available, each with advantages and disadvantages (Fig. 22-9). The conventional hearing aid serves as a simple amplifier. For the patient with bilateral hearing impairment, binaural hearing aids provide the best sound lateralization and speech discrimination. Patients who are motivated and optimistic about using a hearing aid will be more

HEALTHY PEOPLE

Health Impact of Wearing Ear Protection

- Ear protection should be worn during all recreational and work activities involving high noise levels
- Ear protection can greatly reduce the damage to the ear from loud noise
- Periodic audiometric screening is important to detect loss before it progresses

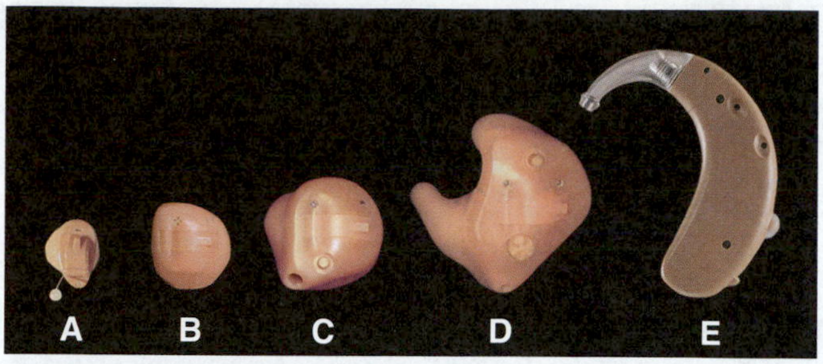

FIG. 22-9 Hearing aids are classified into five basic types. *A,* TRIANO Micro CIC (completely-in-the-canal) hearing aid. *B,* TRIANO ITC (in-the-canal) hearing aid. *C,* TRIANO HS (half shell) hearing aid. *D,* TRIANO ITE (in-the-ear) hearing aid. *E,* TRIANO 3 BTE (behind-the-ear) hearing aid. The TRIANO product family, its fitting philosophy, and its range of accessories were intended to satisfy individuals of all ages, from infants through senior citizens, who have hearing loss. (Image courtesy of Siemens Hearing Solution.)

successful users. The nurse must be prepared to give careful instruction on its use and maintenance and to assist the patient during the period of adjustment.

Initially, use of the hearing aid should be restricted to quiet situations in the home. The patient must first adjust to voices (including the patient's own) and household sounds. The patient should also experiment by increasing and decreasing the volume, as situations require. As adjustment to the increase in sounds and background noise occurs, the patient will be ready to try a different listening environment, such as a small party where several people will be talking simultaneously. Next the environment can be expanded to the outdoors. After adapting to controlled situations, the patient will be ready to encounter environments such as the shopping mall or grocery store. Adjustment to different environments occurs gradually, depending on the individual patient.

When the hearing aid is not being worn, it should be placed in a dry, cool area where it will not be inadvertently damaged or lost. The battery should be disconnected or removed. Battery life averages 1 week, and patients should be advised to purchase only a month's supply at a time. Ear molds should be cleaned weekly or as needed. Toothpicks or pipe cleaners may be used to clear a clogged ear tip.

Speech Reading. *Speech reading,* commonly called *lip reading,* can be helpful in increasing communication. It allows for approximately 40% understanding of the spoken word. The patient is able to use visual cues associated with speech, such as gestures and facial expression, to help clarify the spoken message. In speech reading, many words will look alike to the patient (e.g., rabbit, woman). If the patient wears glasses, the glasses should be used to facilitate speech reading. The nurse can help the patient by using and teaching verbal and nonverbal communication techniques as described in Table 22-19. If a hearing aid is used, it should be readily available to the patient.

Sign Language. *Sign language* is used as a form of communication for deaf people. It is a visual-spatial language that involves gestures and facial features such as eyebrow motion and lip-mouth movements.

Sign language is not universal. American sign language is used in the United States and the English-speaking parts of Canada.

Cochlear Implant. The *cochlear implant* is used as a hearing device for people with severe to profound deafness who get little to no benefit from hearing aids. The implant is an electronic hearing device that stimulates nerves within the inner ear. The system consists of a surgically implanted induction coil beneath the skin behind the ear and an electrode wire placed in the cochlea (Fig. 22-10). The implanted parts interface with an externally worn speech processor. The system stimulates auditory nerve fibers by an electric current so that signals reach the brainstem's auditory nuclei and ultimately the auditory cortex. The implant is intended for the patient whose sensorineural hearing loss is either congenital or acquired. The ideal candidate is one who has become deaf after acquiring speech and language. The adult who was born deaf or became deaf before learning to speak may be considered a candidate for a cochlear implant if she or he has followed an aural/oral educational approach.[34]

The implant offers the profoundly deaf the ability to hear environmental sounds, including speech, at comfortable loudness levels. Multichannel cochlear implants also serve as aids to speech production. Extensive training and rehabilitation are essential to receive maximum benefit from these implants. The positive aspects of a cochlear implant include providing sound to the person who heard none, improving lip reading ability, monitoring the loudness of the person's own speech, improving the sense of security, and decreasing feelings of isolation. With continued research the cochlear implant may offer the possibility of aural rehabilitation for a wider range of hearing-impaired individuals.

The FDA has created an information website on cochlear implants at *www.fda/gov/cdrh/cochlear/index.htm*. The website includes an animated movie to help visualize the implants and how they work.

Assisted Listening Devices. Numerous devices are now available to assist the hearing-impaired person. Direct amplification devices, amplified telephone receivers, alerting systems that flash when activated by sound, an infrared system for amplifying the sound of the television, and a combination FM receiver and hearing aid are all aids that can be explored by the nurse based on patient needs.

TABLE 22-19 Communication with the Hearing-Impaired Patient

Nonverbal Aids
- Draw attention with hand movements.
- Have speaker's face in good light.
- Avoid covering mouth or face with hands.
- Avoid chewing, eating, smoking while talking.
- Maintain eye contact.
- Avoid distracting environments.
- Avoid careless expression that the patient may misinterpret.
- Use touch.
- Move close to better ear.
- Avoid light behind speaker.

Verbal Aids
- Speak normally and slowly.
- Do not overexaggerate facial expressions.
- Do not overenunciate.
- Use simple sentences.
- Rephrase sentence; use different words.
- Write name or difficult words.
- Avoid shouting.
- Speak in normal voice directly into better ear.

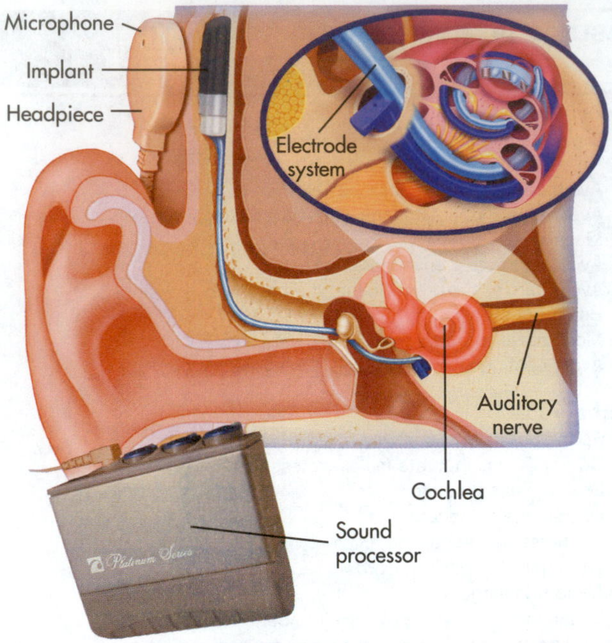

FIG. 22-10 Cochlear implant.

TABLE 22-20 Classification of Presbycusis

Type	Cause	Hearing Change and Prognosis
Sensory	Atrophy of auditory nerve; loss of sensory hair cells	Loss of high-pitched sounds; little effect on speech understanding; good response to sound amplification
Neural	Degenerative changes in cochlea and spinal ganglion	Loss of speech discrimination; amplification alone not sufficient
Metabolic	Atrophy of blood vessels in wall of cochlea with interruption of essential nutrient supply	Uniform loss for all frequencies accompanied by recruitment*; good response to hearing aid
Cochlear	Stiffening of basilar membrane, which interferes with sound transmission in the cochlea	Hearing loss increases from low to high frequencies; speech discrimination affected with higher frequency losses; helped by appropriate forms of amplification

*Abnormally rapid increase in loudness as sound intensity increases.

GERONTOLOGIC CONSIDERATIONS
HEARING LOSS

Presbycusis, hearing loss associated with aging, includes the loss of peripheral auditory sensitivity, a decline in word recognition ability, and associated psychologic and communication issues. Because consonants (high-frequency sounds) are the letters by which spoken words are recognized, the ability of the older person with presbycusis to understand the spoken word is greatly affected. Vowels are heard, but some consonants fall into the high-frequency range and cannot be differentiated. This may lead to confusion and embarrassment because of the difference in what was said and what was heard.

The cause of presbycusis is related to degenerative changes in the inner ear such as loss of hair cells, reduction of blood supply, diminution of endolymph production, decreased basilar membrane flexibility, and loss of neurons in the cochlear nuclei. Noise exposure is thought to be a common factor related to presbycusis. Table 22-20 describes the classification of specific causes and associated hearing changes of presbycusis. Often, more than one type of presbycusis may be present in the same person. The prognosis for hearing depends on the cause of the loss. Sound amplification with the appropriate device is often helpful in improving the understanding of speech. In other situations an audiologic rehabilitation program can be valuable.

The older adult is often reluctant to use a hearing aid for sound amplification. Reasons cited most often include cost, appearance, insufficient knowledge about hearing aids, amplification of competing noise, and unrealistic expectations. Most hearing aids and batteries are small, and neuromuscular changes such as stiff fingers, enlarged joints, and decreased sensory perception often make the care and handling of a hearing aid a difficult and frustrating experience for an older person. Some elderly persons may also tend to accept their losses as part of getting older and believe there is no need for improvement.

CRITICAL THINKING EXERCISE
CASE STUDY

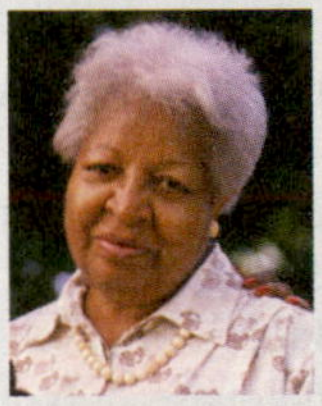

Glaucoma and Diabetic Retinopathy

Patient Profile. Lena Andrews is a 73-year-old African American woman with rheumatoid arthritis and type 2 diabetes mellitus for 20 years with diabetic retinopathy. She returns to the eye clinic for continued evaluation and care of the POAG and reexamination for changes in diabetic retinopathy. Her current medical regimen for POAG includes topical timolol maleate 0.5% extended (Timoptic XE) once daily OU and latanoprost (Xalatan) 0.005% OU hs. At her last examination it was noted that she had microaneurysms and hard exudates of the retina.

Subjective Data

- She can no longer read the newspaper and reports that medication labels are difficult to read.
- States she is not always successful in getting the eyedrops instilled because her hands are gnarled and painful from rheumatoid arthritis.

Objective Data

- Distant and near visual acuity are stable at 20/50 OD and 20/70 OS. This is a reduction from 20/40 OU at her last visit.
- Intraocular pressures are stable at 20 mm Hg OU. There is a new scotoma on visual field testing in the OS.
- Fluorescein angiography reveals diabetic macular edema OU.

Collaborative Care

- Brimonidine (Alphagan) 0.15% OS 15 minutes before and immediately after argon laser trabeculoplasty (ALT)
- Argon laser OU to seal leaking microaneurysms from macular edema

- Postoperative, check intraocular pressure (IOP) 1 hour after ALT
- Continue previous glaucoma drop regimen
- Follow-up examination for glaucoma in 2 weeks for possible ALT OD
- Follow-up examination for diabetic macular edema in 8 weeks

Critical Thinking Questions

1. Explain the etiology of Lena's new scotoma.
2. Why might ALT be an appropriate therapy in this case?
3. What is the purpose of the eyedrops before and immediately after ALT?
4. What topics should the nurse discuss in discharge teaching?
5. What is the etiology of the vision loss from diabetic retinopathy?
6. What should be the priority nursing intervention for Lena?
7. Based on the assessment data, write one or more appropriate nursing diagnoses. Are there any collaborative problems?

NCLEX EXAMINATION REVIEW QUESTIONS

The number of the question corresponds to the same-numbered objective at the beginning of the chapter.

1. Presbyopia occurs in older individuals because
   a. the retina degenerates.
   b. the lens becomes inflexible.
   c. the corneal curvature becomes irregular.
   d. it is associated with cataract development.
2. The most important nursing intervention in patients with epidemic keratoconjunctivitis is
   a. applying patches to the affected eyes.
   b. accurately measuring intraocular pressure.
   c. monitoring near visual acuity every 4 hours.
   d. teaching patient and family members good hygiene techniques.
3. Patients with eye inflammation or an eye infection should be taught
   a. to wear dark glasses to prevent irritation from UV light.
   b. that acute conditions commonly lead to chronic problems.
   c. to apply a cold washcloth with pressure to the inflamed area frequently.
   d. that regular, careful hand washing may prevent the infection from spreading.
4. Rubella can cause hearing problems if
   a. exposure is after 20 weeks of gestation.
   b. exposure is before 16 weeks of gestation.
   c. the mother had rubella before age 18 years.
   d. the mother is vaccinated during the postpartum.
5. In preparing patients for retinal detachment surgery, the nurse should
   a. begin explaining how to care for an ocular prosthesis.
   b. assure patients that they can expect 20/20 vision following surgery.
   c. teach the family how to recognize when the patient is hallucinating.
   d. assess the patient's level of knowledge about retinal detachment and provide information appropriate to the situation.
6. The nurse is teaching an adult patient how to administer antibiotic eardrops. Instructions should include which of the following?
   a. Cool the drops so that they decrease swelling in the canal.
   b. Be careful to avoid touching the tip of the dropper bottle to the ear.
   c. Placement of a cotton wick to assist in administering the drops is not recommended.
   d. Keep the head tilted for 5 to 7 minutes after administering the drops to prevent them from running out of the ear canal.
7. The nurse would suspect otosclerosis from assessment findings of hearing loss in
   a. a 26-year-old woman who has three biologic children under 5 years of age.
   b. a 52-year-old man whose hearing loss is accompanied by vertigo and tinnitus.
   c. a 42-year-old African American woman who has a history of serous otitis media.
   d. a 63-year-old man who can hear high-pitched sounds more effectively than low-pitched sounds.
8. The patient who has a sensorineural hearing loss
   a. has difficulty understanding speech.
   b. experiences clearer sounds with the use of a hearing aid.
   c. may have a reversal of damage caused by ototoxic drugs.
   d. hears low-pitched sounds better than high-pitched sounds.
9. The nurse teaches the patient with extended-wear contact lenses that
   a. the lenses may be moistened with saliva if necessary.
   b. the lenses may be worn for up to 1 week without removal.
   c. any saline solution may be used for moistening as long as it is hypertonic.
   d. the person may continue lens wear if he or she experiences only mild to moderate irritation or redness.
10. The nurse is teaching a patient with a moderate hearing impairment in preparation for hospital discharge. To facilitate communication, the nurse should
    a. use simple sentences.
    b. overenunciate speech.
    c. raise the voice to a higher pitch.
    d. write out all questions and responses.
11. Patients with permanent visual impairment
    a. feel most comfortable with other visually impaired persons.
    b. may feel threatened when others make eye contact during a conversation.
    c. usually need others to speak louder so they can communicate appropriately.
    d. may experience the same grieving process that is associated with other losses.

REFERENCES

1. Thompson JM, et al, editors: *Mosby's clinical nursing,* ed 5, St Louis, 2002, Mosby.
2. Cassin B: *Fundamentals for ophthalmic technical personnel*, Philadelphia, 1995, Saunders.
3. Kanski JJ: *Clinical ophthalmology: a systematic approach*, ed 5, New York, 2003, Butterworth/Heinemann.
4. Chalita M, Krueger R: Correlation of aberrations with visual acuity and symptoms, *Ophthalmol Clin North Am* 17:135, 2004.
5. LASIK for hyperopia, hyperopic astigmatism, and mixed astigmatism: a report by the American Academy of Ophthalmology, *Ophthalmology* 111:1604, 2004.
6. Wilkinson ME: Low vision rehabilitation: a concise overview, *Insight* 28:4, 2003.
7. Brandt JT, Nason FE: Community resources for the ophthalmic practice. In Albert DM, Jakobiec FA, editors: *Principles and practice of ophthalmology: clinical practice,* ed 2, vol 5, Philadelphia, 2000, Saunders.
8. Milligan H: The aetiology of ocular trauma and the ophthalmic nurse's role in its prevention, *Ophthalmic Nurs* 5:4, 2002.

9. Foulks GN: Cornea and external disease, *Ophthalmol Clin North Am* 16:1, 2003.
10. Rietveld R, van Weert HC, ter Riet G, et al: Diagnostic impact of signs and symptoms in acute infectious conjunctivitis: systematic literature search, *BMJ* 327:789, 2003.
11. Ejere H, Alhassan M, Rabiu M: Face washing for preventing active trachoma, *Cochrane Library*, 2005 (#CD003659).
12. Ledgerwood G, D'Arienzo P: Allergic eye disorders: identification and alleviation, *Consultant* 44:785, 2004.
13. Kanski JJ: *Clinical ophthalmology: a synopsis,* New York, 2004, Butterworth/Heinemann.
14. Kohnen T, Koch DD: *Cataract and refractive surgery.* In Krieglstein GK, Weinreb NR, (series editors): *Essentials in ophthalmology,* New York, 2004, Springer.
15. Lee A, Beaver H: Visual loss in the elderly—part I: chronic visual loss, *Clin Geriatr* 11:46, 2003.
16. Snelligen T, et al: Surgical intervention for age-related cataract, *Cochrane Library*, 2005 (#CD001323).
17. Leyland M, Zinicola E: Multifocal vs. monofocal intraocular lenses after cataract extraction, *Cochrane Library*, 2005 (#CD003169).
18. Frank R: Diabetic retinopathy, *N Engl J Med* 350:48, 2004.
19. Wegman-Burns M, et al: Hypertensive retinopathy, *Lancet* 363:456, 2004.
20. Lee A, Beaver H: Visual loss in the elderly—part II: acute visual loss, *Clin Geriatr* 11:41, 2003.
21. Wilkinson C: Interventions for asymptomatic retinal breaks and lattice degeneration for preventing retinal detachment, *Cochrane Library,* 2005, (CD003170).
22. Johns Hopkins University: New strategies for preventing vision loss, *Johns Hopkins Medical Letter* 15:4, 2004.
23. Age-Related Eye Disease Study Research Group: A randomized, placebo-controlled, clinical trial of high-dose supplementation with vitamins C and E, beta-carotene, and zinc for age-related macular degeneration and vision loss, *Arch Ophthalmol* 119:1417, 2001.
24. Kountouras J, Aavos C, Chatzopoulos D: Primary open-angle glaucoma: review article, *Lancet* 363:1711, 2004.
25. Keene WE: Outbreak of *Pseudomonas aeruginosa* infections caused by commercial piercing of upper ear cartilage, *JAMA* 291:901, 2004.
26. Cantrell HF, Lombardy EE, Duncanson FP, et al: Declining susceptibility to neomycin and polymixin B of pathogens recovered in otitis externa clinical trials, *South Med J* 97:465, 2004.
27. Fagan P, Pater N: A hole in the drum: an overview of tympanic membrane perforations, *Aust Fam Physician* 31:707, 2002.
28. Holcomb SS: New guidelines improve treatment of otitis media, *Nurse Pract* 29:6, 2004.
29. Kitahara T, Kondoh K, Morihana T, et al: Surgical management of special cases of intractable Meniere's disease: unilateral cases with intact canals and bilateral cases, *Ann Oto Rhino Laryngol* 11:399, 2004.
30. Flickinger JC, Kondziolka D, Niranjan A, et al: Acoustic neuroma radiosurgery with marginal tumor doses of 12 to 13 Gy, *Int J Rad Onc* 60:225, 2004.
31. Lucas L, Matthews-Flint L: Heed the word about hearing impairment, *Nursing* 33:1, 2003.
32. Duijvestijn JA: Help-seeking behavior of hearing impaired persons aged ≥ 55 years. Effect of complaints, significant others and hearing aid image, *Acta Otolaryngol* 123:846, 2003.
33. Measles, mumps, and rubella—vaccine use and strategies for elimination of measles, rubella, and congenital rubella syndrome and control of mumps: recommendations of the Advisory Committee on Immunization Practices (ACIP), *MMWR* 47:1, 1998. Available at *http://cdc.gov/mmwr/preview/mmwr.html/00053391.htm* (accessed Dec 4, 2004).
34. Morata TC: Chemical exposure as a risk for hearing loss, *Journal of Occupational and Environmental Medicine* 45:676, 2003.

RESOURCES

Alexander Graham Bell Association for the Deaf and Hard of Hearing
202-337-5221 (voice/TTY)
www.agbell.org

American Academy of Audiology
800-AAA-2336 (800-222-2336)
703-790-8466
www.audiology.org

American Academy of Ophthalmology
415-561-8500
www.aao.org

American Foundation for the Blind
212-502-7600
800-AFB-LINE
Email: afbinfo@afb.net
www.afb.org

American Society of Cataract and Refractive Surgery
ASCRS-ASOA
703-591-2220
Email: ascrs@ascrs.org
www.ascrs.org

American Society of Ophthalmic Registered Nurses, Inc.
415-561-8513
www.asorn.org

American Speech-Language-Hearing Association
301-897-5700
800-498-2071 (professionals/students)
800-638-8255 (public)
www.asha.org

Association for Education and Rehabilitation of the Blind and Visually Impaired
703-671-4500
www.aerbvi.org

Ear Foundation
615-627-2724
800-545-HEAR
Email: info@earfoundation.org
www.earfoundation.org

Guide Dogs for the Blind, Inc.
415-499-4000
800-295-4050
www.guidedogs.com

Guide Dog Users, Inc.
301-598-5771
888-858-1008
www.gdui.org

International Hearing Dog, Inc.
303-287-3277
Fax: 303-287-3425
www.ihdi.org

International Hearing Society
734-522-7200
www.ihsinfo.org

National Association for Visually Handicapped
NAVH New York
212-255-2804
www.navh.org

National Association of the Deaf
301-587-1788
301-587-1789 (TTY)
www.nad.org

National Braille Association
585-427-8620
www.nationalbraille.org

National Institute on Deafness and Other Communication Disorders
National Institutes of Health
www.nidcd.nih.gov

Prevent Blindness America
800-331-2020
www.preventblindness.org

Prevention of Blindness Society
202-234-1010
www.youreyes.org

Self-Help for Hard of Hearing People (SHHH)
301-657-2248
301-657-2249 (TTY)
www.shhh.org

Telecommunications for the Deaf
301-589-3006 (TTY)
301-589-3786 (voice)
www.tdi-online.org

For additional Internet resources, see the website for this book at *http://evolve.elsevier.com/Lewis/medsurg.*

Much learning does not teach understanding.

Heraclitus

Nursing Assessment
Integumentary System

23

Barbara Sinni-McKeehen

LEARNING OBJECTIVES

1. Describe the structures and functions of the integumentary system.
2. Describe age-related changes in the integumentary system and differences in assessment findings.
3. Identify the significant subjective and objective data related to the integumentary system that should be obtained from a patient.
4. Describe specific assessments to be made during the physical examination of the skin and appendages.
5. Explain the critical components for describing a lesion.
6. Describe the appropriate techniques used in the physical assessment of the integumentary system.
7. Explain the structural and assessment differences in dark skin color.
8. Differentiate normal from common abnormal findings in a physical assessment of the integumentary system.
9. Describe the purpose, significance of results, and nursing responsibilities related to diagnostic studies of the integumentary system.

KEY TERMS

alopecia, p. 452
apocrine sweat glands, p. 451
dermis, p. 450
eccrine sweat glands, p. 451
epidermis, p. 449
intertriginous, p. 454
keloid, p. 457
keratinocytes, p. 450
melanocytes, p. 449
pruritus, p. 454
sebaceous glands, p. 451

Electronic Resources

Supplemental content related to Chapter 23 can be found . . .

Companion CD

- Stress-Busting Kit for Nursing Students
- NCLEX Examination Review Questions
- Comprehensive Glossary

Evolve Website evolve

http://evolve.elsevier.com/Lewis/medsurg

- Content Updates
- Key Points (Printable and CD/MP3 Download)
- Concept Map Creator
- Expanded Audio Glossary
- Key Term Flash Cards
- Electronic Calculators
- Physical Examination Videos:
  - Head and Face
  - Back and Posterior Chest
  - Feet, Legs, and Hips
- WebLinks

The integumentary system is the largest body organ and is composed of the skin, hair, nails, and glands. The skin is further divided into two layers: the epidermis and dermis. The subcutaneous tissue is immediately under the dermis (Fig. 23-1).

STRUCTURES AND FUNCTIONS OF THE SKIN AND APPENDAGES

Structures

The epidermis is the outermost layer of the skin. The dermis, the second skin layer, contains collagen bundles and supports the nerve and vascular network. The subcutaneous layer is composed primarily of fat and loose connective tissue.

Epidermis. The **epidermis**, the thin avascular superficial layer of the skin, is made up of an outer dead cornified portion that serves as a protective barrier and a deeper, living portion that folds into the dermis. Together these layers measure 0.05 to 0.1 mm in thickness. The epidermis is nourished by blood vessels in the dermis. The epidermis is replaced with new cells every 28 days. The two major types of epidermal cells are the melanocytes (5%) and the keratinocytes (90%).[1]

Melanocytes are contained in the deep, basal layer (stratum germinativum) of the epidermis. They contain melanin, a pigment that gives color to the skin and hair and protects the body from damaging ultraviolet (UV) sunlight. Sunlight and hormones stimulate the melanosome (within the melanocyte) to produce melanin.

Reviewed by Beverly George-Gay, RN, MSN, CCRN, Assistant Professor, Virginia Commonwealth University, Richmond, Va.

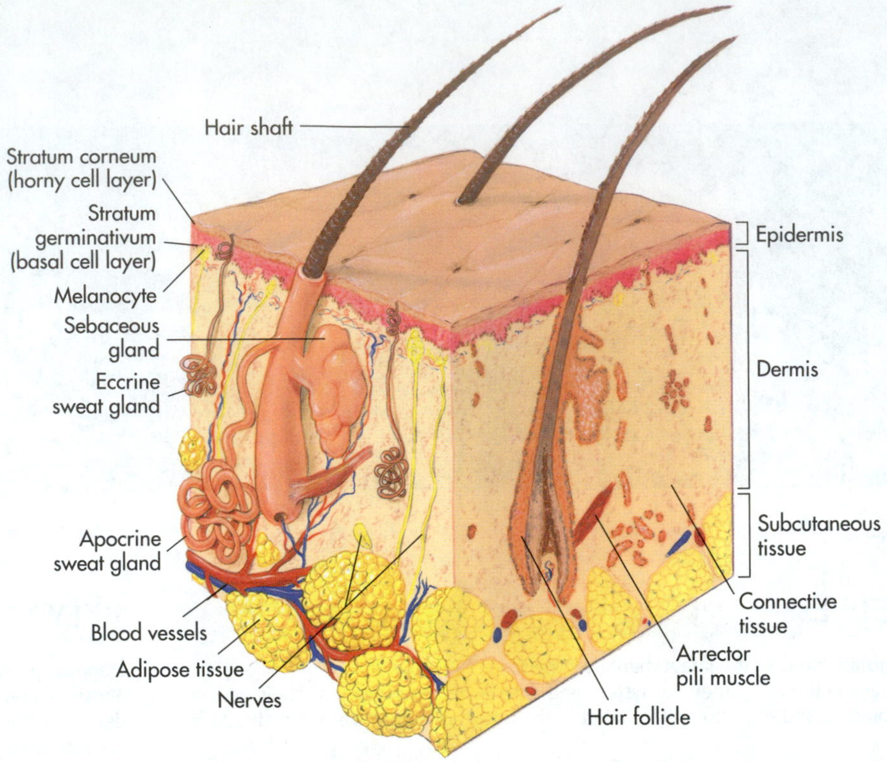

FIG. 23-1 Microscopic view of the skin in longitudinal section.

The wide range of skin color is caused by the amount of melanin produced; more melanin results in darker skin color.[2]

Keratinocytes are synthesized from epidermal cells in the basal layer. Initially these cells are undifferentiated. As they mature (keratinize) they move to the surface where they flatten and die to form the outer skin layer (stratum corneum). Keratinocytes produce a fibrous protein, keratin, which is vital to the protective barrier function of the skin. The upward movement of keratinocytes from the basement membrane to the stratum corneum takes approximately 4 weeks. If dead cells slough off too rapidly, the skin will appear thin and eroded. If new cells form faster than old cells are shed, the skin becomes scaly and thickened. Changes in this cell cycle account for many skin problems, such as psoriasis.

Dermis. The **dermis** is the connective tissue below the epidermis. Dermal thickness varies from 1 to 4 mm. The dermis is highly vascular and assists in body temperature and blood pressure regulation.

The dermis is divided into two layers, an upper thin papillary layer and a deeper, thicker reticular layer. The papillary layer is folded into ridges, or papillae, which extend into the upper epidermal layer. These exposed surface ridges form congenital patterns called fingerprints and footprints. The reticular layer contains collagen and elastic and reticular fibers.

Collagen forms the greatest part of the dermis and is responsible for the mechanical strength of the skin. The primary cell type in the dermis is the *fibroblast.* Fibroblasts produce collagen and elastin fibers and are important in wound healing. Nerves, lymphatic vessels, hair follicles, and sebaceous glands are also found in the dermis.

Subcutaneous Tissue. The subcutaneous tissue lies below the dermis and is not part of the skin. The subcutaneous tissue is often discussed with the skin because it attaches the skin to underlying tissues such as the muscle and bone. The subcutaneous tissue contains loose connective tissue and fat cells that provide insulation. The anatomic distribution of subcutaneous tissue varies according to gender, heredity, age, and nutritional status. This layer also stores lipids, regulates temperature, and provides shock absorption.

Skin Appendages. Appendages of the skin include the hair, nails, and glands (sebaceous, apocrine, and eccrine). These structures develop from the epidermal layer and receive nutrients, electrolytes, and fluids from the dermis. Hair and nails form from specialized keratin that becomes hardened.

Hair grows on most of the body except for the lips, the palms of the hands, and the soles of the feet.[3] The color of the hair is a result of heredity and is determined by the type and amount of melanin in the hair shaft. Hair grows approximately 1 cm per month. On average 100 hairs are lost each day; the rate of growth is not affected by cutting.[2] Baldness results when lost hair is not replaced. This absence of hair may be disease or treatment related or due to heredity, particularly in men.

Nails grow from the matrix. The matrix is commonly called the *lunula,* which is the white crescent-shaped area visible through the nail plate (Fig. 23-2). The nail plate adheres to and is supported by the nail bed. The cuticle is part of the skin that extends a small distance on the nail plate before being shed (like the stratum corneum). Fingernails grow at a rate of 0.7 to 0.84 mm per week, with toenail growth 30% to 50% slower. Nails can be injured by direct trauma. A lost fingernail usually regenerates in 3 to 6 months, whereas a lost toenail may require 12 months or more for regener-

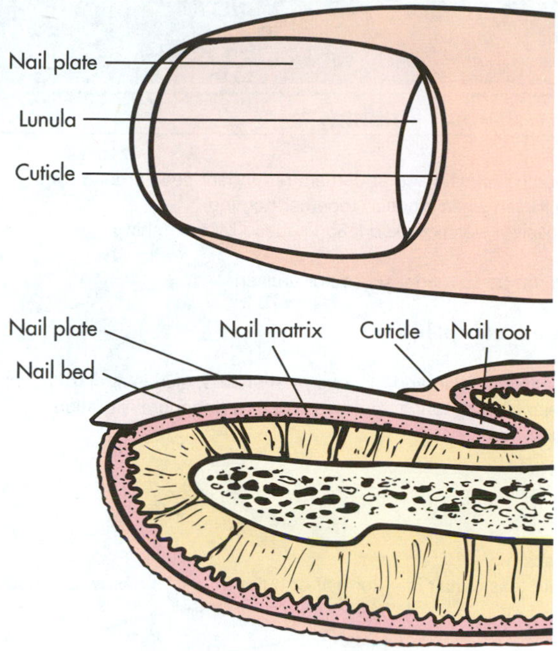

FIG. 23-2 Structure of a nail.

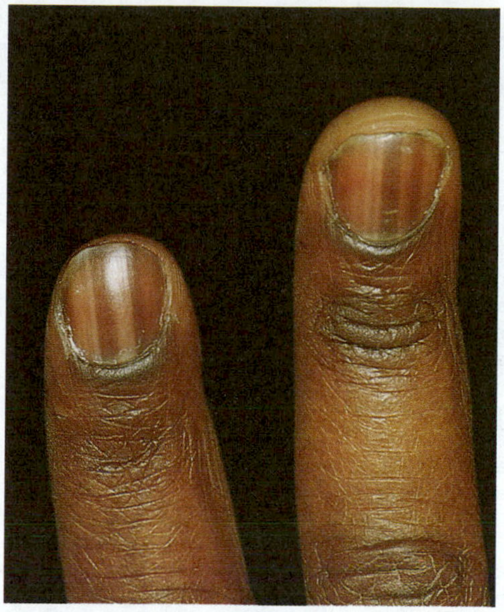

FIG. 23-3 Pigmented nail bed normally seen with dark skin color.

ation. Nail growth may vary according to the person's age and health. Nail color ranges from pink to yellow or brown depending on skin color. Pigmented longitudinal bands (melanonychea striata) may commonly occur in the nail bed in approximately 90% or more of all people with dark skin (Fig. 23-3).

Two major types of glands are associated with the skin: sebaceous and sweat (apocrine and eccrine) glands. The **sebaceous glands** secrete *sebum,* which is emptied into the hair follicles. Sebum prevents the skin and hair from becoming dry. Sebum is somewhat bacteriostatic and consists mainly of lipids. These glands depend on sex hormones, particularly testosterone, to regulate sebum secretion and production. Sebum secretion varies across the life span according to sex hormone levels. Sebaceous glands are present on all areas of the skin except the palms and soles, and are most abundant on the face, scalp, upper chest, and back.

The **apocrine sweat glands** are located in the axillae, breast areolae, umbilical and anogenital areas, external auditory canals, and eyelids. They secrete a thick milky substance of unknown composition that becomes odoriferous when altered by skin surface bacteria. These glands enlarge and become active at puberty because of reproductive hormones.

The **eccrine sweat glands** are widely distributed over the body, except in a few areas, such as the lips. One square inch of skin contains about 3000 of these sweat glands. Sweat is a transparent watery solution composed of salts, ammonia, urea, and other wastes. These glands function to cool the body by evaporation, to excrete waste products through the pores of the skin, and to moisturize surface cells.

Functions of the Integumentary System

The primary function of the skin is to protect the underlying tissues of the body by serving as a surface barrier to the external environment. The skin also acts as a barrier against invasion by bacteria, viruses, and excessive water loss. The fat of the subcutaneous layer insulates the body and provides protection from trauma.

The skin with its nerve endings and special receptors provides sensory perception for environmental stimuli. These highly specialized nerve endings supply information to the brain related to pain, heat and cold, touch, pressure, and vibration. The skin controls heat regulation by responding to changes in internal and external temperature with vasoconstriction or vasodilation. Related to heat regulation is the skin's function of excretion. Between 600 and 900 ml of water is lost daily through insensible perspiration. This function of the skin helps maintain homeostasis through fluid and electrolyte balance. In addition, sebum and sweat are secreted by the skin and lubricate the skin surface. Endogenous synthesis of vitamin D, which is critical to calcium and phosphorus balance, occurs in the epidermis. Vitamin D is synthesized by the action of UV light on vitamin D precursors in epidermal cells.

The esthetic functions of the skin include the expression of various emotions such as anger or embarrassment, as well as displaying the individual identity of a person. The role of absorption at the cutaneous level is well known, and an increasing number of drugs are effectively delivered via patches or creams applied directly to the skin.

GERONTOLOGIC CONSIDERATIONS
EFFECTS OF AGING ON THE INTEGUMENTARY SYSTEM

Many skin changes are associated with aging. Although many changes are not serious except for their cosmetic value, others are more serious and need careful evaluation. Age-related changes of the integumentary system and differences in assessment findings are listed in Table 23-1.

The rate of age-related skin changes is influenced by heredity, a personal history of sun exposure, hygiene practices, nutrition, and general state of health. Skin changes that are related to aging include decreased turgor, thinning, dryness, wrinkling, vascular lesions, increased skin fragility, and benign neoplasms.

The junction between the dermis and the epidermis becomes flattened and the epidermis contains fewer melanocytes. In addition, the dermis loses volume and has fewer blood vessels. Scalp,

TABLE 23-1 GERONTOLOGIC DIFFERENCES IN ASSESSMENT
Integumentary System

Changes	Differences in Assessment Findings
Skin	
• Decreased subcutaneous fat, muscle laxity, degeneration of elastic fibers, collagen stiffening	Increased wrinkling, sagging breasts and abdomen, redundant flesh around eyes, slowness of skin to flatten when pinched together (tenting)
• Decreased extracellular water, surface lipids, and sebaceous gland activity	Dry, flaking skin with possible signs of excoriation caused by scratching
• Decreased activity of apocrine and sebaceous glands	Dry skin with minimal to no perspiration, skin color uneven
• Increased capillary fragility and permeability	Evidence of bruising
• Increased melanocytes in basal layer with pigment accumulation	Solar lentigines on face and back of hands
• Diminished blood supply	Decrease in rosy appearance of skin and mucous membranes; skin is cool to touch; diminished awareness of pain, touch, temperature, and peripheral vibration
• Decreased proliferative capacity	Diminished rate of wound healing
• Decreased immunocompetence	Increase in neoplasms
Hair	
• Decreased melanin and melanocytes	Gray or white hair
• Decreased oil	Dry, coarse hair; scaly scalp
• Decreased density of hair	Thinning and loss of hair; loss of hair in outer half or outer third of eyebrow and back of legs
• Cumulative androgen effect; decreasing estrogen levels	Facial hirsutism; baldness
Nails	
• Decreased peripheral blood supply	Thick, brittle nails with diminished growth
• Increased keratin	Longitudinal ridging
• Decreased circulation	Prolonged return of blood to nails on blanching

pubic, and axillary hair becomes depigmented and thinner. A loss of melanin results in gray or white hair. The nail plate thins and nails become brittle and more prone to splitting and yellowing.

Chronic UV exposure is the major contributor to the photoaging and wrinkling of skin.[4] Sun damage to the skin is cumulative (Fig. 23-4). The wrinkling of sun-exposed areas such as the face is more marked than in sun-shielded areas such as the buttocks. Poor nutrition contributes to aging of the skin resulting from a decreased intake of protein, calories, and vitamins. With aging, collagen fibers stiffen, elastic fibers degenerate, and the amount of subcutaneous tissue decreases. These changes, with the added effects of gravity, lead to wrinkling.

Benign neoplasms related to the aging process can occur on the skin. These growths include seborrheic keratoses, vascular lesions such as cherry angiomas, and skin tags. *Actinic keratoses* appear on areas of chronic sun exposure, especially in the person who has a fair complexion and light eyes (blue, green, or hazel). These premalignant cutaneous lesions place an individual at increased risk for squamous cell and basal cell carcinomas. The photoaged person is more susceptible to skin cancers because there is a decline in the capacity to repair cellular damage (especially DNA) caused by UV exposure. Chronic UV exposure from tanning beds causes the same damage as UV from the sun.

Decreased subcutaneous fat leads to an increased risk of traumatic injury, hypothermia, and skin shearing, which may lead to pressure ulcers. With aging, the apocrine and eccrine sweat glands atrophy, causing dry skin and decreased body odor. The growth rate of the hair and nails decreases as a result of atrophy of the involved structures. Hormonal and vitamin deficiencies can cause dry, thin hair and **alopecia** (partial or complete lack of hair).

The visible effects of aging on the skin and hair may have a profound psychologic effect. A youthful look may be tied to a person's self-image. Although fine wrinkling of the skin, thinning hair, and brittle nails are normal changes with aging, they may result in an altered self-image.[5]

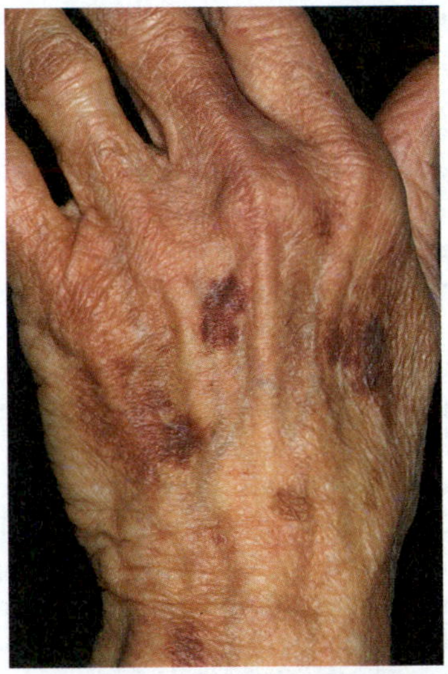

FIG. 23-4 Photoaging. Bleeding occurs with minor injury to the sun-damaged surface of the hand.

ASSESSMENT OF THE INTEGUMENTARY SYSTEM

A general assessment of the skin begins at the initial contact with the patient and continues throughout the examination. Specific areas of the skin are examined during the examination of other body sites unless the chief complaint is that of a dermatologic nature. A general statement about the physical condition of the skin

TABLE 23-2 Normal Physical Assessment of the Integumentary System

Skin	Evenly pigmented and warm; good turgor; no petechiae, purpura, lesions, or excoriations.
Nails	Pink, oval, adhere to nail bed with 160-degree angle.
Hair	Shiny and full; amount and distribution appropriate for age and gender; no flaking of scalp, forehead, or pinna.

should be recorded (Table 23-2), and specific problems should be noted under the appropriate system. In addition, health history questions presented in Table 23-3 should be asked when a skin problem is noted.

Subjective Data

Important Health Information

Past Health History. Past health history will indicate previous trauma, surgery, or prior disease that involves the skin. The nurse should determine if the patient has noticed any dermatologic manifestations of systemic problems such as jaundice (liver disease), delayed wound healing (diabetes mellitus), cyanosis (respiratory disorder), and pallor (anemia). Table 24-10 lists diseases with dermatologic manifestations. Specific information related to food sensitivities, pet or drug allergies, and skin reactions to insect bites and stings should also be obtained. A history of chronic or unprotected exposure to UV light, including tanning bed use and radiation treatments, should be noted.

Medications. The patient should be questioned about skin-related problems that occurred as a result of taking prescription or over-the-counter (OTC) medications. A thorough medication history is important, especially in relation to vitamins, hormones, antibiotics, corticosteroids, and antimetabolites, as these may cause side effects that are manifested in the skin.

The nurse should document the use of prescription or OTC medications used specifically to treat a primary skin problem such as acne or a secondary skin problem such as itching. If a medication is used, the name, length of use, method of application, and effectiveness should be recorded.

Surgery or Other Treatments. It is important to determine if any surgical procedures, including cosmetic surgery, were performed on the skin. If a biopsy was done, the result should be recorded. Any treatments specific for a skin problem, such as phototherapy, or for a health problem, such as radiation therapy, should also be noted. In addition, treatments undergone for primarily cosmetic purposes, such as tanning booth use, laser resurfacing, or cosmetic "peels," should be documented.

Functional Health Patterns

Health Perception–Health Management Pattern. The nurse should ask about the patient's health practices related to the integumentary system, such as self-care habits related to daily hygiene. The frequency of use and sun protection factor (SPF) number of sunscreen products should be documented. Assessment of the use of personal care products (e.g., shampoos, moisturizing agents, cosmetic products), including brand name, quantity, and frequency, should be noted. A description of any current skin problem including onset, symptoms, course, and treatment should be recorded. Medications used for treating hair loss should also be noted.

TABLE 23-3 *HEALTH HISTORY* Integumentary System

Health Perception–Health Management Pattern
- Describe your daily hygiene practices.
- What skin products are you currently using?
- Describe any current skin condition, including onset, course, and treatment (if any).
- Do you have any pets?

Nutritional-Metabolic Pattern
- Describe any changes in the condition of your skin, hair, nails, and mucous membranes.
- Are the conditions related to changes in your diet, including supplemental vitamins and minerals?*
- Have you noticed any recent changes in the way sores or wounds heal?*

Elimination Pattern
- Have you noticed recent changes in your skin related to excessive sweating, dryness, or swelling?

Activity-Exercise Pattern
- Do your leisure activities involve the use of any chemicals that are potentially toxic to the skin?*
- Do you do anything to protect yourself from the sun?

Sleep-Rest Pattern
- Does your skin condition keep you awake or awaken you after you have fallen asleep?

Cognitive-Perceptual Pattern
- Do you have any unusual sensations of heat, cold, or touch?*
- Do you have any pain associated with your skin condition?*
- Do you have any joint pain?*

Self-Perception–Self-Concept Pattern
- How does your skin condition make you feel about yourself?

Role-Relationship Pattern
- Has your skin condition changed your relationships with others?*
- Have you changed your lifestyle because of your skin condition?*
- Are there any environmental skin irritants at your current or previous workplace or home?*

Sexuality-Reproductive Pattern
- Has your skin condition changed your intimate relationships with others?*
- Has your birth control method, if used, caused a skin problem?*

Coping–Stress Tolerance Pattern
- Are you aware of any situation or stressor that changes your skin condition?*
- Do you feel that stress plays a role in your skin condition?*
- How do you handle stress?

Value-Belief Pattern
- Are there any cultural beliefs that influence your thinking or feelings about your skin condition?*
- Are there any treatment options that you would be opposed to using?

*If yes, describe.

Information should be obtained about the family history of any skin diseases, including congenital and familial diseases (e.g., alopecia and psoriasis) and systemic diseases with dermatologic manifestations (e.g., diabetes, thyroid disease, cardiovascular diseases, immune disorders). In addition, a family and personal history of skin cancer, particularly melanoma, should be noted.

Nutritional-Metabolic Pattern. The nurse should question the patient about any changes in the condition of skin, hair, nails, and mucous membranes and whether they are related to dietary changes. A diet history reveals the adequacy of nutrients essential to healthy skin such as vitamins A, D, E, and C; dietary fat; and protein. Food allergies that cause a skin reaction should also be noted. Obese patients should be asked if they have areas of chafing or a rash in **intertriginous** areas, where skin surfaces overlap and rub on each other. Excessive or absent sweating should be noted. Poor or delayed wound healing should also be questioned and recorded.[4]

Elimination Pattern. The patient should be questioned about conditions of the skin such as dehydration, edema, and pruritus, which can indicate alterations in fluid balance. If urinary or fecal incontinence is a problem, the condition of the skin in the anal and perineal areas should be determined.

Activity-Exercise Pattern. Information should be obtained about environmental hazards in relation to hobbies and recreational activities, including exposure to known carcinogens, chemical irritants, and allergens. The patient should be asked if any changes occur in the skin during exercise or other activities.

Sleep-Rest Pattern. The patient should be questioned about disturbances in sleep patterns caused by a skin condition. For example, **pruritus** (itching) can be distressing and cause major alterations in normal sleep patterns. Also, poor sleep and resulting tiredness is often reflected in a patient's face by dark circles under the eyes and a decreased firmness in the facial skin.

Cognitive-Perceptual Pattern. The nurse should ascertain the patient's perception of the sensations of heat, cold, pain, and touch. Discomfort associated with a skin condition should be noted, especially when observed in intact skin. Joint pain related to a patient's skin condition should also be recorded.

Self-Perception–Self-Concept Pattern. Assessment should be made of the feelings related to sadness, anxiety, despair, or altered body image in relation to the patient's skin condition. This can occur with visible skin problems such as acne and psoriasis, which alter a person's physical appearance.

Role-Relationship Pattern. It is important to determine how the patient's skin condition affects relationships with family members, peers, and work associates. The patient should be questioned regarding the effect of environmental factors on the skin such as occupational exposure to irritants, sun, and unusually cold or unhygienic conditions. Contact dermatitis caused by allergies and irritants is a common skin problem associated with occupation.

Sexuality-Reproductive Pattern. The nurse should tactfully question and assess the effect of the patient's skin condition on sexual activity. The nurse should also make note of the reproductive status of the female patient relative to possible therapeutic interventions. For example, isotretinoin (Accutane), used to treat acne, and topical fluorouracil (Efudex, Fluoroplex), used to treat actinic keratoses, are teratogenic drugs that may cause abnormal fetal development. These medications should not be used by pregnant women.

Coping–Stress Tolerance Pattern. It is important for the nurse to assess and question the patient about the role that stress may play in creating or exacerbating the skin condition. The patient should be questioned as to what coping strategies are used to manage the skin condition.

Value-Belief Pattern. The patient should be questioned about cultural or religious beliefs that could influence the perception of self-image as related to the skin condition. Assessment should also be made of values and beliefs that might influence or limit the choice of treatment options.

Objective Data

Physical Examination.

Primary skin lesions develop on previously unaltered skin. The common characteristics of primary skin lesions are shown in Table 23-4. Secondary skin lesions are lesions that change with time or occur because of factors such as scratching or infection. Secondary skin lesions are shown in Table 23-5. General principles when conducting an assessment of the skin are as follows:

1. Have a private examination room of moderate temperature with good lighting; a room with exposure to daylight is preferred.
2. Ensure that the patient is comfortable and in a dressing gown that allows easy access to all skin areas.
3. Be systematic and proceed from head to toe.
4. Compare symmetric parts.
5. Perform a general inspection and then a lesion-specific examination.
6. Use the metric system when taking measurements.
7. Use appropriate terminology and nomenclature when reporting or documenting.

Photographs are useful when accurate findings are needed.

Inspection. The skin is inspected for general color and pigmentation, vascularity, bruising, and the presence of lesions or discolorations. The critical factor in assessment of skin color is change. A skin color that is normal for a particular patient can be a sign of a pathologic condition in another patient. The color of the skin depends on the amount of melanin (brown), carotene (yellow), oxyhemoglobin (red), and reduced hemoglobin (bluish-red) present at a particular time. The most reliable areas in which to assess erythema, cyanosis, pallor, and jaundice are the areas of least pigmentation, such as the sclerae, conjunctivae, nail beds, lips, and buccal mucosa. The true skin color is best observed in photo-protected areas, such as the buttocks. Activity, sun (UV) exposure, emotions, cigarette smoking, and edema, as well as respiratory, renal, cardiovascular, and hepatic disorders, can all directly affect the color of the skin. Table 23-6 describes assessment variations in light- and dark-skinned individuals.

The skin is examined for possible problems related to vascularity, such as areas of bruising, and vascular and purpuric lesions, such as *angioma* (benign tumor of blood or lymph vessels), *petechiae* (tiny purple spots on skin), or *purpura* (bleeding disorder caused by ecchymosis or petechiae). Reaction to direct pressure should be noted. If a lesion blanches on direct pressure and then refills, the redness is due to dilated blood vessels. If the discoloration remains, it is the result of subcutaneous or intradermal bleeding, or the presence of a nonvascular lesion. Any pattern of bruising, for example, in the shape of the hand or fingers or bruises at different stages of resolution should be noted. These may be indications of other health problems or abuse and should be further investigated.

If lesions are found on the skin, the color, size, distribution, location, and shape should be recorded. Skin lesions are usually described in terms related to the lesions' configuration (solitary or pattern in relation to other lesions, Table 23-7) and distribution (arrangement of lesions over an area of skin, Table 23-8).

During systematic inspection it is important to note any unusual odors. Skin sites that contain lesions, such as rashes, that are colonized with yeast or bacteria, as are often found in intertriginous areas (e.g., axillary, overhanging abdominal folds, groin), are often associated with distinctive odors. Tattoos and needle-track marks should be examined and noted for location and the characteristics of the surrounding skin area.

TABLE 23-4 Primary Skin Lesions

Lesion	Description
Macule 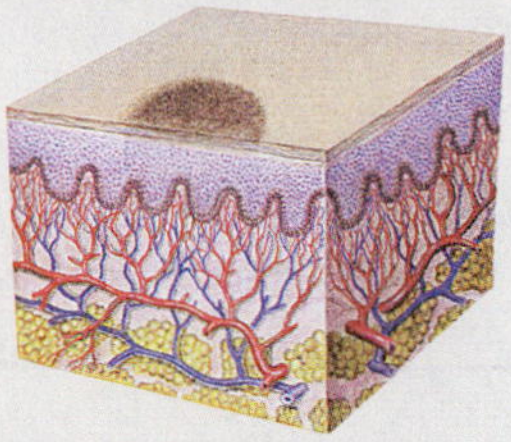	Circumscribed, flat area with a change in skin color; less than 1 cm in diameter *Examples:* freckles, petechiae, measles, flat mole (nevus)
Papule 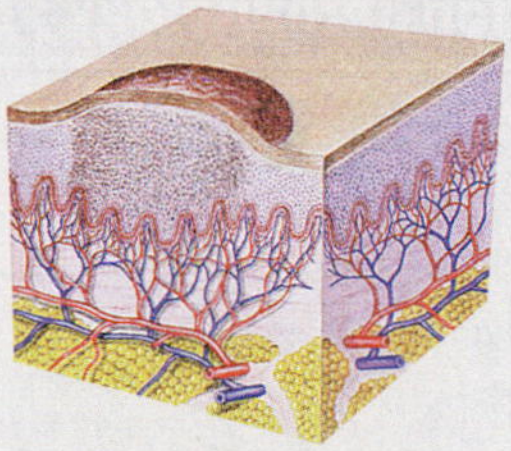	Elevated, solid lesion; less than 1 cm in diameter *Examples:* wart (verruca), elevated moles
Vesicle 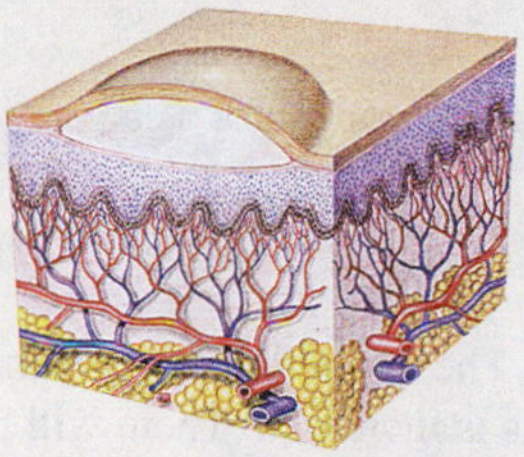	Circumscribed, superficial collection of serous fluid; less than 1 cm in diameter *Examples:* varicella (chickenpox), herpes zoster (shingles), second-degree burn
Plaque 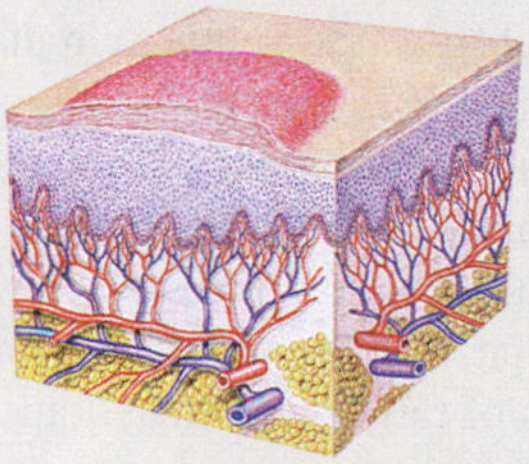	Circumscribed, elevated superficial, solid lesion; greater than 1 cm in diameter *Examples:* psoriasis, seborrheic and active keratoses
Wheal 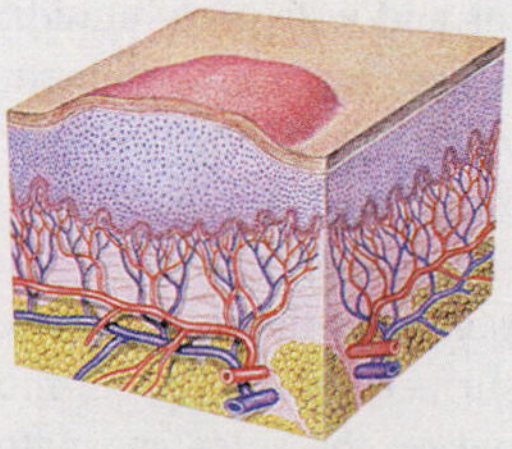	Firm, edematous, irregularly shaped area; diameter variable *Examples:* insect bite, urticaria
Pustule 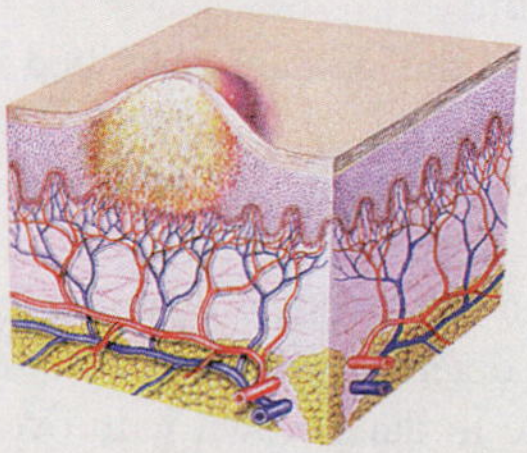	Elevated, superficial lesion filled with purulent fluid *Examples:* acne, impetigo

TABLE 23-5 Secondary Skin Lesions

Lesion	Description
Fissure 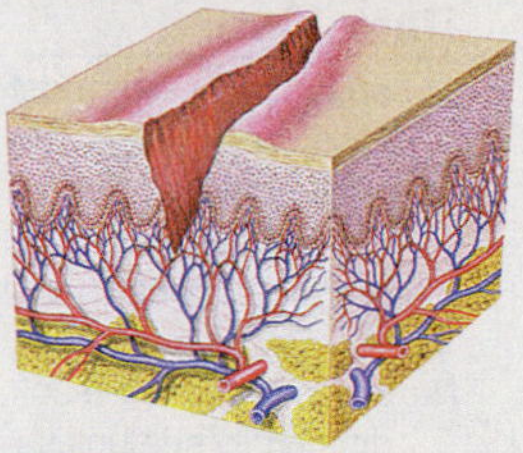	Linear crack or break from the epidermis to dermis; dry or moist *Examples:* athlete's foot, cracks at corner of the mouth
Scale 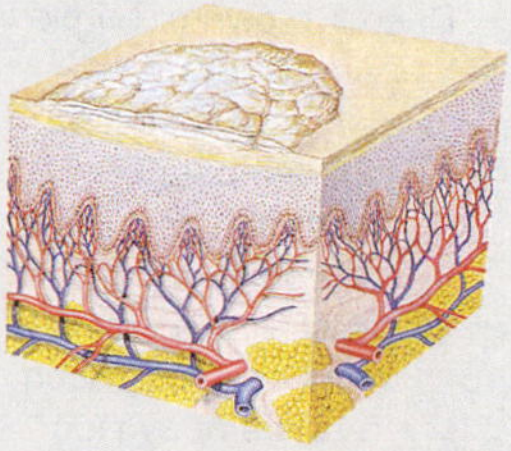	Excess, dead epidermal cells produced by abnormal keratinization and shedding *Examples:* flaking of skin after a drug reaction or scarlet fever
Scar 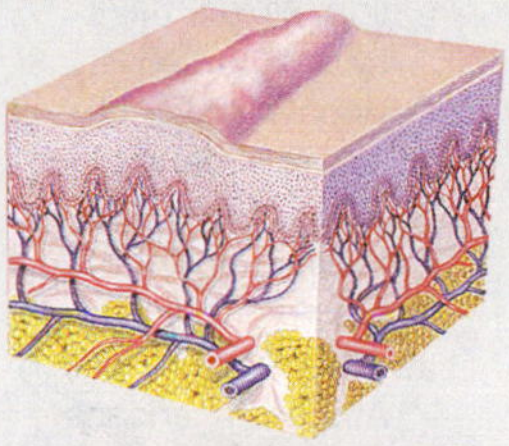	Abnormal formation of connective tissue that replaces normal skin *Examples:* surgical incision or healed wound
Ulcer 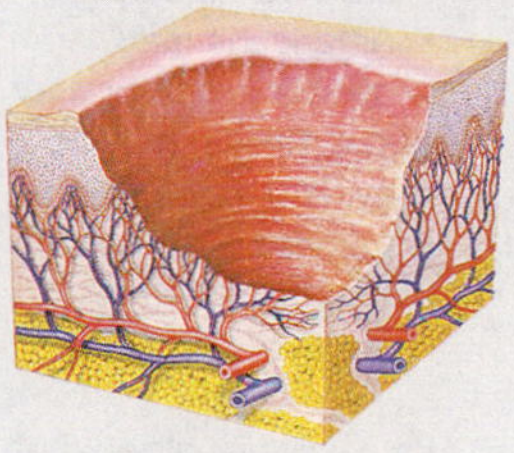	Loss of the epidermis and dermis; crater-like; irregular shape *Examples:* pressure ulcer, chancre
Atrophy 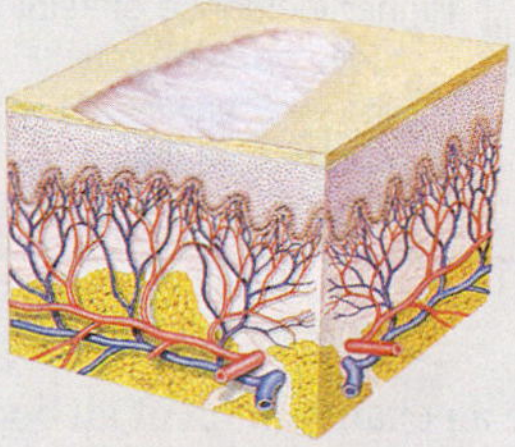	Depression in skin resulting from thinning of the epidermis or dermis *Examples:* aged skin, striae
Excoriation 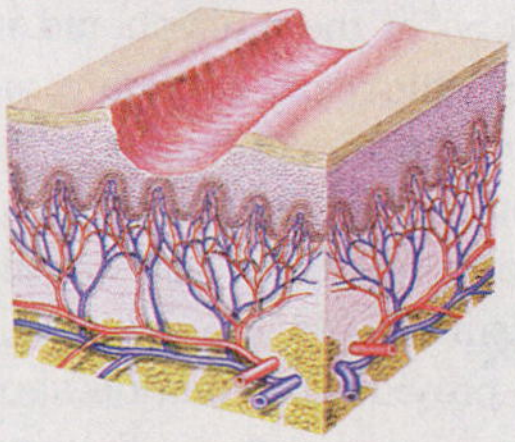	Area in which epidermis is missing, exposing the dermis *Examples:* scabies, abrasion, or scratch

TABLE 23-6 Assessment Variations in Light- and Dark-Skinned Individuals

Clinical Sign	Light Skin	Dark Skin
Cyanosis	Grayish-blue tone, especially in nail beds, earlobes, lips, mucous membranes, and palms and soles of feet	Ashen or gray color most easily seen in the conjunctiva of the eye, mucous membranes, and nail beds
Ecchymosis	Dark red, purple, yellow, or green color, depending on age of bruise	Purple to brownish-black; difficult to see unless occurring in an area of light pigmentation
Erythema	Reddish tone, possibly accompanied by increased skin temperature secondary to localized inflammation	Deeper brown or purple skin tone with evidence of increased skin temperature secondary to inflammation
Jaundice	Yellowish color of skin, sclera, fingernails, palms of hands, and oral mucosa	Yellowish-green color most obviously seen in sclera of eye (do not confuse with yellow eye pigmentation, which may be evident in dark-skinned patients), palms of hands, and soles of feet
Pallor	Pale skin color that may appear white or ashen, also evident on lips, nail beds, and mucous membranes	Underlying red tone in brown or black skin is absent; light-skinned African Americans may have yellowish brown skin; dark-skinned African Americans may appear ashen or gray
Petechiae	Lesions appear as small, reddish-purple pinpoints, best observed on abdomen and buttocks	Difficult to see; may be evident in the buccal mucosa of the mouth or conjunctiva of the eye
Rash	May be visualized, as well as felt with light palpation	Not easily visualized, but may be felt with light palpation
Scar	Generally heals, showing narrow scar line	Higher incidence of keloid development, resulting in a thickened, raised scar (see Fig. 23-5)

Inspection of the hair should include an examination of all body hair. Note the distribution, texture, and quantity of hair. Changes in the normal distribution of body hair and growth may indicate an endocrine or vascular disorder. Inspection of the nails should include a careful examination of nail shape, thickness, curvature, and surface. Any grooves, pitting, ridges, or detachment from nail bed should be noted. Changes in nail smoothness or thickness can occur with anemia, psoriasis, thyroid problems, decreased vascular circulation, and some infectious organisms.

Palpation. The skin is palpated to provide information about temperature, turgor and mobility, moisture, and texture. Temperature of the skin is best assessed by using the backs of the hands. The skin should be warm without being hot. The temperature of the skin increases when blood flow to the dermis is increased. There will be a localized temperature increase with burns and local inflammation. A generalized increase in temperature will result from fever. A decreased body temperature may occur when shock or other circulatory problems, chilling, or emotional distress is present.

TABLE 23-7 Lesion Configuration Terminology

Name	Appearance
Annular	Ring shaped
Gyrate	Spiral shaped
Iris lesions	Concentric rings or "bull's eyes"
Linear	In a line
Nummular, discoid	Coinlike
Polymorphous	Occurring in several forms
Punctate	Marked by points or dots
Serpiginous	Snakelike

TABLE 23-8 Lesion Distribution Terminology

Term	Description
Asymmetric	Unilateral distribution
Confluent	Merging together
Diffuse	Wide distribution
Discrete	Separate from other lesions
Generalized	Diffuse distribution
Grouped	Cluster of lesions
Localized	Limited areas of involvement that are clearly defined
Satellite	Single lesion in close proximity to a large grouping
Solitary	A single lesion
Symmetric	Bilateral distribution
Zosteriform	Bandlike distribution along a dermatome area

Turgor and mobility refer to the elasticity of the skin. The nurse assesses turgor by gently pinching an area of skin under the clavicle or on the back of the hand. Skin with good turgor should move easily when lifted and should immediately return to its original position when released. There is a loss of turgor with dehydration and aging that often causes tenting (Table 23-9).

Moisture of the skin is the dampness or dryness of the skin. Moisture increases in intertriginous areas and with high humidity. The amount of moisture on the skin varies with environmental temperature, muscular activity, body weight, and body temperature. The skin should be intact with no flaking, scaling, or cracking. Skin generally becomes drier with increasing age.

Texture refers to the fineness or coarseness of the skin. The skin should feel smooth and firm with the surface evenly thin in most areas. Thickened callus areas are normal on the soles and palms and relate to weight bearing. Increased thickness is often work related and as a result of excessive pressure.

Common assessment abnormalities of the skin are described in Table 23-9.

Assessment of Dark Skin

A normal range of differences exists in the physical examination of skin, hair, and nails. Genetic factors determine the skin color of the individual and can vary from white to dark brown with overtones of yellow, olive, and red. The darker skin tones result from the reflection of light as it strikes the underlying skin pigment. An

TABLE 23-9 COMMON ASSESSMENT ABNORMALITIES
Integumentary System

Finding	Description	Possible Etiology and Significance
Alopecia	Loss of hair (localized or general)	Heredity, friction, rubbing, traction, trauma, stress, infection, inflammation, chemotherapy, pregnancy, emotional shock, tinea capitis, immunologic factors
Angioma	Tumor consisting of blood or lymph vessels	Normal increase with aging, liver disease, pregnancy, varicose veins
Carotenemia (carotenosis)	Yellow discoloration of skin, no yellowing of sclerae, most noticeable on palms and soles	Vegetables containing carotene (e.g., carrots, squash), hypothyroidism
Comedo (acne lesion)	Enlarged hair follicle plugged with sebum, bacteria, and skin cells; can be open (blackhead) or closed (whitehead)	Heredity, certain drugs, hormonal changes with puberty and pregnancy
Cyanosis	Slightly bluish-gray or dark purple discoloration of the skin and mucous membranes caused by presence of excessive amounts of reduced hemoglobin in capillaries	Cardiorespiratory problems; vasoconstriction, asphyxiation, anemia, leukemia, and malignancies
Cyst	Sac containing fluid or semisolid material	Obstruction of a duct or gland, parasitic infection
Ecchymosis	Large, bruiselike lesion caused by collection of extravascular blood in dermis and subcutaneous tissue	Trauma, bleeding disorders
Erythema	Redness occurring in patches of variable size and shape	Heat, certain drugs, alcohol, ultraviolet rays, any problem that causes dilation of blood vessels to the skin
Hematoma	Extravasation of blood of sufficient size to cause visible swelling	Trauma, bleeding disorders
Hirsutism	Male distribution of hair in women	Abnormality of ovaries or adrenal glands, decrease in estrogen level, familial trait
Hypopigmentation	Congenital or acquired loss of pigment resulting in white, patchy areas	Genetic, chemical agents, nutritional factors, burns, inflammation and infection, vitiligo
Intertrigo	Dermatitis of overlying surfaces of the skin	Moisture, irritation, obesity, may be complicated by *Candida* infection
Jaundice	Yellow (in whites) or yellowish-brown (in African Americans) discoloration of the skin, best observed in the sclera secondary to increased bilirubin in the blood	Liver disease, red blood cell hemolysis; pancreatic cancer, common bile duct obstruction
Keloid	Hypertrophied scar beyond wound margins (see Fig. 23-5)	Predisposition more common in African Americans
Lichenification	Thickening of the skin with accentuated skin markings	Repeated scratching, rubbing, and irritation
Mole (nevus)	Benign overgrowth of melanocytes	Defects of development; excessive numbers and large, irregular moles; often familial
Petechiae	Pinpoint, discrete deposit of blood less than 1 to 2 mm in the extravascular tissues and visible through the skin or mucous membrane	Inflammation, marked dilation, blood vessel trauma, blood dyscrasia that results in bleeding tendencies (e.g., thrombocytopenia)
Telangiectasia	Visibly dilated, superficial, cutaneous small blood vessels, commonly found on face and thighs	Aging, acne, sun exposure, alcohol, liver failure, corticosteroids, radiation, certain systemic diseases, skin tumors
Tenting	Failure of skin to return immediately to normal position after gentle pinching	Aging, dehydration, cachexia
Varicosity	Increased prominence of superficial veins	Interruption of venous return (e.g., from tumor, incompetent valves, inflammation), commonly found on lower legs with aging

increased amount of melanin pigment produced by the melanocytes causes the darker skin color. This increased melanin forms a natural sun shield for dark skin and results in a decreased incidence of skin cancer in these individuals.

The structures of dark skin are no different than those of lighter skin, but they are often more difficult to assess (see Table 23-6). Assessment of color is more easily made in areas where the epidermis is thin and pigmentation is not influenced by sun exposure, such as the lips, mucous membranes, nail beds, and protected areas such as the buttocks. Palmar and plantar surfaces are lighter than other skin areas in darker-skinned individuals. Rashes are often difficult to observe and may need to be palpated. Wrinkling is more apparent in light-skinned individuals than in dark-skinned individuals.[6]

Individuals with dark skin are predisposed to certain skin conditions, including **pseudofolliculitis** (inflammatory response to ingrown hairs that is thought to occur after shaving closely, and is characterized by pustules and papules), **keloid** (overgrowth of collagenous tissue at site of skin injury) (Fig. 23-5), and **mongolian spots** (benign bluish-black macules). Because of the darkness of the skin of some individuals, color often cannot be used as an indicator of systemic conditions (e.g., flushed skin with fever). Cyanosis may be difficult to determine because a normal bluish hue occurs in dark-skinned persons.

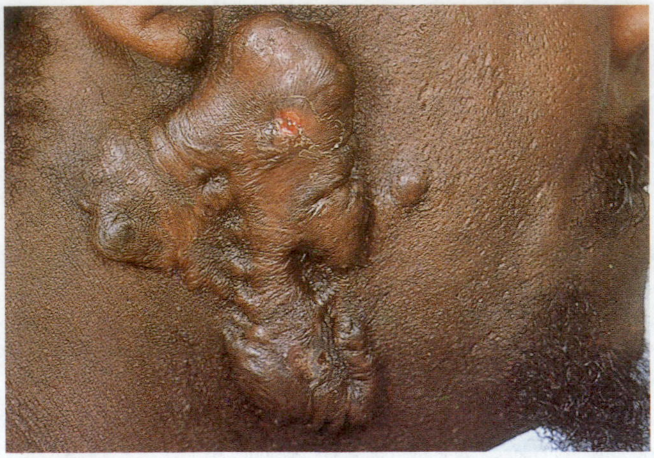

FIG. 23-5 Keloid. Hypertrophic scarring after skin injury, which is more common in dark-skinned individuals.

DIAGNOSTIC STUDIES OF THE INTEGUMENTARY SYSTEM

Diagnostic studies provide important information to the nurse in monitoring the patient's condition and planning appropriate interventions. These studies are considered to be objective data. Table 23-10 contains diagnostic studies common to the integumentary system.

The main diagnostic techniques related to skin problems are inspection of an individual lesion and a careful history related to the problem. If a definitive diagnosis cannot be made by these techniques, additional tests may be indicated.

Biopsy is one of the most common diagnostic tests used in the evaluation of a skin lesion. A biopsy is indicated in all conditions in which a malignancy is suspected or a specific diagnosis is questionable. Techniques include punch, incisional, excisional, and shave biopsies. The method used is related to factors such as the

TABLE 23-10 *DIAGNOSTIC STUDIES* Integumentary System

Study	Description and Purpose	Nursing Responsibility
Biopsy		
Punch	Special punch biopsy instrument of appropriate size used. Instrument rotated to appropriate level to include dermis and some fat. Suturing may or may not be done.	Verify that consent form is signed (if needed). Assist with preparation of site, anesthesia, procedure, and hemostasis. Apply dressing, and give postprocedure instructions to patient. Properly identify specimen.
Excisional	Useful when good cosmetic results and entire removal desired. Skin closed with subcutaneous and skin sutures.	Same as above.
Incisional	Wedge-shaped incision made in lesion too large for excisional biopsy. Useful when larger specimen than shave biopsy is needed.	Same as above.
Shave	Single-edged razor blade used to shave off superficial lesions or small sample of a large lesion. Provides full-thickness specimen of stratum corneum.	Same as above.
Microscopic Tests		
Potassium hydroxide (KOH)	Hair, scales, or nails examined for superficial fungal infection. Specimen is put on a glass slide and 10% to 20% concentration of potassium hydroxide added.	Instruct patient regarding purpose of test. Prepare slide.
Tzanck test (Wright's and Giemsa's stain)	Fluid and cells from vesicles examined. Used to diagnose herpes infections. Specimen put on slide, stained, and examined microscopically.	Inform patient of purpose of test. Use sterile technique for collection of fluid.
Culture	The test identifies fungal, bacterial, and viral organisms. For *fungi,* scraping or swab of skin performed. For *bacteria,* material obtained from intact pustules, bullae, or abscesses. For *viruses,* vesicle/bulla scraped and exudate taken from center of lesion.	Instruct patient regarding purpose and procedure. Properly identify specimen. Follow instructions for storage of specimen if not immediately sent to laboratory.
Mineral oil slides	To check for infestations, scrapings are placed on slide with mineral oil and viewed microscopically.	Instruct patient about purpose of test. Prepare slide.
Immunofluorescent studies	Some cutaneous diseases have specific, abnormal antibody proteins that can be identified by fluorescent studies. Both skin and serum can be examined.	Inform patient about purpose of test. Assist in obtaining specimen.
Miscellaneous		
Wood's lamp (black light)	Examination of skin with long-wave ultraviolet light causes specific substances to fluoresce (e.g., *Pseudomonas* organisms, fungal infections, vitiligo).	Explain purpose of examination. Inform patient it is not painful. Room is darkened for examination.
Patch test	Used to determine whether patient is allergic to any testing material. Small amount of potentially allergenic material applied under occlusion, usually to skin on back.	Explain purpose and procedure to patient. Instruct patient to return in 48 hr for removal of allergens and evaluation. Inform patient if reevaluation is needed at 96 hr.

site of the biopsy, cosmetic result desired, and the type of tissue to be obtained.

Other diagnostic procedures used include stains and cultures for fungal, bacterial, and viral infections. Direct immunofluorescence is a special diagnostic technique used on biopsy specimens and may be indicated in certain conditions such as bullous diseases and systemic lupus erythematosus; indirect immunofluorescence is performed on a sample of blood. Patch testing and photopatch testing may be used in the evaluation of allergic contact dermatitis and photoallergic reactions.[2]

NCLEX EXAMINATION REVIEW QUESTIONS

The number of the question corresponds to the same-numbered objective at the beginning of the chapter.

1. The primary function of the skin is
   a. insulation.
   b. protection.
   c. sensation.
   d. absorption.
2. Age-related changes in the skin include
   a. oily scalp.
   b. a loss of collagen.
   c. thinner, flexible nails.
   d. improved blood supply.
3. When assessing the sleep-rest pattern in relation to the skin, the nurse questions the patient regarding
   a. the presence of dry, flaky skin.
   b. occupational exposure to irritants.
   c. self-care habits related to daily hygiene.
   d. the presence of dark circles under the eyes.
4. During the physical examination of a patient's skin, the nurse would
   a. use a flashlight if the room is poorly lit.
   b. note cool, moist skin as a normal finding.
   c. pinch up a fold of skin to assess for turgor.
   d. perform a lesion-specific examination first and then a general inspection.
5. Skin lesions found by the nurse and described as circumscribed, superficial, elevated, solid, and greater than 1 cm in diameter are called
   a. plaques.
   b. papules.
   c. pustules.
   d. wheals.
6. To assess the skin for temperature and moisture, the most appropriate technique is
   a. palpation.
   b. inspection.
   c. percussion.
   d. auscultation.
7. Individuals with dark skin are more likely to develop
   a. keloids.
   b. wrinkles.
   c. skin rashes.
   d. skin cancer.
8. On inspection of the patient's skin, the nurse notes the complete absence of melanin pigment in patchy areas on the patient's hands. This condition is called
   a. vitiligo.
   b. carotenemia.
   c. telangiectasia.
   d. lichenification.
9. Diagnostic testing is recommended for skin lesions when
   a. a health history cannot be obtained.
   b. a more definitive diagnosis is needed.
   c. percussion reveals an abnormal finding.
   d. treatment with prescribed medication has failed.

REFERENCES

1. Thibodeau GA, Patton KT: *Anatomy and physiology,* ed 6, St Louis, 2007, Mosby.
2. Freedberg I, et al: *Fitzpatrick's dermatology in general medicine,* ed 6, New York, 2003, McGraw-Hill.
3. Thibodeau GA, Patton KT: *Structure and function of the body,* ed 12, St Louis, 2004, Mosby.
4. Hill MJ: *Dermatologic nursing essentials: a core curriculum*, ed 2, New Jersey, 2003, Dermatology Nurses' Association.
5. Jarvis C: *Physical examination and health assessment,* ed 4, Philadelphia, 2004, Saunders.
6. Wilson S, Giddens J: *Health assessment for nursing practice,* ed 3, St Louis, 2005, Mosby.

RESOURCES

Resources for this chapter are listed after Chapter 24 on page 482.
For additional Internet resources, see the website for this book at *http://evolve.elsevier.com/Lewis/medsurg.*

To do the useful thing, to say the courageous thing, to contemplate the beautiful thing, that is enough for one man's life.

Harry S Truman

24 Nursing Management Integumentary Problems

Barbara Sinni-McKeehen and Elise F. Hazzard

LEARNING OBJECTIVES

1. Describe health promotion practices related to the integumentary system.
2. Explain the etiology, clinical manifestations, and nursing and collaborative management of common acute dermatologic problems.
3. Describe the psychologic and physiologic effects of chronic dermatologic conditions.
4. Explain the etiology, clinical manifestations, and collaborative care of malignant dermatologic disorders.
5. Explain the etiology, clinical manifestations, and collaborative care of bacterial, viral, and fungal infections of the integument.
6. Explain the etiology, clinical manifestations, and collaborative care of infestations and insect bites.
7. Explain the etiology, clinical manifestations, and collaborative care of allergic dermatologic disorders.
8. Explain the etiology, clinical manifestations, and collaborative care related to benign dermatologic disorders.
9. Describe the dermatologic manifestations of common systemic diseases.
10. Explain the indications and nursing management related to common cosmetic procedures and skin grafts.

KEY TERMS

actinic keratosis, p. 463
basal cell carcinoma, p. 463
cryosurgery, p. 476
curettage, p. 476
dysplastic nevi, p. 466
lichenification, p. 477
malignant melanoma, p. 465
squamous cell carcinoma, p. 464
sun protection factor (SPF), p. 461

Electronic Resources

Supplemental content related to Chapter 24 can be found . . .

Companion CD

- Stress-Busting Kit for Nursing Students
- NCLEX Examination Review Questions
- Comprehensive Glossary

Evolve Website

http://evolve.elsevier.com/Lewis/medsurg

- Content Updates
- Key Points (Printable and CD/MP3 Download)
- Concept Map Creator
- Expanded Audio Glossary
- Key Term Flash Cards
- Customizable Nursing Care Plan: Chronic Skin Lesions
- Electronic Calculators
- WebLinks

HEALTH PROMOTION

Health promotion practices related to the skin often parallel practices appropriate for general good health. The skin reflects both physical and psychologic well-being. Specific health promotion activities appropriate to good skin health include avoidance of environmental hazards, adequate rest and exercise, proper hygiene and nutrition, and use of self-examination and treatment.

Environmental Hazards

Sun Exposure. Years of exposure to the sun are cumulative and damaging. The ultraviolet (UV) rays of the sun cause degenerative changes in the dermis, resulting in premature aging (e.g., loss of elasticity, thinning, wrinkling, drying of the skin). Prolonged and repeated sun exposure is a major factor in precancerous and cancerous lesions.[1] Actinic keratosis, basal cell carcinoma, squamous cell carcinoma, and malignant melanoma are dermatologic problems that are associated directly or indirectly with sun exposure.

Nurses should be strong advocates of safe sun practices. Specific wavelengths of the sun (Table 24-1) have different effects on the skin. Ultraviolet B (UVB) appears to be the major factor in the development of sunburn and nonmelanoma skin cancer.[2] Ultraviolet A (UVA) contributes to the carcinogenic effects of UVB. Tanning is the skin's response to injury, and is caused by increased

Reviewed by Beverly George-Gay, RN, MSN, CCRN, Assistant Professor, Virginia Commonwealth University, Richmond, Va.

TABLE 24-1 Wavelengths of the Sun and Effects on Skin

Wavelength	Effect
Long (ultraviolet A [UVA])	Can produce elastic tissue damage and actinic skin damage; contributes to formation of skin cancer
Middle (ultraviolet B [UVB])	Causes sunburn and cumulative effect of sun damage; major factor in development of skin cancer
Short (ultraviolet C [UVC])	Does not reach earth; blocked by atmosphere

production of melanin. When sun exposure is excessive, the turnover time of the skin is shortened and results in peeling. Fair-skinned persons should be especially cautious about excessive sun exposure because they have less melanin and thus less natural protection.

Patients should recognize that sun safety guidelines include sun avoidance, especially during the midday hours, protective clothing, and sunscreen. The nurse can also inform the patient about other means of protection from the damaging effects of the sun, such as wearing a large-brimmed hat, sunglasses, and a long-sleeved shirt of a lightly woven fabric or carrying an umbrella. Patients need to know that the rays of the sun are most dangerous between 10 AM and 2 PM standard time or 11 AM and 3 PM daylight saving time, regardless of the latitude. Even on overcast days serious sunburn can occur, because up to 80% of UV rays can penetrate through the clouds. Other factors that increase the possibility of sunburn include being at high altitudes; being in snow, which reflects 85% of the sun's rays; or being in or near water. People should be warned of the dangers of tanning booths and sun lamps, which are predominantly UVA. No presently available sunscreen blocks all UVA.

Sunscreens filter UVA and UVB wavelengths. There are two types of topical sunscreens—chemical and physical. Chemical sunscreens are light creams or lotions designed to absorb or filter UV light, resulting in diminished UV light penetration into the epidermis. Physical sunscreens are thick, opaque, heavy creams that reflect UV radiation. They block all UVA and UVB radiation, as well as all visible light.

The Food and Drug Administration (FDA) has rated popular sunscreen products according to their **sun protection factor (SPF).** This is a method of measuring the effectiveness of a sunscreen in filtering and absorbing UVB radiation. There is no similar rating of products to screen UVA. Patients should be taught to look for the term "broad spectrum" on the packaging that indicates a wide range of absorbance, particularly for UVB wavelengths.

Consumers need to select the sunscreen most appropriate for their needs. Para-aminobenzoic acid (PABA) and PABA esters, cinnamates, salicylates, and methyl anthranilate block UVB rays. PABA has been removed from many sunscreen products because it stains clothing and can cause allergic reactions, including contact dermatitis. Parsol (avobenzone) blocks UVA rays and has been added to most sunscreens. The benzophenones block both UVA and UVB rays.

The general recommendation is that everyone should use a sunscreen with a minimum SPF of 15 daily. Sunscreens with an SPF of 15 or more filter 92% of the UVB rays responsible for erythema and make sunburn unlikely in most individuals when applied appropriately. Sunscreens should be applied 20 to 30 minutes before going outdoors, even in cloudy weather. The SPF value of all sunscreens decreases with time after application and therefore should be reapplied every 2 to 3 hours in a sufficient amount. One ounce per total body application is recommended. The ears, toes, and lips also need sunscreen. Labeling terms such as *water resistant, waterproof,* and *all-day formula* are misleading. All sunscreens should be reapplied immediately after swimming despite the claim of being "waterproof."

Certain topical and systemic medications potentiate the effect of the sun, even with brief exposure. Categories of drug therapy that may contain common photosensitizing medications are listed in Table 24-2. The nurse should be aware that many drugs are included in these categories. The photosensitivity of each individual drug should be examined. The chemicals in these medications absorb light when exposed to natural sunlight and release energy that harms cells and tissues. The clinical manifestations of drug-induced photosensitivity are similar to those of exaggerated sun-

CULTURAL AND ETHNIC HEALTH DISPARITIES

Integumentary Problems

- African Americans and Native Americans have a lower incidence of skin cancer than whites.
- Melanoma can occur in dark-skinned individuals, but often goes unrecognized until the advanced stages.
- Skin assessment may be difficult in individuals with darker skin. The oral mucous membranes and conjunctiva are areas where pallor, cyanosis, and jaundice are more readily detected. The palms of the hands and soles of the feet can also be used for assessment of the skin of darker individuals.
- When darker skin heals following injury or inflammation, it tends to be hypopigmented or hyperpigmented.

TABLE 24-2 *DRUG THERAPY* Drugs That May Cause Photosensitivity

Categories	Examples
Anticancer drugs	methotrexate, vinorelbine (Navelbine)
Antidepressants	amitriptyline (Elavil), clomipramine (Anafranil), doxepin (Sinequan)
Antidysrhythmics	quinidine, amiodarone (Cordarone)
Antihistamines	diphenhydramine (Benadryl), chlorpheniramine, clemastine (Tavist)
Antimicrobials	tetracycline, sulfamethoxazole, azithromycin (Zithromax), ciprofloxacin (Cipro)
Antifungals	griseofulvin, ketoconazole (Nizoral)
Antipsychotics	chlorpromazine (Thorazine), haloperidol (Haldol)
Diuretics	furosemide (Lasix), hydrochlorothiazide (HydroDiuril)
Hypoglycemics	tolbutamide (Orinase), glipizide (Glucotrol), chlorpropamide (Diabinese)
Nonsteroidal antiinflammatory drugs	diclofenac (Voltaren), piroxicam (Feldene), sulindac (Clinoril)

burn. These include swelling, erythema, vesicles, and papular, plaque-like lesions. Skin that is at risk for photosensitivity reactions can be protected by the use of sunscreen products. Nurses have a role in educating patients who are taking these drugs about their photosensitizing effect.

Irritants and Allergens. Patients can seek treatment for irritant or allergic dermatitis, which are two types of contact dermatitis. *Irritant contact dermatitis* is produced by direct chemical injury to the skin. *Allergic contact dermatitis* is an antigen-specific, type IV delayed hypersensitivity response. This response requires sensitization and occurs only in individuals who are predisposed to react to a particular antigen (see Chapter 14).

The nurse should counsel patients to avoid known irritants (e.g., ammonia, harsh detergents). Skin patch testing (application of allergens) can sometimes be helpful in determining the most likely sensitizing agent.[3] Usually the nurse is the first health care provider to detect a contact allergy to various metals, gloves (latex), and adhesives. The nurse must also be aware that prescribed and over-the-counter (OTC) topical and systemic drugs used to treat a variety of conditions may contain fragrances and preservatives that can cause dermatologic reactions.

Radiation. Although most radiology departments are extremely cautious in protecting both themselves and their patients from the effects of excessive radiation, the nurse should help the patient make decisions about radiologic procedures. X-rays can be invaluable in both diagnosis and therapy, but indiscriminate use can cause serious side effects to the skin, including erythema, dry and moist desquamation, edema, and hypo- and hyperpigmentation. In the past (30 years ago), cystic acne was treated with radiation. This information is important for the nurse to obtain because of an increased incidence of basal cell carcinoma for these patients.[2]

Rest and Sleep

Rest and sleep are important health-promotion considerations in relation to the skin. Sleep is restorative. Rest reduces the threshold of itching and the potential skin damage from the resultant scratching.

Exercise

Exercise increases circulation and dilates the blood vessels. In addition to the healthy glow produced by exercise, the psychologic effects can also improve one's appearance and mental outlook. However, caution must be used to avoid or protect from overexposure to heat, cold, and sun during outdoor exercise.

Hygiene

Hygienic practices are influenced by the skin type, lifestyle, and culture of the patient. The normal acidity of the skin and perspiration protect against bacterial overgrowth. Most soaps are alkaline and cause a neutralization of the skin surface and a loss of protection. The use of mild soaps such as Ivory and nonsoap (lipid free) cleansers, as well as avoiding hot water and vigorous scrubbing, can noticeably decrease local irritation and inflammation.

In general, the skin and hair should be washed often enough to remove excess oil and excretions and to prevent odor. Older persons should avoid the use of harsh soaps and shampoos because of the increasing dryness of their skin and scalp. Moisturizers should be used immediately after bath or shower while the skin is still damp to seal in this moisture.

Nutrition

A well-balanced diet adequate in all food groups can produce healthy skin, hair, and nails. Important elements of nutritional skin support include the following:

1. Vitamin A: essential for maintenance of normal cell structure, specifically epithelial cells. It is necessary for normal wound healing. The absence of vitamin A causes dryness of the conjunctiva and poor wound healing.
2. Vitamin B complex: essential for complex metabolic functions. Deficiencies of niacin and pyridoxine (B_6) manifest as dermatologic symptoms such as erythema, bullae, and seborrhea-like lesions.
3. Vitamin C (ascorbic acid): essential for connective tissue formation and normal wound healing. Absence of vitamin C causes symptoms of scurvy, including petechiae, bleeding gums, and purpura.
4. Vitamin K deficiency: essential for synthesizing blood clotting factors. A deficiency interferes with normal prothrombin synthesis in the liver and can lead to bruising.
5. Protein: necessary in amounts adequate for cell growth and maintenance. It is also necessary for normal wound healing.
6. Unsaturated fatty acids: necessary to maintain the function and integrity of cellular and subcellular membranes in tissue metabolism, especially linoleic and arachidonic acids.

Obesity has adverse effects on the skin. The increase in subcutaneous fat can lead to stretching and overheating (see Chapter 41). Overheating secondary to the greater insulation provided by fat causes an increase in sweating, which inflames and dries the skin. Obesity also has an influence on the development of type 2 diabetes mellitus, which may cause skin symptoms such as velvety dark skin of neck and body folds *(acanthosis nigricans),* rash in intertriginous sites *(intertrigo),* skin tags *(acrochordons),* impaired arterial and venous flow, and other skin complications (see Chapter 49). Obesity is also a risk factor for poor wound healing.

Self-Treatment

The nurse must increase the patient's awareness of the dangers of self-diagnosis and treatment. The increasing variety of OTC skin preparations can confuse the consumer.

General instructions that the nurse can discuss with the patient would stress the duration of the treatment and the need to follow package directions closely. Skin problems are generally slow to produce symptoms and slow to resolve. If the package insert of an OTC drug says its use should not exceed 7 days, this warning should be heeded. If the directions say to apply twice daily, the urge to increase the dose and hasten the cure must be avoided. If any systemic signs of inflammation or extension of the skin problem (e.g., an increased number of lesions or increased erythema or swelling) develop, self-care should be stopped and the help of a professional should be enlisted.

Malignant Skin Neoplasms

Cancer of the skin is the most common malignant condition and accounts for 40% of all new cancer diagnoses.[4] The presence of a persistent skin lesion that does not heal is highly suspicious for malignancy and should be examined by a health care provider. Adequate and early treatment can often lead to a highly favorable prognosis. The fact that skin lesions are so visible increases the likelihood of early detection and diagnosis. Patients should be taught to self-examine their skin at least on a monthly basis. The cornerstone of the skin self-examination is the ABCD rule. Examination of skin lesions for ***Asymmetry***, ***Border*** irregularity, ***Color*** change/variation, and ***Diameter*** of 6 mm or more is simple to teach patients and easy to remember. Patients should be aware that lesions once flat and now raised, or once small and recently growing or changing in appearance, should be perceived as warning signs. Many health care providers have now added E to the rule, meaning the lesion is *Evolving* or changing in some way.[5]

Risk Factors

Risk factors for skin malignancies include having a fair skin type (blonde or red hair and blue or green eyes), history of chronic sun exposure, family history of skin cancer, and exposure to tar and systemic arsenicals. Environmental factors that increase the risk of skin malignancies include living near the equator, outdoor occupations, and frequent outdoor recreational activities.[6] Behavioral factors such as professional indoor and outdoor tanning and immunosuppression by smoking are controllable risk factors for skin malignancies. Dark-skinned persons are less susceptible to skin cancer because of the naturally occurring increased melanin, which is an effective sunscreen. However, although dark skin lowers the risk of melanoma, people with dark skin can develop melanoma, most often on the palms, soles, and mucous membranes.

NONMELANOMA SKIN CANCERS

Nonmelanoma skin cancers, either basal cell carcinoma or squamous cell carcinoma, are the most common form of skin cancer. There are more than 1 million new cases yearly in the United States.[6] Nonmelanoma skin cancers do not develop from melanocytes, the skin cells that make melanin, as melanoma skin cancers do. Instead, they are a neoplasm of the epidermis. The most common sites for the development of nonmelanoma skin cancer are in sun-exposed areas and include the face, head, neck, back of the hands, and arms.

Although the number of deaths attributable to nonmelanoma skin cancer is small, the tumors have an inherent potential for severe local destruction, permanent disfigurement, and disability. The most common etiologic factor is sun exposure. Avoidance of exposure to the midday sun and the use of protective clothing and sunscreens beginning early in life can prevent the formation of skin malignancies later in life.[6]

Actinic Keratosis

Actinic keratosis, also known as solar keratosis, consists of hyperkeratotic papules and plaques occurring on sun-exposed areas. Actinic keratosis is a premalignant form of squamous cell carcinoma that affects nearly all of the older white population. It is the most common of all precancerous skin lesions. The clinical appearance of actinic keratosis can be highly varied. The typical lesion is an irregularly shaped, flat, slightly erythematous papule with indistinct borders and an overlying hard keratotic scale or horn (Table 24-3). Many forms of treatment are used, including cryosurgery, fluorouracil (5-FU), surgical removal, tretinoin (Retin-A), imiquimod (Aldara), diclofenac (Solarase), chemical peeling agents, dermabrasion, and laser resurfacing. (These treatments are discussed later in the chapter.) Any lesion that persists should be evaluated for possible biopsy.

EVIDENCE-BASED PRACTICE

Is Retin-A More Effective Than Placebo for Sun-Damaged Skin?

Clinical Question

Is topical tretinoin (Retin-A) (I) more effective than placebo (C) in treating mildly to moderately photodamaged skin (O) on the face and forearms in adults (P)?

Best Available Evidence

Systematic review of randomized controlled trials (RCTs).

Critical Appraisal and Synthesis of Evidence

- Twelve RCTs (n = 1610) found that topical tretinoin cream (0.02% to 0.1%) was superior to placebo.
- Concentrations of less than 0.02% were not effective.
- Treatments lasted 16 to 48 weeks; higher concentrations over longer time showed greater improvement.

Conclusions

- Tretinoin improves the appearance of fine and coarse wrinkles, freckles, and pigmentation associated with overexposure to ultraviolet rays.
- Adverse effects including erythema, scaling/dryness, burning, and stinging may occur in the first few weeks of treatment but decrease with time.

Implications for Nursing

- Tretinoin is an effective and safe method for treating photodamaged skin.
- Greater skin irritation occurs when higher concentrations of tretinoin are applied.
- When using the product, the patient should avoid sun exposure.
- Studies are needed to evaluate the effectiveness of other treatments for photoaged skin including chemical peels, ascorbic acid, hydroxyl acids, and laser (surgical).

Reference for Evidence

Samuel M, Brooke RCC, Hollis S, et al.: Interventions for photodamaged skin, Cochrane Skin Group, *Cochrane Database of Systematic Reviews* 4, 2005.

PICO: P, Patient population of interest; *I*, intervention or area of interest; *C*, comparison of interest or comparison group; *O*, outcome(s) of interest (see p. 6).

Basal Cell Carcinoma

Basal cell carcinoma (BCC) is a locally invasive malignancy arising from epidermal basal cells. It is the most common type of skin cancer and also the least deadly. BCC usually occurs in middle-aged to older adults. Clinical manifestations are described in Table 24-3. The cancerous cells of BCC almost never spread beyond the skin (Fig. 24-1). However, if left untreated, massive tissue destruction may result. Some BCCs are pigmented with curled borders and an opaque appearance and may be misinterpreted as a melanoma. Therefore a tissue biopsy is needed to confirm the diagnosis.

Multiple treatment modalities are used depending on the tumor location and histologic type, history of recurrence, and patient characteristics. Treatment modalities include electrodessication and curettage, excision, cryosurgery, radiation therapy, Mohs' surgery, topical chemotherapy (5-FU or imiquimod), and intralesional α-interferon.[7] (These treatments are discussed later in this chapter.) Electrodessication and curettage, cryosurgery, and excision all have a cure rate of greater than 90% when used correctly on primary lesions. Location and size are important factors in determining the best treatment.

TABLE 24-3 Premalignant and Malignant Conditions of the Skin

Etiology and Pathophysiology	Clinical Manifestations	Treatment and Prognosis
Actinic Keratosis		
Actinic (sun) damage; precursor of squamous cell carcinoma	Flat or elevated, dry, hyperkeratotic scaly papule; possibly flat, rough, or verrucous (wart-like); adherent scale, which returns when removed; often multiple; rough scale on red base; often on erythematous sun-exposed areas; increase in number with age	Cryosurgery, chemical caustics, topical application of 5-FU over entire area for 14-21 days or topical application of imiquimod (Aldara) over 8 or more wks; recurrence possible even with adequate treatment
Dysplastic Nevi		
Morphologically between common acquired nevi and melanoma; may be precursor of cutaneous malignant melanoma	Often larger than 5 mm; irregular border, possibly notched; variegated color mixture of tan, brown, black, red, and pink within single mole; presence of at least one flat portion, often at edge of mole; frequently multiple; uncommon before puberty; most common site on back, but possible in uncommon mole sites such as scalp or buttocks	Marker of increased risk for melanoma; careful monitoring of persons suspected of familial tendency to melanoma or dysplastic nevi; excisional biopsy for suspicious lesions
Basal Cell Carcinoma		
Change in basal cells; no maturation or normal keratinization; continuing division of basal cells and formation of enlarging mass; related to excessive sun exposure, genetic skin type, x-ray radiation, scars, and some types of nevi; basal cells possibly pigmented	*Nodular and ulcerative:* Small, slowly enlarging papule; borders semitranslucent or "pearly," with overlying telangiectasia; erosion, ulceration, and depression of center; normal skin markings lost (see Fig. 24-1) *Superficial:* Erythematous, sharply defined, barely elevated multinodular plaques with varying scaling and crusting; similar to eczema but not pruritic	Excisional surgery, chemosurgery, electrosurgery, cryosurgery; 90% cure rate; slow-growing tumor that invades local tissue; metastasis rare; 5-FU and imiquimod (Aldara) for superficial lesions
Squamous Cell Carcinoma		
Frequent occurrence on previously damaged skin (e.g., from sun, radiation, scar); malignant tumor of squamous (prickle) cell of epidermis; invasion of dermis, surrounding skin; metastasis possible	*Superficial:* Thin, scaly erythematous plaque without invasion into the dermis *Early:* Firm nodules with indistinct borders, scaling and ulceration; opaque *Late:* Covering of lesion with scale or horn from keratinization; most common on sun-exposed areas such as face and hands (see Fig. 24-2)	Surgical removal, cryosurgery, radiation therapy, chemosurgery, Mohs' procedure or microscopically controlled excision, electrodesiccation, and curettage; untreated lesion possibly metastasizes to regional lymph nodes and distant organs; high cure rate with early detection and treatment
Malignant Melanoma		
Neoplastic growth of melanocytes anywhere on skin, eyes, or mucous membranes; classification according to major histologic mode of spread; potential invasion and widespread metastases	Irregular color, surface, and border; variegation of color including red, white, blue, black, gray, brown; flat or elevated; eroded or ulcerated; often under 1 cm in size; most common sites in males are back, then chest; in females are legs, then back (see Fig. 24-3)	Wide surgical excision down to the fascia, and possible sentinal lymph node evaluation depending on the depth; correlation of survival rate with depth of invasion; poor prognosis unless diagnosis and treatment early; spreading by local extension, regional lymphatic vessels, and bloodstream; adjuvant therapy after surgery may be indicated if lesion greater than 1.5 mm in depth
Cutaneous T-Cell Lymphoma (Mycosis Fungoides)		
Origination in skin; chronic, slowly progressing disease, possible etiologies of environmental toxins and chemical exposure	Prevalence is twice as high in men than women in United States; classic presentation involving three stages—patch, plaque, and tumor; history of persistent macular eruption followed by gradual appearance of indurated plaques that appear similar to psoriasis	UVB in patch stage, PUVA, topical nitrogen mustard, radiation therapy, systemic chemotherapy, extracorporeal photopheresis, denileukin diftitox (Ontak); 5-yr life expectancy with only skin manifestations and no treatment; greatly decreased survival rate with generalized erythroderma with exfoliation and abnormal cells in bloodstream (Sézary syndrome)

PUVA, Psoralen ultraviolet A; *UVB,* ultraviolet B.

Squamous Cell Carcinoma

Squamous cell carcinoma (SCC) is a malignant neoplasm of keratinizing epidermal cells (Fig. 24-2). It frequently occurs on sun-exposed skin. SCC is less common than BCC. SCC can be very aggressive, has the potential to metastasize, and may lead to death if not treated early and correctly. Pipe, cigar, and cigarette smoking contribute to the formation of SCC on the mouth and lips.

The clinical manifestations of SCC are described in Table 24-3. A biopsy should always be performed when a lesion is suspected to be SCC. Treatment consists of electrodessication and curettage, excision, radiation therapy, intralesional injection of 5-FU or methotrexate, and Mohs' surgery. There is a high cure rate with early detection and treatment.

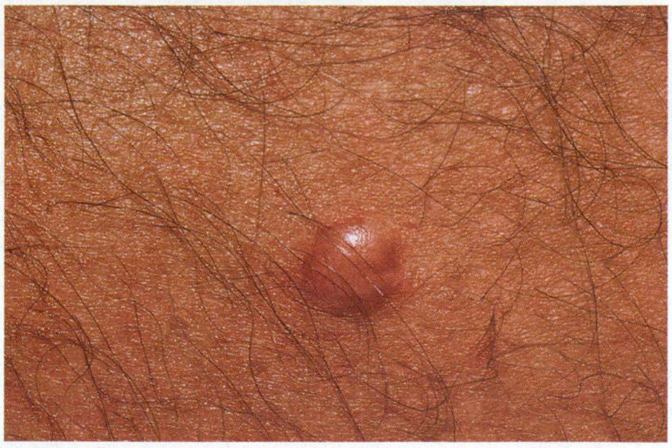

FIG. 24-1 Basal cell carcinoma. Rolled border and central erosion.

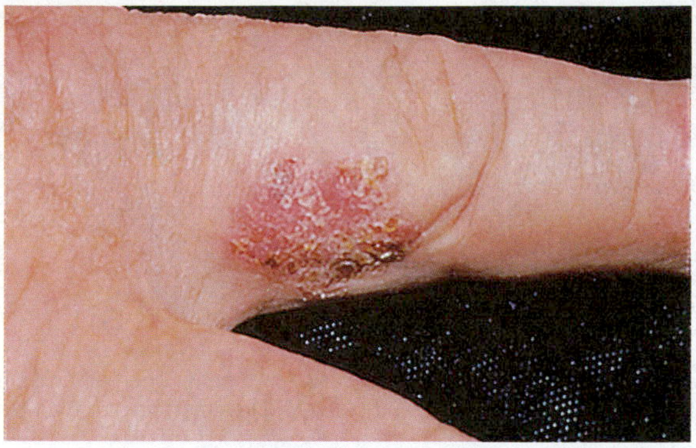

FIG. 24-2 Squamous cell carcinoma of the finger.

EVIDENCE-BASED PRACTICE

What Is the Best Therapy for Basal Cell Carcinoma?

Clinical Question

In adults with basal cell carcinoma (P), is surgery (I), radiation therapy (C_1), or cryotherapy (C_2) more effective in reducing the recurrence at 3 to 5 years (O)?

Best Available Evidence

Systematic review of randomized controlled trials (RCTs).

Critical Appraisal and Synthesis of Evidence

- Only three RCTs were acceptable for comparison: subjects (n = 347) comparing surgery and radiation therapy, subjects (n = 189) comparing surgery, radiation therapy, and cryotherapy.
- Surgery is more effective than radiation therapy; radiation therapy is more effective than cryotherapy.
- Cosmetic results were most favorable with surgery.

Conclusions

- Surgical excision is the recommended treatment based on limited evidence.
- Quality research in this area is very limited. Only low-risk tumors (i.e., superficial and nodular) were consistently studied.

Implications for Nursing Practice

- Provide appropriate educational information, including outcome data on surgery, radiation therapy, and cryotherapy when patients need to make decisions about treatment options.
- More RCTs are needed for evaluating the best therapy for treating basal cell carcinoma, particularly in high-risk populations and for persistent, recurring tumors.

Reference for Evidence

Bath FJ, Bong J, Perkins W, Williams HC: Interventions for basal cell carcinoma of the skin, *Cochrane Database of Systematic Reviews* 2, 2003.

PICO: P, Patient population of interest; *I*, intervention or area of interest; *C*, comparison of interest or comparison group; *O*, outcome(s) of interest (see p. 6).

MALIGNANT MELANOMA

Malignant melanoma is a tumor arising in melanocytes, which are the cells producing melanin. Melanoma has the ability to metastasize to any organ, including the brain and heart. This is the most deadly skin cancer, and its incidence is increasing faster than any other cancer. It accounts for 40,000 deaths a year worldwide. Although it currently accounts for only 4% of all skin cancers, it is responsible for the large majority of skin cancer deaths in the United States.

The exact cause of melanoma is unknown. Risk factors include chronic UV exposure without protection or overexposure to artificial light such as a tanning bed. Persons with fair skin and eyes have less melanin and thus less protection from UV radiation.[8] Genetic factors such as a prior diagnosis of melanoma and having a first-degree relative diagnosed with melanoma increase a person's risk. A mutated gene has been identified in some families who have a high familial incidence of melanoma.[9] Immunosuppression, dysplastic nevi, and exposure to environmental hazards, including herbicides, also increase a person's risk.

Types of Melanoma

The four types of cutaneous melanoma are superficial spreading melanoma (SSM), lentigo malignant melanoma (LMM), acral-lentiginous melanoma (ALM), and nodular melanoma (NM). SSM is the most common type, is the most curable, and often occurs on chronically sun-exposed areas such as the legs and upper back. It frequently arises from a preexisting mole. LMM is commonly located on the face and is often found in elderly patients. Precursor lesions called *lentigines* appear as flat, brown, irregular patches. These patches increase in size for many years before the development of cancer occurs. ALM appears on the soles, palms, mucous membranes, and terminal phalanges. ALM is more common in Asian people and people with dark skin. NM occurs more often in men and can be located anywhere on the body. It is believed to be a more aggressive type of melanoma that develops and invades rapidly. Any of the types of melanoma may be *amelanotic,* or lacking pigment. ALM is the most frequently misdiagnosed melanoma because it may resemble a benign lesion such as a blood blister or polyp, or even a basal cell carcinoma.

Clinical Manifestations

About one third of melanomas occur in existing nevi or moles; about 20% occur in dysplastic nevi (see Table 24-3). Melanoma frequently occurs on the lower legs and backs in women and on the trunk, head, and neck in men. Because most melanoma cells continue to produce melanin, melanoma tumors are often dark brown or black. Individuals should consult their health care provider immediately if their moles or lesions show any of the clinical signs (ABCDs) of melanoma (Fig. 24-3). Any sudden or progressive change or increase in the size, color, or shape of a mole should be evaluated. When melanoma begins in the skin it is called *cutaneous melanoma.* Melanoma can also occur in the eyes, meninges, lymph nodes, digestive tract, and anywhere else in the body where melanocytes are found.

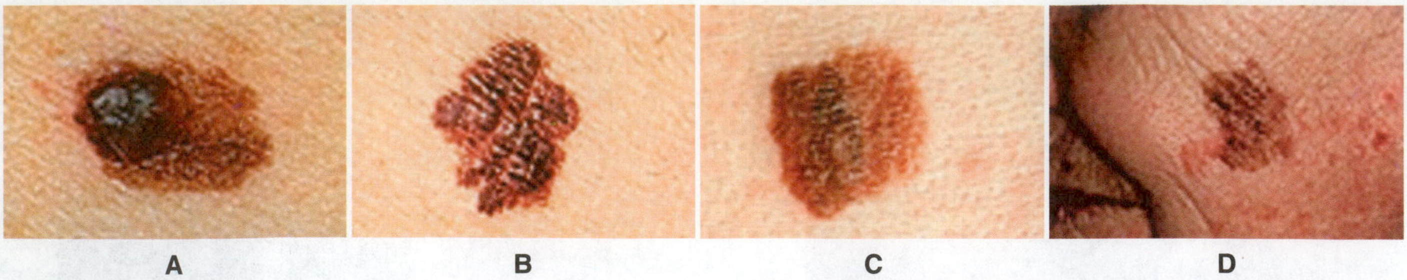

FIG. 24-3 The ABCDs of melanoma. **A,** Asymmetry: one half unlike the other half. **B,** Border irregularity: edges are ragged, notched, or blurred. **C,** Color: varied pigmentation; shades of tan, brown, and black. **D,** Diameter: greater than 6 mm (diameter of a pencil eraser).

Collaborative Care

Pigmented lesions suspected to be melanoma should never be shave-biopsied, shave-excised, or electrocauterized. All suspicious lesions should be biopsied using an excisional biopsy technique. The most important prognostic factor is tumor thickness at the time of diagnosis. Two methods to determine thickness are currently being used. The *Breslow measurement* indicates tumor depth in millimeters, and the *Clark level* indicates the number of skin layers involved (one to five); the higher the number, the deeper the melanoma.

Treatment depends on the site of the original tumor, the stage of the cancer, and the patient's age and general health. The initial treatment of malignant melanoma is surgery. Melanoma that has spread to the lymph nodes or nearby sites usually requires additional therapy such as chemotherapy, biologic therapy (e.g., α-interferon, interleukin-2), and/or radiation therapy. Examples of chemotherapy agents that are used include dacarbazine (DTIC), temozolomide (TMZ), procarbazine (Matulane), carmustine (BCNU), and lomustine (CCNU). Gene and vaccine therapies are currently being examined as additional treatment options (see Chapter 16). Topical immune therapy (imiquimod [Aldara]) is being investigated in the treatment of lentigo malignant melanoma.

The staging of melanoma (stages 0 to IV) is based on tumor size, nodal involvement, and presence of metastasis. In stage 0, the melanoma is confined to one place (in situ) in the epidermis. Melanoma is nearly 100% curable by excision if diagnosed at stage 0. The 5-year survival rate (75% to 95%) in stage I can vary depending on sentinel node biopsy results, which indicate if metastasis has occurred.[10] If spread to regional lymph nodes has occurred (stage III), the patient has a 45% chance of 5-year survival. If metastasis to other organs occurs (stage IV), treatment then becomes mostly palliative.

Dysplastic Nevus

An abnormal nevus pattern called dysplastic nevus syndrome identifies an individual at increased risk of melanoma. Approximately 2% to 8% of the white population has moles classified as dysplastic nevi. **Dysplastic nevi** (DN), or atypical moles, are nevi that are larger than usual (>5 mm across) with irregular borders and various shades of color. These nevi may have the same ABCD characteristics as melanoma, but they are less pronounced. The earliest clinically detectable abnormality associated with DN is an increase in the number of morphologically normal-looking nevi that occurs in children between 2 and 6 years of age. Another proliferation occurs around adolescence, and new nevi continue to appear throughout the person's life. The average number of normal nevi in adults is about 40. Individuals with DN may have over 100 normal-appearing nevi. Obtaining a detailed family history related to melanoma and DN is an important responsibility of the health care provider. The risk of developing melanoma doubles with the presence of one dysplastic nevus, and having multiple DN increases the risk up to twelvefold.

SKIN INFECTIONS AND INFESTATIONS

Bacterial Infections

The skin is covered with numerous microorganisms, especially bacteria. *Staphylococcus aureus* and group A β-hemolytic streptococci are the major types of bacteria responsible for primary and secondary skin infections (Fig. 24-4). The skin provides an ideal environment for bacterial growth with an abundant supply of nutrients, water, and warm temperature.

Bacterial infection occurs when the balance between the host and the microorganisms is altered. This can occur as a primary infection following a break in the skin. It can also occur as a secondary infection to already damaged skin or as a sign of a systemic disease (Table 24-4).

Healthy persons can develop bacterial skin infections. Predisposing factors such as moisture, obesity, skin disease, systemic corticosteroids and antibiotics, and chronic disease such as diabetes mellitus all increase the likelihood of infection (Fig. 24-5). Good hygiene practices and general good health inhibit bacterial infections. If an infection is present, the resulting drainage is infectious. Good skin hygiene and infection control practices are necessary to prevent spread of the infection.

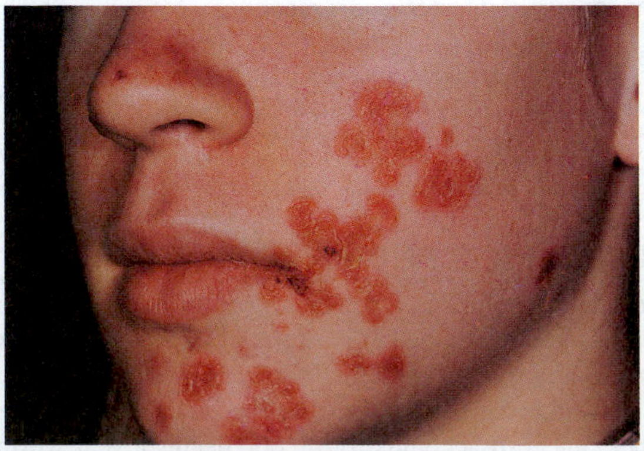

FIG. 24-4 Impetigo. Superficial pustules covered by a thick, honey-yellow colored crust.

TABLE 24-4 Common Bacterial Infections of the Skin

Etiology and Pathophysiology	Clinical Manifestations	Treatment and Prognosis
Impetigo		
Group A β-hemolytic streptococci, staphylococci, or combination of both; associated with poor hygiene and low socioeconomic status; primary or secondary infection; contagious	Vesiculopustular lesions that develop thick, honey-colored crust surrounded by erythema; pruritic; most common on face as primary infection (see Fig. 24-4)	*Systemic antibiotics* Oral penicillin, benzathine penicillin IM, erythromycin *Local treatment* Warm saline or aluminum acetate soaks followed by soap-and-water removal of crusts; topical antibiotic cream (Bactroban); with no treatment, glomerulonephritis possible when streptococcal strain nephritogenic; meticulous hygiene essential
Folliculitis		
Usually staphylococci; present in areas subjected to friction, moisture, rubbing, or oil; increased incidence in patients with diabetes mellitus	Small pustule at hair follicle opening with minimal erythema; development of crusting; most common on scalp, beard, extremities in men; tender to touch	Antistaphylococcal soap (e.g., Hibiclens, Lever 2000, Dial) and water cleansing; topical antibiotics (e.g., Bactroban); warm compresses of water or aluminum acetate solution; healing usually without scarring; if lesions extensive and deep, possible scarring, loss of involved hair follicles, and treatment with systemic antibiotics
Furuncle		
Deep infection with staphylococci around hair follicle, often associated with severe acne or seborrheic dermatitis	Tender erythematous area around hair follicle; draining pus and core of necrotic debris on rupture; most common on face, back of neck, axillae, breasts, buttocks, perineum, thighs; painful	Incision and drainage, packing may be required, antibiotics, meticulous care of involved skin, frequent application of warm, moist compresses
Furunculosis		
Increased incidence in patients who are obese, diabetic, chronically ill, or regularly exposed to moisture, pressure	Lesions as above; malaise, regional adenopathy, elevated body temperature	Warm, moist compresses; systemic antibiotic after culture and sensitivity study of drainage (usually semisynthetic, penicillinase-resistant, oral penicillin such as cloxacillin and oxacillin); measures to reduce surface staphylococci include antimicrobial cream to nares, armpits, and groin and antiseptic to entire skin; often recurrent with scarring; incision and drainage of soft lesions; prevention or correction of predisposing factors; meticulous personal hygiene
Carbuncle		
Multiple, interconnecting furuncles	Many pustules appearing in erythematous area, most common at nape of neck	Treatment same as furuncles; often recurrent despite production of antibodies; healing slow with scar formation
Cellulitis		
Inflammation of subcutaneous tissues; possibly secondary complication or primary infection; often following break in skin; *S. aureus* and streptococci usual causative agents; deep inflammation of subcutaneous tissue from enzymes produced by bacteria	Hot, tender, erythematous, and edematous area with diffuse borders; chills, malaise and fever (see Fig. 24-5)	Moist heat, immobilization and elevation, systemic antibiotic therapy, hospitalization if severe; progression to gangrene possible if untreated
Erysipelas		
Superficial cellulitis primarily involving the dermis; group A β-hemolytic streptococci	Red, hot, sharply demarcated plaque that is indurated and painful; bacteremia possible; most common on face and extremities; toxic signs, such as fever, ↑ white blood cell count, headache, malaise	Systemic antibiotics—usually penicillin; hospitalization often required

IM, Intramuscular.

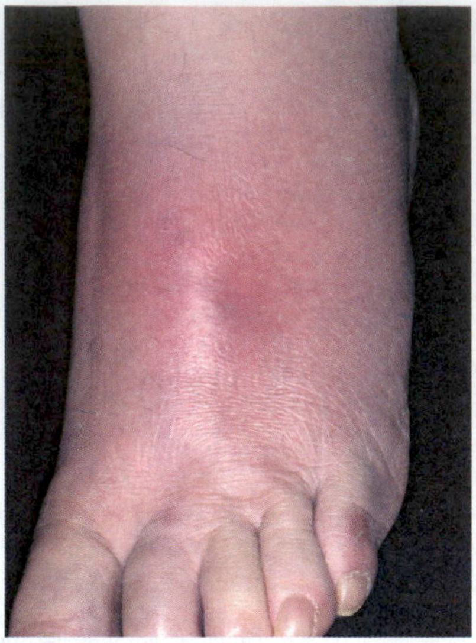

FIG. 24-5 Cellulitis with characteristic erythema, tenderness, and edema.

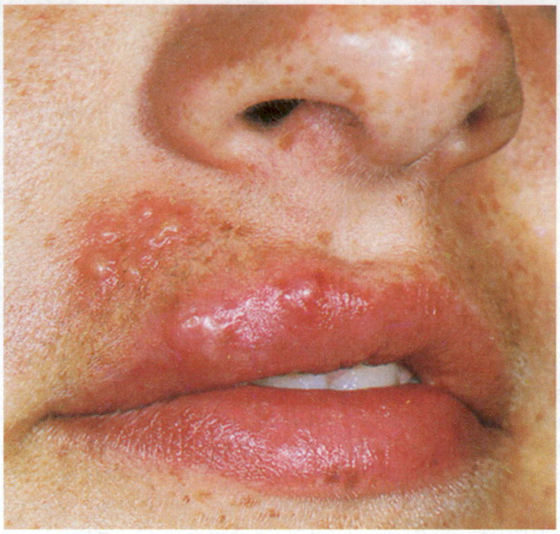

FIG. 24-6 Herpes viral infection on the lips. Typical presentation with vesicles on the lips and extending onto the skin.

TABLE 24-5 Common Viral Infections of the Skin

Etiology and Pathophysiology	Clinical Manifestations	Treatment and Prognosis
Herpes Simplex Virus (HSV) Types 1 and 2		
Oral or genital HSV infections can be serotyped as either HSV1 or HSV2; both are recurrent lifelong viral infections that return to skin and mucous membranes to indicate recurrence when exacerbated by sunlight, trauma, menses, stress, and systemic infection; contagious to those not previously infected; transmission by respiratory droplets or virus-containing fluid, such as saliva or cervical secretions; no protection against subsequent infection in other areas with episodes of infection in one area	**First Episode** Symptoms occurring 3–7 days or more after contact; painful local reaction; single or grouped vesicles on erythematous base; systemic symptoms, such as fever and malaise possible or asymptomatic presentation possible (see Fig. 24-6) **Recurrent** Small; recurrence in similar spot; characteristic grouped vesicles on erythematous base	Symptomatic medication; soothing, moist compresses; white petrolatum to lesions; scarring not usual result; antiviral agents such as acyclovir (Zovirax), famciclovir (Famvir), and valacyclovir (Valtrex)
Herpes Zoster (Shingles)		
Activation of the varicella-zoster virus; frequent occurrence in immunosuppressed patients; potentially contagious to anyone who has not had varicella or who is immunosuppressed	Linear distribution along a dermatome of grouped vesicles on erythematous base; usually unilateral on trunk, face, and lumbosacral areas; burning, pain, and neuralgia preceding outbreak; mild to severe pain during outbreak (see Fig. 24-7)	Symptomatic; antiviral agents such as acyclovir, famciclovir, and valacyclovir; wet compresses, white petrolatum to lesions; analgesia; mild sedation at bedtime; gabapentin (Neurontin) indicated in the treatment of postherpetic neuralgia; usual healing without complications but scarring and postherpetic neuralgia possible; vaccine (Zostavax) to prevent shingles is available in adults ≥60 yr who previously had chickenpox
Verruca Vulgaris		
Caused by HPV; spontaneous disappearance in 1–2 yr possible; mildly contagious by autoinoculation; specific response dependent on body part affected; prevalence greater in youth and immunosuppressed	Circumscribed, hypertrophic, flesh-colored papule limited to epidermis; painful on lateral compression	Multiple treatments, including surgery using blunt dissection with scissors or curette; liquid nitrogen therapy; blistering agent—cantharidin; keratolytic agent—salicylic acid; CO_2 laser destruction
Plantar Warts		
Caused by HPV	Wart on bottom surface of foot, growing inward because of pressure of walking or standing; painful when pressure applied; interrupted skin markings; cone shaped with black dots (thrombosed vessels) when wart removed	Usual treatment is liquid nitrogen or frequent paring followed by application of patches of impregnated chemicals to decrease regrowth; overaggressive destruction possibly resulting in painful, hypertrophic scar

HPV, Human papillomavirus.

Viral Infections

Viral infections of the skin are as difficult to treat as viral infections anywhere in the body. When a virus infects a cell, a skin lesion may develop (Fig. 24-6). Lesions can also result from an inflammatory response to viral infections. Herpes simplex, herpes zoster (Fig. 24-7), and warts are the most common viral infections affecting the skin (Table 24-5).

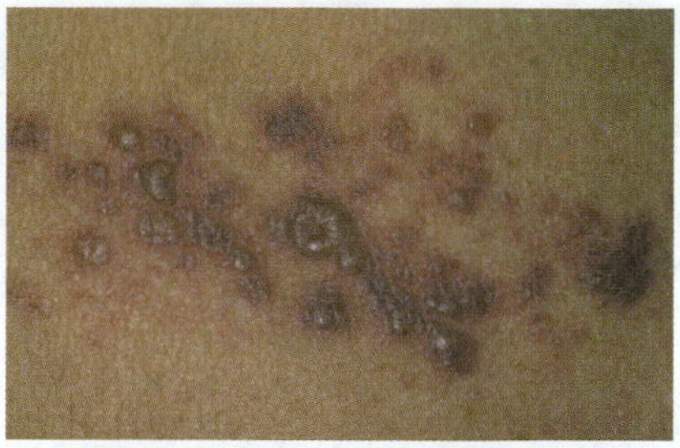

FIG. 24-7 Herpes zoster (shingles) with bullae and vesicles on the anterior chest.

Fungal Infections

Because of the large number of identified fungi, it is almost impossible to avoid exposure to some pathologic varieties in our environment. However, some fungi can cause infections of the skin, hair, and nails, including candidiasis and tinea unguium (Figs. 24-8 and 24-9). Common fungal infections of the skin are presented in Table 24-6.

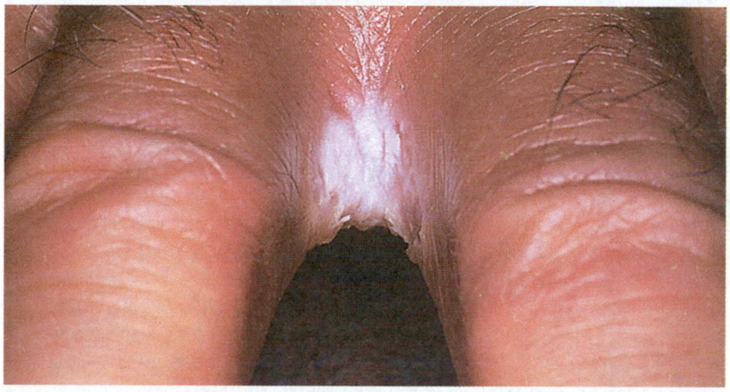

FIG. 24-8 Candidiasis in interdigital cleft. Occurs in workers whose constantly wet hands are not dried often.

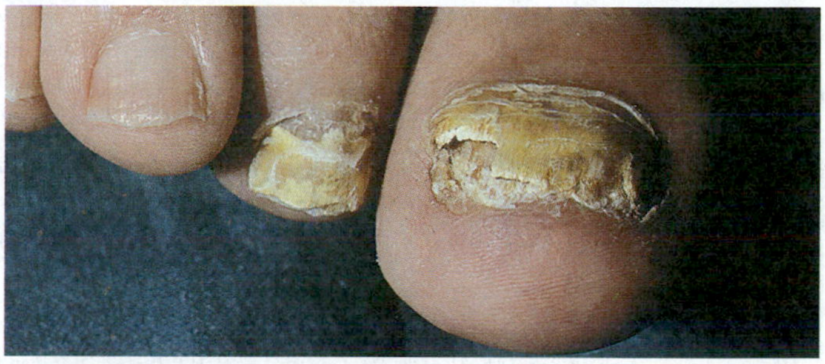

FIG. 24-9 Tinea unguium (onychomycosis). Fungal infection of toenails. Crumbly, discolored, and thickened nails.

TABLE 24-6 Common Fungal Infections of the Skin and Mucous Membranes

Etiology and Pathophysiology	Clinical Manifestations	Treatment and Prognosis
Candidiasis Caused by *Candida albicans;* also known as moniliasis; 50% of adults symptom-free carriers; presenting in warm, moist areas such as groin area, oral mucosa, and submammary folds; HIV infection, chemotherapy, radiation, and organ transplantation related to depression of cell-mediated immunity that allows yeast to become pathogenic	*Mouth* White, cheesy plaque, resembles milk curds *Vagina* Vaginitis with red, edematous, painful vaginal wall, white patches; vaginal discharge; pruritus; pain on urination and intercourse *Skin* Diffuse papular erythematous rash with pinpoint satellite lesions around edges of affected area (see Fig. 24-8)	Microscopic examination and culture; nystatin or other specific medication as vaginal suppository or oral lozenge; abstinence or use of condom; eradication of infection with appropriate medication; skin hygiene to keep it clean and dry; mycostatin powder effective on skin lesions
Tinea Corporis Various dermatophytes, commonly referred to as ringworm	Typical annular (ring-like) scaly appearance, well-defined margins; erythematous	Cool compresses; topical antifungals for isolated patches; creams or solutions of miconazole (Monistat), clotrimazole (Lotrimin), and butenafine (Mentax)
Tinea Cruris Various dermatophytes, commonly referred to as jock itch	Well-defined scaly plaque in groin area; does not affect mucous membranes	Topical antifungal cream or solution
Tinea Pedis Various dermatophytes, commonly referred to as athlete's foot	Interdigital scaling and maceration; scaly plantar surfaces sometimes with erythema and blistering; may be pruritic; possibly painful	Topical antifungal cream, gel, solution, spray, or powder
Tinea Unguium (Onychomycosis) Various dermatophytes; incidence increases with age	Only few nails on one hand may be affected; toenails more commonly affected; scaliness under distal nail plate; brittle, thickened, broken/crumbling nails with yellowish discoloration (see Fig. 24-9)	Topical antifungal cream or solution if unable to tolerate systemic treatment; oral antifungal (terbinafine [Lamisil], itraconazole [Sporanox]); thinning of toenails if needed; nail avulsion (removal) is an option

HIV, Human immunodeficiency virus.

TABLE 24-7 Common Infestations and Insect Bites

Name	Etiology and Pathophysiology	Clinical Manifestations	Treatment and Prognosis
Bees and wasps	*Hymenoptera*	Intense, burning, local pain; swelling and itching; severe hypersensitivity possibly leading to anaphylaxis	Cool compresses; local application of antipruritic lotion; antihistamines if indicated; usually uneventful recovery
Bedbugs	*Cimicidae*; feeding periodic, usually at night; present in furniture, walls during day	Wheal surrounded by vivid flare; firm urticaria transforming into persistent lesion; severe pruritus; often grouped in threes appearing on noncovered parts of body	Bedbug controlled by chlorocyclohexane; lesions usually requiring no treatment; severe itching possibly requiring use of antihistamines or topical corticosteroids
Pediculosis Head lice Body lice Pubic lice	*Pediculus humanus* var. *capitis; Pediculus humanus* var. *corporis; Phthirius pubis;* obligate parasites that suck blood, leave excrement and eggs on skin and hair, live in seams of clothing (if body lice) and in hair as nits; transmission of pubic lice often by sexual contact	Minute, red, noninflammatory; points flush with skin; progression to papular wheal-like lesions; pruritus; secondary excoriation, especially parallel linear excoriations in intrascapular region; firmly attached to hair shaft in head and body lice	γ-Benzene hexachloride or pyrethrins to treat various parts of body; application as directed; contact screening with bed partners, playmates, shared head gear
Scabies	*Sarcoptes scabiei;* mite penetrates stratum corneum, deposits eggs; allergic reaction resulting from presence of eggs, feces, mite parts; transmission by direct physical contact, only occasionally by shared personal items; rarely seen in dark-skinned people	Severe itching, especially at night, usually not on face; presence of burrows, especially in interdigital webs, flexor surface of wrists, genitals, and anterior axillary folds; erythematous papules (may be crusted), possible vesiculation, interdigital web crusting (see Fig. 24-10)	5% permethrin topical lotion, one overnight application with second application 1 wk later may yield 95% eradication; treat environment with plastic covering for 5 days, launder all clothes and linen with bleach; treat sexual partner; antibiotics if secondary infections present; possible residual pruritus up to 4 wk after treatment; recurrence possible if inadequately treated
Ticks	*Borrelia burgdorferi* (spirochete transmitted by ticks in certain areas) causes Lyme disease; endemic areas that include Northeast, Mid-Atlantic states, parts of Midwest and West (see Chapter 65)	Spreading, ring-like rash 3-4 wk after bite; rash commonly in groin, buttocks, axillae, trunk, and upper arms and legs; warm, itchy, or painful rash; flu-like symptoms; cardiac, arthritic, and neurologic manifestations possible; unreliable laboratory test; no acquired immunity	Oral antibiotics, such as doxycycline, tetracycline; intravenous antibiotics for arthritic, neurologic, and cardiac symptoms; rest and healthy diet; most patients recover

Microscopic examination of the scraping of suspicious skin lesions in 10% to 20% potassium hydroxide (KOH) is an easy, inexpensive diagnostic measure to determine the presence of a fungus. The appearance of microscopic hyphae (threadlike structures) is indicative of a fungal infection.[11]

***Drug Alert** - Isotretinoin (Accutane)*
- *Can cause serious damage to fetus.*
- *Should not donate blood while taking drug or for 1 month following treatment.*
- *Contraindicated in women who are pregnant or who are intending to become pregnant while on the drug.*

Infestations and Insect Bites

The possibilities for exposure to *infestations* (harboring insects or worms) and insect bites are numerous. In many instances, an allergy to the venom plays a major role in the reaction. In other cases, the clinical manifestations are a reaction to the eggs, feces, or body parts of the invading organism (Fig. 24-10). Some individuals react with a severe hypersensitivity (anaphylaxis), which can be life threatening. (Anaphylaxis is discussed in Chapter 14.)

Prevention of insect bites by avoidance or by the use of repellents is somewhat effective. Meticulous hygiene related to personal articles, clothing, bedding, and examination and care of pets, as well as careful selection of sexual partners, can reduce the incidence of infestations. Routine inspection is necessary in geographic areas where there is a risk of tick bites and the resulting Lyme disease (Table 24-7).

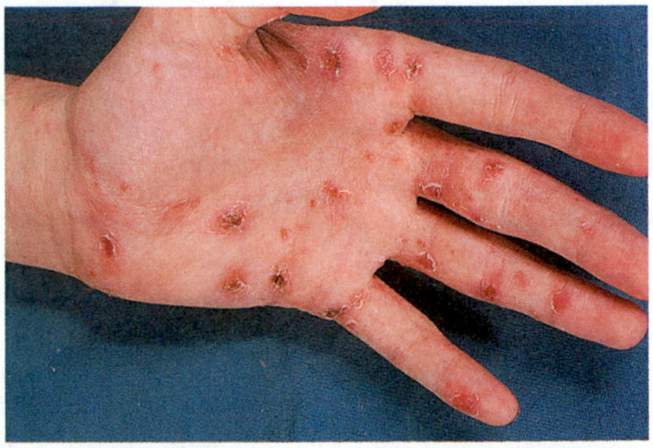

FIG. 24-10 Scabies infestation on hand.

ALLERGIC DERMATOLOGIC PROBLEMS

Dermatologic problems associated with allergies and hypersensitivity reactions may present a challenge to the clinician (Table 24-8). The pathophysiology related to allergic and contact dermatitis is discussed in Chapter 14. A careful family history and discussion of exposure to possible offending agents provide valuable data. Patch testing involves the application of allergens to the patient's skin (usually on the back) for 48 hours with reevaluation at 96 hours; test sites are examined for erythema, papules, vesicles, or all of these. Patch testing is used to aid in determining possible causative agents. The best treatment of allergic dermatitis is avoidance of the causative agent. The extreme pruritus of contact dermatitis and its potential for chronic-

TABLE 24-8 Common Allergic Conditions of the Skin

Etiology and Pathophysiology	Clinical Manifestations	Treatment and Prognosis
Allergic Contact Dermatitis		
Manifestation of delayed hypersensitivity, absorbed agent acting as antigen, sensitization after several exposures, appearance of lesions 2-7 days after contact with allergen	Red papules and plaques; sharply circumscribed with occasional vesicles; usually pruritic; area of dermatitis frequently takes shape of causative agent (e.g., metal allergy and band-like dermatitis on ring finger) (see Fig. 14-13)	Topical corticosteroids, antihistamines; skin lubrication; elimination of contact allergen; avoidance of irritating affected area; systemic corticosteroids if sensitivity severe
Urticaria		
Usually allergic phenomenon; presence of erythema and edema in upper dermis resulting from a local increase in permeability of capillaries (usually from histamine response)	Spontaneously occurring and rounded or arcinate elevations, varying size, usually multiple; a single lesion usually resolves in 24 hr	Removal of source, if known; antihistamine therapy, cool compresses, possibly systemic corticosteroids
Drug Reaction		
Any drug that acts as antigen and causes hypersensitivity reaction is possible cause; certain drugs more prone to reactions (e.g., penicillin)	Rash of any morphology; often red, macular and papular, semiconfluent, generalized rash with abrupt onset; appearance as late as 14 days after cessation of drug; possibly pruritic	Withdrawal of drug if possible; antihistamines, local or systemic corticosteroids possibly necessary
Atopic Dermatitis		
Genetically influenced, chronic, relapsing disease associated with immunologic irregularity involving inflammatory mediators, exaggerated by a cutaneous response to environmental allergens; associated with allergic rhinitis and asthma; most severe in childhood	Multiple presentations include acute, subacute, and chronic stages; all are pruritic; acute stage with bright erythema, oozing vesicles, with extreme pruritus; subacute phase with scaly, light red to red-brown plaques; chronic stage has thickened skin with accentuation of skin markings (lichenification), possible hyperpigmentation; dry skin; common in antecubital and popliteal space in adults	Lubrication of dry (xerotic) skin, topical immunomodulators (pimecrolimus [Elidel], tacrolimus [Protopic]); topical corticosteroids, systemic corticosteroids if severe, phototherapy for relapses; reduction of stress reduces flares; antibiotics for secondary infection as needed

ity make it a frustrating problem for the patient, nurse, and dermatologist, especially if the offending agent cannot be identified.

BENIGN DERMATOLOGIC PROBLEMS

Although the list of benign dermatoses is extensive, some of the most commonly seen and distressing problems are summarized in Table 24-9. Psoriasis is a common benign disorder that currently affects 5.5 million people in the United States.[12] The chronicity of psoriasis can be severe and disabling as people withdraw from social contacts because of visible lesions (Fig. 24-11).

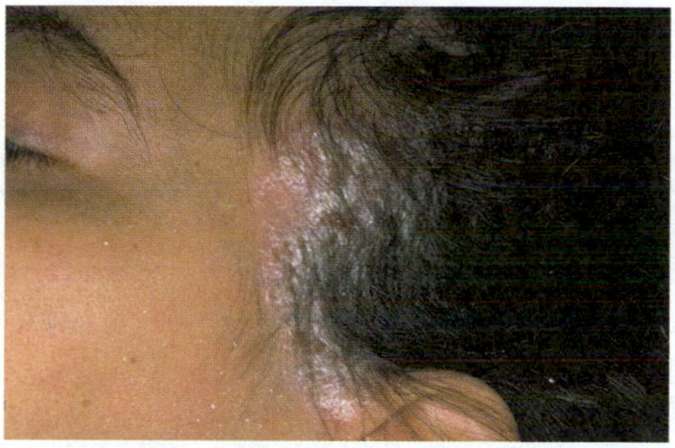

FIG. 24-11 Psoriasis on the scalp.

DISEASES WITH DERMATOLOGIC MANIFESTATIONS

Dermatologic manifestations of various diseases are listed in Table 24-10. The health care provider should always consider the possibility that a particular dermatosis is a clue to an internal, less obvious problem.

Certain life changes have recognized associated dermatoses. At puberty, male- or female-pattern hair growth will be evident as a secondary sex characteristic. Increased apocrine gland activity can lead to body odor. The increased sebaceous gland activity stimulated by androgens can result in seborrhea and acne.

COLLABORATIVE CARE: DERMATOLOGIC PROBLEMS

Diagnostic Studies

A careful history is of prime importance in the diagnosis of skin problems. The clinician must be skilled at detecting any evidence that could lead to the etiology of the extraordinary number of skin diseases/conditions. After a careful history and physical examination, individual lesions are inspected. On the basis of the history, physical examination, and appropriate diagnostic tests, either medical, surgical, or combination therapy is planned.

Collaborative Therapy

Many different treatment methods are used in dermatology. Advances in this field have brought relief to many previously chronic, untreatable conditions. Many of the specific therapeutic treatments require specialized equipment and are usually reserved for use by the dermatologist. Many clinicians prescribe drug therapy. The effectiveness of this therapy can often be related to the base (or vehicle) in which the medication is prepared, if topical. Table 24-11 summarizes the common agents used as bases for topical preparations and their therapeutic considerations.

TABLE 24-9 Common Benign Conditions of the Skin

Etiology and Pathophysiology	Clinical Manifestations	Treatment and Prognosis
Acne		
Inflammatory disorder of sebaceous glands; more common in teenagers but possible development and persistence in adulthood; flare can occur before menses, with use of corticosteroids, and androgen-dominant birth control pills	Noninflammatory lesions, including open comedones (blackheads) and closed comedones (whiteheads); inflammatory lesions, including papules and pustules; most common on face, neck, and upper back	Mechanical removal of multiple lesions with comedo extractor; topical benzoyl peroxide or other antimicrobial; topical retinoids, systemic antibiotics; aim of treatment to suppress new lesions and minimize scarring; spontaneous remission possible; often improvement with exposure to sun Use of isotretinoin (Accutane) for severe nodulocystic acne to possibly provide lasting remission; contraindicated in pregnant women or women intending to become pregnant while on drug; monitoring of liver function and pregnancy tests, cholesterol, and triglycerides essential
Nevi (Moles)		
Grouping of normal cells derived from melanocyte-like precursor cells	Hyperpigmented areas that vary in form and color; flat, slightly elevated, haloid, verrucoid, polypoid, dome-shaped, sessile, or papillomatous; preservation of normal skin markings; hair growth possible	No treatment necessary except for cosmetic reasons; skin biopsy for diagnosis
Psoriasis		
Chronic dermatitis that involves excessively rapid turnover of epidermal cells; family predisposition	Sharply demarcated silvery scaling plaques commonly on the scalp, elbows, knees; palms, soles, and fingernails possibly affected; localized or general, intermittent or continuous (see Fig. 24-11)	Goal is to reduce inflammation and suppress rapid turnover of epidermal cells; topical treatment may be time consuming; usually topical corticosteroids, tar, anthralin; intralesional injection of corticosteroids for chronic plaques; sunlight; UV light; alone or with topical or systemic potentiation (psoralen) and clobetasol propionate 0.05% spray (Clobex); systemic treatments: antimetabolite (methotrexate), immunosuppressant (cyclosporine), retinoid (acitretin), IV or IM administered immunosuppressant (alefacept [Amevive]) for moderate to severe disease; infliximab (Remicade) for severe plaque form of disease; no cure, but control is possible
Seborrheic Keratoses		
Benign, genetically determined superficial growths; found in increasing number with age	Irregularly round or oval, flat-topped papules or plaques; surface often verrucous; well-defined shape, appearance of being stuck on; increase in pigmentation with age of lesion; usually multiple and possibly itchy	Removal by curettage or cryosurgery for cosmetic reasons or to eliminate source of irritation; minimal scarring
Acrochordons (Skin Tags)		
Common after midlife; appearance on neck, axillae, and upper trunk secondary to mechanical friction or redundant skin (associated with obesity)	Small, skin-colored, soft, pedunculated papules; may become irritated	No treatment medically unless for sites of repeated trauma or cosmetic reasons; surgical removal possible; usually just "clipping off" without anesthesia
Lipoma		
Benign tumor of adipose tissue, often encapsulated, most common in 40- to 60-year-old age group	Rubbery, compressible, round mass of adipose tissue; single or multiple; variable in size, possibly extremely large; most common on trunk, back of neck, and forearms	Usually no treatment, biopsy to differentiate from liposarcoma, excision usual treatment (when indicated)
Vitiligo		
Unknown cause; genetically influenced, often precipitated by an event such as illness or a crisis; most noticeable in dark-skinned persons and those with a tan; complete absence of melanocytes; noncontagious	Focal amelanosis (complete loss of pigment); macular; variation in size and location; usually symmetric; may be permanent	Topical steroids often successful in small areas; attempts at repigmentation of larger areas with exposure to UVA and psoralens; depigmentation of pigmented skin with extensive disease (>50% of body involved); cosmetics and stains for camouflage and to deemphasize vitiliginous areas
Lentigo		
Increased number of normal melanocytes in basal layer of epidermis; senile lentigines ("liver spots") related to sun exposure and aging	Hyperpigmented, brown to black macule or patch (flat lesion); usually on sun-exposed areas; potential for progression to lentigo maligna (melanoma in situ) in advanced years	Evaluate carefully for progression; treatment only for cosmetic purposes, liquid nitrogen; laser resurfacing; may recur

TABLE 24-10 Diseases with Dermatologic Manifestations*

Systemic Problem	Dermatologic Manifestations
Endocrine	
Hyperthyroidism	Increased sweating, warm skin with persistent flush, thin nails, vitiligo, alopecia, fine, soft hair
Hypothyroidism	Cold, dry, pale to yellow skin; generalized nonpitting edema; dry, coarse, brittle hair; brittle, slow-growing nails
Glucocorticoid excess (Cushing syndrome)	Atrophy; striae; epidermal thinning; telangiectasia; acne, decreased subcutaneous fat over extremities; thin, loose dermis; impaired wound healing; increased vascular fragility; mild hirsutism; excessive collection of fat over clavicles, back of neck, abdomen, and face
Addison's disease	Loss of body hair (especially axillary), generalized hyperpigmentation (especially in folds)
Androgen excess	Enlarged facial pores, male sex characteristics, acne, acceleration of coarse hair growth
Androgen deficiency—postpuberty	Development of sparse hair; marked reduction in sebum production
Hypoparathyroidism	Opaque, brittle nails with transverse ridges; coarse, sparse hair with patchy alopecia
Hyperpituitarism (acromegaly)	Coarsened skin, deepened lines; increased oiliness and sweating; acne; increased number of nevi, hyperpigmentation; hypertrichosis (excess hair growth)
Diabetes mellitus	Shin spots, delayed wound healing
Gastrointestinal	
Ulcerative colitis, Crohn's disease	Mouth ulcers
Liver disease and biliary tract obstruction	Jaundice, itching, pigmentary abnormalities, alterations in nails and hair, spider angiomas, telangiectasia
Deficiency of essential fatty acids	Scaly skin
Malabsorption syndrome	Acquired ichthyosis (dry, scaly skin)
Cystic fibrosis	Abnormal sweat gland function resulting in failure to conserve sodium
Musculoskeletal and Connective Tissue	
Systemic lupus erythematosus	Maculopapular semiconfluent rash (butterfly rash)
Scleroderma	Leathery hardening and stiffness of skin
Dermatomyositis	Edema; purplish-red upper eyelids; butterfly rash; scaly, macular erythema over knuckles
Metabolic	
Vitamin B_1 (thiamine) deficiency	Edema, redness of soles of feet
Vitamin B_2 (riboflavin) deficiency	Red fissures at corner of mouth, glossitis
Nicotinic acid (niacin) deficiency	Redness of exposed areas of hand or foot; face or neck; infected dermatitis
Vitamin C deficiency	Petechiae, purpura, bleeding gums
Immune	
Hodgkin's disease	Pruritus and nonspecific erythemas
Lymphomas	Papules, nodules, plaques, pruritus
Cardiovascular	
Rheumatic heart disease	Petechiae, urticaria, rheumatoid nodules, erythema nodosum and multiforme
Thromboangiitis obliterans (Buerger's disease)	Superficial migrating thrombophlebitis, pallor or cyanosis, gangrene, ulceration
Peripheral vascular disease	Loss of hair on hands and feet; delayed capillary filling; dependent rubor (redness)
Venous ulcers	Leathery, brownish skin on lower leg; pruritus, concave lesion with edema; scar tissue with healing
Respiratory	
Inadequate oxygenation secondary to respiratory disease	Cyanosis
Hematologic	
Anemia	Pallor, hyperpigmentation, pale mucous membranes, hair loss, nail dystrophy
Clotting disorders	Purpura, petechiae, ecchymosis
Renal	
Chronic kidney disease	Dry skin, pruritus, uremic frost, pallor, dry skin, bruises
Reproductive	
Primary syphilis	Chancre
Secondary syphilis	Generalized skin lesions, alopecia
Tertiary syphilis	Gummas
Paget's disease	Eczematous patch of nipple and areola
Neurologic	
Chronic sensory polyneuropathies Spinal cord trauma	Trophic changes in skin resulting from sensory denervation, pressure ulcers, anesthesia, paresthesias

*Refer to the systemic disease for specific information.

TABLE 24-11 DRUG THERAPY
Common Bases for Topical Medications

Agent	Therapeutic Considerations
Powder	Promotion of dryness, increase in evaporation, absorbing of moisture possible; common base for antifungal preparations; avoid or protect patient from inhaling
Lotion	Suspension of insoluble powders in water; cooling and drying with residual powder film after evaporation of water; useful in subacute pruritic eruptions
Cream	Emulsions of oil and water; most common base for topical medications; lubrication and protection
Ointment	Oil with differing amounts of water added in suspension; lubrication and prevention of dehydration; petrolatum most common
Paste	Mixture of powder and ointment, used when drying effect necessary because moisture is absorbed
Gel	Nongreasy combination of propylene glycol and water; may contain alcohol; used for acute exudative inflammation (e.g., contact dermatitis)

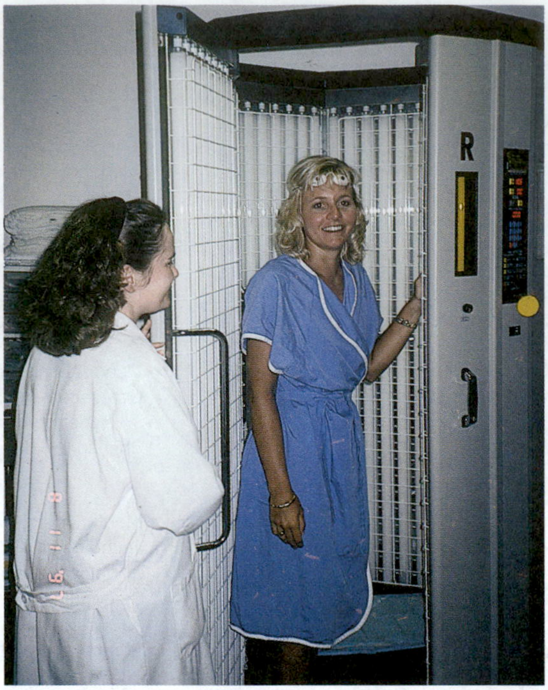

FIG. 24-12 Phototherapy is a method for treating spectrum-specific diseases. The patient's eyes must be protected during the phototherapy session. PUVA unit is illustrated in photo.

Phototherapy. Two types of ultraviolet light (UVL), or a combination of the two types (UVA, UVB), are used to treat many dermatologic conditions. Ultraviolet wavelengths cause erythema, desquamation, and pigmentation and may cause a temporary suppression of basal cell mitosis followed by a rebound increase in cell turnover.

Psoralen plus UVA light (PUVA) is a form of phototherapy. The photosensitizing drug psoralen is given to patients 90 minutes before exposure to UVA to enhance the effect of UVL in the UVA spectrum. Usually a moisturizing agent is applied to the affected area in a thin layer before exposure to UVB. Conditions that are responsive to effective wavelengths with or without drugs include atopic dermatitis, cutaneous T-cell lymphoma, pruritus, psoriasis, vitiligo, and pruritus.

UVL in the specific wavelengths can be produced artificially. Therapeutic doses of UVA and UVB can be measured and used to treat spectrum-specific diseases (Fig. 24-12). Frequent skin assessments must be performed on all patients receiving phototherapy. Inappropriate or excessive exposure to UVL can result in basal or squamous cell carcinoma, as well as severe erythema or burn to the skin. Patients should be cautioned about the potential hazards of using photosensitizing chemicals and further exposure to UV rays from sunlight or artificial UVL during the course of phototherapy. Protective eyewear that blocks 100% of UVL is prescribed for patients receiving PUVA because psoralen is absorbed by the lens of the eye. The eyewear is used to prevent cataract formation. Patients are instructed to use the eyewear for 24 hours after taking the medication when outdoors or near a bright window because UVA penetrates glass. The immunosuppressive effects related to the use of PUVA require careful ongoing monitoring of these patients.

Radiation Therapy. The use of radiation for the treatment of cutaneous malignancies varies greatly according to local practice and availability. Even if radiation therapy is planned, a biopsy must first be performed to obtain a pathologic diagnosis.

Radiation to malignant cutaneous lesions is a painless treatment that is similar in cost to surgery. It produces minimal damage to surrounding tissue. It is a particularly effective treatment for the older adult or debilitated patient who cannot tolerate even a minor surgical procedure and for such areas as the nose, eyelids, and canthal areas, where preservation of the surrounding tissue is of prime consideration. Careful shielding is necessary to prevent ocular lens damage if the irradiated area is around the eyes.

Radiation therapy usually requires multiple visits to a radiology department. It is most effective on lesions above the neck. However, it produces permanent hair loss (alopecia) of the irradiated areas. Other adverse effects include telangiectasia, atrophy, hyperpigmentation, depigmentation, ulceration, chronic radiodermatitis, basal cell carcinoma, and squamous cell carcinoma. (Radiation therapy is discussed in Chapter 16.)

Total-body skin irradiation (body is bombarded with high-energy electrons) may be the treatment of choice or adjunctive therapy for cutaneous T-cell lymphoma. Treatment follows a lengthy course. Patients experience varying degrees of hair loss and radiation dermatitis with transient loss of sweat gland function. This treatment causes premature aging of the skin.

Laser Technology. Laser treatment is expanding rapidly as an efficient surgical tool for many types of dermatologic problems (Table 24-12). Lasers are able to produce measurable, repeatable, consistent zones of tissue damage. They can cut, coagulate, and vaporize tissue to some degree. The wavelength determines the type of delivery system used and the intensity of the energy delivered.

The surgical use of laser energy requires a focusing device to produce a small, high-density spot of energy. This device can be carefully focused on the surgical site and directed to the operative site. Written policies and procedures should cover laser safety and be reviewed by all personnel working with laser equipment.[13] Laser light does not accumulate in body cells and cannot cause cumulative cellular changes or damage.

TABLE 24-12 Use of Laser Treatments for Skin Conditions

• Acne scars	• Port wine stain
• Skin lesions	• Vascular lesions
• Hemangiomas	• Tattoos
• Leg veins	• Resurfacing of skin
• Rosacea	• Psoriasis
• Pigmented nevi	• Wrinkles
• Hair removal	• Epidermal pigment

Several types of lasers are available in most offices and hospitals. The CO_2 laser is the most common treatment. This laser has numerous applications as a vaporizing and cutting tool for most tissues. The argon laser emits light that is primarily absorbed by hemoglobin, and helps in the treatment of vascular and other pigmented lesions. Other, less common, lasers include the use of copper and gold vapors and neodymium:yttrium-aluminum-garnet (Nd:YAG).

Drug Therapy

Antibiotics. Antibiotics are used both topically and systemically to treat dermatologic problems, and they are often used in combination. If used, topical antibiotics should be lightly applied to clean skin. Common OTC topical antibiotics include bacitracin and polymyxin B. Prescription topical antibiotics include mupirocin (used for *Staphylococcus*), gentamicin (used for *Staphylococcus* and most gram-negative organisms), and erythromycin (used for gram-positive cocci [staphylococci and streptococci] and gram-negative cocci and bacilli). Topical erythromycin and clindamycin (Cleocin solutions or gels) are used in the treatment of acne vulgaris. Many of the more popular systemic antibiotics are not used topically because of the danger of allergic contact dermatitis.

If there are signs of systemic infection, a systemic antibiotic should be used. Systemic antibiotics are useful in the treatment of bacterial infections and acne vulgaris. The most frequently used are synthetic penicillin, erythromycin, and tetracycline. These drugs are particularly useful for erysipelas, cellulitis, carbuncles, and severe, infected eczema. Culture and sensitivity of the lesion can guide the choice of antibiotic. Patients require drug-specific instructions on the proper technique of taking or applying antibiotics. For instance, oral tetracycline must be taken on an empty stomach and should never be taken within 1 hour before consuming a dairy product or 2 hours after, which would interfere with absorption.

Corticosteroids. Corticosteroids are particularly effective in treating a wide variety of dermatologic conditions and can be used topically, intralesionally, or systemically. Topical corticosteroids are used for their local antiinflammatory action, as well as for their antipruritic effects. Attempts to diagnose a lesion should be made before a corticosteroid preparation is applied, because corticosteroids will mask the clinical manifestations.[11] Once a sufficient amount of medication is dispensed, limits should be set on the duration and frequency of application. The potency of a particular preparation is related to the concentration of active drug in the preparation. With prolonged use, the more potent corticosteroid formulations can cause adrenal suppression, especially if a large surface area is covered and occlusive dressings are used. High-potency corticosteroids may produce side effects when their use is prolonged, including atrophy of the skin resulting from impaired cell mitosis, capillary fragility, and susceptibility to bruising. In general, dermal and epidermal atrophy does not occur until a corticosteroid has been used for 2 to 3 weeks. If drug use is discontinued at the first sign of atrophy, recovery usually occurs in several weeks. Rosacea eruptions, severe exacerbations of acne vulgaris, and dermatophyte infections may also occur. Rebound dermatitis is not uncommon when therapy is stopped, and this can be reduced by tapering the use of high-potency topical corticosteroids when patient improvement is noted.

Low-potency corticosteroids such as hydrocortisone act more slowly but can be used for a longer period of time without producing serious side effects. Low-potency corticosteroids are safe to use on the face and intertriginous (opposing skin surface) areas, such as the axillae. The potency of a particular preparation is related to the concentration of active drug in the preparation. The ointment form represents the most efficient delivery system. Creams and ointments should be applied in thin layers and slowly massaged into the site one to three times a day as prescribed. Accurate and adequate topical therapy is often the key to a successful outcome.

Intralesional corticosteroids are injected directly into or just beneath the lesion. This method provides a reservoir of medication with an effect lasting several weeks to months. Intralesional injection is commonly used in the treatment of psoriasis, alopecia areata (patchy hair loss), cystic acne, hypertrophic scars, and keloids. Triamcinolone acetonide (Kenalog) is the most common drug used for intralesional injection.

Systemic corticosteroids can have remarkable results in the treatment of dermatologic conditions. However, they often have undesirable systemic effects (see Chapter 50). Corticosteroids can be administered as short-term therapy for acute conditions such as contact dermatitis caused by poison ivy. Long-term corticosteroid therapy for dermatologic conditions is reserved for chronic bullous diseases, for severe systemic effects of collagen and immunologic responses, and as a last resort when other therapies have failed.

Antihistamines. Oral antihistamines are used to treat conditions that exhibit urticaria, angioedema, and pruritus.[14] Dermatologic problems such as atopic dermatitis, contact dermatitis, and other allergic cutaneous reactions can be mediated with the use of histamine blockers. Antihistamines compete with histamine for the receptor site, thus preventing its effect. Antihistamines may have anticholinergic and/or sedative effects. Several different antihistamines may have to be tried before the satisfactory therapeutic effect is achieved. Sedating antihistamines, such as hydroxyzine (Atarax) and diphenhydramine (Benadryl), are often preferred for pruritic conditions because the tranquilizing and sedative effects offer symptomatic relief. The patient should be warned about sedative effects, a particular problem when driving or operating heavy machinery. Antihistamines such as loratidine (Claritin), fexofenadine (Allegra), and cetirizine (Zyrtec) bind to peripheral histamine receptors, providing antihistamine action without sedation. These nonsedating antihistamines are not generally effective for controlling pruritus. Antihistamines should be used with particular caution in older adults because of their long half-life and their anticholinergic effects.

Topical Fluorouracil. Fluorouracil (5-FU) is a topical cytotoxic agent with selective toxicity for sun-damaged cells. 5-FU is available in four strengths (0.5%, 1%, 2%, and 5%) and is used for the treatment of premalignant (especially actinic keratosis) and some malignant skin diseases. Because systemic absorption of the drug is minimal, systemic side effects are virtually nonexistent. Patient compliance is the consideration in the use of 5-FU. The medication produces erythema and pruritus within 3 to 5 days and painful, eroded areas over the damaged skin within 1 to 3 weeks, depending on skin thickness of site. Treatment must continue with applications one to two times a day for 2 to 6 weeks. Healing may take up to 4 weeks after medication is stopped. Because 5-FU is a photosensitizing drug, the patient must be instructed to avoid sunlight during treatment. Patients should be educated about the effect of the medication and should be warned that they will look worse before they look better. Compliance depends on thoroughness of the instruction, and a written handout should always be given. After effective treatment, treated skin is smooth and free of actinic keratosis. Actinic keratosis may recur in treated areas, and multiple courses of chemotherapy may be necessary over the years for individuals with severely sun-damaged skin.

Immunomodulators. Topical immunomodulators, such as pimicromilus (Elidel) and tacrolimus (Protopic), are newer nonsteroidal medications used to treat atopic dermatitis. They work by suppressing an overreactive immune system. The side effects are minimal and may include a transient burning or feeling of heat at the application site. An increased risk of skin cancer and precancerous lesions may be associated with these drugs.

Another topical immunomodulator, imiquimod (Aldara), acts to stimulate the production of α-interferon and other cytokines to enhance cell-mediated immunity. It boosts the immune response only where applied, and is safe for transplant patients. This medication is currently being used for external genital warts, actinic keratoses, and superficial basal cell carcinoma. Most patients using this cream experience skin reactions, including redness, swelling, sore or blister, peeling, itching, and burning.

Diagnostic and Surgical Therapy

Skin Scraping. Scraping is done with a scalpel blade to obtain a sample of surface cells for microscopic inspection and diagnosis. The most common tests of skin scrapings are potassium hydroxide (KOH) for fungus and mineral oil examination for scabies.

Electrodessication and Electrocoagulation. Electrical energy can be converted to heat with the tip of an electrode. This results in tissue being destroyed by burning. The major uses of this type of therapy are coagulation of bleeding vessels to obtain hemostasis and destruction of small *telangiectasias* (dilation of groups of superficial capillaries and venules). *Electrodessication* usually involves more superficial destruction, and a monopolar electrode is used. *Electrocoagulation* has a deeper effect, with better hemostasis an increased possibility of scarring. A dipolar electrode is used for electrocoagulation.

Curettage. **Curettage** is the removal and scooping away of tissue using an instrument with a circular cutting edge attached to a handle (Fig. 24-13). Although the curette is not usually strong enough to cut normal skin, it is useful for removing many types of small, soft skin tumors and superficial lesions, such as warts, actinic keratoses, and small basal and squamous cell carcinomas. The area to be curetted is anesthetized before the procedure. Hemostasis is obtained by use of one of several methods: electrodessication, ferric subsulfate (Monsel's solution), gelatin foam, aluminum chloride (Drysol), or a gauze pressure dressing. A small scar and hypopigmentation can result. The curetted tissue may be sent for biopsy.

Punch Biopsy. Punch biopsy is a common dermatologic procedure used to obtain a tissue sample for histologic study or to remove small lesions. It is generally reserved for lesions smaller than 0.5 cm. Before local anesthesia is used, the biopsy area is outlined so that landmarks will not be obscured by the anesthetizing agent. The biopsy punch instrument cores out a small cylinder of skin when its sharp edge is twirled between the fingers. The core of skin is snipped from the subcutaneous fat and appropriately preserved for examination in a fixative solution. Hemostasis is achieved by using methods similar to curettage, but sites of 4 mm or larger are usually closed with sutures. Other types of biopsies are discussed in Table 23-10 and Chapter 23.

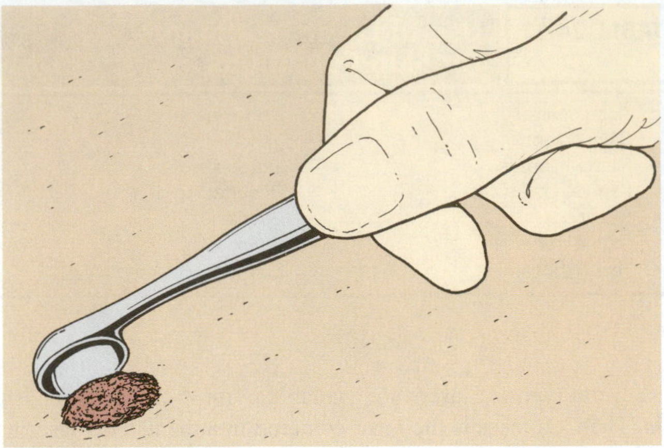

FIG. 24-13 Curettage. The superficial growth is removed by a gentle scooping technique.

Cryosurgery. **Cryosurgery** is the use of subfreezing temperatures to destroy epidermal lesions. Cryosurgery is a useful treatment for common benign, precancerous conditions including common and genital warts, cutaneous tags, thin seborrheic keratosis, lentigines, and actinic keratosis.[15] Topical liquid nitrogen ($-196°$ F) is the agent most commonly used for cryosurgery. The mechanism of injury involves direct cellular freezing, as well as vascular stasis (stoppage or slowdown in the flow of blood), which develops after thawing. Intracellular ice formation causes the cell to rupture during thaw, leading to cell death and necrosis of the treated tissue.

Liquid nitrogen can be applied topically (directly onto the benign or precancerous lesion) with a direct spray or a contact probe with an autoclave tip.[15] Patients are informed that they will feel a stinging cold sensation. The lesion will first become swollen and red, and it may blister. Next, a scab will form and fall off in 1 to 3 weeks. The skin lesion will be sloughed along with the scab. Growth of new skin follows.

Cryosurgery can become expensive if multiple treatments are required to fully destroy a lesion. Because of the temperature of the liquid nitrogen, melanocytes can easily be destroyed, leaving an area of hypopigmentation resembling a scar. The size of an affected area to be treated may limit the use of cryotherapy. The disadvantages of this treatment are (1) the lack of a tissue specimen for histologic confirmation of cell type before destruction and (2) the potential for destruction of adjacent healthy tissue.

Excision. Excision should be considered if the lesion involves the dermis. Complete closure of the excised area usually results in a good cosmetic result.

A specific type of excision is *Mohs' surgery,* which is a microscopically controlled removal of a cutaneous malignancy. This procedure sections the surgical specimen horizontally, so that 100% of the surgical margin can be examined. Tissue is removed in thin layers, and all margins of the specimen are mapped to determine whether tumor remains. Any residual tumor not removed by the first surgical excision can be removed in serial excisions performed the same day. The benefits of this treatment are preservation of normal tissue, producing the smallest possible wound, and complete removal of the cancer before surgical closure. Although this can become a lengthy procedure, it is performed in the outpatient setting under local anesthesia.

NURSING MANAGEMENT
DERMATOLOGIC PROBLEMS

■ *Ambulatory and Home Care*

Dermatologic conditions are not common reasons for hospitalization. Although it may not be the primary reason for hospitalization, many hospitalized patients will exhibit concurrent skin problems that warrant nursing intervention and patient education.

If the patient is in an acute care setting, the nurse will both administer and teach the appropriate treatments. If the patient is in an outpatient setting, the nursing focus is on patient teaching, with opportunities provided for demonstration and repeated demonstration. Subsequent visits provide the opportunity to evaluate patient understanding and treatment effectiveness.

Nursing interventions related to dermatologic conditions fall into broad categories. They are applicable to many skin problems in both inpatient and outpatient settings. A nursing care plan for the patient with chronic skin lesions is available on the Evolve website *http://evolve.elsevier.com/Lewis/medsurg*.

Wet Dressings. Wet dressings are commonly used when there is oozing from the skin. Oozing usually indicates the presence of an infection and/or inflammation. Plain water or a prescribed solution (i.e., Domeboro powder) is used on the skin by soaking (a foot or hand) or applying compresses to a larger area. Wet dressings are also used to relieve itching, suppress inflammation, and debride a wound. In addition, wet dressings increase penetration of topical medications, promote sleep by relieving discomfort, and enhance removal of scales, crusts, and exudate. Such materials as thin sheeting, gauze sponges, thermal underwear, or tube socks can be used for dressings. Ingenuity is sometimes required when odd-shaped parts of the body must be covered.

The prescribed dressing is put into fresh solution, squeezed until it is no longer dripping, and then applied to the affected area, avoiding normal skin tissue. If the desired effect is drying, soaks or compresses are left in place for 20 minutes, three times daily for 2 to 3 days. Care must be taken to avoid overdrying, because new problems may result, such as fissuring. Wet dressings for uses other than drying should be left in place 10 to 30 minutes, two to four times a day as ordered. If the skin appears macerated (softened), the dressings should be discontinued for 2 to 3 hours. The patient should be protected from discomfort and chilling by using linens and bedclothes with pads or plastic.

Wet dressings do not need to be sterile. Tap water at room temperature is the most common solution where water quality is adequate. Filtered or sterile water may be indicated in some locations. Wet dressings should be cool when an antiinflammatory effect is desired and tepid when the purpose is to debride an infected, crusted lesion. These treatments are excellent ways to remove the scabs left by the collection of debris at a wound site.

Baths. Baths are appropriate when large body areas need to be treated. They also have sedative and antipruritic effects. Some medications, such as oilated oatmeal (Aveeno), potassium permanganate, and sodium bicarbonate, can be added directly to the bath water. One cup of the mixture can be added to 2 cups of water and then added to the bath water. The tub should be full enough to cover affected areas. Both the bath water and the prescribed solution should be at a temperature that is comfortable for the patient. The patient can soak for 15 to 20 minutes three to four times a day, depending on the severity of the dermatitis and the patient's discomfort. It is important to stress to the patient that the skin not be rubbed dry with a towel but gently patted to prevent increasing irritation and inflammation. The addition of oils makes the bathtub extremely slippery and should be avoided. If oils are used in the tub, the utmost caution must be used in transferring patients to prevent accidents. To sustain the hydrating effect, cream or ointment emollients (moisturizers) or medications should be applied to the skin directly after the bath. This helps retain the moisture in the hydrated cells.

Topical Medications. A thin layer of ointment, cream, or lotion should be applied to clean skin and spread evenly in a downward motion. Thickly applied topicals waste medication and leave the skin greasy. An alternative method is to apply the medication directly onto a dressing. Pastes are designed to protect the affected area. They should be applied thickly with a tongue blade or a gloved hand. Draining lesions and lesions with oily medication can be covered with a light dressing to prevent soiling clothes. Patients need specific directions on the proper application technique of prescribed topical medications.

Control of Pruritus. Pruritus (itching) can be caused by almost any physical or chemical stimulus to the skin, such as drugs, insects, and dry skin. The itch sensation is carried by the same nonmyelinated nerve fibers as pain. If the epidermis is damaged or absent, the sensation will be felt as pain rather than an itch.

The itch/scratch cycle must be broken to prevent excoriation and lichenification. Control of pruritus is also important because it is difficult to diagnose a lesion that is excoriated and inflamed. Certain circumstances make itching worse. Anything that causes vasodilation, such as heat or rubbing, should be avoided. Dryness of the skin lowers the itch threshold and increases the itch sensation.

The nurse can use or teach the patient various methods to break the itch/scratch cycle.[4] A cool environment may cause vasoconstriction and decrease itching. Topically applied menthol, camphor, or phenol can be used to numb the itch receptors. Systemic antihistamines can be used if necessary to provide relief to a patient while the underlying cause of the pruritus is diagnosed and treated. The principal side effect of most antihistamines is sedation. This may be desirable because pruritus is often worse at night and can interfere with sleep.

Wet dressings can be used effectively to relieve pruritus. Thin, cotton sheets or thermal underwear is placed in warm water, wrung out, and placed over the pruritic area. After 10 to 15 minutes the dressing is removed and the skin is patted dry and a lubricant or medication applied. This procedure can be repeated as necessary for comfort.

Lichenification is a thickening of skin as a result of the proliferation of keratinocytes with accentuation of the normal markings of the skin. Lichenification is caused by chronic scratching or rubbing of the skin and is often associated with atopic dermatoses and pruritic conditions. Although any area of the body may be affected, the hands and forearms are common sites. Treatment of the cause of the itching is the key to prevention of lichenification. Excoriations may be evident in the lichenified skin as a result of persistent pruritus and scratching.

Prevention of Spread. Although most skin problems are not contagious, infection precautions indicate the need for gloves with open or bleeding wounds. Procedures should be explained to the patient in order to avoid demoralizing an already sensitive patient. However, if in doubt, the nurse should wear gloves until a definite diagnosis has been established. The most common contagious lesions that the nurse should be cautious with include impetigo, staphylococcus, pyoderma, primary chancre and secondary syphilis lesions, scabies, and pediculosis. Careful hand washing and safe disposal of soiled dressings are the best means of preventing spread of skin problems.

Prevention of Secondary Infections. Open lesions on the skin are susceptible to invasion by other viral, bacterial, or fungal organisms. Meticulous hygiene, hand washing, and dressing changes are important to minimize potential for secondary infections. Also, the patient should be warned about scratching lesions, which can cause excoriations and create a portal of entry for pathogens. The patient's nails should be trimmed short to minimize trauma from scratching.

Specific Skin Care. Nurses are often in a position to advise patients regarding care of the skin following simple dermatologic surgical procedures, such as skin biopsy, excision, and cryosurgery. Patient follow-up should be individualized. In general, instructions include dressing changes, use of topical antibiotics, and the signs and symptoms of infection. After a dermatologic procedure any oozing wound should be regularly cleansed with a saline solution. An antibiotic ointment may then be applied with a dressing that is both absorbent and nonadherent.

Wounds that are kept moist and covered heal more rapidly and with less scarring. The initial crust that forms should be left undisturbed as a protective coating for the damaged skin beneath it. Healing crusts that have been moisturized and protected will separate naturally from healed epidermis.

A wound that required sutures can be covered with a variety of different dressings. Sutures will generally be removed in 4 to 10 days, depending on the placement site. Sometimes alternating sutures are removed after the third day. Incision lines may require daily cleansing, usually with plain tap water. If necessary, a topical antibiotic is applied and the wound is either covered with a dry sterile dressing or left open to air. The patient may experience some swelling and discomfort in the first 24 hours, during the first phase of wound healing. Ice packs may be applied over the surgical dressing to reduce edema. Mild analgesics such as acetaminophen should control the discomfort. The patient needs to know the manifestations of inflammation such as redness, fever, or increased pain or swelling and signs of infection, such as purulent drainage. If these manifestations occur, they should be reported to the health care provider.

Psychologic Effects of Chronic Dermatologic Problems. Emotional stress can occur for persons who suffer from chronic skin problems such as psoriasis, atopic dermatitis, or acne. The sequelae of chronic skin problems could result in social and employment problems with subsequent financial implications, a poor self-image, problems with sexuality, and increasing and progressive frustration. The usual lack of systemic overt illness coupled with the visibility of the skin lesions often presents a real problem to the patient.

The nurse must continue to be optimistic and help the patient comply with the prescribed regimen. The patient must be allowed to verbalize the "Why me?" question, even though there is no ready answer. Reinforcement of the prescribed hygiene and treatment measures is an important part of the nursing management. Dermatology patient support groups are listed on the American Academy of Dermatology website *(www.aad.org)*. These groups are extremely helpful for patient support and accurate education materials.

Many lesions can be camouflaged with the skillful use of cosmetics. Individual sensitivity to product ingredients must always be considered in the selection of a cosmetic product. Oil-free, hypoallergenic cosmetics are available and may be beneficial to the allergic patient. Rehabilitative cosmetics are available to help camouflage and deemphasize such lesions as *vitiligo* (loss of pigmentation), *melasma* (tan to brown patches on the face), or healed postoperative wound sites. These commercially available products are opaque, smudge resistant, and water resistant.

In addition to specific skin conditions that tend to be chronic, other factors affecting the outcome of long-term dermatologic problems include skin type, history of previous exacerbations, family history, complications, intolerance to therapy, environmental factors, lack of adherence to the prescribed regimen, endocrine factors, and psychologic factors. Lesions that follow a chronic pattern often are associated with lichenification and scarring.

Physiologic Effects of Chronic Dermatologic Problems. Scarring and lichenification are the result of chronic dermatologic problems. Scars occur when ulceration takes place. Scars are pink and vascular at first. With time, they become avascular and white (scars on individuals with darker skin may be hyperpigmented) with increasing strength. Different regions of the body scar differently, such as the face and neck, which heal fairly rapidly because they are well vascularized. Regions of the lower body with less vascularization tend to scar more easily and heal more slowly. Scar formation is described in Chapter 13.

The location of the scar is the determining factor with respect to its cosmetic implications. Facial scars are the most damaging psychologically, because they are so visible. Creative use of cosmetics can do much to mask the scarring of chronic skin conditions. The best treatment is the prevention of scarring by controlling the problem in the acute phase.

COSMETIC PROCEDURES

The vast array of cosmetic procedures is almost limitless. Cosmetic procedures can include chemical peels, toxin injections, collagen fillers, laser surgery, breast enlargement and reduction (see Chapter 52), laser surgery, face-lift, eyelid-lift, and liposuction. Common cosmetic procedures are presented in Tables 24-13 and 24-14.

The reasons for undergoing these procedures are as varied as the techniques. The most common reason that people suffer the discomfort and financial expense (most are not covered by insurance) of a cosmetic procedure is to improve their body image. People project their personal image of themselves. If they feel better about themselves after having cosmetic surgery, they will often act more confident and self-assured. Often social position and economic considerations are part of the decision. Increased longevity provides a larger population to whom cosmetic procedures are especially appealing.

Regardless of the reasons, the nurse should maintain a supportive, nonjudgmental attitude about cosmetic procedures. If the patient wishes to change or enhance a body feature perceived as unattractive, it is a personal decision and the nurse should support this decision.

Elective Surgery

Laser Surgery. When a laser beam enters the skin, the light can affect skin structures by scattering, absorbing, or passing through different layers. The spectrum of clinical application for each laser depends on the depth of the wavelength emitted and the operator technique. Alteration in technique, such as pulse duration and the number of passes over the skin vary the result.[16] New handpiece technology with multiple spot size and cooling device additions have also generated new flexibility in laser technology.

TABLE 24-13 Common Cosmetic Topical Procedures

Procedure	Tretinoin (Retin-A, Renova)	Chemical Peels	Microdermabrasion	Alpha Hydroxy Acids (e.g., glycolic acid, lactic acid)
Indications	Improves appearance of aged and photodamaged skin, especially fine wrinkling and the reduction of actinic keratoses	Improves appearance of aged and photodamaged skin, acne scarring, freckles, actinic and seborrheic keratoses	Smoother appearance of photodamaged and wrinkled skin	Similar indications as microdermabrasion; also called a "mini-peel"
Description	Applied initially QOD, aiming for nightly applications as tolerated; treatment stopped if severe inflammation; maximum response in 8-12 mo	Solution applied (e.g., solid carbon dioxide, trichloracetic acid) in varying amounts to the skin, causing a controlled burn; loss of melanin occurs	Removal of the epidermis and top dermal layer by application of aluminum oxide or baking soda crystals; reepithelialization of abraded surface then occurs	Low concentrations (<10%) found in many skin care products consumers can apply to the skin; higher concentrations (50%-70%) given only by a health care provider
Side effects	Erythema, swelling, flaking, photosensitivity, hypopigmentation and hyperpigmentation; teratogenic; increases phototoxicity if also taking other photosensitive drugs (see Table 24-2)	Moderate swelling and crusting for 1 wk; redness persisting 6-8 wk; pink tone possible for several mo; photosensitivity	Light pink tone that resolves within 24 hr; photosensitivity	Photosensitivity, minimal stinging and redness at lower concentrations, severe redness, oozing, and flaking skin may occur for 1-4 wk at higher concentrations
Patient teaching	Apply emollients (e.g., petroleum jelly) and sunscreen (SPF 15 or higher), use sun-avoidance measures, avoid use of abrasive or drying facial cleansers for severe sensitivity (e.g., excess blistering, peeling); notify health care provider of severe sensitivity	Use sunscreen, avoid sun for 6 mo to prevent hyperpigmentation	Generous application of emollients and sunscreen	Use sunscreen

QOD, Every other day; *SPF*, sun protection factor.

TABLE 24-14 Common Cosmetic Injection Procedures

	Neurotoxin	Fillers
Type	Botulinum toxin (Botox)	Collagen (e.g., Zyplast, CosmoDerm) Hyaluronic acid (Restylane)
Indications	Decreases wrinkles caused by repetitive facial expressions; also used to shape eyebrows into an arch and correct facial asymmetry	Reduces depth and visibility of facial lines and creases (e.g., nasolabial crease, lips)
Description	Tiny amounts injected into and around the targeted muscle; temporarily interferes with neuromuscular transmission thereby paralyzing the affected muscle	Filler substance should be tested on a small patch of skin to assess for allergies; filler substance is injected with a tiny needle under skin surface
Side effects	Transitory and mild redness, pain, bruising, and swelling at injection site; slight headache for several hours	Swelling, bruising, redness, tenderness, and itching; in rare cases an allergic rash may result with hives and flu-like symptoms
Patient teaching	Most people do not notice any unpleasant effects	Ice to relieve discomfort

Lasers can reduce fine wrinkles around the lips or eyes and remove facial lesions (see Table 24-12). Swelling, redness, and bruising are common after treatment. The treated areas usually are kept moist with ointment or occlusive dressings (surgical bandages) for the first few days. The treated skin must be protected from the sun.

Face-Lift. A face-lift *(rhytidectomy)* is the lifting and repositioning of the lower two thirds of the face and neck to improve appearance (Fig. 24-14). Indications for this procedure include the following:

1. Redundant soft tissue resulting from disease (e.g., acne scarring)
2. Asymmetric redundancy of soft tissues (e.g., facial palsy)
3. Redundant soft tissue resulting from trauma
4. Preauricular lesions
5. Redundant soft tissues resulting from *solar elastosis* (sagging of the skin as a result of sun damage), changes in body weight, and the effects of gravity
6. Restoration of body image

The surgical approach and lines of incisions vary according to the nature of the desired correction and the position of the hairline. Eyelid-lifts *(blepharoplasty)* with similar indications are performed to remove redundant tissue and possibly improve the field of vision. Prevention of hematoma formation is the most important postoperative consideration. Application of ice packs is usually used the first 24 to 48 hours to reduce swelling and decrease the possibility of hematoma formation. Complications can occur if the person smokes or is involved in vigorous exercise. Usually there is

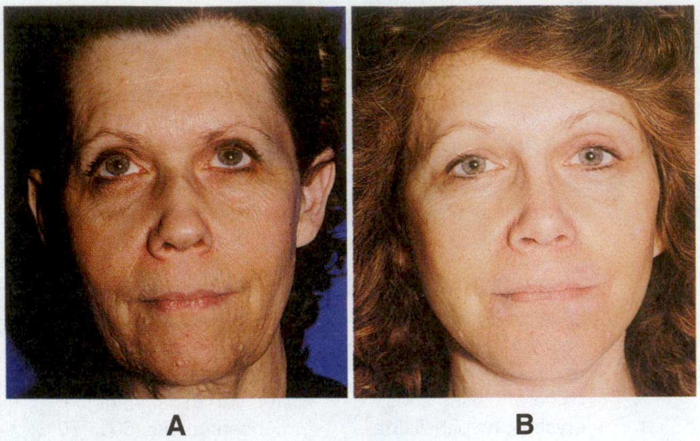

FIG. 24-14 Face-lift. **A,** Preoperative. **B,** Postoperative.

minimal pain. Antibiotics are used at the discretion of the surgeon. Infection is not a common problem.

Liposuction. Liposuction is a technique for removing subcutaneous fat to improve facial and body contours. Although not a substitute for diet and exercise, it can be successful in removing areas of fat from virtually any body area that is resistant to other techniques (Fig. 24-15).

Although relatively free of complications, possible contraindications for the procedure include use of anticoagulants, uncontrolled hypertension, diabetes mellitus, and poor cardiovascular status. Persons under 40 years of age with good skin elasticity are the best candidates. However, patients ranging in age from 16 to 70 years can be treated successfully.

The procedure is usually performed on an outpatient basis with the aid of local anesthesia. One or more sessions may be necessary, depending on the size of the area to be treated. A blunt-tipped cannula is inserted through a 0.5-inch incision and pushed into the fat to break it loose from the fibrous stroma. Multiple repeated thrusts disrupt the fat and create tunnels. The loosened fat is removed with a powerful suction. The area is taped because firm bandaging helps contour the skin and reduce the chance of postoperative bleeding and fluid accumulation. It may take several months for the final results to be evident.

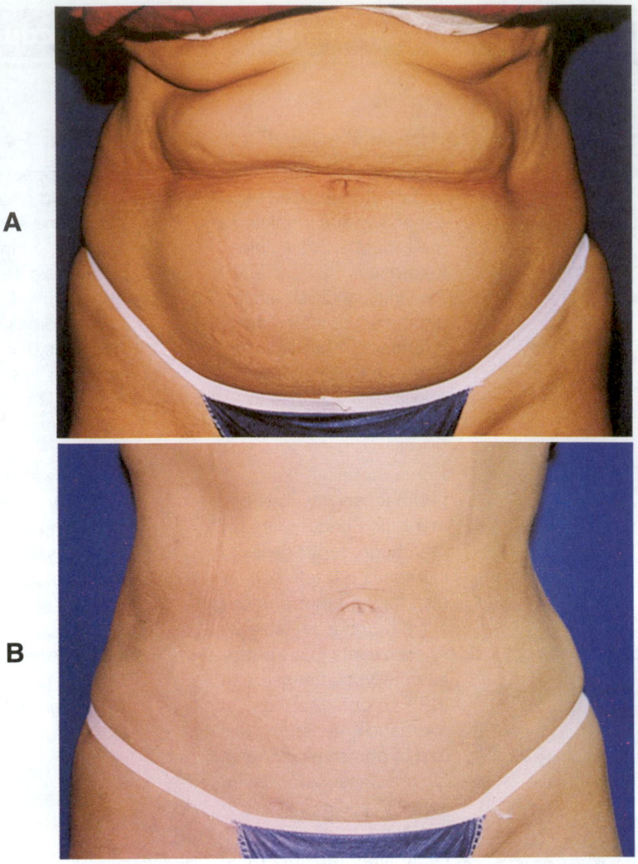

FIG. 24-15 Liposuction. **A,** Preoperative. **B,** Postoperative.

NURSING MANAGEMENT
COSMETIC SURGERY

Many cosmetic surgical procedures are performed in well-equipped day-surgery units or in dermatology surgeons' or plastic surgeons' office surgery suites. Several nursing interventions are appropriate for the patient who has had cosmetic surgery, regardless of where the surgery was done.

Preoperative Management

A major preoperative management consideration relates to informed consent and realistic expectations of what cosmetic surgery can accomplish. Although this information should be provided by the surgeon, the nurse can and should reinforce this information and answer questions and concerns. For instance, a face-lift has little or no effect on deep wrinkling of the forehead and temples, deep nasolabial grooves, or vertical lip wrinkles. Before-and-after treatment photographs of similar cases are often useful in helping the patient to set realistic expectations.

The patient also needs to understand the time frame for healing. Because the third phase of wound healing does not complete for 1 year, immediate, complete results should not be anticipated. The oozing, crusting stage of the abrasive procedure must be explained so the patient can plan time off from work if this seems necessary. The final results of the cosmetic procedure are affected by the patient's age, general state of health, and skin type. If a health problem is present, efforts should be made to correct or control the problem before the procedure is performed.

Postoperative Management

Most of the cosmetic procedures are not extremely painful. Usually mild analgesics are sufficient to keep the patient comfortable.

Although infection is not a common problem after cosmetic surgery, the nurse should assess the surgical sites for signs of infection. The patient should be aware of signs of infection and told to report any such signs and symptoms immediately so that appropriate antibiotic intervention can be started.

If the surgery involved an alteration in the circulation to the skin, such as in a face-lift, a careful monitoring of adequate circulation is necessary. Warm, pink skin that blanches on pressure indicates that adequate circulation is present in the surgical area. Supportive, compressive dressings and ice packs may be necessary early in the postoperative period.

SKIN GRAFTS

Uses

Skin grafts may be necessary to provide protection to underlying structures or to reconstruct areas for cosmetic or functional purposes. Ideally, wounds heal by primary intention. However, large, surgically created wounds, trauma, and chronic wounds can cause extensive tissue destruction, making primary intention healing impossible. In these cases, skin grafting may be necessary to close the defect. Improved surgical techniques make it possible to graft skin, bone, cartilage, fat, fascia, muscles, and nerves. For cosmetically pleasing results, the color, thickness, texture, and hair-growing nature of skin used for grafting must be chosen to match the recipient site. (Skin grafting is also discussed in Chapter 25.)

Types

The two types of skin grafts are free grafts and skin flaps. Free grafts are further classified according to the method of providing a blood supply to the grafted skin. One method is to transfer the graft (epidermis and part or all of the dermis) to the recipient site from the donor site. If the graft is an *autograft* (from the patient's own body) or an *isograft* (from an identical twin), it will revascularize and become fixed to the new site. Chapter 25 discusses full and split skin grafts. Another method of free skin grafting is by *reconstructive microsurgery.* With the use of an operating microscope, circulation is immediately established in the free flap by anastomosis of the blood vessels from the skin flap to the vessels in the recipient site.

Skin flaps involve moving a section of skin and subcutaneous tissue from one part of the body to another without terminating the vascular attachment. The vascular attachment is called a *pedicle.* Skin flaps are used to cover wounds with a poor vascular bed, when padding is needed, and to cover wounds over cartilage and bone. There may be a need for intermediate flap placement if the recipient site is far removed from the donor site. For instance, a skin flap from the thigh to the head would require an intermediate graft. The flap is advanced to the recipient site when circulation is well established at the intermediate site. The type of flap and the route of transfer are determined according to the needs of the patient and the nature of the defect to be repaired.

Soft tissue expansion is a technique for providing skin for resurfacing a defect, such as a burn scar; for removing a disfiguring mark, such as a tattoo; or as a preliminary step in breast reconstruction. A subcutaneous tissue expander of an appropriate size and shape is placed under the skin, usually as an outpatient procedure. Weekly expansion with saline solution can be done in a health care setting or by the patient at home. This expansion procedure is repeated until the skin reaches the size needed for the repair. This may take from several weeks to 3 to 4 months. Once sufficient skin is available, the old incision is opened, the expander is removed, and the soft tissue is ready to be used as an advancement flap. The tissue expander next to a defect retains the primary tissue characteristics such as color and texture.

CRITICAL THINKING EXERCISE

CASE STUDY

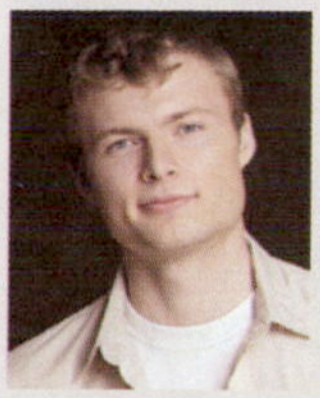

Malignant Melanoma and Dysplastic Nevi

Patient Profile. Michael Patrick, 37, is a white, fair-skinned, blue-eyed Park Ranger who enjoys fishing and river rafting. He comes to the clinic for evaluation of a changing mole.

Subjective Data

- History of a mole on his left lower leg from birth that has become scaly, hard, and lumpy over the last 3 months
- Father and older sister treated for malignant melanoma in the last 10 years
- Anxious that the mole might be cancer and require extensive, disfiguring surgery

Objective Data

Physical Examination

- Has a 6-mm nevus, blue-black in color, scalloped with vaguely defined borders
- Has a large number of small nevi (more than 50) on back, legs, and arms
- Two dysplastic nevi found on back

Diagnostic Studies

- Excisional biopsy confirmed malignant melanoma.
- Further diagnostic tests indicate the melanoma is stage 0.

Critical Thinking Questions

1. What risk factors for malignant melanoma does this patient have?
2. What are the usual manifestations associated with malignant melanoma?
3. What is the prognosis for a patient with this stage of malignant melanoma?
4. What treatment options are available for this patient?
5. How would you address Mr. Patrick regarding his anxiety over the treatment outcomes?
6. What is the priority of care for Mr. Patrick?
7. What would you include in a patient teaching plan to address future sun exposure for this patient?
8. Based on the assessment data presented, write one or more appropriate nursing diagnoses. Are there any collaborative problems?

NCLEX EXAMINATION REVIEW QUESTIONS

The number of the question corresponds to the same-numbered objective at the beginning of the chapter.

1. The nurse advises a patient with photosensitivity to use a sunscreen that contains
   a. cinnamates.
   b. avobenzone.
   c. benzophenones.
   d. para-aminobenzoic acid (PABA).
2. In teaching a patient who is using topical corticosteroids to treat an acute dermatitis, the nurse should tell the patient that
   a. the cream form is the most efficient system of delivery.
   b. topical corticosteroids usually do not cause systemic side effects.
   c. creams and ointments should be applied with a glove in small amounts to prevent further infection.
   d. abruptly discontinuing the use of topical corticosteroids may cause a reappearance of the dermatitis.
3. A patient with psoriasis tells the nurse that she has quit her job as a receptionist because she feels her appearance is disgusting to customers. The nursing diagnosis that best describes this patient response is
   a. ineffective coping related to lack of social support.
   b. impaired skin integrity related to presence of lesions.
   c. anxiety related to lack of knowledge of the disease process.
   d. social isolation related to decreased activities secondary to fear of rejection.

4. In teaching a patient with malignant melanoma about this disorder, the nurse recognizes that the prognosis of the patient is most dependent on
   a. the thickness of the lesion.
   b. the degree of color change in the lesion.
   c. how much the lesion has spread superficially.
   d. the amount of ulceration present in the lesion.
5. The nurse identifies that a patient with a diagnosis of which of the following disorders is most at risk for spreading the disease?
   a. Tinea pedis
   b. Impetigo on the face
   c. Candidiasis of the nails
   d. Psoriasis on the palms and soles
6. A mother and her two children have been diagnosed with pediculosis corporis at a health center. An appropriate measure in treating this condition is
   a. applying pyrethrins to the body.
   b. topical application of griseofulvin.
   c. moist compresses applied frequently.
   d. administration of systemic antibiotics.
7. A common site for the lesions associated with childhood atopic dermatitis is the
   a. buttocks.
   b. temporal area.
   c. antecubital space.
   d. plantar surface of the feet.
8. During assessment of a patient the nurse notes an area of red, sharply defined plaques covered with silvery scales that are mildly itchy on the patient's knees and elbows. The nurse recognizes this finding as
   a. lentigo.
   b. psoriasis.
   c. actinic keratosis.
   d. seborrheic keratosis.
9. A dermatologic manifestation of Cushing syndrome would include
   a. telangiectasia.
   b. thickened skin.
   c. increased sweating.
   d. generalized hyperpigmentation.
10. Important patient teaching after a chemical peel includes
   a. avoidance of sun exposure.
   b. application of firm bandages.
   c. limitation of vigorous exercise.
   d. use of ice to relieve discomfort.

REFERENCES

1. Berger T: Skin, hair, and nails. In Tierney L, et al, editors: *Current medical diagnosis and treatment 2005,* ed 44, New York, 2005, McGraw-Hill.
2. Rigel DS: *Cancer of the skin*, Philadelphia, 2005, Elsevier.
3. Rietschel RL: Clues to an accurate diagnosis of contact dermatitis, *Dermatol Ther* 17:224, 2004.
4. Tsao A, Kim E, Hong W: Chemoprevention of cancer, *CA Cancer J Clin* 54:150, 2004.
5. Skin Cancer Foundation: Melanoma—what to look for. Available at *www.skincancer.org/self-exam* (accessed May 26, 2005).
6. American Cancer Society: *Cancer facts and figures 2005*, Atlanta, 2005, American Cancer Society.
7. Stalberg D, Crandell B, Fawcett R: Diagnosis and treatment of basal cell and squamous cell carcinoma, *Am Fam Physician* 70:1481, 2004.
8. Ayers D: Melanoma, *Nursing* 34:52, 2004.
9. Stahl S, et al: Genetics in melanoma, *Isr Med Assoc J* 6:774, 2004.
10. Balch C: An evidence-based staging system for cutaneous melanoma, *CA Cancer J Clin* 54:131, 2004.
11. Oklota C, Brodell R: Uncovering tinea incognito, *Postgrad Med* 116:65, 2004.
12. Quillen T: Easing the heartbreak of psoriasis, *Nursing* 34:11, 2004.
13. Andersen K: Safe use of lasers in the operating room: what perioperative nurses should know, *AORN J* 79:171, 2004.
14. *Saunders nursing drug handbook 2005,* St Louis, 2005, Elsevier.
15. Habif T: *Clinical dermatology*, ed 4, St Louis, 2004, Elsevier Mosby.
16. Tatum S: Facial plastic surgery, *Curr Opin Otolaryngol Head Neck* 12:316, 2004.

RESOURCES

AcneNet
www.derm-infonet.com/acnenet/index.html

American Academy of Dermatology
847-330-0230
www.aad.org

American Academy of Facial Plastic and Reconstructive Surgery
703-299-9291
www.facial-plastic-surgery.org/index.asp

American Social Health Association
919-361-8400
www.ashastd.org

American Society of Plastic and Reconstructive Surgical Nurses
609-256-2340

Dermatology Foundation
www.dermfnd.org

Dermatology Nurses Association
856-256-2330
www.dnanurse.org

National Alopecia Areata Foundation
www.naaf.org

National Arthritis and Musculoskeletal and Skin Diseases Information Clearinghouse
National Institutes of Health
301-495-4484
877-22-NIAMS
www.niams.nih.gov

National Eczema Association for Science and Education
503-228-4430
800-818-7546
www.nationaleczema.org

National Pediculosis Association
781-449-NITS
www.headlice.org

National Psoriasis Foundation
503-244-7404
800-723-9166
www.psoriasis.org

Skin Cancer Foundation
800-SKIN-490
E-mail: info@skincancer.org
www.skincancer.org

For additional Internet resources, see the website for this book at *http://evolve.elsevier.com/Lewis/medsurg.*

The charity that is a trifle to us can be precious to others.

Homer

Nursing Management Burns

25

Judy A. Knighton

LEARNING OBJECTIVES

1. Describe the causes and prevention of burn injuries.
2. Describe the burn injury classification system.
3. Describe the relationship between the involved structures and the clinical appearance of partial- and full-thickness burns.
4. Identify the parameters used to determine the severity of burns.
5. Describe the pathophysiology, clinical manifestations, complications, and nursing and collaborative management of the three burn phases.
6. Explain fluid and electrolyte shifts during the emergent and acute burn phases.
7. Describe the nutritional therapy of the burn patient during the three burn phases.
8. Describe the interventions that the nurse may use in the management of pain in the burn patient.
9. Explain the physiologic and psychosocial aspects of burn rehabilitation.
10. Describe the nursing management of the emotional needs of the burn patient and family.
11. Discuss the issues involved and rationale for preparing the burn patient to return home.

KEY TERMS

burn, p. 483
chemical burns, p. 484
contracture, p. 504
cultured epithelial autograft, p. 501
debridement, p. 496
electrical burns, p. 485
enzymatic debridement, p. 501
escharotomy, p. 491
excision and grafting, p. 501
full-thickness burns, p. 486
hypermetabolic state, p. 499
partial-thickness burns, p. 486
smoke and inhalation injuries, p. 484
thermal burns, p. 484

Electronic Resources

Supplemental content related to Chapter 25 can be found . . .

Companion CD

- Stress-Busting Kit for Nursing Students
- Interactive Case Study: Burns
- NCLEX Examination Review Questions
- Comprehensive Glossary

Evolve Website evolve

http://evolve.elsevier.com/Lewis/medsurg

- Content Updates
- Key Points (Printable and CD/MP3 Download)
- Concept Map Creator
- Expanded Audio Glossary
- Key Term Flash Cards
- Customizable Nursing Care Plan: Burn Patient
- Electronic Calculators
- WebLinks

A **burn** occurs when there is injury to the tissues of the body caused by heat, chemicals, electric current, or radiation. The resulting effects are influenced by the temperature of the burning agent, duration of contact time, and type of tissue that is injured.

An estimated 1 million Americans and 100,000 Canadians seek medical care each year for burns.[1,2] Approximately 70,000 people are hospitalized in the United States and 5000 in Canada, one third of whom require care in specialized burn units or centers. About 4500 Americans and 450 Canadians die annually as a direct result of their burns. The highest fatality rates occur in children 4 years of age and younger, and adults over the age of 55.

Although burn incidence has decreased slightly in the past few years, burn injuries still occur too frequently. The focus of burn prevention programs has shifted from concentrating on individual blame and changing individual behaviors to include more legislative changes. The aim of these changes is to make improvements in the environment.[3] Coordinated national programs include child-resistant lighters, nonflammable children's clothing, tap water anti-scald devices, fire-safe cigarettes, stricter building codes, smoke detectors/alarms, and fire sprinklers.

Nurses can advocate for scald and fire risk reduction strategies in the home. Occupational health nurses can educate workers to

Reviewed by Mary-Liz Bilodeau, RN, MS, CCRN, CCNS, CS, BC, Acute Care Nurse Practitioner, Critical Care Clinical Nurse Specialist, Massachusetts General Hospital, Boston, Mass.; and Rosie Thompson, RN, MS, CS, Clinical Nurse Specialist, Burn Center, University of Kansas Hospital, Kansas City, Kan.

TABLE 25-1 Common Places and Causes of Burn Injury

Occupational Hazards
- Tar
- Chemicals
- Hot metals
- Steam pipes
- Combustible fuels
- Fertilizers/pesticides
- Electricity from power lines
- Sparks from live electric sources

Home and Recreational Hazards
Kitchen/Bathroom
- Pressure cookers
- Microwaved food
- Hot water heaters set higher than 140° F (60° C)
- Hot grease or liquids from cooking

General Home
- Gas fireplaces
- Open space heaters
- Frayed or defective wiring
- Radiators (home, automobile)
- Improper use of outdoor grills
- Multiple extension cords per outlet
- Carelessness with cigarettes or matches
- Improper use/storage of flammables (e.g., starter fluid, gasoline, kerosene)

TABLE 25-2 Types of Burn Injury and Risk Reduction Strategies

Types	Risk Reduction Strategies
Flame	• Never leave candles unattended or near open windows/curtains. • Encourage use of "child-resistant" lighters. • Install smoke/carbon monoxide detectors. • Encourage use of home fire exit drills. • Never use gasoline or other flammable liquids as accelerants. • Never leave hot oil unattended while cooking. • Do not smoke in bed or if very tired and likely to fall asleep. • Consider a flame-retardant smoking apron for elderly and/or "at-risk" people.
Electrical	• Avoid and/or repair frayed wiring. • Ensure electrical power source is shut off before commencing repairs. • Wear protective eyewear and gloves when conducting electrical repairs.
Scald	• Lower hot water temperature to the "lowest point" or 120° F/40° C. • Utilize "anti-scald" devices with showerhead or faucet fixtures. • Supervise bathing with small children, older adults, or anyone with impaired physical movement/physical sensation/judgment. • After running bath water, check temperature with hand or bath thermometer. • Exercise caution when microwaving food/beverages.
Chemical	• Store chemicals safely in approved containers and label appropriately. • Ensure safety of workers handling chemicals (education, protective eyewear, gloves, masks, clothing).

reduce scald, chemical, electrical, and thermal injuries in the work setting (Tables 25-1 and 25-2).

TYPES OF BURN INJURY

Thermal Burns

Thermal burns, which can be caused by flame, flash, scald, or contact with hot objects, are the most common type of burn (Table 25-2 and Fig. 25-1).

Chemical Burns

Chemical burns result from tissue injury and destruction from acids, alkalis, and organic compounds. Acids are found in many household cleaners and include hydrochloric, oxalic, and hydrofluoric acid. Alkali burns can be more difficult to manage than acid burns since alkaline substances are not neutralized by tissue fluids as readily as acid substances. Alkalis adhere to tissue, causing protein hydrolysis and liquefaction. This damage continues even when the alkali is neutralized. Alkalis are found in oven and drain cleaners, fertilizers, and heavy industrial cleansers. Organic compounds, including phenols and petroleum products, produce contact burns and systemic toxicity. Phenols are found in chemical disinfectants, while petroleum products include creosote and gasoline.

In addition to skin damage, eyes can be injured if they are splashed with a chemical. Respiratory problems and other systemic manifestations, including involvement of the liver and kidney, are also a concern.

With chemical injuries, it is important to remove the person from the burning agent and begin to quickly remove the chemical from the skin. Dry chemical should be brushed from the skin, and then the affected area should be flushed with copious amounts of water to irrigate the skin; this technique is effective when used anywhere from 20 minutes to 2 hours postexposure.[4] Any clothing containing the chemical should be removed, because the burning process will continue as long as the chemical is in contact with the skin. Tissue destruction may continue for up to 72 hours after a chemical injury.

Smoke and Inhalation Injury

Smoke and inhalation injuries result from the inhalation of hot air or noxious chemicals and can cause damage to the tissues of the respiratory tract. Fortunately, gases are cooled to body temperature before they reach the lung tissue. Although damage to the respiratory mucosa can occur, it seldom happens because the vocal cords and glottis close as a protective mechanism. Redness and airway swelling (edema) may result when damage occurs. Smoke inhalation injuries are a major predictor of mortality in burn patients.[5]

There are three types of smoke and inhalation injuries:

1. *Carbon monoxide poisoning.* Carbon monoxide (CO) poisoning and asphyxiation account for the majority of deaths at a fire scene. CO is produced by the incomplete combustion of burning materials. It is subsequently inhaled and displaces oxygen (O_2) on the hemoglobin molecule, causing hypoxia, carboxyhemoglobinemia, and ultimately death when the CO levels are high. Often the victims of fires, especially those who have been trapped in a closed space, will have elevated carboxyhemoglobin levels. If CO intoxication is suspected, the patient should be quickly treated with 100% humidified O_2 and the carboxyhemoglobin level should be measured when feasible. Skin color is often described as "cherry red" in

A

B

C

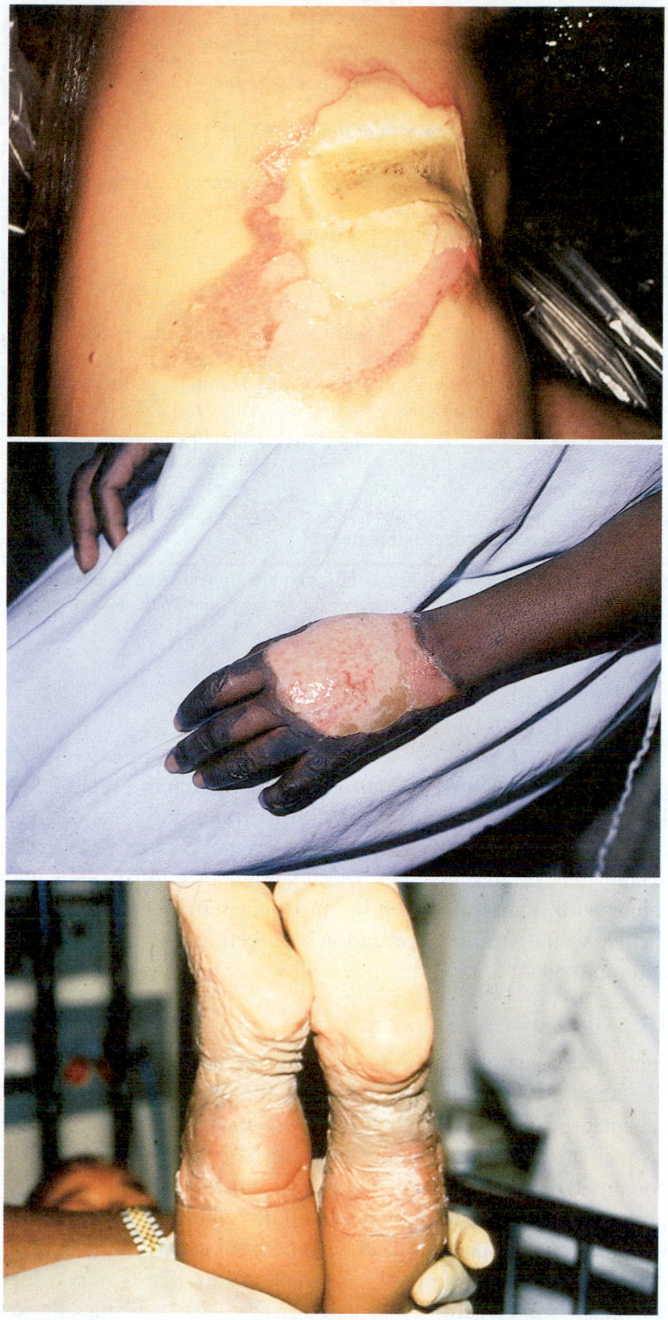

FIG. 25-1 Types of burn injury. **A,** Patient with full-thickness thermal burn. **B,** Partial-thickness burn to the hand. **C,** Partial-thickness burns secondary to immersion in hot water.

appearance with CO poisoning. CO poisoning may occur in the absence of burn injury to the skin.

2. *Inhalation injury above the glottis.* A general principle to remember is that inhalation injury above the glottis is thermally produced, and injury below the glottis is usually chemically produced. Injury above the glottis may be caused by the inhalation of hot air, steam, or smoke. Mucosal burns of the oropharynx and larynx are manifested by redness, blistering, and edema. Mechanical obstruction can occur quickly, presenting a true medical emergency. Reliable clues that this injury is likely include the presence of facial burns, singed nasal hair, hoarseness, painful swallowing, darkened oral and nasal membranes, carbonaceous sputum, history of

A

B

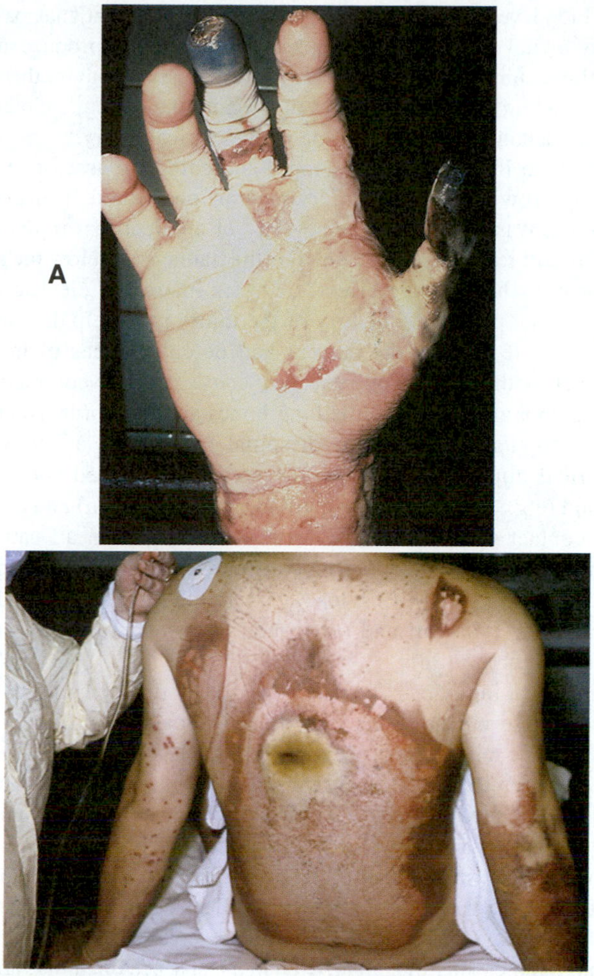

FIG. 25-2 Electrical injury produces heat coagulation of blood supply and contact area as electric current passes through the skin. **A,** Hand. **B,** Back.

being burned in an enclosed space, and clothing burns around the chest and neck.

3. *Inhalation injury below the glottis.* Tissue injury to the lower respiratory tract is related to the duration of exposure to smoke or toxic fumes. Clinical manifestations such as pulmonary edema may not appear until 12 to 24 hours after the burn, and then they may manifest as acute respiratory distress syndrome (ARDS) (see Chapter 68).

Patients with smoke and inhalation injuries must be observed closely for signs of respiratory distress or compromise. They need to be treated quickly and efficiently at the scene by paramedics and emergency department personnel if they are to survive. Patients with both body burns and inhalation injury must be transferred to the nearest burn unit. Respiratory tract complications from burn injury are discussed in detail later in this chapter.

Electrical Burns

Electrical burns are the result of intense heat generated from an electric current (Fig. 25-2). Direct damage to nerves and vessels, causing tissue anoxia and death, can also occur. The severity of the electrical injury depends on the amount of voltage, tissue resistance, current pathways, surface area in contact with the current, and length of time that the current flow was sustained. Tissue densities offer various amounts of resistance to electric current. For example, fat and bone offer the most resistance, whereas nerves and blood vessels offer the least resistance. Current that passes through vital organs (e.g., brain, heart, kidneys) will produce more life-threatening sequelae than that which passes through other tissue. In addition, electric sparks may ignite the patient's clothing, causing a combination of thermal and electrical injury.

As with inhalation injury, rapid and complete assessment of the patient with electrical injury must be performed. Transfer to a burn unit is indicated. The severity of an electrical injury can be difficult to determine as most of the damage is below the skin (known as the "iceberg effect"). Determination of electric current contact points and history of the injury may help determine the probable path of the current and potential areas of injury. Contact with electric current can cause muscle contractions strong enough to fracture the long bones and vertebrae. Another reason to suspect long bone or spinal fractures is a fall. Most electrical injuries occur when the victim is elevated above the ground (e.g., during work as a utility pole lineperson) and comes into contact with a current source. For this reason, all patients with electrical burns should be considered at risk for a potential cervical spine injury. Cervical spine immobilization should be used during transport and subsequent diagnostic testing to rule out any injury.

Electrical injury puts the patient at risk for dysrhythmias or cardiac arrest, severe metabolic acidosis, and myoglobinuria, which can lead to acute renal tubular necrosis (ATN). The electric shock event can cause immediate cardiac standstill or fibrillation. If this occurs, cardiopulmonary resuscitation (CPR) should be initiated immediately. Delayed cardiac dysrhythmias or arrest may also occur without warning during the first 24 hours after injury. Therefore the patient should be monitored continuously. Because of extensive tissue destruction and cell rupture, severe metabolic acidosis develops within minutes after the injury, even in the absence of cardiac arrest. Arterial blood gas (ABG) analysis should be performed as soon as possible by emergency department or burn unit staff to assess the acid-base balance. Fluid resuscitation for an electrical burn includes sodium bicarbonate, administered in amounts sufficient to maintain the serum pH at near-normal levels.

Myoglobin from injured muscle tissue and hemoglobin from damaged red blood cells (RBCs) are released into the circulation whenever massive muscle and blood vessel damage occurs. The released myoglobin pigments are then transported to the kidneys, where they can mechanically block the renal tubules because of their large size. This process can result in ATN and eventual acute renal failure if not appropriately treated (see Chapter 47). Treatment consists of infusing lactated Ringer's solution at a rate sufficient to maintain urinary output at 75 to 100 ml/hr until the urine sample analyses indicate that the myoglobin and hemoglobin have been flushed from the circulatory system. In addition, an osmotic diuretic (e.g., mannitol) may be given to maintain urine output. Sodium bicarbonate may be given to alkalinize the urine.

Cold Thermal Injury

Cold thermal injury, or frostbite, is discussed in Chapter 69.

CLASSIFICATION OF BURN INJURY

The treatment of burns is related to the severity of the injury. Severity is determined by (1) depth of burn, (2) extent of burn calculated in percent of total body surface area (TBSA), (3) location of burn, and (4) patient risk factors. The American Burn Association (ABA) has established referral criteria that recommend which burn injuries should be treated in burn units that have specialized facility and personnel for handling this type of trauma (Table 25-3). Burn injuries that fall outside of the referral criteria can be managed in community hospitals by non–burn unit personnel, either on an inpatient or an outpatient basis. The majority of patients with minor burn injuries are seen in outpatient settings. Goals of care include wound healing, prevention of infection, pain management, and rapid rehabilitation.

TABLE 25-3 Burn Unit Referral Criteria*

Burn injuries that should be referred to a burn unit include the following:

1. Partial-thickness burns greater than 10% total body surface area (TBSA)
2. Burns that involve the face, hands, feet, genitalia, perineum, or major joints
3. Third-degree burns in any age group
4. Electrical burns, including lightning injury
5. Chemical burns
6. Inhalation injury
7. Burn injury in patients with preexisting medical disorders that could complicate management, prolong recovery, or affect mortality
8. Any patients with burns and concomitant trauma (e.g., fractures) in which the burn injury poses the greatest risk of morbidity or mortality. In such cases, if the trauma poses the greater immediate risk, the patient may be initially stabilized in a trauma center before being transferred to a burn unit.
9. Burn injury in patients who will require special social, emotional, or long-term rehabilitative intervention

Source: Guidelines for the operations of burn units. In American College of Surgeons, *Committee on Trauma: Resources for optimal care of the injured patient,* 1999. Available at *www.ameriburn.org.*

*Guidelines from the American Burn Association.

Depth of Burn

Burn injury involves the destruction of the integumentary system. The skin is divided into three layers: the epidermis, dermis, and subcutaneous tissue (Fig. 25-3). The *epidermis,* or nonvascular outer layer of the skin, is approximately as thick as a sheet of paper. It is composed of many layers of nonliving epithelial cells that provide a protective barrier to the skin, hold in fluids and electrolytes, help to regulate body temperature, and keep harmful agents in the external environment from injuring or invading the body. The *dermis,* which lies below the epidermis, is approximately 30 to 45 times thicker than the epidermis. The dermis contains connective tissues with blood vessels and highly specialized structures consisting of hair follicles, nerve endings, sweat glands, and sebaceous glands. Under the dermis lies the subcutaneous tissue, which contains major vascular networks, fat, nerves, and lymphatics. The *subcutaneous tissue* acts as a heat insulator for underlying structures, which include the muscles, tendons, bones, and internal organs.

In the past, burns were defined by degrees: first degree, second degree, and third degree. The ABA now recommends a more precise definition of second- and third-degree burns, categorizing them according to depth of skin destruction: **partial-thickness burns** and **full-thickness burns** (see Fig. 25-3). Table 25-4 shows a comparison of the depth of injury. Skin-reproducing (re-epithelializing) cells are located throughout the dermis and along the shafts of the hair follicles and sebaceous glands. If there is significant damage to the dermis (e.g., a full-thickness burn), there are not enough remaining skin cells to regenerate new skin. A permanent, alternative source of skin then needs to be found.

Extent of Burn

Two commonly used guides for determining the *total body surface area* affected or the extent of a burn wound are the *Lund-Browder chart* (Fig. 25-4, *A*) and the *rule of nines* (Fig. 25-4, *B*). (First-degree burns, equivalent to a sunburn, are not included when calculating BSA.) The Lund-Browder chart is considered more accurate because the patient's age, in proportion to relative body-area size, is taken into account. The rule of nines, which is easy to remember, is considered adequate for initial assessment of an adult burn patient. For irregular- or odd-shaped burns, the palmar surface of the patient's hand is considered to be approximately 1% of the total body surface area (TBSA). The extent of a burn (scald, in particular) is often revised after edema has subsided and a demarcation of the zones of injury has occurred. The *Sage Burn Diagram* is a newer, computerized burn estimation tool (available on the Internet at *www.sagediagram.com*). This tool also calculates fluid resuscitation requirements.

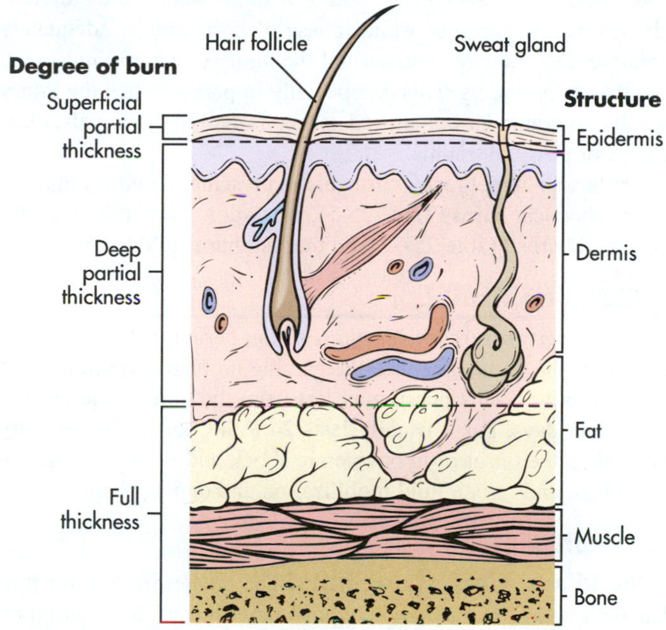

FIG. 25-3 Cross section of skin indicating the degree of burn and structures involved.

Location of Burn

The severity of the burn injury is related to the location of the burn wound. Burns to the face and neck and circumferential burns to the chest/back may inhibit respiratory function due to mechanical obstruction secondary to edema or leathery, devitalized tissue (*es-*

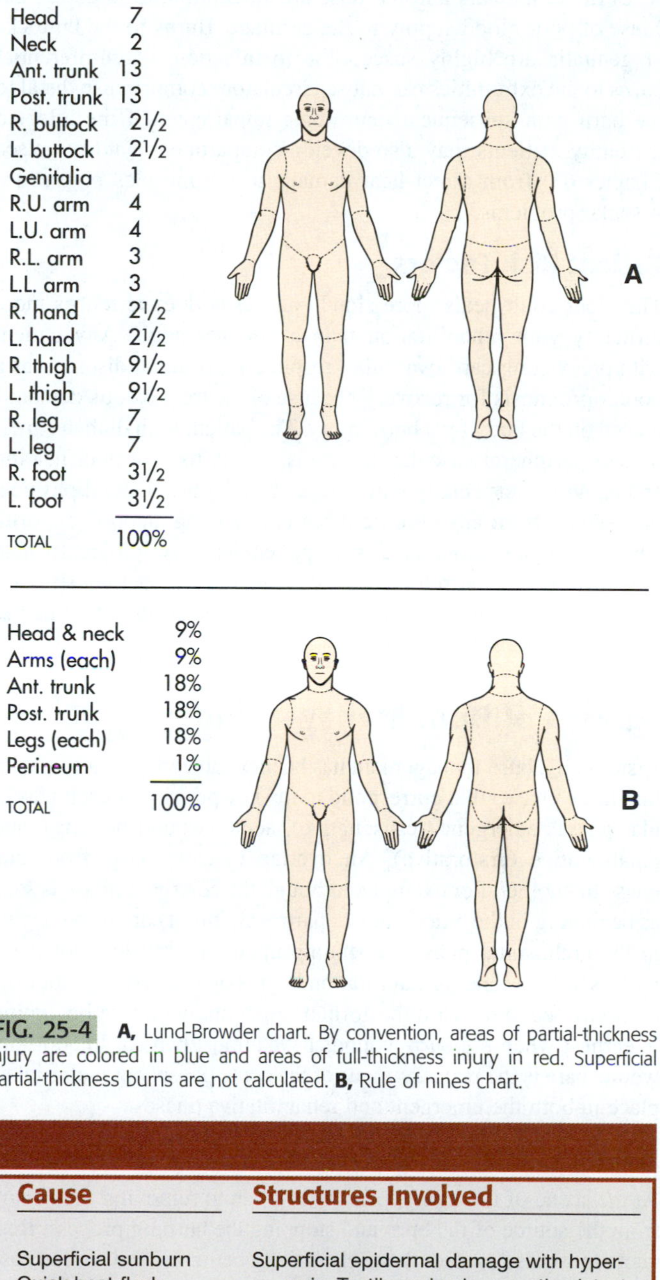
Head 7
Neck 2
Ant. trunk 13
Post. trunk 13
R. buttock 2½
L. buttock 2½
Genitalia 1
R.U. arm 4
L.U. arm 4
R.L. arm 3
L.L. arm 3
R. hand 2½
L. hand 2½
R. thigh 9½
L. thigh 9½
R. leg 7
L. leg 7
R. foot 3½
L. foot 3½
TOTAL 100%
A
Head & neck 9%
Arms (each) 9%
Ant. trunk 18%
Post. trunk 18%
Legs (each) 18%
Perineum 1%
TOTAL 100%
B

FIG. 25-4 **A,** Lund-Browder chart. By convention, areas of partial-thickness injury are colored in blue and areas of full-thickness injury in red. Superficial partial-thickness burns are not calculated. **B,** Rule of nines chart.

TABLE 25-4 Classification of Burn Injury Depth

Classification	Clinical Appearance	Cause	Structures Involved
Partial-Thickness Skin Destruction			
• Superficial (first-degree)	Erythema, blanching on pressure, pain and mild swelling, no vesicles or blisters (although after 24 hr skin may blister and peel)	Superficial sunburn Quick heat flash	Superficial epidermal damage with hyperemia. Tactile and pain sensation intact.
• Deep (second-degree)	Fluid-filled vesicles that are red, shiny, wet (if vesicles have ruptured); severe pain caused by nerve injury; mild to moderate edema	Flame Flash Scald Contact burns Chemical Tar	Epidermis and dermis involved to varying depth. Skin elements, from which epithelial regeneration occurs, remain viable.
Full-Thickness Skin Destruction			
• (Third- and fourth-degree)	Dry, waxy white, leathery, or hard skin; visible thrombosed vessels; insensitivity to pain because of nerve destruction; possible involvement of muscles, tendons, and bones	Flame Scald Chemical Tar Electric current	All skin elements and local nerve endings destroyed. Coagulation necrosis present. Surgical intervention required for healing.

char) formation. These injuries also may signal the possibility of inhalation injury and respiratory mucosal damage.

Burns of the hands, feet, joints, and eyes are of concern because they make self-care very difficult and may jeopardize future function. Burns of the hands and feet are challenging to manage because of superficial vascular and nerve supply systems.

Burns to the ears and the nose are susceptible to infection because of poor blood supply to the cartilage. Burns to the buttocks or genitalia are highly susceptible to infection. Circumferential burns to the extremities can cause circulatory compromise distal to the burn with subsequent neurologic impairment of the affected extremity. Patients may also develop compartment syndrome (see Chapter 63) from direct heat damage to the muscles or preburn vascular problems.

Patient Risk Factors

The older adult heals more slowly and usually experiences more difficulty with rehabilitation than a younger adult. Any patient with preexisting cardiovascular, respiratory, or renal disease has a poorer prognosis for recovery because of the tremendous demands placed on the body by a burn injury. The patient with diabetes mellitus or peripheral vascular disease is at high risk for poor healing and gangrene, especially with foot and leg burns. General physical debilitation from any chronic disease, including alcoholism, drug abuse, or malnutrition, renders the patient less physiologically able to recover from a burn injury. In addition, the burn patient who has concurrently sustained fractures, head injuries, or other trauma has a poorer prognosis for recovery.

Phases of Burn Management

Historically, burn management has been organized chronologically into three phases that correspond to the key priority of each particular phase: emergent (resuscitative), acute (wound healing), and rehabilitative (restorative). An overlap in care exists from one phase to another. For example, although the emergent phase is seen as beginning in the emergency department, initial care often begins in the prehospital phase, depending upon the skill level of paramedics at the scene. Rehabilitation begins on the first day after the burn has occurred, with the formal rehabilitative phase beginning in earnest when the burn wounds have almost healed. In addition, wound care is the primary focus of the acute phase, but it also takes place in both the emergent and rehabilitative phases.

PREHOSPITAL CARE

At the scene of the injury, priority is given to removing the person from the source of the burn and stopping the burning process. Rescuers must also protect themselves from being injured. In the case of electrical injuries, initial management involves removal of the patient from contact with the source of current by a trained individual. Most chemical burns are best treated by brushing solid particles off the skin, followed by thorough lavage with water. (For information on handling specific agents, refer to a hazardous materials text.) Small thermal burns (≤10% TBSA) may be covered with a clean, cool, tap water–dampened towel for the patient's comfort and protection until definitive medical care is instituted. Cooling of the injured area (if small) within 1 minute helps minimize the depth of the injury. Tap water is acceptable for flushing. Time should not be wasted trying to find sterile water, saline solution, or antidotes.

If the thermal burn area is large, attention needs to be focused first on airway, breathing, and circulation (the ABCs):

Airway: check for patency, soot around nares/on the tongue, singed nasal hair, darkened oral or nasal membranes.

Breathing: check for adequacy of ventilation.

Circulation: check for presence and regularity of pulses, and elevate the burned limb above the heart to decrease pain and swelling.

If the burn is large (i.e., >10% TBSA), it is not advisable to immerse the burned body part in cool water since doing so might lead to extensive heat loss. The burn should never be covered in ice as this could cause frostbite. As much burned clothing as possible should be gently removed to prevent further tissue damage. Adherent clothing should be left in place until the patient is transferred to a hospital. The patient should then be wrapped in a dry, clean sheet or blanket to prevent further contamination of the wound and to provide warmth.

The burn patient may also have sustained other injuries that take priority over the burn wound. It is important for the individuals involved in the prehospital phase of burn care to adequately communicate the circumstances of the injury to the hospital-based health care providers. This is especially important when the injury involves entrapment in a closed space, hazardous chemicals, electricity, or possible trauma.

Prehospital emergency burn care is presented in tables that describe chemical burns (Table 25-5), inhalation injury (Table 25-6), electrical burns (Table 25-7), and thermal burns (Table 25-8).

EMERGENT PHASE

The *emergent (resuscitative) phase* is the period of time required to resolve the immediate, life-threatening problems resulting from the burn injury. This phase may last from the time of the burn to 3 or more days, but it usually lasts 24 to 48 hours. The primary concern is the onset of hypovolemic shock and edema formation. The phase ends when fluid mobilization and diuresis begin.

Pathophysiology

Fluid and Electrolyte Shifts. The greatest initial threat to a patient with a major burn is hypovolemic shock.[6] It is caused by a massive shift of fluids out of the blood vessels as a result of increased capillary permeability and can begin as early as 20 minutes postburn. As the capillary walls become more permeable, water, sodium, and later plasma proteins (especially albumin) move into interstitial spaces and other surrounding tissue (Fig. 25-5). The colloidal osmotic pressure decreases with progressive loss of protein from the vascular space. This results in more fluid shifting out of the vascular space into the interstitial spaces. (Fluid accumulation in the interstitium is termed *second spacing.*) Fluid also moves to areas that normally have minimal to no fluid, a phenomenon termed *third spacing.* Examples of third spacing in burn injury are exudate and blister formation, as well as edema in nonburned areas.

The net result of the fluid shift is intravascular volume depletion. Decreased blood pressure (BP), increased pulse rate, and other manifestations of hypovolemic shock are clinically detectable signs (see Chapter 67). If not corrected, irreversible shock and death may result. Another source of fluid loss is insensible loss by evaporation from large, denuded body surfaces. The normal insensible loss of 30 to 50 ml/hr may increase in the severely burned patient.

TABLE 25-5 EMERGENCY MANAGEMENT
Chemical Burns

Etiology	Assessment Findings	Interventions
Acids Alkalis Organic compounds	• Burning • Redness, swelling of injured tissue • Degeneration of exposed tissue • Discoloration of injured skin • Localized pain • Edema of surrounding tissue • Respiratory distress if chemical inhaled • Decreased muscle coordination (if organophosphate) • Paralysis	**Initial** • Ensure patent airway. • Stabilize cervical spine. • Anticipate intubation with significant inhalation injury, circumferential full-thickness burns to the neck/chest, and/or large TBSA burn. • Assess airway, breathing, and circulation before decontamination procedures. • Brush dry chemical from skin before irrigation. • Flush chemical from wound and surrounding area with saline solution or water. • Remove nonadherent clothing, shoes, watches, jewelry, glasses, or contact lenses, if face was exposed. • Establish IV access with 2 large-bore catheters if >15% TBSA burn. • Begin fluid replacement. • Insert urinary catheter if adult burn >15% TBSA. • Elevate burned limbs above heart to decrease edema. • Administer IV analgesia and assess effectiveness frequently. • Cover burned areas with dry dressings or clean sheet. • Contact poison control center for assistance. • Caregiver should protect self from potential exposure. **Ongoing Monitoring** • Monitor airway if exposed to chemicals. • Monitor urine output. • Consider possibility of systemic impact of identified chemical and monitor/treat accordingly.

TBSA, Total body surface area.

TABLE 25-6 EMERGENCY MANAGEMENT
Inhalation Injury

Etiology	Assessment Findings	Interventions
Exposure of respiratory tract to intense heat or flames Inhalation of noxious chemicals, smoke, or carbon monoxide	• History of being burned in an enclosed space or clothing catching fire • Rapid, shallow respirations • Increasing hoarseness • Coughing • Singed nasal or facial hair • Darkened oral/nasal membranes • Smoky breath • Carbonaceous sputum • Productive cough with black, gray, or bloody sputum • Irritation of upper airways or burning pain in throat or chest • Difficulty swallowing • Restlessness, anxiety • Altered mental status, including confusion, coma • Decreased oxygen saturation • Dysrhythmias	**Initial** • Ensure patent airway. • Stabilize cervical spine. • Assess for inhalation injury. • Monitor vital signs, level of consciousness, oxygen saturation, and cardiac rhythm. • Assess airway, breathing, and circulation. • Remove nonadherent clothing, jewelry, glasses, or contact lenses, if face was exposed. • Establish IV access with 2 large-bore catheters if >15% TBSA burn. • Begin fluid replacement and insert urinary catheter. • Elevate burned limbs above heart to decrease edema. • Obtain arterial blood gas, carboxyhemoglobin levels, and chest x-ray. • Administer IV analgesia and assess effectiveness frequently. • Identify and treat other associated injuries (e.g., fractures, pneumothorax, head injury). • Cover burned areas with dry dressings or clean sheet. • Anticipate need for fiberoptic bronchoscopy or intubation. **Ongoing Monitoring** • Monitor airway. • Monitor urine output. • Monitor vital signs, level of consciousness, oxygen saturation, and cardiac rhythm.

Burns

TABLE 25-7 EMERGENCY MANAGEMENT
Electrical Burns

Etiology	Assessment Findings	Interventions
Alternating Current Electric wires Utility wires **Direct Current** Lightning Defibrillator	• Leathery, white, or charred skin • Burn odor • Impaired touch sensation • Minimal or absent pain • Dysrhythmias • Cardiac arrest • Location of contact points • Diminished peripheral circulation in injured extremity • Thermal burns if clothing ignites • Fractures or dislocations from force of current • Head or neck injury if fall occurred • Depth and extent of wound difficult to visualize; assume injury greater than what is seen	**Initial** • Removal from current source must be done by trained personnel with special equipment to prevent injury to rescuer. • Assess and treat patient *after* removal from source of current. • Ensure patent airway. • Stabilize cervical spine. • Monitor vital signs, level of consciousness, respiratory status, oxygen saturation, and cardiac rhythm. • Assess airway, breathing, and circulation. • Check pulses distal to burns. • Remove nonadherent clothing, shoes, watches, jewelry, glasses, or contact lenses, if face was exposed. • Establish IV access with 2 large-bore catheters for >15% TBSA burn. • Begin fluid replacement. • Insert urinary catheter. • Elevate burned limbs above heart to decrease edema. • Administer IV analgesia and assess effectiveness frequently. • Identify and treat other associated injuries (e.g., fractures, pneumothorax, head injury). • Cover burned areas with dry dressing or clean sheet. **Ongoing Monitoring** • Monitor airway. • Monitor vital signs, cardiac rhythm, level of consciousness, respiratory status, oxygen saturation, and neurovascular status of injured limbs. • Monitor urine output to ensure adequate volume replacement. • Monitor urine for development of myoglobinuria secondary to muscle breakdown. • Anticipate administration of mannitol and $NaHCO_3$ for myoglobinuria and hemoglobinuria.

TABLE 25-8 EMERGENCY MANAGEMENT
Thermal Burns

Etiology	Assessment Findings	Interventions
Hot liquids or solids Flash flame Open flame Steam Hot surface Ultraviolet rays	**Partial Thickness (Superficial)** • Redness • Pain • Moderate to severe tenderness • Minimal edema • Blanching with pressure **Partial Thickness (Deep)** • Moist blebs, blisters • Mottled white, pink to cherry red • Hypersensitive to touch or air • Moderate to severe pain • Blanching with pressure **Full Thickness** • Dry, leathery eschar • White waxy, dark brown, or charred appearance • Strong burn odor • Impaired sensation when touched • Absence of pain with severe pain in surrounding tissues • Lack of blanching with pressure	**Initial** • Ensure patent airway. • Stabilize cervical spine. • Assess for inhalation injury. • Monitor vital signs, level of consciousness, respiratory status, oxygen saturation, and cardiac rhythm. • Assess airway, breathing, and circulation. • Remove nonadherent clothing, shoes, watches, jewelry, glasses or contact lenses, if face was exposed. • Establish IV access with 2 large-bore catheters for >15% TBSA burn. • Begin fluid replacement. • Insert urinary catheter. • Elevate burned limbs above heart to decrease edema. • Administer IV analgesia and assess effectiveness frequently. • Identify and treat other associated injuries (e.g., fractures, pneumothorax, head injury). • Cover burned areas with dry dressing or clean sheet. **Ongoing Monitoring** • Monitor airway. • Monitor vital signs, cardiac rhythm, level of consciousness, respiratory status, and oxygen saturation. • Monitor urine output.

TBSA, Total body surface area.

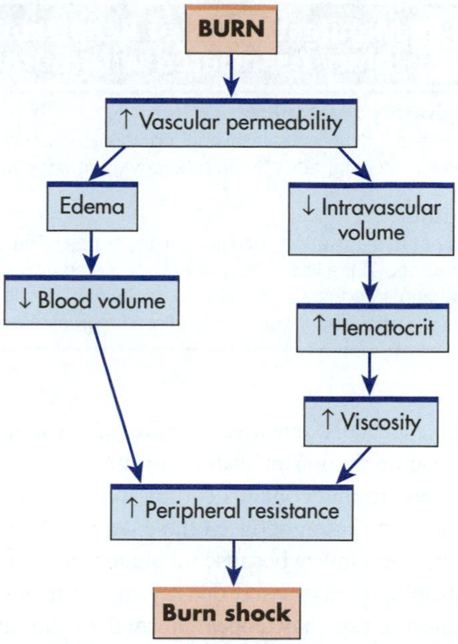

FIG. 25-5 At the time of major burn injury, there is increased capillary permeability. All fluid components of the blood begin to leak into the interstitium, causing edema and a decreased blood volume. The red blood cells and white blood cells do not leak. Therefore the hematocrit increases and the blood becomes more viscous. The combination of decreased blood volume and increased viscosity produces increased peripheral resistance. Burn shock, a type of hypovolemic shock, rapidly ensues and continues for about 24 to 48 hours.

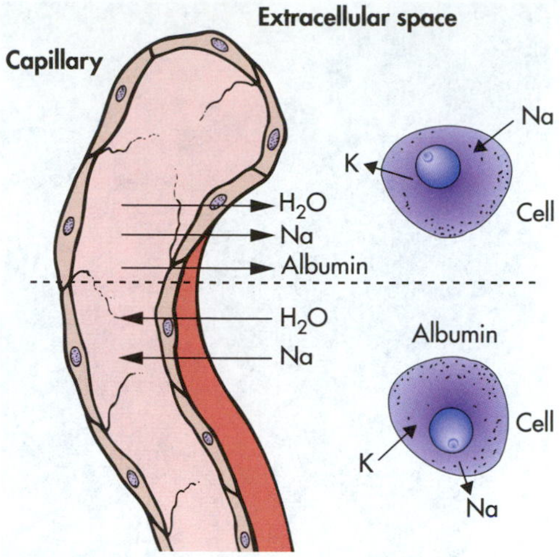

FIG. 25-6 The effects of burn shock during the first 24 to 48 hours are shown above the dotted line. As the capillary seal is lost, the interstitial edema fluid is formed. The cellular integrity is also altered, with sodium (Na) moving into the cell in abnormal amounts and potassium (K) leaving the cell. The shifts after the first 24 to 48 hours are shown below the dotted line. The water and sodium move back into the circulating volume through the capillary. The albumin remains in the interstitium. Potassium is transported into the cell and sodium is transported out as the cellular integrity returns.

The circulatory status is also impaired because of hemolysis of RBCs. The RBCs are hemolyzed by a circulating factor released at the time of the burn as well as by the direct insult of the burn injury. Thrombosis in the capillaries of burned tissue causes an additional loss of circulating RBCs. An elevated hematocrit is commonly caused by hemoconcentration resulting from fluid loss. After fluid balance has been restored, lowered hematocrit levels are found secondary to dilution.

Sodium and potassium are involved in electrolyte shifts. Sodium rapidly shifts to the interstitial spaces and remains there until edema formation ceases (Fig. 25-6). A potassium shift develops initially because injured cells and hemolyzed RBCs release potassium into the circulation.

Toward the end of the emergent phase, capillary membrane permeability will be restored if fluid replacement is adequate. Fluid loss and edema formation cease. Interstitial fluid gradually returns to the vascular space (see Fig. 25-6). Clinically, diuresis is noted with low urine specific gravities.

Inflammation and Healing. Burn injury causes coagulation necrosis, whereby tissues and vessels are damaged or destroyed. Neutrophils and monocytes accumulate at the site of injury. Fibroblasts and newly formed collagen fibrils appear and begin wound repair within the first 6 to 12 hours after injury. (The inflammatory response is discussed in Chapter 13.)

Immunologic Changes. Burn injury causes widespread impairment of the immune system. The skin barrier to invading organisms is destroyed, resulting in bone marrow depression and decreased circulating levels of immunoglobulins. Defects occur in the function of white blood cells (WBCs). The inflammatory cytokine cascade triggered by tissue damage impairs the function of lymphocytes, monocytes, and neutrophils, which puts the patient at greater risk for infection.

Clinical Manifestations

The burn patient is likely to be in shock from pain and hypovolemia. Frequently, areas of full-thickness and deep partial-thickness burns are initially anesthetic because the nerve endings are destroyed. Superficial to moderate partial-thickness burns are painful. Blisters filled with fluid and protein may occur in partial-thickness burns. Fluid is not actually lost from the body as much as it is sequestered in the interstitial spaces and third spaces. It is hard for the nurse to visualize severe dehydration in someone who is so obviously edematous. The patient may have signs of adynamic ileus, such as absent or decreased bowel sounds, as a result of the body's response to massive trauma and potassium shifts. Shivering may occur as a result of chilling that is caused by heat loss, anxiety, or pain.

Most burn patients are quite alert and can provide answers to questions shortly after the injury or until they are intubated. Unconsciousness or altered mental status in a burn patient is usually not a result of the burn. The most common reason for unconsciousness is hypoxia associated with smoke inhalation. Other possibilities include head trauma or excessive amounts of sedation or pain medication.

Complications

The three major organ systems most susceptible to complications during the emergent phase of burn injury are the cardiovascular, respiratory, and urinary systems.

Cardiovascular System. Cardiovascular system complications include dysrhythmias and hypovolemic shock, which may progress to irreversible shock. Circulation to the extremities can be severely impaired by circumferential burns and subsequent edema formation. These processes occlude the blood supply, causing ischemia, paresthesias, necrosis, and eventually gangrene. An **escharotomy** (a scalpel incision through the full-thickness eschar) is frequently performed following transfer to a burn unit to restore circulation to compromised extremities (Fig. 25-7).

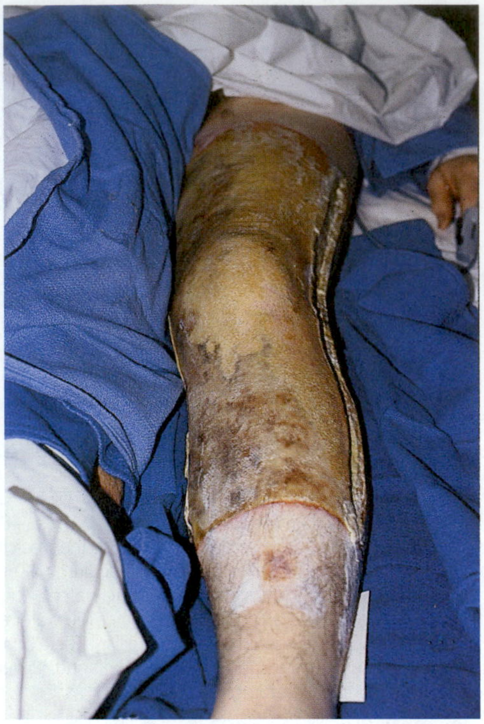

FIG. 25-7 Escharotomy of the lower extremity.

Initially, there is an increase in blood viscosity with burn injuries because of the fluid loss that occurs in the emergent period. Microcirculation is impaired because of the damage to skin structures that contain small capillary systems. These two events result in a phenomenon termed *sludging*. Sludging can be corrected by adequate fluid replacement.

Respiratory System. The respiratory system is especially vulnerable to two types of injury: (1) upper airway burns that cause edema formation and obstruction of the airway and (2) inhalation injury (Table 25-9). Upper airway distress may occur with or without smoke inhalation, and airway injury at either level may occur in the absence of burn injury to the skin.

Upper Respiratory Tract Injury. Upper respiratory tract injury results from direct heat injury or edema formation and can lead to mechanical airway obstruction and asphyxia. The edema associated with an upper respiratory tract burn injury can be massive and the onset insidious, and it occurs in all patients with major thermal burn injuries. Mechanical obstruction of the airway is not limited to the patient with flame burns to the upper airway. Swelling that accompanies scald burns to the face and neck can be lethal, as can pressure from the accumulated edema compressing the airway externally. Flame burns to the neck and chest may contribute to respiratory difficulty because the inelastic eschar becomes tight and constricting due to the underlying edema.

Inhalation Injury. Inhalation injury refers to a direct insult at the alveolar level secondary to the inhalation of chemical fumes or smoke. The result is interstitial edema that prevents the diffusion of oxygen from the alveoli into the circulatory system. The patient with smoke inhalation may not exhibit physical manifestations of injury during the first 24 hours after sustaining a major burn.[7] Fiberoptic bronchoscopy can be used as an early diagnostic tool for suspected inhalation injury. Another diagnostic indicator may be a history of prolonged exposure to smoke or fumes. Therefore the nurse must be especially sensitive to signs of respiratory distress such as increased agitation or change in the rate or character of respirations. Sputum that contains carbon may be present. Generally, there is no correlation between the extent of TBSA burn and severity of inhalation injury because inhalation injury is a factor of time exposure plus the type and density of the material inhaled. The initial chest x-ray may appear normal on admission, with changes noted over the next 24 to 48 hours. ABG values may also be within the normal range on admission and then change during hospitalization.

TABLE 25-9 Manifestations of Respiratory Injury Associated with Burns

Upper Respiratory Tract Injury Edema, hoarseness, difficulty swallowing, copious secretions, stridor, substernal and intercostal retractions, total airway obstruction
Inhalation Injury Initial absence of manifestations possible; high degree of suspicion if patient was trapped in fire in an enclosed space or clothing caught fire, and has facial burns and/or singed nasal or facial hair; dyspnea, carbonaceous sputum, wheezing, hoarseness, altered mental status

Other Respiratory Problems. The patient with preexisting respiratory problems (e.g., chronic obstructive pulmonary disease) is more likely to develop a respiratory infection. Pneumonia is a common complication of major burns (especially in the older adult) because of debilitation, abundant microbial flora, and relative immobility of the patient. If fluid replacement is vigorous, the older adult patient can develop pulmonary edema.

Urinary System. The most common complication of the urinary system in the emergent phase is acute tubular necrosis (ATN). If the patient is allowed to become hypovolemic, blood flow to the kidneys may be decreased, causing renal ischemia. If this continues, acute renal failure may develop.

With full-thickness and electrical burns, myoglobin (from muscle cell breakdown) and hemoglobin (from RBC breakdown) are released into the bloodstream and occlude renal tubules. Adequate fluid replacement and diuretics can counteract myoglobin and hemoglobin obstruction of the tubules.

NURSING *and* COLLABORATIVE MANAGEMENT EMERGENT PHASE

In the emergent phase, patient survival depends on rapid and thorough assessment and intervention.[8] It is usually the nurse, in collaboration with a physician, who makes the initial assessment of depth, degree, and percent of burn, and coordinates the actions of the health care team. In a community hospital, decisions need to be made as to whether the patient requires inpatient or outpatient care, and, in the case of inpatient care, whether the patient remains in that hospital or is transferred to the closest regional burn unit (see Table 25-3). From the onset of the burn event until the patient is stabilized, nursing and collaborative management predominantly consists of airway management, fluid therapy, and wound care (Table 25-10). While the burn management can be chronologically categorized as emergent, acute, and rehabilitative, the overall care requirements are not so easily classified. Depending upon the acuity of the patient, the duration of time spent in each phase varies greatly, and conditions improve and worsen unpredictably on an almost daily basis. Care changes accordingly. Although physiotherapy and occupational therapy are a focus of the acute and rehabilitative phases, proper positioning and splinting begin at the time of admission. Although support and teaching of patients and families begin at the initial contact, they intensify in the rehabilitative phase. See the accompanying nursing care plan (NCP 25-1).

Airway Management

Airway management frequently involves early endotracheal (preferably orotracheal) intubation. Early intubation eliminates the necessity for emergency tracheostomy after respiratory problems have become apparent. In general, the patient with major injuries involving burns to the face and neck requires intubation within 1 to 2 hours after burn injury. (Intubation is discussed in Chapter 66.) After intubation, the patient may be placed on ventilatory assistance, and the delivered oxygen concentration is determined by assessing ABG values. Extubation may be indicated when the edema resolves, usually 3 to 6 days after burn injury, unless severe inhalation injury is involved. Escharotomies of the chest wall may be needed to relieve respiratory distress secondary to circumferential, full-thickness burns of the neck and trunk.

Within 6 to 12 hours after injury in which smoke inhalation is suspected, a fiberoptic bronchoscopy should be performed to assess the lower respiratory tract. Significant findings include the appearance of carbonaceous material, mucosal edema, vesicles, erythema, hemorrhage, and ulceration.

When intubation is not performed, treatment of inhalation injury includes administration of humidified air and supplemental oxygen as required. The patient should be placed in a high Fowler's position unless contraindicated by a possible spinal injury, in which case reverse Trendelenburg may be the position of choice. The patient should also be encouraged to cough and deep breathe every hour, be repositioned every 1 to 2 hours, given chest physiotherapy, and suctioned as necessary. If respiratory failure is impending, intubation should be performed and the patient should be supported with mechanical ventilation. Positive end-expiratory pressure (PEEP) may be used to prevent collapse of the alveoli and progressive respiratory failure (see Chapter 66). Bronchodilators may be administered to treat severe bronchospasm. CO poisoning is treated by administering 100% O_2 until carboxyhemoglobin levels return to normal. The use of hyperbaric oxygen therapy remains controversial.

Fluid Therapy

As soon as the patient (usually with a >15% TBSA burn) arrives at a health care facility, at least one (and usually two) large-bore intravenous (IV) access routes must be obtained. It is critical to establish IV access that can accommodate large volumes of fluid. For burns >30% TBSA, central lines and an arterial line for fluid/medication/blood access should be considered.

The extent of an adult's burn wound should be assessed using the rule of nines or Lund-Browder charts (see Fig. 25-4). These universal standards will allow for the accurate estimation of fluid resuscitation requirements.

IV fluid therapy is usually instituted in the adult patient with burns >15% TBSA. The type of fluid replacement is determined by size and depth of burn, age of the patient, and individual considerations, such as dehydration in the preburn state or preexisting

TABLE 25-10 COLLABORATIVE CARE
Patient with Burns

Emergent Phase

Fluid Therapy
- Assess fluid needs.*
- Begin IV fluid replacement.
- Insert urinary catheter.
- Monitor urine output.

Wound Care
- Start hydrotherapy or wound cleansing.
- Debride as necessary.
- Assess extent and depth of burns.
- Initiate appropriate wound care.
- Administer tetanus toxoid or tetanus antitoxin.

Pain and Anxiety
- Assess and manage pain and anxiety.

Psychosocial Care
- Provide support to patient and family during initial crisis phase.

Physical/Occupational Therapy
- Place patient in position that prevents contracture formation and assess need for splints.

Nutritional Therapy
- Assess nutritional needs and begin feeding patient by most appropriate route as soon as possible.

Acute Phase

Fluid Therapy
- Continue to replace fluids, depending on patient's clinical response.

Wound Care
- Continue hydrotherapy/cleansing.
- Assess wound daily and adjust dressing protocols as necessary.
- Observe for complications.
- Continue debridement (if necessary).
- Continue assessing for and treating pain and anxiety.

Early Excision and Grafting
- Provide temporary homografts.
- Provide permanent autografts.
- Care for donor sites.

Nutritional Therapy
- Continue to assess diet to support wound healing.

Physical/Occupational Therapy
- Begin daily therapy program for maintenance of range of motion.
- Assess need for splints and anti-contracture positioning.
- Counsel and teach patient and family about physical and psychosocial aspects of care.
- Encourage and assist patient with self-care as possible.

Rehabilitation Phase

- Counsel and teach patient and family.
- Encourage and assist patient in resuming self-care.
- Prevent or minimize contractures and assess likelihood for scarring (surgery, physical/occupational therapy, splinting, or pressure garments).
- Discuss possible reconstructive surgery.
- Prepare for discharge home or transfer to rehabilitation hospital.

*See Tables 25-11 and 25-12.
IV, Intravenous.

NURSING CARE PLAN 25-1

Patient with Burns

NURSING DIAGNOSIS **Risk for fluid volume imbalance** *related to* evaporative fluid loss, intracompartmental fluid shifts, and rapid fluid replacement therapy

PATIENT GOALS
1. Maintains fluid and electrolyte balance required for metabolic needs
2. Demonstrates no signs of hypo- or hypervolemia

OUTCOMES (NOC)

Fluid Balance

- Blood pressure ____
- Radial pulse rate ____
- Central venous pressure ____
- Peripheral pulses ____
- Hourly urine output ____
- 24-hr intake and output balance ____
- Serum electrolytes ____
- Hematocrit ____
- Urine specific gravity ____

Measurement Scale
1 = Severely compromised
2 = Substantially compromised
3 = Moderately compromised
4 = Mildly compromised
5 = Not compromised

INTERVENTIONS (NIC) and *RATIONALES*

Fluid/Electrolyte Management

EMERGENT PHASE

- Monitor hemodynamic status, including CVP level, *to determine fluid status.*
- Monitor laboratory results relevant to fluid balance *to determine fluid status.*
- Monitor for abnormal serum electrolyte levels *to determine electrolyte status.*
- Keep an accurate record of intake and output *to monitor fluid loss and gain.*
- Maintain intravenous solution containing electrolyte(s) at constant flow rate *to prevent fluid overload or excessive electrolytes.*
- Monitor for manifestations of electrolyte imbalance *to detect early changes in electrolyte balance.*
- Weigh patient daily and monitor trends *to detect early changes in fluid balance.*
- Consult physician if signs and symptoms of fluid and/or electrolyte imbalance persist or worsen *to provide additional therapy as needed.*

ACUTE PHASE

- Use emergent phase interventions as necessary.
- Obtain laboratory specimens for monitoring of altered fluid or electrolyte levels *to detect changes in fluid/electrolyte balance.*
- Provide oral intake *to promote normal fluid intake and patient comfort.*

NURSING DIAGNOSIS **Acute pain** *related to* burn injury and treatments *as evidenced by* patient's report of pain and nonverbal behaviors indicating pain

PATIENT GOALS
1. Reports pain relief after pain management interventions
2. Reports satisfaction with level of pain control

OUTCOMES (NOC)

Pain Level

- Reported pain ____
- Length of pain episodes ____
- Moaning and crying ____
- Facial expressions of pain ____
- Restlessness ____

Measurement Scale
1 = Severe
2 = Substantial
3 = Moderate
4 = Mild
5 = None

- Blood pressure ____
- Pulse rate ____
- Respiratory rate ____

Measurement Scale
1 = Severely compromised
2 = Substantially compromised
3 = Moderately compromised
4 = Mildly compromised
5 = Not compromised

INTERVENTIONS (NIC) and *RATIONALES*

Pain Management

EMERGENT PHASE

- Provide optimal pain relief with prescribed analgesics *to manage pain.*
- Use pain control measures before pain becomes severe *to avoid pain escalation.*
- Ensure pretreatment analgesia and/or nonpharmacological strategies prior to painful procedures *to prevent breakthrough pain.*
- Evaluate the effectiveness of the pain control measures used through ongoing assessment of the pain experience.
- Observe for nonverbal cues of discomfort, especially in those unable to communicate effectively.
- Institute and modify pain control measures on the basis of the patient's response.

ACUTE PHASE

- Reduce or eliminate factors that precipitate or increase the pain experience (e.g., fear, fatigue, monotony, and lack of knowledge).
- Promote adequate rest/sleep *to facilitate pain relief.*
- Teach the use of nonpharmacological techniques before, after, and, if possible, during painful activities; before pain occurs or increases; and along with other pain relief measures *to augment pain relief.*
- Medicate prior to an activity *to increase participation*, but evaluate the hazard of sedation.
- Encourage patient to monitor own pain and to intervene appropriately.
- Monitor patient satisfaction with pain management at specified intervals.

REHABILITATIVE PHASE

- Determine the impact of the pain experience on quality of life (e.g., sleep, appetite, activity, cognition, mood, relationships, performance of job, and role responsibilities) *to plan long-term pain management.*
- Assist patient and family to seek and obtain support *to manage residual pain.*

CVP, Central venous pressure.

NURSING CARE PLAN 25-1

Patient with Burns—cont'd

NURSING DIAGNOSIS **Imbalanced nutrition: less than body requirements** *related to* hypermetabolic state and inability to ingest increased requirements *as evidenced by* weight loss and negative nitrogen balance

PATIENT GOALS
1. Demonstrates positive nitrogen balance
2. Ingests nutrients sufficient to meet metabolic needs

OUTCOMES (NOC)

Nutritional Status: Nutrient Intake

- Caloric intake ____
- Protein intake ____
- Vitamin intake ____
- Mineral intake ____

Measurement Scale

1 = Not adequate
2 = Slightly adequate
3 = Moderately adequate
4 = Substantially adequate
5 = Totally adequate

INTERVENTIONS (NIC) and *RATIONALES*

Nutrition Therapy

EMERGENT PHASE

- Determine in collaboration with the dietitian the number of calories and type of nutrients needed *to meet nutrition requirements.*
- Administer parenteral fluids *to provide calories and protein until GI system is functional.*
- Administer enteral feedings *to provide nutrition until oral intake can be resumed.*
- Discontinue use of tube feedings, as oral intake is tolerated, *to promote normal nutrition patterns.*
- Monitor food/fluid ingested and calculate daily caloric intake *to assess adequacy of diet.*

ACUTE PHASE

- Provide patient with high-protein, high-calorie, nutritious finger foods and drinks that can be readily consumed *to meet nutritional needs.*
- Select nutritional supplements *to increase nutrient intake.*
- Determine food preferences with consideration of cultural and religious preferences *to promote food intake.*
- Monitor food/fluid ingested and calculate daily caloric intake *to assess adequacy of diet.*

REHABILITATIVE PHASE

- Refer for diet teaching and planning *to meet long-term nutritional needs.*
- Monitor appropriateness of diet orders to meet daily nutritional needs *to prevent excess weight gain.*

NURSING DIAGNOSIS **Risk for infection** *related to* altered skin integrity, endogenous flora, and suppressed immune response

PATIENT GOALS
1. Wound free of debris and necrotic tissue
2. Absence of wound infections

OUTCOMES (NOC)

Wound Healing: Secondary Intention

- Granulation ____
- Scar formation ____
- Decreased wound size ____

Measurement Scale

1 = None
2 = Limited
3 = Moderate
4 = Substantial
5 = Extensive

- Purulent drainage ____
- Wound inflammation ____
- Necrosis ____
- Sloughing ____
- Foul wound odor ____

Measurement Scale

1 = Extensive
2 = Substantial
3 = Moderate
4 = Limited
5 = None

INTERVENTIONS (NIC) and *RATIONALES*

Infection Protection

ALL PHASES

- Monitor for systemic and localized signs and symptoms of infection *to provide early detection and treatment.*
- Administer an immunizing agent (tetanus) *to prevent bacterial colonization.*
- Obtain cultures *to identify infectious agents.*
- Promote sufficient nutritional intake *to promote immune function.*

Wound Care

ALL PHASES

- Shave the hair surrounding the affected area *to reduce contamination.*
- Monitor characteristics of the wound, including drainage, color, size, and odor, *to detect signs of infection.*
- Cleanse with normal saline or a nontoxic cleanser *to remove wound debris and medium for bacterial growth.*
- Apply an appropriate ointment to the skin *to decrease risk of infection.*
- Maintain sterile dressing technique when doing wound care *to prevent wound contamination.*
- Compare and record regularly any changes in the wound *to detect infection.*
- Instruct patient and family member(s) in wound care procedures *to ensure proper technique and increase their sense of control.*
- Instruct patient and family on signs and symptoms of infection *so early treatment can be initiated.*

Continued

NURSING CARE PLAN 25-1

Patient with Burns—cont'd

NURSING DIAGNOSIS **Disturbed body image** *related to* disfigurement secondary to burn *as evidenced by* verbalized negative comments about appearance, unwillingness to look at self or participate in self-care

PATIENT GOALS
1. Sets realistic goals regarding future lifestyle
2. Verbalizes acceptance of altered appearance

OUTCOMES (NOC)

Body Image

- Congruence between body reality, body ideal, and body presentation ____
- Willingness to touch affected body part ____
- Willingness to use strategies to enhance appearance ____

Measurement Scale

1 = Never positive
2 = Rarely positive
3 = Sometimes positive
4 = Often positive
5 = Consistently positive

Adaptation to Physical Disability

- Identifies ways to cope with life changes ____
- Reports decrease in negative body image ____
- Verbalizes ability to adjust to disability ____

Measurement Scale

1 = Never demonstrated
2 = Rarely demonstrated
3 = Sometimes demonstrated
4 = Often demonstrated
5 = Consistently demonstrated

INTERVENTIONS (NIC) and *RATIONALES*

Body Image Enhancement

ALL PHASES

- Determine patient's and family's perceptions of the alteration in body image versus reality *to promote congruence of perceptions.*
- Assist patient to separate physical appearance from feelings of personal worth *to foster sense of support.*
- Use anticipatory guidance to prepare patient for predictable changes in body image *to decrease misconceptions.*
- Monitor whether patient can look at the changed body part *to assess patient's response.*
- Assist patient to identify actions that will enhance appearance *to promote positive perceptions.*
- Identify support groups available to patient *to reduce sense of isolation and the impact of burn event on the patient's life.*

Coping Enhancement

ALL PHASES

- Encourage an attitude of realistic hope as a way of dealing with feelings of helplessness *to promote acceptance of body changes.*
- Encourage the identification of specific life values *to promote decision making.*
- Assist the patient to grieve and work through the losses of chronic illness and/or disability *to enhance adaptation to injury.*
- Assist the patient to identify positive strategies to deal with limitations and manage needed lifestyle or role changes *to facilitate adaptive process.*

chronic illness. Each burn unit has a preference for a replacement regimen. Fluid replacement is accomplished with crystalloid solutions (usually lactated Ringer's), colloids (albumin), or a combination of the two. Paramedics generally give IV saline until the patient's arrival at the hospital.

Of the formulas that are used for fluid replacement, the Brooke and Parkland (Baxter) formulas are the most commonly used (Tables 25-11 and 25-12).[9] It is important to remember that all formulas are estimates and must be titrated based on the patient's physical response. For example, patients with inhalation injury may have greater than normal fluid requirements. The Parkland formula is widely used in North America because it is easy to calculate and monitor using the patient's weight, and it provides a reliable method of fluid replacement for most patients.

Colloidal solutions (e.g., albumin) are also routinely given. The amount is calculated based on the patient's body weight, which predicts the replacement volume (e.g., 0.3 to 0.5 ml/kg/% TBSA burn). Colloid administration is beneficial when capillary permeability returns to normal or near normal. After this time, the plasma remains in the vascular space and expands the circulating volume.

Assessment of the adequacy of fluid replacement is best made by the use of more than one parameter. Urine output is the most commonly used parameter. Assessment parameters include the following:

1. Urine output: 30 to 50 ml/hr in an adult; 75 to 100 ml/hr for electrical burn patient with evidence of hemoglobinuria/myoglobinuria.
2. Cardiopulmonary factors: BP (systolic >90 mm Hg), pulse rate (<120 beats/minute). BP is most appropriately measured by an arterial line. Peripheral measurement is often invalid, because of vasoconstriction and edema.

Wound Care

Wound care should be delayed until a patent airway, adequate circulation, and adequate fluid replacement have been established. Full-thickness wounds will be dry and waxy white to dark brown/black and will have only minor, localized sensation because nerve endings have been destroyed. Partial-thickness wounds are pink to cherry red and wet and shiny with serous exudate. These wounds may or may not have intact blisters and are painful when touched or exposed to air.

Cleansing and gentle debridement, using scissors and forceps, can occur in a hydrotherapy tub, cart shower (Fig. 25-8), shower, or patient bed/stretcher. Extensive, surgical debridement should be performed in the operating room (OR) (Fig. 25-9). During **debridement**, necrotic skin is removed. Releasing escharotomies and fasciotomies can be carried out in the emergent phase, usually in burn units by burn physicians. Care should be taken to accomplish these procedures as quickly and effectively as possible.

Patients find the initial wound care to be both physically and psychologically demanding. Immersion in a tank for longer than 20 to 30 minutes can cause electrolyte loss from open burned areas. Prolonged immersion can lead to chilling after the bath and cross-contamination of wounds from one area of the body to an-

TABLE 25-11 Formulas for Estimating Fluid Replacement

	First 24 Hours	Second 24 Hours	
Formula	**Crystalloids**	**Colloids**	**Glucose In Water**
Brooke (modified)	Lactated Ringer's solution: 2.0 ml/kg/% TBSA burn; ½ given during first 8 hr; ½ given during next 16 hr	0.3-0.5 ml/kg/% TBSA burn	Amount to replace estimated evaporative losses
Parkland (Baxter)	Lactated Ringer's solution: 4 ml/kg/% TBSA burn; ½ given first 8 hr; ¼ given each next 8 hr	20%-60% of calculated plasma volume	Amount to replace estimated evaporative losses

TABLE 25-12 Fluid Resuscitation with the Parkland (Baxter) Formula*

Formula

4 ml lactated Ringer's solution
per
kg body weight
per
% TBSA burn
= total fluid requirements for first 24 hr after burn

Application

½ of total in first 8 hr
¼ of total in second 8 hr
¼ of total in third 8 hr

Example

For a 70-kg patient with a 50% TBSA burn:

4 ml × 70 kg × 50% TBSA burn	= 14,000 ml
	= 14 L in 24 hr
½ of total in first 8 hr	= 7000 ml (875 ml/hr)
¼ of total in second 8 hr	= 3500 ml (436 ml/hr)
¼ of total in third 8 hr	= 3500 ml (436 ml/hr)

*Formulas are guidelines. Fluid is administered at a rate to produce 30 to 50 ml of urine output per hour.
TBSA, Total body surface area.

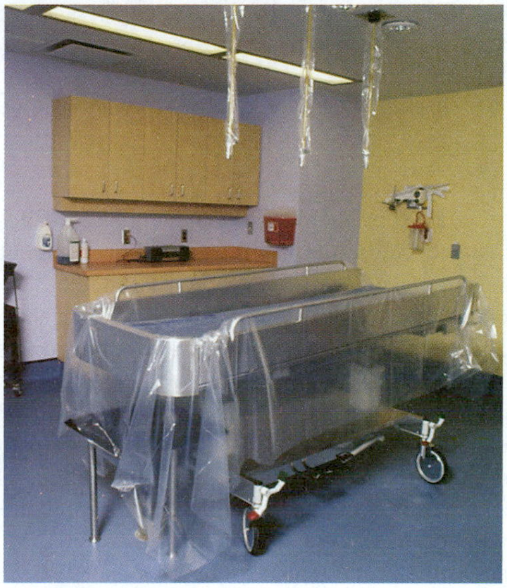

FIG. 25-8 Hydrotherapy cart shower. Showering presents an opportunity for physical therapy as well as wound care.

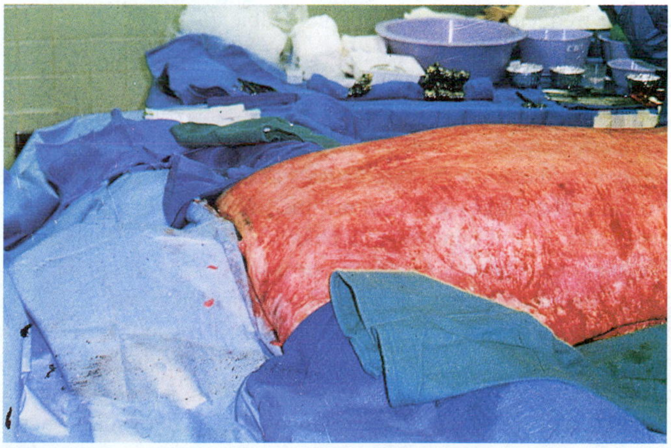

FIG. 25-9 Operative debridement of full-thickness burns is necessary to prepare the wound for grafting.

other. Because of these factors, many institutions no longer submerge or "tub" their burn patients. Instead, they are showered using a cart shower (see Fig. 25-8) or, if the patient is well enough and the TBSA burn is small, a regular shower can be used. The water does not need to be sterile; tap water, not exceeding 104° F (40° C), is acceptable. Because pathogenic organisms are present on the burn wound, a surgical detergent, disinfectant, or cleansing agent may be used. A once-daily shower and dressing change in the morning, followed by a dressing change in the patient's room in the evening, is a common routine in many burn units. Some of the newer antimicrobial dressings can be left in place for up to 3 days, which decreases the frequency of dressing changes.

Infection is the most serious threat to further tissue injury and possible sepsis.[10] Survival is directly related to prevention of wound contamination. The source of infection in burn wounds is the patient's own flora, predominantly from the skin, respiratory tract, and gastrointestinal (GI) tract. The prevention of cross-contamination from one patient to another is a priority for nursing care.

Two types of wound treatment used to control infection are the open method and the use of multiple dressing changes. In the *open method,* the patient's burn is covered with a topical antimicrobial and has no dressing over the wound. In the *multiple dressing change* method, sterile gauze dressings are impregnated with or laid over a topical antimicrobial (Fig. 25-10). These dressings are changed anywhere from every 12 to 24 hours to once every 3 days, depending upon the topical agent and the dressings used. Most burn units support the concept of moist wound healing and use dressings to cover the burned areas, with the exception of the burned face.

When the patient's open burn wounds are exposed, staff must wear disposable hats, masks, gowns, and gloves. When removing contaminated dressings and washing the dirty wound, the nurse may use nonsterile, disposable gloves. Sterile gloves are used when applying ointments and inner, sterile dressings. In addition,

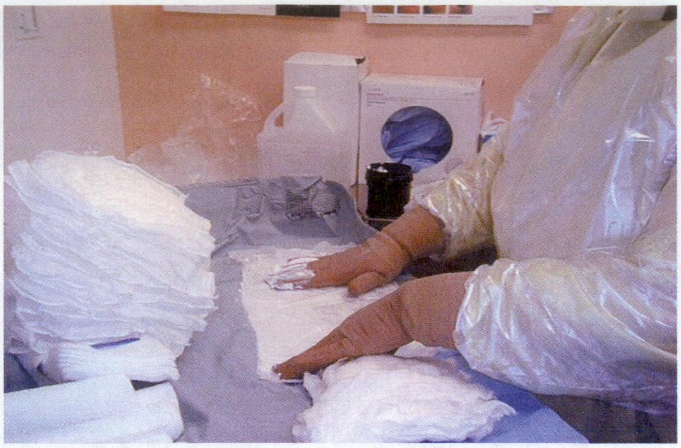

FIG. 25-10 Application of silver sulfadiazine cream to saline-moistened gauze.

the room must be kept warm (approximately 85° F [29.4° C]). All attire is changed before the nurse treats another patient to avoid transmitting organisms from one patient to another, a significant risk especially when there is more than one patient to a room. Careful hand washing and the use of an alcohol hand rinse outside each patient room is also required to prevent cross-contamination. After the patient has been treated in the cart shower, shower, or tub, the equipment and immediate environment are thoroughly cleaned and disinfected with a chemical preparation. The use of plastic liners on this equipment is helpful in reducing the potential contamination of the equipment.

Coverage is the primary goal for burn wounds.[11] Because there is rarely enough unburned skin in the major (>50%) burn patient for immediate skin grafting, other temporary wound closure methods are sometimes used. *Allograft* or *homograft skin* (usually from cadavers) is used, along with newer biosynthetic options, with varying frequency among burn units (Table 25-13).

Other Care Measures

Certain parts of the body (e.g., face, eyes, hands, arms, ears, perineum) require particularly vigilant nursing care. The face is highly vascular and subject to a great amount of edema. Facial care is often performed by the open method since facial dressings cause disorientation and confusion, occlude vision, and slide off easily. Eye care for corneal burns or edema includes antibiotic ointments.[12] An ophthalmology examination should occur soon after admission for all patients with facial burns. Periorbital edema can prevent opening of the eyes and be frightening to the patient. The nurse must provide assurance that the swelling is not permanent. Instillation of methylcellulose drops or artificial tears into the eyes for moisture provides additional comfort for patients.

Hands and arms should be extended and elevated on pillows or in slings to minimize edema. Splints may need to be applied to burned hands and feet to maintain them in functional positions.

Ears should be kept free of pressure because of their poor vascularization and predisposition to infection. The patient with ear burns should not use pillows because pressure on the cartilage may cause chondritis and the ear may stick to the pillowcase, causing pain and bleeding. The patient's head can be elevated using a rolled towel placed under the shoulders, being careful to avoid pressure necrosis. The same holds true for the patient with neck burns. Pillows are removed and a rolled towel is placed under the shoulders to hyperextend the neck and prevent neck wound contraction.

TABLE 25-13 Sources of Grafts

Source	Graft Name	Coverage
Porcine skin	Heterograft or xenograft (different species)	Temporary (3 days to 2 wk)
Cadaveric skin	Homograft or allograft (same species)	Temporary (3 days to 2 wk)
Patient's own skin	Autograft	Permanent
Patient's own skin and cell cultures	Cultured epithelial autograft (CEA)	Permanent
Porcine collagen bonded to silicone membrane	BioBrane	Temporary (10-21 days)
Human, dermal fibroblast-derived matrix with growth factors	TransCyte	Temporary (10-21 days)
Bovine collagen and glycosaminoglycan bonded to silicone membrane	Integra	Permanent
Acellular dermal matrix derived from donated human skin	AlloDerm	Permanent

The perineum must be kept as clean and dry as possible. In addition to providing hourly urine outputs, an indwelling catheter prevents urine contamination of the bowel and perineal area. Regular, once- to twice-daily perineal and catheter care in the presence or absence of a perineal burn wound is essential.

Routine laboratory tests are performed to monitor fluid and electrolyte balance. Blood for the measurement of ABGs is drawn to determine adequacy of ventilation and perfusion in all patients with suspected or confirmed inhalation injury.

Physical therapy is begun immediately, sometimes during hydrotherapy/dressing changes before the new dressings are applied. Early range-of-motion (ROM) exercises are necessary to facilitate mobilization of the extravasated fluid back into the vascular bed. Exercise of body parts also maintains function, prevents contracture, and reassures the patient that movement is still possible.

Drug Therapy

Analgesics and Sedatives. Analgesics are ordered to promote patient comfort. Early in the postburn period, IV pain medications should be given because (1) GI function is slowed or impaired due to shock or paralytic ileus and (2) intramuscular (IM) injections will not be absorbed adequately in burned or edematous areas, causing pooling of medications in the tissues. When fluid mobilization begins, the patient could be inadvertently overdosed from the interstitial accumulation of previous IM medications.

Common narcotics used for pain control are listed in Table 25-14. The need for analgesia must be reevaluated frequently as patients' needs may change and tolerance to medications may develop over time. The drug of choice for pain control is morphine, but hydromorphone and methadone may also be used. When given appropriately, these drugs should provide adequate pain control. Sedative agents should also be given along with analgesics to control the anxiety that patients experience (see Table 25-14). Analgesic requirements can vary tremendously from one patient to another. The extent and depth of burn may not correlate with pain intensity. Hospital pharmacists, psychiatrists,

TABLE 25-14 DRUG THERAPY
Drugs Commonly Used in Burn Treatment

Types and Names of Drugs	Purpose
Nutritional Support	
Vitamins A, C, E, and multivitamins	Promotes wound healing
Minerals: zinc, iron (ferrous sulfate)	Promotes cell integrity and hemoglobin formation
oxandrolone (Oxandrin)	Promotes weight gain and preservation of lean body mass
Analgesia	
morphine	All analgesic drugs
sustained-release morphine (MS Contin)	
hydromorphone (Dilaudid)	
fentanyl (Sublimaze)	
oxycodone (contained in Percocet)	
methadone	
Nonsteroidal antiinflammatory (e.g., ketoprofen [Orudis])	
Adjuvant analgesics (e.g., gabapentin)	
Sedation	
haloperidol (Haldol)	Produces antipsychotic and sedative effects, promotes sleep
lorazepam (Ativan)	Diminishes anxiety
midazolam (Versed)	Has short-acting amnestic properties
Gastrointestinal Support	
ranitidine (Zantac)	Decreases incidence of Curling's ulcer
nystatin (Mycostatin)	Prevents overgrowth of *Candida albicans* in oral mucosa
Mylanta, Maalox	Neutralizes stomach acid

and multidisciplinary pain services are valuable resources for the more complex situations.

Tetanus Immunization. Tetanus toxoid is given routinely to all burn patients because of the likelihood of anaerobic burn wound contamination. If the patient has not received an active immunization within 10 years before the burn injury, tetanus immunoglobulin should be considered.

Antimicrobial Agents. After the wound is cleansed, topical agents are applied (see Fig. 25-10) and covered with a light dressing. Systemic antibiotics are not usually used in controlling burn wound flora because there is little or no blood supply to the burn eschar, and consequently, there is little delivery of the antibiotic to the wound. Some topical burn agents penetrate the eschar, thereby inhibiting bacterial invasion of the wound. Silver sulfadiazine (Silvadene, Flamazine) and mafenide acetate (Sulfamylon) are commonly used. Silver-impregnated dressings (Acticoat, Silverlon, Aquacel Ag) that can be left on for up to 3 days and in some cases longer, are used in some burn units. They are effective against many organisms. Systemic sepsis remains a leading cause of death in the patient with major burns, which may lead to multiple organ dysfunction syndrome (see Chapter 67). Systemic antibiotic therapy is initiated when the clinical diagnosis of invasive burn wound sepsis is made, or when some other source of sepsis is identified (e.g., pneumonia).

Frequently, fungal infections develop in the patient's mucous membranes (mouth and genitalia) as a result of antibiotic therapy and low resistance in the host. The offending organism is usually *Candida albicans.* Oral infection is treated with nystatin (Mycostatin) mouthwash. When a normal diet is resumed, yogurt or *Lactobacillus* (Lactinex) may be given by mouth to reintroduce the normal intestinal flora that have been destroyed by antibiotic therapy.

Nutritional Therapy

Fluid replacement takes priority over nutritional needs in the initial emergent phase. However, early and aggressive nutritional support within several hours of the burn injury can decrease mortality and complications, optimize healing of the burn wound, and minimize the negative effects of hypermetabolism and catabolism. Nonintubated patients with a $<20\%$ TBSA burn will generally be able to eat enough to meet their nutritional requirements. Intubated patients and/or those with larger burns require additional support. Enteral feedings (gastric or intestinal) have almost entirely replaced the need for parenteral feeding. Early enteral feeding preserves GI function, increases intestinal blood flow, and promotes optimal conditions for wound healing. The patient with large ($>20\%$ TBSA) burns frequently develops paralytic ileus within a few hours as a result of the body's response to major trauma. If a large nasogastric tube is inserted on admission, gastric residuals should be checked frequently to rule out a paralytic ileus and delayed gastric emptying. In general, feedings can be commenced slowly at 20 to 40 ml/hr and be increased to the goal rate within 24 to 48 hours.

A **hypermetabolic state** proportional to the size of the wound occurs after a major burn injury. Resting metabolic expenditure may be increased by 50% to 100% above normal in patients with major burns. Core temperature is elevated. Catecholamines, which stimulate catabolism and heat production, are increased. Massive catabolism can occur and is characterized by protein breakdown and increased gluconeogenesis.[13] Failure to supply adequate calories and protein leads to malnutrition and delayed healing. Calorie-containing nutritional supplements and milkshakes are often given because of the great need for calories. Protein powder can also be added to food and liquids. Supplemental vitamins may be given as early as the emergent phase, with iron supplements often started in the acute phase (see Table 25-14).

ACUTE PHASE

The *acute phase* begins with the mobilization of extracellular fluid and subsequent diuresis. This phase is concluded when the burned area is completely covered by skin grafts or when the wounds are healed. This may take weeks or many months.

Pathophysiology

Burn injury involves pathophysiologic changes in many body systems. Diuresis from fluid mobilization occurs, and the patient is less edematous. Areas that are full- or partial-thickness burns are more evident than in the emergent phase. Bowel sounds return. The patient may now become aware of the enormity of the situation. Some healing begins as WBCs surround the burn wound and phagocytosis occurs. Necrotic tissue begins to slough. Fibroblasts lay down matrices of the collagen precursors that eventually form granulation tissue. Kept free from infection and dessication (drying), a partial-thickness burn wound will heal from the edges and from the dermal bed below. However, full-thickness burn wounds, unless extremely small, must be covered by skin grafts. Often, healing time and length of hospitalization are decreased by early excision and grafting.

Clinical Manifestations

Partial-thickness wounds form eschar, which begins separating fairly soon after injury. Once the eschar is removed, re-epithelialization begins at the wound margins and appears as red or pink scar tissue. Epithelial buds from the dermal bed eventually close in the wound, which then heals spontaneously without surgical intervention, usually within 10 to 14 days.

Margins of full-thickness eschar take longer to separate than partial-thickness eschar. As a result, full-thickness wounds require surgical debridement and skin grafting for healing.

Laboratory Values

Because the body is attempting to reestablish fluid and electrolyte homeostasis in the initial acute phase, it is important to follow serum electrolyte levels closely.

Sodium. *Hyponatremia* can occur if hydrotherapy is too lengthy because the hypotonicity of the bath water pulls sodium from open burn areas. Other causes of hyponatremia include excessive GI suction, diarrhea, and excessive water intake. Manifestations of hyponatremia include weakness, dizziness, muscle cramps, fatigue, headache, tachycardia, and confusion. The burn patient may also develop a dilutional hyponatremia called *water intoxication.* To avoid this condition, the patient should drink fluids other than water, such as juice, soft drinks, or nutritional supplements.

Hypernatremia may be seen following successful fluid replacement if copious amounts of hypertonic solutions were required. Other causes of hypernatremia include improper tube feeding therapy or inappropriate fluid administration. Manifestations of hypernatremia include thirst; dried, furry tongue; lethargy; confusion; and possibly seizures.

Potassium. *Hyperkalemia* is noted if the patient has renal failure, adrenocortical insufficiency, or massive deep muscle injury with large amounts of potassium released from damaged cells. Cardiac dysrhythmias and ventricular failure can occur with excessive potassium elevations. Muscle weakness and electrocardiographic (ECG) changes are observed clinically (see Chapter 17).

Hypokalemia occurs with vomiting, diarrhea, prolonged GI suction, and prolonged IV therapy without potassium supplementation. A constant potassium loss occurs through the burn wound.

Complications

Infection. The body's first line of defense, the skin, has been destroyed by burn injury. Pathogens often proliferate before phagocytosis has adequately begun. The burn wound is now colonized with organisms. If the bacterial density at the junction of the eschar with underlying viable tissue rises to greater than 10^5/g of tissue, the patient has a burn wound infection.[14] In the presence of an infection, localized inflammation, induration, and sometimes suppuration can be seen at the burn wound margins. Partial-thickness burns can convert to full-thickness wounds when these organisms invade viable, adjacent, unburned tissue. Invasive wound infections may be treated with systemic antibiotics based on culture results.

Burn wound infection may progress to transient bacteremia as a result of burn wound manipulation (e.g., after hydrotherapy and debridement). The patient may develop sepsis. Manifestations of sepsis include hypo- or hyperthermia, increased pulse and respiratory rate, decreased BP, and decreased urine output. There may be mild confusion, chills, malaise, and loss of appetite. The WBC count will usually be between 10,000/μl (10×10^9/L) and 20,000/μl (20×10^9/L). There are functional defects in the WBCs, and the patient remains immunosuppressed for a period after the burn injury. The causative organisms of sepsis are usually gram-negative bacteria (e.g., *Pseudomonas, Proteus* organisms), putting the patient at further risk for septic shock.

When sepsis is suspected, cultures should be obtained immediately from all possible sources, including blood, urine, the oropharynx, the perineal/rectal region, sputum, the IV site, and the burn wound. However, treatment should not be delayed pending results of the culture and sensitivity studies. Therapy will begin with antibiotics appropriate for the usual residual flora of the particular burn unit. The topical antibiotic in use may be continued or be changed to another agent. At this stage the patient's condition is critical, requiring close monitoring of vital signs.

Cardiovascular and Respiratory Systems. The same cardiovascular and respiratory system complications present in the emergent phase may continue into the acute phase of care. In addition, new problems might arise, requiring timely intervention.

Neurologic System. Neurologically, the patient usually has no physical symptoms, unless severe hypoxia from respiratory injuries or complications from electrical injuries occur. However, some patients may demonstrate certain behaviors that are not completely understood. The patient can become extremely disoriented, may withdraw or become combative, and may have hallucinations and frequent nightmare-like episodes. Delirium is more acute at night and occurs more often in the older patient. This is a transient state, lasting from a day or two to several weeks. Various causes have been considered, including electrolyte imbalance, stress, cerebral edema, sepsis, intensive care unit psychosis syndrome, and the use of analgesics and antianxiety drugs.

Musculoskeletal System. The musculoskeletal system is particularly prone to complications during the acute phase. As the burns begin to heal and scar tissue forms, the skin is less supple and pliant. ROM may be limited, and contractures can occur. Because of pain, the patient will prefer to assume a flexed position for comfort. Splinting can be beneficial to prevent/reduce contracture formation.

Gastrointestinal System. The GI system may also exhibit complications during this phase. Paralytic ileus results from sepsis. Diarrhea may be caused by the use of supplemental feedings or antibiotics. Constipation can occur as a side effect of opioid analgesics, decreased mobility, and a low-fiber diet. *Curling's ulcer,* a type of gastroduodenal ulcer characterized by diffuse superficial lesions (including mucosal erosion), is caused by a generalized stress response resulting in decreased production of mucus and increased gastric acid secretion. This condition is due to the decreased blood flow to the GI tract during the hypovolemic shock phase. The best treatment of Curling's ulcer is prevention. The prophylactic use of antacids and H_2-histamine blockers, such as ranitidine (Zantac), inhibits histamine and the stimulation of hydrochloric acid (HCl acid) secretion. Proton pump inhibitors, such as esomeprazole (Nexium), may be used to reduce gastric acid secretion. Many patients with major burns also have occult blood in their stools during the acute phase.

Endocrine System. An increase in blood glucose levels may be seen transiently because of stress-mediated cortisol and catecholamine release, resulting in the increased mobilization of glycogen stores, gluconeogenesis, and the subsequent production of glucose. There is also an increase in insulin production and release. However, insulin's effectiveness is decreased because of relative insulin insensitivity, leading to an elevated blood glucose level. Later, hyperglycemia can be caused by the increased caloric intake necessary to meet some patients' metabolic requirements. When this occurs, the treatment is supplemental IV insulin, not decreased feeding. Serum glucose levels are checked frequently, and an appropriate amount of insulin is given if hyperglycemia is present. Glucometers may be used to assess blood glucose at the bedside; serum glucose samples are more accurate than capillary blood analysis by glucometer. As the patient's metabolic demands are met and less stress is placed on the entire system, this stress-induced condition is reversed.

NURSING *and* COLLABORATIVE MANAGEMENT ACUTE PHASE

The predominant therapeutic interventions in the acute phase are (1) wound care, (2) excision and grafting, (3) pain management, (4) physical and occupational therapy, (5) nutritional therapy, and (6) psychosocial care.

Wound Care

The goals of wound care are to (1) cleanse and debride the area of necrotic tissue and debris that would promote bacterial growth and (2) promote wound re-epithelialization and/or successful skin grafting.

Wound care consists of daily observation, assessment, cleansing, debridement, and dressing reapplication. Nonsurgical debridement, dressing changes, topical antibiotic therapy, graft care, and donor site care may be performed from 2 times daily to once every few days. Enzymatic debriders made of natural ingredients, such as papain, may be used for the **enzymatic debridement** of burn wounds, which speeds up the removal of dead tissue from the healthy wound bed. When partial-thickness burn wounds have been debrided, a protective, coarse or fine-meshed, greasy gauze dressing is applied to protect the re-epithelializing cells as they resurface and close the open wound bed. If grafting is necessary, the meshed, split-thickness skin graft may be protected with the same greasy gauze dressings next to the graft, followed by middle and outer dressings. These meshed gauze dressings have a greasy base (paraffin or petroleum) that prevents adherence of the graft to the middle/outer, cotton gauze dressings. Dressings often are not applied, so it is possible for *blebs* (serosanguineous exudates) to form between the graft and the recipient bed. Blebs prevent the graft from interfacing and growing to the wound itself. The evacuation of blebs is best performed by aspiration with a tuberculin syringe. Burn unit nurses have the option of pricking the bleb and rolling the skin graft if they have received instruction in this specialized skill. It should not be performed by non–burn unit staff.

Donor site care has been controversial throughout the years. The goals of care are to promote rapid, moist wound healing, decrease pain at the donor site, and prevent infection. Many new methods are being evaluated, and they vary among burn units. The average healing time for a donor site is 10 to 14 days. Several of the newer methods potentially can decrease this healing time, which would facilitate earlier reharvesting of skin at the site. There are many options for donor site dressings. Some units use a transparent dressing (e.g., Opsite, Tegaderm, Biobrane, Aquacel Ag, Acticoat) that permits an occlusive yet visible wound. Pigskin (xenograft), silver sulfadiazine (Silvadene, Flamazine), calcium alginate, and hydrophilic foam dressings are also used with varying degrees of success. Each donor site dressing has specific nursing care aspects, and use varies among units. (Dressings are discussed in Chapter 13 and Table 13-9.)

Excision and Grafting

Current therapeutic management of burn wounds involves early removal of the necrotic tissue followed by application of split-thickness autograft skin.[15] This therapy has changed the management and mortality rate of burn patients. In the past, patients with major burns had low rates of survival because healing and wound coverage took so long that the patient usually died of infection or malnutrition. Due to current earlier intervention, mortality rates have been greatly reduced and morbidity rates have also decreased. Candidates for early excision and grafting are those patients with a stable cardiovascular system after initial fluid resuscitation.

During the procedure of **excision and grafting,** eschar is removed down to the subcutaneous tissue or fascia, depending on the degree of injury. A graft is then placed on clean, viable tissue to achieve good adherence. Hemostasis is achieved by pressure and the application of topical thrombin or epinephrine, after which the wound is covered with *autograft* (person's own) skin (see Table 25-13). With early excision, function is restored and scar tissue formation is minimized. Because the dead tissue is planed off until viable tissue is reached, extensive bleeding is expected to occur, which may pose a problem when grafting is performed. Clots between the graft and the wound keep the graft from adhering to the wound. Frequent observation and appropriate nursing interventions can help identify and manage excessive postoperative bleeding and enhance graft survival.

Donor skin is taken from the patient for grafting by means of a dermatome, which removes a thin (split-thickness) layer of skin from an unburned site (Fig. 25-11). The donor skin can be meshed to allow for greater wound coverage, or it may be applied as a sheet graft for a better cosmetic result when grafting the face, neck, and hands. The donor site now becomes a new open wound. For the thin-skinned elderly patient, healing of the donor site may be a difficult task and requires vigilant care by the health care team.

Cultured Epithelial Autografts. In the patient with large body surface area burns, only a limited amount of unburned skin may be available as donor sites for grafting, and some of that skin may be unsuitable for harvesting. **Cultured epithelial autograft** (CEA) is a method of obtaining permanent skin from a person with limited available skin for harvesting. CEA is grown from biopsy specimens obtained from the patient's own unburned skin.[16] This procedure is performed in burn units as soon as possible after admission on patients who have been identified as suitable candidates. The specimens are sent to a commercial laboratory, where the biopsied keratinocytes are grown in a culture medium containing epidermal growth factor. After approximately 18 to 25 days, the keratinocytes have expanded up to 10,000 times and form confluent sheets that can be used as skin grafts. The cultured skin is returned to the burn unit, where it is placed on the patient's excised burn wounds. Because CEA grafts are made only of epidermal cells, meticulous care is required to prevent shearing injury or infection. CEA grafts generally form a seamless, smooth replacement skin tissue (Fig. 25-12). Problems related to CEA include a poor graft take due to thin epidermal skin graft loss, and contracture development.

Artificial Skin. It is now recognized that any successful artificial skin must replace all functions of the skin and consist of both dermal and epidermal elements. The Integra artificial skin dermal regeneration template is an example of one of the newest and most successful skin replacement systems available in burn care today. Its application requires a high degree of skill. As with CEA, it is indicated for use in the treatment of life-threatening, full-thickness

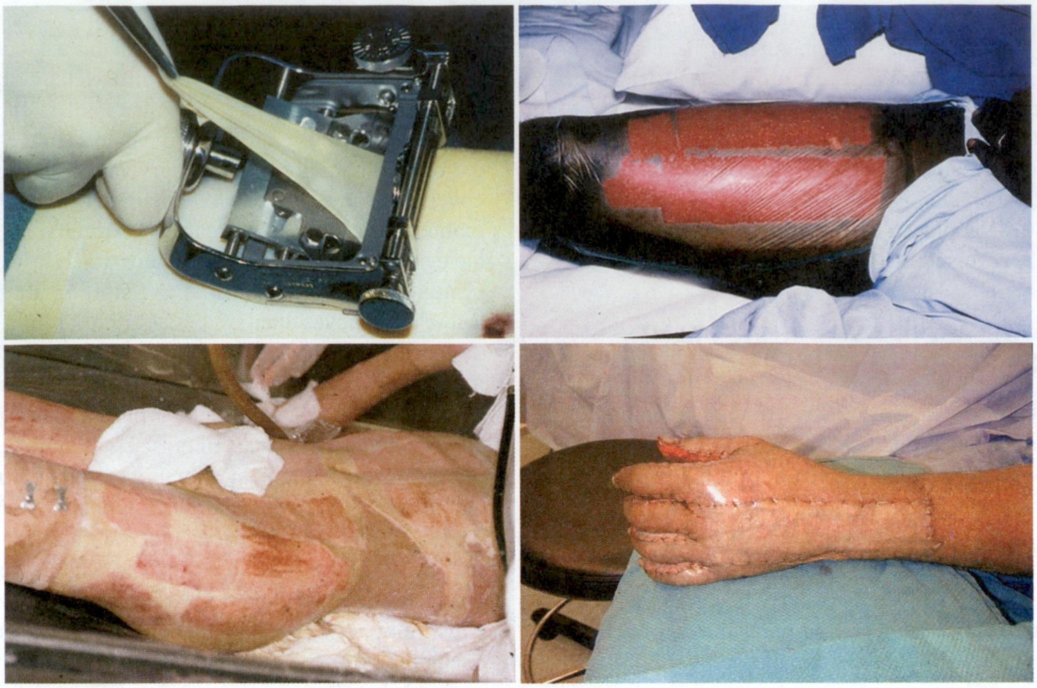

FIG. 25-11 **A,** The surgeon harvests skin from a patient's thigh using a dermatome. **B,** Appearance of donor site after harvesting split-thickness skin graft. Donor site is covered with a transparent occlusive dressing. **C,** Healed donor sites. **D,** Healed split-thickness sheet skin graft to the hand.

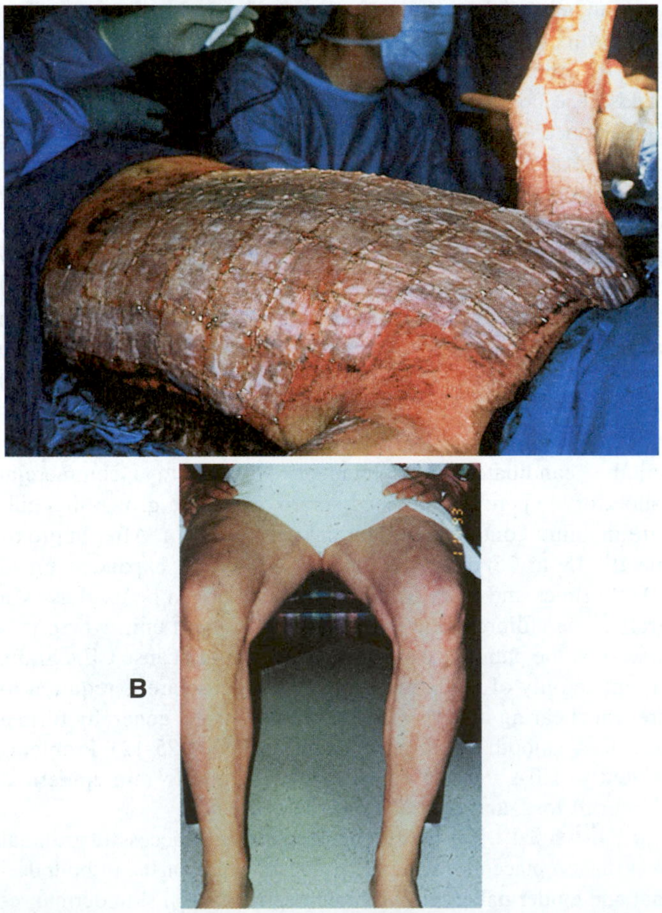

FIG. 25-12 Patient with cultured epithelial autograft (CEA). **A,** Intraoperative application of cultured epithelial autograft. **B,** Appearance of healed cultured epithelial autograft.

or deep partial-thickness burn wounds when conventional autograft is not available or advisable, as in elderly or high-anesthetic-risk patients. It has also been successfully used in reconstructive burn surgery procedures. As with CEA, it may need to be applied within a few days of admission for greatest success.

Integra artificial skin has a bilayer membrane composed of acellular dermis and silicone. In the operating room, the wound is debrided, the bilayer membrane is placed dermal layer down, and the wound is wrapped with dressings. The dermal layer functions as a biodegradable template that induces organized regeneration of new dermis by the body. The silicone layer remains intact for 3 weeks as the dermal layer degrades and epidermal autografts become available. At this point, the silicone is removed during a second surgical procedure and replaced by the patient's own epidermal autografts. In some situations, burn units use CEA as the source of epidermis.

Several other products are currently being evaluated in burn units throughout North America, including AlloDerm, a nonimmunogenic dermal transplant, and LifeSkin, a cultured composite autograft.[17] Clinical evaluations are ongoing to determine the use and effectiveness of these and other new products in burn wound management.

Pain Management

One of the most critical functions a nurse performs on behalf of a burn patient is individualized and consistent pain assessment and management. Many aspects of clinical burn care cause pain. However, patients experience moments of relative comfort if they receive adequate analgesia. A coordinated understanding of both the physiologic and psychologic aspects of pain is essential if the nurse is to intervene with actions that are beneficial. (Pain management is discussed in Chapter 10.) Burn patients experience two kinds of pain: (1) continuous, background pain that exists throughout the day and night and (2) treatment-induced pain associated with dressing changes, ambulation, and rehabilitation activities. The first line of treatment is pharmacologic. With background pain, if the patient has a continuous IV infusion of morphine or hydromorphone, this will allow for a steady, therapeutic level of medication. Breakthrough doses should also be available. If an IV infusion is not present, slow-release twice-a-day opioid medications, such as MS Contin or Dilaudid, are indicated. Around-the-clock oral morphine/hydromorphone can also be used. Again, breakthrough medication needs to be available. Anxiolytics, which frequently potentiate analgesics, are also indicated and include lorazepam (Ativan) or midazolam (Versed).

For treatment-induced pain, premedication with an analgesic and an anxiolytic is required via the IV or oral route. For patients with an IV infusion, a potent, short-acting analgesic, such as fentanyl (Sublimaze), is useful. During treatment/activity, small doses should be given to keep the patient as comfortable as possible. Eradication of all the pain is difficult to achieve, and most patients indicate satisfaction with "tolerable" levels of discomfort. Burn pain management is complex and ever-changing throughout the patient's hospital stay and after discharge.

Pain can also be managed using nonpharmacologic strategies, such as relaxation tapes, visualization, hypnosis, guided imagery, biofeedback, and meditation (see Chapters 8 and 9). These techniques are considered adjuncts to traditional pharmacologic treatments of pain. They are not meant to be used exclusively to control pain in the burn patient.

An important point to remember about pain management is that the more control the patient has in managing the pain, the more successful the chosen strategies. Patient-controlled analgesia (PCA) is used in selected circumstances on some burn units, with varying degrees of success. (PCA is discussed in Chapters 10 and 20.) Active patient participation has also been found to be effective for some patients in anticipating and coping with the pain of dressing changes. Relaxation techniques may help some patients cope with the painful aspects of care, both in the hospital and upon discharge to home. (Relaxation techniques are discussed in Chapter 9.)

Physical and Occupational Therapy

Rigorous physical therapy throughout burn recovery is imperative to maintain optimal joint function. A good time for exercise is during and after wound cleansing, when the skin is softer and bulky dressings are removed. Passive and active ROM should be performed on all joints. The patient with neck burns must sleep without pillows or with the head hanging slightly over the top of the mattress to encourage hyperextension. Custom-fitted splints are designed to keep the joints in functional position and must be reexamined frequently to ensure an optimal fit.

Nutritional Therapy

The goal of nutritional therapy during the acute burn phase is to provide adequate calories and protein to promote healing. The burn patient is in a hypermetabolic and highly catabolic state as a result of the burn injury.[13] Decreasing catecholamine release by minimizing pain, fear, anxiety, and cold can maximize patient comfort and conserve energy. Infection also increases metabolic rate.

Meeting daily caloric requirements is crucial and should begin within the first 1 to 2 days postburn. The daily estimated caloric needs must be regularly calculated by a dietitian and readjusted as the patient's condition changes (e.g., wound healing, sepsis).

If the patient is on a mechanized ventilator or unable to consume adequate calories by mouth, a feeding tube can be placed and a complete liquid diet administered. If caloric requirements cannot be met by enteral feeding alone, parenteral nutrition may be given temporarily while continuing to deliver enteral feedings. When the patient is extubated, a swallowing assessment should be performed by a speech-language pathologist before the oral feeding of liquids or food is commenced. The alert patient should be encouraged to eat high-protein, high-carbohydrate foods to meet increased caloric needs. If family members wish to bring in favorite foods from home, this should be encouraged. Appetite is usually diminished, and constant encouragement may be necessary to achieve adequate intake. Ideally, weight loss should not be more than 10% of preburn weight. The nurse then records the patient's caloric intake daily using calorie count sheets. Calorie intake needs to be monitored by the dietitian on a regular basis. Patients should also be weighed on a regular basis to evaluate progress.

Psychosocial Care

The patient and family have many needs for psychosocial support during the often lengthy, unpredictable, and complex course of care. The social worker and nursing staff have important support and counseling roles to play. Pastoral care may also be helpful for some patients and their families. (Patient and family emotional needs are discussed on p. 505.)

REHABILITATION PHASE

The formal *rehabilitation phase* begins when the patient's burn wounds have healed and the patient is able to resume a level of self-care activity. This can occur as early as 2 weeks or as long as 7 to 8 months after the burn injury. Goals for this period are to assist the patient in resuming a functional role in society and to accomplish functional and cosmetic reconstructive surgery. Rehabilitation-focused activities that have been taking place during the earlier emergent and acute phases now begin in earnest once the patient's wounds have healed.

Pathophysiologic Changes and Clinical Manifestations

Burn wounds heal either by primary intention or by grafting. Layers of epithelialization begin rebuilding the tissue structure destroyed by the burn injury. Collagen fibers, present in the new scar tissue, assist with healing and add strength to weakened areas. The new skin appears flat and pink. In approximately 4 to 6 weeks, the area becomes raised and hyperemic. If adequate ROM is not instituted, the new tissue will shorten, causing a contracture. Mature healing is reached in 6 months to 2 years when suppleness has returned, and the pink or red color has faded to a slightly lighter hue than the surrounding unburned tissue. It takes longer for more heavily pigmented skin to regain its dark color because many of the melanocytes are destroyed. Often, skin never completely regains its original color. Cosmetics can help even out unequal skin tones and improve the patient's overall appearance and self-image.

Scarring has two components: discoloration and contour. The discoloration of scars will fade somewhat with time. However, scar tissue tends to develop altered contours; that is, it is no longer flat or slightly raised but becomes elevated and enlarged above the original burned area. It is believed that pressure can help keep a

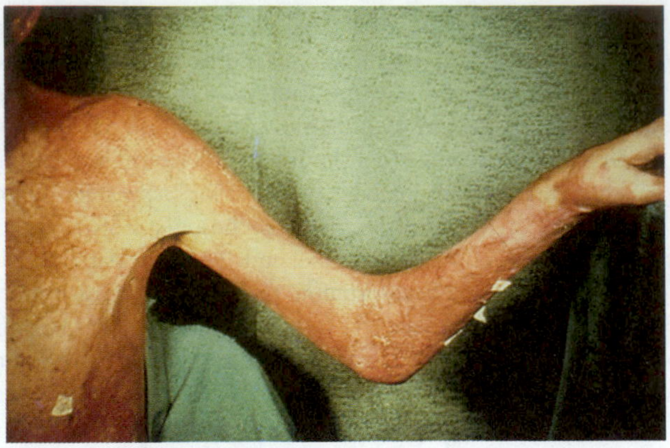

FIG. 25-13 Contracture of the axilla.

scar flat. Gentle pressure can be maintained on the healed burn with custom-fitted pressure garments. These garments are worn up to 24 hours a day for as long as 12 to 18 months. They are removed only for short periods while bathing.

The patient typically experiences discomfort from itching where healing is occurring. Frequent applications of water-based moisturizers and diphenhydramine (Benadryl) help reduce the itching. As "old" epithelium is replaced by new cells, flaking will occur. The newly formed skin is extremely sensitive to trauma. Blisters and skin tears are likely to develop from slight pressure or friction. Additionally, these newly healed areas can be hypersensitive or hyposensitive to cold, heat, and touch. Grafted areas are more likely to be hyposensitive until peripheral nerve regeneration occurs. Healed burn areas must be protected from direct sunlight for 6 to 9 months to prevent hyperpigmentation and sunburn injury.

Complications

The most common complications during the rehabilitative phase are skin and joint contractures and hypertrophic scarring (Fig. 25-13). A **contracture** (an abnormal condition of a joint characterized by flexion and fixation) develops as a result of the shortening of scar tissue in the flexor tissues of a joint.[18] Areas that are most susceptible to contracture formation include the anterior and lateral neck areas, axillae, antecubital fossae, fingers, groin areas, popliteal fossae, knees, and ankles. These areas encompass major joints. Not only does the skin over these areas develop contractures, but the underlying tissues, such as the ligaments and tendons, also have a tendency to shorten during the healing process.

Because of pain, the patient will prefer to assume a flexed position for comfort. This position predisposes wounds to contracture formation. Positioning, splinting, and exercise should be instituted to minimize this complication.[17] These procedures should be continued until the skin matures. Therapy is aimed at the extension of body parts because the flexors are stronger than the extensors. Burned legs may be wrapped with elastic (e.g., tensor/Ace) bandages to assist with circulation to leg graft and donor sites before ambulation. This additional pressure prevents blister formation, promotes venous return, and decreases pain and itchiness. Once the skin is completely healed and less fragile, custom-fitted pressure garments replace the elastic bandages.

NURSING *and* COLLABORATIVE MANAGEMENT
REHABILITATION PHASE

During the rehabilitation phase, both the patient and family are actively encouraged to participate in care. Since the patient may go home with small, unhealed wounds, education and "hands-on" instruction will be needed in dressing changes and wound care. If needed, home care nursing services can be arranged to assist with care for the first few weeks postdischarge. An emollient water-based cream (e.g., Vaseline Intensive Care Extra Strength) that penetrates the dermis should be used routinely on healed areas to keep the skin supple and well moisturized, which will decrease itching and flaking. Oral diphenhydramine (Benadryl) may be used if itching persists. Postburn reconstructive surgery is frequently required following a major burn. It is important for the patient to understand the need for or possibility of further surgery before leaving the hospital.

The continuous role of exercise and physical/occupational therapy cannot be overemphasized. Constant encouragement and reassurance are necessary to maintain a patient's morale, particularly once the patient realizes that recovery can be slow and rehabilitation may need to be a primary focus for at least the next 6 to 12 months.

Because of the tremendous psychologic impact of a burn injury, health care providers should be particularly sensitive and attuned to the patient's emotions and concerns. It is essential that patients be encouraged to discuss their fears regarding loss of their life as they once knew it, loss of function, temporary/permanent deformity and disfigurement, return to work and home life, and financial burdens resulting from a long and costly hospitalization. Care should also be taken to address individual spiritual and cultural needs, as both these facets of a patient's life play a role in recovery. Earlier discussions with family members in the emergent and acute phases have likely identified the different meanings a burn injury can have in different cultures and for their loved one, in particular. Hospital chaplains and cultural community groups may be helpful resources to the patient, family, and health care team. Patients can then be assisted toward a realistic and positive appraisal of their particular situation, emphasizing what they *can* do instead of what cannot be done.

A person's self-esteem is usually adversely affected by a burn injury.[19] In some individuals, an overwhelming fear may be the loss of relationships because of perceived or actual physical disfigurement. In a society that values physical beauty, alterations in body image can result in psychologic distress. Encouraging appropriate independence, an eventual return to preburn activities, and interactions with other burn survivors will involve the patient in familiar activities that may bring comfort and help to restore self-esteem. Counseling should be made available after the patient goes home. Patients need reassurance that their feelings during this period of adjustment are normal, and that their frustration is to be expected as they attempt to resume a normal lifestyle.

GERONTOLOGIC CONSIDERATIONS
BURNS

The older patient presents many challenges for the burn team. The normal aging process puts the patient at risk for injury because of the possibility of an unsteady gait, failing eyesight, and diminished hearing. Once injured, the older adult has more complications in the emergent and acute phases of burn resuscitation because of preexisting medical conditions. For example, older patients with diabetes, heart failure, or chronic obstructive pulmonary disease will have morbidity and mortality rates exceeding those of healthy, younger patients. In older patients, pneumonia is a frequent complication, burn wounds and donor sites take longer to heal, and surgical procedures are less well tolerated. Weaning from a ventilator can be a challenge, and delirium from medication/anesthesia may be a distressing, although usually self-limiting, outcome. It usually takes longer for these patients to rehabilitate to the point where they can safely return home. For some, a return home to independent living may not be possible. As the population ages, developing strategies to prevent burn injuries in this population is particularly important.[20]

EMOTIONAL NEEDS OF THE PATIENT AND FAMILY

For the nurse to adequately manage the enormous range of emotional responses that the burn patient may exhibit, it is important to have an understanding of the circumstances of the burn, family relationships, and previous coping experiences with stressful stimuli. At any time, the various emotions of fear, anxiety, anger, guilt, and depression may be experienced (Table 25-15).

A common emotional response is regression. The patient will revert to behavior that helped in coping with stressful situations in the past. This response can be healthy and is usually short term in nature. Major emotional challenges confront patients and families throughout the burn patient's recovery, and perhaps for years to come. As more and more independence is expected from the patient, new fears must be confronted: "Can I do it?" "Am I a desirable partner/parent?" Open and frequent communication among the patient, family members, close friends, and burn team members is essential.

Burn survivors frequently experience thoughts and feelings that are frightening and disturbing, such as guilt about the burn incident, reliving the experience, fear of death, concern about future therapy and surgery, frustrations with ongoing discomfort and wound breakdown, and, perhaps, hopelessness about the future. Families may share some or all of these feelings. At times, they may feel helpless to assist their loved one. Continued support from trusted and familiar burn team members is essential. Assisting with aspects of care helps family members reconnect with their loved one and assists with the transition home. Many burn survivors and their families remark on the powerful learning experience of the burn and a renewed appreciation of life, despite the ongoing challenges of a prolonged and challenging recovery. Acknowledgment that their many feelings are real and valid can be therapeutic for patients and their families as burn survivors seek to incorporate this life event into their view of themselves and the life they had imagined.

The stress of the burn injury occasionally precipitates a psychiatric/psychologic crisis. Many patients realize this experience is beyond their ability to cope. Assessment by a psychiatrist who can prescribe appropriate medication, if needed, and begin short-term counseling is frequently helpful. Early psychiatric intervention is essential if the patient has been previously treated for a psychiatric illness or if the injury was a suicide attempt. The diagnosis of posttraumatic stress disorder is made in a number of burn patients.[21] Treatment typically begins in the hospital, but links to community resources must be made predischarge to ensure continuity of psychologic care. Once the patient is discharged, referral to a psychiatrist, psychologist, mental health counselor, social worker, or psychiatric clinical nurse specialist may be helpful if concerns are raised at burn clinic follow-up.

The difficult issue of sexuality must be met with honesty.[22] Physical appearance will be altered in the patient who has sustained a major burn. Acceptance of any changes is difficult at first for the patient and significant other. The nature of skin injury in itself causes modifications in processing sexual stimuli. Touch is an important part of sexuality, and immature scar tissue may make the sensation of touch unpleasant or may dull it. This is usually transient, but the patient and family need to know that it is normal and receive anticipatory guidance from health care personnel to avoid undue emotional strain.

Family and patient support groups may be beneficial in meeting the patient's and family's emotional needs at any phase of the recovery process. Speaking with others who have experienced burn trauma can be beneficial, both in terms of reaffirming that what the patient is feeling is normal and in allowing for the sharing of helpful advice. The Phoenix Society *(www.phoenix-society.org)* is an internationally represented burn survivors' support group that has been offering invaluable support to burn survivors, family members, and burn team personnel for many years. A website, yearly conference, newsletter, and one-on-one linking with community-based burn survivor volunteers are just a few of the resources this group has to offer.

TABLE 25-15 Emotional Responses of Burn Patients

Emotion	Possible Verbal Expression
Fear	Will I die? What will happen next? Will I be disfigured? Will my family and friends still love me?
Anxiety	I feel out of control. What's happening to me? When will it end?
Anger	Why did this happen to me? Those nurses enjoy hurting me.
Guilt	If only I'd been more careful. I'm being punished because I did something wrong.
Depression	It's no use going on like this. I don't care what happens to me. I wish people would leave me alone.

SPECIAL NEEDS OF THE NURSING STAFF

Warm, trusting, mutually satisfying relationships frequently develop between burn patients and nursing staff, not only during hospitalization but also during long-term rehabilitation. Sometimes the bond can be so strong that the patient has difficulty separating from the hospital and staff. The frequency and intensity of family contact can also be rewarding as well as draining to the nurse. Nurses new to burn nursing often find it difficult to cope with not only the deformities caused by burn injury but also the odor, the unpleasant sight of the wound, and the reality of the pain that accompanies the burn and its treatment.

Many nurses come to know that the care they provide makes a critical difference in helping patients not only to survive, but to cope with and triumph over a severe and multifaceted injury. It is this belief that allows and inspires nurses to provide such meaningful care to burn patients and their families.

Ongoing support services for the burn nurse or critical incident stress debriefings led by a psychiatrist, psychologist, psychiatric clinical nurse specialist, or social worker may be helpful at times. Peer support groups can serve a similar purpose by helping nursing staff to cope with difficult feelings they may experience when caring for burn patients (e.g., American Burn Association, Canadian Association of Burn Nurses, International Society for Burn Injuries). Burn nursing is physically, psychologically, and intellectually demanding, and therein lie its challenges and its inherent rewards. Attention to self-care is important not only for novice burn nurses, but for seasoned veterans, in order to maintain a positive attitude and healthy work/life balance. Time with family and friends, and rest and relaxation at home is an essential part of self-care and living a life with purpose and fulfillment.

CRITICAL THINKING EXERCISE

CASE STUDY

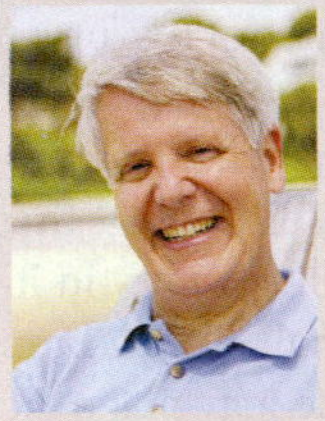

Burn and Inhalation Injury

Patient Profile. Arthur Jefferson, a 65-year-old married white man, is brought to the emergency department with burns to his arm, hand, and face from a kitchen grease fire. He arrives with an 18-gauge IV infusing lactated Ringer's solution at 100 ml/hr, and is receiving 100% humidified oxygen by mask.

Subjective Data

- Complains of impaired vision and having swallowing difficulties
- Cannot remember the accident
- Expresses a great deal of fear

Objective Data

Physical Examination

- Is awake, alert, and oriented, but in obvious distress
- Has irritated eyes, hoarseness, and shivering
- Nasal hair is singed, with blisters on the face and mouth
- Face appears sunburned; arm and hand have shiny, bright red, and wet wounds

Critical Thinking Questions

1. What are the priorities of care in the prehospital environment? How should his airway, breathing, and circulation be managed?
2. What factors place Arthur at high risk for an inhalation injury? What initial interventions can be anticipated?
3. What pain medications might be considered to promote his comfort?
4. Which of the criteria for burn unit referral does Arthur meet for admission to the hospital burn unit?
5. What metabolic disturbances would be expected soon after Arthur's hospitalization? Explain the physiologic basis for these changes.
6. What measures should be taken to support Arthur's family?
7. Based on the assessment data presented, write one or more appropriate nursing diagnoses. Are there any collaborative problems?

NCLEX EXAMINATION REVIEW QUESTIONS

The number of the question corresponds to the same-numbered objective at the beginning of the chapter.

1. In presenting a program on fire and burn prevention for families, the nurse focuses on the most common cause of household fires as
   a. unattended cooking.
   b. frayed or defective wiring.
   c. carelessness with cigarettes.
   d. improper use of inflammables.
2. The injury that is least likely to result in a full-thickness burn is
   a. sunburn.
   b. scald injury.
   c. chemical burn.
   d. electrical injury.
3. When assessing a patient with a partial-thickness burn, the nurse would expect to find
   a. exposed fascia.
   b. dry, waxy appearance.
   c. red, shiny, wet appearance.
   d. absence of blanching with pressure.
4. The extent of burns is assessed by
   a. rating the location of burns at specific body sites.
   b. determining the presence of preexisting risk factors.
   c. estimating the ratio of full-thickness to partial-thickness burns.
   d. using guides to indicate burn location relative to total body surface.
5. An 82-kg patient has a 45% TBSA burn. Using 4 ml/kg/% TBSA burn during the first 24 hours after a burn injury, the nurse would anticipate a fluid replacement of
   a. 3690 ml.
   b. 7380 ml.
   c. 9225 ml.
   d. 14,760 ml.
6. Fluid and electrolyte shifts that occur during the early emergent phase include
   a. adherence of albumin to vascular walls.
   b. movement of potassium into the vascular space.
   c. sequestering of sodium and water in interstitial fluid.
   d. hemolysis of red blood cells from large volumes of rapidly administered fluid.
7. To maintain a positive nitrogen balance in a major burn, the patient must
   a. eat a high-protein, low-fat, low-carbohydrate diet.
   b. increase normal adult caloric intake by about 3 times.
   c. eat at least 1500 calories per day in small, frequent meals.
   d. eat rice and whole wheat for the chemical effect on nitrogen balance.
8. Pain management for the burn patient is most effective when
   a. the nurse administers opioids on a set schedule around the clock.
   b. the patient has as much control over the management of the pain as possible.
   c. the nurse has the flexibility to administer opioids within a dosage and frequency range.
   d. painful dressing changes and repositioning are delayed until the patient's pain is totally relieved.
9. A therapeutic measure used to prevent hypertrophic scarring during the rehabilitative phase of burn recovery is
   a. applying pressure garments.
   b. repositioning the patient every 2 hours.
   c. performing active ROM at least every 4 hours.
   d. massaging the new tissue with water-based moisturizers.

10. It is important for the burn patient and family to
    a. see the burn wound 3 times per day.
    b. talk frequently with the nurse about the patient's progress.
    c. allow nurses to perform total care for the patient to prevent infection.
    d. avoid discussion of the patient's progress to minimize false hope.
11. Discharge planning for the burn patient begins
    a. after grafting.
    b. on admission.
    c. after the emergent phase.
    d. at least 1 week before discharge.

REFERENCES

1. Centers for Disease Control and Prevention: *Burns—injury fact sheet,* Atlanta, 2005, the Centers. Available at *www.bt.cdc.gov.*
2. American Burn Association: *Burn incidence fact sheet—2002.* Available at *www.ameriburn.org.*
3. Thompson NJ, Waterman MB, Sheet DA: Using behavioral science to improve fire escape behaviors in response to a smoke alarm, *J Burn Care Rehabil* 25:179, 2004.
4. Bethel C, Krisands T: Burn care procedures. In Robert J, editor: *Clinical procedures in emergency medicine,* ed 4, St Louis, 2004, Elsevier.
5. Cone J: What's new in general surgery: burns and metabolism, *J Am Coll Surg* 200:607, 2005.
6. Baldwin K, Morris S: Shock, multiple organ dysfunction syndrome, and burns in adults. In McCance KL, Huether SE, editors: *Pathophysiology: the biologic basis for disease in adults and children,* ed 5, St Louis, 2006, Mosby.
7. Miller K, Chang A: Acute inhalation injury, *Emerg Med Clin North Am* 21:533, 2003.
8. Johnson RM, Richard R: Partial-thickness burns: identification and management, *Adv Skin Wound Healing* 16:178, 2003.
9. Gordon MD, Winfree JH: Fluid resuscitation after a major burn. In Carrougher GJ: *Burn care and therapy,* St Louis, 1998, Mosby.
10. Heggars JP, Hawkins H, Edgar P, et al.: Treatment of infection in burns. In Herndon DN: *Total burn care,* ed 2, New York, 2002, Saunders.
11. Carrougher GJ: Burn wound assessment and topical treatment. In Carrougher GJ: *Burn care and therapy,* St Louis, 1998, Mosby.
12. Green J, et al: Eyelid trauma and reconstruction techniques. In Yanoff M, et al, editors: *Ophthalmology,* ed 2, St Louis, 2004, Mosby.
13. Slone DS: Nutritional support of the critically ill and injured patient, *Crit Care Clin* 20:135, 2004.
14. Barillo D, McManus A: Infection in burn patients. In Cohen J, Powderly W, editors: *Infectious diseases,* ed 2, St Louis, 2004, Elsevier.
15. Wolf S, Herndon D: Burns. In Townsend C, et al, editors: *Sabiston textbook of surgery,* ed 17, St Louis, 2004, Elsevier.
16. Jimenez P, Jimenez S: Tissue and cellular approaches to wound repair, *Am J Surg* 187:56S, 2004.
17. Sheridan R, Tompkins R: What's new in burns and metabolism, *J Am Coll Surg* 198:243, 2004.
18. Crowther C, Mourad L: Alterations of musculoskeletal function. In McCance KL, Huether SE, editors: *Pathophysiology: the biologic basis for disease in adults and children,* ed 5, St Louis, 2006, Mosby.
19. Lawrence JW, et al: Visible vs. hidden scars and their relation to body esteem, *J Burn Care Rehabil* 25:25, 2004.
20. Redlick F, et al: A survey of risk factors for burns in the elderly and prevention strategies, *J Burn Care Rehabil* 23:351, 2002.
21. Fauerbach JA, et al: Burden of burn: a norm-based inquiry into the influence of burn size and distress on recovery of physical and psychological function, *J Burn Care Rehabil* 26:21, 2005.
22. Roberts F: Sexuality—the forgotten issue, *Burn Support News: Newsletter of The Phoenix Society* March 14, 2003.

RESOURCES

American Academy of Facial Plastic and Reconstructive Surgery
703-299-9291
www.aafprs.org

American Burn Association
312-642-9260
www.ameriburn.org

American Society of Plastic Surgical Nurses
678-966-3065
info@aspsn.org

Burn Foundation
215-988-9882
www.burnfoundation.org

Burn Surgery.org—Educating Burn Care Professionals World Wide
www.burnsurgery.org

Burn Survivor.org
919-602-6023
www.burnsurvivor.org

Canadian Association of Burn Nurses
c/o Judy Knighton, Reg.N., M.Sc.N.
judy.knighton@sw.ca
www.cabn.ca

Changing Faces
www.changingfaces.org.uk

International Society for Burn Injuries
www.worldburn.org

Phoenix Society for Burn Survivors, Inc.
616-458-2773
800-888-2876
www.phoenix-society.org

For additional Internet resources, see the website for this book at *http://evolve.elsevier.com/Lewis/medsurg.*

Section 5

Problems of Oxygenation: Ventilation

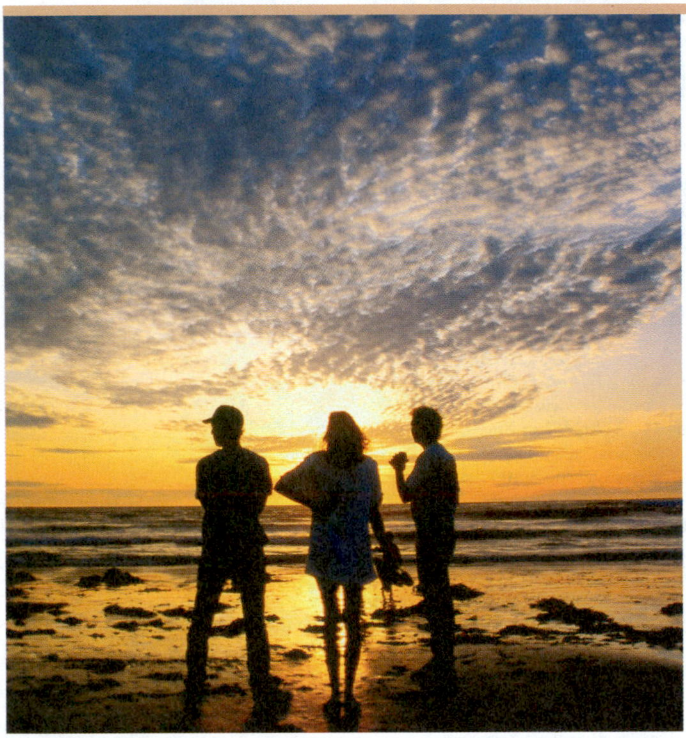

Section Outline

Life becomes harder for us when we live for others, but it also becomes richer and happier.
Albert Schweitzer

Nursing Assessment Respiratory System

26

Jane Steinman Kaufman

LEARNING OBJECTIVES

1. Describe the structures and functions of the upper respiratory tract, the lower respiratory tract, and the chest wall.
2. Describe the process that initiates and controls inspiration and expiration.
3. Describe the process of gas diffusion within the lungs.
4. Identify the respiratory defense mechanisms.
5. Describe the significance of arterial blood gas values and the oxyhemoglobin dissociation curve in relation to respiratory function.
6. Identify the signs and symptoms of inadequate oxygenation and the implications of these findings.
7. Describe age-related changes in the respiratory system and differences in assessment findings.
8. Identify the significant subjective and objective data related to the respiratory system that should be obtained from a patient.
9. Describe the techniques used in physical assessment of the respiratory system.
10. Differentiate normal from common abnormal findings in a physical assessment of the respiratory system.
11. Describe the purpose, significance of results, and nursing responsibilities related to diagnostic studies of the respiratory system.

KEY TERMS

adventitious sounds, p. 524
chemoreceptor, p. 515
compliance, p. 512
crackles, p. 524
dyspnea, p. 512
elastic recoil, p. 512
fremitus, p. 522
mechanical receptors, p. 515
pleural friction rub, p. 524
rhonchi, p. 524
surfactant, p. 511
tidal volume, p. 511
ventilation, p. 512
wheezes, p. 519

Electronic Resources

Supplemental content related to Chapter 26 can be found . . .

Companion CD

- Stress-Busting Kit for Nursing Students
- NCLEX Examination Review Questions
- Comprehensive Glossary
- Animations:
  - Patterns of Respiration
  - Percussion Tones Throughout the Chest
  - Pulmonary Circulation
- Audio Clips:
  - Bronchial Breath Sounds
  - Bronchovesicular Breath Sounds
  - High-Pitched Crackles
  - High-Pitched Wheeze
  - Low-Pitched Crackles
  - Low-Pitched Wheeze
  - Pleural Friction Rub
  - Stridor
  - Vesicular Breath Sounds
- Video Clips:
  - Inspection and Palpation: Breathing and Respiratory Excursion, Anterior Chest
  - Inspection and Palpation: Respirations, Respiratory Excursion, and Tactile Fremitus, Posterior Chest
  - Inspection and Percussion: Diaphragmatic Excursion
  - Inspection: Nose
  - Palpation: Tactile Fremitus, Posterior Chest
  - Percussion: Anterior Thorax

Evolve Website evolve

http://evolve.elsevier.com/Lewis/medsurg

- Content Updates
- Key Points (Printable and CD/MP3 Download)
- Concept Map Creator
- Expanded Audio Glossary
- Key Term Flash Cards
- Electronic Calculators
- Physical Examination Videos
  - Lungs
  - Anterior Chest, Lungs, and Heart
- WebLinks

Reviewed by Christine L. Willis, RN, MSN, ANP-C, Adult Nurse Practitioner, Pulmonary and Critical Care Medicine, Duke University Medical Center, Durham, N.C.

STRUCTURES AND FUNCTIONS OF THE RESPIRATORY SYSTEM

The primary purpose of the respiratory system is gas exchange, which involves the transfer of oxygen and carbon dioxide between the atmosphere and the blood. The respiratory system is divided into two parts: the upper respiratory tract and the lower respiratory tract (Fig. 26-1). The upper respiratory tract includes the nose, pharynx, adenoids, tonsils, epiglottis, larynx, and trachea. The lower respiratory tract consists of the bronchi, bronchioles, alveolar ducts, and alveoli. With the exception of the right and left mainstem bronchi, all lower airway structures are contained within the lungs. The right lung is divided into three lobes (upper, middle, and lower) and the left lung into two lobes (upper and lower) (Fig. 26-2). The structures of the chest wall (ribs, pleura, muscles of respiration) are also essential to respiration.

Upper Respiratory Tract

The nose, made of bone and cartilage, is divided into two nares by the nasal septum. The interior of the nose is shaped into rolling projections called *turbinates* that increase the surface area for warming and moistening air. The internal nose opens directly into the sinuses. The nasal cavity connects with the pharynx, a tubular passageway that is subdivided from above downward into three parts: the nasopharynx, the oropharynx, and the laryngopharynx.

Breathing through the narrow nasal passages (rather than mouth breathing) provides protection for the lower airway. The nose is lined with mucous membrane and small hairs. Air entering the nose is warmed to near body temperature, humidified to nearly 100% water saturation, and filtered of particles larger than 10 μm (e.g., dust, bacteria).

The olfactory nerve endings (receptors for the sense of smell) are located in the roof of the nose. The adenoids and tonsils, which are small masses of lymphatic tissue, are found in the nasopharynx and the oropharynx, respectively.

The epiglottis is a small flap of tissue at the base of the tongue. During swallowing, the epiglottis covers the larynx, preventing solids and liquids from entering the lungs. Conditions such as a stroke, prolonged intubation, or altered level of consciousness may

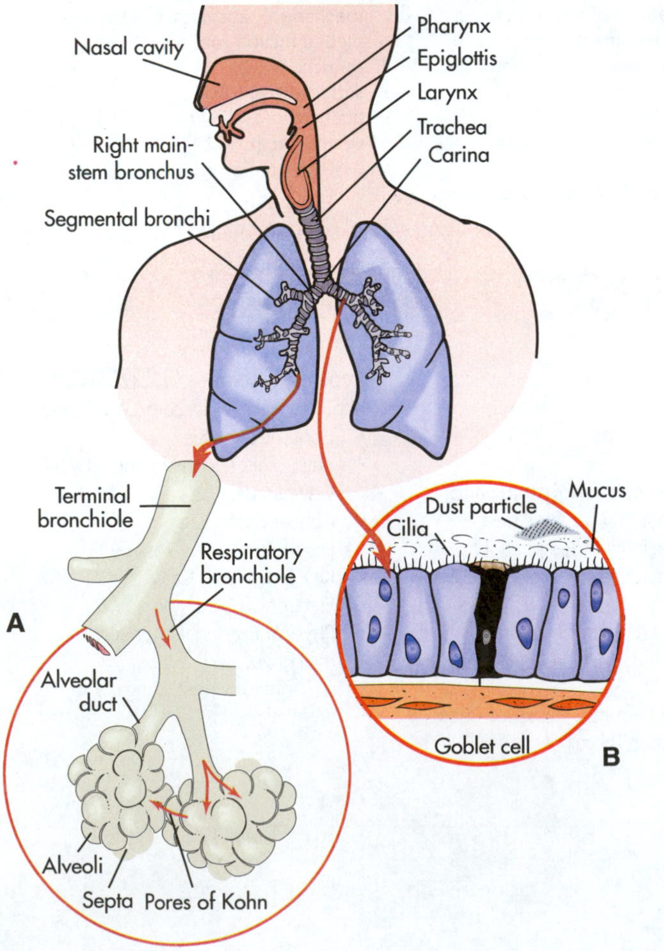

FIG. 26-1 Structures of the respiratory tract. **A,** Pulmonary functional unit. **B,** Ciliated mucous membrane.

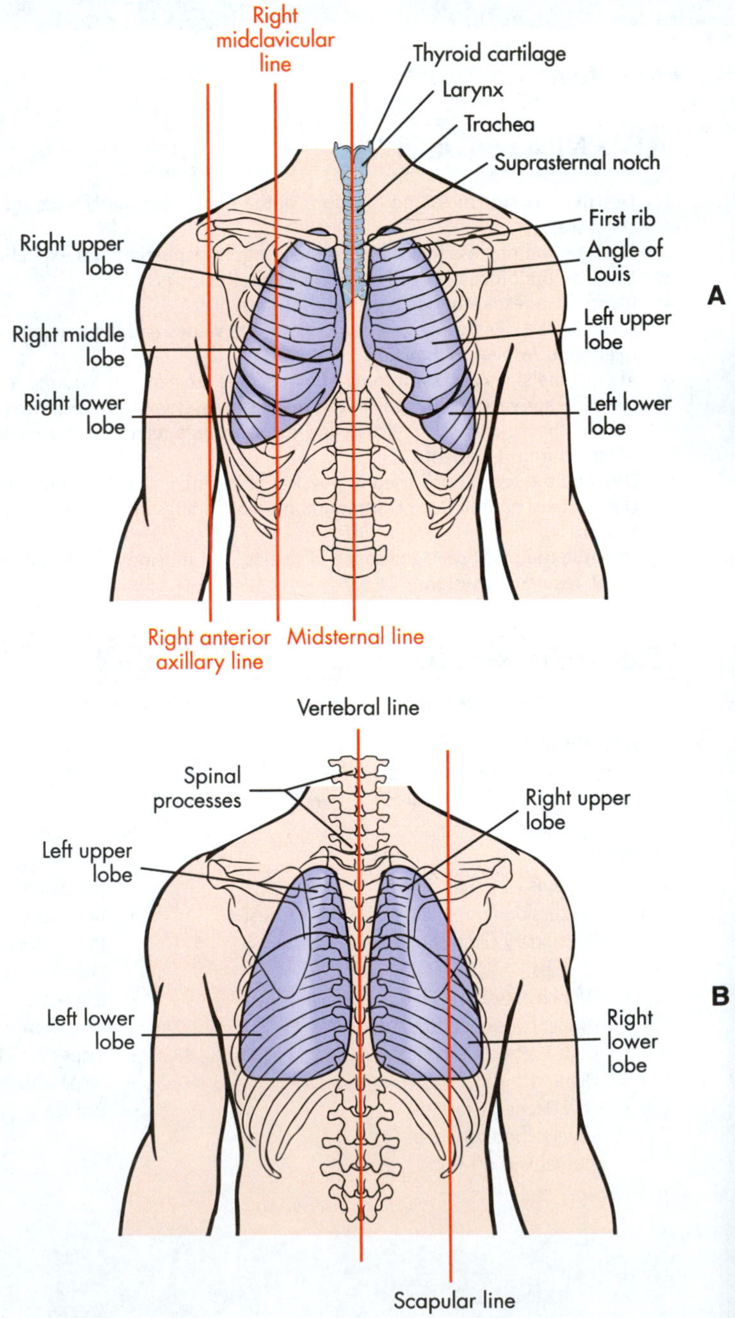

FIG. 26-2 Landmarks and structures of the chest wall. **A,** Anterior view. **B,** Posterior view.

alter the swallowing ability and impair the function of the epiglottis, thus predisposing to aspiration.

After passing through the oropharynx, air moves through the laryngopharynx and the larynx, where the vocal cords are located, and then down into the trachea. The trachea is a cylindric tube about 5 inches (10 to 12 cm) long and 1 inch (1.5 to 2.5 cm) in diameter. The support of U-shaped cartilages keeps the trachea open but allows the adjacent esophagus to expand for swallowing. The trachea bifurcates into the right and left mainstem bronchi at a point called the *carina.* The carina is located at the level of the manubriosternal junction, also called the *angle of Louis.* The carina is highly sensitive, and touching it during suctioning causes vigorous coughing.[1]

Lower Respiratory Tract

Once air passes the carina, it is in the lower respiratory tract. The mainstem bronchi, pulmonary vessels, and nerves enter the lungs through a slit called the *hilus.* The right mainstem bronchus is shorter, wider, and straighter than the left mainstem bronchus. For this reason, aspiration is more likely in the right lung than in the left lung. Lymph nodes in the hilar area, especially when hilar lymphadenopathy is present, may be visible on chest x-ray. These findings may be indicative of sarcoidosis or other conditions associated with inflammation (e.g., cancer, tuberculosis).

The mainstem bronchi subdivide several times to form the lobar, segmental, and subsegmental bronchi. Further divisions form the bronchioles. The most distant bronchioles are called the respiratory bronchioles. Beyond these lie the alveolar ducts and alveolar sacs (Fig. 26-3). The bronchioles are encircled by smooth muscles that constrict and dilate in response to various stimuli. The terms *bronchoconstriction* and *bronchodilation* are used to refer to a decrease or increase in the diameter of the airways caused by contraction or relaxation of these muscles.

No exchange of oxygen or carbon dioxide takes place until air enters the respiratory bronchioles. The area of the respiratory tract from the nose to the respiratory bronchioles serves only as a conducting pathway. It is termed the *anatomic dead space* (VD). This space must be filled with every breath, but the air that fills it is not available for gas exchange. In adults, a normal **tidal volume** (VT), or volume of air exchanged with each breath, is about 500 ml. Of each 500 ml inhaled, about 150 ml is VD. During shallow breathing as seen postoperatively or in an asthma attack, sufficient air (i.e., >150 ml/breath) may not be moving, and hypoxemia can occur quickly during such periods.

After moving through the VD, air reaches the respiratory bronchioles and alveoli (Fig. 26-4). *Alveoli* are small sacs that form the functional unit of the lungs. The alveoli are interconnected by pores of Kohn, which allow movement of air from alveolus to alveolus (see Fig. 26-1). Deep breaths promote air movement through these pores and assist in expelling mucus in respiratory bronchioles. Bacteria can also move through these pores, resulting in an extension of respiratory infection to previously noninfected areas. The 300 million alveoli in the adult have a total volume of about 2500 ml and a surface area for gas exchange that is about the size of a tennis court. The alveolar-capillary membrane (Fig. 26-5) is very thin (less than 1/5000 of an inch, or 5 μm) and is the site of gas exchange. In conditions such as pulmonary edema, excess fluid fills the interstitial space and alveoli, markedly reducing gas exchange.[2,3]

Surfactant. The lung can be conceptualized as a collection of 300 million bubbles (alveoli), each 0.3 mm in diameter. Such a structure is inherently unstable and, as a consequence, the alveoli have a natural tendency to collapse. The alveolar surface is composed of cells that provide structure and cells that secrete surfactant (see Fig. 26-5). **Surfactant,** a lipoprotein that lowers the surface tension in the alveoli, reduces the amount of pressure needed to inflate the alveoli and decreases the tendency of the alveoli to collapse. Normally, each person takes a slightly larger breath, termed a *sigh,* after every five to six breaths. This sigh stretches the alveoli and promotes surfactant secretion.

When insufficient surfactant is present, the alveoli collapse. The term *atelectasis* refers to collapsed, airless alveoli (see Fig. 26-4).

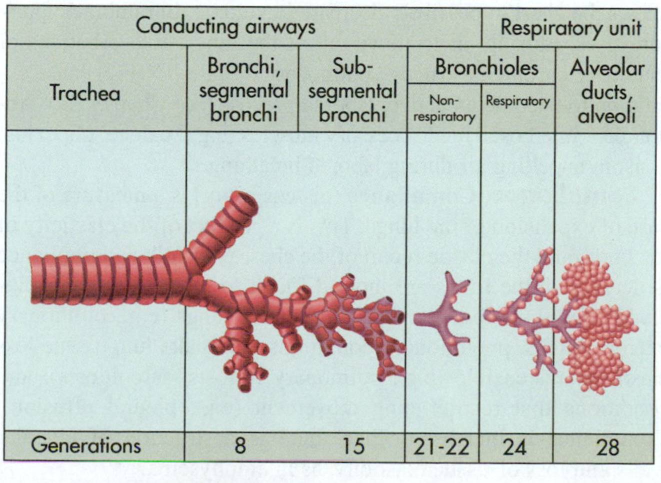

Conducting airways
Respiratory unit
Trachea
Bronchi, segmental bronchi
Sub-segmental bronchi
Bronchioles
Non-respiratory
Respiratory
Alveolar ducts, alveoli
Generations
8
15
21-22
24
28

FIG. 26-3 Structures of lower airways.

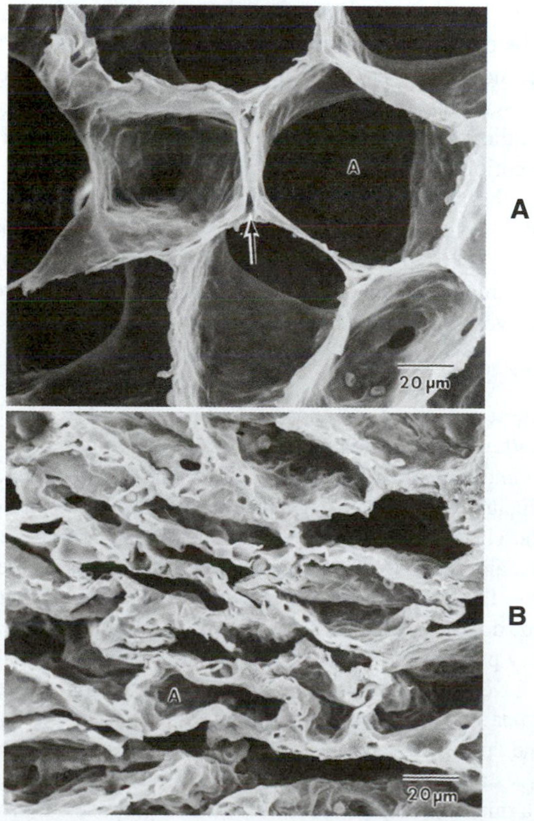

FIG. 26-4 Scanning electron micrograph of lung parenchyma. **A,** Alveoli *(A)* and alveolar-capillary membrane *(arrow).* **B,** Effects of atelectasis. Alveoli *(A)* are partially or totally collapsed.

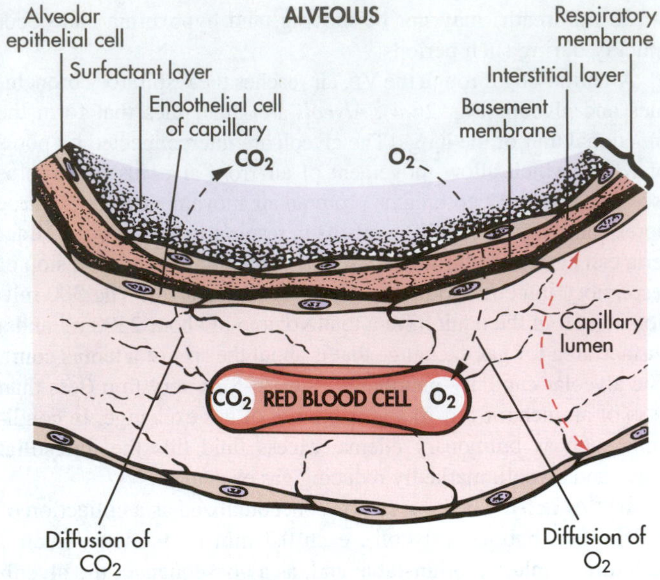

FIG. 26-5 A small portion of the respiratory membrane greatly magnified. An extremely thin interstitial layer of tissue separates the endothelial cell and basement membrane on the capillary side from the epithelial cell and surfactant layer on the alveolar side of the respiratory membrane. The total thickness of the respiratory membrane is less than 1/5000 of an inch.

The postoperative patient is at risk for atelectasis because of the effects of anesthesia and restricted breathing with pain (see Chapter 20). In acute respiratory distress syndrome (ARDS), lack of surfactant contributes to widespread atelectasis[2,4] (see Chapter 68).

Blood Supply. The lungs have two different types of circulation: pulmonary and bronchial. The pulmonary circulation provides the lungs with blood for gas exchange. The pulmonary artery receives deoxygenated blood from the right ventricle of the heart and branches so that each pulmonary capillary is directly connected with many alveoli. Oxygen–carbon dioxide exchange occurs at this point. The pulmonary veins return oxygenated blood to the superior vena cava of the heart.

The bronchial circulation starts with the bronchial arteries, which arise from the thoracic aorta. The bronchial circulation provides oxygen to the bronchi and other pulmonary tissues. Deoxygenated blood returns from the bronchial circulation through the azygos vein into the left atrium.

Chest Wall

The chest wall is shaped, supported, and protected by 24 ribs (12 on each side). The ribs and the sternum protect the lungs and heart from injury and are called the *thoracic cage.* The structures of the chest wall include the thoracic cage, pleura, and respiratory muscles.

The chest cavity is lined with a membrane called the *parietal pleura,* and the lungs are lined with a membrane called the *visceral pleura.* The parietal and visceral pleurae are joined and form a closed, double-walled sac. The visceral pleura does not have any sensory pain fibers or nerve endings. The parietal pleura, however, does have sensory pain fibers. Therefore irritation of the parietal pleura causes pain with each breath.

The space between the pleural layers, termed the *intrapleural space,* is a potential space. In the normal adult, this space is filled with a thin film of fluid, which serves two purposes: it provides lubrication, allowing the layers of pleura to slide over each other during breathing; and it increases cohesion between the pleural layers, thereby facilitating expansion of the pleura and lung during inspiration.

Normally, the pleural space contains 20 to 25 ml of fluid. Fluid is drained from the pleural space by the lymphatic circulation. Several pathologic conditions may cause the accumulation of greater amounts of fluid, termed a *pleural effusion.* Pleural fluid may accumulate because of blockage of lymphatic drainage (e.g., from malignant cells) or when there is an imbalance between intravascular and oncotic fluid pressures, such as occurs in heart failure. Purulent pleural fluid with bacterial infection is called *empyema.*

The diaphragm is the major muscle of respiration. During inspiration, the diaphragm contracts, increasing intrathoracic volume and pushing the abdominal contents downward. At the same time, the external intercostal muscles and scalene muscles contract, increasing the lateral and anteroposterior dimension of the chest. This causes the size of the thoracic cavity to increase and intrathoracic pressure to decrease, so air enters the lungs.

The diaphragm is made up of two hemidiaphragms, each innervated by the right and left phrenic nerves. The phrenic nerves arise from the spinal cord between C3 and C5, the third and fifth cervical vertebrae. Injury to the phrenic nerve results in hemidiaphragm paralysis on the side of the injury. Complete spinal cord injuries above the level of C3 result in total diaphragm paralysis and mechanical ventilator dependence.[5]

Physiology of Respiration

Ventilation. **Ventilation** involves *inspiration* (movement of air into the lungs) and *expiration* (movement of air out of the lungs). Air moves in and out of the lungs because intrathoracic pressure changes in relation to pressure at the airway opening. Contraction of the diaphragm and intercostal and scalene muscles increases chest dimensions, thereby decreasing intrathoracic pressure. Gas flows from an area of higher pressure (atmospheric) to one of lower pressure (intrathoracic). When **dyspnea** (shortness of breath) occurs, neck and shoulder muscles can assist the effort. Some conditions (e.g., phrenic nerve paralysis, rib fractures, neuromuscular disease) may limit diaphragm or chest wall movement and cause the patient to breathe with smaller tidal volumes. As a result, the lungs do not fully inflate, and gas exchange is impaired.

In contrast to inspiration, expiration is passive. **Elastic recoil** is the tendency for the lungs to recoil or reduce in volume after being stretched or expanded. The elasticity of lung tissue is due to the elastin fibers found in the alveolar walls and surrounding the bronchioles and capillaries. The elastic recoil of the chest wall and lungs allows the chest to passively decrease in volume. Intrathoracic pressure rises, causing air to move out of the lungs. Exacerbations of asthma or chronic obstructive pulmonary disease (COPD) cause expiration to become an active, labored process (see Chapter 29). Abdominal, intercostal, and accessory muscles (e.g., scalene, trapezius) assist in expelling air during labored breathing.

Compliance. **Compliance** (distensibility) is a measure of the ease of expansion of the lungs. This is a product of the elasticity of the lungs and the elastic recoil of the chest wall. When compliance is decreased, the lungs are more difficult to inflate. Examples include conditions that increase fluid in the lungs (e.g., pulmonary edema, ARDS, pneumonia); conditions that make lung tissue less elastic or distensible (e.g., pulmonary fibrosis, sarcoidosis); and conditions that restrict lung movement (e.g., pleural effusion). Compliance is increased when there is destruction of alveolar walls and loss of tissue elasticity, as in emphysema.

Diffusion. Oxygen and carbon dioxide move back and forth across the alveolar-capillary membrane by diffusion. The overall direction of movement is from the area of higher concentration to the area of lower concentration. Thus oxygen moves from alveolar gas (atmospheric air) into the arterial blood and carbon dioxide from the arterial blood into the alveolar gas. Diffusion continues until equilibrium is reached (see Fig. 26-5).

The ability of the lungs to oxygenate arterial blood adequately is determined by examination of the partial pressure of oxygen in arterial blood (PaO_2) and arterial oxygen saturation (SaO_2). Oxygen is carried in the blood in two forms: dissolved oxygen and hemoglobin-bound oxygen. The PaO_2 represents the amount of oxygen dissolved in the plasma and is expressed in millimeters of mercury (mm Hg). The SaO_2 is the amount of oxygen bound to hemoglobin in comparison with the amount of oxygen the hemoglobin can carry. The SaO_2 is expressed as a percentage. For example, if the SaO_2 is 90%, this means that 90% of the hemoglobin attachments for oxygen have oxygen bound to them.

Oxygen-Hemoglobin Dissociation Curve. The affinity of hemoglobin for oxygen is described by the *oxygen-hemoglobin dissociation curve* (Fig. 26-6). Oxygen delivery to the tissues depends on the amount of oxygen that can be picked up in the lungs and the ease with which hemoglobin gives up oxygen once it reaches the tissues. In the upper flat portion of the curve, representing the conditions in the lungs, fairly large changes in the PaO_2 cause small changes in hemoglobin saturation. For this reason, if the PaO_2 drops from 100 to 60 mm Hg, the saturation of hemoglobin changes only 7% (from the normal 97% to 90%). Thus the hemoglobin remains 90% saturated despite a 40–mm Hg drop in the PaO_2. This portion of the curve also explains the reason the patient is considered adequately oxygenated when the PaO_2 is greater than 60 mm Hg. Increasing the PaO_2 above this level does little to improve hemoglobin saturation.

The lower portion of the oxyhemoglobin dissociation curve represents oxygen binding by hemoglobin at the level of peripheral tissues. As hemoglobin arrives at the tissues, it is desaturated upon exposure to a tissue PaO_2 of 30 to 40 mm Hg and large amounts of oxygen are released for tissue use. This is an important method of maintaining the oxygen pressure gradient between the blood and the tissues. It also ensures an adequate oxygen supply to peripheral tissues, even if oxygen saturation is reduced.

Many factors alter the affinity of hemoglobin for oxygen. When the oxygen dissociation curve shifts to the left, blood picks up oxygen more readily in the lungs but delivers oxygen less readily to the tissues. This is seen in alkalosis, in hypothermia, and with a decrease in the partial pressure of carbon dioxide in arterial blood ($PaCO_2$) (see Fig. 26-6). The patient with a condition that causes a leftward shift of the curve, such as with hypothermia that follows open heart surgery, may be given higher concentrations of oxygen until the body temperature normalizes. This helps compensate for decreased oxygen unloading in the tissues. When the curve shifts to the right, the opposite occurs. Blood picks up oxygen less rapidly in the lungs but delivers oxygen more readily to the tissues. This is seen in acidosis, in hyperthermia, and when the $PaCO_2$ is increased.

Two methods are used to assess the efficiency of gas transfer in the lung: analysis of *arterial blood gases* (ABGs) and oximetry. These measures are usually adequate if the patient is stable and not critically ill.[6]

Arterial Blood Gases. ABGs are measured to determine oxygenation status and acid-base balance. ABG analysis includes measurement of the PaO_2, $PaCO_2$, acidity (pH), and bicarbonate (HCO_3^-) in arterial blood. The SaO_2 is either calculated or measured during this analysis.

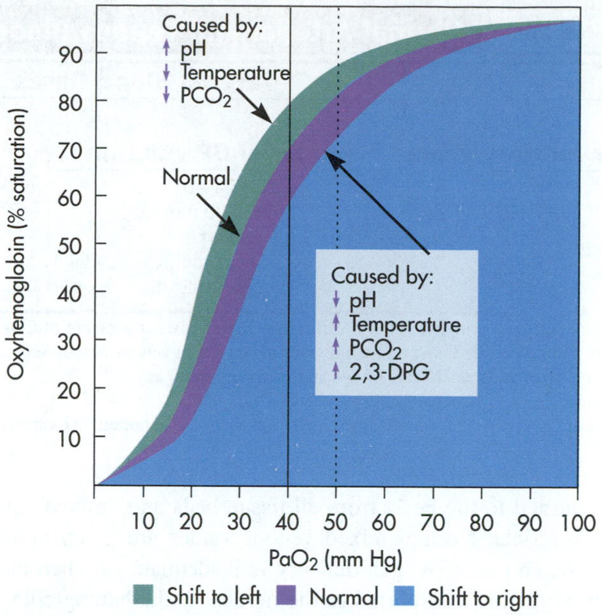

FIG. 26-6 Oxygen-hemoglobin dissociation curve. The effects of acidity and temperature changes are shown. *2,3-DPG,* 2,3-Diphosphoglycerate; *PaO_2,* partial pressure of oxygen in arterial blood; *PCO_2,* pressure of carbon dioxide.

Blood for ABG analysis can be obtained by arterial puncture or from an arterial catheter, usually in the radial or femoral artery. Both techniques are invasive and allow only intermittent analysis. Continuous intraarterial blood gas monitoring is also possible via a fiberoptic sensor or an oxygen electrode inserted into an arterial catheter. An arterial catheter permits ABG sampling without repeated arterial punctures.

Normal values for ABGs are given in Table 26-1. The normal PaO_2 decreases with advancing age. The normal PaO_2 also varies in relation to the distance above sea level. At higher altitudes, the barometric pressure is lower, resulting in a lower inspired oxygen pressure and a lower PaO_2 (see Table 26-1). Most airplanes are pressurized to approximate an altitude of 8000 feet above sea level. A normal person can expect a 16 to 32 mm Hg fall in PaO_2 at this altitude. The patient who is already receiving oxygen therapy or the patient with a PaO_2 less than 72 mm Hg while breathing room air needs a careful evaluation before air travel. Supplemental oxygen or a change in liter flow may be required during the flight. If oxygen is required, the airline should be contacted several weeks in advance to determine the procedures regarding air travel with oxygen.[7,8]

Mixed Venous Blood Gases. For the patient with a normal or near-normal cardiac status, an assessment of PaO_2 or SaO_2 is usually sufficient to determine adequate oxygenation. The patient with impaired cardiac output or hemodynamic instability may have inadequate tissue oxygen delivery or abnormal oxygen consumption. The amount of oxygen delivered to the tissues or consumed can be calculated.

A catheter positioned in the pulmonary artery, termed a *pulmonary artery (PA) catheter,* is used for mixed venous sampling (see Chapter 66). Blood drawn from a PA catheter is termed a *mixed venous blood gas* sample because it consists of venous blood that

TABLE 26-1 Normal Arterial and Venous Blood Gas Values*

Laboratory Value	Arterial Blood Gases: Sea Level BP 760 mm Hg	Arterial Blood Gases: 1 Mile Above Sea Level (5280 ft) BP 629 mm Hg	Venous Blood Gases: Mixed Venous Blood Gases†	
pH	7.35-7.45	7.35-7.45	pH	7.34-7.37
PaO_2	80-100 mm Hg	65-75 mm Hg	PvO_2	38-42 mm Hg
SaO_2	>95%‡	>95%‡	SvO_2	60%-80%‡
$PaCO_2$	35-45 mm Hg	35-45 mm Hg	$PvCO_2$	44-46 mm Hg
HCO_3^-	22-26 mEq/L	22-26 mEq/L	HCO_3^-	24-30 mEq/L

BP, Barometric pressure; *HCO_3^-*, bicarbonate; *$PaCO_2$*, partial pressure of CO_2 in arterial blood; *PaO_2*, partial pressure of oxygen in arterial blood; *$PvCO_2$*, partial pressure of CO_2 in venous blood; *PvO_2*, partial pressure of oxygen in venous blood; *SaO_2*, arterial oxygen saturation; *SvO_2*, venous oxygen saturation.
*Assumes patient is ≤60 years of age and breathing room air.
†Obtained from a pulmonary artery catheter.
‡The same normal values apply when SpO_2 and SvO_2 are obtained by oximetry.

has returned to the heart from all tissue beds and "mixed" in the right ventricle. Normal mixed venous values are given in Table 26-1. When tissue oxygen delivery is inadequate or when inadequate oxygen is transported to the tissues by the hemoglobin, the PvO_2 and SvO_2 fall.

Oximetry. ABG values provide accurate information about oxygenation and acid-base balance. However, they are invasive, require laboratory analysis, and expose the patient to the risk of bleeding from an arterial puncture. Arterial oxygen saturation can be monitored continuously using a *pulse oximetry* probe on the finger, toe, ear, or bridge of the nose (Fig. 26-7).

A pulse oximeter emits two wavelengths of light, one red and one infrared, that pass from a light-emitting diode (positioned on one side of the probe) to a photodetector (positioned on the opposite side). Well-oxygenated blood absorbs light differently than deoxygenated blood does. The oximeter determines the amount of light absorbed by the vascular bed and calculates the saturation. The abbreviation SpO_2 is used to indicate the oxygen saturation value obtained by pulse oximetry. SpO_2 and heart rate are displayed on the monitor as digital readings (Fig. 26-7, *B*). The normal SpO_2 is greater than 95%.

Pulse oximetry is particularly valuable in intensive care and perioperative situations, in which sedation or decreased consciousness might mask hypoxia (Table 26-2). SpO_2 is assessed with each routine vital signs check in many inpatient areas. Changes in SpO_2 can be detected quickly and treated (Table 26-3). Oximetry is also used during exercise testing and when adjusting flow rates during long-term oxygen therapy. Pulse oximetry alone does not provide information about ventilation status and acid-base balance. Therefore ABGs are also needed periodically.

Values obtained by pulse oximetry are less accurate if the SpO_2 is less than 70%. At this level, the oximeter may display a value that is ±4% of the actual value. For example, if the SpO_2 reading is 70%, the actual value can range from 66% to 74%. Pulse oximetry is also inaccurate if hemoglobin variants (e.g., carboxyhemoglobin, methemoglobin) are present. Other factors that can alter the accuracy of pulse oximetry include motion, low perfusion, anemia, cold extremities, bright fluorescent lights, intravascular dyes, thick acrylic nails, and dark skin color. If there is doubt about the accuracy of the SpO_2 reading, an ABG analysis should be obtained to verify accuracy.

Oximetry can also be used to monitor SvO_2 via a PA catheter. A decrease in SvO_2 suggests that less oxygen is being delivered to the tissues or that more oxygen is being consumed. Changes in

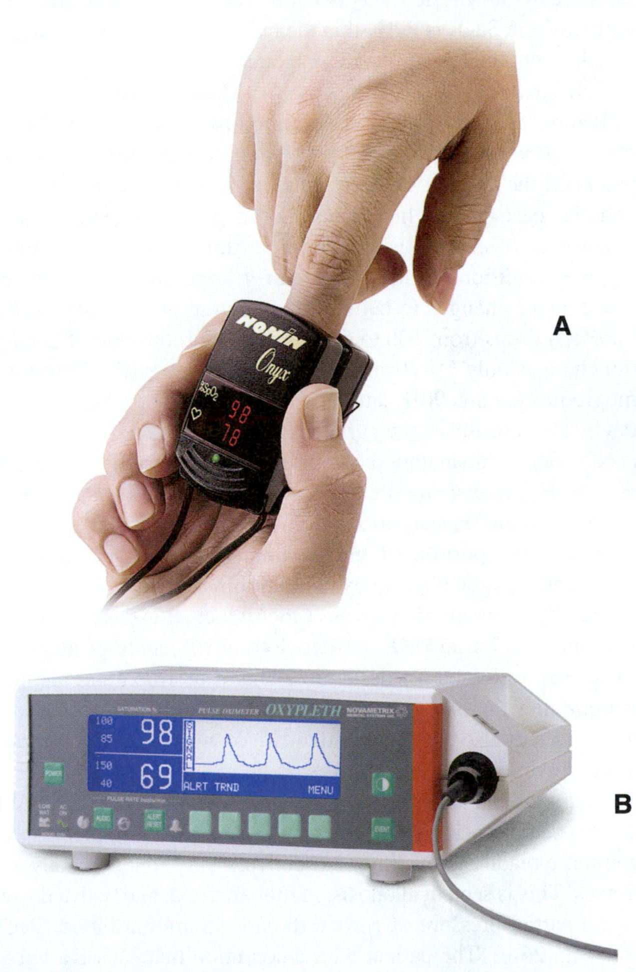

FIG. 26-7 **A,** Portable pulse oximeter displays oxygen saturation (SpO_2) and pulse rate. **B,** A pulse oximeter displays the oxygen saturation and pulse rate as a digital reading.

SvO_2 provide an early warning of a change in cardiac output or tissue oxygen delivery. Normal SvO_2 is 60% to 80%.

Oxygen Delivery. Information from ABGs or oximetry is used to assess adequacy of oxygenation. Several questions must be asked to determine if oxygenation is adequate:

1. What is the patient's SpO_2 or PaO_2 compared with expected normal values? (Normal values are given in Table 26-1.)

TABLE 26-2 Signs and Symptoms of Inadequate Oxygenation

Signs and Symptoms	Onset
Central Nervous System	
Unexplained apprehension	Early
Unexplained restlessness or irritability	Early
Unexplained confusion or lethargy	Early or late
Combativeness	Late
Coma	Late
Respiratory	
Tachypnea	Early
Dyspnea on exertion	Early
Dyspnea at rest	Late
Use of accessory muscles	Late
Retraction of interspaces on inspiration	Late
Pause for breath between sentences, words	Late
Cardiovascular	
Tachycardia	Early
Mild hypertension	Early
Dysrhythmias (e.g., premature ventricular contractions)	Early or late
Hypotension	Late
Cyanosis	Late
Cool, clammy skin	Late
Other	
Diaphoresis	Early or late
Decreased urinary output	Early or late
Unexplained fatigue	Early or late

TABLE 26-3 Critical Values for PaO_2 and SpO_2*

PaO_2 (%)	SpO_2 (%)	Considerations
≥70	≥94	Adequate unless patient is hemodynamically unstable or hemoglobin (Hb) has difficulty releasing oxygen to the tissues (i.e., O_2-Hb dissociation curve shifts to the left). Higher O_2 values may be desired with a low cardiac output, dysrhythmias, a leftward shift of the oxyhemoglobin dissociation curve, or carbon monoxide inhalation. Benefits of a higher blood O_2 value need to be balanced against the risk of O_2 toxicity.
60	90	Adequate in almost all patients. Values are at steep part of O_2-Hb dissociation curve. Provides adequate oxygenation but with less margin for error than above.
55	88	Adequate for patients with chronic hypoxemia if no cardiac problems occur. These values are also used as criteria for prescription of continuous O_2 therapy.
40	75	Inadequate but may be acceptable on a short-term basis if the patient also has CO_2 retention. In this situation, respirations may be stimulated by a low PaO_2. Thus the PaO_2 cannot be raised rapidly. O_2 therapy at a low concentration (24%-28%) will gradually increase the PaO_2. Monitoring for dysrhythmias is necessary.
<40	<75	Inadequate. Tissue hypoxia and cardiac dysrhythmias can be expected.

*The same critical values apply for SpO_2 and SaO_2. Values pertain to rest or exertion.

2. What is the degree of hypoxemia and what is the trend? Has there been a rapid decline in SpO_2 or PaO_2? A sudden drop in blood oxygen level can be life threatening. A gradual decline is tolerated with fewer symptoms. Critical values for SpO_2 and PaO_2 are given in Table 26-3.
3. Are there signs or symptoms of inadequate oxygenation? Changes in central nervous system, respiratory, cardiovascular, and renal function are seen when tissue oxygen delivery is inadequate (see Table 26-2). Because the brain is highly sensitive to a decrease in tissue oxygen delivery, the first evidence of hypoxemia may be apprehension, restlessness, or irritability. If these signs or symptoms are observed, a change in the management plan is needed.
4. What is the oxygenation status with activity or exercise? Pulse oximetry is used to monitor SpO_2 levels during a standardized 6-minute walk test or with activities of daily living to assess for desaturation with activity. An SpO_2 value of 88% or less at rest indicates the need for continuous or supplemental oxygen.[7]

Control of Respiration

The respiratory center in the brainstem medulla responds to chemical and mechanical signals from the body. Impulses are sent from the medulla to the respiratory muscles through the spinal cord and phrenic nerves.

Chemoreceptors. A **chemoreceptor** is a receptor that responds to a change in the chemical composition ($PaCO_2$ and pH) of the fluid around it. Central chemoreceptors are located in the medulla and respond to changes in the hydrogen ion (H^+) concentration. An increase in the H^+ concentration *(acidosis)* causes the medulla to increase the respiratory rate and tidal volume (V_T). A decrease in H^+ concentration *(alkalosis)* has the opposite effect. Changes in $PaCO_2$ regulate ventilation primarily by their effect on the pH of the cerebrospinal fluid. When the $PaCO_2$ level is increased, more CO_2 is available to combine with H_2O and form carbonic acid (H_2CO_3). This lowers the cerebrospinal fluid pH and stimulates an increase in respiratory rate. The opposite process occurs with a decrease in $PaCO_2$ level.

Peripheral chemoreceptors are located in the carotid bodies at the bifurcation of the common carotid arteries and in the aortic bodies above and below the aortic arch. The peripheral chemoreceptors respond to decreases in PaO_2 and pH and to increases in $PaCO_2$. These changes also cause stimulation of the respiratory center.

In a healthy person, an increase in $PaCO_2$ or a decrease in pH causes an immediate increase in the respiratory rate. The process is extremely precise. The $PaCO_2$ does not vary more than about 3 mm Hg if lung function is normal. Conditions such as COPD alter lung function and may result in chronically elevated $PaCO_2$ levels. In these instances, the patient will be relatively insensitive to further increases in $PaCO_2$ as a stimulus to breathe and may be maintaining ventilation largely because of a hypoxic drive from the peripheral chemoreceptors (see Chapter 29).

Mechanical Receptors. **Mechanical receptors** (juxtacapillary and irritant) are located in the lungs, upper airways, chest wall, and diaphragm. They are stimulated by a variety of physiologic factors, such as irritants, muscle stretching, and alveolar wall distortion. Signals from the stretch receptors aid in the control of respiration. As the lungs inflate, pulmonary stretch receptors activate the inspiratory center to inhibit further lung expansion. This is termed the *Hering-Breuer reflex* and it prevents overdistention of the lungs. Impulses from the mechanical sensors are sent through the vagus nerve to the brain. Juxtacapillary (J) receptors are believed to cause the rapid respiration (tachypnea) seen in pulmonary edema. These receptors are stimulated by fluid entering the pulmonary interstitial space.

Respiratory Defense Mechanisms

Respiratory defense mechanisms are efficient in protecting the lungs from inhaled particles, microorganisms, and toxic gases. The defense mechanisms include filtration of air, the mucociliary clearance system, the cough reflex, reflex bronchoconstriction, and alveolar macrophages.

Filtration of Air. Nasal hairs filter the inspired air. In addition, the abrupt changes in direction of airflow that occur as air moves through the nasopharynx and larynx increase air turbulence. This causes particles and bacteria to contact the mucosa lining these structures. Most large particles (greater than 5 μm in diameter) are removed in this manner.

The velocity of airflow slows greatly after it passes the larynx, facilitating the deposition of smaller particles (1 to 5 μm in size). They settle out similar to sand in a river, a process termed *sedimentation.* Particles less than 1 μm in size are too small to settle in this manner and are deposited in the alveoli. An example of small particles that can build up is coal dust, which can lead to pneumoconiosis (see Chapter 28). Particle size is important. Particles greater than 5 μm in size are less dangerous because they are removed in the nasopharynx or bronchi and do not reach the alveoli.

Mucociliary Clearance System. Below the larynx, movement of mucus is accomplished by the mucociliary clearance system, commonly referred to as the *mucociliary escalator.* This term is used to indicate the interrelationship between the secretion of mucus and the ciliary activity. Mucus is continually secreted at a rate of about 100 ml/day by goblet cells and submucosal glands. It forms a mucous blanket that contains the impacted particles and debris from distal lung areas (see Fig. 26-1). The small amount of mucus normally secreted is swallowed without being noticed. Secretory immunoglobulin A (IgA) in the mucus contributes to protection against bacteria and viruses.[9]

Cilia cover the airways from the level of the trachea to the respiratory bronchioles (see Fig. 26-1). Each ciliated cell contains approximately 200 cilia, which beat rhythmically about 1000 times per minute in the large airways, moving mucus toward the mouth. The ciliary beat is slower further down the tracheobronchial tree. As a consequence, particles that penetrate more deeply into the airways are removed less rapidly. Ciliary action is impaired by dehydration, smoking, inhalation of high oxygen concentrations, infection, and ingestion of drugs such as atropine, anesthetics, alcohol, or cocaine. Patients with COPD and cystic fibrosis have repeated upper respiratory infections. Cilia are often destroyed during these infections, resulting in impaired secretion clearance, a chronic productive cough, and chronic colonization by bacteria which leads to frequent respiratory infections.

Cough Reflex. The cough is a protective reflex action that clears the airway by a high-pressure, high-velocity flow of air. It is a backup for mucociliary clearance, especially when this clearance mechanism is overwhelmed or ineffective. Coughing is only effective in removing secretions above the subsegmental level (large or main airways). Secretions below this level must be moved upward by the mucociliary mechanism or by interventions such as postural drainage before they can be removed by coughing.

Reflex Bronchoconstriction. Another defense mechanism is reflex bronchoconstriction. In response to the inhalation of large amounts of irritating substances (e.g., dusts, aerosols), the bronchi constrict in an effort to prevent entry of the irritants. A person with hyperreactive airways, such as a person with asthma, may experience bronchoconstriction after inhalation of triggers such as cold air, perfume, or other strong odors.

Alveolar Macrophages. Because ciliated cells are not found below the level of the respiratory bronchioles, the primary defense mechanism at the alveolar level is alveolar macrophages. *Alveolar macrophages* rapidly phagocytize inhaled foreign particles such as bacteria. The debris is moved to the level of the bronchioles for removal by the cilia or removed from the lungs by the lymphatic system. Particles (e.g., coal dust, silica) that cannot be adequately phagocytized tend to remain in the lungs for indefinite periods and can stimulate inflammatory responses (see Chapter 28). Because alveolar macrophage activity is impaired by cigarette smoke, the smoker who is employed in an occupation with heavy dust exposure (e.g., mining, foundries) is at an especially high risk for lung disease.

GERONTOLOGIC CONSIDERATIONS
EFFECTS OF AGING ON THE RESPIRATORY SYSTEM

Age-related changes in the respiratory system can be divided into alterations in structure, in defense mechanisms, and in respiratory control. Structural alterations include a decrease in elastic recoil of the lung, a decrease in chest wall compliance, and a stiffening of the chest wall. The anterior-posterior diameter of the thoracic cage increases and the residual volume increases. The costal cartilages calcify with aging and interfere with chest expansion. The outward curvature of the spine is marked, especially with osteoporosis, and the lumbar curve flattens. Therefore the chest may appear barrel shaped and the elderly may need to use accessory muscles to breathe. Many elders lose subcutaneous fat, and bony prominences are pronounced. Within the lung, there is a decrease in the number of functional alveoli and they become less elastic. Small airways in the lung bases close earlier in expiration. As a consequence, more inspired air is distributed to the lung apices and ventilation is less well matched to perfusion, causing a lowering of the PaO_2. Therefore older adults have less tolerance for exertion. Dyspnea can occur if their activity exceeds their normal exercise.[10,11]

Respiratory defense mechanisms are less effective because of a decline in cell-mediated immunity and formation of antibodies. The alveolar macrophages are less effective at phagocytosis. An elderly patient has a less forceful cough and fewer and less functional cilia. Mucous membranes tend to be drier. Retained mucus predisposes the elderly to respiratory infections. Formation of secretory IgA, an important mechanism in neutralizing the effect of viruses, is diminished. Swallowing is slower because of transit time in the pharyngeal area, and there is reduced sensation in the pharynx. If the elderly patient has a superimposed neurologic condition, aspiration is likely.

Respiratory control is altered, resulting in a more gradual response to changes in blood oxygen or carbon dioxide level. The PaO_2 drops to a lower level and the $PaCO_2$ rises to a higher level before the respiratory rate changes.

TABLE 26-4 GERONTOLOGIC DIFFERENCES IN ASSESSMENT
Respiratory System

Changes	Differences in Assessment Findings
Structures	
Chest wall stiffening Costal cartilage calcification ↓ Elastic recoil ↓ Chest wall compliance ↑ Anteroposterior diameter ↓ Functioning alveoli ↓ Expiratory muscle strength	Barrel chest appearance; kyphotic posture; ↓ chest wall movement; ↓ deep breathing; mucus thickened; ↓ vital capacity; ↑ residual volume; ↑ functional residual capacity; diminished breath sounds, particularly at lung bases; ↓ PaO_2 and SaO_2; normal pH and $PaCO_2$.
Defense Mechanisms	
↓ Cell-mediated immunity ↓ Specific antibodies ↓ Cilia function ↓ Cough force ↓ Alveolar macrophage function ↓ Sensation in pharynx	↓ Cough effectiveness; ↓ secretion clearance; ↑ risk of upper respiratory aspiration, infection, influenza, pneumonia. Respiratory infections may be more severe and last longer.
Respiratory Control	
↓ Response to hypoxemia ↓ Response to hypercapnia	Greater ↓ in PaO_2 and ↑ in $PaCO_2$ before respiratory rate changes. ↓ Ability to maintain acid-base balance. Significant hypoxemia or hypercapnia may develop from relatively small incidents. Retained secretions, excessive sedation, or positioning that impairs chest expansion may substantially alter PaO_2 or SpO_2 values.

There is much variability in the extent of these changes in persons of the same age. The elderly patient who has a significant smoking history, is obese, and is diagnosed with a chronic illness is at greatest risk of adverse outcomes.[12,13] Age-related changes in the respiratory system and differences in assessment findings are presented in Table 26-4.

ASSESSMENT OF THE RESPIRATORY SYSTEM

Correct diagnosis depends on an accurate health history and a thorough physical examination. A respiratory assessment can be done as part of a comprehensive physical examination or as an examination in itself. Judgment must be used in determining whether all or part of the history and physical examination will be completed based on problems presented by the patient and the degree of respiratory distress. If respiratory distress is severe, only pertinent information should be obtained and a thorough assessment should be deferred until the patient's condition stabilizes.

Subjective Data

Important Health Information

Past Health History. The nurse should determine the frequency of upper respiratory problems (e.g., colds, sore throats, sinus problems, allergies) and if seasonal changes affect these problems. The patient with allergies should be questioned about possible precipitating factors or triggers such as medications, pollen, smoke, mold, or pet exposure. Characteristics and severity of the allergic reaction, such as runny nose, wheezing, scratchy throat, or chest tightness, should be documented. The frequency of asthma exacerbations and triggers if known should also be determined. A past history of lower respiratory problems, such as asthma, COPD, pneumonia, and tuberculosis, should also be elicited. Respiratory symptoms are often manifestations of problems that involve other body systems. Therefore the patient should be asked if there is a history of additional health problems other than just those involving the respiratory system. For example, the patient with cardiac dysfunction may experience dyspnea (shortness of breath) as a consequence of heart failure. The patient with human immunodeficiency virus (HIV) infection may experience frequent respiratory infections because immune function is compromised.

Medications. The patient should be questioned carefully about prescription and over-the-counter drugs used to manage respiratory problems, such as antihistamines, bronchodilators, corticosteroids, cough suppressants, and antibiotics. Information about the reason for taking the medication, its name, the dose and frequency, length of time taken, its effect, and any side effects should be obtained. Overuse of short-term bronchodilators should be assessed as a key indicator of symptom control. It will help to guide management. Inquire about the use of an angiotensin-converting enzyme (ACE) inhibitor as cough is a relatively common side effect of this class of drugs.

If the patient is using oxygen to ease a breathing problem, the fraction of inspired oxygen concentration (FIO_2), liter flow, method of administration, the number of hours used per day, and effectiveness of the therapy should be documented. Safety practices, including the patient's mechanical and cognitive ability related to using oxygen, should also be assessed.

Surgery or Other Treatments. The nurse should determine if the patient has been hospitalized for a respiratory problem. If so, the dates, therapy (including surgery), and current status of the problem should be recorded. Determine if the patient has ever been intubated because of a respiratory problem. The nurse should ask about the use and the response to respiratory treatments such as a nebulizer, humidifier, and airway clearance modalities (e.g., Flutter valve), high-frequency chest oscillation, postural drainage, and percussion.

Functional Health Patterns. Health history questions to ask a patient with a respiratory problem are presented in Table 26-5.

Health Perception–Health Management Pattern. The patient should be asked if there has been a perceived change in health status within the last several days, months, or years. In COPD, lung function declines slowly over many years. The patient may not notice this decline because activity is altered to accommodate reduced exercise tolerance. If an upper respiratory infection is superimposed on a chronic problem, dyspnea and decreased exercise tolerance may occur very quickly. In asthma, symptoms may occur or worsen in the presence of exercise, animals, or change in temperature, causing the patient to avoid these activities or exposures.

Common cues that should alert the nurse to the possibility of respiratory problems should be explored and documented (Table 26-6). The course of the patient's illness, including when it began,

TABLE 26-5 HEALTH HISTORY
Respiratory System

Health Perception–Health Management Pattern
- Describe your daily activities. Have breathing problems changed activities that you can perform in the last several days?* Months?* Years?* Are your breathing problems better, worse, or about the same compared to 6 months ago?
- How do your breathing problems affect your self-care abilities?
- Have you ever smoked? Do you smoke now? If yes, how many cigarettes each day and for how long? Are you interested in stopping smoking? Are there aids we can tell you about that would assist your quitting? Would you be willing to come back for a visit so we can explore your quitting? If you stopped smoking, did you do so because of your health?* How did you stop?
- Have you ever smoked street drugs?*
- Have you had a Pneumovax vaccination? When was your last flu shot?
- What equipment helps you manage your respiratory problems? How often do you use it? Does it help? Cause problems?

Nutritional-Metabolic Pattern
- Have you recently lost weight because of difficulty eating secondary to a respiratory problem? How much? Voluntarily?
- Do any particular foods affect your sputum production or breathing?*

Elimination Pattern
- Does your respiratory problem make it difficult for you to get to the toilet?*
- Are you inactive because of dyspnea to the point where it causes constipation?*

Activity-Exercise Pattern
- Are you ever short of breath during exercise?* At rest?*
- Do you get too short of breath to do the things you want to do?*
- Is your home one story? Two stories? How many steps from the street to your door?
- Can you walk up a flight of steps without stopping?
- Are you able to maintain your typical activity pattern? If not, explain.
- What do you do when you get short of breath?

Sleep-Rest Pattern
- Do breathing problems cause you to awaken during the night?*
- Can you lie flat at night? If not, how many pillows do you use?
- Do you need to sleep upright in a chair?*
- Are you or your sleep partner aware of any snoring?
- Do you awaken in the morning feeling rested?
- Do you have a morning headache?*
- Do you fall asleep easily during the day?*

Cognitive-Perceptual Pattern
- Do you have any pain associated with breathing?* On a scale from 0 to 10, with 10 being the worst pain you can imagine, where would you rate your pain? Does it hurt more on inspiration?*
- Do you ever feel restless, irritable, or confused without a reason?*
- Do you have difficulty remembering things?*

Self-Perception–Self-Concept Pattern
- Describe how your respiratory problems have changed your life.
- Do you ever go out without bringing your oxygen? When and why?

Role-Relationship Pattern
- Has your respiratory problem caused any difficulties in your work, family, or social relationships?*

Sexuality-Reproductive Pattern
- Has your respiratory problem caused a change in your sexual activity?*
- Do you want to discuss ways to decrease dyspnea during sexual activity?

Coping–Stress Tolerance Pattern
- How often do you leave your home?
- Would you want to join a support group? Pulmonary rehabilitation program?
- Does stress have an effect on your breathing?*
- What effect does your respiratory problem have on your emotions?

Value-Belief Pattern
- What do you believe causes your respiratory problems?
- Do you think the things you have been told to do for your respiratory problems really help? If not, why?

*If yes, describe.

the type of symptoms, and factors that alleviate or aggravate these symptoms, should be described. Because of the chronic nature of respiratory problems, the patient may relate a change in symptoms rather than the onset of new symptoms when describing the present illness. Such changes should be carefully documented because they often suggest the cause of illness. For example, increased shortness of breath, or a change in the volume or increased purulence of sputum may suggest the onset of an acute exacerbation of COPD.

If a cough is present, the nurse should evaluate the quality of the cough. For example, a loose-sounding cough indicates the presence of secretions; a dry, hacking cough indicates airway irritation or obstruction; a harsh, barky cough suggests upper airway obstruction from inhibited vocal cord movement related to subglottic edema. The nurse should assess whether the cough is strong enough to clear secretions and note if it is productive or nonproductive of secretions. Determining if a cough is acute or chronic (>3 weeks in duration) or if it first began with an upper respiratory infection is helpful in the differential diagnosis process. The pattern and etiology of the cough are determined by asking questions such as the following: What has been the pattern of coughing? Has it been regular or paroxysmal (i.e., sudden, periodic onset), or related to a time of day or weather, certain activities, talking, or deep breaths? Any change over time? Is the throat cleared a lot? What efforts have been tried to alleviate the coughing? Were any prescription or over-the-counter drugs tried?

If the patient has a productive cough, the following characteristics of sputum should be evaluated: amount, color, consistency, and odor. The amount should be quantified in teaspoons, tablespoons, or cups per day. The nurse should note any recent increases or decreases in the amount. The normal color is clear or slightly whitish. If a patient is a cigarette smoker, the sputum is usually clear to gray with occasional specks of brown. The patient with COPD may exhibit clear, whitish, or slightly yellow sputum, especially in the morning on rising. If the patient reports any change from baseline color, pulmonary complications should be suspected. Changes in consistency of sputum to thick, thin, or frothy and pink tinged should be noted. These changes may indicate dehydration, postnasal drip or sinus drainage, or possible pulmonary edema. Normally sputum should be odorless. A foul odor or ex-

TABLE 26-6 Cues to Respiratory Problems

Manifestation	Description
Shortness of breath (dyspnea)	Distressful sensation of uncomfortable breathing. Most common complaint of people with respiratory problems. Person may become accustomed to sensation and not recognize its presence. Difficult to evaluate because it is a subjective experience.
Wheezing	May or may not be heard by patient. May be described as chest tightness.
Pleuritic chest pain	Described on a continuum from discomfort during inspiration to intense, sharp pain at the end of inspiration. Pain is usually aggravated by deep breathing and coughing. Pain is very localized versus diffuse.
Cough	Characteristics of cough are important diagnostic cues.
Sputum production	Material coughed up from lungs. Contains mucus, cellular debris, or microorganisms, and may contain blood or pus. Amount, color, and constituents of sputum are important diagnostic information.
Hemoptysis	Coughing up of blood; either gross, frankly bloody sputum or blood-tinged sputum. Precipitating events should be investigated.
Voice change	Hoarseness, stridor (whistling sound during inspiration), muffling, or a barking cough may indicate abnormalities of upper airway, vocal cord dysfunction, or gastroesophageal reflux disease (GERD).
Fatigue	Sense of overwhelming tiredness not completely relieved by sleep or rest.

ceptionally bad breath or taste in the mouth suggests an infectious process. The patient should be asked if the sputum was produced along with a position change (e.g., increased with lying down) or a change in activity.

The patient should be questioned about a history of coughing up blood *(hemoptysis),* which can range from slight streaking of blood in the mucus to massive coughing up of blood, in which the patient loses 100 to 600 ml of blood in a 24-hour period.[14] This situation is a medical emergency.

Frequently the patient cannot differentiate between hemoptysis and *hematemesis* (vomiting blood). Carefully questioning and then testing for an acidic pH (which is present with hematemesis) can differentiate between the two. Hemoptysis can be found with a variety of conditions such as pneumonia, tuberculosis, lung cancer, and severe bronchiectasis.

A history of wheezing should be assessed. **Wheezes** are musical sounds that can be audible to the patient and the nurse. Wheezing indicates some degree of airway obstruction, such as asthma, foreign body aspiration, and postnasal drip.

The patient should be questioned about a family history of respiratory problems that may be genetic or have familial tendencies, such as asthma, emphysema resulting from α_1-antitrypsin deficiency, or cystic fibrosis. Any history of family exposure to *Mycobacterium tuberculosis* should be assessed.

The nurse should ask where the patient has lived and traveled. Risk factors for tuberculosis include prior residence in Asia, Africa, the former Soviet Republic, Latin America, or any third-world country. Risk factors for fungal infections of the lung include living or traveling in the Southwest (coccidioidomycosis) and the Mississippi River Valley (histoplasmosis).

The nurse should also ask about current and past smoking habits and quantify exposure in pack-years. This is done by multiplying the number of packs smoked per day by the number of years smoked. For example, a person who smoked 1 pack per day for 15 years has a 15 pack-year history. The risk of lung cancer rises in direct proportion to the number of cigarettes smoked. Smoking is the most important risk factor for COPD and lung cancer. In addition to asking about cigarette use, it is important to find out the use of any tobacco products, including cigars, pipes, chewing tobacco, and smokeless tobacco products. It is also important to know about exposure to secondhand smoke. The nurse should also ask if efforts have been made to quit using these tobacco products, including prescription, over-the-counter, and herbal remedies.

The nurse should ask if the patient received immunization for influenza (flu) and pneumococcal pneumonia (Pneumovax). Influenza vaccine should be administered yearly in the fall. Pneumovax administered any time during the year is recommended for persons 65 years or older or those individuals with certain chronic diseases (e.g., cardiovascular disease, COPD, immunocompromised state, or diabetes mellitus). Revaccination is currently advised only if the patient received the vaccine more than 5 years previously and was less than 65 years old at the time of vaccination. In immunocompromised persons (e.g., transplant recipient), who are at the highest risk for serious pneumocccal infection, an initial vaccine is recommended followed by revaccination once every 5 years.[15]

The patient should be asked about the use of equipment to manage respiratory symptoms (e.g., home oxygen therapy equipment, metered-dose inhaler [MDI] with spacer or nebulizer for medication administration, positive airway pressure device for relief of sleep apnea). The patient should be questioned about the type of equipment used, cleaning of the device, frequency of use, its effect, and any side effects. The patient should be asked to demonstrate use of the MDI or dry powder inhalers. Many patients do not know how to use these devices correctly (see Chapter 29).

Nutritional-Metabolic Pattern. Weight loss is a symptom of many respiratory diseases. The nurse should determine if weight loss was intentional and, if not, if food intake is altered by anorexia (from medications), fatigue (from hypoxemia, increased work of breathing), feeling full quickly (from lung hyperinflation), or social isolation. Anorexia, weight loss, and chronic malnutrition are common symptoms in patients with COPD, acquired immunodeficiency syndrome (AIDS), lung cancer, tuberculosis, and chronic severe infection (bronchiectasis). Fluid intake should also be noted. Dehydration can result in thickened mucus, which can cause airway obstruction.

Excessive weight interferes with normal ventilation and may cause sleep apnea (see Chapter 27). Morbidly obese individuals may hypoventilate while awake or asleep, and weight loss can improve ABGs. Rapid weight gain from fluid retention may decrease pulmonary gas exchange.

Elimination Pattern. Healthy elimination habits depend on the ability to reach a toilet when necessary. Activity intolerance secondary to dyspnea could result in incontinence. Dyspnea can also be the cause of limited mobility, which can cause constipation. The patient with dyspnea should be questioned about both of these possibilities. Patients, especially females, with a chronic cough may be troubled with urinary incontinence during paroxysms of coughing.

Activity-Exercise Pattern. The nurse should determine if the patient's activity is limited by dyspnea at rest or during exercise. The nurse should also note whether the patient's housing (e.g., number of steps, levels) poses a problem that increases social isolation. The nurse should record and objectively measure the degree of the patient's dyspnea. For example, can the patient walk up one flight of stairs without stopping because of dyspnea? Is dyspnea that is associated with an activity better, worse, or about the same in the last few months? The nurse should explore if the patient has difficulty breathing in a certain position, or if relief of dyspnea can be obtained by assuming a different position (e.g., tripod position in COPD). To determine the intensity of dyspnea, the use of a Borg scale or visual analog scale (VAS) may be helpful[16] (Fig. 26-8).

The nurse should also inquire if the patient is able to carry out activities of daily living without dyspnea or other respiratory symptoms. If unable, the amount and type of care needed should be documented. Self-care strategies to minimize dyspnea should be reinforced. Immobility and sedentary habits can be risk factors for hypoventilation leading to atelectasis or pneumonia.

Sleep-Rest Pattern. The nurse should ask if the patient wakes up because of pulmonary problems. The patient with asthma or COPD may awaken at night with chest tightness, wheezing, or coughing. This suggests a need for a longer acting bronchodilator or other medication change. The patient with cardiovascular disease (e.g., heart failure) may sleep with the head elevated on several pillows to avoid respiratory problems brought on by lying flat *(orthopnea).* The patient with sleep apnea may have snoring, insomnia, abrupt awakenings, daytime drowsiness, and early morning headaches. Night sweats may be a manifestation of tuberculosis.

Cognitive-Perceptual Pattern. Because hypoxia can cause neurologic symptoms, the nurse should ask about apprehension, restlessness, irritability, and memory changes, which can indicate inadequate cerebral oxygenation (see Table 26-2). Hypoxemia interferes with the ability to learn and retain information. For this reason, teaching may be more effective if another person is present during the teaching session to provide reinforcement at a later date.

The patient's cognitive ability and functional capacity to cooperate with treatment should be assessed. Failure or inability to participate in needed therapy can result in exacerbation of respiratory problems.

The nurse should inquire about any discomfort or pain with breathing. A complaint of chest pain must be explored carefully to rule out cardiac involvement. Problems such as pleurisy, fractured ribs, and costochondritis cause chest pain. Pleuritic pain is described as a sharp, localized, stabbing pain associated with movement or deep breathing. Fractured ribs cause localized sharp pain associated with breathing. The pain of costochondritis is located along the borders of the sternum and is associated with breathing.

Self-Perception–Self-Concept Pattern. Dyspnea limits activity, impairs ability to fulfill normal developmental role functions, and often alters self-esteem. One example could be concern about a highly visible nasal cannula and the difficulty of managing equipment, which may cause the patient to resist using oxygen in public. The nurse should ask how the patient views his or her personal body image. A barrel chest, clubbed fingers, pursed-lip breathing, and frequent expectoration of sputum or throat clearing can be embarrassing and can lead to social isolation. Referral to a support group or pulmonary rehabilitation program may be beneficial in developing a support system and coping strategies.

Role-Relationship Pattern. Acute or chronic respiratory problems can seriously affect performance in work or other activities. The nurse should ask about the impact of medications, oxygen, and special routines (e.g., pulmonary hygiene for cystic fibrosis) on the patient's family, job, and social life.

The nurse should document the nature of the patient's work and the frequency and intensity of exposure to fumes, toxins, asbestos, coal, fibers, or silica. Inquire whether symptoms are worse in specific situations (e.g., home vs. work environments). Patient-specific allergens such as dust or fumes, which could be present in the work environment, should be investigated. Hobbies such as woodworking (sawdust) or pottery (silica) and exposure to animals (allergies) may also cause respiratory problems. Because of hyperreactive airways, exposure to fumes, smoke, and other chemicals may trigger wheezing in the asthmatic patient.

Sexuality-Reproductive Pattern. Most patients can continue to have satisfactory sexual relationships despite marked physical limitations. In a tactful manner, the nurse should determine whether breathing difficulties have caused alterations in sexual activity. If so, teaching can be provided about positions that decrease dyspnea during sexual activity and alternative strategies for sexual fulfillment. Many patients will need to perform good pulmonary hygiene (bronchodilators, coughing and deep breathing) prior to intimacy. This is similar to what they would do prior to strenuous physical activity. They may need to wear oxygen therapy equipment during intercourse.

Coping–Stress Tolerance Pattern. Dyspnea causes anxiety, and anxiety exacerbates dyspnea. The result is a vicious cycle—the patient avoids activities that cause dyspnea, becoming more deconditioned and more dyspneic. The outcome is often physical and social isolation. The nurse should ask how often the patient leaves home and interacts with others. Referral to a support group or pulmonary rehabilitation program may be beneficial.

	Breathlessness
0	Nothing at all
0.5	Very, very slight
1	Very slight
2	Slight
3	Moderate
4	Somewhat severe
5	Severe
6	
7	Very severe
8	
9	Very, very severe (almost maximal)
10	Maximal

FIG. 26-8 Borg category-ratio scale. This scale can be used in assessment of dyspnea (e.g., "Using this scale from 0 to 10, how much shortness of breath do you have right now?").

The chronic nature of many respiratory problems such as COPD and asthma can cause prolonged stress. Inquiry should be made into the patient's coping strategies to manage this stress.

Value-Belief Pattern. The nurse should determine the patient's adherence to the management regimen. Reasons for lack of adherence should be explored, including conflict with culturally specific beliefs, financial constraints (costs of prescriptions), failure to note benefit, or other reasons.[10] Including the patient and family in the planning of care can improve compliance.

Objective Data

Physical Examination. Vital signs, including temperature, pulse, respirations, blood pressure, and SpO_2 (oxygen saturation obtained by pulse oximetry), are important data to collect before examination of the respiratory system.

Nose. The nose is inspected for patency, inflammation, deformities, symmetry, and discharge. Each naris is checked for air patency with respiration while the other naris is briefly occluded. The nurse tilts the patient's head backward and pushes the tip of the nose upward gently. With a nasal speculum and a good light, the interior of the nose is inspected. The mucous membrane should be pink and moist, with no evidence of edema (bogginess), exudate, or bleeding. The nasal septum should be observed for deviation, perforations, and bleeding. Some nasal deviation is normal in an adult. The turbinates should be observed for polyps, which are abnormal, fingerlike projections of swollen nasal mucosa. Polyps may result from long-term irritation of the mucosa, as from allergies. Any discharge should be assessed for color and consistency. The presence of purulent and malodorous discharge could indicate the presence of a foreign body. Watery discharge could be secondary to allergies or from cerebrospinal fluid. Bloody discharge could be from trauma or dryness. Thick mucosal discharge could indicate the presence of infection.

Mouth and Pharynx. Using a good light source, the nurse inspects the interior of the mouth for color, lesions, masses, gum retraction, bleeding, and poor dentition. The tongue is inspected for symmetry and presence of lesions. The nurse observes the pharynx by pressing a tongue blade against the middle of the back of the tongue. If the oropharynx is tight, having the patient yawn will usually allow more structures to be visible. The pharynx should be smooth and moist, with no evidence of exudate, ulcerations, swelling, or postnasal drip. The color, symmetry, and any enlargement of the tonsils are noted. The nurse stimulates the gag reflex by placing a tongue blade along the side of the pharynx behind the tonsil. A normal response (gagging) indicates that cranial nerves IX (glossopharyngeal) and X (vagus) are intact and that the airway is protected.

Neck. The nurse inspects the neck for symmetry and presence of tender or swollen areas. The lymph nodes are palpated while the patient is sitting erect with the neck slightly flexed. Progression of palpation is from the nodes around the ears, to the nodes at the base of the skull, and then to those located under the angles of the mandible to the midline. The patient may have small, mobile, nontender nodes *(shotty nodes),* which are not a sign of a pathologic condition. Tender, hard, or fixed nodes indicate disease. The location and characteristics of any palpable nodes are described.

Thorax and Lungs. Imaginary lines can be pictured on the chest to help in identifying abnormalities (see Fig. 26-2). Abnormalities can be described in relation to their location relative to these lines (e.g., 2 cm from the right midclavicular line).

Chest examination is best performed in a well-lighted, warm room with measures taken to ensure the patient's privacy. All physical assessment maneuvers (inspection, palpation, percussion, auscultation) should be performed on either the anterior or the posterior chest rather than moving from anterior to posterior or vice versa with each maneuver. It is best to begin on the posterior chest, particularly with females, as more information can be obtained without the breast tissue interfering with the exam. In addition, if the patient tires or the nurse is interrupted, baseline data with the most information will have been obtained as the posterior chest has been examined.

Inspection. The patient's anterior chest should be exposed while sitting upright or with the head of the bed upright. The patient may need to lean forward for support on the bedside table to facilitate breathing. First, the nurse observes the patient's appearance and notes any evidence of respiratory distress, such as tachypnea or use of accessory muscles. Next, the nurse determines the shape and symmetry of the chest. Chest movement should be equal on both sides, and the anterior-posterior (AP) diameter should be less than the side-to-side or transverse diameter by a ratio of 1:2. An increase in AP diameter (e.g., barrel chest) may be a normal aging change or result from lung hyperinflation. The nurse observes for abnormalities in the sternum (e.g., *pectus carinatum* [a prominent protrusion of the sternum] and *pectus excavatum* [an indentation of the lower sternum above the xiphoid process]).

Next the respiratory rate, depth, and rhythm should be observed. The normal rate is 12 to 20 breaths/minute; in the elderly, it is 16 to 25 breaths/minute. Inspiration (I) should take half as long as expiration (E) (I:E = 1:2). The nurse should observe for abnormal breathing patterns, such as Kussmaul (rapid, deep breathing), Cheyne-Stokes (abnormal pattern of respiration characterized by alternating periods of apnea and deep, rapid breathing), or Biot's (irregular breathing with apnea every four to five cycles) respirations.[10,11]

Skin color provides clues to respiratory status. Cyanosis, a late sign of hypoxemia, is best observed in a dark-skinned patient in the conjunctivae, lips, palms, and under the tongue. Causes of cyanosis include hypoxemia or decreased cardiac output. The fingers should be inspected for evidence of long-standing hypoxemia known as *clubbing* (an increase in the angle between the base of the nail and the fingernail to 180 degrees or more, usually accompanied by an increase in the depth, bulk, and sponginess of the end of the finger).

When the nurse is inspecting the posterior chest, the patient should be asked to lean forward with arms folded. This position moves the scapulae away from the spine, so there is more exposure of the area to be examined. The same sequence of observations that were done on the anterior part of the chest is performed on the posterior part. In addition, any spinal curvature is noted. Spinal curvatures that affect breathing include kyphosis, scoliosis, and kyphoscoliosis.

Palpation. The nurse determines tracheal position by gently placing the index fingers on either side of the trachea just above the suprasternal notch and gently pressing backward. Normal tracheal position is midline; deviation to the left or right is abnormal. Tracheal deviation occurs away from the side of a tension pneumothorax or a neck mass, but toward the side of a pneumonectomy or lobar atelectasis.[17]

The nurse determines symmetry of chest expansion and extent of movement at the level of the diaphragm. The nurse places the hands over the lower anterior chest wall along the costal margin and moves them inward until the thumbs meet at midline. The patient is asked to breathe deeply, and the nurse observes the movement of the thumbs away from each other. Normal expansion is 1 inch (2.5 cm). On the posterior side of the chest, the nurse places the hands at the level of the tenth rib and moves the thumbs until they meet over the spine (Fig. 26-9). The nurse can check for expansion anteriorly or posteriorly, but it is not necessary to check both.

Normal chest movement is equal. Unequal expansion occurs when air entry is limited by conditions involving the lung (e.g., atelectasis, pneumothorax) or the chest wall (e.g., incisional pain). Equal but diminished expansion occurs in conditions that produce a hyperinflated or barrel chest or in neuromuscular diseases (e.g., amyotrophic lateral sclerosis, spinal cord lesions). Movement may be absent or unequal over a pleural effusion, an atelectasis, or a pneumothorax.

Fremitus is vibration of the chest wall produced by vocalization. To elicit tactile fremitus, the nurse places the palmar surface of the hands with hyperextended fingers against the patient's chest and asks the patient to repeat a phrase such as "ninety-nine" in a deeper, louder than normal voice. The nurse moves the hands from side to side at the same time from top to bottom on the patient's chest (Fig. 26-10). In clinical practice, checking for fremitus has limited value. However, when it is done, all areas of the chest should be palpated and vibrations compared from similar areas. Tactile fremitus is most intense adjacent to the sternum and between the scapulae because these areas are closest to the major bronchi. Fremitus is less intense farther away from these areas.

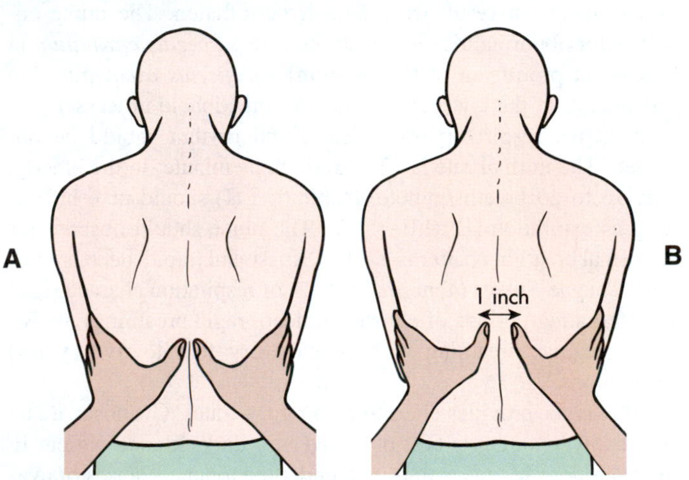

FIG. 26-9 Estimation of thoracic expansion. **A,** Exhalation. **B,** Maximal inhalation.

An increase, decrease, or absence of fremitus should be noted. Increased fremitus occurs when the lung becomes filled with fluid or more dense. As the patient's voice moves through a dense tissue or fluid, the vibration felt by the examiner is increased. This is noted in pneumonia, in lung tumors, with thick bronchial secretions, and above a pleural effusion (the lung is compressed upward). Fremitus is decreased if the hand is farther from the lung (e.g., pleural effusion) or the lung is hyperinflated (e.g., barrel chest). Absent fremitus may be noted with pneumothorax or atelectasis. The anterior of the chest is more difficult to palpate for fremitus because of the presence of large muscles and breast tissue.

Percussion. Percussion is done to assess density or aeration of the lungs. Percussion sounds are described in Table 26-7. (The technique for percussion is described in Chapter 4.)

The anterior chest is usually percussed with the patient in a semi-sitting or supine position. Starting above the clavicles, the nurse percusses downward, interspace by interspace (see Fig. 26-10). The area over lung tissue should be resonant, with the exception of the area of cardiac dullness (Fig. 26-11). For percussion of the posterior chest, the patient should sit leaning forward with arms folded. The posterior chest should be resonant over lung tissue to the level of the diaphragm (Fig. 26-12).

Auscultation. During chest auscultation, the patient is instructed to breathe slowly and a little deeper than normal through the mouth. The nurse should proceed from the lung apices to the bases, comparing opposite areas of the chest, unless it is possible the patient will tire; if so, one should start at the bases (see Fig. 26-10). The stethoscope should be placed over lung tissue, not over bony prominences. At each placement of the stethoscope, the nurse should listen to at least one cycle of inspiration and expira-

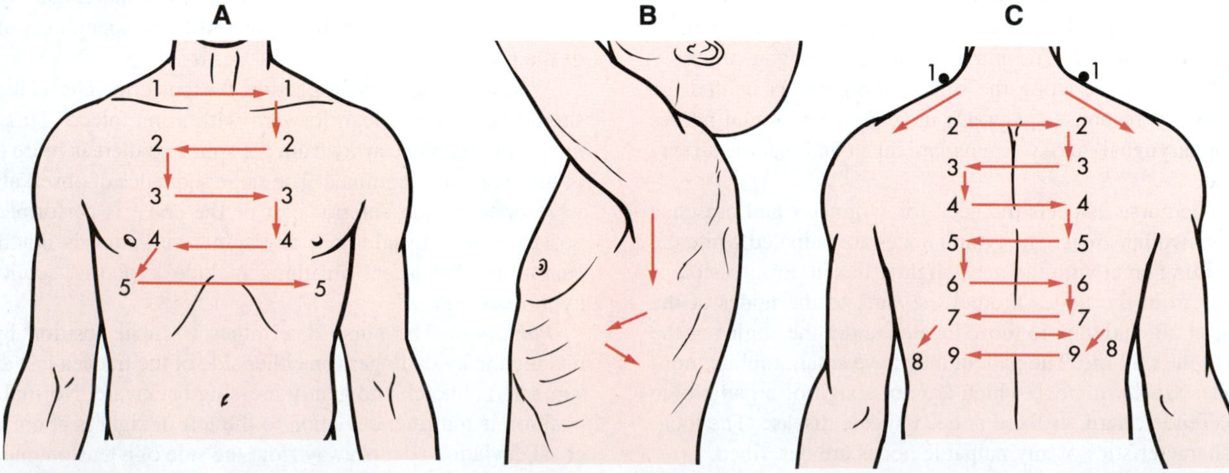

FIG. 26-10 Sequence for examination of the chest. **A,** Anterior sequence. **B,** Lateral sequence. **C,** Posterior sequence. For palpation, place the palms of the hands in the position designated as "1" on the right and left sides of the chest. Compare the intensity of vibrations. Continue for all positions in each sequence. For percussion, tap the chest at each designated position, moving downward from side to side. Compare percussion sounds at all positions. For auscultation, place the stethoscope at each position and listen to at least one complete inspiratory and expiratory cycle. Keep in mind that, with a female patient, the breast tissue will modify the completeness of the anterior examination.

tion. Note the pitch (e.g., high, low), duration of sound, and presence of adventitious or abnormal sounds. The location of normal auscultatory sounds is more easily understood by visualization of a lung model (Fig. 26-13).

TABLE 26-7 Percussion Sounds

Sound	Description
Resonance	Low-pitched sound heard over normal lungs
Hyperresonance	Loud, lower pitched sound than normal resonance heard over hyperinflated lungs, such as in chronic obstructive lung disease and acute asthma
Tympany	Sound with drumlike, loud, empty quality heard over gas-filled stomach or intestine, or pneumothorax
Dull	Sound with medium-intensity pitch and duration heard over areas of "mixed" solid and lung tissue, such as over top area of liver, partially consolidated lung tissue (pneumonia), or fluid-filled pleural space
Flat	Soft, high-pitched sound of short duration heard over very dense tissue where air is not present, such as posterior chest below level of diaphragm

The lung sounds are heard anteriorly from a line drawn perpendicular to the xiphoid process lateral to the midclavicular line. Then the nurse should palpate inferiorly (down) two ribs in the midaxillary line and around to the posterior chest. This gives the examiner a fairly accurate and easy way to determine the lung fields to be auscultated. When documenting the location of the lung sounds, the nurse can arbitrarily divide the anterior and posterior lung into thirds (upper, mid, and lower) and note, for example, "crackles posterior right lower lung field." It is not expected that the nurse should define which lobe of the lung has particular lung sounds.

There are three normal breath sounds: vesicular, bronchovesicular, and bronchial. *Vesicular sounds* are relatively soft, low-pitched, gentle, rustling sounds. They are heard over all lung areas except the major bronchi. Vesicular sounds have a 3:1 ratio, with inspiration 3 times longer than expiration. *Bronchovesicular sounds* have a medium pitch and intensity and are heard anteriorly over the mainstem bronchi on either side of the sternum and posteriorly between the scapulae. Bronchovesicular sounds have a 1:1 ratio, with inspiration equal to expiration. *Bronchial sounds* are louder and higher pitched and resemble air blowing through a hollow pipe. Bronchial sounds have a 2:3 ratio, with a gap between inspiration and expiration, reflecting the short pause between these respiratory cycles. To hear the likeness of bronchial breath sounds, the nurse can place the stethoscope alongside the trachea in the neck.

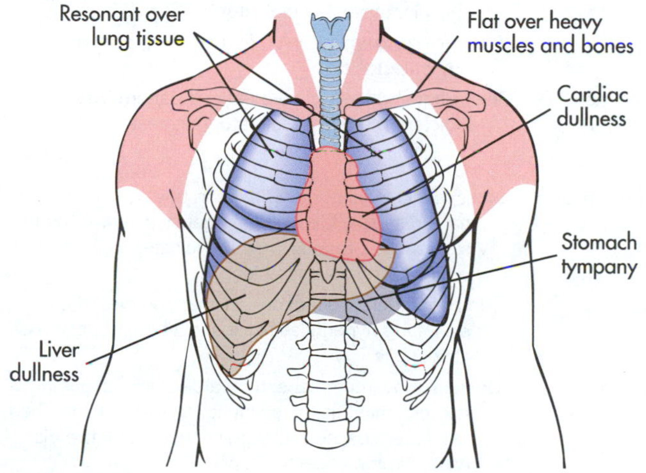

FIG. 26-11 Diagram of percussion areas and sounds in the anterior side of the chest.

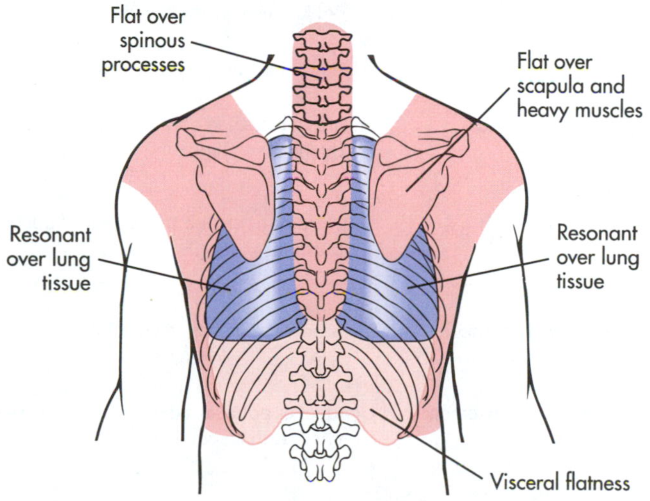

FIG. 26-12 Diagram of percussion areas and sounds in the posterior side of the chest. Percussion proceeds from the lung apices to the lung bases, comparing sounds in opposite areas of the chest.

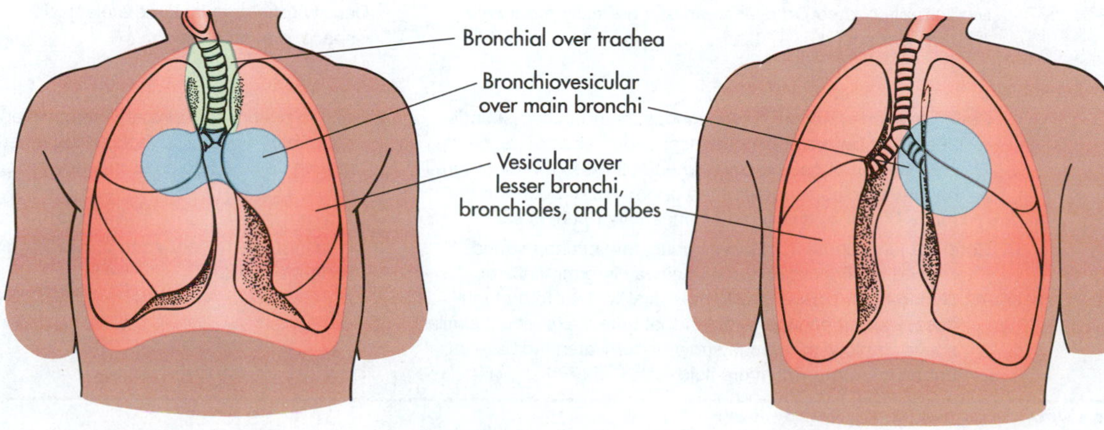

FIG. 26-13 Normal auscultatory sounds.

The term *abnormal breath sounds* is used to describe bronchial or bronchovesicular sounds heard in the peripheral lung fields. **Adventitious sounds** are extra breath sounds that are abnormal. Adventitious breath sounds include **crackles, rhonchi, wheezes,** and **pleural friction rub** (described in Table 26-8).

The terminology for assessing lung sounds is not well standardized despite guidelines from the American Thoracic Society and American College of Chest Physicians published in 1975. The nurse will find a variety of terms used to describe breath sounds.[18-20] The spoken voice can be auscultated over the thorax just as it can

TABLE 26-8 *COMMON ASSESSMENT ABNORMALITIES* Respiratory System

Finding	Description	Possible Etiology and Significance*
Inspection		
Pursed-lip breathing	Exhalation through mouth with lips pursed together to slow exhalation	COPD, asthma. Suggests ↑ breathlessness. Strategy taught to slow expiration, ↓ dyspnea
Tripod position; inability to lie flat	Learning forward with arms and elbows supported on overbed table	COPD, asthma in exacerbation, pulmonary edema. Indicates moderate to severe respiratory distress
Accessory muscle use; intercostal retractions	Neck and shoulder muscles used to assist breathing. Muscles between ribs pull in during inspiration	COPD, asthma in exacerbation, secretion retention. Indicates severe respiratory distress, hypoxemia
Splinting	Voluntary ↓ in tidal volume to ↓ pain on chest expansion	Thoracic or abdominal incision. Chest trauma, pleurisy
↑ AP diameter	AP chest diameter equal to lateral. Slope of ribs more horizontal (90 degrees) to spine	COPD, asthma, cystic fibrosis. Lung hyperinflation. Advanced age
Tachypnea	Rate >20 breaths/min; >25 breaths/min in elderly	Fever, anxiety, hypoxemia, restrictive lung disease. Magnitude of ↑ above normal rate reflects increased work of breathing
Kussmaul respirations	Regular, rapid, and deep respirations	Metabolic acidosis; ↑ in rate aids body in ↑ CO_2 excretion
Cyanosis	Bluish color of skin best seen in lips and on the palpebral conjunctiva (inside the lower eyelid)	Reflects 5-6 g of hemoglobin not bound with oxygen. ↓ Oxygen transfer in lungs, ↓ cardiac output. Nonspecific, unreliable indicator
Clubbing of fingers	↑ Depth, bulk, sponginess of distal portion of finger	Chronic hypoxemia. Cystic fibrosis, lung cancer, bronchiectasis
Abdominal paradox	Inward (rather than normal outward) movement of abdomen during inspiration	Inefficient and ineffective breathing pattern. Nonspecific indicator of severe respiratory distress
Palpation		
Tracheal deviation	Leftward or rightward movement of trachea from normal midline position	Nonspecific indicator of change in position of mediastinal structures. Medical emergency if caused by tension pneumothorax. Trachea deviates to the side opposite the collapsed lung
Altered tactile fremitus	Increase or decrease in vibrations	↑ In pneumonia, pulmonary edema; ↓ in pleural effusion, lung hyperinflation; absent in pneumothorax, atelectasis
Altered chest movement	Unequal or equal but diminished movement of two sides of chest with inspiration	Unequal movement caused by atelectasis, pneumothorax, pleural effusion, splinting; equal but diminished movement caused by barrel chest, restrictive disease, neuromuscular disease
Percussion		
Hyperresonance	Loud, lower-pitched sound over areas that normally produce a resonant sound	Lung hyperinflation (COPD), lung collapse (pneumothorax), air trapping (asthma)
Dullness	Medium-pitched sound over areas that normally produce a resonant sound	↑ Density (pneumonia, large atelectasis), ↑ fluid pleural space (pleural effusion)
Auscultation		
Fine crackles	Series of short-duration, discontinuous, high-pitched sounds heard just before the end of inspiration; result of rapid equalization of gas pressure when collapsed alveoli or terminal bronchioles suddenly snap open; similar sound to that made by rolling hair between fingers just behind ear	Idiopathic pulmonary fibrosis, interstitial edema (early pulmonary edema), alveolar filling (pneumonia), loss of lung volume (atelectasis), early phase of heart failure
Coarse crackles	Series of long-duration, discontinuous, low-pitched sounds caused by air passing through airway intermittently occluded by mucus, unstable bronchial wall, or fold of mucosa; evident on inspiration and, at times, expiration; similar sound to blowing through straw under water; increase in bubbling quality with more fluid	Heart failure, pulmonary edema, pneumonia with severe congestion, COPD

AP, Anterior-posterior; *COPD,* chronic obstructive pulmonary disease.
*Limited to common etiologic factors. (Further discussion of conditions listed may be found in Chapters 27 through 29.)

TABLE 26-8 COMMON ASSESSMENT ABNORMALITIES Respiratory System—cont'd

Finding	Description	Possible Etiology and Significance*
Auscultation—cont'd		
Rhonchi	Continuous rumbling, snoring, or rattling sounds from obstruction of large airways with secretions; most prominent on expiration; change often evident after coughing or suctioning	COPD, cystic fibrosis, pneumonia, bronchiectasis
Wheezes	Continuous high-pitched squeaking or musical sound caused by rapid vibration of bronchial walls; first evident on expiration but possibly evident on inspiration as obstruction of airway increases; possibly audible without stethoscope	Bronchospasm (caused by asthma), airway obstruction (caused by foreign body, tumor), COPD
Stridor	Continuous musical or crowing sound of constant pitch; result of partial obstruction of larynx or trachea	Croup, epiglottitis, vocal cord edema after extubation, foreign body
Absent breath sounds	No sound evident over entire lung or area of lung	Pleural effusion, mainstem bronchi obstruction, large atelectasis, pneumonectomy, lobectomy
Pleural friction rub	Creaking or grating sound from roughened, inflamed surfaces of the pleura rubbing together; evident during inspiration, expiration, or both and no change with coughing; usually uncomfortable, especially on deep inspiration	Pleurisy, pneumonia, pulmonary infarct
Bronchophony, whispered pectoriloquy	Spoken or whispered syllable more distinct than normal on auscultation	Pneumonia
Egophony	Spoken "e" similar to "a" on auscultation because of altered transmission of voice sounds	Pneumonia, pleural effusion

TABLE 26-9 Normal Physical Assessment of the Respiratory System

Nose	• Symmetric with no deformities. Nasal mucosa pink, moist with no edema, exudate, blood, or polyps. Nasal septum straight. Nares patent bilaterally.
Oral mucosa	• Light pink, moist, with no exudate or ulcerations.
Tonsils	• Not inflamed or enlarged.
Pharynx	• Smooth, moist, and pink.
Neck	• Trachea midline. No cervical nodes palpable.
Chest	• Anterior-posterior (AP) to lateral diameter 1:2. Respirations nonlabored at 14/min. Excursion equal bilaterally with no increase in tactile fremitus. Percussion resonant throughout. Breath sounds vesicular without crackles, rhonchi, or wheezes.

be palpated for fremitus. *Egophony* is positive when the person says "E" but it is heard as "A." *Bronchophony* is positive when a person says "ninety-nine" and the voice is not muffled and indistinct, but is clear and louder. *Whispered pectoriloquy* is positive when the patient whispers "one-two-three" and the almost inaudible voice is transmitted quite clearly and distinctly. Conditions that increase lung density or when the lung is consolidated, as in pneumonia, will have positive voice sounds.[10]

A record of the normal physical assessment of the respiratory system is shown in Table 26-9. Common assessment abnormalities of the thorax and lungs are presented in Table 26-8. Chest examination findings in common pulmonary problems are presented in Table 26-10. Age-related changes in the respiratory system and assessment findings are presented in Table 26-4.

DIAGNOSTIC STUDIES OF THE RESPIRATORY SYSTEM

Blood Studies

Common blood studies used to assess the respiratory system are the hemoglobin (Hb), hematocrit (Hct), and arterial blood gas (ABG) determinations. Table 26-11 describes nursing responsibilities associated with these tests.

Oximetry

Oximetry is used to noninvasively monitor SpO_2 and SvO_2 (see Tables 26-1 and 26-2). Nursing care associated with oximetry is discussed in Table 26-11.

Sputum Studies

Sputum samples can be obtained by expectoration, tracheal suction, or bronchoscopy, a technique in which a flexible scope is inserted into the airways. When the patient is unable to expectorate spontaneously, sputum may also be collected by inhalation of an irritating aerosol, usually hypertonic saline. This is called sputum induction. The specimens may be examined for culture and sensitivity to identify an infecting organism (e.g., *Mycobacterium, Pneumocystis jiroveci*) or to confirm a diagnosis (e.g., malignant cells). Regardless of whether specimen tests are ordered, it is important to observe the sputum for color, blood, volume, and viscosity. Nursing responsibilities for specimen collection are given in Table 26-11.

Skin Tests

Skin tests may be performed to test for allergic reactions or exposure to tuberculosis (TB) bacilli or fungi. Skin tests involve the intradermal injection of an antigen. A positive result on a TB skin test indicates that the patient has been exposed to the antigen. It

TABLE 26-10 Chest Examination Findings in Common Pulmonary Problems

Problem	Inspection	Palpation	Percussion	Auscultation
Chronic obstructive pulmonary disease	Barrel chest; cyanosis; tripod position; use of accessory muscles	↓ Movement	Hyperresonant or dull if consolidation	Crackles; rhonchi; wheezes; distant breath sounds
Asthma				
• In exacerbation	Prolonged expiration; tripod position; pursed lips	↓ Movement	Hyperresonance	Wheezes; ↓ breath sounds ominous sign if no improvement (severely diminished air movement)
• Not in exacerbation	Normal	Normal	Normal	Normal
Pneumonia	Tachypnea; use of accessory muscles; duskiness or cyanosis	↑ Fremitus over affected area	Dull over affected areas	Early: Bronchial sounds Later: Crackles; rhonchi; egophony; whispered pectoriloquy
Atelectasis	No change unless involves entire segment, lobe	If small, no change If large, ↓ movement; ↑ fremitus	Dull over affected areas	Crackles (may disappear with deep breaths); absent sounds if large
Pulmonary edema	Tachypnea; labored respirations; cyanosis	↓ Movement or normal movement	Dull or normal depending on amount of fluid	Fine or coarse crackles at bases moving upward as condition worsens
Pleural effusion	Tachypnea; use of accessory muscles	↑ Movement ↑ Fremitus above effusion; absent fremitus over effusion	Dull	Diminished or absent over effusion; egophony over effusion
Pulmonary fibrosis	Tachypnea	↓ Movement	Normal	Crackles or "Velcro" rales (sounds like Velcro being pulled apart)

does not indicate that TB is currently present. A negative result indicates that there has been no exposure or there is depression of cell-mediated immunity such as occurs in HIV infection.

Nursing responsibilities are similar for all skin tests. First, to prevent a false-negative reaction, the nurse should be certain that the injection is intradermal and not subcutaneous. After the injection, the sites should be circled and the patient instructed not to remove the marks. When charting administration of the antigen, the nurse should draw a diagram of the forearm and hand and label the injection sites. The diagram is especially helpful when more than one test is administered.

When reading test results, the nurse should use a good light. If an induration is present, a marking pen should be used to indicate the periphery on all four sides of the induration. As the pen touches the raised area, a mark should be made. The nurse then determines the diameter of the induration in millimeters. Reddened, flat areas are not measured. Table 26-12 presents a description of reactions that indicate a positive TB skin test.[21]

Radiologic Studies

Chest X-Ray. A chest x-ray is the most commonly used test for assessment of the respiratory system. It is also used to assess progression of disease and response to treatment. The most common views used are the posterior-anterior (PA) and lateral. (See Table 26-11 for nursing responsibilities related to chest x-rays.)

Computed Tomography. A computed tomography (CT) scan, which exposes a patient to radiation, may be used to examine cross sections of the entire body. CT scans of the chest are used to evaluate areas that are difficult to assess by conventional x-ray, such as the mediastinum, hilum, and pleura. Common types of CT scans are helical or spiral CT, in which contrast dye is usually used, and high-resolution CT scan, in which contrast is not used. Spiral CT is the most common noninvasive imaging procedure used to diagnose a pulmonary embolism (PE). Nursing responsibilities related to chest CT are presented in Table 26-11.

Magnetic Resonance Imaging. While in a strong magnetic field, the alignment of spinning nuclei can be changed with a superimposed radiofrequency and the rate at which they return to alignment with the field can be measured. Magnetic resonance imaging (MRI) uses this technique to produce images of body structures, so the patient is not exposed to radiation. MRI has limited indications in pulmonary diagnoses. It is most useful when evaluating images near the lung apex or spine and for distinguishing vascular from nonvascular structures. Nursing responsibilities related to MRI are presented in Table 26-11.

Ventilation-Perfusion Scan. A ventilation-perfusion scan is used primarily to check for the presence of a PE. However, it cannot determine with 100% certainty the presence of a PE, only the probability. An intravenous (IV) radioisotope is given for the perfusion portion of the test, and the pulmonary vasculature is outlined and photographed. For the ventilation portion, the patient inhales a radioactive gas (xenon or krypton), which outlines the alveoli, and another photograph is taken. Normal scans show homogeneous radioactivity. Diminished or absent radioactivity suggests lack of perfusion or airflow.[22,23] Nursing responsibilities related to ventilation-perfusion scans are presented in Table 26-11.

Pulmonary Angiography. Pulmonary angiography is the most specific examination used to confirm the diagnosis of a PE. However, chest CT is replacing angiography as it is less invasive. A series of x-rays is taken after radiopaque dye is injected into the pulmonary artery. This test also detects congenital and acquired lesions of the pulmonary vessels. Nursing responsibilities related to pulmonary angiography are presented in Table 26-11.

Positron Emission Tomography. Positron emission tomography (PET) scans involve the use of radionuclides with short half-lives. PET scans are used to distinguish benign and malignant

TABLE 26-11 *DIAGNOSTIC STUDIES* Respiratory System

Study	Description and Purpose	Nursing Responsibility
Blood Studies		
Hemoglobin	Test reflects amount of hemoglobin available for combination with oxygen. Venous blood is used. *Normal level* for adult man is 13.5-18 g/dl (135-180 g/L); *normal level* for adult woman is 12-16 g/dl (120-160 g/L).	Explain procedure and its purpose.
Hematocrit	Test reflects ratio of red blood cells to plasma. Increased hematocrit (polycythemia) found in chronic hypoxemia. Venous blood is used. *Normal* for adult man is 40%-54% (0.40-0.54); *normal* for adult woman is 38%-47% (0.38-0.47).	Explain procedure and its purpose.
ABGs	Arterial blood is obtained through puncture of radial or femoral artery or through arterial catheter. ABG tests are performed to assess acid-base balance, ventilation status, need for oxygen therapy, change in oxygen therapy, or change in ventilator settings.* Continuous ABG monitoring is also possible via a sensor or electrode inserted into the arterial catheter.	Indicate whether patient is using O_2 (percentage, L/min). Avoid change in oxygen therapy or interventions (e.g., suctioning, position change) for 20 min before obtaining sample. Assist with positioning (e.g., palm up, wrist slightly hyperextended if radial artery is used). Collect blood into heparinized syringe. To ensure accurate results, expel all air bubbles, and place sample in ice, unless it will be analyzed in less than 1 min. Apply pressure to artery for 5 min after specimen is obtained to prevent hematoma at the arterial puncture site.
Oximetry	Test monitors arterial or venous oxygen saturation. Probe attaches to the earlobe, finger, or nose for SpO_2 monitoring or is contained in a pulmonary artery catheter for SvO_2 monitoring. Oximetry is used for intermittent or continuous monitoring and exercise testing.*	Apply probe. When interpreting SpO_2 and SvO_2 values, first assess patient status and presence of factors that can alter accuracy of pulse oximeter reading. For SpO_2 these include motion, low perfusion, cold extremities, bright lights, use of intravascular dyes, acrylic nails, dark skin color, carbon monoxide, and disease states of anemia. For SvO_2, these include change in O_2 delivery or O_2 consumption. For SpO_2, notify health care provider of $\pm 4\%$ change from baseline or ↓ to $<90\%$. For SvO_2, notify health care provider of $\pm 10\%$ change from baseline or ↓ to $<60\%$.
Sputum Studies		
Culture and sensitivity	Single sputum specimen is collected in a sterile container. Purpose is to diagnose bacterial infection, select antibiotic, and evaluate treatment. Takes 48-72 hr for results.	Instruct patient on how to produce a good specimen (see Gram stain). If patient cannot produce specimen, bronchoscopy may be used (see Fig. 26-15).
Gram stain	Staining of sputum permits classification of bacteria into gram-negative and gram-positive types. Results guide therapy until culture and sensitivity results are obtained.	Instruct patient to expectorate sputum into the container after coughing deeply. Obtain sputum (mucoidlike), not saliva. Obtain specimen in early morning, after mouth care, because secretions collect during night. If unsuccessful, try increasing oral fluid intake unless fluids are restricted. Collect sputum in sterile container (sputum trap) during suctioning or by aspirating secretions from the trachea. Send specimen to laboratory promptly.
Acid-fast smear and culture	Test is performed to collect sputum for acid-fast bacilli (e.g., *Mycobacterium tuberculosis*). A series of three early morning specimens is used.	Instruct patient how to produce a good specimen (see Gram stain). Cover specimen and send to laboratory for analysis.
Cytology	Single sputum specimen is collected in special container with fixative solution. Purpose is to determine presence of abnormal cells that may indicate malignant condition.	Send specimen to laboratory promptly. Instruct patient on to produce a good specimen (see Gram stain). If patient cannot produce specimen, bronchoscopy may be used (see Fig. 26-15).
Radiology		
Chest x-ray	Test is used to screen, diagnose, and evaluate change. Most common views are PA and lateral.	Instruct patient to undress to waist, put on gown, and remove any metal between neck and waist.
Computed tomography (CT)	Test is performed for diagnosis of lesions difficult to assess by conventional x-ray studies. Images show structures in cross section.	Same as for chest x-ray. Contrast media may be given IV. Evaluation of BUN and serum creatinine is done prior to contrast to assess renal function. Assess if patient is allergic to shellfish (iodine) as the contrast is iodine based. Be sure the patient is well hydrated before and after procedure (to excrete the dye). Know that contrast injection may cause a feeling of being warm and flushed. Instruct patient that he/she will need to lie very still on a hard table and the scanner will revolve around the body with clicking noises. Some patients may require sedation before the procedure. Most scanners have weight limits, so check with radiology before sending obese patients for scanning.

ABGs, Arterial blood gases; *BUN,* blood urea nitrogen; *IV,* intravenous(ly); *PA,* posterior-anterior; *SpO_2,* arterial oxygen saturation by pulse oximetry; *SvO_2,* venous oxygen saturation.

*For normal values, see Table 26-1.

TABLE 26-11 DIAGNOSTIC STUDIES
Respiratory System—cont'd

Study	Description and Purpose	Nursing Responsibility
Radiology—cont'd		
Magnetic resonance imaging (MRI)	Test is used for diagnosis of lesions difficult to assess by CT scan (e.g., lung apex near the spine).	Same as for chest x-ray and CT scan, except contrast media are not iodine based. If patient has claustrophobia, provide patient with relaxation or other modes to cope as the table is guided into a tube until the chest is within the magnetic field and the face may be very close to tube. Patient must remove all metal (e.g., jewelry, watch) on the body before test. Patients with pacemakers and implantable cardioverter-defibrillators cannot undergo MRI. Patients with metal implants should be screened to determine if they can undergo MRI.
Ventilation-perfusion (V/Q) **scan**	Test is used to identify areas of the lung not receiving airflow (ventilation) or blood flow (perfusion). Ventilation without perfusion suggests the probability of a pulmonary embolus.	Same as for chest x-ray. No precautions needed afterward because the gas and isotope transmit radioactivity for only a brief interval.
Pulmonary angiogram	Study is used to visualize pulmonary vasculature and locate obstruction or pathologic conditions such as pulmonary embolus. Contrast medium is injected through a catheter into the pulmonary artery or right side of the heart.	Same as for chest x-ray. (See CT scan for contrast media precautions.) Check pressure dressing site after procedure. Monitor blood pressure, pulse, and circulation distal to injection site. Report and record significant changes.
Positron emission tomography (PET)	Test is used to distinguish benign and malignant lung nodules. It involves IV injection of a radioisotope with short half-life.	Same as for chest x-ray study. No precautions needed afterward because isotope only transmits radioactivity for brief interval. Encourage fluids afterward to excrete radioactive substance.
Endoscopic Examinations		
Bronchoscopy	Flexible fiberoptic scope is used for diagnosis, biopsy, specimen collection, or assessment of changes. It may also be done to suction mucous plugs, lavage the lungs, or remove foreign objects.	Instruct patient to be on NPO status for 6-12 hr prior to the test. Obtain signed permission. Give sedative if ordered. After procedure, keep patient NPO until gag reflex returns and monitor for laryngeal edema; monitor for recovery from sedatives. Blood-tinged mucus is not abnormal. If biopsy was done, monitor for hemorrhage and pneumothorax.
Mediastinoscopy	Test is used for inspection and biopsy of lymph nodes in mediastinal area.	Prepare patient for surgical intervention. Obtain signed permission. Afterward, monitor as for bronchoscopy.
Biopsy		
Lung biopsy	Specimens may be obtained by transbronchial, percutaneous or transthoracic needle aspiration (TTNA), video-assisted thoracic surgery (VATS), or open lung biopsy. Transbronchial and VATS biopsy can be performed in the bronchoscopy suite. TTNA is done under CT guidance in radiology. Open lung biopsy is performed in the operating room (OR). VATS can also be done in the OR. These tests are used to obtain specimens for laboratory analysis.	Same as bronchoscopy if procedure done with bronchoscope, and same as thoracotomy if open-lung biopsy done. With a TTNA, check breath sounds q4hr for 24 hr and report any respiratory distress. Check incision site for bleeding. A chest x-ray should be done after TTNA or transbronchial biopsy to check for pneumothorax. With VATS, a chest tube may be kept in postprocedure until lung has reexpanded. Monitor breath sounds to follow chest reexpansion. Encourage deep breathing for lung reinflation. Obtain signed permission for all procedures.
Other		
Thoracentesis	Test is used to obtain specimen of pleural fluid for diagnosis, to remove pleural fluid, or to instill medication. Chest x-ray is always obtained after procedure to check for pneumothorax.	Explain procedure to patient and obtain signed permission before procedure, which is usually performed in the patient's room. Position patient upright with elbows on an overbed table and feet supported. Instruct the patient not to talk or cough, and assist during procedure. Observe for signs of hypoxia and pneumothorax and verify breath sounds in all fields after procedure. Encourage deep breaths to expand lungs. Send labeled specimens to laboratory.
Pulmonary function tests	Tests are used to evaluate lung function. Involves use of a spirometer to diagram air movement as patient performs prescribed respiratory maneuvers.†	Avoid scheduling immediately after mealtime. Avoid administration of inhaled bronchodilator 6 hr before procedure. Explain procedure to patient. Assess for respiratory distress prior to procedure and report. Provide rest after procedure.

NPO, Nothing by mouth.
†For normal values, see Tables 26-13 and 26-14.

solitary pulmonary nodules. Because malignant lung cells have an increased uptake of glucose, the PET scan, which uses an IV radioactive glucose preparation, can demonstrate increased uptake of glucose in malignant lung cells.[23] Nursing responsibilities related to PET scans are presented in Table 26-11.

Endoscopic Examinations

Bronchoscopy. *Bronchoscopy* is a procedure in which the bronchi are visualized through a fiberoptic tube. Bronchoscopy may be used for diagnostic purposes to obtain biopsy specimens and assess changes resulting from treatment. Small amounts

TABLE 26-12 Interpreting Responses to Tuberculin Skin Testing

Types of Responses	Consider Positive in the Following Groups
Positive Reactions	
≥5-mm induration	• HIV-positive persons • Suspected HIV infection • Recent close contact with person diagnosed with infectious TB • Persons with fibrotic lesions on chest x-ray consistent with old healed TB • Patients with organ transplants and other immunosuppressed patients (receiving the equivalent of ≥15 mg/day of prednisone for ≥1 mo)
≥10-mm induration	• Persons with clinical conditions (e.g., diabetes mellitus, end-stage renal disease, prolonged corticosteroid therapy, cancer of oropharynx or upper GI tract) that place them at high risk • Recent immigrants (within the last 5 yr) from high-prevalence countries • Medically underserved groups, homeless • Residents of long-term care facilities, prisons, homeless shelters, and other congregate settings • IV drug users • Mycobacteriology laboratory personnel
≥15-mm induration	• All other persons who are at low risk
False Reactions	**Possible Causes**
False-Negative Reactions	• Anergy, immunosuppression • Testing too soon after exposure to TB (up to 12 wk may be required to develop immune response). 25% of persons with active TB have a negative reaction • Overwhelming TB infection • Poor nutrition and poor health • Aging (may result in decrease in delayed-type hypersensitivity) • Long time since TB infection. Sensitivity to tuberculin may wane over the years, resulting in a negative reaction. However, the tuberculin test may stimulate (boost) ability to react to tuberculin, causing a positive reaction to future tests. *Two-step testing* is therefore recommended for individuals likely to be tested often (e.g., health care providers and individuals who may have decrease in delayed hypersensitivity).
False-Positive Reactions	• Nontuberculous mycobacteria (e.g., *Mycobacterium avium-intracellulare* [MAI] or *Mycobacterium avium* complex [MAC]) • BCG vaccine

Sources: American Thoracic Society, 2000 and *www.cdc.gov/nchstp/tb/pubs/corecurr/Chapter4/Chapter_4_Skin_Testing.htm.*
BCG, Bacille Calmette-Guérin; *GI,* gastrointestinal; *HIV,* human immunodeficiency virus; *IV,* intravenous; *TB,* tuberculosis.

(30 ml) of sterile saline may be injected through the scope and withdrawn and examined for cells, a technique termed *bronchoalveolar lavage* (BAL). BAL is used to diagnose a variety of conditions, including *Pneumocystis* pneumonia (Fig. 26-14). Bronchoscopy is also used for treatment. For example, mucous plugs or foreign bodies can be removed. Laser therapy, electrocautery, cryotherapy, and stents may be placed through a bronchoscope to achieve patency of an airway that has been completely or partially obstructed by tumors.[24]

A

B

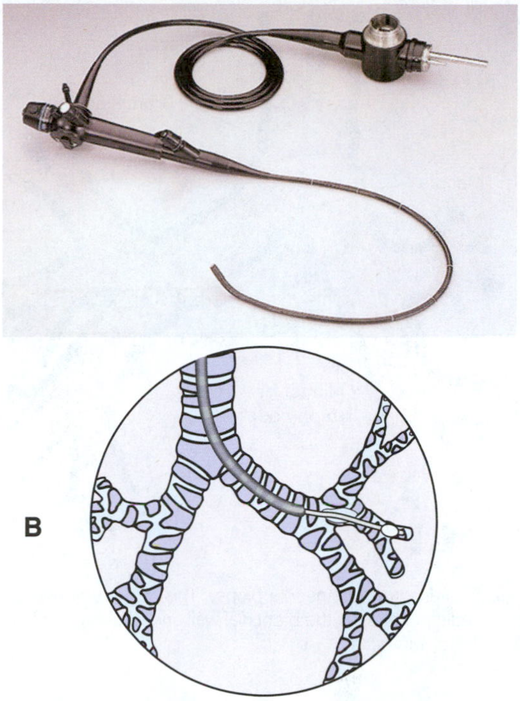

FIG. 26-14 Fiberoptic bronchoscope. **A,** The transbronchoscopic balloon-tipped catheter and the flexible fiberoptic bronchoscope. **B,** The catheter is introduced into a small airway and the balloon inflated with 1.5 to 2 ml of air to occlude the airway. Bronchoalveolar lavage is performed by injecting and withdrawing 30-ml aliquots of sterile saline solution, gently aspirating after each instillation. Specimens are sent to the laboratory for analysis.

Bronchoscopy can be performed in an outpatient procedure room, in a surgical suite, or at the bedside in the intensive care unit or on a medical-surgical floor, with the patient lying down or seated. After the nasal pharynx and oral pharynx are anesthetized with local anesthetic, the bronchoscope is coated with lidocaine (Xylocaine) and inserted, usually through the nose, and threaded down into the airways. Bronchoscopy can be done on mechanically ventilated patients through the endotracheal tube. The nursing care for the patient undergoing this procedure is described in Table 26-11.

Mediastinoscopy. For *mediastinoscopy,* a scope is inserted through a small incision in the suprasternal notch and advanced into the mediastinum to inspect and biopsy lymph nodes. The test is used to diagnose carcinoma, non-Hodgkin's lymphoma, granulomatous infections, and sarcoidosis. The procedure is performed in the operating room and the patient is given a general anesthetic. Nursing responsibilities related to mediastinoscopy are presented in Table 26-11.

Lung Biopsy

Lung biopsy may be done (1) transbronchially, (2) percutaneously or via transthoracic needle aspiration (TTNA), (3) by video-assisted thoracic surgery (VATS), or (4) as an open lung biopsy. The purpose of a lung biopsy is to obtain tissue, cells, or secretions for evaluation. Transbronchial lung biopsy involves passing a forceps or needle through the bronchoscope for a specimen (Fig. 26-15). Specimens can be cultured or examined for malignant cells. A

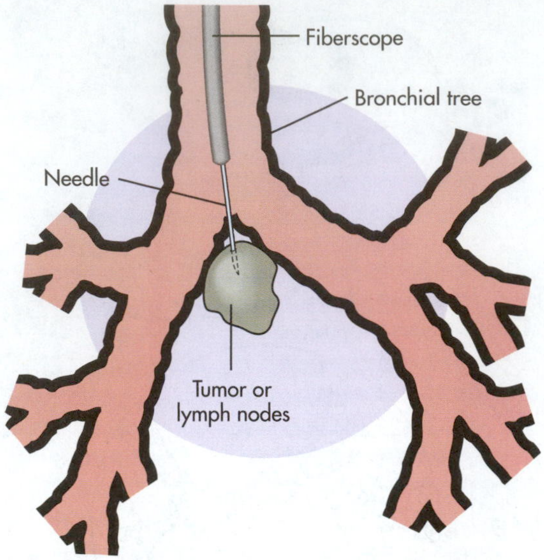

FIG. 26-15 Transbronchial needle biopsy. The diagram shows a transbronchial biopsy needle penetrating the bronchial wall and entering a mass of subcarinal lymph nodes or tumor.

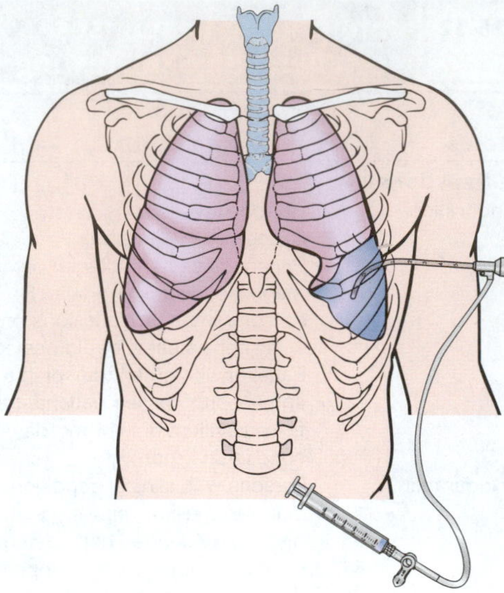

FIG. 26-16 Thoracentesis. A catheter is positioned in the pleural space to remove accumulated fluid.

combination of transbronchial lung biopsy and BAL is used to differentiate infection and rejection in lung transplant recipients. Percutaneous needle aspiration or TTNA involves inserting a needle through the chest wall, usually under CT guidance. Because of the risk of a pneumothorax, a chest x-ray is ordered after TTNA. In VATS, a rigid scope with a lens is passed through a trocar placed into the pleura via one or two small incisions in the intercostal muscles. The physician views the lesions on a monitor directly via the lens, and biopsy specimens can be taken. A chest tube is kept in place until the lung reexpands. Lesions in the pleura or peripheral lung are biopsied via VATS. VATS is much less invasive than open lung biopsy and is the procedure of choice when appropriate.[25] Open lung biopsy is used when pulmonary disease cannot be diagnosed by other procedures. The patient is anesthetized, the chest is opened with a thoracotomy incision, and a biopsy specimen is obtained. Nursing care for the procedure is the same as after thoracotomy (see Chapter 28). (See Table 26-11 for nursing responsibilities related to lung biopsy.)

Thoracentesis

Thoracentesis is the insertion of a large-bore needle through the chest wall into the pleural space to obtain specimens for diagnostic evaluation, remove pleural fluid, or instill medication into the pleural space (Fig. 26-16). The patient is positioned sitting upright with elbows on an overbed table and feet supported. The skin is cleansed and a local anesthetic (Xylocaine) is instilled subcutaneously. A chest tube may be inserted to permit further drainage of fluid. Nursing care is described in Table 26-11.

Pulmonary Function Tests

Pulmonary function tests (PFTs) measure lung volumes and airflow. The results of PFTs are used to diagnose pulmonary disease, monitor disease progression, evaluate disability, and evaluate response to bronchodilators. Airflow is measured by a spirometer and administered by trained personnel. The patient inserts a mouthpiece, takes as deep a breath as possible, and exhales as hard, fast, and long as possible. Verbal coaching is given to ensure that the patient continues blowing out until exhalation is complete.

The computer calculates the patient's percentage of predicted values in terms of how well the performance compares to an average based on age, gender, race, and height. Normal values are approximately 80% to 120% of the predicted value. Whites have been shown to have higher forced vital capacity (FVC) and forced expiratory volume in 1 second (FEV_1) than Mexican Americans or African Americans.[26] Normal values for PFTs are shown in Tables 26-13 and 26-14 and Fig. 26-17.

Spirometry may be ordered before and after the administration of a bronchodilator to determine the degree of the response. This may help to document reversibility of airway obstruction (e.g., asthma). A positive response to the bronchodilator is >200 ml increase or >12% increase between pre- and postadministration values.

PFTs cannot be interpreted in isolation; the entire clinical presentation must be considered. Trends in airflow, lung volume, and diffusion capacity over time are useful in assessment of disease progression and/or response to treatment.

Home spirometry may be used to monitor lung function in persons with asthma or cystic fibrosis, as well as before and after lung transplantation. A peak flow meter is the instrument used at home. It is a handheld device through which one blows forcefully and quickly after taking a deep breath. It measures milliliters of volume. Spirometry changes at home can warn of early lung transplant rejection or infection. Feedback from a peak flow meter can increase the sense of control when persons with asthma learn to modify activities and medications in response to changes in PEF rates (see Chapter 29).

Pulmonary function parameters can also be used to determine the need for mechanical ventilation or the readiness to be weaned from ventilatory support. Measurements of vital capacity, maximum inspiratory pressure, and minute ventilation are used to make this determination (see Table 26-13). (See Table 26-11 for nursing responsibilities related to pulmonary function.)

Exercise Testing

Exercise testing is used in diagnosis, in determining exercise capacity, and for disability evaluation. A complete exercise test involves walking on a treadmill while expired oxygen and carbon dioxide, respiratory rate, heart rate, and heart rhythm are monitored. A modi-

TABLE 26-13 Lung Volumes and Capacities

Parameter	Definitions	Normal Values*
Volumes		
Tidal volume (V_T)	Volume of air inhaled and exhaled with each breath; only a small proportion of total capacity of lungs	0.5 L
Expiratory reserve volume (ERV)	Additional air that can be forcefully exhaled after normal exhalation is complete	1.0 L
Residual volume (RV)	Amount of air remaining in lungs after forced expiration; air available in lungs for gas exchange between breaths	1.5 L
Inspiratory reserve volume (IRV)	Maximum volume of air that can be inhaled forcefully after normal inhalation	3.0 L
Capacities		
Total lung capacity (TLC)	Maximum volume of air that lungs can contain ($TLC = IRV + V_T + ERV + RV$)	6.0 L
Functional residual capacity (FRC)	Volume of air remaining in lungs at end of normal exhalation ($FRC = ERV + RV$); increase or decrease possible with lung disease	2.5 L
Vital capacity (VC)	Maximum volume of air that can be exhaled after maximum inspiration ($VC = IRV + V_T + ERV$); higher VC for men (generally)	4.5 L
Inspiratory capacity (IC)	Maximum volume of air that can be inhaled after normal expiration ($IC = V_T + IRV$)	3.5 L

*Normal values vary with height, weight, age, race, and gender of patient.

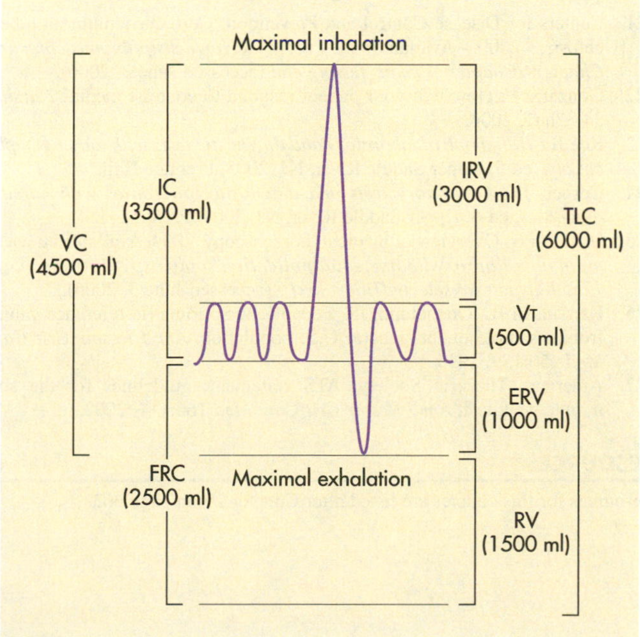

FIG. 26-17 Relationship of lung volumes and capacities. (For abbreviations used, see Table 26-13.)

TABLE 26-14 Common Measures of Pulmonary Function Airflow

Measure	Description	Normal Value*
Forced vital capacity (FVC)	Amount of air that can be quickly and forcefully exhaled after maximum inspiration	Over 80% of predicted
Forced expiratory volume in first second of expiration (FEV_1)	Amount of air exhaled in first second of FVC; grades severity of airway obstruction	Over 80% of predicted
FEV1/FVC ratio	Dividing of value for FEV_1 by value for FVC; useful in differentiating obstructive and restrictive pulmonary dysfunction	Age <50: ≥75% of predicted; Age ≥50: ≥70% of predicted
Forced midexpiratory flow rate ($FEF_{25\%-75\%}$)	Measurement of airflow rate in middle half of forced expiration; early indicator of disease of small airways	Age <50: ≥75% of predicted; Age ≥50: ≥70% of predicted
Maximal voluntary ventilation (MVV)	Deep breathing as rapidly as possible for specified period; fairly nonspecific test that gives information about exercise capacity. Used in conjunction with exercise stress test	About 170 L/min
Peak expiratory flow rate (PEFR)	Maximum airflow rate during forced expiration; aids in monitoring bronchoconstriction in asthma; can be measured with peak flow meter	Up to 600 L/min

*Normal values vary with height, age, race, and gender of patient.

fied test (desaturation test) may also be used. In this case, only SpO_2 is monitored. A desaturation test can also be used to determine the oxygen flow needed to maintain the SpO_2 at a safe level during activity or exercise in patients who use home oxygen therapy.

A 6-minute walk test can also be used to measure functional capacity and response to medical interventions in patients with moderate to severe heart or lung disease. The patient is instructed by a trained practitioner to walk as far as possible during 6 minutes, stopping when short of breath and continuing when able. Pulse oximetry is usually monitored during the walk. The distance walked is measured and used to monitor progression of disease or improvement after rehabilitation.[27]

NCLEX EXAMINATION REVIEW QUESTIONS

The number of the question corresponds to the same-numbered objective at the beginning of the chapter.

1. The mechanism that stimulates the release of surfactant is
   a. fluid accumulation in the alveoli.
   b. alveolar collapse from atelectasis.
   c. alveolar stretch from deep breathing.
   d. air movement through the alveolar pores of Kohn.

2. During inspiration, air enters the thoracic cavity as a result of
   a. contraction of the accessory abdominal muscles.
   b. increased carbon dioxide and decreased oxygen in the blood.
   c. stimulation of the respiratory muscles by the chemoreceptors.
   d. decreased intrathoracic pressure relative to pressure at the airway.
3. The ability of the lungs to adequately oxygenate the arterial blood is best determined by examination of the
   a. heart rate.
   b. hemoglobin level.
   c. arterial oxygen tension.
   d. arterial carbon dioxide tension.
4. The most important respiratory defense mechanism distal to the respiratory bronchioles is the
   a. alveolar macrophage.
   b. impaction of particles.
   c. reflex bronchoconstriction.
   d. mucociliary clearance mechanism.
5. A rightward shift of the oxygen-hemoglobin dissociation curve
   a. is caused by metabolic alkalosis.
   b. is seen in postoperative hypothermia.
   c. facilitates release of oxygen at the tissue level.
   d. causes blood to pick up more oxygen in the lungs.
6. Very early signs or symptoms of inadequate oxygenation include
   a. dyspnea and hypotension.
   b. apprehension and restlessness.
   c. cyanosis and cool, clammy skin.
   d. increased urine output and diaphoresis.
7. During the respiratory assessment of the older adult, the nurse would expect to find
   a. a vigorous cough.
   b. increased chest expansion.
   c. increased anterior-posterior chest diameter.
   d. increased breath sounds in the lung apices.
8. When assessing activity-exercise patterns related to respiratory health, the nurse inquires about
   a. dyspnea during rest or exercise.
   b. recent weight loss or weight gain.
   c. willingness to wear oxygen in public.
   d. ability to sleep through the entire night.
9. When auscultating the chest of an elderly patient in respiratory distress, it is best to
   a. begin listening at the apices.
   b. begin listening at the lung bases.
   c. begin listening on the anterior chest.
   d. ask the patient to breathe through the nose with the mouth closed.
10. Which of the following is an abnormal assessment finding of the respiratory system?
    a. Inspiratory chest expansion of 1 inch
    b. Percussion resonance over the lung bases
    c. Symmetric chest expansion and contraction
    d. Bronchial breath sounds in the lower lung fields
11. A diagnostic procedure done to remove pleural fluid for analysis is
    a. thoracentesis.
    b. bronchoscopy.
    c. pulmonary angiography.
    d. sputum culture and sensitivity.

REFERENCES

1. Thibodeau GA, Patton KT: *Structure and function of the body,* ed 12, St Louis, 2004, Mosby.
2. Nowak TJ, Handford AG: *Pathophysiology: concepts and applications for health care professionals*, ed 3, New York, 2004, McGraw-Hill.
3. Weinberger SE: *Principles of pulmonary medicine,* ed 4, Philadelphia, 2004, Saunders.
4. Huether SE, McCance KL: *Understanding pathophysiology*, ed 3, St Louis, 2004, Mosby.
5. Snell RS: *Clinical anatomy*, ed 7, Philadelphia, 2004, Lippincott, Williams & Wilkins.
6. Porth CM: *Pathophysiology: concepts of altered health states,* ed 7, Philadelphia, 2004, Lippincott, Williams & Wilkins.
7. McCance KL, Huether SE: *Pathophysiology: the biologic basis for disease in adults and children,* ed 5, St Louis, 2006, Mosby.
8. West JB: *Respiratory physiology: the essentials,* ed 7, Philadelphia, 2004, Lippincott, Williams & Wilkins.
9. Ho JC, et al: The effect of aging on nasal mucociliary clearance, beat frequency, and ultrastructure of respiratory cilia, *Am J Respir Crit Care Med* 163:983, 2001.
10. Jarvis C: *Physical examination and health assessment,* ed 4, Philadelphia, 2004, Saunders.
11. Seidel HM, et al: *Mosby's guide to physical examination,* ed 6, St Louis, 2006, Mosby.
12. Taffett GE: Physiology of aging. In Cassel CK, et al, editors: *Geriatric medicine: an evidence based approach*, ed 4, New York, 2003, Springer.
13. Webster JR: Pulmonary disease. In Cassel CK, et al, editors: *Geriatric medicine: an evidence based approach,* ed 4, New York, 2003, Springer.
14. Weinberger SE: Cough and hemoptysis. In Kaspar DL, et al, editors: *Harrison's principles of internal medicine*, ed 16, New York, 2005, McGraw-Hill.
15. Centers for Disease Control and Prevention: MMWR recommendations and reports. Prevention of pneumococcal disease: recommendations of the Advisory Committee on Immunization Practices (ACIP), April 4, 1997. Available at: *www.cdc.gov/mmwr/preview/mmwrhtml/00047135.htm* (accessed June 30, 2005).

*16. Heinzer MM, Bish C, Detwiler R: Acute dyspnea as perceived by patients with chronic obstructive pulmonary disease, *Clin Nurs Res* 12:85, 2003.

17. Wilson SF, Giddens JF: *Health assessment for nursing practice,* ed 3, St Louis, 2005, Mosby.
18. Goolsby MJ, Grubbs L: *Advanced assessment: interpreting findings and formulating differential diagnoses,* Philadelphia, 2006, FA Davis.
19. American College of Chest Physicians & American Thoracic Society: Pulmonary terms and symbols, *Chest* 67:583, 1975.
20. Wilkins RL, et al: Lung sound nomenclature survey, *Chest* 98:886, 1990.
21. Centers for Disease Control and Prevention: Core curriculum on tuberculosis, 2000. Available at: *www.cdc.gov/nchstp/tb/pubs/corecurr/Chapter4/Chapter_4_Skin_Testing.htm* (accessed June 3, 2006).
22. Gonzalez F: How will your patient respond to contrast media? *Nursing* 34:32hn1, 2004.
23. Kee JL: *Handbook of laboratory and diagnostic tests with nursing implications,* ed 5, Upper Saddle River, NJ, 2005, Prentice Hall.
24. Corbett JV: *Laboratory tests and diagnostic procedures with nursing diagnoses,* ed 6, Upper Saddle River, NJ, 2004, Prentice Hall.
25. Mathur PN: Overview of medical thoracoscopy, 2004. Available at: *www.utdol.com.libproxy.lib.unc.edu/application/topic.asp?file=misclung/17559&type=A&selectedTitle=1~16* (accessed June 3, 2006).
26. Hankinson JL, Odencrantz JR, Fedan KB: Spirometric reference values from a sample of the general U.S. population, *Am J Respir Crit Care Med* 150:179, 1999.
27. American Thoracic Society: ATS statement: guidelines for the six-minute walk test, *Am J Respir Crit Care Med* 166:111, 2002.

RESOURCES

Resources for this chapter are listed after Chapter 29 on page 663.

*Nursing research–based reference.

Whenever you are asked if you can do a job, tell 'em, "Certainly I can!" Then get busy and find out how to do it.

Theodore Roosevelt

Nursing Management Upper Respiratory Problems 27

Valerie Bender Howard

LEARNING OBJECTIVES

1. Describe the clinical manifestations and nursing management of problems of the nose.
2. Describe the clinical manifestations and nursing management of problems of the paranasal sinuses.
3. Describe the clinical manifestations and nursing management of problems of the pharynx and larynx.
4. Discuss the nursing management of the patient who requires a tracheostomy.
5. Identify the steps involved in performing tracheostomy care and suctioning an airway.
6. Describe the risk factors and warning symptoms associated with head and neck cancer.
7. Discuss the nursing management of the patient with a laryngectomy.
8. Describe the methods used in voice restoration for the patient with temporary or permanent loss of speech.

KEY TERMS

Electronic Resources

Supplemental content related to Chapter 27 can be found . . .

Companion CD

- Stress-Busting Kit for Nursing Students
- Interactive Case Study: Head and Neck Cancer: Laryngectomy with Tracheostomy
- NCLEX Examination Review Questions
- Comprehensive Glossary
- Animation: Anatomic Location of Sinuses

Evolve Website

http://evolve.elsevier.com/Lewis/medsurg

- Content Updates
- Key Points (Printable and CD/MP3 Download)
- Concept Map Creator
- Expanded Audio Glossary
- Key Term Flash Cards
- Customizable Nursing Care Plans:
  - Tracheostomy
  - Total Laryngectomy and/or Radical Neck Surgery
- Patient and Family Instruction Guides in English and Spanish:
  - Acute or Chronic Sinusitis
  - How to Reduce Symptoms of Allergic Rhinitis
- Electronic Calculators
- WebLinks

Structural and Traumatic Disorders of the Nose

DEVIATED SEPTUM

Deviated septum is a deflection of the normally straight nasal septum. It is most commonly caused by trauma to the nose or congenital disproportion, a condition in which the size of the septum is not proportional to the size of the nose. On inspection, the septum is bent to one side, altering the air passage. Symptoms are variable. The patient may experience obstruction to nasal breathing, nasal edema, or dryness of the nasal mucosa with crusting and bleeding *(epistaxis)*. There is conflicting evidence to support that a severely deviated septum may block drainage of mucus from the sinus cavities, resulting in infection *(sinusitis)*.[1]

Medical management of deviated septum includes nasal allergy control as in allergic rhinitis (see pp. 535 to 536). For patients with severe symptoms, a nasal septoplasty is performed to reconstruct and properly align the deviated septum.

NASAL FRACTURE

Nasal fractures account for approximately 40% of bone injuries in cases of facial trauma. They are most often caused by a substantial blow to the middle of the face. Some cases of facial trauma can be prevented by using protective sports equipment

Reviewed by Christine L. Willis, RN, MSN, ANP-C, Adult Nurse Practitioner, Pulmonary and Critical Care Medicine, Duke University Medical Center, Durham, N.C.

and protecting against falls. Complications of the fracture include airway obstruction, epistaxis, meningeal tears, septal hematoma, and cosmetic deformity. Nasal fractures can be classified as unilateral, bilateral, or complex. A unilateral fracture typically produces little or no displacement. Bilateral fractures, the most common fractures, give the nose a flattened look. Powerful frontal blows cause complex fractures, which may also involve subsequent damage to adjacent facial structures such as the teeth, eyes, or other facial bones.

Diagnosis is based on the health history and physical examination. Although obvious facial deformity with a nasal fracture is common, often epistaxis may be the only presenting sign.[2] Plain radiographic imaging is rarely indicated when an uncomplicated nasal fracture is suspected. On inspection, the nurse should assess the patient's ability to breathe through each side of the nose and note the presence of edema, bleeding, or hematoma. There may be ecchymosis under one or both eyes. Ecchymosis involving both eyes is often termed *raccoon eyes.* The nose is inspected internally for evidence of septal deviation, hemorrhage, or clear drainage, which suggests leakage of cerebrospinal fluid (CSF). If clear drainage is observed, a quick test may be done at the bedside or a specimen may be sent to the laboratory to determine if glucose is present, indicating that the fluid is CSF. Injury of sufficient force to fracture nasal bones results in considerable swelling of soft tissues. With extensive swelling, it may be necessary to wait 5 to 10 days to repair the fracture when the edema subsides.

The goals of nursing management are to maintain the airway, reduce edema, prevent complications, and provide emotional support. The airway can best be maintained by keeping the patient in an upright position. Ice may be applied to the face and nose to reduce edema and bleeding. When a fracture is confirmed, the goal of medical management is to realign the fracture using closed or open reduction (septoplasty, rhinoplasty) and to assure that a septal hematoma does not develop as this increases the patient's risk for infection. These procedures reestablish cosmetic appearance and proper function of the nose and provide an adequate airway.[2]

RHINOPLASTY

Rhinoplasty, the surgical reconstruction of the nose, is performed for cosmetic reasons or to improve airway function when trauma or developmental deformities result in nasal obstruction. Assessment of the patient's expectations is a critical aspect of preparation for rhinoplasty. Any actual or perceived alteration in body image (e.g., a deformed or enlarged nose) can affect self-esteem and interactions with others. The patient's expectations concerning surgical results should be assessed with regard to the expected change. Computerized photographs made to life-size measurements can be used to simulate appearance after the surgery and may help the patient decide whether to undergo rhinoplasty. Expected results of surgery should be explained frankly and truthfully to avoid disappointment.

Collaborative Care

Rhinoplasty is performed as an outpatient procedure using regional anesthesia. Nasal tissue may be added or removed, and the nose may be lengthened or shortened. Plastic implants are sometimes used to reshape the nose. After surgery, nasal packing may be inserted to apply pressure and prevent bleeding or septal hematoma formation. Nasal septal splints (small pieces of plastic or Silastic) may be inserted to help prevent scar tissue formation between the surgical site and lateral nasal wall. An external plastic splint is molded to the new shape of the nose and placed on the nose. Steri-Strips are placed to hold the skin against the septal cartilage. Typically, nasal packing is removed the day after surgery, and the splint is removed in 3 to 5 days.

NURSING MANAGEMENT
NASAL SURGERY

Examples of nasal surgery include rhinoplasty, septoplasty, and nasal fracture reductions. Before surgery, the patient should be instructed to not take aspirin-containing drugs or nonsteroidal anti-inflammatory drugs (NSAIDs) for 2 weeks to reduce the risk of bleeding. Nursing interventions during the immediate postoperative period include maintenance of the airway, assessment of respiratory status, pain management, and observation of the surgical site for bleeding, infection, and edema. Teaching is important because the patient must be able to detect early and late complications at home. There is an interim period while edema and ecchymosis resolve before the final cosmetic effect can be achieved.

EPISTAXIS

Epistaxis (nosebleed) occurs in a bimodal distribution, with children less than 10 years of age and adults over the age of 50 most affected.[3] Epistaxis may be caused by trauma, foreign bodies, topical corticosteroid use, nasal spray abuse, street drug use, anatomic malformation, allergic rhinitis, or tumors. Any condition that prolongs bleeding time or alters platelet counts will predispose the patient to epistaxis. Bleeding time may also be prolonged if the patient takes aspirin or NSAIDs. Although hypertension may not increase the risk of epistaxis, elevated blood pressure makes bleeding more difficult to control.[3]

Children and young adults have a tendency to develop anterior nasal bleeding, whereas older adults more commonly have posterior nasal bleeding. Anterior bleeding usually stops spontaneously or can be self-treated; posterior bleeding may require medical treatment.[3]

NURSING *and* COLLABORATIVE MANAGEMENT
EPISTAXIS

Simple first aid measures should be used first to control epistaxis. The nurse should (1) keep the patient quiet; (2) place the patient in a sitting position, leaning forward, or if not possible, in a high Fowler's position; (3) apply direct pressure by pinching the entire soft lower portion of the nose for 10 to 15 minutes; (4) apply ice compresses to the nose; (5) partially insert a small gauze pad into the bleeding nostril, and apply digital pressure if bleeding continues; and (6) obtain medical assistance if bleeding does not stop.

If first aid is not effective, medical management involves identification of the bleeding site and application of a vasoconstrictive agent, cauterization, or anterior packing by a health care provider. Anterior packing may consist of ribbon gauze or a nasal tampon impregnated with antibiotic ointment and/or vasoconstrictive agents such as oxymetazoline or cocaine that is wedged firmly in the desired location and remains in place for 48 to 72 hours. If posterior packing is required, the elderly patient or those with other comorbid conditions should be hospitalized. Inflatable balloons similar to a urinary catheter may be used as a nasal pack or gauze rolls may be inserted (Fig. 27-1). Strings attached to the packing are brought to the outside and taped to the cheek for ease

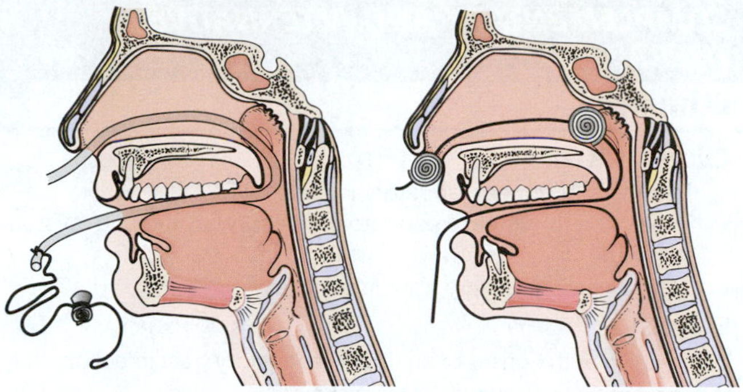

FIG. 27-1 Method for placing posterior nasal pack. **A,** Catheter is passed through the bleeding side of the nose and pulled out through the mouth with a hemostat. Strings are tied to the catheter, and the pack is pulled up behind the soft palate and into the nasopharynx. **B,** Nasal pack in position in the posterior nasopharynx. Dental roll at the nose helps maintain correct position.

of removal. A nasal sling (a folded 2 × 2–inch gauze pad) should be taped over the nares to absorb drainage.

Nasal packing may alter respiratory status, especially in older adults. Some patients experience *hypoventilation* (increase in partial pressure of carbon dioxide in arterial blood [$PaCO_2$]) and *hypoxemia* (decrease in partial pressure of oxygen in arterial blood [PaO_2]), which may lead to cardiac dysrhythmias or respiratory arrest. The nurse should closely monitor respiratory rate, heart rate and rhythm, oxygen saturation using pulse oximetry (SpO_2), and level of consciousness and observe for signs of aspiration. Because of the risk of complications, the patient may be admitted to a monitored unit to permit closer observation.

Packing is painful because sufficient pressure must be applied to stop the bleeding. Nasal packing predisposes to infection from bacteria (e.g., *Staphylococcus aureus*) present in the nasal cavity. Another complication of nasal packing is a septal hematoma. The patient should receive a mild opioid analgesic for pain (e.g., acetaminophen with codeine) and an antibiotic effective against staphylococci to protect against infection.

Nasal packing is left in place for a minimum of 3 days. Before removal, the patient should be medicated for pain, because this procedure is very uncomfortable. After removal, the nares may be gently cleaned and lubricated with water-soluble jelly.

Failure of posterior packing to control epistaxis indicates the need for surgery or radiologic embolization of the affected artery. The most common surgical procedure involves ligation of the internal maxillary artery performed through an incision under the upper lip to gain access to the artery.

The patient can be discharged after being taught about home care. The patient should be instructed to avoid vigorous nose blowing, strenuous activity, lifting, and straining for 4 to 6 weeks. The patient should be taught to sneeze with the mouth open and to avoid the use of aspirin-containing products or NSAIDs.

Inflammation and Infection of the Nose and Paranasal Sinuses

ALLERGIC RHINITIS

Allergic rhinitis is the reaction of the nasal mucosa to a specific allergen. Although "seasonal" and "perennial" are still widely used to describe the two types of allergic rhinitis, the use of the terms *intermittent* and *persistent* is preferred. *Intermittent* means that the symptoms are present less than 4 days a week or less than 4 weeks per year. *Persistent* means that the symptoms are present more than 4 days a week and for more than 4 weeks per year. Attacks of intermittent rhinitis usually occur in the spring and fall and are caused by allergy to pollens from trees, flowers, or grasses. The typical attack lasts for several weeks during times when pollen counts are high, disappears, and recurs at the same time the following year. Persistent rhinitis is present intermittently or constantly.

Symptoms of allergic rhinitis are usually caused by specific environmental triggers such as pet saliva, dust mites, molds, or cockroaches. Symptoms of allergic rhinitis can occur whenever a patient is exposed to a specific allergen. Sensitization to an allergen occurs with initial allergen exposure, which results in the production of antigen-specific immunoglobulin E (IgE). After exposure, mast cells and basophils release histamine, prostaglandins, and leukotrienes, which cause the early symptoms of sneezing, itching, rhinorrhea, and moderate congestion. Two to 4 hours after exposure, there is infiltration of inflammatory cells into the nasal tissues causing and maintaining the inflammatory response.[4] Because symptoms of perennial rhinitis resemble the common cold, the patient may believe the condition is a continuous or repeated cold.

Clinical Manifestations

Manifestations of allergic rhinitis are initially sneezing; watery, itchy eyes and nose; altered sense of smell; and thin, watery nasal discharge that can lead to a more sustained nasal congestion. The nasal turbinates appear pale, boggy, and swollen. The turbinates may fill the air space and press against the nasal septum. The posterior ends of the turbinates can become so enlarged that they obstruct sinus aeration or drainage and result in sinusitis. With chronic exposure to allergens, the patient's responses include headache, congestion, pressure, nasal polyps, and postnasal drip as the most common cause of cough. The patient may complain of cough, hoarseness, and/or the recurrent need to clear the throat. Congestion may cause snoring.

NURSING *and* COLLABORATIVE MANAGEMENT ALLERGIC RHINITIS

Several steps are used in managing allergic rhinitis. The most important step involves identifying and avoiding triggers of allergic reactions (Table 27-1). The patient should be instructed to keep a diary of times when the allergic reaction occurs and the activities that precipitate the reaction. Patients may be more aware of intermittent exposure to an allergen such as pets, rather than a more perennial exposure such as to dust mites, cockroaches, or mold.[4] Steps can then be taken to avoid these triggers.

The goal of medication therapy is to reduce inflammation associated with allergic rhinitis and reduce nasal symptoms so that the patient has no adverse effects and can sleep well at night to avoid daytime somnolence. This involves the use of antihistamines, intranasal corticosteroids, and leukotriene receptor antagonists (LTRAs) to manage symptoms[5] (Table 27-2). Second-generation (nonsedating) antihistamines are preferred over first-generation antihistamines due to their selectivity and nonsedating effects.[3] While taking antihistamines, patients need to be reminded to have adequate fluid intake to reduce adverse symptoms. Intranasal corticosteroids and cromolyn sprays are effective for allergic rhinitis. Nasal corticosteroid sprays are used to decrease inflammation locally with little absorption in

TABLE 27-1 PATIENT AND FAMILY TEACHING GUIDE
How to Reduce Symptoms of Allergic Rhinitis

1. **Avoidance** is the best treatment.
2. **Avoid house dust.** Use the approach "less is best." Focus on the bedroom. Remove carpeting. Limit furniture. Enclose the pillows, mattress, and springs in airtight vinyl encasements. Limit clothing in the bedroom to items used frequently. Place clothing in airtight, zipper-sealed vinyl clothes bags. Install an air filter. Close the air-conditioning vent into the room. Use blinds rather than draperies.
3. **Avoid house dust mites.** Wash bedding in hot water (130° F [54° C]) weekly. Wear a mask when vacuuming. Double-bag the vacuum cleaner. Install a filter on the outlet port of the vacuum cleaner. Avoid sleeping or lying on upholstered furniture. Remove carpets that are laid on concrete. If possible, have someone else clean the house. Keep house temperature and conditions cool and dry.
4. **Avoid mold spores.** The three *D*s that promote growth of mold spores are darkness, dampness, and drafts. Avoid places where humidity is high (e.g., basements, camps on the lake, clothes hampers, greenhouses, stables, barns). Dehumidifiers are rarely helpful. Ventilate closed rooms, open doors, and install fans. Consider adding windows to dark rooms. Consider keeping a small light on in closets. A basement light with a timer that provides light several hours a day may decrease mold growth.
5. **Avoid pollens.** Stay inside with closed doors and windows during high-pollen season. Avoid the use of fans. Install an air conditioner with a good air filter. Wash filters weekly during high-pollen season. Put the car air conditioner on "recirculate" when driving. Get someone else to tend to your yard. Avoid having plants, especially in the bedroom.
6. **Avoid pet allergens.** Remove pets from the interior of the home. Clean the living area thoroughly. Do not expect instant relief. Symptoms usually do not improve significantly for 2 months following pet removal.
7. **Avoid smoke.** The presence of a smoker will sabotage the best of all possible symptom reduction programs.

the systemic circulation. Therefore systemic side effects are rare. Relief may require combining a nasal corticosteroid spray and an antihistamine. The patient should begin the intranasal corticosteroid 2 to 3 weeks prior to the allergy season, if possible. The patient using intranasal inhalers needs careful instructions about proper use (Fig. 27-2). Immunotherapy ("allergy shots") may be used if drugs are not tolerated, or are not effective, when a specific unavoidable allergen is identified. Immunotherapy involves controlled exposure to small amounts of the known allergen through frequent (at least weekly) injections with the goal to decrease sensitivity. (Immunotherapy is discussed in Chapter 14.)

ACUTE VIRAL RHINITIS

Acute viral rhinitis (common cold or acute coryza) is caused by an adenovirus that invades the upper respiratory tract and often accompanies an acute upper respiratory infection (URI). It is the most prevalent infectious disease and is spread by airborne droplet sprays emitted by the infected person while breathing, talking, sneezing, or coughing or by direct hand contact. This virus can survive on inanimate objects for up to 3 days. Frequency of the infection increases in the winter months when people stay indoors and overcrowding is more common. Other factors, such as fatigue, physical and emotional stress, and compromised immune status, may increase susceptibility. The patient with acute viral rhinitis typically first experiences tickling, irritation, sneezing, or dryness of the nose or nasopharynx, followed by copious nasal secretions, some nasal obstruction, watery eyes, elevated temperature, general malaise, and headache. After the early profuse secretions, the nose becomes more obstructed, and the discharge is thicker. Within a few days the general symptoms improve, nasal passages reopen, and normal breathing is established.

COMPLEMENTARY AND ALTERNATIVE THERAPIES
Echinacea

Clinical Uses
- Treatment of upper respiratory infections*
- Prevention of upper respiratory infections, immune system stimulation†
- Wound healing, urinary tract infections‡

Effects
When taken at the onset of an upper respiratory tract infection, may reduce length and severity of symptoms.

Nursing Implications
Echinacea is considered safe when used in recommended doses. May interfere with drugs that suppress the immune system. Caution is advised in patients with conditions affecting the immune system. May lead to liver inflammation. Caution is advised when used with drugs, herbs, and supplements that may damage the liver. Unclear evidence related to safety during pregnancy or lactation. Short-term use (10 to 14 days) is recommended. Should not be taken for more than 8 weeks.

Adapted from Ulbricht CE, Basch EM: *Natural standard herb and supplement reference: evidence-based clinical reviews,* St Louis, 2005, Mosby *(www.naturalstandard.com).*
*Good scientific evidence for its use.
†Unclear scientific evidence for its use.
‡Uses based on tradition, theory, or limited scientific evidence.

COMPLEMENTARY AND ALTERNATIVE THERAPIES
Goldenseal

Clinical Uses
Heart failure, immunostimulant, infectious diarrhea, upper respiratory tract infection*

Effects
Commonly used to treat inflamed mucosal tissue. Little scientific evidence is available to determine effectiveness. Appears safe in recommended doses for short-term use. Commonly combined with echinacea in preparations.

Nursing Implications
Should not be used for longer than 2 to 3 weeks. Use with caution in patients with cardiovascular disease. May increase risk of bleeding. Should not be used concurrently with anticoagulants. Contraindicated in pregnancy and lactation.

Adapted from Ulbricht CE, Basch EM: *Natural standard herb and supplement reference: evidence-based clinical reviews,* St Louis, 2005, Mosby *(www.naturalstandard.com).*
*Unclear scientific evidence for its use.

NURSING *and* COLLABORATIVE MANAGEMENT ACUTE VIRAL RHINITIS

Rest, fluids, proper diet, antipyretics, and analgesics are recommended. Complications of acute viral rhinitis include pharyngitis, sinusitis, otitis media, tonsillitis, and lung infections. Unless

TABLE 27-2 DRUG THERAPY
Allergic Rhinitis and Sinusitis

Preparation	Mechanism of Action	Side Effects	Nursing Actions
Corticosteroids ***Nasal Spray*** beclomethasone (Vancenase) budesonide (Rhinocort) flunisolide (Nasalide) fluticasone (Flonase) mometasone (Nasonex) triamcinolone (Nasacort)	Inhibits inflammatory response. At recommended dose, systemic side effects are unlikely because of low systemic absorption. Systemic effects may occur with greater than recommended doses.	Mild transient nasal burning and stinging. In rare instances, localized fungal infection with *Candida albicans*.	• Teach patient correct use (see Fig. 27-2). • Begin 2 wk before pollen season starts and use throughout pollen season. • Instruct patient to use on regular basis and not prn. • Reinforce that spray acts to decrease inflammation and effect is not immediate, as with decongestant sprays. • Discontinue use if nasal infection develops.
Mast Cell Stabilizer ***Nasal Spray*** cromolyn spray (NasalCrom)	Inhibits degranulation of sensitized mast cells, which occurs after exposure to specific antigens.	Minimal side effects. Occasional burning or nasal irritation.	• Teach patient correct use (see Fig. 27-2). • Reinforce that spray prevents symptoms. • Begin 2 wk before pollen season starts and use throughout pollen season. • If isolated allergy, such as cat, use prophylactically (i.e., 10-15 min before exposure to allergen).
Leukotriene Receptor Antagonists (LTRAs) and Inhibitors ***Antagonists*** zafirlukast (Accolate) montelukast (Singulair) ***Inhibitors*** zileuton (Zyflo)	Antagonize or inhibit leukotriene activity, thereby inhibiting airway edema and bronchoconstriction, and decreasing inflammatory process (see Fig. 13-5).	Headaches, dizziness, rash, altered liver function tests, abdominal pain. Zafirlukast and zileuton: Monitor PT levels and theophylline levels if patient is taking coumadin or theophylline. Zafirlukast: rare Churg-Strauss syndrome (flu-like syndrome: fever, muscle aches and pain, worsening respiratory symptoms, loss of weight).	• Monitor liver function tests periodically while on therapy. Discontinue if elevated. • Administer on empty stomach. • Do not discontinue therapy without consulting health care professional. • Not to be used for acute attacks. • Advise patient to notify health care professional immediately if symptoms of Churg-Strauss occur.
Anticholinergic ***Nasal Spray*** ipratropium bromide (Atrovent)	Blocks hypersecretory effects by competing for binding sites on the cell. Reduces rhinorrhea in the common cold and nonallergic rhinitis.	Dryness of the mouth and nose may occur. Does not cause systemic side effects.	• Teach patient correct use (see Fig. 27-2). • Reinforce that spray prevents symptoms with onset of action within 1 hr of use. • May reduce the need for other rhinitis medications.
Antihistamines ***First-Generation Agents*** *Ethanolamines* clemastine (Tavist) diphenhydramine (Benadryl) *Ethylenediamines* tripelennamine (PBZ) *Alkylamines* brompheniramine (Dimetane) chlorpheniramine (Chlor-Trimeton) dexchlorpheniramine (Polaramine) *Piperidine* azatadine (Optimine)	Bind with H_1 receptors on target cells, blocking histamine binding. Relieve acute symptoms of allergic response (itching, sneezing, excessive secretions, mild congestion).	**First-generation agents** cross blood-brain barrier, bind to H_1 receptors in brain, cause *sedation* (diminished alertness, slow reaction time, somnolence) and *stimulation* (restless, nervous, insomnia). Some drugs (e.g., ethanolamines) are more likely to cause sedation. Patients vary in their sensitivity to these side effects. The next most common side effects involve the GI system and include loss of appetite, epigastric distress, constipation, or diarrhea. May cause palpitations, tachycardia, urinary retention or frequency.	**First-generation agents:** • Warn patient that operating machinery and driving may be dangerous because of sedative effect. Drowsiness usually passes after 2 wk of treatment. • Teach patient to report palpitations, change in heart rate, change in bowel, bladder habits. • Instruct patient not to use alcohol with antihistamines because of additive depressant effect. • Rapid onset of action, no drug tolerance with prolonged use. • Limited use with sinusitis.

PT, prothrombin time.

Continued

TABLE 27-2 *DRUG THERAPY*
Allergic Rhinitis and Sinusitis—cont'd

Preparation	Mechanism of Action	Side Effects	Nursing Actions
Antihistamines—cont'd			
Second-Generation Agents			
loratadine (Claritin) cetirizine (Zyrtec) fexofenadine (Allegra) desloratadine (Clarinex)		**Second-generation agents** have limited affinity for brain H_1 receptors. Cause minimal sedation, few effects on psychomotor activities, bladder function.	**Second-generation agents:** • Teach patient to expect few, if any, side effects. • More expensive than classic antihistamines. • Rapid onset of action, no drug tolerance with prolonged use. • Limited use with sinusitis. *General interactions:* • Do not take with alcohol or any form of tranquilizer or sedative. • Do not take with any monoamine oxidase inhibitor.
Decongestants			
Oral			
pseudoephedrine (Sudafed)	Stimulate adrenergic receptors on blood vessels, promote vasoconstriction, and reduce nasal edema and rhinorrhea.	CNS stimulation, causing insomnia, excitation, headache, irritability, increased blood and ocular pressure, dysuria, palpitations, tachycardia.	• Advise patient of adverse reactions. • Advise that some preparations are contraindicated for patients with cardiovascular disease, hypertension, diabetes, glaucoma, prostate hyperplasia, hepatic and renal disease.
Topical (Nasal Spray)			
oxymetazoline (Dristan) phenylephrine (Neo-Synephrine)	Same as above.	Same as above, plus rhinitis medicamentosa (rebound nasal congestion).	• Teach patient that these drugs should not be used for >3 days or more than 3-4 times a day.
azelastine (Astelin)	Blocks action of histamine.	Headache, bitter taste, somnolence, nasal irritation.	• Longer use increases risk of rebound vasodilation, which can increase congestion.

CNS, Central nervous system.

symptoms of complications are present, antibiotic therapy is not indicated. Antibiotics have no effect on viruses and, if taken injudiciously, may produce antibiotic-resistant bacteria. If symptoms remain for at least 7 days with no improvement, acute bacterial sinusitis may be present and antibiotics will be prescribed.[6]

During the cold season, the patient with a chronic illness or a compromised immune status should be advised to avoid crowded, close situations and other persons who have obvious cold symptoms. Frequent hand washing and avoiding hand-to-face contact may help prevent direct spread.

Interventions are directed toward relieving annoying symptoms. The patient should be encouraged to drink increased amounts of fluids to liquefy secretions. Antihistamine or decongestant therapy reduces postnasal drip and significantly decreases severity of cough, nasal obstruction, and nasal discharge. Patients should be cautioned to use the intranasal decongestant sprays for no more than 3 days to prevent rebound congestion from occurring. The patient should also be taught to recognize the symptoms of secondary bacterial infection, such as a temperature higher than 100.4° F (38° C); purulent nasal exudate; tender, swollen glands; and a sore, red throat. In the patient with pulmonary disease, signs of infection include a change in consistency, color, or volume of the sputum. Because infection can progress rapidly, the patient with chronic respiratory disease may be taught to begin antibiotics for sputum changes, increased shortness of breath, and chest tightness.

INFLUENZA

Each year influenza (flu) causes significant morbidity and mortality. Influenza-related deaths average 36,000 per year in the United States.[7] Most deaths occur in persons over 60 years of age with underlying heart or lung disease, but could be prevented with vaccination of high-risk groups[7] (Table 27-3).

There are two main groups of influenza viruses (A and B). Influenza viruses have a remarkable ability to change over time. This accounts for widespread disease and the need for annual vaccination against new strains. Fewer cases of influenza result when a minor change in the virus occurs because most persons have partial immunity.[7]

Clinical Manifestations

The onset of flu is typically abrupt, with systemic symptoms of cough, fever, and myalgia often accompanied by a headache and sore throat. Milder symptoms, similar to the common cold, may also occur. Physical findings are usually minimal, with normal assessment on chest auscultation. Dyspnea and diffuse crackles are

Before using the inhaler, gently blow your nose, making sure your nostrils are clear.

Then follow these steps:

1. Remove the protective cap from the nasal inhaler.
2. Shake the canister well.
3. Hold the inhaler between the thumb and forefinger.
4. Tilt the head back slightly and insert the end of the inhaler into one nostril, pointing it slightly toward the outside nostril wall. Hold the other nostril closed with one finger.
5. Press down on the canister to release one dose and, at the same time, inhale gently.
6. Hold your breath for a few seconds, then breathe out slowly through the mouth.
7. Withdraw the inhaler from the nostril and repeat the process for the other nostril. If more than one puff is prescribed per nostril, repeat steps 4-6. To avoid irritation, direct the spray at a different area of the mucosa for each puff.
8. Replace the protective cap on the inhaler.

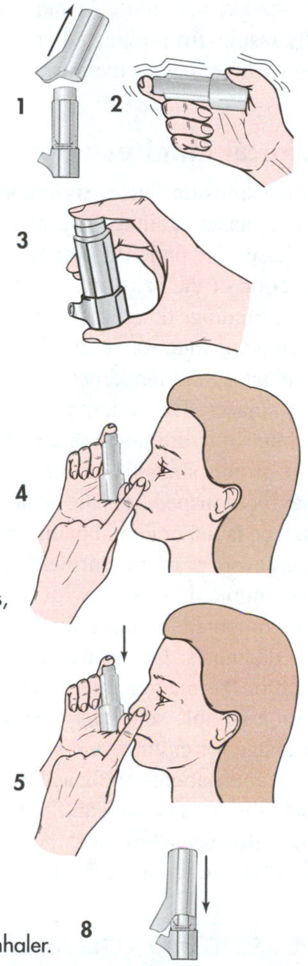

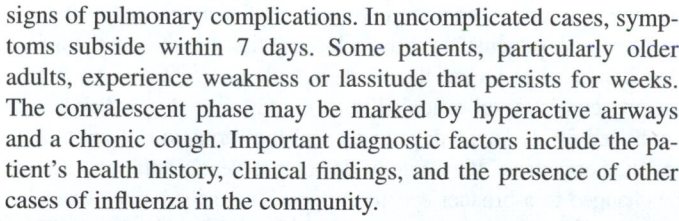

FIG. 27-2 Method for using an intranasal inhaler.

COMPLEMENTARY AND ALTERNATIVE THERAPIES

Zinc

Clinical Uses

Common cold, upper respiratory tract infections, wound healing, dermatitis, acne, herpes simplex

Effects

May prevent replication of viruses. May stimulate the immune system. Severe zinc deficiency results in severely depressed immune function and frequent infections.

Nursing Implications

Zinc supplements are available as oral tablets and lozenges. Oral zinc should not be taken with foods that will reduce its absorption, such as coffee, bran, protein, or calcium. Long-term use of zinc supplements over 15 mg/day is not recommended without medical supervision.

TABLE 27-3 Target Groups for Influenza Immunization

Inactivated Vaccine

Groups at High Risk

- Anyone ≥50 years old
- Adults of any age with chronic cardiac or pulmonary disease
- Adults who had regular medical follow-up or were hospitalized during the preceding year
- Residents of long-term care facilities
- Immunocompromised adults
- Women who will be in second or third trimester of pregnancy during influenza season

Groups Who Can Transmit Influenza to High-Risk Persons

- Health care workers
- Providers of home care to high-risk persons
- Household members of high-risk persons

Live, Attenuated Influenza Vaccine (LAIV)

- All persons 5–49 years of age
- Given intranasally

signs of pulmonary complications. In uncomplicated cases, symptoms subside within 7 days. Some patients, particularly older adults, experience weakness or lassitude that persists for weeks. The convalescent phase may be marked by hyperactive airways and a chronic cough. Important diagnostic factors include the patient's health history, clinical findings, and the presence of other cases of influenza in the community.

The most common complication of influenza is pneumonia. The patient who develops secondary bacterial pneumonia experiences gradual improvement of influenza symptoms, then worsening cough and purulent sputum. Treatment with antibiotics is usually effective if started early.

NURSING *and* COLLABORATIVE MANAGEMENT INFLUENZA

There are two types of flu vaccines available: inactivated and live, attenuated. The nurse should advocate the use of inactivated influenza vaccination in all patients >50 years of age or who are at high risk during routine office visits or, if hospitalized, at the time of discharge (see Table 27-3). The vaccine is 70% to 90% effective in preventing influenza in adults. To be most effective, the vaccine should be given in the fall (mid-October) before exposure occurs, but it can be given later if needed. As long as there is adequate availability, the present policy in the United States is for routine vaccination of persons over 50 years old.[7] High priority should also be given to groups that can transmit influenza to high-risk persons, such as health care workers. By being vaccinated, the nurse can decrease the risk of transmitting influenza to those who have less ability to cope with the effects of this illness. Despite obvious benefits, many persons are reluctant to be vaccinated. Current vaccines are highly purified, and reactions are extremely uncommon. Soreness at the injection site is usually the only side effect. The contraindications are history of Guillain-Barré syndrome and hypersensitivity to eggs, because the vaccine is produced in eggs. New guidelines suggest that nurses should encourage all healthy patients between the ages of 5 and 49 years of age (and not pregnant) to receive the live, attenuated influenza vaccine (LAIV; FluMist), which is given intranasally.

The primary goals in nursing management are supportive measures directed toward relief of symptoms and prevention of secondary infection. Unless at high risk or complications develop, the patient with influenza usually requires only symptomatic therapy. Older adults and those with a chronic illness may require hospitalization. Antivirals such as amantadine (Symmetrel) or rimantadine (Flumadine) can be given for chemoprophylaxis if an outbreak occurs. These drugs are given orally to prevent or decrease symptoms of flu. Other antivirals, including zanamivir (Relenza) and oseltamivir (Tamiflu), are used in both the prevention and treatment of influenza A and B. These drugs are neuraminidase inhibitors that prevent the virus from budding and spreading to other cells. For maximum benefit in the treatment of influenza, they should be initiated as soon as possible and ideally within 2 days of the onset of symptoms. They shorten the course of influenza. Zanamivir is administered using an inhaler. Oseltamivir is available as an oral capsule. Both zanamivir and oseltamivir have been effectively shown to reduce symptom duration and severity of influenza. Both drugs can be used prophylactically for control of outbreaks of influenza.[8]

***Drug Alert** - Pseudoephedrine (Sudafed)*
- *Large doses may produce tachycardia and palpitations, especially in patients with cardiac disease.*
- *Overdosage in those over 60 years of age may result in central nervous system depression, seizures, and hallucinations.*

SINUSITIS

Sinusitis develops when the ostia (exit) from the sinuses are narrowed or blocked by inflammation or hypertrophy (swelling) of the mucosa (Fig. 27-3). The secretions that accumulate behind the obstruction provide a rich medium for growth of bacteria, viruses, and fungi, all of which may cause infection. Bacterial sinusitis is most commonly caused by *Streptococcus pneumoniae, Haemophilus influenzae,* or *Moraxella catarrhalis.*[6] Viral sinusitis follows an upper respiratory infection in which the virus penetrates the mucous membrane and decreases ciliary transport. Fungal sinusitis is uncommon and is usually found in patients who are debilitated or immunocompromised.

Acute sinusitis usually results from an upper respiratory infection, allergic rhinitis, swimming, or dental manipulation, all of which can cause inflammatory changes and retention of secretions. When acute sinusitis follows viral rhinitis, symptoms worsen after 5 to 7 days and are worse than the original rhinitis. *Chronic sinusitis* (lasting longer than 3 weeks) is a persistent infection usually associated with allergies and nasal polyps. Chronic sinusitis generally results from repeated episodes of acute sinusitis that result in irreversible loss of the normal ciliated epithelium lining the sinus cavity.

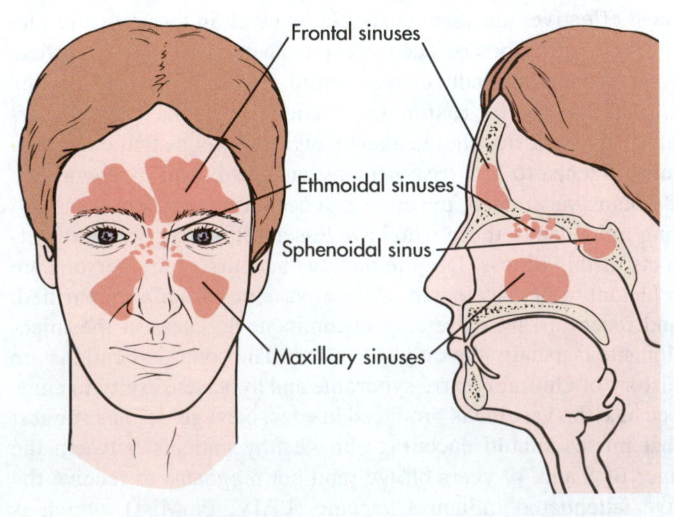

FIG. 27-3 Location of the sinuses.

Clinical Manifestations

Acute sinusitis causes significant pain over the affected sinus, purulent nasal drainage, nasal obstruction, congestion, fever, and malaise. The patient looks and feels sick. Assessment involves inspection of the nasal mucosa and palpation of the sinus points for pain. Findings that indicate acute sinusitis include a hyperemic and edematous mucosa, a discolored purulent nasal drainage, enlarged turbinates, and tenderness over the involved frontal and/or maxillary sinuses. The patient may have recurrent headaches that change in intensity with position changes or when secretions drain.

Chronic sinusitis is difficult to diagnose because symptoms may be nonspecific. The patient is rarely febrile. Although there may be facial or dental pain, nasal congestion, and increased drainage, severe pain and purulent drainage are often absent. Symptoms may mimic those seen with allergies. X-rays of the sinuses or a sinus computed tomography (CT) scan may be performed to confirm the diagnosis. CT scans may show the sinuses to be filled with fluid or the mucous membrane to be thickened. Nasal endoscopy with a flexible scope may be used to examine the sinuses, obtain drainage for culture, and restore normal drainage.

Many patients with asthma have sinusitis. The link between these diseases is unclear. Sinusitis may trigger asthma by stimulating reflex bronchospasm. Appropriate treatment of sinusitis often causes a reduction in asthma symptoms.[9]

NURSING *and* COLLABORATIVE MANAGEMENT SINUSITIS

If allergies are the precipitating cause of sinusitis, the patient needs to be instructed in ways to reduce sinus inflammation and infection, including environmental control of allergies and appropriate drug therapy (see section on allergic rhinitis, earlier in this chapter).

Treatment of acute sinusitis includes antibiotics to treat the infection if it persists longer than 7 days without treatment. Antibiotic therapy consisting of amoxicillin as the first-line drug of choice is continued for 10 to 14 days to prevent the formation of antibiotic-resistant organisms. If symptoms do not resolve, the antibiotic should be changed to a broader spectrum agent such as sulfamethoxazole/trimethoprim (Bactrim) or erythromycin. With chronic sinusitis, mixed bacterial flora are often present and infections are difficult to eliminate. Broad-spectrum antibiotics may be used for 4 to 6 weeks. The use of the following ancillary medications can also relieve symptoms: oral or topical decongestants to promote drainage, nasal corticosteroids to decrease inflammation, and antihistamines (Table 27-4). Patients using topical decongestants must be instructed to use the medication for no longer than 3 days to prevent rebound congestion due to vasodilation. Classic (first-generation) antihistamines increase the viscosity of mucus and promote continued symptoms, so they should be avoided. Nonsedating (second-generation) antihistamines do not cause this problem, but research does not support their use with infectious sinusitis.[10]

TABLE 27-4 PATIENT AND FAMILY TEACHING GUIDE
Acute or Chronic Sinusitis

1. Keep well hydrated by drinking 6 to 8 glasses of water to loosen secretions.
2. Take hot showers twice daily; use a steam inhaler (15-min vaporization of boiled water), bedside humidifier, or nasal saline spray to promote secretion drainage.
3. Report temperature of 100.4° F (38° C), which may indicate infection.
4. Follow prescribed medication regimen:
   - Take analgesics to relieve pain.
   - Take decongestants/expectorants to relieve swelling and thin mucus.
   - Take antibiotics, as prescribed, for infection. Be sure to take entire prescription and report continued symptoms or a change in symptoms.
   - Administer nasal sprays correctly.
5. Do not smoke and avoid exposure to smoke. Smoke is an irritant and may worsen symptoms.
6. If allergies predispose to sinusitis, follow instructions regarding environmental control, drug therapy, and immunotherapy to reduce the inflammation and prevent sinus infection.

Drug Alert - *Antihistamines*

- *First-generation antihistamines (e.g., chlorpheniramine [Chlor-Trimeton]) can cause drowsiness and sedation.*
- *Patients should be warned that operating machinery and driving may be dangerous because of sedative effect.*

The patient should be encouraged to increase fluid intake (6 to 8 glasses daily) and use nasal cleaning techniques. This many include taking a hot shower in the morning and evening followed by blowing the nose thoroughly. Other interventions that may provide symptomatic relief include irrigating the nose with saline nasal spray or steam inhalations.

Saline nasal spray is available over the counter as sterile physiologic saline solution in spray bottles. Alternatively, saline solution may be prepared at home with ¼ tsp of salt dissolved in 8 oz of tap water. A pinch of baking soda may be added. The patient should place the solution in a spray bottle or ear bulb syringe for lavage. Two to four puffs of nasal saline should be administered at least 3 times a day. The alternative, more aggressive method is lavage with a bulb syringe while leaning over the sink with the mouth open. Repeated full-syringe wash and aspiration is recommended at least 3 times daily to wash out the secretions if they cannot be effectively removed with saline spray alone. Alternatively, a Water Pik device (set on the lowest setting) may be used.

The patient with persistent or recurrent sinus complaints not alleviated by medical therapy may require nasal endoscopic surgery to relieve blockage caused by hypertrophy or septal deviation. This is an outpatient procedure usually performed under local anesthesia.

Obstruction of the Nose and Paranasal Sinuses

POLYPS

Nasal polyps are benign mucous membrane masses that form slowly in response to repeated inflammation of the sinus or nasal mucosa. Polyps, which appear as bluish, glossy projections in the naris, can exceed the size of a grape. The patient may be anxious, fearing they are malignant. Clinical manifestations include nasal obstruction, nasal discharge (usually clear mucus), and speech distortion. Nasal polyps can be removed with endoscopic or laser surgery, but recurrence is common. Topical or systemic corticosteroids may slow polyp growth.

FOREIGN BODIES

A variety of foreign bodies may lodge in the upper respiratory tract. Inorganic foreign bodies such as buttons and beads may cause no symptoms, lie undetected, and be accidentally discovered on routine examination. Organic foreign bodies such as wood, cotton, beans, peas, and paper produce a local inflammatory reaction and nasal discharge, which may become purulent and foul smelling. Foreign bodies should be removed from the nose through the route of entry. Sneezing with the opposite nostril closed may be effective in assisting the removal of foreign bodies. Irrigation of the nose or pushing the object backward should not be done, because either could cause aspiration and airway obstruction. If sneezing or blowing the nose does not remove the object, the patient should see a health care provider.

Problems Related to the Pharynx

ACUTE PHARYNGITIS

Acute pharyngitis is an acute inflammation of the pharyngeal walls. It may include the tonsils, palate, and uvula. It can be caused by a viral, bacterial, or fungal infection. Viral pharyngitis accounts for approximately 70% of cases. Acute follicular pharyngitis ("strep throat") results from β-hemolytic streptococcal invasion and accounts for an additional 5% to 15% of episodes in adults.[11] Fungal pharyngitis, especially candidiasis, can develop with prolonged use of antibiotics or inhaled corticosteroids or in immunosuppressed patients, especially those with human immunodeficiency virus (HIV).

Clinical Manifestations

Symptoms of acute pharyngitis range in severity from complaints of a "scratchy throat" to pain so severe that swallowing is difficult. Both viral and strep infections appear as a red and edematous pharynx, with or without patchy yellow exudates. Appearance is not always diagnostic. Cultures or a rapid strep antigen test is done to establish the cause and direct appropriate management. Inadequate treatment of acute streptococcal pharyngitis can result in rheumatic heart disease or glomerulonephritis as a sequela to the infection.

White, irregular patches suggest fungal infection with *Candida albicans.* In diphtheria, a gray-white false membrane, termed a *pseudomembrane,* is seen covering the oropharynx, nasopharynx, and laryngopharynx and sometimes extends to the trachea.

NURSING *and* COLLABORATIVE MANAGEMENT ACUTE PHARYNGITIS

The goals of nursing management are infection control, symptomatic relief, and prevention of secondary complications. The patient with documented strep throat is treated with antibiotics. *Candida* infections are treated with nystatin (Mycostatin), an antifungal antibiotic. The preparation should be swished in the mouth as long as possible before it is swallowed, and treatment should continue until symptoms are gone. Those taking inhaled corticosteroids are at risk for infection with *Candida,* which can be prevented by thoroughly rinsing the mouth out with water after dosing. The patient with pharyngitis should be encouraged to increase fluid intake. Cool, bland liquids and gelatin will not irritate the pharynx; citrus juices can be irritating.

PERITONSILLAR ABSCESS

Peritonsillar abscess is a complication of acute pharyngitis or acute tonsillitis when bacterial infection invades one or both tonsils. The tonsils may enlarge sufficiently to threaten airway patency. The patient experiences a high fever, leukocytosis, "hot potato voice," and chills.[11] Intravenous (IV) antibiotic therapy is given along with needle aspiration or incision and drainage of the abscess. An emergency tonsillectomy may be performed, or an elective tonsillectomy may be scheduled after the infection has subsided.

OBSTRUCTIVE SLEEP APNEA

Obstructive sleep apnea (OSA), also called obstructive sleep apnea-hypopnea syndrome (OSAHS), is a condition characterized by partial or complete upper airway obstruction during sleep.[12] **Apnea** is the cessation of spontaneous respirations lasting longer than 20 seconds. *Hypopnea* is a condition characterized by shallow (30% to 50% reduction in airflow) respirations. Airflow obstruction occurs when the tongue and the soft palate fall backward and partially or completely obstruct the pharynx (Fig. 27-4). The obstruction may last from 15 to 90 seconds. During the apneic period, the patient can experience severe *hypoxemia* (decreased PaO_2 or SpO_2) and *hypercapnia* (increased $PaCO_2$). These changes are ventilatory stimulants and cause the patient to partially awaken. The patient has a generalized startle response, snorts, and gasps, which causes the tongue and soft palate to move forward and the airway to open. Apnea and arousal cycles occur repeatedly, as many as 200 to 400 times during 6 to 8 hours of sleep.[12]

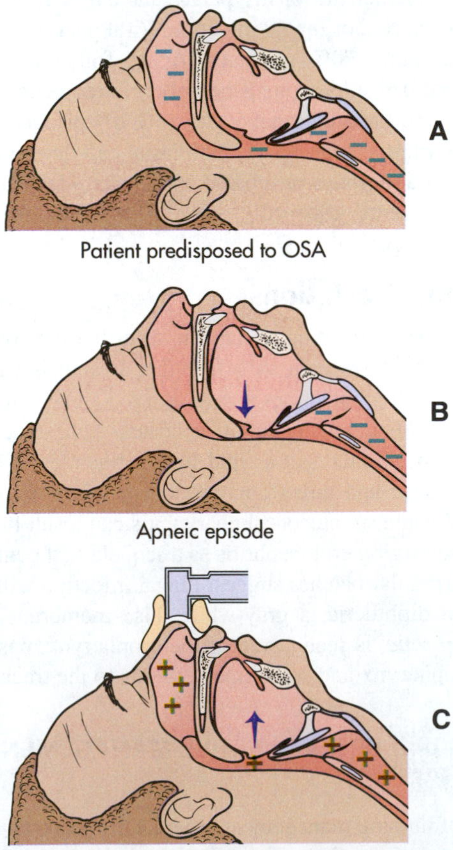

FIG. 27-4 How sleep apnea occurs. **A,** The patient predisposed to obstructive sleep apnea (OSA) has a small pharyngeal airway. **B,** During sleep, the pharyngeal muscles relax, allowing the airway to close. Lack of airflow results in repeated apneic episodes. **C,** With CPAP, continuous positive airway pressure splints the airway open, preventing airflow obstruction.

Sleep apnea occurs in 2% to 10% of the population but is considered to be underreported. The risk increases with obesity (body mass index >28 kg/m²), age >65, neck circumference >17 inches, and craniofacial abnormalities that impact the upper airway. Obstructive sleep apnea is more common in men than women.[12]

Clinical Manifestations and Diagnostic Studies

Clinical manifestations of sleep apnea include frequent awakening at night, insomnia, excessive daytime sleepiness, and witnessed apneic episodes. The patient's bed partner may complain about the patient's loud snoring. The snoring may be so disruptive that both persons cannot sleep in the same room. Other symptoms include morning headaches (from hypercapnia, which causes vasodilation of cerebral blood vessels), personality changes, and irritability. Complications that can result from untreated sleep apnea include hypertension, right-sided heart failure from pulmonary hypertension caused by chronic nocturnal hypoxemia, and cardiac dysrhythmias.[13] Symptoms of sleep apnea alter many aspects of the patient's lifestyle. Chronic sleep loss predisposes to diminished ability to concentrate, impaired memory, failure to accomplish daily tasks, and interpersonal difficulties. The male patient may experience impotence. Driving accidents are more common in habitually sleepy persons.[13] Family life and the patient's ability to maintain employment are also often compromised. As a result, the patient may experience severe depression. Appropriate referral should be made if problems are identified. Cessation of breathing reported by the bed partner is usually a source of great anxiety because of the fear that breathing may not resume.

Diagnosis of sleep apnea is made by polysomnography. The patient's chest and abdominal movement, oral airflow, nasal airflow, SpO_2, ocular movement, and heart rate and rhythm are monitored. Progression through each sleep stage is determined by monitoring brain waves through electroencephalography (EEG). A diagnosis of sleep apnea requires documentation of apneic events (no airflow with respiratory effort) or hypopnea (airflow diminished 30% to 50% with respiratory effort). Generally, more than 10 events an hour with oxygen desaturation below 90% is considered a positive test for OSA. Typically, polysomnography is carried out in a sleep laboratory with sleep technicians monitoring the patient. In some instances, portable sleep studies are conducted in the home setting. Overnight pulse oximetry assessment may be an alternative to determine if nocturnal O_2 supplementation is indicated.

NURSING *and* COLLABORATIVE MANAGEMENT SLEEP APNEA

Mild sleep apnea may respond to simple measures. The patient should be instructed to avoid sedatives and alcoholic beverages for 3 to 4 hours before sleep. Referral to a weight loss program may help, because excessive weight worsens sleep apnea.[14] Symptoms resolve in up to half of patients with OSA who use an oral appliance during sleep to prevent airflow obstruction. Oral appliances bring the mandible and tongue forward to enlarge the airway

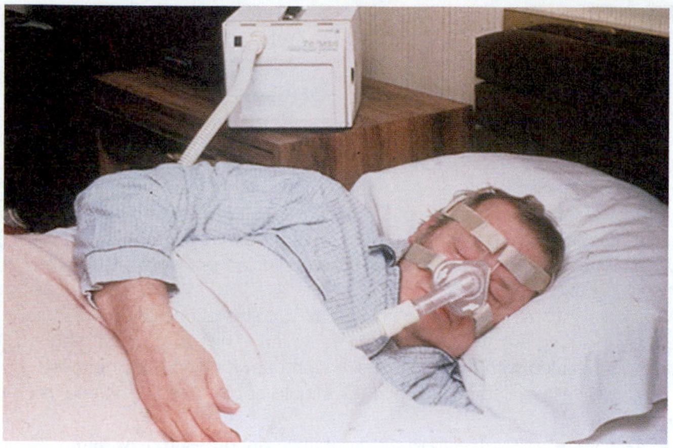

FIG. 27-5 Management of sleep apnea often involves sleeping with a nasal mask in place. The pressure supplied by air coming from the compressor opens the oropharynx and nasopharynx.

space, thereby preventing airway occlusion. Some individuals find a support group beneficial, where concerns and feelings can be expressed and strategies for resolving problems can be discussed.

In patients with more severe symptoms, continuous positive airway pressure (CPAP) by mask is the treatment of choice.[12,13] With CPAP, the patient applies a nasal mask that is attached to a high-flow blower (Fig. 27-5). The blower is adjusted to maintain sufficient positive pressure (5 to 20 cm H_2O) in the airway during inspiration and expiration to prevent airway collapse. Some patients cannot adjust to exhaling against the high pressure. A technologically more sophisticated therapy, bilevel positive airway pressure (BiPAP), can deliver a higher inspiration pressure and a lower pressure during expiration. With BiPAP the apnea can be relieved with a lower mean pressure and may be better tolerated. Although CPAP is highly effective, compliance may be poor even if symptoms of sleep apnea are relieved.[12-14] When patients with a history of OSA are hospitalized, the nurse must be aware that the use of opioid pain medications may worsen the symptoms by depressing respiration, necessitating that the patient wear the CPAP or BiPAP when resting or sleeping.

If other measures fail, sleep apnea may be managed surgically. The two most common procedures are uvulopalatopharyngoplasty (UPPP or UP3) and genioglossal advancement and hyoid myotomy (GAHM). UPPP involves excision of the tonsillar pillars, uvula, and posterior soft palate with the goal of removing the obstructing tissue. GAHM involves advancing the attachment of the muscular part of the tongue on the mandible. When GAHM is performed, UPPP is generally performed as well. Symptoms are relieved in up to 60% of patients.[15] Laser-assisted uvulopalatoplasty (LAUP) is a new surgical procedure that has been used to treat OSA. Complications of airway obstruction or hemorrhage occur most often in the immediate postoperative period. Therefore patients can usually be discharged to home within 1 day following the procedure.[16]

Problems Related to the Trachea and Larynx

AIRWAY OBSTRUCTION

Airway obstruction may be complete or partial. Complete airway obstruction is a medical emergency. Partial airway obstruction may occur as a result of aspiration of food or a foreign body. In addition, partial airway obstruction may result from laryngeal edema following extubation, laryngeal or tracheal stenosis, central nervous system depression, and allergic reactions. Symptoms include stridor, use of accessory muscles, suprasternal and intercostal retractions, wheezing, restlessness, tachycardia, and cyanosis. Prompt assessment and treatment are essential because partial obstruction may quickly progress to complete obstruction. Interventions to reestablish a patent airway include the obstructed airway (Heimlich) maneuver (see Appendix A), cricothyroidotomy, endotracheal intubation, and tracheostomy. Unexplained or recurrent symptoms indicate the need for additional tests, such as a chest x-ray, pulmonary function tests, and bronchoscopy.

TRACHEOSTOMY

A **tracheotomy** is a surgical incision into the trachea for the purpose of establishing an airway. A **tracheostomy** is the stoma (opening) that results from the tracheotomy. Indications for a tracheostomy are to (1) bypass an upper airway obstruction, (2) facilitate removal of secretions, (3) permit long-term mechanical ventilation, and (4) permit oral intake and speech in the patient who requires long-term mechanical ventilation. Most patients who require mechanical ventilation are initially managed with an endotracheal tube, which can be quickly inserted in an emergency. (Care of the patient with an endotracheal tube is discussed in Chapter 66.) Previously, a tracheostomy required surgical dissection and was therefore not typically an emergency procedure. A newer procedure, a *percutaneous tracheostomy,* can be performed emergently at the bedside, and has been reported to be a valid alternative to a surgically inserted tracheostomy, with reports of less bleeding and fewer postoperative infections.[17]

Several advantages make a tracheostomy the better option for long-term care. With a tracheostomy, there is less risk of long-term damage to the airway. Patient comfort may be increased because no tube is present in the mouth. The patient can eat with a tracheostomy because the tube enters lower in the airway (Fig. 27-6). Because the tracheostomy tube is more secure, mobility may be increased.[18]

NURSING MANAGEMENT TRACHEOSTOMY

Providing Tracheostomy Care

Before the tracheotomy procedure, the nurse should explain to the patient and the family the purpose of the procedure. They should also be informed that the patient will not be able to speak while an inflated cuff is used.

A variety of tubes are available to meet individual patient needs (Table 27-5). All tracheostomy tubes contain a faceplate or flange, which rests on the neck between the clavicles and outer cannula. In addition, all tubes have an obturator, which is used when inserting the tube (see Fig. 27-6, *C*). During surgical insertion of the tube, the obturator is placed inside the outer cannula with its rounded tip protruding from the end of the tube to ease insertion. After insertion, the obturator must be immediately removed so air can flow through the tube. The obturator should be kept in an easily accessible place at the bedside (e.g., taped to the wall) so that it can be used quickly in case of accidental decannulation.[19]

Some tracheostomy tubes also have an inner cannula, which can be removed for cleaning (see Fig. 27-6, *B*). The cleaning procedure removes mucus from the inside of the tube. If humidification is adequate, mucus may not accumulate and a tube with-

TABLE 27-5 Characteristics and Nursing Management of Tracheostomies

Tube	Characteristics	Nursing Management
Tracheostomy tube with cuff and pilot balloon (see Fig. 27-6, *A* and *B*)	When properly inflated, low-pressure, high-volume cuff distributes cuff pressure over large area, minimizing pressure on tracheal wall.	**Procedure for cuff inflation** • *Mechanically ventilated patient:* Inflate the cuff to *minimal occlusion pressure* by slowly injecting air into the cuff until no leak (sound) is heard at peak inspiratory pressure (end of ventilator inspiration) when a stethoscope is placed over the trachea. Use cuff pressure monitor to determine cuff inflation pressure. An alternative approach, termed *minimal leak technique* (MLT), involves inflating the cuff to minimal occlusion pressure and then withdrawing 0.1 ml of air. • *Spontaneously breathing patient:* Inflate cuff to minimal occlusion pressure by slowly injecting air into the cuff until no sound is heard after deep breath or during inhalation with manual resuscitation bag. If using MLT, remove 0.1 ml of air while maintaining seal. MLT should not be used if there is risk of aspiration. • *Immediately after cuff inflation (both groups):* Verify pressure is within accepted range ($\leq$20 mm Hg or $\leq$25 cm H_2O) with a manometer. Record cuff pressure and volume of air used for cuff inflation in chart. **Care of patients with an inflated cuff** • Monitor and record cuff pressure q8hr. Cuff pressure should be $\leq$20 mm Hg or $\leq$25 cm H_2O to allow adequate tracheal capillary perfusion. If needed, remove or add air to the pilot tubing using a syringe and stopcock. Afterward, verify cuff pressure is within accepted range with manometer. • Report inability to keep the cuff inflated or need to use progressively larger volumes of air to keep cuff inflated. Potential causes include tracheal dilation at the cuff site or a crack or slow leak in the housing of the one-way inflation valve. If the leak is due to tracheal dilation, the physician may intubate the patient with a larger tube. Cracks in the inflation valve may be temporarily managed by clamping the small-bore tubing with a hemostat. The tube should be changed within 24 hr.
Fenestrated tracheostomy tube (Shiley, Portex) with cuff, inner cannula, and decannulation plug (see Fig. 27-6, *B*; Fig. 27-9, *A*)	When inner cannula is removed, cuff deflated, and decannulation plug inserted, air flows around tube, through fenestration in outer cannula, and up over vocal cords. Patient can then speak.	• Assess risk of aspiration before removing inner cannula. Deflate cuff. Note coughing. Have patient swallow a small amount of clear liquid (grape juice) or 30 ml of water with a few drops of blue food coloring. Observe secretions after patient coughs or when suctioned for presence of colored secretions. If no aspiration is noted, a fenestrated tube may be used. • ***Never*** insert decannulation plug in tracheostomy tube until cuff is deflated and inner cannula removed. Prior insertion will prevent patient from breathing (no air inflow). This may precipitate a respiratory arrest. • Assess for signs of respiratory distress when a fenestrated cannula is first used. If this occurs, the cap should be removed, the inner cannula replaced, and the cuff reinflated. • Cuff management as described above.
Speaking tracheostomy tube (Portex, National) with cuff, two external tubings (see Fig. 27-9, *B*)	Has two tubings, one leading to cuff and second to opening above the cuff. When port is connected to air source, air flows out of opening and up over the vocal cords, allowing speech with cuff inflated.	• Once tube is inserted, wait 2 days before use so that the stoma can close around the tube and prevent leaks. • When patient desires to speak, connect port to compressed air (or oxygen). Be certain to identify correct tubing. If gas enters the cuff, it will overinflate and rupture, requiring an emergency tube change. Use lowest flow (typically 4–6 L/min) that results in speech. High flows dehydrate mucosa. • Cover port adapter. This will cause the air to flow upward. Instruct patient to speak in short sentences because voice becomes a whisper with long sentences. • Disconnect flow when patient does not want to speak to prevent mucosal dehydration. • Cuff management as described above.
Tracheostomy tube (Bivona Fome-Cuf) with foam-filled cuff (see Fig. 27-6, *C*)	Cuff is filled with plastic foam. Before insertion, cuff is deflated. After insertion, cuff is allowed to fill passively with air. Pilot tubing is not capped, and no cuff pressure monitoring is required.	• Before insertion, withdraw all air from the cuff using a 20-ml syringe. Cap pilot balloon tubing to prevent reentry of air. After tracheostomy is inserted, remove cap from pilot tubing, allowing cuff to passively reinflate. • Do not inject air into tubing or cap pilot balloon tubing while in patient. Air will flow in and out in response to pressure changes (head turning). Place tag on tubing alerting staff not to cap or inflate cuff. • Deflate cuff daily via pilot balloon to evaluate integrity of cuff. Also assess ability to easily deflate cuff. Difficulty deflating cuff indicates a need for tube change. If aspirate returns with air, the cuff is no longer intact. • Tube can be used for up to 1 mo in patients on home mechanical ventilation. • Good choice for patients who require inflated cuff at home since teaching about cuff pressure is simplified.

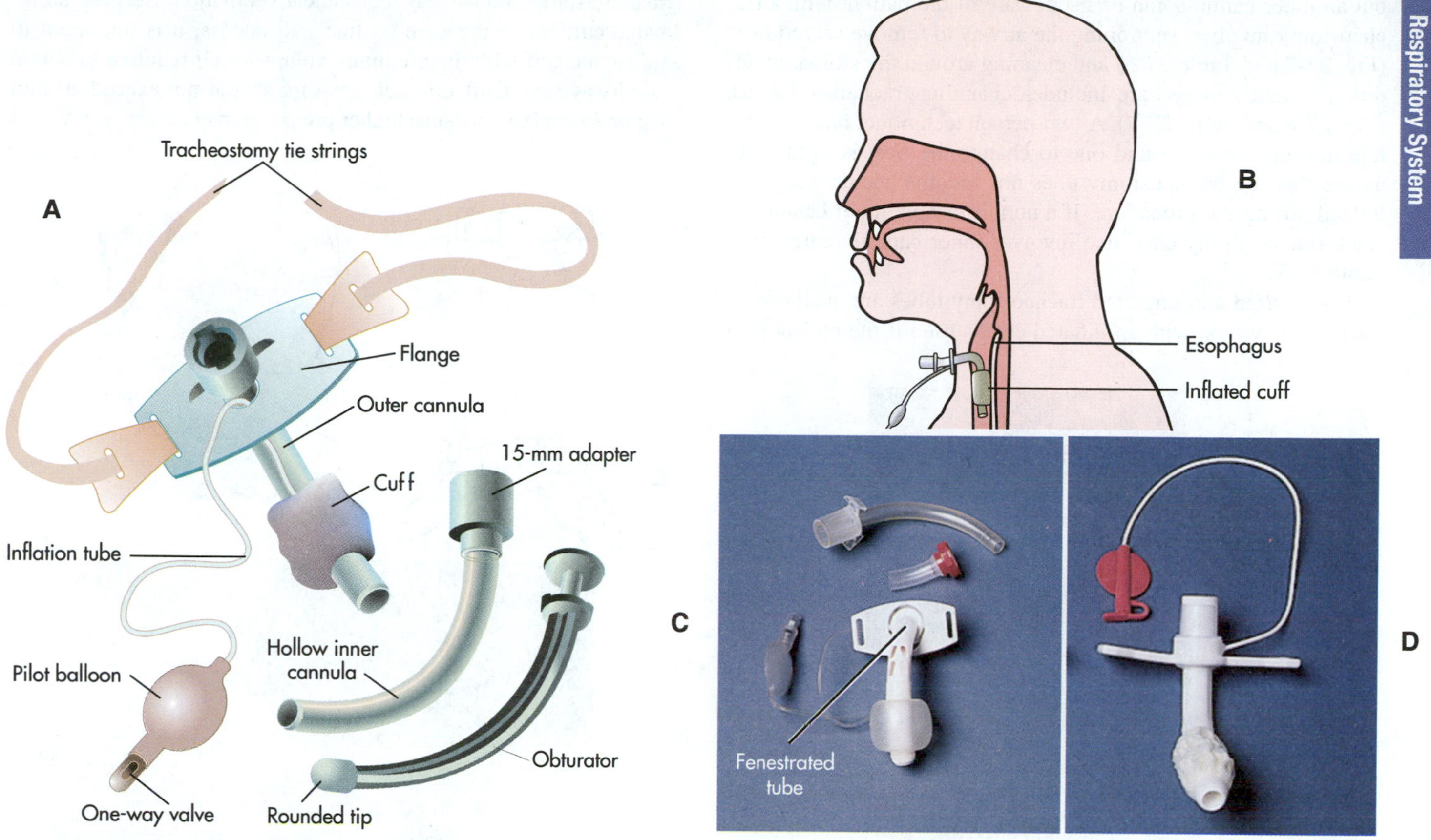

FIG. 27-6 Types of tracheostomy tubes. **A,** Parts of a tracheostomy tube. **B,** Tracheostomy tube inserted in airway with inflated cuff. **C,** Fenestrated tracheostomy tube with cuff, inner cannula, decannulation plug, and pilot balloon. **D,** Tracheostomy tube with foam cuff and obturator (one cuff is deflated on tracheostomy tube). (See Table 27-5 and NCP 27-1 for related nursing management.)

TABLE 27-6 Procedure for Suctioning a Tracheostomy Tube

1. Assess the need for suctioning q2hr. Indications include coarse crackles or rhonchi over large airways, moist cough, increase in peak inspiratory pressure on mechanical ventilator, and restlessness or agitation if accompanied by decrease in SpO_2 or PaO_2. Do not suction routinely or if patient is able to clear secretions with cough.
2. If suctioning is indicated, explain procedure to patient.
3. Collect necessary sterile equipment: suction catheter (no larger than half the lumen of the tracheostomy tube), gloves, water, cup, and drape. If a closed tracheal suction system is used, the catheter is enclosed in a plastic sleeve and reused. No additional equipment is needed.
4. Check suction source and regulator. Adjust suction pressure until the dial reads −120 to −150 mm Hg pressure with tubing occluded.
5. Assess SpO_2, heart rate and rhythm to provide baseline for detecting change during suctioning.
6. Wash hands. Put on goggles and gloves.
7. Use sterile technique to open package, fill cup with water, put on gloves, and connect catheter to suction. Designate one hand as contaminated for disconnecting, bagging, and operating the suction control. Suction water through the catheter to test the system.
8. Provide preoxygenation by (1) adjusting ventilator to deliver 100% O_2; (2) using a reservoir-equipped manual resuscitation bag (MRB) connected to 100% oxygen; or (3) asking the patient to take 3-4 deep breaths while administering oxygen. The method chosen will depend on the patient's underlying disease and acuity of illness. The patient who has had a tracheostomy for an extended period of time and is not acutely ill may be able to tolerate suctioning without use of an MRB or the ventilator.
9. Gently insert catheter *without suction* to minimize the amount of oxygen removed from the lungs. Insert the catheter the length of the artificial airway. Stop if an obstruction is met.
10. Withdraw the catheter ½–¾ inch (1–2 cm) and apply suction intermittently, while withdrawing catheter in a rotating manner. If secretion volume is large, apply suction continuously.
11. *Limit suction time to 10 seconds.* Discontinue suctioning if heart rate decreases from baseline by 20 beats/minute, increases from baseline by 40 beats/minute, a dysrhythmia occurs, or SpO_2 decreases to less than 90%.
12. After each suction pass, oxygenate with 3–4 breaths by ventilator, MRB, or deep breaths with oxygen.
13. Rinse catheter with sterile water (if in suction kit).
14. Repeat procedure until airway is clear. Limit insertions of suction catheter to as few as needed.
15. Return oxygen concentration to prior setting.
16. Rinse catheter and suction the oropharynx or use mouth suction.
17. Dispose of catheter by wrapping it around fingers of gloved hand and pulling glove over catheter. Discard equipment in proper waste container.
18. Auscultate to assess changes in lung sounds. Record time, amount, and character of secretions and response to suctioning.

out an inner cannula can be used. Care of the patient with a tracheostomy involves suctioning the airway to remove secretions[20] (Fig. 27-7 and Table 27-6) and cleaning around the stoma. In addition, tracheostomy care includes changing tracheostomy ties (Fig. 27-8 and Table 27-7). A two-person technique, one to stabilize the tracheostomy and one to change the ties, is optimal to assure that the tracheostomy does not become accidentally dislodged during the procedure. If a nondisposable inner cannula is used, tracheostomy care also involves inner cannula care[21] (see Table 27-7).

Both cuffed and uncuffed tracheostomy tubes are available. A tracheostomy tube with an inflated cuff is used if the patient is at risk of aspiration or needs mechanical ventilation. Because an inflated cuff exerts pressure on tracheal mucosa, it is important to inflate the cuff with the minimum volume of air required to obtain an airway seal. Cuff inflation pressure should not exceed 20 mm Hg or 25 cm H_2O because higher pressures may compress tracheal

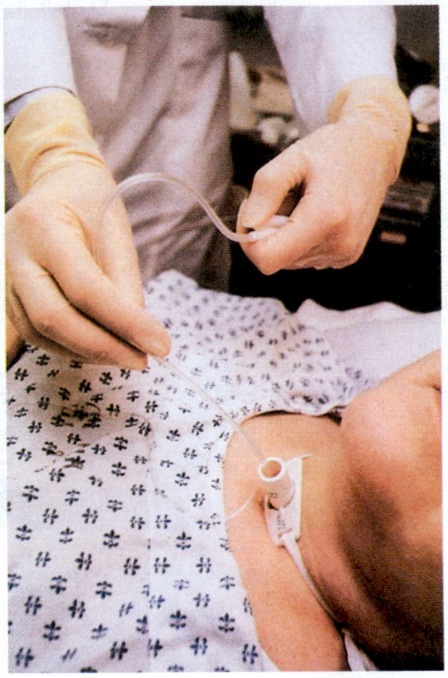

FIG. 27-7 Suctioning a tracheostomy. Using sterile technique, the suction catheter is being withdrawn from the airway while suction is applied. The pilot balloon tubing may be seen lying on the patient's chest.

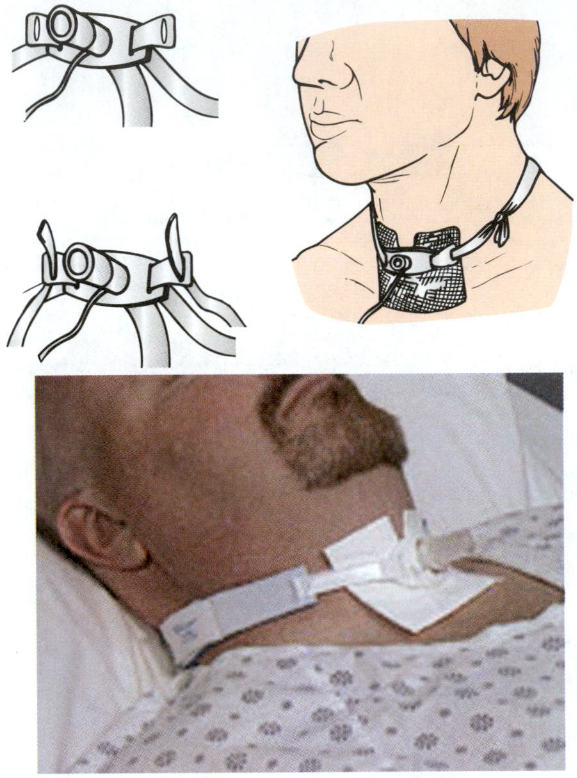

FIG. 27-8 Changing tracheostomy ties. **A,** A slit is cut about 1 inch (2.5 cm) from the end. The slit end is put into the opening of the cannula. **B,** A loop is made with the other end of the tape. **C,** The tapes are tied together with a double knot on the side of the neck. **D,** A tracheostomy tube holder can be used in place of twill ties to make tracheostomy tube stabilization more secure.

TABLE 27-7 Tracheostomy Care

1. Explain procedure to patient.
2. Use tracheostomy care kit or collect necessary sterile equipment (e.g., suction catheter, gloves, water, basin, drape, tracheostomy ties, tube brush or pipe cleaners, 4 × 4 gauze pads, hydrogen peroxide [3%], sterile water, and tracheostomy dressing [optional]). *Note:* Clean rather than sterile technique is used at home.
3. Position patient in semi-Fowler's position.
4. Assemble needed materials on bedside table next to patient.
5. Wash hands. Put on goggles and clean gloves.
6. Auscultate chest sounds. If rhonchi or coarse crackles are present, suction the patient if unable to cough up secretions (see Table 27-6). Remove soiled dressing and clean gloves.
7. Open sterile equipment, pour sterile H_2O and hydrogen peroxide in basins, and put on sterile gloves.
8. Unlock and remove inner cannula, if present. Many tracheostomy tubes do not have inner cannulas. Care for these tubes includes all steps except for inner cannula care.
9. If disposable inner cannula is used, replace with new cannula. If a nondisposable cannula is used:
   a. Immerse inner cannula in 3% hydrogen peroxide and clean inside and outside of cannula using tube brush or pipe cleaners.
   b. Drain hydrogen peroxide from cannula. Immerse cannula in sterile water. Remove from sterile water and shake to dry.
   c. Insert inner cannula into outer cannula with the curved part downward and lock in place.
10. Remove dried secretions from stoma using 4 × 4 gauze pad soaked in hydrogen peroxide. Rinse with another 4 × 4 soaked in sterile water. Gently pat area around the stoma dry. Be sure to clean under the tracheostomy faceplate, using cotton swabs to reach this area.
11. Maintain position of tracheal retention sutures, if present, by taping above and below the stoma.
12. Change tracheostomy ties. Use two-person change technique or secure new ties to flanges before removing the old ones. Tie tracheostomy ties securely with room for one finger between ties and skin (see Fig. 27-8). To prevent accidental tube removal, secure the tracheostomy tube by gently applying pressure to the flange of the tube during the tie changes. *Do not change tracheostomy ties for 24 hr after the tracheotomy procedure.*
13. As an alternative, some patients prefer tracheostomy ties made of Velcro, which are easier to adjust.
14. If drainage is excessive, place dressing around tube (see Fig. 27-8). A tracheostomy dressing or unlined gauze should be used. Do not cut the gauze because threads may be inhaled or wrap around the tracheostomy tube. Change the dressing frequently. Wet dressings promote infection and stoma irritation.
15. Repeat care 3 times a day and as needed.

capillaries, limit blood flow, and predispose to tracheal necrosis. An alternative approach, termed the *minimal leak technique* (MLT), involves inflating the cuff with the minimum amount of air to obtain a seal and then withdrawing 0.1 ml of air. A disadvantage of MLT is risk of aspiration from secretions leaking around the cuff. MLT should not be used when the tracheostomy was placed to bypass an upper airway obstruction, such as with head and neck surgical patients.[20]

In some patients, cuff deflation is performed to remove secretions that accumulate above the cuff. Before deflation, the patient should cough up secretions, if possible, and the tracheostomy tube and mouth should be suctioned (see Fig. 27-7 and Table 27-6). This step is important to prevent secretions from being aspirated during deflation. The cuff is deflated during exhalation because the exhaled gas helps propel secretions into the mouth. The patient should also cough or be suctioned after cuff deflation. The cuff should be reinflated during inspiration. The volume of air required to inflate the cuff should be monitored daily because this volume may increase if there is tracheal dilation from cuff pressure. The nurse should assess the ability of the patient to protect the airway from aspiration and remain with the patient when the cuff is initially deflated unless the patient can protect the airway from aspiration and breathe without respiratory distress. When the patient can protect the airway from aspiration and does not require mechanical ventilation, a cuffless tracheostomy tube should be used.

Retention sutures are often placed in the tracheal cartilage when the tracheostomy is performed. The free ends should be taped to the skin in a place and manner that leaves them accessible if the tube is dislodged. Care should be taken not to dislodge the tracheostomy tube during the first few days when the stoma is not mature (healed). Because tube replacement can be difficult, several precautions are required: (1) a replacement tube of equal or smaller size is kept at the bedside, readily available for emergency reinsertion; (2) tracheostomy tapes are not changed for at least 24 hours after the insertion procedure; and (3) the first tube change is performed by a physician usually no sooner than 7 days after the tracheostomy.

If the tube is accidentally dislodged, the nurse should immediately attempt to replace it. The retention sutures (if present) are grasped and the opening is spread. A hemostat can also be used to spread the opening to facilitate replacing the tube. The obturator is inserted in the replacement tube, lubricated with saline poured over the tip, and the tube is inserted in the stoma at a 45-degree angle to the neck. If insertion is successful, the obturator is removed immediately so that air can flow through the tube. Another method is to insert a suction catheter to allow passage of air and to serve as a guide for insertion. The tracheostomy tube should be threaded over the catheter and the suction catheter removed. If the tube cannot be replaced, assess the level of respiratory distress. Minor dyspnea may be alleviated by use of the semi-Fowler's position until assistance arrives. Severe dyspnea may progress to respiratory arrest. If this situation occurs, the stoma should be covered with a sterile dressing, and the patient should be ventilated with bag-mask ventilation until help arrives, unless the patient has experienced a total laryngectomy and has complete separation between the upper airway and the trachea.

Initially, tracheostomy patients should receive humidified air to compensate for the loss of the upper airway to warm and moisturize secretions. After the first tube change, the tube should be changed approximately once a month. When a tracheostomy has been in place for several months, the healed tract will be well formed. The patient can then be taught to change the tube using a clean technique at home (Fig. 27-9). Teaching will vary, depending on the illness of the patient and the device selected.

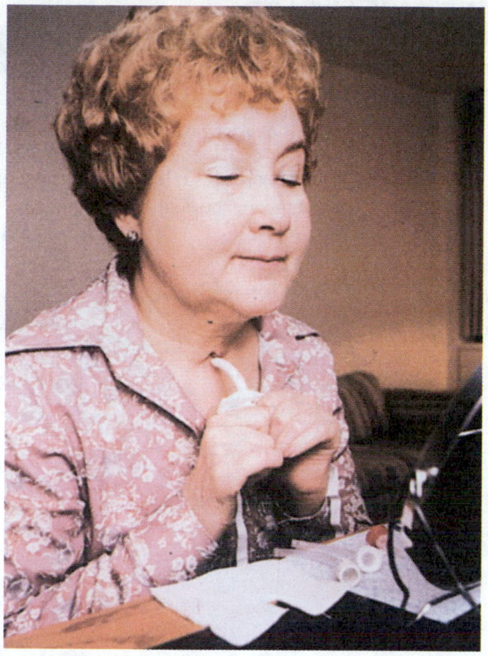

FIG. 27-9 Changing the tracheostomy tube at home. When a tracheostomy has been in place for several months, the tract will be well formed. The patient can then be taught to change the tube using a clean technique at home.

Nursing diagnoses for the patient with a tracheostomy include, but are not limited to, those presented in NCP 27-1.

Swallowing Dysfunction

The patient with a tracheostomy who cannot protect the airway from aspiration requires an inflated cuff. However, an inflated cuff may result in swallowing dysfunction because the cuff interferes with the normal function of muscles used to swallow. For this reason, it is important to evaluate the risk for aspiration with the cuff deflated. The patient may be able to swallow without aspirating when the cuff is deflated but not when it is inflated. The cuff may then be left deflated or a cuffless tube substituted (see Fig. 27-10).

There are two ways to evaluate aspiration: adding blue food coloring to a clear liquid or testing of tracheobronchial secretions for glucose. In the first method, the cuff is deflated and the patient is instructed to swallow a small amount of clear liquid such as grape juice or 30 ml of water that has blue food coloring added. Any coughing and secretions are noted. If needed, the trachea is suctioned to check for the presence of blue-colored secretions. If there is no indication of aspiration, the patient is judged to have adequate epiglottic function without risk for aspiration. This method may place the patient at risk for allergic reactions to the food coloring, and is also very subjective.[20] In the second method, tracheobronchial secretions are tested for glucose with the understanding that mucus generally has a low glucose content. Limitations of this method include false-positive results if the mucus is blood-tinged.[20] A formal swallowing evaluation may be done by a speech therapist.

Respiratory System

NURSING CARE PLAN 27-1

Patient with a Tracheostomy

NURSING DIAGNOSIS **Ineffective airway clearance** *related to* presence of tracheostomy tube and difficulty expectorating sputum *as evidenced by* adventitious breath sounds, tenacious secretions, increase in restlessness, ineffective or absent cough

PATIENT GOALS
1. Demonstrates effective coughing and secretion clearance
2. Maintains normal breath sounds

OUTCOMES (NOC)

Respiratory Status: Airway Patency

- Ease of breathing ____
- Respiratory rate ____
- Respiratory rhythm ____
- Moves sputum out of airway ____
- Moves blockage out of airway ____

Measurement Scale

1 = Severely compromised
2 = Substantially compromised
3 = Moderately compromised
4 = Mildly compromised
5 = Not compromised

- Adventitious breath sounds ____

Measurement Scale

1 = Severe
2 = Substantial
3 = Moderate
4 = Mild
5 = None

INTERVENTIONS (NIC) and *RATIONALES*

Airway Management

- Auscultate breath sounds, noting areas of decreased or absent ventilation and presence of adventitious sounds.
- Remove secretions by encouraging coughing or by suctioning *to clear airway.*
- Encourage slow deep breathing, turning, and coughing *to assist in mobilizing secretions.*
- Position to alleviate dyspnea (e.g., head of bed elevated 30-40 degrees) *to allow maximum lung expansion and a more forceful cough.*
- Monitor respiratory and oxygenation status *to determine effectiveness of interventions.*

Artificial Airway Management

- Provide 100% humidification of inspired gas/air *because normal upper airway humidification not present.*
- Provide adequate systemic hydration via oral or intravenous fluid administration *to liquefy secretions.*
- Suction oropharynx and secretions from top of tube cuff before deflating cuff *to prevent aspiration of upper airway secretions.*
- Tape a second tracheostomy tube (same type and size) and forceps to head of bed to replace tube *to maintain airway in case of accidental decannulation.*
- Maintain inflation of endotracheal/tracheostoma cuff at 15 to 20 mm Hg during mechanical ventilation and during and after feeding *to minimize pressure on trachea.*

NURSING DIAGNOSIS **Ineffective therapeutic regimen management** *related to* lack of knowledge about care of tracheostomy at home *as evidenced by* questioning about care (patient and/or family), agitation, and restlessness when planning for discharge

PATIENT GOALS
1. Demonstrates satisfactory tracheostomy care, including suctioning and stoma care
2. Verbalizes key elements of the therapeutic regimen, including knowledge of disease and treatment plan

OUTCOMES (NOC)

Knowledge: Treatment Procedure(s)

- Description of treatment procedure(s) ____
- Description of steps in procedure(s) ____
- Description of use of equipment ____

Measurement Scale

1 = None
2 = Limited
3 = Moderate
4 = Substantial
5 = Extensive

Knowledge: Disease Process

- Description of cause or contributing factors ____
- Description of usual disease course ____
- Description of signs and symptoms of complications ____

Measurement Scale

1= None
2= Limited
3= Moderate
4= Substantial
5= Extensive

INTERVENTIONS (NIC) and *RATIONALES*

Teaching: Psychomotor Skill

- Demonstrate skill for patient.
- Give clear, step-by-step directions *so patient can care for self at home.*
- Provide practice sessions (spaced to avoid fatigue, but often enough to prevent excessive forgetting).
- Provide frequent feedback to patient on what he/she is doing correctly and incorrectly *so patient can care for self at home.*
- Provide written information/diagrams *for reference.*
- Observe patient return demonstrate skill *to assess skill level and need for additional teaching.*

Teaching: Disease Process

- Identify possible etiologies *so patient understands rationale for tracheostomy.*
- Describe the disease process *to allow patient to plan treatment routine.*
- Instruct the patient on which signs and symptoms (e.g., changes in secretion [yellow to green or blood-tinged] and/or elevated body temperature) to report to health care provider *as these may be early signs of respiratory infection.*
- Refer patient to local community agencies/support groups *to provide ongoing assistance and support.*

NURSING CARE PLAN 27-1

Patient with a Tracheostomy—cont'd

NURSING DIAGNOSIS **Impaired verbal communication** *related to* use of cuffed artificial airway *as evidenced by* inability to speak and signs of frustration

PATIENT GOAL Uses effective written and nonverbal communication techniques to exchange messages with others

OUTCOMES (NOC)

Communication

- Use of written language ____
- Use of pictures and drawings ____
- Use of nonverbal language ____
- Exchanges messages accurately with others ____

Measurement Scale

1 = Severely compromised
2 = Substantially compromised
3 = Moderately compromised
4 = Mildly compromised
5 = Not compromised

INTERVENTIONS (NIC) and *RATIONALES*

Communication Enhancement: Speech Deficit

- Listen attentively.
- Use picture board.

Teaching: Disease Process

- Provide information to patient about condition.
- Provide reassurance about patient's condition *to allay fear and frustration.*
- Instruct patient on measures to control/minimize symptoms (e.g., small cuffless tube, fenestrated tube, speaking valve, speaking tracheostomy tube) *to permit speech.*

NURSING DIAGNOSIS **Risk for infection** *related to* bypass of upper airway defense mechanisms and impaired skin integrity

PATIENT GOAL Demonstrates no signs or symptoms of infection

OUTCOMES (NOC)

Infection Severity

- Purulent sputum ____
- Fever ____
- Pain/tenderness ____
- Malaise ____
- Chilling ____
- Lethargy ____
- Sputum culture colonization ____
- White blood cell count elevation ____

Measurement Scale

1 = Severe
2 = Substantial
3 = Moderate
4 = Mild
5 = None

INTERVENTIONS (NIC) and *RATIONALES*

Infection Protection

- Monitor for systemic and localized signs and symptoms of infection *to promote early detection of infection.*
- Monitor absolute granulocyte count, WBC count, and differential results *to promote early detection of infection.*

Artificial Airway Management

- Maintain sterile technique when suctioning and providing tracheostomy care *to reduce occurrence of infection.*
- Provide trachea care every 4 to 8 hours as appropriate: clean inner cannula, clean and dry the area around the stoma, and change tracheostomy ties.

Tube Care

- Inspect the area around the tube insertion site for redness and skin breakdown *to detect infection.*
- Change tube routinely, as indicated by agency protocol, *to prevent contaminated tubing from being a source of infection.*

NURSING DIAGNOSIS **Impaired swallowing** *related to* tracheostomy tube *as evidenced by* inability to swallow without difficulty and/or without aspiration

PATIENT GOAL Demonstrates adequate swallowing of oral foods without aspiration

OUTCOMES (NOC)

Swallowing Status

- Maintains food in mouth ____
- Handles oral secretions ____
- Ability to clear oral cavity ____
- Timely swallow reflex ____
- Swallow study findings: oral phase ____

Measurement Scale

1 = Severely compromised
2 = Substantially compromised
3 = Moderately compromised
4 = Mildly compromised
5 = Not compromised

INTERVENTIONS (NIC) and *RATIONALES*

Swallowing Therapy

- Determine patient's ability to focus attention on learning/performing eating and swallowing tasks *to evaluate patient's potential for oral intake.*
- Provide/monitor consistency of food/liquid based on findings of swallowing study *to ease swallowing and minimize aspiration.*
- Monitor for signs and symptoms of aspiration *that indicate swallowing dysfunction.*
- Monitor body weight *to determine need for enteral feedings to maintain nutrition.*

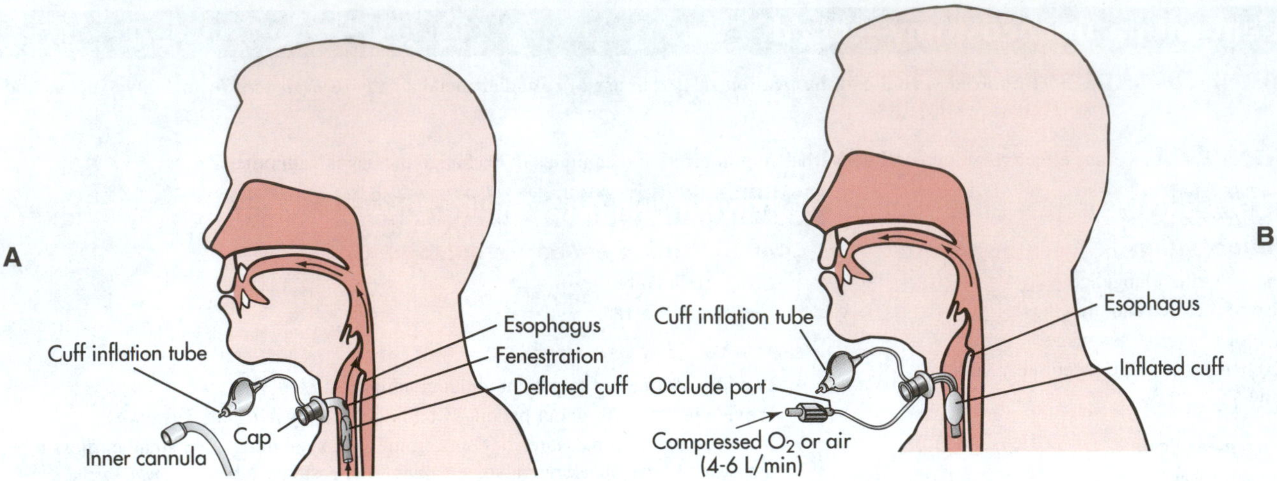

FIG. 27-10 Speaking tracheostomy tubes. **A,** Fenestrated tracheostomy tube with cuff deflated, inner cannula removed, and tracheostomy tube capped to allow air to pass over the vocal cords. **B,** Speaking tracheostomy tube. One tube is used for cuff inflation. The second tube is connected to a source of compressed air or oxygen. When the port on the second tube is occluded, air flows up over the vocal cords, allowing speech with an inflated cuff. (See Table 27-5 and NCP 27-1 for related nursing management.)

Speech with a Tracheostomy Tube

A number of techniques promote speech in the patient with a tracheostomy. The spontaneously breathing patient may be able to talk by deflating the cuff, which allows exhaled air to flow upward over the vocal cords. This can be enhanced by the patient occluding the tube. Frequently, a small cuffless tube is inserted so exhaled air can pass freely around the tube. If the patient is on mechanical ventilation, speech may be possible by allowing a constant air leak around the cuff. In addition, tracheostomy tubes and valves have been designed to facilitate speech. The nurse can be an advocate in promoting use of these specialized devices. Their use can provide great psychologic benefit and facilitate self-care for the patient with a tracheostomy.

A fenestrated tube has openings on the surface of the outer cannula that permit air from the lungs to flow over the vocal cords (see Fig. 27-6, *C,* and Fig. 27-10, *A*). A fenestrated tube allows the patient to breathe spontaneously through the larynx, speak, and cough up secretions while the tracheostomy tube remains in place. It can be used by the patient who can swallow without risk of aspiration but requires suctioning for secretion removal. It may also be used by the patient who requires mechanical ventilation for fewer than 24 hours a day (e.g., during sleep).

Before the fenestrated tube is used, the patient's ability to swallow without aspiration is determined (see Table 27-5 and NCP 27-1). If there is no aspiration, (1) the inner cannula is removed, (2) the cuff is deflated, and (3) the decannulation cap is placed in the tube (see Fig. 27-10, *A*). It is important to perform the steps in order because severe respiratory distress may result if the tube is capped before the inner cannula is removed and the cuff deflated. When a fenestrated cannula is first used, the nurse should frequently assess the patient for signs of respiratory distress. If the patient is not able to tolerate the procedure, the cap should be removed, the inner cannula replaced, and the cuff reinflated. A disadvantage of fenestrated tubes is the potential for development of tracheal polyps from tracheal tissue granulating into the fenestrated openings.[22] A speaking tracheostomy tube has two pigtail tubings. One tubing connects to the cuff and is used for cuff inflation, and the second connects to an opening just above the cuff (see Fig. 27-10, *B*). When the second tubing is connected to a low-flow (4 to 6 L/min) air source, sufficient air moves up over the vocal cords to permit speech. The patient can then speak, although the cuff is inflated.

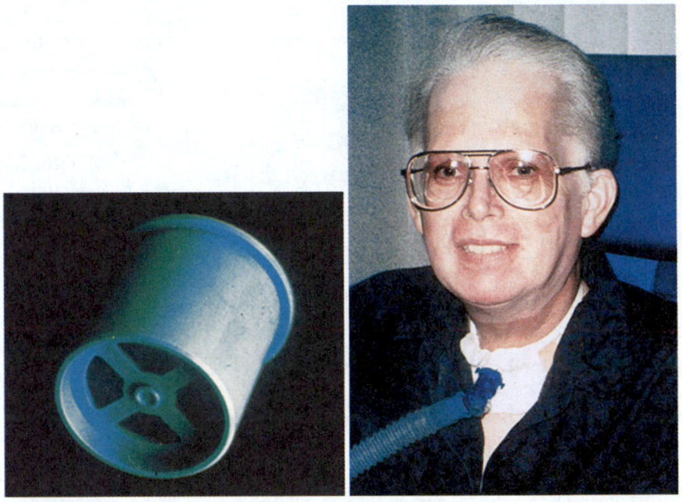

FIG. 27-11 Passy-Muir™ Tracheostomy & Ventilator Swallowing and Speaking Valves (PMVs). The PMV™ is placed over the hub of the tracheostomy tube after the cuff is deflated. The valve contains a one-way diaphragm that allows air to enter the lungs during inspiration and redirects air upward over the vocal cords into the mouth during expiration. The PMV 007 (Aqua) (shown) is designed for use with disposable ventilator tubing. The PMV 2000 (Clear) & PMV 2001 (Purple) can also be used on the ventilator with non-disposable tubing. All PMVs (with the exception of the PMV 2020 for metal trach tubes) can be used on or off the ventilator with the appropriate ventilator tubing.

When a speaking tracheostomy valve is used, a cuffless tube must be in place or the cuff needs to be deflated to allow exhalation (Fig. 27-11). Ability to tolerate cuff deflation without aspiration or respiratory distress must also be evaluated in patients using this device. If there is no aspiration, the cuff is deflated and the valve is placed over the tracheostomy tube opening. The speaking valve contains a thin plastic diaphragm that opens on inspiration and closes on expiration. During inspiration, air flows in through the valve. During expiration, the diaphragm prevents exhalation and air flows upward over the vocal cords and into the mouth.

If speaking devices are not used, the patient should be provided with a paper and pencil or Magic Slate. A word (communication) board can usually be obtained from speech therapy or one can be devised with pictures of common needs and an alphabet for spelling words.

Decannulation

When the patient can adequately exchange air and expectorate secretions, the tracheostomy tube can be removed. The stoma is closed with tape strips and covered with an occlusive dressing. The dressing must be changed if it gets soiled or wet. The patient should be instructed to splint the stoma with the fingers when coughing, swallowing, or speaking.[23] Epithelial tissue begins to form in 24 to 48 hours, and the opening will close in several days. Surgical intervention to close the tracheostomy is not required.

LARYNGEAL POLYPS

Laryngeal polyps may develop on the vocal cords from vocal abuse (e.g., excessive talking, singing) or irritation (e.g., intubation, cigarette smoking). The most common symptom is hoarseness. Polyps may be treated conservatively with voice rest and adequate hydration. Surgical removal may be indicated for large polyps, which may cause dyspnea and stridor. Polyps are usually benign but may be removed because they may later become malignant.

HEAD AND NECK CANCER

Head and neck cancer arises from mucosal surfaces and is typically squamous cell in origin. This category of tumors includes the paranasal sinuses, the oral cavity, and the nasopharynx, oropharynx, and larynx. (Cancer of the oral cavity is discussed in Chapter 42.) An estimated 8300 new cases of oral and pharyngeal cancer are diagnosed each year in the United States, with nearly 2000 deaths each year. Although this type of cancer is not common, disability is great because of the potential loss of voice, disfigurement, and social consequences. Most (90%) head and neck cancers occur in individuals 50 years or older after prolonged use of tobacco and alcohol. Other risk factors include consumption of a diet poor in fruits and vegetables and infection by the human papillomavirus (HPV). Males are affected at a 2 to 5 times greater rate than women.[24]

Clinical Manifestations

Early signs and symptoms of head and neck cancer vary with the tumor location. Cancer of the oral cavity may be a painless growth in the mouth, an ulcer that does not heal, or a change in fit of dentures. Pain is a late symptom that may be aggravated by acidic food. Cancers of the oropharynx, hypopharynx, and supraglottic larynx are almost always squamous cell carcinoma. They rarely produce early symptoms and are usually diagnosed in late stages.[24] The patient may complain of persistent unilateral sore throat or otalgia (ear pain). Hoarseness may be a symptom of early laryngeal cancer. Some patients experience what feels like a lump in the throat or a change in voice quality. If a lump in the neck or hoarseness lasts longer than 2 weeks, a medical evaluation is indicated.

Late stages of head and neck cancers have easily detectable signs and symptoms, including pain, dysphagia, decreased mobility of the tongue, airway obstruction, and cranial nerve neuropathies. The nurse should thoroughly examine the oral cavity, including the area under the tongue and dentures, with a flashlight. The floor of the mouth, tongue, and lymph nodes in the neck should be bimanually palpated. There may be thickening of the normally soft and pliable oral mucosa. *Leukoplakia* (white patch) or *erythroplakia* (red patch) may be seen and should be noted for later biopsy. Both leukoplakia and carcinoma in situ (localized to a defined area) may precede invasive carcinoma by many years.

Diagnostic Studies

If lesions are suspected, the upper airways may be examined using indirect laryngoscopy, which involves using a laryngeal mirror to visualize the laryngeal area, or a flexible nasopharyngoscope may be used. The larynx and vocal cords are visually inspected for lesions and tissue mobility. A CT scan or magnetic resonance imaging (MRI) may be performed to detect local and regional spread. Neoplastic tissue is identifiable because it contains tissue of greater density or because it distorts, displaces, or destroys normal anatomic structures. The use of positron emission tomography (PET) scanning along with CT has been successful in diagnosing recurring cases of head and neck cancer.[25] Typically, multiple biopsy specimens are obtained to determine the extent of the disease.

Collaborative Care

The stage of the disease will be determined based on tumor size (T), number and location of involved nodes (N), and extent of metastasis (M). TNM staging classifies disease as stage I to stage IV and guides treatment. Choice of treatment is based on medical history, extent of disease, cosmetic considerations, urgency of treatment, and patient choice. Approximately one third of patients with head and neck cancers have highly confined lesions that are stage I or II at diagnosis. Such patients can undergo radiation therapy or surgery with the goal of cure. Radiation therapy may be effective in curing early vocal cord lesions. This therapy is usually successful in eliminating the tumor while preserving the quality of the voice, but hypothyroidism can occur after treatment. Chemotherapy is being investigated as an adjuvant treatment with radiation for later stages.[26]

If radiation therapy is not successful or the lesion is too advanced for this therapy, surgery may be performed. A *cordectomy* (partial removal of one vocal cord) is used when there is a superficial tumor involving one cord (Fig. 27-12). A *hemilaryngectomy* involves removal of one vocal cord or part of a cord and requires a temporary tracheostomy. A *supraglottic laryngectomy* involves removing structures above the true cords—the false vocal cords and epiglottis. The patient is left at high risk of aspiration following

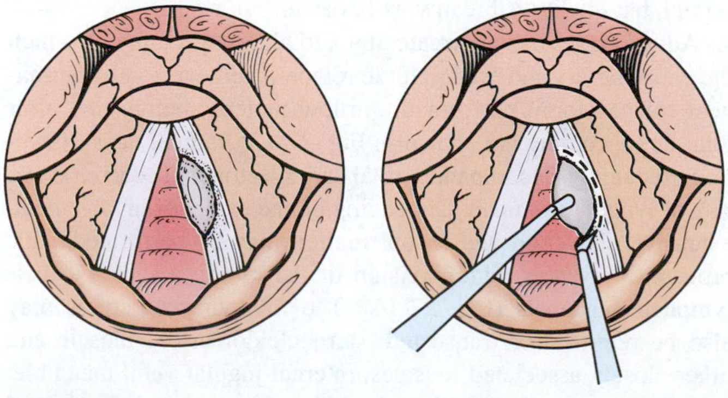

FIG. 27-12 Excision of laryngeal cancer. This cancer of the right vocal cord meets criteria for resection by transoral cordectomy. The cord is fully mobile and the lesion can be fully exposed. It does not approach or cross the anterior commissure.

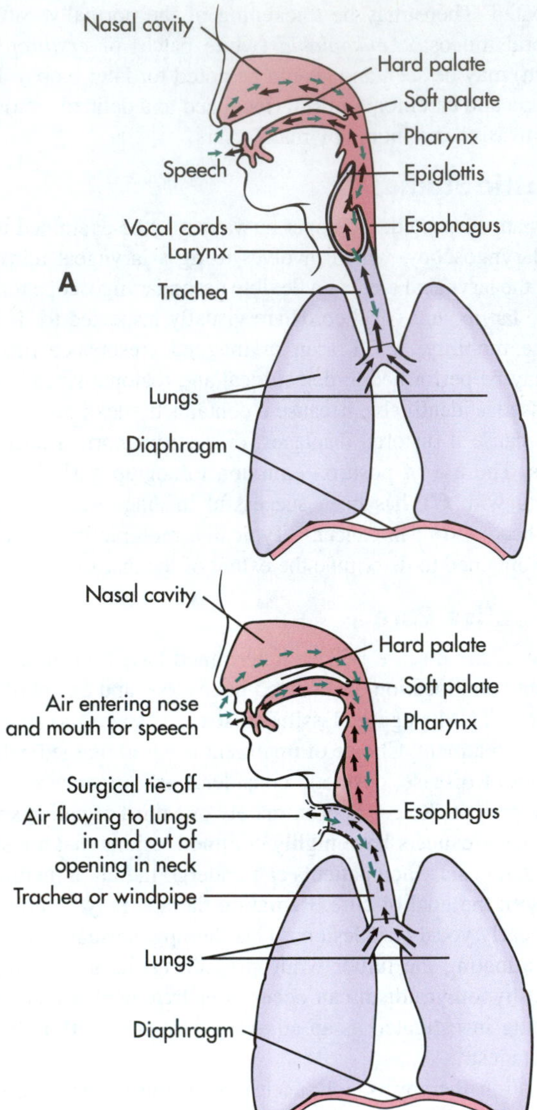

FIG. 27-13 **A,** Normal airflow in and out of the lungs. **B,** Airflow in and out of the lungs after total laryngectomy. Patients using esophageal speech trap air in the esophagus and release it to create sound.

surgery and requires a temporary tracheostomy. Both a hemilaryngectomy and supraglottic laryngectomy allow the voice to be preserved, but quality is breathy and hoarse.

Advanced lesions are treated by a total laryngectomy, in which the entire larynx and preepiglottic region is removed and a permanent tracheostomy performed. Airflow patterns before and after total laryngectomy are shown in Fig. 27-13. *Radical neck dissection* frequently accompanies total laryngectomy to decrease the risk of lymphatic spread. Depending on the extent of involvement, extensive dissection and reconstruction may be performed. This procedure involves wide excision of the lymph nodes and their lymphatic channels (Fig. 27-14). The following structures may also be removed or transected: sternocleidomastoid muscle and other closely associated muscles, internal jugular vein, mandible, submaxillary gland, part of the thyroid and parathyroid glands, and spinal accessory nerve.

A *modified neck dissection* is performed whenever possible as an alternative to a radical neck dissection. The dissection is modified by sparing as many structures as possible to limit disfigurement and functional loss. A modified neck dissection usually involves dissection of the major cervical lymphatic vessels and lateral cervical space with preservation of nerves and vessels, including the sympathetic and vagus nerves, spinal accessory nerves, and internal jugular vein. Neck dissection with vocal cord cancer usually involves one side of the neck. However, if the lesion is midline, a bilateral neck dissection may be performed. When a bilateral neck dissection is performed, it is always modified on at least one side to minimize structural and functional deficits.

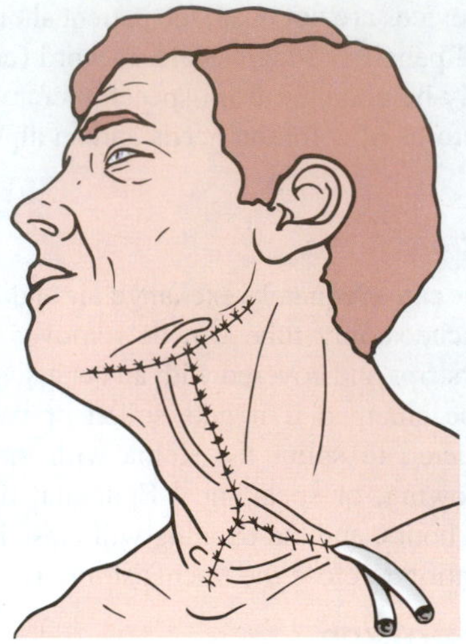

FIG. 27-14 Radical neck incision with suction tubing in place.

In addition, brachytherapy, a concentrated and localized method of delivering radiation that involves placing a radioactive source into or near the tumor, may be used to treat head and neck cancer. The goal is to deliver high doses of radiation to the target area while limiting exposure of surrounding tissues. Thin, hollow, plastic needles are inserted into the tumor area, and radioactive iridium seeds are placed in the needles. The seeds emit continuous radiation. Brachytherapy can be used alone or combined with external radiation or surgical intervention. (Radiation therapy and brachytherapy are discussed in Chapter 16.)

The patient may refuse surgical intervention for advanced lesions because of the extent of the procedure and the potential risk to the patient. In this situation, external radiation therapy may be used as the sole treatment or in combination with a clinical trial of chemotherapy. Patient support and counseling by the nurse is extremely important in this situation.

Cetuximab (Erbitux), a targeted therapy, is used in combination with radiation therapy for patients with unresectable cancers. It is also used as monotherapy for treatment of squamous cell cancer of the head and neck that has metastasized following standard chemotherapy.[26] (Targeted therapy is discussed in Chapter 16 and Table 16-17.)

Nutritional Therapy. After radical neck surgery, the patient may be unable to take in nutrients through the normal route of ingestion because of swelling, the location of sutures, or difficulty with swallowing. Parenteral fluids will be given for the first 24 to 48 hours. Tube feedings are usually given via a nasogastric, nasointestinal, or gastrostomy tube that was placed during surgery. (Tube feedings are described in Chapter 40.) The nurse must observe for tolerance of the feedings and adjust the amount, time, and formula if nausea, vomiting, diarrhea, or distention occurs. The

TABLE 27-8 PATIENT AND FAMILY TEACHING GUIDE
Steps for Performing the Supraglottic Swallow

1. Take a deep breath to aerate lungs.
2. Perform Valsalva maneuver to close vocal cords.
3. Place food in mouth and swallow. Some food will enter airway and remain on top of closed vocal cords.
4. Cough to remove food from top of vocal cords.
5. Swallow so food is moved from top of vocal cords.
6. Breathe after cough-swallow sequence to prevent aspiration of food collected on top of vocal cords.

patient and family are instructed about the tube feedings. When the patient can swallow, small amounts of water are given with the patient in high Fowler's position. Close observation for choking is essential. Suctioning may be necessary to prevent aspiration.

Swallowing problems should be anticipated when the patient resumes eating. The type and degree of difficulty vary, depending on the procedure. When a supraglottic laryngectomy is performed, the surgeon excises the upper portion of the larynx, including the epiglottis and false vocal cords. The patient can speak because the true vocal cords remain intact. However, a new technique, the *supraglottic swallow,* must be learned to compensate for removal of the epiglottis and minimize risk of aspiration (Table 27-8). When learning this technique, it may be helpful to start with carbonated beverages because the effervescence provides cues about the liquid's position. With this exception, thin, watery fluids should be avoided because they are difficult to swallow and increase the risk of aspiration. A better choice is nonpourable pureed foods, which are thicker and allow more control during swallowing. Swallowing can be enhanced by thickening liquids through the use of a commercially available thickening agent (Thick It).

Good nutrition is important during radiation therapy because calories and protein are needed for tissue repair. Antiemetics or analgesics may be given before meals to reduce nausea and mouth pain. Bland foods may be better tolerated. Caloric intake may be increased by adding dry milk to foods during preparation, selecting foods high in calories, and using oral supplements. It is helpful to add sauces and gravies to food, which adds calories and moistens food so it is more easily swallowed. If an adequate intake cannot be maintained, enteral feedings may be used. The patient should always be in a position with the head elevated.

NURSING MANAGEMENT HEAD AND NECK CANCER

Nursing Assessment

Subjective and objective data that should be obtained from a person with head and neck cancer are presented in Table 27-9.

Nursing Diagnoses

Nursing diagnoses for the patient with head and neck cancer include, but are not limited to, those presented in NCP 27-2.

Planning

The overall goals are that the patient will have (1) a patent airway, (2) no spread of cancer, (3) no complications related to therapy, (4) adequate nutritional intake, (5) minimal to no pain, (6) the ability to communicate, and (7) an acceptable body image.

TABLE 27-9 NURSING ASSESSMENT
Head and Neck Cancer

Subjective Data

Important Health Information

Past health history: Positive family history; prolonged tobacco use (cigarettes, pipes, cigars, chewing tobacco, smokeless tobacco); prolonged, heavy alcohol use; poor intake of fruits and vegetables

Medications: Prolonged use of over-the-counter medication for sore throat, decongestants

Functional Health Patterns

Health perception–health management: Does not participate in preventive health measures, long history of alcohol and tobacco use

Nutritional-metabolic: Mouth ulcer that does not heal, change in fit of dentures, change in appetite, weight loss, swallowing difficulty (e.g., sensation of lump in throat, pain with swallowing, aspiration when swallowing)

Activity-exercise: Fatigue with minimal exertion

Cognitive-perceptual: Sore throat, pain on swallowing, referred ear pain

Objective Data

Respiratory

Hoarseness, change in voice quality, chronic laryngitis, nasal voice, palpable neck mass and lymph nodes (tender, hard, fixed), tracheal deviation; dyspnea, stridor (late sign)

Gastrointestinal

White (leukoplakia) or red (erythoplakia) patches inside mouth, ulceration of mucosa, asymmetric tongue, exudate in mouth or pharynx, mass or thickening of mucosa

Possible Findings

Mass on direct or indirect laryngoscopy; tumor on soft tissue x-ray, computed tomography (CT) scan, or magnetic resonance imaging (MRI); positive biopsy

Nursing Implementation

Health Promotion. Development of head and neck cancer is closely related to personal habits, primarily tobacco use, including the use of cigarettes, cigars, chewing tobacco, and snuff. "Snuff dipping," or the placement and retention of tobacco in the cheek, is common among young people. Long-term snuff users and cigar smokers are at increased risk of oral cancer. Prolonged alcohol use has been implicated as a cause of head and neck cancer.

The nurse should include information about risk factors in health teaching. If cancer has been diagnosed, tobacco cessation is still important. The patient with head and neck cancer who continues to smoke during radiation therapy has a lower rate of response and survival than the patient who does not smoke during radiation therapy. Additionally, risk of a second primary cancer is significantly increased in patients who continue to smoke. Patients should be given information about smoking cessation programs and techniques for success.

Acute Intervention. The patient and the family must be taught about the type of therapy to be performed and care required. Assessment of concerns is integral to the care plan. The patient and family must deal with the psychologic impact of the diagnosis of cancer, alteration of physical appearance, and possible need for altered methods of communication due to a loss of voice. The care plan should include assessment of the patient's support system. The patient may not have someone to provide assistance after discharge, may not be employed, or may be employed in a job that cannot be continued.

NURSING CARE PLAN 27-2

Patient Having Total Laryngectomy and/or Radical Neck Surgery

NURSING DIAGNOSIS **Ineffective airway clearance***

NURSING DIAGNOSIS **Impaired swallowing***

NURSING DIAGNOSIS **Risk for infection***

NURSING DIAGNOSIS **Anxiety** *related to* lack of knowledge regarding surgical procedure, pain management, and prevention of complications *as evidenced by* questioning about impending surgery, postoperative care, agitation, and restlessness

PATIENT GOALS
1. Verbalizes that information provided preoperatively reduced anxiety
2. Demonstrates effective use of relaxation techniques

OUTCOMES (NOC)

Anxiety Self-Control

- Seeks information to reduce anxiety __
- Uses effective coping strategies __
- Uses relaxation techniques to reduce anxiety __
- Controls anxiety response __

Measurement Scale

1 = Never demonstrated
2 = Rarely demonstrated
3 = Sometimes demonstrated
4 = Often demonstrated
5 = Consistently demonstrated

INTERVENTIONS (NIC) and *RATIONALES*

Anxiety Reduction

- Encourage verbalization of feelings, perceptions, and fears *to understand patient's perspective of situation, treatment, and prognosis to begin adjustment and acceptance.*
- Provide factual information concerning diagnosis, treatment, and prognosis *to reduce patient's sense of helplessness and increase sense of control.*
- Assist patient to articulate a realistic description of upcoming event.
- Encourage family to stay with patient *to provide caring and support.*

NURSING DIAGNOSIS **Acute pain** *related to* surgical procedure *as evidenced by* report of discomfort; facial mask of pain; changes in blood pressure, pulse, and respiratory rate

PATIENT GOALS
1. Reports satisfaction with pain relief
2. Uses pain relief techniques effectively

OUTCOMES (NOC)

Pain Control

- Uses analgesics appropriately __
- Uses nonanalgesic relief measures appropriately __
- Reports pain controlled __

Measurement Scale

1 = Never demonstrated
2 = Rarely demonstrated
3 = Sometimes demonstrated
4 = Often demonstrated
5 = Consistently demonstrated

INTERVENTIONS (NIC) and *RATIONALES*

Pain Management

- Observe for nonverbal cues of discomfort, especially in those unable to communicate effectively (e.g., facial expression, reluctance to cough or move) *to plan appropriate interventions.*
- Perform a comprehensive assessment of pain to include location, characteristics, onset/duration, frequency, quality, intensity, or severity of pain and precipitating factors.
- Teach use of nonpharmacological techniques (e.g., relaxation, guided imagery, music therapy, distraction, and massage) before, after, and, if possible, during painful activities; before pain occurs or increases; and along with other pain relief measures *to manage pain.*
- Provide the person optimal pain relief with prescribed analgesics *to determine if it is effective.*
- Use pain control measures before pain becomes severe.

NURSING DIAGNOSIS **Impaired verbal communication** *related to* removal of vocal cords *as evidenced by* inability to speak

PATIENT GOAL Communicates basic needs using written and nonverbal communication techniques

OUTCOMES (NOC)

Communication

- Use of written language __
- Use of pictures and drawings __
- Use of sign language __
- Use of nonverbal language __
- Exchanges messages accurately with others __

Measurement Scale

1 = Severely compromised
2 = Substantially compromised
3 = Moderately compromised
4 = Mildly compromised
5 = Not compromised

INTERVENTIONS (NIC) and *RATIONALES*

Communication Enhancement: Speech Deficit

- Instruct patient and family on use of speech aids (e.g., tracheal-esophageal prosthesis and artificial larynx).
- Use picture board.
- Listen attentively.
- Reinforce need for follow-up with speech pathologist after discharge *to learn use of voice prosthesis, electrolarynx, or esophageal speech.*

*Because a tracheostomy is usually performed for the patient with a total laryngectomy and/or radical neck surgery, see the related nursing care plan, NCP 27-1, on pp 548-549 for these nursing diagnoses.

Continued

NURSING CARE PLAN 27-2

Patient Having Total Laryngectomy and/or Radical Neck Surgery—cont'd

NURSING DIAGNOSIS **Imbalanced nutrition: less than body requirements** *related to* surgical procedure, edema, and dysphagia *as evidenced by* absence of or inadequate oral intake

PATIENT GOALS
1. Maintains body weight
2. Consumes adequate fluids and nutrients to meet metabolic needs in the postoperative period

OUTCOMES (NOC)

Nutritional Status

- Nutrient intake __
- Weight/height ratio __
- Food intake __
- Fluid intake __

Measurement Scale

1 = Severe deviation from normal range
2 = Substantial deviation from normal range
3 = Moderate deviation from normal range
4 = Mild deviation from normal range
5 = No deviation from normal range

INTERVENTIONS (NIC) and *RATIONALES*

Nutrition Therapy

- Complete a nutritional assessment.
- Administer enteral feedings *to provide adequate nutrients while wound heals.*
- Ensure availability of progressive therapeutic diet *to allow patient time to adjust to initiation of oral intake.*
- Instruct patient and family about prescribed diet.
- Monitor food/fluid ingested and calculate daily caloric intake *to evaluate effectiveness of therapy.*

NURSING DIAGNOSIS **Disturbed body image** *related to* disfiguring surgery and loss of speaking ability *as evidenced by* withdrawal, depression, isolation, unwillingness to look at self or assist with care, and refusal to see other visitors

PATIENT GOALS
1. Acknowledges changes in body image
2. Discusses feelings about and the meaning of changes in physical appearance
3. Participates in self-care

OUTCOMES (NOC)

Body Image

- Adjustment to changes in physical appearance __
- Adjustment to changes in body function __
- Willingness to use strategies to enhance function __

Measurement Scale

1 = Never positive
2 = Rarely positive
3 = Sometimes positive
4 = Often positive
5 = Consistently positive

INTERVENTIONS (NIC) and *RATIONALES*

Body Image Enhancement

- Use anticipatory guidance to prepare patient for predictable changes in body image *to facilitate effective coping mechanisms.*
- Assist patient to discuss changes caused by illness or surgery.
- Identify means of reducing the impact of any disfigurement through clothing or cosmetics *to aid in successful adjustment.*
- Assist patient to separate physical appearance from feelings of personal worth *to increase acceptance of altered physical appearance.*

Socialization Enhancement

- Encourage enhanced involvement in already established relationships *as acceptance by significant others is a critical factor in patient's own acceptance.*

Self-Care Assistance

- Encourage patient to perform normal activities of daily living to level of ability *as participation in self-care is a sign of successful adjustment.*

Continued

Radiation Therapy. The nurse can suggest interventions to reduce side effects of radiation therapy. Dry mouth *(xerostomia),* the most frequent and annoying problem, typically begins within a few weeks of treatment. The patient's saliva decreases in volume and becomes thick. The change may be temporary or permanent. Pilocarpine hydrochloride (Salagen) can be effective in increasing saliva production and should be started before the initiation of radiation therapy and continued for 90 days. Symptom relief can also be obtained by increasing fluid intake, chewing sugarless gum or sugarless candy, using nonalcoholic mouth rinses (baking soda or glycerin solutions), and using artificial saliva. Instruct patients to always carry a water bottle with them.

Fatigue is one of the most common side effects of radiation therapy and usually begins a few weeks into therapy. Patients should be encouraged to take frequent rest periods during the day. Also, light, regular exercise such as walking may help to give the patient more energy.

The patient may also complain of stomatitis, especially if the oral cavity is in the field of therapy. Irritation, ulceration, and pain are common complaints. Patients should be encouraged to eat soft, bland foods during this time. Frequent rinses with water or sucking on ice chips can help with the pain. Commercial mouthwashes and hot or spicy foods should be avoided because they are irritating. If the problem is severe, a mixture of equal parts of antacid, diphenhydramine (Benadryl), and topical lidocaine can be used. The patient should be instructed to rinse the mouth with the mixture without swallowing the liquid.

Skin over the radiated area often becomes reddened and sensitive to touch. Patients should be instructed to only use prescribed lotions and skin products while undergoing radiation therapy, and to not use

NURSING CARE PLAN 27-2

Patient Having Total Laryngectomy and/or Radical Neck Surgery—cont'd

NURSING DIAGNOSIS **Ineffective therapeutic regimen management** *related to* lack of knowledge about home care after discharge *as evidenced by* verbalized concern about ability to manage self-care at home

PATIENT GOALS
1. Demonstrates satisfactory care of tubes and incisions
2. Verbalizes key elements of the therapeutic regimen and speech rehabilitation, including knowledge of disease, complications, and treatment plan

OUTCOMES (NOC)	INTERVENTIONS (NIC) and *RATIONALES*
Discharge Readiness: Independent Living • Seeks assistance appropriately __ • Uses available social support __ • Describes signs and symptoms to health care professional __ • Describes prescribed treatments __ • Describes risks for complications __ • Manages own medications __ **Measurement Scale** 1 = Never demonstrated 2 = Rarely demonstrated 3 = Sometimes demonstrated 4 = Often demonstrated 5 = Consistently demonstrated	***Teaching: Psychomotor Skill*** • Provide written information/diagrams *as an accurate reference reduces error.* • Demonstrate skill for the patient. • Observe patient return demonstrate the skill *to ensure correct performance of technique.* ***Teaching: Disease Process*** • Instruct patient on which signs and symptoms to report to health care provider *to detect possible recurrence of tumor or tracheal stenosis.* • Refer patient to local community agencies/support groups.

any lotions within 2 hours prior to treatment. If a moist skin reaction occurs, the health care provider should be notified immediately. All exposure to the sun should be avoided to reduce discomfort, and sunscreen should be applied daily.

Surgical Therapy. Preoperative care for the patient who is to have a radical neck dissection involves consideration of the patient's physical and psychosocial needs. Physical preparation is the same as for any major surgery, with special emphasis on oral hygiene. Explanations and emotional support are of special significance and should include postoperative measures relating to communication and feeding. The surgical procedure should be explained to the patient and family, and the nurse should make sure that the information is understood.

Teaching must be tailored to the planned surgical procedure. For surgeries that involve a laryngectomy, teaching should include information about expected changes in speech. The nurse or speech pathologist should demonstrate means of communicating other than speaking that can be used temporarily or permanently. This may include some type of communication board.

After surgery, maintenance of a patent airway is essential. The inflammation in the surgical area may compress the trachea. A tracheostomy tube will be in place. The patient will be placed in a semi-Fowler's position to decrease edema and limit tension on the suture lines. Vital signs should be monitored frequently because of the risk of hemorrhage and respiratory compromise. Pressure dressings, packing, or drainage tubes (Hemovac, Jackson-Pratt) may be used for wound management, depending on the type of surgical procedure. When a radical neck dissection is performed, wound suction using a portable system, such as a Hemovac, is usually used. If skin flaps are employed, dressings are typically not used. This allows better visualization of the incision and avoids excessive pressure on tissue (see Fig. 27-14). The drainage should be serosanguineous and gradually decrease in volume over 24 hours. Patency of drainage tubes should be monitored every 4 hours to ensure that they are properly removing serous drainage and for the amount and character of drainage. If the tubing becomes obstructed, fluid will accumulate under the skin flap and predispose to impaired wound healing and infection. After drainage tubes are removed, the area should be closely monitored to detect any swelling. If fluid continues to accumulate, aspiration may be necessary.

Immediately after surgery, the patient with a laryngectomy requires frequent suctioning via the laryngectomy tube. Secretions typically change in amount and consistency over time. The patient may initially have copious blood-tinged secretions that diminish and thicken. Normal saline bolus via the tracheostomy tube is not recommended to assist with removal of thickened secretions as this causes hypoxia and damage to the epithelial cells.[20] However, the patient will benefit from the use of a humidifier while hospitalized and at home.

Following a neck dissection, the patient should be taught to use the upper extremities to assist with support and movement of the head. Following the immediate postoperative period, an exercise program should be instituted to maintain strength and movement in the affected shoulder and neck. This is especially important when the spinal accessory nerve and sternocleidomastoid muscles are removed or damaged. Without exercise, the patient will be left with a "frozen" shoulder and limited range of neck motion. This exercise program should be continued following discharge to prevent future functional disabilities.

Voice Rehabilitation. A speech therapist should meet with the patient following a total laryngectomy to discuss voice restoration options. The International Association of Laryngectomees, an association of laryngectomy patients, focuses on assisting patients to reestablish speech. Local groups, called Lost Cord Clubs, often provide member volunteers to visit the patient, preferably preoperatively. Several options are available to restore speech. These include the use of voice prosthesis, esophageal speech, and an electrolarynx.

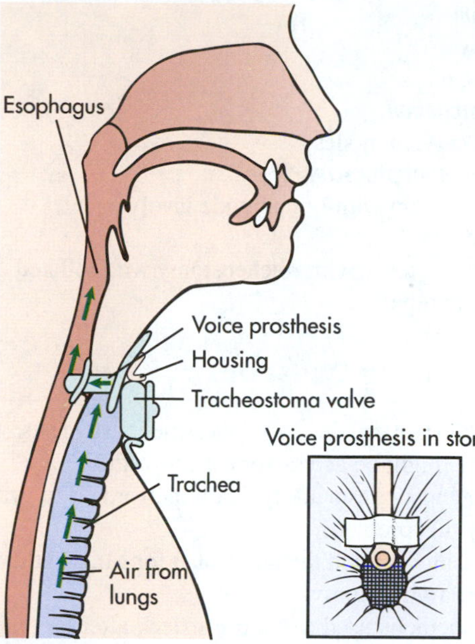

FIG. 27-15 Blom-Singer voice prosthesis and tracheostoma valve. With this prosthesis and valve, patients with a laryngectomy can speak normally. *Inset* shows laryngectomy stoma and voice prosthesis with tracheostoma valve removed.

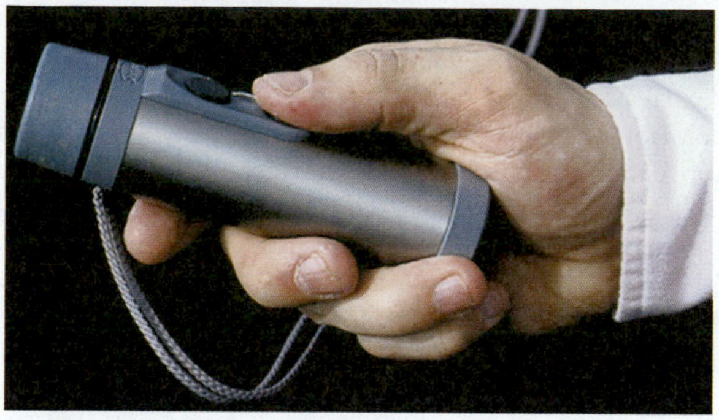

FIG. 27-16 Artificial larynx. Battery-powered electronic artificial larynx for patient who has had a total laryngectomy.

The most commonly used voice prosthesis is the Blom-Singer prosthesis (Fig. 27-15). This soft plastic device is inserted into a fistula made between the esophagus and the trachea. The puncture may be created at the time of surgery or afterward, depending on the preference of the surgeon. A red rubber catheter is placed in the tracheoesophageal puncture and must remain intact until a tract is formed. Once the tract is formed, the speech prosthesis is inserted. This prosthesis allows air from the lungs to enter the esophagus by way of the tracheal stoma. A one-way valve prevents aspiration of food or saliva from the esophagus into the tracheostomy. To speak, the patient manually blocks the stoma with the finger. Air moves from the lungs, through the prosthesis, into the esophagus, and out the mouth. Speech is produced by the air vibrating against the esophagus and is formed into words by moving the tongue and lips. A valve may also be used with this device. When the valve is in place, the stoma does not need to be closed with the finger to speak. The prosthesis must be cleaned regularly and replaced when it becomes blocked with mucus.

An electrolarynx is a handheld, battery-powered device that creates speech with the use of sound waves. One device, the Cooper-Rand artificial larynx, uses a plastic tube placed in the corner of the roof of the mouth to create vibrations. To create the most normal sound when using this device, the patient should (1) avoid trying to use the tongue to hold the tube in place; (2) compress the tone generator for short intervals and speak in phrases, rather than full sentences; (3) speak using large movements of the lips, tongue, and jaw, rather than keeping the mouth partially closed; (4) talk face-to-face with the listener; and (5) practice, because development of skill takes time.

An artificial larynx is placed against the neck rather than in the mouth. This device is used after surgical healing is complete and there is no edema remaining (Fig. 27-16). With experience, the patient can learn to move the lips in ways that create normal-sounding speech. With both devices, voice pitch is low and the sound is mechanical.

Esophageal Speech. Esophageal speech involves swallowing air, trapping it in the esophagus, and releasing it to create sound. The air causes vibration of the pharyngoesophageal segment and sound (which initially is similar to a belch). With practice, 50% of patients develop some speech skills, but only 10% develop fluent speech.

Stoma Care. Before discharge, the patient should be instructed in the care of the laryngectomy stoma. The area around the stoma should be washed daily with a moist cloth. If a laryngectomy tube is in place, the entire tube must be removed at least daily and cleaned in the same manner as a tracheostomy tube. The inner cannula may need to be removed and cleaned more frequently. A scarf, a loose shirt, or a crocheted shield can be used to shield the stoma.

The patient should cover the stoma when coughing (because mucus may be expectorated) and during any activity (e.g., shaving, applying makeup) that might lead to inhalation of foreign materials. Because water can easily enter the stoma, the patient should wear a plastic collar when taking a shower. Swimming is contraindicated. Initially, humidification will be administered via a tracheostomy mask. After discharge, a bedside humidifier can be used. A high oral fluid intake must be maintained, especially in dry weather.

The patient should be told the importance of wearing a Medic Alert bracelet or other identification that alerts people in an emergency situation of the use of neck breathing. Because the patient no longer breathes through the nose, the ability to smell smoke and food may be lost. Advise the patient to install smoke and carbon monoxide detectors in the home. It is important for food to be colorful, attractively prepared, and nutritious because taste may also be diminished secondary to the loss of smell as well as radiation therapy.

Depression. Depression is common in the patient who has had a radical neck dissection. The patient may not be able to speak because of the laryngectomy and cannot control saliva. The neck and shoulders may be numb because of the transected nerves. The facial appearance may be significantly altered, with swelling, edema, and deformities. The patient must understand that many of the physical changes are reversible as the edema subsides and the tracheostomy tube is removed. Depression may also be related to concern about the prognosis. The nurse can help the patient through the depression by allowing verbalization of feelings, conveying acceptance, and helping the patient regain an acceptable self-concept. Sometimes it is appropriate to obtain a psychiatric referral for the patient who is experiencing prolonged or severe depression.[27]

Sexuality. Surgery and the presence of foreign attachments such as tracheostomy and gastrostomy tubes may affect body image dramatically. The patient may feel less desirable sexually. The nurse can assist the patient by allowing discussions regarding sexuality and encouraging the patient to discuss this problem with the sexual partner. It may be difficult for the patient to orally discuss sexual problems because of the alteration in communication. The nurse can allow the patient to plan how to communicate with the sexual partner and offer support and guidance to the sexual partner. Helping the patient see that sexuality involves much more than appearance may relieve some anxiety.

Ambulatory and Home Care. The patient is often discharged with a tracheostomy and a nasogastric or gastrostomy feeding tube. Home health care may need to be provided initially to evaluate the family's or the patient's ability to perform self-care activities. The patient and the family must be taught how to manage tubes and who to call if there are problems.

The patient can resume exercise, recreation, and sexual activity when able. Most patients can return to work 1 to 2 months after surgery. However, many never return to full-time employment. The changes that follow a total laryngectomy can be upsetting. Loss of speech, loss of the ability to taste and smell, inability to produce audible sounds (including laughing and weeping), and the presence of a permanent tracheal stoma that produces undesirable mucus are often overwhelming to the patient. Although changes are discussed before surgery, the patient may not be prepared for the extent of these changes. If the patient has a significant other, the reaction of this person to the patient's altered appearance is important. Acceptance by another person can promote an improved self-image. Encouraging the patient to participate in self-care is another important part of rehabilitation.

Reconstructive surgery may be performed at the time of the initial surgery or soon after the tumor is removed. Various types of flaps and grafts are used. It may be necessary to rebuild the nose or the mandible or to close oral cutaneous openings. Prosthetic materials, such as Silastic and Plastigel (which is soft), are often used to reconstruct various deformities.

Despite the use of surgical interventions and radiation therapy, the cure rate is disappointingly low for advanced head and neck cancer. Metastatic cancer is often painful, leaving the affected person in a severely debilitated state. If pain is a problem, a pain control regimen should be identified to provide comfort, and referral should be made to palliative care services or hospice if indicated.

■ *Evaluation*

Expected outcomes for the patient with head and neck cancer who is treated surgically are addressed in NCP 27-2.

CRITICAL THINKING EXERCISE

CASE STUDY

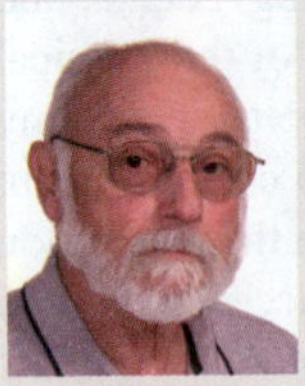

Laryngeal Cancer

Patient Profile. Mr. Matthews, a 60-year-old white male, was admitted for evaluation of mild pain on swallowing and a persistent sore throat over the past year. He has a history of type 2 diabetes mellitus.

Subjective Data

- States that his symptoms worsened in the last 2 months
- Has used various cold remedies to relieve symptoms without relief
- Has lost weight because of decrease in appetite and difficulty swallowing
- Has smoked 3 packs of cigarettes a day for 40 years
- Consumes 6 cans of beer a day

Objective Data

Laryngoscopy

- Subglottic mass

Physical Examination

- Enlarged cervical nodes

Computed Tomography Scan

- Subglottic lesion with lymph node involvement

Collaborative Care

- Total laryngectomy with tracheostomy with inflated cuff
- Nasogastric tube

Critical Thinking Questions

1. What information in the assessment suggests that Mr. Matthews might be at risk for cancer of the larynx?
2. What diagnostic tests are typically performed to evaluate the extent of this problem?
3. What teaching should the nurse plan for Mr. Matthews before and after laryngectomy?
4. Discuss methods used to restore speech after laryngectomy.
5. Is there anything in his history that may affect wound healing after surgery?
6. While in the recovery room, Mr. Matthews develops shortness of breath. Prioritize your nursing interventions.
7. What teaching is required to assist this patient to assume self-care after his surgery? What precautions should the patient take because of his stoma?
8. While on the medical surgical unit, Mr. Matthews is tearful and is staring toward the wall. What should you do?
9. Based on the assessment data presented, write one or more nursing diagnoses. Are there any collaborative problems?

NCLEX EXAMINATION REVIEW QUESTIONS

The number of the question corresponds to the same-numbered objective at the beginning of the chapter.

1. A patient was seen in the clinic for an episode of epistaxis, which was controlled by placement of anterior nasal packing. During discharge teaching, the nurse instructs the patient to
   a. use aspirin for pain relief.
   b. remove the packing later that day.
   c. skip the next dose of antihypertensive medication.
   d. avoid vigorous nose blowing and strenuous activity.
2. A patient with allergic rhinitis reports severe nasal congestion, sneezing, and watery, itchy eyes and nose at various times of the year. To teach the patient to control these symptoms, the nurse advises the patient to
   a. avoid all intranasal sprays and oral antihistamines.
   b. limit the duration of use of nasal decongestant spray to 10 days.
   c. use oral decongestants at bedtime to prevent symptoms during the night.
   d. keep a diary of when the allergic reaction occurs and what precipitates it.
3. A patient with sleep apnea would like to avoid using a nasal CPAP device, if possible. To help him reach this goal, the nurse suggests that he
   a. lose excess weight.
   b. take a nap during the day.
   c. eat a high-protein snack at bedtime.
   d. use mild sedatives or alcohol at bedtime.
4. A type of tracheostomy tube that prevents speech is
   a. a cuffless tracheostomy tube.
   b. a fenestrated tracheostomy tube.

c. a tube with an inflated foam cuff.
d. a cuffed tube with the cuff deflated.

5. To prevent excessive pressure on tracheal capillaries, pressure in the cuff on a tracheostomy tube should be
   a. monitored every 2 to 3 days.
   b. less than 20 mm Hg or 25 cm H_2O.
   c. less than 30 mm Hg or 35 cm H_2O.
   d. sufficient to fill the pilot balloon until it is tense.
6. Which of the following is a late symptom of head and neck cancer?
   a. Hoarseness
   b. Change in fit of dentures
   c. Mouth ulcers that do not heal
   d. Decreased mobility of the tongue
7. While in the recovery room, a patient with a total laryngectomy is suctioned and has bloody mucus with some clots. Which of the following nursing interventions would apply?
   a. Notify the physician immediately.
   b. Place the patient in the prone position to facilitate drainage.
   c. Instill 3 ml of normal saline into the tracheostomy tube to loosen secretions.
   d. Continue your assessment of the patient, including oxygen saturation, respiratory rate, and breath sounds.
8. When using a voice prosthesis, the patient
   a. swallows air using a Valsalva maneuver.
   b. places a vibrating device in the mouth.
   c. places a speaking valve over the stoma.
   d. blocks the stoma entrance with a finger.

REFERENCES

1. Kieff DA, Busaba NY: Isolated chronic maxillary sinusitis of non-dental origin does not correlate per se with ipsilateral intranasal structural abnormalities, *Ann Otol Rhinol Laryngol* 113:474, 2004.
2. Kucik CJ, Clenney T, Phelan J: Management of acute nasal fractures, *Am Fam Physician* 70:1315, 2004.
3. Kucik CJ, Clenney T: Management of epistaxis, *Am Fam Physician* 71:305, 2005.

*4. Hayden ML: Allergic rhinitis: proper management benefits concomitant diseases, *Nurse Pract* 29(12):26, 35, 2004.

*5. Banasiak NC, Meadows-Oliver M: Leukotrienes: their role in the treatment of asthma and seasonal allergic rhinitis, *Pediatr Nurs* 31(1):35, 2005.

6. Leggett JE: Acute sinusitis: when—and when not—to prescribe antibiotics, *Postgrad Med* 115:13, 2004.
7. Centers for Disease Control and Prevention: Prevention and control of influenza: recommendations of the Advisory Committee on Immunization Practices (ACIP), *MMWR Recomm Rep* 53(RR06):1, 2004. Available at *www.cdc.gov/mmwr/preview/mmwrhtml/rr5306a1.htm.*
8. Centers for Disease Control and Prevention: Influenza antiviral medications: 2004-2005 interim chemoprophylaxis and treatment guidelines, Department of Health and Human Services. Available at *www.cdc.gov/flu/professionals/pdf/0405antiviralguide.pdf* (accessed August 20, 2005).
9. Scheid DC, Hamm RM: Acute bacterial rhinosinusitis in adults: part I. Evaluation, *Am Fam Physician* 70:1697, 2004.
10. Scheid DC, Hamm RM: Acute bacterial rhinosinusitis in adults: part II. Treatment, *Am Fam Physician* 70:1685, 2004.
11. Vincent MT, Celestin N, Hussain AN: Pharyngitis, *Am Fam Physician* 69:1465, 2004.

*12. Merritt SL, Berger BE: Obstructive sleep apnea-hypopnea syndrome, *Am J Nurs* 104(7):49, 2004.

13. Caples SM, Gami AS, Somers VK: Obstructive sleep apnea, *Ann Intern Med* 142:187, 2005.
14. Trupp R: The heart of sleep: sleep-disordered breathing and heart failure, *J Cardiovasc Nurs* 19(6 Suppl):S67, 2004.
15. Attarian HP, Sabri AN: When to suspect obstructive sleep apnea syndrome: symptoms may be subtle, but treatment is straightforward, *Postgrad Med* 111:70, 2002.
16. Overnight stay not required for most performed surgeries for sleep disorder, *Managed Care Weekly Digest*, May 24, 2004.
17. Kluge S, Meyer A, Kuhnelt P, et al: Percutaneous tracheostomy is safe in patients with severe thrombocytopenia, *Chest* 126:547, 2004.
18. Thelan LA, et al: *Critical care nursing: diagnosis and management*, ed 5, St Louis, 2006, Mosby.
19. Seay SJ, Gray SL, Strauss M: Tracheostomy emergencies, *Am J Nurs* 102(3):59, 2002.
20. St. John R: Airway management, *Crit Care Nurse* 24(2):93, 2004.
21. Russell C: High-dependency nursing: providing the nurse with a guide to tracheostomy care and management, *Br J Nurs* 14(8):428, 2005.
22. St. John RE, Malen JF: Contemporary issues in adult tracheostomy management, *Crit Care Nurs Clin North Am* 16:413, 2004.
23. Barnett M: Tracheostomy management and care, *J Community Nurs* 19(1):4, 2005.
24. National Cancer Institute: Oropharyngeal treatment guide for the health professional 2005. Available at *www.cancer.gov/cancertopics/pdq/treatment/oropharyngeal/healthprofessional* (accessed August 20, 2005).
25. Zimmer L, et al: The use of combined PET/CT for localizing recurrent head and neck cancer: the Pittsburgh experience, *ENT J* 84:104, 2005.
26. National Cancer Institute: Stage 3 oropharyngeal cancer 2005. Available at *www.cancer.gov/cancertopics/pdq/treatment/oropharyngeal/HealthProfessional/page7.*
27. National Cancer Institute: Support for people with cancer of the larynx 2005. Available at *www.cancer.gov/cancertopics/wyntk/larynx/page23.*

RESOURCES

American Academy of Sleep Medicine
708-492-0930
www.asda.org

American Sleep Apnea Association
202-293-3650
www.sleepapnea.org

International Association of Laryngectomees
866-IAL-FORU (425-3678)
www.larynxlink.com

National Cancer Institute
www.cancer.gov

National Sleep Foundation
202-347-3471
www.sleepfoundation.org

For additional Internet resources, see the website for this book at *http://evolve.elsevier.com/Lewis/medsurg.*

*Nursing research–based reference.

Do your best every day, and your life will gradually expand into satisfying fullness.

Alexander Graham Bell

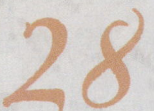

28 Nursing Management
Lower Respiratory Problems

Janet T. Crimlisk

LEARNING OBJECTIVES

1. Describe the pathophysiology, types, clinical manifestations, and collaborative care of pneumonia.
2. Explain the nursing management of the patient with pneumonia.
3. Describe the pathogenesis, classification, clinical manifestations, complications, diagnostic abnormalities, and nursing and collaborative management of tuberculosis.
4. Identify the causes, clinical manifestations, and nursing and collaborative management of pulmonary fungal infections.
5. Explain the pathophysiology, clinical manifestations, and nursing and collaborative management of lung abscesses.
6. Identify the causative factors, clinical features, and management of environmental lung diseases.
7. Describe the causes, risk factors, pathogenesis, clinical manifestations, and nursing and collaborative management of lung cancer.
8. Identify the mechanisms involved and the clinical manifestations of pneumothorax, fractured ribs, and flail chest.
9. Describe the purpose, methods, and nursing responsibilities related to chest tubes.
10. Explain the types of chest surgery and appropriate preoperative and postoperative care.
11. Compare and contrast extrapulmonary and intrapulmonary restrictive lung disorders in terms of causes, clinical manifestations, and collaborative management.
12. Describe the pathophysiology, clinical manifestations, and management of pulmonary embolism, pulmonary hypertension, and cor pulmonale.
13. Discuss the use of lung transplantation as a treatment for pulmonary disorders.

KEY TERMS

acute bronchitis, p. 561
atelectasis, p. 597
community-acquired pneumonia, p. 562
cor pulmonale, p. 602
flail chest, p. 588
hemothorax, p. 587
hospital-acquired pneumonia, p. 563
lung abscess, p. 576
pleural effusion, p. 595
pleurisy (pleuritis), p. 597
pneumoconiosis, p. 577
pneumonia, p. 561
pneumothorax, p. 585
pulmonary edema, p. 597
pulmonary embolism, p. 598
pulmonary hypertension, p. 600
tension pneumothorax, p. 586
thoracentesis, p. 595
thoracotomy, p. 592
tuberculosis, p. 569

Electronic Resources

Supplemental content related to Chapter 28 can be found . . .

Companion CD

- Stress-Busting Kit for Nursing Students
- Interactive Case Studies:
  - Lung Cancer
  - Pulmonary Embolism
- NCLEX Examination Review Questions
- Comprehensive Glossary

Evolve Website

http://evolve.elsevier.com/Lewis/medsurg

- Content Updates
- Key Points (Printable and CD/MP3 Download)
- Concept Map Creator
- Expanded Audio Glossary
- Key Term Flash Cards
- Customizable Nursing Care Plans:
  - Pneumonia
  - Thoracotomy
- Electronic Calculators
- WebLinks

A wide variety of problems affect the lower respiratory system. Lung diseases that are characterized primarily by an obstructive disorder, such as asthma, emphysema, chronic bronchitis, and cystic fibrosis, are discussed in Chapter 29. All other lower respiratory tract diseases are discussed in this chapter.

Respiratory tract infections are common. Lower respiratory tract infections are the most common cause of death in the world. Chronic lower respiratory disease is the fourth leading cause of death in the United States, and pneumonia ranks as the seventh leading cause of death despite the availability of antimicrobial

Reviewed by Christine L. Willis, RN, MSN, ANP-C, Adult Nurse Practitioner, Pulmonary and Critical Care Medicine, Duke University Medical Center, Durham, N.C.

agents.[1] Tuberculosis, although potentially curable and preventable, is a worldwide public health threat.

ACUTE BRONCHITIS

Acute bronchitis is an inflammation of the bronchi in the lower respiratory tract, usually due to infection. It is one of the most common conditions seen in primary care. It usually occurs as a sequela to an upper respiratory tract infection. A type of acute bronchitis seen in chronic obstructive pulmonary disease (COPD) is acute exacerbation of chronic bronchitis (AECB). AECB represents an acute infection superimposed on chronic bronchitis. AECB is a potentially serious condition that may lead to respiratory failure. (Chronic bronchitis is discussed in Chapter 29.)

The cause of most cases of acute bronchitis is viral (rhinovirus, influenza). However, bacterial causes are also common both in smokers (e.g., *Streptococcus pneumoniae, Haemophilus influenzae*) and in nonsmokers (e.g., *Mycoplasma pneumoniae, Chlamydia pneumoniae*). In acute bronchitis, persistent cough following an acute upper airway infection (e.g., rhinitis, pharyngitis) is the most common symptom. Cough is often accompanied by production of clear, mucoid sputum, although some patients produce purulent sputum. Associated symptoms include fever, headache, malaise, and shortness of breath on exertion. Physical examination may reveal mildly elevated temperature, pulse, and respiratory rate with either normal breath sounds or rhonchi and expiratory wheezing. Chest x-rays can differentiate acute bronchitis from pneumonia because there is no evidence of consolidation or infiltrates on x-ray with bronchitis.

Acute bronchitis is usually self-limiting, and the treatment is generally supportive, including fluids, rest, and antiinflammatory agents. Cough suppressants or bronchodilators may be prescribed for symptomatic treatment of nocturnal cough or wheezing. Antibiotics generally are not prescribed unless the person has a prolonged infection associated with constitutional symptoms. If this is an acute bronchitis due to an influenza virus, treatment with antiviral drugs—either zanamivir (Relenza) or oseltamivir (Tamiflu)—can be started, but the antiviral drug must be initiated within 48 hours of the onset of symptoms.

The COPD patient with severe AECB is usually treated empirically with broad-spectrum antibiotics for 5 to 7 days.[2] Early initiation of antibiotic treatment in COPD patients has resulted in a decrease in relapses and a decrease in hospital admissions. (See Chapter 29 for a discussion of COPD.)

PNEUMONIA

Pneumonia is an acute inflammation of the lung parenchyma caused by a microbial organism. Until 1936, pneumonia was the leading cause of death in the United States. The discovery of sulfa drugs and penicillin was pivotal in the treatment of pneumonia. Since that time, there has been remarkable progress in the development of antibiotics to treat pneumonia. However, despite the new antimicrobial agents, pneumonia is still common and is associated with significant morbidity and mortality. Pneumonia and influenza are the seventh leading cause of death in the United States. Data indicate that the mortality from pneumonia and influenza is increasing (3.2%). Pneumonia is currently the leading cause of death from an infectious disease in the United States.

Etiology

Normal Defense Mechanisms. Normally, the airway distal to the larynx is sterile because of protective defense mechanisms. These mechanisms include the following: filtration of air, warming and humidification of inspired air, epiglottis closure over the trachea, cough reflex, mucociliary escalator mechanism, secretion of immunoglobulin A, and alveolar macrophages (see Chapter 26).

Factors Predisposing to Pneumonia. Pneumonia is more likely to result when defense mechanisms become incompetent or are overwhelmed by the virulence or quantity of infectious agents. Decreased consciousness depresses the cough and epiglottal reflexes, which may allow aspiration of oropharyngeal contents into the lungs. Tracheal intubation interferes with the normal cough reflex and the mucociliary escalator mechanism. It also bypasses the upper airways, in which filtration and humidification of air normally take place. The mucociliary mechanism is impaired by air pollution, cigarette smoking, viral upper respiratory infections (URIs), and normal changes of aging. In cases of malnutrition, the functions of lymphocytes and polymorphonuclear (PMN) leukocytes are altered. Diseases such as leukemia, alcoholism, and diabetes mellitus are associated with an increased frequency of gram-negative bacilli in the oropharynx. (Gram-negative bacilli are not normal flora in the respiratory tract.) Altered oropharyngeal flora can also occur secondary to antibiotic therapy given for an infection elsewhere in the body. The factors predisposing to pneumonia are listed in Table 28-1.

Acquisition of Organisms. Organisms that cause pneumonia reach the lung by three methods:

1. *Aspiration* from the nasopharynx or oropharynx. Many of the organisms that cause pneumonia are normal inhabitants of the pharynx in healthy adults.
2. *Inhalation* of microbes present in the air. Examples include *Mycoplasma pneumoniae* and fungal pneumonias.
3. *Hematogenous spread* from a primary infection elsewhere in the body. An example is *Staphylococcus aureus.*

TABLE 28-1 Factors Predisposing to Pneumonia

- Aging
- Air pollution
- Altered consciousness: alcoholism, head injury, seizures, anesthesia, drug overdose, stroke
- Altered oropharyngeal flora secondary to antibiotics
- Bed rest and prolonged immobility
- Chronic diseases: chronic lung disease, diabetes mellitus, heart disease, cancer, end-stage renal disease
- Debilitating illness
- Human immunodeficiency virus (HIV) infection
- Immunosuppressive drugs (corticosteroids, cancer chemotherapy, immunosuppressive therapy after organ transplant)
- Inhalation or aspiration of noxious substances
- Intestinal and gastric feedings via nasogastric or nasointestinal tubes
- Malnutrition
- Smoking
- Tracheal intubation (endotracheal intubation, tracheostomy)
- Upper respiratory tract infection

Respiratory System

TABLE 28-2 Organisms Associated with Pneumonia

Community-Acquired Pneumonia

- *Streptococcus pneumoniae**
- *Mycoplasma pneumoniae*
- *Haemophilus influenzae*
- Respiratory viruses
- *Chlamydia pneumoniae*
- *Legionella pneumophila*
- Oral anaerobes
- *Moraxella catarrhalis*
- *Staphylococcus aureus*
- *Nocardia*
- Enteric aerobic gram-negative bacteria (e.g., *Klebsiella*)
- Fungi
- *Mycobacterium tuberculosis*

Hospital-Acquired Pneumonia

- *Pseudomonas aeruginosa*
- *Enterobacter*
- *Escherichia coli*
- *Proteus*
- *Klebsiella*
- *Staphylococcus aureus*
- *Streptococcus pneumoniae*
- Oral anaerobes

*Most common cause of community-acquired pneumonia (CAP).

Types of Pneumonia

Pneumonia can be caused by bacteria, viruses, *Mycoplasma,* fungi, parasites, and chemicals. Although pneumonia can be classified according to the causative organism, a clinically effective way is to classify pneumonia as community-acquired or hospital-acquired pneumonia. Classifying pneumonia is important because of differences in the likely causative organisms and the selection of appropriate antibiotics (Table 28-2).

Community-Acquired Pneumonia. **Community-acquired pneumonia** (CAP) is defined as a lower respiratory tract infection of the lung parenchyma with onset in the community or during the first 2 days of hospitalization. More than 4 million adults are diagnosed with CAP yearly in the United States, and more than 1 million are hospitalized.[3] The number of cases of pneumococcal pneumonia peaks in midwinter. Smoking is an important risk factor. The causative organism is identified only 50% of the time. Organisms that are commonly implicated in CAP include *S. pneumoniae* (35%), *H. influenza* (10%), and atypical organisms (e.g., *Legionella, Mycoplasma, Chlamydia,* viruses) (see Table 28-2). Once the patient is diagnosed with CAP, a three-step approach is recommended in initiating therapy.[4] The Infectious Disease Society of America (IDSA) and the American Thoracic Society (ATS) are working jointly on updated CAP management guidelines. The three-step approach identifies where to treat the patient:

Step 1: Assessment of the ability to treat the patient at home (e.g., evaluate comorbidities, hemodynamic stability, etc.).

Step 2: Calculation of the pneumonia PORT (Pneumonia Patient Outcomes Research Team) Severity Index (PSI), with recommendations for home care and clinical judgment. This scale, produced by the Agency for Healthcare Research and Quality (AHRQ), is based on multiple factors and the score indicates the patient's risk class[5] (Table 28-3). (The PSI calculator is available for PDA download at *http://pda.ahrq.gov.*)

TABLE 28-3 PORT (Pneumonia Patient Outcomes Research Team) Severity Index (PSI)

Identifying the Level of Risk

This tool may be used as a supplement to clinical judgment.

Pneumonia Severity Index (PSI)

Patient Characteristic	Points Assigned
Demographic Factors	
Age: Males	Age in years
Age: Females	Age in years − 10
Nursing home resident	+10
Comorbid Diseases	
Neoplastic disease	+30
Liver disease	+20
Heart failure	+10
Cerebrovascular disease	+10
Renal disease	+10
Physical Examination Findings	
Altered mental status	+20
Respiratory rate ≥30 breaths/min	+20
Systolic BP <90 mm Hg	+20
Temperature <95° F (35° C) or >104° F (40° C)	+15
Pulse ≥125 beats/min	+10
Laboratory Results	
pH <7.35	+30
BUN >10.7 mmol/L	+20
Sodium <130 mEq/L	+20
Glucose >13.9 mmol/L	+10
Hematocrit <30%	+10
PaO_2 <60 mm Hg	+10
Pleural effusion	+10

Scoring the Risk Levels

Based on PSI score, patient's risk level is identified and site to treat is indicated.

Risk	Risk Class	Based on*	Recommended Treatment Site
Low	I	None	Outpatient
Low	II	70 or fewer points	Outpatient
Low	III	71–90 total points	Outpatient
Moderate	IV	91–130 total points	Inpatient
High	V	>130 total points	Inpatient

Adapted and reprinted with permission from Stanton MA: *Improving treatment decisions for patients with community-acquired pneumonia,* AHRQ Research In Action, Number 7 (AHRQ Publication No. 02-0033). Rockville, Md, 2002, Agency for Healthcare Research and Quality.

*A risk score (total point score) for a given patient is obtained by summing the patient age in years (age − 10 for females) and the points for each applicable patient characteristic.

BUN, Blood urea nitrogen.

Step 3: Clinician judgment in the final decision to treat, either as an outpatient or in the hospital.

Specific antibiotics for empiric treatment have been recommended by the ATS, the IDSA (Table 28-4 presents the IDSA comprehensive guide for immunocompetent adults), and the Canadian Infectious Disease Society/Canadian Thoracic Society (CIDS/CTS). These guidelines provide an evidence-based consensus approach to initial empiric management of CAP for both outpatients and inpatients. The IDSA CAP guidelines are available online at *www.AHRQ.gov.*

TABLE 28-4 DRUG THERAPY
Initial Therapy for Suspected Bacterial Community-Acquired Pneumonia in Immunocompetent Adults

Patient Variable	Preferred Treatment Options*
Outpatient	
Previously healthy	
• No recent antibiotic therapy	A macrolide or doxycycline
• Recent antibiotic therapy (last 3 mo)	A respiratory fluoroquinolone alone, an advanced macrolide plus high-dose amoxicillin, or an advanced macrolide plus high-dose amoxicillin/clavulanate
Comorbidities (COPD, diabetes, renal disease, HF, malignancy)	
• No recent antibiotic therapy	An advanced macrolide or a respiratory fluoroquinolone
• Recent antibiotic therapy	A respiratory fluoroquinolone alone or an advanced macrolide plus a β-lactam
Suspected aspiration with infection	Amoxicillin-clavulanate or clindamycin
Influenza with bacterial superinfection	A β-lactam or a respiratory fluoroquinolone
Inpatient	
Medical Unit	
• No recent antibiotic therapy	A respiratory fluoroquinolone alone or an advanced macrolide plus a β-lactam
• Recent antibiotic therapy	An advanced macrolide plus a β-lactam or a respiratory fluoroquinolone (antibiotic selected based on previous antibiotic history)
ICU	
• *Pseudomonas* infection not an issue	• A β-lactam plus an advanced macrolide or a respiratory fluoroquinolone
• *Pseudomonas* infection not an issue but patient has β-lactam allergy	• A respiratory fluoroquinolone with or without clindamycin
• *Pseudomonas* is an issue	• Either an antipseudomonal agent plus ciprofloxacin or an antipseudomonal agent plus an aminoglycoside plus a respiratory fluoroquinolone or a macrolide
• *Pseudomonas* is an issue but patient has β-lactam allergy	• Either aztreonam plus levofloxacin or aztreonam plus moxifloxacin or gatifloxacin, with or without an aminoglycoside

Source: Adapted from the Infectious Disease Society of America *(www.idsociety.org)*.

*__Macrolides:__ erythromycin, azithromycin (Zithromax), clarithromycin (Biaxin); **respiratory fluoroquinolones:** moxifloxacin (Avelox, Vigamox), gatifloxacin (Tequin), levofloxacin (Levaquin), gemifloxacin (Factive); **advanced macrolides:** azithromycin, clarithromycin; **β-lactams:** high-dose amoxicillin, amoxicillin/clavulanate (Augmentin), cefpodoxime (Vantin), cefprozil (Cefzil), cefuroxime (Ceftin); **antipseudomonal agents:** piperacillin (Pipracil), imipenem/cilastatin (Primaxin), meropenem (Merrem IV), cefepime (Maxipime), piperacillin/tazobactam (Zosyn).

COPD, Chronic obstructive pulmonary disease; *HF*, heart failure; *ICU*, intensive care unit.

Therapy for pneumonia is empiric because specific pathogens are not identified at the time treatment is initiated. The specific antibiotics recommended from the IDSA, ATS, and CIDS/CTS for empiric treatment are all fairly similar and start with either a macrolide (erythromycin, azithromycin [Zithromax], clarithromycin [Biaxin]) or doxycycline (Vibramycin). If comorbidities are present, a β-lactam antibiotic (e.g., amoxicillin/clavulanate [Augmentin]) may be added. If patients are hospitalized, intravenous antibiotics are initiated and may include two or three drugs. The specific antibiotic choice must be guided by each institution's *antibiogram,* which is an antimicrobial susceptibility trending chart designed by each health care facility to guide antibiotic use. The antibiotic prescribed needs to be started "door to dose," within 4 hours of arrival at the hospital. The timing of initial therapy is crucial. Data have shown that early treatment reduces mortality.[6] Once specific pathogens are identified, antibiotic therapy can be pathogen specific. With appropriate antibiotic therapy, some improvement in clinical course is seen in 48 to 72 hours. Fever, cough, crackles, and chest x-rays will all start to improve but may take 3 days to 3 weeks to resolve.[7] While the guidelines do not address length of time of antibiotic therapy, many experts suggest 10 to 14 days for the majority of patients and extended therapy for atypical CAP caused by atypical organisms.[3]

The IDSA recommends hospital discharge criteria for patients with CAP. During the 24 hours prior to discharge to home, the patient should have no more than one of the following (unless it represents the patient's baseline status): temperature >100.4° F (37.8° C); pulse >100 beats/minute; respiratory rate >24 breaths/minute; systolic blood pressure (BP) <90 mm Hg; oxygen saturation in arterial blood by pulse oximetry (SpO_2) <90%; and inability to maintain oral intake.[4]

Hospital-Acquired, Ventilator-Associated, and Health Care–Associated Pneumonia. **Hospital-acquired pneumonia** (HAP) is pneumonia occurring 48 hours or longer after hospital admission and not incubating at the time of hospitalization.[8] *Ventilator-associated pneumonia* (VAP) refers to pneumonia that occurs more than 48 to 72 hours after endotracheal intubation. *Health care–associated pneumonia* (HCAP) includes any patient with a new-onset pneumonia who (1) was hospitalized in an acute care hospital for 2 or more days within 90 days of the infection; (2) resided in a long-term care facility; (3) received recent intravenous antibiotic therapy, chemotherapy, or wound care within the past 30 days of the current infection; or (4) attended a hospital or hemodialysis clinic. HAP is estimated to occur at a rate of 5 to 15 cases per 1000 hospital admissions, with the rate increasing by 6 to 20 times in patients requiring mechanical ventilation.[8] HAP is the second most common nosocomial infection, second only to urinary tract infection. It costs $1.3 billion annually in hospital charges.[9]

The microorganisms responsible for HAP, VAP, and HCAP are usually bacterial and rarely viral or fungal (see Table 28-2). Many of the organisms enter the lungs after aspiration of particles from the patient's own oropharynx. Immunosuppressive therapy, general debility, and endotracheal intubation are risk factors predisposing to pneumonia (see Table 28-1), while contaminated health care devices and the general environment are potential sources of pathogens.

Once the diagnosis is made, empiric treatment of the pneumonia is initiated based on known risk factors, early versus late onset, and disease severity. A major problem in treating infectious diseases is multidrug-resistant (MDR) organisms, which means that the pathogen has developed resistance to multiple antibiotics. MDR organisms are identified by antibiotic susceptibility tests. The virulence of these organisms can severely limit the available and appropriate antimicrobial therapy. In addition, MDR organisms can increase the morbidity and mortality associated with pneumonia. (MDR organisms are discussed in Chapter 15.)

Fungal Pneumonia. Fungi may also be a cause of pneumonia (see the section on Pulmonary Fungal Infections later in this chapter).

Aspiration Pneumonia. *Aspiration pneumonia* refers to the sequelae occurring from abnormal entry of secretions or substances into the lower airway. It usually follows aspiration of material from the mouth or stomach into the trachea and subsequently the lungs. The person who has aspiration pneumonia usually has a history of loss of consciousness (e.g., as a result of seizure, anesthesia, head injury, stroke, or alcohol intake). With loss of consciousness, the gag and cough reflexes are depressed, and aspiration is more likely to occur. Another risk factor is tube feedings. The dependent portions of the lung are most often affected, primarily the superior segments of the lower lobes and the posterior segments of the upper lobes, which are dependent in the supine position.

The aspirated material—food, water, vomitus, or toxic fluids—is the triggering mechanism for the pathology of this type of pneumonia. There are three distinct forms of aspiration pneumonia. If the aspirated material is an inert substance (e.g., barium), the initial manifestation is usually caused by mechanical obstruction of airways. When the aspirated materials contain toxic fluids such as gastric juices, there is chemical injury to the lung with infection as a secondary event, usually 48 to 72 hours later; this is identified as *chemical (noninfectious) pneumonitis.* The most important form of aspiration pneumonia is bacterial infection. The infecting organism is usually one of the normal oropharyngeal flora, and multiple organisms, including both aerobes and anaerobes, are isolated from the sputum of the patient with aspiration pneumonia. Antibiotic therapy is based on an assessment of the severity of illness, where the infection was acquired (community vs. hospital), and the type of organism present.

Opportunistic Pneumonia. Certain patients with altered immune responses are highly susceptible to respiratory infections. Individuals considered at risk include (1) those who have severe protein-calorie malnutrition; (2) those who have immune deficiencies; (3) those who have received transplants and been treated with immunosuppressive drugs; and (4) patients who are being treated with radiation therapy, chemotherapy drugs, and corticosteroids (especially for a prolonged period). The individual has a variety of altered parameters, including altered B- and T-lymphocyte function, depressed bone marrow function, and decreased levels or function of neutrophils and macrophages. In addition to the bacterial and viral causative agents (especially gram-negative bacteria), other agents that cause pneumonia in the immunocompromised patient are *Pneumocystis jiroveci* (formerly *carinii*) and other fungi, and cytomegalovirus (CMV).

Pneumocystis jiroveci is an opportunistic pathogen; this fungus rarely causes pneumonia in the healthy individual. *Pneumocystis jiroveci* pneumonia (PCP) has been identified as the most common acquired immunodeficiency syndrome (AIDS)–defining opportunistic infection in the United States and is a common cause of AIDS-associated pneumonia. In this type of pneumonia, the chest x-ray usually shows a diffuse bilateral alveolar pattern of infiltration. In widespread disease, the lungs are massively consolidated.

Clinical manifestations are insidious and include fever, tachypnea, tachycardia, dyspnea, nonproductive cough, and hypoxemia. Pulmonary physical findings are minimal in proportion to the serious nature of the disease. Bacterial and viral pneumonias must first be ruled out because of the vague presentation of PCP. Treatment consists of a course of trimethoprim/sulfamethoxazole (Bactrim) as the primary agent. An alternative medication for the Bactrim-intolerant patient is dapsone.[10] In populations at risk for development of PCP (e.g., patients with hematologic malignancies or human immunodeficiency virus [HIV]–positive patients with $CD4^+$ T-lymphocyte counts $<200/\mu l$), prophylactic therapy with trimethoprim/sulfamethoxazole may be used. Aerosolized pentamidine (NebuPent), although less commonly used, is an alternative for prophylaxis in Bactrim-intolerant patients. (PCP is also discussed in Chapter 15.)

Cytomegalovirus (CMV) is a cause of viral pneumonia in the immunocompromised patient, particularly in transplant recipients. CMV is a member of the herpesvirus family, which includes Epstein-Barr virus, herpes simplex virus, and varicella-zoster virus.[6-8] This virus is not highly contagious, but it is a prevalent virus, with 40% to 100% of the population generally exposed in childhood.[11] CMV gives rise to latent infections and reactivation with shedding of infectious virus. It can be a serious lung pathogen in transplant patients. CMV interstitial pneumonia can be a mild disease, or it can result in severe pulmonary insufficiency with high mortality rates. Ganciclovir (Cytovene) is recommended for treatment of CMV pneumonia.

Pathophysiology

Pneumococcal pneumonia is the most common cause of bacterial pneumonia and is caused by the *Streptococcus pneumoniae* organism. *S. pneumoniae,* also called pneumococcus, can infect the upper respiratory tract, the blood, and the nervous system. The organism is generally found in the nose and throat. When it invades the lung, pneumonia can occur. The Centers for Disease Control and Prevention (CDC) estimates that 40,000 deaths and 500,000 cases of pneumococcal pneumonia occur annually in the United States. There are twice as many cases in African Americans compared to whites.[12]

The pathophysiology related to this type of pneumonia is discussed here. (The pathophysiology of other types of pneumonia is similar.) There are four characteristic stages of the disease process:

1. *Congestion.* After the pneumococcus organisms reach the alveoli, there is an outpouring of fluid into the alveoli. The organisms multiply in the serous fluid, and the infection is spread. The pneumococci damage the host by their overwhelming growth and by interfering with lung function.
2. *Red hepatization.* There is massive dilation of the capillaries, and alveoli are filled with organisms, neutrophils, red blood cells (RBCs), and fibrin (Fig. 28-1). The lung appears red and granular, similar to the liver, which is why the process is called hepatization.

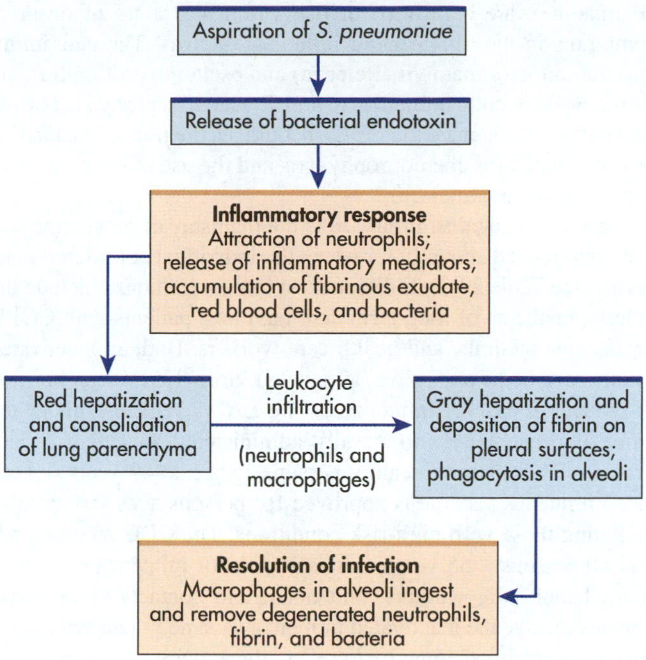

FIG. 28-1 Pathophysiologic course of pneumococcal pneumonia.

3. *Gray hepatization.* Blood flow decreases, and leukocytes and fibrin consolidate in the affected part of the lung.
4. *Resolution.* Complete resolution and healing occur if there are no complications. The exudate becomes lysed and is processed by the macrophages. The normal lung tissue is restored, and the person's gas-exchange ability returns to normal.

Clinical Manifestations

Patients with pneumonia usually have a sudden onset of symptoms, including fever, shaking chills, shortness of breath, cough productive of purulent sputum (rust-colored sputum can be seen in pneumococcal pneumonia), and pleuritic chest pain (in some cases). In the elderly or debilitated patient, confusion or stupor (possibly related to hypoxia) may be the only finding. On physical examination, signs of pulmonary consolidation, such as dullness to percussion, increased fremitus, bronchial breath sounds, and crackles, may be found. The typical pneumonia syndrome is usually caused by the most common pathogen, *S. pneumoniae,* but can also be due to other bacterial pathogens, such as *H. influenzae.*

Pneumonia may also manifest atypically with a more gradual onset, a dry cough, and extrapulmonary manifestations such as headache, myalgias, fatigue, sore throat, nausea, vomiting, and diarrhea. On physical examination, crackles are often heard. This presentation of manifestations is classically produced by *M. pneumoniae* but can also be caused by *Legionella* and *C. pneumoniae.*

The initial manifestations of viral pneumonia are highly variable. Viruses also cause pneumonia that is usually characterized by an atypical presentation with chills; fever; dry, nonproductive cough; and extrapulmonary symptoms. Primary viral pneumonia can be caused by influenza virus infection. Viral pneumonia is also found in association with systemic viral diseases such as measles, varicella-zoster, and herpes simplex.

Complications

Most cases of pneumonia generally run an uncomplicated course. However, complications can occur, and they develop more frequently in individuals with underlying chronic diseases and other risk factors. Complications may include the following:

1. *Pleurisy* (inflammation of the pleura) is relatively common.
2. *Pleural effusion* (transudate fluid in the pleural space) can occur. It develops in 40% of hospitalized patients with pneumococcal pneumonia. Usually the effusion is sterile and is reabsorbed in 1 to 2 weeks; occasionally, effusions require aspiration by means of thoracentesis.
3. *Atelectasis* (collapsed, airless alveoli) of one or part of one lobe may occur. These areas usually clear with effective coughing and deep breathing.
4. *Bacteremia* (bacterial infection in the blood) occurs in 30% of patients with pneumococcal pneumonia and is associated with a 20% mortality rate. The rate can go as high as 60% in elderly patients.[12]
5. *Lung abscess* is not a common complication of pneumonia. It is seen with pneumonia caused by *S. aureus* and gram-negative pneumonias (see the section on Lung Abscess later in this chapter).
6. *Empyema* (accumulation of purulent exudate in the pleural cavity) is relatively infrequent (occurs in $<5\%$ of cases) but requires antibiotic therapy and drainage of the exudate by a chest tube or open surgical drainage.
7. *Pericarditis* results from spread of the infecting organism from an infected pleura or via a hematogenous route to the pericardium (fibroserous sac around the heart).
8. *Meningitis* can be caused by *S. pneumoniae.* The patient with pneumonia who is disoriented, confused, or somnolent should have a lumbar puncture to evaluate the possibility of meningitis.
9. *Endocarditis* can develop when the organisms attack the endocardium and the valves of the heart. The clinical manifestations are similar to those of acute bacterial endocarditis (see Chapter 37).

Diagnostic Studies

The common diagnostic measures for pneumonia are presented in Table 28-5. History, physical examination, and chest x-ray often provide enough information to make management decisions without costly laboratory tests.

Chest x-ray often shows a typical pattern characteristic of the infecting organism and is invaluable in the diagnosis of pneumonia. Lobar or segmental consolidation suggests a bacterial cause, usually *S. pneumoniae* or *Klebsiella.* Diffuse pulmonary infiltrates are most commonly caused by infection with viruses, *Legionella,* or pathogenic fungi. Cavitary shadows suggest the presence of a necrotizing infection with destruction of lung tissue commonly caused by *S. aureus,* gram-negative bacteria, and *M. tuberculosis.* Pleural effusions, which can occur in up to 30% of patients with CAP, can also be seen on x-ray.

Sputum Gram stain and cultures are not always obtainable. The interpretation of a Gram stain is not standardized, and atypical pathogens are missed. However, obtaining a lower respiratory tract sputum specimen for culture is recommended before initiating antibiotic therapy in the hospitalized patient.[6] If a delay in the time from collecting the sputum to incubation exceeds 2 to 5 hours, results are less reliable. Sputum needs to be sent for culture as soon

TABLE 28-5 COLLABORATIVE CARE Pneumonia

Diagnostic
History and physical examination
Chest x-ray
Gram stain of sputum
Sputum culture and sensitivity test (if drug-resistant pathogen or organism not covered by empiric therapy)
Pulse oximetry or ABGs (if indicated)
Complete blood count, differential, and routine blood chemistries (if indicated)
Blood cultures (if indicated)
Collaborative Therapy
Appropriate antibiotic therapy (see Tables 28-3 and 28-4)
Increased fluid intake (at least 3 L/day)
Limited activity and rest
Antipyretics
Analgesics
Oxygen therapy (if indicated)

ABGs, Arterial blood gases.

as it is collected. Before antibiotic treatment is begun, two blood cultures may be done for patients who are seriously ill. Although microbial studies are expected before treatment, initiation of antibiotics should not be delayed. Empiric therapy is generally started without culture results in order to maximize treatment effectiveness. Empiric therapy is based on observation and experience, and the exact cause of the infection may not be known. Pulse oximetry is measured routinely and can reveal oxygen desaturation. Arterial blood gases (ABGs) may be obtained and can reveal hypoxemia (partial pressure of oxygen in arterial blood [PaO_2] <80 mm Hg), hypercapnia (partial pressure of carbon dioxide in arterial blood [$PaCO_2$] >45 mm Hg), and acidosis. Leukocytosis is found in the majority of patients with bacterial pneumonia, usually with a white blood cell (WBC) count greater than 15,000/μl (15×10^9/L) with the presence of bands (immature neutrophils).

Collaborative Care

Prompt treatment with the appropriate antibiotic almost always cures bacterial and mycoplasma pneumonia. In uncomplicated cases, the patient responds to drug therapy within 48 to 72 hours. Indications of improvement include decreased temperature, improved breathing, and reduced chest pain. Abnormal physical findings can last for more than 7 days.

In addition to antibiotic therapy, supportive measures may be used, including oxygen therapy to treat hypoxemia, analgesics to relieve the chest pain for patient comfort, and antipyretics such as aspirin or acetaminophen for significantly elevated temperature. During the acute febrile phase, the patient's activity should be restricted, and rest should be encouraged and planned.

Most individuals with mild to moderate illness who have no other underlying disease process can be treated on an outpatient basis. If there is a serious underlying disease or if the pneumonia is accompanied by severe dyspnea, hypoxemia, or other complications, the patient should be hospitalized. Guidelines for hospitalization for CAP are presented in Table 28-3.

Currently, there is no definitive treatment for viral pneumonia. Two antiviral drugs, amantadine (Symmetrel) and rimantadine (Flumadine), are approved for use within 48 hours of onset of symptoms in the treatment of influenza A virus. The neuraminidase inhibitors, zanamivir (Relenza) and oseltamivir (Tamiflu), are active against both influenza A and B (see Chapter 27). During outbreaks of influenza, the CDC encourages the use of amantadine or rimantadine for chemoprophylaxis and the use of oseltamivir or zanamivir for treatment.[13]

Vaccination against influenza is the mainstay of prevention and is recommended annually for use in the individual considered to be at risk (see Table 27-3). Individuals at risk for influenza include the elderly, residents of long-term care facilities, patients with COPD or diabetes mellitus, and health care workers. Both an inactivated influenza vaccine and a live, attenuated virus (LAIV) can be used to reduce the risk of influenza.[14] The LAIV, marketed under the name FluMist, is an intranasally administered vaccine only approved for use among healthy persons ages 5 to 49 years. Inactivated influenza vaccine is approved for persons ages ≥6 months, including those with high-risk conditions. The CDC recommends that all persons ≥65 years, others at risk for influenza complications, health care workers, and household contacts of high-risk persons receive the inactivated influenza vaccine.[14] The inactivated vaccine is modified annually to reflect the anticipated strains in the upcoming season. This vaccine is 30% to 40% effective in preventing clinical illness.

Pneumococcal Vaccine. Pneumococcal vaccine is indicated primarily for the individual considered at risk who (1) has chronic illnesses such as lung and heart disease and diabetes mellitus, (2) is recovering from a severe illness, (3) is 65 years of age or older, or (4) is in a long-term care facility. This is particularly important because the rate of drug-resistant *S. pneumoniae* infections is increasing. The vaccine is 50% to 80% effective in preventing bacteremic pneumococcal disease.[15] In the immunosuppressed individual at risk for development of fatal pneumococcal infection (e.g., asplenic patient; patient with nephrotic syndrome, renal failure, or AIDS; transplant recipient), a second dose is recommended after 5 years, although the efficacy of revaccination is unknown.[4] All persons ≥65 years of age who have not received vaccine within 5 years (and were <65 years of age at the time of vaccination) should receive another dose of vaccine. Pneumococcal vaccine and influenza vaccine can be given at the same time in different arms.[4]

Drug Therapy. The main problems with the use of antibiotics in pneumonia are the development of multidrug-resistant (MDR) organisms and the patient's hypersensitivity or allergic reaction to certain antibiotics.

Most cases of CAP in otherwise healthy adults do not require hospitalization. The oral antibiotic therapy administered is frequently empiric treatment with broad-spectrum antibiotics. Once the patient is categorized (see Table 28-3), empiric therapy can be based on the likely infecting organism.

For HAP, VAP, and HCAP, the American Thoracic Society (ATS) recommends that empiric antibiotic therapy be based on whether the patient has risk factors for MDR organisms. The antibiotic regimen needs to be adapted to the local patterns of antibiotic resistance.

When using empiric therapy, it is important to recognize the nonresponding patient. Therapy may require modification based on the patient's sputum culture results or clinical response. Clinical response is evaluated by factors such as a change in fever, sputum purulence, leukocytosis, oxygenation, and chest x-ray patterns. Clinical improvement after adequate VAP treatment can be seen by day 3 to 5. Patients with VAP may experience rapid deterioration. Patients who deteriorate or fail to respond to therapy will require aggressive evaluation to assess for noninfectious etiologies, complications, other coexisting infectious processes, or pneumonia caused by a drug-resistant pathogen.[16] While monotherapy (one-drug therapy) with selected agents can be used with severe HAP and VAP in the absence of resistant organisms, patients in risk groups initially receive combination therapy until the culture results are known and it is confirmed that one agent can be used. Aerosolized antibiotics have not proven to have value in the treatment of VAP, but they may be considered adjunctive therapy for patients with MDR gram-negative organisms not responding to systemic therapy.[8]

Nutritional Therapy. Fluid intake of at least 3 L/day is important in the supportive treatment of pneumonia. If the patient has heart failure, fluid intake must be individualized. If oral intake cannot be maintained, intravenous (IV) administration of fluids and electrolytes may be necessary for the acutely ill patient. Weight loss often occurs in patients with pneumonia because of increased metabolic needs and difficulty eating due to shortness of breath and pleuritic pain. Therefore it is important to provide nutritional intake to meet the needs of the patient. Small, frequent meals are better tolerated by the dyspneic patient.

TABLE 28-6 NURSING ASSESSMENT
Pneumonia

Subjective Data

Important Health Information

Past health history: Lung cancer, COPD, diabetes mellitus, chronic debilitating disease, malnutrition, altered consciousness, AIDS, exposure to chemical toxins, dust, or allergens

Medications: Use of antibiotics; corticosteroids, chemotherapy, or any other immunosuppressants

Surgery or other treatments: Recent abdominal or thoracic surgery, splenectomy, endotracheal intubation, or any surgery with general anesthesia; tube feedings

Functional Health Patterns

Health perception–health management: Cigarette smoking, alcoholism; recent upper respiratory tract infection, malaise

Nutritional-metabolic: Anorexia, nausea, vomiting; chills

Activity-exercise: Prolonged bed rest or immobility; fatigue, weakness; dyspnea, cough (productive or nonproductive); nasal congestion

Cognitive-perceptual: Pain with breathing, chest pain, sore throat, headache, abdominal pain, muscle aches

Objective Data

General

Fever, restlessness or lethargy; splinting of affected area

Respiratory

Tachypnea; pharyngitis; asymmetric chest movements or retraction; decreased excursion; nasal flaring; use of accessory muscles (neck, abdomen); grunting; crackles, friction rub on auscultation; dullness on percussion over consolidated areas, increased tactile fremitus on palpation; pink, rusty, purulent, green, yellow, or white sputum (amount may be scant to copious)

Cardiovascular

Tachycardia

Neurologic

Changes in mental status, ranging from confusion to delirium

Possible Findings

Leukocytosis; abnormal ABGs with ↓ or normal PaO_2, ↓ $PaCO_2$, and ↑ pH initially, and later ↓ PaO_2, ↑ $PaCO_2$, and ↓ pH; positive sputum Gram stain and culture; patchy or diffuse infiltrates, abscesses, pleural effusion, or pneumothorax on chest x-ray*

*In the elderly dehydrated patient, chest x-ray may not be indicative of pneumonia until patient is rehydrated.

ABGs, Arterial blood gases; *AIDS,* acquired immunodeficiency syndrome; *COPD,* chronic obstructive pulmonary disease.

NURSING MANAGEMENT PNEUMONIA

Nursing Assessment

Subjective and objective data that should be obtained from a patient with pneumonia are presented in Table 28-6.

Nursing Diagnoses

Nursing diagnoses for the patient with pneumonia may include, but are not limited to, those presented in NCP 28-1.

Planning

The overall goals are that the patient with pneumonia will have (1) clear breath sounds, (2) normal breathing patterns, (3) no signs of hypoxia, (4) normal chest x-ray, and (5) no complications related to pneumonia.

Nursing Implementation

Health Promotion. There are many nursing interventions to help prevent the occurrence of, as well as the morbidity associated with, pneumonia. Teaching the individual to practice good health habits, such as proper diet and hygiene, adequate rest, and regular exercise, can maintain the natural resistance to infecting organisms. If possible, exposure to URIs should be avoided. If a URI occurs, it should be treated promptly with supportive measures (e.g., rest, fluids). If symptoms persist for more than 7 days, the person should obtain medical care. The individual at risk for pneumonia (e.g., the chronically ill, older adult) should be encouraged to obtain both influenza and pneumococcal vaccines.

In the hospital, the nursing role involves identifying the patient at risk (see Tables 28-1 and 28-3) and taking measures to prevent the development of pneumonia. The patient with altered consciousness should be placed in positions (e.g., side-lying, upright) that will prevent or minimize the risk of aspiration. The patient should be turned and repositioned at least every 2 hours to facilitate adequate lung expansion and to discourage pooling of secretions. In VAP, a significant reduction in pneumonia incidence is found when patients are placed in a semirecumbent position (45 degrees). The ATS recommends that intubated patients be in a semirecumbent position (30 to 45 degrees), particularly during enteral feeding.[8] In intubated patients, the ATS also recommends continuous aspiration of subglottic secretions above the tracheal tube cuff using a specially designed endotracheal tube to prevent the risk of VAP.

The patient who has a feeding tube generally requires attention to measures to prevent aspiration (see Chapter 40). Although the feeding tube is small, an interruption in the integrity of the lower esophageal sphincter still exists, which can allow reflux of gastric and intestinal contents. The ATS recommends that oral tubes be placed, rather than nasal tubes, to prevent nosocomial sinusitis.[8]

The patient who has difficulty swallowing (e.g., stroke patient) needs assistance in eating, drinking, and taking medication to prevent aspiration. The patient who has recently had surgery and oth-

NURSING CARE PLAN 28-1

Patient with Pneumonia

NURSING DIAGNOSIS **Ineffective breathing pattern** *related to* inflammation and pain *as evidenced by* dyspnea, tachypnea, nasal flaring, altered chest excursion

PATIENT GOAL Demonstrates an effective respiratory rate, rhythm, and depth of respirations

OUTCOMES (NOC)

Respiratory Status: Ventilation

- Respiratory rate ___
- Respiratory rhythm ___
- Ease of breathing ___
- Symmetrical chest expansion ___

Measurement Scale

1 = Severely compromised
2 = Substantially compromised
3 = Moderately compromised
4 = Mildly compromised
5 = Not compromised

INTERVENTIONS (NIC) and *RATIONALES*

Ventilation Assistance

- Monitor respiratory and oxygenation status *to determine change in status.*
- Position to minimize respiratory efforts (e.g., elevate the head of the bed and provide overbed table for patient to lean on) *to reduce oxygen needs.*
- Encourage slow deep breathing, turning, and coughing *to promote effective breathing pattern.*
- Monitor for respiratory muscle fatigue *to provide additional support if needed.*
- Initiate and maintain supplemental oxygen *to improve respiratory status.*
- Administer medications (e.g., bronchodilators and inhalers) *that promote airway patency and gas exchange.*

NURSING DIAGNOSIS **Ineffective airway clearance** *related to* retained secretions and excessive mucus *as evidenced by* ineffective cough, adventitious breath sounds, dyspnea

PATIENT GOALS
1. Demonstrates effective coughing and increased air exchange
2. Experiences normal breath sounds

OUTCOMES (NOC)

Respiratory Status: Airway Patency

- Respiratory rate ___
- Ease of breathing ___
- Moves sputum out of airway___

Measurement Scale

1 = Severely compromised
2 = Substantially compromised
3 = Moderately compromised
4 = Mildly compromised
5 = Not compromised

INTERVENTIONS (NIC) and *RATIONALES*

Airway Management

- Auscultate breath sounds, noting areas of decreased/absent ventilation, and presence of adventitious sounds *to obtain ongoing data on patient's response to therapy.*
- Remove secretions by encouraging coughing or by suctioning *to clear airway.*
- Regulate fluid intake *to optimize fluid balance and liquefy secretions.*

Cough Enhancement

- Assist patient to a sitting position with head slightly flexed, shoulders relaxed, and knees flexed *to improve respiratory status.*
- Instruct patient to inhale deeply several times, to exhale slowly, and to cough at the end of exhalation *to promote effective coughing.*
- Encourage use of incentive spirometry *to aid in lung expansion and prevent atelectasis.*

NURSING DIAGNOSIS **Acute pain** *related to* inflammation and ineffective pain management and/or comfort measures *as evidenced by* patient report of pleuritic chest pain and presence of pleural friction rub, shallow respirations

PATIENT GOAL Reports control of pain following relief measures

OUTCOMES (NOC)

Pain Control

- Reports pain controlled ___
- Described causal factors ___
- Uses nonanalgesic relief measures ___
- Uses analgesics appropriately ___

Measurement Scale

1 = Never demonstrated
2 = Rarely demonstrated
3 = Sometimes demonstrated
4 = Often demonstrated
5 = Consistently demonstrated

INTERVENTIONS (NIC) and *RATIONALES*

Pain Management

- Perform a comprehensive assessment of pain to include location, characteristics, onset/duration, frequency, quality, intensity or severity of pain, and precipitating factors *to determine appropriate interventions.*
- Encourage patient to monitor own pain and to intervene appropriately *to allow independence and prepare for discharge.*
- Teach use of nonpharmacological techniques (e.g., relaxation, guided imagery, music therapy, distraction, and massage) before, after, and, if possible, during painful activities; before pain occurs or increases; and along with other pain relief measures *to relieve pain and reduce the need for analgesia.*
- Use pain control measures before pain becomes severe *because mild to moderate pain is controlled more quickly.*
- Medicate prior to an activity to increase participation, but evaluate the hazard of sedation *to help minimize pain that will be experienced.*

ers who are immobile need assistance with turning and deep-breathing measures at frequent intervals (see Chapter 20). The nurse must be careful to avoid overmedication with opioids or sedatives, which can cause a depressed cough reflex and accumulation of fluid in the lungs. The gag reflex should be present in the individual who has had local anesthesia to the throat before the administration of fluids or food.

Strict medical asepsis and adherence to infection control guidelines should be practiced by the nurse to reduce the incidence of nosocomial infections. Poor hand-washing practices allow spread of pathogens via the hands of the health care worker. Staff should wash their hands each time before and after they provide care to a patient and whenever removing gloves. Respiratory devices can harbor microorganisms and have been associated with outbreaks of pneumonia. Strict sterile aseptic technique should be used when suctioning the trachea of a patient, and caution is required when handling ventilator circuits, tracheostomy tubing, and nebulizer circuits that can become contaminated from patient secretions.

Acute Intervention. Although many patients with pneumonia are treated on an outpatient basis, the nursing care plan for a patient with pneumonia (see NCP 28-1) is applicable to both these individuals and in-hospital patients. It is important for the nurse to remember that pneumonia is an acute, infectious disease. Although most cases of pneumonia are potentially completely curable, complications can result. The nurse must be aware of these complications and their manifestations. The essential components of nursing care for patients with pneumonia include monitoring physical assessment parameters, facilitating laboratory and diagnostic tests, providing treatment, and monitoring the patient's response to treatment (see Table 28-6). Along with physical assessment (including pulse oximetry monitoring), prompt collection of specimens and prompt initiation of antibiotics (within 4 hours of arriving at the hospital) are critical. Oxygen therapy, administration of bronchodilators, hydration, nutritional support, and therapeutic positioning are part of the management of the patient.

Therapeutic positioning identifies the best position for the patient to assure stable oxygenation status. The concepts of therapeutic positioning are based on type of lung disease and patient response to positioning. The "good lung down" position is utilized for patients with unilateral lung disease, in whom better oxygenation is achieved when the unaffected lung (good lung) is placed in the down (lateral) position.[17-19] For bilateral lung disease, research indicates that positioning the patient with the right lung down provides the best ventilation and perfusion.[17] The use of bronchial hygiene techniques (postural drainage, percussion, vibration) is generally not warranted unless the patient is producing large volumes of sputum (>30 ml/day) or has x-ray evidence of mucous plugging and lobar collapse.[19] Incentive spirometry, turning, coughing, and deep breathing all increase lung volume, mobilize secretions, and prevent atelectasis. Exercise and early ambulation augment bronchial hygiene and are encouraged as tolerated.

Ambulatory and Home Care. The patient needs to be reassured that complete recovery from pneumonia is possible. It is extremely important to emphasize the need to take all of the prescribed drug and to return for follow-up medical care and evaluation. The patient needs to be taught about any drug-drug and food-drug interactions for the prescribed antibiotic. Adequate rest is needed to maintain progress toward recovery and to prevent a relapse. The patient should be told that it may be weeks before the usual vigor and sense of well-being are felt. A prolonged period of convalescence may be necessary for the older adult or chronically ill patient.

The patient considered to be at risk for pneumonia should be told about available vaccines and should discuss them with the health care provider. Deep-breathing exercises or incentive spirometry therapy should be practiced for 6 to 8 weeks after the patient is discharged from the hospital.

> ***HEALTHY PEOPLE***
> **Prevention of Respiratory Diseases**
>
> - Avoid cigarette smoking and exposure to environmental smoke
> - Avoid exposure to allergens, indoor pollutants, and ambient air pollutants
> - Wear proper protection when working in an occupation with prolonged exposure to dust, fumes, or gases

Evaluation

The expected outcomes for the patient with pneumonia are presented in NCP 28-1.

TUBERCULOSIS

Tuberculosis (TB) is an infectious disease caused by *Mycobacterium tuberculosis.* It usually involves the lungs, but it also occurs in the larynx, kidneys, bones, adrenal glands, lymph nodes, and meninges and can be disseminated throughout the body. TB is the world's second most common cause of death from infectious disease, after HIV/AIDS. An estimated 2 billion people (one third of the world's population) are infected with the *M. tuberculosis* bacteria. There are an estimated 8 to 9 million cases a year, and approximately 2 million people die annually.[20] The highest incidence is seen in the developing countries of Africa and Asia, with a recent increase seen in the former Soviet Union.[21] Although a decline has been seen in TB rates in the United States, over 14,000 new cases of TB per year are still being reported. Despite the decline in TB nationwide, rates have increased in certain states and high rates continue to be reported in certain populations (e.g., foreign-born persons, ethnic minorities [see Cultural and Ethnic Health Disparities Box]). Targeted interventions for these at-risk populations and efforts toward a worldwide attack against TB are needed.

The major factors that have contributed to the resurgence of TB have been (1) high rates of TB among patients with HIV infection and (2) the emergence of multidrug-resistant (MDR) strains of *M. tuberculosis.* Once a strain of *M. tuberculosis* develops resistance to isoniazid and rifampin, it is defined as multidrug-resistant tuberculosis (MDR-TB). MDR-TB developed because patients had poor compliance with drug therapy, leading to treatment failure; were lost to follow-up treatment; or were placed on drug regimens to which their infections were no longer susceptible.

TB is seen disproportionately in the poor, the underserved, and minorities. Individuals at risk for TB include homeless persons, residents of inner-city neighborhoods, foreign-born persons, older adults, those in institutions (long-term care facilities, prisons), injection drug users, persons at poverty level, and those with poor access to health care. Immunosuppression from any etiology (e.g.,

CULTURAL AND ETHNIC HEALTH DISPARITIES

Tuberculosis

- Of the reported TB cases in the United States, 82% occur in racial and ethnic minorities.
- Asians have the highest TB rate of any ethnic group (29.3%) in the United States. Native Hawaiian and other Pacific Islanders have the second highest TB rate (21.8%).
- African Americans have 45% of the TB cases in U.S.-born persons.
- Hispanics equaled African Americans (28%) as the racial/ethnic group with the largest percentage of cases.
- The case rate of TB among foreign-born persons in the United States is 53% which is more than 8 times higher than among U.S.-born persons.
- Eleven U.S. states (California, Connecticut, Hawaii, Iowa, Massachusetts, Minnesota, Nebraska, New Hampshire, New Jersey, Utah, and Vermont) had ≥70% of their annual total cases of TB among foreign-born persons.

Source: Centers for Disease Control and Prevention: Reported Tuberculosis in the United States.

HIV infection, malignancy) increases the risk of TB infection. The prevalence of TB is high in areas of the United States where there is a large population of Native Americans, such as Arizona and New Mexico. Higher TB rates are found in non-Hispanic whites in seven southeastern states of the Unites States compared with the rest of the country. In the United States, African Americans have TB rates 8 times higher than non-Hispanic whites. Health care workers with increased exposure to TB are considered at high risk.

Etiology and Pathophysiology

M. tuberculosis is a gram-positive, acid-fast bacillus that is usually spread from person to person via airborne droplets. These droplets are produced when the infected individual with pulmonary or laryngeal TB coughs, sneezes, speaks, or sings. Brief exposure to a few tubercle bacilli rarely causes an infection. Rather, TB is more commonly spread by repeated close contact (within 6 inches of the person's mouth) with the infected person. TB is not highly infectious, and transmission usually requires close, frequent, or prolonged exposure. The disease cannot be spread by hands, books, glasses, or dishes.

The very small droplet nuclei, 1 to 5 μm in size, contain *M. tuberculosis.* Because they are so small in size, the particles remain airborne for minutes to hours. Once inhaled, these small nuclei lodge in alveoli in the small distal airways of the lung. *M. tuberculosis* replicates slowly and spreads via the lymphatic system. The organisms find favorable environments for growth primarily in the upper lobes of the lungs, kidneys, epiphyses of the bone, cerebral cortex, and adrenal glands.

Cellular immunity limits further multiplication and spread of the infection. After the cellular immune system is activated, a characteristic tissue *granuloma,* formed from alveolar macrophages, contains the bacteria and prevents further replication. At this point the person has TB infection, which can be detected by using the tuberculin skin test. (It may take 2 to 10 weeks for the infected person to develop a positive reaction to the tuberculin skin test.) The granuloma is usually not viable and, as a result, the infection remains contained and active disease may never occur.[21] Persons who are infected with *M. tuberculosis,* but who do not have TB disease, cannot spread the infection to other people.

TB infection occurs when the bacteria are inhaled but there is an effective immune response and the bacteria become inactive. The majority of people mount effective immune responses to encapsulate these organisms for the rest of their lives, preventing primary infection from progressing to disease. TB infection in a person who does not have the active TB disease is not considered a case of TB and is often referred to as *latent TB infection* (LTBI).[22] If the initial immune response is not adequate, control of the organisms is not maintained and active primary disease results. *TB disease* is defined as active bacteria that multiply and cause clinically active disease. Certain individuals are at a higher risk of active disease, including those who are immunosuppressed for any reason (e.g., patients with HIV infection, those receiving cancer chemotherapy or long-term corticosteroid therapy) or have diabetes mellitus.

Dormant but viable *M. tuberculosis* organisms persist for years. Once infected with TB, 3% to 5% of individuals develop TB disease within 1 year, and another 3% to 5% develop TB disease within their lifetime.[23] Reactivation of LTBI can occur if the host's defense mechanisms become impaired. The reasons for reactivation of latent infection are not well understood, but they are related to decreased resistance found in older adults, individuals with concomitant diseases, and those who receive immunosuppressive therapy.

Classification

The American Thoracic Association and American Lung Association have adopted a classification system that covers the entire population (Table 28-7).

Clinical Manifestations

In the early stages of TB, the person is usually free of symptoms. People with LTBI have a positive skin test but are asymptomatic. Active TB disease may initially present with fatigue, malaise, anorexia, unexplained weight loss, low-grade fevers, and night sweats. A characteristic pulmonary manifestation is a cough that becomes frequent and produces white, frothy sputum. Dyspnea is unusual. Hemoptysis is not a common finding and is usually associated with more advanced cases. Sometimes TB has more acute, sudden manifestations; the patient has high fever, chills, generalized flu-like symptoms, pleuritic pain, and a productive cough.

The HIV-infected patient with TB often has atypical physical examination and chest x-ray findings. Classic signs such as fever, cough, and weight loss may be attributed to *Pneumocystis jiroveci* pneumonia (PCP) or other HIV-associated opportunistic diseases. Clinical manifestations of respiratory problems in patients with HIV must be carefully investigated to determine the cause.

Complications

Miliary TB. Large numbers of organisms can invade the bloodstream and spread to all body organs. This hematogenous disseminated spread with involvement of many organs simultaneously is called *miliary TB.* It can occur as a result of primary disease or reactivation of latent infection.[21] The patient may be either acutely ill with fever, dyspnea, and cyanosis or chronically ill with systemic manifestations of weight loss, fever, and gastrointestinal (GI) disturbance. Hepatomegaly, splenomegaly, and generalized lymphadenopathy may be present.

TABLE 28-7 Classification of Tuberculosis (TB)

Class 0	No TB exposure	No TB exposure, not infected (no history of exposure, negative tuberculin skin test)
Class 1	TB exposure, no infection	TB exposure, no evidence of infection (history of exposure, negative tuberculin skin test)
Class 2	Latent TB infection, no disease	TB infection without disease (significant reaction to tuberculin skin test, negative bacteriologic studies, no x-ray findings compatible with TB, no clinical evidence of TB)
Class 3	TB clinically active	TB infection with clinically active disease (positive bacteriologic studies or both a significant reaction to tuberculin skin test and clinical or x-ray evidence of current disease)
Class 4	TB, but not clinically active	No current disease (history of previous episode of TB or abnormal, stable x-ray findings in a person with a significant reaction to tuberculin skin test; negative bacteriologic studies if done; no clinical or x-ray evidence of current disease)
Class 5	TB suspect	TB suspect (diagnosis pending); person should not be in this classification for more than 3 months

Source: American Thoracic Society, 2000.

Pleural Effusion and Empyema. Pleural TB can result from either primary disease or reactivation of latent infection. A pleural effusion is caused by the bacteria in the pleural space triggering an inflammatory reaction and a pleural exudate of protein-rich fluid. Empyema is less common than effusion but may occur from large numbers of tubercular organisms in the pleural space.

Tuberculosis Pneumonia. Acute pneumonia may result when large amounts of tubercle bacilli are discharged from granulomas into the lung or lymph nodes. The clinical manifestations are similar to those of bacterial pneumonia, including chills, fever, productive cough, pleuritic pain, and leukocytosis.

Other Organ Involvement. Although the lungs are the primary site of TB, other body organs may also be involved. The most serious is involvement of the central nervous system with inflammation of the meninges. Bone (Pott's disease of the spine) and joint tissue may be involved in the infectious disease process. The kidneys, adrenal glands, lymph nodes, and both female and male genital tracts may also be infected.

Diagnostic Studies

TB Skin Test. The intradermal administration of tuberculin as a diagnostic test for tuberculous infection has been used for over 100 years.[21] The tuberculin skin test (TST) (Mantoux test) using purified protein derivative (PPD) is the best way to diagnose latent *M. tuberculosis* infection. Induration (not redness) at the injection site 48 to 72 hours after the test means the person has been exposed to TB and has developed antibodies. The reaction occurs 2 to 12 weeks after the initial exposure. The induration is measured and, based on the size of the induration and the population risk, an interpretation is made according to diagnostic standards for determining a positive test reaction.[24] (The procedure for performing the tuberculin skin test is described in Chapter 26.) If a person has a positive reaction, he or she should not be tested again since the sensitivity to tuberculin tends to persist throughout life.

Guidelines for targeted tuberculin testing emphasize targeting only high-risk groups and discourage testing low-risk individuals. Because the response to TST may be decreased in the immunocompromised patient, smaller induration reactions (≥ 5 mm) are considered positive. Two-step testing is recommended for initial testing for health care workers, who get repeated testing, and for individuals who have a decreased response to allergens. In these people, a second TST may cause an accelerated response ("booster effect") that may be misinterpreted as a new conversion.[24] (See Table 26-12 for guidelines in interpreting the TST.)

Chest X-Ray. Although the findings on chest x-ray examination are important, it is not possible to make a diagnosis of TB solely on the basis of this examination. This is because other diseases can mimic the x-ray appearance of TB. The chest x-ray findings suggestive of TB include upper lobe infiltrates, cavitary infiltrates, and lymph node involvement.

Bacteriologic and Other Studies. The diagnosis of TB disease requires demonstration of tubercle bacilli bacteriologically. The initial testing involves a microscopic examination of stained sputum smears for acid-fast bacilli (AFB test), confirming tubercle bacilli. Three consecutive sputum specimens collected on different days are obtained and sent for smear and culture. The culture to grow the organisms for confirmatory diagnosis can take up to 8 weeks. Samples for other suspected TB sites can be collected from gastric washings, cerebrospinal fluid, (CSF), or fluid from an effusion or abscess.

A new test for TB, QuantiFERON-TB (QFT), is a rapid diagnostic test. Blood is obtained from the patient and placed in chambers along with mycobacterial antigens. If the patient is infected with tuberculosis organisms, the lymphocytes in the blood will recognize these antigens and secrete γ-interferon, a cytokine produced by lymphocytes. Test results are available in a few hours. This test does not replace routine sputum smears and cultures, but it offers an option in detecting TB and may be used in place of TST in TB screening programs in health care settings.[23,25]

Collaborative Care

Hospitalization for initial treatment of TB is generally not necessary. Most patients are treated on an outpatient basis (Table 28-8). Many people can continue to work and maintain their lifestyles with few changes. Hospitalization may be used for the severely ill or debilitated. The mainstay of TB treatment is drug therapy (Table 28-9). Drug therapy is used to treat an individual with active disease and to prevent disease in a TB-infected person. Promoting and monitoring compliance is critical for treatment to be successful.

Drug Therapy

Active Disease. In view of the growing prevalence of multidrug-resistant TB, the patient with active TB should be managed aggressively. Because of the high number of patients with organisms resistant to isoniazid (INH), four drugs are necessary in the initial phase for the 6-month regimen to be maximally effective. Four drug regimen options have been identified by the CDC for previously untreated TB (Table 28-10). In most circumstances, the treatment regimen for patients with previously untreated TB consists of a 2-month initial phase with four-drug therapy (INH, rifampin [Rifadin], pyrazinamide [PZA], and ethambutol). If drug suscepti-

TABLE 28-8 COLLABORATIVE CARE Pulmonary Tuberculosis

Diagnostic
History and physical examination
Tuberculin skin test (TST)
QuantiFERON-TB test
Chest x-ray
Bacteriologic studies
Sputum smear for acid-fast bacilli (AFB)
Sputum culture
Collaborative Therapy
Long-term treatment with antimicrobial drugs (see Tables 28-9 and 28-10)
Follow-up bacteriologic studies and chest x-rays

bility test results indicate the bacteria are susceptible to all drugs, ethambutol may be discontinued. If PZA cannot be included in the initial phase (due to liver disease, pregnancy, etc.), option 4 is recommended.

***Drug Alert** - Isoniazid (INH)*
- *Alcohol may increase hepatotoxicity of drug. Instruct patient to avoid drinking alcohol during treatment.*
- *Monitor for signs of liver damage before and while taking drug.*

Other drugs are primarily used for treatment of resistant strains or if the patient develops toxicity to the primary drugs. The newer rifamycins, rifabutin and rifapentine, should be considered first line in special situations: rifabutin for patients receiving medications that have interactions with rifampin or who have an intolerance to rifampin, and rifapentine with INH in once-weekly dosing for selected patients.[26]

Directly observed therapy (DOT) involves providing the antituberculous drugs directly to the patient and watching as he or she swallows the medications. It is the preferred strategy for all patients with TB to assure adherence.[26] When DOT is not being used, fixed-dose combination antituberculous drugs may enhance adherence to treatment recommendations. Combinations of isoniazid and rifampin (Rifamate) and of isoniazid, rifampin, and pyrazinamide (Rifater) are available to simplify therapy. The therapy for persons with HIV follows the same therapy options outlined in Table 28-10 except that alternative regimens that include once-weekly INH plus rifapentine continuation dosing in any HIV-infected patient and twice-weekly INH plus rifampin or rifabutin should not be used if $CD4^+$ counts are $<100/\mu l$. Health care providers must be alert for possible drug interactions between antiretrovirals and rifamycins.

Many second-line drugs for treatment of TB carry a greater risk of toxicity and require closer monitoring. Newer drugs for the treatment of TB that have been placed in categories of second-line drugs include the quinolones, such as levofloxacin, moxifloxacin, and gatifloxacin.

An important reason for follow-up care in the patient with TB is to ensure adherence to the treatment regimen. Noncompliance is a major factor in the emergence of multidrug resistance and treatment failures. Many individuals do not adhere to the treatment program in spite of understanding the disease process and the value of treatment. DOT is recommended for patients known to be at risk for noncompliance with therapy. DOT is an expensive but essential public health issue. Completing therapy is important because of the danger of reactivation of TB and MDR-TB seen in patients who do not complete the full course of therapy. In many areas, the public health nurse administers DOT at a clinic site.

Teaching patients about the side effects of these drugs and when to seek prompt medical attention is critical. The major side effect of isoniazid, rifampin, and pyrazinamide is nonviral hepatitis. Liver function tests should be monitored. Baseline liver function tests are done at the start of treatment. Monthly monitoring of liver function tests is done if baseline tests are abnormal.

Latent Tuberculosis Infection. *Latent TB infection* (LTBI) occurs when an individual becomes infected with *M. tuberculosis.* Drug therapy can be used to prevent a TB infection from developing into *active disease.* The indications for treatment of LTBI are presented in Table 28-11.

The drug generally used in treatment of LTBI is isoniazid (INH). It is effective and inexpensive and can be administered orally. Isoniazid is usually administered once daily for 6 to 9 months. INH can be given daily or twice weekly with DOT. The 9-month regimen is more effective, but compliance issues may make the 6-month regimen preferable. For HIV patients and those with fibrotic lesions on chest x-ray, INH is given for 9 months. An alternative 4-month therapy with rifampin may be indicated if the patient is resistant to INH.

Vaccine. Immunization with bacille Calmette-Guérin (BCG) vaccine, a live, attenuated strain of *Mycobacterium bovis,* to prevent TB is in use in many parts of the world. Although millions of people have been vaccinated with BCG, the efficacy of the vaccine in preventing TB in adults is not clear. BCG was found to reduce the incidence of TB, particularly fatal disseminated TB, in infants and young children.[23] Thus BCG is being offered at birth for children in high-prevalence areas in developing countries. The BCG vaccination can result in a positive reaction on the TST. This reaction will wane over time. Recent advances in DNA sequencing hold promise for an *M. tuberculosis* vaccine. The development of a TB vaccine is an urgent worldwide public health priority.

NURSING MANAGEMENT TUBERCULOSIS

■ *Nursing Assessment*

It is important to determine whether the patient was ever exposed to a person with TB. The patient should be assessed for productive cough, night sweats, afternoon temperature elevation, weight loss, pleuritic chest pain, and crackles over the apices of the lungs. If the patient has a productive cough, an early-morning sputum specimen will be required for an acid-fast bacillus (AFB) smear to detect the presence of mycobacteria.

■ *Nursing Diagnoses*

Nursing diagnoses for the patient with TB may include, but are not limited to, the following:

- Ineffective breathing pattern *related to* decreased lung capacity
- Imbalanced nutrition: less than body requirements *related to* chronic poor appetite, fatigue, and productive cough
- Noncompliance *related to* lack of knowledge of disease process, lack of motivation, and long-term nature of treatment

TABLE 28-9 DRUG THERAPY
Tuberculosis (TB)

Drug	Mechanisms of Action	Side Effects	Comments
First-Line Drugs			
• isoniazid (INH)	Bacteriocidal against rapidly dividing cells	Asymptomatic elevation of aminotransferases, clinical hepatitis, fulminant hepatitis, peripheral neurotoxicity, hypersensitivity (skin rash, arthralgia, fever)	Metabolism primarily by liver and excretion by kidneys, pyridoxine (vitamin B_6) administration during high-dose therapy as prophylactic measure; routine monthly monitoring of liver tests not necessary unless preexisting liver disease or abnormal liver tests; safe in pregnancy.
• rifampin (Rifadin)	Bacteriocidal against rapidly dividing cells and against semidormant bacteria	Cutaneous reactions, GI disturbance (nausea, anorexia, abdominal pain), flulike syndrome, hepatotoxicity, immunologic reactions, orange discoloration of bodily fluids (sputum, urine, sweat, tears); drug interactions	Most common use with isoniazid; safe in pregnancy; low incidence of side effects; suppression of effect of oral contraceptives; possible orange urine.
• ethambutol (Myambutol)	Bacteriostatic for the tubercle bacillus	Retrobulbar neuritis (decreased red-green color discrimination), peripheral neuritis (rare), skin rash	Side effects uncommon and reversible with discontinuation of drug; most common use as substitute drug when toxicity occurs with isoniazid or rifampin; safe in pregnancy; baseline Snellen test and color discrimination and monthly if dose >15-25 mg/kg.
• rifabutin (Mycobutin)	Bacteriocidal against rapidly dividing cells and against semidormant bacteria	Hematologic toxicity, uveitis (rare), GI symptoms, polyarthralgias, hepatotoxicity (<1%); pseudojaundice (usually resolves), rash (rare), orange discoloration of bodily fluids	Used as a substitute for rifampin; reserved for patients unable to take rifampin. Patients should be warned of the orange discoloration. Soft contact lenses and clothing may be permanently stained. Drug used with caution in pregnancy.
• pyrazinamide (PZA)	Bacteriocidal effect against dormant or semidormant organisms	Hepatotoxicity, GI symptoms (nausea, vomiting), polyarthralgias, skin rash, hyperuricemia, dermatitis	No data on safety of PZA in pregnancy; World Health Organization recommends it for use in pregnancy.
• rifapentine (Priftin)	Bacteriocidal against rapidly dividing cells and against semidormant bacteria	Similar to those of rifampin	No sufficient data to recommend it in pregnancy; monitoring similar to rifampin.
Second-Line Drugs			
• cycloserine (Seromycin)	Bacteriocidal or bacteriostatic; inhibits cell wall synthesis	Central nervous system effects (headache, restless, seizures, psychosis); given with pyridoxine to prevent neurotoxic effects	Neuropsychiatric monitoring monthly; used for drug-resistant organisms that are susceptible to this drug; use in pregnancy only when no other alternative; contraindicated if history of psychosis.
• ethionamide (Trecator)	Exact mechanism of action unknown	Hepatotoxicity, neurotoxicity, GI effects (metallic taste, nausea, vomiting), endocrine effects (hypothyroid, impotence)	Liver function tests should be obtained at baseline and monitored monthly if there is underlying liver disease; thyroid-stimulating hormone should be measured at baseline and at monthly intervals.
• streptomycin	Bacteriocidal; inhibits protein synthesis	Ototoxicity, neurotoxicity, nephrotoxicity	Contraindicated in pregnancy; baseline hearing, Romberg test, serum creatinine measurements.
• capreomycin (Capastat)	Bacteriocidal; inhibits protein synthesis	Ototoxicity, nephrotoxicity	Cautious use in older adults; avoid in pregnancy; monitoring as for streptomycin.
• kanamycin (Kantrex) and amikacin	Bacteriocidal; inhibits protein synthesis	Ototoxicity, nephrotoxicity	Use in selected cases for treatment of resistant strains; contraindicated in pregnancy.
• *para*-aminosalicylic acid (PAS)	Interferes with metabolism of tubercle bacillus	Hepatotoxicity, GI distress, malabsorption syndrome, coagulopathy	Use in selected cases for treatment of resistant strains.
• Fluoroquinolones: levofloxacin (Levaquin), moxifloxacin (Avelox, Vigamox), gatifloxacin (Tequin)	Bacteriocidal	GI disturbance, neurologic effects (dizzy, headache), rash	Preferred oral agent for drug-resistant TB caused by organisms sensitive to this drug; avoid in pregnancy due to teratogenic effects.

Source: Centers for Disease Control and Prevention: *MMWR Recomm Rep* 52(RR-11), 2003.

TABLE 28-10 DRUG THERAPY
Regimen Options for the Initial Treatment of Tuberculosis

Tuberculosis Previously Untreated: Initial Phase and Continuation Phase	
Option 1	**Initial phase:** 4-drug regimen consisting of INH, rifampin, pyrazinamide, ethambutol. Given daily for 56 doses **OR** 5 days/wk DOT for 40 doses. Ethambutol may be discontinued if susceptibility to INH or rifampin is documented. **Continuation phase:** INH, rifampin daily for 126 doses **OR** 5 days/wk DOT for 90 doses.
Option 2	**Initial phase:** 4-drug regimen consisting of INH, rifampin, pyrazinamide, ethambutol. Given daily for 14 doses, followed by twice weekly for 12 doses **OR** 5 days/wk DOT for 10 doses, then twice weekly for 12 doses. **Continuation phase:** INH, rifampin twice weekly for 36 doses **OR** once weekly for 18 doses.
Option 3	**Initial phase:** 4-drug regimen consisting of INH, rifampin, pyrazinamide, ethambutol. Given 3 times weekly for 24 doses. **Continuation phase:** INH, rifampin 3 times weekly for 54 doses.
Option 4	**Initial phase:** 3-drug regimen consisting of INH, rifampin, ethambutol. Given daily for 56 doses **OR** 5 days/wk DOT for 40 doses. **Continuation phase:** INH, rifampin daily for 217 doses **OR** 5 days/wk DOT for 155 doses.

Source: Centers for Disease Control and Prevention: *MMWR Recomm Rep* 52(RR-11), 2003.
DOT, Directly observed therapy; *INH,* isoniazid.

TABLE 28-11 Indications for Treatment of Latent Tuberculosis Infection

- Newly infected patient at high risk
- Person with known or suspected HIV infection and positive tuberculin skin test
- Exposure of household members and other close associates to newly diagnosed patient
- Significant tuberculin skin test reactors with abnormal chest x-ray
- Significant tuberculin skin test reactors in special clinical situations (immunosuppression therapy, use of corticosteroids, diabetes mellitus, silicosis, gastrectomy, end-stage renal disease, head and neck cancer)
- Other significant tuberculin skin test converters (10-mm increase within a 2-yr period regardless of age)
- Other significant tuberculin skin test reactors (persons born outside of the United States from high-prevalence countries; medically underserved low-income populations, including high-risk racial or ethnic populations [e.g., Asian/Pacific Islanders, American Indian/Alaskan Native, African Americans, Hispanics], residents in long-term care facilities, health care workers, mycobacteriology laboratory technicians)

Source: American Thoracic Society, 2000.
HIV, Human immunodeficiency virus.

- Ineffective health maintenance *related to* lack of knowledge about the disease process and therapeutic regimen
- Activity intolerance *related to* fatigue, decreased nutritional status, and chronic febrile episodes

Planning

The overall goals are that the patient with TB will (1) comply with the therapeutic regimen, (2) have no recurrence of disease, (3) have normal pulmonary function, and (4) take appropriate measures to prevent the spread of the disease.

Nursing Implementation

Health Promotion. The ultimate goal related to TB in the United States is eradication. Selective screening programs in known risk groups are of value in detecting individuals with TB. The person with a positive tuberculin skin test should have a chest x-ray to assess for the presence of TB. Another important measure is to identify the contacts of the individual who has TB. These contacts should be assessed for the possibility of infection and the need for chemoprophylaxis.

Acute Intervention. Acute in-hospital care is seldom required for the patient with TB. If hospitalization is needed, it is usually for a brief period. Patients strongly suspected of having TB should (1) be placed on airborne isolation, (2) receive appropriate drug therapy, and (3) receive an immediate medical workup, including chest x-ray, sputum smear, and culture. Airborne infection isolation is indicated for the patient with pulmonary or laryngeal TB until the patient is considered to be noninfectious (effective drug therapy, improving clinically, three negative AFB smears). *Airborne infection isolation* refers to isolation of patients infected with organisms spread by the airborne route in a single-occupancy room with negative pressure and an airflow of 6 to 12 exchanges per hour. Ultraviolet radiation of the air in the upper part of the room is another approach to reduce airborne TB organisms. Ultraviolet lights are commonly seen in clinics and homeless shelters. Masks are needed to filter out droplet nuclei. High-efficiency particulate air (HEPA) masks are worn whenever entering the patient's room because they can remove almost 100% of the small particles >3 μm in diameter. The mask must be molded to fit tightly around the nose and mouth.

The patient should be taught to cover the nose and mouth with paper tissue every time he or she coughs, sneezes, or produces sputum. The tissues should be thrown into a paper bag and disposed of with the trash, burned, or flushed down the toilet. The patient should also be taught careful hand-washing techniques after handling sputum and soiled tissues. If the patient needs to be out of the negative-pressure room, the patient wears a standard isolation mask to prevent coughing tubercular organisms into the environment. Special precautions should be taken during high-risk procedures that induce coughing, such as sputum induction, aerosolized pentamidine treatments, intubation, bronchoscopy, or endoscopy.

Ambulatory and Home Care. Patients who have responded clinically are discharged home despite positive smears if their household contacts have already been exposed and the patient is not posing a risk to susceptible persons. Determination of absolute noninfectiousness requires negative cultures. Most treatment failures occur because the patient neglects to take the drug, discontinues it prematurely, or takes it irregularly.

The nurse should teach the patient so that the need for compliance with the prescribed regimen is fully understood by the patient and family. Notification of the public health department is essential if drug compliance is questionable so that follow-up of close contacts can be accomplished. In some cases, the public health nurse will be responsible for DOT. When the chemotherapy regimen has been completed and there is evidence of negative cultures, the patient is improving clinically, and there is radiologic evidence of improvement, most individuals can be considered adequately treated. Follow-up care may be indicated during the subsequent 12 months, including bacteriologic studies and chest x-ray.

Because approximately 5% of individuals experience relapses, the patient should be taught to recognize the symptoms that indicate recurrence of TB. If these symptoms occur, immediate medical attention should be sought. The patient needs to be instructed about certain factors that could reactivate TB, such as immunosuppressive therapy, malignancy, and prolonged debilitating illness. If the patient experiences any of these events, the health care provider must to be told so that reactivation of TB can be closely monitored. In some situations, it may be necessary to put the patient on anti-TB therapy.

Evaluation

The expected outcomes are that the patient with TB will have

- complete resolution of the disease
- normal pulmonary function
- absence of any complications
- no transmission of TB

ATYPICAL MYCOBACTERIA

Pulmonary disease that closely resembles TB may be caused by atypical acid-fast mycobacteria. This type of pulmonary disease is indistinguishable from TB clinically and radiologically but can be differentiated by bacteriologic culture. These organisms are not believed to be airborne and thus are not transmitted by droplet nuclei.

There are many atypical mycobacteria that can affect the lung. *M. avium* complex (MAC), an opportunistic mycobacterium found in water, causes pulmonary infection due to exposure to aerosols generated from baths, hot spas, and swimming pools. This is one of the most common of the atypical mycobacteria presently encountered. However, only a small number of people exposed to the organism will actually develop MAC lung disease. These are people who are immunosuppressed (e.g., HIV, cancer) or have underlying lung disease (e.g., cystic fibrosis).[27] Other mycobacteria include *M. kansasii, M. scrofulaceum, M. intracellulare,* and *M. xenopi.* Treatment depends on identification of the causative agent and determination of drug sensitivity. Many of the drugs used in treating TB are used in combating infections from atypical mycobacteria.

PULMONARY FUNGAL INFECTIONS

Pulmonary fungal infections are increasing in incidence. They are found frequently in seriously ill patients being treated with corticosteroids, antineoplastic and immunosuppressive drugs, or multiple antibiotics. They are also found in patients with AIDS and cystic fibrosis. Community-acquired pulmonary lung infections include aspergillosis, cryptococcosis, and candidiasis.[28] Types of fungal infections are presented in Table 28-12. These infections are not transmitted from person to person, and the patient does not have to be placed in isolation. The clinical manifestations are similar to those of bacterial pneumonia. Skin testing, serology, and biopsy methods are available to assist in identifying the infecting organism.

ETHICAL DILEMMAS
Patient Adherence

Situation

The health clinic for the homeless discovers that an African American man with tuberculosis (TB) has not been complying with taking his medication. He tells the nurse that it is hard for him to get to the clinic to obtain the medication, much less to keep on a schedule. The nurse is concerned not only about this patient, but also about the risks for the other people at the shelter, in the park, and at the meal sites.

Important Points for Consideration

- Adherence is a complex issue involving a person's culture and values, perceived risk of disease, availability of resources, access to treatment, and perceived consequences of available choices.
- Nurses in the community are concerned not only with providing benefits and supporting decision making for individual patients, but also the health and well-being of the entire community.
- Greater harm may result for the community when more virulent multidrug-resistant strains of microorganisms develop as a consequence of partial treatment or inability of the patient to complete a course of therapy.
- Advocacy for the patient and the community obliges the nurse to involve other members of the health care team, such as social services, to assist in obtaining the necessary resources or support to facilitate completing the course of treatment by the patient.
- If the patient is unable to comply with the treatment program even with necessary supports in place, concern for the public's health would take priority and necessitate placing him in a supervised living situation until his treatment is completed.

Critical Thinking Questions

1. Under what circumstances are health care providers justified in overriding a patient's autonomy or decision making?
2. How would you determine if there were cultural beliefs interfering with this man's ability to understand the importance of completing the treatment? What would you do about it?

Collaborative Care

Amphotericin B remains the standard therapy for treating serious systemic fungal infections. It must be given intravenously to achieve adequate blood and tissue levels because it is poorly absorbed from the GI tract. Amphotericin B is considered a toxic drug with many possible side effects, including hypersensitivity reactions, fever, chills, malaise, nausea and vomiting, thrombophlebitis at the injection site, and abnormal renal function. Many of the side effects during infusion can be avoided by premedicating with an antiinflammatory and/or diphenhydramine (Benadryl) 1 hour before the infusion. Inclusion of a small amount of hydrocortisone in the infusion helps decrease the irritation of the veins. Monitoring of renal function and ensuring adequate hydration is essential while a person is receiving this drug. Renal changes are

TABLE 28-12 Fungal Infections of the Lung

Infection	Characteristics
Histoplasmosis	
Histoplasma capsulatum	Indigenous to soil of North American river valleys, inhalation of mycelia into lungs, infected individual often free of symptoms, generally self-limiting, chronic disease similar to TB
Coccidioidomycosis	
Coccidioides immitis	Indigenous to semiarid regions of southwestern United States, inhalation of arthrospores into lungs, suppurative and granulomatous reaction in lungs, symptomatic infection in one third of individuals
Blastomycosis	
Blastomyces dermatitidis	Indigenous to southeastern and midwestern United States, inhalation of fungus into lungs, progression of disease often insidious, possible involvement of skin
Cryptococcosis	
Cryptococcus neoformans	True yeast, indigenous worldwide in soil and pigeon excreta, inhalation of fungus into lungs, possible meningitis
Aspergillosis	
Aspergillus niger or *Aspergillus fumigatus*	True mold inhabiting mouth, widely distributed, invasion of lung tissue resulting in possible necrotizing pneumonia; in individual with asthma, allergic bronchopulmonary aspergillosis may require corticosteroid therapy
Candidiasis	
Candida albicans	Leading cause of mycotic infections in hospitalized and immunocompromised hosts, ubiquitous and frequent colonization of upper respiratory and GI tracts, infections often following broad-spectrum antibiotic therapy (systemic or inhaled), possible development of localized pulmonary infiltrate to widespread bilateral consolidation with hypoxemia
Actinomycosis	
Actinomyces israelii	Not a true fungus, pseudohyphae present; anaerobic; gram-positive, higher bacteria with branching hyphae; presence of necrotizing pneumonia after aspiration; pneumonitis, commonly in lower lobes with abscess or empyema formation
Nocardiosis	
Nocardia asteroides	Not a true fungus; aerobic, higher bacteria with branching hyphae; soil saprophyte widely distributed in nature; acquisition of infection from nature; rarely present in sputum without accompanying disease
***Pneumocystis* Pneumonia (PCP)**	
Pneumocystis jiroveci (formerly *carinii*)	This organism rarely causes pneumonia in the healthy individual; fungus present in the environment; common opportunistic pneumonia in persons with AIDS and impaired immune systems

AIDS, Acquired immunodeficiency syndrome.

at least partially reversible. Amphotericin infusions are incompatible with most other drugs. Amphotericin is frequently administered every other day after an initial period of several weeks of daily therapy. Total treatment with the drug may range from 4 to 12 weeks.

Oral imidazole and triazole compounds with antifungal activity, such as ketoconazole (Nizoral), fluconazole (Diflucan), voriconazole (Vfend), and itraconazole (Sporanox), have been successful in the treatment of fungal infections. Their effectiveness in treatment allows an alternative to the use of amphotericin B in many cases. Effectiveness of therapy can be monitored with fungal serology titers.

Flucytosine (Ancobon) has also been used in selected types of pulmonary fungal infections. It is given orally. Common adverse reactions include nausea, vomiting, diarrhea, and abdominal discomfort. Antiemetics may be helpful. Hepatotoxicity and bone marrow suppression may occur. Frequent blood monitoring, including complete blood count, (CBC), potassium levels, and renal and hepatic function, is done.

LUNG ABSCESS

Etiology and Pathophysiology

Lung abscess is a pus-containing lesion of the lung parenchyma that gives rise to a cavity. The cavity is formed by necrosis of the lung tissue. In many cases the causes and pathogenesis of lung abscess are similar to those of pneumonia. Most lung abscesses are caused by aspiration of material from the GI tract into the lungs. Risk factors for aspiration include alcoholism, seizure disorders, neuromuscular diseases, drug overdose, general anesthesia, and stroke. The areas of the lung most commonly affected are the superior segments of the lower lobes and the posterior segments of the upper lobes. Fibrous tissue usually forms around the abscess in an attempt to wall it off. The abscess may erode into the bronchial system, causing the production of foul-smelling or sour-tasting sputum. It may grow toward the pleura and cause pleuritic pain. Multiple small abscesses can occur within the lung.

Infectious agents generally cause lung abscesses. The organisms involved cause infection and necrosis of the lung tissue. Examples include enteric gram-negative organisms (e.g., *Klebsiella*), *S. aureus,* and anaerobic bacilli (e.g., *Bacteroides*). Putrid, offensive sputum is associated with anaerobic bacteria. Lung abscess can also result from malignant growth, TB, and various parasitic and fungal diseases of the lung.

Clinical Manifestations and Complications

The onset of a lung abscess is usually insidious, especially if anaerobic organisms are the primary cause. A more acute onset occurs with aerobic organisms. The most common manifestation is cough-producing purulent sputum (often dark brown) that is foul smelling and foul tasting. Hemoptysis is common, especially at the time that an abscess ruptures into a bronchus. Other common manifestations are fever, chills, prostration, pleuritic pain, dyspnea, cough, and weight loss.

Physical examination of the lungs indicates dullness to percussion and decreased breath sounds on auscultation over the segment of lung involved. There may be transmission of bronchial breath sounds to the periphery if the communicating bronchus becomes patent and drainage of the segment begins. Crackles may also be present in the later stages as the abscess drains. Oral examination often reveals dental caries, gingivitis, and periodontal infection.

Complications that can occur include chronic pulmonary abscess, bronchiectasis, brain abscess as a result of the hematogenous spread of infection, bronchopleural fistula, and empyema from abscess perforation into the pleural cavity.

Diagnostic Studies

A chest x-ray may reveal a solitary cavitary lesion with fluid that is identified as an air-fluid level. Computed tomography (CT) scanning is very helpful if there is a question of cavitation not clearly seen on chest x-ray. Lung abscess, in contrast to other types of abscesses, does not require assisted drainage, as long as there is drainage via the bronchus. Routine sputum cultures can be collected. However, contaminants can confuse the results, and it is difficult to isolate anaerobic bacteria. Pleural fluid and blood cultures may be obtained. Bronchoscopy may be used in cases of abscess in which drainage is delayed or in which there are factors that suggest an underlying malignancy.

NURSING *and* COLLABORATIVE MANAGEMENT LUNG ABSCESS

Antibiotics given for a prolonged period (up to 2 to 4 months) are usually the primary method of treatment. Penicillin has historically been the drug of choice because of the frequent presence of anaerobic organisms. However, recent studies suggest that there is β-lactamase production by the anaerobic bacteria involved in abscesses of the lung, and they are resistant to penicillin. Clindamycin (Cleocin) has been shown to be superior to penicillin and is the standard treatment for an anaerobic lung infection. Patients with putrid lung abscesses usually show clinical improvement with decreased fever within 3 to 4 days of beginning antibiotics.

Because of the need for prolonged antibiotic therapy, the patient must be aware of the importance of continuing the medication for the prescribed period. The patient needs to know about untoward side effects that need to be reported to the health care provider. Sometimes the patient is asked to return periodically during the course of antibiotic therapy for repeat cultures and sensitivity tests to ensure that the infecting organism is not becoming resistant to the antibiotic. When antibiotic therapy is completed, the patient is reevaluated.

The patient should be taught how to cough effectively (see Table 29-25). Chest physiotherapy and postural drainage are sometimes used to drain abscesses located in the lower or posterior portions of the lung. Postural drainage to the lung area involved will aid the removal of secretions (see Fig. 29-17). Rest, good nutrition, and adequate fluid intake are all supportive measures to facilitate recovery. If dentition is poor and dental hygiene is not adequate, the patient should be encouraged to obtain dental care.

Surgery is rarely indicated but occasionally may be necessary when reinfection of a large cavitary lesion occurs or to establish a diagnosis when there is evidence of an underlying neoplasm or chronic associated disease. The usual procedure in such cases is a lobectomy or pneumonectomy. An alternative to surgery is percutaneous drainage, but there is a potential risk of contamination of the pleural space.

ENVIRONMENTAL LUNG DISEASES

Environmental or occupational lung diseases are caused or aggravated by workplace or environmental exposure and are preventable.[29] They result from inhaled dust or chemicals. The duration of exposure and the amount of inhalant have a major influence on whether the exposed individual will have lung damage. Occupational and environmental asthma is especially prevalent and is discussed in Chapter 29. The other major groups of diseases are pneumoconiosis, chemical pneumonitis, and hypersensitivity pneumonitis.

Pneumoconiosis is a general term for a group of lung diseases caused by inhalation and retention of dust particles. The literal meaning of *pneumoconiosis* is "dust in the lungs." Examples of this condition are silicosis, asbestosis, and berylliosis. The classic response to the inhaled substance is diffuse parenchymal infiltration with phagocytic cells. This eventually results in diffuse *pulmonary fibrosis* (excess connective tissue). Fibrosis is the result of tissue repair after inflammation. Pneumoconiosis and other environmental lung diseases are presented in Table 28-13. Hantavirus, a potentially fatal disease with outbreaks reported in the United States and Canada, is transmitted by inhalation of aerosolized rodent excreta particles.

Chemical pneumonitis results from exposures to toxic chemical fumes. Acutely, there is diffuse lung injury characterized as pulmonary edema. Chronically, the clinical picture is that of *bronchiolitis obliterans* (obstruction of the bronchioles due to inflammation and fibrosis), which is usually associated with a normal chest x-ray or one that shows hyperinflation. An example is silo filler's disease.

Hypersensitivity pneumonitis or extrinsic allergic alveolitis is a form of parenchymal lung disease seen when antigens are inhaled to which an individual is allergic. Examples include bird fancier's lung and farmer's lung.

Lung cancer, either squamous cell carcinoma or adenocarcinoma, is the most frequent cancer associated with asbestos exposure. People with more exposure are at a greater risk of disease. There is a minimum lapse of 15 to 19 years between first exposure and development of lung cancer. Mesotheliomas, both pleural and peritoneal, are also associated with asbestos exposure.

Clinical Manifestations

Acute symptoms of pulmonary edema may be seen following early exposures to chemical fumes. However, symptoms of many environmental lung diseases may not occur until at least 10 to 15 years after the initial exposure to the inhaled irritant. Dyspnea and cough are often the earliest manifestations. Chest pain and cough with sputum production usually occur later. Pulmonary function studies often show reduced vital capacity. A chest x-ray will often reveal lung involvement specific to the primary problem. CT scans have been shown to be useful in detecting early lung involvement. Cor pulmonale (described later in this chapter) is a late complication, especially in conditions characterized by diffuse pulmonary fibrosis. Complications that often result are pneumonia, chronic bronchitis, emphysema, and lung cancer. Manifestations of these complications can be the reason the patient seeks health care.

Collaborative Care

The best approach to management of environmental lung diseases is to try to prevent or decrease environmental and occupational risks. Well-designed, effective ventilation systems can reduce ex-

TABLE 28-13 Environmental Lung Diseases

Disease	Agents/Industries	Description	Complications
Asbestosis	Asbestos fibers present in insulation, construction material (roof tiling, cement products), shipyards, textiles (for fireproofing), automobile clutch and brake linings	Disease appears 15–35 yr after first exposure. Interstitial fibrosis develops. Pleural plaques, which are calcified lesions, develop on pleura. Dyspnea, basal crackles, and decreased vital capacity are early manifestations.	Diffuse interstitial pulmonary fibrosis; lung cancer, especially in cigarette smokers; mesothelioma (rare type of cancer affecting pleura and peritoneal membrane)
Berylliosis	Beryllium dust present in aircraft manufacturing, metallurgy, rocket fuels	Formation of noncaseating granulomas. Acute pneumonitis occurs after heavy exposure. Interstitial fibrosis can also occur.	Progress of disease possible after removal of stimulating inhalant
Bird fancier's, breeder's, or handler's lung	Bird droppings or feathers	Hypersensitivity pneumonitis is present.	Progressive fibrosis of lung
Byssinosis	Cotton, flax, and hemp dust (textile industry)	Airway obstruction is caused by contraction of smooth muscles. Chronic disease results from severe airway obstruction and decreased elastic recoil.	Progression of chronic disease after cessation of dust exposure
Coalworker's pneumoconiosis (black lung)	Coal dust	Incidence is high (20%-30%) in coal workers. Deposits of carbon dust cause lesions to develop along respiratory bronchioles. Bronchioles dilate because of loss of wall structure. Chronic airway obstruction and bronchitis develop. Dyspnea and cough are common early symptoms.	Progressive, massive lung fibrosis; increased risk of chronic obstructive pulmonary disease with smoking
Farmer's lung	Inhalation of airborne material from moldy hay or similar matter	Hypersensitivity pneumonitis occurs. *Acute* form is similar to pneumonia, with manifestations of chills, fever, and malaise. *Chronic,* insidious form is type of pulmonary fibrosis.	Progressive fibrosis of lung
Hantavirus pulmonary syndrome (HPS)	Rodent droppings inhaled while in rodent-infested areas	Acute hemorrhagic fever associated with severe pulmonary and cardiovascular collapse and death. Incubation period is 1-4 wk with prodrome (3-5 days) of flulike symptoms. No cure or specific treatment exists.	CDC recommends rapid transfer to ICU with supportive therapy and early intervention vital; research on this virus is done in high-level biocontainment facilities
Silicosis	Silica dust present in quartz rock in mining of gold, copper, tin, coal, lead; also present in sandblasting, foundries, quarries, pottery making, masonry	In *chronic disease,* dust is engulfed by macrophages and may be destroyed, resulting in fibrotic nodules. *Acute disease* results from intense exposure in short time period. Within 5 yr, it progresses to severe disability from lung fibrosis.	Increased susceptibility to tuberculosis; progressive, massive fibrosis; high incidence of chronic bronchitis
Silo filler's disease	Nitrogen oxides from fermentation of vegetation in freshly filled silo	Chemical pneumonitis occurs.	Progressive bronchiolitis obliterans

CDC, Centers for Disease Control and Prevention; *ICU,* intensive care unit.

posure to irritants. Wearing masks is appropriate in some occupations. Periodic inspections and monitoring of workplaces by agencies such as the Occupational Safety and Health Administration (OSHA) and the National Institute for Occupational Safety and Health (NIOSH) reinforce the obligations of employers to provide a safe work environment. NIOSH is responsible for workplace safety and health regulations in the United States *(www.cdc.gov/niosh/homepage.html).*

Active and passive smoking increases the insult to the lungs. Patients need to be advised that they should not smoke and to avoid passive smoke as well. Passive smoke, inhalation of environmental tobacco smoke by a nonsmoker, is an important source of occupational exposure with increased risk for development of lung cancer. This has led to regulations requiring a smoke-free workspace for all employees.

Early diagnosis is essential if the disease process is to be halted. There is no specific treatment for most environmental lung diseases. The best treatment is to decrease or stop exposure to the harmful agent. Strategies are directed toward providing symptomatic relief. If there are coexisting problems, such as pneumonia, chronic bronchitis, emphysema, or asthma, they need to be treated.

LUNG CANCER

Lung cancer is the leading cause of cancer-related deaths in the United States. Lung cancer accounts for 28% of all cancer deaths. There are about 172,570 new cases of lung cancer every year in the United States. It is the leading cause of cancer death among men; 58% of the lung cancer deaths are in men. African Americans have the highest death rate and Hispanics the lowest.[30]

Lung cancer is now the leading cause of death in women, surpassing breast cancer. The Surgeon General's report, *Women and Smoking: A Report of the Surgeon General—2001,* identified a 600% increase in women's death rates from lung cancer since

GENDER DIFFERENCES

Lung Cancer

Men

- Men with lung cancer have a worse prognosis than women.
- Lung cancer incidence and deaths are decreasing in men.

Women

- Women who smoke are at 2 times greater risk of developing lung cancer than men who smoke.
- Women:
  - Develop lung cancer after fewer years of smoking as compared to men.
  - Develop lung cancer at a younger age than men.
  - Are more likely to develop small cell carcinoma than men.
- Nonsmoking women are at greater risk of developing lung cancer than men.

1950 and attributes this to smoking.[31] The CDC compared lung cancer death rates between the genders. They found that mortality rates increased from 1968 to 1999 for women (266%) versus men (15%), highlighting the need for smoking prevention strategies targeting women.[32] In addition, a total of 36.5% of teenagers (male and female) smoke. The overall 5-year survival rate from lung cancer is 15%. Lung cancer most commonly occurs in individuals more than 50 years of age who have a long history of cigarette smoking. The disease is found most in persons 40 to 75 years of age, with peak incidence between 55 and 65 years of age.

Etiology

Cigarette smoking is the most important risk factor in the development of lung cancer. Smoking is responsible for approximately 80% to 90% of all lung cancers. Tobacco smoke contains 60 carcinogens in addition to substances (carbon monoxide, nicotine) that interfere with normal cell development. Cigarette smoking, a lower airway irritant, causes a change in the bronchial epithelium, which usually returns to normal when smoking is discontinued. The risk of lung cancer is gradually lowered when smoking ceases, and continues to decline with time. Ten years following cessation of smoking, lung cancer mortality risk is reduced 30% to 50%. The Memorial Sloan-Kettering Cancer Center has developed a tool that calculates risk for developing lung cancer for older smokers and ex-smokers *(www.mskcc.org/PredictionTools/LungCancer)*.

The risk of developing lung cancer is directly related to total exposure to cigarette smoke, measured by total number of cigarettes smoked in a lifetime, age of smoking onset, depth of inhalation, tar and nicotine content, and the use of unfiltered cigarettes. Sidestream smoke (smoke from burning cigarettes, cigars) contains the same carcinogens found in mainstream smoke (smoke inhaled and exhaled from the smoker). This environmental tobacco smoke inhaled by nonsmokers poses a 35% increased risk of the development of lung cancer in nonsmokers.[33] This exposure, called passive smoking, can occur early in life for children of smokers. Children are more vulnerable to environmental smoke than adults because their respiratory and immune systems are not fully developed. Childhood exposure to cigarette smoke is associated with increased prevalence of asthma among adults. Children exposed to cigarette smoke are more likely to become smokers.

Those who smoke pipes and cigars also have an increased risk of developing lung cancer; their risk is slightly higher than that of nonsmokers. Cigar smokers are at higher risk for lung cancer than are pipe smokers. However, heavy smoking of cigars and inhalation of smoke from small cigars correlate with the rates of lung cancer observed in cigarette smokers.

CULTURAL AND ETHNIC HEALTH DISPARITIES

Lung Cancer

- Lung cancer occurs more frequently in men than women.
- African American men get lung cancer at a higher rate than men of other ethnic groups. Asian/Pacific Islander and Hispanic men have the lowest rate.
- White women have a higher rate of lung cancer than women of other ethnic groups. Asian/Pacific Islander and Hispanic women have the lowest rate.
- Cigarette consumption has decreased dramatically in developed countries such as the United States and Canada; however, it is increasing in developing countries (e.g., nations in Africa, Asia, Latin America).
- Close to 60% of the 5.7 billion cigarettes smoked each year and 75% of tobacco users are in developing countries.

Source: *www.cdc.gov/cancer/lung/statistics.htm* and *www.who.int/tobacco/wntd/2004rationale/en.*

Another major risk factor for lung cancer is inhaled carcinogens. These include asbestos, radon, nickel, iron and iron oxides, uranium, polycyclic aromatic hydrocarbons, chromates, arsenic, and air pollution. Exposure to these substances is common for employees of industries involved in mining, smelting, or chemical or petroleum manufacturing. The cigarette smoker who is also exposed to one or more of these chemicals or to high amounts of air pollution is at significantly higher risk for lung cancer.

There are marked variations in a person's propensity to develop lung cancer. To date no genetic abnormality has conclusively been identified for lung cancer. It is known that the carcinogens in cigarette smoke directly damage DNA. One theory is that people have different genetic carcinogen-metabolizing pathways.

Pathophysiology

The pathogenesis of primary lung cancer is not well understood. Lung cancer is thought to arise from bronchial epithelial cells (bronchogenic). These cells grow slowly, and it takes 8 to 10 years for a tumor to reach 1 cm in size, which is the smallest lesion detectable on an x-ray. Lung cancers occur primarily in the segmental bronchi or beyond and have a preference for the upper lobes of the lungs (Fig. 28-2). Pathologic changes in the bronchial system show nonspecific inflammatory changes with hypersecretion of mucus, desquamation of cells, reactive hyperplasia of the basal cells, and metaplasia of normal respiratory epithelium to stratified squamous cells. Pathologic types of lung cancer are presented in Fig. 28-3.

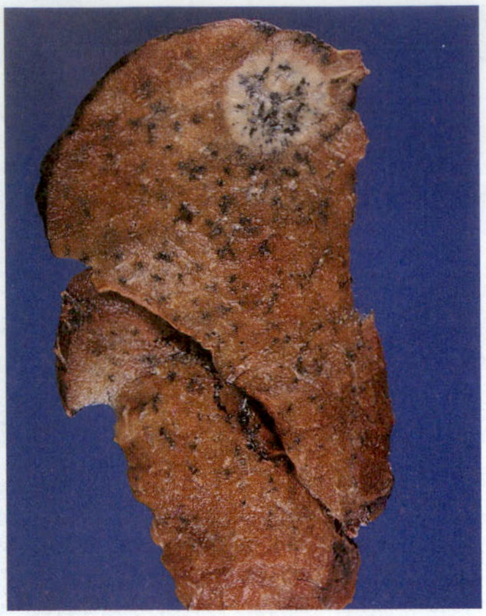

FIG. 28-2 Lung cancer (peripheral adenocarcinoma). The tumor shows prominent black pigmentation, suggestive of having evolved in an anthracotic scar.

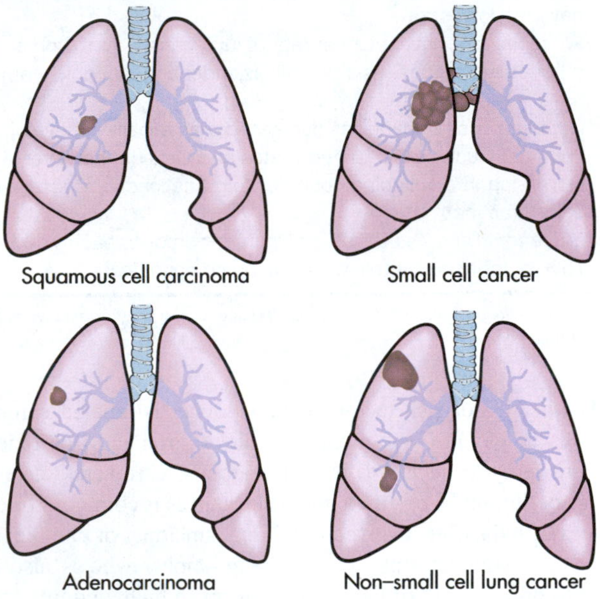

FIG. 28-3 Predominant sites of types of lung cancer.

Primary lung cancers are often categorized into two broad subtypes (Table 28-14), non–small cell lung cancer (NSCLC) (80%) and small cell lung cancer (SCLC) (20%).[34] Lung cancers metastasize primarily by direct extension and via the blood circulation and the lymph system. The common sites for metastatic growth are the liver, brain, bones, scalene lymph nodes, and adrenal glands.

Paraneoplastic Syndrome. Certain lung cancers cause the *paraneoplastic syndrome,* which results from production of active substances (e.g., hormones, enzymes, antigens) either by the tumor itself or in response to the tumor. SCLCs are most commonly associated with the paraneoplastic syndrome. The systemic manifestations seen are hormonal, dermatologic, neuromuscular, vascular, hematologic, and connective tissue syndromes. These syndromes can respond temporarily to symptomatic treatment, but they are impossible to control without successful treatment of the underlying lung cancer.

Clinical Manifestations

Lung cancer is clinically silent for most individuals for the majority of its course. Asymptomatic patients whose cancer is found on routine chest x-ray account for about 10% of new cases. The clinical manifestations of lung cancer are usually nonspecific and appear late in the disease process. Manifestations depend on the type of primary lung cancer, its location, and metastatic spread. Persistent pneumonitis that is a result of obstructed bronchi may be one of the earliest manifestations, causing fever, chills, and cough.

One of the most common symptoms, and often the one reported first, is a persistent cough that may be productive of sputum. Blood-tinged sputum may be produced because of bleeding caused by malignancy, but hemoptysis is not a common symptom. Chest pain may be present and localized or unilateral, ranging from mild to severe. Dyspnea and an auscultatory wheeze may be present if there is bronchial obstruction.

Later manifestations may include nonspecific systemic symptoms such as anorexia, fatigue, weight loss, and nausea and vomiting. Hoarseness may be present as a result of involvement of the laryngeal nerve. Unilateral paralysis of the diaphragm, dysphagia, and superior vena cava obstruction may occur because of intrathoracic spread of the malignancy. There may be palpable lymph nodes in the neck or axilla. Mediastinal involvement may lead to pericardial effusion, cardiac tamponade, and dysrhythmias.

Diagnostic Studies

Chest x-rays may initially identify a lung mass or infiltrate. The findings may show obstructive features of the tumor such as atelectasis and pneumonia. The x-ray can also show evidence of metastasis to the ribs or vertebrae and the presence of pleural effusion. CT scanning is the single most effective noninvasive technique for evaluating lung cancer. CT scans of the brain and bone scans complete the evaluation for metastatic disease. With CT scans, the location and extent of masses in the chest can be identified, as well as any mediastinal involvement or lymph node enlargement. Magnetic resonance imaging (MRI) may be used in combination with or instead of CT scans. Positron emission tomography (PET) promises to be a useful diagnostic tool in early clinical staging. PET allows measurement of differential metabolic activity in normal and diseased tissues.

Sputum cytology can identify malignant cells, but results are positive in only 20% to 30% of specimens because the malignant cells may not be present in the sputum.[35] Biopsy is necessary for a definitive diagnosis. If the mass is well visualized on CT scan and accessible, cells can be aspirated using guided percutaneous fine-needle biopsy technique. If it is too small or difficult to access, an alternative is a bronchoscopy to obtain transbronchial aspirations, brushings, and washings. Mediastinoscopy is another technique that involves the insertion of a scope via a small anterior chest incision into the mediastinum. This is done to obtain tissue from the mediastinal lymph nodes to assess for metastasis. Video-assisted thoracoscopy (VAT) involves inserting a scope via a small thoracic incision in the chest wall to obtain tissue samples inaccessible by mediastinoscopy. If a thoracentesis is performed to relieve a pleural effusion, the fluid should be analyzed for malignant cells. Table 28-15 summarizes the diagnostic management of lung cancer.

Staging. Staging of non–small cell lung cancer (NSCLC) is performed according to the TNM staging system (see Table 16-5). Assessment criteria are T, which denotes tumor size, location, and degree of invasion; N, which indicates regional lymph node involvement; and M, which represents the presence or absence of

TABLE 28-14 Comparison of the Types of Primary Lung Cancer

Cell Type	Risk Factors	Characteristics	Response to Therapy
Non–Small Cell Lung Cancer (NSCLC)			
• Adenocarcinoma	Has been associated with lung scarring and chronic interstitial fibrosis; is not related to cigarette smoking	Most common type; Accounts for approximately 30%-40% of lung cancers; more common in women; often has no clinical manifestations until widespread metastasis is present; usually begins in mucous glandular tissue; is most commonly located in peripheral portions of lungs*	Surgical resection is often attempted; cancer does not respond well to chemotherapy
• Squamous cell carcinoma	Almost always associated with cigarette smoking; is associated with exposure to environmental carcinogens (e.g., uranium, asbestos)	Second most common type of lung cancer; accounts for 30%-35% of lung cancers; is more common in men; arises from the bronchial epithelium (surface cells) of the lungs or bronchus, slow-growing cancer that usually begins in the bronchial tubes; disease nodules tend to be clumped together; produces earlier symptoms because of bronchial obstructive characteristics; does not have a strong tendency to metastasize	Surgical resection is often attempted; life expectancy is better than for small cell lung cancer
• Large cell (undifferentiated) carcinoma	High correlation with cigarette smoking and exposure to environmental carcinogens	The least common form of NSCLS; accounts for 5%-15% of lung cancers; composed of large-sized cells that are anaplastic and often arise in the bronchi; commonly causes cavitation; is highly metastatic via lymphatics and blood; commonly peripheral rather than central location in lungs	Surgery is not usually attempted because of high rate of metastases; tumor may be radiosensitive but often recurs
Small Cell Lung Cancer (SCLC)			
• Small cell carcinoma	Associated with cigarette smoking, exposure to environmental carcinogens	Accounts for 15%-25% of lung cancers; is most malignant form; tends to spread early via lymphatics and bloodstream; is frequently associated with endocrine disturbances; predominantly central and can cause bronchial obstruction and pneumonia	Cancer has poorest prognosis; however, chemotherapy advances have been substantial; radiation is used as adjuvant therapy as well as palliative measure; average median survival is 16 mo

*See Fig. 28-3.

distant metastases. Depending on the TNM designation, the tumor is then staged, which assists in estimating prognosis and determining the appropriate therapy. A simplified version of staging of NSCLC is presented in Table 28-16. Patients with stages I, II, and IIIA disease may be surgical candidates. However, stage IIIB or IV disease is usually inoperable and has a poor prognosis.

Staging of small cell lung cancer (SCLC) by TNM has not been useful because this cancer is very aggressive and always considered systemic. The stages of SCLC are *limited* and *extensive*. Limited means that the tumor is confined to the chest and to regional lymph nodes. Only 10% of patients who receive aggressive treatment for this type of cancer survive 2 years or longer after diagnosis. Extensive SCLC means that some of the cancer extends to the chest wall or to other parts of the body. On average, patients with extensive SCLC survive only 7 to 10 months.[35]

Screening for Lung Cancer. Early screening for lung cancer is very controversial. The U.S. Preventive Services Task Force *(www.preventiveservices.ahrq.gov)* found fair evidence that screening (chest x-ray, low-dose CT, sputum cytology) can detect lung cancer at an earlier stage. However, there is poor evidence that it decreased lung cancer mortality. Overall, there is insufficient evidence to recommend for or against screening asymptomatic persons.[36] The American College of Chest Physicians recommends against ongoing screening for asymptomatic, low-risk individuals. The Early Lung Cancer Action Project is being conducted to deter-

TABLE 28-15 COLLABORATIVE CARE Lung Cancer

Diagnostic
- History and physical examination
- Chest x-ray
- Sputum for cytologic study
- Bronchoscopy
- Computed tomography (CT) scan
- Magnetic resonance imaging (MRI)
- Positron emission tomography (PET)
- Spirometry (preoperative)
- Mediastinoscopy
- Video-assisted thoracoscopy (VAT)
- Pulmonary angiography
- Lung scan
- Fine-needle aspiration

Collaborative Therapy
- Surgery
- Radiation therapy
- Chemotherapy
- Biologic and targeted therapy
- Prophylactic cranial radiation
- Bronchoscopic laser therapy
- Photodynamic therapy
- Airway stenting
- Cryotherapy

TABLE 28-16 Staging of Non–Small Cell Lung Cancer

Stages	Characteristics
I	Tumor is small and localized to lung. No lymph node involvement
A	Tumor <3 cm
B	Tumor >3 cm and invading surrounding local areas
II	
A	Tumor <3 cm with invasion of lymph nodes on same side of chest
B	Tumor >3 cm involving the bronchus and lymph nodes on same side of chest and tissue of other local organs
III	
A	Tumor spread to the nearby structures (chest wall, pleura, pericardium) and regional lymph nodes
B	Extensive tumor involving heart, trachea, esophagus, mediastinum, malignant pleural effusion, contralateral lymph nodes, scalene or supraclavicular lymph nodes
IV	Distant metastasis

mine the usefulness of CT in early lung cancer detection. The National Screening Trial is examining the effectiveness of single-view chest x-ray and CT to detect early-stage lung cancer.[37] The Canadian Task force *(www.ctfphc.org)* states there is insufficient evidence to recommend screening for lung cancer with chest x-ray or CT and that smoking cessation should be emphasized to the patient as the preferred modality for reducing lung cancer mortality. A new noninvasive blood test that could detect lung cancer in its earliest stages is being studied at Duke University Medical Center.[38]

The nurses' role in screening for lung cancer includes educating patients on the strengths and limitations of the proposed screening measures for early detection of lung cancer. Smoking cessation and prevention are essential in decreasing morbidity and mortality associated with lung cancer. Nurses play a vital role in counseling patients in tobacco cessation and prevention. (Smoking cessation is discussed in Chapter 12.)

Collaborative Care

Surgical Therapy. Surgical resection is the treatment of choice in NSCLC stages I and II, because the disease is potentially curable with resection. The 5-year survival in stage I disease with complete resection is 60% to 80%; in patients with stage II disease, it is 40% to 60%.[35] For other NSCLC stages, surgery may be indicated in conjunction with radiation therapy and/or chemotherapy. Fifty percent of all NSCLC lung cancers are not resectable at the time of diagnosis. In limited-stage SCLC (which is rare), surgical resection, chemotherapy, and radiation therapy may be recommended. The surgical procedures that may be performed include pneumonectomy (removal of one entire lung), lobectomy (removal of one or more lobes of the lung), or lung-conserving resection or segmental or wedge resection procedures. When the tumor is considered operable, the patient's cardiopulmonary status must be evaluated to determine the ability to withstand surgery. This is done by clinical studies of pulmonary function, arterial blood gases (ABGs), and other tests, as indicated by the individual's status.

Radiation Therapy. Radiation therapy may be used with the intent to cure in the individual who is unable to tolerate surgical resection due to comorbidities. It may also be used as adjuvant therapy after resection of the tumor. Recent guidelines indicate that radiation therapy is useful as part of the treatment for locally advanced, unresectable NSCLC.[39] Improved survival and symptom control have been achieved with combination treatments (radiation therapy, surgery, chemotherapy).[40] Complications of radiation therapy include esophagitis, skin irritation, and radiation pneumonitis. Hyperfractionated radiation, given twice daily, has improved response and survival rates in SCLC. However, there is increased toxicity, particularly esophagitis.[41]

Radiation therapy is also used to relieve symptoms of dyspnea and hemoptysis resulting from bronchial obstructive tumors and to treat superior vena cava syndrome. It can also be used to treat pain that is caused by metastatic bone lesions or cerebral metastasis. Radiation may be used preoperatively to reduce tumor mass prior to resection or postoperatively as an adjuvant measure.

Chemotherapy. Chemotherapy may be used in the treatment of nonresectable tumors or as adjuvant therapy to surgery in NSCLC. A variety of chemotherapy drugs and multidrug regimens (i.e., protocols), including combination chemotherapy, have been used. These drugs include etoposide (VePesid), carboplatin (Paraplatin), cisplatin (Platinol), paclitaxel (Taxol), vinorelbine (Navelbine), cyclophosphamide (Cytoxan), ifosfamide (Ifex), docetaxel (Taxotere), gemcitabine (Gemzar), topotecan (Hycamtin), and irinotecan (Camptosar).[34,35]

Chemotherapy has improved survival in patients with advanced NSCLC and is now considered standard treatment. Treatment of limited-stage SCLC includes combination chemotherapy and radiation therapy.[42]

Biologic and Targeted Therapy. Targeted therapy uses drugs that specifically block the growth of molecules involved in specific aspects of tumor growth (see Chapter 16). Therefore there are usually fewer toxicities than with chemotherapy. One type of targeted therapy that is approved for patients with locally advanced and metastatic NSCLC is erlotinib (Tarceva). It inhibits an enzyme, tyrosine kinase, associated with epidermal growth factor receptor. Thus this drug blocks the growth-stimulatory signals in the cancer cells. Erlotinib is used to treat patients whose cancer has progressed despite other treatments. Gefitinib (Iressa), which has a mechanism of action similar to that of erlotinib, is available on a limited basis in the United States to patients who have shown a response to the drug in the past, and to current users who are responding to it now.

Other Therapies

Prophylactic Cranial Radiation. Intracranial metastasis occurs in up to 39% of patients with SCLC. Most chemotherapy drugs do not adequately penetrate the blood-brain barrier. Prophylactic cranial radiation is effective in preventing metastasis (20%), although it is not known if it increases survival.[42] Toxicities of this therapy may include scalp erythema, fatigue, and alopecia.

Bronchoscopic Laser Therapy. Bronchoscopic laser therapy makes it possible to remove obstructing bronchial lesions. The neodymium:yttrium-aluminum-garnet (Nd:YAG) laser is most commonly used for laser resection using either the flexible or the rigid bronchoscope. The thermal energy of the laser is transmitted to the target tissue. It is a safe and effective treatment of endobronchial obstructions from tumors.[40] Relief of the symptoms from airway obstruction as a result of thermal necrosis and shrinkage of the tumor can be dramatic.

Photodynamic Therapy. Photodynamic therapy is a safe, bronchoscopic laser therapy for lung cancer. Porfimer (Photofrin) is injected intravenously and selectively concentrates in tumor cells. After a set time period (usually 48 hours), the tumor is exposed to laser light, producing a toxic form of oxygen that destroys tumor cells. Necrotic tissue is removed through a bronchoscope.

Airway Stenting. Stents can be used alone or in combination with other techniques for palliation of dyspnea, cough, or respiratory insufficiency. The advantage of an airway stent is that it supports the airway wall against collapse or external compression and can impede extension of tumor into the airway lumen.

Cryotherapy. Cryotherapy is a technique in which tissue is destroyed as a result of freezing. Bronchoscopic cryotherapy is used to ablate (destroy) bronchogenic carcinomas, especially polypoid lesions. There is insufficient evidence that supports its success in the treatment of early-stage lung cancer.[40]

NURSING MANAGEMENT
LUNG CANCER

Nursing Assessment

It is important to determine the understanding of the patient and the family concerning the diagnostic tests (those completed as well as those planned), the diagnosis or potential diagnosis, the treatment options, and the prognosis. At the same time, the nurse can assess the level of anxiety experienced by the patient and the support provided and needed by the patient's significant others. Subjective and objective data that should be obtained from a patient with lung cancer are presented in Table 28-17.

Nursing Diagnoses

Nursing diagnoses for the patient with lung cancer may include, but are not limited to, the following:

- Ineffective airway clearance *related to* increased tracheobronchial secretions and presence of tumor
- Anxiety *related to* lack of knowledge of diagnosis or unknown prognosis and treatments
- Acute pain *related to* pressure of tumor on surrounding structures and erosion of tissues
- Imbalanced nutrition: less than body requirements *related to* increased metabolic demands, increased secretions, weakness, and anorexia
- Ineffective health maintenance *related to* lack of knowledge about the disease process and therapeutic regimen

EVIDENCE-BASED PRACTICE

Do Noninvasive Interventions Improve Quality of Life in Patients with Lung Cancer?

Clinical Question

In lung cancer patients (P), does receiving noninvasive interventions (I) compared to receiving no additional treatment (C) improve symptoms, psychologic functioning, and quality of life (O)?

Best Available Evidence

Systematic review of randomized controlled trials (RCTs)

Critical Appraisal and Synthesis of Evidence

- Meta-analysis of 9 RCTs ($n = 833$)
- Interventions studied included nursing interventions to manage breathlessness, nursing care programs, nutritional interventions, psychotherapeutic interventions, exercise, and reflexology.

Conclusions

- Nursing interventions to manage breathlessness showed improved symptom control, performance status, and emotional functioning.
- Nursing programs were effective in delaying clinical deterioration, dependency, and symptom distress, as well as improving emotional functioning and satisfaction with care.
- Exercise had a beneficial effect on self-empowerment.
- Nutritional interventions only showed positive results in increasing energy.
- Psychologic interventions and reflexology had some short-lasting positive effects on quality of life.

Implications for Nursing Practice

- It is important to develop and maintain a supportive and empathetic relationship with the patient with lung cancer.
- Offer patients supportive multidisciplinary interventions that may benefit their emotional, psychologic, and physical well-being.
- These interventions may also help patients with other types of cancers.

Reference for Evidence

Sola I, Thompson E, Subirana M, et al: Non-invasive interventions for improving well-being and quality of life in patients with lung cancer, Cochrane Lung Cancer Group, *Cochrane Database of Systematic Reviews* 4, 2005.

PICO: P, Patient population of interest; *I*, intervention or area of interest; *C*, comparison of interest or comparison group; *O*, outcome(s) of interest (see p. 6).

TABLE 28-17 NURSING ASSESSMENT Lung Cancer

Subjective Data

Important Health Information

Past health history: Exposure to secondhand smoke, airborne carcinogens (e.g., asbestos, radon, hydrocarbons), or other pollutants; urban living environment; chronic lung disease, including TB, COPD, bronchiectasis

Medications: Use of cough medicines or other respiratory medications

Functional Health Patterns

Health perception–health management: Smoking history; family history of lung cancer; frequent respiratory infections

Nutritional-metabolic: Anorexia, nausea, vomiting, dysphagia (late); weight loss; chills

Activity-exercise: Fatigue; persistent cough (productive or nonproductive); dyspnea, hemoptysis (late symptom)

Cognitive-perceptual: Chest pain or tightness, shoulder and arm pain, headache, bone pain (late symptom)

Objective Data

General

Fever, neck and axillary lymphadenopathy, paraneoplastic syndromes (e.g., syndrome of inappropriate ADH secretion)

Integumentary

Jaundice (liver metastasis); edema of neck and face (superior vena cava syndrome), digital clubbing

Respiratory

Wheezing, hoarseness, stridor, unilateral diaphragm paralysis, pleural effusions (late signs)

Cardiovascular

Pericardial effusion, cardiac tamponade, dysrhythmias (late signs)

Neurologic

Unsteady gait (brain metastasis)

Musculoskeletal

Pathologic fractures, muscle wasting (late)

Possible Findings

Observance of lesion on chest x-ray, CT scan, or PET scan; MRI findings of vertebral, spinal cord, or mediastinal invasion; positive sputum or bronchial washings for cytologic studies; positive fiberoptic bronchoscopy and biopsy findings

ADH, Antidiuretic hormone; *COPD,* chronic obstructive pulmonary disease; *CT,* computed tomography; *MRI,* magnetic resonance imaging; *PET,* positron emission tomography; *TB,* tuberculosis.

- Ineffective breathing pattern *related to* decreased lung capacity

Planning

The overall goals are that the patient with lung cancer will have (1) effective breathing patterns, (2) adequate airway clearance, (3) adequate oxygenation of tissues, (4) minimal to no pain, and (5) a realistic attitude toward treatment and prognosis.

Nursing Implementation

Health Promotion. The best way to halt the epidemic of lung cancer is for people to stop smoking. Important nursing activities to assist in the progress toward this goal include promoting smoking cessation programs and actively supporting education and policy changes related to smoking. Important changes have occurred as the result of the recognition that passive smoke is a health hazard; laws require designation of nonsmoking areas or prohibiting smoking in most public places and a ban on smoking on airline flights. Other actions aimed at controlling tobacco use include restrictions on tobacco advertising on television and warning label requirements for cigarette packaging. For the individual who does have a smoking habit, efforts should be made to assist the smoker to stop smoking. The updated evidence-based guideline, *Treating Tobacco Use and Dependence: Clinical Practice Guideline,* describes a framework (the five *A*s) for approaching patients who are willing to attempt to quit smoking.[33] The five *A*s stand for the five strategies: ask, advise, assess, assist, and arrange (see Chapter 12, Table 12-5). The four stages of change identified in smokers attempting to quit include precontemplation ("I want"), contemplation ("I might"), preparation ("I will"), and action ("I am"). (The stages of change in relationship to patient teaching are discussed in Chapter 5 and Table 5-3.) Each stage requires specific actions to progress to the next stage. Nurses working with patients at their individual stage of change will help them progress to the next stage. For patients unwilling to quit, motivational interviewing is recommended (discussed in Chapter 12 on p. 188).

The evidence-based guideline also offers the five *R*s strategy for motivating smokers to quit: relevance, risk, reward, roadblocks, and repetition (see Table 12-5). Because some patients relapse months or years after having stopped smoking, nurses need to continually provide assistance to prevent relapse. (Agents and strategies to assist patients to stop smoking are discussed in Chapter 12 and Tables 12-4, 12-5, and 12-6.)

In addition, the 2004 Surgeon General's Report on Smoking and Health *(www.cdc.gov/tobacco/sgr)* offers tips to quit, strategies to use, and an online interactive visual animation of the effects of smoking and the benefits in quitting ("The Health Consequences of Smoking on The Human Body"). Nicotine's addictive properties make quitting a difficult task that requires much support. Nicotine replacement significantly lessens the urge to smoke and increases the percentage of smokers who successfully quit smoking. All patients should be offered some form of nicotine replacement. (Nicotine replacement therapy products are presented in Table 12-4.) Research into smoking behaviors and successful strategies to promote smoking cessation is ongoing. A combination of behavioral techniques and nicotine replacement products is the most effective strategy to help smokers quit.[43] The advice and motivation of health care professionals can be a powerful force in smoking cessation. Nurses are in a unique position to promote smoking cessation because they see large numbers of smokers who may be reluctant to seek help. Support for the smoker includes education that smoking a few cigarettes during a cessation attempt (a slip) is much different than resuming the full smoking habit (a relapse). Despite the slip, smokers should be encouraged to continue the attempt at cessation without viewing the effort as a failure. The nurse needs to be aware of resources in the community to assist the individual who is interested in quitting.

Acute Intervention. Care of the patient with lung cancer will initially involve support and reassurance during the diagnostic evaluation. (Specific nursing measures related to the diagnostic studies are outlined in Chapter 26.)

Another major responsibility of the nurse is to help the patient and family cope with the diagnosis of lung cancer. The patient may feel guilty about cigarette smoking having caused the cancer and need to discuss this feeling with someone who has a nonjudgmental attitude. Counseling from a social worker, psychologist, or member of the clergy may be needed. Nursing research focusing on the effects of spirituality on the sense of well-being of people with lung cancer found that people with more meaning in their lives had decreased symptom distress. Additionally, prayer was associated positively with psychologic well-being.[44] This validates the impact of spiritual care for these patients and helps guide nurses' practice in spiritual needs. Research on the role of the family found that family disagreements about treatment decisions for patients with advanced lung cancer were common.[45] For nurses, these findings suggest the need to be aware of differences of opinion in order to facilitate family communication and improve patient satisfaction with treatment decisions.

Specific care of the patient will depend on the treatment plan. Providing symptom management is critical. The nurse needs to monitor for signs and symptoms of progressive or recurrent disease and notify the physician if this is suspected. Postoperative care for the patient having surgery is discussed later in this chapter. Care of the patient undergoing radiation therapy and chemotherapy is discussed in Chapter 16. The nurse has a major role in providing patient comfort, teaching methods to reduce pain, monitoring for side effects of prescribed medications, fostering appropriate coping strategies for the patient and family, assessing smoking cessation readiness, and helping access resources to deal with the illness. The nurse coordinates care with members of the interdisciplinary team and keeps the patient and family informed.

Ambulatory and Home Care. The patient who has had a surgical resection with intent to cure should be followed up carefully for manifestations of metastasis. The patient and family should be told to contact the physician if symptoms such as hemoptysis, dysphagia, chest pain, and hoarseness develop.

For many individuals who have lung cancer, little can be done to significantly prolong their lives. Radiation therapy and chemotherapy can be used to provide palliative relief from distressing symptoms. Constant pain becomes a major problem. (Measures used to relieve pain are discussed in Chapter 10. Care of the patient with cancer is discussed in Chapter 16.)

Evaluation

The expected outcomes are that the patient with lung cancer will have

- adequate breathing patterns
- minimal to no pain
- realistic attitude about prognosis

OTHER TYPES OF LUNG TUMORS

Other types of primary lung tumors include sarcomas, lymphomas, and bronchial adenomas. Bronchial adenomas are small tumors that arise from the lower trachea or major bronchi and are considered malignant because they are locally invasive and frequently metastasize. Clinical manifestations of bronchial adenomas include hemoptysis, persistent cough, localized obstructive wheezing, and pneumonia. Bronchial adenomas can usually be treated successfully with surgical resection.

The lungs are a common site for secondary metastases and are more often affected by metastatic growth than by primary lung tumors. The pulmonary capillaries, with their extensive network, are ideal sites for tumor emboli. In addition, the lungs have an extensive lymphatic network. The primary malignancies that spread to the lungs often originate in the GI or genitourinary (GU) tracts and in the breast. General symptoms of lung metastases are chest pain and nonproductive cough.

Benign tumors of the lung are rare. *Hamartomas* of the lung are the most common benign tumor. These tumors, composed of fibrous tissue, fat, and blood vessels, are congenital malformations of the connective tissue of the bronchiolar walls. Hamartomas are slow-growing tumors. *Chondromas* are rare benign tumors that arise in the bronchial cartilage; *leiomyomas* are myomas of smooth, nonstriated muscle. *Mesotheliomas* may be malignant or benign and originate from the visceral pleura. Benign mesotheliomas are localized lesions.

Chest Trauma and Thoracic Injuries

Thoracic injuries are the cause of death in 20% to 25% of all trauma victims; injury to the chest wall is found in 45% of these thoracic trauma victims.[46] Traumatic injuries fall into two major categories: (1) blunt trauma and (2) penetrating trauma. *Blunt trauma* occurs when the body is struck by a blunt object, such as a steering wheel. The types of forces involved in blunt chest trauma injuries include deceleration, acceleration, shearing, and compression. The external injury may appear minor, but the impact may cause severe, life-threatening internal injuries, such as a ruptured spleen. *Contrecoup trauma,* a type of blunt trauma, is caused by the impact of parts of the body against other objects. This type of injury differs from blunt trauma primarily in the velocity of the impact. Internal organs are rapidly forced back and forth (acceleration-deceleration injury) within the bony structures that surround them so that internal injury is sustained not only on the side of the body impacted but also on the opposite side, where the organ or organs hit bony structures. If the velocity of impact is great enough, organs and blood vessels can literally be torn from their points of origin. This is the shearing injury that can cause transection of the aorta, hemothorax, and diaphragmatic rupture injuries. Compression injury occurs when the body cannot handle the degree of external pressure during blunt trauma, resulting in contusions, crush injuries, and organ rupture.

Penetrating trauma occurs when a foreign body impales or passes through the body tissues (e.g., gunshot wounds, stabbings). Table 28-18 describes selective traumatic injuries as they relate to the categories of trauma and the mechanism of injury. Emergency care of the patient with a chest injury is presented in Table 28-19.

Thoracic injuries range from simple rib fractures to life-threatening tears of the aorta, vena cava, and other major vessels.

TABLE 28-18 Common Traumatic Chest Injuries and Mechanisms of Injury

Mechanism of Injury	Common Related Injury
Blunt Trauma	
Blunt steering-wheel injury to chest	Rib fractures, flail chest, pneumothorax, hemopneumothorax, myocardial contusion, pulmonary contusion, cardiac tamponade, great vessel tears
Shoulder-harness seat belt injury	Fractured clavicle, dislocated shoulder, rib fractures, pulmonary contusion, pericardial contusion, cardiac tamponade
Crush injury (e.g., heavy equipment, crushing thorax)	Pneumothorax and hemopneumothorax, flail chest, great vessel tears and rupture, decreased blood return to heart with decreased cardiac output
Penetrating Trauma	
Gunshot or stab wound to chest	Open pneumothorax, tension pneumothorax, hemopneumothorax, cardiac tamponade, esophageal damage, tracheal tear, great vessel tears

The most common thoracic emergencies and their management are described in Table 28-20.

PNEUMOTHORAX

A **pneumothorax** is air in the pleural space. As a result of the air in the pleural space, there is partial or complete collapse of the lung. This condition should be suspected after any blunt trauma to the chest wall. Pneumothorax may be closed or open. Pneumothorax associated with trauma may be accompanied by hemothorax, a condition called *hemopneumothorax.*

Types of Pneumothorax

Closed Pneumothorax. *Closed pneumothorax* has no associated external wound. The most common form is a spontaneous pneumothorax, which is accumulation of air in the pleural space without an apparent antecedent event. It is caused by rupture of small blebs on the visceral pleural space. The cause of the blebs is unknown. This condition occurs most commonly in underweight male cigarette smokers between 20 and 40 years of age. There is a tendency for this condition to recur.

Other causes of closed pneumothorax include the following:

1. Injury to the lungs from mechanical ventilation
2. Injury to the lungs from insertion of a subclavian catheter
3. Perforation of the esophagus
4. Injury to the lungs from broken ribs
5. Ruptured blebs or bullae in a patient with COPD

Open Pneumothorax. *Open pneumothorax* occurs when air enters the pleural space through an opening in the chest wall (Fig. 28-4, *B*). Examples include stab or gunshot wounds and surgical thoracotomy. A penetrating chest wound is often referred to as a sucking chest wound.

An open pneumothorax should be covered with a vented dressing. (A vented dressing is one secured on three sides with the fourth side left untaped.) This allows air to escape from the vent and decreases the likelihood of tension pneumothorax developing.

TABLE 28-19 EMERGENCY MANAGEMENT
Chest Trauma

Etiology	Assessment Findings	Interventions
Blunt Motor vehicle accident Pedestrian accident Fall Assault with blunt object Crush injury Explosion **Penetrating** Knife Gunshot Stick Arrow Other missiles	**Respiratory** • Dyspnea, respiratory distress • Cough with or without hemoptysis • Cyanosis of mouth, face, nail beds, mucous membranes • Tracheal deviation • Audible air escaping from chest wound • Decreased breath sounds on side of injury • Decreased O_2 saturation • Frothy secretions **Cardiovascular** • Rapid, thready pulse • Decreased BP • Narrowed pulse pressure • Asymmetric BP values in arms • Distended neck veins • Muffled heart sounds • Chest pain • Crunching sound synchronous with heart sounds • Dysrhythmias **Surface Findings** • Bruising • Abrasions • Open chest wound • Asymmetric chest movement • Subcutaneous emphysema	**Initial** • Ensure patent airway. • Administer high-flow O_2 with non-rebreather mask. • Establish IV access with two large-bore catheters. Begin fluid resuscitation as appropriate. • Remove clothing to assess injury. • Cover sucking chest wound with nonporous dressing taped on three sides. • Stabilize impaled objects with bulky dressings. *Do not remove.* • Assess for other significant injuries and treat appropriately. • Stabilize flail rib segment with hand followed by application of large pieces of tape horizontal across the flail segment. • Place patient in a semi-Fowler's position or position patient on the injured side if breathing is easier *after* cervical spine injury has been ruled out. **Ongoing Monitoring** • Monitor vital signs, level of consciousness, oxygen saturation, cardiac rhythm, respiratory status, and urinary output. • Anticipate intubation for respiratory distress. • Release dressing if tension pneumothorax develops after sucking chest wound is covered.

TABLE 28-20 EMERGENCY MANAGEMENT
Thoracic Injuries

Injury	Definition	Clinical Manifestations	Emergency Management
Pneumothorax	Air in pleural space (see Fig. 28-4).	Dyspnea, decreased movement of involved chest wall, diminished or absent breath sounds on the affected side, hyperresonance to percussion	Chest tube insertion with chest drainage system
Hemothorax	Blood in the pleural space, usually occurs in conjunction with pneumothorax.	Dyspnea, diminished or absent breath sounds, dullness to percussion, shock	Chest tube insertion with chest drainage system; autotransfusion of collected blood, treatment of hypovolemia as necessary
Tension pneumothorax	Air in pleural space that does not escape. Continued increase in amount of air shifts intrathoracic organs and increases intrathoracic pressure (see Fig. 28-5).	Cyanosis, air hunger, violent agitation, tracheal deviation away from affected side, subcutaneous emphysema, neck vein distention, hyperresonance to percussion	Medical emergency: needle decompression followed by chest tube insertion with chest drainage system
Flail chest	Fracture of two or more adjacent ribs in two or more places with loss of chest wall stability (see Fig. 28-6).	Paradoxic movement of chest wall, respiratory distress, associated hemothorax, pneumothorax, pulmonary contusion	Stabilize flail segment with intubation in some patients; taping in others; oxygen therapy; treat associated injuries; analgesia
Cardiac tamponade	Blood rapidly collects in pericardial sac, compresses myocardium because the pericardium does not stretch, and prevents heart from pumping effectively.	Muffled, distant heart sounds, hypotension, neck vein distention, increased central venous pressure	Medical emergency: pericardiocentesis with surgical repair as appropriate

If the object that caused the open chest wound is still in place, it should not be removed until a physician is present. The impaled object should be stabilized with a bulky dressing.

Tension Pneumothorax. **Tension pneumothorax** is a pneumothorax with rapid accumulation of air in the pleural space, causing severely high intrapleural pressures with resultant tension on the heart and great vessels. It may result from either an open or a closed pneumothorax (Fig. 28-5). In an open chest wound, a flap may act as a one-way valve; thus air can enter on inspiration but cannot escape. The intrathoracic pressure increases, the lung collapses, and the mediastinum shifts toward the unaffected side, which is subsequently compressed. As the pressure increases, cardiac output is altered because of decreased venous return and compression of the vena cava and aorta. Tension pneumothorax

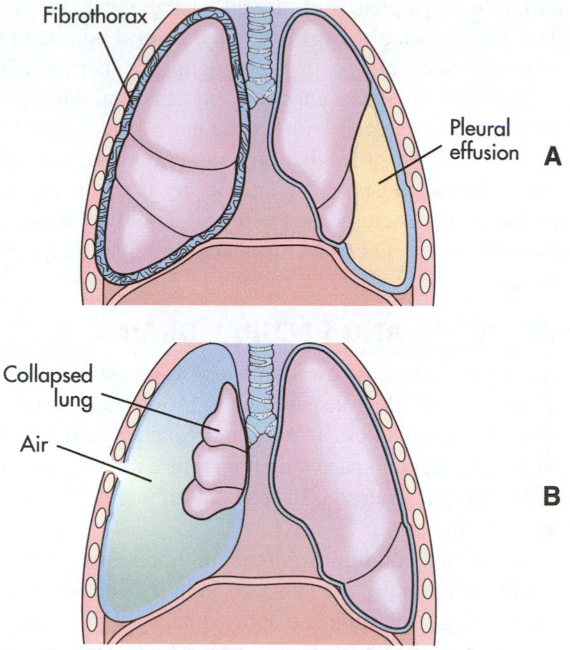

FIG. 28-4 Disorders of the pleura. **A,** Fibrothorax resulting from an organization of inflammatory exudate, and pleural effusion. **B,** Open pneumothorax resulting from collapse of lung due to disruption of chest wall and outside air entering.

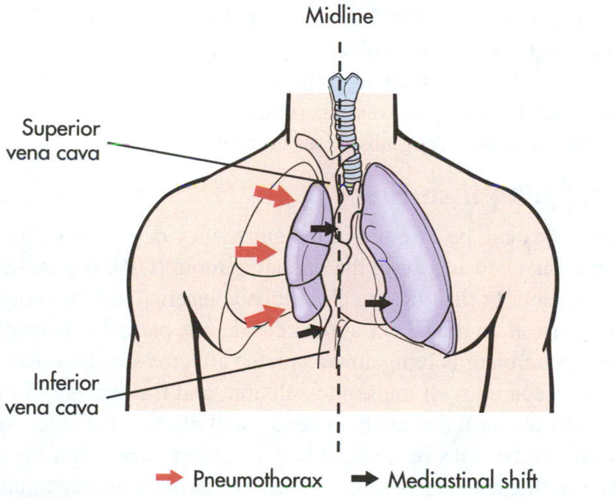

FIG. 28-5 Tension pneumothorax. As pleural pressure on the affected side increases, mediastinal displacement ensues with resultant respiratory and cardiovascular compromise.

can occur with mechanical ventilation and resuscitative efforts. It can also occur if chest tubes are clamped or become blocked in a patient with a pneumothorax. Unclamping the tube or relief of the obstruction will remedy this situation.

Tension pneumothorax is a medical emergency, with both the respiratory and circulatory systems affected. If the tension in the pleural space is not relieved, the patient is likely to die from inadequate cardiac output or severe hypoxemia. The emergency management is to insert a large-bore needle into the chest wall to release the trapped air.

Hemothorax. **Hemothorax** is an accumulation of blood in the intrapleural space. It is frequently found in association with open pneumothorax and is then called a *hemopneumothorax.* Causes of hemothorax include chest trauma, lung malignancy, complications of anticoagulant therapy, pulmonary embolus, and tearing of pleural adhesions.

Chylothorax. **Chylothorax** is lymphatic fluid in the pleural space due to a leak in the thoracic duct. Causes include trauma, surgical procedures, and malignancy. The thoracic duct is disrupted and the chylous fluid, milky white with high lipid content, fills the pleural space. Total lymphatic flow through the thoracic duct is 1500 to 2400 ml/day. Fifty percent of cases will heal with conservative treatment (chest drainage, bowel rest, and parenteral nutrition). Surgery and pleurodesis are options if conservative therapy fails. *Pleurodesis* is the artificial production of adhesions between the parietal and visceral pleura, usually done with a chemical sclerosing agent.

Clinical Manifestations

If the pneumothorax (hemothorax or chylothorax) is small, mild tachycardia and dyspnea may be the only manifestations. If the pneumothorax (hemothorax or chylothorax) is large, respiratory distress may be present, including shallow, rapid respirations; dyspnea; air hunger; and oxygen desaturation. Chest pain and a cough with or without hemoptysis may be present. On auscultation, there are no breath sounds over the affected area. A chest x-ray shows the presence of air or fluid in the pleural space.

If a tension pneumothorax develops, severe respiratory distress, tachycardia, and hypotension occur. Mediastinal displacement can occur with a tracheal shift to the unaffected side. The patient is hemodynamically unstable in this medical emergency.

Collaborative Care

Treatment depends on the severity of the pneumothorax (hemothorax or chylothorax) and the nature of the underlying disease. If the patient is stable, and the amount of air and fluid accumulated in the intrapleural space is minimal, no treatment may be needed as the pneumothorax will resolve spontaneously. If the amount of air or fluid is minimal, the pleural space also can be aspirated with a large-bore needle. As a lifesaving measure, needle venting (using a large-bore needle) of the pleural space may be used. A Heimlich valve may also be used to evacuate air from the pleural space. The Heimlich valve is a portable, lightweight, one-way flutter valve device similar to a water-seal drain. The most definitive and common form of treatment of pneumothorax and hemothorax is to insert a chest tube and connect it to water-seal drainage. Repeated spontaneous pneumothorax may need to be treated surgically by a partial pleurectomy, stapling, or pleurodesis to promote adherence of the pleurae to one another.

FRACTURED RIBS

Rib fractures are the most common type of chest injury resulting from trauma. Ribs 5 through 10 are most commonly fractured because they are least protected by chest muscles. If the fractured rib is splintered or displaced, it may damage the pleura and lungs.

Clinical manifestations of fractured ribs include pain (especially on inspiration) at the site of injury. The patient splints the affected area and takes shallow breaths to try to decrease the pain. Because the patient is reluctant to take deep breaths, atelectasis may develop because of decreased ventilation.

The main goal in treatment is to decrease pain so that the patient can breathe adequately to promote good chest expansion. Strapping the chest with tape or using a binder is not generally done. Most physicians believe that these measures should be avoided because they reduce lung expansion and predispose the individual to atelectasis. Opioid drug therapy must be individualized and used with caution because these drugs can depress respirations.

FLAIL CHEST

Flail chest results from multiple rib fractures, causing an unstable chest wall (Fig. 28-6). The diagnosis of flail chest is made on the basis of fracture of two or more ribs, in two or more separate locations, causing an unstable segment.[47] The flail segment usually involves anterior (sternal separation) or lateral rib fractures. The chest wall cannot provide the bony structure necessary to maintain bellows action and ventilation. The affected (flail) area will move paradoxically with respect to the intact portion of the chest during respiration. During inspiration the affected portion is sucked in, and during expiration it bulges out. This paradoxical chest movement prevents adequate ventilation of the lung in the injured area and increases the work of breathing. The underlying lung may have a pulmonary contusion aggravating hypoxemia. The associated pain, fractures, and lung injury give rise to an alteration in breathing pattern and hypoxemia.

A flail chest is usually apparent on visual examination of the unconscious patient. The patient manifests rapid, shallow respirations and tachycardia. A flail chest may not be initially apparent in the conscious patient as a result of splinting of the chest wall. The patient moves air poorly, and movement of the thorax is asymmetric and uncoordinated. Palpation of abnormal respiratory movements, evaluation for crepitus near the rib fractures, chest x-ray, and ABGs all assist in the diagnosis.

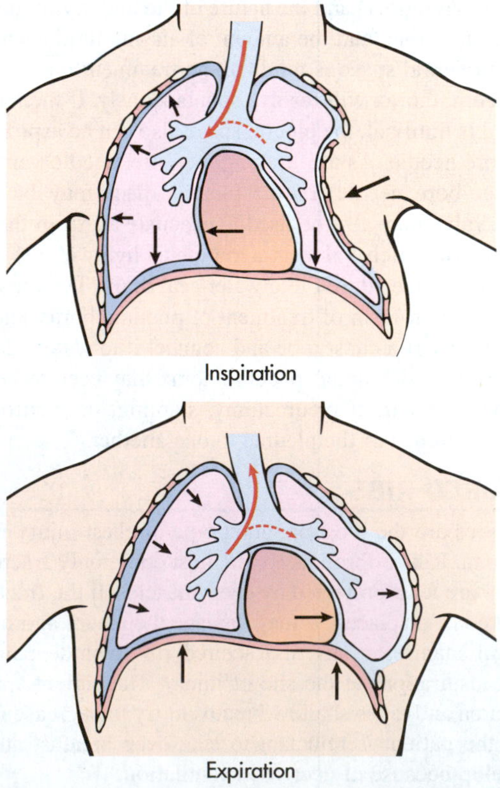

FIG. 28-6 Flail chest produces paradoxic respiration. On inspiration, the flail section sinks in with mediastinal shift to the uninjured side. On expiration, the flail section bulges outward with mediastinal shift to the injured side.

Initial therapy consists of airway management, adequate ventilation, supplemental oxygen therapy, careful administration of IV solutions, and pain control. The definitive therapy is to reexpand the lung and ensure adequate oxygenation. Although many patients can be managed without the use of mechanical ventilation, a short period of intubation and ventilation may be necessary until the diagnosis of the lung injury is complete. The lung parenchyma and fractured ribs will heal with time. Some patients continue to experience intercostal pain after the flail chest has resolved.

CHEST TUBES AND PLEURAL DRAINAGE

The purpose of chest tubes and pleural drainage is to remove air and fluid from the pleural space and to restore normal intrapleural pressure so that the lungs can reexpand. Small accumulations of air or fluid in the pleural space may not require removal by thoracentesis or chest tube insertion. Instead, the air and fluid may be reabsorbed over time.

Under normal conditions, intrapleural pressure is below atmospheric pressure (approximately 4 to 5 cm H_2O below atmospheric pressure during expiration and approximately 8 to 10 cm H_2O below atmospheric pressure during inspiration). (Intrapleural pressure and the intrapleural space are described in Chapter 26.) If intrapleural pressure becomes equal to atmospheric pressure, the lungs will collapse (pneumothorax). Air can enter the intrapleural space by a variety of mechanisms, including traumatic chest injury (e.g., gunshot wound, fractured rib), thoracotomy, and spontaneous pneumothorax. Fluid can accumulate in the pleural space *(pleural effusion)* as a result of impaired lymphatic drainage (e.g., from malignancy) or changes in the colloidal osmotic pressure (e.g., heart failure). *Empyema* is purulent pleural fluid, which may be associated with lung abscesses or pneumonia.

Chest Tube Insertion

Chest tubes can be inserted in the emergency department (ED), at the patient's bedside, or in the operating room (OR), depending on the situation. In the OR, the chest tube is inserted via the thoracotomy incision. In the ED or at the bedside, the patient is placed in a sitting position or is lying down with the affected side elevated. The area is prepared with antiseptic solution, and the site is infiltrated with a local anesthetic agent. After a small incision is made, one or two chest tubes may be inserted into the pleural space. If air is to be removed, the catheter is placed anteriorly through the second intercostal space to remove air (Fig. 28-7). If fluid is to be drained, a chest tube is placed posteriorly through the eighth or ninth intercostal space to drain fluid and blood. Some clinicians are using the fourth or fifth anterior or midaxillary line as the recommended site since the anterior approach requires dissection of the pectoral muscles. In this instance, the tube is directed apically for air evacuation and inferiorly and posteriorly for fluid removal.[48]

The tubes are sutured to the chest wall, and the puncture wound is covered with a dressing. Some clinicians prefer to use an airtight seal with petroleum gauze. However, continued use of petroleum gauze or ointment can irritate the skin.[49] During insertion, the tubes are kept clamped. After the tubes are in place in the pleural space, they are connected to drainage tubing and pleural drainage and the clamp is removed. Each tube may be connected to a separate drainage system and suction. More commonly, a Y-connector is used to attach both chest tubes to the same drainage system.

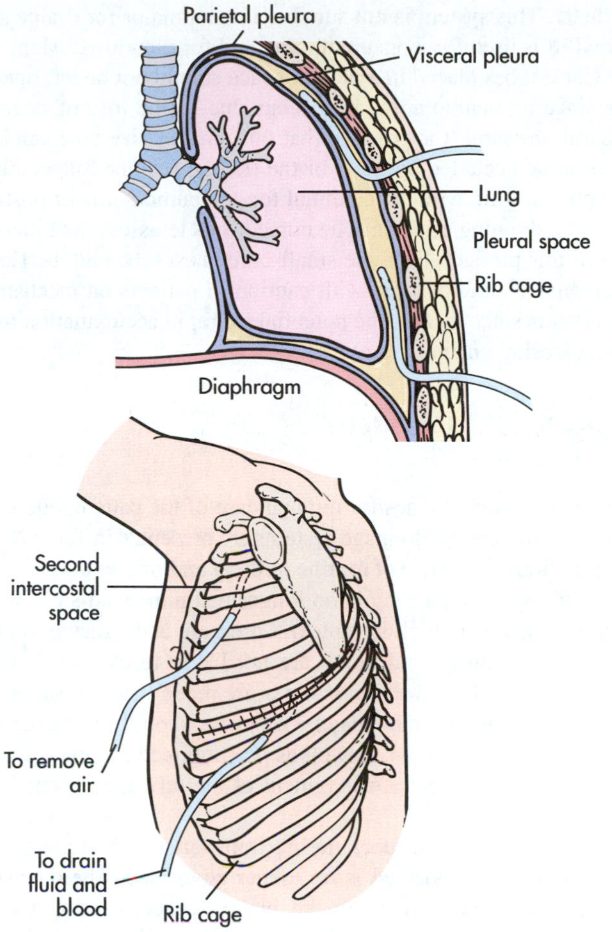

FIG. 28-7 Placement of chest tubes.

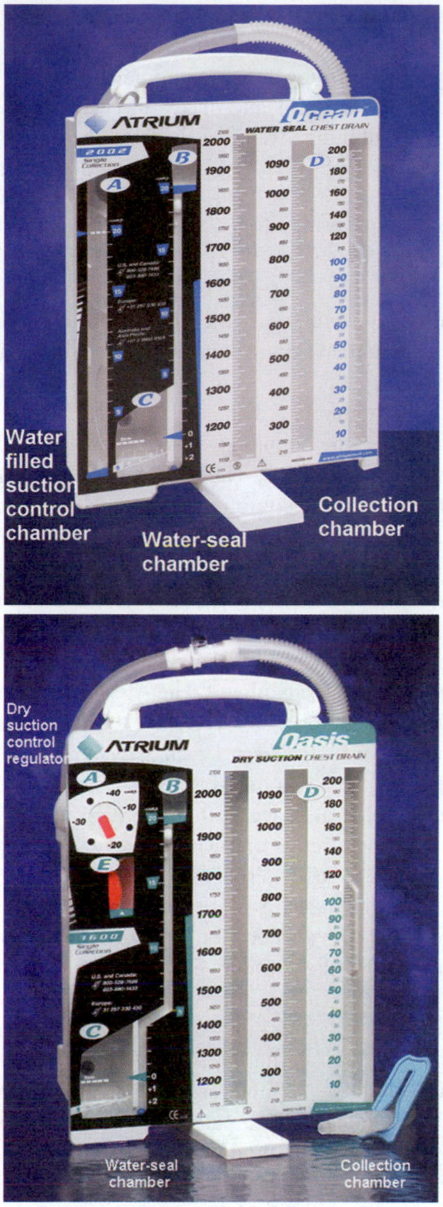

FIG. 28-8 Chest drainage unit. Both units have three chambers: (1) collection chamber; (2) water-seal chamber; and (3) suction control chamber. Suction control chamber requires a connection to a wall suction source that is dialed up higher than the prescribed suction for the suction to work. **A,** Water suction. This unit uses water in the suction control chamber to control the wall suction pressure. **B,** Dry suction. This unit controls wall suction by using a regulator control dial.

Pleural Drainage

Most pleural drainage systems have three basic compartments, each with its own separate function (Fig. 28-8). The *first compartment,* or collection chamber, receives fluid and air from the chest cavity. The fluid drains through the 6-foot connecting tube into this collection chamber. The chamber holds up to 2000 ml. The fluid stays in this chamber while the air vents to the second compartment. The *second compartment,* called the water-seal chamber, contains 2 cm of water, which acts as a one-way valve. The incoming air enters from the collection chamber and bubbles up through the water. (The water acts as a one-way valve to prevent backflow of air into the patient from the system.) Initial bubbling of air is seen in this chamber when a pneumothorax is evacuated. Intermittent bubbling can also be seen during exhalation, coughing, or sneezing due to an increase in the patient's intrathoracic pressure. In this chamber fluctuations, or "tidaling," will be seen that reflect the pressures in the pleural space. If tidaling is not seen, either the lungs have reexpanded or there is a kink or obstruction in the tubing. The air exits the water seal and enters the suction control chamber.

The *third compartment,* the suction control chamber, applies controlled suction to the chest drainage system. The classic suction control chamber uses a column of water with the top end vented to the atmosphere to control the amount of suction from the wall regulator. The chamber is typically filled with 20 cm of water. When the negative pressure generated by the suction source exceeds the set 20 cm, air from the atmosphere enters the chamber through the vent on top and the air bubbles up through the water, causing a suction-breaker effect. As a result, excess pressure is relieved. The amount of suction applied is regulated by the amount of water in this chamber and not by the amount of suction applied to the system. An increase in suction does not result in an increase in negative pressure to the system because any excess suction merely draws in air through the vent on the top of the third chamber. The suction pressure is usually ordered to be −20 cm H_2O, although higher pressures (−40 cm H_2O) are sometimes necessary to evacuate the pleural space.

Two types of suction control chambers are available on the market: water and dry (see Fig. 28-8). The water suction control chamber system is the classic system outlined previously. Bubbling in this third compartment indicates if the suction is functioning. To start the suction, the vacuum source is turned up until gentle bubbling appears. Turning the vacuum source higher just makes the bubbling more vigorous and makes the water evaporate faster. Even at gentle bubbling, water evaporates in this chamber, and water must be added periodically. The dry suction control chamber system contains no water. It has a visual alert that indicates if the suction is working, so bubbling is not seen in a third chamber. It uses either a restrictive device or a regulator to dial the desired negative pressure; this is internal in the chest drainage system. To increase the suction pressures, the dial is turned on the drainage system. Increasing the vacuum suction source will not increase the pressure.

A variety of commercial disposable plastic chest drainage systems are available. One popular system is the Atrium Chest Drainage Unit shown in Fig. 28-8. The manufacturer's suggestions for use are included with the equipment. Another chest drainage unit, a portable unit, can be used to allow the patient more mobility. This unit (Fig. 28-9) allows for a maximum of 500 ml drainage and offers a dry seal system to prevent air leaks, and can be used for long-term drainage. If a patient is discharged home with this device, patient and family teaching includes how to use the system and empty the drainage chamber.[50] The Atrium Medical Company offers online educational videos of these products *(www.atriummed.com/Products/Chest_Drains/education.asp)*.

Heimlich Valves. Another device that may be used to evacuate air from the pleural space is the Heimlich valve. This device consists of a rubber flutter one-way valve within a rigid plastic tube. It is attached to the external end of the chest tube. The valve opens whenever the pressure is greater than atmospheric pressure and closes when the reverse occurs. The Heimlich valve is a flutter valve, and functions like a water seal. The device can be used for emergency transport, in an emergency pneumothorax kit, when placing small-bore chest drains (pigtail catheters), and for home care or long-term care nursing units.

Small Chest Tubes. Small-size (<14 F) chest tubes ("pigtail catheters") are used in selected patients because they are less traumatic. They drain air and fluid equally well as large-bore chest tubes. The drains may be straight catheters or "pigtail" catheters (curled at the distal end to look like a pig's tail). Curled catheters are considered to be less traumatic than straight catheters. These catheters, if occluded, can be irrigated using sterile water. Irrigation of these tubes is generally performed by physicians. Chemical pleurodesis (adding an abrasive product into the pleural space to obliterate the pleural space) can be performed using this small-size catheter. This system is not suitable for trauma or for drainage of blood. It is used for a pneumothorax and for pleural effusions.

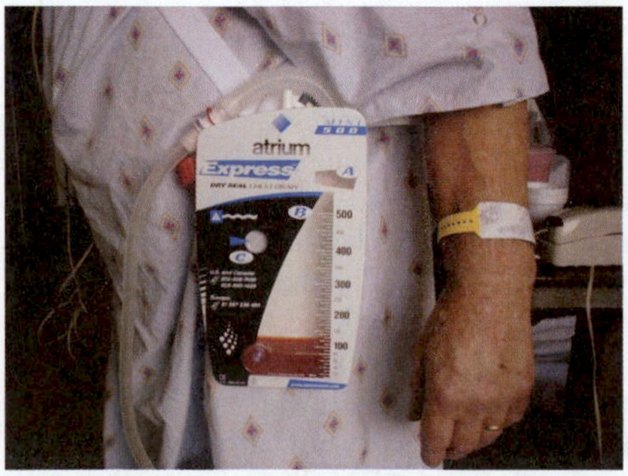

FIG. 28-9 Portable chest drainage unit allows the patient more mobility.

Chest tubes placed in a pleural space should not be left open to air since a pneumothorax can occur due to the loss of negative pleural pressure. It is possible that this smaller size tube can kink or become occluded by fluid, or the tip can become lodged along the pleural wall, with the potential for a pneumothorax or obstruction of a draining effusion. The nurse needs to assess the functioning of this product. Both the small-bore chest tube and the Heimlich valve should be used with caution in patients on mechanical ventilators since there is the potential for rapid accumulation of air and a tension pneumothorax.[51]

NURSING MANAGEMENT
CHEST DRAINAGE

Some general guidelines for nursing care of the patient with chest tubes and water-seal drainage systems are presented in Table 28-21. The traditional practice of routine milking and/or stripping of chest tubes to maintain patency is no longer recommended since it can cause dangerously high intrapleural pressure and damage to pleural tissue. Drainage and blood are not likely to clot inside chest tubes because the newer chest tubes are made with a coating that makes them nonthrombogenic. The nurse should remember that insertion of a chest tube, as well as its continued presence, can be painful for the patient. Dislodgment of the tube may occur if the tube is not stabilized.

Clamping of chest tubes during transport or when the tube is accidentally disconnected is no longer advocated. The danger of rapid accumulation of air in the pleural space, causing tension pneumothorax, is far greater than that of a small amount of atmospheric air entering the pleural space. Chest tubes may be momentarily clamped to change the drainage apparatus or to check for air leaks. Clamping for more than a few moments is indicated only in assessing how the patient will tolerate chest tube removal. The physician may want to do this to simulate chest tube removal and identify if there will be clinical problems with tube removal. Generally this is done 4 to 6 hours before the tube is removed, and the patient is monitored closely. If a chest tube becomes disconnected, the most important intervention is reestablishment of the water-seal system immediately and attachment of a new drainage system as soon as possible. In some hospitals, when disconnection occurs, the chest tube is immersed in sterile water (about 2 cm) until the system can be reestablished. It is important for the nurse to know the unit protocol, individual clinical situation (whether an air leak exists), and physician preference before resorting to prolonged chest tube clamping.

Complications

Chest tube malposition is the most common complication. Routine monitoring is done by the nurse to evaluate if the chest drainage is successful by observing for tidaling in the water-seal chamber, listening for breath sounds over the lung fields, and measuring the amount of fluid drainage. Reexpansion pulmonary edema can occur after rapid expansion of a collapsed lung in patients with a pneumothorax or evacuation of large volumes of pleural fluid (>1 to 1.5 L). A vasovagal response with symptomatic hypotension can occur from too rapid removal of fluid.

Infection at the skin site is also possible. Meticulous sterile technique during dressing changes can reduce the incidence of infected

TABLE 28-21 Clinical Guidelines for Care of Patient with Chest Tubes and Water-Seal Drainage

Drainage System

1. Keep all tubing as straight as possible and coiled loosely below chest level. Do not let the patient lie on it.
2. Keep all connections between chest tubes, drainage tubing, and the drainage collector tight and tape at connections.
3. Observe for air bubbling in the water-seal chamber and fluctuations (tidaling).
   - If no tidaling is observed (rising with inspiration and falling with expiration in the spontaneously breathing patient), the drainage system is blocked, the lungs are reexpanded, or the system is attached to suction.
   - If bubbling increases, there may be an air leak in the drainage system or a leak from the patient (bronchopleural leak).
4. If the chest tube is connected to suction, disconnect from wall suction to check for tidaling.
5. Bubbling in the water seal may occur intermittently.
   - When bubbling is continuous and constant, the source of the air leak may be determined by momentarily clamping the tubing at successively distal points, starting at the patient's chest site and ending at the drainage set, until the bubbling ceases.
   - When bubbling ceases, the leak is above the clamp.
   - Retaping tubing connections, replacing the drainage apparatus, or securing the chest tube with air-occlusive dressing may be necessary to correct the air leak.
6. Keep the water-seal chamber at the appropriate water level by adding sterile water as needed due to evaporation of water.
7. High fluid levels in the water seal indicate residual negative pressure.
   - The chest system may need to be vented by using the high-negativity release valve available on the drainage system to release residual pressure from the system.
   - Do not lower water-seal column when wall suction is not operating or when patient is on gravity drainage.

Patient's Clinical Status

1. Monitor the patient's clinical status.
   - Take and document vital signs, auscultate lungs, observe chest wall. Document pain level.
2. Assess every shift for manifestations of reaccumulation of air and fluid in the chest (↓ or absent breath sounds), significant bleeding (>100 ml/hr), chest drainage site infection (drainage, erythema, fever, ↑ WBC), or poor wound healing. Notify physician for management plan. Evaluate for subcutaneous emphysema at chest tube site.
3. Encourage the patient to breathe deeply periodically to facilitate lung expansion and encourage range-of-motion exercises to the shoulder on the affected side. Incentive spirometry every hour while awake may be necessary to prevent atelectasis or pneumonia.
4. Chest tubes are *not routinely clamped.* They are not clamped for transport. A physician may require clamping for 24 hr to evaluate for reaccumulation of fluid or air prior to discontinuing the chest tube. A physician order is required.

Chest Drainage

1. Never elevate the drainage system to the level of the patient's chest because this will cause fluid to drain back into the lungs. Secure the unit to the drainage stand. If the drainage chambers are full, change the system. Do not try to empty it.
2. Mark the time of measurement and the fluid level on the drainage bottle according to the prescribed orders. Marking intervals may range from once per hour to q8hr. Any change in the quantity or characteristics of drainage (e.g., clear yellow to bloody) should be reported to the physician and recorded. Notify physician if >100 ml/hr drainage.
3. Monitor the fluid drainage and evacuate no more than 1000 to 1200 ml of pleural fluid from the pleural space at one time to prevent rebound hypotension or reexpansion pulmonary edema.
4. Check the position of the chest drainage container. If the drainage system is overturned and the water seal is disrupted, return it to an upright position and encourage the patient to take a few deep breaths, followed by forced exhalations and cough maneuvers.
5. If the drainage system breaks, place the distal end of the chest tubing connection in a sterile water container at a 2-cm level as an emergency water seal.
6. Do not strip or milk chest tubes routinely since this dangerously increases pleural pressures.
   Stripping: pinch tubing close to chest with one hand and, using a thumb and forefinger, compress and slide fingers down toward receptacle; release pressure on tube and repeat stripping action down tube.
   Milking: alternately folding or squeezing and then releasing drainage tubing. Milk only if drainage and evidence of clots/obstruction. Take 15-cm strips of the chest tube and squeeze and release starting close to the chest and repeating down the tube distally.

Monitoring Wet vs. Dry Suction Chest Drainage Systems

Suction Control Chamber in Wet Suction System

1. Keep the suction control chamber at the appropriate water level by adding sterile water as needed due to evaporation
2. Keep the muffler in place covering the suction control chamber opening to prevent more rapid evaporation of water and to decrease the noise of the bubbling.
3. After filling the suction control chamber to the ordered suction amount (generally 20 cm water suction), connect the suction tubing to the wall suction.
4. Dial the wall suction regulator higher than the ordered suction amount until bubbling is seen in the suction control chamber (generally 80-120 mm Hg). Vigorous bubbling is not necessary and will cause quicker evaporation of the water in the chamber. Use gentle bubbling.
5. This suction control chamber should have constant bubbling. This indicates the suction is functioning.
6. If there is no bubbling seen in the suction control chamber, this indicates (1) no suction/suction loss, (2) suction not high enough, or (3) pleural air leak so large that suction not high enough to evacuate it.

Suction Control Chamber in Dry Suction System (Atrium Dry System)

1. After connecting patient to system, turn the dial on the chest drainage system to amount ordered (generally 20 cm pressure), connect suction tubing to wall suction source, and increase the suction until all of the orange float valve is seen in the window.
2. The orange float valve is a visual indicator of suction. The orange bellows needs to be extended to the arrow (delta mark) or further. Wall suction must be set from 80 to 120 mm Hg. There is no water, bubbling, or evaporation. This system can be dialed up to 40 cm suction if needed for a patient.
3. If suction is to be decreased, turn the dial down. There will still be high negative pressure in the system, as evidenced by high water-seal manometer pressure, and it needs to be vented by using the high-negativity release valve.

WBC, White blood cells.

Continued

Respiratory System

TABLE 28-21 Clinical Guidelines for Care of Patient with Chest Tubes and Water-Seal Drainage—cont'd

Chest Tube Dressings
1. Change dressing when wet; change routinely Monday, Wednesday, and Friday unless ordered more frequently by physician.
2. Remove old dressing carefully to avoid removing unsecured chest tube. Evaluate the site and culture site if necessary.
3. Clean site with sterile normal saline. Apply sterile 4 × 4 gauze and tape to secure the dressing. Vaseline gauze may be used around the tube to prevent air leak. Date the dressing and document dressing change.

Obtaining a Sample from the Chest Tube
1. Form a loop in the tubing in an area to get the most recently drained fluid.
2. Swab an area of the tubing with alcohol and allow to air dry.
3. Insert a 20-gauge or smaller syringe needle at an angle and aspirate the sample; do not puncture the other side of the tubing.
4. Place sample in appropriate, labeled container and send to lab.

sites. Other complications include (1) pneumonia (from not turning, coughing, and taking deep breaths and/or not using incentive spirometers) and (2) shoulder disuse ("frozen shoulder") from lack of range-of-motion exercises. Poor patient compliance or lack of patient teaching can contribute to these complications. Nurses can make a tremendous impact on preventing these complications.

Chest Tube Removal

The patient with a chest tube has frequent chest x-rays to evaluate for reexpansion and for evacuation of drainage. The chest tubes are removed when the lungs are reexpanded and fluid drainage has ceased. Generally suction is discontinued and the patient is placed on gravity drainage 24 hours before the tube is removed. Explain the procedure to the patient and premedicate the patient at least 15 minutes before tube removal. The tube is removed by cutting the sutures; applying sterile petroleum jelly gauze dressing; having the patient take a deep breath, exhale, and bear down (Valsalva maneuver); and then removing the tube. The site is covered with an airtight dressing; the pleura will seal itself off, and the wound is healed in several days. A chest x-ray is done after the chest tube is removed to evaluate for pneumothorax and/or reaccumulation of fluid. The wound is observed for drainage and the dressing reinforced if necessary. The patient is observed for respiratory distress, which may signify a recurrent or new pneumothorax.

CHEST SURGERY

Chest surgery is performed for a variety of reasons, some of which are unrelated to primary lung problems. For example, a thoracotomy may be performed for heart and esophageal surgery. The types of chest surgery are compared in Table 28-22.

Preoperative Care

Before chest surgery, baseline data are obtained on the respiratory and cardiovascular systems. Diagnostic studies performed are pulmonary function studies, chest x-rays, electrocardiogram (ECG), ABGs, blood urea nitrogen (BUN), serum creatinine, blood glucose, serum electrolytes, and complete blood count. An anesthesia consult is done preoperatively. Additional studies of cardiac function may be done for the patient who is to undergo a pneumonectomy. A careful physical assessment of the lungs, including percussion and auscultation, should be done. This will allow the nurse to compare preoperative and postoperative findings.

The patient should be encouraged to stop smoking before surgery to decrease secretions and increase O_2 saturation. In the anxious period before surgery, this is not an easy thing for the habitual smoker to do. Preoperative teaching should include exercises for effective deep breathing and incentive spirometry. If the patient practices these techniques before surgery, the techniques will be easier to perform postoperatively. The patient should be told that adequate medication will be given to reduce the pain, and the patient is helped to splint the incision with a pillow to facilitate deep breathing.

For most types of chest surgery, chest tubes are inserted and connected to water-sealed drainage systems. The purpose of these tubes should be explained to the patient. In addition, supplemental oxygen is frequently given the first 24 hours after surgery. Range-of-motion exercises on the surgical side similar to those for the mastectomy patient should be taught (see Chapter 52).

The thought of losing part of a vital organ is frequently frightening. The patient should be reassured that the lungs have a large degree of functional reserve. Even after the removal of one lung, there is enough lung tissue to maintain adequate oxygenation.

The nurse should be available to deal with the questions asked by the patient and the family. Questions should be answered honestly. The nurse should try to facilitate the expression of concerns, feelings, and questions. (General preoperative care and teaching are discussed in Chapter 18.)

Surgical Therapy

Thoracotomy (surgical opening into the thoracic cavity) surgery is considered major surgery because the incision is large, cutting into bone, muscle, and cartilage. The two types of thoracic incisions are median sternotomy, performed by splitting the sternum, and lateral thoracotomy. The median sternotomy is primarily used for surgery involving the heart. The two types of lateral thoracotomy are posterolateral and anterolateral. The posterolateral thoracotomy is used for most surgeries involving the lung. The incision is made from the anterior axillary line below the nipple level posteriorly at the fourth, fifth, or sixth intercostal space. It is rarely necessary to remove the ribs. Strong mechanical retractors are used to gain access to the lung. The anterolateral incision is made in the fourth or fifth intercostal space from the sternal border to the midaxillary line. This procedure is commonly used for surgery or trauma victims, mediastinal operations, and wedge resections of the upper and middle lobes of the lung.

The extensiveness of the thoracotomy incision often results in severe pain for the patient after surgery. Because muscles have been severed, the patient is reluctant to move the shoulder and arm on the surgical side. Chest tubes are placed in the pleural space except in pneumonectomy surgery. In a pneumonectomy, the space from which the lung was removed gradually fills with serosanguineous fluid.

Video-Assisted Thoracic Surgery (VATS). VATS is a thoracoscopic surgical procedure that in many cases can avoid

TABLE 28-22 Chest Surgeries

Type and Description	Indication	Comments
Lobectomy Removal of one lobe of lung	Lung cancer, bronchiectasis, TB, emphysematous bullae, benign lung tumors, fungal infections	Most common lung surgery; postoperative insertion of two chest tubes; removal of lobe and closure of bronchial stump; expansion of remaining lung tissue to fill up space left by resected lobe
Pneumonectomy Removal of entire lung	Lung cancer (most common)	Done only when lobectomy or segmental resection will not remove all diseased lung; no drainage tubes (generally), fluid gradually filling space where lung has been removed; position patient on operative side to facilitate expansion of remaining lung
Segmental resection Removal of one or more lung segments	Lung cancer, bronchiectasis	Done to remove bronchovascular lung segment; insertion of chest tubes; expansion of remaining lung tissue to fill space; indicated for a patient unable to handle more extensive surgery
Wedge resection Removal of small, localized lesion that occupies only part of a segment	Lung biopsy, excision of small nodules	Most conservative approach; need chest tubes postoperatively; done to remove small peripheral nodules or for patients unable to handle more extensive surgery; mortality low (3%), but reoccurrence rate of cancer 15%
Decortication Removal or stripping of thick, fibrous membrane from visceral pleura	Empyema unresponsive to conservative management	Use of chest tubes and drainage postoperatively
Exploratory thoracotomy Incision into thorax to look for injured or bleeding tissues	Chest trauma	Use of chest tubes and drainage postoperatively
Thoracotomy not involving lungs Incision into thorax for surgery on other organs	Hiatal hernia repair, open heart surgery, esophageal surgery, tracheal resection, aortic aneurysm repair	Postoperative care related to thoracotomy as well as primary reason for surgical procedure
Video-assisted thoracic surgery (VATS)	VATS under general anesthesia in OR. Procedures performed using VATS include lung biopsy, lobectomy, resection of nodules, repair of fistulas	Video-assisted technique with a rigid scope with a distal lens inserted into the pleura and image shown on a monitor screen; allows surgeon to manipulate instruments passed into the pleural space through separate small intercostal incisions
Lung volume reduction surgery (LVRS)	Advanced bullous emphysema, α_1-antitrypsin emphysema	Involves reducing lung volume by multiple wedge excisions or VATS (see p. 644)

the impact of a full thoracotomy. The procedure involves three or four 1-inch incisions made on the chest that allow the thoracoscope (a special fiberoptic camera) and instruments to be inserted and manipulated. Video-assisted thoracoscopy improves visualization because the surgeon can view the thoracic cavity on the video monitor. The thoracoscope is equipped with a camera that magnifies the image on the monitor. Thoracoscopy can be used to diagnose and treat a variety of conditions of the lung, pleura, and mediastinum.

The candidate for this type of procedure should not have a prior history of conventional thoracic surgery because the probability of adhesion formation would make access more difficult. The patient whose lesions are in the lung periphery or the mediastinum is a better candidate because of better accessibility. The patient considered for thoracoscopic surgery should have sufficient pulmonary function preoperatively to allow the surgeon to perform conventional thoracotomy if complications occur. Complications that may occur are bleeding, diaphragmatic perforation, air emboli, persistent pleural air leaks, and tension pneumothorax.

There are many benefits of VATS when compared with a conventional thoracotomy procedure. These include less adhesion formation, minimal blood loss, less time under anesthesia, shorter hospitalization, faster recovery, less pain, and less need for postoperative rehabilitation therapy because of minimal disruption of thoracic structures.

Chest tubes are placed at the end of the procedure through one of the incisions. The incisions are closed with sutures or a wound-approximating adhesive bandage. Nursing assessment and care postoperatively include monitoring respiratory status and lung re-expansion with the chest tubes and checking the incisions for drainage or dehiscence. The most common complication is prolonged air leak. A return to prior activities should be encouraged as quickly as possible. The hospital stay averages from 1 to 5 days, depending on the type of surgery.

Postoperative Care

Specific measures related to patient care after a thoracotomy are presented in NCP 28-2. The specific follow-up care depends on the type of surgical procedure. General postoperative care is discussed in Chapter 20.

Restrictive Respiratory Disorders

Restrictive respiratory disorders are characterized by a restriction in lung volume (caused by decreased compliance of the lungs or chest wall) as opposed to obstructive disorders, which are characterized by increased resistance to airflow. Pulmonary function tests are the best means of differentiating between restrictive and obstructive respiratory disorders (Table 28-23). Mixed obstructive and restrictive disorders can be seen together.

NURSING CARE PLAN 28-2

Patient After Thoracotomy

NURSING DIAGNOSIS **Impaired gas exchange** *related to* air and/or fluid collection in lungs and pleural space *as evidenced by* drainage from chest tube(s), decreased breath sounds, abnormal pulse oximetry

PATIENT GOAL Demonstrates full lung expansion with normal oxygen saturation

OUTCOMES (NOC)

Respiratory Status: Gas Exchange

- Cognitive status ____
- Ease of breathing ____
- Oxygen saturation ____

Respiratory Status: Ventilation

- Auscultated breath sounds ____
- Symmetrical chest expansion ____

Measurement Scale

1 = Severely compromised
2 = Substantially compromised
3 = Moderately compromised
4 = Mildly compromised
5 = Not compromised

INTERVENTIONS (NIC) and *RATIONALES*

Ventilation Assistance

- Monitor respiratory and oxygenation status to allow early recognition of significant changes in respiratory function.
- Initiate and maintain supplemental oxygen to treat hypoxemia.
- Position to alleviate dyspnea to increase patient's comfort and to facilitate aeration of the lungs.

Tube Care: Chest

- Monitor for bubbling of the suction chamber of the chest tube drainage system and tidaling in water-seal chamber *to assure adequate ventilation.*
- Ensure that all tubing connections are securely attached and taped *to prevent air leaks.*
- Keep the drainage container below chest level *to prevent tension pneumothorax.*

NURSING DIAGNOSIS **Ineffective breathing pattern** *related to* pain and position *as evidenced by* shortness of breath, shallow respirations

PATIENT GOAL Demonstrates an effective respiratory rate, rhythm, and depth of respirations

OUTCOMES (NOC)

Respiratory Status: Ventilation

- Respiratory rate ____
- Respiratory rhythm ____
- Depth of inspiration ____
- Ease of breathing ____

Measurement Scale

1 = Severely compromised
2 = Substantially compromised
3 = Moderately compromised
4 = Mildly compromised
5 = Not compromised

INTERVENTIONS (NIC) and *RATIONALES*

Respiratory Monitoring

- Monitor rate, rhythm, depth, and effort of respirations to evaluate the rate, quality, and depth of patient's respirations, and the need for tracheal suctioning.
- Auscultate breath sounds, noting areas of decreased/absent ventilation and presence of adventitious sounds.

Pain Management

- Provide the patient optimal pain relief with prescribed analgesics *to promote deep breathing, turning, and coughing.*
- Use pain control measures before pain becomes severe *to provide continuous pain control.*
- Institute and modify pain control measures on the basis of the patient's response.

Ventilation Assistance

- Position to alleviate dyspnea to increase compliance with respiratory treatments.
- Assist with incentive spirometer to provide visual feedback to the patient on effectiveness of respirations.

TABLE 28-23 Relationship of Lung Volumes to Type of Ventilatory Disorder

Lung Volumes	Restrictive	Obstructive	Restrictive and Obstructive
Vital capacity (VC)	↓	Normal or ↓	↓
Total lung capacity (TLC)	↓	↑	Variable
Residual volume (RV)	Normal or ↓	↑	Variable
Forced expiratory volume in 1 second (FEV_1)	Normal or ↓	↓	↓
FEV_1/functional vital capacity (FVC)	Normal or ↑	↓	↓

For example, a patient may have both chronic bronchitis (an obstructive problem) and pulmonary fibrosis (a restrictive problem).

Restrictive problems are generally categorized into extrapulmonary and intrapulmonary disorders. Extrapulmonary causes of restrictive lung disease include disorders involving the central nervous system (CNS) or the neuromuscular system, and chest wall disorders that limit chest wall expansion. (Some of these disorders are listed in Table 28-24.) In this group of extrapulmonary causes, the lung tissue is normal. Intrapulmonary causes of restrictive lung disease are intrinsic lung diseases involving the pleura or the lung tissue. This damage can be caused by inflammation and scarring of lung tissue (interstitial lung disease), air spaces (pneumonitis), or pleura (empyema) (Table 28-25).

TABLE 28-24 Extrapulmonary Causes of Restrictive Lung Disease

Disease or Alteration	Description	Comments
Central Nervous System		
• Head injury, CNS lesion (e.g., tumor, stroke)	Injury to or impingement on respiratory center, causing hypoventilation or hyperventilation; relationship of manifestations to increased intracranial pressure (see Chapters 57 and 58)	Management is directed toward treating the underlying cause, maintaining the airway, using mechanical ventilation for supportive care, and assessing for manifestations of increased intracranial pressure.
• Opioid and barbiturate use	Depression of respiratory center, respiratory rate of <12 breaths/min	Respiratory depression is caused by drug overdose or inadvertent administration of drugs to a person with respiratory difficulty. These drugs should not be administered to a person with a respiratory rate of <12 breaths/min.
Neuromuscular System		
• Spinal cord injury	Complete cervical-level injuries and complete upper thoracic–level injuries have restrictive ventilation. The lung volumes are reduced due to inspiratory muscle weakness	Patient with a cervical injury may need mechanical ventilator support initially.
• Guillain-Barré syndrome	Acute inflammation of peripheral nerves and ganglia; paralysis of intercostal nerves leading to diaphragmatic breathing; paralysis of vagal preganglionic and postganglionic fibers leading to reduced ability of bronchioles to constrict, dilate, and respond to irritants	Patient often has to be put on mechanical ventilation for supportive care (see Chapter 61).
• Amyotrophic lateral sclerosis	Progressive degenerative disorder of the motor neurons in the spinal cord, brainstem, and motor cortex; respiratory system involvement as a result of interruption of nerve transmission to respiratory muscles, especially diaphragm	See Chapter 59 for clinical manifestations and management.
• Myasthenia gravis	Defect in neuromuscular junction, respiratory system involvement as a result of interruption of nerve transmission to respiratory muscles	See Chapter 59 for clinical manifestations and management.
• Muscular dystrophy	Hereditary disease; eventual involvement of all skeletal muscles; paralysis of respiratory muscles, including intercostals, diaphragm, and accessory muscles	Pulmonary problems develop late in disease process.
Chest Wall		
• Chest wall trauma (e.g., flail chest, fractured rib)	Rib fracture causing inspiratory pain; voluntary splinting of chest, resulting in shallow, rapid breathing; impaired ventilatory ability caused by paradoxical breathing	Strapping the chest wall to stabilize the fractures is not recommended because this increases the restrictive defect.
• Obesity-hypoventilation syndrome (OHS) (pickwickian syndrome)	Excess adipose tissue interfering with chest-wall and diaphragmatic excursion, somnolence from hypoxemia and CO_2 retention, polycythemia from chronic hypoxia; common to have obstructive sleep apnea (OSA) contributing to OHS	Weight loss generally causes reversal of symptoms. Prevention and prompt treatment of respiratory infections are important. Condition is worsened in supine position.
• Kyphoscoliosis	Posterior and lateral angulation of the spine; restriction of ventilation as a result of alteration in thoracic excursion; increase in work of breathing; pattern of rapid, shallow breathing; reduction of lung volume; compression of alveoli and blood vessels	Only small number of persons with condition develop severe respiratory problems. Atelectasis and pneumonia are common complications.

PLEURAL EFFUSION

Types

The pleural space lies between the lung and chest wall and normally contains a very thin layer of fluid. **Pleural effusion** is a collection of fluid in the pleural space (see Fig. 28-5, *A*). It is not a disease but rather a sign of a serious disease. Pleural effusion is frequently classified as transudative or exudative according to whether the protein content of the effusion is low or high, respectively.[51] A *transudate* occurs primarily in noninflammatory conditions and is an accumulation of protein-poor, cell-poor fluid. Transudative pleural effusions (also called *hydrothoraces*) are caused by (1) increased hydrostatic pressure found in heart failure (HF), which is the most common cause of pleural effusion, or (2) decreased oncotic pressure (from hypoalbuminemia) found in chronic liver or renal disease. In these situations, fluid movement is facilitated out of the capillaries and into the pleural space.

An *exudative effusion* is an accumulation of fluid and cells in an area of inflammation. An exudative pleural effusion results from increased capillary permeability characteristic of the inflammatory reaction. This type of effusion occurs secondary to conditions such as pulmonary malignancies, pulmonary infections, pulmonary embolization, and GI disease (e.g., pancreatic disease, esophageal perforation).

The type of pleural effusion can be determined by a sample of pleural fluid obtained via **thoracentesis** (a procedure done to remove fluid from the pleural space). Exudates have a high protein content, and the fluid is generally dark yellow or amber.[52] Transu-

TABLE 28-25 Intrapulmonary Causes of Restrictive Lung Disease

Disease or Alteration	Description
Pleural Disorders	Inflammation, scarring, or fluid in the pleural space causing restriction
• Pleural effusion	Accumulation of fluid in pleural space secondary to altered hydrostatic or oncotic pressure; fluid collection >250 ml showing up on chest x-ray
• Pleurisy (pleuritis)	Inflammation of pleura; classification as fibrinous (dry) or serofibrinous (wet); wet pleurisy accompanied by an increase in pleural fluid and possibly resulting in pleural effusion
• Pneumothorax	Accumulation of air in pleural space with accompanying lung collapse
Parenchymal Disorders	Inflammation, collapse, or scarring of the lung tissue
• Atelectasis	Condition of lung characterized by collapsed, airless alveoli; possibly acute (e.g., in postoperative patient) or chronic (e.g., in patient with malignant tumor)
• Pneumonia	Acute inflammation of lung tissue caused by bacteria, viruses, fungi, chemicals, dusts, and other factors
• Interstitial lung diseases (ILDs)	General term that includes a variety of chronic lung disorders characterized by some type of injury, inflammation, and scarring (or fibrosis); this process occurs in the interstitium (tissue between the alveoli) and the lung becomes stiff (fibrotic); can be caused by occupational and environmental exposures (see Table 28-13), infections (e.g., TB), and connective tissue disorders (e.g., rheumatoid arthritis); when all known causes of ILDs are ruled out, the condition is termed *idiopathic pulmonary fibrosis* (IPF)
• ARDS*	Atelectasis, pulmonary edema, congestion, and hyaline membrane lining the alveolar wall; result of variety of conditions, including shock lung, O_2 toxicity, gram-negative sepsis, cardiopulmonary bypass, and aspiration pneumonia

*See Chapter 68 for clinical manifestations and management.
ARDS, Acute respiratory distress syndrome.

dates have a low protein content or contain no protein, and the fluid is clear or pale yellow. The fluid can also be analyzed for RBCs and WBCs, malignant cells, bacteria, and glucose.

An **empyema** is a pleural effusion that contains pus. It is caused by conditions such as pneumonia, TB, lung abscess, and infection of surgical wounds of the chest. A complication of empyema is *fibrothorax,* in which there is fibrous fusion of the visceral and parietal pleurae (see Fig. 28-4, *A*).

Clinical Manifestations

Common clinical manifestations of pleural effusion are progressive dyspnea and decreased movement of the chest wall on the affected side. There may be pleuritic pain from the underlying disease. Physical examination of the chest will indicate dullness to percussion and absent or decreased breath sounds over the affected area. The chest x-ray will indicate an abnormality if the effusion is greater than 250 ml. Manifestations of empyema include the manifestations of pleural effusion, as well as fever, night sweats, cough, and weight loss. A thoracentesis reveals an exudate containing thick, purulent material.

Thoracentesis

If the cause of the pleural effusion is not known, a diagnostic thoracentesis is needed to obtain pleural fluid for analysis (see Fig. 26-16). If the degree of pleural effusion is severe enough to impair breathing, a therapeutic thoracentesis is done to improve breathing and to remove fluid for analysis.

A thoracentesis is performed by having the patient sit on the edge of a bed and lean forward over a bedside table. The puncture site is determined by chest x-ray, and percussion of the chest is used to assess the maximum degree of dullness. The skin is cleaned with an antiseptic solution and anesthetized locally. The thoracentesis needle is inserted into the intercostal space. Fluid can be aspirated with a syringe, or tubing can be connected to allow fluid to drain into a sterile collecting bottle. After the fluid is removed, the needle is withdrawn, and a bandage is applied over the insertion site.

Usually only 1000 to 1200 ml of pleural fluid are removed at one time. Because high volumes are removed, rapid removal can result in hypotension, hypoxemia, or pulmonary edema. A follow-up chest x-ray should be done to detect a possible pneumothorax that could have been induced by perforation of the visceral pleura. During and after the procedure, vital signs and pulse oximetry are monitored, and the patient should be observed for any manifestations of respiratory distress.

Collaborative Care

The main goal of management of pleural effusions is to treat the underlying cause. For example, adequate treatment of HF with diuretics and sodium restriction will result in decreased pleural effusions. The treatment of pleural effusions secondary to malignant disease represents a more difficult problem. These types of pleural effusions are frequently recurrent and accumulate quickly after thoracentesis. Chemical pleurodesis may be used to sclerose the pleural space and prevent reaccumulation of effusion fluid. Although doxycycline (Vibramycin) and bleomycin (Blenoxane) have been used for sclerosing with good results, talc appears to be the most effective agent for pleurodesis.[53] Thoracoscopy can be used to perform talc pleurodesis after inspection of the pleural space. After instillation of the sclerosing agent, patients may be instructed to rotate their positions to spread the agent uniformly throughout the pleural space. The decision to rotate the patient from side to side to back depends on physician preference and the patient's ability to tolerate turning.[53] Chest tubes are left in place after pleurodesis until fluid drainage is less than 150 ml/day and no air leaks are noted. A more rapid completion of the pleurodesis procedure, in less than 24 hours, is reported in the literature with good results,[54] and this limited admission for symptomatic malignant effusions may become more frequent.

Treatment of empyema is generally with chest tube drainage. Appropriate antibiotic therapy is also needed to eradicate the causative organism. A condition called *trapped lung* can occur with effusions and empyemas. This is a fibrous peel around the pleura that can cause severe pulmonary restriction. A *decortication* surgical procedure to remove the pleural peel may need to be performed.

PLEURISY

Pleurisy (pleuritis) is an inflammation of the pleura. The most common causes are pneumonia, TB, chest trauma, pulmonary infarctions, and neoplasms. The inflammation usually subsides with adequate treatment of the primary disease. The pain of pleurisy is typically abrupt and sharp in onset and is aggravated by inspiration. The patient's breathing is shallow and rapid to avoid unnecessary movement of the pleura and chest wall. A pleural friction rub may occur, which is the sound over areas where inflamed visceral pleura and parietal pleura rub over one another during inspiration. This sound is usually loudest at peak inspiration but can be heard during exhalation as well.

Treatment of pleurisy is aimed at treating the underlying disease and providing pain relief. Taking analgesics and lying on or splinting the affected side may provide some relief. The patient should be taught to splint the rib cage when coughing. Intercostal nerve blocks may be done if the pain is severe.

ATELECTASIS

Atelectasis is a condition of the lungs characterized by collapsed, airless alveoli. The most common cause of atelectasis is airway obstruction that results from retained exudates and secretions. This is frequently observed in the postoperative patient. Normally the pores of Kohn (see Fig. 26-1) provide for collateral passage of air from one alveolus to another. Deep inspiration is necessary to open the pores effectively. For this reason, deep-breathing exercises are important in preventing atelectasis in the high-risk patient (e.g., postoperative, immobilized patient). (The prevention and treatment of atelectasis are discussed in Chapter 19.)

Interstitial Lung Diseases

Many acute and chronic lung disorders with variable degrees of pulmonary inflammation and fibrosis are collectively referred to as *interstitial lung diseases* (ILD) or *diffuse parenchymal lung diseases.* ILDs have been difficult to classify because more than 200 known diseases have diffuse lung involvement. The lung involvement may occur either from the primary condition or as a significant part of a multiorgan process, as may occur in connective tissue disorders (e.g., systemic lupus erythematosus, rheumatoid arthritis).

Among the ILDs of known cause, the largest group comprises occupational and environmental exposures, especially the inhalation of dusts and various fumes or gases. The most common ILDs of unknown etiology are idiopathic pulmonary fibrosis and sarcoidosis.

IDIOPATHIC PULMONARY FIBROSIS

Idiopathic pulmonary fibrosis (IPF) is characterized by scar tissue in the connective tissue of the lungs as a sequela to inflammation or irritation. A common risk factor for IPF is environmental or occupational inhalation of organic and inorganic substances (see the section on Environmental Lung Diseases earlier in this chapter). Other risk factors include cigarette smoking and history of chronic aspiration. There also may be genetic risk factors.

Clinical manifestations of IPF include exertional dyspnea, nonproductive cough, and inspirational crackles with or without clubbing. Chest x-ray shows changes characteristic of IPF. High-resolution CT scan is the most definitive diagnostic study. Pulmonary function tests show a typical pattern characteristic of restrictive lung disease (see Table 28-23). Open lung biopsy using VATS may help to differentiate the specific pathology.

The clinical course is variable and the prognosis poor, with a 5-year survival rate of 30% to 50% after diagnosis. Treatment includes corticosteroids, cytotoxic agents (azathioprine [Imuran], cyclophosphamide [Cytoxan]), and antifibrotic agents (colchicine). However, there is no good evidence that any of these treatments improves survival or quality of life. Lung transplantation is an option that should be considered for those who meet the criteria. (Lung transplantation is discussed later in this chapter.)

SARCOIDOSIS

Sarcoidosis is a chronic, multisystem granulomatous disease of unknown cause that primarily affects the lungs. The disease may also involve the skin, eyes, liver, kidney, heart, and lymph nodes. It is seen worldwide, can be familial, and is 3 to 4 times more common among African Americans. The lifetime risk of sarcoidosis in African Americans in the United States is 2.4%, compared to a risk of 0.85% for whites.[55] Spontaneous resolution of the disease is common, but progressive and disabling organ failure can occur in up to 10% of patients. The disease is often acute or subacute and self-limiting, but in other patients it is chronic, with remissions and exacerbations.

Marked pulmonary fibrosis can be present with severe restrictive lung disease. Cor pulmonale (right-sided heart failure) and bronchiectasis can develop in the advanced stages. Corticosteroids are the most commonly used agents for the treatment of pulmonary sarcoidosis. A trial of methotrexate may be considered if the patient does not respond to or cannot tolerate corticosteroid therapy. If this is ineffective or not tolerated, cyclophosphamide (Cytoxan) or azathioprine (Imuran) may be initiated.[55] Nonsteroidal antiinflammatory agents, such as ibuprofen (Motrin), may help decrease acute inflammation or relieve symptoms but are not a treatment of sarcoidosis. Disease progression is monitored by pulmonary function tests, chest x-ray, and CT scan.

Vascular Lung Disorders

PULMONARY EDEMA

Pulmonary edema is an abnormal accumulation of fluid in the alveoli and interstitial spaces of the lungs. It is a complication of various heart and lung diseases (Table 28-26). It is considered a medical emergency and may be life threatening.

Normally, there is a balance between the hydrostatic and colloidal oncotic pressures in the pulmonary capillaries. If the hydrostatic pressure increases or the colloidal oncotic pressure decreases, the net effect will be fluid leaving the pulmonary capillaries

TABLE 28-26 Causes of Pulmonary Edema

- Heart failure
- Overhydration with intravenous fluids
- Hypoalbuminemia: nephrotic syndrome, hepatic disease, nutritional disorders
- Altered capillary permeability of lungs: inhaled toxins, inflammation (e.g., pneumonia), severe hypoxia, near-drowning
- Malignancies of the lymph system
- Respiratory distress syndrome (e.g., O_2 toxicity)
- Unknown causes: neurogenic condition, opioid overdose, reexpansion pulmonary edema, high altitude

and entering the interstitial space. This stage is referred to as *interstitial edema.* At this stage, the lymphatics can usually drain away the excess fluid. If fluid continues to leak from the pulmonary capillaries, it will enter the alveoli. This stage is referred to as *alveolar edema.* Pulmonary edema interferes with gas exchange by causing an alteration in the diffusing pathway between the alveoli and the pulmonary capillaries. The most common cause of pulmonary edema is left-sided HF. (The clinical manifestations and management of pulmonary edema are described in Chapter 35.)

PULMONARY EMBOLISM

Etiology and Pathophysiology

Pulmonary embolism (PE) is the blockage of pulmonary arteries by a thrombus, fat or air embolus, or tumor tissue. The word *embolus* derives from a Greek word meaning "plug" or "stopper." A pulmonary embolus consists of material that gains access to the venous system and then to the pulmonary circulation. The material eventually reaches a section of the pulmonary arterial vessels, where it lodges, thus obstructing perfusion (Fig. 28-10). More than 500,000 patients a year are diagnosed with PE in the United States, resulting in approximately 200,000 deaths.[56] Of the people who die, approximately 13,000 die because of lack of response to treatment. The vast majority die because of failure of diagnosis.[57] Without treatment, the mortality rate is 30%; with treatment there is a 2% to 8% mortality rate.[56] It is one of the most common causes of preventable death in hospitalized patients.[58]

Most pulmonary emboli arise from thrombi in the deep veins of the legs. Other sites of origin include the right side of the heart (especially with atrial fibrillation), the upper extremities (rare), and the pelvic veins (especially after surgery or childbirth). Lethal pulmonary emboli most commonly originate in the femoral or iliac veins. *Emboli* are mobile clots that generally do not stop moving until they lodge at a narrowed part of the circulatory system. The lungs are an ideal location for emboli to lodge because of their extensive arterial and capillary network. The lower lobes are most frequently affected because they have a higher blood flow than the other lobes.

Thrombi in the deep veins can dislodge spontaneously. However, a more common mechanism is jarring of the thrombus by mechanical forces, such as sudden standing, and by changes in the rate of blood flow, such as those that occur with the Valsalva maneuver. The majority of patients with PE due to deep vein thrombosis (DVT) have no leg symptoms at the time of diagnosis.[56]

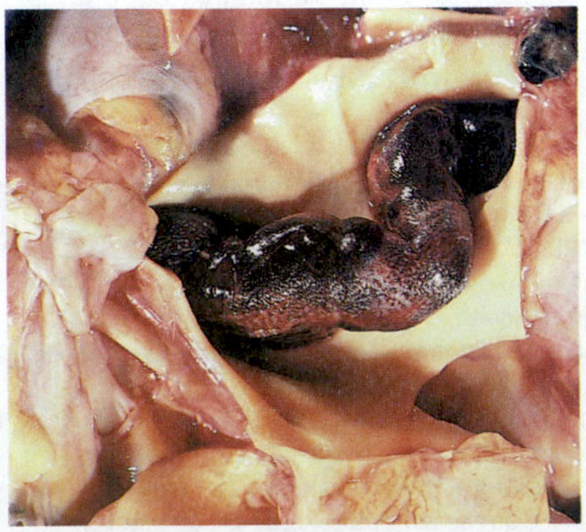

FIG. 28-10 Large embolus from the femoral vein lying in the main left and right pulmonary arteries.

In addition to dislodged thrombi, less common causes of PE include fat emboli (from fractured long bones), air emboli (from improperly administered IV therapy), bacterial vegetations, amniotic fluid, and tumors. Tumor emboli may originate from primary or metastatic malignancies.

The most common risk factors for PE are immobilization, surgery within the last 3 months, stroke, history of DVT, and malignancy.[56] The Nurses' Health Study reported an increased risk of PE in women associated with obesity, heavy cigarette smoking, and hypertension.[56] More than 95% of pulmonary emboli arise from thrombi in the deep veins of the lower extremity. Generally the DVTs that are below the knee have not been considered a risk factor for PE since they rarely migrate to the pulmonary circulation without first extending above the knee. Upper extremity DVT occasionally occurs in the presence of central venous catheters or cardiac pacing wires. These cases may resolve with removal of the catheter. The highest rate of DVT is seen in spinal cord injury patients (67% to 100%).[59]

Clinical Manifestations

The signs and symptoms of PE are generally subtle and nonspecific, making diagnosis difficult. The classic triad of dyspnea, chest pain, and hemoptysis occurs in only about 20% of patients. The most common manifestations of PE are anxiety and the sudden onset of unexplained dyspnea, tachypnea, or tachycardia. A mild to moderate hypoxemia with a low $PaCO_2$ is a common finding. Other manifestations are cough, pleuritic chest pain, hemoptysis, crackles, fever, accentuation of the pulmonic heart sound, and sudden change in mental status as a result of hypoxemia.

Massive emboli may produce sudden collapse of the patient with shock, pallor, severe dyspnea, hypoxemia, and crushing chest pain. However, some patients with massive PE do not have pain. The pulse is rapid and weak, the BP is low, and an ECG indicates right ventricular strain. When rapid obstruction of 50% or more of the pulmonary vascular bed occurs, acute cor pulmonale may result because the right ventricle can no longer pump blood into the lungs.[57] The mortality rate of persons with massive PE and shock is approximately 33%.

Medium-sized emboli often cause pleuritic chest pain, dyspnea, slight fever, and a productive cough with blood-streaked sputum. A physical examination may reveal tachycardia and a pleural friction rub. Small emboli frequently are undetected or produce vague, transient symptoms. The exception to this is the patient with underlying cardiopulmonary disease, in whom even small- or medium-sized emboli may result in severe cardiopulmonary compromise. However, repeated small emboli gradually cause a reduction in the capillary bed and eventual pulmonary hypertension. An ECG and chest x-ray may indicate right ventricular hypertrophy secondary to pulmonary hypertension.

Complications

Pulmonary infarction (death of lung tissue) is most likely when the following factors are present: (1) occlusion of a large- or medium-sized pulmonary vessel (>2 mm in diameter), (2) insufficient collateral blood flow from the bronchial circulation, or (3) preexisting lung disease. Infarction results in alveolar necrosis and hemorrhage. Occasionally the infarced tissue becomes infected, and an abscess may develop. Concomitant pleural effusion is frequently found.

Pulmonary hypertension occurs when more than 50% of the area of the normal pulmonary bed is compromised. Pulmonary hypertension also results from hypoxemia. As a single event, an embolus does not cause pulmonary hypertension unless it is massive. However, recurrent small- to medium-sized emboli may result in chronic pulmonary hypertension. Pulmonary hypertension eventually results in dilation and hypertrophy of the right ventricle. Depending on the degree of pulmonary hypertension and its rate of development, outcomes can vary, with some patients dying within months of the diagnosis and others living for decades.

Diagnostic Studies

A ventilation-perfusion lung scan is the most frequently used test to aid in the diagnosis of PE. The lung scan has two components and is most accurate when both are performed:

1. Perfusion scanning involves IV injection of a radioisotope. A scanning device detects the adequacy of the pulmonary circulation.
2. Ventilation scanning involves inhalation of a radioactive gas such as xenon. Scanning reflects the distribution of gas through the lung. The ventilation component requires the cooperation of the patient and may be impossible to perform in the critically ill patient, particularly if the patient is intubated.

D-dimer testing may be recommended when a PE is initially suspected. D-dimer is a degradation product rarely found in healthy individuals. However, levels of D-dimer are elevated in any condition involving degradation of fibrin (infection, cancer, surgery, heart failure). They are elevated 8 times higher in venous thromboembolism.[60] When D-dimer levels are normal (<250 mcg/L), it is highly unlikely that the patient has a PE. Thus a normal or near-normal D-dimer level can rule out a PE. In the event that the D-dimer levels are elevated, a noninvasive venous study (see Table 38-8) is indicated to look for a DVT as the likely source of a PE. If a DVT is located by *venous ultrasound,* the index of suspicion for PE is very high and anticoagulant treatment should be initiated immediately. Patients with an elevated D-dimer level but normal venous ultrasound need a lung scan or spiral CT scan.

If the lung scan is inconclusive, *pulmonary angiography* is recommended. Pulmonary angiography is an invasive procedure that involves the insertion of a catheter through the antecubital or femoral vein, advancement to the pulmonary artery, and injection of contrast medium. This allows visualization of the pulmonary vascular system and location of the embolus.

The use of computed tomography (CT) has revolutionized the diagnosis of PE. A *spiral (or helical) CT* scan, a noninvasive diagnostic test, may also be used to diagnose PE. Conventional CT scans rotate a frame 360 degrees in one direction, stop, make an image (called a slice), and then spin back in the opposite direction to make another slice after again stopping. The spiral CT scan is able to continuously rotate while obtaining slices and does not have to start and stop between each slice. This allows visualization of entire anatomic regions such as the lungs. The data can be computer reconstructed to allow for a three-dimensional picture of the area being imaged and assist in emboli visualization.

ABG analysis is important, but not diagnostic. The PaO_2 is low because of inadequate oxygenation secondary to an occluded pulmonary vasculature. The $PaCO_2$ is usually low because of hyperventilation. The pH remains normal unless respiratory alkalosis develops as a result of prolonged hyperventilation or to compensate for lactic acidosis caused by shock. Abnormal findings are usually reported on the chest x-ray (atelectasis, pleural effusion) and the ECG (ST segment and T wave changes), but they are not diagnostic for PE. Serum troponin levels are elevated in 30% to 50% of patients with PE, and, although not diagnostic, they are predictive of an adverse prognosis.[56] Serum b-type natriuretic peptide (BNP) levels, while not diagnostic, may be helpful in identifying the severity of the clinical course.[60]

Collaborative Care

When the diagnosis of PE has been made, treatment should be instituted immediately (Table 28-27). The objectives of treatment are to (1) prevent further growth or multiplication of thrombi in the lower extremities, (2) prevent embolization from the upper or lower extremities to the pulmonary vascular system, and (3) provide cardiopulmonary support if indicated.

Conservative Therapy. Supportive therapy for the patient's cardiopulmonary status varies according to the severity of the PE. The administration of supplemental O_2 by mask or cannula may be adequate for some patients. Oxygen is given in a concentration determined by ABG analysis. In some situations, endotracheal intubation and mechanical ventilation may be needed to maintain adequate oxygenation. Respiratory measures such as turning, coughing, and deep breathing are necessary to prevent or treat atelectasis. If symptoms of shock are present, vasopressor agents may be necessary to support the systemic circulation (see Chapter 67). If heart failure is present, diuretics are used (see Chapter 35). Pain resulting from pleural irritation or reduced coronary blood flow is treated with opioids, usually morphine.

TABLE 28-27 COLLABORATIVE CARE Acute Pulmonary Embolism

Diagnostic
History and physical examination
Chest x-ray
Continuous ECG monitoring
ABGs
Venous ultrasound
CBC count with WBC differential
D-dimer level
Troponin level, BNP level
Ventilation-perfusion lung scan
Spiral CT
Pulmonary angiography
Collaborative Therapy
Supplemental oxygen, intubation may be necessary
IV for medications and fluid replacement
Continuous IV heparin for acute treatments
Warfarin (Coumadin) for long-term therapy
Monitoring of aPTT and INR levels
Bed rest
Opioids for pain relief
Inferior vena cava filter
Thrombolytic agent may be considered
Pulmonary embolectomy in life-threatening situation

ABGs, Arterial blood gases; *aPTT,* activated partial thromboplastin time; *BNP,* b-type natriuretic peptide; *CBC,* complete blood count; *CT,* computed tomography; *ECG,* electrocardiogram; *INR,* international normalized ratio; *IV,* intravenous; *WBC,* white blood cell.

Drug Therapy. Properly managed anticoagulant therapy is effective in the treatment of many patients with PE. Although unfractionated heparin has been traditionally used for PE, low-molecular-weight heparin (e.g., enoxaparin [Lovenox]) is becoming more commonly used in the treatment of PE. Warfarin (Coumadin) should be initiated within the first 24 hours and is typically administered for 3 to 6 months. Factor Xa inhibitors and direct thrombin inhibitors (see Table 38-9) are also being used in the treatment of PE.

The dosage of heparin is adjusted according to the activated partial thromboplastin time (aPTT), while warfarin dose is determined by the international normalized ratio (INR). Frequent changes and titrations of heparin doses are needed initially in order to obtain a therapeutic aPTT level. The heparin works to prevent future clots, but does not dissolve existing clots. Anticoagulant therapy may be contraindicated if the patient has blood dyscrasias, hepatic dysfunction causing alteration in the clotting mechanism, injury to the intestine, overt bleeding, a history of hemorrhagic stroke, or neurologic conditions.

Fibrinolytic agents, such as tissue plasminogen activator (tPA) or alteplase (Activase), dissolve the pulmonary embolus and the source of the thrombus in the pelvis or deep leg veins, thereby decreasing the likelihood of recurrent emboli. Indications for thrombolytic therapy in PE include hemodynamic instability and right ventricular dysfunction.[60] (Fibrinolytic therapy is discussed in Chapter 34.)

Surgical Therapy. If the degree of pulmonary arterial obstruction is severe and the patient does not respond to conservative therapy, an immediate embolectomy may be indicated. Pulmonary embolectomy, a rare procedure, has a 50% mortality rate. Preoperative pulmonary angiography is necessary to identify and locate the site of the embolus. When a pulmonary embolectomy is performed, the patient also has placement of a vena cava filter.

To prevent further pulmonary embolization, an inferior vena cava (IVC) filter may be warranted. This device prevents migration of large clots into the pulmonary system, is easily and safely placed percutaneously, is biocompatible, and does not require the patient be anticoagulated. It can be used for patients who have an absolute contraindication to anticoagulant therapy. In addition, it may be used as a prophylactic measure for patients at high risk of PE (e.g., those with spinal cord injury or cor pulmonale). The complications associated with this device are rare and include misplacement, migration, and perforation. The spinal cord injury patient with an IVC filter cannot have assisted cough ("quad cough") to mobilize secretions since the quad cough procedure can displace the filter.

NURSING MANAGEMENT
PULMONARY EMBOLISM

■ Nursing Implementation

Health Promotion. Nursing measures aimed at prevention of PE parallel those for prophylaxis of deep vein thrombosis (see Chapter 38, p. 911).

Acute Intervention. The prognosis of a patient with PE is good if therapy is promptly instituted. The patient should be kept on bed rest in a semi-Fowler's position to facilitate breathing. An IV line should be maintained for medications and fluid therapy. The nurse should know the side effects of medications and observe for them. Oxygen therapy should be administered as ordered. Careful monitoring of vital signs, cardiac dysrhythmia monitoring, pulse oximetry, ABGs, and lung sounds is critical to assess the patient's status. Laboratory results are monitored to assure normal ranges of aPTT and INR. Nursing care includes assessing for the complications of anticoagulant therapy (e.g., bleeding, hematomas, bruising) and PE (e.g., atelectasis, pneumonia). The nursing care plan includes interventions related to immobility and fall precautions.

The patient is usually anxious because of pain, sense of doom, inability to breathe, and fear of death. The nurse should carefully explain the situation and provide emotional support and reassurance to help relieve the patient's anxiety.

Ambulatory and Home Care. The patient affected by thromboembolic processes may require psychologic and emotional support. In addition to the thromboembolic problems, the patient may have an underlying chronic illness requiring long-term treatment. To provide supportive therapy, the nurse must understand and differentiate between the various problems caused by the underlying disease and those related to thromboembolic disease. Patient teaching regarding long-term anticoagulant therapy is critical. The anticoagulant therapy continues for at least 3 to 6 months; patients with recurrent emboli are treated indefinitely. Warfarin blood levels are initially drawn monthly, and patients may have follow-up appointments at a nurse-managed anticoagulation clinic to monitor their medication and adjust dosages.

Long-term management is similar to that for the patient with DVT (see discussion of DVT in Chapter 38 on p. 916). Discharge planning is aimed at limiting progression of the condition and preventing complications and recurrence. The nurse must reinforce the need for the patient to return to the health care provider for regular follow-up examination.

■ Evaluation

The expected outcomes are that the patient who has a PE will have

- adequate tissue perfusion and respiratory function
- adequate cardiac output
- increased level of comfort
- no recurrence of PE

Pulmonary Hypertension

Pulmonary hypertension is elevated pulmonary pressures resulting from an increase in pulmonary vascular resistance to blood flow. The disease commonly presents with shortness of breath and fatigue. Pulmonary hypertension can occur as a primary disease (primary pulmonary hypertension) or as a secondary complication of a respiratory, cardiac, autoimmune, hepatic, or connective tissue disorder (secondary pulmonary hypertension).

PRIMARY PULMONARY HYPERTENSION

Primary pulmonary hypertension (PPH) is a severe and progressive disease. PPH is characterized by mean pulmonary arterial pressure greater than 25 mm Hg at rest (normal, 12 to 16 mm Hg) or greater than 30 mm Hg with exercise in the absence of a demonstrable cause. Until the last decade, this disorder was rapidly progressive with right-sided heart failure and death. The median survival if untreated was 2.8 years. Epoprostenol (Flolan) therapy, introduced in the 1990s, greatly improved survival rates. Unfortunately, the disease remains incurable despite these advances.

Etiology and Pathophysiology

The exact etiology of PPH is unknown. It is a rare and potentially fatal disease. PPH has been linked to the use of fenfluramine in the drug Fen-Phen, which was used as an appetite suppressant to treat obesity.

The drug was withdrawn from the market in 1996. PPH affects more women than men; the mean age at diagnosis is 36 years old. It may have a genetic component as the incidence is higher in families.

Normally the pulmonary circulation is characterized by low resistance and low pressure. In pulmonary hypertension, the pulmonary pressures are elevated. Until recently the pathophysiology of PPH was poorly understood. Recently it was discovered that a key mechanism involved in PPH is a deficient release of vasodilator mediators from the pulmonary epithelium, with a resultant cascade of injury (Fig. 28-11). Vasoconstriction, remodeling of the walls of the pulmonary vessels, and thrombosis in situ are the three elements that combine to cause the increased vascular resistance.[61] The remodeling process is a complex set of events involving endothelial cell injury that results in intimal/medial wall thickening.

Clinical Manifestations

Classic symptoms of pulmonary hypertension are dyspnea on exertion and fatigue. Exertional chest pain, dizziness, and exertional syncope are other symptoms. These symptoms are related to the inability of cardiac output to increase in response to increased oxygen demand. Eventually, as the disease progresses, dyspnea occurs at rest. Pulmonary hypertension increases the workload of the right ventricle and causes right ventricular hypertrophy (a condition called *cor pulmonale*) and eventually heart failure. A chest x-ray generally shows enlarged central pulmonary arteries and clear lung fields. An enlarged right heart may be seen. Echocardiogram usually reveals right ventricular hypertrophy. The mean time between onset of symptoms and the diagnosis is 2 years. By the time patients become symptomatic, the disease is already in the advanced stages and the pulmonary artery pressure is 2 to 3 times normal.

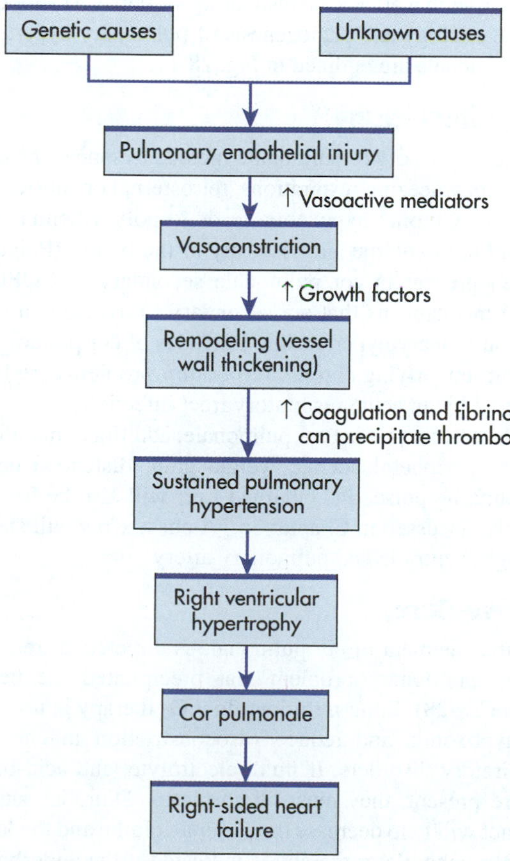

FIG. 28-11 Pathogenesis of pulmonary hypertension and cor pulmonale.

Collaborative Care

PPH is a diagnosis of exclusion. All other conditions must be ruled out. Diagnostic evaluation includes ECG, chest x-ray, pulmonary function tests, echocardiogram, and spiral CT. Cardiac catheterization is done to measure pulmonary artery pressure, cardiac output, and left ventricular filling pressure. Early recognition of pulmonary hypertension is essential to interrupt the vicious cycle responsible for the progression of the disease (see Fig. 28-11). Patients are classified using the New York Heart Association functional classification (see Chapter 35, Table 35-4).

Although there is no cure for PPH, treatment can relieve symptoms, increase quality of life, and prolong life. Diuretic therapy relieves dyspnea and peripheral edema and may be useful in reducing right ventricular volume overload. Anticoagulation therapy is recommended for patients with severe pulmonary hypertension to prevent in situ thrombus formation and venous thrombosis. Warfarin is given to keep the INR in the 2 to 3 range. Hypoxia is a potent pulmonary vasoconstrictor, and use of low-flow oxygen provides symptomatic relief. The goal is to keep oxygen saturation at ≥90%.

Vasodilator therapy is used to reduce right ventricular overload by dilating pulmonary vessels and reversing remodeling. Some patients with pulmonary hypertension can be effectively managed with calcium channel blocker therapy, such as sustained-release nifedipine (Procardia) or diltiazem (Cardizem).

Epoprostenol (Flolan) has revolutionized the management of PPH. It is a prostacyclin that promotes pulmonary vasodilation and reduces pulmonary vascular resistance. Continuous epoprostenol has been shown to result in significant improvement in clinical symptoms and long-term survival. It is now the treatment of choice for selected patients who are unresponsive to calcium channel blockers. Its administration requires the placement of an indwelling central line catheter and continuous infusion pump. The patient and family must be trained to use the portable intravenous infusion pump, mix medications, manage the central line, and monitor for complications (Fig. 28-12). The half-life of the drug is less than 6 minutes. If the central line is disrupted, stopped, or dislodged for any reason, clinical deterioration from abrupt withdrawal of epoprostenol can occur. This is a serious event with potential rebound pulmonary hypertension and clinical deterioration developing within minutes. The patient will have signs and symptoms of right-sided heart failure, including dyspnea, cyanosis, cough, syncope,

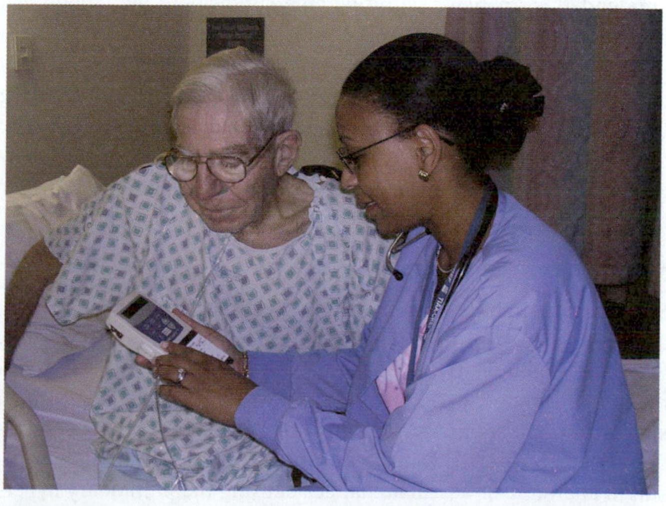

FIG. 28-12 A patient with pulmonary hypertension who is on continuous epoprostenol infusion is being taught how to use the portable infusion pump.

and weakness. If the patient loses significant weight, the dosage, which is weight based, may become excessive. Symptoms of overdose include flushing, hypotension, and tachycardia. The major problems have been infections related to vascular access and broken central lines.

Epoprostenol has been successful in improving the quality of life of patients with PPH. The drug was developed as a bridge to lung transplantation but is now a standard of care. Although the patient and family teaching is extensive, the patient on continuous epoprostenol therapy can be successfully managed with an interdisciplinary health care team.

Treprostinil (Remodulin), a prostacyclin, is used as a continuous subcutaneous injection. It causes vasodilation of the pulmonary arterial system and inhibits platelet aggregation. The subcutaneous route has drawbacks, including needles that could dislodge and infusion site pain and reactions. The drug has recently been approved for continuous intravenous use. This drug is stable at room temperature and has a longer half-life than epoprostenol. It may be a reasonable alternative to epoprostenol for some patients.

Bosentan (Tracleer), a form of prostacyclin, is the only oral vasodilator currently approved for the treatment of pulmonary hypertension. It is an active endothelin receptor antagonist and works by blocking the hormone endothelin, which causes blood vessels to constrict. Monthly liver function tests are needed since there is a risk of hepatotoxicity. Sildenafil (Revatio) is an oral phosphodiesterase inhibitor that prolongs the vasodilatory effect of nitric oxide and appears to be as effective in decreasing pulmonary vascular resistance.[62] It should not be taken by patients using nitrates because severe hypotension may develop. Iloprost (Ventavis) is an inhaled form of prostacyclin in an aerosolized preparation. It is taken 6 to 9 times a day using a disk inserted into a nebulizer. Because of the risk of orthostatic hypotension, iloprost should not be taken by patients with low systolic blood pressure (<85 mm Hg). Beraprost (an oral formulation of prostacyclin) is undergoing clinical trials for the treatment of early-stage pulmonary hypertension.

Surgical interventions for pulmonary hypertension include atrial septostomy (AS), pulmonary thromboendarterectomy (PTE), and lung transplantation.[63] AS involves the creation of an intra-atrial right-to-left shunt to decompress the right ventricle. It is indicated for a select group of patients awaiting lung transplantation. PTE may provide a potential cure for those patients suffering from chronic thromboembolic pulmonary hypertension. It is only recommended for patients with operable sites where the emboli can be surgically removed by embolectomy.

Lung transplantation has been the mainstay of treatment for pulmonary hypertension for those patients who do not respond to drug therapy and progress to severe right-sided heart failure. Recurrence of the disease has not been reported in individuals who have undergone transplantation. A patient education and support website for pulmonary hypertension is located at *www.phassociation.org.*

SECONDARY PULMONARY HYPERTENSION

Secondary pulmonary hypertension (SPH) occurs when a primary disease causes a chronic increase in pulmonary artery pressures. Secondary pulmonary hypertension can develop as a result of parenchymal lung disease, left ventricular dysfunction, intracardiac shunts, chronic pulmonary thromboembolism, or systemic connective tissue disease. The specific primary disease pathology can result in anatomic or vascular changes causing the pulmonary hypertension. Anatomic changes causing the increased pulmonary vascular resistance include (1) loss of capillaries as a result of alveolar wall damage (e.g., COPD), (2) stiffening of the pulmonary vasculature (e.g., pulmonary fibrosis connective tissue disorders), and (3) obstruction of blood flow (chronic emboli).

Vasomotor increases in pulmonary vascular resistance are found in conditions characterized by alveolar hypoxia. Hypoxia causes localized vasoconstriction and shunting of blood away from poorly ventilated alveoli. Alveolar hypoxia can be caused by a wide variety of conditions. It is possible to have a combination of both anatomic changes and vasomotor constriction. This is found in the patient with long-standing chronic bronchitis who has chronic hypoxia in addition to loss of lung tissue.

The symptoms can reflect the underlying disease, but some are directly attributable to SPH, including dyspnea, fatigue, lethargy, and chest pain. The initial physical findings can include right ventricular hypertrophy and signs of right ventricular failure (increased pulmonic heart sound, right-sided fourth heart sound, peripheral edema, hepatomegaly). Diagnosis of SPH is similar to that of PPH. Treatment of SPH consists mainly of treating the underlying primary disorder. When irreversible pulmonary vascular damage has occurred, therapies used for PPH are initiated. The efficacy of treatment for pulmonary hypertension has been primarily evaluated for PPH, and there are limited data on the effectiveness of these therapies for SPH.[64] Epoprostenol is used in the management of SPH. More studies are ongoing into effective therapies for SPH.

COR PULMONALE

Cor pulmonale is enlargement of the right ventricle secondary to diseases of the lung, thorax, or pulmonary circulation. Pulmonary hypertension is usually a preexisting condition in the individual with cor pulmonale. Cor pulmonale may be present with or without overt cardiac failure. The most common cause of cor pulmonale is COPD. Almost any disorder that affects the respiratory system can cause cor pulmonale. The etiology and pathogenesis of pulmonary hypertension and cor pulmonale are outlined in Fig. 28-11.

Clinical Manifestations

Clinical manifestations of cor pulmonale include dyspnea, chronic productive cough, wheezing respirations, retrosternal or substernal pain, and fatigue. Chronic hypoxemia leads to polycythemia and increased total blood volume and viscosity of the blood. (Polycythemia is often present in cor pulmonale secondary to COPD.) Compensatory mechanisms that are secondary to hypoxemia can aggravate the pulmonary hypertension. Episodes of cor pulmonale in a person with underlying chronic respiratory problems are frequently triggered by an acute respiratory tract infection.

If heart failure accompanies cor pulmonale, additional manifestations such as peripheral edema; weight gain; distended neck veins; full, bounding pulse; and enlarged liver will also be found. (Heart failure is discussed in Chapter 35.) A chest x-ray will show an enlarged right ventricle and pulmonary artery.

Collaborative Care

The primary management of cor pulmonale is directed at treating the underlying pulmonary problem that precipitated the heart problem (Table 28-28). Long-term low-flow O_2 therapy is used to correct the hypoxemia and reduce vasoconstriction in chronic states of respiratory disorders. If fluid, electrolyte, and acid-base imbalances are present, they must be corrected. Diuretics and a low-sodium diet will help decrease the plasma volume and the load on the heart. Bronchodilator therapy is indicated if the underlying respiratory problem is due to an obstructive disorder. Digoxin use

TABLE 28-28 COLLABORATIVE CARE
Cor Pulmonale

Diagnostic
History and physical examination
ABGs
Serum and urine electrolytes
Monitoring with ECG
Chest x-ray
Collaborative Therapy
O_2 therapy
Bronchodilators
Diuretics
Low-sodium diet
Fluid restriction
Antibiotics (if indicated)
Digitalis (if left-sided heart failure)
Vasodilators (if indicated)
Calcium channel blockers (if indicated)

ABGs, Arterial blood gases; *ECG*, electrocardiogram.

is controversial. However, studies have confirmed a modest effect of digoxin on the failing right ventricle in chronic cor pulmonale.[65] Other treatments include those for pulmonary hypertension, such as vasodilator therapy, calcium channel blockers, and anticoagulants. Theophylline may help due to its weak inotropic effect on the heart.[65] When medical treatment fails, lung transplantation is an option for some patients.

Chronic management of cor pulmonale resulting from COPD is similar to that described for COPD (see Chapter 28). Continuous low-flow O_2 during sleep, exercise, and small, frequent meals may allow the patient to feel better and be more active.

LUNG TRANSPLANTATION

Lung transplantation has become an important mode of therapy for patients with a variety of end-stage lung diseases. A variety of pulmonary disorders are potentially treatable with some type of lung transplantation (Table 28-29). Improved patient selection criteria, technical advances, and better methods of immunosuppression have resulted in improved survival rates. Four types of transplant procedures are available: single-lung transplantation, bilateral lung transplantation, heart-lung transplantation, and transplantation of lobes from a living related donor.[66]

Single-lung transplantation involves an incision on the side of the chest. The opposite lung is ventilated while the diseased lung is excised. The lung is removed and the donor lung implanted. Three anastomoses are done: the bronchus, pulmonary artery, and pulmonary veins. In a bilateral lung transplantation, the incision is made across the sternum and the donor lungs are implanted separately. A median sternotomy incision is used for a heart-lung transplant procedure. Chest tubes are placed around the donor lungs to help them reexpand with air. Lobar transplantation from living donors is reserved for candidates who urgently need transplantation and are unlikely to survive until a donor becomes available. The majority of these transplant recipients are patients with cystic fibrosis, and their parents or relatives are donors.

Patients being considered for lung transplantation need to undergo extensive evaluation. The candidate for lung transplantation should not have a malignancy or recent history of malignancy (within the last 2 years), renal or liver insufficiency, or HIV. Typically patients wait an average of 12 to 18 months for a donor lung.

TABLE 28-29 Indications for Lung Transplantation

- α_1-Antitrypsin deficiency
- Bronchiectasis
- Cystic fibrosis
- Emphysema
- Idiopathic pulmonary fibrosis
- Interstitial lung disease
- Pulmonary fibrosis secondary to other diseases (e.g., sarcoidosis)
- Pulmonary hypertension

The candidate and the family undergo psychologic screening to determine the ability to cope with a postoperative regimen that requires strict adherence to immunosuppressive therapy, continuous monitoring for early signs of infection, and prompt reporting of manifestations of infection for medical evaluation. Many transplant centers require preoperative outpatient pulmonary rehabilitation to maximize physical conditioning.

Early postoperative care includes ventilatory support, fluid and hemodynamic management, immunosuppression, detection of early rejection, and prevention or treatment of infection. Pulmonary clearance measures, including aerosolized bronchodilators, chest physiotherapy, and deep-breathing and coughing techniques, minimize potential complications. Maintenance of fluid balance is vital in the postoperative phase.

Lung transplant recipients are at high risk for bacterial, viral, fungal, and protozoal infections. Infections are the leading cause of death in the early period after the transplant. Gram-negative bacterial pneumonia is common. Among potential causes of viral infections, cytomegalovirus (CMV) is the most important in lung transplantation patients, usually seen 4 to 8 weeks postoperatively. Clinical manifestations of CMV infection include fever, bone marrow suppression, hepatitis, enteritis, and pneumonitis. *Aspergillus* is the most common fungal infection.

Immunosuppressive therapy usually includes a three-drug regimen of cyclosporine or tacrolimus, azathioprine (Imuran) or mycophenolate mofetil (CellCept), and prednisone. (The mechanisms of action of these drugs are discussed in Tables 14-18 and Fig. 14-18.) However, because of an array of potential adverse effects and drug interactions, there are limitations to immunosuppressive therapy. Drug levels are monitored on a regular basis. Lung transplant recipients are usually maintained on higher levels of immunosuppressive therapy than other organ recipients.[67] Immunosuppressive drugs are discussed in Chapter 14.

Acute rejection is fairly common in lung transplantation and can be seen as soon as 5 to 7 days after surgery. It is characterized by low-grade fever, fatigue, and oxygen desaturation with exercise. Accurate diagnosis is by transtracheal biopsy. Treatment is high doses of corticosteroids administered IV for 3 days. In patients with persistent or recurrent acute rejection, other strategies may include antilymphocyte antibodies or changing maintenance immunosuppressive drugs.

Bronchiolitis obliterans (an obstructive airway disease causing progressive occlusion) is thought to be a manifestation of chronic rejection in lung transplant patients. The onset is often subacute, with gradual onset of progressive obstructive airflow defect, including cough, dyspnea, and recurrent lower respiratory tract infection. Treatment involves optimum maintenance immunosuppression.

Discharge planning begins in the preoperative phase. Prior to discharge, the patient needs to be able to perform self-care activities, including medication management and activities of daily living, and to accurately identify when to call the transplant team physician. Patients are placed in an outpatient rehabilitation program to improve physical endurance. Home spirometry has been useful in monitoring trends in lung function. Patients are taught to keep medication logs, laboratory results, and spirometry records. The average lung transplant patient takes 13 medications (range, 5 to 24) a day.[68] After discharge, the patients are followed by the transplant team for transplant-related issues. The patients return to their primary care team for their health maintenance and routine illnesses. As transplant procedures become more frequent, transplant patients will return to hospitals for other routine procedures. Coordination of care between the transplant team, primary care team, and inpatient teams is essential for ongoing successful management of these patients. (Organ transplantation, histocompatibility, rejection, and immunosuppressive therapy are discussed in Chapter 14.)

CRITICAL THINKING EXERCISE

CASE STUDY

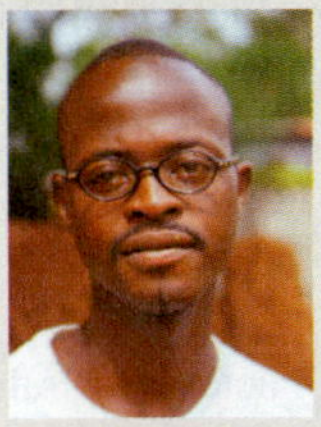

Aspiration Pneumonia

Patient Profile. Sam, a 27-year-old African American man, was admitted to the hospital because of an uncontrollable fever. He was transferred from a long-term care facility. He has a history of a gunshot wound to his left chest. Following a cardiac arrest after the accident, he developed hypoxic encephalopathy. He has a tracheostomy and gastrostomy tube. He has a history of methicillin-resistant *Staphylococcus aureus* (MRSA) in his sputum.

Subjective Data

- Family says that they visit him regularly and are very devoted to him.

Objective Data

Physical Examination

- Thin, cachectic African American man in moderate respiratory distress
- Unresponsive to voice, touch, or painful stimuli
- Vital signs: temperature 104° F (40° C), heart rate 120, respiratory rate 30, O_2 saturation 90%
- Chest auscultation revealed crackles and scattered rhonchi in the left upper lobe

Diagnostic Studies

- Serum albumin 2.8 g/dl (28 g/L)
- White blood cell (WBC) count 18,000/µl (18×10^9/L)
- Sputum specimen: thick, green colored, foul smelling; cultures pending
- Arterial blood gases: pH 7.29, PaO_2 80 mm Hg, $PaCO_2$ 40 mm Hg, bicarbonate 16 mEq/L
- Stool culture positive for *Clostridium difficile*
- Chest x-ray: infiltrate in left upper lobe; no pleural effusions noted

Critical Thinking Questions

1. What types of infectious disease precautions should be taken related to Sam's hospitalization?
2. Using the PORT Pneumonia Severity Index tool (see Table 28-3), what is Sam's PSI score and risk level?
3. What clinical manifestations of aspiration pneumonia did Sam exhibit? Explain their pathophysiologic bases.
4. What antibiotic medication is likely to be prescribed?
5. What is his acid-base balance and oxygenation status?
6. What other clinical issues must be addressed in Sam's plan of care? What is his priority of care?
7. What family interventions would you initiate?
8. Based on the assessment data presented, write one or more appropriate nursing diagnoses. Are there any collaborative problems?

NCLEX EXAMINATION REVIEW QUESTIONS

The number of the question corresponds to the same-numbered objective at the beginning of the chapter.

1. In assessing a patient with pneumococcal pneumonia, the nurse recognizes that clinical manifestations of this condition include
   a. fever, chills, and a productive cough with rust-colored sputum.
   b. a nonproductive cough and night sweats that are usually self-limiting.
   c. a gradual onset of nasal stuffiness, sore throat, and purulent productive cough.
   d. an abrupt onset of fever, nonproductive cough, and formation of lung abscesses.
2. An appropriate nursing intervention for a patient with pneumonia with the nursing diagnosis of ineffective airway clearance related to thick secretions and fatigue would be to
   a. perform postural drainage every hour.
   b. provide analgesics as ordered to promote patient comfort.
   c. administer oxygen as prescribed to maintain optimal oxygen levels.
   d. teach the patient how to cough effectively to bring secretions to the mouth.
3. A patient with TB has been admitted to the hospital and is placed in an airborne infection isolation room. The patient is taught all the following to prevent spread of the disease except
   a. expect routine TST to evaluate infection.
   b. take all medications for the full length of time to prevent multidrug-resistant TB.
   c. wear a standard isolation mask if leaving the airborne infection isolation room.
   d. maintain precautions in airborne infection isolation room by coughing into a paper tissue.
4. A patient has been receiving high-dose corticosteroids and broad-spectrum antibiotics for treatment secondary to a traumatic injury and infection. The nurse plans care for the patient knowing that the patient is most susceptible to
   a. candidiasis.
   b. aspergillosis.
   c. histoplasmosis.
   d. coccidioidomycosis.
5. Which of the following statements best describes the treatment of lung abscess?
   a. It is best treated with surgical excision and drainage.
   b. Antibiotics given for a prolonged period are the usual treatment of choice.
   c. The abscess is difficult to treat and frequently results in pulmonary fibrosis.
   d. Penicillin can effectively eradicate the anaerobic organisms causing the abscess.
6. A common complication of many types of environmental lung diseases is
   a. pulmonary fibrosis.
   b. liquefactive necrosis.

c. benign tumor growth.
d. diffuse airway obstruction.

7. The patient with lung cancer needs to receive influenza vaccine and pneumococcal vaccines. The nurse will
   a. administer both vaccines at the same time in the same arm.
   b. administer both vaccines at the same time in different arms.
   c. administer the flu shot and tell the patient to come back 1 week later to receive the pneumococcal vaccine.
   d. administer the pneumococcal vaccine and suggest Flumist (nasal vaccine) instead of the influenza injection.
8. The nurse identifies a flail chest in a trauma patient when
   a. multiple rib fractures are determined by x-ray.
   b. a tracheal deviation to the unaffected side is present.
   c. paradoxic chest movement occurs during respiration.
   d. there is decreased movement of the involved chest wall.
9. The nurse notes tidaling of the water level in the tube submerged in the water-seal chamber in a patient with closed chest tube drainage. The nurse should
   a. continue to monitor this normal finding.
   b. check all connections for a leak in the system.
   c. lower the drainage collector further from the chest.
   d. clamp the tubing at progressively distal points away from the patient until the tidaling stops.
10. A nursing measure that should be instituted after a pneumonectomy is
    a. monitoring chest tube drainage and functioning.
    b. positioning the patient on the unaffected side or back.
    c. range-of-motion exercises on the affected upper extremity.
    d. auscultating frequently for lung sounds on the affected side.
11. Guillain-Barré syndrome causes respiratory problems primarily by
    a. depressing the CNS.
    b. deforming chest wall muscles.
    c. paralyzing the diaphragm secondary to trauma.
    d. interrupting nerve transmission to respiratory muscles.
12. A patient is on a continuous epoprostenol infusion pump. The alarm goes off indicating an obstruction in the intravenous line downstream. The nurse should
    a. check vital signs and oxygen saturation.
    b. auscultate the lungs for pulmonary congestion.
    c. assess the central line immediately for any obstruction or accidental clamping of tubing.
    d. monitor for flushing and hypotension due to rebound from no medication and the short half-life of the drug.
13. Which of the following statements does not describe the follow-up management of lung transplantation?
    a. The lung is biopsied using a transtracheal method.
    b. High doses of oxygen are administered around the clock.
    c. The use of a home spirometer will help to monitor lung function.
    d. Immunosuppressant therapy usually involves a three-drug regimen.

REFERENCES

1. Centers for Disease Control and Prevention: National Center for Health Statistics, 2004. Available at *www.cdc.gov/nchs/fastats* (accessed August 18, 2005).
2. Bartlett JG: Exacerbations of chronic bronchitis. In Rose BD, editor: *UpToDate,* Waltham, Mass., 2006. Available at *www.uptodate.com* (accessed August 9, 2005).
3. Regueiro CR: The latest approaches to managing pneumonia, *The Clinical Advisor* 25, 2004.
4. Mandell LA, Bartlett JG, Dowell SC, et al: Update of practice guidelines for the management of community-acquired pneumonia for immunocompetent adults, *Clin Infect Dis* 37:1405, 2003.
5. Stanton MW: *Improving treatment decisions for patients with community acquired pneumonia,* AHRQ Research in Action, Number 7 (AHRQ Publication No. 02-0033), Rockville, MD, 2002, Agency for Healthcare Research and Quality.
6. Kleinpell RM, Elpern EH: Community-acquired pneumonia, *Crit Care Nurs Q* 27:231, 2004.
7. Adelson-Mitty J, Zaleznik DF: Treatment of community-acquired pneumonia. In Rose BD, editor: *UpToDate,* Waltham, Mass., 2006. Available at *www.uptodate.com* (accessed October 14, 2005).
8. American Thoracic Society: Guidelines for the management of adults with hospital-acquired, ventilator-associated, and healthcare-associated pneumonia, *Am J Respir Crit Care Med* 171:388, 2005.
9. Dent MR: Hospital-acquired pneumonia, the "gift" that keeps on giving, *Nursing* 34:48, 2004.
10. Shuey KM: Persistent fever and cough with nonspecific lower lung lobe consolidation, *Clin J Oncol Nurs* 7:463, 2003.
11. Taylor GH: Cytomegalovirus, *Am Fam Physician* 67:524, 2003.
12. National Institute of Allergy and Infectious Diseases, National Institutes of Health: Pneumococcal pneumonia: NIAID Fact Sheet, December 2004. Available at *www.niaid.nih.gov/factsheets/pneumonia.htm* (accessed August 17, 2005).
13. Centers for Disease Control and Prevention: Influenza antiviral medications: 2004-05 interim chemoprophylaxis and treatment guidelines, November 3, 2004. Available at *www.cdc.gov/flu/professionals/treatment* (accessed August 20, 2005).
14. Centers for Disease Control and Prevention: Revised interim guidance for late-season influenza vaccination, January 27, 2005. Available at *www.cdc.gov/flu/professionals/vaccination* (accessed August 20, 2005).
15. Karnath B, Agyeman A, Lai A: Pneumococcal pneumonia: update on therapy in the era of antibiotic resistance, *Consultant* 43:321, 2003.
16. Donowitz GR: Are care guidelines useful in community-acquired pneumonia? *Postgrad Med* 118:13, 2005.
17. Doering LV: The effect of positioning on hemodynamics and gas exchange in the critically ill: a review, *Am J Crit Care* 2:208, 1993.
18. Wong WP: Use of body positioning in the mechanically ventilated patient with acute respiratory failure: application of Sackett's rules of evidence, *Physiother Theory Pract* 15:25, 1999.
19. Fink JB: Positioning versus postural drainage, *Respir Care* 47:769, 2002.
20. Centers for Disease Control and Prevention: Trends in tuberculosis—United States, 1998–2003, *MMWR Morb Mortal Wkly Rep* 53:1, 2004.
21. Frieden TR, Sterling TR, Munsiff SS, et al: Tuberculosis, *Lancet* 362:887, 2003.
22. Centers for Disease Control and Prevention: Core curriculum on tuberculosis, 2000. Available at *www.cdc.gov* (accessed August 20, 2005).
23. Lauzardo M, Ashkin D: Phthisiology at the dawn of the new century: a review of tuberculosis and the prospects for its elimination, *Chest* 117:1455, 2000.
24. Centers for Disease Control and Prevention: Diagnostic standards and classification of tuberculosis in adults and children. Available at *www.cdc.gov/nchstp/tb/pubs/PDF/1376.pdf.*
25. Taggart EW, Hill HR, Ruegner RG, et al: Evaluation of an in vitro assay for gamma interferon production in response to *Mycobacterium tuberculosis* infections, *Clin Diagn Lab Immunol* 11:1089, 2004.
26. Neff M: ATS,CDC, and IDSA update recommendations on the treatment of tuberculosis, *Am Fam Physician* 68:1854, 2003.
27. Falkinham KO: Mycobacterial aerosols and respiratory disease, *Emerg Infect Dis* 9:763, 2003.
28. Chen K, Shiann-Chin K, Hsueh P, et al: Pulmonary fungal infection, *Chest* 120:177, 2001.
29. Kuschner WG, Stark P: Occupational lung disease. Part 2, *Postgrad Med* 113:81, 2003.
30. Centers for Disease Control and Prevention: Lung cancer statistics. Available at *www.cdc.gov/cancer/lung/statistics.htm#trends* (accessed October 26, 2005).
31. Centers for Disease Control and Prevention: Women and smoking: a report of the Surgeon General—2001. Available at *www.cdc.gov/tobacco/sgr/sgr_forwomen/ataglance.htm* (accessed April 10, 2006).
32. Kazerouni N, Alverson CIJ, Redd SC, et al: Sex differences in COPD and lung cancer mortality trends—United States, 1968-1999. *J Womens Health* 13:17, 2003.
33. Fiore MC, Bailey WC, Cohen SJ, et al: Treating tobacco use and dependence, clinical practice guideline, Rockville, Md., 2000, U.S. Public Health Service.
34. Baldwin PD: Lung cancer, *Clin J Oncol Nurs* 7:699, 2003.
35. Kreamer KM: Getting the lowdown on lung cancer, *Nursing* 33:36, 2003.
36. U.S. Preventive Services Task Force: Lung cancer screening: recommendation statement, *Ann Intern Med* 140:738, 2004.

*37. Mahon SM: Screening for lung cancer: what is the evidence? *Clin J Oncol Nurs* 8:188, 2004.
38. New noninvasive test may detect lung cancer at earlier stages, *Clin J Oncol Nurs* 8:24, 2004.
39. Inzeo D, Haughney A: Laser therapy in the management of lung cancer, *Clin J Oncol Nurs* 8:94, 2004.
40. National Comprehensive Cancer Network: Non-small cell lung cancer. In: *Clinic practice guidelines in oncology,* vol 2, Jenkintown, Pa., 2005, The Network. Available at *www.nccn.org* (accessed August 24, 2005).
41. Walker S: Updates in small cell lung cancer treatment, *Clin J Oncol Nurs* 7:563, 2003.
42. National Comprehensive Cancer Network: Small cell lung cancer. In *Clinic practice guidelines in oncology,* vol 2, Jenkintown, Pa., 2005, The Network. Available at *www.nccn.org* (accessed August 3, 2005).
43. Prochaska AV: New developments in smoking cessation, *Chest* 117:169S, 2000.
*44. Meraviglia MG: The effects of spirituality on well-being of people with lung cancer, *Oncol Nurs Forum* 31:89, 2004.
*45. Zhang AY, Siminoff LA: The role of the family in treatment decision making by patients with cancer, *Oncol Nurs Forum* 30:1022, 2003.
46. Yeo TP: Long-term sequelae following blunt thoracic trauma, *Orthop Nurs* 20:35, 2001.
47. Yamamoto L, Schroeder C, Beliveau C: Thoracic trauma: the deadly dozen, *Crit Care Nurs Q* 28:22, 2005.
48. Jantz MA, Sahn SA: Tube thoracostomy. In Rose BD, editor: *UpToDate,* Waltham, Mass., 2006. Available at *www.uptodate.com* (accessed August 9, 2005).
49. Lazzara D: Eliminate the air of mystery from chest tubes, *Nursing* 32:36, 2002.
50. Andrs K: Chest drainage to go, *Nursing* 34:54, 2004.
*51. Behnia MM, Garrett K: Association of tension pneumothorax with use of small-bore chest tubes in patients receiving mechanical ventilation, *Crit Care Nurse* 24:64, 2004.
52. Pleural effusion, *Nursing* 34:64, 2004.
53. Roman M, Weinstein A, Macaluso S: Primary spontaneous pneumothorax, *MEDSURG Nurs* 12:161, 2003.
54. Spiegler PA, Hurewitz AN, Groth ML: Rapid pleurodesis for malignant pleural effusions, *Chest* 123:1895, 2003.
55. King T: Overview of sarcoidosis. In Rose BD, editor: *UpToDate,* Waltham, Mass., 2006. Available at *www.uptodate.com* (accessed August 20, 2005).
56. Thompson BT, Hales CA: Clinical manifestation of and diagnostic strategies for acute pulmonary embolism. In Rose BD, editor: *UpToDate,* Waltham, Mass., 2006. Available at *www.uptodate.com* (accessed August 14, 2005).
57. Dalen JE: Pulmonary embolism: what have we learned since Virchowz? *Chest* 122:1440, 2002.
58. Valentine KA, Hull RD: Treatment of acute pulmonary embolism. In Rose BD, editor: *UpToDate,* Waltham, Mass., 2006. Available at *www.uptodate.com* (accessed August 14, 2005).
59. Yang JC: Prevention and treatment of deep vein thrombosis and pulmonary embolism in critically ill patients, *Crit Care Nurs Q* 28:72, 2005.
60. Cardin T, Marinelli A: Pulmonary embolism, *Crit Care Nurs Q* 27:310, 2004.
61. Berkowitz DS, Coyne NG: Understanding primary pulmonary hypertension, *Crit Care Nurs Q* 26:28, 2003.
62. Rubin LJ: Prognosis and treatment of primary pulmonary hypertension. In Rose BD, editor: *UpToDate,* Waltham, Mass., 2006. Available at *www.uptodate.com* (accessed August 10, 2005).
63. Doyle RL, McCrory D, Channick RN, et al: Surgical treatments/interventions for pulmonary arterial hypertension, *Chest* 126:63S, 2004.

*Nursing research–based reference.

64. Dauerman HL, Morgan JP: Treatment of secondary pulmonary hypertension. In Rose BD, editor: *UpToDate,* Waltham, Mass., 2006. Available at *www.uptodate.com* (accessed August 10, 2005).
65. Yunis NA: Cor pulmonale. New York, 2006, eMedicine. Available at *www.emedicine.com* (accessed August 26, 2005).
66. Trulock EP: Procedure and postoperative management in lung transplantation. In Rose BD, editor: *UpToDate,* Waltham, Mass., 2006. Available at *www.uptodate.com* (accessed August 24, 2005).
67. Faro A: Lung transplantation. New York, 2006, eMedicine. Available at *www.emedicine.com* (accessed August 26, 2005).
68. Petty M: Lung and heart-lung transplantation: implications for nursing care when hospitalized outside the transplant center, *MEDSURG Nurs* 12:250, 2003.

RESOURCES

American Cancer Society
800-ACS-2345
www.cancer.org

American Lung Association
212-315-8700
800-586-4872
www.lungusa.org

American Society of Clinical Oncology
703-299-0150
www.asco.org

Cancer Care Ontario
Lung Cancer Clinical Practice Guidelines
416-971-9800
www.ccopebc.ca/lungcpg.html

Cancer Information Service
NCI Public Inquiries Office
800-422-6237
www.nci.nih.gov

Centers for Disease Control and Prevention
National Center for Chronic Disease Prevention and Health Promotion
Tobacco Information and Prevention Source (TIPS)
800-311-3435
www.cdc.gov/tobacco

Centers for Disease Control and Prevention
National Center for Health Statistics
301-458-4000
www.cdc.gov/nchs/fastats

Centers for Disease Control and Prevention
Surgeon General's Report on Smoking and Health—2005
404-639-3311
www.cdc.gov/tobacco/sgr/sgr

Pulmonary Hypertension Association (PHA)
301-565-3004
www.phassociation.org

Smoking Cessation Consumer Tool Kit
Agency for Healthcare Research and Quality (AHRQ)
301-427-1364
www.ahrq.gov

Try To Stop
Massachusetts Department of Public Health
800-TRY-TO-STOP (800-879-8678)
www.trytostop.org

For additional Internet resources, see the website for this book at *http://evolve.elsevier.com/Lewis/medsurg.*

Never doubt that a small group of committed citizens can change the world. Indeed, it is the only thing that ever has.

Margaret Mead

Nursing Management Obstructive Pulmonary Diseases 29

Jane Steinman Kaufman

LEARNING OBJECTIVES

1. Describe the etiology, pathophysiology, clinical manifestations, and collaborative care of asthma.
2. Describe the nursing management of the patient with asthma.
3. Differentiate between the etiology, pathophysiology, clinical manifestations, and collaborative care of the patient with chronic obstructive pulmonary disease (COPD).
4. Describe the effects of cigarette smoking on the lungs.
5. Identify the indications for O_2 therapy, methods of delivery, and complications of O_2 administration.
6. Explain the nursing management of the patient with COPD.
7. Describe the pathophysiology, clinical manifestations, collaborative care, and nursing management of the patient with cystic fibrosis.
8. Describe the pathophysiology, clinical manifestations, collaborative care, and nursing management of the patient with bronchiectasis.

KEY TERMS

α_1-antitrypsin (AAT) deficiency, p. 632
asthma, p. 608
bronchiectasis, p. 659
chronic bronchitis, p. 629
chronic obstructive pulmonary disease, p. 629
cor pulmonale, p. 635
cystic fibrosis, p. 655
emphysema, p. 629
pursed-lip breathing, p. 646
status asthmaticus, p. 612

Electronic Resources

Supplemental content related to Chapter 29 can be found . . .

Companion CD

- Stress-Busting Kit for Nursing Students
- Audio Lecture: Asthma
- Interactive Case Studies:
  - Asthma
  - Chronic Obstructive Pulmonary Disease
  - Cystic Fibrosis
- NCLEX Examination Review Questions
- Comprehensive Glossary

Evolve Website evolve

http://evolve.elsevier.com/Lewis/medsurg

- Content Updates
- Key Points (Printable and CD/MP3 Download)
- Concept Map Creator
- Expanded Audio Glossary
- Key Term Flash Cards
- Customizable Nursing Care Plans:
  - Asthma
  - Chronic Obstructive Pulmonary Disease
- Patient and Family Instruction Guides in English and Spanish:
  - Home Oxygen Use
  - How to Use a Dry Powder Inhaler (DPI)
  - How to Use a Peak Flow Meter
- Asthma Action Plan (Spanish)
- Electronic Calculators
- WebLinks

"When you can't breathe, nothing else matters," is the mantra of the American Lung Association. More than 35 million Americans are living with chronic lung disease. Obstructive pulmonary diseases, the most common chronic lung diseases, include diseases characterized by increased resistance to airflow as a result of airway obstruction or airway narrowing. Airway obstruction may result from accumulated secretions, edema, and swelling of the inner lumen of airways, bronchospasm, or destruction of lung tissue. Types of obstructive lung diseases are asthma, chronic obstructive pulmonary disease (COPD), cystic fibrosis, and bronchiectasis.

Reviewed by Elizabeth A. Palmer, RN, PhD, Associate Professor, Department of Nursing and Allied Health Professions, Indiana University of Pennsylvania, Indiana, Pa.; and Christine L. Willis, RN, MSN, ANP-C, Adult Nurse Practitioner, Pulmonary and Critical Care Medicine, Duke University Medical Center, Durham, N.C.

Asthma is a chronic inflammatory lung disease that results in recurrent episodes of airflow obstruction, but it is usually reversible. *COPD* is an obstructive pulmonary disease that includes *chronic bronchitis* and *emphysema* and is characterized by limitation in airflow that is not fully reversible.[1,2]

The patient with asthma has variations in airflow over time, usually with normal lung function between exacerbations, whereas the limitation in expiratory airflow in the patient with COPD is generally more constant. The pathology of asthma and response to therapy differ from COPD. However, the patient with a diagnosis of obstructive pulmonary disease may have distinguishing features of both asthma and COPD. Patients with asthma who have less responsive reversible airflow obstruction are very difficult to distinguish from COPD patients.[3]

Cystic fibrosis, another form of obstructive pulmonary disease, is a genetic disorder that produces airway obstruction because of changes in exocrine glandular secretions. *Bronchiectasis* is an obstructive disease characterized by dilated bronchioles resulting from years of pulmonary infections that cause an increase in sputum production.

ASTHMA

Asthma is a chronic inflammatory disorder of the airways. The chronic inflammation causes an increase in airway hyperresponsiveness that leads to recurrent episodes of wheezing, breathlessness, chest tightness, and cough, particularly at night or in the early morning. These episodes are associated with widespread but variable airflow obstruction that is usually reversible, either spontaneously or with treatment.[4] The clinical course of asthma is unpredictable, ranging from periods of adequate control to exacerbations of dyspnea, wheezing, and chest tightness.

Asthma affects an estimated 20 million Americans. Among adults, women have a 30% greater prevalence of asthma than men (see Gender Differences box). The asthma prevalence rates are 39% higher in African Americans than in whites and are increasing in African Americans while decreasing in whites. Prevalence rates in Hispanics are significantly lower than in whites. Persons with the highest incidence of asthma are white women, 18 to 44 years of age, from the southern United States.[5] Older adults may be underdiagnosed with asthma primarily because their symptoms are similar to those of COPD and pulmonary function testing is limited in this age-group.[1]

After a long period of a steady increase in rates, it appears that mortality and morbidity rates from asthma have plateaued and/or decreased. Yet there are over 4000 deaths per year from asthma. The death rate is 42% greater in women than in men and three times higher in African Americans than in whites, with the highest death rate in African American women. The ethnic health disparities are likely due to the low income levels of these populations, the inability to access medical care, and inability to afford the primary treatment for asthma (i.e., inhaled corticosteroids).

Asthma affects school attendance, occupational choices, physical activity, and other quality-of-life issues. The economic impact of asthma is significant at $14 billion, which accounts for health care costs and lost productivity.[5] The significant morbidity rates related to asthma may be attributed to limited access to health care, an inaccurate assessment of disease severity, a delay in seeking help, inadequate medical treatment, nonadherence to prescribed therapy (especially antiinflammatory therapy), and an increase in allergens in the environment, especially in the inner city.

Triggers of Asthma Attacks

Although the exact mechanisms that cause asthma remain unknown, triggers are involved (Table 29-1). These triggers are discussed in this section.

Allergens. Approximately 40% of all cases of asthma are related to an allergic response.[4] Allergic asthma may be seasonal and related to allergies such as tree or weed pollen. It is seen mainly in young adults and children. Nonseasonal forms of asthma may be year round (perennial) and related to allergens such as dust mites, molds, animals, feathers, and cockroaches. Exposure to cockroach allergen might be the most important risk factor for asthma in inner-city households.[6]

Exercise. Asthma that is induced or exacerbated during physical exertion is called *exercise-induced asthma* (EIA). Typically, EIA occurs after vigorous exercise, not during it (e.g., jogging, aerobics, walking briskly, and climbing stairs). Symptoms of EIA are pronounced during activities where there is exposure to cold air. For example, swimming in an indoor heated pool is less likely to produce symptoms than downhill skiing. Airway obstruction may occur due to changes in the airway mucosa caused by the hyperventilation occurring during exercise with either cooling or rewarming of air and capillary leakage in the airway wall. Cromolyn (Intal), nedocromil (Tilade), and β_2-adrenergic agonists have successfully maintained bronchodilation during exercise when these drugs are inhaled 10 to 20 minutes before exercise. Long-acting β_2-adrenergic agonists with inhaled corticosteroids (e.g., fluticasone/salmeterol [Advair]) may also be of value. The patient should perform a brief warm-up of stretching for 2 to 3 minutes before exercise. When exercising in cold or dry climate conditions, breathing through a scarf or mask may decrease the likelihood of symptoms.

GENDER DIFFERENCES

Asthma

Men

- Before puberty, boys are more affected than girls.

Women

- After puberty and into adulthood, more women are affected than men.
- Women who are admitted to the emergency department are more likely to need hospitalization.
- Women have an increased risk of death from asthma compared with men.

CULTURAL AND ETHNIC HEALTH DISPARITIES

Obstructive Pulmonary Diseases

- Female African Americans have the highest mortality rates from asthma among all ethnic/gender groups.
- Whites have the highest incidence of chronic obstructive pulmonary disease despite high rates of smoking among other ethnic groups.
- Whites have the highest incidence of cystic fibrosis.
- Cystic fibrosis is uncommon among African Americans, Hispanics, and Asian Americans.

TABLE 29-1 Triggers of Acute Asthma Attacks

Allergen inhalation
- Animal danders (e.g., cats, mice, guinea pigs)
- House dust mite
- Cockroaches
- Pollens
- Molds

Air pollutants
- Exhaust fumes
- Perfumes
- Oxidants
- Sulfur dioxides
- Cigarette smoke
- Aerosol sprays

Viral upper respiratory infection
Sinusitis
Exercise and cold, dry air
Stress
Drugs
- Aspirin
- Nonsteroidal antiinflammatory drugs
- β-Adrenergic blockers

Occupational exposure
- Metal salts
- Wood and vegetable dusts
- Industrial chemicals and plastics
- Pharmaceutical agents

Food additives
- Sulfites (bisulfites and metabisulfites)
- Beer, wine, dried fruit, shrimp, processed potatoes
- Monosodium glutamate
- Tartrazine

Hormones/menses
Gastroesophageal reflux disease (GERD)

Air Pollutants. Various air pollutants, cigarette or wood smoke, vehicle exhaust, elevated ozone levels, sulfur dioxide, and nitrogen dioxide can trigger asthma attacks. In heavily industrialized or densely populated areas, climatic conditions often lead to concentrated pollution in the atmosphere, especially with thermal inversions and stagnant air masses.[4,7] Ozone alert days are regularly noted on the news reports, and patients should minimize outdoor activity during these times.

Occupational Factors. Occupational asthma is the most common form of occupational lung disease, with an estimated 15% to 23% of new-onset adult asthma cases in the United States caused by occupational exposures. These exposures in the workplace can also aggravate preexisting asthma.[8] These agents are diverse, such as wood and vegetable dusts (flour), pharmaceutical agents, laundry detergents, animal and insect dusts, secretions and serums (e.g., chickens, crabs), metal salts, chemicals, paints, solvents, and plastics. Individuals can become sensitized to these agents. Characteristically, patients will give a history of arriving at work feeling well but experience gradual development of symptoms by the end of the day. The nurse should obtain a history and ascertain if the patient is symptom free over a period of time (e.g., the weekend) when he or she is not at work. Inquire if co-workers are also developing similar symptoms. Occupational health measures, such as the use of masks and proper ventilation, have lessened the exposure for many individuals.

Respiratory Infections. Respiratory infections (i.e., viral and not bacterial) or allergy to microorganisms is the major precipitating factor of an acute asthma attack. Influenza and rhinovirus are the major pathogens in older children and adults. Infections cause inflammatory changes in the tracheobronchial system and alter the mucociliary mechanism. Therefore they increase the hyperresponsiveness of the bronchial system. Increased airway responsiveness can last from 2 to 8 weeks after the infection in both normal and asthmatic persons. It is thought that viruses cause asthma exacerbations by activating the immune system. This ultimately results in production of inflammatory mediators leading to the onset of asthma symptoms (Fig. 29-1).

The patient with asthma should avoid people with colds or flu, get yearly influenza vaccinations, and avoid taking over-the-counter (OTC) cold remedies unless approved by the health care provider. Influenza vaccines are safe for individuals with asthma regardless of the severity of their asthma.[9]

Nose and Sinus Problems. Some patients with asthma have chronic sinus and nasal problems. Nasal problems include allergic rhinitis, which can be seasonal or perennial, and nasal polyps. Treatment of allergic rhinitis may reduce the frequency of asthma exacerbations.[10] Sinus problems are usually related to inflammation of the mucous membranes, most commonly from noninfectious causes such as allergies. Bacterial sinusitis may also be a cause. Sinusitis must be treated and large nasal polyps removed for the asthma patient to have good control. (Sinusitis is discussed in Chapter 27.)

EVIDENCE-BASED PRACTICE

Can Physical Training Improve Respiratory and General Health in Persons with Asthma?

Clinical Question

In patients with asthma (P), does physical training (I) as compared with a control group (C) improve respiratory and general health (O)?

Best Available Evidence

Systemic review of randomized controlled trials (RCTs)

Critical Appraisal and Synthesis of Evidence

- Meta-analysis of 13 RCTs ($n = 455$).
- Subjects with any degree of asthma severity and who were 8 years and older were included. Physical training (aerobic exercise) had to be undertaken for at least 20 to 30 minutes, two to three times a week, over a minimum of 4 weeks.
- No adverse effects were noted on lung function and wheeze in asthmatic patients.
- Physical training was found to have no effect on resting lung function or the number of days of wheeze.
- Physical training can improve cardiopulmonary fitness in individuals with asthma.

Conclusions

- Physical training can improve cardiopulmonary fitness without changing lung function.
- The benefit of improved fitness on quality of life is unknown.

Implications for Nursing Practice

- Patients with asthma should be encouraged to engage in regular physical exercise.
- Patients should be advised about prevention and treatment of exercise-induced asthma.

Reference for Evidence

Ram FSF, Robinson SM, Black PN, et al: Physical training for asthma, Cochrane Airways Group, *Cochrane Database of Systematic Reviews* 4, 2005.

PICO: P, Patient population of interest; *I*, intervention or area of interest; *C*, comparison of interest or comparison group; *O*, outcome(s) of interest (see p. 6).

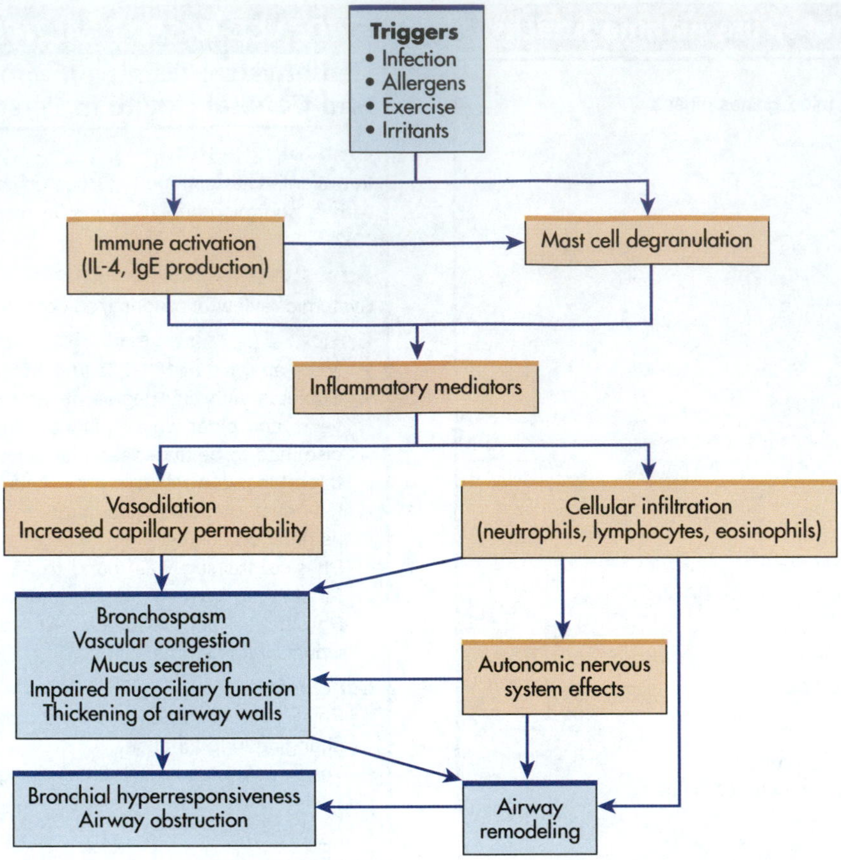

FIG. 29-1 Pathophysiology of asthma. *IL,* Interleukin.

Drugs and Food Additives. Sensitivity to specific drugs may occur in some asthmatic persons, especially those with nasal polyps and sinusitis. Some people with asthma have what is termed the *asthma triad*—nasal polyps, asthma, and sensitivity to aspirin and nonsteroidal antiinflammatory drugs (NSAIDs). Salicylic acid can be found in many OTC drugs and some foods, beverages, and flavorings. In some asthmatics who ingest aspirin or NSAIDs (e.g., ibuprofen [Motrin], indomethacin [Indocin]), wheezing will develop within 2 hours. In addition, there is usually profound rhinorrhea, congestion, and tearing. Facial flushing, gastrointestinal symptoms, and angioedema can occur. Some patients are also sensitive to salicylates, which are found in many foods, beverages, and flavorings.

Although sensitivity to salicylates persists for many years, the nature and severity of the reaction can change over time. Avoidance of aspirin and NSAIDs are required. However, patients with aspirin sensitivity under the care of an allergist can be desensitized by daily administration of the drug.

β-Adrenergic blockers in oral form (e.g., propranolol [Inderal]) or topical eyedrops (e.g., timolol [Timoptic]) may trigger asthma because they inhibit adrenergic stimulation of the bronchioles and thus prevent bronchodilation. Angiotensin-converting enzyme (ACE) inhibitors may produce cough in susceptible individuals, thus making asthma symptoms worse. Other agents that may precipitate asthma in the susceptible patient are tartrazine (yellow dye no. 5, found in many foods) and sulfiting agents widely used in the food and pharmaceutical industries as preservatives and sanitizing agents. Sulfiting agents are commonly found in fruits, beer, and wine and used extensively in salad bars to protect vegetables from oxidation. Asthma exacerbations have been reported after the use of sulfite-containing preservatives found in topical ophthalmic solutions, IV corticosteroids, and some inhaled bronchodilator solutions. The mechanism of action causing the asthma symptoms is unknown.[7]

Food allergies may cause asthma symptoms. Avoidance diets may be needed to prevent asthma. However, food allergies triggering asthma in adults are rare.

Gastroesophageal Reflux Disease. The exact mechanism by which gastroesophageal reflux disease (GERD) triggers asthma is unknown. It is postulated that reflux of stomach acid into the esophagus can be aspirated into the lungs, causing reflex vagal stimulation and bronchoconstriction. Although GERD is primarily involved in nocturnal asthma, it can trigger daytime asthma as well. Patients with hiatal hernia, delayed gastric emptying, and a prior history of reflux or peptic ulcer disease may have acid reflux as an asthma trigger. Trials of H_2-histamine blockers or proton pump inhibitors are given to ameliorate symptoms. (GERD is discussed in Chapter 42.)

Psychologic Factors. Another factor often discussed in relationship to the etiology of asthma is psychologic or emotional stress. Asthma is not a psychosomatic disease. However, psychologic factors can interact with the asthmatic response to worsen or ameliorate the disease process. Crying, laughing, anger, and fear can lead to hyperventilation and hypocapnia, which can cause airway narrowing.[4] An asthma attack caused by any trigger can produce panic, stress, and anxiety, which are not unexpected emotions during this experience. Anxiety is a very normal response to not being able to breathe. The extent to which psychologic factors contribute to the induction and continuation of any given acute exacerbation is unknown, but it probably varies from patient to patient and in the same patient from episode to episode.

Pathophysiology

The primary pathophysiologic process in asthma is chronic inflammation, which leads to airway hyperresponsiveness (hyperreactivity) and acute airflow limitation. Exposure to allergens or irritants initiates the inflammatory cascade (see Fig. 29-1). A variety of inflammatory cells are involved in asthma. Examples of inflammatory cells in asthma are mast cells, macrophages, eosinophils, neutrophils, T and B lymphocytes, and epithelial cells of the airways.[11]

As the inflammatory process begins, mast cells (found beneath the basement membrane of the bronchial wall) degranulate and release multiple inflammatory mediators (Fig. 29-2). Common inflammatory mediators are leukotrienes, histamine, cytokines (e.g., interleukins 4 and 5), prostaglandins, and nitric oxide. Some inflammatory mediators have effects on the blood vessels, causing vasodilation and increasing capillary permeability. Some mediators result in the airways being infiltrated by eosinophils, lymphocytes, and neutrophils. The resulting inflammatory process results in vascular congestion; edema formation; production of thick, tenacious mucus; bronchial muscle spasm; thickening of airway walls; and increased bronchial hyperresponsiveness[12] (Fig. 29-3). This whole process is sometimes referred to as the *early-phase response* in asthma. Clinically it can occur within 30 to 60 minutes after exposure to the allergen or irritant.

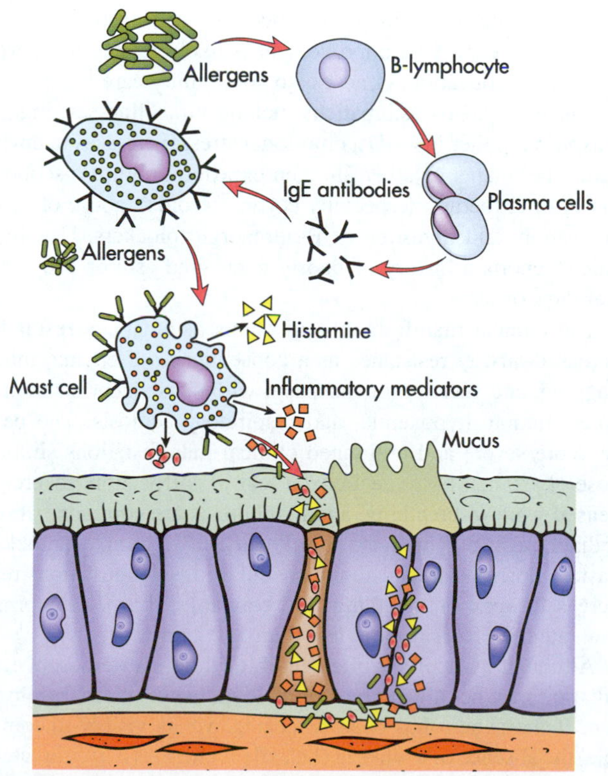

FIG. 29-2 Allergic asthma is triggered when an allergen cross-links IgE receptors on mast cells, which are then activated to release histamine and other inflammatory mediators (early-phase response). A late-phase response may occur due to further inflammation.

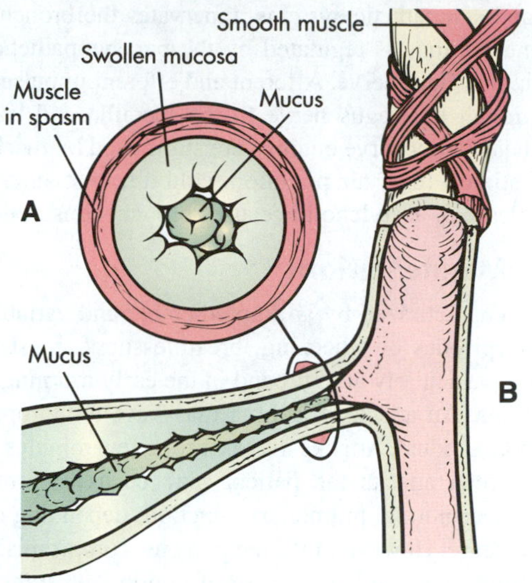

FIG. 29-3 Factors causing obstruction (especially expiratory obstruction) in asthma. **A,** Cross section of a bronchiole occluded by muscle spasm, swollen mucosa, and mucus in the lumen. **B,** Longitudinal section of a bronchiole.

Symptoms can recur 4 to 10 hours after the initial attack because of eosinophil and lymphocyte activation and further release of more inflammatory mediators. The epithelial cells also produce cytokines and other inflammatory mediators. This delayed response is called the *late-phase response* in asthma. Only about 30% to 50% of patients experience this delayed response. It can be more severe than the early-phase response and persist for 24 hours or more. It is characterized by a self-sustaining cycle of inflammation. Airflow may be limited from the swelling of the airways with or without bronchoconstriction. Corticosteroids are effective in treating this inflammation.

Untreated inflammation can lead to long-term damage that is irreversible. Chronic inflammation resulting in structural changes in the bronchial wall is known as *remodeling.* The bronchial smooth muscle hypertrophies and collagen is deposited in the airway walls. The mechanisms responsible for remodeling are thought to be related to chronic or recurrent inflammation of the airways. The combination of damage to the epithelium of the airways, prolonged repair of the epithelium, fibrosis, and increased types of fibroblasts are central to remodeling. The airway smooth muscles hypertrophy and mucus-secreting cells undergo hyperplasia in remodeling. There is some evidence that remodeling can occur even in mild asthma of recent onset, but it can be prevented by early introduction of inhaled corticosteroids.[4]

Hyperventilation occurs during an asthma attack as lung receptors respond to increased lung volume from trapped air and airflow limitation. Decreased perfusion and ventilation of the alveoli and increased alveolar gas pressure lead to ventilation-perfusion abnormalities in the lungs. The patient will be hypoxemic early on with decreased $PaCO_2$ and increased pH (respiratory alkalosis) as he or she is hyperventilating. As the airflow limitation worsens with air trapping, the patient works much harder to breathe. The $PaCO_2$ will normalize as the patient tires, and then it will rise to produce respiratory acidosis, which is an ominous sign signifying respiratory failure.[12]

Alterations in the neural control of the airways also occur in asthma. The autonomic nervous system, consisting of the parasympathetic and sympathetic systems, innervates the bronchi. Airway smooth muscle tone is regulated by the parasympathetic nervous system via the vagus nerve. Afferent and efferent impulses are conducted through the vagus nerve to the medulla and back to the lungs. When airway nerve endings are stimulated by mechanical or chemical stimuli (e.g., air pollution, cold air, dust, allergens), increased release of acetylcholine causes bronchoconstriction.[13]

Clinical Manifestations

Asthma is characterized by an unpredictable and variable course. Recurrent episodes of wheezing, breathlessness, chest tightness, and cough, particularly at night and in the early morning, are typical in asthma. An attack of asthma may have an abrupt onset or may be more gradual. Attacks may last for a few minutes to several hours. Between attacks the patient may be asymptomatic with normal or near-normal pulmonary function, depending on the severity of disease. However, in some persons, compromised pulmonary function may result in a state of continuous symptoms and chronic debilitation characterized by irreversible airway disease.

The characteristic clinical manifestations of asthma are wheezing, cough, dyspnea, and chest tightness after exposure to a precipitating factor or trigger. Expiration may be prolonged. Instead of a normal inspiratory-expiratory ratio of 1:2, it may be prolonged to 1:3 or 1:4. Normally the bronchioles constrict during expiration. However, as a result of bronchospasm, edema, and mucus in the bronchioles, the airways become narrower than usual. Thus it takes longer for the air to move out of the bronchioles. This produces the characteristic wheezing, air trapping, and hyperinflation.

Wheezing is an unreliable sign to gauge the severity of an attack. Many patients with minor attacks wheeze loudly, whereas others with severe attacks do not wheeze. The patient with severe asthmatic attacks may have no audible wheezing because of the marked reduction in airflow. For wheezing to occur, the patient must be able to move enough air to produce the sound. Wheezing usually occurs first on exhalation. As asthma progresses, the patient may wheeze during inspiration and expiration.

In some patients with asthma, cough is the only symptom, and this is termed *cough variant asthma.* The bronchospasm may not be severe enough to cause airflow obstruction, but it can increase bronchial tone and cause irritation with stimulation of the cough receptors. The cough may be nonproductive. Secretions may be thick, tenacious, white, gelatinous mucus, which makes their removal difficult.

The person with asthma has difficulty with air movement in and out of the lungs, which creates a feeling of suffocation. Therefore during an acute attack, the person with asthma usually sits upright or slightly bent forward using the accessory muscles of respiration to try to get enough air. The more difficult the breathing becomes, the more anxious the patient feels.

Examination of the patient during an acute attack usually reveals signs of hypoxemia, which may include restlessness, increased anxiety, inappropriate behavior, increased pulse and blood pressure, and *pulsus paradoxus* (a drop in systolic pressure during the inspiratory cycle greater than 10 mm Hg). As the patient worsens, it becomes difficult to speak in complete sentences. The respiratory rate is significantly increased (usually greater than 30 breaths per minute) with the use of accessory muscles. Percussion of the lungs indicates hyperresonance, and auscultation indicates the presence of inspiratory or expiratory wheezing. As the episode resolves, coughing produces thick, stringy mucus.

Diminished or absent breath sounds may indicate a significant decrease in air movement resulting from exhaustion and an inability to generate enough muscle force to ventilate. Severely diminished breath sounds, often referred to as the "silent chest," are an ominous sign, indicating severe obstruction and impending respiratory failure. Diminished or absent breath sounds may also indicate atelectasis or pneumothorax.

Classification of Asthma

Asthma can be classified as mild intermittent, mild persistent, moderate persistent, or severe persistent[14] (Table 29-2). Patients may move to different asthma categories over the course of their disease. Good asthma control correlates with minimal symptoms, ability to sleep through the night, and ability to participate in sports, exercise, and strenuous activity.

Complications

Severe acute asthma can result in complications such as rib fractures, pneumothorax, pneumomediastinum, atelectasis, pneumonia, and status asthmaticus.

Status Asthmaticus. **Status asthmaticus** is a severe, life-threatening asthma attack that is refractory to usual treatment and places the patient at risk for developing respiratory failure. An axiom describes status asthmaticus: "The longer it lasts, the worse it gets, and the worse it gets, the longer it lasts." Acute asthmatic attacks account for nearly 1 million emergency department (ED) visits a year in the United States and nearly 500,000 hospital admissions each year.[5]

Of the persons with asthma admitted to the hospital, approximately 10% require intensive care unit (ICU) monitoring or ventilatory assistance for status asthmaticus.[13] However, there appears to be a significant decline in patients with status asthmaticus over the past 10 years. This improvement is likely related to improved medication, education, or access to community care.[14]

Causes of status asthmaticus include viral illnesses, ingestion of aspirin or other NSAIDs, emotional stress, increases in environmental pollutants or other allergen exposure, abrupt discontinuation of drug therapy (especially corticosteroids), abuse of aerosol medication, and ingestion of β-adrenergic blockers. Usually the patient reports a history of poorly controlled asthma progressing over days or weeks.

The clinical manifestations of status asthmaticus result from increased airway resistance as a consequence of edema, mucous plugging, and severe bronchospasm with subsequent air trapping, hyperinflation, hypoxemia, and respiratory acidosis. The patient has more severe and prolonged clinical manifestations similar to those of asthma. Extreme anxiety, fear of suffocation, severely increased work of breathing, and diaphoresis are common. Absence of diaphoresis may indicate significant dehydration. Sternocleidomastoid, intercostal, and supraclavicular muscle retractions reflect increased work of breathing. If obtainable, the peak expiratory flow rate (PEFR) is usually less than 150 L/min.

Although wheezing is often audible without a stethoscope, auscultation may not always be a reliable indicator of airway obstruction. If the patient has been wheezing, yet is visibly uncomfortable, the absence of a wheeze (i.e., silent chest) is a life-threatening situation that may require mechanical ventilation. The chest appears fixed in a hyperinflated position and is often described as "tight," indicating severely decreased movement of air through the constricted bronchial airways.

TABLE 29-2 Classification of Asthma Severity

Classification	Symptoms	Nighttime Symptoms	Pulmonary Function*
Step 1 Mild intermittent	Symptoms ≤2 times/wk Asymptomatic and normal PEFR between exacerbations Exacerbations brief (hours to days) Intensity of exacerbations varies	≤2 times/mo	FEV_1/PEFR ≥80% of predicted PEFR variability <20%
Step 2 Mild persistent	Symptoms >2 times/wk but <1 time/day Exacerbations may affect activity	>2 times/mo	FEV_1/PEFR ≥80% of predicted PEFR variability 20%-30%
Step 3 Moderate persistent	Daily symptoms Daily use of inhaled short-acting β_2-agonist Exacerbations affect activity Exacerbations at least 2 times/wk and may last for days	>1 time/wk	FEV_1/PEFR >60% but <80% of predicted PEFR variability >30%
Step 4 Severe persistent	Continual symptoms Limited physical activity Frequent exacerbations	Frequent	FEV_1/PEFR ≤60% of predicted PEFR variability >30%

Source: *Practical guide for the diagnosis and management of asthma, based on Expert Panel Report 2: guidelines for the diagnosis and management of asthma,* Washington, DC, 1997, National Institutes of Health.

*Percent predicted values for forced expiratory volume in 1 second (FEV_1) and percent of personal best for peak expiratory flow rate (PEFR).

NOTES:

- Patients should be assigned to the most severe step in which any feature occurs. Clinical features for individual patients may overlap across steps.
- An individual's classification may change over time.
- Patients at any level of severity of chronic asthma can have mild, moderate, or severe exacerbations of asthma. Some patients with intermittent asthma experience severe and life-threatening exacerbations separated by long periods of normal lung function and no symptoms.
- Patients with two or more asthma exacerbations per week (i.e., progressively worsening symptoms that may last hours or days) tend to have moderate to severe persistent asthma.

Forced exhalation with the use of the abdominal musculature can result in increased intrathoracic pressure transmitted to the great vessels and heart. Neck vein distention and a pulsus paradoxus of 40 mm Hg or higher may result. Usually it is difficult to auscultate pulsus paradoxus secondary to a noisy chest or increased work of breathing. (Pulsus paradoxus is described in Chapter 37 and Table 37-8.) Hypertension, sinus tachycardia, and ventricular dysrhythmias may occur. These three conditions are related to hypoxemia, catecholamine release caused by an endogenous response to hypoxia, and underlying coronary artery disease in the older adult population. Electrocardiogram (ECG) results may show sinus tachycardia or signs of strain on the right side of the heart secondary to pulmonary vasoconstriction, which may be seen as P pulmonale (right atrial hypertrophy) and a right axis deviation.

Hypoxemia with hypocapnia usually occurs initially as the patient attempts to hyperventilate to maintain adequate oxygenation and ventilation. Arterial blood gases (ABGs) initially show hypocapnia caused by increased respiratory rate. Respiratory alkalosis may develop. As the severity of the attack increases, the work of breathing increases and the patient tires, making it more difficult for the patient to overcome the increased resistance to breathing. The patient becomes fatigued, resulting in more CO_2 retention. The patient must move greater than 150 ml of air to have air participating in gas exchange. From the nares to the alveoli (where gas exchange occurs) are areas that do not participate in the exchange of gases (e.g., nares, trachea, mainstem bronchi). The area not participating in gas exchange is called *dead space.* If the patient has a slight respiratory alkalosis and hypocarbia early in the attack because the patient is hyperventilating, diffusion is occurring. If the blood gases normalize (i.e., CO_2 is normal) but the patient is still very uncomfortable as he or she tires, and the lung sounds are quiet, the patient can be on the verge of respiratory failure. Ultimately, the patient deteriorates to hypercapnia and hypoxemia (Table 29-3). A moderate elevation in $PaCO_2$ may be tolerated without intubation and mechanical ventilation if the patient remains alert and cooperative and continues to improve during the first 2 to 3 hours of treatment.[14]

Complications of status asthmaticus include pneumothorax, pneumomediastinum, acute cor pulmonale with right ventricular failure, and severe respiratory muscle fatigue leading to respiratory arrest. Death from status asthmaticus is usually the result of respiratory arrest or cardiac failure.

Diagnostic Studies

Underdiagnosis of asthma is common. Wheezing and cough are seen with a variety of disorders, including asthma, COPD, pulmonary embolism, GERD, obesity, and pulmonary infections. Also, the elderly may have asthma symptoms confused with other comorbidities, such as heart failure. There is some controversy about how to best diagnose asthma. Common diagnostic measures are presented in Table 29-4. In general, the health care provider should consider the diagnosis of asthma if various indicators (i.e., clinical manifestations, health history, and peak flow variability) are positive. Pulmonary function tests can be used to determine the reversibility of bronchoconstriction and thus establish the diagnosis of asthma.

A detailed history is important in determining if a person has had previous attacks of a similar nature, often precipitated by a

TABLE 29-3 Arterial Blood Gas Results Correlated with Clinical Manifestations During an Acute Asthmatic Attack

Time Frame	pH	$PaCO_2$	PaO_2	Physiologic Event	Clinical Manifestations
Early in attack	↑	↓	↓	Alveolar hyperventilation → hypocarbia Respiratory alkalosis Hypoxemia secondary to ventilation-perfusion mismatch	Use of all accessory muscles of ventilation to overcome increased airway resistance Increased heart rate, diaphoresis, chest tightness, cough, wheezing
Increasing severity	N	N	↓	Adequate alveolar ventilation CO_2 not being eliminated as well Decrease in effective alveolar ventilation	Tiring of patient and difficulty with increased work of breathing
Prolonged attack, status asthmaticus	↓	↑	↓	Hypercarbia indicating that ventilation is no longer adequate Alveolar hypoventilation → respiratory acidosis Worsening hypoxemia as result of hypoventilation and ventilation-perfusion mismatch Respiratory acidosis	Exhaustion, diminished breath sounds, intubation and mechanical ventilation necessary

N, Normal.

TABLE 29-4 *COLLABORATIVE CARE* Asthma

Diagnostic

History and physical examination
Pulmonary function studies including response to bronchodilator therapy
Peak expiratory flow rate (PEFR)
Chest x-ray
Measurement of ABGs or oximetry (if severe exacerbation)
Allergy skin testing (if indicated)
Blood level of eosinophils and IgE (if indicated)
Nitric oxide levels

Collaborative Therapy

Mild Intermittent or Persistent Asthma

Identification and avoidance/elimination of triggers
Desensitization (immunotherapy) if indicated
Patient and family teaching
Drug therapy (see Tables 29-5, 29-6, and 29-7)
Asthma action plan (see Table 29-13)

Status Asthmaticus

SaO_2 monitoring
ABGs
Inhaled β_2-adrenergic agonists or anticholinergic agents
O_2 by mask or nasal prongs
IV or oral corticosteroids
IV fluids
IV magnesium
Intubation and assisted ventilation

ABGs, Arterial blood gases; *IgE*, immunoglobulin E; *SaO_2*, oxygen saturation.

known cause. Seasonal attacks may indicate pollen or other environmental triggers. Attacks that occur at night may be caused by sleeping with a cat, sleep apnea, GERD, or dust mites present in the bed linen. It is important to determine whether the patient can sleep through the night or participate in an aerobic exercise program. Finding out if the patient works in occupations (e.g., exposure to paints, chemicals) where sensitization may occur would give clues to possible triggers. Noting if there is a family history of allergies and skin rashes assists in determining if the person is prone to allergies.

The PEFR correlates with forced expiratory volume (FEV) and is a helpful tool for the health care provider to diagnose and manage asthma. A variety of peak flow meters are on the market, but there are no standardized PEFR reference values. In general, however, peak flow meters are best designed as monitoring, and not diagnostic, devices.[13]

Pulmonary function tests (PFTs) are usually within normal limits between attacks if the patient has no other underlying pulmonary disease. Pulmonary function tests are frequently used to diagnose asthma and are an objective measurement of airflow obstruction. The patient with asthma usually has a decrease in forced vital capacity (FVC), forced expiratory volume in 1 second (FEV_1), PEFR, FEV_1 to FVC ratio (FEV_1/FVC), and forced expiratory flow rate measured during the middle of FVC ($FEF_{25\%-75\%}$), with the degree of obstruction depending on the values obtained. (The normal values for pulmonary function tests are discussed in Chapter 26.)

Reversibility of lung function is key to diagnosing asthma. The patient is asked to withhold taking any bronchodilator medications for 6 to 12 hours before the scheduled PFTs. Spirometry is then performed before bronchodilator use. The patient inhales a short-acting bronchodilator (e.g., albuterol), waits 15 minutes, and the spirometry is repeated. If the patient has a 12% increase in spirometry values and 200 ml increased volume, he or she is considered to have reversibility. When correlated with classic asthma symptoms, the diagnosis is virtually confirmed. The patient may also be placed on a trial of oral corticosteroids and spirometry taken before and after steroid use to determine reversibility.[13] A PEFR improvement of 15% post–inhaled bronchodilator correlates with FEV_1 and is a helpful tool for the health care provider to diagnose asthma if office spirometry is unavailable.

Lung function parameters decrease from their baseline levels during an exacerbation. Some patients may have symptoms of asthma, but have normal lung function. Therefore measures of airway responsiveness to known bronchial irritants, such as methacholine, histamine, or exercise, may assist in establishing the diagnosis of asthma. However, a positive test does not always mean a patient has asthma. The patient may have other conditions such as allergic rhinitis. But a negative test is useful to determine that the patient does not have asthma.[4]

An elevated serum eosinophil count and elevated serum immunoglobulin E (IgE) levels are highly suggestive of *atopy* (allergic tendency), which may be the etiology of a person's asthma. Allergy skin testing may be of some value to determine sensitivity to specific allergens. However, a positive skin test does not necessarily mean that the allergen is causing the asthma attack. On the other hand, a negative allergy test does not mean that the asthma is not allergy related. A radioallergosorbent test (RAST), which is a blood test, is sometimes used to identify allergic causes in certain patients who show negative skin tests and in those who should not be skin tested (e.g., patients with severe eczema). (Allergy testing is discussed in Chapter 14.)

A chest x-ray in an asymptomatic patient with asthma is usually normal, but needs to be obtained as a baseline on initial diagnosis. A chest x-ray obtained during an acute attack usually shows hyperinflation and may reveal other complications of asthma such as mucoid impaction, pneumothorax, atelectasis, or pneumomediastinum.

If the patient has wheezing and acute distress, it is not feasible to obtain a detailed health history (although a family member may supply some pertinent information). During an acute attack of asthma, bedside spirometry (specifically FEV_1 or FVC, but usually PEFR) may be used to monitor obstruction. Pulmonary function test results, serial spirometric parameters, oximetry, and measurement of ABGs help provide information about the severity of the attack and the response to therapy. A complete blood cell count (CBC) and serum electrolytes are also obtained to help monitor the course of therapy.

A sputum specimen for culture and sensitivity may be obtained to rule out the presence of bacterial infection, especially if the patient has purulent sputum, a history of upper respiratory tract infection, a fever, or an elevated white blood cell (WBC) count. However, the vast majority of asthma exacerbations are viral in nature and sputum cultures are rarely done on an outpatient basis.

Nitric oxide levels are increased in the breath of people with asthma, and changes in nitric oxide levels may indicate whether or not treatment for asthma is working. A noninvasive test monitors a patient's response to medication by measuring the concentration of nitric oxide in exhaled breath. A decrease in exhaled nitric oxide concentration suggests that the treatment may be decreasing the lung inflammation associated with asthma.

The NIOX Nitric Oxide Test System combines equipment that detects nitric oxide and equipment that analyzes exhaled breath with a special computer system. To use this new device, the patient places a mouthpiece, connected by a breathing tube to the computer, over her or his mouth. The person inhales nitric oxide–free air to total lung capacity, and then slowly exhales into the mouthpiece. The nitric oxide concentration is displayed immediately on the computer screen.

Collaborative Care

The National Asthma Education and Prevention Program (NAEPP) of the National Heart, Lung, and Blood Institute (NHLBI) have convened expert panels to prepare guidelines for the diagnosis and management of asthma.[13,15] Principles addressed in the first NAEPP report served as a foundation for the development of reports prepared by asthma experts worldwide, and the Global Initiative for Asthma (GINA) was created. The goals of GINA are to decrease asthma morbidity and mortality rates and improve the management of asthma worldwide. The evidence in both reports is quite similar. The NAEPP guidelines are noted in several tables in the chapter (e.g., Tables 29-2 and 29-5).

Education remains the cornerstone of asthma management and should be carried out by health care providers delivering asthma care. Education should start at the time of asthma diagnosis and be integrated into every step of clinical asthma care. Asthma self-management should be tailored to the needs of each patient, maintaining sensitivity to cultural beliefs and practices. Desirable therapeutic outcomes include (1) control or elimination of chronic symptoms such as cough, dyspnea, and nocturnal awakenings; (2) attainment of normal or nearly normal lung function; (3) restoration or maintenance of normal levels of activity; (4) reduction in the number of, or elimination of, recurrent exacerbations; (5) reduction in the number of, or elimination of, ED visits and acute care hospitalizations; and (6) elimination or reduction of side effects of medications.[13] A description of asthma education programs for adults can be accessed through the American Lung Association website at *www.lungusa.org*.

Mild Intermittent and Persistent Asthma. The patient who has persistent airflow obstruction and frequent attacks of asthma should be taught to avoid triggers of acute attacks and to premedicate before exercising. The choice of drug therapy depends on the severity of symptoms (see Tables 29-4 and 29-5). The patient with mild intermittent asthma or EIA should use inhaled β_2-adrenergic agonists, cromolyn (Intal), or nedocromil (Tilade) before exercising or when anticipating exposure to allergens known to cause asthma. In all three classifications of persistent asthma, inhaled corticosteroids (ICS) are the preferred treatment as the daily long-term control medication. In mild persistent asthma, cromolyn, nedocromil, or one of the leukotriene receptor blockers (e.g., montelukast [Singulair]) is an alternative treatment if the desired effect is not reached with low-dose ICS. Moderate persistent asthma requires daily use of inhaled low- or medium-dose ICS. The lowest dose of ICS is always used when possible to minimize adverse reactions. Low- or medium-dose ICS may be combined with a long-acting inhaled β_2 agonist (e.g., salmeterol [Serevent]) either as a separate medication or in combination (e.g., fluticasone/salmeterol [Advair]). Alternatively, in conjunction with the ICS, montelukast (Singulair) or theophylline can be used. For severe persistent asthma, a combination of high-dose ICS and inhaled β_2 agonists (e.g., Advair) is used to alleviate symptoms. Some persons may require continuous oral corticosteroids, which should be maintained at the lowest dosage possible and administered on alternate days (if possible) to reduce systemic side effects.[15]

Drug Alert* - *Long-Acting β_2-Adrenergic Agonists

- *Should not be the first medicine used to treat asthma.*
- *Should be added to the treatment plan only if other controller medicines do not control asthma.*
- *Do not use these drugs to treat wheezing that is getting worse.*
- *Always use a short-acting β_2-agonist to treat sudden wheezing.*

Acute Asthma Episode. A patient frequently comes to the ED or a health care provider's office in acute respiratory distress. The choice of treatment of acute asthma depends on the severity of the attack and response to initial therapy. Severity can be measured objectively by measuring FEV_1 or PEFR. Assessing the degree or amount of change from the patient's personal best PEFR (if known) and the patient's baseline pulse oximetry results can help determine the severity of the attack. O_2 therapy should be started immediately, and the administration should be monitored by pulse oximetry to keep the SpO_2 >90% (or >95% in pregnant women and patients with coexisting heart disease). In more severe cases, oxygenation status is measured by ABGs. Initial therapy should include inhaled β_2-adrenergic agonists administered by metered-

TABLE 29-5 DRUG THERAPY
Stepwise Approach for Managing Asthma

Classification of Asthma	Long-Term Control Drugs (Taken Daily)	Quick-Relief Drugs (prn)*
Step 1 Mild intermittent	No daily medication is needed. For severe exacerbations a course of systemic corticosteroids is recommended.	Short-acting inhaled β_2-agonists
Step 2 Mild persistent	*Preferred treatment:* low-dose inhaled corticosteroids. *Alternative treatment:* cromolyn, leukotriene modifier, nedocromil, or sustained-release theophylline.	Short-acting inhaled β_2-agonists
Step 3 Moderate persistent	*Preferred treatment:* low- to medium-dose inhaled corticosteroids and long-acting inhaled β_2-agonists. *Alternative treatment:* increase inhaled corticosteroids within medium-dose range or low- to medium-dose inhaled corticosteroids and either leukotriene modifier or theophylline. If needed (particularly in patients with recurring severe exacerbations): *Preferred treatment:* increase inhaled corticosteroids within medium-dose and add long-acting inhaled β_2-agonists. *Alternative treatment:* increase inhaled corticosteroids within medium-dose range and add either leukotriene modifier or theophylline.	Short-acting inhaled β_2-agonists
Step 4 Severe persistent	*Preferred treatment:* high-dose inhaled corticosteroids and long-acting inhaled β_2-agonists and, if needed, oral corticosteroids.	Short-acting inhaled β_2-agonists

Panel Report: *Guidelines for the diagnosis and management of asthma—update on selected topics.*
Source: Quick reference of the National Asthma Education and Prevention Program (NAEPP) expert, 2002. Available at *www.nhlbi.nih.gov/guidelines/asthma/asthsumm.htm.*
*Intensity of treatment will depend on severity of exacerbation; up to three treatments at 20-minute intervals or a single nebulizer treatment as needed. Course of systemic corticosteroids may be needed. Use of short-acting β-agonists >2 times a week in intermittent asthma (daily, or increasing use in persistent asthma) may indicate the need to initiate (increase) long-term control therapy.

dose inhaler (MDI) using spacer devices or a nebulizer. Generally, aerosolized medications by nebulizer therapy or by MDI with a spacer are given every 20 minutes for 1 hour. If the exacerbation is severe, anticholinergic medication (ipratropium [Atrovent]) is nebulized with the β_2-adrenergic agonist every 20 minutes or continuously for 1 hour.

Systemic corticosteroids speed the resolution of asthma exacerbations and are integral to the management of all but the mildest of exacerbations. Corticosteroids are indicated if the initial response to the β_2-adrenergic agonist is insufficient (e.g., no response within 30 to 60 minutes), if the patient has had several recent asthma attacks, or if the patient is receiving oral corticosteroid therapy. Oral routes are usually as effective as intravenous (IV) routes and less invasive and less expensive. If there are concerns about compliance, intramuscular administration can be given. If there are concerns of impending respiratory arrest, IV administration is needed. Therapy should be continued until the patient is breathing comfortably, wheezing has disappeared, and pulmonary function study results are near baseline values.[16]

Status Asthmaticus. An important predictor of whether the patient develops status asthmaticus from severe asthma is a prior history of intubation and mechanical ventilation. Management of the patient with status asthmaticus focuses on correcting hypoxemia and improving ventilation. Most of the therapeutic measures are the same as those for acute asthma. It may be necessary, however, to increase the frequency and dose of inhaled bronchodilators. An inhaled β_2-adrenergic agonist, usually albuterol, is given hourly or continuously via nebulizer and may be mixed with an anticholinergic (ipratropium). This combination of medications will provide better bronchodilation than either drug alone. Therapy with inhaled agents is usually initiated despite prior home use because drug delivery at home may have been submaximal and higher doses given under supervision may be beneficial.

Continuous monitoring of the patient is critical. Obtaining a PEFR during a severe asthma attack is usually not possible. However, if it can be obtained and it is <200 L/min, it indicates severe obstruction in all but very small adults. IV corticosteroids (methylprednisolone) are administered every 4 to 6 hours, although their peak effect is not apparent for 4 to 12 hours. Oral corticosteroids are often as effective as IV. In selected groups of patients IV magnesium sulfate is given as a one-time infusion to act as a bronchodilator. Although it is no longer listed in the guidelines for asthma management, subcutaneous epinephrine is occasionally administered if selective β_2-adrenergic agonists are not available. If administered, patients need their blood pressure (BP) and ECG monitored closely.[4]

Supplemental O_2 is given by mask or nasal prongs to achieve a PaO_2 of at least 60 mm Hg or an O_2 saturation >90%. An arterial catheter may be inserted to facilitate frequent ABG monitoring. Because the patient's insensible loss of fluids is increased and the metabolic rate is increased, moderate rates of IV fluids are given to provide optimal hydration. Sodium bicarbonate administration is usually limited to treatment of severe metabolic or respiratory acidosis (pH <7.29) in the mechanically ventilated patient because effective bronchodilation by β-adrenergic agonists is not possible if the patient has extreme acidosis. Bronchoscopy, although rarely performed during an acute attack, may be necessary to remove thick mucous plugs.

Occasionally, asthma attacks are so severe that the patient requires intubation and mechanical ventilation if there is no response to treatment. Indications for mechanical ventilation are persistent or progressive CO_2 retention >42 to 45 mm Hg; clinical deterioration indicated by fatigue; declining mental clarity, such as hypersomnolence; hypoxemia (PaO_2 <60 mm Hg) despite supplemental oxygen; and cardiopulmonary arrest.[13] In status asthmaticus, the goals of initiating mechanical ventilation are to achieve a PaO_2 ≥60 mm Hg, an O_2 saturation ≥90%, and a normal pH.

Louder wheezing may actually occur in the airways that are responding to the therapy as airflow in the airways increases. As improvement continues and airflow increases, breath sounds increase and wheezing decreases. As the patient begins to respond to therapy and symptoms begin to subside, it is important to remember that despite the disappearance of most of the bronchospasm, the edema and cellular infiltration of the airway mucosa and the viscous mucous plugs may take several days to improve. Thus intensive therapy must be continued even after clinical improvement has occurred.

IV corticosteroids are usually tapered rapidly and the patient is started on the oral form. The length of oral prednisone treatment is usually about 14 days. Inhaled corticosteroids are usually added while the patient is still in the hospital. High-dose inhaled corticosteroids prevent asthma relapse and may be prescribed until the patient can step down to lower doses. Nebulized medications are continued for several days even after clinical improvement is noted. Antibiotics are not recommended for asthma treatment unless there are signs of bacterial pneumonia, fever, and purulent sputum, suggesting bacterial infections. Chest physiotherapy has no role and is generally not recommended for asthma because it is too stressful for the breathless patient.[13] The patient's cough often becomes productive of mucous plugs, and breath sounds improve. If the patient is asked to perform a forced expiratory maneuver, a faint wheeze may still be heard. The patient can be switched to a β_2-adrenergic agonist administered via MDI before discharge.

Drug Therapy

A stepwise approach to drug therapy is based on the asthma severity (see Table 29-5). Persistent asthma requires daily long-term therapy in addition to appropriate medications to manage acute asthma exacerbations. Medications are divided into two general classifications: (1) long-term–control medications to achieve and maintain control of persistent asthma and (2) quick-relief medications to treat symptoms and exacerbations[15] (Table 29-6).

Antiinflammatory Drugs

Corticosteroids. Because chronic inflammation is a primary component of asthma, corticosteroids, which suppress the inflammatory response, are the most potent and effective antiinflammatory medication currently available to treat asthma (Table 29-7). The inhaled form of corticosteroids is the preferred treatment in the long-term control of persistent asthma. Systemic corticosteroids are used to gain prompt control of asthma in exacerbations and also to manage severe persistent asthma that is not controlled with maximal inhaled therapy.[13]

Corticosteroids reduce symptoms of asthma by suppressing the inflammatory response.[17] By decreasing the inflammation, corticosteroids reduce bronchial hyperresponsiveness. They also decrease mucus production and increase the number of bronchial β_2 receptors, as well as their responsiveness to β_2-adrenergic agonists.

TABLE 29-6 DRUG THERAPY
Long-Term Control versus Quick Relief of Asthma

Long-Term Control Medications
Antiinflammatory Drugs
Corticosteroids (inhaled or oral)
Cromolyn (Intal) and nedocromil (Tilade)
Leukotriene modifiers
Omalizumab (Xolair)
Bronchodilators
Long-acting inhaled β_2-adrenergic agonists
Long-acting oral β_2-adrenergic agonists
Theophylline
Quick-Relief Medications
Bronchodilators
Short-acting inhaled β_2-adrenergic agonists
Anticholinergics (inhaled)
Antiinflammatory Drugs
Corticosteroids (systemic)*

*Considered quick-relief drugs when used in a short burst (3 to 10 days) at the start of therapy or during a period of gradual deterioration. Corticosteroids are not used for immediate relief of an ongoing attack.

Corticosteroids are used for prophylaxis of chronic asthma. Administration of these drugs needs to be done on a fixed schedule. Inhaled corticosteroids are first-line therapy for patients with asthma. All patients with moderate-to-severe asthma should use these drugs[18] (see Table 29-5). Usually, inhaled corticosteroids must be administered for 1 to 2 weeks before maximum therapeutic effects can be seen. Some inhaled corticosteroids (e.g., fluticasone [Flovent], budesonide [Pulmicort]) begin to have a therapeutic effect in 24 hours.

When corticosteroids are administered in the inhaled form as MDIs or dry powder inhalers (DPIs), asthma can usually be controlled without significant systemic side effects because little systemic drug absorption occurs from these devices. However, inhaled corticosteroids, particularly at the highest dosage levels, have been associated with the development of side effects such as easy bruising, accelerated bone loss, and suppression of the hypothalamic-pituitary-adrenal axis.[17] Oropharyngeal candidiasis, hoarseness, and dry cough are local side effects caused by inhalation of corticosteroids. These problems can be reduced or prevented by using a spacer (Fig. 29-4) with the MDI and by gargling with water or mouthwash after each use. Using a spacer or holding device for inhalation of inhaled corticosteroids can be helpful in getting more medication into the lungs.

Short courses of orally administered corticosteroids are indicated for acute exacerbations of asthma. Side effects associated with short-term therapy include insomnia, heartburn, mood swings, blurry vision, headache, increased appetite, and weight gain. Maintenance doses of oral corticosteroids may be necessary to control asthma in a minority of patients with severe chronic asthma when long-term therapy is required. A single dose in the morning to coincide with endogenous cortisol production and alternate-day dosing are associated with fewer side effects. (Side effects of long-term corticosteroid therapy are discussed in Chapter 50.) Women, especially postmenopausal women, who have asthma and who use corticosteroids should take adequate amounts of calcium and vitamin D and participate in regular weight-bearing exercise. (Osteoporosis is discussed in Chapter 64.)

TABLE 29-7 ***DRUG THERAPY*** **Asthma and Chronic Obstructive Pulmonary Disease**

Drug	Route of Administration	Side Effects	Comments
Antiinflammatory Agents			
Corticosteroids			
hydrocortisone (Solu-Cortef)	IV	Cushingoid appearance, skin changes (acne, striae, bruising), osteoporosis, increased appetite, obesity; peptic ulcer, hypertension, hypokalemia, cataracts, menstrual irregularities, muscle weakness, immunosuppression, catabolism, dysphonia, growth retardation	Alternate-day therapy minimizes side effects. Oral dose should be taken in morning with food or milk. When given in high doses, observe for epigastric distress. The patient taking long-term corticosteroids may be given vitamin D and calcium to prevent osteoporosis. Discontinue gradually over time to prevent adrenal insufficiency. If during tapering symptoms recur, health care provider should be notified.
methylprednisolone (Medrol, Solu-Medrol)	Oral IV		
prednisone	Oral		
beclomethasone (Vanceril, Beclovent, Vanceril DS, Qvar, Qvar HFA)	MDI, nasal spray	Oral thrush infections, hoarseness, irritated throat, dry mouth, cough, few systemic effects	Not recommended for acute asthma attack. Rinse mouth with water or mouthwash after use to prevent oral fungal infections. Use of spacer device with MDI may decrease incidence of thrush. Nasal spray is used for allergic rhinitis.
triamcinolone (Azmacort)	MDI	Same as above	Same as above. Advantage is that it has a built-in spacer device.
flunisolide (AeroBid, AeroBid-M)	MDI	Same as above	AeroBid-M contains menthol.
fluticasone (Flovent HFA, Flovent Diskus)	MDI, DPI	High incidence of yeast infections	Same as beclomethasone.
budesonide (Pulmicort Turbuhaler, Pulmicort Respules)	DPI, oral	Same as above	
mometasone (Asmanex Twisthaler)	DPI	Same as above	
Mast Cell Stabilizers			
cromolyn (Intal)	Nebulizer, MDI	Irritation of throat, relatively nontoxic effects, bronchospasm	Used for asthma (e.g., before exercise) prophylactically if allergen is causative agent. Instruct patient in correct use of inhaler. May follow treatment with glass of water to reduce pharyngeal irritation. Maximal effects may take several weeks before clinical response occurs.
nedocromil (Tilade)	MDI	Same as above; transient unpleasant taste, rhinitis	Same as above.
Anticholinergics			
Short-Acting			
ipratropium (Atrovent)	Nebulizer, MDI	Drying of oral mucosa, cough, flushing of skin, bad taste	Alternating schedules of β-adrenergic agonists and atropine administration may be helpful in some patients. Temporary blurred vision will occur if sprayed in eyes. Use cautiously in patients with narrow-angle glaucoma or prostatic enlargement.
Long-Acting			
tiotropium (Spiriva)	DPI	Dry mouth, upper respiratory infection	May have blurred vision if powder comes in contact with eyes. Must discontinue use of ipratropium while on Spiriva. Patient must use short-acting β-adrenergic agonists for quick relief medication.
IgE Antagonist			
omalizumab (Xolair)	Subcutaneous injection	Injection site reaction (e.g., bruising, redness, warmth, pain)	Only for moderate to severe persistent allergic asthma with symptoms not adequately controlled by ICS. Not for acute bronchospasm. Serum IgE and body weight are used to determine doses of drug.

DPI, Dry powder inhaler; *GI,* gastrointestinal; *HFA,* hydrofluoroalkane (propellant); *IV,* intravenous; *MDI,* metered-dose inhaler.

TABLE 29-7 DRUG THERAPY
Asthma and Chronic Obstructive Pulmonary Disease—cont'd

Drug	Route of Administration	Side Effects	Comments
Leukotriene Modifiers			
Leukotriene Receptor Blocker			
zafirlukast (Accolate)	Oral tablets	Headache, dizziness; nausea, vomiting, diarrhea, fatigue, abdominal pain	Take at least 1 hr before or 2 hr after meals. Affects metabolism of erythromycin and theophylline. Not to be used to treat acute asthma episodes.
montelukast (Singulair)	Oral tablets, chewable tablets, oral granules	Well tolerated	Not to be used to treat acute asthma episodes.
Leukotriene Inhibitor			
zileuton (Zyflo)	Oral tablets	↑ liver enzymes; dizziness, insomnia, dyspepsia, abdominal pain	Monitor liver enzymes. May interfere with metabolism of warfarin (Coumadin) and theophylline. Not to be used to treat acute asthma episodes.
β_2-Adrenergic Agonists			
Inhaled: Short-Acting*			
metaproterenol (Alupent, Metaprel)	Nebulizer, oral tablets, elixir, MDI	Tachycardia, BP changes, nervousness, palpitations, muscle tremors, nausea, vomiting, vertigo, insomnia, dry mouth, headache, hypokalemia	Should not be used in patient with angina or other cardiac disorders. Has fairly rapid onset of action (5-10 min). Duration of action is 3-4 hr. Oral lasts up to 8 hr.
albuterol (Proventil, Proventil HFA, Ventolin, Ventolin HFA, Salbutamol, Volmax)	Nebulizer, MDI, oral tablets, rotahaler	Same as above but cardiac effects are less	Has rapid onset of action (1-3 min). Duration of action is 4-8 hr.
levalbuterol (Xopenex, Xopenex HFA)	Nebulizer, MDI	Tachycardia, nervousness, tremor	Too frequent use can result in loss of effectiveness.
pirbuterol (Maxair)	MDI	Same as metaproterenol but cardiac effects are less	
terbutaline (Bricanyl, Brethine)	Oral tablets, nebulizer, subcutaneous, MDI	Same as above	Has slow onset of action (except nebulized and subcutaneous route). Duration of action is 4-6 hr.
bitolterol (Tornalate)	MDI, nebulizer	Same as above	Duration of action is 4-8 hr.
Inhaled: Long-Acting			
salmeterol (Serevent)	DPI	Headache, throat dryness, tremor, dizziness, pharyngitis	Not to exceed 2 puffs every 12 hours. Not to be used for acute exacerbations.
formoterol (Foradil)	DPI	Angina, tachycardia, nervousness, headache, tremor, dizziness	Can affect blood glucose levels. Should be used with caution in patients with diabetes.
Immediate-Acting			
epinephrine (Adrenalin)	Subcutaneous	Headache, dizziness, palpitations, hypertension, dysrhythmias, tachycardia	Used primarily to treat severe asthma attacks. Should not be used in patient with dysrhythmias or hypertension.
Methylxanthines			
IV agent: aminophylline (rarely used) *Oral:* Elixophyllin, Quibron, Slo-bid, Slo-Phyllin, Theochron, Theolair, Theo-24, Uniphyl	Oral tablets, IV, elixir, sustained-release tablets	Tachycardia, BP changes, dysrhythmias, anorexia, nausea, vomiting, nervousness, irritability, headache, muscle twitching, flushing, epigastric pain, diarrhea, insomnia, palpitations	Wide variety of response to drug metabolism exists. Half-life is decreased by smoking and is increased by heart failure and liver disease. Cimetidine, ciprofloxacin, erythromycin, and other drugs may rapidly increase theophylline levels. Taking drug with food or antacids may help GI effects. Patient must be encouraged to take drugs even when feeling well.

BP, Blood pressure; *DPI,* dry powder inhaler; *GI,* gastrointestinal; *HFA,* hydrofluoroalkane (propellant); *IV,* intravenous; *MDI,* metered-dose inhaler.
*Although these drugs are available in oral preparations, they are classified in this table based on their onset and duration of action as an inhaled drug.

Continued

TABLE 29-7 DRUG THERAPY
Asthma and Chronic Obstructive Pulmonary Disease—cont'd

Drug	Route of Administration	Side Effects	Comments
Combination Agents			
ipratropium and albuterol (Combivent, DuoNeb)	MDI, nebulizer	Chest pain, pharyngitis, diarrhea, nausea	Patients must be careful not to overuse. Must take as prescribed.
fluticasone/salmeterol (Advair)	DPI	Headache, pharyngitis, oral candidiasis	See salmeterol and fluticasone.
budesonide/formoterol (Symbicort)	MDI	Dysrhythmias, hypertension, paradoxic bronchospasm	See budesonide and formoterol

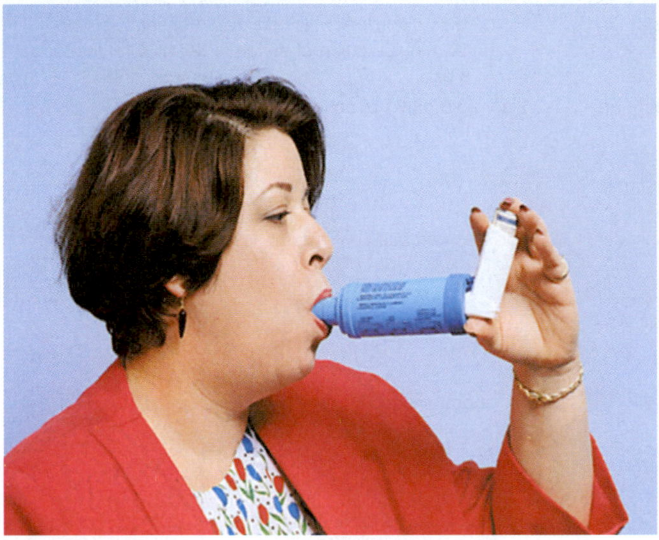

FIG. 29-4 Example of an AeroChamber spacer used with a metered-dose inhaler.

Mast Cell Stabilizers. Cromolyn (Intal) and nedocromil (Tilade) are classified as mast cell stabilizers. These nonsteroidal antiinflammatory drugs inhibit the IgE-mediated release of inflammatory mediators from mast cells and suppress other inflammatory cells (e.g., eosinophils). They inhibit the immediate response related to exercise and allergens, but are not used to treat acute bronchospasm. Long-term administration can reduce bronchial hyperresponsiveness and prevent the increased bronchial hyperresponsiveness associated with pollens in susceptible asthmatics. These drugs can be used successfully for seasonal asthma and if someone is anticipating encountering a trigger in a few days (e.g., visit a home where a cat resides). They are particularly effective in exercise-induced asthma when used 10 to 20 minutes before exercise. Cromolyn can be nebulized or inhaled via a Spinhaler device whereas nedocromil is only inhaled. Few adverse effects are associated with these drugs.[16]

Leukotriene Modifiers. Leukotriene modifiers include leukotriene receptor blockers (antagonists) (zafirlukast [Accolate], montelukast [Singulair]) and leukotriene synthesis inhibitors (zileuton [Zyflo]). These drugs interfere with the synthesis or block the action of leukotrienes. Leukotrienes are inflammatory mediators that are produced from arachidonic acid metabolism (see Chapter 13, Fig. 13-5). Leukotrienes are potent bronchoconstrictors, and some also cause airway edema and inflammation, thus contributing to the symptoms of asthma. Because these drugs block the release of some substances from mast cells and eosinophils, they have both bronchodilator and antiinflammatory effects. These drugs are not indicated for use in the reversal of bronchospasm in acute asthma attacks. They are used for prophylactic and maintenance therapy. One advantage of leukotriene modifiers is that they are only administered orally.[19] Leukotriene modifiers can successfully be used as add-on therapy to reduce (not substitute for) the doses of inhaled corticosteroids. They are less effective than long-acting β_2-adrenergic agonists as add-on therapy. There are few adverse effects from these drugs, but liver functions should be monitored during treatment with zileuton.

Monoclonal Antibody to IgE. Omalizumab (Xolair) is a monoclonal antibody to IgE that decreases circulating free IgE levels. Omalizumab prevents IgE from attaching to mast cells, thus preventing the release of chemical mediators. A reduction in corticosteroids and improved asthma control have been found with the administration of omalizumab. The indication for the drug is moderate to severe persistent, allergic asthma that cannot be controlled with inhaled corticosteroids. Omalizumab is administered subcutaneously every 2 to 4 weeks and costs about $10,000 per year but most medical insurance will cover it.[4] The drug has a small risk of anaphylaxis and cancer.

Bronchodilators. Three classes of bronchodilator drugs currently used in asthma therapy are β_2-adrenergic agonists (also referred to as β_2 agonists), methylxanthines and derivatives, and anticholinergics (see Table 29-7).

β_2-Adrenergic Agonist Drugs. Short-acting inhaled β_2-adrenergic agonists are the most effective drugs for relieving acute bronchospasm. They are also used for acute exacerbations of asthma.[17] Examples of these drugs include albuterol (Proventil, Proventil HFA, Ventolin), metaproterenol (Alupent), bitolterol (Tornalate), and pirbuterol (Maxair). These drugs have an onset of action within minutes and are effective for 4 to 8 hours. These drugs act by stimulating β-adrenergic receptors in the bronchioles, thus producing bronchodilation. They also increase mucociliary clearance.

Drug Alert - *β_2-Adrenergic Agonists*
- *Should not be used in patients with angina or cardiac disorders.*
- *Overuse may cause rebound bronchospasm.*

β_2-Adrenergic agonists are also useful in preventing bronchospasm precipitated by exercise and other stimuli because they prevent the release of inflammatory mediators from mast cells. They do not inhibit the late-phase response of asthma or have antiinflammatory effects. If used frequently, inhaled β_2-adrenergic agonists may produce tremors, anxiety, tachycardia, palpitations, and nausea. Overuse of β_2-adrenergic agonists may cause rebound bronchospasm, which is especially common with albuterol. Too frequent use of β_2-adrenergic agonists indicates poor asthma control, may mask asthma severity, and may lead to reduced drug effectiveness. Inhaled β_2 agonists are not first-choice drugs for long-term control, and they should not be used alone. They should be added to the treatment regimen when control has been inadequate with a preferred long-acting drug (e.g., inhaled corticosteroid). Oral β_2 agonists are used for long-term control. However, they should not be used alone or as first-line therapy in treating asthma.

Long-acting (12 hours) inhaled β_2-adrenergic agonists include salmeterol (Serevent) and formoterol (Foradil). They should not be the first medications used to treat asthma. Long-acting β_2 agonists should be used only in patients taking a recommended medication for long-term control, and only if that medication has been inadequate by itself.[20,21] Salmeterol should not be initiated in patients with significantly worsening or acutely deteriorating asthma. Patients should have a short-acting β_2 agonist available for acute breathing problems. If patients need more medicine than short-acting β_2 agonists, inhaled corticosteroids should be added first and then salmeterol added if the other drugs are not enough to control symptoms.

Long-acting inhaled β_2 agonists may increase the risk of severe asthma and asthma-related death, but only when used incorrectly (i.e., as first-line monotherapy for long-term control). When used as recommended, they are safe.[20] Patients should be told that salmeterol should not be used for acute symptoms. Patient teaching should stress that these drugs are used only once every 12 hours and are not used to obtain quick relief from bronchospasm.

Combination therapy using an inhaled corticosteroid (fluticasone) and an inhaled long-acting β_2-adrenergic agonist (salmeterol) is available as Advair Diskus. Adding an inhaled corticosteroid to an inhaled long-acting β_2-adrenergic agonist results in improved lung function, decreased nocturnal asthma, decreased need for short-acting β_2-adrenergic agonists, decreased asthma symptoms, and reduced number of exacerbations. Patients should receive this combination drug only if they are not responding to low or medium doses of inhaled corticosteroids.

Methylxanthines. Methylxanthine (theophylline) preparations are less effective long-term control bronchodilators than β_2-adrenergic agonists. The trend in the United States is now toward introducing theophylline as an alternative bronchodilator if other agents are not effective. Theophylline is not effective as an inhalant. Sustained-release theophylline preparations are preferred for maintenance therapy. Although the exact mechanism of action is unknown, the main therapeutic action of theophylline is bronchodilation.

Drug Alert - *Theophylline*
- *Instruct patient to report signs of toxicity:*
  - *Nausea, vomiting, seizures, insomnia.*
- *Avoid caffeine to prevent intensifying adverse effects.*

Theophylline alleviates the early phase of asthma attacks and the bronchoconstrictive component of the late-phase asthmatic response. However, it has little or no effect on bronchial hyperresponsiveness. Long-acting theophylline products administered at bedtime may be used to treat the patient with nocturnal asthma. The main problem with theophylline is the relatively high incidence of interaction with other drugs and the occurrence of side effects, which include nausea, headache, insomnia, gastrointestinal distress, tachycardia, dysrhythmias, and seizures. Theophylline has a narrow margin of safety, and serum blood levels should be monitored regularly to determine if the drug is within therapeutic range.[13]

Anticholinergic Drugs. Airway diameter is predominantly controlled by the parasympathetic division of the autonomic nervous system. The effects of acetylcholine on the airways are increased mucus secretion and smooth muscle contraction, resulting in bronchoconstriction. Anticholinergic agents (e.g., ipratropium [Atrovent]) block the bronchoconstricting influence of the parasympathetic nervous system. In asthma these drugs are less effective than β_2-adrenergic agonists and are usually used in combination with other bronchodilators. Because anticholinergics and β_2 agonists promote bronchodilation by different mechanisms, their beneficial effects are additive. Anticholinergics are also used in combination with β_2-adrenergic agonists (e.g., ipratropium and albuterol [Combivent]).

The onset of action of ipratropium is slower than β_2-adrenergic agonists, peaking at 30 minutes to 1 hour and lasting up to 4 to 6 hours. Systemic side effects of inhaled anticholinergics are uncommon because they are poorly absorbed. The most common side effect of anticholinergic drugs is a dry mouth.

Patient Teaching Related to Drug Therapy. Information about medications should include the name, dosage, method of administration, and schedule, taking into consideration meal times and other activities of daily living (ADLs). Teaching should also include purpose, side effects, appropriate action if side effects occur, consequences of improper use, and the importance of refilling the prescription before the medication runs out.

One of the major factors determining success in asthma management is the correct administration of drugs. There are multiple devices for asthma drug administration, and it can be confusing. The majority of asthma drugs are administered only or preferably by inhalation. Inhalation of drugs is often preferred to oral administration because systemic side effects are reduced. In addition, the onset of action of bronchodilators is faster. Inhalation devices include metered-dose inhalers (MDIs), dry powder inhalers (DPIs), and nebulizers. MDIs are small, handheld, pressurized devices that deliver a measured dose of drug with each activation. Dosing is usually accomplished with one or two puffs. Nebulizers are small machines used to convert drug solutions into mists. Inhalation of the mist can be done through a face mask or mouthpiece held between the teeth. They are usually used for severe asthma or for individuals who have difficulty with the MDI inhalation.

Individuals who have poor coordination can solve this problem by using a spacer device (AeroChamber, InspirEase) (see Fig. 29-4). Adding a spacer to an MDI also improves inhalation of the drug.[22] If an MDI uses hydrofluoroalkane (HFA) as a propellant, it may be incompatible with a spacer.

The MDI should be cleaned by removing the dust cap and rinsing it in warm water at least two times per week (Fig. 29-5). The patient who needs to use several MDIs is often unclear about the

Using an inhaler seems simple, but most patients do not use it the right way. When you use your inhaler the wrong way, less medicine gets to your lungs. (Your doctor may give you other types of inhalers.)

For the next 2 weeks, read these steps aloud as you do them or ask someone to read them to you. Ask your doctor or nurse to check how well you are using your inhaler.

Use your inhaler in one of the three ways pictured below (**A** or **B** are best, but **C** can be used if you have trouble with **A** and **B**).

Steps for Using Your Inhaler

Getting ready

1. Take off the cap and shake the inhaler.
2. Breathe out all the way.
3. Hold your inhaler the way your doctor said (**A, B,** or **C** below).

Breathe in slowly

4. As you start breathing in **slowly** through your mouth, press down on the inhaler **one** time. (If you use a holding chamber, first press down on the inhaler. Within 5 sec, begin to breathe in slowly.)
5. Keep breathing in **slowly,** as deeply as you can.

Hold your breath

6. Hold your breath as you count to 10 slowly, if you can.
7. For inhaled quick-relief medicine (β_2 agonists), wait about 1 min between puffs. There is no need to wait between puffs for other medicines.

A. Hold inhaler 1 to 2 in in front of your mouth (about the width of two fingers).

B. Use a spacer/holding chamber. These come in many shapes and can be useful to any patient.

C. Put the inhaler in your mouth. Do not use for steroids.

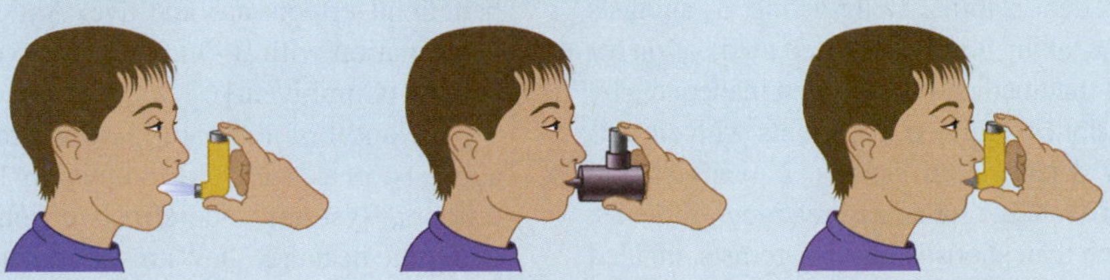

Clean Your Inhaler as Needed

Look at the hole where the medicine sprays out from your inhaler. If you see "powder" in or around the hole, clean the inhaler. Remove the metal canister from the L-shaped plastic mouthpiece. Rinse only the mouthpiece and cap in warm water. Let them dry overnight. In the morning, put the canister back inside. Put the cap on.

Know When to Replace Your Inhaler

For medicines you take each day (an example):
Say your new canister has 200 puffs (number of puffs is listed on canister) and you are told to take 8 puffs per day.

$$8 \text{ puffs per day}\overline{\big) \; 200 \text{ puffs in canister}} = 25 \text{ days}$$

So this canister will last 25 days. If you started using this inhaler on May 1, replace it on or before May 25.

You can write the date on your canister.

For **quick-relief medicine take as needed** and count each puff.

Do not put your canister in water to see if it is empty. This does not work.

FIG. 29-5 How to use your metered-dose inhaler correctly.

order in which to take the medications. Historically it has been recommended that short-term β_2-adrenergic agonists should be used first to open up the airway and improve the delivery of subsequent medications. However, this is no longer recommended because there is no evidence demonstrating that it is beneficial, and it is a potential source of confusion to patients because the short-term β_2-adrenergic agonists are usually used on an as-needed (prn) basis.[23]

One of the major problems with metered-dose drugs is the potential for overuse, that is, using them much more frequently than prescribed (>2 canisters/month), rather than seeking needed medical care (Table 29-8). As a patient develops additional asthmatic symptoms, she or he may use the β_2-adrenergic agonist MDI re-

TABLE 29-8 Problems Encountered with Metered-Dose Inhaler (MDI) Use

1. Failing to coordinate activation with inspiration
2. Activating MDI in the mouth while breathing through nose
3. Inspiring too rapidly
4. Not holding the breath for 10 sec (or as close to 10 sec as possible)
5. Holding MDI upside down or sideways
6. Inhaling more than 1 puff with each inspiration
7. Not shaking MDI before use
8. Not waiting a sufficient amount of time between each puff
9. Not opening mouth wide enough, causing medication to bounce off teeth, tongue, or palate
10. Not having adequate strength to activate MDI
11. Unable to understand and incorporate directions

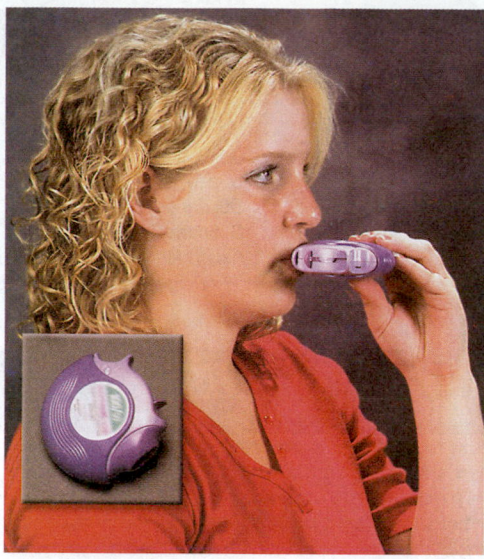

FIG. 29-6 Example of a dry powder inhaler (DPI).

TABLE 29-9 ***PATIENT AND FAMILY TEACHING GUIDE*** **How to Use a Dry Powder Inhaler (DPI)**

1. Remove mouthpiece cap or open the device according to manufacturer's instructions. Check for dust or dirt. If there is an external counter, note the number of doses remaining.
2. Load the medicine into the inhaler or engage the lever to allow the medicine to become available. Some DPIs should be held upright while loading. Others should be held sideways or in a horizontal position.
3. Do not shake your medicine.
4. Tilt your head back slightly and breathe out, getting as much air out of your lungs as you can. Do not breathe into your inhaler because this could affect the dose.
5. Close your lips tightly around the mouthpiece of the inhaler.
6. Breathe in deeply and quickly. This will ensure that the medicine moves down deeply into your lungs. You may not taste or sense the medicine going into your lungs.
7. Hold your breath for 10 seconds or as long as you can to disperse the medicine into your lungs.
8. If there is an external counter, note the number of doses remaining. It should be one less than the number in step 1 above.
9. Do not keep your DPI in a humid place such as a shower room because the medicine may clump.

TABLE 29-10 Comparison of Metered-Dose and Dry Powder Inhalers

	Metered-Dose Inhaler (MDI)*	Dry Powder Inhaler (DPI)
Shaking before use	Yes, shake well	No
Inspiration	Slow	Rapid
Spacer	Yes, at least with inhaled corticosteroids	None permitted
Counting device	No external device	Most preloaded forms include counter
Inhalations/dose	Often 2/dose	Often 1/dose
Cleaning	Use water for plastic case	Avoid moisture

*Some MDIs use hydrofluoroalkane (HFA) as a propellant and shaking or a spacer may not be needed.

peatedly. β_2-Adrenergic agonists help by relieving bronchospasm; they do not treat the inflammatory response. Therefore the patient must receive explicit instructions in the correct therapeutic use of these drugs. Also the patient needs to know the correct way to determine if the MDI is empty (see Fig. 29-5). In the past, floating the MDI in water was an appropriate way to determine if medication remained in the MDI. That is not recommended because it is not accurate and water can enter the MDI. Patients should be taught that shaking the canister is not an accurate way to determine if the MDI is empty because they may be hearing only the propellant when the MDI is nearly empty.

DPIs are simpler to use than MDIs (Fig. 29-6 and Table 29-9). The DPI contains dry, powdered medication and is breath activated. No propellant is used; instead an aerosol is created when the patient inhales through a reservoir containing a dose of powder. The convenient-to-carry diskus has several advantages over MDIs: (1) less manual dexterity is needed; (2) there is no need to coordinate device puffs with inhalation; (3) an easily visible color or number system indicates the number of doses left in the diskus; and (4) no spacer is required. Disadvantages are that commonly prescribed drugs are not yet available in DPIs and the medication may clump if exposed to humidity. Since the medicine is only delivered by the patient's inspiratory effort, patients with a low FEV_1 (<1 L) may not be able to inspire the medication adequately.

Differences between MDIs and DPIs are presented in Table 29-10. Aerosolized medication delivery systems, when used with comparable drug doses, provide equivalent efficacy. Therefore the device should be best suited to the individual patient.

Poor adherence with asthma therapy is a major challenge in the long-term management of chronic asthma. Lack of adherence often occurs because the patient has no symptoms. Thus the patient does not realize that the inflammatory process is ongoing at all times and the patient needs inhaled corticosteroids. In addition, the inhaled drugs are expensive and patients may not be able to afford them. The patient will use β_2-adrenergic agonist inhalers because they provide immediate relief of symptoms. However, if the patient is symptom free, he or she often does not use the long-term therapy (inhaled corticosteroids or cromolyn) regularly because no immediate benefit is felt. It is important to explain to the patient the importance and purpose of taking the long-term therapy regularly, emphasizing that maximum improvement may take more than 1 week. It is important to emphasize that without regular use, the swelling in the airways may progress and the asthma will likely worsen over time. The nurse needs to become familiar with the vast array of compassionate use programs offered by the pharmaceutical companies to help lower-income patients obtain medications (e.g., *www.needymeds.com*).

In addition to the typical MDI and DPI devices, a variety of other devices are used to deliver inhalant pulmonary medications. The nurse must be certain that the patient understands exactly how to use the device, and printed instructions should be given. (See *http://asthma.nationaljewish.org/treatments/devices* for instructions.) Most inhalant drugs have very clear patient instructions, but the nurse needs to either use a placebo device or the actual drug to assess the patient's ability to deliver the medication. The patient's understanding of how to deliver the drugs needs to be reassessed at every visit.

Nonprescription Combination Drugs. Several nonprescription combination drugs are available over the counter (OTC). They are usually combinations of a bronchodilator and an expectorant (Table 29-11). These agents are advertised as drugs to re-

TABLE 29-11 Nonprescription Combination Asthma Drugs

Drug Product	Ingredients: Sympathomimetic	Ingredients: Xanthine	Ingredients: Other
Bronkaid Dual Action Caplets	Ephedrine	Xanthine	Guaifenesin
Dynafed Two-Way Tablets	Ephedrine	Xanthine	Guaifenesin
Mini Two-Way Action Tablets	Ephedrine	Xanthine	Guaifenesin
Primatene tablets	Ephedrine	Xanthine	Guaifenesin
Primatene Mist Inhaler	Epinephrine	Xanthine	Ascorbic acid, alcohol

lieve bronchospasm. In general they should be avoided. Many persons consider these drugs safe because they can be obtained without a prescription. Some of the dangers of these drugs are as follows:

1. Epinephrine, found in Primatene spray, acts only for a short time and may increase the patient's heart rate and blood pressure. This drug is not recommended for use.
2. Ephedrine (found in many OTC decongestants) causes stimulation of the central nervous and cardiovascular systems. Side effects include nervousness, heart palpitations and dysrhythmias, tremors, insomnia, and increases in blood pressure. In February 2004 the Food and Drug Administration (FDA) banned dietary supplements containing ephedrine because they pose a risk of serious adverse events, including stroke and heart attack. This ban did not include OTC respiratory products, but many of the OTC aids containing ephedrine are no longer on the market.[24]

An important teaching responsibility is to warn the patient about the dangers associated with nonprescription combination drugs. These drugs are especially dangerous to a patient with underlying cardiac problems because elevated blood pressure and tachycardia often occur. The patient who persists in taking one of these medications should be cautioned to read and follow the accompanying directions on the label. Another way of discouraging the use of these drugs is to carefully monitor and reevaluate the effectiveness of the prescribed drug therapy. The drug regimen may have to be adjusted to help the patient obtain maximum relief from bronchospasm. An attitude of understanding and caring will often reassure the patient that the health care professional is concerned. This may prevent the patient from attempting to find relief at the local drugstore.

NURSING MANAGEMENT ASTHMA

Nursing Assessment

If a patient can speak and is not in acute distress, a detailed health history, including identification of any precipitating factors and what has helped alleviate attacks in the past, can be taken. Subjective and objective data that should be obtained from a patient with asthma are presented in Table 29-12.

Nursing Diagnoses

Nursing diagnoses for the patient with asthma may include, but are not limited to, those presented in NCP 29-1.

Planning

The overall goals are that the patient with asthma will (1) maintain >80% of personal best PEFR or FEV_1, (2) have minimal symptoms during the day and night, (3) maintain acceptable activity

TABLE 29-12 *NURSING ASSESSMENT* Asthma

Subjective Data

Important Health Information

Past health history: Allergic rhinitis, sinusitis, or skin allergies; previous asthma attack and hospitalization or intubation; symptoms worsened by pollen, danders, feathers, mold, dust, inhaled irritants, weather changes, exercise, smoke, menses; gastroesophageal reflux; occupational exposure to chemical irritants (e.g., paints, dust)

Medications: Use of and compliance with corticosteroids, bronchodilators, cromolyn, anticholinergics, antibiotics; pattern and amount of short-acting β-adrenergic agonist used per week; medications that may precipitate an attack in susceptible asthmatics such as aspirin, nonsteroidal antiinflammatory drugs, β-adrenergic blockers

Functional Health Patterns

Health perception–health management: Family history of allergies or asthma; recent upper respiratory infection or sinus infection

Activity-exercise: Fatigue, decreased or absent exercise tolerance; dyspnea, cough (especially at night), productive cough with yellow or green sputum or sticky sputum; chest tightness, feelings of suffocation, air hunger, talk in sentences or words/phrases, sitting upright in order to breathe

Sleep-rest: Awakened from sleep because of cough or breathing difficulties, insomnia

Coping–stress tolerance: Emotional distress, stress in work environment or in the home

Objective Data

General

Restlessness or exhaustion, confusion, upright or forward-leaning body position

Integumentary

Diaphoresis, cyanosis (circumoral, nail bed), eczema

Respiratory

Nasal discharge, nasal polyps, mucosal swelling; wheezing, crackles, diminished or absent breath sounds, and rhonchi on auscultation; hyperresonance on percussion; sputum (thick, white, tenacious), ↑ work of breathing with use of accessory muscles; intercostal and supraclavicular retractions; tachypnea with hyperventilation; prolonged expiration

Cardiovascular

Tachycardia, pulsus paradoxus, jugular venous distention, hypertension or hypotension, premature ventricular contractions

Possible Findings

Abnormal ABGs during attacks, ↓ O_2 saturation, serum and sputum eosinophilia, ↑ serum IgE, positive skin tests for allergens, chest x-ray demonstrating hyperinflation with attacks, abnormal pulmonary function tests showing ↓ flow rates; FVC, FEV_1, PEFR, and FEV_1/FVC ratio that improve between attacks and with bronchodilators

FEV_1, Forced expiratory volume in 1 second; *FVC,* forced vital capacity; *PEFR,* peak expiratory flow rate.

NURSING CARE PLAN 29-1

Patient with Asthma

NURSING DIAGNOSIS **Ineffective airway clearance** *related to* bronchospasm, excessive mucus production, tenacious secretions, and fatigue *as evidenced by* ineffective cough, inability to raise secretions, adventitious breath sounds

PATIENT GOALS
1. Maintains clear airway with removal of excessive secretions
2. Experiences normal breath sounds and respiratory rate

OUTCOMES (NOC)

Respiratory Status: Airway Patency

- Respiratory rate ____
- Respiratory rhythm ____
- Moves sputum out of airway ____
- Ease of breathing ____

Measurement Scale

1 = Severely compromised
2 = Substantially compromised
3 = Moderately compromised
4 = Mildly compromised
5 = Not compromised

INTERVENTIONS (NIC) and *RATIONALES*

Asthma Management

- Determine baseline respiratory status *to use as a comparison point.*
- Monitor rate, rhythm, depth, and effort of respiration *to determine need for intervention and evaluate effectiveness of interventions.*
- Observe chest movement, including symmetry, use of accessory muscles, and supraclavicular and intercostal muscle retractions, *to evaluate respiratory status.*
- Auscultate breath sounds, noting areas of decreased/absent ventilation and adventitious sounds, *to evaluate respiratory status.*
- Administer medication as appropriate and/or per policy and procedural guidelines *to improve respiratory function.*
- Coach in breathing/relaxation techniques *to improve respiratory rhythm and rate.*
- Offer warm fluids to drink *to liquefy secretions and promote bronchodilation.*

NURSING DIAGNOSIS **Anxiety** *related to* difficulty breathing, perceived or actual loss of control, and fear of suffocation *as evidenced by* restlessness, elevated pulse, respiratory rate, and blood pressure

PATIENT GOALS
1. Reports decreased anxiety with increased control of respirations
2. Experiences vital signs within normal limits

OUTCOMES (NOC)

Anxiety Level

- Restlessness ____
- Increased blood pressure ____
- Increased pulse rate ____
- Increased respiratory rate ____

Measurement Scale

1 = Severe
2 = Substantial
3 = Moderate
4 = Mild
5 = None

INTERVENTIONS (NIC) and *RATIONALES*

Anxiety Reduction

- Identify when level of anxiety changes *to determine possible precipitating factors.*
- Use calm, reassuring approach *to provide reassurance.*
- Stay with patient *to promote safety and reduce fear.*
- Encourage verbalization of feelings, perceptions, and fears *to identify problem areas so appropriate planning can take place.*
- Instruct patient in the use of pursed-lip breathing and relaxation techniques *to relieve tension and to promote ease of respirations.*

Continued

levels (including exercise and other physical activity), (4) have no recurrent exacerbations of asthma or decreased incidence of asthma attacks, and (5) have adequate knowledge to participate in and carry out management.

Nursing Implementation

Health Promotion. The nursing role in preventing asthma attacks or decreasing the severity focuses primarily on teaching the patient and family. The patient should be taught to identify and avoid known personal triggers for asthma (e.g., cigarette smoke, pet dander) and irritants (e.g., cold air, aspirin, foods, cats, indoor air pollution) (see Table 29-1). Use of special dust covers on mattresses and pillows is thought to significantly reduce exposure to dust mites and improve symptoms, and some evidence supports this.[25] However, other large-scale reviews of studies show that chemical and/or physical methods aimed at reducing house dust mites did not change the asthma symptoms.[26] Further studies are needed to determine methods that can reduce dust mite exposure and thus reduce symptoms in allergy-prone individuals.

If cold air cannot be avoided, dressing properly with scarves or using a mask helps reduce the risk of an asthma attack. Aspirin and NSAIDs should be avoided if they are known to precipitate an attack. Many OTC drugs contain aspirin. Therefore the patient should be instructed to read the labels carefully. Nonselective β blockers (e.g., propranolol [Inderal]) are contraindicated because they inhibit bronchodilation. Selective β blockers (e.g., atenolol) should be used with caution. Desensitization (immunotherapy) may be partially effective in decreasing the patient's sensitivity to known allergens (see Chapter 14).

Prompt diagnosis and treatment of upper respiratory tract infections and sinusitis may prevent an exacerbation of asthma. If occupational irritants are involved as etiologic factors, the patient may need to consider changing jobs. The patient should be encouraged to maintain a fluid intake of 2 to 3 L per day, good nutrition, and adequate rest. If exercise is planned, administering a β_2-adrenergic

NURSING CARE PLAN 29-1

Patient with Asthma—cont'd

NURSING DIAGNOSIS **Deficient knowledge** *related to* lack of information and education about asthma and its treatment *as evidenced by* frequent questioning regarding all aspects of long-term management

PATIENT GOALS
1. Describes the disease process and treatment regimen
2. Demonstrates correct administration of aerosol medications
3. Expresses confidence in ability for long-term management of asthma

OUTCOMES (NOC)	INTERVENTIONS (NIC) and *RATIONALES*
Asthma Self-Management	***Asthma Management***
• Describes causal factors ____ • Initiates action to avoid and manage personal triggers ____ • Monitors peak flow routinely ____ • Monitors peak flow when symptoms occur ____ • Makes appropriate medication choices ____ • Demonstrates appropriate use of inhalers, spacers, and nebulizers ____ • Self-manages exacerbations ____ • Reports uncontrolled symptoms to health care provider ____ **Measurement Scale** 1 = Never demonstrated 2 = Rarely demonstrated 3 = Sometimes demonstrated 4 = Often demonstrated 5 = Consistently demonstrated	• Determine patient/family understanding of disease and management *to assess learning needs.* • Teach patient to identify and avoid triggers as possible *to prevent asthma attacks.* • Encourage verbalization of feelings about diagnosis, treatment, and impact on lifestyle *to offer support and increase compliance with treatment.* • Educate patient about the use of the peak expiratory flow rate (PEFR) meter at home *to promote self-management of symptoms.* • Instruct patient/family on antiinflammatory and bronchodilator medications and their appropriate use *to promote understanding of effects.* • Teach proper techniques for using medication and equipment (e.g., inhaler, nebulizer, peak flow meter)* *to promote self-care.* • Establish a written plan with the patient for managing exacerbations *to plan adequate treatment of future exacerbations.*

*See Tables 29-9 and 29-14 and Fig. 29-6.

agonist, cromolyn, or nedocromil 10 to 20 minutes before the activity should prevent bronchospasm.

Acute Intervention. A goal in asthma care is to maximize the ability of the patient to safely manage acute asthma episodes via an asthma action plan developed in conjunction with the health care provider (Table 29-13). During an acute attack of asthma it is important to monitor the patient's respiratory and cardiovascular systems. This includes auscultating lung sounds; taking the pulse rate, respiratory rate, and BP; and monitoring ABGs, pulse oximetry, and PEFR. Red flags that warrant urgent medical intervention to prevent respiratory failure in a severe asthma attack would be heart rate >120 beats per minute, pulsus paradoxus, respiratory rate >30 breaths per minute, wheezes heard on chest auscultation that turn silent, patient speaks in words (not sentences), oxygen saturation <90%, PaO_2 <60 mm Hg, $PaCO_2$ >45 mm Hg, PEFR <100 L/min, and agitation.[4] The patient can take two to four puffs of a short-acting β_2 agonist every 20 minutes three times or one nebulized treatment as a rescue plan.[15] Depending on the response with alleviation of symptoms or improved peak flow, continued short-acting β_2-adrenergic agonist use and/or oral corticosteroids may be a part of the home management plan. The patient's work of breathing (i.e., use of accessory muscles, degree of fatigue) and response to therapy should also be evaluated. If the patient's condition deteriorates, the health care provider must be notified immediately to initiate prompt medical intervention in a hospital setting. Nursing interventions include administering O_2, bronchodilators, and medications (as ordered) and ongoing patient monitoring (especially lung auscultation), including the effectiveness of these interventions.

An important nursing goal during an acute attack is to decrease the patient's sense of panic. A calm, quiet, reassuring attitude may help the patient relax. The patient should be positioned comfortably (usually sitting) to maximize chest expansion. The nurse needs to stay with the patient and be available to provide additional comfort. A technique called "talking down" can help the patient to remain calm. In "talking down" the nurse gains eye contact with the patient. In a firm, calm voice the nurse coaches the patient to use pursed-lip breathing, which keeps the airways open by maintaining positive pressure, and abdominal breathing, which slows the respiratory rate and encourages deeper breaths. The nurse or family member should stay with the patient until the respiratory rate (with the assistance of the medications) has slowed. (Pursed-lip breathing is explained on p. 646.)

When the acute attack subsides, the nurse should provide rest and a quiet, calm environment for the patient. When the patient has recovered from exhaustion, the nurse should attempt to obtain information about the patient's health history and pattern of asthma. If family members are present, they may be able to provide information about the patient's health history. A thorough physical assessment should be completed (see Table 29-12). This information is important in planning an individualized nursing care plan for the patient. Well thought out, written plans involving the patient and significant others increase the patient's knowledge and control of the situation and may help improve confidence and compliance.

Ambulatory and Home Care. It is important to remember that asthma is potentially controllable and that every effort should be made to keep the patient free of symptoms. The patient with asthma usually takes several medications with different routes of

TABLE 29-13 Asthma Action Plan*

General Information:
- Name ______
- Emergency contact ______ Phone numbers ______
- Physician/health care provider ______ Phone numbers ______
- Physician signature ______ Date ______

Severity Classification	Triggers	Exercise
❍ Mild intermittent ❍ Moderate persistent ❍ Mild persistent ❍ Severe persistent	❍ Colds ❍ Smoke ❍ Weather ❍ Exercise ❍ Dust ❍ Air pollution ❍ Animals ❍ Food ❍ Other ______	1. Premedication (how much and when) ______ 2. Exercise modifications ______

■ Green Zone: Doing Well

Symptoms
- Breathing is good
- No cough or wheeze
- Can work and play
- Sleeps all night

Peak Flow Meter
More than 80% of personal best or ______

Peak Flow Meter Personal Best =

Control Medications

Medicine	How Much to Take	When to Take It

■ Yellow Zone: Getting Worse

Symptoms
- Some problems breathing
- Cough, wheeze, or chest tight
- Problems working or playing
- Wake at night

Peak Flow Meter
Between 50% and 80% of personal best or ______ and ______

Contact Physician if Using Quick Relief More Than 2 Times per Week

Continue Control Medicines and Add:

Medicine	How Much to Take	When to Take It

IF your symptoms (and peak flow, if used) return to Green Zone after 1 hour of the quick-relief treatment, THEN
- ❍ Take quick-relief medication every 4 hours for 1 to 2 days
- ❍ Change your long-term control medicines by ______
- ❍ Contact your physician for follow-up care

IF your symptoms (and peak flow, if used) DO NOT return to the GREEN ZONE after 1 hour of the quick-relief treatment, THEN
- ❍ Take quick-relief treatment again
- ❍ Change your long-term control medicines by ______
- ❍ Call your physician/health care provider within ______ hours of modifying your medication routine

■ Red Zone: Medical Alert

Symptoms
- Lots of problems breathing
- Cannot work or play
- Getting worse instead of better
- Medicine is not helping

Peak Flow Meter
Between 0% and 50% of personal best or ______ and ______

Ambulance/Emergency Phone Number:

Continue Control Medicines and Add:

Medicine	How Much to Take	When to Take It

Go to the hospital or call for an ambulance if
- ❍ Still in the red zone after 15 minutes
- ❍ You have not been able to reach your physician/health care provider for help

Call an ambulance immediately if the following danger signs are present
- ❍ Trouble walking/talking due to shortness of breath
- ❍ Lips or fingernails are blue

Source: American Lung Association, available at *www.lungusa.org.*
*Available in Spanish on Evolve Website.

administration and time frames for dosage (e.g., tapering corticosteroid schedules, using several different inhalers with different indications). The drug regimen itself can be confusing and complex. The patient with asthma must learn about the numerous medications and develop self-management strategies. The patient and the health professional need to monitor the patient's responsiveness to medication. It is easy to undermedicate or overmedicate a patient with asthma unless careful monitoring is ongoing. Some patients may benefit from keeping a diary to record medication use, the presence of wheezing or coughing, PEFR, the drug's side effects, and the activity level. This information will be valuable in helping the health care provider adjust the medication. The patient must understand the importance of continuing the medication even when symptoms are not present. If worsening bronchospasm or severe side effects of the drugs occur, the patient should seek medical attention.

Good nutrition is important. Physical exercise (e.g., swimming, walking, stationary cycling) within the patient's limit of tolerance is also beneficial. If dyspnea occurs on exertion, it can often be prevented with pretreatment of short-acting β_2-adrenergic agonist MDI, cromolyn, or nedocromil. Sleep that is uninterrupted by asthma symptoms is an important goal. If patients with asthma wake up because of asthma symptoms, their asthma is not under good control and their therapeutic plan should be reevaluated.

Written asthma action plans (see Table 29-13) should be developed together with the patient and family, especially with

TABLE 29-14 ***PATIENT AND FAMILY TEACHING GUIDE***
How to Use Your Peak Flow Meter

A peak flow meter helps you check how well your asthma is controlled. Peak flow meters are most helpful for people with moderate or severe asthma. This guide will tell you (1) how to find your personal best peak flow number, (2) how to use your personal best number to set your peak flow zones, (3) how to take your peak flow, and (4) when to take your peak flow to check your asthma each day.

Starting Out: Find Your Personal Best Peak Flow Number

To find your personal best peak flow number, take your peak flow each day for 2 to 3 weeks. Your asthma should be under good control during this time. Take your peak flow as close to the times listed below as you can.

- Between noon and 2:00 PM each day.
- Each time you take your quick-relief medicine to relieve symptoms. (Measure your peak flow *after* you take your medicine.)
- Any other time your health care provider suggests.

(These times for taking your peak flow are *only* for finding your personal best peak flow. To check your asthma each day, you will take your peak flow in the morning.)

Write down the number you get for each peak flow reading. The highest peak flow number you had during the 2 to 3 weeks is your personal best.

Your personal best can change over time. Ask your health care provider when to check for a new personal best.

Your Peak Flow Zones

Your peak flow zones are based on your personal best peak flow number. The zones will help you check your asthma and take the right actions to keep it controlled. The colors used with each zone come from the traffic light. Electronic peak flow meters can be programmed with green, yellow, and red zones.

Green Zone (80%-100% of your personal best) signals **good control.** Take your usual daily long-term–control medicines, if you take any. Keep taking these medicines even when you are in the yellow or red zones.

Yellow Zone (50%-79% of your personal best) signals **caution: your asthma is getting worse.** Add quick-relief medicines. You might need to increase other asthma medicines as directed by your doctor.

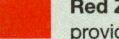

Red Zone (below 50% of your personal best) signals **MEDICAL ALERT!** Add or increase quick-relief medicines and call your health care provider ***now***.

Ask Your Health Care Provider to Write an Action Plan for You that Tells You

- The peak flow numbers for *your* green, yellow, and red zones. Mark the zones on your peak flow meter with colored tape or a marker.
- The medicines you should take while in each peak flow zone.

How to Take Your Peak Flow

1. Move the marker to the bottom of the numbered scale.
2. Stand up or sit up straight.
3. Take a deep breath. Fill your lungs all the way.
4. Hold your breath while you place the mouthpiece in your mouth, between your teeth. Close your lips around it. Do ***not*** put your tongue inside the hole.
5. Blow out as hard and fast as you can. Your peak flow meter will measure how fast you can blow out air.
6. Write down the number you get. But if you cough or make a mistake, do not write down the number. Do it over again.
7. Repeat steps 1 through 6 two more times. Write down the highest of the three numbers. This is your peak flow number.
8. Check to see which peak flow *zone* your peak flow number is in. Do the actions your doctor told you to do while in that zone.

Your health care provider may ask you to write down your peak flow numbers each day. You can do this on a calendar or other paper. This will help you and your health care provider see how your asthma is doing over time.

Checking Your Asthma: When to Use Your Peak Flow Meter

- **Every morning** when you wake up, *before* you take medicine. Make this part of your daily routine.
- **When you are having asthma symptoms or an attack.** And after taking medicine for the attack. This can tell you how bad your asthma attack is and whether your medicine is working.
- Any other time your health care provider/doctor suggests.

If you use more than one peak flow meter (such as at home and at school), be sure that both meters are the same brand.

Bring to Each of Your Health Care Provider's Visits

- Your peak flow meter.
- Your peak flow numbers if you have written them down each day.

Also, ask your health care provider or nurse to check how you use your peak flow meter—just to be sure you are doing it right.

Source: *Practical guide for the diagnosis and management of asthma, based on Expert Panel Report 2: guidelines for the diagnosis and management of asthma,* Washington, DC, 1997, National Institutes of Health.

moderate or severe persistent asthma or a history of severe exacerbations. Most plans are developed based on the patient's asthma symptoms and peak flow readings. A management plan can be established when the patient's best peak flow is established and the patient has good asthma control (e.g., not waking up at night with asthma symptoms, able to perform some type of aerobic exercise or strenuous activity, not having frequent daily symptoms).

To follow the management plan, the patient must measure his or her peak flow at least daily. Some patients may desire to just follow symptoms for self-management. Patients with asthma frequently do not perceive changes in their breathing. Therefore peak flow monitoring when done correctly can be a reliable objective measurement of asthma (Table 29-14).

If a patient's PEFR is within the green zone (usually 80% to 100% of the person's personal best), the patient should remain on her or his usual medications. If the PEFR is within the yellow zone (usually 50% to 80% of personal best), it indicates caution. Something is triggering the patient's asthma. Patients who get a cold or sinus infection, which may trigger asthma, should have a written asthma action plan that prescribes an increase in medications during the acute phase of the infection. The dose is usually decreased once the cold subsides. Different strategies may be employed by the patient based on the asthma management plan. For example, the patient could use the β_2-adrenergic agonist inhaler more frequently.

If the PEFR is in the red zone (50% or less of personal best), it indicates a serious problem. A rescue plan should be a part of the asthma action plan. Definitive action must be taken. The NAEPP suggests a rescue plan of two to four puffs of a short-acting inhaled β_2-adrenergic agonist for up to three treatments at 20-minute intervals or a single nebulizer treatment, depending on symptoms.[15] In addition to increasing the use of β_2-adrenergic agonist inhalers, oral corticosteroids may be indicated. The patient needs to contact or be seen by the health care provider.

Electronic peak flow monitors are available that store patient readings (some up to 30 readings or days) so that they do not need to write them down. They are also small and portable. In addition, they can be programmed with the patient's personal best scores and set to display whether a reading is in the green, yellow, or red zone.

It is important to emphasize to the patient the need to monitor PEFR daily to have an objective measure that can be correlated with symptoms. Although it may occur, it is unusual for a patient's PEFR to drop from the green zone to the red zone quickly. Usually the patient has time to make changes in medications, avoid triggers, and notify the health care provider.

When developing a management plan, it is important to involve the patient's family or caregiver. Often the family member feels frustrated and does not know how to help. The family member or significant other should be taught what can be done to help the patient during an asthmatic attack. This person should know where the patient's inhalers, oral medications, and emergency phone numbers are located. The significant other can also be instructed on how to decrease the patient's anxiety if an asthma attack occurs. When the patient is stabilized or controlled, the significant other can gently remind the patient about doing daily PEFR by asking questions such as, "What zone are you in? How's your peak flow today?"

An increased number of older adults are diagnosed with asthma, and they have more complicated health issues than younger patients with asthma. Issues that older adults (particularly urban, minority), caregivers, and health professionals have identified as problematic in this group are the negative impact of asthma on the quality of life, costly medications, nonadherence to medical regimen, and difficulty in accessing the health system. These factors should be kept in mind when implementing a management plan for older adults.[27]

Counseling may be indicated to help the patient and the family resolve personal, family, social, and occupational problems that have resulted from asthma. Relaxation therapies (e.g., yoga, meditation, relaxation techniques, breathing techniques) may be of value in helping a patient relax respiratory muscles and decrease the respiratory rate. (Chapter 9 discusses relaxation breathing and other relaxation strategies.) A healthy emotional outlook can also be important in preventing future asthma attacks. A variety of websites have excellent resources for patient teaching (see Resources at the end of the chapter). Some communities have asthma support groups. Table 29-15 is a patient and family teaching guide for the patient with asthma.

Evaluation

The expected outcomes for the patient with asthma are presented in NCP 29-1.

CHRONIC OBSTRUCTIVE PULMONARY DISEASE

Chronic obstructive pulmonary disease (COPD) is a preventable and treatable disease state characterized by airflow limitation that is not fully reversible. The airflow limitation is usually progressive and associated with an abnormal inflammatory response of the lungs to noxious particles or gases, primarily caused by cigarette smoking. Although COPD affects the lungs, systemic consequences also develop.[1,2]

The term *chronic obstructive pulmonary disease* encompasses two types of obstructive airway diseases, chronic bronchitis and emphysema. **Chronic bronchitis** is the presence of chronic productive cough for 3 months in each of 2 consecutive years in a patient in whom other causes of chronic cough have been excluded. **Emphysema** is an abnormal permanent enlargement of the air spaces distal to the terminal bronchioles, accompanied by destruction of their walls and without obvious fibrosis. Only about 10% of patients with COPD have pure emphysema. Patients with COPD may have a predominance of one of these conditions, but in reality it is often difficult to determine because the conditions usually coexist. COPD is discussed in this section as one disease state from the standpoint of pathophysiology and management.

Patients with COPD may have asthma, and some patients with asthma may go on to develop fixed or irreversible airflow obstruction. It may be nearly impossible to differentiate asthma from COPD, especially if the individual has a history of cigarette smoking.[2]

An estimated 10.7 million adults in the United States over age 18 have COPD. Persons with COPD are greatly underestimated because the disease is usually not diagnosed until it is moderately advanced. The number of women with COPD is on the rise because of the increased number of women smoking cigarettes. COPD is the fourth leading cause of death in the United States. Since 2000 more women than men have died from COPD. COPD is the only lung disease in which whites have more deaths than African Americans. Death rates related to COPD for Hispanics are significantly lower than other ethnic groups.[28] More than one half

GENDER DIFFERENCES
Chronic Obstructive Pulmonary Disease

Men
- More common in men than women, but trend for men is not increasing.
- Fewer men are dying from COPD than women.

Women
- Number of women with disease is increasing.
- Increase is probably due to increased number of women smoking cigarettes and increased susceptibility (e.g., smaller lungs and airways, lower elastic recoil).
- Women with disease have lower quality of life, more exacerbations, increased dyspnea, and better response to O_2 therapy.

TABLE 29-15 PATIENT AND FAMILY TEACHING GUIDE
Asthma

Goal
To assist patient in improving quality of life through education, increased understanding, and promotion of lifestyle practices that support successful living with asthma.

Teaching Topic	Resources
What Is Asthma? • Basic anatomy and physiology of lung • Pathophysiology of asthma • Relationship of pathophysiology to signs and symptoms • Measurement and correlation of pulmonary function tests and peak expiratory flow rate	*What Is Asthma?* (NIH/NHLBI) Available at *www.nhlbi.nih.gov/health/dci/Diseases/Asthma/Asthma_WhatIs.html* Q & A: What Is Asthma? (Global Initiative for Asthma). Available under patient section at *www.ginasthma.org* Understanding Asthma (National Jewish Research and Medical Center). Available at *www.nationaljewish.org/disease-info/diseases/asthma/index.aspx*
What Is Good Asthma Control?	Resource for patient on personal ideas of good control *Asthma Control Test* (American Lung Association). Also in Spanish. Available at *www.asthmacontrol.com*
Hindrances to Asthma Treatment and Control • Intermittent nature of symptoms • Role of denial • Poor perception of asthma severity by patient	Discussion with patient and family about possible hindrances
Environmental/Trigger Control • Identifications of possible triggers and possible preventive measures • Avoidance of allergens and other triggers • Need to maintain good hydration	*Home Control of Asthma and Allergies* (American Lung Association). Available under asthma section at *www.lungusa.org* *Pollen count report. Sign up for daily notification about a particular area* (American Academy of Asthma Allergy and Immunology.) Available at *www.aaaai.org/nab* Trigger diary kept by patient
Medications Types (include mechanism of action) • β_2 agonists • Cromolyn/nedocromil • Corticosteroids • Methylxanthines • Leukotriene modifiers	*Pocket Guide for Asthma Management and Prevention* (Global Initiative for Asthma). Available under Guidelines and Resources at *www.ginasthma.org*
Establishing medication schedule Use of preventive/maintenance agents (e.g., antiinflammatory agents)	Asthma Action Plan (see Table 29-13) Write out medication list and schedule
Correct Use of Metered-Dose Inhaler, Dry Powder Inhaler, Spacer, and Nebulizer	Demonstration–return demonstration with placebo devices (see Figs. 29-4, 29-5, and 29-6; see Tables 29-8, 29-9, and 29-10) *Instructions for Inhaler and Spacer Use* (Global Initiative for Asthma). Available under Guidelines and Resources at *www.ginasthma.org*
Breathing Techniques • Pursed-lip breathing	Demonstration–return demonstration
Correct Use of Peak Flow Meter	See Table 29-14 *What Is a Peak Flow Meter?* (American Lung Association). Available under asthma section at *www.lungusa.org*
Asthma Action Plan • Peak flow zones • Individualize plan • Early recognition of infection • Keeping a partnership with your health care provider • Questions patients may have about asthma, but patient cannot reach the provider	See Table 29-13 Patient completes asthma action plan and discusses it with health care provider Asthma research and new items via Internet (American Lung Association). Available at *www.lungusa.org*—click on MyLUNG USA *Asthma: Nex Profiler Treatment Option Tool.* Online decision support tool assists patient in understanding treatment options and side effects and provides them with personalized questions to ask the provider in addition to research reports (American Lung Association). Available at *www.lungusa.org* *Lung Line:* Ask a specialized nurse questions about early detection, care, and prevention of respiratory, allergic, and immune diseases (National Jewish Research and Medical Center). Telephone: 1-800-222-LUNG (5864) or (outside the United States) 303-388-4461 (7700) or *www.nationaljewish.org/ll1.html*

of COPD patients die within 10 years of diagnosis. The decrease in cigarette smoking in the United States should lead to a decrease in COPD mortality rates in the future. However, there has been a marked increase in cigarette smoking in developing countries, which will increase COPD mortality rates worldwide.[1]

Etiology

Cigarette Smoking. The major risk factor for developing COPD is cigarette smoking. Although the prevalence of cigarette smoking in the United States has decreased since 1964, it is still a major public health concern, especially among young people. Nearly all first-time use of tobacco occurs before high school graduation, and each day 2000 teens will become regular, daily smokers, with one third of them eventually dying because of a smoking-related disease.[29]

Clinically significant airway obstruction develops in approximately 15% to 20% of smokers, and 80% to 90% of COPD deaths in the United States are related to tobacco smoking.[1] For most Americans who die of lung diseases related to cigarette smoking, death is preceded by a long period of debilitation characterized by frequent hospitalizations and loss of many years of productivity. Cigarette smoking costs over $150 billion in health-related costs. Cigarette smoking remains the most preventable cause of premature death in the United States. In addition to being linked with COPD and lung cancer, cigarette smoking has also been implicated as a factor in cancers of the mouth, pharynx, larynx, esophagus, pancreas, kidney, stomach, colon, cervix, uterus, and bladder. When cigarettes are smoked, tar is inhaled, which contains approximately 4000 chemicals. Over 60 carcinogens have been isolated from cigarette smoke, including cyanide, formaldehyde, and ammonia.[29]

Nicotine is probably not a carcinogen, but it has other deleterious effects. It acts by stimulating the sympathetic nervous system, resulting in increased heart rate, increased peripheral vasoconstriction, increased BP, and increased cardiac workload. Nicotine also decreases the amount of functional hemoglobin and increases platelet aggregation. These effects of nicotine compound the problems in a person with coronary artery disease. (The effects of nicotine are discussed in Chapter 12.)

Cigarette smoke has several direct effects on the respiratory tract (Table 29-16). The irritating effect of the smoke causes hyperplasia of cells, including goblet cells, which subsequently results in increased production of mucus. Hyperplasia reduces airway diameter and increases the difficulty in clearing secretions. Smoking reduces the ciliary activity and may cause actual loss of ciliated cells. Smoking also produces abnormal dilation of the distal air space with destruction of alveolar walls. Many cells develop large, atypical nuclei, which are considered a precancerous condition.

After a short time of smoking, changes in small airway function can develop. In the early stages these changes are mostly inflammatory with mucosal edema and an influx of inflammatory cells. In later stages, however, thickening of the airway wall occurs by a remodeling process related to tissue repair and the inability of cilia to clear mucus, thus resulting in accumulation of inflammatory exudates in the airway lumen. Quitting smoking can prevent or delay the development of airflow limitation or reduce its progression.[1]

Carbon monoxide (CO) is a component of tobacco smoke. CO has a high affinity for hemoglobin and combines with it more readily than does O_2, thereby reducing the smoker's O_2-carrying capacity. The smoker inhales a lower percentage of O_2 than normal, resulting in less O_2 available at the alveolar level. The heart's need for O_2 is increased because of the stimulatory effect of nicotine on the sympathetic nervous system. Because the blood's O_2-carrying capacity is reduced, the heart must pump more rapidly to adequately supply tissues with O_2. CO also seems to impair psychomotor performance and judgment.

Passive smoking is the exposure of nonsmokers to cigarette smoke, also known as *environmental tobacco smoke* (ETS) or secondhand smoke. In adults, involuntary smoke exposure is associated with decreased pulmonary function, increased respiratory symptoms, and severe lower respiratory tract infections such as pneumonia. ETS also is associated with increased risk for lung cancer and nasal sinus cancer. The cardiovascular system is affected by ETS with increased heart rate and blood pressure and decreased levels of high-density lipoproteins (HDLs). Approximately 40,000 people die each year from cardiovascular disease related to secondhand smoke.[30]

Occupational Chemicals and Dusts. If a person has intense or prolonged exposure to various dusts, vapors, irritants, or fumes in the workplace, COPD can develop independently of cigarette smoking. If the person smokes, the risk of COPD increases. Exposure to these irritants causes the airways to be hyperresponsive.[1]

Air Pollution. High levels of urban air pollution are harmful to persons with existing lung disease. However, the effect of outdoor air pollution as a risk factor for COPD appears to be small compared to the effect of cigarette smoking. Another risk factor for COPD development is fossil fuels that are used for indoor heating and cooking. Many women, particularly worldwide who have never smoked, are developing COPD because of cooking with these fuels in poorly ventilated areas.[1]

Infection. Infections are a risk factor for developing COPD. Severe recurring respiratory tract infections in childhood have been associated with reduced lung function and increased respiratory symptoms in adulthood. Recurring infections impair normal defense mechanisms, making the bronchioles and alveoli more

TABLE 29-16 Effects of Tobacco Smoke on the Respiratory System

Area of Defect	Acute Effects	Long-Term Effects
Respiratory mucosa		
• Nasopharyngeal	↓ Sense of smell	Cancer
• Tongue	↓ Sense of taste	Cancer
• Vocal cords	Hoarseness	Chronic cough, cancer
• Bronchus and bronchioles	Bronchospasm, cough	Chronic bronchitis, asthma, cancer
Cilia	Paralysis, sputum accumulation, cough	Chronic bronchitis, cancer
Mucous glands	↑ Secretions, ↑ cough	Hyperplasia and hypertrophy of glands, chronic bronchitis
Alveolar macrophages	↓ Function	↑ Incidence of infection
Elastin and collagen fibers	↑ Destruction by proteases, ↓ function of antiproteases (α_1-antitrypsin), ↓ synthesis and repair of elastin	Emphysema

GENETICS IN CLINICAL PRACTICE

α_1-Antitrypsin (AAT) Deficiency

Genetic Basis

- Autosomal codominant disorder
- Mutations in SERPINA1 gene (located on chromosome 14) cause AAT
- Gene provides instructions for making the protein AAT

Incidence

- 1 in 1700 to 3500 live births in the United States
- Persons of northern European descent most affected

Genetic Testing

- DNA testing available
- Screening of siblings useful
- Serum assay available to measure the amount of α_1-antitrypsin

Clinical Implications

- α_1-Antitrypsin produced mainly in liver; deficiency can cause lung and liver disease
- Onset of disease appears between ages 20 and 40 years
- Treatment includes α_1-antitrypsin replacement (Prolastin)
- Predisposes to early-onset emphysema

susceptible to injury. The person with COPD is prone to acute exacerbations of the disease, with 50% to 75% of cases thought to be caused by bacteria. These respiratory infections subsequently intensify the pathologic destruction of lung tissue and the progression of COPD. The most common causative organisms are *Haemophilus influenzae, Streptococcus pneumoniae,* and *Moraxella catarrhalis.*[31]

Heredity. **α_1-Antitrypsin (AAT) deficiency** is the genetic risk factor that leads to COPD (see the Genetics in Clinical Practice box). AAT deficiency, an autosomal recessive disorder, accounts for 1% to 2% of COPD cases in the United States. Also known as α_1-protease inhibitor, AAT is a serum protein produced by the liver and normally found in the lungs. Severe AAT deficiency leads to premature bullous emphysema in the lungs found via radiologic testing. Normally AAT inhibits the lysis of lung tissues by proteolytic enzymes from neutrophils and macrophages. Emphysema occurs because of the AAT deficiency. Lower levels of AAT result in insufficient inactivation and subsequent destruction of lung tissue. Smoking greatly exacerbates the disease process in these patients.[32]

The level of AAT is controlled by a pair of autosomal codominant genes. Low levels of AAT are related to homozygosity for the deficiency gene (ZZ), intermediate levels to heterozygosity (MZ), and normal values to homozygosity for the normal gene (MM). In the recessive gene homozygous group (ZZ), many individuals may have relatively normal lung function, especially those who never smoked. However, those with ZZ have the most severe disease. Clues to AAT deficiencies are the onset of symptoms often occurring by age 40, minimal to no tobacco use, and family history of emphysema. Chronic liver disease as an infant or adult with increased liver enzyme tests may also be seen. The people with this type of emphysema are primarily of northern European origin. A simple blood test can determine low levels of AAT. Those with borderline or low levels can then be genetically tested.[32]

IV-administered AAT (Prolastin) augmentation therapy is approved for persons with AAT deficiency. The infusions are administered weekly. Its effectiveness in slowing the progression of the disease continues to be evaluated.

Aging. Some degree of emphysema is common in the lungs of the older person, even a nonsmoker. Aging results in changes in the lung structure, the thoracic cage, and the respiratory muscles. As people age there is gradual loss of the elastic recoil of the lung. The lungs become more rounded and smaller. The number of functional alveoli decreases as a result of the loss of the alveolar supporting structures and loss of the intraalveolar septum. These changes are similar to those seen in the patient with emphysema. Clinically significant emphysema, however, is usually not caused by aging alone.

Thinner alveolar walls contribute to loss of alveolar septal tissue and alveolar capillaries. With fewer capillaries available for gas exchange, arterial O_2 (PaO_2) levels decrease from 80 mm Hg at 20 years of age to 65 to 70 mm Hg by 70 years of age.[33]

Thoracic cage changes result from osteoporosis and calcification of the costal cartilages. The thoracic cage becomes stiff and rigid, and the ribs are less mobile. The shape of the rib cage gradually changes because of the increased residual volume (RV), causing it to expand and become rounded. Decreased chest compliance and elastic recoil of the lungs caused by aging affects the mechanical aspects of ventilation and increases the work of breathing. Changes in the elasticity of the lungs reduce the ventilatory reserve, and ability to clear secretions decreases with age.[34]

Pathophysiology

COPD is characterized by chronic inflammation found in the airways, lung parenchyma (gas-exchanging surfaces of the lung [respiratory bronchioles and alveoli]), and pulmonary vasculature (Fig. 29-7). The pathogenesis of COPD is complex and involves many mechanisms. However, the primary process is inflammation.

The inflammatory process starts with inhalation of noxious particles and gases (e.g., cigarette smoke, air pollution). The predominant inflammatory cells, macrophages and lymphocytes (primarily CD8 cells), increase and release inflammatory mediators, including leukotrienes, interleukins, and tumor necrosis factor. These mediators cause damage to the lung tissue. Later, neutrophils infiltrate into the lungs and release more inflammatory mediators.

The airways become inflamed, resulting in increased numbers of enlarged goblet cells. This results in excess mucus production (or chronic bronchitis). Peripheral airways (small bronchi and bronchioles with internal diameter <2 mm) undergo repeated cycles of injury and repair of the airway walls with resultant structural remodeling. Increased collagen and scar tissue formation in the walls cause fibrosis.

Destruction of the lung parenchyma in COPD patients results in emphysema with significant loss of attachments, which could be likened to rubber bands connecting airways and keeping the airways open. With loss of attachments ("rubber bands"), the peripheral airways collapse. One type of emphysema, called *centrilobular,* involves dilation and destruction of the respiratory bronchioles and is the most commonly seen in upper lobes in mild disease (Fig. 29-8). The pathologic changes may occur throughout the lungs in severe disease and the pulmonary capillary bed may also be destroyed. The second type of emphysema involves destruction of the alveolar ducts, alveolar sacs, and respiratory bronchioles and is called *panlobular* (Fig. 29-8). It is most prominent in the lower lobes and is seen with α_1-antitrypsin deficiency.[1,2]

Destruction of the lung parenchyma is thought to be due to an imbalance of proteinases/antiproteinases. This occurs as a consequence of inflammation, but there can be a genetic basis to the proteinase imbalance. Individuals have elastin, which provides the

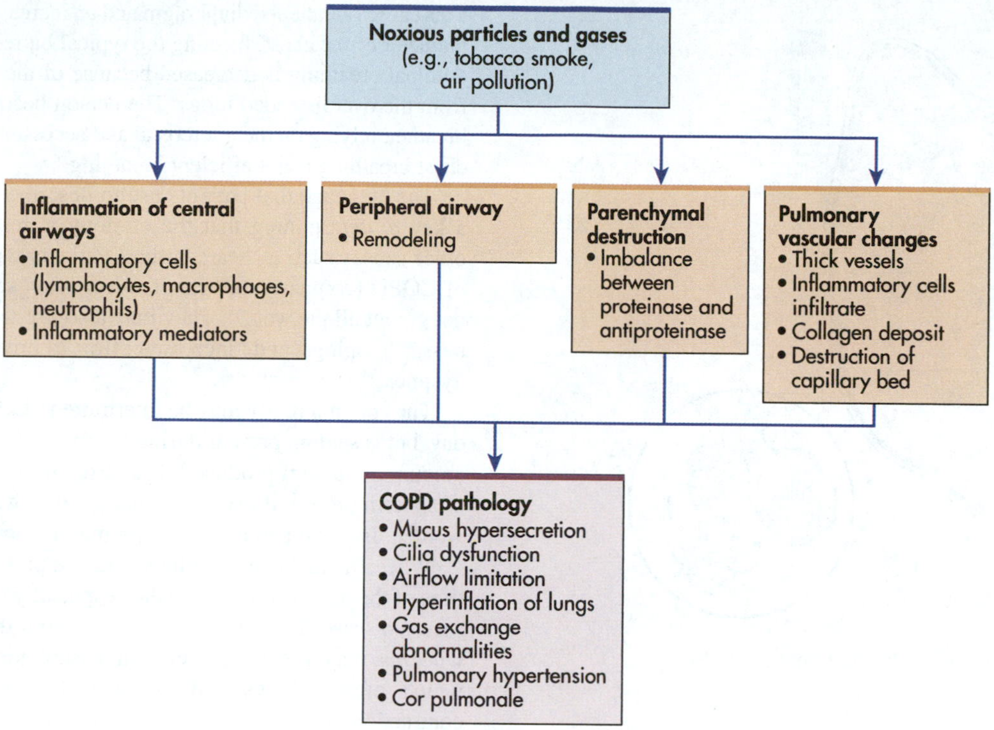

FIG. 29-7 Pathophysiology of COPD.

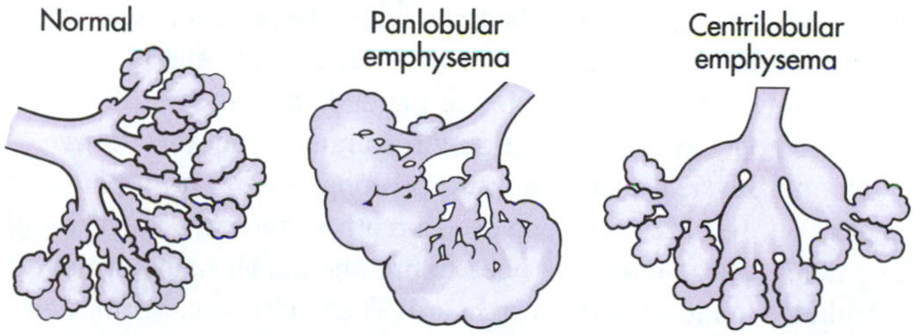

FIG. 29-8 Morphologic types of COPD. In panlobular emphysema the entire primary lobule is involved, with destruction and distention distal to the respiratory bronchioles. In centrilobular emphysema, destruction is central, involving primarily the respiratory bronchioles.

structural makeup of the connective tissue of the alveolar wall. In a healthy person, proteinases (elastase is the main component) in the parenchyma function to break down the alveolar walls (elastin). Normally, proteinase inhibitors (called α_1-antitrypsin [AAT]) prevent this destructive process. In smokers the numbers of neutrophils, macrophages, and other inflammatory cells are increased and with the inflammatory process overwhelm the body's normal AAT defense. Therefore there is destruction of the basic elastin structure of the parenchyma. In addition, inflammatory cells in COPD release a variety of inflammatory mediators such as leukotrienes and interleukins. In the genetic form of emphysema there is a deficiency of AAT, and an imbalance of proteinases/antiproteinases occurs. As the disease progresses, these microscopic lesions may progress to bullae in the lung parenchyma or blebs in the visceral pleura. These anatomic changes can be likened to a balloon that has been blown up too many times (Fig. 29-9). Bullae and blebs are areas with greatly reduced diffusion of gases as the alveolar capillary bed is destroyed.

In COPD, as the supporting structures of the lung are destroyed, there is no pull or traction on the walls of the bronchioles. Like air being blown into a paper bag, air goes into the lungs easily but is unable to come out on its own; it remains in the lung. Thus the bronchioles tend to collapse (especially on expiration) and air is trapped in the distal alveoli, resulting in hyperinflation and overdistention of the alveoli. This trapped air in the lungs gives the patient the typical barrel-chested appearance. In COPD the lungs can be inflated easily but can only partially deflate.

Pulmonary vascular changes can begin early in the disease. Inflammatory cells infiltrate the smooth muscle of the blood vessels causing thickening as the disease advances. Because of the loss of alveolar walls and the capillaries surrounding them, the amount of surface area that is available for diffusion of O_2 decreases. The patient with COPD compensates for this problem by increasing the respiratory rate to increase alveolar ventilation. Typically, the patient does not have difficulty with hypoxemia at rest until late in the disease. However, hypoxemia may develop during exercise, and the patient may benefit from supplemental O_2. Air can move into the lungs, thus there is ventilation. However, because of the anatomic changes noted previously, perfusion of gases is affected, and thus there is a ventilation/perfusion imbalance. Hypercapnia and respiratory acidosis do not develop until late in the disease process. In severe cases, collagen deposition in the vessels along with emphysematous destruction of the capillary bed occurs, leading to pulmonary hypertension and cor pulmonale; the prognosis is poor.[35]

These changes in the lungs result in the following characteristic disease manifestations: mucus hypersecretion, dysfunction of the cilia, airflow limitation and hyperinflation of the lungs, gas exchange abnormalities, pulmonary hypertension, and cor pulmonale (see Fig. 29-7). Mucus hypersecretion and dysfunction of cilia lead to chronic cough and sputum production. Inability to expire air (largely irreversible) is the main characteristic of COPD. The main site of the airflow limitation is in the smaller airways and is due to remodeling. Because of the loss of alveolar walls and attachments,

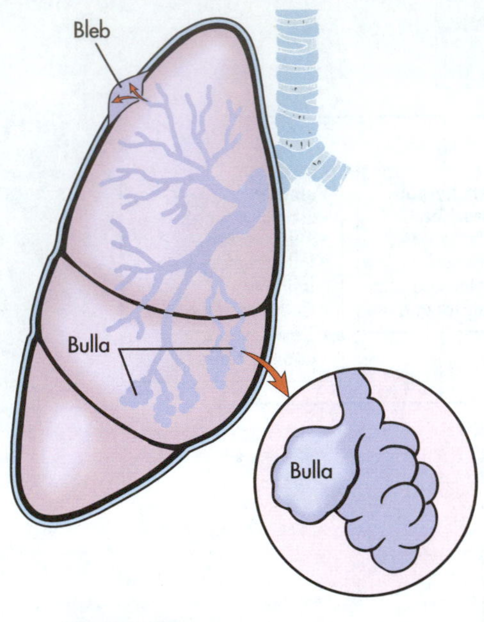

FIG. 29-9 Pulmonary blebs and bullae.

the elastic recoil of the lung is decreased. Recoil is also affected by the influx of inflammatory cells and exudates in the bronchi together with hyperinflation of the lungs.

COPD has been shown to have systemic effects with inflammation (oxidative stress and inflammatory cells) and skeletal muscle wasting. Cigarette smoking begins the process of inflammation via oxidative stress, but inflammation appears to be sustained years after smoking ceases. This mechanism is being investigated. These effects limit the exercise abilities of the patient and worsen the prognosis.[36]

Clinically it is common to find a combination of emphysema and chronic bronchitis in the same person, often with one condition predominating. Patients with COPD may also have asthma, and if they experience poorly reversible airflow limitation, the symptoms may be indistinguishable from COPD, but clinically are treated as asthma. Pathologically, the types of inflammatory cells are quite different between COPD and asthma.

Clinical Manifestations

Clinical manifestations of COPD typically develop slowly around 50 years of age after 20 pack-years of cigarette smoking.[32] A diagnosis of COPD should be considered in any patient who has symptoms of cough, sputum production, or dyspnea, and/or a history of exposure to risk factors for the disease. An intermittent cough, which is the earliest symptom, usually occurs in the morning with the expectoration of small amounts of sticky mucus resulting from bouts of coughing. Patients usually seek medical help when they have an acute respiratory infection, with dyspnea being the main concern.

Dyspnea is often progressive, and usually occurs with exertion. However, patients may dismiss the importance of this symptom as they rationalize, "I'm just getting older." They change behaviors to avoid dyspnea, such as taking the elevator. Gradually the dyspnea interferes with daily activities, such as carrying grocery bags, and they cannot walk as fast as their spouse or peers.

In late stages of COPD, dyspnea may be present at rest. As more alveoli become overdistended, increasing amounts of air are trapped. This causes a flattened diaphragm and an increased anterior-posterior diameter of the chest, forming the typical barrel chest. Effective abdominal breathing is decreased because of the flattened diaphragm from the overdistended lungs. The person becomes more of a chest breather, relying on the intercostal and accessory muscles. However, chest breathing is not efficient breathing.

The language that patients use to describe the dyspnea may be a key to determining that the etiology is respiratory rather than other causes such as heart failure. Patients with dyspnea because of COPD (compared to heart failure) often say, "My breath does not go out all the way."[37] They may also use words such as "heaviness," "gasping," and "increased effort to breathe" to describe the dyspnea.[38]

The cough initially may be intermittent. Later it is present every day, but is seldom present during the night. There are ranges in the amount of sputum produced. It is difficult to quantify the amount of sputum produced because many people swallow it, particularly women. In some people the cough may be nonproductive.

Wheezing and chest tightness may be present, but may vary by time of the day or from day to day, especially in patients with more severe disease. The wheeze may arise from the laryngeal area, or wheezes may not be present on auscultation. Chest tightness, which often follows activity, may feel similar to muscular contraction.

The person with advanced COPD frequently experiences weight loss and anorexia. The exact cause for this is not well understood. One possibility is that the patient is in a hypermetabolic state with increased energy requirements. Even when the patient has adequate caloric intake, weight loss is still experienced. Fatigue is a highly prevalent symptom that affects the patient's activities of daily living.[39] Hemoptysis can occur during respiratory tract infections.

During physical examination a prolonged expiratory phase of respiration, wheezes, or decreased breath sounds are noted in all lung fields. The patient may need to breathe louder than normal for auscultated breath sounds to be heard. The anterior-posterior diameter of the chest is increased ("barrel chest") from the chronic air trapping. The patient may sit upright with arms supported on a fixed surface such as an overbed table *(tripod position)*. The patient may naturally purse lips on expiration (pursed-lip breathing) and use accessory muscles, such as those in the neck, to aid with inspiration. Edema in the ankles may be the only clue to right-sided heart involvement.

Over time, hypoxemia (PaO_2 <60 mm Hg or O_2 saturation <88%) may develop with hypercapnia ($PaCO_2$ >45 mm Hg) later in the disease. The bluish-red color of the skin results from polycythemia and cyanosis. Polycythemia develops as a result of increased production of red blood cells as the body attempts to compensate for chronic hypoxemia. Hemoglobin concentrations may reach 20 g/dl (200 g/L) or more. Cyanosis develops when there is at least 5 g/dl (50 g/L) or more of circulating unoxygenated hemoglobin.

As noted previously, it is sometimes quite difficult for the health care provider to distinguish COPD from asthma. However, there are some clinical features that are different (Table 29-17).

Classification of COPD. COPD should be considered in any person with an exposure to risk factors such as cigarettes and/or environmental or occupational pollutants and/or chronic cough and dyspnea. The diagnosis is confirmed by spirometry. COPD can be classified as at risk, mild, moderate, severe, and very severe (Table 29-18). The FEV_1/FEV <70% establishes the diagnosis of

TABLE 29-17 Comparison of Asthma and COPD*

	Asthma	COPD
Clinical Features		
Age	Usually <40 yr (onset)	Usually 40-50 yr (onset)
Smoking history	Not causal	Long history (>10-20 pack-years)
Health and family history	Presence of allergy, rhinitis, eczema; family history of asthma	Infrequent allergies. May have exposure to environmental pollutants; with α_1-antitrypsin deficiency, a family history of lung or liver disease without smoking history
Clinical symptoms	Intermittent, vary day to day, at night or early morning	Slowly progressive and persistent
Dyspnea	Absent except in exacerbations or poor control	Dyspnea during exercise
Sputum	Infrequent	Often
Disease course	Stable (with exacerbations)	Progressive worsening (with exacerbations)
Diagnostic Study Results		
ABGs	Normal between attacks	
pH	N→↑ during attack	N→↓
PaO_2	N→↓ during attack	N→↓
$PaCO_2$	N→↓ during attack	N→↑
Chest x-ray	May reveal hyperinflation	Hyperinflation; may have cardiac enlargement, flattened diaphragm
Lung volumes	Often normalizes	Never normalizes
Total lung capacity	Increased	Increased
Residual volume	Increased	Increased
FEV_1	Decreased	Decreased
FEV_1/FVC	Normal to decreased	Decreased (<70%)

Adapted from Braman SS, Peters SG: COPD: will early detection and aggressive intervention control disease progression? Maximizing positive outcomes in COPD, *CE-Today for Nurse Practitioners* 4:7, 2005. Available at *www.np.ce-today.com*.
*Persons may have features of both asthma and COPD.
ABGs, Arterial blood gases; *FEV_1*, forced expiratory volume in 1 second; *FVC,* forced vital capacity.

TABLE 29-18 Classification of Severity of COPD

		Pulmonary Function Tests	
Stage	**Symptoms**	**FEV_1/FVC**	**FEV_1 % Predicted**
Stage 0 At Risk	Chronic symptoms (cough, sputum production)	Normal spirometry	
Stage I Mild COPD	With or without chronic symptoms	<70%	≤80%
Stage II Moderate COPD	With or without chronic symptoms	<70%	50%-80%
Stage III Severe COPD	With or without chronic symptoms	<70%	30%-50%
Stage IV Very Severe COPD	With or without chronic symptoms	<70%	<30% or <50% and chronic respiratory failure

Adapted from *Global Initiative for Chronic Obstructive Lung Disease (GOLD)* workshop report. Available at *www.goldcopd.org*.

COPD, and the severity of obstruction (as indicated by FEV_1) determines the stage of COPD. The management of COPD is primarily based on the patient's symptoms, but the staging provides a general guideline for the type of interventions.

Complications

Cor Pulmonale. Cor pulmonale is hypertrophy of the right side of the heart, with or without heart failure, resulting from pulmonary hypertension. It is caused by diseases affecting the lungs or pulmonary blood vessels (Fig. 29-10). Cor pulmonale is a late manifestation of chronic pulmonary heart disease. The patient benefits most when a diagnosis of pulmonary heart disease can be made early so therapy can be instituted. In patients with severe COPD, 40% demonstrate cor pulmonale, and the prognosis is poor.[40] In COPD, pulmonary hypertension is caused primarily by constriction of the pulmonary vessels in response to alveolar hypoxia, with acidosis further potentiating the vasoconstriction. Chronic alveolar hypoxia causes vascular remodeling. Chronic hypoxia also stimulates erythropoiesis, which causes polycythemia. This results in increased viscosity of the blood. In COPD there may be an anatomic reduction of the pulmonary vascular bed as seen in emphysema with bullae. These patients would have increased pulmonary vascular resistance.

Normally the right ventricle and pulmonary circulatory system are low-pressure systems compared with the left ventricle and systemic circulation. When pulmonary hypertension develops, the pressures on the right side of the heart must increase to push blood into the lungs. Eventually, right-sided heart failure develops.

The clinical manifestations of chronic pulmonary heart disease and cor pulmonale are related to dilation and failure of the right ventricle with subsequent intravascular volume expansion and systemic venous congestion. Dyspnea is a usual symptom, and is associated with hypoxemia and hypercarbia. Lung sounds are normal or crackles may be heard in the bases of the lungs bilaterally. Heart

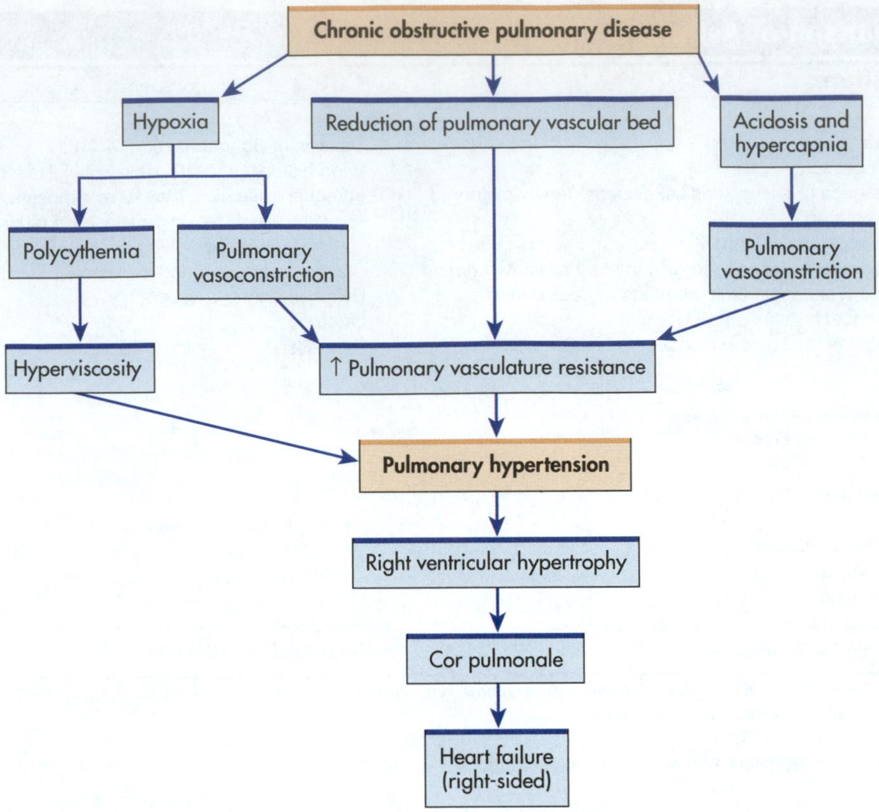

FIG. 29-10 Mechanisms involved in the pathophysiology of cor pulmonale secondary to chronic obstructive pulmonary disease.

sound changes include accentuation of the pulmonic component of the second heart sound, right-sided ventricular diastolic S_3 gallop, and a loud pulmonic component of S_2 along the left sternal border. ECG changes include increased P wave amplitude (P pulmonale), a tendency for right axis deviation, and incomplete right bundle branch block. Overt manifestations of right-sided heart failure may develop, which include distended neck veins (jugular venous distention), hepatomegaly with right upper quadrant tenderness, ascites, epigastric distress, peripheral edema, and weight gain.

Management of cor pulmonale includes continuous low-flow O_2. Long-term O_2 therapy improves survival of hypoxemic patients, especially when used $>$15 hours per day.[41] Vasodilator therapy has not demonstrated sustained benefit and is not recommended on a routine basis. Although the use of digitalis is not indicated for right-sided heart failure, it may be used when left-sided heart failure is present. Diuretics are generally used, but serum creatinine and blood urea nitrogen (BUN) are needed to monitor renal function as diuretics can cause volume depletion.[40] (Cor pulmonale is discussed further in Chapter 28.) Electrolytes must be monitored to assess for hypokalemia, which can predispose to dysrhythmias.

Exacerbations of COPD. Exacerbations of COPD are signaled by a change in the patient's usual dyspnea, cough, and/or sputum that is different from the usual daily patterns. These flares require changes in management. Patients have an increase in dyspnea, sputum volume, and/or sputum purulence. They may also have nonspecific complaints of malaise, insomnia, fatigue, depression, confusion, decrease in exercise tolerance, increased wheezing, increased cough, or fever without other causes.[42]

As the severity of COPD increases, exacerbations of COPD are associated with poorer outcomes. Exacerbations of COPD may be treated at home or in the hospital intermediate care unit or intensive care unit, depending on the severity. The primary causes of exacerbations of COPD are tracheobronchial infection and air pollution. Bacteria account for 33% to 75% of the cases of infection.[2, 31] The most common organisms causing exacerbations are *H. influenzae, M. catarrhalis,* and *S. pneumoniae.* Other causes of COPD exacerbations include viruses.

Medications used to decrease airway resistance during exacerbations of COPD are bronchodilators and oral systemic corticosteroids.[35] If a patient has clinical signs of airway infection (e.g., increased volume and change in color of sputum and/or fever, especially in the severe stages of COPD with more than three to four exacerbations per year), antibiotic treatment is usually used. Therapies used to treat exacerbations of COPD in the hospital are similar to home management, except supplemental oxygen therapy titrated by ABG measurement may be used.[1] Attempts are made to use noninvasive mechanical methods (e.g., continuous positive airway pressure [CPAP] to support ventilation rather than invasive ventilatory support [e.g., intubation]).[43] Teaching the patient and family early recognition of signs and symptoms of exacerbations is important to promote early treatment to prevent hospitalization and possible respiratory failure.

Acute Respiratory Failure. Patients with severe COPD who have exacerbations are at risk for the development of respiratory failure.[44] Frequently, COPD patients wait too long to contact their health care provider when they develop fever, increased cough and dyspnea, or other symptoms suggestive of exacerbations of COPD. An exacerbation of cor pulmonale may also lead to acute respiratory failure. Discontinuing bronchodilator or corticosteroid medication may also precipitate respiratory failure. The use of β-adrenergic blockers (e.g., propranolol [Inderal]) may also exacerbate acute respiratory failure in the patient with a reversible component to the COPD. However, cardioselective β-adrenergic blockers (e.g., atenolol, metoprolol) should not be withheld from patients with mild to moderate diseases because they do not produce clinically significant problems with respiration.[45]

The indiscriminate use of sedatives, benzodiazepines, and opioids, especially in the preoperative or postoperative patient who retains CO_2, may suppress the ventilatory drive and lead to respiratory failure. The person with COPD who retains CO_2 should be treated with low flow rates of O_2 with careful monitoring of ABGs to avoid hypercarbia to ensure that adequate oxygenation occurs, and to monitor for acidosis. It has been thought that high flow rates of O_2 depress the respiratory center and that the patient's respirations will diminish or cease. However, it is vital to provide adequate oxygen while assessing the ABGs, rather than not providing O_2 because of the fear of CO_2 narcosis (discussed on p. 643).

Surgery or severe, painful illness involving the chest or abdominal organs may lead to splinting and ineffective ventilation and respiratory failure. To prevent postoperative pulmonary complications, careful preoperative screening, which includes pulmonary function tests and ABG assessment, is important in the patient with a heavy smoking history and/or COPD. (Respiratory failure is discussed in Chapter 68.)

Peptic Ulcer and Gastroesophageal Reflux Disease. The incidence of peptic ulcer disease is increased in persons with COPD. The reason for this occurrence is partly explained by hypersecretion of gastric acid resulting from increased arterial CO_2 and decreased arterial O_2 tension. This occurs only in patients who chronically retain CO_2. The ulcers are more commonly in the duodenum rather than stomach and do not cause pain.[46] It is important to test gastric aspirates and feces for occult blood.

Gastroesophageal reflux disease (GERD), which may or may not be associated with a hiatal hernia, occurs frequently in patients with COPD and may aggravate respiratory symptoms. The reflux and accompanying heartburn may be aggravated or even precipitated by theophylline or β_2-adrenergic agonists. However, patients with severe COPD and GERD have also been found to have asymptomatic GERD.[47] (Treatment of GERD is discussed in Chapter 42.)

Depression/Anxiety. Patients with COPD experience many losses as the disease progresses over time. They can feel helpless with low self-esteem and unable to vent their emotions for fear of compromising their breathing. The reported prevalence of depression in COPD varies, but may be four times more frequent in COPD than in the general population. Anxiety can complicate respiratory compromise and may precipitate dyspnea and hyperventilation. When a person is exceptionally dyspneic, particularly if it occurs suddenly, the person becomes anxious and tries to breathe faster, thus affecting his or her oxygenation status. Proper screening for anxiety and depression by health care providers is needed for a proper diagnosis.

After diagnosis, treatment consists of cognitive and behavioral psychotherapy and/or pharmacotherapy. Selective serotonin reuptake inhibitors (SSRIs) are often used for both depression and anxiety. Buspirone, which is one medication used to treat anxiety, has few if any respiratory depression effects. Benzodiazepines are avoided because they may depress the respiratory drive and may be habit forming. The nurse should explore the psychologic realm of the patient's disease and the impact it has on the patient's quality of life. Providing sufficient time for nursing interventions during an acute exacerbation is important to help reduce anxiety.[35] When the patient becomes anxious because of dyspnea, the use of pursed-lip breathing (discussed later in chapter) and short-acting bronchodilators may be appropriate.

ETHICAL DILEMMAS

Advance Directives

Situation

A 79-year-old man with COPD is admitted to the hospital in respiratory failure. He is placed on a ventilator and responds occasionally by opening his eyes. His advance directives were executed 5 years ago and copies were given to his wife and health care provider at that time. The wife brings the documents to the intensive care unit and tells the nurse that the hospital must stop treating her husband and allow him to die as he requested. However, the oldest son is threatening the hospital with a lawsuit if the staff does not provide full care to his father.

Important Points for Consideration

- The first advance directive was the living will (lay term), which was provided for under the Patient Self-Determination Act of 1991.
- Advance directives are prepared by the person indicating his or her treatment wishes should the person become terminally ill or in a situation where there is no hope of recovery.*
- A determination needs to be made whether this is a respiratory crisis that is reversible or whether the patient is terminally ill.
- Durable power of attorney for health care is a form of an advance directive in which a person names another to make health care decisions in the event the person is no longer able.
- Directives to physicians and medical power of attorney are additional types of advance directives that protect and respect the patient's autonomy; that is, the right to self-determination regarding health care at the end of life.
- Advance directives are legally binding in most states.
- Health care providers are obligated to follow the patient's advance directives when a patient is no longer able to speak for himself or herself.
- Health care providers are protected from liability when they adhere to advance directives.

Critical Thinking Questions

1. What should the nurse do next with the information provided by the wife?
2. How should the nurse address the needs of each member of this family in the patient's plan of care?
3. What resources can the nurse use to facilitate decision making in this situation?

*Table 11-4 explains common documents used in end-of-life care.

Diagnostic Studies

The diagnosis of COPD is confirmed by pulmonary function tests. Goals of the diagnostic workup are to confirm the diagnosis of COPD via spirometry, evaluate the severity of the disease, and determine the impact of the disease on the patient's quality of life. These factors enable the health care provider to design an individualized treatment plan. In addition to pulmonary function tests, other diagnostic studies are performed (Table 29-19). Chest x-rays taken early in the disease are seldom diagnostic unless bullous disease is present. Patients may have significant airflow limitation as demonstrated by spirometry but not chronic cough. Most patients seek medical help because of dyspnea that starts affecting

TABLE 29-19 COLLABORATIVE CARE COPD

Diagnostic
History and physical examination
Pulmonary function tests
Chest x-ray
Serum α_1-antitrypsin levels
Sputum specimen for Gram stain and culture
ABGs
ECG
Exercise testing with oximetry
Echocardiogram or cardiac nuclear scans
Collaborative Therapy
Cessation of cigarette smoking
Treatment of exacerbations
Bronchodilator therapy (see Table 29-7)
β_2-Adrenergic agonists
Anticholinergic agents
Long-acting theophylline preparations and blood levels
Corticosteroids (oral for exacerbations, inhaled corticosteroids)
Chest physiotherapy and postural drainage
Breathing exercises and retraining
Hydration of 3 L/day (if not contraindicated)
Appropriate rest periods
Patient and family teaching
Influenza immunization yearly
Pneumovax immunization
Long-term O_2 (if indicated)
Progressive plan of exercise, especially walking and upper body strengthening
Pulmonary rehabilitation program
Nutritional supplementation if low BMI
Surgery
Lung volume reduction
Lung transplantation

ABGs, Arterial blood gases; *BMI,* body mass index; *ECG,* electrocardiogram.

their daily activities. Later in the disease the findings presented in Table 29-17 may be present.[48]

A history and physical examination are extremely important in a diagnostic workup. Pulmonary function studies are useful in diagnosing and assessing the severity of COPD. Usually spirometry is ordered before and after bronchodilation. The most significant findings are related to increased resistance to expiratory airflow. Typical findings include the following:

- Reduced FEV_1, $FEF_{25\%-75\%}$, FEV_1/FVC ratio, diffusing capacity for carbon monoxide
- Increased residual volume, functional residual capacity (FRC)

When the FEV_1/FVC ratio is less than 70%, it suggests the presence of obstructive lung disease. The value of FEV_1 in milliliters can provide a guideline to determine the severity of the patient's lung disease and the degree of disease progression (Table 29-20; see Table 29-18).

The body mass index (BMI) and degree of dyspnea are useful in predicting outcomes, such as survival. Current practice guidelines recommend that the BMI and dyspnea be evaluated in all patients. BMI is obtained by dividing weight (in kilograms [kg]) by height (in square meters [m^2]). A BMI below 21 kg/m^2 is associated with an increase in mortality rate. Functional dyspnea can be assessed with the Medical Research Council Dyspnea Scale from level 0 (no trouble with breathlessness except with strenuous exercise) to level 4 (too breathless to leave the house or breathless when dressing or undressing).[2]

TABLE 29-20 Correlation of FEV_1 with Probable Clinical Manifestations

Approximate FEV_1	Probable Clinical Manifestation
1500 ml	Shortness of breath just beginning to be noticed
1000 ml	Shortness of breath with activity
500 ml	Shortness of breath at rest

ABGs are usually assessed in the severe stages and monitored in patients hospitalized with acute exacerbations. In the later stages of COPD, typical findings are low PaO_2, elevated $PaCO_2$, decreased or low-normal pH, and increased bicarbonate (HCO_3^-) levels. In the early stages there may be a normal or only slightly decreased PaO_2 and a normal $PaCO_2$. A 6-minute walk test to determine O_2 saturation in the blood with pulse oximetry may be performed to evaluate the degree of O_2 desaturation that occurs with exercise. An ECG may be normal or show signs indicative of right ventricular failure (e.g., low voltage, right-axis deviation, P pulmonale). An echocardiogram or gated pool nuclear blood study (see Chapter 32) can be used to evaluate right-sided ventricular and left ventricular function. Sputum for culture and sensitivity may be obtained if the patient is hospitalized for an acute exacerbation and has not responded to empiric therapy with antibiotics.

Collaborative Care

The *Global Initiative for Chronic Obstructive Lung Disease (GOLD)* workshop report lists a summary of recommended treatment by each stage (Table 29-21). The primary goals of care for the COPD patient are to (1) prevent disease progression, (2) relieve symptoms and improve exercise tolerance, (3) prevent and treat complications, (4) promote patient participation in care, (5) prevent and treat exacerbations, and (6) improve quality of life and reduce mortality risk (see Evidence-Based Practice box). The majority of patients are treated as outpatients. They are hospitalized for exacerbations of COPD and potential complications when respiratory failure, pneumonia, and heart failure and/or cor pulmonale are also present.

Environmental or occupational irritants should be evaluated for their possible negative effect, and ways to control or avoid them should be determined. For example, aerosol hair sprays and smoke-filled rooms should be avoided. The patient with COPD is extremely susceptible to pulmonary infections. The patient with COPD should have a vaccination with influenza virus vaccine yearly and with pneumococcal vaccine. Pneumococcal revaccination is recommended once if the patient is ≥65 years of age, the vaccination was ≥5 years previously, and the patient was <65 years of age at the time of the primary vaccination.[49]

Exacerbations of COPD should be treated as soon as possible, especially if the patient is in the severe stages of COPD. Often the best indication of the presence of a bacterial infection is the increasing quantity, viscosity, or purulence of sputum. Some patients are given a prescription for a 7- to 10-day supply of antibiotics and are instructed to begin taking them at the first signs of change in sputum. The most common antibiotics given for outpatients are macrolides (e.g., azithromycin [Zithromax]), doxycy-

TABLE 29-21 Therapy at Each Stage of COPD

Stage 0 At Risk	Stage I Mild COPD	Stage II Moderate COPD	Stage III Severe COPD	Stage IV Very Severe COPD
Avoidance of risk factor(s); influenza vaccination				
	Add short-acting bronchodilator when needed			
		Add regular treatment with one or more long-acting bronchodilators *Add* rehabilitation		
			Add inhaled corticosteroids if repeated exacerbations	
				Add long-term oxygen if chronic respiratory failure *Consider* surgical treatments

Adapted from Global initiative for chronic obstructive lung disease (GOLD) workshop report. Available at *www.goldcopd.org*.

EVIDENCE-BASED PRACTICE

Managing Stable Chronic Obstructive Pulmonary Disease

Key Points	Level of Evidence
• Health education can play a role in improving skills, ability to cope with illness, and health status. It is effective in accomplishing certain goals, including smoking cessation.	A
• None of the existing medications for COPD has been shown to modify long-term decline in lung function.	A
• Therefore drug therapy for COPD is used to decrease symptoms and/or complications.	A
• Bronchodilator medications are central to the symptomatic management of COPD. They are used to prevent or reduce symptoms.	A
• The principal bronchodilator treatments are β_2 agonists, anticholinergics, theophylline, and a combination of one or more of these drugs.	A
• Regular treatment with long-acting bronchodilators is more effective and convenient than treatment with short-acting bronchodilators.	A
• The addition of regular treatment with inhaled corticosteroids to bronchodilator treatment is appropriate for symptomatic COPD patients with an FEV_1 <50% predicted and repeated exacerbations.	A
• Chronic treatment with systemic corticosteroids should be avoided.	A
• All COPD patients benefit from exercise training programs.	A
• The long-term administration of oxygen (>15 hr/day) to patients with chronic respiratory failure has been shown to increase survival.	A

Levels of Evidence: *A*, Evidence is from endpoints of well-designed randomized controlled trials (RCTs) that provide a consistent pattern of findings in the population for which the recommendations is made.
Source: *Global Initiative for Chronic Obstructive Lung Disease (GOLD)* workshop report. Available at *www.goldcopd.com*.
FEV_1, Forced expiratory volume in 1 second.

cline, and newer cephalosporins (e.g., cefpodoxime [Vantin]). Amoxicillin may be used, but patterns of antibiotic resistance are limiting its use. If the patient has failed prior antibiotic therapy or is hospitalized, common antibiotics are amoxicillin/clavulanate (Augmentin), or respiratory fluoroquinolones (e.g., levofloxacin [Levaquin]).[31]

Smoking Cessation. Cessation of cigarette smoking in all stages of COPD is the single most effective and cost-effective intervention to reduce the risk of developing COPD and stop the progression of the disease. After discontinuation of smoking, the accelerated decline in pulmonary function slows and pulmonary function usually improves. Normally individuals after age 35 lose approximately 20 to 25 ml (as measured by FEV_1) of lung function per year as measured by spirometry. Persons with COPD who continue to smoke lose approximately 50 ml per year. With the cessation of smoking, the loss can fall to almost nonsmoking levels at 35 ml per year.[50] Thus the sooner the smoker stops, the less pulmonary function is lost and the sooner the symptoms decrease, especially cough and sputum production (see Evidence-Based Practice box). (Smoking cessation techniques are discussed in Chapter 12 and in Tables 12-4, 12-5, and 12-6.)

Drug Therapy. Medications for COPD can reduce or abolish symptoms, increase the capacity to exercise, improve overall health, and reduce the number and severity of exacerbations. Presently no drug modifies the decline of lung function with COPD. Bronchodilator drug therapy relaxes smooth muscles in the airway and improves the ventilation of the lungs, thus reducing the degree of breathlessness. Although patients with COPD do not respond as dramatically as those with asthma to bronchodilator therapy, a reduction in dyspnea and an increase in FEV_1 are usually achieved. The inhaled route of medication is preferred and given on a prn or regular basis. Medications are given in a stepwise fashion (see Table 29-21).

Bronchodilator medications commonly used are β_2-adrenergic agonists, anticholinergic agents, and methylxanthines (see Table 29-7). The choice of bronchodilator depends on the availability and the patient's response. However, when the patient has mild COPD or intermittent symptoms, a short-acting bronchodilator is

EVIDENCE-BASED PRACTICE

Reducing Risk Factors for Chronic Obstructive Pulmonary Disease

Key Points	Level of Evidence
• Smoking cessation is the single most effective—and cost-effective—intervention to reduce the risk of developing COPD and stop its progression.	A
• Brief tobacco dependence treatment is effective, and every tobacco user should be offered at least this treatment at every visit to the health care provider.	A
• Several effective nicotine replacement therapies (see Table 12-4) for tobacco dependence are available.	A
• At least one of these should be added to counseling if necessary.	
• Progression of many occupationally induced respiratory disorders can be reduced or controlled through a variety of strategies aimed at reducing the burden of inhaled particles and gases.	B

Levels of Evidence: *A*, Evidence is from well-designed randomized controlled trials (RCTs) that provide a consistent pattern of findings in the population for which the recommendation is made. *B*, Evidence is from the endpoints of intervention studies that include only a limited number of patients, posthoc or subgroup analysis of RCTs, or meta-analysis of RCTs.
Source: *Global Initiative for Chronic Obstructive Lung Disease (GOLD)* workshop report. Available at *www.goldcopd.com.*

used as needed. Short-acting bronchodilators increase exercise tolerance. Albuterol or ipratropium (Atrovent) may be used as single agents, but combining bronchodilators improves their effect and decreases the risk of adverse effects, compared with the use of a single agent. As a single agent, ipratropium (Atrovent) is superior to albuterol because the only side effect is usually dry mouth. These two agents can be nebulized together (DuoNeb) or delivered by one MDI (Combivent).

As symptoms persist or moderate stages of COPD develop, a long-acting bronchodilator is used in addition to a short-acting bronchodilator (see Table 29-7). Salmeterol (Serevent) is a widely used long-acting β_2-adrenergic agonist, and unlike in drug therapy for asthma, it can be used in COPD as monotherapy. Formoterol (Foradil) is another long-acting β_2 agonist.

Tiotropium (Spiriva), a long-acting anticholinergic, can be used for daily therapy of bronchospasm and dyspnea in COPD. Tiotropium also improves bronchodilation, results in less dyspnea, improves quality of life, and decreases the number of COPD exacerbations when compared with ipratropium (Atrovent).[51] Tiotropium is the first inhaled drug for COPD to be dosed once a day.[52]

The use of long-acting theophylline in the treatment of COPD is controversial because it interacts with many drugs. Although it has some action as a mild bronchodilator in the patient with partial reversibility of airflow obstruction, its main value may be to improve contractility of the diaphragm and decrease diaphragmatic fatigue.

Inhaled corticosteroid therapy may be beneficial for patients with moderate-to-severe COPD. However, inhaled corticosteroids (ICS) do not appear to help patients with mild COPD.[53] ICS combined with long-acting β_2-adrenergic agonists (e.g., fluticasone/salmeterol [Advair]) are more effective than the single-drug therapy. Oral corticosteroids should not be used for long-term therapy in COPD.

O_2 Therapy. O_2 therapy is frequently used in the treatment of COPD and other problems associated with hypoxemia. Long-term O_2 therapy (LTOT) improves survival, exercise capacity, cognitive performance, and sleep in hypoxemic patients.[2] O_2 is a colorless, odorless, tasteless gas that constitutes 20.95% of the atmosphere. Administering supplemental O_2 raises the partial pressure of O_2 (PO_2) in inspired air. Used clinically it is considered a drug. For reimbursement purposes, it is considered durable medical equipment, which Medicare covers when certain clinical criteria are met (i.e., the patient's O_2 saturation needs to be $\leq$88%, $PaO_2 \leq 55$ mm Hg).

Indications for Use. Goals for O_2 therapy are to reduce the work of breathing, maintain the PaO_2, and/or reduce the workload on the heart, keeping the SaO_2 >90% during rest, sleep, and exertion, or PaO_2 >60 mm Hg.[54] O_2 is usually administered to treat hypoxemia caused by (1) respiratory disorders such as COPD, pulmonary hypertension, cor pulmonale, pneumonia, atelectasis, lung cancer, and pulmonary emboli; (2) cardiovascular disorders such as myocardial infarction, dysrhythmias, angina pectoris, and cardiogenic shock; and (3) central nervous system disorders such as overdose of opioids, head injury, and disordered sleep (sleep apnea).

Methods of Administration. The goal of O_2 administration is to supply the patient with adequate O_2 to maximize the O_2-carrying ability of the blood. There are various methods of O_2 administration (Table 29-22 and Figs. 29-11 through 29-14). The method selected depends on factors such as the fraction of inspired O_2 (FIO_2) required by the patient and delivered by the device, the mobility of the patient, humidification required, patient cooperation, comfort, cost, and available financial resources.

O_2 delivery systems are classified as low- or high-flow systems. Most methods of O_2 administration are low-flow devices that deliver O_2 in concentrations that vary with the person's respiratory pattern. In contrast, the Venturi mask is a high-flow device that delivers fixed concentrations of O_2 independent of the patient's respiratory pattern. With the Venturi mask, O_2 is delivered to a small jet (Venturi device) in the center of a wide-based cone (see Fig. 29-11, *C*). Air is entrained (pulled through) openings in the cone as O_2 flows through the small jet. The mask has large vents through which exhaled air can escape. The degree of restriction or narrowness of the jet determines the amount of entrainment and dilution of pure O_2 with room air, and thus the concentration of O_2 delivered can be precise. Mechanical ventilators are another example of a high-flow O_2 delivery system. Because room air is mixed with O_2, in low-flow systems, the percentage of O_2 delivered to the patient is not as precise as with high-flow systems.

Humidification and Nebulizers. O_2 obtained from cylinders or wall systems is dry. Dry O_2 has an irritating effect on mucous membranes and dries secretions. Therefore it is important that O_2 be humidified when administered, either by humidification or nebulization. A common device used for humidification when the patient has a catheter, cannula, or low-flow mask is a bubble-through humidifier. It is a small plastic jar filled with sterile distilled water that is attached to the O_2 source by means of a flow

TABLE 29-22 Methods of Oxygen Administration

Advantages	Disadvantages	Nursing Interventions
Low-Flow Delivery Devices		
Nasal Cannula		
Most commonly used device. It is a safe and simple method that is relatively comfortable and acceptable. It is useful for a patient requiring low O_2 concentrations (e.g., those with chronic CO_2 retention). It allows patient to move about in bed. Patient can eat, talk, or cough while wearing device (see Fig. 29-11, *F*).	Cannula is difficult to maintain in position and can be easily dislodged. Patient must be alert and cooperative to keep cannula in proper place. High flow rates (>5 L/min) dry nasal membranes and may cause pain in frontal sinuses. Can irritate nares and skin around ears.	Nasal cannula should be stabilized when caring for a restless patient. O_2 concentrations of 24% (at 1 L/min) to 44% (at 6 L/min) can be obtained. Amount of O_2 inhaled depends on room air and patient's breathing pattern. Most patients with COPD can tolerate 2 L/min via cannula. May need to pad the cannula where it sits on the ears.
Simple Face Mask		
O_2 can be given quickly for short periods. Useful when transporting patients. O_2 concentrations of 35%-50% can be achieved with flow rates of 6-12 L/min. Mask provides adequate humidification of inspired air (see Fig. 29-11, *A*).	Lack of patient tolerance results in inadequate therapy. Mask may be uncomfortable because tight seal must be maintained between face and mask. Mask may produce pressure necrosis of the skin and confines heat radiating from the face about nose and mouth. It must be removed to eat or drink.	Wash and dry under mask q2hr. Mask must fit snugly. Nasal cannula may be provided while patient is eating. Watch for pressure necrosis at the top of ears from elastic straps. (Gauze or other padding may be used to alleviate this problem.) Method requires at least 5 L/min flow to prevent accumulation of expired air in the mask.
Partial Rebreathing Mask		
Mask is lightweight and easy to use. Reservoir bag conserves O_2. Useful for short-term (24 hr) therapy for patients needing higher O_2 concentrations.	Mask cannot be used with a high degree of humidity. Patient may find mask uncomfortable and refuse to wear it.	Method is useful when blood O_2 concentrations must be raised. It is not recommended for patient with COPD and should never be used with a nebulizer. Bag should not be allowed to deflate during inspiration, so make sure the reservoir does not kink, which results in bag deflation.
Non-Rebreathing Mask		
High concentrations of O_2 can be delivered accurately. O_2 flows into bag and mask during inhalation. Valve prevents expired air from flowing back into bag. Good for short-term (24 hr) therapy for patients needing higher O_2 concentrations.	Mask cannot be used with a high degree of humidity. Patient may find mask uncomfortable and refuse to wear it.	Mask should fit snugly. Flow rate must be sufficient to keep bag from collapsing during inspiration. Bag should not be allowed to deflate during inspiration. Make sure valves are open during expiration and closed during inhalation to prevent drastic decrease in FIO_2. Monitor closely because patient may require intubation as the next step.
Oxygen-Conserving Cannula		
Cannula has a built-in reservoir that increases O_2 concentration delivered and allows patient to use lower flow, usually 30%-50%, which increases comfort, lowers cost, and can be increased with activities (see Fig. 29-12). It can deliver up to 8 L/min of O_2. It is reportedly more comfortable than standard cannulas.	Cannula cannot be cleaned; manufacturer recommends changing cannula every week. It is more expensive than standard cannulas and requires evaluation with ABGs and oximetry to determine correct flow for patient. Cannula is highly visible. Cannula heavy on ears.	Method is generally indicated for patient requiring long-term O_2 therapy at home versus during hospitalization. It may be "moustache" or "pendant" type. May cause necroses over the tops of the ears; can be padded.
Transtracheal Catheter		
Catheter is less visible. Flow requirement may be reduced approximately 50%-70%, which greatly increases amount of time available from portable source of O_2. Less nasal irritation occurs (see Fig. 29-13).	Patient and family must learn entire program of care for tracheostoma and how to replace catheter. Procedure is invasive. Procedure and replacement add costs to O_2 therapy.	Method may not be appropriate for patient with excessive mucus production from mucous plugging because the catheter may frequently become obstructed.
Face Tent		
Tent is ideal for providing moderate- to high-density aerosol. O_2 concentration administered varies with O_2 flow rate (see Fig. 29-11, *E*).	Amount of O_2 delivered is imprecise.	Open plastic mask fits under chin. Temperature of aerosol must be checked to maintain at or near body temperature. It is rarely used.
Tracheostomy Collar		
Collar can deliver high humidity and O_2 via tracheostomy.	Condensed fluid in tubing may drain into tracheostomy. Water traps are usually put in. Secretions collect inside collar and around tracheostomy. O_2 concentration is lost into atmosphere because collar does not fit tightly.	Collar attaches to neck with elastic strap and should be removed and cleaned at least q4hr to prevent aspiration of fluid and infection.

ABGs, Arterial blood gases; *COPD,* chronic obstructive pulmonary disease.

Continued

TABLE 29-22 Methods of Oxygen Administration—cont'd

Advantages	Disadvantages	Nursing Interventions
Low-Flow Delivery Devices—cont'd		
Tracheostomy T Bar		
Tight fit allows better O_2 and humidity delivery than tracheostomy collar.	Condensed fluid in tubing may drain into tracheostomy. Water traps are usually put in.	T bar must be removed for suctioning. Mörch swivel may be used to eliminate the need for removal. It should be emptied as necessary.
High-Flow Delivery Devices		
Venturi Mask		
Mask can deliver precise, high flow rates of O_2. Lightweight plastic, cone-shaped device is fitted to face. Masks are available for delivery of 24%, 28%, 31%, 35%, 40%, and 50% O_2. Adaptors can be applied to increase humidification (see Fig. 29-11, *C*).	Mask is uncomfortable and must be removed when patient eats. Patient can talk but voice may be muffled. Other disadvantages are the same as those discussed for the simple face mask.	Entrainment device on mask must be changed to deliver higher concentrations of O_2. Method is especially helpful for administering low, constant O_2 concentrations to patients with COPD. Air entrainment ports must not be occluded.

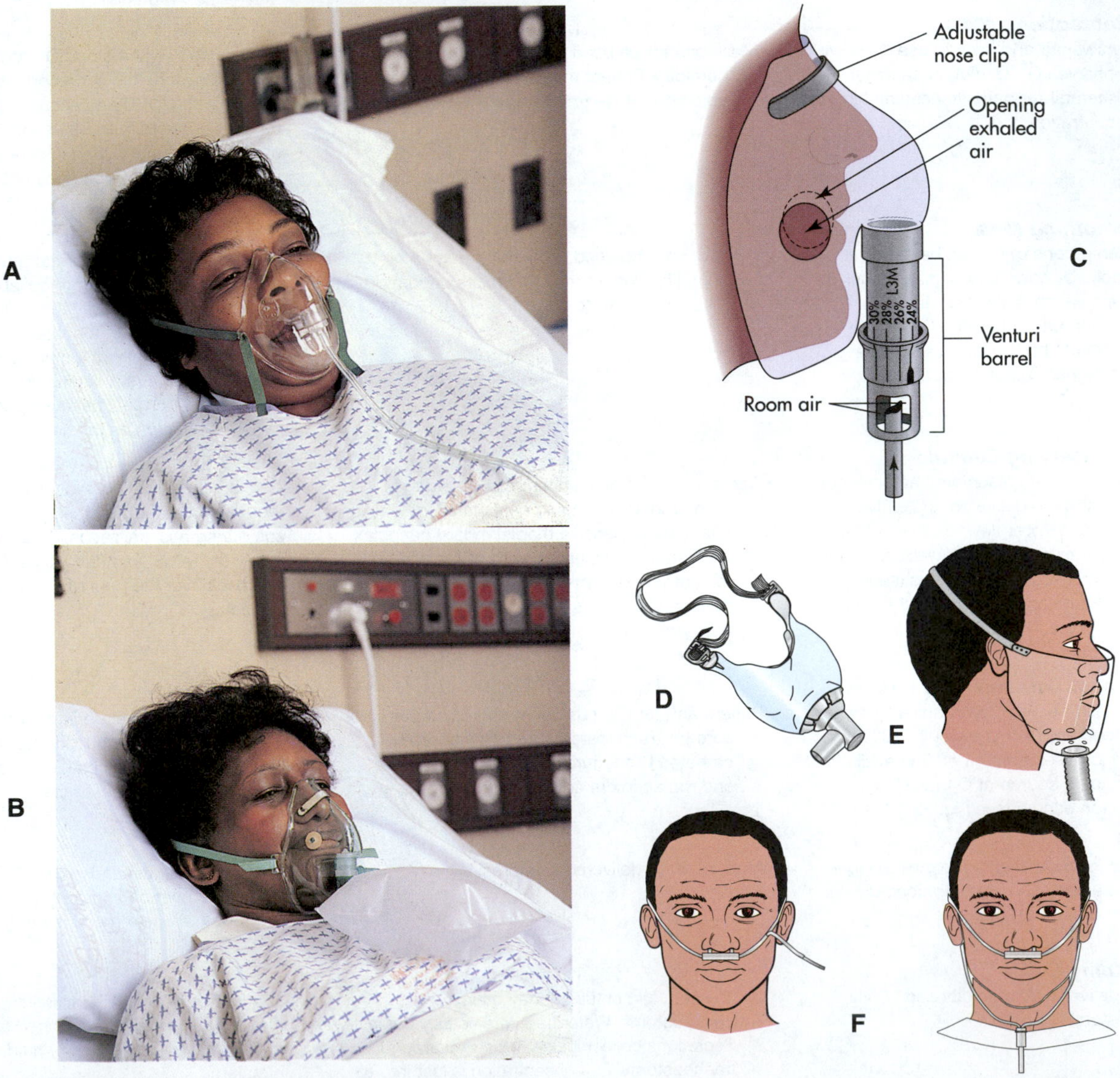

FIG. 29-11 Methods of oxygen administration. **A,** Simple face mask. **B,** Plastic face mask with reservoir bag. **C,** Venturi mask. **D,** Tracheostomy mask. **E,** Face tent. **F,** Standard nasal cannulas.

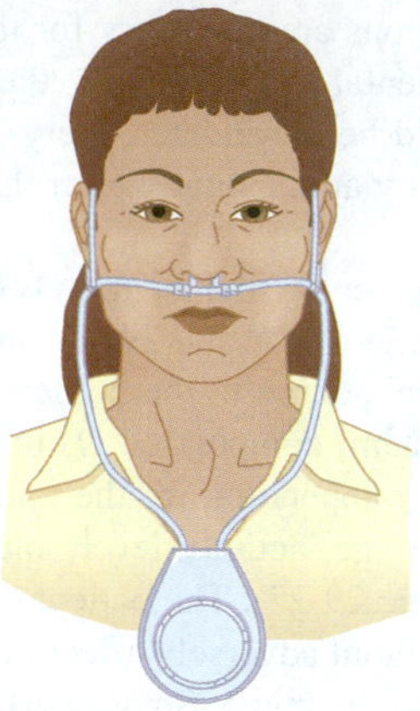

FIG. 29-12 Pendant-type oxygen-conserving cannula.

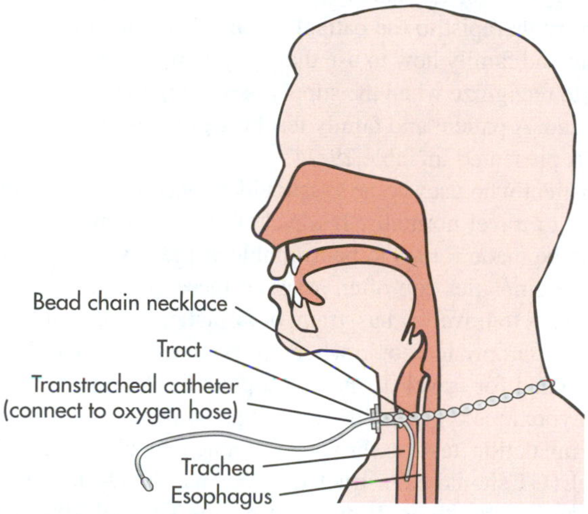

FIG. 29-13 Transtracheal catheter for oxygen administration.

meter. O_2 passes into the jar, bubbles through the water, and then goes through tubing to the patient's catheter, cannula, or mask. The purpose of the bubble-through humidifier is to restore the humidity conditions of room air. However, the need for bubble-through humidifiers at flow rates between 1 and 4 L per minute is dependent on patient preference.

Another means of administering humidified O_2 is via a nebulizer. It delivers particulate water mist (aerosols) with nearly 100% humidity. The humidity can be raised by heating the water, which increases the ability of the gas to hold moisture. Heated (98.6° F [37° C]) and humidified (100%) gas is required when the upper airway is bypassed in acute care. However, patients with established tracheotomies do not always require 100% humidity. When nebulizers are used, large-size tubing should be employed to connect the device to a face mask or T bar. If small-size tubing is used, condensation can occlude the flow of O_2. Vapotherm can deliver high flows (15 to 20 L/min) of warm humidified air (either sterile air or O_2) to the patient through a nasal cannula or transtracheal cannula using technology to warm and saturate the gas stream.

Complications

Combustion. O_2 supports combustion and increases the rate of burning. This is why it is important that smoking be prohibited in the area in which O_2 is being used. A "No Smoking" sign should be prominently displayed on the patient's door. The patient should

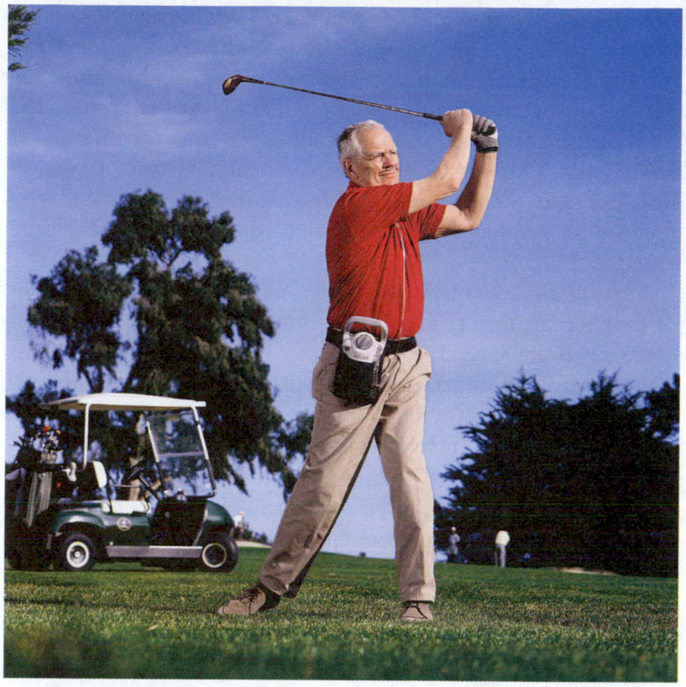

FIG. 29-14 Golfer uses Helios liquid portable oxygen system.

also be cautioned against smoking cigarettes with O_2 cannula in place.

CO_2 Narcosis. The two chemoreceptors in the respiratory center that control the drive to breathe respond to CO_2 and O_2. Normally, CO_2 accumulation is the major stimulant of the respiratory center. Over time some COPD patients develop a tolerance for high CO_2 levels (the respiratory center loses its sensitivity to the elevated CO_2 levels). Theoretically, for these individuals the "O_2 drive" to breathe is hypoxemia. Thus there has been concern regarding the dangers of administering O_2 to COPD patients and reducing their drive to breathe. This has been a pervasive myth but is not a serious threat. In fact, not providing adequate O_2 to these patients is much more detrimental. Although O_2 administration should be titrated to the lowest effective dose, many patients who have end-stage COPD require high flow rates and higher concentrations for survival. They may, in fact, exhibit higher than normal levels of CO_2 in their blood, but this is of little concern. What is important is careful, ongoing assessment when providing O_2 to these patients, monitoring both physical and cognitive effects of O_2.

It is critical to start O_2 at low flow rates until ABGs can be obtained. ABGs are used as a guide to determine what FIO_2 level is sufficient and can be tolerated. The patient's mental status and vital signs should be assessed before starting O_2 therapy and frequently thereafter.

O_2 Toxicity. Pulmonary **O_2 toxicity** may result from prolonged exposure to a high level of O_2 (PaO_2). The development of O_2 toxicity is relatively rare, but is determined by patient tolerance, exposure time, and effective dose. High concentrations of O_2 damage alveolar-capillary membranes, inactivate pulmonary surfactant, cause interstitial and alveolar edema, and decrease compliance. These individuals develop acute respiratory distress syndrome (ARDS)[34] (see Chapter 68). Prevention of O_2 toxicity is important for the patient who is receiving O_2. The amount of O_2 administered should be just enough to maintain the PaO_2 within a normal or acceptable range for the patient. ABGs should be monitored frequently to evaluate the effectiveness of therapy and to guide the tapering of supplemental O_2. A safe limit of O_2 concentrations has not yet been established. All levels above 50% and used for longer than 24 hours should be considered potentially toxic. Levels of 40% and below may be regarded as relatively nontoxic and may not result in development of significant O_2 toxicity if the exposure period is short.

Absorption Atelectasis. Normally, nitrogen, which constitutes 79% of the air that is breathed, is not absorbed into the bloodstream. This prevents alveolar collapse. When high concentrations of O_2 are given, nitrogen is washed out of the alveoli and replaced with O_2. If airway obstruction occurs, the O_2 is absorbed into the bloodstream and the alveoli collapse. This process is called **absorption atelectasis.**

Infection. Infection can be a major hazard of O_2 administration. Heated nebulizers present the highest risk. The constant use of humidity supports bacterial growth, with the most common infecting organism being *Pseudomonas aeruginosa.* Disposable equipment that operates as a closed system should be used. There should be a hospital policy stating the required frequency of equipment changes based on the type of equipment used at that particular institution.

Chronic O_2 Therapy at Home. Improved survival occurs in patients with COPD who receive long-term O_2 therapy (LTOT) (>15 hours/day) to treat hypoxemia.[41] The improved prognosis results from preventing progression of the disease and subsequent cor pulmonale. The benefits of long-term O_2 therapy include improved mental acuity, lung mechanics, sleep, and exercise tolerance; decreased hematocrit; and reduced pulmonary hypertension. Some patients believe they will become "addicted" to O_2 and are very reluctant to use it. They need to be educated that it is not "addicting" and that it needs to be used for the prescribed times during the day because of the positive effects on the heart, lungs, and brain. The need for LTOT should be evaluated when the patient's condition has stabilized. The goal of O_2 therapy is to maintain SaO_2 >90% during rest, sleep, and exertion.

Short-term home O_2 therapy (1 to 30 days) may be indicated for the patient in whom hypoxemia persists after discharge from the hospital. For example, the patient with underlying COPD who develops a serious respiratory infection may continue to have clearing of the infection after completion of antibiotic therapy and discharge from the hospital. This patient may demonstrate continued hypoxemia for 4 to 6 weeks after discharge. It is important to measure the patient's oxygenation status by ABGs 30 to 90 days after an acute episode to determine if the O_2 is still warranted.

Patients whose disease is stable with a PaO_2 of 55 mm Hg or less (corresponding to an SaO_2 of 88% or less) should receive LTOT. A patient whose PaO_2 is between 55 and 60 mm Hg (SaO_2 89%) and who exhibits signs of tissue hypoxia, such as cor pulmonale, erythrocytosis, peripheral edema from right-sided heart failure, or impaired mental status, should also receive LTOT. Desaturation only during exercise or sleep suggests consideration of O_2 therapy specifically under those conditions. Patients may receive O_2 only during exercise and/or sleep. The need for O_2 during these periods should be evaluated with a 6-minute walk test or overnight oximetry. (Pulse oximetry is discussed in Chapter 26.) Sleep-disordered breathing may be seen in some of these patients, and they will require a full sleep study.

Periodic reevaluations are necessary for the patient who is using chronic supplemental O_2. Generally the recommendation is that the patient should be reevaluated every 30 to 90 days during the first year of therapy and annually after that, as long as the patient remains stable.

Nasal cannulas, either regular or the O_2-conserving type (see Table 29-22 and Figs. 29-11, *F,* and 29-13), are usually used to deliver O_2 from a central source in the home. The source may be a liquid O_2 storage system, compressed O_2 in tanks, or an O_2 concentrator or extractor, depending on the patient's home environment, insurance coverage, activity level, and proximity to an O_2 supply company (Table 29-23). The patient can use extension tubing (up to 50 feet) without adversely affecting the O_2 flow delivery to increase mobility in the home. Small, portable systems, such as liquid O_2, may be provided for the patient who remains active outside the home (Fig. 29-15).

Home O_2 systems are usually rented from a company that sends a respiratory therapist to the patient's home. The therapist teaches the patient and family how to use the O_2 system, how to care for it, and how to recognize when the supply is running low and needs to be reordered. A patient and family teaching guide for the use of O_2 at home is presented in Table 29-24.

The patient who uses home O_2 should be encouraged to remain active and to travel normally. If travel is by automobile, arrangements can be made for O_2 to be available at the destination point. O_2 supply companies can often assist in these arrangements. If a patient wishes to travel by bus, train, or airplane, the patient should inform the appropriate people when reservations are made that O_2 will be needed for travel. If there is a potential for the patient to become hypoxic, oxygen needs for flying can be determined via a hypoxia inhalation test or through a mathematical formula. Patients on LTOT should be instructed to increase the O_2 flow by 1 to 2 L/min during the flight. Those with resting PaO_2 of 70 mm Hg are likely to be safe to fly without O_2. However, they may become hypoxemic as PaO_2 may fall an average of 25 mm Hg. If patients have other comorbidities, such as certain cardiac disease or anemia, they may also become hypoxemic. Patients should be warned that walking along the aisles on an airplane at high altitude can worsen hypoxemia. Because airplane cabins are pressurized to an elevation of 7000 or 8000 feet, the patient who uses supplemental O_2 should have it provided during flight. The airline's O_2 system must be used. Patients may not use their own O_2 system during flight because it is not properly pressurized. Airlines allow patients to bring their O_2 system to be carried in the baggage compartment for use at the point of destination, but the reservoirs (liquid or tank) must be empty and the valves left open. Some patients may need to avoid prolonged exposure to high elevations during travel unless they are instructed by their health care provider regarding adjustments in their O_2 flow to attempt to compensate for altitude.

Surgical Therapy for COPD. Three different surgical procedures have been used in severe COPD. One type of surgery is *lung volume reduction surgery* (LVRS).[55] The goal of therapy is to reduce the size of the lungs by removing about 30% of the most diseased lung tissue so the remaining healthy lung tissue can perform better. The rationale for this type of surgery is that by reducing the size of the hyperinflated emphysematous lungs, there is decreased airway obstruction and increased room for the remaining normal alveoli to expand and function. The procedure reduces lung volume and improves lung and chest wall mechanics. There are different types of LVRS. In one approach a median sternotomy

TABLE 29-23 Home Oxygen Delivery Systems

System	Advantages	Disadvantages	Comments
Liquid oxygen	Portable* unit (see Fig. 29-14) can be refilled by patient from reservoir (see Fig. 29-15). Portable unit holds 6-8 hr supply at 2 L/min; reservoir will last approximately 7-10 days at 2 L/min continuously.	Liquid system slightly more expensive, depending on location; not available everywhere; generally limited to urban areas.	As liquid warms to gas, some is vented from the system. In summer, evaporation is accelerated and may decrease reservoir duration to <1 wk.
Compressed O_2 cylinders	Portability possible with cart. Aluminum cylinders available that are light and easy to maneuver. Duration will vary with cylinder size and liter flow.	Duration of H or J tank at 2 L/min flow about 50 hr; storage of 4-5 large cylinders in the home necessary to have 1-wk to 10-day supply; portable cylinder on cart is cumbersome and heavy. Duration of E cylinder at 2 L/min approximately 4-5 hr; a cylinder at 2 L/min will last approximately 8-10 hr.	Some smaller tanks (D or M) may be used; these can be refilled from large cylinders and weigh about 10 lb. Tank can be carried on shoulder strap, backpack, or fanny pack or placed on portable cart.
Concentrator or extractor	Because the O_2 supply is made from room air, they never need to be "filled." On wheels, movable from room to room. Compact, excellent system for rural or homebound patient. Convenient, safe, and reliable.	Increase in electricity bill not reimbursable by insurance; >3 L flow results in significant decrease in concentration. Patient will need backup O_2 tank in case electricity fails.	Concentrator should be kept in room other than bedroom; extension tubing should be used if noise disturbs sleep.
O_2 conserving or pulsed devices	Delivers a pulse of O_2 only during inhalation to conserve O_2. Allows patient increased mobility. Devices are relatively lightweight, varying from approximately 3-6 lb with a supply of oxygen up to 20 hr. System may clip on belt or be contained in a backpack or shoulder bag.	Device may not be able to provide sufficient oxygen during exertion. Audible pulses may be annoying. Some devices may require batteries. Although rare, mechanical failure can occur. Device is costly. Becomes less efficient at higher O_2 flow rates. Usually best for low activity levels.	Monitor patient's O_2 saturation during rest and exercise to determine if oxygenation is acceptable. Will need to speak with vendor and/or respiratory therapist if O_2 saturation is below desired level.

**Portable* usually refers to units weighing more than 10 lb (4.5 kg) and ambulatory units weighing less than 10 lb.

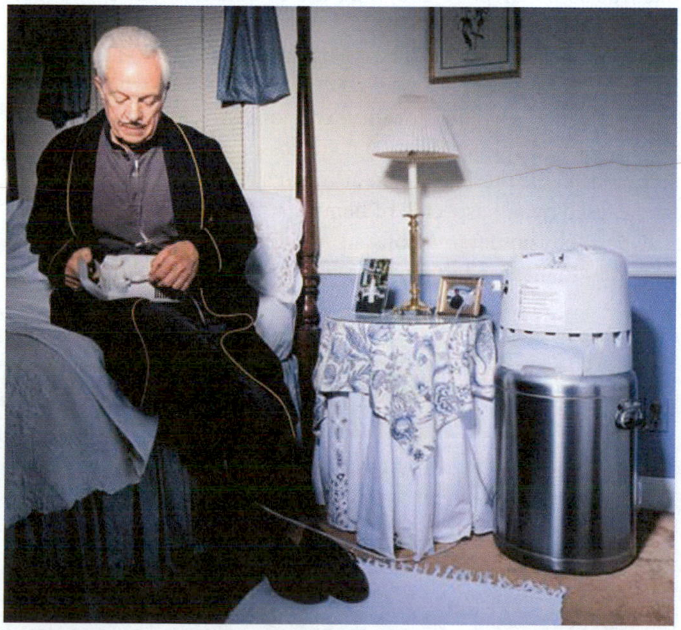

FIG. 29-15 A portable liquid O_2 unit can be refilled from a liquid O_2 reservoir unit.

TABLE 29-24 *PATIENT AND FAMILY TEACHING GUIDE* Home Oxygen Use

Mask/Cannula
- Ensure that the straps are not too tight
- Remove 2-3 times/day to wash and dry skin where straps touch the skin; massage skin
- Pad any pressure points
- Observe tops of ears for skin breakdown from pressure points

Oral and Nasal Mucous Membranes
- Assess oral and nasal mucous membranes 2-3 times/day
- Use water-based gel on lips and nasal mucosa
- Provide frequent oral hygiene
- Provide humidification via humidifier or nebulizing device

Decreasing Risk for Infection
- Remove mask or collar and cleanse with water 2-3 times/day
- Cleanse skin carefully at this time and observe for cuts, scratches, and bruises
- Change disposable equipment frequently
- Remove secretions that are coughed out

Decreasing Risk of Fire Injuries
- Post "No Smoking" warning signs in home where they can be seen
- Do not use electric razors, portable radios, open flames, wool blankets, or mineral oils in the area where oxygen is in use
- Do not allow smoking in the home

A good resource is Patient information series: oxygen therapy by American Thoracic Society. Available at *www.thoracic.org/patiented/patedmaterials.asp*.

is performed and parts of each lung are removed and tissue reattached using a stapling device. Another approach is a video-assisted thoracoscopy that can be performed unilaterally or bilaterally. In this approach either a stapling or laser procedure can be done, or they can be done together. The most common postoperative complication is pneumonia. Another technique for LVRS is a minimally invasive technique via a bronchoscope.[56,57] In certain patients LVRS has been shown to improve breathing, lung capacity, and quality of life.[55] However, it does not cure COPD. It is best used for patients with upper lobe emphysema.[55] However, hospital costs of LVRS are high and it is still considered experimental.[1]

The second surgical procedure is *bullectomy.* This procedure is used for patients with emphysematous COPD who have large bullae (>1 cm). The bullae are usually resected via thoracoscope. In certain patients this procedure has resulted in improved lung function and reduction in dyspnea.

The third surgical procedure is *lung transplantation.* COPD patients are the largest group of patients on waiting lists for lung transplantation. Although single-lung transplant is the most commonly used technique because of a shortage of donors, bilateral transplantation can be performed. In some cases LVRS is a bridge until transplantation. In appropriately selected patients with very advanced COPD, lung transplantation improves functional capacity and enhances quality of life.[58] However, rejection and effects of immunosuppressive therapy remain an obstacle. (Lung transplantation is discussed in Chapters 14 and 28.)

Respiratory and Physical Therapy. Respiratory therapy (RT) and physical therapy (PT) rehabilitation activities are performed by respiratory therapists or physical therapists depending on the institution. RT and/or PT activities include breathing retraining, effective cough techniques, and chest physiotherapy. RT is responsible for aerosol-nebulization therapy.

Breathing Retraining. The patient with COPD develops an increased respiratory rate with a prolonged expiration to compensate for the obstruction to airflow resulting in dyspnea. In addition, the accessory muscles of breathing in the neck and upper part of the chest are used excessively to promote chest wall movement. These muscles are not designed for long-term use, and as a result the patient experiences increased fatigue. Breathing exercises may assist the patient during rest and activity (e.g., lifting, walking, stair climbing) by decreasing dyspnea, improving oxygenation, and slowing the respiratory rate. The main types of breathing exercises commonly taught are (1) pursed-lip breathing and (2) diaphragmatic breathing.

The proposed rationale for using **pursed-lip breathing** (PLB) is to prolong exhalation and thereby prevent bronchiolar collapse and air trapping. Often instinctively patients will perform this technique. The patient should be taught PLB before, during, and after any activity causing dyspnea or tachypnea. The patient is taught to inhale slowly through the nose and then to exhale slowly through pursed lips, almost as if whistling. Exhalation should be at least three times as long as inhalation. It is helpful to have the nurse demonstrate the breathing exercises so the patient can imitate the action. The following techniques can be used to teach PLB:

1. Blow through a straw in a glass of water with the intent of forming small bubbles.
2. Blow at a lit candle enough to bend the flame without blowing it out.
3. Steadily blow a table-tennis ball across a table.
4. Blow a tissue held in the hand until it gently flaps.

Patients should be taught to use "just enough" positive pressure with the pursed lips because excessive resistance may increase the work of breathing. The issue of whether and how extensively PLB affects dyspnea is still questioned, but current evidence seems to support the use of PLB to improve the breathing of patients with COPD.[59,60]

Diaphragmatic (abdominal) breathing focuses on using the diaphragm instead of the accessory muscles of the chest to (1) achieve maximum inhalation and (2) slow the respiratory rate. To date, evidence from controlled studies does not support the use of diaphragmatic breathing in patients with COPD patients.[61] For patients with severe COPD, diaphragmatic breathing may result in hyperinflation because of increased fatigue and dyspnea and abdominal paradoxic breathing (the inward movement of the abdomen and the outward movement of the upper chest during inspiration) rather than with normal chest wall motion (the outward movement of the abdomen and upper chest simultaneously during inspiration).

PLB slows the respiratory rate and is much easier to learn than diaphragmatic breathing. In the setting of extreme acute dyspnea when the patient is hospitalized for infection or heart failure, it is more important to focus on helping the patient slow the respiratory rate by using the principles of PLB.

PLB is simple and easy to teach and learn. PLB should be practiced for 8 to 10 repetitions three or four times a day. PLB gives the patient more control over breathing, especially during exercise and periods of dyspnea.

Effective Coughing. Many patients with COPD have developed ineffective coughing patterns that do not adequately clear their airways of sputum. In addition, they fear they may develop spastic coughing, resulting in increased dyspnea. Guidelines for effective coughing are presented in Table 29-25. *Huff coughing* is an effective technique that the patient can be easily taught. The main goals of effective coughing are to conserve energy, reduce fatigue, and facilitate removal of secretions.

Chest Physiotherapy. Chest physiotherapy (CPT) is indicated in the patient with (1) excessive bronchial secretions who has difficulty clearing secretions with expectorated sputum production greater than 25 ml per day, (2) evidence or suggestion of retained secretions in the presence of an artificial airway, or (3) lobar atelectasis caused by or suspected of being caused by mucous plugging.

Chest physiotherapy consists of percussion, vibration, and postural drainage (Table 29-26). Percussion and vibration are

TABLE 29-25 ***PATIENT AND FAMILY TEACHING GUIDE***
Guidelines for Effective Coughing

1. Patient assumes a sitting position with head slightly flexed, shoulders relaxed, knees flexed, and forearms supported by pillow, and if possible, with feet on the floor.
2. Patient then drops head and bends forward while using slow, pursed-lip breathing to exhale.
3. Sitting up again, patient uses diaphragmatic breathing to inhale slowly and deeply.
4. Patient repeats steps 2 and 3 three to four times to facilitate mobilization of secretions.
5. Before initiating a cough, patient should take a deep abdominal breath, bend slightly forward, and then huff cough (cough three to four times on exhalation). Patient may need to support or splint thorax or abdomen to achieve a maximum cough.

manual or mechanical techniques used to augment postural drainage. **Postural drainage** uses the principle of gravity to assist in bronchial drainage. Percussion and vibration are used after the patient has assumed a postural drainage position to assist in loosening the mobilized secretions. Percussion, vibration, and postural drainage may assist in bringing secretions into larger, more central airways. Effective coughing is then necessary to help raise these secretions. After each drainage position change, the patient should be given time to cough and deep breathe. These techniques are individualized based on the patient's pulmonary condition and response to the initial treatment. Sometimes it takes several hours after CPT for secretions to be expectorated. It is important to evaluate CPT for both its effectiveness and relief of the patient's symptoms. CPT should be performed by an individual who has been properly trained. Complications associated with improperly performed CPT include fractured ribs, bruising, hypoxemia, and discomfort to the patient. CPT may not be beneficial and may be stressful for some patients. Some patients may develop hypoxemia and bronchospasms with CPT.

Percussion. Percussion is performed in the appropriate postural drainage position with the hands in a cuplike position (Fig. 29-16). The hands are cupped, and the fingers and thumbs are closed. The cupped hand should create an air pocket between the patient's chest and the hand. Both hands are cupped and used in an alternating rhythmic fashion. Percussion is accomplished with flexion and extension of the wrists. If it is performed correctly, a hollow sound should be heard. The air-cushion impact facilitates the movement of thick mucus. A thin towel should be placed over the area to be percussed, or the patient may choose to wear a T-shirt or hospital gown. The patient's face should be in clear view when percussing in case a mucous plug occludes the airway and the patient is unable to speak. Percussion should not be performed over the kidneys, sternum, spinal cord, bony prominences, or any tender or painful area. Other contraindications to percussion include hemoptysis, carcinoma, and induced bronchospasm. Commercial devices that percuss are available if the patient lives alone and has no one to help with the therapy.

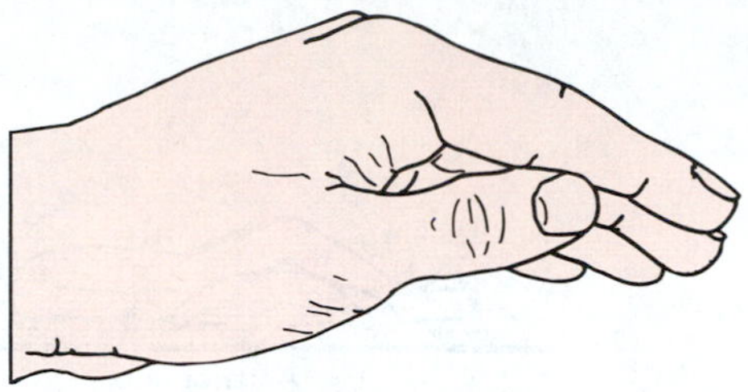

FIG. 29-16 Cupped-hand position for percussion. The hand should be cupped as though scooping up water.

Vibration. Vibration is accomplished by tensing the hand and arm muscles repeatedly and pressing mildly with the flat of the hand on the affected area while the patient slowly exhales a deep breath. Isometric contractions of the arms and hands are also appropriate. The vibrations facilitate movement of secretions to larger airways. Mild vibration is tolerated better than percussion and can be used in situations where percussion may be contraindicated. Commercial vibrators are available for hospital and home use.

Postural Drainage. The lungs are divided into five lobes, with three on the right side and two on the left side. There are 18 segments in the lungs, which can be drained by 18 positions. Fig. 29-17 shows the modified postural drainage positions most often used in clinical practice. The purpose of various positions in postural drainage is to drain each segment toward the larger airways. The postural drainage positions are determined by the areas of involved lung, which are assessed by chest x-rays, percussion, palpation, and auscultation. Aerosolized bronchodilators and hydration therapy are frequently administered before postural drainage. The chosen postural drainage position is maintained for 5 to 15 minutes or during percussion/vibration. The degree of slope can be obtained with pillows, blocks, books, or a tilt board.

The frequency and choice of postural drainage positions depend on the location of retained secretions and patient tolerance to dependent positions. A common order is two to four times a day. In acute situations, postural drainage may be performed as frequently as every 1 to 2 hours. The procedure should be planned to occur and be completed at least 1 hour before meals or 3 hours after meals.

If a patient has difficulty in assuming various positions, adaptations will be needed to reduce the angle or length of time of the procedure. A side-lying position can be used for the patient who cannot tolerate a head-down position. There are also beds on the market that can rotate and percuss in various postural drainage positions. Some positions for postural drainage (e.g., Trendelenburg) should not be performed on the patient with chest trauma, hemoptysis, heart disease, or head injury, and in other situations where the patient's condition is not stable.

TABLE 29-26 Steps in Chest Physiotherapy

1. Perform procedure 1 hr before meals or 1-3 hr after meals.
2. Administer bronchodilator approximately 15 min before procedure.
3. Collect needed equipment such as tissues, emesis basin, paper bag, and pillows.
4. Help patient assume correct position for postural drainage based on findings from x-ray, auscultation, palpation, and percussion of chest. If patient's tolerance is limited, start with the lower lung fields. Position should be maintained for 5-15 min to mobilize secretions via gravity.
5. Observe patient during treatment to assess tolerance. Particularly observe breathing and color changes, especially duskiness in face.
6. Have patient take several deep abdominal breaths.
7. Percuss appropriate area for 1-2 min keeping the patient's face in full view.
8. Vibrate the same area while the patient exhales 4-5 deep breaths.*
9. Assist patient to cough while assuming same position. Splinting with towel or hands may be necessary to aid in effective coughing. Patient may have to assume sitting position to generate enough airflow to expel secretions. (Coughing productively may be a long waiting process that may occur 30 min after procedure.) Suction may be necessary if coughing is not effective.
10. Repeat percussion, vibration, and coughing until patient no longer expectorates mucus.
11. Repeat same procedure in all necessary positions.
12. After procedure, help patient assume a comfortable position, assist with oral hygiene, and discard used tissues.
13. Monitor for hypoxemia if patient is having any respiratory difficulty during the procedure.
14. Evaluate and chart effectiveness of treatment by amount of sputum produced and the results of auscultation. Also chart patient tolerance.

*If using an electronic vibrator, use for periods of 5-20 min in each position according to the patient's tolerance.

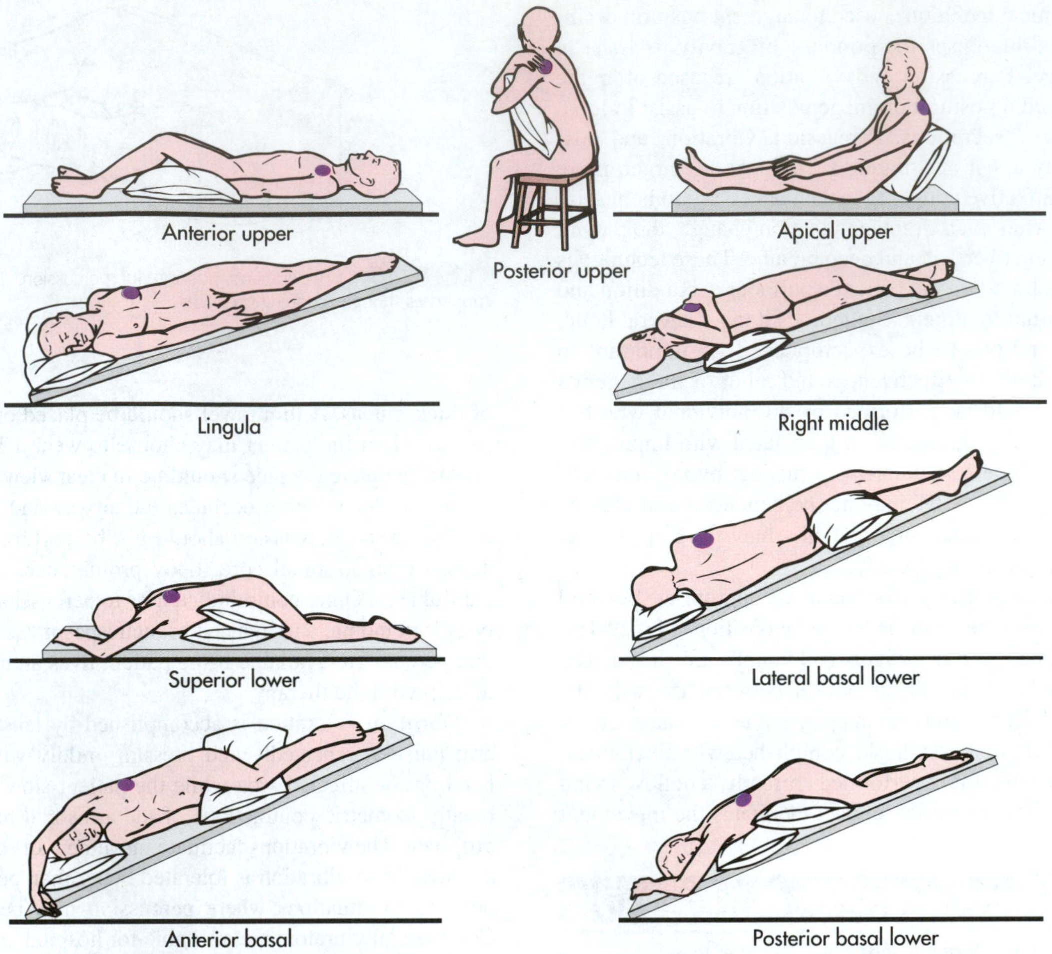

FIG. 29-17 Representative positions for postural drainage. *Shaded areas* in each drawing indicate the segment of the lung in which drainage is promoted.

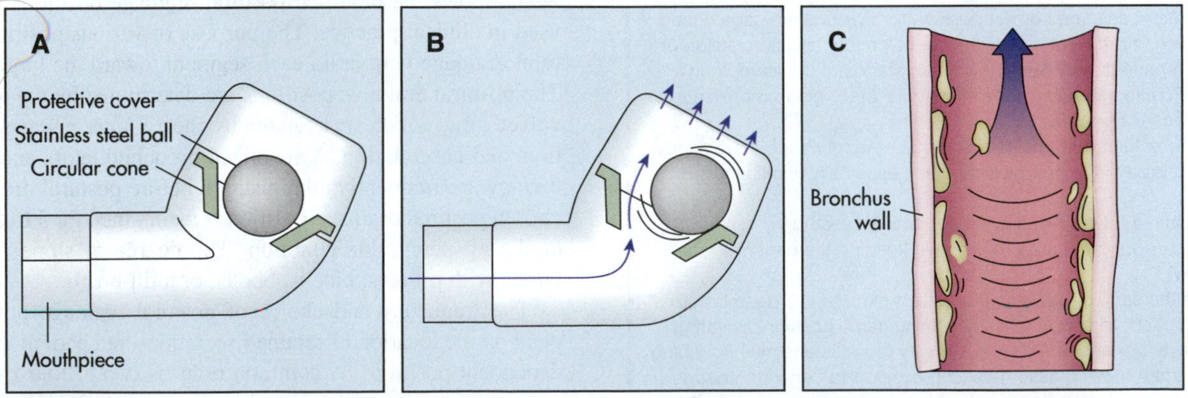

FIG. 29-18 Flutter mucus clearance device is a small handheld device that provides positive expiratory pressure (PEP) therapy. It is used to facilitate removal of mucus from the lungs. **A,** It consists of a hard plastic mouthpiece, a plastic perforated cover, and a high-density stainless steel ball resting in a circular cone. **B,** The Flutter effects occur during expiration. Before exhalation, the steel ball blocks the conical canal of the Flutter. During exhalation, the position of the steel ball is the result of an equilibrium between the pressure of the exhaled air, the force of gravity on the ball, and the angle of the cone where the contact with the ball occurs. As the steel ball rolls and moves up and down, it creates an opening and closing cycle that repeats itself many times throughout each exhalation. The net result is that vibrations occur in the airways resulting in the "fluttering" sensation. **C,** These vibrations loosen mucus from the airway walls and facilitate their movement up the airways.

Flutter Mucus Clearance Device. The Flutter mucus clearance device is a handheld device that is shaped like a small, fat pipe (Fig. 29-18). It provides positive expiratory pressure (PEP) treatment for patients with mucus-producing conditions. The Flutter has a mouthpiece, a high-density stainless steel ball, and a cone that holds the ball. When the patient exhales through the Flutter, the steel ball moves, which causes vibrations in the lungs and loosens mucus. It helps move mucus up through the airways to the mouth where the mucus can be expectorated. Although the Flutter valve is mostly used in patients with cystic fibrosis, it has been effectively used in patients with excessive secretions with COPD and bronchiectasis.

High-Frequency Chest Compression (ThAIRaphy Vest). High-frequency chest compression uses an inflatable vest (ThAIRaphy vest) with hoses connected to a high-frequency pulse generator. The pulse generator delivers air to the vest, which vibrates the chest. The high-frequency air waves clear all lobes of the lungs. The vest has been found to be more effective than conventional CPT in clearing mucus, and it can be done without the aid of another person. The unit weighs only 30 lb and is quiet. It comes in its own suitcase and is portable.

Acapella. Acapella is a small handheld device that combines the benefits of both PEP therapy and airway vibrations of the Flutter valve to mobilize pulmonary secretions. It works by using oscillating vibrations that travel to the lung, shaking free mucous plugs that the patient can then cough up. It can be used in virtually any setting as the patients are free to sit, stand, or recline. It improves clearance of secretions, is easier to tolerate than CPT, takes less than half the time of conventional CPT sessions, and facilitates opening of airways.

Aerosol Nebulization Therapy. Medications for COPD patients are most often delivered via metered-dose or dry powder inhalers. This is the preferred delivery route, although devices that deliver a suspension of fine particles of liquid in a gas, called nebulizers, may also be used to deliver medications to the COPD patient. Nebulizers are usually powered by a compressed air or O_2 generator. At home the patient may have an air-powered compressor; in the hospital, wall O_2 or compressed air is used to power the nebulizer.

Aerosolized medication orders must include the medication, dose, diluent, and whether it is to be nebulized with O_2 or compressed air. Medication is nebulized or reduced to a fine spray, and depending on several factors, including droplet size, it can be inhaled into the patient's tracheobronchial tree. The advantage to aerosol-nebulization therapy is that it is easy to use. Medications that are routinely nebulized include albuterol and ipratropium.

The patient is placed in an upright position that allows for most efficient breathing to ensure adequate penetration and deposition of the aerosolized medication. The patient must breathe slowly and deeply through the mouth and hold inspiration for 2 to 3 seconds. Deep diaphragmatic breathing helps ensure deposition of the medication. The patient is instructed to do normal breathing in between these large forced breaths to prevent alveolar hypoventilation and dizziness. After the treatment the patient should be instructed to cough effectively. Postural drainage and CPT are ideally done after bronchodilator medications are given.

A disadvantage of nebulizer equipment use is the potential for bacterial growth. Because home nebulization is used for the patient with COPD, it is important for the health care professional in the hospital and home care setting to review cleaning procedures for home respiratory equipment with the patient. A frequently used, effective home-cleaning method is to wash the nebulizer daily in soap and water, rinse it with water, and soak it for 20 to 30 minutes in a 1:1 white vinegar–water solution followed by a water rinse and air drying. Commercial respiratory cleaning agents may also be used if directions are followed carefully. Cleaning the nebulizer in the top shelf of an automatic dishwasher saves time, and the hot water destroys most organisms.

Nutritional Therapy. Weight loss and malnutrition are commonly seen in the patient with severe emphysematous COPD. The cause of this weight loss is not entirely known but is likely multifactorial. Eating becomes an effort because of dyspnea and O_2 desaturation, especially in the later stages of COPD. Patients may require more caloric expenditure than calories ingested. A full stomach presses up on the flattened diaphragm, causing increased dyspnea and discomfort. It is difficult for some patients to eat and breathe at the same time; therefore inadequate amounts of food are eaten. Also large amounts of energy are expended to breathe and maintain even normal activities. Therefore weight loss and muscle wasting are likely.[62] Excessive weight loss is also related to increased energy consumption, stress, and the burden and devastation of the inflammatory processes occurring in the lung, which may lead to a cachectic state.

The patient with COPD should try to keep body mass index (BMI) between 21 and 25 kg/m^2. Being either overweight or underweight can be a problem with COPD. However, a reduced BMI or weight loss is associated with poor outcomes in acute exacerbations and increased morbidity and mortality rates in COPD patients.[35]

To decrease dyspnea and conserve energy, the patient should rest for at least 30 minutes before eating, use a bronchodilator before meals, and select foods that can be prepared in advance. The patient should eat five to six small, frequent meals to avoid feelings of bloating and early satiety when eating. Liquid, blenderized, or commercial diets may be helpful. Foods that require a great deal of chewing should be avoided or served in another manner (e.g., grated, pureed). Cold foods may give less of a sense of fullness than hot foods. Exercises and treatments should be avoided for at least 1 hour before and after eating. The exertion involved in the preparation and eating of food is often fatiguing. The use of frozen foods and a microwave oven may help conserve the patient's energy in food preparation. The patient's dentition should be assessed because broken, missing teeth or loose dentures make eating more difficult. Activity such as walking or getting out of bed during the day can stimulate the appetite and promote weight gain. Many patients with COPD have feelings of bloating and early satiety when eating. This sensation can be attributed to swallowing air while eating, side effects of medication (especially corticosteroids and theophylline), and the abnormal position of the diaphragm relative to the stomach in association with hyperinflation. Intestinal gas–forming foods should be avoided, such as cabbage, brussels sprouts, and beans.

Underweight patients with emphysematous COPD have a greater than normal nutritional requirement for protein and calories. They may need 25 to 45 kcal/kg and 1.2 to 1.9 g of protein per kilogram to even maintain their weight. A high-calorie, high-protein diet is recommended and can be divided into five or six small meals a day. High-protein, high-calorie nutritional supplements can be offered between meals. Ice cream added to these supplements can help increase calories. Drinking skim or 1% milk rather than whole milk may cause less mucus production. (Nutritional supplements are discussed in Chapter 40.) Nonprotein calories should be divided evenly between fat and carbohydrate while not overfeeding the patient.[62] In most cases just getting the patients to eat adequate amounts of any foods can be difficult. The oral anabolic steroid, oxandrolone (Oxandrin), has shown promise in helping patients gain weight and improve muscle strength.[63] Megestrol (Megace) has also been used to stimulate and increase appetite. If the patient has O_2 prescribed, use of supplemental O_2 by nasal cannulas while eating may also be beneficial, because eating expends energy. Fluid intake should be at least 3 L per day unless contraindicated for other medical conditions, such as heart or renal failure. Fluids should be taken between meals (rather than with them) to prevent excess stomach distention and to decrease pressure on the diaphragm. Sodium restriction may be indicated if there is accompanying heart failure.

NURSING MANAGEMENT
CHRONIC OBSTRUCTIVE PULMONARY DISEASE

▪ Nursing Assessment

Subjective and objective data that should be obtained from a person with COPD are presented in Table 29-27.

▪ Nursing Diagnoses

The nursing diagnoses for the patient with COPD may include, but are not limited to, those presented in NCP 29-2.

▪ Planning

The overall goals are that the patient with COPD will have (1) prevention of disease progression, (2) ability to perform ADLs and improved exercise tolerance, (3) relief from symptoms, (4) no complications related to COPD, (5) knowledge and ability to implement a long-term treatment regimen, and (6) overall improved quality of life.[1]

▪ Nursing Implementation

Health Promotion. The incidence of COPD would decrease dramatically if people would not begin smoking or would stop smoking. (Techniques to help patients stop smoking are discussed in Chapter 12 and Tables 12-4, 12-5, and 12-6.) Avoiding or controlling exposure to occupational and environmental pollutants and irritants is another preventive measure to maintain healthy lungs. (These factors are discussed in the section on nursing management of lung cancer in Chapter 28.)

Early detection of small-airway disease is important. The person who has smoked for only a few years may have early evidence of obstructive airway disease on spirometry testing as it is the first test to show abnormal results. It is extremely important for the person to stop smoking because it is the only way to stop the progression of COPD. Therefore, when patients are confronted with an abnormal test (FEV_1), they can often be motivated to stop smoking if they realize how much lung function they can regain.[64] As health care professionals, nurses who smoke should reevaluate their own smoking behavior and its relationship to their health. Nurses, health care providers, and respiratory therapists who smoke and smell of cigarette smoke should be aware that the odor of their clothes can be offensive or tempting to patients.

Early diagnosis and treatment of respiratory tract infections and exacerbations of COPD are other ways to decrease the incidence of COPD. Avoiding exposure to large crowds in the peak periods for influenza may be necessary, especially for the older adult and the person with a history of respiratory problems. Influenza and pneumococcal pneumonia vaccines are recommended for the patient with COPD.

Families with a history of COPD, as well as AAT deficiency, should be aware of the genetic nature of the disease. Genetic counseling is appropriate for the patient with AAT deficiency who is planning to have children.

Acute Intervention. The patient with COPD will require acute intervention for complications such as exacerbations of COPD, pneumonia, cor pulmonale, and acute respiratory failure. (The nursing care for these conditions is discussed in Chapters 28 and 68.) Once the crisis in these situations has been resolved, the nurse can assess the degree and severity of the underlying respiratory problem. The information obtained will help plan the nursing care.

TABLE 29-27 NURSING ASSESSMENT COPD

Subjective Data

Important Health Information

Past health history: Long-term exposure to chemical pollution, respiratory irritants, occupational fumes, dust; recurrent respiratory infections; previous hospitalizations

Medications: Use of O_2 and duration of O_2 use, bronchodilators, corticosteroids, antibiotics, anticholinergics, OTC drugs, herbs, medications purchased from outside United States or Canada

Functional Health Patterns

Health perception–health management: Smoking (pack-years, including passive smoking, willingness to stop smoking, and previous attempts); family history of respiratory disease (especially α_1-antitrypsin deficiency)

Nutritional-metabolic: Anorexia, weight loss or gain

Activity-exercise: Fatigue, ability to perform ADLs; swelling of feet; progressive dyspnea, especially on exertion; ability to walk up one flight of stairs without stopping; wheezing; recurrent cough; sputum production (especially in the AM) with changes in color, odor, viscosity, amount; orthopnea

Elimination: Constipation, gas, bloating

Sleep-rest: Insomnia; sitting up position for sleeping, paroxysmal nocturnal dyspnea

Cognitive-perceptual: Headache, chest or abdominal soreness

Coping-stress tolerance: Anxiety, depression

Objective Data

General

Debilitation, restlessness, assumption of upright position

Integumentary

Cyanosis (bronchitis), pallor or ruddy color, poor skin turgor, thin skin, digital clubbing, easy bruising; peripheral edema (cor pulmonale)

Respiratory

Rapid, shallow breathing; inability to speak; prolonged expiratory phase; pursed-lip breathing; wheezing; rhonchi, crackles, diminished or bronchial breath sounds; ↓ chest excursion and diaphragm movement; use of accessory muscles; hyperresonant or dull chest sounds on percussion

Cardiovascular

Tachycardia; dysrhythmias, jugular vein distention, distant heart tones, right-sided S_3 (cor pulmonale), edema (especially in feet)

Gastrointestinal

Ascites, hepatomegaly (cor pulmonale)

Musculoskeletal

Muscle atrophy, ↑ anterior-posterior diameter (barrel-chest)

Possible Findings

Abnormal ABGs (compensated respiratory acidosis, $\downarrow PaO_2$ or SaO_2, $\uparrow PaCO_2$), polycythemia, pulmonary function tests showing expiratory airflow obstruction (e.g., low FEV_1, low FEV_1/FVC, large RV, chest x-ray showing flattened diaphragm and hyperinflation or infiltrates

ABGs, Arterial blood gases; *ADLs,* activities of daily living; *FEV_1,* forced expiratory volume in 1 second; *FVC,* forced vital capacity; *OTC,* over-the-counter; *RV,* residual volume.

Ambulatory and Home Care. By far the most important aspect in the long-term care of the patient with COPD is teaching. (A patient and family teaching guide is presented in Table 29-28.) With the rising cost of health care in the United States, nurses will likely be caring for patients in communities and in patients' homes.

Pulmonary Rehabilitation. Pulmonary rehabilitation should be included in the clinical management of all patients with

NURSING CARE PLAN 29-2

Patient with COPD

NURSING DIAGNOSIS **Ineffective airway clearance** *related to* expiratory airflow obstruction, ineffective cough, decreased airway humidity, and infection in airways *as evidenced by* ineffective or absent cough, presence of abnormal breath sounds, or absence of breath sounds

PATIENT GOALS
1. Maintains clear airway by effectively coughing
2. Experiences clear breath sounds

OUTCOMES (NOC)

Respiratory Status: Airway Patency

- Ease of breathing ____
- Respiratory rate ____
- Respiratory rhythm ____
- Moves sputum out of airway ____

Measurement Scale

1 = Severely compromised
2 = Substantially compromised
3 = Moderately compromised
4 = Mildly compromised
5 = Not compromised

- Adventitious breath sounds ____

Measurement Scale

1 = Severe
2 = Substantial
3 = Moderate
4 = Mild
5 = None

INTERVENTIONS (NIC) and *RATIONALES*

Cough Enhancement

- Assist patient to sitting position with head slightly flexed, shoulders relaxed, and knees flexed *to allow for adequate chest expansion.*
- Instruct patient to inhale deeply, bend forward slightly, and perform three or four huffs (against an open glottis) *to prevent airway collapse during exhalation.*
- Instruct the patient to follow coughing with several maximal inhalation breaths *to reoxygenate the lungs.*

Airway Management

- Encourage slow, deep breathing; turning; and coughing *to mobilize pulmonary secretions.*
- Position patient *to maximize ventilation potential.*
- Regulate fluid intake to optimize fluid balance *to liquefy secretions for easier expectoration.*
- Perform chest physiotherapy *to use effect of gravity in removing secretions.*
- Administer bronchodilators and aerosol treatments *to facilitate clearance of retained secretions and increase ease of breathing.*

NURSING DIAGNOSIS **Impaired gas exchange** *related to* alveolar hypoventilation *as evidenced by* headache on awakening, $PaCO_2 \geq 45$ mm Hg, $PaO_2 < 60$ mm Hg, or $SaO_2 < 90\%$ at rest

PATIENT GOALS
1. Returns to baseline respiratory function
2. $PaCO_2$ and PaO_2 return to levels normal for patient

OUTCOMES (NOC)

Respiratory Status: Gas Exchange

- Ease of breathing ____
- PaO_2 ____
- $PaCO_2$ ____
- Oxygen saturation ____

Measurement Scale

1 = Severely compromised
2 = Substantially compromised
3 = Moderately compromised
4 = Mildly compromised
5 = Not compromised

INTERVENTIONS (NIC) and *RATIONALES*

Airway Management

- Monitor respiratory and oxygenation status *to assess need for intervention.*
- Teach patient how to use prescribed inhalers.

Oxygen Therapy

- Administer supplemental oxygen as ordered.
- Set up oxygen equipment and administer through a heated, humidified system.
- Periodically check oxygen delivery device *to ensure that the prescribed concentration is being delivered.*
- Observe for signs of oxygen-induced hypoventilation *because this occurs with carbon dioxide narcosis.*
- Instruct patient and family about use of oxygen at home *to promote safe long-term oxygen therapy.*

Continued

COPD.[65] Research has validated the benefits of rehabilitation in patients with COPD, including increased exercise performance, reduced dyspnea, and health-related quality of life.[35] Pulmonary rehabilitation should no longer be viewed as a "last ditch" effort for patients with severe COPD.

The components of pulmonary rehabilitation, which can be done inpatient, outpatient, or in home settings, include physical therapy (e.g., bronchial hygiene, exercise conditioning, breathing retraining, energy conservation), nutrition, and education.[66] Other important topics in the structured program include smoking cessation, environmental factors, health promotion, psychologic counseling, and vocational rehabilitation. Nurses who have experience in pulmonary care are often responsible for the management of pulmonary rehabilitation centers. A large part of the nurse's role is to teach patients with COPD self-management of their disease. The minimum length of an effective program should be 2 months, but the longer the program,

NURSING CARE PLAN 29-2

Patient with COPD—cont'd

NURSING DIAGNOSIS **Imbalanced nutrition: less than body requirements** *related to* poor appetite, lowered energy level, shortness of breath, gastric distention, sputum production, and depression *as evidenced by* weight loss >10% of ideal body weight, serum albumin level below normal laboratory values, lack of interest in food

PATIENT GOALS 1. Maintains body weight within normal range for height and age
2. Consumes adequate nutrients for metabolic needs

OUTCOMES (NOC)

Appetite

- Desire to eat ____
- Enjoyment of food ____
- Reports energy to eat ____
- Food intake ____

Measurement Scale

1 = Severely compromised
2 = Substantially compromised
3 = Moderately compromised
4 = Mildly compromised
5 = Not compromised

Nutritional Status: Nutrient Intake

- Caloric intake ____
- Protein intake ____
- Vitamin intake ____
- Mineral intake ____

Measurement Scale

1 = Not adequate
2 = Slightly adequate
3 = Moderately adequate
4 = Substantially adequate
5 = Totally adequate

INTERVENTIONS (NIC) and *RATIONALES*

Nutrition Therapy

- Monitor food/fluid ingested and calculate daily caloric intake *to determine adequacy of intake.*
- Monitor laboratory values *for evidence of malnutrition.*
- Provide oral care before meals *to moisten and clean the mouth of sputum taste.*
- Provide patient with high-protein, high-calorie, nutritious finger foods and drinks that can be readily consumed *to provide adequate calories and protein that do not require much energy to consume.*
- Select nutritional supplements *to provide nutritional between-meal snacks.*

Nutrition Management

- Weigh patient at appropriate intervals *to assess nutritional status.*
- Provide food selection *to stimulate the appetite.*
- Adjust diet to patient's lifestyle *to reduce bloating.*
- Provide appropriate information about nutritional needs and how to meet them *to ensure nutritional adequacy after discharge.*

NURSING DIAGNOSIS **Insomnia** *related to* anxiety, dyspnea, depression, hypoxemia and/or hypercapnia, paroxysmal nocturnal dyspnea, and orthopnea *as evidenced by* frequent awakening, prolonged onset of sleep, lethargy, fatigue, irritability

PATIENT GOALS 1. Reports feeling rested upon awakening from sleep
2. Reports sleeping at least 6 hours a night

OUTCOMES (NOC)

Sleep

- Hours of sleep (at least 5 hr/24 hr) ____
- Sleep pattern ____
- Sleep quality ____
- Sleeps through the night consistently ____
- Feel rejuvenated after sleep ____

Measurement Scale

1 = Severely compromised
2 = Substantially compromised
3 = Moderately compromised
4 = Mildly compromised
5 = Not compromised

INTERVENTIONS (NIC) and *RATIONALES*

Sleep Enhancement

- Determine patient's sleep/activity pattern *to provide baseline data.*
- Monitor patient's sleep pattern, and note physical (e.g., sleep apnea, obstructed airway, and pain/discomfort and urinary frequency) and/or psychologic (e.g., fear or anxiety) circumstances that interrupt sleep *so appropriate interventions can be initiated.*
- Initiate/implement comfort measures of massage, positioning, and affective touch *to foster sleep.*
- Adjust environment (e.g., light, noise, temperature, mattress, and bed) *to promote sleep.*
- Monitor bedtime food and beverage intake for items that facilitate or interfere with sleep *to reduce interference with sleep.*
- Assist patient to limit daytime sleep by providing activity that promotes wakefulness.

the more effective the results. Exercise training, which includes upper and lower extremity work, should include a minimum of 20 sessions, 3 times per week to achieve results.

Activity Considerations. Exercise training leads to energy conservation which is an important component in COPD rehabilitation. This patient is typically an upper thoracic and neck breather who uses accessory muscles rather than the diaphragm. Thus the patient has difficulty performing upper-extremity activities, particularly those activities that require arm elevation above the head. Exercise training of the upper extremities may improve muscle function and help to reduce dyspnea. Frequently the patient has already adapted alternative energy-saving practices for ADLs. Alternative methods of hair care, shaving, showering, and reaching may need to be explored. An occupational therapist may help with ideas in these areas. Assuming a tripod posture (elbows supported on a table, chest in fixed position) and a mirror placed on the table

NURSING CARE PLAN 29-2

Patient with COPD—cont'd

NURSING DIAGNOSIS **Risk for infection** *related to* decreased pulmonary function, possible corticosteroid therapy, ineffective airway clearance, and lack of knowledge regarding signs and symptoms of infection and preventive measures

PATIENT GOALS
1. Uses behaviors that minimize risk of infection
2. Experiences no infection

OUTCOMES (NOC)

Knowledge: Infection Control

- Description of mode of transmission ____
- Description of factors contributing to transmission ____
- Description of practices that reduce transmission ____
- Description of monitoring procedures ____
- Description of signs and symptoms ____
- Description of treatment for diagnosed infection ____

Measurement Scale

1 = None
2 = Limited
3 = Moderate
4 = Substantial
5 = Extensive

INTERVENTIONS (NIC) and *RATIONALES*

Infection Protection

- Monitor for systemic and localized signs and symptoms of infection *to determine if an infection is present.*
- Monitor WBC count and differential results *to detect presence of infection.*
- Teach patient and family members how to avoid infections.
- Teach the patient and family about signs and symptoms of infection and when to report them to the health care provider *so treatment can be started promptly.*
- Administer vaccine *to decrease occurrence or severity of influenza or pneumonia.*

Infection Control

- Instruct patient on appropriate hand-washing techniques *to prevent spread of infection.*
- Encourage deep breathing and coughing *to prevent stasis of respiratory secretions.*

during use of an electric razor or hair dryer conserves much more energy than when the patient stands in front of a mirror to shave or blow-dry hair. If the patient uses home O_2 therapy, it is essential that the patient use the O_2 during activities of hygiene, because these are energy consuming. The patient should be encouraged to make a schedule and plan daily and weekly activities so as to leave plenty of time for rest periods. The patient should also try to sit as much as possible when performing activities. Another energy-saving tip is to exhale when pushing, pulling, or exerting effort during an activity and inhale during rest.

Walking or other endurance exercises such as cycling combined with strength training is likely the best intervention to strengthen muscles and improve the patient's endurance. Coordinated walking with slow, pursed-lip breathing without breath holding is a difficult task that requires conscious effort and frequent reinforcement. During coordinated walking and breathing, the patient is taught to breathe in through the nose while taking one step, then to breathe out through pursed lips while taking two to four steps (the number depends on the patient's tolerance). Walking should occur at a slow pace with rest periods when necessary so the patient can sit or lean against an object such as a tree or post. The patient may need to ambulate using O_2. The patient may be able to successfully perform coordinated walking with pursed-lip breathing, The nurse should walk with the patient, giving verbal reminders when necessary regarding breathing (inhalation and exhalation) and steps. Walking with the patient helps decrease anxiety and helps maintain a slow pace. It also enables the nurse to observe the patient's actions and physiologic responses to the activity. Many patients with moderate or severe COPD are anxious and fearful of walking or performing exercise. These patients and their families require much support while they build the confidence they need to walk or to perform daily exercises.

The patient should be encouraged to walk 15 to 20 minutes a day at least three times a week with gradual increases. Severely disabled patients can begin at a slow pace by walking for 2 to 5 minutes three times a day and slowly building up to 20 minutes a day, if possible. Adequate rest periods should be allowed. Some patients benefit from using their β_2-adrenergic agonist approximately 10 minutes before exercise. Parameters that may be monitored in the patient with mild COPD are resting pulse and pulse rate after walking. Pulse rate after walking should not exceed 75% to 80% of the maximum heart rate (maximum heart rate is age in years subtracted from 220). In the patient with other than mild COPD and without significant heart disease, it is usually dyspnea and the limitation in breathing rather than increased heart rate that limits the exercise. Thus it is better to use the patient's perceived sense of dyspnea as an indication of exercise tolerance. The Borg scale (see Chapter 26, Fig. 26-9) can be used to have the patient determine the intensity of dyspnea.

The patient should be told that shortness of breath will probably increase during exercise (as it does for a healthy individual) but that the activity is not being overdone if this increased shortness of breath returns to baseline within 5 minutes after the cessation of exercise. The patient should be told to wait 5 minutes after completion of exercise before using the β_2-adrenergic agonist to allow a chance to recover. During this time, slow, pursed-lip breathing should be used. If it takes longer than 5 minutes to return to baseline, the patient most likely has overdone it and should proceed at a slower pace during the next exercise period. The patient may benefit from keeping a diary or log of the exercise program. The diary can help provide a realistic evaluation of the patient's progress. In addition, the diary can help motivate the patient and add to the patient's sense of accomplishment. Stationary cycling can also be used either alone or with walking. Cycles and treadmills are particularly good when weather prevents walking outside.

Fatigue, sleep disturbances, and dyspnea are common complaints of patients with COPD. Of these symptoms, dyspnea appears to be the only symptom that affects the patient's ability to

TABLE 29-28 PATIENT AND FAMILY TEACHING GUIDE
Chronic Obstructive Pulmonary Disease

Goal:
To assist a patient and family in improving quality of life through education and promotion of lifestyle practices that support successful living with chronic obstructive pulmonary disease (COPD).

Teaching Topic	Resources
Overall guide including topics below	Global Initiative for Lung Disease (GOLD) Patient Guide: What You and Your Family Can Do about COPD. Available at *www.goldcopd.org.*
What Is COPD? • Basic anatomy and physiology of lung • Basic pathophysiology of COPD • Signs and symptoms of COPD, exacerbation, cold, flu, pneumonia • Tests to assess breathing	*COPD statement: Patient Education Section* (American Thoracic Society [ATS]). Available at *www.thoracic.org.* *Human Respiratory System* and *Learn about Your Respiratory System* (American Lung Association [ALA]). Available under Your Lungs at *www.lungsusa.org.*
Breathing Retraining • Pursed-lip breathing	Demonstration and return demonstration
Energy Conservation Techniques • Daily activities (e.g., waking up, bathing, grooming, shopping, traveling)	Consult with physical therapist and occupational therapist. *Around the Clock with COPD: Helpful Hints for Respiratory Patients* (ALA). Available in COPD Center at *www.lungusa.org.*
Medications Types (include mechanism of action and types of devices) • Methylxanthines • β_2-adrenergic agonists • Corticosteroids • Anticholinergics • Antibiotics • Other medications Establishing medication schedule	*COPD statement: Patient Education Section: Medications and Other Treatments* (ATS). Available at *www.thoracic.org.* **OR** *COPD Medicines Chart* (ALA). Available in COPD Center at *www.lungusa.org* **OR** *COPD Medications (National Jewish Medicine and Research Center).* Available at *www.nationaljewish.org/medfacts.html.* Write out medication list and schedule.
Correct Use of Metered-Dose Inhaler, Dry Powder Inhaler, Spacer, and Nebulizer	See Figs. 29-4, 29-5, and 29-6. See Tables 29-8, 29-9, and 29-10.
Home Oxygen • Explanation of rationale for use • Guide for home O_2 use and equipment	*Around the Clock with COPD: Helpful Hints for Respiratory Patients and Traveling with Oxygen* (ALA). Available in COPD Center at *www.lungusa.org.*
Psychosocial/Emotional Issues Concerns about interpersonal relationships • Dependency • Intimacy Problems with emotions • Depression • Anxiety • Panic Effects of medications Treatment decisions • Support and rehabilitation groups End-of-life issues	Open discussion (sharing with patient, significant other, and family) COPD Lung NexProfiler (interactive decision support tool via ALA). Available at *www.lungusa.org.* *Questions about Pulmonary Rehabilitation* (English and Spanish) (ATS). Available at *www.thoracic.org.* *Better Breathers Clubs* and *Living with Lung Disease* (online support group) (ALA). Available at *www.lungusa.org.*
COPD Management Plan • Focusing on self-management • Need to report changes • Cause of flare-ups or exacerbation • Recognition of signs and symptoms of respiration infection, heart failure • Reduce risk factors, especially smoking cessation • Exercise program of walking and arm strengthening • Yearly follow-up	Nurse and patient develop and write up COPD management plan that meets individual needs.
Healthy Nutrition • Strategies to lose weight (if overweight) • Strategies to gain weight (if underweight)	Consultation with dietitian.

ETHICAL DILEMMAS

Durable Power of Attorney for Health Care

Situation

A 50-year-old woman is being treated for complications of COPD. She is currently on a ventilator and not coherent because of the drugs she is receiving. Her life partner, another woman, has been with her throughout this hospitalization. The patient had executed a valid durable power of attorney for health care decisions before this admission and had named her partner as her primary agent. However, the patient's parents and siblings have arrived and demand to be in charge of her treatment decisions. They do not accept the partner or the patient's appointment of this woman to make decisions for her.

Important Points for Consideration

- Durable power of attorney for health care is one type of advance directive in which the person, when she or he is competent, identifies someone else to make decisions for the person, should the person lose her or his decision-making ability in the future.
- The surrogate decision maker, who is named as durable power of attorney for health care, is often selected because the person believes that personal values, beliefs, and wishes will be respected when making treatment decisions for her or him.
- Advance directives are legal documents. However, it is often difficult for health care providers when family members or designated surrogates do not agree.
- State laws may differ regarding surrogate decision makers, so it is imperative to be familiar with the statutes in the state in which one practices.

Critical Thinking Questions

1. How would you handle a situation in which the family and surrogate decision maker disagree?
2. What resources would you consult or seek assistance from under these circumstances?

carry out daily activities. Therefore it is suggested that the nurse and other health team members should focus their interventions on improving dyspnea, which would then improve the patient's functional performance.[67] In addition to a traditional pulmonary rehabilitation program, preliminary studies show that an Internet-based self-management program decreases the dyspnea associated with ADLs.[68]

Sexual Activity. Modifying but not abstaining from sexual activity can also contribute to a healthy psychologic well-being. Using an inhaled bronchodilator before sexual activity can help ventilation. The patient with COPD will also use less energy if these guidelines are followed: (1) plan sexual activity during the part of the day when breathing is best, (2) use slow pursed-lip breathing, (3) refrain from sexual activity after eating or strenuous activity, (4) do not assume a dominant position, (5) use O_2 if prescribed, and (6) do not prolong foreplay. These aspects of sexual activity require open communication between partners regarding their needs and expectations and the changes that may be necessary as the result of a chronic disease (e.g., changes in body image, role reversal).

Sleep. Adequate sleep is extremely important. Getting adequate amounts of sleep can be difficult for the COPD patient. Medications may cause restlessness and insomnia. Many patients with COPD have postnasal drip or nasal congestion that may cause coughing and wheezing at night. Nasal saline sprays or rinses before sleep and in the morning may help. The health care provider may also prescribe a nasal decongestant or nasal corticosteroid inhaler that may be used at bedtime. Long-acting theophylline preparations frequently aid in promoting sleep by decreasing bronchospasm and airway obstruction. If the patient is a restless sleeper, snores, stops breathing while asleep, and has a tendency to fall asleep during the day, the patient may need to be tested for sleep apnea (see Chapter 27).

Psychosocial Considerations. Healthy coping is often the most difficult task for a patient with COPD to accomplish. People with COPD frequently have to deal with many lifestyle changes that may involve decreased ability to care for themselves, decreased energy for social activities, and loss of a job.

When a patient with COPD is first diagnosed or when a patient has complications that require hospitalization, the nurse should expect a variety of emotional responses. Emotions frequently encountered include guilt, depression, anxiety, social isolation, denial, and dependence. Guilt may result from the knowledge that the disease was caused largely by cigarette smoking. There is a lack of research concerning the effects of stopping smoking on the quality of life in the late stages of the disease.[69] Therefore the nurse must personally decide what advice to give the patient in the terminal stage of COPD. Depression affects approximately 40% of patients with COPD as the severity and chronicity of the disease are realized. The nurse should convey a sense of understanding and caring to the patient.[70] The patient with COPD may benefit from stress management techniques (e.g., massage, progressive muscle relaxation) (see Chapter 9). Acupressure has demonstrated some promise in decreasing dyspnea.[71] Support groups at local American Lung Associations, hospitals, and clinics can also be helpful.

Patients frequently ask whether moving to a warmer or drier climate will help. In general, such a move is not significantly beneficial. Moving to places with an elevation of 4000 feet or more should be discouraged because of the lower partial pressure of O_2 found in the air at higher elevations. A disadvantage of moving may be that a person leaves an occupation, friends, and familiar environment, which could be psychologically stressful. Any advantage gained from a different climate may be outweighed by the psychologic effects of the move.

Patients need to know that symptoms can be controlled for the most part, but COPD cannot be cured. End-of-life issues and advance directives are important topics for discussion in the terminal stages of COPD. However, this may be difficult for the patient and family to consider because of the uncertainty of the disease.

■ *Evaluation*

The expected outcomes for the patient with COPD are presented in NCP 29-2.

CYSTIC FIBROSIS

Cystic fibrosis (CF) is an autosomal recessive, multisystem disease characterized by altered function of the exocrine glands primarily involving the lungs, pancreas, and sweat glands.[72] (Autosomal recessive disorders are discussed in Chapter 14.) Abnormally thick, abundant secretions from mucous glands can lead to a chronic, diffuse, obstructive pulmonary disorder in almost all patients. Exocrine pancreatic insufficiency is associated with most cases of CF. Sweat glands excrete increased amounts of sodium and chloride.

Of the over 22,000 CF patients in the Cystic Fibrosis Registry, 41.8% were ≥18 years of age.[73] There may be up to 7000 adults in the United States who have CF but are not in the registry. In adults, the ethnic breakdown is 95.3% white, 6.7% Hispanic, and 4% African American. Nearly 52% of the patients with CF are males.[73] The first signs and symptoms typically occur in children, but approximately 4% of patients are not diagnosed until they are adults.[74] The severity and progression of the disease vary from person to person. With early diagnosis and improvements in therapy, the prognosis has been significantly improved. The median predicted survival in 1970 was 16 years, but as of 2004 it was 35 years of age. Approximately 12% of adults with CF live past age 40. Patients with CF can live until their seventies.[73]

Etiology and Pathophysiology

The CF gene is located on chromosome 7 and produces a protein called CF transmembrane regulator (CFTR). The CFTR protein localizes to the lining of the exocrine portion of particular organs such as airways, pancreatic duct, sweat gland duct, and reproductive tract. CFTR regulates sodium and chloride channels. Mutations in the CFTR gene alter this protein in such a way that the channels are blocked.[75] As a result, cells that line the passageways of the lungs, pancreas, and other organs produce abnormally thick, sticky mucus. This mucus obstructs the airways and glands. The glands distal to the duct eventually undergo fibrosis.[76] The high concentrations of sodium and chloride in the sweat of the patient with CF result from decreased chloride reabsorption in the sweat duct.

In the respiratory system, both upper and lower respiratory tracts can be affected. Upper respiratory tract manifestations may be present and include chronic sinusitis and nasal polyposis. The hallmark of respiratory involvement in CF is its effect on the airways. Obstruction of the exocrine glands by mucus is the main reason for morbidity and mortality in patients with CF.[72] The disease progresses from being a disease of the small airways *(chronic bronchiolitis)* to involvement of the larger airways, and finally causes destruction of lung tissue. Thick secretions obstruct bronchioles and lead to air trapping and hyperinflation of the lungs. The stasis of mucus provides an excellent growth medium for bacteria. CF is characterized by chronic airway infection that is difficult to eradicate. Organisms commonly cultured from the sputum of a patient with CF are *S. aureus, H. influenzae, Burkholderia cepacia,* and *P. aeruginosa,* with the latter being by far the most common. Pulmonary inflammation may precede the chronic infection and can cause respiratory decline. Inflammatory mediators such as interleukins, tumor necrosis factor, and leukotrienes have also been found to be elevated and cause the progression of lung disease.[77]

Lung disorders that initially occur are chronic bronchiolitis and bronchitis, but after months or years changes in the bronchial walls lead to bronchiectasis (Fig. 29-19). Over a long period of time, pulmonary vascular remodeling occurs because of local hypoxia and arteriolar vasoconstriction with pulmonary hypertension and cor pulmonale resulting in the later phases of the disease. Blebs and large cysts in the lung are also severe manifestations of lung destruction. Other pulmonary complications include hemoptysis occurring because of erosion of enlarged pulmonary arteries, which develops in response to inflammation with bronchiectasis. Hemoptysis may range from scant streaking to major bleeding; it can sometimes be fatal.

GENETICS IN CLINICAL PRACTICE
Cystic Fibrosis (CF)

Genetic Basis
- Autosomal recessive disorder
- Mutations in CFTR gene cause CF
- Gene location on chromosome 7
- Many different mutations of the gene have been identified

Incidence
- In the United States 1 in 3000 white births
- Uncommon in other ethnic populations
- 1 in 20-25 are carriers of the gene
- If both parents carry the affected gene, there is a 25% chance each offspring will have the disease (see Figs. 14-2 and 14-4, *A*)

Genetic Testing
- Blood-based DNA testing for disease and carrier states
- Testing usually done in children if CF is suspected or if parents are possible carriers
- In parents who are known carriers, amniocentesis or chorionic villus sampling in pregnant women may be useful for prenatal testing

Clinical Implications
- Most common autosomal recessive disease in whites
- Wide range of clinical expression of disease
- Requires long-term medical management
- Advances in medical care have improved life expectancy
- Current recommendations are that CF screening be offered to individuals with a family history of CF and reproductive partners of individuals who have CF

Initially, CF is an obstructive lung disease caused by the overall obstruction of the airways with mucus. Later, CF also progresses to a restrictive lung disease because of the fibrosis, lung destruction, and thoracic wall changes.

Pancreatic insufficiency is caused primarily by mucous plugging of the pancreatic duct and its branches, which results in fibrosis of the acinar glands of the pancreas. The exocrine function of the pancreas is altered and may be lost completely. Pancreatic enzymes such as lipase, amylase, and the proteases (trypsin, chemotrypsin) do not reach the intestine to digest ingested nutrients. There is malabsorption of fat, protein, and fat-soluble vitamins (vitamins A, D, E, and K). Fat malabsorption results in steatorrhea, and protein malabsorption results in failure to grow and gain weight.

Diabetes mellitus may occur if the islets of Langerhans become fibrotic. Cystic fibrosis–related diabetes mellitus affects approximately 18% of patients 18 to 42 years of age and approximately 27% of patients 35 to 44 years of age.[73] It differs from type 1 diabetes in that some insulin is secreted, it is nonketotic, and it is slow in onset. It differs from type 2 diabetes in that individuals are underweight (as opposed to being overweight), the onset is in a younger age population, and the individual is hypoinsulinemic. Routine screening is indicated to follow serum glucose levels. Insulin may be required for treatment of CF-related diabetes.

The sweat glands of CF patients secrete normal volumes of sweat, but sodium chloride cannot be absorbed from sweat as it moves through the sweat duct. Therefore they excrete four times the normal amount of sodium and chloride in sweat. This abnormality usually does not affect the general health of the person, but it is useful in diagnosis (explained later in the diagnostic studies section).

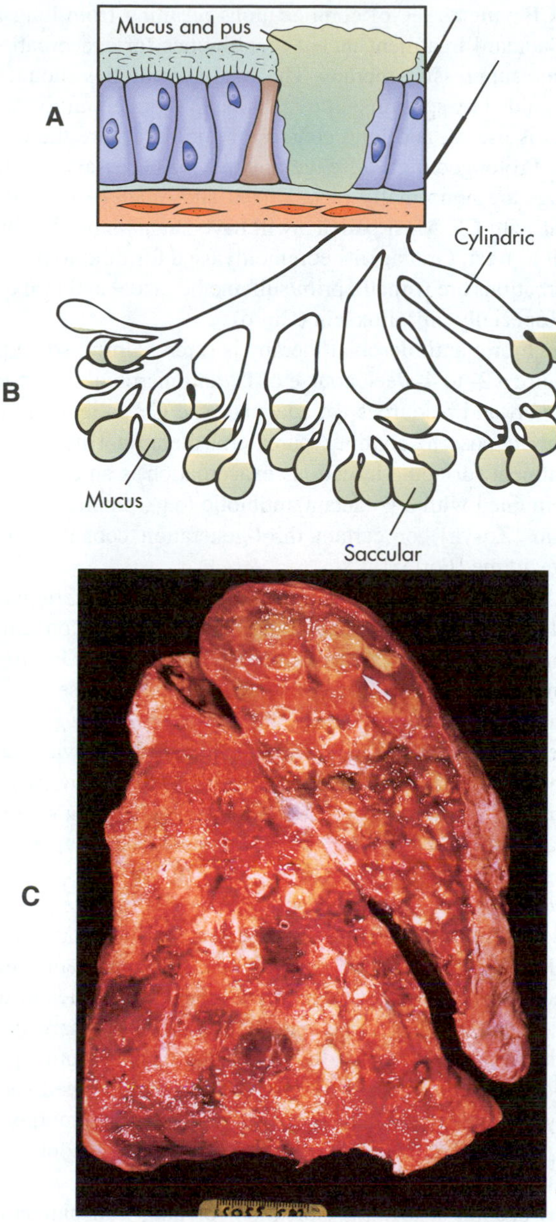

FIG. 29-19 Pathologic changes in bronchiectasis. **A,** Longitudinal section of bronchial wall where chronic infection has caused damage. **B,** Collection of purulent material in dilated bronchioles, leading to persistent infection. **C,** Bronchiectasis in a patient with cystic fibrosis who underwent lung transplantation. Cut surfaces of lung show markedly distended peripheral bronchi filled with mucopurulent secretions.

Individuals with CF often have gastrointestinal problems, including abdominal pain, which may be caused by conditions such as GERD or gastritis. GERD is a major problem in individuals with CF, particularly in those with pulmonary disease. The cause of the relationship between reflux and exacerbation of respiratory disease is not known, but it is known that these two entities enhance each other.

Distal intestinal obstruction syndrome (DIOS) is a syndrome that results from intermittent obstruction commonly in the ileal-cecal area in patients with pancreatic insufficiency. The degree to which the bowel is obstructed may vary with each episode, and a partial obstruction may progress rapidly to a life-threatening complete obstruction. Complete obstruction requires gastric decompression and a surgical consultation; partial and uncomplicated episodes of DIOS are treated with ingestion of a balanced polyethylene glycol (PEG) electrolyte solution (MiraLax, GoLYTELY) or contrast solution used to thin bowel contents. If the bowel obstruction is severe, a hypertonic enema may be administered. Constipation develops in the sigmoid colon and progresses proximally, whereas DIOS develops in the ileal-cecal area and progresses distally. Osmotic cathartics are used to prevent DIOS. Careful monitoring of bowel habits and patterns is essential for CF patients.

The liver may become involved, occurring most commonly between ages 10 and 20 and less commonly after age 20. Biliary cirrhosis may not be recognized until late in the disease. Gallstones, pancreatitis, and portal hypertension can also occur.[76]

Clinical Manifestations

The clinical manifestations of CF vary depending on the severity of the disease. The manifestations of the disorder are caused by the production of abnormally thick, sticky mucus in the body's organs.

An initial finding of meconium ileus in the newborn infant is present in 10% to 15% of persons with CF. Early manifestations in childhood are failure to grow, clubbing, persistent cough with mucus production, tachypnea, and large, frequent bowel movements. A large, protuberant abdomen may develop with an emaciated appearance of the extremities.

Problems with breathing are among the most serious symptoms. The first symptom of CF in the adult is frequent cough. With time the cough becomes persistent and produces viscous, purulent, often greenish-colored sputum as the prevalence of *Pseudomonas* occurs in up to 80% of adolescents with CF.[76] Other respiratory problems that may be indicative of CF are recurring lung infections such as bronchiolitis, bronchitis, and pneumonia. As the disease progresses, periods of clinical stability are interrupted by exacerbations characterized by increased cough, weight loss, increased sputum, and decreased pulmonary function. Over time the exacerbations become more frequent, bronchiectasis develops, and the recovery of lost lung function is less complete, ultimately leading to respiratory failure.

DIOS causes right lower quadrant pain, loss of appetite, emesis, and often a palpable mass. Insufficient pancreatic enzyme release causes the typical pattern of protein and fat malabsorption with frequent, bulky, foul-smelling stools.

The function of the reproductive system is altered. This finding is important because more persons with CF are living to adulthood. The male adult is usually sterile (although not impotent) as a result of glandular obstruction of the vas deferens in utero, and some men have a congenital absence of the vas deferens.[72] The female adult usually has delayed menarche. During exacerbations, menstrual irregularities and secondary amenorrhea are fairly common. The woman may be unable to become pregnant because of generally poor health or the increased viscosity of the cervical mucus. Women with CF do become pregnant, but the fertility rate is lower than in healthy women.[73] The baby is heterozygous (and hence a carrier) for CF if the father is not a carrier. If the father is a carrier, there is a 50% chance that the baby will have CF. (See Chapter 14, Figs. 14-2 and 14-4, *A,* for explanation of the genetic transmission of CF.)

Complications

Pneumothorax is common, with approximately 20% of adults with CF experiencing it in their lifetime.[79] The presence of small amounts of blood in sputum is common in the CF patient with lung infection. Massive hemoptysis is life threatening. With advanced lung disease, digital clubbing becomes evident in almost all patients with CF. Respiratory failure and cor pulmonale are late complications of CF.

Diagnostic Studies

The diagnostic criteria for CF are evidence of CFTR malfunction assessed by the sweat chloride test and characteristic respiratory or gastrointestinal symptoms. The sweat chloride test is performed with the pilocarpine iontophoresis method, which is abnormal in >90% of adults diagnosed with CF.[74] Pilocarpine is placed on the skin and carried by a small electric current to stimulate sweat production. This part of the process takes about 5 minutes and the patient will feel a slight tingling or warmth. The sweat is collected on filter paper or gauze and then analyzed for sweat chloride concentrations. The test takes approximately 1 hour. Values greater than 60 mEq/L for sweat chloride are consistent with the diagnosis of CF, especially in a person who has other clinical features of the disease. The degree of sweat chloride elevation does not necessarily correlate with the severity of the disease. The sweat chloride test will be positive from birth and remain so throughout a patient's life. Other diagnostic studies used to support the diagnosis include chest x-ray, pulmonary function tests, and fecal analysis for fat.

Because of the large number of CF mutations, DNA (CFTR) analysis or genotype is not used for the primary diagnostic test. DNA analysis may be performed in CF patients to corroborate the diagnosis.[74] Fetal diagnosis can be done from samples obtained by amniocentesis or chorionic villus sampling.

Collaborative Care

For improved patient outcomes a multidisciplinary team should be involved in the patient's care. Team members should include nurse, physician, respiratory therapist, dietitian, and social worker who ideally have specialized training in CF. The major objectives of therapy in CF are to (1) promote clearance of secretions, (2) control infection in the lungs, and (3) provide adequate nutrition. Management of pulmonary problems in CF aims at relieving airway obstruction and controlling infection. Drainage of thick bronchial mucus is assisted by aerosol and nebulization treatments of medications used to liquefy mucus and to facilitate coughing. The abnormal viscoelastic properties of CF secretions are primarily caused by mucus glycoproteins and DNA from degenerated neutrophils. Agents that degrade the high concentrations of DNA in CF sputum (e.g., DNase [Pulmozyme]) decrease sputum viscosity and increase airflow. Bronchodilators (e.g., β_2-adrenergic agonists, theophylline) and mucolytics may be used.

Airway clearance techniques are critical in reducing mucus. These techniques include CPT, positive expiratory pressure (PEP) devices, and breathing and high-frequency chest wall oscillation systems (e.g., Flutter device [see Fig. 29-18], ThAIRaphy vest, Acapella). Individuals with CF may have a preference for a certain technique that works well for them in a daily routine.[74] (These airway clearance techniques are discussed in the section on respiratory therapy for COPD earlier in this chapter on pp. 646 to 649.)

Aerobic exercise seems to be effective in clearing the airways. Important needs to consider when planning an aerobic exercise program for the patient with CF are (1) frequent rest periods interspersed throughout the exercise regimen, (2) meeting increased nutritional demands of exercise, (3) observing for manifestations of hyperthermia, and (4) drinking large amounts of fluid and replacing salt losses.

Most CF patients die of complications resulting from lung infection. Standard treatment includes antibiotics for exacerbations and chronic suppressive therapy. The use of antibiotics should be carefully guided by sputum culture results. Early intervention with antibiotics is useful, and long courses of antibiotics are the usual treatment. Prolonged high-dose therapy may be necessary because many drugs are abnormally metabolized and rapidly excreted in the patient with CF. Most patients will have *Pseudomonas,* which is difficult to treat. Oral agents commonly used for mild to moderate exacerbations are trimethoprim/sulfamethoxazole and oral quinolones, especially ciprofloxacin (Cipro).

Although oral antimicrobial therapy is often helpful, some patients require a 2- to 4-week course of IV antimicrobial therapy. If home support and resources are adequate, the CF patient and the family may choose to continue parenteral therapy at home. The usual treatment for acute infectious exacerbation is an aminoglycoside combined with a β-lactam antibiotic (e.g., piperacillin and tazobactam [Zosyn]) or certain third-generation cephalosporins (e.g., ceftazidime [Fortaz]).

Adult patients who are chronically infected with *P. aeruginosa* may need to receive chronic suppressive antibiotics. The concern of using long-term antibiotics is antimicrobial resistance. One treatment found to significantly improve lung function, decrease number of days in the hospital, and decrease the density of *P. aeruginosa* is aerosolized tobramycin (TOBI). TOBI is administered twice daily for 28 days on and 28 days off the medication until improvement is noticed. In addition, azithromycin (Zithromax) has been shown to be effective against *P. aeruginosa*.[80] There is no evidence to support the chronic use of oral antibiotics in adults with CF.

Aerosolized bronchodilators and antiinflammatory agents (e.g., inhaled corticosteroids) are used in selected patients, particularly before CPT. The patient with cor pulmonale or hypoxemia may require home O_2 therapy. (O_2 therapy is discussed earlier in this chapter.) Patients with a large pneumothorax will require chest tube drainage, perhaps repeatedly. Sclerosing of the pleural space or partial pleural stripping and pleural abrasion performed surgically may be indicated for recurrent episodes of pneumothorax. However, sclerosing makes subsequent surgical procedures for transplant more difficult.[79]

CF has become a leading indication for lung transplantation. (Lung transplants are discussed in Chapter 28.) Lung transplantations for the patient with CF have resulted in significant improvement of pulmonary function and prolonging of life.

The management of pancreatic insufficiency includes pancreatic enzyme replacement of lipase, protease, and amylase (e.g., Pancrease, Creon, Ultrase) administered before each meal and snack. Adequate intake of fat, calories, protein, and vitamins is important. Fat-soluble vitamins (vitamins A, D, E, and K) must be supplemented. Use of caloric supplements improves nutritional status. Added dietary salt is indicated whenever sweating is excessive, such as during hot weather, when fever is present, or from intense physical activity.

Gene therapy has been used in clinical trials, but has yet to show clinical usefulness.[76] (Gene therapy is discussed in Chapter 14.)

NURSING MANAGEMENT CYSTIC FIBROSIS

■ *Nursing Assessment*

Subjective and objective data that should be obtained from the patient with cystic fibrosis are presented in Table 29-29.

TABLE 29-29 NURSING ASSESSMENT
Cystic Fibrosis

Subjective Data

Important Health Information

Past health history: Recurrent respiratory and sinus infections, persistent cough with excessive sputum production

Medications: Use of and compliance with corticosteroids, bronchodilators, antibiotics, herbs

Functional Health Patterns

Health perception–health maintenance: Family history of cystic fibrosis; diagnosis of cystic fibrosis in childhood

Nutritional-metabolic: Dietary intolerances, voracious appetite, weight loss, heartburn

Elimination: Intestinal gas; large, frequent bowel movements, constipation

Activity-exercise: Fatigue, ↓ exercise tolerance, amount/type of exercise; dyspnea, cough, excessive mucus or sputum production, coughing up blood

Cognitive-perceptual: Abdominal pain

Sexuality-reproductive: Delayed menarche, menstrual irregularities, and secondary amenorrhea; problems conceiving or fathering a child

Coping-stress tolerance: Anxiety, depression, problems adapting to diagnosis

Objective Data

General

Restlessness; failure to thrive

Integumentary

Cyanosis (circumoral, nail bed), digital clubbing; salty skin

Eyes

Scleral icterus

Respiratory

Sinus difficulties; persistent runny nose; diminished breath sounds, sputum (thick, white or green, tenacious), hemoptysis, ↑ work of breathing, use of accessory muscles of respiration, barrel chest

Cardiovascular

Tachycardia

Gastrointestinal

Protuberant abdomen; abdominal distention; foul, fatty stools

Possible Findings

Abnormal ABGs and pulmonary function tests; abnormal sweat chloride test, chest x-ray, fecal fat analysis

Nursing Diagnoses

Nursing diagnoses for the patient with CF may include, but are not limited to, the following:

- Ineffective airway clearance *related to* abundant, thick bronchial mucus, weakness, and fatigue
- Ineffective breathing pattern *related to* bronchoconstriction, anxiety, and airway obstruction
- Impaired gas exchange *related to* recurring lung infections
- Imbalanced nutrition: less than body requirements *related to* dietary intolerances, intestinal gas, and altered pancreatic enzyme production

Planning

The overall goals are that the patient with CF will have (1) adequate airway clearance, (2) reduced risk factors associated with respiratory infections, (3) adequate nutritional support to maintain appropriate BMI, (4) ability to perform ADLs, (5) no complications related to CF, and (6) active participation in planning and implementing a therapeutic regimen.

Nursing Implementation

The nurse and other health professionals can assist young adults to gain independence by helping them assume responsibility for their care and for their vocational or school goals. An important issue that should be discussed is sexuality. Delayed or irregular menstruation is not uncommon. There may be delayed development of secondary sex characteristics such as breasts in girls. The person may use the illness to avoid certain events or relationships. The healthy person may hesitate to make friends with someone who is sick. Other crises and life transitions that must be dealt with in the young adult include building confidence and self-respect on the basis of achievements, persevering with employment goals, developing motivation to achieve, learning to cope with the treatment program, and adjusting to the need for dependence if health fails. Disclosing the CF diagnosis to friends, potential spouses, or employers may pose challenges emotionally and financially.

The issue of marrying and having children is difficult. Genetic counseling may be an appropriate suggestion for the couple considering having children. Most men with CF are sterile. Women with the disease may have difficulty becoming pregnant. In addition, any children produced will either be carriers of CF or have the disease. Another concern is the shortened life span of the parent with CF, and the parent's ability to care for the child must be taken into consideration.

Acute intervention for the patient with CF includes relief of bronchoconstriction, airway obstruction, and airflow limitation. Interventions include aggressive CPT, antibiotics, O_2 therapy, and corticosteroids in severe disease. Good nutrition is important to support the immune system. Advances in long-term vascular access (e.g., implanted ports) have made IV access and administration of medication much easier. This has also eased the transition for IV treatment at home.

CPT is the mainstay of intervention for ineffective airway clearance for these patients. Home management of cystic fibrosis includes an aggressive plan of postural drainage with percussion and vibration, use of mucus-clearing devices and techniques (discussed earlier in the chapter), aerosol-nebulization therapy, and breathing retraining. The patient is taught controlled coughing techniques, deep-breathing exercises, and progressive exercise conditioning such as a bicycling program.

The family and the person with CF have a great financial and emotional burden. The cost of drugs, special equipment, and health care is often a financial hardship. Because most CF patients live to childbearing age, family planning and genetic counseling are important. The burden of living with a chronic disease at a young age can be emotionally overwhelming. Community resources are often available to help the family. In addition, the Cystic Fibrosis Foundation can be of assistance. As the person continues toward and into adulthood, the nurse and other skilled health professionals should be available to help the patient and family cope with complications resulting from the disease.

BRONCHIECTASIS

Etiology and Pathophysiology

Bronchiectasis is characterized by permanent, abnormal dilation of one or more large bronchi. The pathophysiologic change that results in dilation is destruction of the elastic and muscular structures supporting the bronchial wall. The disease process results in a reduced ability to clear mucus from the lungs and decreased expiratory airflow. Thus bronchiectasis is classified as an obstructive lung disease.

A variety of pathophysiologic processes can result in bronchiectasis. There can be primary disorders of structures in the bronchi (cartilage defects), diseases of mucus clearance (CF), infectious etiologies (severe childhood bronchial infections), and inflammatory diseases (ulcerative colitis).[81] Bronchiectasis can cause generalized effects on the lungs, as seen with CF, or the pattern may be more localized in a segment of the lung. Most frequently infection is the primary reason for the continuing cycle of inflammation, airway damage, and remodeling. Bronchiectasis can follow a severe pneumonia, with a wide variety of infectious agents initiating bronchiectasis, including adenovirus, influenza virus, *S. aureus, Klebsiella,* and anaerobes. Infections cause the bronchial walls to weaken, and pockets of infection begin to form (see Fig. 29-19). When the walls of the bronchial system are injured, the mucociliary mechanism is damaged, allowing bacteria and mucus to accumulate within the pockets. The infection becomes worse and results in bronchiectasis.

Clinical Manifestations

The hallmark of bronchiectasis is persistent or recurrent cough with production of large amounts of purulent sputum that may exceed 500 ml/day. However, some patients with severe disease and upper lobe involvement may have no sputum production and little cough. The other manifestations of bronchiectasis are dyspnea, wheezing, pleuritic chest pain, and hemoptysis. On auscultation of the lungs, crackles are the most common finding, but wheezing is also found in about one third of the patients. Hemoptysis may occur during the frequent infections and it can be massive, thus necessitating immediate medical care.

Diagnostic Studies

An individual with a chronic productive cough with copious purulent sputum (which may be blood streaked) should be suspected of having bronchiectasis. Chest x-rays are usually done and may show some nonspecific abnormalities. High-resolution CT (HRCT) scan of the chest is the gold standard for diagnosing bronchiectasis. Bronchoscopy as a diagnostic tool is now largely obsolete with the advent of the noninvasive HRCT. Sputum may provide additional information regarding the severity of impairment and the presence of active infection. Patients are frequently colonized with *H. influenzae* or *P. aeruginosa.* Pulmonary function studies usually show an obstructive pattern including a decrease in FEV_1 and FEV_1/FVC.[81]

Collaborative Care

Bronchiectasis is difficult to treat. Therapy is aimed at treating acute flare-ups and preventing decline in lung function. Antibiotics are the mainstay of treatment and are often given empirically, but attempts are made to culture the sputum. Long-term suppressive therapy with antibiotics is reserved for those patients who have symptoms that recur a few days after stopping antibiotics. There has been some success with rotating antibiotics prophylactically to reduce exacerbation frequency to prevent antibiotic resistance. Antibiotics may be given orally, intravenously, or inhaled. Inhaled tobramycin (TOBI) is quite effective in patients with *P. aeruginosa.* Concurrent bronchodilator therapy is given to prevent bronchospasm. β_2 Agonists have been shown to stimulate mucociliary clearance. Other forms of drug therapy may include mucolytic agents and antiinflammatory agents such as ICS. Maintaining good hydration is important to liquefy secretions. Chest physiotherapy and other airway clearance techniques are important to facilitate expectoration of sputum. (These techniques are discussed earlier in the chapter.) The individual should reduce exposure to excessive air pollutants and irritants, avoid cigarette smoking, and obtain pneumococcal and influenza vaccinations.

Surgical resection of parts of the lungs, although not used as often as previously, may be done if more conservative treatment is not effective. Surgical resection of an affected lobe or segment may be indicated for the patient with repeated bouts of pneumonia, hemoptysis, and disabling complications. Surgery is not advisable when there is diffuse or widespread involvement. For selected patients who are disabled in spite of maximal therapy, lung transplantation is an option.

NURSING MANAGEMENT
BRONCHIECTASIS

The early detection and treatment of lower respiratory tract infections will help prevent complications such as bronchiectasis. Any obstructing lesion or foreign body should be removed promptly. Other measures to decrease the occurrence or progression of bronchiectasis include avoiding cigarette smoking and decreasing exposure to pollution and irritants.

An important nursing goal is to promote drainage and removal of bronchial mucus. Various airway clearance techniques can be effectively used to facilitate secretion removal. The patient should be taught effective deep-breathing exercises and effective ways to cough (see Table 29-25). Chest physiotherapy with postural drainage should be done on affected parts of the lung (see Fig. 29-17). Some individuals require elevation of the foot of the bed by 4 to 6 inches to facilitate drainage. Pillows may be used in the hospital and at home to help the patient assume postural drainage positions. A Flutter mucus clearance device is a handheld device that provides airway vibration during the expiratory phase of breathing (see Fig. 29-18). Two to four 15-minute sessions daily by a patient who has been properly trained can provide satisfactory mucus clearance. Positive expiratory pressure (PEP) therapy is a breathing maneuver against an expiratory resistance often used in conjunction with nebulized medications. (Respiratory therapy procedures are explained previously in this chapter.)

Administration of the prescribed medications is important. The patient needs to understand the importance of taking the prescribed regimen of drugs to obtain maximum effectiveness. The patient should be aware of possible side effects or adverse effects that must be reported to the physician.

Rest is important to prevent overexertion. Bed rest may be indicated during the acute phase of the illness. Chilling and excess fatigue should be avoided.

Good nutrition is important and may be difficult to maintain because the patient is often anorexic. Oral hygiene to cleanse the mouth and remove dried sputum crusts may improve the patient's appetite. Offering foods that are appealing may also increase the desire to eat. Adequate hydration to help liquefy secretions and thus make it easier to remove them is extremely important. Unless there are contraindications, such as renal disease, the patient should be instructed to drink at least 3 L of fluid daily. To accomplish this, the patient should be advised to increase fluid consumption from the baseline by increasing intake by one glass per day until the goal is reached. Generally the patient should be counseled to use low-sodium fluids to avoid systemic fluid retention.

Direct hydration of the respiratory system may also prove beneficial in the expectoration of secretions. Usually a bland aerosol with normal saline solution delivered by a jet-type nebulizer is used. Alternatively, hypertonic saline may be used for a more aggressive effect. At home a steamy shower can prove effective; expensive equipment that requires frequent cleaning is usually unnecessary. The patient and family should be taught to recognize significant clinical manifestations to be reported to the health care provider. These manifestations include increased sputum production, grossly bloody sputum, increasing dyspnea, fever, chills, and chest pain.

CRITICAL THINKING EXERCISE

CASE STUDY

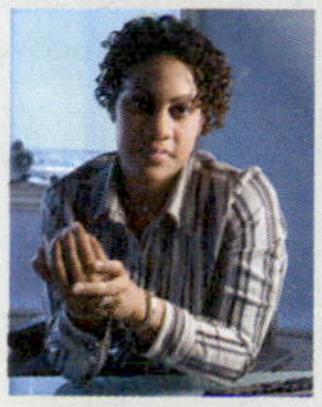

Asthma

Patient Profile. Mrs. S., a 30-year-old African American mother of two preschoolers, comes to the emergency department (ED) with severe wheezing, dyspnea, and anxiety. She was in the ED only 6 hours ago with an acute asthma attack.

Subjective Data

- Treated in the ED previously with nebulized albuterol and responded quickly.
- Can speak only one- to three-word sentences.
- Is allergic to cigarette smoke.
- Began to experience increased shortness of breath and tightness in her chest when she returned home.
- Given albuterol in the ED and used it (without a spacer) repeatedly at home with no relief.
- Coughing at night wakes her up three or four times a week.
- Has no health care provider she sees regularly. On no medications. Was diagnosed with asthma 2 years ago.

Objective Data

Physical Examination

- Uses accessory muscles to breathe
- Has audible wheezing
- Respiratory rate 34 breaths/min
- Auscultation reveals no air movement in lower lobes
- Heart rate 126 beats/min

Diagnostic Studies

- ABGs: PaO_2 80 mm Hg, $PaCO_2$ 35 mm Hg, pH 7.46
- PEFR: 150 L/min (personal best: 400 L/min)

Critical Thinking Questions

1. Why did Mrs. S. return to the ED? Explain the pathophysiology of this exacerbation of asthma.
2. What are the nursing care priorities for Mrs. S.?
3. What are the complications that the nurse must be ready for based on her assessment of Mrs. S.?
4. What should be included in her discharge plan of care? Include discussions with the health care provider.
5. Based on the assessment data presented, write one or more nursing diagnoses. Are there any collaborative problems?

NCLEX EXAMINATION REVIEW QUESTIONS

The number of the question corresponds to the same-numbered objective at the beginning of the chapter.

1. Asthma is best characterized as
   a. an inflammatory disease.
   b. a steady progression of bronchoconstriction.
   c. an obstructive disease with loss of alveolar walls.
   d. a chronic obstructive disorder characterized by mucus production.
2. In evaluating the asthmatic patient's knowledge of self-care, the nurse recognizes that additional instruction is needed when the patient says,
   a. "I use my corticosteroid inhaler when I feel short of breath."
   b. "I get a flu shot every year and see my health care provider if I have an upper respiratory infection."
   c. "I use my bronchodilator inhaler before I visit my aunt who has a cat, but I only visit for a few minutes because of my allergies."
   d. "I walk 30 minutes every day but sometimes I have to use my bronchodilator inhaler before walking to prevent me from getting short of breath."
3. A plan of care for the patient with COPD could include
   a. exercise such as walking.
   b. chronic oral corticosteroid therapy.
   c. high flow rate of O_2 administration.
   d. breathing exercises that involve inhaling longer than exhaling.
4. The effects of cigarette smoking on the respiratory system include
   a. increased proliferation of ciliated cells.
   b. hypertrophy of the alveolar membrane.
   c. destruction of all alveolar macrophages.
   d. hyperplasia of goblet cells and increased production of mucus.
5. The major advantage of a Venturi mask is that it can
   a. deliver up to 80% O_2.
   b. provide continuous 100% humidity.
   c. deliver a precise concentration of O_2.
   d. be used while a patient eats and sleeps.
6. One of the most important things that a nurse can teach a patient with COPD is to
   a. move to a hot, dry climate.
   b. perform chest physiotherapy.
   c. obtain adequate rest in the supine position.
   d. know the early signs/symptoms of COPD exacerbation.
7. Diagnostic studies that the nurse would expect to be abnormal in a person with CF are
   a. insulin tolerance and blood glucose.
   b. pancreatic enzymes and hormones.
   c. sweat test and vitamin B tolerance test.
   d. pulmonary function test and sweat test.
8. A primary goal for the patient with bronchiectasis is that the patient will
   a. have no recurrence of disease.
   b. have normal pulmonary function.
   c. maintain removal of bronchial secretions.
   d. avoid environmental agents that precipitate attacks.

REFERENCES

1. Global Initiative for Chronic Obstructive Lung Disease (GOLD) Workshop Report. Available at *www.goldcopd.org* (accessed June 1, 2006).
2. Celli BR, MacNee W, Agusti A, et al: Standards for the diagnosis and treatment of patients with COPD: a summary of the ATS/ERS position paper, *Eur Respir J* 23:932, 2004.
3. American Thoracic Society and European Respiratory Society: Standards for the diagnosis and treatment of patients with COPD. Available at *www.thoracic.org* (accessed May 20, 2006).

4. Global Initiative for Asthma (GINA) Workshop Report. Available at *www.ginasthma.org* (accessed May 20, 2006).
5. American Lung Association: Trends in asthma morbidity and mortality. Epidemiology and Statistics Unit. Research and Scientific Affairs. April 2004. Available at *www.lungusa.org* (accessed May 20, 2006).
6. National Institute of Environmental Health Sciences (NIEHS): Asthma research at NIEHS, February 14, 2003. Available at *www.niehs.nih.gov/airborne/research/cockroach.html* (accessed May 20, 2006).
7. McFadden ER: Stimuli that incite asthma. In Kaspar DL, et al, editors: *Harrison's principles of internal medicine,* ed 16, New York, 2005, McGraw-Hill.
8. National Institute for Occupational Safety and Health: Respiratory diseases. In *Worker health chartbook,* 2004, Publication No. 2004-146. Available at *www.cdc.gov/niosh/docs/chartbook* (accessed May 20, 2006).
9. CDC National Center for Environmental Health: Asthma and flu shots, January 14, 2005. Available at *www.cdc.gov/asthma/flushot.htm* (accessed May 20, 2006).
10. Corren J, Manning BE, Thompson SF, et al: Rhinitis therapy and the prevention of hospital care for asthma: case-control study, *J Allergy Clin Immunol* 113:415, 2004.
11. Barnes PJ: Pathophysiology of asthma. In Crapo JD, Glassroth J, Karlinsky JB, et al, editors: *Baum's textbook of pulmonary disease,* ed 7, Philadelphia, 2004, Lippincott Williams & Wilkins.
12. Brashers VL: Alterations of pulmonary function. In Huether SE, McCance KL, editors: *Understanding pathophysiology,* ed 3, St Louis, 2004, Mosby.
13. National Institutes of Health: *Highlights of the Expert Panel Report 2: guidelines for the diagnosis and management of asthma,* Publication No. 97-4051A, 1997, U.S. Department of Health and Human Services.
14. Han P, Cole RP: Evolving differences in the presentation of severe asthma requiring intensive care unit admission, *Respiration* 71:458, 2004.
15. National Institutes of Health: *Guidelines for the diagnosis and management of asthma—update on selected topics,* 2002, Publication No. 02-5075, 2002, U.S. Department of Health and Human Services.
16. Kallstrom TJ: Evidence-based asthma management, *Respir Care* 49:783, 2004.
17. Sutherland ER, Kraft M, Crapo JD: Diagnosis and treatment of asthma. In Crapo JD, Glassroth J, Karlinsky JB, et al, editors: *Baum's textbook of pulmonary disease,* ed 7, Philadelphia, 2004, Lippincott Williams & Wilkins.
18. Gibson PG, Powell H: Initial corticosteroid therapy for asthma, *Curr Opin Pulm Med* 12(1):48, 2006.
19. Dahlen SE: Treatment of asthma with antileukotrienes: first line or last resort therapy? *Eur J Pharmacol* 533:40, 2006.
20. Food and Drug Administration: The FDA safety information and adverse event reporting program. MedWatch, 2003. Safety alert—Serevent (salmeterol xinafoate). Available at *www/fda/gov/medwatch/SAFETY/2003/serevent.htm* (accessed May 20, 2006).
21. Fisher AA, Davis MW, McGill DA: Acute myocardial infarction associated with albuterol, *Ann Pharmacother* 38:2045, 2004.
22. Melani AS, Zanchetta D, Barbato N, et al: Inhalation technique and variables associated with misuse of conventional metered-dose inhalers and newer dry powder inhalers in experienced adults, *Ann Allergy Asthma Immunol* 93:439, 2004.
23. Williams DM, Self TH: Drugs for asthma. In Bernardi RR, editor: *Handbook of nonprescription drugs: an interactive approach to self care,* ed 14, Washington, DC, 2004, American Pharmacists Association.
24. Food and Drug Administration: *Federal Register Rules and Regulations,* February 11, 2004, vol 69, no 28, pp 6787-6845. Available at *www.cfsan.fda.gov/~lrd/fr040211.html* (accessed May 20, 2006).
25. van den Bemt L, van Knapen L, de Vries MP, et al: Clinical effectiveness of a mite allergen impermeable bed-covering system in asthmatic mite-sensitive patients, *J Allergy Clin Immunol* 114:858, 2004.
26. Gøtzsche PC, Johansen HK, Schmidt LM, et al: House dust mite control measures for asthma, *Cochrane Database Syst Rev* 2004. Available at *www.thecochranelibrary.com* (accessed May 20, 2006).
*27. Cortes T, Lee A, Boal J, et al: Using focus groups to identify asthma care and education issues for elderly urban-dwelling minority individuals, *Appl Nurs Res* 17:207, 2004.
28. American Lung Association: *Trends in chronic bronchitis and emphysema: morbidity and mortality.* Epidemiology and Statistics Unit. Research and Scientific Affairs. November 2004. Available at *www.lungusa.org* (accessed May 20, 2006).
29. American Cancer Society: *Child and teen tobacco use,* January 7, 2005. Available at *www.cancer.org/docroot/PED/content/PED_10_2X_Child_and_Teen_Tobacco_Use.asp?sitearea=PED* (accessed May 20, 2006).
30. Kaufman JS: Smoking cessation. In Davis LL, editor: *Cardiovascular nursing secrets,* St Louis, 2004, Mosby.
31. Niederman MS, et al: NATIONALISE: National American Taskforce on Improving Outcomes in AECB and LRTIs—implementation, strategies, and education, *Consultant* 42:S2, 2002.
32. Desai TJ, Karlinsky JB: COPD: clinical manifestations, diagnosis, and treatment. In Crapo JD, Glassroth J, Karlinsky JB, et al, editors: *Baum's textbook of pulmonary disease,* ed 7, Philadelphia, 2004, Lippincott Williams & Wilkins.
33. Porth CM: *Pathophysiology: concepts of altered health state,* ed 7, Philadelphia, 2004, Lippincott Williams & Wilkins.
34. Brashers V, Huether SE: Structure and function of the pulmonary system. In Huether SE, McCance KL: *Understanding pathophysiology,* ed 3, St Louis, 2004, Mosby.
35. Gronkiewicz C, Borkgren-Okonek M: Acute exacerbation of COPD: nursing application of evidence-based guidelines, *Crit Care Nurs Q* 27:336, 2004.
36. Shapiro SD: COPD unwound, *N Engl J Med* 352:2016, 2005.
37. De Souza A, Lareau SC: Descriptors of dyspnea by patients with chronic obstructive pulmonary disease versus congestive heart failure, *Heart Lung* 33:102, 2004.
*38. Michaels C, Meek P: The language of breathing among individuals with chronic obstructive pulmonary disease, *Heart Lung* 33:390, 2004.
*39. Theander K, Unosson M: Fatigue in patients with chronic obstructive pulmonary disease, *J Adv Nurs* 45:172, 2004.
40. Rubin L: Pulmonary heart disease. In Crapo JD, Glassroth J, Karlinsky JB, et al, editors: *Baum's textbook of pulmonary disease,* ed 7, Philadelphia, 2004, Lippincott Williams & Wilkins.
41. Nocturnal Oxygen Therapy Trial Group: Continuous or nocturnal oxygen therapy in hypoxemic chronic obstructive lung disease, *Ann Intern Med* 93:391, 1980.
42. Anthonisen NE, et al: Antibiotic therapy in exacerbations of chronic obstructive pulmonary disease, *Ann Intern Med* 106:196, 1987.
43. Locke DL: Establishing a GOLD standard for managing COPD in your practice. In *Maximizing positive outcomes in COPD, CE-Today for Nurse Practitioners* 4:17, 2005. Available at *www.np.ce-today.com* (accessed May 20, 2006).
44. Hill NS: Chronic respiratory failure and noninvasive ventilation. In Crapo JD, Glassroth J, Karlinsky JB, et al, editors: *Baum's textbook of pulmonary disease,* ed 7, Philadelphia, 2004, Lippincott Williams & Wilkins.
45. Salpeter SR, Ormiston TM, Salpeter EE: Cardioselective β-blockers in patients with reactive airway disease: a meta-analysis, *Ann Intern Med* 137:715, 2002.
46. Prakash UBS, King TE: Gastrointestinal diseases. In Crapo JD, Glassroth J, Karlinsky JB, et al, editors: *Baum's textbook of pulmonary disease,* ed 7, Philadelphia, 2004, Lippincott Williams & Wilkins.
47. Casanova C, Baudet JS, del Valle Velasco M, et al: Increased gastroesophageal reflux disease in patients with severe COPD, *Eur Respir J* 23:841, 2004.
48. Braman SS, Peters SG: COPD: will early detection and aggressive intervention control disease progression? In *Maximizing positive outcomes in COPD, CE-Today for Nurse Practitioners* 4:17, 2005. Available at *www.np.ce-today.com* (accessed May 20, 2006).
49. Centers for Disease Control and Prevention: Recommended adult immunization schedule by vaccine and age group United States, Oct 2004-Sept 2005. Available at *www.cdc.gov/nip/recs/adult-schedule-2page.pdf* (accessed May 20, 2006).
50. Piquette CA, Rennard SI, Snider GL: Chronic bronchitis and emphysema. In Murray JF, Nadel JA, editors: *Textbook of respiratory medicine,* ed 3, Philadelphia, 2000, Saunders.
51. Lausten G, Wimmett L: 2004 drug approval highlights FDA update, *Nurse Pract* 30:14, 2005.
52. Tashkin DP: Is a long-acting inhaled bronchodilator the first agent to use in stable chronic obstructive pulmonary disease? *Curr Opin Pulm Med* 11:121, 2005.
53. Gartlehner EG, Hansen RA, Carson SS, et al: Efficacy and safety of inhaled corticosteroids in patients with COPD: a systematic review and meta-analysis of health outcomes, *Ann Fam Med* 4:253, 2006.
54. Harkreader H, Hogan MA: *Fundamentals of nursing: caring and clinical judgment,* ed 2, St Louis, 2004, Elsevier Saunders.
55. National Emphysema Treatment Trial Research Group: A randomized trial comparing lung volume reduction surgery with medical therapy for severe emphysema, *N Engl J Med* 348:2059, 2003.

*Nursing research–based reference.

56. Maxfield RA: New and emerging minimally invasive techniques for lung volume reduction, *Chest* 125:777, 2004.
57. Miller JD, Berger RL, Malthaner RA, et al: Lung volume reduction surgery vs medical treatment: for patients with advanced emphysema, *Chest* 127:1166, 2005.
58. Huang M, Singer LG: Surgical interventions for COPD, *Geriatrics Aging* 8:40, 2005.
59. Bianchi R, Gigliotti F, Romagnoli I, et al: Chest wall kinematics and breathlessness during pursed-lip breathing in patients with COPD, *Chest* 125:459, 2004.
60. Dechman G, Wilson CR: Evidence underlying breathing retraining in people with stable chronic obstructive pulmonary disease, *Phys Ther* 84:1189, 2004.
61. Nici L, Donner C, Wouters E, et al: American Thoracic Society/European Respiratory Society statement on pulmonary rehabilitation, *Am J Respir Crit Care Med* 173(12):1390, 2006.
62. Grodner M, Long S, DeYoung S*: Foundations and clinical applications of nutrition: a nursing approach,* ed 3, St Louis, 2004, Elsevier Mosby.
63. ONeill P: Nutrition for a patient with COPD can be complicated, *Nursing* 34:32hn6, 2004.
64. Hyatt RE, Scanlon PD, Nakamura M, editors: *Interpretation of pulmonary function tests: a practical guide,* Philadelphia, 1997, Lippincott Williams & Wilkins.
65. American Thoracic Society: Pulmonary rehabilitation: official statement of the American Thoracic Society, *Am J Respir Crit Care Med* 159:1666, 1999.
66. Rossi G, Florini F, Romagnoli M, et al: Length and clinical effectiveness of pulmonary rehabilitation in outpatients with chronic airway obstruction, *Chest* 127(1):105, 2005.
*67. Reishtein JL: Relationship between symptoms and functional performance in COPD, *Res Nurs Health* 28:39, 2005.
*68. Nguyen HQ, Carrieri-Kohlman V, Rankin SH, et al: Is Internet-based support for dyspnea self-management in patients with chronic obstructive pulmonary disease possible? Results of a pilot study, *Heart Lung* 34:51, 2005.
69. Blackler L, Mooney C, Jones CH: Palliative care in the management of chronic obstructive pulmonary disease, *Br J Neurosurg* 13:528, 2004.
70. Yohannes AM: Depression and COPD in older people: a review and discussion, *Br J Community Nurs* 10:42, 2005.
*71. Wu H, Wu S, Lin J, et al: Effectiveness of acupressure in improving dyspnea in chronic obstructive pulmonary disease, *J Adv Nurs* 45:252, 2004.
72. Rowe SM, Miller S, Sorscher EJ: Cystic fibrosis, *N Engl J Med* 352:1992, 2005.
73. Cystic Fibrosis Foundation Patient Registry: *Annual data report 2004,* Bethesda, Md., Cystic Fibrosis Foundation. Available at *www.cff.org*.
74. Yankaskas JR, Marshall BC, Sufian B, et al: Cystic fibrosis adult care: consensus conference report, *Chest* 125(suppl):1S, 2004.
75. Stutts MJ, Boucher RC: Cystic fibrosis gene and functions of CFTR. In Yankaskas JR, et al., editors: *Cystic fibrosis in adults*, Philadelphia, 1999, Lippincott-Raven.
76. Yankaskas JR: Cystic fibrosis. In Crapo JD, Glassroth J, Karlinsky JB, et al, editors: *Baum's textbook of pulmonary disease*, ed 7, Philadelphia, 2004, Lippincott Williams & Wilkins.
77. Huether SE, McCance KL, editors: *Understanding pathophysiology,* ed 3, St Louis, 2004, Mosby.
78. Orenstein D: *Cystic fibrosis: a guide for patients and families,* ed 3, Philadelphia, 2004, Lippincott.
79. Yankaskas JR, Egan TM, et al.: Major complications. In Yankaskas JR, Knowles MR, editors: *Cystic fibrosis in adults,* Philadelphia, 1999, Lippincott-Raven.
80. Baumann U, King M: Long term azithromycin therapy in cystic fibrosis patients: a study on drug levels and sputum properties, *Can Respir J* 11:151, 2004.
81. O'Regan AW, Berman JS: Bronchiectasis. In Crapo JD, Glassroth J, Karlinsky JB, et al, editors: *Baum's textbook of pulmonary disease,* ed 7, Philadelphia, 2004, Lippincott Williams & Wilkins.

*Nursing research–based reference.

RESOURCES

Alpha-1 Association
410-216-6916
800-521-3025
www.alpha1.org

American College of Allergy, Asthma and Immunology
847-427-1200
www.acaai.org

American Lung Association
212-315-8700
www.lungusa.org

American Thoracic Society
212-315-8600
www.thoracic.org

Association of Asthma Educators
888-988-7747
www.asthmaeducators.org/web_resources.htm

Asthma Action America
888-825-5249
www.asthmaactionamerica.org

Cystic Fibrosis Foundation
301-951-4422 or 800-344-4823
www.cff.org

Global Initiative for Asthma (GINA)
www.ginasthma.com

Global Initiative for Chronic Obstructive Lung Disease (GOLD)
www.goldcopd.com

National Heart, Lung, and Blood Institute (NHLBI)
301-592-8573
www.nhlbi.nih.gov/index.htm

NHLBI Clinical Guidelines
301-592-8573
www.nhlbi.nih.gov/guidelines/index.htm

National Institute of Allergy and Infectious Diseases (NIAID)
301-496-5717
www.niaid.nih.gov

National Institute of Environmental Health Sciences (NIEHS)
919-541-3345
www.niehs.nih.gov/airborne/home.htm

National Jewish Medical and Research Center
800-222-LUNG (5864)
www.nationaljewish.org

National Respiratory Training Center
919-832-3539
www.nrtc-usa.org/resources.htm

For additional Internet resources, see the website for this book at *http://evolve.elsevier.com/Lewis/medsurg*.

Section 6

Problems of Oxygenation: Transport

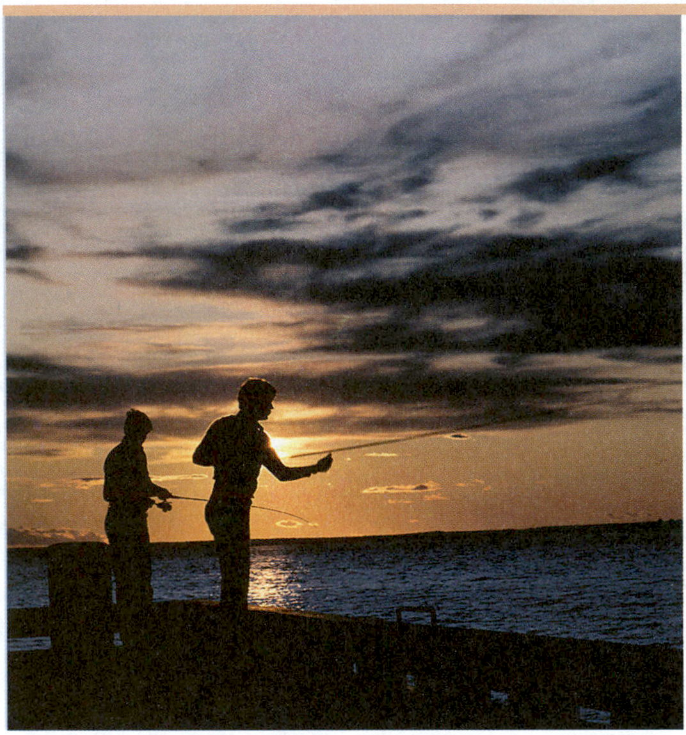

Section Outline

We learn by example and by direct experience because there are real limits to the adequacy of verbal instruction.

Malcolm Gladwell

Nursing Assessment Hematologic System

30

Brenda K. Shelton, Sandra Irene Rome, and Sharon L. Lewis

LEARNING OBJECTIVES

1. Describe the structures and functions of the hematologic system.
2. Differentiate among the different types of blood cells and their functions.
3. Explain the process of hemostasis.
4. Describe the age-related changes in the hematologic system and differences in hematologic studies.
5. Describe the significant subjective and objective assessment data related to the hematologic system that should be obtained from a patient.
6. Describe the components of a physical assessment of the hematologic system.
7. Differentiate normal from common abnormal findings of a physical assessment of the hematologic system.
8. Describe the purpose, significance of results, and nursing responsibilities related to diagnostic studies of the hematologic system.

KEY TERMS

ecchymoses, p. 677
erythropoiesis, p. 667
fibrinolysis, p. 670
hematology, p. 665
hematopoiesis, p. 665
hemoglobin, p. 667
hemolysis, p. 667
leukopenia, p. 678
pancytopenia, p. 677
petechiae, p. 677
thrombocytosis, p. 678

Electronic Resources

Supplemental content related to Chapter 30 can be found …

Companion CD

- Stress-Busting Kit for Nursing Students
- NCLEX Examination Review Questions
- Comprehensive Glossary

Evolve Website evolve

http://evolve.elsevier.com/Lewis/medsurg

- Content Updates
- Key Points (Printable and CD/MP3 Download)
- Concept Map Creator
- Expanded Audio Glossary
- Key Term Flash Cards
- Electronic Calculators
- Physical Examination Video Clips
  - Precordium and Jugular Veins
  - Neck
  - Upper Extremities
  - Anterior Chest
  - Abdominal Reflexes, Abdominal Muscles, and Inguinal Area
- WebLinks

Hematology is the study of blood and blood-forming tissues. This includes the bone marrow, blood, spleen, and lymph system. A basic knowledge of hematology is useful in clinical settings to evaluate the patient's ability to transport oxygen and carbon dioxide, coagulate blood, and combat infections. Assessment of the hematologic system is based on the patient's health history, physical examination, and results of diagnostic studies.

STRUCTURES AND FUNCTIONS OF THE HEMATOLOGIC SYSTEM

Bone Marrow

Blood cell production **(hematopoiesis)** occurs within the bone marrow. **Bone marrow** is the soft material that fills the central core of bones. Although there are two types of bone marrow (yellow

Reviewed by Joyce A. Marrs, APRN-BC, MS, AOCNP, Nurse Practitioner, Hematology and Oncology of Dayton, Dayton, Ohio; and Dana Reeves, RN, MSN, Assistant Professor, University of Arkansas–Fort Smith, Forth Smith, Ark.

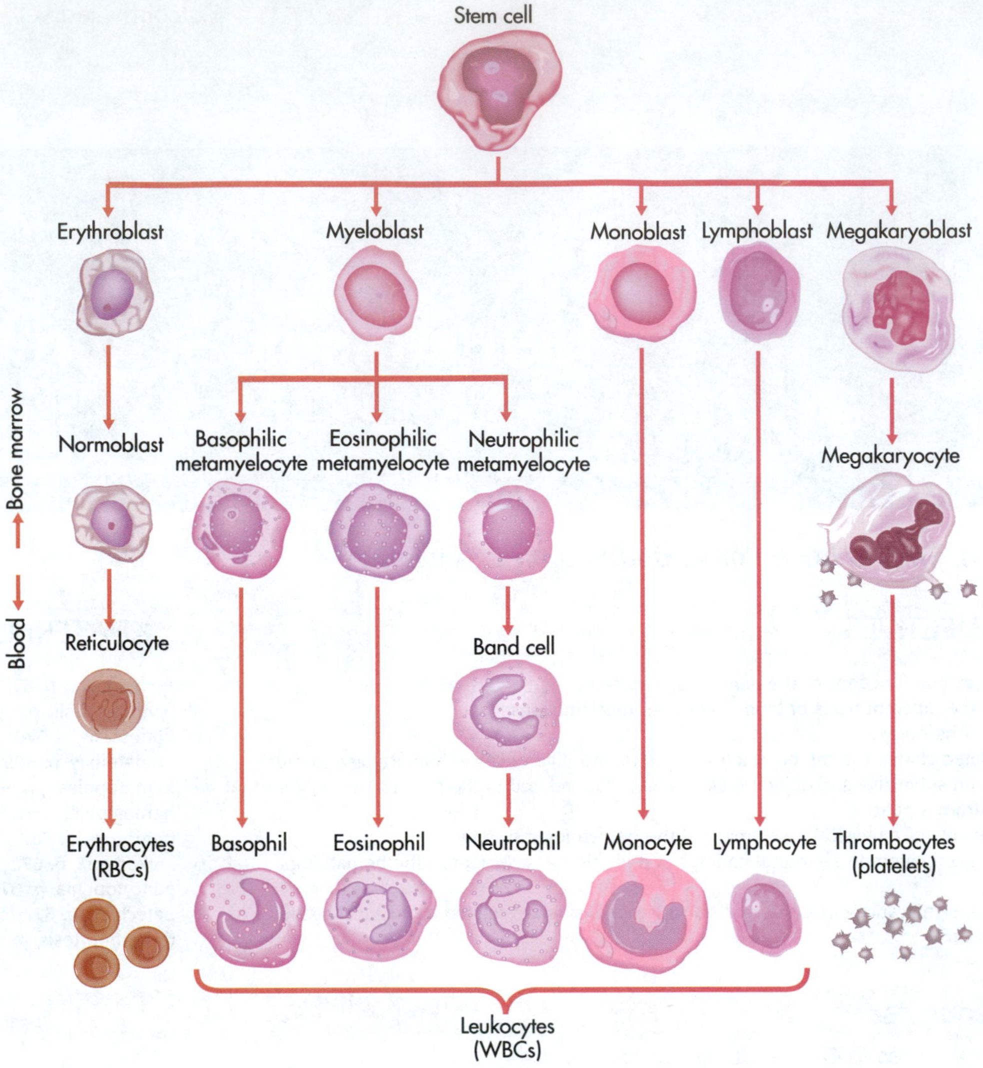

FIG. 30-1 Development of blood cells. *RBCs,* Red blood cells; *WBCs,* white blood cells.

[adipose] and red [hematopoietic]), it is the red marrow that actively produces blood cells. In the adult, the red marrow is found primarily in the flat and irregular bones, such as the ends of long bones, pelvic bones, vertebrae, sacrum, sternum, ribs, flat cranial bones, and scapulae.

All three types of blood cells (red blood cells [RBCs], white blood cells [WBCs], and platelets) develop from a common hematopoieitic stem cell within the bone marrow. The hematopoietic **stem cell** is best described as a nondifferentiated immature blood cell found in the bone marrow. As the cells mature and differentiate, several different types of blood cells are formed (Fig. 30-1). The marrow is able to respond to increased demands for various types of blood cells by increasing production via a negative feedback system. The bone marrow is stimulated by various factors (e.g., erythropoietin) that cause differentiation of the stem cells into one of the committed hematopoietic cells (e.g., RBC).

Blood

Blood is a type of connective tissue that performs three major functions: transportation, regulation, and protection (Table 30-1). The blood is responsible for the *transportation* of oxygen, nutrients, hormones, and waste products around the body. Blood also plays a role in the *regulation* of fluid, electrolyte, and acid-base balance. Finally, the blood has a *protective role* in its ability to clot and combat infections. There are two major components to blood: plasma and blood cells.

TABLE 30-1 Functions of Blood

Function	Examples
Transportation	• Oxygen from lungs to cells • Nutrients from gastrointestinal tract to cells • Hormones from endocrine glands to tissues and cells • Metabolic waste products (e.g., CO_2, NH_3, urea) from cells to lungs, liver, and kidneys
Protection	• Combating invasion of pathogens and other foreign substances • Maintaining homeostasis of blood coagulation
Regulation	• Fluid and electrolyte balance • Acid-base balance • Body temperature

Plasma. Approximately 55% of blood is plasma (Fig. 30-2). Plasma is composed primarily of water, but it also contains pro-

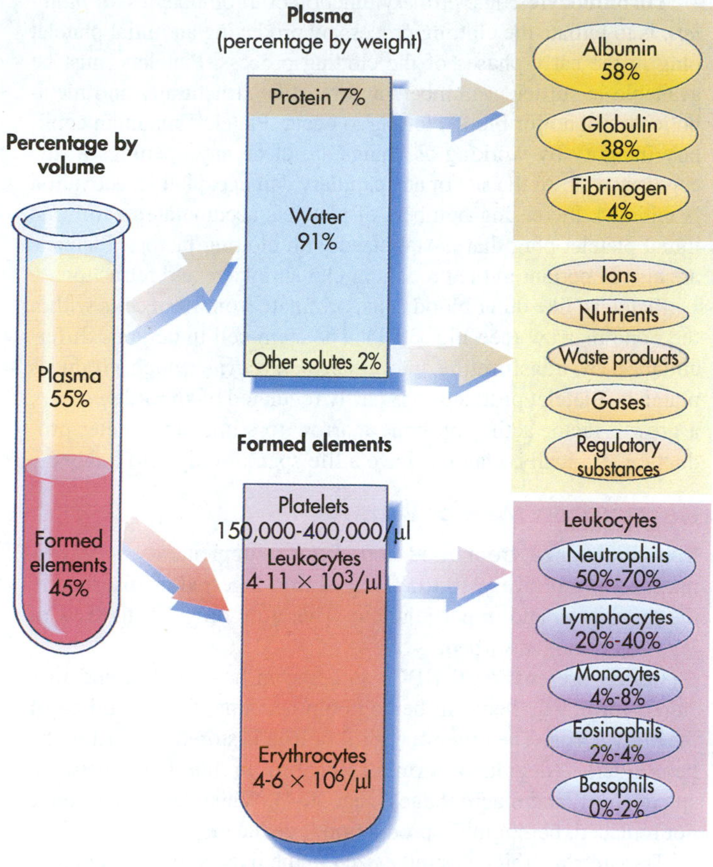

FIG. 30-2 Approximate values for the components of blood in the adult. Normally, 45% of the blood is composed of blood cells, and 55% is composed of plasma.

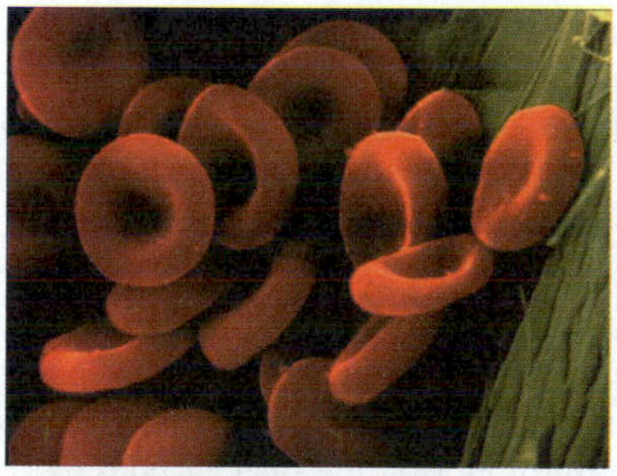

FIG. 30-3 Mature erythrocytes.

teins, electrolytes, gases, nutrients, and waste. The term *serum* refers to plasma minus its clotting factors.[1] Plasma proteins include albumin, globulin, and clotting factors, mostly fibrinogen.

Blood Cells. About 45% of the blood (see Fig. 30-2) is composed of formed elements, or blood cells. There are three types of blood cells: **erythrocytes** (RBCs), **leukocytes** (WBCs), and **thrombocytes** (platelets). The primary function of erythrocytes is oxygen transportation, whereas the leukocytes are involved in protection of the body from infection. Platelets function to promote blood coagulation.

Erythrocytes. The primary functions of RBCs include transport of gases (both oxygen and carbon dioxide) and assistance in maintaining acid-base balance. The composition and features of an erythrocyte are ideal for its gas transportation role. It is a flexible cell with a unique biconcave shape (Fig. 30-3). Flexibility enables the cell to alter its shape so that it can easily pass through tiny capillaries. The cell membrane is very thin to facilitate the diffusion of gases. Erythrocytes are primarily composed of a large molecule called hemoglobin. **Hemoglobin,** a complex protein-iron compound composed of heme (an iron compound) and globin (a simple protein), functions to bind with oxygen and carbon dioxide. As RBCs circulate through the capillaries surrounding alveoli within the lung, oxygen attaches to the iron on the hemoglobin. The oxygen-bound hemoglobin is referred to as *oxyhemoglobin* and is responsible for giving arterial blood its bright red appearance. As RBCs flow to body tissues, oxygen detaches from the hemoglobin and diffuses from the capillary into tissue cells. Carbon dioxide diffuses from tissue cells into the capillary, attaches to the globin portion of hemoglobin, and is transported to the lungs for removal. Hemoglobin also acts as a buffer and plays a role in maintaining acid-base balance. This buffering function is described further in Chapter 17.

Erythropoiesis (the process of RBC production) is regulated by cellular oxygen requirements and general metabolic activity. Erythropoiesis is stimulated by hypoxia and controlled by *erythropoietin,* a glycoprotein growth factor synthesized and released by the kidney. Erythropoietin stimulates the bone marrow to increase erythrocyte production. Normally the bone marrow releases 3×10^9 RBCs/kg of body weight per day. Erythropoiesis is also influenced by the availability of nutrients. Many essential nutrients are necessary for erythropoiesis, including protein, iron, folate (folic acid), cobalamin (vitamin B_{12}), riboflavin (vitamin B_2), and pyridoxine (vitamin B_6).[2] Erythrocyte production is also affected by endocrine hormones, such as thyroxine, corticosteroids, and testosterone. For example, hypothyroidism can be the cause of a microcytic anemia.[3]

Several distinct cell types evolve during erythrocyte maturation (see Fig. 30-1). The **reticulocyte** is an immature erythrocyte. The reticulocyte count measures the rate at which new RBCs appear in the circulation. Reticulocytes can develop into mature RBCs within 48 hours of release into circulation. Therefore assessing the number of reticulocytes is a useful means of evaluating the rate and adequacy of erythrocyte production.

Hemolysis (destruction of RBCs) by monocytes and macrophages removes abnormal, defective, damaged, and old RBCs from circulation. Hemolysis normally occurs in the bone marrow, liver, and spleen. Hemolysis of RBCs results in increased bilirubin to be processed by the body. When hemolysis occurs via normal mechanisms, the liver is able to conjugate and excrete all bilirubin that is released (see Fig. 31-2). The normal life span of an erythrocyte is 120 days.

Leukocytes. Leukocytes (WBCs) appear white when separated from blood. Like the RBCs, leukocytes originate from stem cells within the bone marrow (see Fig. 30-1). There are five different types of leukocytes, each of which has a different function. Leukocytes containing granules within the cytoplasm are called *granulocytes* (also known as polymorphonuclear leukocytes). Granulocytes include three types: neutrophils, basophils, and eosinophils. Leukocytes that do not have granules within the cytoplasm are called *agranulocytes* and include lymphocytes and monocytes (Table 30-2). Lymphocytes and monocytes are also referred to as mononuclear cells because they have only one discrete nucleus. Leukocytes have a widely variable life span. Granulocytes may only live for hours, yet some T lymphocytes may live for years.

Granulocytes. The primary function of the granulocytes is **phagocytosis,** a process by which WBCs ingest or engulf any un-

TABLE 30-2 Types and Functions of Leukocytes

Type	Cell Function
Granulocytes	
Neutrophil	Phagocytosis, especially during the early phase of inflammation
Eosinophil	Phagocytosis (not as effective as neutrophil); allergic response; protection from parasitic infections
Basophil	Inflammatory response and allergic response; release of bradykinin, heparin, histamine, serotonin; limited phagocytosis
Agranuloctyes	
Lymphocyte	Cellular and humoral immune response
Monocyte	Phagocytosis; cellular immune response

wanted organism and then digest and kill it. The *neutrophil* is the most common type of granulocyte, accounting for 50% to 70% of all WBCs. Neutrophils are the primary phagocytic cells involved in acute inflammatory responses. A mature neutrophil is called a *segmented neutrophil* or "seg" or "polysegmented neutrophil" because the nucleus is segmented into two to five lobes connected by strands. An immature neutrophil is called a *band* (for the band appearance of the nucleus). Although band cells are sometimes found in the peripheral circulation of normal persons and are capable of phagocytosis, the mature neutrophil is much more effective.

Eosinophils account for only 2% to 4% of all WBCs. They have a similar but reduced ability for phagocytosis. One of their primary functions is to engulf antigen-antibody complexes formed during an allergic response. They also are able to defend against parasitic infections. *Basophils* make up less than 2% of all leukocytes. They have a limited role in phagocytosis. These cells have cytoplasmic granules that contain heparin, serotonin, and histamine. If a basophil is stimulated by an antigen or by tissue injury, it will respond by releasing substances within the granules. This is part of the response seen in allergic and inflammatory reactions.

Lymphocytes. Lymphocytes, one of the agranular leukocytes, constitute 20% to 40% of the WBCs. The main function of lymphocytes is related to the immune response (see Chapter 14). Lymphocytes form the basis of the cellular and humoral immune responses. Two lymphocyte subtypes are B cells and T cells. Although T-cell precursors originate in the bone marrow, these cells migrate to the thymus gland for further differentiation into T cells. (Details of lymphocyte function are presented in Chapter 14.)

Monocytes. Monocytes are the other type of agranular leukocytes. These cells account for approximately 4% to 8% of the total WBCs. Monocytes are potent phagocytic cells. They can ingest small or large masses of matter, such as bacteria, dead cells, tissue debris, and old or defective RBCs. Monocytes are the second type of WBCs to arrive at the scene of an injury. These cells are only present in the blood for a short time before they migrate into the tissues and become macrophages (see Chapter 13). In addition to macrophages that have differentiated from monocytes, resident macrophages can also be found in tissues. These resident macrophages are given special names (e.g., Kupffer cells in the liver, osteoclasts in the bone, alveolar macrophages in the lung). These macrophages protect the body from pathogens at these entry points and are more phagocytic than monocytes. Macrophages also interact with lymphocytes to facilitate the humoral and cellular immune responses (see Chapter 14).

Thrombocytes. The primary function of thrombocytes, or *platelets,* is to initiate the clotting process by producing an initial platelet plug in the early phases of the clotting process. Platelets must be available in sufficient numbers and must be structurally and metabolically sound for blood clotting to occur. Platelets maintain capillary integrity by working as "plugs" to close any openings in the capillary wall. At the site of any capillary damage, platelet activation is initiated. Increasing numbers of platelets accumulate to form an initial platelet plug that is stabilized with clotting factors. Platelets are also important in the process of clot shrinkage and retraction.

Platelets, like other blood cells, originate from stem cells within the bone marrow (see Fig. 30-1). The stem cell undergoes differentiation by transforming into a *megakaryocyte,* which produces platelets. Platelet production is partly regulated by *thrombopoietin,* a growth factor acting on bone marrow to stimulate platelet production. Typically, platelets have a life span of only 5 to 9 days.

Normal Iron Metabolism

Iron is obtained from food and dietary supplements. Approximately 1 mg of every 10 to 20 mg of iron ingested is absorbed in the duodenum and upper jejunum. Therefore only 5% to 10% of ingested iron is absorbed.

Iron is present in all RBCs as heme in hemoglobin and in a stored form. The heme in hemoglobin accounts for two thirds of the body's iron. The other one third of iron is stored as ferritin and hemosiderin (degraded form of ferritin) in the bone marrow, spleen, liver, and macrophages (Fig. 30-4). When the stored iron is not replaced, hemoglobin production is reduced.

Transferrin, which is synthesized in the liver, serves as a carrier plasma protein for iron. The degree to which transferrin is saturated with iron is a reliable indicator of the iron supply for developing red blood cells.

As part of normal iron metabolism, iron is recycled after macrophages in the liver and spleen phagocytize, or ingest and destroy, old and damaged red blood cells. Iron binds to transferrin in the plasma or is stored as ferritin or hemosiderin (see Fig. 30-4).

Normal Clotting Mechanisms

Hemostasis is a term used to describe the blood clotting process. This process is important in minimizing blood loss when various body structures are injured. Four components contribute to normal hemostasis: vascular response, platelet plug formation, the development of the fibrin clot on the platelet plug by plasma clotting factors, and the ultimate lysis of the clot.

Vascular Response. When a blood vessel is injured, an immediate local vasoconstrictive response occurs. Vasoconstriction reduces the leakage of blood from the vessel not only by restricting the

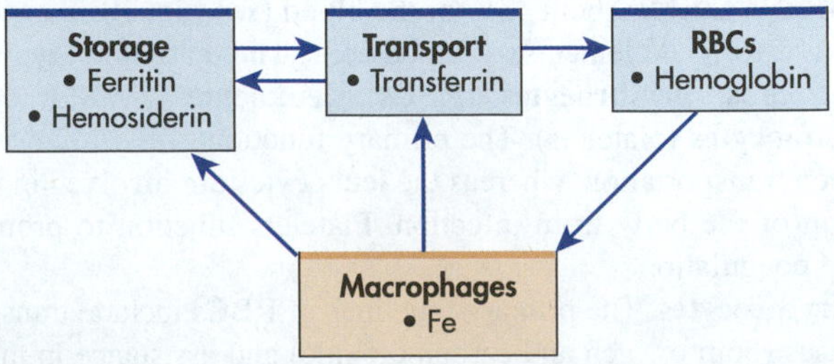

FIG. 30-4 Normal iron metabolism. Macrophages break down ingested RBCs. Iron is returned to blood bound to transferrin or stored as ferritin or hemosiderin.

vessel size but also by pressing the endothelial surfaces together. The latter reaction enhances vessel wall stickiness and maintains closure of the vessel even after the vasoconstriction subsides. Vascular spasm may last for 20 to 30 minutes, allowing time for the platelet response and plasma clotting factors to be activated. The platelet response and plasma clotting factors are triggered by endothelial injury and the release of substances such as tissue factor (TF).[4]

Platelet Plug Formation. Platelets are activated when they are exposed to interstitial collagen from an injured blood vessel. Platelets stick to one another and form clumps. The stickiness is termed *adhesiveness,* and the formation of clumps is termed *aggregation* or *agglutination.* When a blood vessel is injured, the circulating platelets are exposed to the collagen from the inner lining of the vessel. This interaction causes the platelets to release substances such as platelet factor 3 and serotonin, which facilitate coagulation. At the same time, platelets release adenosine diphosphate, which increases platelet adhesiveness and aggregation, thereby enhancing the formation of a platelet plug.

In addition to their independent contribution to clotting, platelets also facilitate the reactions of the plasma clotting factors. As Fig. 30-5 shows, platelet lipoproteins stimulate necessary conversions in the clotting process.

Plasma Clotting Factors. The formation of a visible fibrin clot on the platelet plug is the conclusion of a complex series of reactions involving different clotting factors. The plasma clotting factors are labeled with both names and Roman numerals (Table 30-3). Plasma proteins circulate in inactive forms until stimulated to initiate clotting through one of two pathways, intrinsic or extrin-

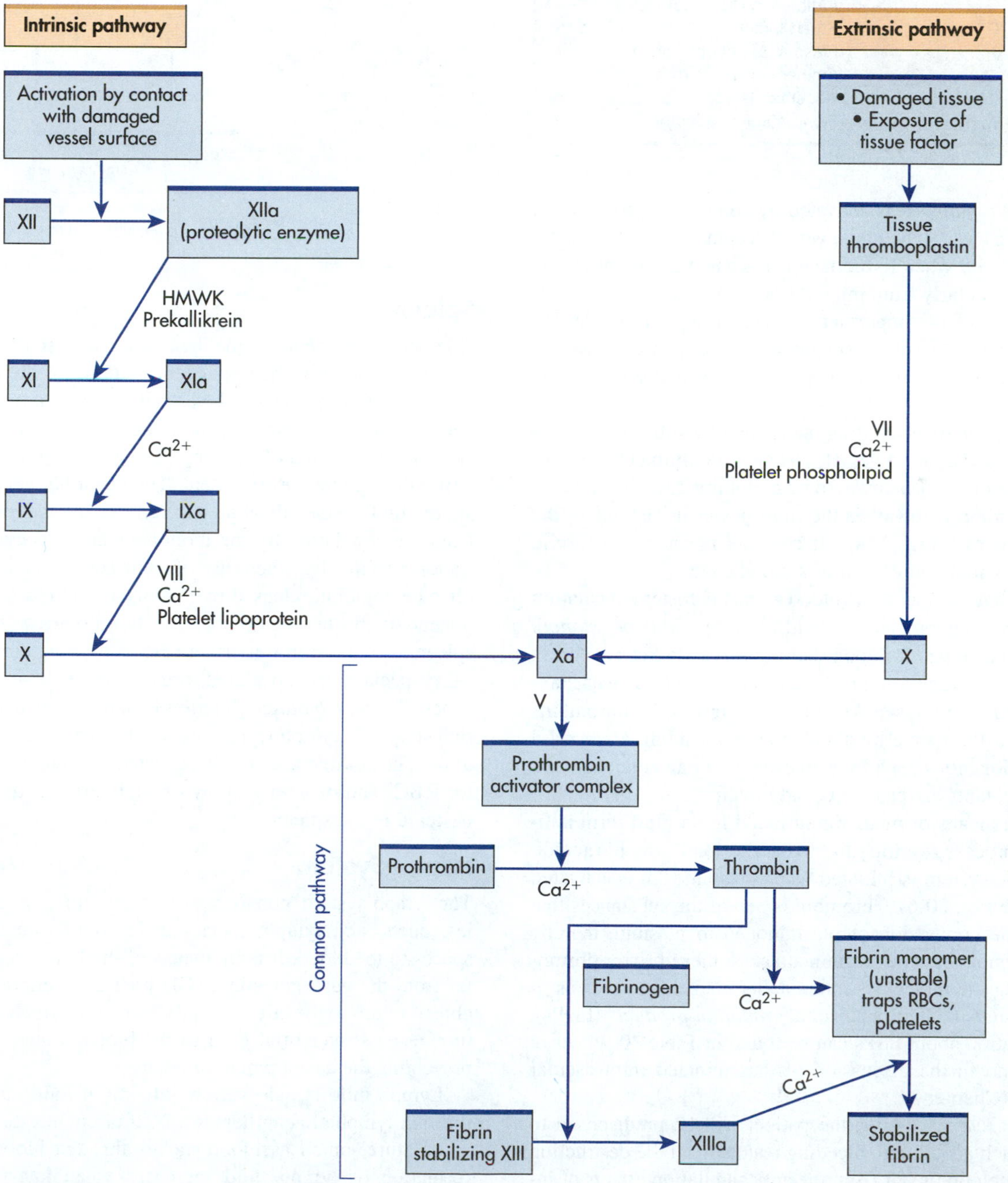

FIG. 30-5 Coagulation mechanism showing steps in the intrinsic pathway and extrinsic pathway as it would occur in the test tube. *HMWK,* High-molecular-weight kininogen; *RBCs,* red blood cells.

TABLE 30-3 Coagulation Factors

Coagulation Factor	Names
I	Fibrinogen
II	Prothrombin
III	Thromboplastin Thrombokinase Tissue factor
IV	Calcium
V	Proaccelerin Labile factor Ac globulin
VI	Not in use (now obsolete)
VII	Prothrombin conversion accelerator
VIII	Antihemophilic globulin Antihemophilic factor
IX	Plasma thromboplastin component Antihemophilic factor B
X	Stuart factor
XI	Plasma thromboplastin antecedent Antihemophilic factor C
XII	Hageman factor
XIII	Fibrin-stabilizing factor

sic. The *intrinsic pathway* is activated by collagen exposure from endothelial injury when the blood vessel is damaged. The *extrinsic pathway* is initiated when tissue factor or tissue thromboplastin is released extravascularly from injured tissues. In addition, von Willebrand factor (vWF) is important in forming an adhesive bridge between platelets and vascular subendothelial structures. It is synthesized in endothelial cells and megakaryocytes and acts as a carrier for factor VIII.[5]

Regardless of whether clotting is initiated by substances internal or external to the blood vessel, coagulation ultimately follows the same final common pathway of the clotting cascade. Thrombin, in the common pathway, is the most powerful enzyme in the coagulation process (Fig. 30-6). It converts fibrinogen to fibrin, which is an essential component of a blood clot.

Lysis of Clot. Just as some blood elements foster coagulation *(procoagulants),* others interfere with clotting *(anticoagulants).* This countermechanism to blood clotting serves to keep blood in its fluid state. Anticoagulation may be achieved by two means, antithrombins and fibrinolysis. As the name implies, antithrombins keep blood in a fluid state by antagonizing thrombin, a powerful coagulant. Endogenous heparin is an example of an anticoagulant. Other anticoagulants are protein C and protein S.

The second means of maintaining blood in its fluid form is **fibrinolysis,** a process resulting in the dissolution of the fibrin clot. The fibrinolytic system is initiated when plasminogen is activated to plasmin (see Fig. 30-6). Thrombin is one of the substances that can activate the conversion of plasminogen to plasmin, thereby promoting fibrinolysis. The plasmin attacks either fibrin or fibrinogen by splitting the molecules into smaller elements known as *fibrin split products* (FSPs) or *fibrin degradation products* (FDPs). (More information about FSPs can be found in Table 30-9 later in this chapter and in the discussion of disseminated intravascular coagulation in Chapter 31.)

If fibrinolysis is excessive, the patient will be predisposed to bleeding. In such a situation, bleeding results from the destruction of fibrin in platelet plugs or from the anticoagulation effects of increased FSPs. Increased FSPs lead to impaired platelet aggregation, reduced prothrombin, and an inability to stabilize fibrin.

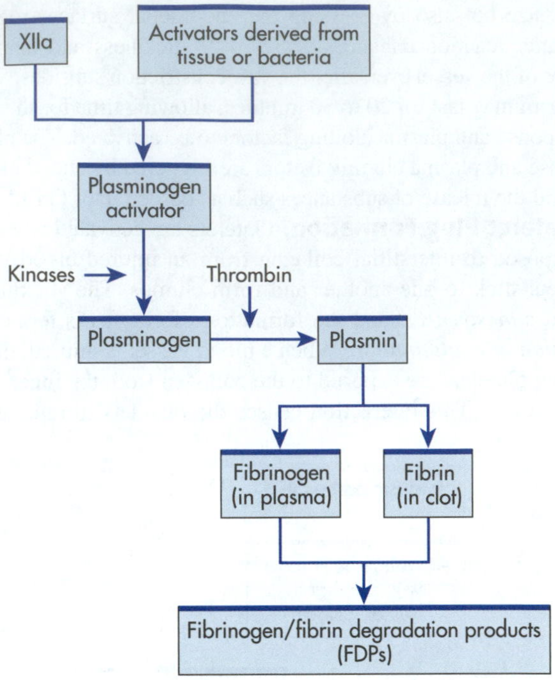

FIG. 30-6 Fibrinolytic system.

Spleen

Another component of the hematologic system is the spleen, which is located in the upper left quadrant of the abdomen. The functions of the spleen can be classified into four major functions: hematopoietic, filtration, immunologic, and storage. *Hematopoietic function* is manifested by the spleen's ability to produce RBCs during fetal development. The *filtration function* is demonstrated by the spleen's ability to remove old and defective RBCs from the circulation by the mononuclear phagocyte system. Filtration also involves the reuse of iron. The spleen is able to catabolize hemoglobin released by hemolysis and return the iron component of the hemoglobin to the bone marrow for reuse. The spleen also plays an important role in filtering circulating bacteria, especially encapsulated organisms such as gram-positive cocci. The *immunologic function* is demonstrated by the spleen's rich supply of lymphocytes, monocytes, and stored immunoglobulins. The *storage function* is reflected in its role as a storage site for RBCs and platelets. Approximately 30% of the platelet mass is stored in the spleen.

Lymph System

The lymph system, consisting of lymph fluid, lymphatic capillaries, ducts, and lymph nodes, carries fluid from the interstitial spaces to the blood. It is by means of the lymph that proteins and fat from the gastrointestinal (GI) tract and certain hormones are able to return to the circulatory system. The lymph system also returns excess interstitial fluid to the blood, which is important in preventing the development of edema.

Lymph fluid is pale yellow interstitial fluid that has diffused through lymphatic capillary walls. It circulates through a special vasculature, much as blood moves through blood vessels. The formation of lymph fluid increases when interstitial fluid increases, thereby forcing more fluid into the lymph system. When too much interstitial fluid develops or when something interferes

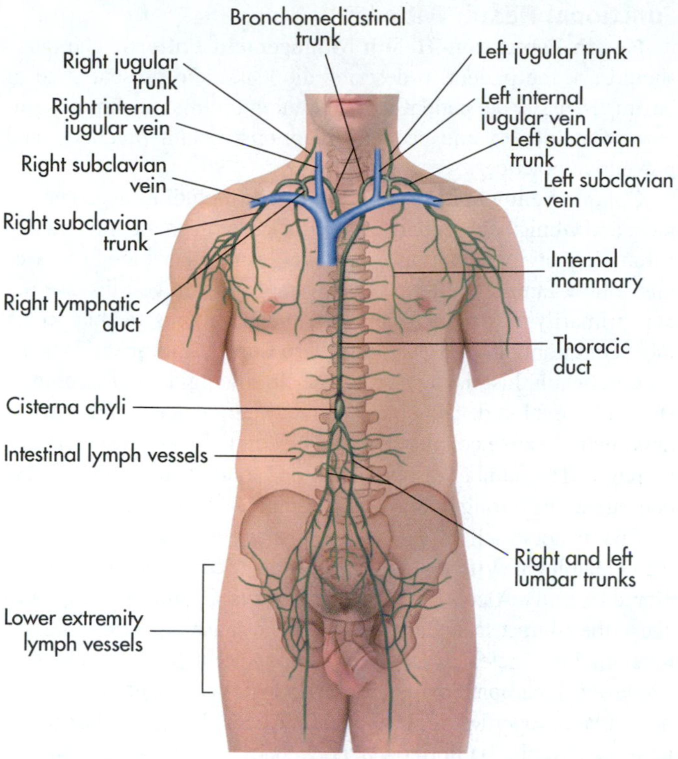

FIG. 30-7 Lymphatic drainage. Lymph fluid drains from tiny lymph vessels. Lymph vessels drain into large lymph ducts. Lymph ducts merge into the venous system at the subclavian veins.

with the reabsorption of lymph, lymphedema develops. The lymphedema that may occur as a complication of mastectomy or lumpectomy with dissection of axillary nodes is often caused by the obstruction of lymph flow from the removal of lymph nodes.

The lymphatic capillaries are thin-walled vessels that have an irregular diameter. They are somewhat larger than blood capillaries and do not contain valves. Lymphatic capillaries unite to form lymphatic vessels (also called lymphatic channels) that carry all lymph fluid to either the right lymphatic duct or the thoracic duct. These large lymphatic ducts drain into subclavian veins in the neck (Fig. 30-7).

The lymph nodes are also a part of the lymphatic system. Structurally, the nodes are small clumps of lymphatic tissue and are found in groups along lymph vessels at various sites. There are over 200 lymph nodes throughout the body, with the greatest predominance being in the abdomen surrounding the GI tract. Lymph nodes are situated both superficially and deep. The superficial nodes can be palpated, but evaluation of the deep nodes requires radiologic examination.[6] A primary function of lymph nodes is filtration of pathogens and foreign particles that are carried by lymph to the nodes.

Liver

The liver functions as a filter. It also produces all the procoagulants that are essential to hemostasis and blood coagulation. Additionally, it stores iron that is in excess of tissue needs. Hepcidin, produced by the liver, is a key regulator of iron balance. The synthesis of hepcidin is stimulated by iron overload or inflammation.[7,8] Other functions of the liver are described in Chapter 44.

GERONTOLOGIC CONSIDERATIONS
EFFECTS OF AGING ON THE HEMATOLOGIC SYSTEM

Physiologic aging is a gradual process that involves cell loss and organ atrophy. The amount of red marrow and the number of stem cells decrease with aging. However, there does not appear to be a complete depletion even in very old adults.[9] The remaining stem cells maintain their functional capacity to divide, but they decrease in number because they are gradually replaced by nonfunctional fat cells. Although the older adult is still capable of maintaining adequate blood cell levels, the reserve capacity leaves the older adult more vulnerable to possible problems with clotting, oxygen transport, and fighting infection, especially during periods of increased demand. This results in a diminished ability of an older adult to compensate for an acute or chronic illness.[9]

Hemoglobin levels begin to decrease in both men and women after middle age, with the low normal levels seen in most older people. Estimates of the prevalence of anemia in the elderly range from a low of 2% among the upper socioeconomic class of independently living elderly to a high of 40% among institutionalized elderly.[10] Although iron deficiency is usually responsible for the low hemoglobin levels, the cause of anemia in many older patients is unknown. However, hematopoietic defects in the older adult during illness may in part be explained by impaired production of growth factors (e.g., erythropoietin, granulocyte-macrophage colony-stimulating factor [GM-CSF]) and thus a reduced response of hematopoiesis in illness.[11]

Iron absorption is not impaired in the older patient, but adequate nutritional intake of iron may be decreased. It is essential to assess for signs of disease processes such as GI bleeding before concluding that decreased hemoglobin levels are caused solely by aging.

The osmotic fragility of RBCs is increased in the older person. This may account for a slight increase in mean corpuscular volume (MCV) and a slight decrease in mean corpuscular hemoglobin concentration (MCHC) of RBCs in some older individuals.

The total WBC count and differential are generally not affected by aging.[9] Leukocyte function is also well preserved. However, during an infection, the older adult may have only a minimal elevation in the total WBC count. These laboratory findings suggest a diminished bone marrow reserve of granulocytes in older adults and reflect the possible impaired stimulation of hematopoiesis. Platelets are unaffected by the aging process. However, changes in vascular integrity from aging can manifest as easy bruising.

The effects of aging on hematologic studies are presented in Table 30-4. Immune changes related to aging are presented in Chapter 14.

ASSESSMENT OF THE HEMATOLOGIC SYSTEM

Much of the evaluation of the hematologic system is based on a thorough health history. Consequently, the nurse must be knowledgeable about what to include in the health history so that questions may be phrased in a manner eliciting the most information related to the hematologic problem. Key questions to ask a patient with a hematologic problem are presented in Table 30-5.

Subjective Data

Important Health Information

Past Health History. It is important to learn whether the patient has had prior hematologic problems. Specifically the nurse

TABLE 30-4 GERONTOLOGIC DIFFERENCES IN ASSESSMENT
Effects of Aging on Hematologic Studies

Study	Changes
CBC Studies	
Hb	Normal; possibly slight decrease in men
MCV	May be slightly increased
MCHC	May be slightly decreased
WBC count	Diminished response to infection
Platelets	Unchanged
Clotting Studies	
Partial thromboplastin time	Decreased
Fibrinogen	May be elevated
Factors V, VII, VIII, IX	May be elevated
ESR	Increased significantly
Iron Studies	
Serum iron	Decreased
Total iron-binding capacity	Decreased
Ferritin	Increased
Erythropoietin	May be decreased

CBC, Complete blood count; *ESR,* erythrocyte sedimentation rate; *Hb,* hemoglobin; *MCHC,* mean corpuscular hemoglobin concentration; *MCV,* mean corpuscular volume; *WBC,* white blood cell.

needs to ask about previous problems with anemia, bleeding disorders, and blood diseases such as leukemia. Other related medical conditions such malabsorption, liver (e.g., hepatitis, cirrhosis), kidney, or spleen disorders should also be documented. Patients may have received a kidney transplant, may have lost a spleen to traumatic injury, or may have a history of intravenous drug use that may affect their risk for hematologic disorders. A history of recurrent infections or problems with blood clotting are also important to note.

Medications. A complete medication history of prescription and over-the-counter drugs is an important component of a hematologic assessment. The use of vitamins, herbal products, or dietary supplements should specifically be addressed because many patients may not consider these to be drugs. Many drugs may interfere with normal hematologic function (Table 30-6). Herbal therapy can interfere with clotting (see Complementary and Alternative Therapies box in Chapter 38 on p. 903). Antineoplastic agents used to treat malignant disorders (see Chapter 16) and antiretroviral agents used to treat human immunodeficiency virus (HIV) infection (see Chapter 15) may cause depression of the bone marrow (see Chapter 16). A patient previously treated with chemotherapy agents, particularly alkylating agents, is at a higher risk of developing a secondary malignancy of leukemia or lymphoma.

Surgery or Other Treatments. Specific past surgical procedures to ask the patient about include splenectomy, tumor removal, prosthetic heart valve placement, surgical excision of the duodenum (where iron absorption occurs), partial or total gastrectomy (which removes parietal cells, thus reducing intrinsic factor needed for the absorption of cobalamin [vitamin B_{12}]), and ileal resection (where cobalamin absorption takes place). The nurse should also ascertain how wound healing progressed postoperatively and if and when any bleeding problems occurred in relation to the surgery. Wound healing and bleeding should be discussed as responses to past injuries (including minor trauma) and to dental extractions. The number of previous blood transfusions and possible complications during administration should also be determined.

Functional Health Patterns

Health Perception–Health Management Pattern. The nurse should ask the patient to describe the usual and present state of health. To assist the patient in maintaining optimal health, it is important to identify the health perceptions, health practices, and preventive practices.

Complete biographic data are needed, including age, gender, race, and ethnic background. There is a known genetic influence in certain hematologic conditions, as well as in other blood diseases that follow familial patterns. For example, sickle cell disease occurs primarily in African Americans, and pernicious anemia occurs most commonly in persons of northern European descent. When a family health history is taken, the following health problems should be explored: jaundice, anemia, malignancies, RBC disorders such as sickle cell disease, and bleeding disorders such as hemophilia. The number of previous blood transfusions and possible complications during administration should be determined.

Risk factors such as alcohol and cigarette use that might disrupt the hematologic system must be assessed. Alcohol use must be explored tactfully. Alcohol is a caustic agent to GI mucosa, and damage to the GI tract secondary to alcohol can cause GI bleeding. Cigarette smoking increases low-density lipoprotein (LDL) cholesterol and levels of carbon dioxide, leading to hypoxia and altering the anticoagulant properties of the endothelium. Smoking increases platelet reactivity, plasma fibrinogen, hematocrit, and blood viscosity.

Hematemesis (bright red, brown, or black vomitus) can be a symptom of this problem and should be investigated. Chronic alcohol abusers frequently have vitamin deficiencies. Alcohol also exerts a damaging effect on platelet function and the liver, where clotting factors are produced. Consequently, bleeding problems can develop and should be anticipated in cases of known alcohol abuse. Illicit drug use is important to document, as many of these drugs may affect hematopoiesis.

Nutritional-Metabolic Pattern. During the patient interview and assessment, the nurse should obtain the patient's weight and determine if the patient has experienced anorexia, nausea, vomiting, or oral discomfort. A dietary history may provide clues about the cause of anemia. Iron, cobalamin, and folic acid are necessary for the development of RBCs. Iron and folic acid deficiencies are associated with inadequate intake of foods such as liver, meat, eggs, whole-grain and enriched breads and cereals, potatoes, leafy green vegetables, dried fruits, legumes, and citrus fruits. Folic acid deficiencies may be offset by a diet including foods that are also high in iron.[12]

Any changes in the skin's texture or color should be explored. The patient should be asked about any bleeding of gum tissue. Any *petechiae* or *ecchymotic* areas on the skin should be noted. If present, the frequency, size, and cause should be documented. The location of petechiae can indicate an accumulation of blood in the skin or mucous membranes. Small vessels leak under pressure, and the platelet numbers are insufficient to stop the bleeding. Petechiae are more likely to occur where clothing constricts the circulation.

The patient should also be questioned about any lumps or swelling in the neck, armpits, or groin. Specifically, the patient needs to be asked what the lumps feel like (i.e., hard or soft, tender or nontender) and if they are mobile or fixed. Primary lymph tumors are usually not painful. A nontender swollen lymph node may be a sign of Hodgkin's lymphoma or non-Hodgkin's lymphoma. Lymph nodes that are enlarged and tender are usually associated with an acute infection.[13] Any incidents of fever should be explored thoroughly. It should be determined if the patient currently has a fever, recurring fevers, chills, or night sweats.

TABLE 30-5 HEALTH HISTORY Hematologic System

Health Perception–Health Management Pattern
- Do you have any difficulty performing daily activities because of a lack of energy?*
- Do you smoke or drink alcohol?*
- Do you take any prescribed or over-the-counter medications?*
- Are you taking any herbal products?* Home remedies?*
- Have you in the past or are you currently consuming illegal drugs? What agents? What route? How frequently? When did you last use?*
- Have you ever received a blood transfusion?*
- Is there any family history of anemia, cancer, bleeding, or clotting problems?*
- Have you had any surgeries?*

Nutritional-Metabolic Pattern
- Do you have any difficulties with eating, chewing, or swallowing?*
- Have you had any mouth sores, sore tongue, swollen or sore gums, excessive oral bleeding?*
- What kind of diet do you follow? If a vegetarian, do you eat eggs, milk products, fish, chicken?
- How has your appetite been?
- Have you had any changes in your weight in the past year?*
- Do you take any vitamins, nutritional supplements, or iron?*
- Is nausea and vomiting a problem for you?*
- Have you ever experienced any unusual bleeding or bruising?*
- Have there been recent changes in the condition or color of your skin?*
- Have you experienced night sweats or cold intolerance?*
- Have you noticed any swelling in your armpits, neck, or groin?*

Elimination Pattern
- Have you had black or tarry stools?* Have you had light, clay-colored stools?*
- Have you noticed any blood or dark "tea color" in your urine?*
- Has your urine had a foul odor or cloudiness?
- Have you had any decrease in urinary output?*
- Do you ever have diarrhea or change in bowel patterns?*

Activity-Exercise Pattern
- Do you have any shortness of breath at rest? With activity?*
- Do you have any limitations in joint motion?* Have any of your joints been swollen?*
- Do you have a problem with unsteady gait? Have you fallen recently?*
- After activity, do you ever notice bleeding or bruising?*

Sleep-Rest Pattern
- Have you experienced excessive fatigue recently?*
- Are you more fatigued than usual?*
- Do you feel rested on awakening? If no, explain.

Cognitive-Perceptual Pattern
- Have you experienced any numbness or tingling?*
- Have you had any problems with your vision, hearing, or taste?*
- Have you noticed any changes in your mental function?*
- Do you have any pain, such as bone, joint, or abdominal pain, or abdominal fullness?*
- Do you have pain when moving your joints?*
- Have your muscles been sore or achy recently?*

Self-Perception–Self-Concept Pattern
- Does your health problem make you feel differently about yourself?*
- Do you have any physical changes that cause you distress?*

Role-Relationship Pattern
- Does your occupation bring you into contact with hazardous substances?*
- Has your present illness caused a change in your roles and relationships?*

Sexuality-Reproductive Pattern
- Has your hematologic problem caused any sexual problems that concern you?*
- Women: When was your last menses? Do you consider your cycle normal? How long does your bleeding usually last? Have you had any increase in cramping or clotting?* Have there been any changes in the amount of flow?*
- Men: Do you experience impotence?*
- Have you had unprotected sex in the past 6 mo?* Was your partner someone new or a person with whom you have had a long-term sexual relationship?

Coping–Stress Tolerance Pattern
- Do you have a support system to assist you when needed?
- What coping strategies do you use during exacerbation of symptoms?
- Do you experience any specific symptoms when you feel stressed?

Value-Belief Pattern
- Do you have any personal or religious objection to receiving blood or blood products?*
- Do you have any conflicts between your planned therapy and your value-belief system?*

*If yes, describe.

Patients should be asked if they have a history of cardiac or pulmonary diseases. Cardiovascular disorders such as valvular disease or hypertension may predispose patients to hemolysis. Many of the medications used to treat cardiovascular disease can also cause abnormalities in hematopoietic cell production or coagulation. Pulmonary disorders that lead to hypoxemia may cause chronic stimulation of erythropoietin and result in **polycythemia** (excessive RBCs).

Elimination Pattern. The patient should be asked if blood has been noted in the urine or stool or if black, tarry stools have occurred. In addition, any decrease in urinary output or diarrhea should be documented.

Activity-Exercise Pattern. Because fatigue is a prominent symptom in many hematologic disorders, the patient should be asked about feelings of tiredness. Weakness and complaints of heavy extremities should also be determined. Symptoms of apathy, malaise, dyspnea, or palpitations should be documented. Any change in the patient's ability to perform activities of daily living (ADLs) should be noted, especially as they relate to patient safety and a possible history of falling.

Sleep-Rest Pattern. The patient's feeling of being rested after a night's sleep should be determined. Fatigue secondary to a hematologic problem often will not be resolved following sleep.

Cognitive-Perceptual Pattern. *Arthralgia* (joint pain) may be caused by a hematologic problem and should be assessed. Pain in the joint may indicate an autoimmune disorder or may be caused by gout secondary to increased uric acid production as a result of a hematologic malignancy or hemolytic anemia. Aching bones may result from pressure of expanding bone marrow with diseases

TABLE 30-6 Drugs Affecting Hematologic Function and Laboratory Values*

Drug Class	Hematologic Effects
Antidysrhythmics (e.g., procainamide [Pronestyl], quinidine)	Agranulocytosis, anemia, hemolytic anemia, thrombocytopenia
Antiseizure (e.g., phenytoin [Dilantin], carbamazepine [Tegretol])	Anemia
Antihypertensives (e.g., methyldopa [Aldomet])	Hemolytic anemia
Antimicrobials	
aminoglycosides	Interfere with platelet function
amphotericin B (Fungizone)	Anemia
chloramphenicol (Chloromycetin)	Anemia, neutropenia, thrombocytopenia
flucytosine (Ancobon)	Anemia, neutropenia, thrombocytopenia
isoniazid (INH)	Neutropenia
trimethoprim-sulfamethoxazole (Bactrim, Septra)	Anemia, leukopenia, neutropenia, thrombocytopenia
Antineoplastics (e.g., alkylating agents, antitumor antibiotics, platinol agents)	Anemia, neutropenia, leukopenia, thrombocytopenia
Antiretrovirals (e.g., zidovudine [AZT, Retrovir])	Neutropenia, anemia
Corticosteroids (e.g., dexamethasone [Decadron], hydrocortisone, prednisolone)	Lymphopenia, neutrophilia
Diuretics (e.g., loop diuretics, thiazide diuretics)	Interfere with platelet function
Histamine H_2-blocking agents (e.g., ranitidine [Zantac], cimetidine [Tagamet])	Interfere with platelet production
Hormonal agents (e.g., diethylstilbestrol, [DES], megestrol acetate, oral contraceptives)	Increase in factors II, V, VII, VIII, IX, X; increase in fibrinogen; increase in thrombin; decrease in prothrombin and partial thromboplastin times; increase in coagulation and thromboemboli formation
Immunosuppressants (e.g., azathioprine [Imuran], cyclosporine, tacrolimus [Prograf])	Lymphopenia
Nonsteroidal antiinflammatory agents (e.g., ibuprofen [Motrin, Advil], phenylbutazone [Butazolidin])	Anemia, leukopenia, neutropenia, thrombocytopenia, inhibit platelet aggregation
Phenothiazines (e.g., chlorpromazine [Thorazine], prochlorperazine [Compazine])	Interfere with platelet function
Salicylates (e.g., aspirin and aspirin-containing compounds [e.g., Percodan])	Interfere with platelet function
Sympathomimetics (e.g., dopamine [Intropin], epinephrine)	Leukocytosis
Tricyclic antidepressants	Interfere with platelet function
Miscellaneous	
allopurinol	Neutropenia
dextran	Interfere with platelet function

*This represents only a partial listing of drugs affecting the hematologic system.

such as leukemia. *Hemarthrosis* (blood in a joint) occurs in the patient with bleeding disorders and can be painful.

Paresthesias, numbness, and tingling may be related to a hematologic disorder and should be noted. Any changes in vision, hearing, taste, or mental status should also be assessed carefully.

Self-Perception–Self-Concept Pattern. The effect of the health problem on the patient's perception of self and personal abilities should be determined. The effect of certain problems, such as bruising, petechiae, and lymph node swelling, on the patient's personal appearance should also be assessed.

Role-Relationship Pattern. The patient should be questioned about any past or present occupational or household exposures to radiation or chemicals. If such exposure has occurred, the type, amount, and duration of the exposure should be determined.

It is known that a person who has been exposed to radiation, as a treatment modality or by accident, has a higher incidence of certain hematologic problems. The same is true of a person who has been exposed to chemicals (e.g., benzene, lead, naphthalene, phenylbutazone). These chemicals are commonly used by potters, dry cleaners, and individuals involved with occupations that use adhesives. The patient should also be questioned about a history in the military. Many Vietnam War veterans were exposed to a dioxin-containing defoliant (Agent Orange), which has been linked with leukemia and lymphoma. The nurse also should assess the effect of the present illness on the patient's usual roles and responsibilities.

Sexuality-Reproductive Pattern. A careful menstrual history should be obtained from women, including the age at which menarche and menopause began, duration and amount of bleeding, incidence of clotting and cramping, and any associated problems. Any intrapartum or postpartum bleeding problems should also be documented. Men should be asked if they have any problems related to impotence because this is not uncommon in men with hematologic problems. The patient should also be questioned about sexual behavior because HIV infection is potentially a concern, particularly among high-risk groups.[14]

Coping–Stress Tolerance Pattern. The patient with a hematologic problem often needs assistance with ADLs. The patient should be asked if adequate support is available to meet daily needs. The patient's usual methods of handling stress should also be determined. In the patient with platelet disorders or hemophilia, the potential for hemorrhage can be so frightening that usual life patterns may be drastically curtailed, affecting the person's quality of life. The nurse should explore the accuracy of the patient's understanding of the problem.

Value-Belief Pattern. Some hematologic problems are treated with blood transfusions or a bone marrow transplant. The nurse should determine if these types of treatments cause any conflicts with the patient's value-belief system, including the patient's cultural and religious beliefs related to blood and blood transfusions. If conflicts are identified, the health care provider should be notified.

Objective Data

Physical Examination. A complete physical examination is necessary to accurately examine all systems that affect or are affected by the hematologic system (see Chapter 4). The nurse must be aware that disorders of the hematologic system can manifest in various ways; thus a patient's presenting symptoms may not immediately point to a hematologic problem[14] (Table 30-7). For ex-

TABLE 30-7 COMMON ASSESSMENT ABNORMALITIES
Hematologic System

Finding	Description	Possible Etiology and Significance
Skin		
Pallor of skin or nail beds	Paleness; decreased or absence of skin coloration	Low Hb level (anemia)
Flushing	Transient, episodic redness of skin (usually around face and neck)	Increase in Hb (polycythemia), congestion of capillaries Flushing of the palms of the hands or soles of the feet may indicate anemia
Jaundice	Yellow appearance of skin and mucous membranes	Accumulation of bile pigment caused by rapid or excessive hemolysis or liver damage
Cyanosis	Bluish discoloration of skin and mucous membranes	Reduced Hb, excessive concentration of deoxyHb in blood
Excoriation	Scratch or abrasion of skin	Scratching from intense pruritus
Pruritus	Unpleasant cutaneous sensation that provokes the desire to rub or scratch the skin	Hodgkin's lymphoma, cutaneous lymphomas, infiltrative leukemias, increased bilirubin
Leg ulcers	Prominent on the malleoli on the ankles	Sickle cell disease
Angioma	Benign tumor consisting of blood or lymph vessels	Most are congenital; some may disappear spontaneously
Telangiectasia	Small angioma with tendency to bleed; focal red lesions, coarse or fine red lines	Dilation of small vessels
Spider nevus	Form of telangiectasia characterized by a round red central portion and branching radiations resembling the profile of a spider; usually develop on face, neck, or chest	Elevated estrogen levels as in pregnancy or liver disease
Purpura	Any of a small group of conditions characterized by ecchymosis or other small hemorrhages in skin and mucous membranes	Decreased platelets or clotting factors resulting in hemorrhage into the skin; vascular abnormalities; break in blood vessel walls resulting from trauma
Petechiae	Pinpoint, nonraised, perfectly round area >2 mm; purple, dark red, or brown in color	Same as above
Ecchymosis (bruise)	Small hemorrhagic spot, larger than petechiae; nonelevated; round or irregular	Same as above
Hematoma	A localized collection of blood, usually clotted	Same as above
Chloroma	A tumor arising from myeloid tissue and containing a pale green pigment	Acute myelogenous leukemia that has infiltrated the skin
Plasmacytoma	A tumor arising from abnormal plasma cells	Multiple myeloma that has infiltrated tissue
Eyes		
Jaundiced sclera	Yellow appearance of the sclera	Accumulation of bile pigment resulting from rapid or excessive hemolysis or liver disease or infiltration
Conjunctival pallor	Paleness; decreased or absence of coloration in the conjunctiva	Low Hb level (anemia)
Blurred vision, diplopia, visual field cuts	Decreased visual acuity or areas of blindness (field cuts)	Anemia, extreme leukocytosis, polycythemia may cause visual abnormalities Thrombocytopenia may cause intraocular hemorrhage with visual abnormalities Excessive clotting may cause thromboses in the circulation to the brain that cause visual field cuts
Nose		
Epistaxis	Spontaneous bleeding from the nares	May occur with low platelet counts, especially if the patient bends down for a long time period, tries to lift a heavy item, or with an intense Valsalva maneuver
Mouth		
Gingival and mucous membrane changes	Pallor Gingival/mucosal ulceration, swelling, or bleeding	Low Hb level (anemia) Neutropenia; inability of impaired leukocytes to combat oral infections; thrombocytopenia Gingival hyperplasia may be present with some types of leukemia
Smooth tongue	Tongue surface is smooth and shiny; mucosa is thin and red from decreased papillae	Pernicious anemia, iron-deficiency anemia
Lymph Nodes		
Lymphadenopathy	Lymph nodes are enlarged (>1 cm); may be tender to touch	Infection, foreign infiltrations, or systemic disease such as leukemia, lymphoma, Hodgkin's lymphoma, and metastatic cancer

Hb, Hemoglobin.

Continued

TABLE 30-7 COMMON ASSESSMENT ABNORMALITIES Hematologic System—cont'd

Finding	Description	Possible Etiology and Significance
Heart and Chest		
Tachycardia	Heart rate >100 beats/min	Compensatory mechanism in anemia to increase cardiac output
Palpitations	Sensation of feeling the heart beat, flutter, or pound in the chest	Anemia, fluid volume overload, hypotension with impending syncope, hypertension, and dysrhythmias may cause palpitations
Altered blood pressure	Orthostasis: heart rate >20/min increase or blood pressure >20 mm Hg decrease from baseline when moving from a lying position to either sitting or standing Hypotension: <90 mm Hg systolic or >40 mm Hg drop from baseline Hypertension: >130/90 mm Hg	Orthostasis is a common manifestation in anemia, especially if also accompanied by low blood volume Hypotension may indicate an infectious process, blood loss, or compromised cardiovascular compensatory mechanisms Hypertension may occur initially when patients are anemic as a compensatory mechanism for anemia
Sternal tenderness	Abnormal sensitivity to touch or pressure on sternum	Leukemia resulting from increased bone marrow cellularity, causing increase in pressure and bone erosion; multiple myeloma as a result of stretching of periosteum
Low oxygen saturation	Oxygen-carrying capacity is reflected by the oxygen saturation by pulse oximetry	Oxygen saturation may be decreased in cases of severe anemia
Abdomen		
Hepatomegaly	Palpable liver	Leukemia, cirrhosis, or fibrosis secondary to iron overload from sickle cell disease or thalassemia
Splenomegaly	Palpable spleen	Anemia, thrombocytopenia, leukemia, lymphomas, leukopenia, mononucleosis, malaria, cirrhosis, trauma, portal hypertension
Distended abdomen	Distended abdomen is a larger than normal abdominal profile; it may be soft or firm, tender or nontender, and accompanied by other symptoms such as nausea, vomiting, or rebound tenderness	Lymphoma may manifest as abdominal adenopathy, mass(es), or bowel obstruction
Nervous System		
Paresthesias of feet and hands; ataxia	Numbness sensation and extreme sensitivity experienced in central and peripheral nerves; impaired muscle movement	Cobalamin (vitamin B_{12}) deficiency or folate deficiency
Weakness	Lacking physical strength or energy	Low Hb level (anemia)
Headache, nuchal rigidity	Pain in the cranium, potentially involving one area or extending from the frontal area to the back of the neck	Generalized headache is a common manifestation of mild to moderate anemia Severe headache with or without visual disturbances may signal intracranial hemorrhage due to thrombocytopenia Headache with nuchal rigidity may indicate meningitis carcinomatosis that may accompany certain types of leukemia
Musculoskeletal System		
Bone pain	Pain in pelvis, ribs, spine, sternum	Multiple myeloma related to enlarged tumors that stretch periosteum; bone invasion by leukemia cells; bone demineralization resulting from various malignancies; sickle cell disease
Joint swelling	Fluid-filled spaces surrounding the joints	Occurs with sickle cell anemia as bleeding occurs into the joint (hemarthria) causing inflammation
Arthralgia	Joint pain	Sickle cell disease from hemarthrosis

ample, paresthesias of the lower extremities may not immediately appear to reflect a hematologic problem, but when combined with other clinical findings or risk factors, nutritional anemia may be suspected. Although a full examination should be performed on patients suspected of a hematologic disorder, certain aspects of the physical examination are specifically relevant in hematologic disorders. These include the skin, lymph nodes, spleen, and liver. Examination of the skin is discussed in Chapter 23; spleen and liver examination is found in Chapter 39.

Lymph Node Assessment. Lymph nodes are distributed throughout the body. Superficial lymph nodes can be evaluated by light palpation (Fig. 30-8). Deep lymph nodes cannot be palpated and are best evaluated by radiologic examination. Lymph nodes should be assessed symmetrically with regard to location, size (in centimeters), degree of fixation (e.g., movable, fixed), tenderness, and texture. To assess superficial lymph nodes, the examiner should lightly palpate the nodes using the pads of the fingers. The examiner should gently roll the skin over the area and concentrate

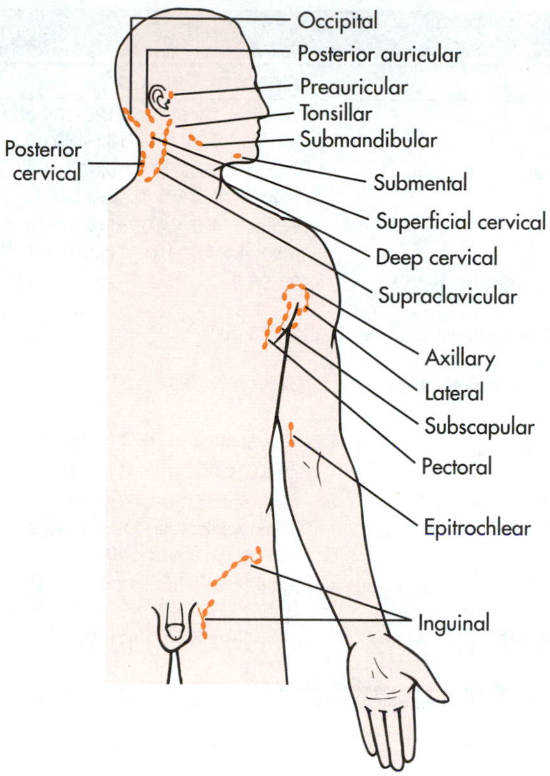

FIG. 30-8 Palpable superficial lymph nodes.

on feeling for possible lymph node enlargement. Ordinarily, lymph nodes are not palpable in adults. If a node is palpable, it should be small (0.5 to 1 cm), mobile, firm, and nontender to be considered a normal finding. Abnormal findings, warranting further investigation, include any of the following: tender, hard, fixed, or enlarged (regardless if they are tender or not). Tender nodes are usually a result of inflammation, whereas hard or fixed nodes suggest malignancy.[13]

It is important to develop a sequence when examining the lymph nodes. A convenient sequence for examination is to start at the head and neck. First the preauricular, posterior auricular, occipital, tonsillar, submaxillary, submental, superficial cervical, posterior cervical chain, deep cervical chain, and supraclavicular nodes are palpated. Next the axillary lymph nodes and pectoral, subscapular, and lateral groups of nodes are palpated. The epitrochlear nodes, located in the antecubital fossa between the biceps and triceps muscles, are then examined. The inguinal lymph nodes, found in the groin, are palpated last.

Palpation of the Liver or Spleen. Both the liver and spleen are normally not detectable by palpating the abdomen. When they are enlarged, they may be detectable by percussion or palpation. The degree of enlargement of the liver is measured by the number of fingerbreadths it extends below the rib border. The spleen may be more difficult to detect because of its deep location in the left abdomen. Specific techniques for palpating the liver and spleen are described in Chapter 39.

Skin Assessment. In hematologic disorders, assessment of the skin may be a valuable source of information about the hematologic system. The skin should be examined over the entire body in a systematic manner (e.g., starting with the face and oral cavity and moving downward over the body). In patients with RBC disorders the skin may be pale or have pasty skin tones, or have a cyanotic tinge in severe anemia. Erythrocytosis often produces small vessel occlusions causing a purple, mottled appearance of the face, nose, fingers, or toes. Clubbing of the fingers can be seen with chronic anemia such as in patients with sickle cell disease. Leukocyte disorders may cause infectious skin lesions or malignant nodular lesions. These may occur anywhere and have a variable distribution pattern. During the physical assessment of the skin, the nurse needs to look carefully for **petechiae** (small purplish-red lesions), **ecchymoses** (bruising), and **spider nevus** (a form of **telangiectasia**) (see Table 30-7) because these can indicate bleeding disorders.

DIAGNOSTIC STUDIES OF THE HEMATOLOGIC SYSTEM

The most direct means of evaluating the hematologic system is through laboratory analysis and other diagnostic studies. Repeated acquisition of blood specimens may be distressing for the patient. Some patients may become concerned that the amount of blood withdrawn for tests could lead to adverse effects. Although multiple blood studies may be uncomfortable, it is only in rare situations that diagnostic blood withdrawal predisposes the patient to significant loss of blood. For patients requiring frequent blood studies for several months, a central venous catheter may be recommended for venous access. Diagnostic tests of the hematologic system are presented in Tables 30-8 through 30-12.

Laboratory Studies

Complete Blood Count. The complete blood count (CBC) involves several laboratory tests (Table 30-8), each of which serves to assess the three major blood cells formed in the bone marrow. Although the status of each cell type is important, the entire system may be disrupted by diseases, as well as by treatment of diseases. When the entire CBC is suppressed, a condition termed **pancytopenia** (marked decrease in the number of RBCs, WBCs, and platelets) exists. In such cases the patient needs care directed toward the management of anemia, infection, and hemorrhage (see Chapter 31). The effects of aging on hematologic studies are presented in Table 30-4.

Red Blood Cells. Normal values of some RBC tests are reported separately for men and for women because normal values are based on body mass and men usually have a larger body mass than women.

The *hemoglobin (Hb) value* is reduced in cases of anemia, hemorrhage, and states of hemodilution, such as those that occur when the fluid volume is excessive. Increases in hemoglobin are found in polycythemia or in states of hemoconcentration, which can develop from volume depletion (dehydration).

The *hematocrit (Hct) value* is determined by spinning blood in a centrifuge, which causes RBCs and plasma to separate. The RBCs, being the heavier elements, settle to the bottom. The hematocrit value represents the percentage of RBCs compared with the total blood volume. Reductions and elevations of hematocrit value are seen in the same conditions that raise and lower the hemoglobin value. The hematocrit value generally is three times the hemoglobin value.

The total RBC count is reported as RBC $\times 10^6/\mu l$. However, total RBC count is not always reliable in determining the adequacy of RBC function. Consequently, other data, such as hemoglobin, hematocrit, and RBC indices, must also be evaluated. The RBC

TABLE 30-8 Complete Blood Count Studies

Study	Description and Purpose	Normal Values
Hb	Measurement of gas-carrying capacity of RBC	Women: 12-16 g/dl (120-160 g/L) Men: 13.5-18 g/dl (135-180 g/L)
Hct	Measure of packed cell volume of RBCs expressed as a percentage of the total blood volume	Women: 38%-47% (0.38-0.47) Men: 40%-54% (0.40-0.54)
Total RBC count	Count of number of circulating RBCs	Women: 4-5 × 10^6/μl (4-5 × 10^{12}/L) Men: 4.5-6 × 10^6/μl (4.5-6 × 10^{12}/L)
Red cell indices	Determination of relative size of RBCs; low MCV reflection of microcytosis, high MCV reflection of macrocytosis	82-98 fl
	Measurement of average weight of Hb/RBCs; low MCH indication of microcytosis or hypochromia, high MCH indication of macrocytosis	27-33 pg
	Evaluation of RBC saturation with Hb; low MCHC indication of hypochromia, high MCHC evident in spherocytosis	32%-36% (0.32-0.36)
RBC morphology	Examination of the shape and size of RBCs	No variation in RBC morphology
WBC count	Measurement of total number of leukocytes	4000-11,000/μl (4–11 × 10^9/L)
WBC differential	Determination of whether each kind of WBC is present in proper proportion Absolute value of each type of WBC can be determined by multiplying the percentage of cell type by total WBC count and dividing by 100	Neutrophils: 50%-70% (0.50-0.70) Eosinophils: 2%-4% (0.02-0.04) Basophils: 0%-2% (0-0.02) Lymphocytes: 20%-40% (0.20-0.40) Monocytes: 4%-8% (0.04-0.08)
Platelet count	Measurement of number of platelets available to maintain platelet clotting functions (not measurement of quality of platelet function)	150,000-400,000/μl (150–400 × 10^9/L)

Hb, Hemoglobin; *Hct,* hematocrit; *MCH,* mean corpuscular hemoglobin; *MCHC,* mean corpuscular hemoglobin concentration; *MCV,* mean corpuscular volume; *RBC,* red blood cell; *WBC,* white blood cell.

count is altered by the same conditions that raise and lower the hemoglobin and hematocrit values.

RBC indices are special indicators that reflect RBC volume, color, and hemoglobin saturation (see Table 30-8). These parameters may provide insight into the cause of anemia. (The significance of these parameters is discussed further in Chapter 31.)

The shape and appearance of cells is called *morphology.* Cell morphology can provide clues to the presence of specific disease states. Examples of RBC morphologies that may be reported include Dohl bodies, Heinz bodies, anistocytes, schistocytes, and sickled cells (discussed in Chapter 31).

White Blood Cells. The WBC count provides two different sets of information. The first is a total count of WBCs in 1 μl of peripheral blood. Elevations in WBC count over 11,000/μl are associated with infection, inflammation, tissue injury or death, and malignancies (e.g., leukemia, lymphoma). Although the degree of WBC elevation does not necessarily predict the severity of illness, it can provide clues to the etiology. Certain types of leukemias are more likely to produce extremely high WBC counts (e.g., greater than 25,000/μl). A total WBC count less than 4000/μl **(leukopenia)** is associated with bone marrow depression, severe or chronic illness, and/or some types of leukemia.

The second aspect of the WBC count, the differential count, measures the percentage of each type of leukocyte. The information from the WBC differential provides valuable clues in determining the cause of illness. An important concept related to neutrophil counts is the *shift to the left.* When infections are severe, more granulocytes are released from the bone marrow as a compensatory mechanism. To meet the increased demand, many young, immature polymorphonuclear neutrophils (bands) are released into circulation. The usual laboratory procedure is to report the WBCs in order of maturity, with the less mature forms on the left side of the written report. Consequently, the existence of many immature cells is termed a "shift to the left."

The WBC differential is of considerable significance because it is possible for the total WBC count to remain essentially normal despite a marked change in one type of leukocyte. For example, a patient may have a normal WBC count of 8800/μl, whereas the differential count may show a relative proportion of lymphocytes to be reduced to 10%. This is an abnormal finding that warrants further investigation.

When there is a low lymphocyte count, an absolute lymphocyte count (ALC) may be tabulated. If the ALC is low, other diagnostic tests may be performed to investigate for an underlying reason.

When the bone marrow does not produce enough neutrophils, neutropenia occurs. **Neutropenia** is a condition associated with a neutrophil count (absolute neutrophil count [ANC]) less than 1000 cells/μl; severe neutropenia is associated with an ANC of less than 500 cells/μl. The ANC is determined by multiplying the total WBC count by the percentage of neutrophils. Neutropenia results from a number of disease processes, such as leukemia, or from bone marrow depression (see Chapter 31), and is associated with a high risk of infection.

Platelet Count. The platelet count is the number of platelets per microliter of blood. Normal platelet counts are between 150,000 and 400,000/μl; counts below 100,000/μl signify a condition termed **thrombocytopenia.** Bleeding may occur with thrombocytopenia. Spontaneous hemorrhage is possible once platelet counts fall below 20,000/μl.[15] A more extensive description of clotting studies is presented in Table 30-9. **Thrombocytosis** is defined as excessive platelets, a disorder that occurs with inflammation and some malignant disorders (see Chapter 31). The most likely complication related to thrombocytosis is excessive clotting.

Erythrocyte Sedimentation Rate. Erythrocyte sedimentation rate (ESR or "sed rate") measures the sedimentation or settling of RBCs and is used as a nonspecific measure of many diseases, especially inflammatory conditions. Increased ESR is

TABLE 30-9 Clotting Studies

Study	Description and Purpose	Normal Values
Platelet count	Count of number of circulating platelets	150,000-400,000/μl
Prothrombin time (PT)	Assessment of extrinsic coagulation by measurement of factors I, II, V, VII, X	12-15 sec
International normalized ratio (INR)	Standardized system of reporting PT based on a reference calibration model and calculated by comparing the patient's PT with a control value	2-3*
Activated partial thromboplastin time (aPTT)	Assessment of intrinsic coagulation by measuring factors I, II, V, VIII, IX, X, XI, XII; longer with use of heparin	30-45 sec
Automated coagulation time (ACT)	Evaluation of intrinsic coagulation status; more accurate than aPTT; used during dialysis, coronary artery bypass procedure, arteriograms	150-180
Thromboplastin generation test (TGT)	Reflection of generation of thromboplastin; if abnormal, second stage done to identify missing coagulation factor	<12 sec (100%)
Bleeding time	Measurement of timed, small skin incision bleeds; reflection of ability of small blood vessels to constrict	1-6 min
Thrombin time	Reflection of adequacy of thrombin; prolonged thrombin time indicates that coagulation is inadequate secondary to decreased thrombin activity	8-12 sec
Fibrinogen	Reflection of level of fibrinogen; increase in fibrinogen possible indication of enhancement of fibrin formation, making patient hypercoagulable; decrease in fibrinogen indicates that patient possibly predisposed to bleeding	200-400 mg/dl (2-4 g/L)
Fibrin split products† (FSP)	Reflection of degree of fibrinolysis and predisposition to bleed (if present); screening test for DIC; elevated levels associated with DIC, advanced malignancy, severe inflammation	<10 mg/L (<10 mcg/ml)
D-dimer	Assay to measure a fragment of fibrin that is formed as a result of fibrin degradation and clot lysis; used in diagnosis of hypercoagulable conditions (e.g., DIC)	<250 ng/ml (250 mcg/L)
Antithrombin III (AT-III)	Naturally occurring protein synthesized by liver that inhibits coagulation through inactivation of thrombin and other factors; is depleted in DIC	21-30 mg/dl (210-300 mg/L) or 85%-115% of standard
Clot retraction	Reflection of clot shrinkage or retraction from sides of test tube after 24 hours; used to confirm a platelet problem	50%-100% in 24 hr
Capillary fragility test (tourniquet test, Rumpel-Leede test)	Reflection of capillary integrity when positive or negative pressure is applied to various areas of the body; positive test indication of thrombocytopenia, toxic vascular reactions	No petechiae or negative
Protamine sulfate tests	Reflection of presence of fibrin monomer (portion of fibrin remaining after elements that polymerize and stabilize clot detach); positive test indication of predisposition to bleed and possible presence of DIC	Negative

DIC, Disseminated intravascular coagulation.
*Desired level for anticoagulation regimens.
†Also called fibrin degradation products (FDPs).

common during acute and chronic inflammatory reactions when cell destruction is increased. ESR is also increased in people with malignancy, myocardial infarction, and end-stage renal disease. Although the ESR is a nonspecific test, it is often used as a routine screening procedure.

Blood Typing and Rh Factor. Blood group antigens (A and B) are found only on RBC membranes and form the basis for the ABO blood typing system. The presence or absence of one or both of the two inherited antigens is the basis for the four blood groups: A, B, AB, and O. Blood group A has A antigens, group B has B antigens, group AB has both antigens, and group O has neither A nor B antigens. Each person has antibodies in the serum termed *anti-A* and *anti-B* that react with A or B antigens. These antibodies are found when the corresponding antigen is absent from the RBC surface. For example, B antibodies are found in the serum of persons with blood group A (Table 30-10).

Blood reactions based on ABO incompatibilities result from intravascular hemolysis of the RBCs.[15] RBCs *agglutinate* (or clump) when a serum antibody is present to react with the antigens on the RBC membrane. For example, agglutination would occur in the blood of a person with type A blood when blood is transfused from a person with B antigens (i.e., type B or AB) into the person with type A blood. The anti-B antibodies in the type A blood would react with the B antigens, thus initiating the process that results in RBC hemolysis.

The Rh system is based on a third antigen, D, which is also found on the RBC membrane. Rh-positive persons have the D antigen, whereas Rh-negative persons do not. As a result of transfusion therapy or during childbirth, an Rh-negative person may be exposed to Rh-positive blood. Such exposure results in formation of an antibody, anti-D, which acts against Rh antigens. (Rh-positive persons normally have no anti-D.) The person is then sensitized to Rh-positive blood, and a second exposure to Rh positive blood will cause a severe hemolytic reaction. A Coombs test can be used to evaluate the person's Rh status (Table 30-11).

Iron Metabolism. The laboratory tests used in evaluating iron metabolism include serum iron, total iron-binding capacity (TIBC), serum ferritin, and transferrin saturation. Additional tests for nutritional deficiencies leading to defective RBC production may also be done[16-18] (see Table 30-11).

Serum iron is a measurement of the amount of protein-bound iron circulating in the serum. TIBC provides a measurement of all proteins that act to bind or transport iron between the tissues and bone marrow. Although this indirect measurement is a general reflection of the amount of transferrin present in the circulation, it

TABLE 30-10 ABO Blood Groups and Compatibilities*

Recipient's Blood Group	RBC Antigen	Serum Antibody	Compatible Donors for RBC Transfusions
A	A	Anti-B	A and O
B	B	Anti-A	B and O
AB (universal recipient)	A and B	Neither anti-A nor anti-B	A, B, AB, and O
O	Neither	Anti-A and anti-B	O (universal donor)

RBC, Red blood cell.
*ABO blood groups are named for the antigen found on the RBCs. Compatibility is based on the antibodies present in the serum.

TABLE 30-11 Miscellaneous Laboratory Blood Studies

Study	Description and Purpose	Normal Values
Bilirubin	Measurement of degree of RBC hemolysis or liver's inability to excrete normal quantities of bilirubin; increase in indirect bilirubin with hemolytic problems	Total: 0.2-1.3 mg/dl (3.4-22 μmol/L) Direct: 0.1-0.3 mg/dl (1.7-5.1 μmol/L) Indirect: 0.1-1 mg/dl (1.7-17 μmol/L)
Coombs test	Differentiation among types of hemolytic anemias; detection of immune antibodies; detection of Rh factor	Negative
Direct	Detection of antibodies that are attached to RBCs	Negative
Indirect	Detection of antibodies in serum	Negative
Cobalamin (vitamin B_{12})	Level of vitamin B_{12} available for production of new RBCs	160 pg/ml (118-701 pmol/L)
Erythropoietin	Measurement of degree of hormonal stimulation to the bone marrow to stimulate the release of RBCs	5-36 IU/L
Erythrocyte sedimentation rate (ESR)	Measurement of sedimentation or settling of RBCs in 1 hr; inflammatory process causes an alteration in plasma proteins, resulting in aggregation of RBCs and making them heavier; the faster the sedimentation rate, the higher the ESR	Women: 1-20 mm in 1 hr Men: 1-15 mm in 1 hr 11-263 ng/ml (11-263 μl/L)
Ferritin	Major iron storage protein; is normally present in blood in concentrations directly related to iron storage	10-300 ng/ml (10-300 mcg/L)
Folic acid (folate)	Amount of folic acid/folate available for RBC production	3-25 ng/ml (7-57 nmol/L)
Hemoglobin (Hb) **electrophoresis**	Proteins involved in development of the hemoglobin molecule have a definitive pattern of separation on electrophoresis; this pattern is altered with abnormal hemoglobin synthesis such as occurs in thalassemia or in sickle cell anemia where Hb S is increased	Normal Hb A_1: 95%-98% Hb A_2: 2%-3% Hb F: 0.8%-2% Hb S: 0% Hb C: 0%
Homocysteine	Homocysteine is an amino acid formed from methionine; rapidly metabolized through pathways that require vitamin B_{12} and folic acid; increased in cobalamin (vitamin B_{12}) and folic acid deficiency	8-20 μmol/L
Iron		
Serum iron	Reflection of amount of iron combined with proteins in serum; accurate indication of status of iron storage and use	50-150 mcg/dl (9-26.9 μmol/L)
Total iron-binding capacity (TIBC)	Measurement of all proteins available for binding iron; transferrin represents the largest quantity of iron-binding proteins; therefore TIBC is an indirect measure of transferrin; evaluation of amount of extra iron that can be carried	250-410 mcg/dl (45-73 μmol/L)
Methylmalonic acid	Methylmalonic acid metabolism requires cobalamin; helps differentiate cobalamin deficiency from folic acid deficiency	80-560 μmol/L
Reticulocyte count	Measurement of immature RBCs; reflection of bone marrow activity in producing RBCs	0.5%-1.5% of RBC count (0.005-0.015 of RBC count)
Serum protein electrophoresis (SPEP)	Separates proteins in the blood on basis of electrical charge; helps detect hyperglobulinemic states, such as in multiple myeloma or some lymphomas	Normal banding pattern of albumin and globulins; an increase in any protein ("protein spike") is abnormal
Transferrin	The largest of proteins that bind to iron; increased in majority of people with iron deficiency anemia	215-380 mg/dl (2.15-3.8 g/L)
Transferrin saturation (%)	$\frac{\text{Serum iron level}}{\text{TIBC}} \times 100\%$ Decreased in iron deficiency anemia and increased in hemolytic and megaloblastic anemia	15%-50%

RBCs, Red blood cells.

overestimates transferrin levels by 16% to 20% because it also measures other proteins that can bind iron. These alternative proteins only bind iron when transferrin is more than half saturated. Also, TIBC varies inversely with tissue iron stores; it is higher when iron stores are low and lower when iron stores are high.

Transferrin saturation is a better indicator of the availability of iron for erythropoiesis than serum iron because, unlike serum iron, the iron bound to transferrin is readily available for the body to use. Transferrin saturation is calculated by dividing serum iron by TIBC and multiplying by 100. For example, a patient with a serum iron level of 100 mcg/dl and a TIBC of 300 mcg/dl would have a transferrin saturation of about 33%.

Under normal conditions, the serum ferritin concentration correlates closely with body iron stores. In normal patients, 1 ng/ml of ferritin corresponds to 8 to 10 mg of stored iron.

Radiologic Studies

Radiologic studies for the hematology system involve primarily the use of computed tomography (CT) or magnetic resonance imaging (MRI) for evaluating the spleen, liver, and lymph nodes. In the past, lymphangiography with the use of contrast media was a common procedure used to evaluate deep lymph nodes. However, its use has been replaced with the more sensitive CT and MRI tests. Spiral (helical) CT scans are used to evaluate lymph nodes.

Positron emission tomography (PET) scanning has become an invaluable diagnostic tool to detect active malignancy because of its ability to highlight areas with increased metabolism. This test has permitted more accurate diagnosis and monitoring of lymphoid malignant diseases. PET/CT scanning, either with fusion software (separate scans are taken and fused via computer) or a combined PET/CT scanner, may also be used.[19,20]

Nursing responsibilities related to these studies are presented in Table 30-12.

Biopsies

Biopsy procedures specific to hematologic assessment are bone marrow examination and lymph node biopsy. In general, these procedures are done because a peripheral blood smear is nonspecific and usually a diagnosis cannot be established from a peripheral blood smear. Furthermore, a biopsy provides additional information about a hematologic problem that is needed for diagnostic purposes, as well as planning treatment options.

Bone Marrow Examination. Bone marrow examination is important in the evaluation of many hematologic disorders. The examination of the marrow may involve aspiration only or aspiration with biopsy. The benefits gained from bone marrow examination are (1) a full evaluation of hematopoiesis and (2) the ability to obtain specimens for cytopathology and chromosomal abnormalities.[21]

The preferred site for both aspiration and biopsy of bone marrow is the posterior iliac crest.[10] The anterior iliac crest and sternum are alternative sites; however, the sternum is usually used only for aspiration. Bone marrow aspiration and biopsy are performed by a physician or specially credentialed nurse. Conscious sedation may be used to minimize anxiety and pain that the patient may experience. For bone marrow aspiration, the skin over the puncture site is cleansed with a bactericidal agent. The skin, subcutaneous tissue, and periosteum are infiltrated with a local anesthetic agent. The patient may be uncomfortable when the periosteum is penetrated. Once the area is anesthetized, a bone marrow needle is inserted through the cortex of the bone. The stylet of the needle is then removed, the hub is attached to a 10-ml syringe, and 0.2 to 0.5 ml of the fluid marrow is aspirated (Fig. 30-9). The patient experiences pain with aspiration. Although it lasts for only a few seconds, the pain may be quite uncomfortable. After the marrow aspiration, the needle is removed. Pressure is applied over the aspiration site to ensure hemostasis. If the patient is thrombocytopenic, pressure may be required for 5 to 10 minutes or longer.

If a bone biopsy is required, the preparatory procedure remains the same, but a different needle is used. The needle has a cutting blade that allows a specimen of the bone to be removed. When either a marrow aspirate or a biopsy specimen is acquired, a glass slide is carefully prepared with a thin film of the marrow.

Although complications of bone marrow aspiration are minimal, there is a possibility of damaging underlying structures. This hazard is greatest in aspiration procedures involving the sternum.[22] Other complications include hemorrhage (particularly if the patient is thrombocytopenic) and infection (particularly if the patient is leukopenic).[9] The needle aspiration or biopsy site is covered with a sterile pressure dressing. If bleeding is present, the nurse should advise the patient to lie on the side for 30 to 60 minutes to maintain pressure on the site. If the bed is too soft, have the patient lie on a rolled towel to provide additional pressure.

Lymph Node Biopsy. Lymph node biopsy involves obtaining lymph tissue for histologic examination to determine the diagnosis and to help for planning therapy. This may be accomplished by either an open biopsy or a closed (needle) biopsy. In the *open biopsy procedure,* an incision is made, and the lymph node and surrounding tissue are dissected (excised) whenever possible. Care must be taken because neoplastic cells can be disseminated during the biopsy procedure if the scalpel passes through tissues containing cancerous cells. An open biopsy is performed in the operating room or procedure area using either local or general anesthesia.

A *closed (needle) biopsy* or *fine needle aspiration* may also be performed to analyze lymph tissue. This procedure is performed by a physician at the bedside or in an outpatient area. Sterile technique is essential throughout the procedure. An extremely small needle is used to reduce the risk of tracking malignant cells through normal subcutaneous tissue. Nursing personnel must recognize the possibility of insidious bleeding, and direct pressure should be applied to the area after the biopsy procedure to achieve hemostasis. Frequent observations of the site for bleeding and monitoring of vital signs should be done, especially if the platelet count is low. The sterile dressing should be changed as ordered, and the wound should be inspected for healing and infection. It is important to recognize that if the results from a needle biopsy are negative, it may only indicate that the cancer cells were not part of the tissue in the biopsy specimen. However, a positive finding is sufficient evidence for confirming a diagnosis. This technique is rarely used to confirm an initial diagnosis because larger specimens are usually required in order to perform cytopathologic tests, but it may be used to validate disease recurrence or a new site of disease.

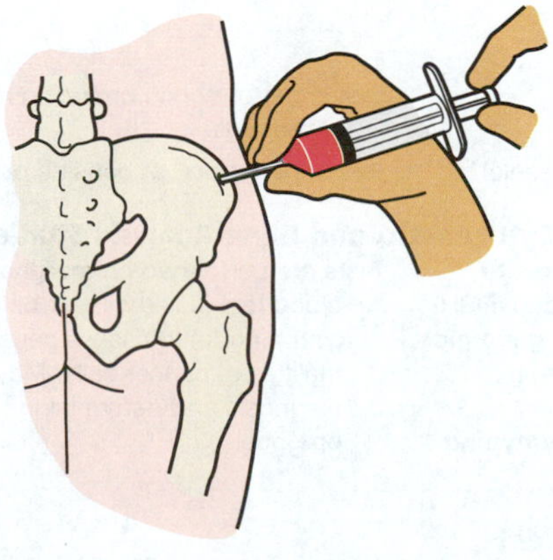

FIG. 30-9 Bone marrow aspiration from the posterior iliac crest.

TABLE 30-12 DIAGNOSTIC STUDIES
Hematologic System

Study	Description and Purpose	Nursing Responsibility
Urine Studies		
Bence Jones protein	An electrophoretic measurement is used to detect the presence of the Bence Jones protein, which is found in most cases of multiple myeloma. Negative finding is considered normal.	Acquire random urine specimen.
Radioisotope Studies		
Liver/spleen scan	Radioactive isotope is injected intravenously. Images from the radioactive emissions are used to evaluate the structure of the spleen and liver. Patient is not a source of radioactivity.	No specific nursing responsibilities.
Bone scan	Same procedure as for the spleen scan except used for evaluating the structure of the bones.	No specific nursing responsibilities.
Radiologic Studies		
Skeletal x-ray	X-rays done as a bone survey to determine the presence of lytic lesions associated with multiple myeloma. Bone scans do not identify lesions in this condition because there is no uptake of radioactive isotopes due to lack of blood supply.	No specific nursing responsibilities.
Liver, spleen, or abdominal ultrasound	Noninvasive probe is lubricated and slid across the abdomen to detect the density and borders of the abdominal organs. Irregular borders, masses, vascular structure, and biliary tree can be detected.	Patients must be comfortable lying flat and having the probe compress the abdomen.
Positron emission tomography (PET)	A nuclear tracer substance is injected and is taken up by metabolically active cells. The follow-up scan shows different-colored tissues based on the metabolic rate. "Hot spots" reflect increased glucose consumption that is typical of tumors.	Intravenous access is required for injection of the tracer substance. Patients should have nothing by mouth, except water and medications, for at least 4 hr before the test. IV solutions containing glucose may be held. Patients who are glucose intolerant or diabetic may need adjustments in their medications. Bowel preparation may also be needed, depending on the area being studied.
Computed tomography (CT)	Noninvasive radiologic examination using computer-assisted x-ray evaluates the lymph nodes. Contrast medium often is used in abdominal studies of the liver or spleen.	Investigate iodine sensitivity if contrast medium is used.
Magnetic resonance imaging (MRI)	Noninvasive procedure produces sensitive images of soft tissue without using contrast media. No ionizing radiation is required. Technique is used to evaluate spleen, liver, and lymph nodes.	Instruct patient to remove all metal objects and ask about any history of surgical insertion of staples, plates, or other metal appliances. Inform patient of need to lie still in small chamber.
Biopsies		
Bone marrow	Technique involves removal of bone marrow through a locally anesthetized site to evaluate the status of the blood-forming tissue. It is used to diagnose multiple myeloma, all types of leukemia, and some lymphomas and to stage some solid tumors (e.g., breast cancer). It is also done to assess efficacy of leukemia therapy.*	Explain procedure to patient. Obtain signed consent form. Consider preprocedure analgesic administration to enhance patient comfort and cooperation. Apply pressure dressing after procedure. Assess biopsy site for bleeding.
Lymph node biopsy	Purpose is to obtain lymph tissue for histologic examination to determine diagnosis and therapy.	Explain procedure to patient. Obtain signed consent form. Use sterile technique in dressing changes after procedure. Carefully evaluate wound for healing. Assess patient for complications, especially bleeding and edema.
• Open	Test is performed in operating room with direct visualization of the area.	
• Closed (needle)	Test is performed at bedside or in office.	
Molecular, Cytogenetic, and Gene Analysis Studies		
Fluorescent in situ hybridization (FISH) **Comparative genomic hybridization** (CGH) **Spectral karyotyping** (SKY)	Tests are performed on malignant cells, either peripheral blood (e.g., leukemia) or biopsy specimen (bone marrow, lymph node) to assess genetic or chromosomal abnormalities of cancer cells. May be useful in confirming diagnosis and determining treatment modalities and prognosis.	No specific nursing responsibilities. Explain purpose of testing to patient.
Blood Studies†		

*See Chapter 31.
†See Tables 30-8, 30-9, and 30-11.

Molecular Cytogenetics and Gene Analysis

Testing for specific genetic or chromosomal variations in hematologic conditions is often helpful in assisting in diagnosis and staging. These results also help determine the treatment options and prognosis. If a large number of abnormal cells are circulating in the blood, such as in acute leukemia, these tests may be done by obtaining peripheral blood. However, testing is usually done on samples from bone marrow and lymph node biopsies. For example, fluorescent in situ hybridization (FISH) can identify specific areas by attaching a probe to a targeted region of DNA. It may be used to illuminate an abnormal extra chromosome 8 that is common in certain leukemias. Spectral karyotyping (SKY) allows for each set of chromosomes to be painted different colors. It can be used to identify the chromosomal translocation of 22 to 9 in the Philadelphia chromosome of chronic myelogenous leukemia.[23] More information on genetics is in Chapter 14.

NCLEX EXAMINATION REVIEW QUESTIONS

The number of the question corresponds to the same-numbered objective at the beginning of the chapter.

1. An individual who lives at a high altitude may normally have an increased RBC count because
   a. high altitudes cause vascular fluid loss, leading to hemoconcentration.
   b. hypoxia caused by decreased atmospheric oxygen stimulates erythropoiesis.
   c. the function of the spleen in removing old RBCs is impaired at high altitudes.
   d. impaired production of leukocytes and platelets leads to proportionally higher red cell counts.
2. Malignant disorders that arise from granulocytic cells in the bone marrow will have the primary effect of causing
   a. risk for hemorrhage.
   b. altered oxygenation.
   c. decreased production of antibodies.
   d. decreased phagocytosis of bacteria.
3. An anticoagulant such as warfarin (Coumadin) that interferes with the production of prothrombin will alter the clotting mechanism during
   a. platelet aggregation.
   b. activation of thrombin.
   c. the release of tissue thromboplastin.
   d. stimulation of factor activation complex.
4. When reviewing laboratory results of an 83-year-old patient with an infection, the nurse would expect to find
   a. minimal leukocytosis.
   b. decreased platelet count.
   c. increased hemoglobin and hematocrit levels.
   d. decreased erythrocyte sedimentation rate (ESR).
5. Significant information obtained from the patient's health history that relates to the hematologic system includes
   a. jaundice.
   b. bladder surgery.
   c. early menopause.
   d. multiple pregnancies.
6. While assessing the lymph nodes, the nurse
   a. applies gentle, firm pressure to deep lymph nodes.
   b. palpates the deep cervical and supraclavicular nodes last.
   c. lightly palpates superficial lymph nodes with the pads of the fingers.
   d. uses the tips of the second, third, and fourth fingers to apply deep palpation.
7. If a lymph node is palpated, which of the following is a normal finding?
   a. Hard, fixed nodes.
   b. Firm, mobile nodes.
   c. Enlarged, tender nodes.
   d. Hard, nontender nodes.
8. Immediately following a bone marrow biopsy and aspiration, the nurse should instruct the patient to
   a. expect to receive a blood transfusion.
   b. lie still with a sterile pressure dressing intact.
   c. lie with knees slightly bent and head elevated.
   d. cleanse the site immediately with povidone-iodine.

REFERENCES

1. Thibodeau GA, Patton KT: *The human body in health and disease,* ed 4, St Louis, 2005, Mosby.
2. McCance KL, Huether SE, editors: *Pathophysiology: the biologic basis for disease in adults and children,* ed 4, St Louis, 2006, Mosby.
3. Marks PW, Glader B: Approach to anemia in the adult and child. In Hoffman R, et al, editors: *Hematology: basic principles and practice,* ed 4, Philadelphia, 2005, Elsevier.
4. Chu AJ: Tissue factor mediates inflammation, *Arch Biochem Biophys* 440(2):123, 2005.
5. Dahlback B: Blood coagulation and its regulation by anticoagulant pathways: genetic pathogenesis of bleeding and thrombotic diseases, *J Intern Med* 257(3):209, 2005.
6. Powell LD, Baum LG: Overview and compartmentalization of the immune system. In Hoffman R, et al, editors: *Hematology: basic principles and practice,* ed 4, Philadelphia, 2005, Elsevier.
7. Andrews NC: Pathology of iron metabolism. In Hoffman R, Benz R, Shattil S, et al, editors: *Hematology: basic principles and practice,* ed 4, Philadelphia, 2005, Elsevier.
8. Means RT: Hepcidin and anaemia, *Blood Rev* 18:219, 2005.
9. Lichtman MA, Williams WJ: Hematology in the aged. In Beutler E, editor: *Williams hematology,* ed 7, New York, 2006, McGraw-Hill.
10. Kane RL, Ouslander JG, Abrass IB: *Essentials of clinical geriatrics,* New York, 2004, McGraw-Hill.
11. Rothstein G: Hematologic problems. In Cassel CK, editor: *Geriatric medicine: an evidence based approach,* ed 4, New York, 2003, Springer-Verlag.
12. Grodner M, Anderson SL, DeYoung S: *Foundations and clinical applications of nutrition: a nursing approach,* ed 3, St Louis, 2004, Mosby.
13. Wilson SF, Giddens JF: *Health assessment for nursing practice,* ed 3, St Louis, 2005, Mosby.
14. Beutler E, et al: Approach to the patient. In Beutler E, editor: *Williams hematology,* ed 7, New York, 2006, McGraw-Hill.
15. Pagana KD, Pagana TJ: *Mosby's diagnostic and laboratory test reference,* ed 7, 2005, Mosby.
16. Linker CA: Blood. In Tierney LM, McPhee SJ, Papadakis MA, editors: *Current medical diagnosis and treatment,* ed 44, New York, 2005, McGraw-Hill.
17. Antony AA: Megaloblastic anemias. In Hoffman R, Benz R, Shattil S, et al, editors: *Hematology: basic principles and practice,* ed 4, Philadelphia, 2005, Elsevier.
18. Schnell ZB, Van Leeuwen AM, Kranpitz TR: *Davis's comprehensive handbook of laboratory and diagnostic tests with nursing implications,* Philadelphia, 2003, FA Davis.
19. Yap JT, Carney JP, Hall NC, et al: Image-guided cancer therapy using PET/CT, *Cancer J* 10:221, 2004.
20. Lobrano MB, Singha P: Positron emission tomography in oncology, *Clin J Oncol Nurs* 7:379, 2003.
21. Trewhitt KG: Bone marrow aspiration and biopsy: collection and interpretation, *Oncol Nurs Forum* 28:1409, 2001.
22. Ryan DH: Examination of the marrow. In Beutler E, editor: *Williams hematology,* ed 7, New York, 2006, McGraw-Hill.
23. Stoltzfus PK, Rust D, Ried T: Molecular cytogenetics and gene analysis: implications for oncology nurses, *Clin J Oncol Nurs* 5:201, 2001.

RESOURCES

Resources for this chapter are listed in Chapter 31 on p. 737.

It is one of the beautiful compensations of this life that no one can sincerely try to help another without helping himself.

Charles Dudley Warner

31 Nursing Management Hematologic Problems

Sandra Irene Rome

LEARNING OBJECTIVES

1. Describe the general clinical manifestations and complications of anemia.
2. Describe the etiologies, clinical manifestations, diagnostic findings, and nursing and collaborative management of iron deficiency, megaloblastic, and aplastic anemias and anemia of chronic disease.
3. Explain the nursing management of anemia secondary to blood loss.
4. Describe the pathophysiology, clinical manifestations, and nursing and collaborative management of anemia caused by increased erythrocyte destruction, including sickle cell disease and acquired hemolytic anemias.
5. Describe the pathophysiology and nursing and collaborative management of polycythemia.
6. Explain the pathophysiology, clinical manifestations, and nursing and collaborative management of various types of thrombocytopenia.
7. Describe the types, clinical manifestations, diagnostic findings, and nursing and collaborative management of hemophilia and von Willebrand disease.
8. Explain the pathophysiology, diagnostic findings, and nursing and collaborative management of disseminated intravascular coagulation.
9. Describe the etiology, clinical manifestations, and nursing and collaborative management of neutropenia.
10. Describe the pathophysiology, clinical manifestations, and nursing and collaborative management of myelodysplastic syndrome.
11. Compare and contrast the major types of leukemia regarding distinguishing clinical and laboratory findings.
12. Explain the nursing and collaborative management of acute and chronic leukemias.
13. Compare Hodgkin's lymphoma and non-Hodgkin's lymphomas in terms of clinical manifestations, staging, and nursing and collaborative management.
14. Describe the pathophysiology, clinical manifestations, and nursing and collaborative management of multiple myeloma.
15. Describe the spleen disorders and related collaborative care.
16. Describe the nursing management of the patient receiving transfusions of blood and blood components.

KEY TERMS

anemia, p. 685
aplastic anemia, p. 693
disseminated intravascular coagulation, p. 710
hemochromatosis, p. 699
hemolytic anemia, p. 695
hemophilia, p. 707
Hodgkin's lymphoma, p. 723
iron-deficiency anemia, p. 687
leukemia, p. 717
lymphomas, p. 723
megaloblastic anemias, p. 691
multiple myeloma, p. 728
myelodysplastic syndrome, p. 716
neutropenia, p. 713
non-Hodgkin's lymphomas, p. 724
pernicious anemia, p. 692
polycythemia, p. 700
sickle cell disease, p. 696
thalassemia, p. 691
thrombocytopenia, p. 701

Electronic Resources

Supplemental content related to Chapter 31 can be found . . .

Companion CD
- Stress-Busting Kit for Nursing Students
- Interactive Case Studies:
  - Chronic Myelogenous Leukemia
  - Sickle Cell Anemia
- NCLEX Examination Review Questions
- Comprehensive Glossary

Evolve Website
http://evolve.elsevier.com/Lewis/medsurg
- Content Updates
- Key Points (Printable and CD/MP3 Download)
- Concept Map Creator
- Expanded Audio Glossary
- Key Term Flash Cards
- Customizable Nursing Care Plans:
  - Anemia
  - Neutropenia
  - Thrombocytopenia
- Electronic Calculators
- WebLinks

Reviewed by Joyce A. Marrs, APRN-BC, MS, AOCNP, Nurse Practitioner, Hematology and Oncology of Dayton, Dayton, Ohio; and Dana Reeves, RN, MSN, Assistant Professor, University of Arkansas–Fort Smith, Forth Smith, Ark.

Anemia

Definition and Classification

Anemia is a deficiency in the number of erythrocytes (red blood cells [RBCs]), the quantity of hemoglobin, and/or the volume of packed RBCs (hematocrit). It is a prevalent condition with many diverse causes such as blood loss, impaired production of erythrocytes, or increased destruction of erythrocytes (Fig. 31-1). Because RBCs transport oxygen (O_2), erythrocyte disorders can lead to tissue hypoxia. This hypoxia accounts for many of the signs and symptoms of anemia. Anemia is not a specific disease; it is a manifestation of a pathologic process. Anemia is identified by a thorough history and physical examination, and then classified by laboratory review of the complete blood count (CBC), reticulocyte count, and peripheral blood smear. Once anemia is identified, further investigation is done to determine its cause.[1,2]

Anemia can result from primary hematologic problems or can develop as a secondary consequence of defects in other body systems. The various types of anemia can be grouped according to either a *morphologic* (cellular characteristic) or an *etiologic* (underlying cause) classification. Morphologic classification is based on descriptive, objective laboratory information about erythrocyte size and color. (The terms used in this classification system are explained in Chapter 30.) Etiologic classification is related to the clinical conditions causing the anemia, such as decreased erythrocyte production, blood loss, or increased erythrocyte destruction (Table 31-1). Although the morphologic system is the most accurate means of classifying anemias, it is easier to discuss patient care by focusing on the etiology of the anemia. Table 31-2 relates morphologic classifications to various etiologies.

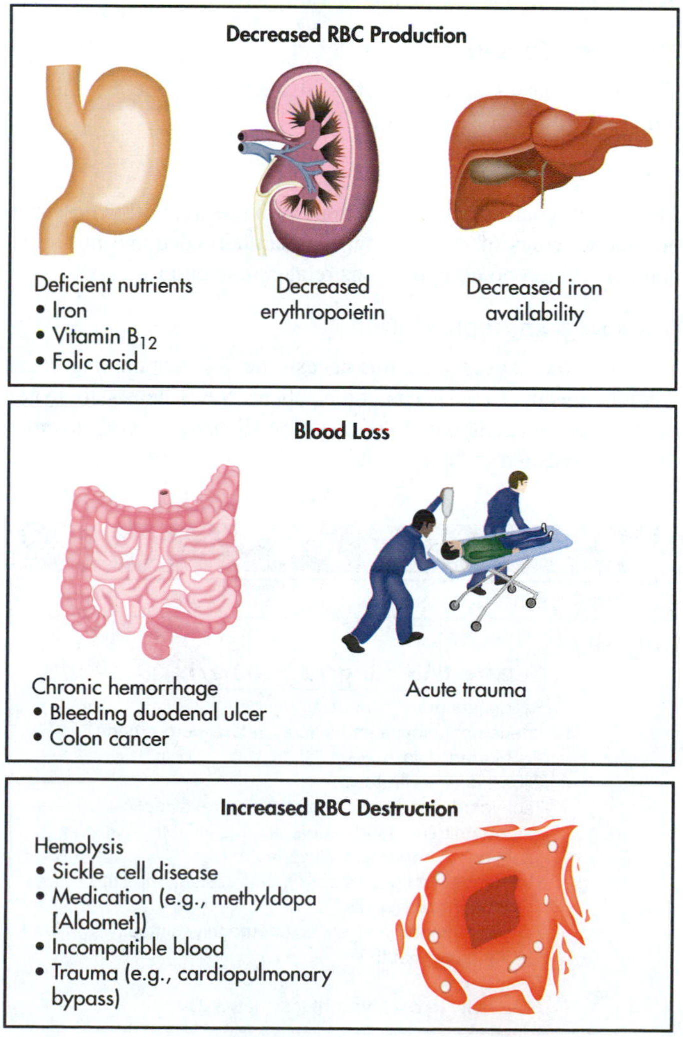

FIG. 31-1 Causes of anemia.

CULTURAL AND ETHNIC HEALTH DISPARITIES

Hematologic Problems

- Sickle cell disease has a high incidence among African Americans.
- Thalassemia has a high incidence among African Americans and people of Mediterranean origin.
- Tay-Sachs disease has the highest incidence in families of Eastern European Jewish origin, especially the Ashkenazi Jews.
- Pernicious anemia has a high incidence among Scandinavians and African Americans.

TABLE 31-1 Etiologic Classification of Anemia

Decreased Erythrocyte Production
Decreased Hemoglobin Synthesis
Iron deficiency
Thalassemias (decreased globin synthesis)
Sideroblastic anemia (decreased porphyrin)
Defective DNA Synthesis
Cobalamin (vitamin B_{12}) deficiency
Folic acid deficiency
Decreased Number of Erythrocyte Precursors
Aplastic anemia
Anemia of myeloproliferative diseases (e.g., leukemia) and myelodysplasia
Chronic diseases or disorders
Chemotherapy
Blood Loss
Acute
Trauma
Blood vessel rupture
Chronic
Gastritis
Menstrual flow
Hemorrhoids
Increased Erythrocyte Destruction*
Intrinsic
Abnormal hemoglobin (Hb S–sickle cell anemia)
Enzyme deficiency (G6PD)
Membrane abnormalities (paroxysmal nocturnal hemoglobinuria, hereditary spherocytosis)
Extrinsic
Physical trauma (prosthetic heart valves, extracorporeal circulation)
Antibodies (isoimmune and autoimmune)
Infectious agents, medications, and toxins (malaria)

DNA, Deoxyribonucleic acid; *G6PD*, glucose-6-phosphate dehydrogenase; *Hb S*, hemoglobin S.
*Hemolytic anemias.

Clinical Manifestations

The clinical manifestations of anemia are caused by the body's response to tissue hypoxia. Specific manifestations can vary depending on the rate at which it has evolved, the severity of the anemia, and the presence of coexisting disease. Hemoglobin (Hb) levels are often used to determine the severity of anemia. Mild states of anemia (Hb 10 to 14 g/dl [100 to 140 g/L]) may exist without causing symptoms. If symptoms develop, it is because the patient has an underlying disease or is experiencing a compensatory response to heavy exercise. Symptoms include palpitations, dyspnea, and diaphoresis. In cases of moderate anemia (Hb 6 to 10 g/dl [60 to 100 g/L]), the cardiopulmonary symptoms are increased and the patient may experience them while resting, as well as with activity. The patient with severe anemia (Hb less than 6 g/dl [60 g/L]) has many clinical manifestations involving multiple body systems (Table 31-3).

Integumentary Changes. Integumentary changes include pallor, jaundice, and pruritus. Pallor results from reduced amounts of hemoglobin and reduced blood flow to the skin. Jaundice occurs when hemolysis of RBCs results in an increased concentration of serum bilirubin. Pruritus occurs because of increased serum and skin bile salt concentrations. In addition to the skin, the sclera of the eyes and mucous membranes should be evaluated for jaundice because they reflect the integumentary changes more accurately, especially in a dark-skinned individual.

Cardiopulmonary Manifestations. Cardiopulmonary manifestations of severe anemia result from additional attempts by the heart and lungs to provide adequate amounts of oxygen to the tissues. Cardiac output is maintained by increasing the heart rate and stroke volume. The low viscosity of the blood contributes to the development of systolic murmurs and bruits. In extreme cases or when concomitant heart disease is present, angina pectoris and myocardial infarction (MI) may occur if myocardial O_2 needs cannot be met. Heart failure (HF), cardiomegaly, pulmonary and systemic congestion, ascites, and peripheral edema may develop if the heart is overworked for an extended period of time.

TABLE 31-2 Relationship of Morphologic Classification and Etiologies of Anemia

Morphology	Etiology
Normocytic, normochromic (normal size and color)	Acute blood loss, hemolysis, chronic kidney disease, chronic disease, cancers, sideroblastic anemia, refractory anemia, diseases of endocrine dysfunction, aplastic anemia, sickle cell anemia, pregnancy
Macrocytic, normochromic (large size, normal color)	Cobalamin (vitamin B_{12}) deficiency, folic acid deficiency, liver disease (including effects of alcohol abuse), postsplenectomy
Microcytic, hypochromic (small size, pale color)	Iron-deficiency anemia, thalassemia, lead poisoning

NURSING MANAGEMENT
ANEMIA

This section discusses general nursing management of anemia. Specific care related to various types of anemia is discussed later in this chapter.

■ *Nursing Assessment*

Subjective and objective data that should be obtained from a patient with anemia are presented in Table 31-4.

■ *Nursing Diagnoses*

Nursing diagnoses for the patient with anemia include, but are not limited to, those presented in NCP 31-1.

■ *Planning*

The overall goals are that the patient with anemia will (1) assume normal activities of daily living, (2) maintain adequate nutrition, and (3) develop no complications related to anemia.

■ *Nursing Implementation*

The numerous causes of anemia necessitate different nursing interventions specific to the needs of the patient. Nevertheless, there are certain general components of care for all patients with anemia that are presented in NCP 31-1.

TABLE 31-3 Clinical Manifestations of Anemia

	Severity of Anemia		
Body System	**Mild (Hb 10-14 g/dl [100-140 g/L])**	**Moderate (Hb 6-10 g/dl [60-100 g/L])**	**Severe (Hb <6 g/dl [<60 g/L])**
Integument	None	None	Pallor, jaundice,* pruritus*
Eyes	None	None	Icteric conjunctiva and sclera,* retinal hemorrhage, blurred vision
Mouth	None	None	Glossitis, smooth tongue
Cardiovascular	Palpitations	Increased palpitations, "bounding pulse"	Tachycardia, increased pulse pressure, systolic murmurs, intermittent claudication, angina, HF, MI
Pulmonary	Exertional dyspnea	Dyspnea	Tachypnea, orthopnea, dyspnea at rest
Neurologic	None	"Roaring in the ears"	Headache, vertigo, irritability, depression, impaired thought processes
Gastrointestinal	None	None	Anorexia, hepatomegaly, splenomegaly, difficulty swallowing, sore mouth
Musculoskeletal	None	None	Bone pain
General	None	Fatigue	Sensitivity to cold, weight loss, lethargy

Hb, Hemoglobin; *HF,* heart failure; *MI,* myocardial infarction.
*Caused by hemolysis.

TABLE 31-4 NURSING ASSESSMENT
Anemia

Subjective Data	Objective Data
Important Health Information *Past health history:* Recent blood loss or trauma; chronic liver, endocrine, or renal disease (including dialysis); GI disease (malabsorption syndrome, ulcers, gastritis, or hemorrhoids); inflammatory disorders (especially Crohn's disease); smoking, exposure to radiation or chemical toxins (arsenic, lead, benzenes, copper); infectious diseases (HIV) or recent travel suggesting exposure to infection; angina, myocardial infarction; history of falling *Medications:* Use of vitamin and iron supplements; aspirin, anticoagulants, oral contraceptives, phenobarbital, penicillins, nonsteroidal antiinflammatory drugs, phenacetin, quinine, quinidine, phenytoin (Dilantin), methyldopa (Aldomet), sulfonamides, herbal products *Surgery or other treatments:* Recent surgery, small bowel resection, gastrectomy, prosthetic heart valves, chemotherapy, radiation therapy *Dietary history:* General dietary patterns, consumption of alcohol, pica **Functional Health Patterns** *Health perception–health management:* Family history of anemia; malaise *Nutritional-metabolic:* Nausea, vomiting, anorexia, weight loss; dysphagia, dyspepsia, heartburn, night sweats, cold intolerance *Elimination:* Hematuria, decreased urinary output; diarrhea, constipation, flatulence, tarry stools, bloody stools *Activity-exercise:* Fatigue, muscle weakness and decreased strength; dyspnea, orthopnea, cough, hemoptysis; palpitations; shortness of breath with activity *Cognitive-perceptual:* Headache; abdominal, chest, and bone pain; painful tongue; paresthesias of feet and hands; pruritus; disturbances in vision, taste, or hearing; vertigo; hypersensitivity to cold; dizziness *Sexuality-reproductive:* Menorrhagia, metrorrhagia; recent or current pregnancy; male impotence	**General** Lethargy, apathy, general lymphadenopathy, fever **Integumentary** Pale skin and mucous membranes; blue, pale white, or icteric sclera; cheilitis; poor skin turgor; brittle, spoon-shaped fingernails; jaundice; petechiae; ecchymoses; nose or gingival bleeding; poor healing; dry, brittle, thinning hair **Respiratory** Tachypnea **Cardiovascular** Tachycardia, systolic murmur, dysrhythmias; postural hypotension, widened pulse pressure, bruits (especially carotid); intermittent claudication, ankle edema **Gastrointestinal** Hepatosplenomegaly; glossitis; beefy, red tongue; stomatitis; abdominal distention; anorexic **Neurologic** Headache, roaring in the ears, confusion, impaired judgment, irritability, ataxia, unsteady gait, paralysis, loss of vibration sense **Possible Findings** ↓ RBCs, ↓ Hb; ↓ Hct; ↑ or ↓ reticulocytes, MCV, serum iron, ferritin, folate, or cobalamin (vitamin B_{12}); heme (guaiac)–positive stools; ↓ serum erythropoietin level; ↑ or ↓ LDH, bilirubin, transferrin (see Table 31-6).

GI, Gastrointestinal; *Hb*, hemoglobin; *Hct*, hematocrit; *LDH*, lactic dehydrogenase; *MCV*, mean corpuscular volume; *RBCs*, red blood cells.

Correcting the cause of the anemia is ultimately the goal of therapy. Acute interventions may include blood or blood product transfusions, drug therapy (e.g., erythropoietin, vitamin supplements), volume replacement, and oxygen therapy to stabilize the patient. Dietary and lifestyle changes (described with specific types of anemia) can reverse some anemias so that the patient can return to the former state of health. Ongoing assessment of the patient's knowledge regarding adequate nutritional intake and compliance with safety precautions to prevent falls and injury and drug therapies should be included in the plan of care.

GERONTOLOGIC CONSIDERATIONS
ANEMIA

Modest changes in red blood cell mass occur in older adults. In healthy older men, there is a modest decline in hemoglobin with age of about 1 g/dl between ages 70 and 88 years, in part because of the decreased production of androgens. Only a minimal decrease in hemoglobin occurs between these ages in healthy women (about 0.2 g/dl).[1] Cobalamin (vitamin B_{12}) deficiency may occur in more than 20% of elderly people because of pernicious anemia, insufficient dietary intake, and malabsorption.[3] Multiple comorbid conditions in older adults increase the likelihood of occurrence of many types of anemia. Signs and symptoms of anemia in the older adult may include pallor, confusion, ataxia, fatigue, worsening angina, and HF. Unfortunately, anemia may go unrecognized in the older adult because manifestations of anemia may be mistaken as normal aging changes or overlooked because of another health problem. By recognizing signs of anemia, the nurse can play a pivotal role in appropriate health assessment and related interventions for the older adult.

Anemia Caused By Decreased Erythrocyte Production

Normally RBC production (termed *erythropoiesis*) is in equilibrium with RBC destruction and loss. This balance ensures that an adequate number of erythrocytes are available at all times. The normal life span of an RBC is 120 days. Three alterations in erythropoiesis may occur that decrease RBC production: (1) decreased hemoglobin synthesis may lead to iron-deficiency anemia, thalassemia, and sideroblastic anemia; (2) defective DNA synthesis in RBCs (e.g., cobalamin [vitamin B_{12}] deficiency, folic acid deficiency) may lead to megaloblastic anemias; and (3) diminished availability of erythrocyte precursors may result in aplastic anemia and anemia of chronic disease (see Table 31-1).

IRON-DEFICIENCY ANEMIA

Iron-deficiency anemia, one of the most common chronic hematologic disorders, is found in up to 30% of the world's population. In the United States, it occurs in about 5% to 10% of people over 45. In addition, those most susceptible to iron-deficiency anemia are the very young, those on poor diets, and women in their reproductive years.[4]

NURSING CARE PLAN 31-1

Patient with Anemia

NURSING DIAGNOSIS **Activity intolerance** *related to* weakness and imbalance between oxygen supply/demand *as evidenced by* increased pulse and blood pressure in response to activity and patient report of weakness

PATIENT GOALS
1. Participates in normal activities of daily living without abnormal increases in blood pressure and pulse
2. Reports less weakness and fatigue

OUTCOMES (NOC)

Activity Tolerance

- Pulse rate with activity ____
- Respiratory rate with activity ____
- Oxygen saturation with activity ____
- Ease of performing ADLs ____

Measurement Scale

1 = Severely compromised
2 = Substantially compromised
3 = Moderately compromised
4 = Mildly compromised
5 = Not compromised

INTERVENTIONS (NIC) and *RATIONALES*

Energy Management

- Encourage alternate rest and activity periods *to provide activity without tiring the patient.*
- Limit number of visitors and interruptions by visitors.
- Limit environmental stimuli *to reduce demands placed on the patient.*
- Plan activities for periods when patient has the most energy.
- Assist with regular physical activities (e.g., ambulation, transfers, personal care).
- Monitor cardiorespiratory response to activity (e.g., tachycardia, dyspnea, diaphoresis) *to evaluate activity intolerance.*
- Determine patient's physical limitations.
- Determine what and how much activity is required to build endurance.

NURSING DIAGNOSIS **Altered nutrition: less than body requirements** *related to* inadequate nutritional intake and anorexia *as evidenced by* weight loss, low serum albumin, decreased iron levels, vitamin deficiencies

PATIENT GOALS
1. Maintains dietary intake that provides minimum daily requirements of nutrients
2. Experiences normal blood values of nutrients necessary to prevent anemia

OUTCOMES (NOC)

Nutritional Status

- Nutrient intake ____
- Weight/height ratio ____

Nutritional Status: Biochemical Measures

- Serum albumin ____
- Hemoglobin ____
- Hematocrit ____
- Total iron-binding capacity ____

Measurement Scale

1 = Severe deviation from normal range
2 = Substantial deviation from normal range
3 = Moderate deviation from normal range
4 = Mild deviation from normal range
5 = No deviation from normal range

INTERVENTIONS (NIC) and *RATIONALES*

Nutrition Management

- Determine, in collaboration with dietitian, number of calories and type of nutrients needed to meet nutritional requirements *to plan interventions.*
- Teach patient how to keep a food diary *to help evaluate nutritional intake.*
- Monitor recorded intake for nutritional content and calories *to evaluate nutritional status.*
- Encourage increased intake of protein, iron, and vitamin C *to provide nutrients needed for hemoglobin production.*
- Provide appropriate information about nutritional needs and how to meet them *to increase intake of essential nutrients needed.*

Normally, 1 mg of iron is lost daily through feces, sweat, and urine in the adult male and 1.5 mg/day in normal menstruating women. The median total iron loss with pregnancy is about 500 mg, or almost 2 mg/day over the 280 days of gestation.[5]

Etiology

Iron-deficiency anemia may develop from inadequate dietary intake, malabsorption, blood loss, or hemolysis. (Normal iron metabolism is discussed in Chapter 30 on p. 668.) Dietary iron is adequate to meet the needs of men and older women, but it may be inadequate for those individuals who have higher iron needs (e.g., menstruating or pregnant women). Table 31-5 lists nutrients needed for erythropoiesis.[6]

Malabsorption of iron may occur after certain types of gastrointestinal (GI) surgery and in malabsorption syndromes. Surgical procedures may involve removal or bypass of the duodenum (see Chapter 42). As iron absorption occurs in the duodenum, malabsorption syndromes may involve disease of the duodenum in which the absorption surface is altered or destroyed.

Blood loss is a major cause of iron deficiency in adults. Two milliliters of whole blood contain 1 mg of iron. The major sources of chronic blood loss are from the GI and genitourinary (GU) systems. GI bleeding is often not apparent and therefore may exist for a considerable time before the problem is identified. Loss of 50 to 75 ml of blood from the upper GI tract is required for stools to appear black *(melena).* The black color results from the iron in the RBCs. Common causes of GI blood loss are peptic ulcer, gastritis, esophagitis, diverticuli, hemorrhoids, and neoplasia. GU blood loss occurs primarily from menstrual bleeding. The average monthly menstrual blood loss

NURSING CARE PLAN 31-1

Patient with Anemia—cont'd

NURSING DIAGNOSIS **Ineffective management of therapeutic regimen** *related to* lack of knowledge about appropriate nutrition and medication regimen *as evidenced by* questioning about lifestyle adjustments, diet, medications

PATIENT GOAL Verbalizes knowledge necessary to maintain adequate nutrition and management of medication regimen

OUTCOMES (NOC)

Knowledge: Diet

- Description of diet ____
- Description of foods allowed in diet ____
- Description of rationale for diet ____
- Description of how to select foods ____

Knowledge: Medication

- Identification of correct name of medication(s) ____
- Description of correct administration of medication(s) ____
- Description of actions of medication(s) ____
- Description of side effects of medication(s) ____

Measurement Scale

1 = None
2 = Limited
3 = Moderate
4 = Substantial
5 = Extensive

INTERVENTIONS (NIC) and *RATIONALES*

Nutritional Counseling

- Facilitate identification of eating behaviors to be changed.
- Discuss patient's knowledge of the four basic food groups, as well as perceptions of the needed diet modification.
- Discuss food buying habits and budget constraints.
- Use accepted nutritional standards to assist patient in evaluating adequacy of dietary intake *to evaluate adequacy.*
- Discuss nutritional requirements and patient's perceptions of prescribed/recommended diet.
- Provide referral/consultation with other members of the health care team *to help patient maintain gains and adjustments throughout recovery.*
- Review with patient measurements of fluid intake and output, hemoglobin values, blood pressure readings, or weight gains and losses.

Teaching: Prescribed Medication

- Instruct the patient on the purpose and action of each medication.
- Instruct the patient on dosage, route, and duration of each medication *to improve compliance.*
- Instruct the patient on possible adverse effects of each medication.

TABLE 31-5 *NUTRITIONAL THERAPY* **Nutrients Needed for Erythropoiesis**

Nutrient	Role in Erythropoiesis	Food Sources
Cobalamin (vitamin B_{12})	RBC maturation	Red meats, especially liver
Folic acid	RBC maturation	Green leafy vegetables, liver, meat, fish, legumes, whole grains
Iron	Hemoglobin synthesis	Liver and muscle meats, eggs, dried fruits, legumes, dark green leafy vegetables, whole-grain and enriched bread and cereals, potatoes
Vitamin B_6	Hemoglobin synthesis	Meats (especially pork and liver), wheat germ, legumes, potatoes, cornmeal, bananas
Amino acids	Synthesis of nucleoproteins	Eggs, meat, milk and milk products (cheese, ice cream), poultry, fish, legumes, nuts
Vitamin C	Conversion of folic acid to its active forms, aids in iron absorption	Citrus fruits, leafy green vegetables, strawberries, cantaloupe

RBC, Red blood cell.

is about 45 ml and causes the loss of about 22 mg of iron. Postmenopausal bleeding can contribute to anemia in a susceptible older woman.

Pregnancy contributes to iron deficiency because of the diversion of iron to the fetus for erythropoiesis, blood loss at delivery, and lactation. In addition to anemia of chronic renal failure, dialysis treatment may induce iron-deficiency anemia because of the blood lost in the dialysis equipment and frequent blood sampling.

Clinical Manifestations

In the early course of iron-deficiency anemia, the patient may be free of symptoms. As the disease becomes chronic, any of the general manifestations of anemia may develop (see Table 31-3). In addition, specific clinical symptoms may occur related to iron deficiency anemia. Pallor is the most common finding, and *glossitis* (inflammation of the tongue) is the second most common; another finding is *cheilitis* (inflammation of the lips). In addition, the patient may report headache, paresthesias, and a burning sensation of the tongue, all of which are caused by lack of iron in the tissues.

Diagnostic Studies

Laboratory abnormalities characteristic of iron-deficiency anemia are presented in Table 31-6. Other diagnostic studies are done to determine the cause of the iron deficiency (e.g., stool guaiac test). Endoscopy and colonoscopy may be used to detect GI bleeding. A bone marrow biopsy may be done if other tests are inconclusive.

TABLE 31-6 Laboratory Study Findings in Anemias

	Hb/Hct	MCV	Reticulocytes	Serum Iron	TIBC	Transferrin	Ferritin	Bilirubin
Iron deficiency	↓	↓	N or slight ↓ or ↑	↓	↑	N or ↓	↓	N or ↓
Thalassemia major	↓	N or ↓	↑	↑	↓	↓	N or ↑	↑
Cobalamin deficiency	↓	↑	N or ↓	N or ↑	N	Slight ↑	↑	N or slight ↑
Folic acid deficiency	↓	↑	N or ↓	N or ↑	N	Slight ↑	↑	N or slight ↑
Aplastic anemia	↓	N or slight ↑	↓	N or ↑	N or ↑	N	N	N
Chronic disease	↓	N or ↓	N or ↓	N or ↓	↓	N or ↓	N or ↑	N
Acute blood loss	↓	N or ↓	N or ↑	N	N	N	N	N
Chronic blood loss	↓	↓	N or ↑	↓	↓	N	N	N or ↓
Sickle cell anemia	↓	N	↑	N or ↑	N or ↓	N	N	↑
Hemolytic anemia	↓	N or ↑	↑	N or ↑	N or ↓	N	N or ↑	↑

Hb, Hemoglobin; *Hct,* hematocrit; *MCV,* mean corpuscular volume; *N,* normal; *TIBC,* total iron-binding capacity.

Collaborative Care

The main goal of collaborative care of iron-deficiency anemia is to treat the underlying disease that is causing reduced intake (e.g., malnutrition, alcoholism) or absorption of iron. In addition, efforts are directed toward replacing iron (Table 31-7). The patient should be taught which foods are good sources of iron (see Table 31-5). If nutrition is already adequate, increasing iron intake by dietary means may not be practical. Consequently, oral or occasionally parenteral iron supplements are used. If the iron deficiency is from acute blood loss, the patient may require a transfusion of packed RBCs.

Drug Therapy. Oral iron should be used whenever possible because it is inexpensive and convenient. Many iron preparations are available. The following five factors should be considered in the administration of iron:

1. Iron is absorbed best from the duodenum and proximal jejunum. Therefore enteric-coated or sustained-release capsules, which release iron farther down in the GI tract, are counterproductive and expensive.
2. The daily dosage should provide 150 to 200 mg of elemental iron. This can be ingested in three or four daily doses, with each tablet or capsule of the iron preparation containing between 50 and 100 mg of iron (e.g., a 300-mg tablet of ferrous sulfate contains 60 mg of elemental iron).
3. Iron is best absorbed as ferrous sulfate (Fe^{2+}) in an acidic environment. For this reason and to avoid binding the iron with food, iron should be taken about an hour before meals, when the duodenal mucosa is most acidic. Taking iron with vitamin C (ascorbic acid) or orange juice, which contains ascorbic acid, also enhances iron absorption. Gastric side effects, however, may necessitate ingesting iron with meals.
4. Undiluted liquid iron may stain the patient's teeth; therefore it should be diluted and ingested through a straw.
5. GI side effects of iron administration may occur, including heartburn, constipation, and diarrhea. If side effects develop, the dose and type of iron supplement may be adjusted. For example, many individuals who need supplemental iron cannot tolerate ferrous sulfate because of the effects of the sulfate base. However, ferrous gluconate may be an acceptable substitute. All patients should know that the use of iron preparations will cause their stools to become black because the GI tract excretes excess iron. Constipation is common, and the patient should be started on stool softeners and laxatives when started on iron.

TABLE 31-7 COLLABORATIVE CARE Iron-Deficiency Anemia

Diagnostic
- History and physical examination
- Hct and Hb levels
- RBC count, including morphology
- Reticulocyte count
- Serum iron
- Serum ferritin
- Serum transferrin
- Total iron-binding capacity (TIBC)
- Stool examination for occult blood

Collaborative Therapy
- Identification and treatment of underlying cause
- Ferrous sulfate or ferrous gluconate
- Iron dextran, iron sucrose, sodium ferric gluconate IM or IV
- Nutritional and diet therapy (see Table 31-5)
- Transfusion of packed RBCs (symptomatic patient only)

Hb, Hemoglobin; *Hct,* hematocrit; *IM,* intramuscular; *IV,* intravenous; *RBC,* red blood cell.

***Drug Alert** - Iron*
- *Enteric-coated or sustained-release iron should not be used.*
- *Iron should be taken about 1 hour before meals.*
- *Vitamin C (ascorbic acid) enhances iron absorption.*

In some situations, it may be necessary to administer iron parenterally. Parenteral use of iron is indicated for malabsorption, intolerance of oral iron, a need for iron beyond oral limits, or poor patient compliance in taking the oral preparations of iron. Parenteral iron can be given intramuscularly (IM) or intravenously (IV). An iron-dextran complex (INFeD) contains 50 mg/ml of elemental iron in 2 ml and has the longest use historically. Sodium ferrous gluconate and iron sucrose are alternatives, and may provide less risk of life-threatening anaphylaxis (0.5% to 1% of patients receiving iron dextran) and delayed serum sickness. A test dose of parenteral iron is often done to assess for a potential allergic reaction.

Because IM iron solutions may stain the skin, separate needles should be used for withdrawing the solution and for injecting the medication. Approximately 0.5 ml of air should be left in the syringe to clear the iron completely from the syringe. Iron should be given deep IM in the upper outer quadrant of the buttocks, with a 2- to 3-inch, 19- to 20-gauge needle. Preferably, no more than 2 ml of iron is given in a single injection. A Z-track technique should be used for injection to prevent leakage of the iron solution to the subcutaneous tissue. The site should not be massaged after the injection is given. IV administration of iron dextran should not be mixed with other medications or added to parenteral nutrition solutions. It should be given undiluted and at a rate of no more than 1 ml/min. The IV line should be flushed with normal saline.

NURSING MANAGEMENT
IRON-DEFICIENCY ANEMIA

It is important to recognize groups of individuals who are at an increased risk for the development of iron-deficiency anemia. These include premenopausal and pregnant women, persons from low socioeconomic backgrounds, older adults, and individuals experiencing blood loss. Diet teaching, with an emphasis on foods high in iron, is important for these groups. Supplemental iron is especially important for the pregnant woman. Appropriate nursing measures are presented in NCP 31-1. It is important to discuss with the patient the need for diagnostic studies to identify the cause. The hemoglobin and RBC counts are reassessed to evaluate the response to therapy. Compliance with dietary and drug therapy is emphasized. To replenish the body's iron stores, the patient needs to continue to take iron therapy for 2 to 3 months after the hemoglobin level returns to normal. Patients who require lifelong iron supplementation should be monitored for potential liver problems related to the iron storage.

THALASSEMIA

Etiology

Another cause of decreased erythrocyte production is thalassemia. **Thalassemia** is a group of diseases that have an autosomal recessive genetic basis involving inadequate production of normal hemoglobin. Hemolysis also occurs in thalassemia, but insufficient production of normal Hb is the predominant problem. In contrast to iron-deficiency anemia, in which heme synthesis is the problem, thalassemia is due to an absent or reduced globulin protein. α-Globin chains are absent or reduced in α-thalassemia, and β-globin chains are absent or reduced in β-thalassemia. Therefore the basic defect of thalassemia is abnormal Hb synthesis.

Thalassemia is commonly found in members of ethnic groups whose origins are near the Mediterranean Sea and equatorial or near-equatorial regions of Asia, the Middle East, and Africa. An individual with thalassemia may have a heterozygous or homozygous form of the disease. A person who is heterozygous has one thalassemic gene and one normal gene and is said to have *thalassemia minor* (or thalassemic trait), which is a mild form of the disease. A homozygous person has two thalassemic genes, causing a severe condition known as *thalassemia major.*[7,8]

Clinical Manifestations

Thalassemia major is a life-threatening disease in which growth, both physical and mental, is often retarded. The person who has thalassemia major is pale and displays other general symptoms of anemia (see Table 31-3). The symptoms develop in childhood by 2 years of age and can cause growth and development deficits. In addition, the person has pronounced splenomegaly and hepatomegaly. Jaundice from RBC hemolysis is prominent. As the bone marrow responds to the deficit of oxygen-carrying capacity of the blood, red blood cell production is stimulated and the marrow becomes packed with immature erythroid precursors that die. This stimulates further erythropoiesis, leading to the chronic bone marrow hyperplasia and expansion of the marrow space. This may cause thickening of the cranium and maxillary cavity. The patient with thalassemia minor is frequently asymptomatic. The patient has mild to moderate anemia with *microcytosis* (small cells) and *hypochromia* (pale cells).

Collaborative Care

The laboratory abnormalities of thalassemia major are summarized in Table 31-6. No specific drug or diet therapies are effective in treating thalassemia. Thalassemia minor requires no treatment because the body adapts to the reduction of normal hemoglobin. The symptoms of thalassemia major are managed with blood transfusions or exchange transfusions in conjunction with IV deferoxamine (Desferal) (a chelating agent that binds to iron) to reduce the iron overloading (hemochromatosis) that occurs with chronic transfusion therapy. Transfusions are administered to keep the Hb level at approximately 10 g/dl (100 g/L). This level is low enough to maintain the patient's own erythropoiesis without enlarging the spleen. Zinc supplementation may be needed (it is reduced with the chelation therapy), as well as ascorbic acid supplementation during the chelation therapy (increases urine excretion of iron; it should not be taken otherwise as it increases the absorption of dietary iron). Iron supplements should not be given. Because RBCs are sequestered in the enlarged spleen, thalassemia may be treated by splenectomy.

Hepatitis C is present in the majority of patients older than 25 years because of having received blood transfusions before they were screened for hepatitis C virus. Hepatitis C may result in cirrhosis and hepatocellular carcinoma. Cardiac complications from iron overload are reported to cause 71% of the deaths. Pulmonary disease and hypertension also contribute to early death. Thus hepatic, cardiac, and pulmonary organ function should be monitored and treated as appropriate. Endocrinopathies (hypogonadotrophic hypogonadism) and thrombosis may also be complications of the disease. Deferoxamine can cause side effects such as visual blurring, hearing loss, tinnitus, and knock-knees.[8]

MEGALOBLASTIC ANEMIAS

Megaloblastic anemias are a group of disorders caused by impaired DNA synthesis and characterized by the presence of large RBCs. When DNA synthesis is impaired, defective RBC maturation results. The RBCs are large (macrocytic) and abnormal and are referred to as *megaloblasts.* Macrocytic RBCs are easily destroyed because they have fragile cell membranes. Although the overwhelming majority of megaloblastic anemias result from cobalamin (vitamin B_{12}) and folic acid deficiencies, this type of RBC deformity can also occur from suppression of DNA synthesis by drugs, from inborn errors of cobalamin and folic acid metabolism, and from *erythroleukemia* (malignant blood disorder characterized by a proliferation of erythropoietic cells in bone marrow). Two common forms of megaloblastic anemia are cobalamin deficiency and folic acid deficiency[9] (Table 31-8).

COBALAMIN (VITAMIN B_{12}) DEFICIENCY

Normally, a protein termed *intrinsic factor* (IF) is secreted by the parietal cells of the gastric mucosa. IF is required for cobalamin (extrinsic factor) absorption. Therefore if IF is not secreted, cobalamin will not be absorbed. (Cobalamin is normally absorbed in the

TABLE 31-8 Classification of Megaloblastic Anemias

Cobalamin (Vitamin B_{12}) Deficiency
Dietary deficiency
Deficiency of gastric intrinsic factor
Pernicious anemia
Gastrectomy
Intestinal malabsorption
Increased requirement
Chronic alcoholism
Folic Acid Deficiency
Dietary deficiency
Impaired absorption
Increased requirement
Alcohol abuse
Drug-Induced Suppression of DNA Synthesis
Folate antagonists
Metabolic inhibitors
Alkylating agents
Inborn Errors
Defective folate metabolism
Defective transport of cobalamin
Erythroleukemia

distal ileum.) There are many causes of cobalamin deficiency. The most common cause is **pernicious anemia,** a disease in which the gastric mucosa is not secreting IF because of antibodies being directed against the gastric parietal cells and/or IF itself. Other causes of cobalamin deficiency include gastrectomy, gastritis, nutritional deficiency, chronic alcoholism, and hereditary enzymatic defects of cobalamin utilization (see Table 31-8).

Pernicious anemia is a disease of insidious onset that begins in middle age or later (usually after age 40) with 60 years being the most common age at diagnosis. Pernicious anemia occurs frequently in persons of Northern European ancestry (particularly Scandinavians) and African Americans. In African Americans, the disease tends to begin early, occurs with higher frequency in women, and is often severe.

Etiology

Cobalamin deficiency can occur in patients who have had GI surgery such as gastrectomy; patients who have had a small bowel resection involving the ileum; and patients with Crohn's disease, ileitis, diverticuli of the small intestine, and/or chronic atrophic gastritis. In these cases, cobalamin deficiency results from the loss of IF-secreting gastric mucosal cells or impaired absorption of cobalamin in the distal ileum. Cobalamin deficiency is also found in long-term users of H_2-histamine receptor blockers.

Pernicious anemia is caused by an absence of IF, from either gastric mucosal atrophy or autoimmune destruction of parietal cells. This results in a decrease of hydrochloric acid secretion by the stomach. An acid environment in the stomach is required for the secretion of IF.

Clinical Manifestations

General symptoms of anemia related to cobalamin deficiency develop because of tissue hypoxia (see Table 31-3). GI manifestations include a sore tongue, anorexia, nausea, vomiting, and abdominal pain. Typical neuromuscular manifestations include weakness, paresthesias of the feet and hands, reduced vibratory and position senses, ataxia, muscle weakness, and impaired thought processes ranging from confusion to dementia. Because cobalamin deficiency–related anemia has an insidious onset, it may take several months for these manifestations to develop.

Diagnostic Studies

Laboratory data reflective of cobalamin deficiency anemia are presented in Table 31-6. The RBCs appear large (macrocytic) and have abnormal shapes. This structure contributes to erythrocyte destruction because the cell membrane is fragile. Serum cobalamin levels are reduced. Serum folate levels are also obtained. If they are normal and cobalamin levels are low, it suggests that megaloblastic anemia is due to a cobalamin deficiency. Because the potential for gastric cancer is increased in patients with pernicious anemia, a gastroscopy and biopsy of the gastric mucosa may also be done.

Another means of assessing parietal cell function is by a Schilling test. After radioactive cobalamin is administered to the patient, the amount of cobalamin excreted in the urine is measured. An individual who cannot absorb cobalamin excretes only a small amount of this radioactive form. The same procedure may be followed with the parenteral administration of IF. Absorption of cobalamin when IF is added is diagnostic of pernicious anemia. Additional testing of serum methylmalonic acid (MMA) and serum homocysteine can be used if the other tests are not definitive.

Collaborative Care

Regardless of how much is ingested, the patient is not able to absorb cobalamin if intrinsic factor is lacking or if there is impaired absorption in the ileum. For this reason, increasing dietary cobalamin does not correct the anemia. However, the patient should be instructed on adequate dietary intake to maintain good nutrition (see Table 31-5). Parenteral (cyanocobalamin or hydroxocobalamin) or intranasal (Nascobal) administration of cobalamin is the treatment of choice. Without cobalamin administration, these individuals will die in 1 to 3 years. The dosage and frequency of cobalamin administration may vary. A typical treatment schedule consists of 1000 mg of cobalamin IM daily for 2 weeks and then weekly until the hematocrit is normal, then monthly for life. High-dose oral cobalamin and sublingual cobalamin are also available. As long as supplemental cobalamin is used, the anemia can be reversed. However, if the person has had long-standing neuromuscular complications, they may not be reversible.

FOLIC ACID DEFICIENCY

Folic acid (folate) deficiency also causes megaloblastic anemia. Folic acid is required for DNA synthesis leading to RBC formation and maturation. Common causes of folic acid deficiency include the following:

1. Poor nutrition, especially a lack of leafy green vegetables, liver, citrus fruits, yeast, dried beans, nuts, and grains
2. Malabsorption syndromes, particularly small bowel disorders
3. Drugs that impede the absorption and use of folic acid (e.g., methotrexate), antiseizure drugs (e.g., phenobarbital, diphenylhydantoin [Dilantin]), and others (e.g., trimethoprim, sulfasalazine)
4. Alcohol abuse and anorexia
5. Hemodialysis patients because folic acid is lost during dialysis

The clinical manifestations of folic acid deficiency are similar to those of cobalamin deficiency. The disease develops insidiously, and the patient's symptoms may be attributed to other coexisting problems such as cirrhosis or esophageal varices. GI disturbances include dyspepsia and a smooth, beefy red tongue. The absence of neurologic problems is an important diagnostic finding. This lack of neurologic involvement differentiates folic acid deficiency from cobalamin deficiency.

The diagnostic findings for folic acid deficiency are presented in Table 31-6. In addition, the serum folate level is low (normal is 3 to 25 mg/ml [7 to 57 mol/L]), the serum cobalamin level is normal, and the gastric analysis is positive for hydrochloric acid.

Folic acid deficiency is treated by replacement therapy. The usual dose is 1 mg per day by mouth. In malabsorption states, up to 5 mg per day may be required. The duration of treatment depends on the reason for the deficiency. The patient should be encouraged to eat foods containing large amounts of folic acid (see Table 31-5).

NURSING MANAGEMENT
MEGALOBLASTIC ANEMIA

Because there is a familial predisposition for pernicious anemia, the most common type of cobalamin deficiency, patients who have a positive family history of pernicious anemia should be evaluated for symptoms. Although disease development cannot be prevented, early detection and treatment can lead to reversal of symptoms. Signs and symptoms of other possible megaloblastic anemias should also be considered and brought to the attention of the primary health care provider.

The nursing measures presented in the nursing care plan for the patient with anemia (see NCP 31-1) are appropriate for the patient with cobalamin or folic acid deficiency anemia. In addition to these measures, the nurse should ensure that injuries are not sustained because of the diminished sensations to heat and pain resulting from the neurologic impairment. The patient must be protected from falling, burns, and trauma. If heat therapy is required, the patient's skin must be evaluated at frequent intervals to detect redness.

Ongoing care is focused on ensuring good patient compliance with treatment. There must also be careful follow-up to assess for neurologic difficulties that were not fully corrected by adequate replacement therapy. Because the potential for cancer may be increased (e.g., gastric carcinoma is increased in patients with atrophic gastritis–related pernicious anemia, alcohol increases the likelihood of oral and esophageal cancers), the patient should have frequent and careful appropriate screenings.

ANEMIA OF CHRONIC DISEASE

Chronic inflammatory, autoimmune, infectious, or malignant diseases can lead to anemia of chronic disease. Anemia of chronic disease is associated with an underproduction of RBCs and mild shortening of RBC survival. The RBCs are usually normocytic, normochromic, and hypoproliferative. The anemia is usually mild, but it can be more severe. This type of anemia is primarily immune driven. The cytokines released by these conditions cause an increased uptake and retention of iron within macrophages. This leads to a diversion of iron from the circulation into storage sites, subsequent limitation of the availability of iron for erythroid progenitor cells, and iron-restricted erythropoiesis. For any chronic disease, there may also be additional factors. For example, with renal disease, the primary factor causing anemia is decreased erythropoietin, a hormone made in the kidneys that stimulates erythropoiesis. With impaired renal function, erythropoietin production is decreased (see Chapter 47).

Any condition that causes increased RBC destruction (e.g., autoimmune hemolysis) accompanied by the failure to augment erythropoiesis will contribute to anemia. Myelosuppression and decreased erythropoiesis caused by disease, medications (e.g., chemotherapy), or radiation will contribute to the anemia of chronic disease. Human immunodeficiency virus (HIV) and its treatments, hepatitis, malaria, and bleeding episodes are other contributors to this type of anemia.[10]

Hypopituitary and hypothyroid states both lead to reduced tissue metabolism; therefore tissue oxygen needs are diminished, leading to a reduced production of erythropoietin by the kidneys. Adrenal dysfunction caused by either adrenalectomy or Addison's disease also results in anemia.

Anemia of chronic disease must first be recognized and differentiated from anemias of other etiologies. Findings of elevated serum ferritin and increased iron stores distinguish it from iron-deficiency anemia. Normal folate and cobalamin blood levels distinguish it from those types of anemias. The best treatment of anemia of chronic disease is correction of the underlying disorder. If the anemia is severe, blood transfusions may be indicated, but are not recommended for long-term treatment. Erythropoietin therapy (Epogen, Procrit) is used for anemia related to renal disease (see Chapter 47) or anemia related to cancer therapies (see Chapter 16 and Table 16-18). Darbepoetin (Aranesp) is a newer formulation of erythropoietin. It has a longer duration of action than erythropoietin. Intravenous iron should only be administered, if necessary, to improve the response to therapy with erythropoietin.

APLASTIC ANEMIA

Aplastic anemia is a disease in which the patient has peripheral blood *pancytopenia* (decrease of all blood cell types—RBCs, white blood cells [WBCs], and platelets) and hypocellular bone marrow. The signs and symptoms can range from a chronic condition managed with erythropoietin or blood transfusions to a critical condition with hemorrhage and sepsis.

Etiology

The incidence of aplastic anemia is low, affecting approximately 4 of every 1 million persons. There are various etiologic classifications for aplastic anemia, but they can be divided into two major groups: congenital or acquired (Table 31-9).

1. *Congenital origin* is caused by chromosomal alterations. Approximately 30% of the aplastic anemias that appear in childhood are inherited.
2. *Acquired aplastic anemia* results from exposure to ionizing radiation, chemical agents (e.g., benzene, insecticides, arsenic, alcohol), viral and bacterial infections (e.g., hepatitis, parvovirus, biliary tuberculosis), and prescribed medications (e.g., alkylating agents, antiseizure agents, antimetabolites, antimicrobials, gold). Approximately 70% of the acquired aplastic anemias are idiopathic.[11]

Clinical Manifestations

Aplastic anemia can present abruptly (over days) or insidiously over weeks to months and can vary from mild to severe.[12] Clinically the patient may have symptoms caused by suppression of any or all bone marrow elements. General manifestations of anemia such as fatigue and dyspnea, as well as cardiovascular and cerebral

TABLE 31-9 Causes of Aplastic Anemia

Congenital	• Fanconi syndrome • Congenital dyskeratosis • Amegakaryocytic thrombocytopenia • Schwachman-Diamond syndrome
Acquired	• Chemical agents and toxins • Drugs • Idiopathic • Pregnancy • Radiation • Viral and bacterial infections

responses, may be seen (see Table 31-3). The patient with neutropenia (low neutrophil count) is susceptible to infection and may be febrile. Thrombocytopenia is manifested by a predisposition to bleeding (e.g., petechiae, ecchymosis, epistaxis).

Diagnostic Studies

The diagnosis is confirmed by laboratory studies. Because all marrow elements are affected, hemoglobin, WBC, and platelet values are often decreased in aplastic anemia. Other RBC indices are generally normal (see Table 31-6). The condition is therefore classified as a normocytic, normochromic anemia. The reticulocyte count is low. Bleeding time is prolonged.

Aplastic anemia can be further evaluated by assessing various iron studies. The serum iron and total iron-binding capacity (TIBC) may be elevated as initial signs of erythropoiesis suppression. Bone marrow biopsy, aspiration, and pathologic examination may be done for any anemic state. However, the findings are especially important in aplastic anemia because the marrow is hypocellular with increased yellow marrow (fat content).

NURSING *and* COLLABORATIVE MANAGEMENT APLASTIC ANEMIA

Management of aplastic anemia is based on identifying and removing the causative agent (when possible) and providing supportive care until the pancytopenia reverses. Nursing interventions appropriate for the patient with pancytopenia from aplastic anemia are presented in the nursing care plan for the patient with anemia (see NCP 31-1) earlier in this chapter and the nursing care plans for thrombocytopenia (see NCP 31-2) and neutropenia (see NCP 31-3) later in this chapter. Nursing actions are directed at preventing complications from infection and hemorrhage.

The prognosis of severe untreated aplastic anemia is poor (approximately 75% fatal). However, advances in medical management, including hematopoietic stem cell transplant (HSCT) and immunosuppressive therapy with antithymocyte globulin (ATG) and cyclosporine or high-dose cyclophosphamide (Cytoxan), have improved outcomes significantly. ATG is a horse serum that contains polyclonal antibodies against human T cells. It can cause anaphylaxis and a serum sickness. The rationale for this therapy is that aplastic anemia is an immune-mediated disease.[1,2,13] (ATG and cyclosporine are discussed in Chapter 14 and Table 14-18.)

The treatment of choice for adults less than 45 years of age who do not respond to the immunosuppressive therapy and who have a human leukocyte antigen (HLA)–matched donor is an HSCT. The best results occur in a younger patient who has not had previous blood transfusions. Prior transfusions increase the risk of graft rejection. (HSCT is discussed in Chapter 16.)

For the older adult or the patient without an HLA-matched donor, the treatment of choice is immunosuppression with ATG or cyclosporine or high-dose cyclophosphamide. Although this therapy may be only partially beneficial, transfusions usually can be avoided.

Anemia Caused by Blood Loss

Anemia resulting from blood loss may be caused by either acute or chronic problems.

ACUTE BLOOD LOSS

Acute blood loss occurs as a result of sudden hemorrhage. Causes of acute blood loss include trauma, complications of surgery, and conditions or diseases that disrupt vascular integrity. There are two clinical concerns in such situations. First, there is a sudden reduction in the total blood volume that can lead to hypovolemic shock. Second, if the acute loss is more gradual, the body maintains its blood volume by slowly increasing the plasma volume. Although the circulating fluid volume is preserved, the number of RBCs available to carry oxygen is significantly diminished.

Clinical Manifestations

The clinical manifestations of anemia from acute blood loss are caused by the body's attempts to maintain an adequate blood volume and meet oxygen requirements. Table 31-10 summarizes the clinical manifestations of patients with varying degrees of blood volume loss. It is essential to understand that the clinical signs and symptoms the patient is experiencing are more important than the laboratory values. For example, an adult with a bleeding peptic ulcer who had a 750-ml hematemesis (15% of a normal total blood volume) within the past 30 minutes may have postural hypotension, but have normal values for Hb and Hct. Over the ensuing 36 to 48 hours, most of the volume deficit will be repaired by the movement of fluid from the extravascular into the intravascular space. Only at these later times will the hemoglobin and hematocrit reflect the blood loss.[2]

The nurse should be alert to the patient's expression of pain. Internal hemorrhage may cause pain because of tissue distention, organ displacement, and nerve compression. Pain may be localized or referred. In the case of retroperitoneal bleeding, the patient may not experience abdominal pain. Instead, the patient may have numbness and pain in a lower extremity secondary to compression of the lateral cutaneous nerve, which is located in the region of the first to third lumbar vertebrae. The major complication of acute blood loss is shock (see Chapter 67).

Diagnostic Studies

When blood volume loss is sudden, plasma volume has not yet had a chance to increase, the loss of RBCs is not reflected in laboratory data, and values may seem normal or high for 2 to 3 days. However, once the plasma is replaced by endogenous and exogenous means, the RBC mass is less concentrated. At this time, RBC, hemoglobin, and hematocrit levels are low and reflect the blood loss.

TABLE 31-10 Clinical Manifestations of Acute Blood Loss

Volume Lost (%)	Clinical Manifestations
10	None
20	No detectable signs or symptoms at rest, tachycardia with exercise and slight postural hypotension
30	Normal supine blood pressure and pulse at rest, postural hypotension and tachycardia with exercise
40	Blood pressure, central venous pressure, and cardiac output below normal at rest; rapid, thready pulse and cold, clammy skin
50	Shock and potential death

Collaborative Care

Collaborative care is initially concerned with (1) replacing blood volume to prevent shock and (2) identifying the source of the hemorrhage and stopping the blood loss. IV fluids used in emergencies include dextran, hetastarch, albumin, and/or crystalloid electrolyte solutions such as lactated Ringer's. The amount of infusion varies with the solution used. (Management of shock is discussed in Chapter 67.)

Once volume replacement is established, attention can be directed to correcting the RBC loss. The body needs 2 to 5 days to manufacture more RBCs in response to increased erythropoietin. Consequently, blood transfusions (packed RBCs) may be needed if the blood loss is significant. In addition, if the bleeding is related to a platelet or clotting disorder, replacement of that deficiency is addressed.

The patient may also need supplemental iron because the availability of iron affects the marrow production of erythrocytes. When anemia exists after acute blood loss, dietary sources of iron will probably not be adequate to maintain iron stores. Therefore oral or parenteral iron preparations are administered.

NURSING MANAGEMENT ACUTE BLOOD LOSS

In the case of trauma, it may be impossible to prevent the situation leading to the blood loss. For the postoperative patient, the nurse carefully monitors the blood loss from various drainage tubes and dressings and implements appropriate actions. The nursing care plan for the patient with anemia resulting from acute blood loss will most likely include administration of blood products (described at the end of this chapter).

Once the source of hemorrhage is identified, blood loss is controlled, and fluid and blood volumes are replaced, the anemia should begin to correct itself. There should be no need for long-term treatment of this type of anemia.

CHRONIC BLOOD LOSS

The sources of chronic blood loss are similar to those of iron-deficiency anemia (e.g., bleeding ulcer, hemorrhoids, menstrual and postmenopausal blood loss). The effects of chronic blood loss are usually related to the depletion of iron stores and are usually considered as iron-deficiency anemia. Management of chronic blood loss anemia involves identifying the source and stopping the bleeding. Supplemental iron may be required. The nursing measures presented in NCP 31-1 are relevant to anemia of chronic blood loss.

Anemia Caused by Increased Erythrocyte Destruction

The third major cause of anemia is termed **hemolytic anemia,** a condition caused by the destruction or hemolysis of RBCs at a rate that exceeds production. Hemolysis can occur because of problems intrinsic or extrinsic to the RBCs. *Intrinsic hemolytic anemias* result from defects in the RBCs themselves caused by abnormal hemoglobin (e.g., sickle cells), enzyme deficiencies that alter glycolysis (glucose-6-phosphate dehydrogenase [G6PD] deficiency), or RBC membrane abnormalities. Intrinsic hemolytic anemias are usually hereditary. More common are the *extrinsic hemolytic anemias,* which are acquired. In this type of anemia the patient's RBCs are normal, but damage is caused by external factors such as trapping of cells within the sinuses of the liver or spleen, antibody-mediated destruction, toxins, or mechanical injury (e.g., prosthetic heart valves).

The two sites of hemolysis are classified as intravascular or extravascular. *Intravascular* destruction occurs within the circulation; *extravascular* hemolysis takes place in the macrophages of the spleen, liver, and bone marrow. The spleen is the primary site of the destruction of RBCs that are old, defective, or moderately damaged. Fig. 31-2 indicates the sequence of events involved in extravascular hemolysis.

The patient with hemolytic anemia manifests the general symptoms of anemia and clinical manifestations specific to this type of anemia (see Table 31-3). Jaundice is likely because the increased destruction of RBCs causes an elevation in bilirubin levels. The spleen and liver may enlarge because of their hyperactivity, which is related to macrophage phagocytosis of the defective erythrocytes.

In all causes of hemolysis a major focus of treatment is to maintain renal function. When an RBC is hemolyzed, the hemoglobin

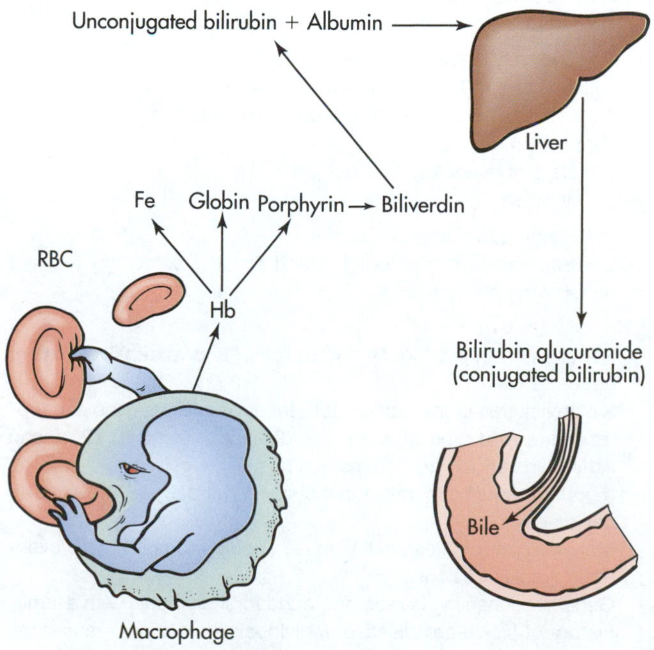

FIG. 31-2 Sequence of events in extravascular hemolysis.

molecule is released and filtered by the kidneys. The accumulation of hemoglobin molecules can obstruct the renal tubules and lead to acute tubular necrosis (see Chapter 47).

SICKLE CELL DISEASE

Sickle cell disease (SCD) is a group of inherited, autosomal recessive disorders characterized by the presence of an abnormal form of hemoglobin in the erythrocyte. (Autosomal recessive genetic disorders are discussed in Chapter 14 and Table 14-2.) This abnormal hemoglobin, *hemoglobin S* (Hb S), causes the erythrocyte to stiffen and elongate taking on a sickle shape in response to low oxygen levels. Hemoglobin S results from substitution of valine for glutamic acid on the β-globin chain of hemoglobin. Because this is a genetic disorder, SCD is usually identified during infancy or early childhood. It is an incurable disease that is often fatal by middle age from renal and pulmonary failure.[14]

SCD affects more than 50,000 Americans and is predominant in African Americans, occurring in an estimated prevalence of 1 in about 400 live births. It can also affect people of Mediterranean, Caribbean, South and Central American, Arabian, or East Indian ancestry.[14]

Etiology and Pathophysiology

Types of Sickle Cell Disease. Types of SCD disorders include sickle cell anemia, sickle cell–thalassemia, sickle cell Hb C disease, and sickle cell trait. *Sickle cell anemia* is the most severe of the SCD syndromes. This occurs when a person is homozygous for hemoglobin S (Hb SS); the person has inherited Hb S from both parents. *Sickle cell–thalassemia* and *sickle cell Hb C* occur when a person inherits Hb S from one parent and another type of abnormal hemoglobin (such as thalassemia or hemoglobin C) from the other parent. Both of these forms of SCD are less common and less severe than sickle cell anemia. *Sickle cell trait* occurs when a person is heterozygous for hemoglobin S (Hb AS); the person has inherited hemoglobin S from one parent and normal hemoglobin (hemoglobin A) from the other parent. Sickle cell trait is typically a very mild to asymptomatic condition.

Sickling Episodes. The major pathophysiologic event of SCD is the sickling of RBCs. Sickling episodes are most commonly triggered by low oxygen tension in the blood. Hypoxia or deoxygenation of the RBCs can be caused by viral or bacterial infection, high altitude, emotional or physical stress, surgery, and blood loss. Infection is the most common precipitating factor. Other events that can trigger or sustain a sickling episode include dehydration, increased hydrogen ion concentration (acidosis), increased plasma osmolality, decreased plasma volume, and low body temperature. A sickling episode can also occur without an obvious cause.

Sickled RBCs become rigid and take on an elongated, crescent shape (Fig. 31-3). Sickled cells cannot easily pass through capillaries or other small vessels and can cause vascular occlusion, leading to acute or chronic tissue injury. The resulting hemostasis promotes a self-perpetuating cycle of local hypoxia, deoxygenation of more erythrocytes, and more sickling. Circulating sickled cells are hemolyzed by the spleen, leading to anemia. Initially the sickling of cells is reversible with reoxygenation, but it eventually becomes irreversible because of cell membrane damage from recurrent sickling. Thus vasoocclusive phenomena and hemolysis are the clinical hallmarks of sickle cell disease.[15]

Sickle cell crisis is a severe, painful, acute exacerbation of RBC sickling causing a vasoocclusive crisis. As blood flow is impaired by sickled cells, vasospasm occurs, further restricting blood flow. Severe capillary hypoxia causes changes in membrane permeability, leading to plasma loss, hemoconcentration, the development of thrombi, and further circulatory stagnation. Tissue ischemia, infarction, and necrosis eventually occur from lack of oxygen. Shock is a possible life-threatening consequence of sickle cell crisis because of severe oxygen depletion of the tissues and a reduction of the circulating fluid volume. Sickle cell crisis can begin suddenly and persist for days to weeks.

The frequency, extent, and severity of sickling episodes are highly variable and unpredictable, but are largely dependent on the percentage of Hb S present. Individuals with sickle cell anemia have the most severe form because the erythrocytes contain a high percentage of Hb S.

GENETICS IN CLINICAL PRACTICE
Sickle Cell Disease

Genetic Basis
- Autosomal recessive disorder
- Mutation in β-globin gene located on chromosome 11
- Hb S variant involves substitution of valine for glutamic acid in the β-globin gene

Incidence
- 1 in 350 to 500 African Americans
- 1 in 1000 to 1400 Hispanic Americans
- Also affects people of Mediterranean, Caribbean, Arabian, and East Indian descent
- Affects 8 of every 100,000 people

Genetic Testing
- DNA testing available but costly
- Electrophoresis of hemoglobin and sickling screening test are more commonly used

Clinical Implications
- Requires ongoing continuity of care and extensive patient education.
- Sickle cell trait is the carrier state for sickle cell disease and represents a mild type of sickle cell disease; 1 in 10 to 12 African Americans and 1 in 25 Hispanics has sickle cell trait.
- If both parents have trait, 1 in 4 chance that baby will have sickle cell disease.
- Management of sickle cell disease should focus on the prevention of sickle cell crisis.
- Genetic counseling is recommended for individuals with a family history of sickle cell disease. Individuals should understand the risks of transmitting the genetic mutation.

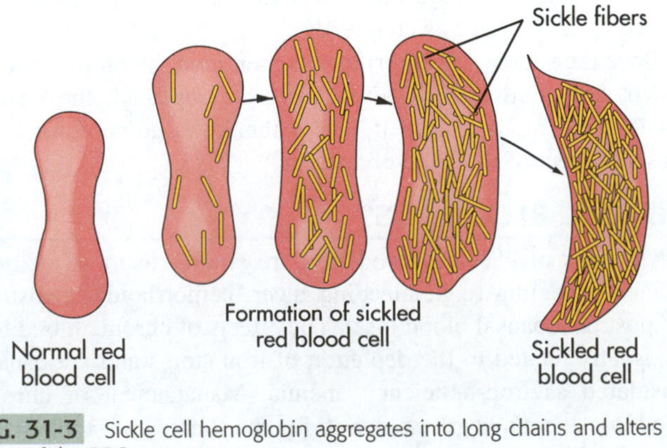

FIG. 31-3 Sickle cell hemoglobin aggregates into long chains and alters the shape of the RBC.

Clinical Manifestations

The effects of sickle cell disease vary greatly from person to person. Many people with sickle cell anemia are in reasonably good health the majority of the time. However, they may have chronic health problems and pain because of organ tissue hypoxia and damage (e.g., involving the kidneys and/or liver). The typical patient is anemic but asymptomatic except during sickling episodes. Clinical manifestations of chronic anemia include pallor of mucous membranes, fatigue, and decreased exercise tolerance. Because most individuals with sickle cell anemia have dark skin, pallor is more readily detected by examining the mucous membranes. The skin may have a grayish cast. Because of the hemolysis, jaundice is common and patients are prone to gallstones (cholelithiasis).

The primary symptom associated with sickling is pain. During sickle cell crisis the pain is severe because of ischemia of tissue. The episodes can affect any area of the body or several sites simultaneously, with the back, chest, extremities, and abdomen being most commonly affected. The pain severity can range from trivial to excruciating. Approximately one half of episodes are accompanied by objective clinical signs such as fever, swelling, tenderness, tachypnea, hypertension, nausea, and vomiting.[16]

Complications

With repeated episodes of sickling there is gradual involvement of all body systems, especially the spleen, lungs, kidneys, and brain. Organs that have a high need for oxygen are most often affected and form the basis for many of the complications of sickle cell disease (Fig. 31-4). Infection is a major cause of morbidity and mortality in patients with sickle cell disease. One reason for this is the failure of the spleen to phagocytize foreign substances as it becomes infarcted and dysfunctional (usually by 2 to 4 years of age) from the sickled red cells. The spleen becomes small because of repeated scarring, a phenomenon termed *autosplenectomy.* Pneumonia is the most common infection and often is of pneumococcal origin. Infections can be so severe that they can cause an aplastic and hemolytic crisis and gallstones. *Acute chest syndrome* is a term used to describe acute pulmonary complications that include pneumonia, tissue infarction, and fat embolism. It is characterized by fever, chest pain, cough, pulmonary infiltrates, and dyspnea. Pulmonary infarctions may cause pulmonary hypertension, MI, HF, and ultimately cor pulmonale. The heart may become ischemic and enlarged, leading to HF. Retinal vessel obstruction may result in hemorrhage, scarring, retinal detachment, and blindness. The kidneys may be injured from the increased blood viscosity and the lack of oxygen and can lead to renal failure. Stroke can result from

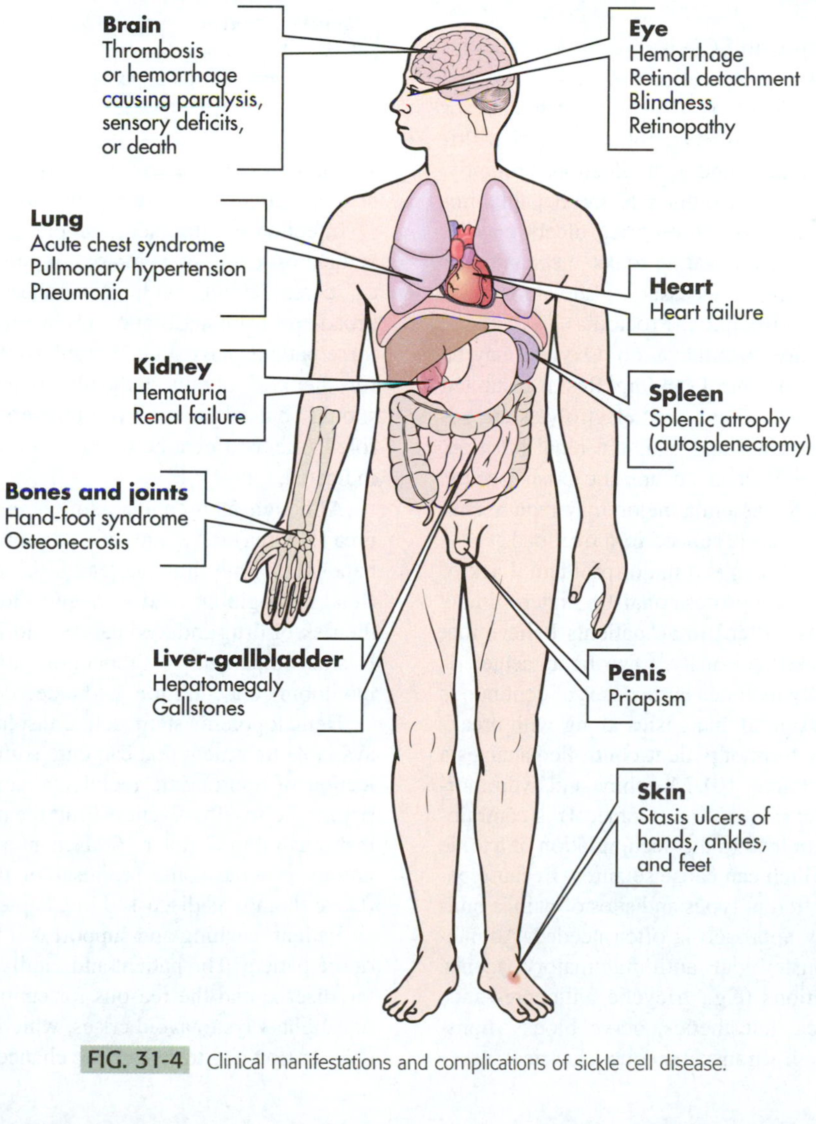

FIG. 31-4 Clinical manifestations and complications of sickle cell disease.

thrombosis and infarction of cerebral blood vessels. Bone changes may include osteoporosis and osteosclerosis after infarction. Chronic leg ulcers can result from the hypoxia and are especially prevalent around the ankles. *Priapism* (persistent penile erection) may occur if penile veins become occluded.

Diagnostic Studies

A peripheral blood smear may reveal sickled cells and abnormal reticulocytes. The presence of sickle hemoglobin can be diagnosed by the sickling test, which uses RBCs (in vitro) and exposes them to a deoxygenation agent. Electrophoresis of hemoglobin readily identifies the presence of abnormal hemoglobin. DNA testing can be done, but is costly.

As a result of the accelerated RBC breakdown, the patient has characteristic clinical findings of hemolysis (jaundice, elevated serum bilirubin levels) and abnormal laboratory test results (see Table 31-6). Skeletal x-rays will demonstrate bone and joint deformities and flattening. Magnetic resonance imaging may be used to diagnose a stroke caused by blocked cerebral vessels from sickled cells. Doppler studies may be used to assess for deep vein thromboses. Other tests may be indicated, such as a chest x-ray, to diagnose infection or organ malfunction.

NURSING *and* COLLABORATIVE MANAGEMENT SICKLE CELL DISEASE

Collaborative care for a patient with SCD is directed toward alleviating the symptoms from the complications of the disease and minimizing end-organ damage. There is no specific treatment for the disease. Patients with SCD should be taught to avoid high altitudes, maintain adequate fluid intake, and treat infections promptly. Pneumovax, *Haemophilus influenzae,* influenza, and hepatitis immunizations should be administered. Chronic leg ulcers may be treated with bed rest, antibiotics, warm saline soaks, mechanical or enzyme debridement, and grafting if necessary. Priapism is managed with pain medication and nifedipine (Procardia).

Sickle cell crises may require hospitalization. Oxygen may be administered to treat hypoxia and control sickling. Rest is instituted to reduce metabolic requirements. Fluids and electrolytes are administered to reduce blood viscosity and maintain renal function. Transfusion therapy is indicated when an aplastic crisis occurs. These patients, like those with thalassemia major, may require chelation therapy to reduce transfusion-produced iron overload.

Undertreatment of sickle cell pain is a major problem. Lack of understanding can lead health care professionals to underestimate how much pain these patients suffer. Some patients believe that their reports of pain are not taken seriously.[17] During an acute crisis, optimal pain control usually includes large doses of continuous (rather than as-needed [prn]) opioid analgesics along with breakthrough analgesia, often in the form of patient-controlled analgesia (PCA) (PCA is discussed in Chapter 10). Morphine and hydromorphone are the drugs of choice; meperidine (Demerol) is contraindicated because high doses can lead to the accumulation of a toxic metabolite, normeperidine, which can cause seizures. Because patients may be experiencing different types and sites of pain, a multimodal and multidisciplinary approach is often needed. Adjunctive measures, such as nonsteroidal antiinflammatory agents, antineuropathic pain medications (e.g., tricyclic antidepressants, antiseizure medications), local anesthetics, nerve blocks, transelectrodermal nerve stimulator (transcutaneous electrical nerve stimulation [TENS]), and/or acupuncture may be used. After discharge, patients will often continue on oral opioid analgesics.[17,18]

ETHICAL DILEMMAS
Pain Management

Situation

A 21-year-old African American man is admitted to the emergency department in sickle cell crisis with complaints of excruciating pain. He is known to several of the nurses and physicians in the department. One of the nurses remarks to you that it must be time for his "fix" of pain medications.

Important Points for Consideration

- The experience of pain is subjective, and experts in pain management agree that "pain is what the patient says it is."
- Acute or chronic pain can have serious and debilitating physical and psychologic effects for patients.
- Persons experiencing chronic pain have different physiologic and psychologic responses to pain and to pain medications.
- The nurse's duty to prevent harm and provide benefit to patients is undermined when a patient's complaints of unrelieved pain are attributed to attention-seeking or drug-seeking behavior.
- People with chronic pain are often stigmatized because of lack of knowledge on the part of health care providers or long-term use of opioids or other pain medications.
- The nurse's obligation to provide holistic individualized care to patients is compromised when stereotypes or myths interfere with the ability to accurately assess a patient's problems.

Critical Thinking Questions

1. How would you respond to the nurse's negative remark?
2. What important factors would need to be included in your assessment of this patient?

Infection is a frequent complication and must be treated. Pain is the most common symptom of patients with SCD seeking medical care. Patients with acute chest syndrome are treated with broad-spectrum antibiotics, O_2 therapy, and fluid therapy. Because these patients have an increased need for folic acid, it is important for them to obtain daily supplementation. Blood transfusions should be used judiciously to treat a crisis. They have little if any role in the treatment between crises. In general, iron therapy is not indicated.

Although many antisickling agents have been tried, hydroxyurea (Hydrea) is the only one that has been shown to be clinically beneficial. This drug increases the production of hemoglobin F (fetal hemoglobin) and is given in low enough doses to minimize the risk of drug-induced cancer and leukemia. The increase in Hb F is accompanied by a reduction in hemolysis, an increase in hemoglobin concentration, and a decrease in sickled cells.[19]

Hematopoietic stem cell transplantation (HSCT) is the only available treatment that can cure some patients with SCD. The selection of appropriate recipients, scarcity of appropriate donors, risk, and cost-effectiveness limit the use of HSCT for SCD. (HSCT is discussed in Chapter 16.) Recent advances in gene therapy technology provide some promise for the future treatment of SCD. (Gene therapy is discussed in Chapter 14.)

Patient teaching and support is important in the long-term care of the patient. The patient and family must understand the basis of the disease and the reasons for supportive care. The patient must be taught ways to avoid crises, which include taking steps to avoid dehydration and to reduce the chance of developing hypoxia, such as avoiding high altitudes and seeking medical attention quickly to counteract problems such as upper respiratory tract infections. Education on pain control is also needed because the pain during a crisis may be severe and often requires considerable analgesia. Minor pain episodes that are not associated with infection or other symptoms warranting medical attention can sometimes be managed at home.

Recurrent episodes of severe acute pain and unrelenting chronic pain can be profoundly disabling and depressing. Occupational therapists and physiotherapists can help the patient achieve optimum physical functioning and independence; a psychologist may be able to use cognitive-behavioral therapy to help patients with SCD cope with anxiety and depression. Because there are often these additional quality-of-life issues, the nurse can play an important role in ensuring that these needs are met through appropriate referrals.[17]

ACQUIRED HEMOLYTIC ANEMIA

Extrinsic causes of hemolysis can be separated into three categories: (1) physical factors, (2) immune reactions, and (3) infectious agents and toxins.

Physical destruction of RBCs results from the exertion of extreme force on the cells. Traumatic events causing disruption of the RBC membrane include hemodialysis, extracorporeal circulation used in cardiopulmonary bypass, and prosthetic heart valves. In addition, the force needed to push blood through abnormal vessels, such as those that have been burned or affected by angiopathic disease (e.g., diabetes mellitus), may also physically damage RBCs.

Antibodies may destroy RBCs by the mechanisms involved in antigen-antibody reactions. The reactions may be of an isoimmune or autoimmune type. *Isoimmune reactions* occur when antibodies develop against antigens from another person of the same species. Blood transfusion reactions typify this response, when the recipient's antibodies hemolyze donor cells.

Autoimmune reactions result when individuals develop antibodies against their own RBCs. Autoimmune hemolytic reactions may be idiopathic, developing with no prior hemolytic history as a result of the immunoglobulin IgG covering the RBCs, or secondary to other autoimmune diseases (e.g., systemic lupus erythematosus), leukemia, lymphoma, or medications (penicillin, indomethacin [Indocin], phenylbutazone [Butazolidine], phenacetin, quinidine, quinine, and methyldopa [Aldomet]).

Infectious agents and toxins cause the third category of acquired hemolytic disorders. Infectious agents foster hemolysis in four ways: (1) by invading the RBC and destroying its contents (e.g., parasites such as in malaria); (2) by releasing hemolytic substances (e.g., *Clostridium perfringens*); (3) by generating an antigen-antibody reaction; and (4) by contributing to splenomegaly as a means of increasing removal of damaged RBCs from the circulation. Various agents may be toxic to RBCs and cause hemolysis. These hemolytic toxins involve chemicals such as oxidative drugs, arsenic, lead, copper, and snake venom.

Laboratory findings in hemolytic anemia are presented in Table 31-6. Treatment and management of acquired hemolytic anemias involve general supportive care until the causative agent can be eliminated or at least rendered less injurious to the RBCs. Because a hemolytic crisis is a potential consequence, the nurse needs to be ready to institute appropriate emergent therapy. Supportive care may include administering corticosteroids and blood products or removing the spleen.

GENETICS IN CLINICAL PRACTICE

Hemochromatosis

Genetic Basis

- Autosomal recessive trait
- Most common mutations: C282Y and H63D
- Genetic defect located in close proximity to the major histocompatibility complex on chromosome 6

Incidence

- Most common genetic disease in people of European ancestry
- Affects 1 in 200 to 500 in the United States
- Very low prevalence in other ethnic populations

Genetic Testing

- Genetic testing recommended for all first-degree relatives of people with disease
- American Hemochromatosis Society recommends genetic testing regardless of family history
- Useful diagnostic tests include serum iron concentration, total iron-binding capacity, and transferrin saturation
- Liver biopsy, once considered the gold standard diagnostic test, is primarily used to quantify iron deposition and estimate the prognosis and extent of disease

Clinical Implications

- Early treatment can prevent serious complications.
- Clinical expression is variable depending on dietary iron, blood loss, and other modifying factors.
- If untreated, progressive iron deposits can lead to multiple organ failure.

HEMOCHROMATOSIS

Hemochromatosis is an autosomal recessive disease characterized by increased intestinal iron absorption and, as a result, increased tissue iron deposition (see the Genetics in Clinical Practice box). It is the most common genetic disorder among whites, with an incidence of 3 to 5 per 1000 whites of European ancestry. The normal range for total body iron is 2 to 6 g. Individuals with hemochromatosis accumulate iron at a rate of 0.5 to 1.0 g each year and may exceed total iron concentrations of 50 g. Symptoms of hemochromatosis usually develop between 40 and 60 years of age. In addition to the primary genetic defect, hemochromatosis occurs secondary to diseases such as thalassemia and sideroblastic anemia. It may also be caused by liver disease and multiple blood transfusions.[20]

Early symptoms are nonspecific and include fatigue, arthralgia, impotence, abdominal pain, and weight loss. Later, the excess iron accumulates in the liver and causes liver enlargement and eventually cirrhosis. Then other organs become affected, resulting in diabetes mellitus, skin pigment changes (bronzing), cardiac changes (e.g., cardiomyopathy), arthritis, and testicular atrophy. Physical examination reveals an enlarged liver and spleen and pigmentation changes in the skin. Laboratory values demonstrate an elevated serum iron, TIBC, and serum ferritin. Molecular testing for known genetic mutations is clinically used to confirm the diagnosis. If this testing is not definitive, a liver biopsy can quantify the amount of iron and establish the diagnosis.

The goal of treatment is to remove excess iron from the body and minimize any symptoms the patient may have. Iron removal is achieved by removing 500 ml of blood each week for 2 to 3 years until the iron stores in the body are depleted. Then less frequent removal of blood is needed to maintain iron levels within normal limits. Management of organ involvement (e.g., diabetes mellitus, HF) is the same as conventional treatment for these problems. Dietary modifications may also assist in the reduction of iron accumulation, such as avoidance of vitamin C and iron supplements, uncooked seafood, and iron-rich foods. The most common causes of death are cirrhosis, liver failure, hepatic carcinoma, and cardiac failure. With early diagnosis and treatment, life expectancy is normal. However, many cases go undetected and untreated.

POLYCYTHEMIA

Polycythemia is the production and presence of increased numbers of RBCs. The increase in RBCs can be so great that blood circulation is impaired as a result of the increased blood viscosity *(hyperviscosity)* and volume *(hypervolemia).*

Etiology and Pathophysiology

The two types of polycythemia are primary polycythemia, or polycythemia vera, and secondary polycythemia (Fig. 31-5). Their etiologies and pathogenesis differ, although their complications and clinical manifestations are similar. *Polycythemia vera* is considered a chronic myeloproliferative disorder arising from a chromosomal mutation in a single pluripotent stem cell. Therefore not only are RBCs involved but also white blood cells and platelets, leading to increased production of each of these blood cells. The disease develops insidiously and follows a chronic, vacillating course. The median age at diagnosis is 60 years old with a slightly male predominance. No strong evidence supports disease association with environmental exposure, although some have been suggested. With this myeloproliferative disorder the patient has enhanced blood viscosity and blood volume and congestion of organs and tissues with blood. These patients have hypercoagulopathies that predispose them to clotting. Splenomegaly and hepatomegaly are common.[21]

Secondary polycythemia can be either hypoxia driven or hypoxia independent. In the former, hypoxia stimulates erythropoietin (EPO) production in the kidney, which in turn stimulates erythrocyte production. The need for O_2 may be due to high altitude, pulmonary disease, cardiovascular disease, alveolar hypoventilation, defective O_2 transport, or tissue hypoxia. EPO levels may return to normal once the hemoglobin is stabilized at a higher level. In this situation, secondary polycythemia is a physiologic response in which the body tries to compensate for a problem rather than a pathologic response. (Hypoxia-driven secondary polycythemia is discussed in the section on chronic obstructive pulmonary disease in Chapter 29.) In hypoxia-independent secondary polycythemia, EPO is produced by a malignant or benign tumor tissue. Serum EPO levels often remain elevated in these situations.[21]

Clinical Manifestations and Complications

Circulatory manifestations of polycythemia vera occur because of the hypertension caused by hypervolemia and hyperviscosity. They are often the first symptoms and include subjective complaints of headache, vertigo, dizziness, tinnitus, and visual disturbances. Generalized pruritus (often exacerbated by a hot bath) may be a striking symptom and is related to histamine release from an increased number of basophils. Paresthesias and *erythromelalgia* (painful burning and redness of the hands and feet) may also be present. In addition, the patient may experience angina, heart failure, intermittent claudication, and thrombophlebitis, which may be complicated by embolization. These manifestations are caused by blood vessel distention, impaired blood flow, circulatory stasis, thrombosis, and tissue hypoxia caused by the hypervolemia and hyperviscosity. The most common serious acute complication is stroke secondary to thrombosis.[21]

Hemorrhagic phenomena caused by either vessel rupture from overdistention or inadequate platelet function may result in petechiae, ecchymoses, epistaxis, or GI bleeding. Hemorrhage can be acute and catastrophic. Hepatomegaly and splenomegaly from organ engorgement may contribute to patient complaints of satiety and fullness. The patient may also experience pain from peptic ulcer caused by either increased gastric secretions or liver and spleen engorgement. *Plethora* (ruddy complexion) may also be present. Hyperuricemia is caused by the increase in RBC destruction that accompanies excessive RBC production. Uric acid is one of the products of cell destruction. As RBC destruction increases, uric acid production also increases, thus leading to hyperuricemia. This problem may cause a form of gout.

Diagnostic Studies

The following laboratory manifestations are seen in a patient with polycythemia vera: (1) elevated hemoglobin and RBC count with microcytosis; (2) low to normal EPO level (secondary polycythe-

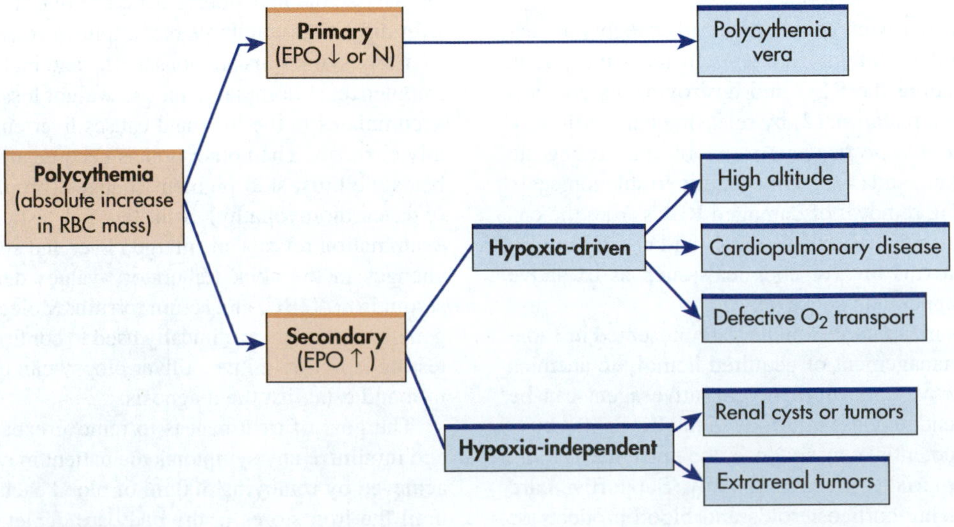

FIG. 31-5 Differentiating between primary and secondary polycythemia. *EPO,* Erythropoietin; *N,* normal.

mia will have a high level); (3) elevated WBC count with basophilia; (4) elevated platelets (thrombocytosis) and platelet dysfunction; (5) elevated leukocyte alkaline phosphatase, uric acid, and cobalamin levels; and (6) elevated histamine levels. Bone marrow examination in polycythemia vera shows hypercellularity of RBCs, WBCs, and platelets. Splenomegaly is found in 90% of patients with primary polycythemia but does not accompany secondary polycythemia.

Collaborative Care

Once the diagnosis of polycythemia vera is made, treatment is directed toward reducing blood volume and viscosity and bone marrow activity. Phlebotomy is the mainstay of treatment. The aim of phlebotomy is to reduce the hematocrit and keep it less than 45% to 48%. Generally, at the time of diagnosis 300 to 500 ml of blood may be removed every other day until the hematocrit is reduced to normal levels. An individual managed with repeated phlebotomies eventually becomes deficient in iron, although this effect is rarely symptomatic. Iron supplementation should be avoided. Hydration therapy is used to reduce the blood's viscosity. Myelosuppressive agents such as busulfan (Myleran), hydroxyurea (Hydrea), melphalan (Alkeran), and radioactive phosphorus may be given to inhibit bone marrow activity. However, because of their side effects, these treatments are usually reserved for patients at high risk for complications (e.g., thromboses). Paroxetine (Paxil) or low-dose aspirin may be used adjunctively to alleviate symptoms of *erythromelalgia* (paroxysmal peripheral dilation of peripheral blood vessels). Interferon alpha (IFN-α) is of particular use in women of childbearing age or those with intractable pruritus. Anagrelide (Agrylin) may be used to reduce the platelet count and inhibit platelet aggregation. Allopurinol may reduce the number of acute gouty attacks.[21,22]

NURSING MANAGEMENT
POLYCYTHEMIA VERA

Primary polycythemia vera is not preventable. However, because secondary polycythemia is generated by any source of hypoxia, maintaining adequate oxygenation may prevent problems. Therefore controlling chronic pulmonary disease, stopping smoking, and avoiding high altitudes may be important.

When acute exacerbations of polycythemia vera develop, the nurse has several responsibilities. Depending on the institution's policies, the nurse may either assist with or perform the phlebotomy. Fluid intake and output must be evaluated during hydration therapy to avoid fluid overload (which further complicates the circulatory congestion) and underhydration (which can cause the blood to become even more viscous). If myelosuppressive agents are used, the nurse must administer the drugs as ordered, observe the patient, and teach the patient about medication side effects.

Assessment of the patient's nutritional status in collaboration with the dietitian may be necessary to offset the inadequate food intake that can result from GI symptoms of fullness, pain, and dyspepsia. Activities must be instituted to decrease thrombus formation. The relative immobility normally imposed by hospitalization puts the patient at risk for thrombus formation. Active or passive leg exercises and ambulation when possible should be initiated.

Because of its chronic nature, polycythemia vera requires ongoing evaluation. Phlebotomy may need to be done every 2 to 3 months, reducing the blood volume by about 500 ml each time. The nurse must evaluate the patient for the development of complications.

Although the incidence is low, myelofibrosis and leukemia develop in some patients with polycythemia vera (10% and 5%, respectively). These occurrences may be caused by the chemotherapeutic drugs used to treat the disease, or they may be secondary to a disorder in the stem cells that progresses to erythroleukemia. The major cause of morbidity and mortality from polycythemia vera is related to thrombosis (e.g., stroke).

Problems of Hemostasis

The homeostatic process involves the vascular endothelium, platelets, and coagulation factors, which normally function together to arrest hemorrhage and repair vascular injury. (These mechanisms are described in Chapter 30.) Disruption in any of these components may result in bleeding or thrombotic disorders.

Three major disorders of hemostasis discussed in this section are (1) thrombocytopenia (low platelet count), (2) hemophilia and von Willebrand disease (inherited disorders of specific clotting factors), and (3) disseminated intravascular coagulation (DIC).

THROMBOCYTOPENIA

Etiology and Pathophysiology

Thrombocytopenia is a reduction of platelets below 150,000/μl (150×10^9/L). Acute, severe, or prolonged decreases from this normal range can result in abnormal hemostasis that manifests as prolonged bleeding from minor trauma to spontaneous bleeding without injury.

Platelet disorders can be inherited (e.g., Wiskott-Aldrich syndrome), but the vast majority are acquired. The causes of acquired disorders include autoimmune diseases, increased platelet consumption, splenomegaly, marrow suppression (infectious or drug mediated), and bone marrow failure (Table 31-11). Most acquired abnormalities occur following ingestion of certain foods, herbs, or drugs (Table 31-12). Although some agents are directly myelosuppressive (e.g., chemotherapy, ganciclovir [Cytovene]), the usual mechanism of thrombocytopenia caused by foods, herbs, or drugs is accelerated platelet destruction caused by drug-dependent antibodies. Antibodies attack the platelets when the offending agent binds to a platelet surface glycoprotein. A careful review of the patient's history helps distinguish these causes versus one of the causes mentioned below. For example, quinine is in tonic water and in many herbal preparations. In addition, some drugs can affect platelet aggregation. Aspirin doses as low as 81 mg (a baby aspirin) can alter platelet aggregation. Normal function is restored with the generation of newly formed platelets.[23-25]

Immune Thrombocytopenic Purpura. The most common acquired thrombocytopenia is a syndrome of abnormal destruction of circulating platelets termed *immune thrombocytopenic purpura* (ITP). It was originally termed *idiopathic thrombocytopenic purpura* because its cause was unknown. However, it is now known that ITP is an autoimmune disease. In ITP, platelets are coated with antibodies. Although these platelets function normally, when they reach the spleen, the antibody-coated platelets are recognized as foreign and are destroyed by macrophages.

Platelets normally survive 8 to 10 days. However, in ITP survival of platelets is only 1 to 3 days. Chronic ITP occurs most commonly in women between 20 and 40 years of age. Chronic ITP has a gradual onset, and transient remissions occur.[23]

TABLE 31-11 Causes of Thrombocytopenia

Inherited

Fanconi syndrome (pancytopenia)
Hereditary thrombocytopenia

Acquired

Immune

Immune thrombocytopenic purpura (ITP)
Neonatal alloimmune thrombocytopenia

Nonimmune

Shortened circulation

- Thrombotic thrombocytopenic purpura (TTP)
- Disseminated intravascular coagulation (DIC)
- Heparin-induced thrombocytopenia (HIT)
- Splenomegaly/splenic sequestration

Turbulent blood flow (hemangiomas, abnormal cardiac valves, intra-aortic balloon pumps)

Decreased production

- Drug-induced marrow suppression
- Chemotherapy
- Viral infection (hepatitis C virus, HIV, cytomegalovirus)
- Bacterial infection (sepsis)
- Alcoholism/bone marrow suppression
- Myelodysplastic syndrome (MDS)
- Myelofibrosis
- Aplastic anemia
- Hematologic malignancy (leukemias, lymphomas, myeloma)
- Solid tumor infiltrating bone marrow
- Radiation to the bone

HIV, Human immunodeficiency virus.

TABLE 31-12 Food, Drug, and Herbal Causes of Thrombocytopenia*

- Thiazide diuretics
- Alcohol
- Estrogen
- Chemotherapeutic drugs
- Digoxin
- Nonsteroidal antiinflammatory drugs: ibuprofen (Advil, Motrin), indomethacin (Indocin), naproxen (Naproxyn, Aleve)
- Antibiotics: penicillins, cephalosporins, sulfonamides
- Other antiinfectives: rifampin (Rifadin), ganciclovir (Cytovene), amphotericin B
- Analgesics: aspirin and aspirin-containing drugs, acetaminophen
- Antipsychotics and antiseizures: haloperidol (Haldol), valproate (Depakene), lithium
- Platelet glycoprotein inhibitors: abciximab (ReoPro), tirofiban (Aggrastat), eptifibatide (Integrilin)
- H_2 antagonists: cimetidine (Tagamet), ranitidine (Zantac)
- Gold compounds: auranofin (Ridaura)
- Spices: ginger, cumin, turmeric, cloves
- Vitamins: vitamin C, vitamin E
- Heparin
- Herbs: angelica, bilberry, evening primrose, feverfew, garlic, ginger, ginkgo biloba, ginseng, goldenseal
- Quinine compounds: tonic water, china bark, Peruvian bark, yellow cinchona

*List is not all-inclusive.

Thrombotic Thrombocytopenic Purpura. *Thrombotic thrombocytopenic purpura* (TTP) is an uncommon syndrome characterized by hemolytic anemia, thrombocytopenia, neurologic abnormalities, fever (in the absence of infection), and renal abnormalities; not all features are always present in all patients. Because it is almost always associated with hemolytic-uremic syndrome, it is often referred to as TTP-HUS. The disease is associated with enhanced agglutination of platelets, which form microthrombi that deposit in arterioles and capillaries. In most cases, the cause is due to the deficiency of a plasma enzyme (ADAMTS13) that usually breaks down the von Willebrand (vWF) clotting factor (vWF is the most important protein mediating platelet adhesion to damaged endothelial cells) into normal size. Without the enzyme, unusually large vWF multimers attach to activated platelets, thereby promoting platelet aggregation.

TTP is seen primarily in adults between 20 and 50 years of age, with a slight female predominance. The syndrome may be idiopathic (thought to be due to an autoimmune disorder against ADAMTS13), but may be due to certain drug toxicities (e.g., chemotherapy, cyclosporine, quinine, oral contraceptives, valacyclovir [Valtrex]), pregnancy, infection, or the result of a known autoimmune disorder such as systemic lupus erythematosus or scleroderma. TTP is a medical emergency because bleeding and clotting occur simultaneously.[26]

Heparin-Induced Thrombocytopenia and Thrombosis Syndrome. One of the risks associated with the broad and increasing use of heparin is the development of the life-threatening condition called *heparin-induced thrombocytopenia and thrombosis syndrome* (HITTS), also called white clot syndrome or HIT. HITTS can be mild (type I) or severe (type II). An estimated 5% to 25% of patients on heparin therapy develop HITTS. A lower incidence is seen in patients receiving porcine preparations of heparin as compared with other types. The major clinical problem of HITTS is venous thrombosis; arterial thrombosis can also develop. Deep vein thromboses and pulmonary emboli most commonly result as a complication of the thromboses. Additional complications may include arterial vascular infarcts resulting in skin necrosis, stroke, and end-organ damage, such as to the kidneys. There are rarely symptoms of bleeding because the platelet count rarely drops below 60,000/μl.

Type I HITTS is usually of no clinical consequence. In type II HITTS, platelet destruction and vascular endothelial injury are the two major responses to what is believed to be an immune-mediated response to heparin. Platelet factor 4 (PF4) binds to heparin; this complex then binds to the platelet surface, leading to further platelet activation and release of more PF4, thus creating a positive feedback loop. Antibodies are created against this complex and they are removed prematurely from circulation, leading to thrombocytopenia and platelet-fibrin thrombi. Platelet aggregation also induces heparin to be neutralized. Thus more heparin is required to maintain therapeutic activated partial thromboplastin times.[27-29]

Clinical Manifestations

Many patients with thrombocytopenia are usually asymptomatic. The most common symptom is bleeding, usually mucosal or cutaneous. Mucosal bleeding may manifest as epistaxis and gingival bleeding, and large bullous hemorrhages may appear on the buccal mucosa because of the lack of vessel protection by the submucosal tissue. Bleeding into the skin is manifested as petechiae, purpura, or superficial ecchymoses (Fig. 31-6). *Petechiae* are small, flat, pinpoint, red or reddish-brown microhemorrhages. When the platelet count is low, RBCs may leak out of the blood vessels and into the skin to cause petechiae. When petechiae are numerous, the resulting reddish skin bruise is called *purpura*. Larger purplish lesions caused by hemorrhage are termed *ecchymoses*. Ecchymoses may be flat or raised; pain and tenderness sometimes are present.

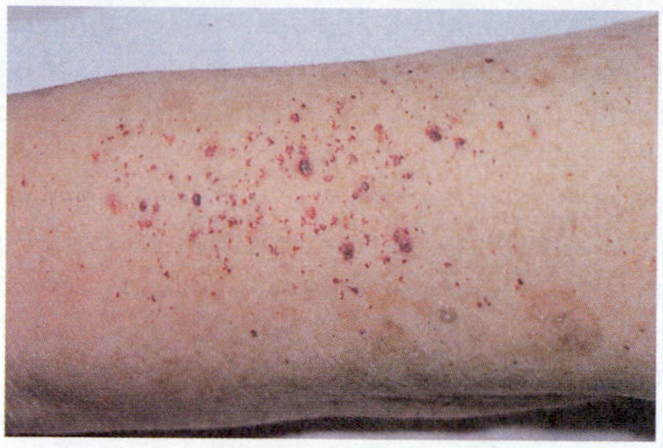

FIG. 31-6 Acute idiopathic thrombocytopenic purpura commonly manifests with purpuric lesions of this kind, although they may often be more widespread by the time medical attention is sought.

Prolonged bleeding after routine procedures such as venipuncture or IM injection may also indicate thrombocytopenia. Because the bleeding may be internal, the nurse must also be aware of manifestations that reflect this type of blood loss, including weakness, fainting, dizziness, tachycardia, abdominal pain, and hypotension.

The major complication of thrombocytopenia is hemorrhage. The hemorrhage may be insidious or acute and internal or external. It may occur in any area of the body, including the joints, retina, and brain. Cerebral hemorrhage may be fatal in persons with ITP. Insidious hemorrhage may first be detected by discovering the anemia that accompanies blood loss.

Because thrombocytopenia can be accompanied by vascular thromboses in some of these disorders, signs and symptoms of vascular ischemic problems can manifest (see Chapter 38). For example, subtle confusion, headache, or even serious manifestations such as seizures and coma due to TTP-related thrombosis may be seen. Because signs and symptoms may be subtle, astute and thorough assessment of the patient is essential.

Diagnostic Studies

The platelet count is decreased in cases of thrombocytopenia. Any reduction below 150,000/μl (150×10^9/L) may be termed *thrombocytopenia.* However, prolonged bleeding from trauma or injury does not usually occur until platelet counts are less than 50,000/μl (50×10^9/L). When the count drops below 20,000/μl (20×10^9/L), spontaneous, life-threatening hemorrhages (e.g., intracranial bleeding) can occur. Platelet transfusions are generally not recommended until the count is below 10,000/μl (20×10^9/L) unless the patient is actively bleeding. Examination of the peripheral blood smear may assist in distinguishing acquired disorders such as ITP and TTP from congenital disorders, which may be indicated by abnormally sized platelets.

Laboratory tests that assess secondary hemostasis or coagulation, such as the prothrombin time (PT) and activated partial thromboplastin time (aPTT), can be normal even in severe thrombocytopenia. If they are elevated, this may point toward *disseminated intravascular coagulation* (DIC). Bone marrow examination is done to rule out production problems as the cause of thrombocytopenia (e.g., leukemia, aplastic anemia, other myeloproliferative disorders). Specific assays, such as ITP-positive antigen specific assay or 14C-serotonin release assay for HIT, can be done to assist with the diagnosis. In TTP, testing for deficiency of ADAMTS13 is not widely clinically available, so an increase of lactic dehydrogenase (LDH) is used to help establish the diagnosis. Bone marrow analysis is done if other tests are inconclusive, especially in older patients because of a higher suspicion of an underlying bone marrow disorder. When destruction of circulating platelets is the etiology, bone marrow analysis shows *megakaryocytes* (precursors of platelets) to be normal or increased, even though circulating platelets are reduced. The absence or decreased numbers of megakaryocytes on bone marrow biopsy is consistent with thrombocytopenia caused by decreased bone marrow production (e.g., aplastic anemia). Special blood analyses using flow cytometry and other techniques can detect antiplatelet antibodies as the source of destruction.

The nurse needs to closely monitor the platelet count and other coagulation studies. In addition, the nurse should monitor the patient's hemoglobin and hematocrit levels and observe the patient for cardiopulmonary distress and other manifestations of anemia. When thrombocytopenia occurs with anemia characterized by altered RBC morphology, including *spherocytes* (small, globular, completely hemoglobinated erythrocytes), fragmented cells (schistocytes), and pronounced reticulocytosis, a diagnosis of TTP should be suspected. These findings are partially a result of intravascular fibrin deposition causing a "slicing" of RBCs. In TTP, thrombocytopenia may be severe, but coagulation studies are normal.

Collaborative Care

Collaborative care of thrombocytopenia differs based on the etiology of the thrombocytopenia. Discussion of management strategies for these different etiologies follows (Table 31-13).

Immune Thrombocytopenic Purpura. Multiple therapies are used to manage the patient with ITP. If the patient is asymptomatic, therapy may not be used unless the patient's platelet count is less than 30,000/μl. Corticosteroids (e.g., prednisone) are used initially to treat ITP because of their ability to suppress the phagocytic response of splenic macrophages. This alters the spleen's recognition of platelets and increases the life span of the platelets. In addition, corticosteroids depress antibody formation. Corticosteroids also reduce capillary fragility and bleeding time. The mechanism of action for this response is poorly understood. If there are neurologic manifestations related to intracranial bleeding, high-dose methylprednisolone (Solu-Medrol) can be administered IV. Methylprednisolone has also been used when patients are resistant to prednisone.

Splenectomy is indicated if the patient does not respond to prednisone initially or requires unacceptably high doses to maintain an adequate platelet count. Approximately 80% of patients benefit from splenectomy, resulting in a complete or partial remission. The effectiveness of splenectomy is based on four factors. First, the spleen contains an abundance of the macrophages that sequester and destroy platelets. Second, structural features of the spleen enhance antibody-coated platelets and macrophage interaction. Third, some antibody synthesis occurs in the spleen; thus antiplatelet antibodies decrease after splenectomy. Fourth, the spleen normally sequesters approximately one third of the platelets, so its removal increases the number of platelets in circulation. Post-splenectomy refractory patients should be evaluated for an accessory spleen and have subsequent medical therapies tailored to the individual.

High doses of IV immunoglobulin (IVIG) and a component of IVIG, anti-Rh_o(D) (anti-D, WinRho) may be used in the patient who is unresponsive to corticosteroids or splenectomy. These agents work by competing with the antiplatelet antibodies for macrophage receptors. They effectively raise the platelet count, but the beneficial effects may be temporary.

Hematology System

TABLE 31-13 ***COLLABORATIVE CARE*** **Thrombocytopenia**

Diagnostic
History and physical examination
Bone marrow aspiration and biopsy
CBC including platelet count
Specific studies (e.g., ITP antibody)

Collaborative Therapy
Immune Thrombocytopenic Purpura
Corticosteroids
Platelet transfusions
Splenectomy
Intravenous immunoglobulin
Anti-Rh_o(D)
Danazol
Immunosuppressives (e.g., rituximab [Rituxan], cyclosporine, cyclophosphamide [Cytoxan], azathioprine [Imuran], mycophenolate mofetil [CellCept])
High-dose cyclophosphamide or combination chemotherapy
Thrombotic Thrombocytopenic Purpura
Plasmapheresis (plasma exchange)
High-dose prednisone
Splenectomy
Dextran
Chemotherapy (vincristine [Oncovin], vinblastine [Velban])
Immunosuppressives (cyclophosphamide [Cytoxan], rituximab [Rituxan])
Heparin-Induced Thrombocytopenia and Thrombosis Syndrome
Direct thrombin inhibitor (lepirudin [Refludan], argatroban [Acova])
Indirect thrombin inhibitor (fondaparinux [Arixtra])
Plasmapheresis (plasma exchange)
Protamine sulfate
Coumadin
Thrombolytic agents
Decreased Platelet Production
Identification and treatment of cause
Corticosteroids
Platelet transfusions
Oprelvekin (Neumega)

CBC, Complete blood count; *ITP*, idiopathic thrombocytopenic purpura.

Danazol (Danocrine), an androgen, is often used along with steroids in some patients. Although the mechanism is not totally understood, it is suggested that danazol increases CD4 T cells, thereby reducing the immune response. Immunosuppressive therapy used in refractory cases includes rituximab (Rituxan), cyclophosphamide (Cytoxan), azathioprine (Imuran), cyclosporine, and mycophenolate mofetil (CellCept). High-dose cyclophosphamide and combination chemotherapy is third-line therapy.[24]

Drug Alert - *Rituximab (Rituxan)*
- *Monitor patient for signs of severe hypersensitivity infusion reactions, especially with first infusion.*
- *Manifestations may include hypotension, bronchospasm, dysrhythmias, angioedema, and cardiogenic shock.*

Platelet transfusions may be used to increase platelet counts in cases of life-threatening hemorrhage. Platelets should not be administered prophylactically because of the possibility of antibody formation. The usual indication for administering platelets is for a platelet count ≤10,000/μl or if there is bleeding before a procedure. Several studies indicate that the risk of bleeding may not be substantial until the count is ≤5000/μl.[30] ABO compatibility is not a necessary prerequisite for platelet transfusions. However, after multiple platelet transfusions, a patient may develop anti-HLA antibodies to the transfused platelets.

By using lymphocyte typing to match HLA types of the donor and the recipient, multiple platelet transfusions can be given with fewer complications. In addition, the patient may be premedicated with an antihistamine (e.g., diphenhydramine [Benadryl]) and hydrocortisone to decrease the possibility of reacting to platelet transfusions. Aminocaproic acid (Amicar), an antifibrinolytic agent, may be used for severe bleeding. Aspirin and aspirin-containing compounds should be avoided in the patient with thrombocytopenia.[23]

Thrombotic Thrombocytopenic Purpura. TTP may be treated in a variety of ways. The first step is to treat the underlying disorder (e.g., infection) or remove the causative agent, if identified. If untreated, TTP usually results in irreversible renal failure and death. Corticosteroids are used initially. Plasma exchange or plasmapheresis (see Chapter 14) may be needed to aggressively reverse the process. This reverses platelet consumption by supplying the appropriate vWF and enzyme (ADAMTS13) and removing the large vWF molecules binding with platelets. Treatment should be continued daily until the patient's platelet counts normalize and hemolysis has ceased. Splenectomy, corticosteroids, dextran (antiplatelet agent), and vincristine (Oncovin) or vinblastine (Velban) have also been used with success. Recently, immunosuppressive therapy such as cyclophosphamide and rituximab has been used. The administration of platelets is generally contraindicated because this may lead to new vWF-platelet complexes and increased clotting.[31]

Heparin-Induced Thrombocytopenia and Thrombosis Syndrome. Heparin must be discontinued when HITTS is first recognized, which is usually if the patient's platelet count has fallen 50% or more from its baseline or if a thrombus forms while the patient is on heparin therapy. Heparin flushes for vascular catheters should also be stopped.

To maintain anticoagulation, the patient should be started on a direct thrombin inhibitor, such as lepirudin (Refludan) or argatroban. Fondaparinux (Arixtra), a factor Xa inhibitor (indirect thrombin inhibitor), has also been used. Coumadin may be started when the platelet count has reached 100,000/μl. If the clotting is severe, the most commonly used treatment modalities are plasmapheresis to clear the platelet-aggregating IgG from the blood, protamine sulfate to interrupt the circulating heparin, thrombolytic agents to treat the thromboembolic events, and surgery to remove clots. Platelet transfusions are not effective because they may enhance thromboembolic events.[29,32,33] Patients who have had HITTS should never be given heparin or low-molecular-weight heparin. This should be clearly marked on the patient's medical record.

Acquired Thrombocytopenia from Decreased Platelet Production. The management of acquired thrombocytopenia is based on identifying the cause and treating the disease or removing the causative agent. If the precipitating factor is unknown, the patient may receive corticosteroids. Platelet transfusions are given if life-threatening hemorrhage develops. Splenectomy is not used because the spleen is not contributing to this type of thrombocytopenia.

Often, acquired thrombocytopenia is caused by another underlying condition (e.g., aplastic anemia, leukemia) or therapy used to treat another problem. For example, in acute leukemia all blood cell types may be depressed. Additionally, the patient may receive chemotherapeutic drugs that cause bone marrow suppression. If the patient can be adequately supported throughout the course of chemotherapy-induced thrombocytopenia, the thrombocytopenia will also resolve.

Oprelvekin (Neumega), a platelet growth factor that is a recombinant form of interleukin-11, stimulates the bone marrow to produce platelets. It may be used to treat chemotherapy-induced thrombocytopenia. (Oprelvekin is discussed in Chapter 16 and Table 16-18.)

Since thrombopoietin (a hematopoietic growth factor that stimulates the bone marrow to make platelets) was discovered in 1994, there has been much progress in the development of recombinant thrombopoietin. However, no thrombopoietin product has yet been approved for clinical use.

NURSING MANAGEMENT THROMBOCYTOPENIA

Nursing Assessment

Subjective and objective data that should be obtained from a patient with thrombocytopenia are presented in Table 31-14.

Nursing Diagnoses

Nursing diagnoses for the patient with thrombocytopenia may include, but are not limited to, those presented in NCP 31-2.

Planning

The overall goals are that the patient with thrombocytopenia will (1) have no gross or occult bleeding, (2) maintain vascular integrity, and (3) manage home care to prevent any complications related to an increased risk for bleeding.

Nursing Implementation

Health Promotion. It is important for the nurse to discourage excessive use of over-the-counter (OTC) medications known to be possible causes of acquired thrombocytopenia. Many medications contain aspirin as an ingredient. Aspirin reduces platelet adhesiveness, thus contributing to bleeding.

It is also important for the nurse to encourage persons to have a complete medical evaluation if manifestations of bleeding tendencies (e.g., prolonged epistaxis, petechiae) develop. In addition, the nurse must observe for early signs of thrombocytopenia in the patient receiving cancer chemotherapy drugs.

Acute Intervention. The goal during acute episodes of thrombocytopenia is to prevent or control hemorrhage[34] (see NCP 31-2). In the patient with thrombocytopenia, bleeding is usually from superficial sites; deep bleeding (into muscles, joints, and abdomen) usually occurs only when clotting factors are diminished. It is important to emphasize that a seemingly minor nosebleed or new petechiae may indicate potential hemorrhage and the health care provider should be notified. Bleeding from the posterior nasopharynx may be difficult to detect because the blood may be swallowed. If an IM or subcutaneous injection is unavoidable, the use of a small-gauge needle and application of direct pressure for at least 5 to 10 minutes after injection is indicated or application of an ice pack may be helpful. The patient needs to understand the importance of adherence to self-care measures that reduce the risk of bleeding (Table 31-15).

In a woman with thrombocytopenia, menstrual blood loss may exceed the usual amount and duration. Counting sanitary napkins used during menses is another important intervention to detect excess blood loss. Fifty milliliters of blood will completely soak a sanitary napkin. Suppression of menses with hormonal agents may be indicated during predictable periods of thrombocytopenia to reduce blood loss from menses (e.g., during chemotherapy and hematopoietic stem cell transplantation).

TABLE 31-14 NURSING ASSESSMENT Thrombocytopenia

Subjective Data

Important Health Information

Past health history: Recent hemorrhage, excessive bleeding, or viral illness; HIV infection; cancer (especially leukemia or lymphoma); aplastic anemia; systemic lupus erythematosus; cirrhosis; exposure to radiation or toxic chemicals; disseminated intravascular coagulation

Medications: Use of thiazide diuretics, furosemide (Lasix), aspirin, acetaminophen, estrogens, gold salts, nonsteroidal antiinflammatory drugs, phenylbutazone (Butazolidine), penicillins, cephalothin, streptomycin, sulfonamides, quinidine, quinine, phenobarbital, methyldopa (Aldomet), phenytoin (Dilantin), chlorpropamide (Diabinese), meprobamate (Equanil), chemotherapy drugs, other drugs listed in Table 31-12

Functional Health Patterns

Health perception–health management: Family history of bleeding problems; malaise

Nutritional-metabolic: Bleeding gingiva; coffee-ground or bloody vomitus; easy bruising

Elimination: Hematuria, dark or bloody stools

Activity-exercise: Fatigue, weakness, fainting; epistaxis, hemoptysis; dyspnea

Cognitive-perceptual: Pain and tenderness in bleeding areas (e.g., abdomen, head, extremities); headache

Sexuality-reproductive: Menorrhagia, metrorrhagia

Objective Data

General

Fever, lethargy

Integumentary

Petechiae, ecchymoses, purpura

Gastrointestinal

Splenomegaly, abdominal distention; guaiac-positive stools

Possible Findings

Platelet count $<150{,}000/\mu l$ ($150 \times 10^9/L$), prolonged bleeding time, ↓ hemoglobin and hematocrit; normal or ↑ megakaryocytes in bone marrow examination

HIV, Human immunodeficiency virus.

The proper administration of platelet transfusions is an important nursing responsibility. Platelet concentrates, derived from fresh whole blood, can increase the platelet level effectively. Centrifuging 500 ml of whole blood derives 1 unit of platelets, a yellow liquid that is usually 30 to 50 ml in volume. Platelet concentrates from multiple units of blood (usually from six to eight different donors) can be pooled together for a single administration. The degree of increase or increment from a pooled platelet product varies widely and is usually measured by performing a platelet count within 1 hour following the transfusion.

Platelet transfusions can also be prepared by pheresing or removing the platelets from a single donor. This may be indicated when HLA-matched platelets are needed, especially for patients requiring multiple platelet transfusions. In this procedure, blood is removed from the donor, the platelets are removed, and the rest of the blood is reinfused into the donor. This procedure results in 200 to 400 ml of platelets and plasma. Once acquired from a donor, platelets can

NURSING CARE PLAN 31-2

Patient with Thrombocytopenia

NURSING DIAGNOSIS **Impaired oral mucous membrane** *related to* low platelet counts and/or effects of pathologic conditions and treatment *as evidenced by* oral bleeding and blood-filled bullae

PATIENT GOAL Experiences lesion-free oral mucosa without bleeding

OUTCOMES (NOC)

Oral Hygiene

- Bleeding ____
- Oral mucosa lesions ____

Measurement Scale

1 = Severe
2 = Substantial
3 = Moderate
4 = Mild
5 = None

INTERVENTIONS (NIC) and *RATIONALES*

Oral Health Restoration

- Monitor lips, tongue, mucous membranes, tonsillar fossae, and gums for moisture, color, texture, presence of debris and infection using good lighting and a tongue blade *to provide information for planning interventions.*
- Assist the patient to select soft, bland, and nonacidic foods *to decrease irritation of oral mucosa.*
- Use a soft toothbrush for removal of dental debris.
- Use toothettes or disposable foam swabs *to stimulate and clean cavity with minimal trauma to gingiva.*
- Instruct and assist patient to perform oral hygiene after eating and as often as needed *to avoid breakdown of oral mucosa.*
- Avoid use of lemon-glycerin swabs *to prevent excessive drying of the mucosa.*

NURSING DIAGNOSIS **Risk for injury** *related to* low platelet counts and treatments

PATIENT GOALS
1. Maintains tissue integrity
2. Has no evidence of bleeding or bruising

OUTCOMES (NOC)

Blood Coagulation

- Bleeding ____
- Bruising ____
- Petechiae ____
- Ecchymosis ____
- Purpura ____
- Hematuria ____
- Hemoptysis ____

Measurement Scale

1 = Severe
2 = Substantial
3 = Moderate
4 = Mild
5 = None

INTERVENTIONS (NIC) and *RATIONALES*

Bleeding Precautions

- Monitor for signs and symptoms of persistent bleeding (e.g., check all secretions for frank or occult blood) *to detect internal bleeding.*
- Monitor coagulation studies, including prothrombin time (PT), partial thromboplastin time (PTT), fibrinogen, fibrin degradation/split products, and platelet counts *to determine bleeding risk.*
- Avoid injections (IV, IM, or subcutaneous) *to prevent bleeding into tissue surrounding puncture site.*
- Use electric razor instead of straight-edge razor for shaving *to reduce potential for skin nicks.*
- Protect patient from trauma that may cause bleeding *to reduce tissue trauma and subsequent bleeding into tissue.*
- Administer blood products (e.g., platelets, fresh frozen plasma) *to replace coagulation factors.*
- Teach patient to avoid aspirin or other anticoagulants *to prevent additional bleeding risk.*

NURSING DIAGNOSIS **Ineffective management of therapeutic regimen** *related to* lack of knowledge of disease process, activity, and medication *as evidenced by* frequent questioning about disease management, anxiety, restlessness

PATIENT GOAL Verbalizes required knowledge and skills to manage disease process at home

OUTCOMES (NOC)

Knowledge: Disease Process

- Description of specific disease process ____
- Description of signs and symptoms ____
- Description of usual disease course ____
- Description of signs and symptoms of complications ____

Measurement Scale

1 = None
2 = Limited
3 = Moderate
4 = Substantial
5 = Extensive

INTERVENTIONS (NIC) and *RATIONALES*

Teaching: Disease Process

- Appraise patient's current level of knowledge related to specific disease process *to plan appropriate interventions.*
- Describe disease process.
- Describe common signs and symptoms of the disease.
- Discuss treatment/therapy options *to decrease anxiety and prevent complications.*
- Discuss lifestyle changes that may be required to prevent future complications and/or control the disease process *so patient will be knowledgeable and able to manage own care or direct others in care.*
- Refer patient to local community agencies/support groups.
- Provide the phone numbers to call if complications occur.

TABLE 31-15 PATIENT AND FAMILY TEACHING GUIDE
Thrombocytopenia

This instruction sheet explains precautions you should take to protect yourself when your platelet count is low. Please make sure to ask your health care provider specific precautions you should take that relate to your bleeding risk factors.

- Notify your health care provider of any manifestations of bleeding. These include the following:
  - Black, tarry, or bloody bowel movements
  - Black or bloody vomit, sputum, or urine
  - Bruising or small red or purple spots on the skin
  - Bleeding from the mouth or anywhere in the body
  - Headache or changes in how well you can see
  - Difficulty talking, sudden weakness of an arm or leg, or feeling confused
- Ask your health care provider regarding restrictions in your normal activities, such as vigorous exercise, lifting weights, etc. Generally, walking can be done safely and should be done with sturdy shoes or slippers. If you are weak and at risk for falling, get help or supervision when getting out of bed.
- Do not blow your nose forcefully; gently pat it with a tissue if needed. For a nosebleed, keep your head up and apply firm pressure to the nostrils and bridge of your nose. If bleeding continues, place an ice bag over the bridge of your nose and the nape of your neck. If you are unable to stop a nosebleed after 10 min, call your health care provider.
- Do not bend down with your head lower than your waist.
- Prevent constipation by drinking plenty of fluids and do not strain when having a bowel movement. Your health care provider may prescribe a stool softener. Do not use a suppository, an enema, or a rectal thermometer without the permission of your health care provider.
- Shave only with an electric razor; do not use blades.
- Do not pluck your eyebrows or other body hair.
- Do not puncture your skin, such as getting tattoos or body piercing.
- Avoid using any medication that can prolong clotting, such as aspirin. Other medications and herbs can have similar effects. If you are unsure about any medication, ask your health care provider or pharmacist about it in relation to your thrombocytopenia.
- Use a soft-bristle toothbrush to prevent injuring the gums. Flossing is also usually safe if it is done gently using the thin tape floss. Do not use alcohol-based mouthwashes as they can dry your gums and increase bleeding.
- Women who are menstruating should keep track of the number of pads that are used per day. When you start using more pads per day than usual or bleed more days, notify your health care provider. Do not use tampons; use sanitary pads only.
- Ask your health care provider before you have any invasive procedures done, such as a dental cleaning, manicure, or pedicure.

be stored at room temperature for 1 to 5 days. Gentle agitation of the bag is useful to prevent the platelets from adhering to the plastic. In a severely immunocompromised patient, these products are also irradiated to further ensure WBC removal and prevent the complication of graft-versus-host disease (see Chapter 14).

Again, it should be noted that many of these disorders may be accompanied by vascular clotting and appropriate assessment and management should be taken (see Chapter 38).

Ambulatory and Home Care. The patient with ITP who is receiving corticosteroids should be monitored frequently for the response to therapy. If the ITP is reversed by splenectomy, there is usually no recurrence. The person with acquired thrombocytopenia must be taught to avoid causative agents when possible (see Table 31-12). If the causative agents cannot be avoided (e.g., chemotherapy), the patient should learn to avoid injury or trauma during these periods and to detect the clinical signs and symptoms of bleeding caused by thrombocytopenia (see Table 31-15). The patient with either ITP or acquired thrombocytopenia should have planned periodic medical evaluations to assess the patient's status and to intercede in situations in which exacerbations and bleeding are likely to occur.

GENETICS IN CLINICAL PRACTICE
Hemophilia A and B

Genetic Basis
- X-linked recessive disorder
- Mutations in gene that encodes clotting factor VIII (hemophilia A) or clotting factor IX (hemophilia B)

Incidence
- 1 in 5000 to 10,000 male births (hemophilia A)
- 1 in 30,000 to 50,000 male births (hemophilia B)

Genetic Testing
- Possible with DNA technology

Clinical Implications
- Female carriers will transmit the genetic defect to 50% of their sons, and 50% of their daughters will be carriers.
- Males with hemophilia will not transmit the genetic defect to their sons, but all of their daughters will be carriers.
- Female hemophilia can occur if a male with hemophilia mates with a female carrier. However, this is a rare situation.
- Clinical manifestations of hemophilia A and B are very similar.
- Replacement therapy is available for factors VIII and IX (see Table 31-18).

Evaluation

The expected outcomes for the patient with thrombocytopenia are presented in NCP 31-2.

HEMOPHILIA AND VON WILLEBRAND DISEASE

Hemophilia is a sex-linked recessive genetic disorder caused by defective or deficient coagulation factor (see the Genetics in Clinical Practice box and Fig. 14-4). (Sex-linked genetic disorders are discussed in Chapter 14.) The two major forms of hemophilia, which can occur in mild to severe forms, are hemophilia A (classic hemophilia, factor VIII deficiency) and hemophilia B (Christmas disease, factor IX deficiency). von Willebrand's disease is a related disorder involving a deficiency of the von Willebrand coagulation protein. Factor VIII is synthesized in the liver and circulates as a complex with von Willebrand factor (vWF).[35,36]

Hemophilia A is the most common form of hemophilia; it makes up approximately 80% of all cases. The incidence of hemophilia A is approximately 1 in 5000 to 10,000 males; hemophilia B is seen in 1 in 30,000 to 50,000 males. von Willebrand's disease is considered the most common congenital bleeding disorder in humans, with estimates as high as 1 or 2 in 100. However, because this disease can exist in mild to severe forms, life-threatening hemorrhage in patients is rare.[36-38] The deficiency and inheritance patterns of these three forms of inherited coagulopathies are compared in Table 31-16.

Clinical Manifestations and Complications

Clinical manifestations and complications related to hemophilia include (1) slow, persistent, prolonged bleeding from minor trauma and small cuts (Figs. 31-7 and 31-8); (2) delayed bleeding after

TABLE 31-16 Comparison of Types of Hemophilia

Disorder	Deficiency	Inheritance Pattern
Hemophilia A	Factor VIII	Recessive sex-linked (transmitted by female carriers, displayed almost exclusively in men)
Hemophilia B	Factor IX	Recessive sex-linked (transmitted by female carriers, displayed almost exclusively in men)
von Willebrand's disease	vWF, variable factor VIII deficiencies and platelet dysfunction	Autosomal dominant, seen in both sexes Recessive (in severe forms of the disease)

vWF, von Willebrand factor.

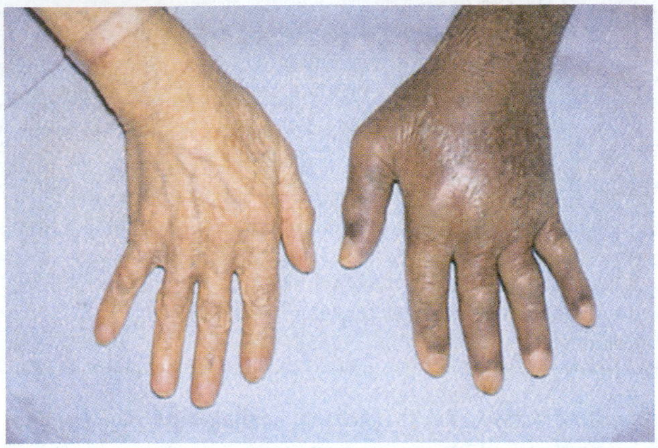

FIG. 31-7 Severe ecchymosis of the left hand in a person with hemophilia following a minor cut.

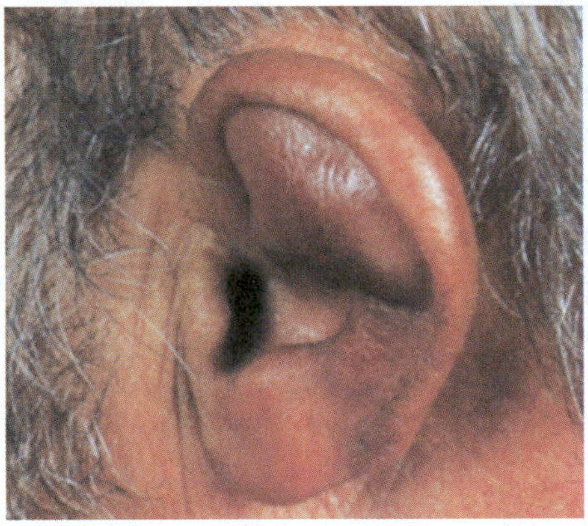

FIG. 31-8 Hematoma that developed in a person with hemophilia after trauma to the ear.

minor injuries (the delay may be several hours or days); (3) uncontrollable hemorrhage after dental extractions or irritation of the gingiva with a hard-bristle toothbrush; (4) epistaxis, especially after a blow to the face; (5) GI bleeding from ulcers and gastritis; (6) hematuria from GU trauma and splenic rupture resulting from falls or abdominal trauma; (7) ecchymoses and subcutaneous hematomas; (8) neurologic signs, such as pain, anesthesia, and paralysis, which may develop from nerve compression caused by hematoma formation; and (9) hemarthrosis (bleeding into the joints) (Fig. 31-9), which may lead to joint injury and deformity severe enough to cause crippling (most commonly in the knees, elbows, shoulders, hips, and ankles).

In children these symptoms may lead to the diagnosis. In adults, these developments may be the first sign of a newly diagnosed mild form of the disease that escaped detection through a

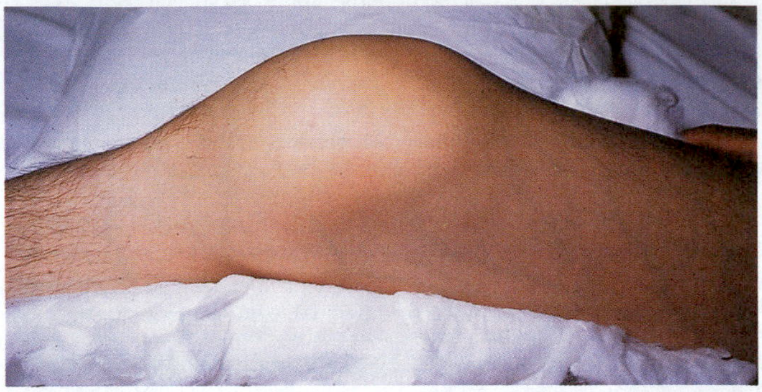

FIG. 31-9 Acute hemarthrosis of the knee is a common complication of hemophilia.

childhood free of major injuries, dental procedures, or surgeries. All clinical manifestations relate to bleeding, and any bleeding episode in persons with hemophilia may lead to a life-threatening hemorrhage.

Historically, hemophilia was a disease of childhood because of early death from complications. In the early 1900s the average life expectancy was 11 years. By the 1970s, advances in treatment enabled persons with hemophilia to have an average life expectancy of 68 years. Unfortunately, the acquired immunodeficiency syndrome (AIDS) epidemic and the HIV contamination of blood products in the 1980s caused the majority of hemophilia deaths in the late 1980s. However, longer-term survival (up to 72 years old) is now being observed because of improved preparation of replacement products, improved screening of blood donor populations, and use of recombinant replacement factors. The development of hepatitis C in hemophilia patients was also common for many years because of lack of an available test to detect it and the use of pooled blood products. However, hepatitis C antibody screening is now routinely done on all donated blood and blood products.[35]

Diagnostic Studies

Laboratory studies are used to determine the type of hemophilia present. Any factor deficiency within the intrinsic system (factors VIII, IX, XI, or XII or vWF) will yield the laboratory results presented in Table 31-17.

Collaborative Care

The goals of collaborative care are to prevent and treat bleeding. Collaborative care for persons with hemophilia or von Willebrand's disease requires the provision of preventive care, the use of replacement therapy during acute bleeding episodes and as prophylaxis, and the treatment of the complications of the disease and its therapy.

Replacement of deficient clotting factors is the primary means of supporting a patient with hemophilia. In addition to treating

TABLE 31-17 Laboratory Results in Hemophilia

Test	Comments
Prothrombin time	No involvement of extrinsic system
Thrombin time	No impairment of thrombin-fibrinogen reaction
Platelet count	Adequate platelet production
Partial thromboplastin time	Prolonged because of deficiency in any intrinsic clotting system factor
Bleeding time	Prolonged in von Willebrand's disease because of structurally defective platelets; normal in hemophilia A and B because platelets not affected
Factor assays	Reduction of factor VIII in hemophilia A, vWF in von Willebrand's disease; reduction of factor IX in hemophilia B

vWF, von Willebrand factor.

TABLE 31-18 *DRUG THERAPY* Replacement Factors Used in Treating Hemophilia

Factor VIII	Factor IX
Advate	Bebulin VH
Alphanate	Benefix
Autoplex	Konyne 80
Bioclate	Mononine
Feiba VH Immuno	Profilnine SD
Helixate FS	Thrombate III
Hemofil M	
Humate P	
Hyate: C	
Koāte-DVI, Koāte-HP	
Kogenate	
Monarc M	
Monoclate P	
Recombinate	
ReFacto	

acute crises, replacement therapy may be given before surgery and dental care as a prophylactic measure. Examples of replacement therapy are listed in Table 31-18. Fresh frozen plasma, once commonly used for replacement therapy, is rarely used today.

For mild hemophilia A and certain subtypes of von Willebrand's disease, desmopressin acetate (also known as DDAVP), a synthetic analog of vasopressin, may be used to stimulate an increase in factor VIII and vWF. This drug acts on endothelial cells to cause the release of vWF, which subsequently binds with factor VIII, thus increasing their concentration. It can be administered intravenously, subcutaneously, or by intranasal spray. Beneficial effects (e.g., decreased bleeding time) of DDAVP, when administered IV, are seen within 30 minutes and can last for more than 12 hours. Because the effect of DDAVP is relatively short-lived, the patient must be closely monitored and repeated doses may be necessary. It is an appropriate therapy for minor bleeding episodes and dental procedures. The intranasal form may be indicated for home therapy for some patients with mild to moderate forms of the disease.[36]

Antifibrinolytic therapy (tranexamic acid [Cyklokapron] and epsilon aminocaproic acid [EACA, Amicar]) inhibits fibrinolysis by inhibiting plasminogen activation in the fibrin clot, thereby enhancing clot stability. These agents are useful therapeutic adjuncts to stabilize clots in areas of increased fibrinolysis, such as the oral cavity, and in patients with difficult episodes of epistaxis and menorrhagia. They are contraindicated in patients with hematuria because lack of fibrinolysis in the kidneys could lead to renal failure.

Complications of treatment of hemophilia include development of inhibitors to factors VIII or IX, transfusion-transmitted infectious disorders, allergic reactions, and thrombotic complications with the use of factor IX because it contains activated coagulation factors. Patients with vWF may also develop alloantibodies against vWF, the infusion of which could cause life-threatening anaphylaxis; thus replacement factors for these patients should be devoid of vWF. Because of the improved viral-detecting processes and donor screening practices, the risk of HIV and hepatitis B and C transmission is greatly reduced.

The most common difficulties with acute management are starting factor replacement therapy too late and stopping it too soon. Generally, minor bleeding episodes should be treated for at least 72 hours. Surgery and traumatic injuries may need support for 10 to 14 days. Because of the short half-life of the factors, regular intermittent or continuous infusions have been used to manage bleeding episodes or expected traumatic procedures. Chronically, development of inhibitors to the factor products has occurred and requires individualized expert patient management by the health care team.

Designated treatment centers have been established in the United States and many other countries to provide multidisciplinary care of hemophilia and related disorders. The multidisciplinary team provides optimal chronic disease management.

Gene therapy has been used on an experimental basis to treat hemophilia. These clinical trials have involved (1) removing cells from the patient and genetically modifying them to secrete factor VIII or IX and (2) injecting vectors with the genes for factors VIII and IX.[35-37] (Gene therapy is discussed in Chapter 14.)

NURSING MANAGEMENT HEMOPHILIA

Nursing Implementation

Health Promotion. Because of the hereditary nature of hemophilia, referral for genetic counseling is essential when considering preventive measures. This is especially important because many persons with hemophilia live into adulthood. Reproductive concerns and long-term effects are issues that the nurse should include in the patient's care plan.

Acute Intervention. Interventions are related primarily to controlling bleeding and include the following:

1. Stop the topical bleeding as quickly as possible by applying direct pressure or ice, packing the area with Gelfoam or fibrin foam, and applying topical hemostatic agents such as thrombin.
2. Administer the specific coagulation factor to raise the patient's level of the deficient coagulation factor. Monitor the patient for signs and symptoms, such as hypersensitivity.
3. When joint bleeding occurs, in addition to administering replacement factors, it is important to totally rest the involved joint to prevent crippling deformities from hemarthrosis. The joint may be packed in ice. Analgesics (e.g., acetaminophen, codeine) are given to reduce severe pain. However, aspirin and aspirin-containing compounds should never be used. As soon as bleeding ceases, it is important to encourage mobilization of the affected area through range-of-motion exercises

and physical therapy. Weight bearing is avoided until all swelling has resolved and muscle strength has returned.

4. Manage any life-threatening complication that may develop as a result of hemorrhage or side effects from coagulation factors or other medications, such as hyponatremia, by desmopressin. Examples include nursing interventions to prevent or treat airway obstruction from hemorrhage into the neck and pharynx, as well as early assessment and treatment of intracranial bleeding.

Ambulatory and Home Care. Home management is a primary consideration for the patient with hemophilia because the disease follows a progressive, chronic course. The quality and the length of life may be significantly affected by the patient's knowledge of the illness and how to live with it. The patient and family can be referred to a local chapter of the National Hemophilia Society to encourage associations with other individuals who are dealing with the problems of hemophilia. The nurse must provide ongoing assessment of the patient's adaptation to the illness. Psychosocial support and assistance should be readily available as needed.

Most of the long-term care measures are related to patient teaching. The patient with hemophilia must be taught to recognize disease-related problems and to learn which problems can be resolved at home and which require hospitalization. Immediate medical attention is required for severe pain or swelling of a muscle or joint that restricts movement or inhibits sleep and for a head injury, a swelling in the neck or mouth, abdominal pain, hematuria, melena, and skin wounds in need of suturing.

Daily oral hygiene must be performed without causing trauma. Understanding how to prevent injuries is another consideration. This is no easy task; there are many potential sources of trauma. The patient can learn to participate in noncontact sports (e.g., golf) and wear gloves when doing household chores to prevent cuts or abrasions from knives, hammers, and other tools. The patient should wear a Medic Alert tag to ensure that health care providers know about the hemophilia in case of an accident.

The patient needs information about routine follow-up care, and the compliance with scheduled visits must be assessed. A reliable person can be taught to self-administer some of the factor replacement therapies at home.

Evaluation

The overall expected outcomes are similar to those for the patient with thrombocytopenia and are presented in NCP 31-2.

DISSEMINATED INTRAVASCULAR COAGULATION

Disseminated intravascular coagulation (DIC) is a serious bleeding and thrombotic disorder. It results from abnormally initiated and accelerated clotting. Subsequent decreases in clotting factors and platelets ensue, which may lead to uncontrollable hemorrhage. The term *disseminated intravascular coagulation* can be misleading because it suggests that blood is clotting. However, the paradox of this condition is characterized by the profuse bleeding that results from the depletion of platelets and clotting factors. DIC is always caused by an underlying disease or condition. The underlying problem must be treated for the DIC to resolve.

Etiology and Pathophysiology

DIC is not a disease; it is an abnormal response of the normal clotting cascade stimulated by a disease process or disorder. The diseases and disorders known to predispose a patient to DIC are listed in Table 31-19. DIC can occur as an acute, catastrophic condition, or it may exist at a subacute or chronic level. Each condition may have one or multiple triggering mechanisms to start the clotting cascade. For example, tumors and traumatized or necrotic tissue release tissue factors into circulation. Endotoxin from gram-negative bacteria activates several steps in the coagulation cascade.[39]

TABLE 31-19 Predisposing Conditions to Disseminated Intravascular Coagulation

Acute DIC

Shock
- Hemorrhagic
- Cardiogenic
- Anaphylactic

Septicemia

Hemolytic processes
- Transfusion of mismatched blood
- Acute hemolysis from infection or immunologic disorders

Obstetric conditions
- Abruptio placentae
- Amniotic fluid embolism
- Septic abortion

Malignancies
- Acute leukemia
- Lymphoma
- Tumor lysis syndrome

Tissue damage
- Extensive burns and trauma
- Heatstroke
- Severe head injury
- Transplant rejections
- Postoperative damage, especially after extracorporeal membrane oxygenation
- Fat and pulmonary emboli
- Snakebites
- Glomerulonephritis
- Acute anoxia (e.g., after cardiac arrest)
- Prosthetic devices
- Fulminant hepatitis

Subacute DIC

Malignant disease
- Myeloproliferative/lymphoproliferative malignancies
- Metastatic cancer

Obstetric
- Retained dead fetus

Chronic DIC

Liver disease

Systemic lupus erythematosus

Localized malignancy

DIC, Disseminated intravascular coagulation.

Tissue factor is released at the site of tissue injury and by some malignancies, such as leukemia, and causes normal coagulation mechanisms to be enhanced. Abundant intravascular thrombin, the most powerful coagulant, is produced (Fig. 31-10). It catalyzes the conversion of fibrinogen to fibrin and enhances platelet aggregation. There is widespread fibrin and platelet deposition in capillaries and arterioles, resulting in thrombosis; this can lead to multiorgan failure. In addition, clotting inhibitory mechanisms, such as antithrombin III (AT III) and protein C, are depressed. This excessive clotting activates the fibrinolytic system, which in turn breaks down the newly formed clot, creating fibrin split (fibrin degradation) products. These products have anticoagulant properties and

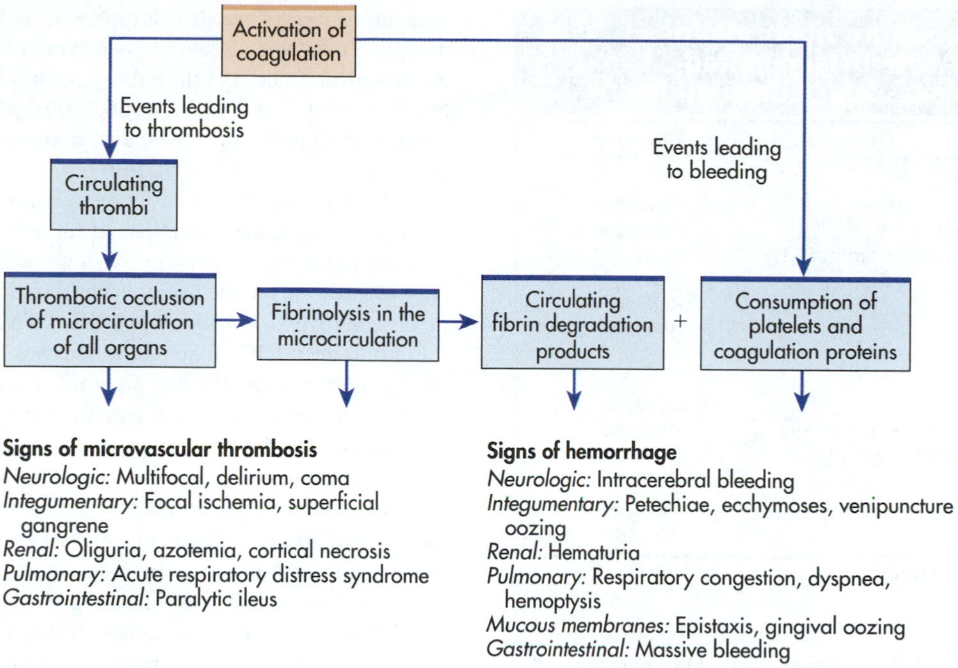

FIG. 31-10 The sequence of events that occur during disseminated intravascular coagulation (DIC).

inhibit normal blood clotting. Ultimately with fibrin split products accumulating and clotting factors being depleted, the blood loses its ability to clot. Therefore a stable clot cannot be formed at injury sites. This situation predisposes the patient to hemorrhage.[39-41]

Chronic and subacute DIC is most commonly seen in patients with long-standing illnesses such as malignant disorders or autoimmune diseases. The incidence of DIC associated with malignancy ranges from 10% to 75%. Occasionally these patients have subclinical disease manifested only by laboratory abnormalities.[39,40] However, the clinical spectrum ranges from easy bruising to hemorrhage and from hypercoagulability to thrombosis.

Clinical Manifestations

There is no well-defined sequence of events in acute DIC. Bleeding in a person with no previous history or obvious cause should be questioned because it may be one of the first manifestations of acute DIC. Other nonspecific manifestations can include weakness, malaise, and fever.

There are both bleeding and thrombotic manifestations in DIC. Bleeding manifestations of DIC are multifactorial (see Fig. 31-10) and result from consumption and depletion of platelets and coagulation factors, as well as clot lysis and formation of fibrin split products that have anticoagulant properties.

Bleeding manifestations include integumentary manifestations, such as pallor, petechiae, purpura (Fig. 31-11), oozing blood, venipuncture site bleeding, hematomas, and occult hemorrhage; respiratory manifestations, such as tachypnea, hemoptysis, and orthopnea; cardiovascular manifestations, such as tachycardia and hypotension; GI manifestations, such as upper and lower GI bleeding, abdominal distention, and bloody stools; urinary manifestations, such as hematuria; neurologic changes, such as vision changes, dizziness, headache, changes in mental status, and irritability; and musculoskeletal complaints, such as bone and joint pain.

Thrombotic manifestations are a result of fibrin or platelet deposition in the microvasculature (see Fig. 31-10) and include integumentary changes, such as cyanosis, ischemic tissue necrosis (e.g., gangrene), and hemorrhagic necrosis; respiratory changes, such as tachypnea, dyspnea, pulmonary emboli, and acute respiratory distress syndrome (ARDS); cardiovascular changes, such as electrocardiogram (ECG) changes and venous distention; GI changes, such as abdominal pain and paralytic ileus; and kidney damage and oliguria, leading to failure.

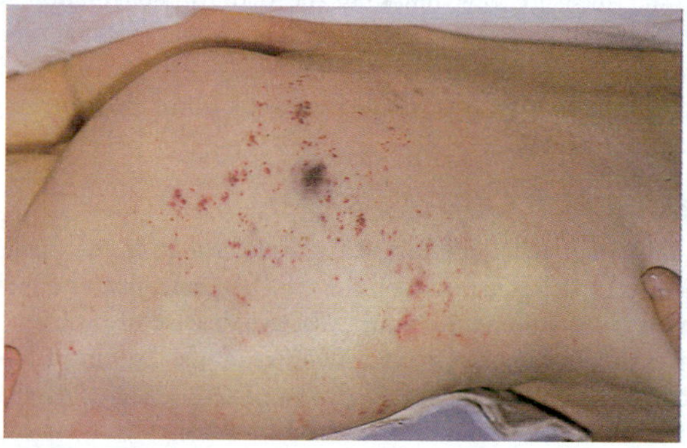

FIG. 31-11 Disseminated intravascular coagulation resulting from staphylococcal septicemia. Note the characteristic skin hemorrhage ranging from small purpuric lesions to larger ecchymoses.

Diagnostic Studies

Tests used to diagnose acute DIC and their findings are listed in Table 31-20. As more clots are made in the body, more breakdown products from fibrinogen and fibrin are also formed. These are termed *fibrin split products* (FSPs) or *fibrin degradation products* (FDPs), and they work in three ways to interfere with blood coagulation. First, they coat the platelets and interfere with platelet function. Second, they interfere with thrombin and thereby disrupt coagulation. Third, the FSPs attach to fibrinogen, which interferes with the polymerization process necessary to form a stable clot. A

TABLE 31-20 Laboratory Abnormalities in Acute Disseminated Intravascular Coagulation

Test	Finding
Screening Tests	
Prothrombin time (PT)	Prolonged
Partial thromboplastin time (PTT)	Prolonged
Activated partial thromboplastin time (aPTT)	Prolonged
Thrombin time	Prolonged
Fibrinogen	Reduced
Platelets	Reduced
Special Tests	
Fibrin split products (FSPs)*	Elevated
Factor assays (for factors V, VII, VIII, X, XIII)	Reduced
D-dimers (cross-linked fibrin fragments)	Elevated
Antithrombin III (AT III)	Reduced
Protein S	Reduced
Protein C	Reduced

*Fibrin degradation products (FDP).

much more specific test is the D-dimer assay. D-dimer, a specific polymer resulting from the breakdown of fibrin (and not fibrinogen), is a specific marker for the degree of fibrinolysis. In general, tests that measure raw materials needed for coagulation (e.g., platelets, fibrinogen) are reduced, and values that measure times to clot are prolonged. Fragmented erythrocytes (schistocytes), indicative of partial occlusion of small vessels by fibrin thrombi, may be found on blood smears.

Collaborative Care

It is important to diagnose DIC quickly, stabilize the patient if needed (e.g., oxygenation, volume replacement), institute therapy that will resolve the underlying causative disease or problem, and provide supportive care for the manifestations resulting from the pathology of DIC itself. The treatment of DIC remains controversial and under investigation as researchers attempt to determine the most suitable means of managing this dangerous syndrome. Consequently, it is imperative that the nurse maintain an ongoing awareness of current modes of therapy and that each patient is managed on the basis of his or her particular clinical manifestations. Diagnosing and treating the primary disease process is essential to the resolution of DIC.

Depending on its severity, a variety of different methods are used to provide supportive and symptomatic management of DIC (Fig. 31-12). First, if chronic DIC is diagnosed in a patient who is not bleeding, no therapy for DIC is necessary. Treatment of the underlying disease may be sufficient to reverse the DIC (e.g., antineoplastic therapy when DIC is caused by malignancy). Second, when the patient with DIC is bleeding, therapy is directed toward providing support with necessary blood products while treating the primary disorder. The blood products are administered cautiously on the basis of specific component deficiencies to patients who have serious bleeding, are at high risk for bleeding (e.g., surgery), or require invasive procedures. Blood product support with platelets, cryoprecipitate, and fresh frozen plasma (FFP) is usually reserved for a patient with life-threatening hemorrhage. The concern is that one is adding "fuel to the fire" of already activated coagulation. However, it may be the only method to avoid fatal hemorrhage in some patients. Therapy will stabilize a patient, prevent exsanguination or massive thrombosis, and permit institution of definitive therapy to treat the underlying cause. In general, platelets are given to correct thrombocytopenia if the platelet count is less than 20,000/μl or less than 50,000/μl with bleeding. Cryoprecipitate replaces factor VIII and fibrinogen and is given if the fibrinogen is below 100 mg/dl. FFP replaces all clotting factors except platelets and provides a source of antithrombin.

A patient with manifestations of thrombosis is often treated by anticoagulation with heparin or low-molecular-weight heparin (LMWH). However, the use of heparin in the treatment of DIC remains controversial. Antithrombin III (ATnativ) is sometimes useful in fulminant DIC, although it increases the risk of bleeding. A recombinant human activated protein C (drotrecogin alfa [Xigris]) has been shown to have both anticoagulant and antiinflammatory effects and has reduced the relative risk of death from sepsis. However, because it causes increased bleeding, it is contraindicated in patients with a platelet count less than 30,000/μl. Hirudin, a thrombin inhibitor, is also being studied as a blocker of the abnormal coagulation process. Epsilon aminocaproic acid (EACA, Amicar) is generally contraindicated because of its ability to inhibit fibrinolysis and enhancement of thrombosis.[40-42]

Chronic DIC does not respond to oral anticoagulants, but it can be controlled with long-term use of heparin. Some patients with indolent (inactive and slowly developing) tumors and severe, chronic DIC may need continuous infusion of heparin with portable pumps.

NURSING MANAGEMENT
DISSEMINATED INTRAVASCULAR COAGULATION

Nursing Diagnoses

Nursing diagnoses for the patient with DIC may include, but are not limited to, the following:

- Ineffective tissue perfusion (cerebral, cardiopulmonary, renal, GI, and peripheral) *related to* bleeding and sluggish or diminished blood flow secondary to thrombosis
- Acute pain *related to* bleeding into tissues and diagnostic procedures
- Decreased cardiac output *related to* fluid volume deficit and hypotension
- Anxiety *related to* fear of the unknown, disease process, diagnostic procedures, and therapy

Nursing Implementation

Nurses must be alert to the possible development of DIC and especially to the precipitating factors listed in Table 31-19. This may be difficult because the nurse is focusing on the complex care often required by the primary problem that precipitated the DIC. The nurse must also remember that because DIC is secondary to an underlying disease, appropriate care for managing the causative problem must be provided while providing supportive care related to the manifestations of DIC.[43]

Appropriate nursing interventions are essential to the survival of a patient with acute DIC. Astute, ongoing assessment, active attention to manifestations of the syndrome, and institution of appropriate treatment measures are challenging and sometimes paradoxic nursing responsibilities (e.g., administering heparin to a bleeding patient). Table 31-14 and NCP 31-2 provide assessments and interventions appropriate for the patient with DIC. Early detection of bleeding, both occult and overt, must be a primary goal.

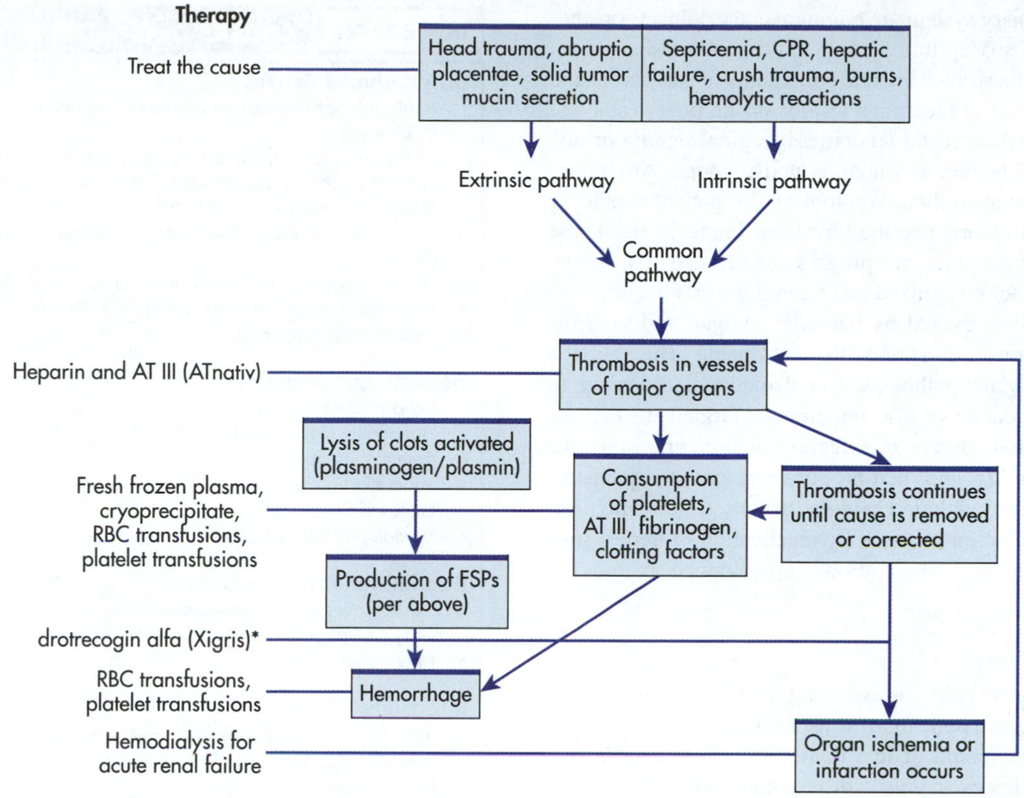

FIG. 31-12 Intended sites of action for therapies in disseminated intravascular coagulation. *AT III,* Antithrombin III; *CPR,* cardiopulmonary resuscitation; *FSPs,* fibrin split products. *Recombinant form of activated protein C.

The patient is assessed for signs of external bleeding (e.g., petechiae, oozing at IV or injection sites) and signs of internal bleeding (e.g., increased heart rate, changes in mental status, increasing abdominal girth, pain). Any sites of bleeding are carefully monitored for continued bleeding. Tissue damage should be minimized and the patient protected from additional foci of bleeding.

An additional nursing responsibility is to administer blood products and medications correctly. Blood product transfusion is discussed later in this chapter.

NEUTROPENIA

Leukopenia refers to a decrease in the total WBC count (granulocytes, monocytes, and lymphocytes). *Granulocytopenia* is a deficiency of granulocytes, which include neutrophils, eosinophils, and basophils. The neutrophilic granulocytes, which play a major role in phagocytizing pathogenic microbes, are closely monitored in clinical practice as an indicator of a patient's risk for infection. A reduction in neutrophils is termed **neutropenia.** (Some clinicians use the terms *granulocytopenia* and *neutropenia* interchangeably because the largest constituency of granulocytes is the neutrophils.) The absolute neutrophil count is determined by multiplying the total WBC count by the percentage of neutrophils. *Neutropenia* is defined as a neutrophil count of less than 1000 to 1500/μl (1 to 1.5×10^9/L). Severe neutropenia is defined as a neutrophil count of less than 500/μl. Normally, neutrophils range from 4000 to 11,000/μl. However, in considering the clinical significance of neutropenia it is important to know the rapidity of the decrease in the neutrophil count (gradual or rapid), degree of neutropenia, and the duration. The faster the drop and the longer the duration, the greater the likelihood of developing life-threatening infection, sepsis, and death. Other factors and comorbid conditions, such as being older than 60, the presence of an existing infection, being in the hospital, having diabetes, and other factors, can increase the risk of a serious infection.[44-47]

Neutropenia is a clinical consequence that occurs with a variety of conditions or diseases (see Table 31-20). It can also be an expected effect, a side effect, or an unintentional effect of taking certain drugs. The most common cause of neutropenia is iatrogenic, resulting from widespread use of chemotherapeutic and immunosuppressive therapy in the treatment of malignancies and autoimmune diseases.[48]

Clinical Manifestations

The patient with neutropenia is predisposed to infection with nonpathogenic organisms that constitute normal body flora, as well as opportunistic pathogens. When the WBC count is depressed or immature WBCs are present, normal phagocytic mechanisms are impaired. Also because of the diminished phagocytic response, the classic signs of inflammation—redness, heat, and swelling—may not occur. WBCs are the major component of pus. Therefore in the patient with neutropenia, pus formation (e.g., as a visible skin lesion or as pulmonary infiltrates on a chest x-ray) is also absent. Because neutropenia masks some of the signs and symptoms of infection, the presence of even a low-grade fever is of great significance.[44]

When fever occurs in a neutropenic patient, it is assumed to be caused by infection and requires immediate attention. The immunocompromised, neutropenic patient has little or no ability to fight infection. Thus minor infections can lead rapidly to sepsis. The mucous membranes of the throat and mouth, the skin, the perianal area, and the pulmonary system are common entry points for pathogenic organisms in susceptible hosts. Clinical manifestations related to infection at these sites include complaints of sore throat and dysphagia, appearance of ulcerative lesions of the pharyngeal and buccal mucosa, diarrhea, rectal tenderness, vaginal itching or discharge, shortness of breath, and nonproductive cough. Any minor complaint of pain or any other symptom by the patient should be taken seriously and reported to the physician immediately. These seemingly minor complaints can progress to fever, chills, sepsis, and septic shock if not recognized and treated in early stages.

Systemic infections caused by bacterial, fungal, and viral organisms are common in patients with neutropenia. The patient's own flora (normally nonpathogenic) contributes significantly to life-threatening infections such as pneumonia. Organisms that are known to be common sources of infection include gram-positive *Staphylococcus aureus* and aerobic gram-negative organisms. Fungi that are involved include *Candida* (usually *C. albicans*) and *Aspergillus.* Viral infections caused by reactivation of herpes simplex and zoster are common following prolonged periods of neutropenia.[47,48]

Diagnostic Studies

The primary diagnostic tests for assessing neutropenia are the peripheral WBC count and bone marrow aspiration and biopsy (Table 31-21). A total WBC count of less than 4000/μl (4×10^9/L) reflects leukopenia. However, only a differential count can confirm the presence of neutropenia (neutrophil count 1000 to 1500/μl [1 to 1.5×10^9/L]). If the differential WBC count reflects an absolute neutropenia of 500 to 1000/μl (0.5 to 1.0×10^9/L), the patient is at moderate risk for a bacterial infection. An absolute neutropenia of less than 500/μl (0.5×10^9/L) places the patient at severe risk.

A peripheral blood smear is used to assess for immature forms of WBCs (e.g., bands). The hematocrit level, reticulocyte count, and platelet count are done to evaluate bone marrow function. A review of the patient's recent past and current drug history should also be done. If the cause of neutropenia is unknown, bone marrow aspirations and biopsies are done to examine cellularity and cell morphology. Additional studies may be done as indicated to assess spleen and liver function.

TABLE 31-21 Causes of Neutropenia

Drug-Induced Causes
• Antitumor antibiotics (daunorubicin [Cerubidine], doxorubicin [Adriamycin])
• Alkylating agents (nitrogen mustards, busulfan [Myleran])
• Antimetabolites (methotrexate [Folex], 6-mercaptopurine [6-MP])
• Antiinflammatory drugs (phenylbutazone)
• Psychotropics and antidepressants (clozapine, imipramine [Tofranil])
• Miscellaneous (gold, penicillamine, mepacrine, amodiaquine)
• Antimicrobial agents (zidovudine [AZT, Retrovir], trimethoprim-sulfamethoxazole [Bactrim])
Hematologic Disorders
• Idiopathic neutropenia
• Congenital (cyclic neutropenia)
• Aplastic anemia
• Fanconi anemia
• Leukemia
• Myelodysplastic syndrome
Autoimmune Disorders
• Systemic lupus erythematosus
• Felty's syndrome
• Rheumatoid arthritis
Infections
• Viral (e.g., hepatitis, influenza, HIV, measles)
• Fulminant bacterial infection (e.g., typhoid fever, miliary tuberculosis)
• Parasitic
• Rickettsial
Miscellaneous
• Severe sepsis
• Bone marrow infiltration (e.g., carcinoma, tuberculosis, lymphoma)
• Hypersplenism (e.g., portal hypertension, Felty's syndrome, storage diseases [e.g., Gaucher's disease])
• Nutritional deficiencies (cobalamin, folic acid)
• Transfusion reaction
• Hemodialysis

HIV, Human immunodeficiency virus.

NURSING *and* COLLABORATIVE MANAGEMENT NEUTROPENIA

The factors involved in the nursing and collaborative care of neutropenia include (1) determining the cause of the neutropenia; (2) identifying the offending organisms if an infection has developed; (3) instituting prophylactic, empiric, or therapeutic antibiotic therapy; (4) administering hematopoietic growth factors (e.g., granulocyte colony-stimulating factor [G-CSF] and granulocyte-macrophage colony-stimulating factor [GM-CSF]); and (5) instituting protective environmental practices, such as strict hand washing, visitor restrictions, and a private room if hospitalized; a positive-pressure room or high-efficiency particulate air (HEPA) filtration may be used for HSCT patients (Table 31-22).

Occasionally the cause of the neutropenia can be easily treated (e.g., nutritional deficiencies). However, neutropenia can also be a side effect that must be tolerated as a necessary step in therapy (e.g., chemotherapy, radiation therapy). In some situations the neutropenia resolves when the primary disease is treated (e.g., tuberculosis).

The nurse needs to monitor the neutropenic patient for signs and symptoms of infection (e.g., any fever ≥100.4° F [38° C]) and early septic shock. Early identification of a potentially infective organism depends on acquiring cultures from various sites. Serial blood cultures (at least two) or one from a peripheral site and one from a venous access device should be done promptly and antibiotics started immediately. Additionally, cultures of sputum, throat, lesions, wounds, urine, and feces are essential in the surveillance of the patient. It may also be necessary to do a tracheal aspiration, bronchoscopy with bronchial brushings, or lung biopsy to diagnose the cause of pneumonic infiltrates. However, invasive diagnostic studies are often contraindicated because of the concern of introducing infection and the fact that these patients are also often thrombocytopenic. Despite these many tests, the causative organism is identified only in approximately one half of neutropenic patients.

When a febrile episode occurs in a neutropenic patient, antibiotic therapy must be initiated immediately (within 1 hour) even before the determination of a specific causative organism by culture. Administration of broad-spectrum antibiotics is usually by the IV route because of the rapidly lethal effects of infection. However, some oral antibiotics are highly effective and routinely used for prophylaxis

TABLE 31-22 COLLABORATIVE CARE
Neutropenia

Diagnostic
History and physical examination
WBC count with differential count
WBC morphology
Hct and Hb values
Reticulocyte and platelet count
Bone marrow aspiration or biopsy
Cultures of nose, throat, sputum, urine, stool, obvious lesions, blood (as indicated)
Chest x-ray

Collaborative Therapy
Identification and removal of cause of neutropenia (if possible)
Identification of site of infection (if present) and causative organism
Antibiotic therapy
Hematopoietic growth factors (G-CSF, GM-CSF, pegfilgrastim [Neulasta])
Strict hand washing and patient hygiene
Single-patient room, positive-pressure or high-efficiency particulate air (HEPA) filtration, depending on risk
Community isolation and home precautions if outpatient

G-CSF, Granulocyte colony-stimulating factor; *GM-CSF,* granulocyte-macrophage colony-stimulating factor; *Hb,* hemoglobin; *Hct,* hematocrit; *WBC,* white blood cell.

TABLE 31-23 PATIENT AND FAMILY TEACHING GUIDE
Neutropenia

This instruction sheet explains precautions you should take to protect yourself when your neutrophil count is low. Please make sure to ask your health care provider specific precautions you should take that relate to your infection risk factors.

- WASH YOUR HANDS frequently and make sure those around you wash their hands frequently, particularly if they help with your care. An antibacterial hand gel may also be used.
- Notify your nurse or health care provider if you have any of the following:
  - If you have a fever greater than 100.4° F (38° C)
  - Have any chills or feel hot
  - Notice any redness, swelling, discharge, or new pain on or in your body
  - Have changes in urination or bowel movements
  - Have a cough, sore throat, mouth sores, or blisters
- If you are at home, take your temperature as directed and follow instructions on what to do if you have a fever.
- Avoid crowds and people with colds, flu, or infections. If you are in a public area, wear a mask.
- Avoid raw foods, such as sushi, Caesar salad dressing (may have raw eggs), blue cheese, and fruits that cannot be peeled or vegetables that cannot be well cleaned. Ask your health care provider about specific dietary guidelines for you.
- Bathe or shower daily. A moisturizer may be used to prevent skin from drying and cracking.
- Do not perform gardening or clean up after pets. Feeding and petting your dog or cat are fine as long as you wash your hands well after handling.

against infection in some neutropenic patients. The use of a third- or fourth-generation cephalosporin (e.g., cefepime [Maxipime], ceftazidime [Ceptaz]), a carbapenem (e.g., imipenem/cilastatin [Primaxin]), or a combination of an aminoglycoside plus an antipseudomonal offers broad-spectrum coverage for initial management.[49] Regardless of the combination, the nurse must initiate therapy promptly and observe the patient for side effects of antimicrobial agents. Side effects common to aminoglycosides include nephrotoxicity and ototoxicity; side effects common to cephalosporins include rashes, fever, and pruritus.

The duration of the neutropenia also increases the infection risk of the patient. The longer the neutropenia, the greater the risk of a fungal infection. Antifungal therapy is initiated whenever a culture is positive, or in patients who do not become afebrile with broad-spectrum antibiotic coverage.

G-CSF (filgrastim [Neupogen], pegfilgrastim [Neulasta]) and GM-CSF (sargramostim [Leukine, Prokine]) can be used to treat a neutropenic patient. G-CSF stimulates the production and function of neutrophils. GM-CSF stimulates the production and function of neutrophils and monocytes. These agents can be given IV or subcutaneously. The nurse can teach the patient and family how to administer the subcutaneous medication. These factors are especially beneficial in enhancing granulocyte recovery after chemotherapy and shorten the period of vulnerability to fatal infections. Keratinocyte growth factor (palifermin [Kepivance]) may also be used to reduce the duration and severity of mucositis which may contribute to infection.[50] (G-CSF, GM-CSF, and Kepivance are discussed in Chapter 16 and Table 16-18.)

An important consideration in the care of a neutropenic patient is the determination of the best means to protect the patient whose own defenses against infection are compromised. To accomplish this goal, the following principles must be kept in mind: (1) the patient's normal flora is the most common source of microbial colonization and infection; (2) transmission of organisms from humans most commonly occurs by direct contact with the hands; (3) air, food, water, and equipment provide additional opportunities for infection transmission; and (4) health care providers with transmittable illnesses and other patients with infections can also be sources of infection transmission under certain conditions.

Hand washing is the single most important preventive measure in minimizing the risk of infection in the neutropenic patient. Strict hand washing by all persons coming in contact with the compromised patient is the major method to prevent transmission of harmful pathogens. The Centers for Disease Control and Prevention (CDC)[51] advocates hand washing before, during, and after care. This seemingly routine technique has a significant effect in reducing infection. It must be emphasized and enforced despite its seeming simplicity.

The CDC also encourages separating immunocompromised patients from those who are infected or who have conditions that increase the probability of transmitting infections (e.g., poor hygiene caused by lack of understanding or cognitive dysfunction). Often, patients can be managed on an outpatient basis if the patient and family can astutely monitor for fevers and other signs of infection and then report promptly to a nearby health care facility (Table 31-23). If the patient is hospitalized, private rooms should be used. High-efficiency particulate air (HEPA) filtration is an air-handling method with a high-flow filtering system that can reduce or eliminate the number of aerosolized pathogens in the environment. Although it is expensive to install, it is often used for a patient with severe prolonged neutropenia (e.g., bone marrow transplant patients). Care routines in an HEPA environment are essentially the same as care in any other private room. Additional neutropenic precaution guidelines may also be employed, such as avoidance of tap water, fresh fruits and vegetables, and prophylactic antibiotics and antifungals. The nursing measures presented in NCP 31-3 are important in the treatment of the patient with neutropenia.[51]

Hematology System

NURSING CARE PLAN 31-3
Patient with Neutropenia

NURSING DIAGNOSIS **Risk for infection** *related to* decreased neutrophils, altered response to microbial invasion, and presence of environmental pathogens

PATIENT GOALS
1. Adheres to infection control and protection practices
2. Experiences no signs or symptoms of infection

OUTCOMES (NOC)

Infection Severity
- Purulent sputum ____
- Purulent drainage ____
- Chest x-ray infiltration ____
- Fever ____
- Pain/tenderness ____
- Blood culture colonization ____
- Unexplained cognitive impairment ____
- White blood count elevation ____

Measurement Scale
1 = Severe
2 = Substantial
3 = Moderate
4 = Mild
5 = None

INTERVENTIONS (NIC) and *RATIONALES*

Infection Control
- Institute designated isolation precautions.
- Wash hands before and after each patient care activity *to prevent transmission of pathogens.*
- Use antimicrobial soap for hand washing.
- Limit number of visitors.
- Instruct visitors to wash hands on entering and leaving patient's room *to prevent the transmission of harmful pathogens to patient.*

Infection Protection
- Provide private room.
- Maintain asepsis for patient at risk.
- Screen all visitors for communicable disease.
- Monitor for systemic and localized signs and symptoms of infection.
- Monitor absolute granulocyte count and WBC count and differential results *to identify signs of and potential for infection.*
- Inspect skin and mucous membranes for redness, extreme warmth, or drainage.
- Instruct patient to take antibiotics as prescribed *to prevent microbial resistance.*
- Eliminate fresh fruits, vegetables, and pepper from diet of patients with neutropenia *to avoid introduction of pathogens.*
- Remove fresh flowers and plants from patient areas *to avoid introduction of pathogens.*
- Report suspected infections to infection control personnel *in order to promptly initiate antibiotic therapy due to the rapidly lethal effects of infection.*
- Teach patient and family how to avoid infections (e.g., personal hygiene techniques of hand washing, oral care, skin hygiene, and pulmonary hygiene).
- Teach patient and family about signs and symptoms of infection and when to report them to the health care provider.

Quality-of-life issues for the patient with neutropenia should not be overlooked in these patients. Potential patient experiences of fatigue, malaise, a decrease in functioning, social isolation, and depression, as well as family support, require appropriate interventions.[45,52]

The value of effective nursing care in reducing the development of infection or limiting its extent cannot be overemphasized. Regular assessment and early detection of infectious sources are key roles for the nurse in reducing morbidity and mortality rates from infection.

GERONTOLOGIC CONSIDERATIONS
THROMBOCYTOPENIA AND NEUTROPENIA

About 55% to 60% of cancers are currently diagnosed in individuals older than 65 years of age. This proportion is expected to further increase in the next two decades. Age-related changes of bone marrow function are rather subtle and probably not significant for the hematopoietic function of normal older individuals. These changes, however, may become clinically evident under conditions of severe hematopoietic stress, such as the administration of repeated courses of chemotherapy and/or radiation therapy.[53] The use of supportive therapies, such as hematopoietic growth factors, increases the likelihood that older individuals will be treated with standard and even aggressive therapies, leading to neutropenia and thrombocytopenia. The nurse also needs to be aware that older individuals may have signs and symptoms different from those of a younger individual. For example, the older adult may have delirium as compared with cough as a clinical manifestation of pneumonia. (Refer to Chapter 6 on older adults.)

MYELODYSPLASTIC SYNDROME

Myelodysplastic syndrome (MDS) is a group of related hematologic disorders characterized by a change in the quantity and quality of bone marrow elements. Peripheral blood cytopenias in combination with a hypercellular bone marrow exhibiting dysplastic changes are the hallmark of MDS. It is estimated that 7000 to 12,000 new cases of MDS are diagnosed each year in the United States. Although it can occur in all age-groups, the highest prevalence is in people over 60 years of age.

Etiology and Pathophysiology

The etiology of MDS is unknown. Its manifestations result from neoplastic transformation of the pluripotent hematopoietic stem cells within the bone marrow. Occasionally one type of MDS transforms into another. In some cases, MDS will progress to acute myelogenous leukemia.

MDS is referred to as a *clonal disorder* because some bone marrow stem cells continue to function normally whereas others (a specific clone) do not. The abnormal clone of the stem cells is usually found in the bone marrow but eventually may be found in circulation. In contrast to acute myelogenous leukemia (AML), in which the leukemic cells show little normal maturation, the clonal cells in MDS always display some degree of maturity. Disease progression is slower than in AML. However, eventually the abnormal cells replace the bone marrow. Typically, life-threatening anemia, thrombocytopenia, and neutropenia occur during the advanced stage of MDS.

Clinical Manifestations

MDS commonly manifests as infection and bleeding caused by inadequate numbers of ineffective functioning circulating granulocytes or platelets. MDS is often discovered in the elderly as a result of testing for the symptoms of anemia, thrombocytopenia, or neutropenia. It may also be diagnosed incidentally from a routine complete blood count (CBC).

Diagnostic Studies

Bone marrow biopsy with aspirate analysis is essential for both the diagnosis and the classification of the specific types of myelodysplasia. In MDS the bone marrow is normocellular, hypocellular, or hypercellular and the patient has peripheral cytopenia. Laboratory data and bone marrow studies will help rule out other causes of the dysplasia, such as nonmalignant disorders, cobalamin and folate deficiencies, and infectious causes. MDS is staged according to clinical and laboratory findings. The relationship between the number of circulating blast cells and the number of blast cells in the bone marrow serves as the main indicator of prognosis in this disease. The findings of the biopsy also help in deciding how aggressive the treatment will be.

NURSING *and* COLLABORATIVE MANAGEMENT MYELODYSPLASTIC SYNDROME

Supportive treatment of MDS is based on the premise that the aggressiveness of treatment should match the aggressiveness of the disease. Supportive treatment consists of hematologic monitoring (serial bone marrow and peripheral blood examinations), antibiotic therapy, or transfusions with blood products. Side effects and toxicities from supportive treatment include anemia, thrombocytopenia, and blood transfusion reactions. The overall goal is to improve hematopoiesis and ensure age-related quality of life.

Low-risk patients can often be treated with erythropoietin and G-CSF. Only about one third of high-risk patients are treated with intensive chemotherapy and/or hematopoietic stem cell transplantation (HSCT). Azacitidine (Vidaza) is the first effective treatment for patients with MDS. It helps restore normal growth control and differentiation of hematopoietic cells. It has a response rate of up to 64% and reduces the frequency of transformation of MDS to acute leukemia. Side effects include myelosuppression, nausea, vomiting, constipation or diarrhea, renal dysfunction, and injection site erythema. Lenalidomide (Revimid) is used to treat patients with a subtype of MDS. This drug is similar in structure to thalidomide. Other treatments for MDS include cytarabine (Cytosar, Ara-C) with or without antitumor antibiotics (anthracyclines), decitabine (Dacogen), antithymocyte globulin, cyclosporine, and thalidomide. High-dose chemotherapy and allogeneic HSCT have been used in an attempt to treat bone marrow dysfunction of MDS and restore it with normal hematopoiesis. However, because of the aggressiveness of this treatment, it is generally recommended for patients less than 55 to 60 years old.[54,55]

Nursing care of a patient with MDS is similar to that of a patient with manifestations of anemia (see nursing care plan for the patient with anemia [NCP 31-1]), thrombocytopenia (see nursing care plan for the patient with thrombocytopenia [NCP 31-2]), and neutropenia (see nursing care plan for the patient with neutropenia [NCP 31-3]).

LEUKEMIA

Leukemia is the general term used to describe a group of malignant disorders affecting the blood and blood-forming tissues of the bone marrow, lymph system, and spleen. Leukemia occurs in all age-groups. It results in an accumulation of dysfunctional cells because of a loss of regulation in cell division. It follows a progressive course that is eventually fatal if untreated. An estimated 34,810 new cases are diagnosed each year. Although often thought of as a disease of children, the number of adults affected with leukemia is approximately 10 times that of children.[56]

Etiology and Pathophysiology

Regardless of the specific type of leukemia, there is generally no single causative agent in the development of leukemia. Most leukemias result from a combination of factors, including genetic and environmental influences. Chromosomal changes, first recognized in chronic myelogenous leukemia, have led to discoveries of how normal genes, once transformed, can result in abnormal genes (oncogenes) capable of causing many types of cancers, including leukemias (see Chapter 16). Chemical agents (e.g., benzene), chemotherapeutic agents (e.g., alkylating agents), viruses, radiation, and immunologic deficiencies have all been associated with the development of leukemia in susceptible hosts. There is an increased incidence of leukemia in radiologists, persons who have lived near nuclear bomb test sites or nuclear reactor accidents (e.g., Chernobyl), survivors of the bombing of Nagasaki and Hiroshima, and persons previously treated with radiation therapy or chemotherapy. Although RNA retroviruses cause a number of leukemias in animals, a viral cause for a human leukemia has been established only for some patients with adult T-cell leukemia. This form of leukemia is endemic in southwestern Japan and parts of the Caribbean and central Africa and is caused by the human T-cell leukemia virus type 1 (HTLV-1).

Classification

Classification of leukemia can be done based on acute versus chronic and on the type of WBC involved. The terms *acute* and *chronic* refer to cell maturity and nature of disease onset. Acute leukemia is characterized by the clonal proliferation of immature hematopoietic cells. The leukemia develops following malignant transformation of a single type of immature hematopoietic cell, followed by cellular replication and expansion of that malignant clone. Chronic leukemias involve more mature forms of the WBC, and the disease onset is more gradual.

Leukemia can also be classified by identifying the type of leukocyte involved, whether it is of myelogenous origin or of lymphocytic origin. By combining the acute and chronic categories with the cell type involved, specific types of leukemia can be identified. Four major types of leukemia are acute lymphocytic leukemia (ALL), acute myelogenous leukemia (AML), chronic myelogenous (granulocytic) leukemia (CML), and chronic lymphocytic

TABLE 31-24 Types of Leukemia

Type	Age of Onset	Clinical Manifestations	Diagnostic Findings
Acute myelogenous leukemia (AML)	Increase in incidence with advancing age, peak incidence between 60-70 yr of age	Fatigue and weakness, headache, mouth sores, anemia, bleeding, fever, infection, sternal tenderness, gingival hyperplasia, minimal hepatosplenomegaly and lymphadenopathy	Low RBC count, Hb, Hct; low platelet count; low to high WBC count with myeloblasts; high LDH, greatly hypercellular bone marrow with myeloblasts
Acute lymphocytic leukemia (ALL)	Before 14 yr of age, peak incidence between 2-9 yr of age and in older adults	Fever; pallor; bleeding; anorexia; fatigue and weakness; bone, joint, and abdominal pain; generalized lymphadenopathy; infections; weight loss; hepatosplenomegaly; headache; mouth sores; neurologic manifestations, including CNS involvement, increased intracranial pressure (nausea, vomiting, lethargy, cranial nerve dysfunction), secondary to meningeal infiltration	Low RBC count, Hb, Hct; low platelet count; low, normal, or high WBC count; high LDH; transverse lines of rarefaction at ends of metaphysis of long bones on x-ray; hypercellular bone marrow with lymphoblasts; lymphoblasts also possible in cerebrospinal fluid; presence of Philadelphia chromosome (20%-25% of patients)
Chronic myelogenous leukemia (CML)	25-60 yr of age, peak incidence around 45 yr of age	No symptoms early in disease, fatigue and weakness, fever, sternal tenderness, weight loss, joint pain, bone pain, massive splenomegaly, increase in sweating	Low RBC count, Hb, Hct; high platelet count early, lower count later; increase in polymorphonuclear neutrophils, normal number of lymphocytes, and normal or low number of monocytes in WBC differential; low leukocyte alkaline phosphatase; presence of Philadelphia chromosome in 90% of patients
Chronic lymphocytic leukemia (CLL)	50-70 yr of age, rare below 30 yr of age, predominance in men	No symptoms frequently, detection of disease often during examination for unrelated condition, chronic fatigue, anorexia, splenomegaly and lymphadenopathy, hepatomegaly; may progress to fever, night sweats, weight loss, fatigue, and frequent infections	Mild anemia and thrombocytopenia with disease progression; total WBC count >100,000/μl; increase in peripheral lymphocytes; increase in presence of lymphocytes in bone marrow; hypogammaglobulinemia; may have autoimmune hemolytic anemia (4%-11%), idiopathic thrombocytopenia purpura (2%-4%)

CNS, Central nervous system; *Hb,* hemoglobin; *Hct,* hematocrit; *LDH,* lactic dehydrogenase; *RBC,* red blood cell; *WBC,* white blood cell.

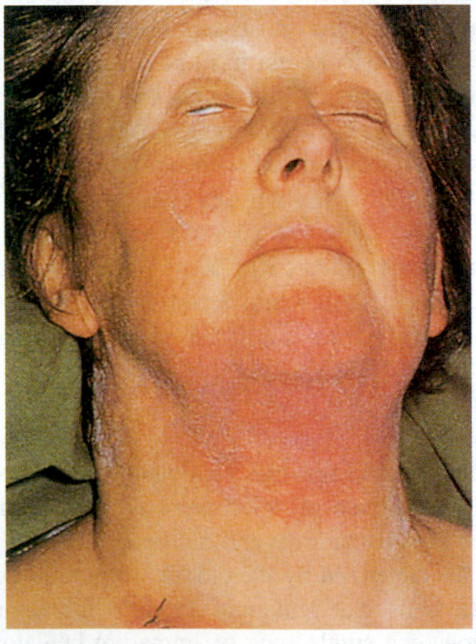

FIG. 31-13 Complications of acute leukemia. Spreading cellulitis of the neck and chin in this woman with acute myelogenous leukemia results from streptococcal and candidal infection. She was at risk because of previous chemotherapy and prolonged neutropenia.

leukemia (CLL). Other defining features of these leukemic subtypes are presented in Table 31-24.

Acute Myelogenous Leukemia. AML represents only one fourth of all leukemias, but it makes up approximately 85% of the acute leukemias in adults. Its onset is often abrupt and dramatic. A patient may have serious infections and abnormal bleeding from the onset of the disease (Fig. 31-13).

AML is characterized by uncontrolled proliferation of myeloblasts, the precursors of granulocytes. There is hyperplasia of the bone marrow. The clinical manifestations are usually related to replacement of normal hematopoietic cells in the marrow by leukemic myeloblasts and, to a lesser extent, to infiltration of other organs and tissue[57] (see Table 31-22).

Acute Lymphocytic Leukemia. ALL is the most common type of leukemia in children and accounts for about 15% of acute leukemia in adults. The 5-year event-free survival rate is nearly 80% for children and approximately 40% for adults.[58] In ALL, immature lymphocytes proliferate in the bone marrow; most are of B-cell origin. Fever is present in the majority of patients at the time of diagnosis. Signs and symptoms may appear abruptly with bleeding or fever, or they may be insidious with progressive weakness, fatigue, bone and/or joint pain, and bleeding tendencies.

Central nervous system (CNS) manifestations are especially common in ALL and represent a serious problem. Leukemic meningitis caused by arachnoid infiltration occurs in many patients with ALL.[59]

Chronic Myelogenous Leukemia. CML is caused by excessive development of mature neoplastic granulocytes in the bone marrow. The excess neoplastic granulocytes move into the peripheral blood in massive numbers and ultimately infiltrate the liver and spleen. These cells contain a distinctive cytogenetic abnormality, the *Philadelphia chromosome,* which serves as a disease marker and results from translocation of genetic material between chromosomes 9 and 22.

The natural history of CML is a chronic stable phase, followed by the development of a more acute, aggressive phase referred to as the *blastic phase.* The chronic phase of CML can last for several years and can usually be well controlled with treatment. Even with treatment, the chronic phase of the disease will eventually progress to the accelerated phase, ending in a blastic phase. Once CML transforms to an acute or blastic phase, it is often refractory to therapy and the patient may live for only a few months.

Chronic Lymphocytic Leukemia. CLL is the most common leukemia in adults. CLL is characterized by the production and accumulation of functionally inactive but long-lived, small, mature-appearing lymphocytes. The type of lymphocyte involved is usually the B cell. The lymphocytes infiltrate the bone marrow, spleen, and liver. Lymph node enlargement (lymphadenopathy) is present throughout the body, and there is an increased incidence of infection because of T-cell deficiencies or hypogammaglobulinemia. B-cell CLL is considered to be identical to the mature B-cell small-lymphocytic lymphoma, a type of non-Hodgkin's lymphoma, and 5% to 8% of these patients will experience a transformation to a diffuse, large B-cell non-Hodgkin's lymphoma, called Richter's syndrome.[60] Complications from early-stage CLL are rare but may develop as the disease advances. Pressure on nerves from enlarged lymph nodes causes pain and even paralysis. Mediastinal node enlargement leads to pulmonary symptoms. Because CLL is usually a disease of older adults, treatment decisions must be made by considering the progression of the disease and the side effects of treatment. Many individuals in the early stages of CLL require no treatment. Fifty percent of patients with early-stage CLL experience rapid progressive disease and will require some therapy.[61]

Hairy Cell Leukemia. *Hairy cell leukemia* accounts for approximately 2% of all adult leukemias. Hairy cell leukemia is usually seen in male patients over 40 years of age. It is a chronic disease of lymphoproliferation predominantly involving B lymphocytes that infiltrate the bone marrow and spleen. Cells have a "hairy" appearance under the microscope. The spleen sequesters increasing numbers of normal hematopoietic cells, making splenomegaly a common finding. Liver infiltration may also occur, although hepatomegaly is less common.

A patient with hairy cell leukemia usually has symptoms from splenomegaly, pancytopenia, infection caused by impaired host defense, or vasculitis. Many asymptomatic patients are detected on routine CBC. The disease is often indolent, and some patients may not need therapy for up to 10 years. For patients needing treatment, α-interferon, pentostatin (Nipent), cladribine (Leustatin), and rituximab (Rituxan) are effective agents for this type of leukemia.[62,63]

Unclassified Leukemias. Occasionally the subtype of leukemia cannot be identified. The malignant leukemic cells may have lymphoid, myeloid, or mixed characteristics. Frequently these patients do not respond to treatment and have a poor prognosis.

Clinical Manifestations

The clinical manifestations of leukemia are varied (see Table 31-24). Essentially they relate to problems caused by bone marrow failure and the formation of leukemic infiltrates. Bone marrow failure results from (1) bone marrow overcrowding by abnormal cells and (2) inadequate production of normal marrow elements. The patient is predisposed to anemia, thrombocytopenia, and decreased number and function of WBCs.

As leukemia progresses, fewer normal blood cells are produced. The abnormal WBCs continue to accumulate because they do not go through the normal cell life cycle to death *(apoptosis).* The leukemic cells infiltrate the patient's organs, leading to problems such as splenomegaly, hepatomegaly, lymphadenopathy, bone pain, meningeal irritation, and oral lesions. Solid masses resulting from collections of leukemic cells called *chloromas* can also occur.

Diagnostic Studies

Peripheral blood evaluation and bone marrow examination are the primary methods of diagnosing and classifying the subtypes of leukemia. Morphologic, histochemical, immunologic, and cytogenetic methods are all used to identify cell subtypes and the stage of development of leukemic cell populations. This is important because different subtypes have different natural histories, prognoses, and chemotherapeutic regimens. Other studies such as lumbar puncture and computed tomography (CT) scan can determine the presence of leukemic cells outside of the blood and bone marrow.

The malignant cells in most patients with AML and ALL have chromosomal abnormalities. In some cases, specific cytogenetic abnormalities are associated with distinct subsets of the disease. In addition to establishing the type of AML or ALL, specific cytogenetic abnormalities have diagnostic, prognostic, and therapeutic importance. In CML, the finding of the Philadelphia chromosome has diagnostic value.

Collaborative Care

Once a diagnosis of leukemia has been made, collaborative care is focused on the initial goal of attaining remission. Age and chromosome analysis often help form the basis of important treatment decisions. Because cytotoxic chemotherapy is the mainstay of the treatment, the nurse must understand the principles of cancer chemotherapy, including cellular kinetics, the use of multiple drugs rather than single agents, and the cell cycle. (See the section on chemotherapy in Chapter 16.)

In some cases, such as nonsymptomatic patients with CLL, watchful waiting with active supportive care may be appropriate. Although a patient may not be cured, attaining remission or disease control is a realistic option for the majority of patients. In some cases, cure is a realistic goal. In *complete remission* there is no evidence of overt disease on physical examination, and the bone marrow and peripheral blood appear normal. A lesser state of control is known as partial remission. *Minimal residual* disease is defined as tumor cells that cannot be detected by morphologic examination, but can be identified by molecular testing. *Partial remission* is characterized by a lack of symptoms and a normal peripheral blood smear, but there is still evidence of disease in the bone marrow. *Molecular remission* is defined as $<0.01\%$ (1 out of 10,000) blasts in the bone marrow.[59] The patient's prognosis is directly related to the ability to maintain a remission. The patient's prognosis becomes more unfavorable with each relapse. Each time there is a relapse, the succeeding remission may be more difficult to achieve and shorter in duration.

Sometimes patients have such a high WBC count (e.g., $\geq 100{,}000/\mu l$) that initial emergent treatment may employ the use of leukapheresis and hydroxyurea. The purpose of these treatments is to reduce the WBC count and risk of leukemia-induced thrombosis.

The chemotherapeutic treatment of acute leukemia is often divided into stages. The first stage, *induction therapy,* is the attempt to induce or bring about a remission. Induction is aggressive treatment that seeks to destroy leukemic cells in the tissues, peripheral blood, and bone marrow in order to eventually restore normal hematopoiesis on bone marrow recovery. During induction therapy a patient may become critically ill because the bone marrow is severely depressed by the chemotherapeutic agents. Throughout the induction phase, nursing interventions focus on neutropenia, thrombocytopenia, and anemia, as well as providing psychosocial support to the patient and family. Common chemotherapy agents for induction of AML include cytarabine (Ara-C, Cytosar) and antitumor antibiotics (anthracyclines) such as daunorubicin (Cerubidine), doxorubicin (Adriamycin), idarubicin (Idamycin), amsacrine, or mitoxantrone (Novantrone). After one course of induction therapy, approximately 70% of newly diagnosed patients achieve complete remission. There is one subtype of AML, called promyelocytic leukemia (M3), in which tretinoin (Vesanoid) is used along with chemotherapy to induce a remission. It is generally assumed that leukemic cells persist undetected after induction therapy. This could lead to relapse within a few months if no further therapy is administered.

Drug Alert *- Daunorubucin (Cerubidine)*
- *Avoid contact with people who have had live virus vaccinations.*
- *Do not have immunizations without physician's approval.*

Terms used to describe postinduction or postremission chemotherapy include intensification, consolidation, and maintenance. *Intensification therapy,* or high-dose therapy, may be given immediately after induction therapy for several months. This therapy may use the same drugs as those used in induction but at higher dosages. Other drugs that target the cell in a different way than those administered during induction may also be added.

Consolidation therapy is started after a remission is achieved. It may consist of one or two additional courses of the same drugs given during induction or involve high-dose therapy (intensive consolidation). The purpose of consolidation therapy is to eliminate remaining leukemic cells that may not be clinically or pathologically evident.

Maintenance therapy is treatment with lower doses of the same drugs used in induction or other drugs given every 3 to 4 weeks for a prolonged period of time. Like consolidation or intensification, the goal is to keep the body free of leukemic cells. Each leukemia requires different maintenance therapy. In AML, maintenance therapy is rarely effective and therefore rarely administered.

In addition to chemotherapy, corticosteroids and radiation therapy can also have a role in the complex therapeutic plans for the patient with leukemia. Total body radiation may be used to prepare a patient for bone marrow transplantation, or it may be restricted to certain areas (fields) such as the liver and spleen or other organs affected by infiltrates. In ALL, prophylactic intrathecal methotrexate or cytarabine is given to decrease the chance of CNS involvement, which is common in this particular type of leukemia. When CNS leukemia does occur, cranial radiation may be given. Biologic and targeted therapy may be indicated for specific leukemias. (Biologic and targeted therapy is discussed in Chapter 16 and Table 16-17.)

Drug Therapy Regimens. The therapeutic agents used to treat leukemia vary. Table 31-25 lists various agents used to treat leukemia. Table 31-26 gives examples of treatment regimens used in various types of leukemia.[57,59,61,64-67]

TABLE 31-25 DRUG THERAPY
Agents Used to Treat Leukemia

Drug Classification	Drug Name
Alkylating agents	busulfan (Myleran) chlorambucil (Leukeran) cyclophosphamide (Cytoxan)
Antitumor antibiotics (anthracyclines)	daunorubicin (Cerubidine) doxorubicin (Adriamycin) mitoxantrone (Novantrone) idarubicin (Idamycin)
Antimetabolites	cytarabine (Cytosar, Ara-C) 6-mercaptopurine (Purinethol) methotrexate (Folex) 6-thioguanine (6-TG) fludarabine (Fludara) nelarabine (Arranon)
Corticosteroid	prednisone dexamethasone (Decadron)
Nitrosoureas	carmustine (BCNU)
Mitotic inhibitors/ Vinca alkaloids	vincristine (Oncovin) vinblastine (Velban)
Biologic/targeted therapy	rituximab (Rituxan) alemtuzumab (Campath) gemtuzumab ozogamicin (Mylotarg) imatinib (Gleevec) dasatinib (Sprycel)
Podophyllotoxin	etoposide (VePesid)
Retinoid	tretinoin (Vesanoid)
Miscellaneous	L-asparaginase (Elspar) pegaspargase (Oncaspar) hydroxyurea (Hydrea) arsenic trioxide (Trisenox) pentostatin (Nipent)

Combination therapy is the mainstay of treatment for leukemia. The three purposes for using multiple drugs are to (1) decrease drug resistance, (2) minimize the drug toxicity to the patient by using multiple drugs with varying toxicities, and (3) interrupt cell growth at multiple points in the cell cycle.

Acronyms made from the letters of the drugs used in combination chemotherapy are used to identify the regimen. For example, COAP stands for cyclophosphamide, Oncovin, arabinoside, and prednisone. This combination of drugs is used to treat ALL.

Newer therapeutic drugs are aimed at affecting small molecules that promote the growth and differentiation of leukemic cells. For example, arsenic trioxide (Trisenox) is used in the treatment of acute promyelocytic leukemia. It causes morphologic changes and DNA fragmentation and programmed cell death. In addition, it inhibits proliferation and angiogenesis. Imatinib (Gleevec) represents a new class of drugs that specifically target an abnormal cell. (Targeted therapy is discussed in Chapter 16.) Imatinib targets an abnormal version of a normal cell protein (the Bcr-Abl protein) that is present in nearly all patients with CML. This abnormal protein is probably the cause of the disease. The Bcr-Abl gene is located on the Philadelphia chromosome. Thus this drug kills only cancer cells, leaving healthy cells alone.

The use of specific targeted therapy in the form of monoclonal antibodies is an exciting new treatment modality in hematopoietic malignancies (see Table 16-17 and Fig. 16-21). Rituximab (Rituxan) binds to the B-cell antigen (CD 20) and has been used

TABLE 31-26 DRUG THERAPY
Treatments Used in Leukemia*

Drug Therapy	Other Therapy
Acute Myelogenous Leukemia	
cytarabine, daunorubicin, doxorubicin, idarubicin, 6-thioguanine, mitoxantrone, thioguanine, arsenic trioxide,† tretinoin (Vesanoid),† gemtuzumab ozogamicin, etoposide, combination chemotherapy of cytarabine and antitumor antibiotic (most common) or cytosine arabinoside and another drug	Autologous or allogeneic hematopoietic stem cell transplant (see Chapter 16)
Acute Lymphocytic Leukemia	
daunorubicin, doxorubicin, vincristine, prednisone, dexamethasone, L-asparaginase, pegaspargase, dasatinib, cyclophosphamide, methotrexate, 6-mercaptopurine, cytarabine, combination chemotherapy of cyclophosphamide and vincristine and prednisone and antitumor antibiotic and L-asparaginase, combination chemotherapy of daunorubicin and cytarabine and 6-mercaptopurine and vincristine and prednisone, nelarabine	Cranial radiation therapy, intrathecal methotrexate or cytarabine Allogeneic hematopoietic stem cell transplant (see Chapter 16)
Chronic Myelogenous Leukemia	
imatinib, dasatinib, hydroxyurea, combination chemotherapy including any of the following: cytarabine, thioguanine, daunorubicin, methotrexate, prednisone, vincristine, L-asparaginase, carmustine, 6-mercaptopurine	Radiation (total body or spleen), hematopoietic stem cell transplant, α-interferon, leukapheresis
Chronic Lymphocytic Leukemia	
chlorambucil, cyclophosphamide, prednisone, CVP protocol (cyclophosphamide, vincristine, and prednisone), fludarabine, rituximab, alemtuzumab, pentostatin	Radiation (total body, lymph nodes, or spleen), splenectomy, colony-stimulating factors, α-interferon; allogeneic hematopoietic stem cell transplant

*Trade names for drugs listed on this table are given on Table 31-25.
†Used for acute promyelocytic leukemia.

with CLL. Alemtuzumab (Campath) binds to CD52, a panlymphocyte antigen present on both T and B cells, and is used to treat CLL. Gemtuzumab ozogamicin (Mylotarg) is an anti-CD33 monoclonal antibody conjugated with an antitumor antibiotic (calicheamicin) that binds to myeloid cells. After the monoclonal antibodies bind to the lymphocytes, the drug induces antibody-dependent lysis (killing). This causes the removal of malignant lymphocytes or myelocytes from the blood, bone marrow, and other affected organs.[57,61,67]

Hematopoietic Stem Cell Transplantation. Hematopoietic stem cell transplantation (HSCT) is another type of therapy used for patients with different forms of leukemia. The goal of HSCT is to totally eliminate leukemic cells from the body using combinations of chemotherapy with or without total body irradiation. This treatment also eradicates the patient's hematopoietic stem cells, which are then replaced with those of an HLA-matched sibling or volunteer donor (allogeneic), an identical twin (syngeneic), or the patient's own (autologous) stem cells that were removed (harvested) before the intensive therapy. (HSCT is discussed in Chapter 16.)

The primary complications of patients with allogeneic HSCT are graft-versus-host disease (GVHD), relapse of leukemia (especially ALL), and infection (especially interstitial pneumonia). GVHD is discussed in Chapter 14. Because HSCT has serious associated risks, the patient must weigh the significant risks of treatment-related death or treatment failure (relapse) with the hope of cure.

NURSING MANAGEMENT LEUKEMIA

Nursing Assessment

Subjective and objective data that should be obtained from a patient with leukemia are presented in Table 31-27.

Nursing Diagnoses

Nursing diagnoses for the patient with leukemia include those appropriate for anemia, thrombocytopenia, and neutropenia (see the appropriate nursing care plans [NCPs 31-1, 31-2, and 31-3] in this chapter).

Planning

The overall goals are that the patient with leukemia will (1) understand and cooperate with the treatment plan, (2) experience minimal side effects and complications associated with both the disease and its treatment, and (3) feel hopeful and supported during the periods of treatment, relapse, or remission.

Nursing Implementation

Acute Intervention. The nursing role during acute phases of leukemia is extremely challenging because the patient has many physical and psychosocial needs. As with other forms of cancer, the diagnosis of leukemia can evoke great fear and be equated with death. It may be viewed as a hopeless, horrible disease with many painful and undesirable consequences. For each patient, it is important that the nurse has an understanding of the patient's type of leukemia, the prognosis, the treatment plan, and the goals. By doing this, the nurse can help the patient realize that although the future may be uncertain, one can have a meaningful quality of life while in remission or with disease control, and that, in some cases, there is reasonable hope for cure. The family also needs help in adjusting to the stress of this abrupt onset of serious illness (e.g., dependence, withdrawal, changes in role responsibilities, alterations in body image) and the losses imposed by the sick role. The diagnosis of leukemia often brings with it the need to make difficult decisions at a time of profound stress for the patient and family. As the majority of patients are older than 65 years old, patients may have comorbid conditions that affect treatment decisions. In

TABLE 31-27 NURSING ASSESSMENT
Leukemia

Subjective Data

Important Health Information

Past health history: Exposure to chemical toxins (e.g., benzene, arsenic), radiation, or viruses (Epstein-Barr, HTLV-1); chromosome abnormalities (Down syndrome, Klinefelter syndrome, Fanconi syndrome), immunologic deficiencies; organ transplantation; frequent infections; bleeding tendencies

Medications: Use of phenylbutazone (Butazolidine), chloramphenicol, chemotherapy

Surgery or other treatments: Radiation exposure; prior radiation and chemotherapy for cancer

Functional Health Patterns

Health perception–health management: Family history of leukemia; malaise

Nutritional-metabolic: Mouth sores, weight loss; chills, night sweats; nausea, vomiting, anorexia, dysphagia, early satiety; easy bruising

Elimination: Hematuria, decreased urine output; diarrhea, dark or bloody stools

Activity-exercise: Fatigue with progressive weakness; dyspnea, epistaxis, cough

Cognitive-perceptual: Headache; muscle cramps; sore throat; generalized sternal tenderness, bone, joint, abdominal pain; paresthesias, numbness, tingling, visual disturbances

Sexuality-reproductive: Prolonged menses, menorrhagia, impotence

Objective Data

General

Fever, generalized lymphadenopathy, lethargy

Integumentary

Pallor or jaundice; petechiae, ecchymoses, purpura, reddish-brown to purple cutaneous infiltrates, macules, and papules

Cardiovascular

Tachycardia, systolic murmurs

Gastrointestinal

Gingival bleeding and hyperplasia; oral ulcerations, herpes and *Candida* infections; perirectal irritation and infection; hepatomegaly, splenomegaly

Neurologic

Seizures, disorientation, confusion, decreased coordination, cranial nerve palsies, papilledema

Musculoskeletal

Muscle wasting, bone pain, joint pain

Possible Findings

Low, normal, or high WBC count with shift to the left (↑ blast cells); anemia, ↓ hematocrit and hemoglobin, thrombocytopenia, Philadelphia chromosome; hypercellular bone marrow aspirate or biopsy with myeloblasts, lymphoblasts, and markedly ↓ normal cells

HTLV-1, Human T-cell leukemia virus, type 1; *WBC,* white blood cell.

addition, although older adults have often learned to live with periods-of-life hardships, disappointments, and loss, health care providers need to assess all patients for potential symptoms of depression and provide appropriate care and referrals.[68]

The nurse is an important advocate in helping the patient and family understand the complexities of treatment decisions and manage the side effects and toxicities. A patient empowered by knowledge of the disease and treatment can have a more positive outlook and improved quality of life. A patient may require hospitalization or may need to temporarily relocate to an appropriate treatment center. These situations can lead a patient to feel deserted and isolated at a time when support is most needed. The nurse has contact with a patient 24 hours a day, and can help reverse feelings of abandonment and loneliness by balancing the demanding technical needs with a humanistic, caring approach. Nurses face special challenges when meeting the intense psychosocial needs of a patient with leukemia while continuing to offer the complex physical care that is required. The needs of the patient with leukemia are best met by a multidisciplinary team (e.g., psychiatric and oncology clinical nurse specialists, case managers, dietitians, chaplains, and social workers).

From a physical care perspective, the nurse is challenged to make astute assessments and plan care to help the patient manage the severe side effects of chemotherapy. The life-threatening results of bone marrow suppression (neutropenia, thrombocytopenia, and anemia) require aggressive nursing interventions (see NCPs 31-1, 31-2, and 31-3). Additional complications of chemotherapy may affect the patient's GI tract, nutritional status, skin and mucosa, cardiopulmonary status, liver, kidneys, and neurologic system. (Nursing interventions related to chemotherapy are discussed in Chapter 16.)

The nurse must be knowledgeable about all drugs being administered. This includes the mechanism of action, purpose, routes of administration, usual doses, potential side effects, safe-handling considerations, and toxic effects of the drugs. In addition, the nurse must know how to assess laboratory data reflecting the effects of the drugs. Patient survival and comfort during aggressive chemotherapy are significantly affected by the quality of nursing care.

Ambulatory and Home Care. Ongoing care for the patient with leukemia is necessary to monitor for signs and symptoms of disease control or relapse. For a patient requiring long-term or maintenance chemotherapy, the fatigue of long-term chronic disease management can become arduous and discouraging. Therefore a patient and the significant other must be taught to understand the importance of the continued diligence in disease management and the need for follow-up care. The patient and significant other must be taught about the drugs, self-care measures, and when to seek medical attention.

The goals of rehabilitation for long-term survivors of childhood and adult leukemia are to manage the physical, psychologic, social, and spiritual consequences and delayed effects from the disease and its treatment. (Delayed effects are discussed in Chapter 16.) Assistance may be needed to reestablish the various relationships that are a part of the patient's life. Friends and family may not know how to interact with the patient. The patient and family must learn to regain attitudes of health and life while facing the real fear of relapse of disease. Involving the patient in survivor networks, support groups, or services such as Can Surmount and Make Today Count may help the patient adapt to living after a life-threatening illness. Exploring resources in the community (e.g., American Cancer Society, Leukemia-Lymphoma Society, Meals-on-Wheels) may reduce the financial burden and the feelings of dependence. Spiritual support may give the patient inner strength and peace.

The patient will need support in adapting to any physical limitations or changes imposed by the illness. Vigilant follow-up care by providers who are aware of the unique needs of a cancer survivor is of the utmost importance for early recognition and treatment of long-term or delayed physical, psychologic, and social effects. The nurse may involve other health care providers in meeting the patient's needs. However, often these needs will require the initiation of a referral or consultation. For example, physical therapy

TABLE 31-28 Comparison of Hodgkin's Lymphoma and Non-Hodgkin's Lymphoma

	Hodgkin's Lymphoma	Non-Hodgkin's Lymphoma
Cellular origin	B lymphocytes	B lymphocytes (90%) T lymphocytes (10%)
Extent of disease	Localized to regional, but may be bulky	Disseminated
B symptoms*	Common	40%
Extranodal involvement	Rare	Common
Histopathologic classification	Five	Many different classifications

*B symptoms include fever, night sweats, and weight loss.

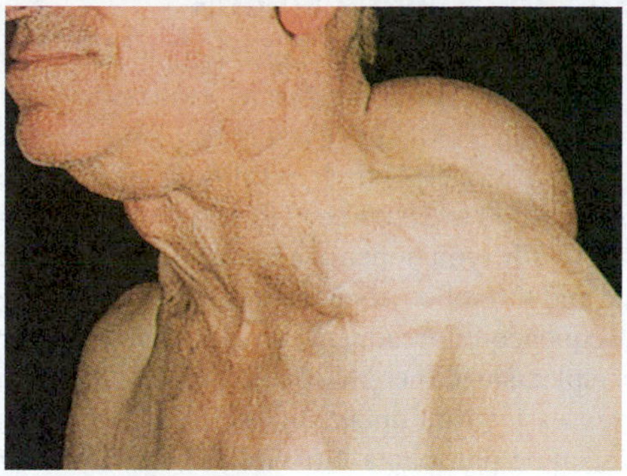

FIG. 31-14 Hodgkin's lymphoma (stage IIA). This patient has enlargement of the cervical lymph nodes.

personnel may be asked to develop an exercise program to prevent posttreatment deficits caused by drug-induced peripheral neuropathy. Most patients should receive the pneumococcal vaccine (Pneumovax) at diagnosis and every 5 years, and an annual influenza vaccine. These needs can also include other concerns such as growth and development concerns for childhood survivors, vocational retraining, and reproductive concerns for a patient of child-bearing age. The long-term recovery following treatment for leukemia affects the quality of the patient's life.

■ Evaluation

The expected outcomes are that the patient with leukemia will (1) cope effectively with diagnosis, treatment regimen, and prognosis; (2) attain and maintain adequate nutrition; (3) experience no complications related to the disease or its treatment; and (4) feel comfortable and supported throughout treatment.

Lymphomas

Lymphomas are malignant neoplasms originating in the bone marrow and lymphatic structures resulting in the proliferation of lymphocytes. Lymphomas are the fifth most common type of cancer in the United States.[56,69] Two major types of lymphoma—Hodgkin's lymphoma and non-Hodgkin's lymphoma (NHL)—are discussed in this chapter. A comparison of these two types of lymphoma is presented in Table 31-28.

HODGKIN'S LYMPHOMA

Hodgkin's lymphoma, also called Hodgkin's disease, makes up about 12% of all lymphomas. It is a malignant condition characterized by proliferation of abnormal giant, multinucleated cells, called *Reed-Sternberg cells,* which are located in lymph nodes. The disease has a bimodal age-specific incidence, occurring most frequently in persons from 15 to 35 years of age and above 50 years of age. In adults, it is twice as prevalent in men as in women. Approximately 7350 new cases of Hodgkin's lymphoma are diagnosed each year, and approximately 1410 deaths occur each year.[56]

Etiology and Pathophysiology

Although the cause of Hodgkin's lymphoma remains unknown, several key factors are thought to play a role in its development. The main interacting factors include infection with Epstein-Barr virus (EBV), genetic predisposition, and exposure to occupational toxins. The incidence of Hodgkin's lymphoma is increased among human immunodeficiency virus (HIV)–infected patients.[70]

Normally, the lymph nodes are composed of connective tissues that surround a fine mesh of reticular fibers and cells. In Hodgkin's lymphoma the normal structure of lymph nodes is destroyed by hyperplasia of monocytes and macrophages. The main diagnostic feature of Hodgkin's lymphoma is the presence of Reed-Sternberg cells in lymph node biopsy specimens. The disease is believed to arise in a single location (it originates in lymph nodes in 90% of patients) and then spreads along adjacent lymphatics. However, in recurrent disease, it may be more diffuse, and not necessarily contiguous. It eventually infiltrates other organs, especially the lungs, spleen, and liver. In approximately two thirds of patients the cervical lymph nodes are the first to be affected. When the disease begins above the diaphragm, it remains confined to lymph nodes for a variable period of time. Disease originating below the diaphragm frequently spreads to extralymphoid sites such as the liver.

Clinical Manifestations

The onset of symptoms in Hodgkin's lymphoma is usually insidious. The initial development is most often enlargement of cervical, axillary, or inguinal lymph nodes (Fig. 31-14); a mediastinal node mass is the second most common location. This lymphadenopathy affects discrete nodes that remain movable and nontender. The enlarged nodes are not painful unless they exert pressure on adjacent nerves.

The patient may notice weight loss, fatigue, weakness, fever, chills, tachycardia, or night sweats. A group of initial findings including fever, night sweats, and weight loss (termed *B symptoms*) correlates with a worse prognosis. After the ingestion of even small amounts of alcohol, individuals with Hodgkin's lymphoma may complain of a rapid onset of pain at the site of disease. The cause for the alcohol-induced pain is unknown. Generalized pruritus without skin lesions may develop. Cough, dyspnea, stridor, and dysphagia may all reflect mediastinal node involvement.

In more advanced disease there may be hepatomegaly and splenomegaly. Anemia results from increased destruction and decreased production of erythrocytes. Other physical signs vary depending on where the disease is located. For example, intrathoracic involvement may lead to superior vena cava syndrome, enlarged retroperitoneal nodes may cause palpable abdominal masses or interfere with renal function, jaundice may occur from liver involvement, and spinal cord compression leading to paraplegia may occur with extradural involvement. Bone pain occurs as a result of bone involvement.

Diagnostic and Staging Studies

Peripheral blood analysis, excisional lymph node biopsy, bone marrow examination, and radiologic evaluation are important means of evaluating Hodgkin's lymphoma. Peripheral blood analysis often reveals a microcytic hypochromic anemia, neutrophilic leukocytosis (15,000 to 28,000/μl [15 to 28 × 10^9/L]), which may be associated with lymphopenia and an increased platelet count. Leukopenia and thrombocytopenia may develop, but they are usually a consequence of treatment, advanced disease, or superimposed hypersplenism. Other blood studies may show hypoferremia caused by excessive iron uptake by the liver and spleen, elevated leukocyte alkaline phosphatase from liver and bone involvement, hypercalcemia from bone involvement, and hypoalbuminemia from liver involvement.

Excisional lymph node biopsy offers a definitive means of diagnosis. The removed peripheral lymph node is examined for the presence of the diagnostic Reed-Sternberg cells and to identify the subtype (the most common is nodular sclerosing). Bone marrow biopsy is performed as an important aspect of staging. Reed-Sternberg cells may also be found in the bone marrow of patients.

Radiologic evaluation can help define all sites and determine the clinical stage of the disease. CT or magnetic resonance imaging (MRI) scans are used as initial staging tools. Positron emission tomography (PET) with or without CT scans are used to assess the response to therapy and to differentiate residual tumor from fibrotic masses after treatment. These scans may show increased uptake (by PET) and masses (by CT) such as mediastinal lymphadenopathy, renal displacement caused by retroperitoneal node enlargement, abdominal lymph node enlargement, and liver, spleen, bone, and brain infiltration.[70]

NURSING *and* COLLABORATIVE MANAGEMENT
HODGKIN'S LYMPHOMA

Using all of the information from the various diagnostic studies, a clinical stage of disease is determined (Fig. 31-15). The final staging is based on the clinical stage (extent of the disease), as well as the presence of B symptoms. Treatment depends on the nature and extent of the disease. The nomenclature used in staging involves an A or B classification, depending on whether symptoms are present when the disease is found, and a Roman numeral (I to IV) that reflects the location and extent of the disease. Additional features, such as an elevated sedimentation rate; age ≥50 years; and the presence of a large mediastinal mass and low serum albumin, hemoglobin, and lymphocyte counts may move an early stage (I or II) to an unfavorable prognosis, warranting more aggressive therapy.[71,72]

Once the stage of Hodgkin's lymphoma is established, management focuses on selecting a treatment plan. The standard for chemotherapy is the ABVD regimen: doxorubicin (Adriamycin), bleomycin, vinblastine, and dacarbazine. Patients with favorable early-stage disease will receive two to four cycles of chemotherapy. Patients with early-stage but unfavorable prognostic features (e.g., the presence of B symptoms) or intermediate-stage disease will be treated with four to six cycles of chemotherapy. Advanced-stage Hodgkin's lymphoma is treated more aggressively using six to potentially eight cycles of chemotherapy. Other chemotherapy regimens include MOPP alternating with ABVD. MOPP consists of mechlorethamine, vincristine (Oncovin), procarbazine, and prednisone. Other, more aggressive, regimens are Stanford V and BEACOPP and ICE. The role of radiation as a supplement to chemotherapy varies depending on sites of disease and the presence of resistant disease after chemotherapy.[71,73]

Intensive chemotherapy with or without the use of autologous or allogeneic HSCT and hematopoietic growth factors is the treatment of choice for advanced, refractory or relapsed Hodgkin's lymphoma (stages IIIB and IV). HSCT has allowed patients to receive higher, potentially curative doses of chemotherapy while reducing life-threatening leukopenia (see Chapter 16). Combination chemotherapy works well because, as in leukemia, drugs are used that have an additive antitumor effect without increasing side effects. As with leukemia, therapy must be aggressive. Therefore potentially life-threatening problems are encountered in an attempt to achieve a remission.

Maintenance chemotherapy does not contribute to increased survival once a complete remission is achieved. Occasionally, single drugs may be administered palliatively to patients who cannot tolerate intensive combination therapy. A serious consequence of the treatment for Hodgkin's lymphoma is the later development of secondary malignancies (see Chapter 16), as well as potential long-term toxicities from the treatment, such as endocrine, cardiac, and pulmonary dysfunction.[71] The estimated risk of a secondary cancer is approximately 18% at 15 years after treatment for Hodgkin's lymphoma. The most common secondary malignancies are acute myelogenous leukemia, non-Hodgkin's lymphoma, and solid tumors.

The nursing care for Hodgkin's lymphoma is largely based on managing problems related to the disease (e.g., pain due to tumor), pancytopenia, and other side effects of therapy. Because the survival of patients with Hodgkin's lymphoma depends on their response to treatment, supporting the patient through the consequences of treatment is extremely important.

The patient undergoing radiation therapy has special nursing needs. The skin in the radiation field requires attention. Also, the nurse must understand the concepts related to administration of radiation therapy (see Chapter 16).

Psychosocial considerations are just as important as they are with leukemia. However, the prognosis for Hodgkin's lymphoma is better than that for many forms of cancer or leukemia. Early-stage Hodgkin's lymphoma has a 10-year survival rate near 90%, and advanced-stage Hodgkin's lymphoma has a 10-year survival rate of more than 50%. The physical, psychologic, social, and spiritual consequences of the patient's disease must be addressed. Fertility issues may be of particular concern because this disease is frequently seen in adolescents and young adults. The nurse must help ensure that these issues have been addressed soon after diagnosis. Evaluation of patients for long-term effects of therapy is important because delayed consequences of disease and treatment may not be apparent for many years.[69,71] (Secondary malignancies and delayed effects are discussed in Chapter 16.)

NON-HODGKIN'S LYMPHOMA

Non-Hodgkin's lymphomas (NHLs) are a heterogeneous group of malignant neoplasms of primarily B- or T-cell origin affecting all ages. B-cell lymphomas constitute about 90% of all NHLs. They are classified according to different cellular and lymph node characteristics. A variety of clinical presentations and courses are recognized, from indolent (slowly developing) to rapidly progressive disease. NHL is the most commonly occurring hematologic cancer and the fifth leading cause of cancer death. Approximately

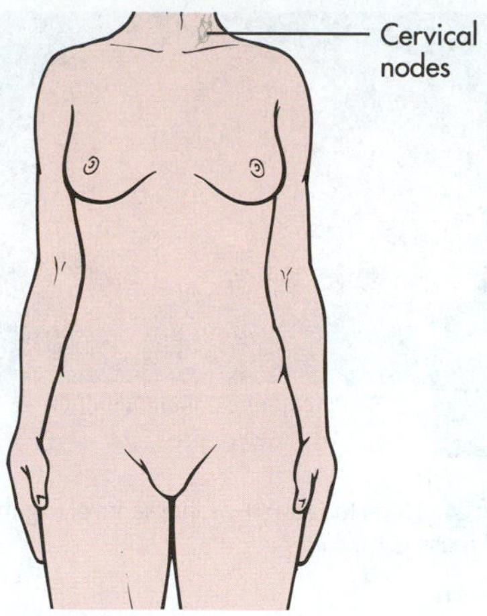

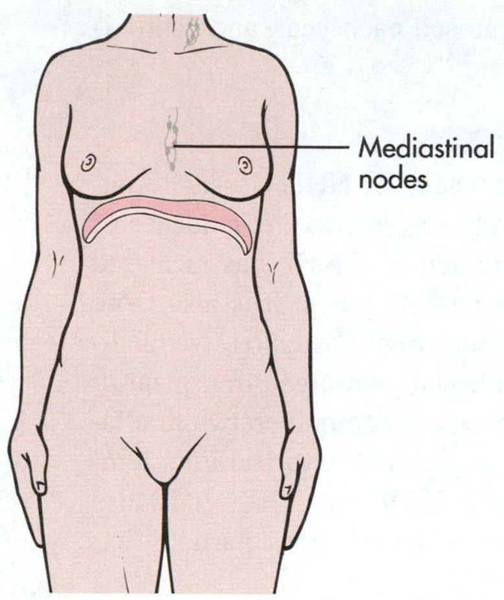

Stage I
Involvement of a single lymph node or a single extranodal site

Stage II
Involvement of two or more lymph node regions on the same side of the diaphragm or localized involvement of an extranodal site and one or more lymph node regions of the same side of the diaphragm

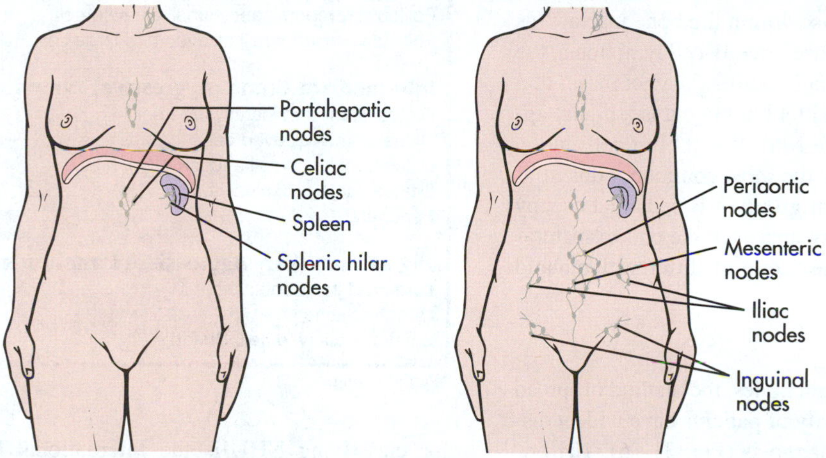

Stage III
Involvement of lymph node regions on both sides of the diaphragm. May include a single extranodal site, the spleen, or both; now subdivided into lymphatic involvement of the upper abdomen in the spleen (splenic, celiac, and portal nodes) (*Stage* III_1) and the lower abdominal nodes in the periaortic, mesenteric, and iliac regions (*Stage* III_2)

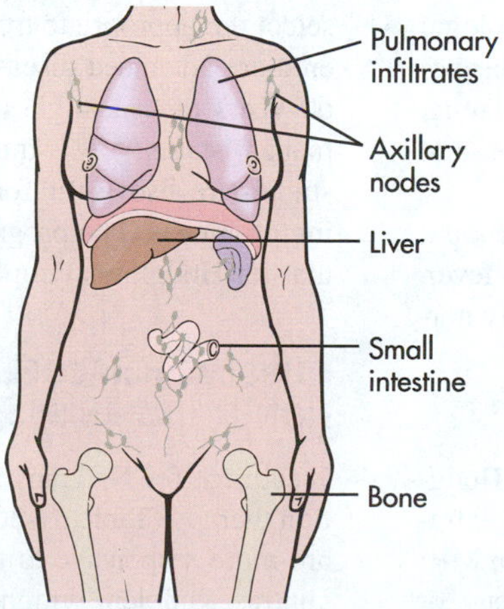

Stage IV
Diffuse or disseminated disease of one or more extralymphatic organs or tissues with or without associated lymph node involvement; the extranodal site is identified as *H*, hepatic; *L*, lung; *P*, pleura; *M*, marrow; *D*, dermal; *O*, osseous

FIG. 31-15 Staging system for Hodgkin's lymphoma and non-Hodgkin's lymphoma.

56,000 new cases of NHL are diagnosed each year, and approximately 19,200 deaths occur each year.[56]

Etiology and Pathophysiology

As with Hodgkin's lymphoma, the cause of NHL is usually unknown. However, as the population has aged and the incidence of HIV infection has increased, the incidence of NHL has increased 2% to 3% per year for at least the past 30 years. It is also more common in individuals who have used immunosuppressive medications (e.g., to prevent rejection following an organ transplant or to treat autoimmune disorders) or received chemotherapy or radiation therapy. Epstein-Barr virus is associated with Burkitt's lymphoma, but not all individuals with EBV get NHL. It is also thought that occupational exposure to carcinogens partially explains the increased incidence.[56,74,75]

There is no hallmark feature in NHL that parallels the Reed-Sternberg cell of Hodgkin's lymphoma. However, all NHLs involve lymphocytes arrested in various stages of development. For example, lymphoblastic lymphoma and lymphoblastic leukemia result from malignant proliferation of small naïve B lymphocytes, the latter having a majority of disease within the bone marrow (as compared to the lymph nodes). Diffuse large B-cell lymphoma, the most common aggressive lymphoma in adults, is a neoplasm that originates in the lymph nodes. Burkitt's lymphoma is a highly aggressive disease thought to originate from B-cell blast cells in the lymph nodes. Follicular lymphoma, the most common indolent or low-grade lymphoma, is a malignant group of B cells that occupy the center of the lymph node as they approach the end of maturation.[74] Thus NHL comprises a large group of different lymphoid malignancies.

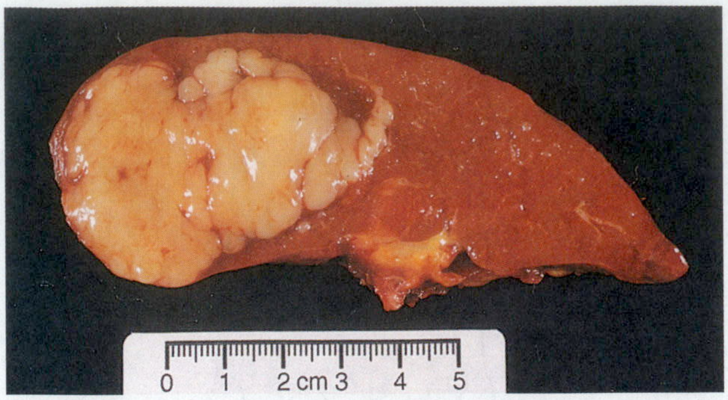

FIG. 31-16 Non-Hodgkin's lymphoma involving the spleen. The presence of an isolated mass is typical.

TABLE 31-29 Non-Hodgkin's Lymphoma Classification*

Low-Grade (Indolent) Lymphomas
Small lymphocytic, plasmacytoid
Follicular, predominantly small cleaved cell
Follicular, mixed small cleaved and large cell
Intermediate-Grade (Aggressive) Lymphomas
Follicular, predominantly large cell
Diffuse, small cleaved cell
Diffuse, mixed, small and large cell
Diffuse, large cell; cleaved cell
Peripheral T cell
High-Grade (Very Aggressive) Lymphomas
Large cell immunoblastic
Lymphoblastic
Small noncleaved cell; Burkitt's

*Partial listing.

Clinical Manifestations

NHLs can originate outside the lymph nodes, the method of spread can be unpredictable, and the majority of patients have widely disseminated disease at the time of diagnosis (Fig. 31-16). The primary clinical manifestation is painless lymph node enlargement. The lymphadenopathy can wax and wane in indolent disease. Because the disease is usually disseminated when it is diagnosed, other symptoms will be present depending on where the disease has spread (e.g., hepatomegaly with liver involvement, neurologic symptoms with CNS disease). NHL can also manifest in nonspecific ways, such as an airway obstruction, hyperuricemia and renal failure from tumor lysis syndrome, pericardial tamponade, and gastrointestinal complaints.

Patients with high-grade lymphomas may have lymphadenopathy and constitutional symptoms (B symptoms) such as fever, night sweats, and weight loss. The peripheral blood is usually normal, but some lymphomas manifest in a "leukemic" phase.

Diagnostic and Staging Studies

Diagnostic studies used for NHL resemble those used for Hodgkin's lymphoma. However, because NHL is more often in extranodal sites, more diagnostic studies may be done, such as an MRI to rule out CNS or bone marrow infiltration, or a barium enema or CT to visualize suspected GI involvement. Clinical staging, as described for Hodgkin's lymphoma, is used to help guide therapy (see Fig. 31-15), but establishment of the precise histologic subtype is extremely important. Lymph node biopsy establishes the cell type and pattern. NHL is classified based on morphologic, genetic, immunophenotypic, and clinical features. A useful system for classifying NHL is the International Working Formulation (IWF) that simply divides each subtype of lymphoma into low grade (indolent), intermediate grade (aggressive), and high grade (very aggressive) (Table 31-29). Additional factors, known as the International Prognostic Index (IPI), may be considered to help select the appropriate treatment for these patients. Factors considered are advanced disease, number of extranodal sites, older than 60 years of age, high serum lactate dehydrogenase, and performance status.[69,74,75] Immunologic, cytogenetic, and molecular studies are also useful for making therapeutic decisions and assessing prognosis. The prognosis for NHL is generally not as good as that for Hodgkin's lymphoma.

NURSING *and* COLLABORATIVE MANAGEMENT
NON-HODGKIN'S LYMPHOMA

Treatment for NHL involves chemotherapy and sometimes radiation therapy (Table 31-30). Ironically, more aggressive lymphomas are more responsive to treatment and more likely to be cured. In contrast, indolent lymphomas have a naturally long course but are difficult to effectively treat.[73,74,76,77]

Patients with low-grade (indolent) lymphoma have a median overall survival of 9 years. However, most patients relapse several times and cure is very unlikely. A previous approach was that patients who were asymptomatic were followed with "watchful waiting" to assess the progress of the disease. However, some initial

TABLE 31-30 Guidelines for Treatment of Non-Hodgkin's Lymphoma

Grade	Recommended Therapies	Common Combination Regimens
Low (indolent)	Observation until disease progression for asymptomatic patients with low-volume tumors and normal blood counts External beam irradiation for local, limited disease Single-agent rituximab weekly × 4 and then maintenance Rituximab with another agent (cyclophosphamide, fludarabine, cladribine, pentostatin, chlorambucil, denileukin diftitox) and/or: Combination chemotherapy (CHOP [or "CHOP-R"], FMC, CVP, FCD) Radioimmunotherapy Autologous hematopoietic stem cell transplant	**CHOP-R** = **c**yclophosphamide, doxorubicin **h**ydrochloride, **o**ncovin, **p**rednisone, **r**ituximab **CVP** = **c**yclophosphamide, **v**incristine, **p**rednisone **FMC** = **f**ludarabine, **m**itoxantrone, **c**yclophosphamide **FCD** = **f**ludarabine, **c**yclophosphamide, **d**examethasone, rituximab **FMD** = **f**ludarabine, **m**itoxantrone, **d**examethasone *Aggressive combination chemotherapy regimens:* **CHOP-14** = **c**yclophosphamide, doxorubicin, **h**ydrochloride, **o**ncovin, **p**rednisone, rituximab every 14 days with G-CSF support **ACVBP** = doxorubicin (**A**driamycin), **c**yclophosphamide, **v**indesine, **b**leomycin, **p**rednisone **ICE** (or "RICE" with rituximab) = **i**fosfamide, **c**yclophosphamide, **e**toposide **EPOCH** = **e**toposide, **p**rednisone, vincristine, **c**yclophosphamide, doxorubicin **DHAP** = **d**examethasone, cytarabine (**A**ra-c), cis**p**latin **ESHAP** = **e**toposide, prednisone, high-dose cytarabine (**A**ra-c), cis**p**latin **Hyper-CVAD** = hyperfractionated **c**ytoxan, vincristine, doxorubicin (**A**driamycin), **d**examethasone alternating with high-dose methotrexate and cytarabine **High-dose methotrexate with leucovorin rescue**
Intermediate (aggressive)	Combination chemotherapy with localized radiation if needed Aggressive combination chemotherapy for 3-8 cycles with rituximab with local radiation if needed Intrathecal chemotherapy if needed Autologous hematopoietic stem cell transplant	
High (very aggressive)	Combination chemotherapy (high dose), aggressive with rituximab and with localized radiation if needed Intrathecal chemotherapy if needed Autologous hematopoietic stem cell transplant	

G-CSF, Granulocyte colony-stimulating factor.

therapies can be well tolerated and have shown to reduce the time to progression of the disease. Therapy for these patients would be indicated if the patient has local symptoms from progressive, bulky, or painful disease or a compromise of normal organ function. An option for these patients is rituximab every week and then every 2 months as maintenance therapy. Rituximab, a genetically engineered monoclonal antibody against the CD20 antigen on the surface of normal and malignant B lymphocytes, is used to treat NHL. Once bound to the cells, rituximab causes lysis and cell death. Once the disease is symptomatic, rituximab with chemotherapy, such as cyclophosphamide (Cytoxan) with or without prednisone or even the CHOP regimen (cyclophosphamide, doxorubicin [Adriamycin], vincristine [Oncovin], prednisone, and rituximab [Rituxan]) may be used.[74,78] Complete remissions are uncommon, but the majority of patients will respond with improvement in adenopathy and symptoms. Numerous chemotherapy combinations have been used to try to overcome the resistant nature of this disease.

Intermediate-grade (aggressive) and high-grade (very aggressive) lymphomas may be treated similarly, depending on the extent of the disease and the patient's prognostic factors. Diffuse large B-cell NHL is the most common high-grade lymphoma and the most common subtype. The most common standard chemotherapeutic regimen is CHOP-R. Other combination therapies may be used for very aggressive or refractory disease. These include RICE, EPOCH, DHAP, and ESHAP (see Table 31-30). Dose-dense (intensified) treatment with CHOP-14 every 2 weeks (versus every 3 to 4 weeks) with hematopoietic growth factor support may be used in patients with aggressive disease. High-dose chemotherapy with autologous HSCT has shown a better outcome than conventional chemotherapy in the treatment of patients with relapsed, aggressive NHL who are still responding to salvage chemotherapy. The role of allogeneic transplant in NHL is uncertain, but it is thought that it may have some benefit in certain subtypes with aggressive or refractory lymphoma.[74,76,77,79]

Because NHL represents a large variety of neoplasms, some subtypes may be treated differently than the general standards described previously. For example, cutaneous T-cell lymphoma may be treated with topical corticosteroids or topical chemotherapy for limited-stage disease. For more diffuse disease, treatment may include phototherapy, α-interferon, oral bexarotene (Targretin), a retinoid, or denileukin diftitox (Ontak), which is a novel fusion protein consisting of interleukin-2 and diphtheria toxin.[80,81] (Biologic and targeted therapy is discussed in Chapter 16.)

Other therapies for NHL include the monoclonal antibodies ibritumomab tiuxetan (Zevalin) and tositumomab (Bexxar). These antibodies are linked to a radioactive isotope (yttrium-90 and iodine-131, respectively) (see Table 16-17). The monoclonal antibody targets the CD20 antigen, which is on the surface of mature B cells and B-cell tumors. This allows for the delivery of radiation directly to the malignant cells. Currently, these therapies are primarily used for patients with indolent lymphomas, particularly those with chemotherapy-refractory disease. Side effects of this type of treatment include pancytopenia.[82,83] The nurse needs to be aware of the necessary precautions in caring for these patients, both to educate patients about safety issues and to minimize the risk of radiation exposure to staff and others.[84]

The nursing care for NHL is similar to that for Hodgkin's lymphoma. Nursing care is largely based on managing problems related to the disease (e.g., pain due to the tumor, spinal cord compression, tumor lysis syndrome), pancytopenia, and other side effects of therapy. However, because NHL can be more extensive and involve specific organs (e.g., CNS, spleen, liver, GI tract, bone marrow), it is important that the nurse have an understanding of the subtype and extent of the disease. For example, a patient with known involvement of the colon may complain of acute abdominal pain. The patient most likely would have abdominal guarding and an enlarged and tympanic abdomen. This could indicate a bowel perforation and be considered a medical emergency. A patient with a Burkitt's NHL starting chemotherapy would be at high risk for tumor lysis syndrome, and would have to have frequent laboratory parameters drawn and monitored, as well as being on strict intake and output. For oncologic problems, refer to Chapter 16. Because most of these patients receive therapy that is potentially myelosuppressive, the NCPs 31-1, 31-2, and 31-3 would apply to these patients as well.

The patient undergoing radiation therapy has special nursing needs. The skin in the radiation field requires attention. In addition, the nurse needs to understand the concepts related to administration of and safety issues regarding radiation therapy (see Chapter 16).

Psychosocial considerations are very important. Helping the patient and family understand the disease, treatment, and expected and potential untoward side effects is paramount in enlisting their help in the patient's well-being and safety. Fertility issues may be of concern in young patients. As in Hodgkin's lymphoma, evaluation of patients with NHL for long-term effects of therapy is important because delayed consequences of disease and treatment may not be apparent for many years. (Secondary malignancies and delayed effects are discussed in Chapter 16.)

MULTIPLE MYELOMA

Multiple myeloma, or *plasma cell myeloma,* is a condition in which neoplastic plasma cells infiltrate the bone marrow and destroy bone. A patient usually lives for approximately 2 years after diagnosis if untreated. The incidence of multiple myeloma is approximately 4 per 100,000 people. The disease is twice as common in men as in women and usually develops after 40 years of age, with an average age of 65 years. Multiple myeloma occurs in African Americans more commonly than in whites.[56,85]

Etiology and Pathophysiology

The cause of multiple myeloma is unknown. Exposure to radiation, organic chemicals (such as benzene), herbicides, and insecticides may play a role. Genetic factors and viral infection may also influence the risk of developing multiple myeloma.

The disease process involves excessive production of plasma cells. Plasma cells are activated B cells, which produce immunoglobulins (antibodies) that normally serve to protect the body. However, in multiple myeloma the malignant plasma cells infiltrate the bone marrow and produce abnormal and excessive amounts of immunoglobulin (usually IgG [most common], IgA, IgD, or IgE). This abnormal immunoglobulin is termed a *myeloma protein* or *M protein.* Furthermore, plasma cell production of excessive and abnormal amounts of cytokines (interleukins [ILs]; IL-4, IL-5, and IL-6) also plays an important role in the pathologic process of bone destruction. As myeloma protein increases, normal plasma cells are reduced, which further compromises the body's normal immune response. In some patients, excessive production and secretion of free light-chain proteins (called *Bence Jones* proteins) from the myeloma cell is also seen and can be detected in the urine. Proliferation of malignant plasma cells and the overproduction of immunoglobulin and proteins result in the end-organ effects of myeloma to the bone marrow, bone, and kidneys and possibly the spleen, lymph nodes, liver, and even heart muscle.

Clinical Manifestations

Multiple myeloma develops slowly and insidiously. The patient often does not manifest symptoms until the disease is advanced, at which time skeletal pain is the major manifestation. Pain in the pelvis, spine, and ribs is particularly common. The pain is triggered by movement. Diffuse osteoporosis develops as the myeloma protein destroys bone. Osteolytic lesions are seen in the skull, vertebrae, and ribs. Vertebral destruction can lead to collapse of vertebrae with ensuing compression of the spinal cord. Loss of bone integrity can lead to the development of pathologic fractures; about 30% of patients have pathologic fractures.

Bony degeneration also causes calcium to be lost from bones, eventually causing hypercalcemia. Hypercalcemia may cause renal, GI, or neurologic manifestations such as polyuria, anorexia, confusion, and ultimately seizures, coma, and cardiac problems. High protein levels caused by the presence of the myeloma protein can result in renal failure, from renal tubular obstruction by the myeloma protein, and interstitial nephritis. The patient may also display manifestations of anemia, thrombocytopenia, and neutropenia, all of which are related to the replacement of normal bone marrow with plasma cells.

Diagnostic Studies

Evaluating multiple myeloma involves laboratory, radiologic, and bone marrow examination. The presence of a monoclonal (M) antibody protein can be found in the blood and urine. Pancytopenia, hypercalcemia, the presence of Bence Jones protein in the urine, and an elevated serum creatinine are possible findings.

X-rays show distinct lytic areas of bone erosions, generalized thinning of the bones, and/or fractures, especially in the vertebrae, ribs, pelvis, and bones of the thigh and upper arms. Bone marrow analysis shows significantly increased numbers of plasma cells in the bone marrow. The simplest measure of prognosis in multiple myeloma is based on blood levels of two markers: β_2-microglobulin and albumin. In general, higher levels of β_2-microglobulin and lower levels of albumin are associated with a poorer prognosis.

Collaborative Care

Collaborative care involves managing both the disease and its symptoms. The current treatment options include watchful waiting (for early multiple myeloma), corticosteroids, chemotherapy, biologic therapy, and hematopoietic stem cell transplantation (HSCT). Multiple myeloma is seldom cured, but treatment can relieve symptoms, produce remission, and prolong life. Ambulation and adequate hydration are used to treat hypercalcemia, dehydration, and potential renal damage. Weight bearing helps the bones reabsorb some calcium, and fluids dilute calcium and prevent protein precipitates from causing renal tubular obstruction. Control of pain and prevention of pathologic fractures are other goals of management. Analgesics, orthopedic supports, and localized radiation help reduce the skeletal pain. Bisphosphonates, such as pamidronate (Aredia), zoledronic acid (Zometa), and etidronate (Didronel), inhibit bone breakdown and are used for the treatment of skeletal pain and hypercalcemia. They inhibit bone resorption without inhibiting bone formation and mineralization. They are given monthly by IV infusion. Radiation therapy is another important component of treatment, primarily because of its effect on localized lesions. Surgical procedures, such as vertebroplasty, may be done to support degenerative vertebrae.

***Drug Alert** - Zoledronic Acid (Zometa)*
- *Patient should be adequately rehydrated before administering drug.*
- *Renal toxicity may occur if IV infusion of drug is administered in <15 minutes.*

Chemotherapy is usually the first treatment recommended for multiple myeloma. It is used to reduce the number of plasma cells. The agents most frequently used are the alkylating drugs, including melphalan (Alkeran), cyclophosphamide (Cytoxan), vincristine (Oncovin), and doxorubicin (Adriamycin). Corticosteroids (prednisone, dexamethasone [Decadron]) may be added because they exert an antitumor effect in some patients. A common regimen is VAD—vincristine, doxorubicin (Adriamycin), and dexamethasone—given once a month over several months before an autologous HSCT. Because of improved response rates and survival rates, high-dose chemotherapy, such as melphalan, followed by autologous HSCT has evolved as the standard of care in eligible patients. Some patients may also benefit from a tandem transplant (e.g., two transplants). The role of allogeneic HSCT has yet to be determined, but may also be effective for some patients.[85,86]

Other medications may also be used to keep the myeloma under control for some time. Bortezomib (Velcade) is a new targeted therapy known as a proteasome inhibitor (see Table 16-17). Proteasomes are present in all cells and regulate cell growth. Normal cells are capable of recovery from proteasome inhibition, but cancer cells undergo death when proteasomes are inhibited.[87] Bortezomib is indicated for patients whose disease has relapsed after two prior treatments and who have demonstrated resistance to their last treatment. Thalidomide (Thalomid) is an immune-modulating and antiangiogenic drug that may slow the growth of plasma cells and reduce their numbers. Thalidomide may be given alone or with corticosteroids or chemotherapy drugs. The use of thalidomide is contraindicated in pregnant women because it is known to cause birth defects. It is also associated with an increase in deep vein thrombosis, neuropathies, and excess somnolence, so it may not be tolerated by some patients. α-Interferon therapy has been used following chemotherapy. It works by altering the receptors for IL-6, which is a growth factor for myeloma cells.

Drugs may be used to treat complications of multiple myeloma. For example, allopurinol (Zyloprim) may be given to reduce hyperuricemia, and IV furosemide (Lasix) promotes renal excretion of calcium. Calcitonin can be used to decrease the risk of fractures and reduce bone pain.

NURSING MANAGEMENT
MULTIPLE MYELOMA

A major focus of care relates to the bone involvement and sequelae from bone breakdown. Maintaining adequate hydration is a primary nursing consideration to minimize problems from hypercalcemia. Fluids are administered to attain a urinary output of 1.5 to 2 L per day. This may require an intake of 3 to 4 L. In addition, weight bearing helps bones reabsorb some of the circulating calcium, and corticosteroids may augment the excretion of calcium. Once chemotherapy is initiated, the uric acid levels may rise because of the increased cell destruction. Hyperuricemia is treated by ensuring adequate hydration and using allopurinol to prevent any renal damage. Because of the myeloma proteins, the patient is at additional risk of renal dysfunction. The nurse needs to monitor electrolytes and fluid balance.

Because of the potential for pathologic fractures, the nurse must be careful when moving and ambulating the patient. A slight twist or strain in the wrong area (e.g., a weak area in the patient's bones) may be sufficient to cause a fracture. In addition, the development of peripheral neuropathy is common with several therapies for multiple myeloma and can contribute to discomfort, the inability to perform basic activities of daily living, and the risk of injury from falling.

Pain management requires innovative and knowledgeable nursing interventions. Analgesics, such as nonsteroidal antiinflammatory drugs, acetaminophen, or an acetaminophen/opioid combination, may be more effective than opioids alone in diminishing bone pain. Braces, especially for the spine, may also help control pain. As in any pain management situation, the nurse is responsible for assessing the patient and for implementing necessary measures to alleviate the pain. (Pain management is discussed in Chapter 10.)

Assessment and prompt treatment of infection is important in the care of patients with multiple myeloma. Some 50% to 70% of patients will die as a result of bacterial infections. These recurrent infections may be due to a decrease in the production of normal immunoglobins, the ineffectiveness of the overproduced and abnormal immunoglobins, and/or neutropenia as a result of the bone marrow infiltration or side effects of treatment.[85] Nursing care plans for anemia (NCP 31-1), thrombocytopenia (NCP 31-2), and neutropenia (NCP 31-3) apply to the patient with multiple myeloma.

The patient's psychosocial needs require sensitive, skilled management. It is important to help the patient and significant others adapt to changes fostered by chronic sickness, deal with reality, and adjust to the losses related to the disease process. The symptoms of multiple myeloma remit and exacerbate. Consequently, acute care is needed at various times during the course of the illness. The final, acute phase is unresponsive to treatment and usually short in duration. The way in which patients and families deal with confronting death may be affected by the manner in which they have learned to accept and live with the chronic nature of the disease.

DISORDERS OF THE SPLEEN

The spleen can be affected by many illnesses, most of which can cause some degree of *splenomegaly* (enlarged spleen) (Table 31-31). The term *hypersplenism* refers to the occurrence of splenomegaly and peripheral cytopenias (anemia, leukopenia, and thrombocytopenia). The degree of splenic enlargement varies with the disease. For example, massive splenic enlargement occurs with chronic myelogenous leukemia, hairy cell leukemia, and thalassemia major. Mild splenic enlargement occurs with heart failure and systemic lupus erythematosus. The normal spleen contains 20 to 40 ml of blood and does not usually serve as a reservoir for blood volume or erythrocytes.[88,89]

When the spleen enlarges, its normal filtering and sequestering capacity increases. Consequently, there is often a reduction in the number of circulating blood cells. In addition, there are unusual findings in the peripheral smear, such as pitted or pocked erythrocytes or Howell-Jolly bodies. These findings assist with diagnosing a malfunctioning spleen. A slight to moderate enlargement of the spleen is usually asymptomatic and found during a routine examination of the abdomen. Even massive splenomegaly can be well tolerated, but the patient may complain of abdominal discomfort and early satiety. In addition to physical examination, other techniques to assess the size of the spleen include ^{99m}Tc-sulfur colloid liver-spleen scan, CT scan, MRI, and ultrasound scan.[89]

Occasionally laparoscopy or open laparotomy and splenectomy are indicated in the evaluation or treatment of splenomegaly. Splenectomy can have a dramatic effect in increasing peripheral RBC, WBC, and platelet counts. Another major indication for splenectomy is splenic rupture. The spleen may rupture from trauma, inadvertent tearing during other surgical procedures, and diseases such as mononucleosis, malaria, and lymphoid neoplasms.

TABLE 31-31 Causes of Splenomegaly

Hereditary Hemolytic Anemias
Sickle cell disease
Thalassemia
Autoimmune Cytopenias
Acquired hemolytic anemia
Immune thrombocytopenia
Infections and Inflammations
Bacterial infections: endocarditis
Mycobacterial infections: tuberculosis
Spirochetes: syphilis, Lyme disease
Viral infections: hepatitis, human immunodeficiency virus, cytomegalovirus, mononucleosis
Parasitic infections: malaria, trypanosomiasis, schistosomiasis, leishmaniasis, toxoplasmosis, echinococcosis
Rickettsial infections: Rocky Mountain spotted fever, typhoid fever, kala-azar
Fungal infections: histoplasmosis
Systemic lupus erythematosus, rheumatoid arthritis
Infiltrative Diseases
Acute and chronic leukemia
Lymphomas
Polycythemia vera
Multiple myeloma, amyloidosis
Other primary or secondary neoplasms and cysts
Sarcoidosis
Others: Gaucher disease, Niemann-Pick disease
Congestion
Cirrhosis of the liver
Heart failure
Portal or splenic vein thrombosis

ETHICAL DILEMMAS

Religious Interest

Situation

An elderly woman is transferred from a nursing home because of gastrointestinal bleeding from an unknown cause. Some of her family members tell the nurse that she is a Jehovah's Witness and must not receive blood products. If she does not have exploratory surgery and transfusions, the surgeon believes that she will die.

Important Points for Consideration

- Competent adults have the right to make health care decisions based on their religious beliefs, including the right to refuse treatment.
- Health care professionals should make every effort to incorporate the patient's values and beliefs into the treatment plan. When the extent of the patient's beliefs is not clear, members of the health care team should consult other available resources, such as family, friends, or church officials, in an attempt to ascertain the patient's commitment to his or her faith.
- Jehovah's Witnesses believe that if they receive blood or blood products there are eternal consequences.
- When a clear determination of the patient's beliefs cannot be made, the patient is unable to communicate his or her wishes, and there are no advance directives, a decision by the health care team to perform the lifesaving surgery and transfusion would be acceptable.

Critical Thinking Questions

1. What resources do you have available to consult on religious practices?
2. How could you make a determination if the family were acting in the patient's best interest or their own?

Nursing responsibilities for the patient with spleen disorders vary depending on the nature of the problem. Splenomegaly may be painful and may require analgesic administration; care in moving, turning, and positioning; and evaluation of lung expansion because spleen enlargement may impair diaphragmatic excursion. If anemia, thrombocytopenia, or leukopenia develops from splenic enlargement, nursing measures must be instituted to support the patient and prevent life-threatening complications. If splenectomy is performed, the nurse must provide the meticulous care warranted after any surgery. In addition, there must be special observation for hemorrhage, which could lead to shock, fever, and abdominal distention.

After splenectomy, immunologic deficiencies may develop. IgM levels are reduced, and IgG and IgA values remain within normal limits. Postsplenectomy patients have a lifelong risk for infection, especially from encapsulated organisms such as pneumococcus. This risk is reduced by immunization with pneumococcal vaccine (e.g., Pneumovax).

BLOOD COMPONENT THERAPY

Blood component therapy is frequently used in managing hematologic diseases. Many therapeutic and surgical procedures depend on blood product support. However, blood component therapy only temporarily supports the patient until the underlying problem is resolved. Because transfusions are not free from hazards, they should be used only if necessary. The research regarding red blood cell substitutes is ongoing. To reduce the use of blood products, antifibrinolytic agents and other products may be used in some situations.[90] Nurses must be careful to avoid developing a complacent attitude about this common but potentially dangerous therapy. The nurse also needs to make sure that the physician has discussed the risks, benefits, and alternatives with the patient and that this is documented in the patient's medical record.

Traditionally, the term *blood transfusion* meant the administration of whole blood. Blood transfusion now has a broader meaning because of the ability to administer specific components of blood such as platelets, packed red blood cells (PRBCs), or plasma. Usually a specific component is ordered, although whole blood may be used rarely with massive hemorrhage or for an exchange transfusion[91] (Table 31-32). (See Chapter 16 for discussion of hematopoietic stem cell transplants.)

Administration Procedure

Blood components can be administered safely through a 23-gauge needle, but this usually impedes flow and could cause hemolysis, particularly if using a pressured infusion device. If a small gauge is to be used, it is best to have the unit split (the blood bank issues half of the unit at a time) or diluted with normal saline during administration to ensure that it does not run over the maximum time of 4 hours. Therefore a larger gauge of at least 19 is preferred, running the unit into a free-flowing IV line. Larger needles (e.g., 18 or 16 gauge) may be preferred if rapid transfusions are given. Smaller needles can be used for platelets, albumin, and clotting factor replacement. Most blood product administration tubing is of a "Y type" with a microaggregate filter (filters out particulate) with one Y for the isotonic saline solution and the other Y for the blood

TABLE 31-32 Blood Products*

Description	Special Considerations	Indications for Use
Packed RBCs Packed RBCs are prepared from whole blood by sedimentation or centrifugation. One unit contains 250-350 ml.	Use of RBCs for treatment allows remaining components of blood (e.g., platelets, albumin, plasma) to be used for other purposes. There is less danger of fluid overload. Packed RBCs are preferred RBC source because they are more component specific. Leukocyte depletion (by the blood bank or filter) may be used to reduce hemolytic febrile reactions in patients who receive frequent transfusions.	Severe or symptomatic anemia, acute blood loss. In general, one unit of packed red blood cells can be expected to increase a patient's hemoglobin level by 1 g/dl or Hct by 30%.
Frozen RBCs Frozen RBCs are prepared from RBCs using glycerol for protection and frozen. They can be stored for 10 yr at −188.6° F (−87 C°).	They must be used within 24 hr of thawing. Successive washings with saline solution remove majority of WBCs and plasma proteins.	Autotransfusion; stockpiling or rare donors for patients with alloantibodies. Infrequently used because filters remove most WBCs.
Platelets Platelets are prepared from fresh whole blood within 4 hr after collection. One unit contains 30-60 ml of platelet concentrate.	Multiple units of platelets can be obtained from one donor by plateletpheresis. They can be kept at room temperature for 1-5 days depending on type of collection and storage bag used. Bag should be agitated periodically. Expected increase is 10,000/μl/U. Failure to have a rise may be due to fever, sepsis, splenomegaly, or DIC. For patients who receive frequent transfusions or do not respond to previous platelet transfusions, may give leukocyte reduced, HLA, or type specific to prevent alloimmunization to HLA antigens.	Bleeding caused by thrombocytopenia, platelet levels $<$10,000-20,000/μl (10-20 × 10^9/L); may be contraindicated in immune thrombocytopenic purpura, thrombotic thrombocytopenic purpura, and heparin-induced thrombocytopenia except in life-threatening hemorrhage.
Fresh Frozen Plasma Liquid portion of whole blood is separated from cells and frozen. One unit contains 200-250 ml. Plasma is rich in clotting factors but contains no platelets. It may be stored for 1 yr. It must be used within 2 hr after thawing.	Use of plasma in treating hypovolemic shock is being replaced by pure preparations such as albumin plasma expanders.	Bleeding caused by deficiency in clotting factors (e.g., DIC, hemorrhage, massive transfusion, liver disease, vitamin K deficiency, excess warfarin).
Albumin Albumin is prepared from plasma. It can be stored for 5 yr. It is available in 5% or 25% solution.	Albumin 25 g/100 ml is osmotically equal to 500 ml of plasma. Hyperosmolar solution acts by moving water from extravascular to intravascular space. It is heat treated and does not transmit viruses.	Hypovolemic shock, hypoalbuminemia.
Cryoprecipitates and Commercial Concentrates Cryoprecipitate is prepared from fresh frozen plasma, with 10-20 ml/bag. It can be stored for 1 yr. Once thawed, must be used.	See Table 31-18.	Replacement of clotting factors, especially factor VIII, von Willebrand disease, and fibrinogen.

DIC, Disseminated intravascular coagulation; *Hct,* hematocrit; *HLA,* human leukocyte antigen; *RBCs,* red blood cells; *WBCs,* white blood cells.
*Component therapy has replaced the use of whole blood, which accounts for less than 10% of all transfusions. Granulocyte transfusions are not included here because they are rarely used.

product. Dextrose solutions or lactated Ringer's should not be used because they induce RBC hemolysis. No other additives (including medications) should be given via the same tubing as the blood unless the tubing is cleared with saline solution.[92]

When the blood or blood components have been obtained from the blood bank, positive identification of the donor blood and recipient must be made. Improper product-to-patient identification causes 90% of hemolytic transfusion reactions, thus placing a great responsibility on nursing personnel to carry out the identification procedure appropriately. The nurse must follow the policy and procedures at the place of employment. The blood bank is responsible for typing and crossmatching the donor's blood with the recipient's blood; the result of the compatibility testing should be noted on the product bag or tag, if pertinent.

Make sure that the patient understands the procedure and the signs and symptoms to report, and that he or she agrees with the treatment plan. Take the patient's vital signs before the beginning of the transfusion so that you have a baseline measure; if the patient has abnormal vital signs, such as an elevated fever, call the physician to clarify when the blood component may be administered. The blood should be administered as soon as it is brought to the patient. It should not be refrigerated on the nursing unit. If the blood is not used within 30 minutes, it should be returned to the blood bank. During the first 15 minutes or 50 ml of blood infusion, the nurse should remain with the patient. If there are any untoward reactions, they are most likely to occur at this time. The rate of infusion during this period should be no more than 2 ml/min. PRBCs should not be infused quickly unless an emergency exists. Rapid infusion of cold blood may cause the patient to become chilled. If rapid replacement of large amounts of blood is necessary, a blood-warming device may be used. Other blood components, such as fresh frozen plasma and platelets, may be infused over 15 to 30 minutes.

After the first 15 minutes, vital signs are usually retaken, and the rate of infusion is governed by the clinical condition of the patient and the product being infused. Most patients not in danger of fluid overload can tolerate the infusion of 1 unit of PRBCs over 2 hours. The transfusion should not take more than 4 hours to administer because of the increased risk of bacterial growth in the product once it is out of refrigeration. Blood unrefrigerated for 4 hours or longer should not be infused and should be returned to the blood bank.

Blood Transfusion Reactions

A *blood transfusion reaction* is an adverse reaction to blood transfusion therapy that can range in severity from mild symptoms to a life-threatening condition. Because complications of transfusion therapy may be significant, judicious evaluation of the patient is required. Blood transfusion reactions can be classified as acute or delayed (Tables 31-33 and 31-34).

If an acute transfusion reaction occurs, the following steps should be taken: (1) stop the transfusion; (2) maintain a patent IV line with saline solution; (3) notify the blood bank and the health care provider immediately; (4) recheck identifying tags and numbers; (5) monitor vital signs and urine output; (6) treat symptoms per physician order; (7) save the blood bag and tubing and send them to the blood bank for examination; (8) complete transfusion reaction reports; (9) collect required blood and urine specimens at intervals stipulated by hospital policy to evaluate for hemolysis; and (10) document on transfusion reaction form and patient chart. The blood bank and laboratory are responsible for identifying the type of reaction.

Acute Transfusion Reactions

Acute Hemolytic Reactions. The most common cause of hemolytic reactions is transfusion of ABO-incompatible blood (see Table 31-33). This is an example of a type II cytotoxic hypersensitivity reaction (see Chapter 14). Severe hemolytic reactions are rare. Mislabeling specimens and administering blood to the wrong individual cause most acute hemolytic reactions. This again points to the importance of the use of proper patient identifiers when drawing blood samples and when administering medications and blood products.

When an acute hemolytic reaction occurs, antibodies in the recipient's serum react with antigens on the donor's RBCs. This results in agglutination of cells, which can obstruct capillaries and block blood flow. Hemolysis of the RBCs releases free hemoglobin into the plasma. The hemoglobin is filtered by the kidney and may be found in the urine (hemoglobinuria). Hemoglobin may obstruct the renal tubules, leading to acute renal failure, DIC, and death (see Chapter 47).

The clinical manifestations of an acute hemolytic reaction may be mild or severe and usually develop within the first 15 minutes of transfusion. Free hemoglobin in blood and urine specimens obtained at the onset of the reaction will provide evidence of an acute hemolytic reaction. Delayed transfusion reactions occur 2 to 14 days after the administration of blood.[91] (The clinical manifestations and nursing management for the patient with a hemolytic reaction are presented in Table 31-33.)

Febrile Reactions. Febrile reactions are most commonly caused by leukocyte incompatibility. Many individuals who receive five or more transfusions develop circulating antibodies to the small amount of WBCs in the blood product. Febrile reactions can often be prevented by using additional filters in the tubing to leukocyte-deplete RBCs and platelets. Leukocyte-poor blood products (filtered, washed, or frozen) can also be used to prevent febrile reactions.

Allergic Reactions. Allergic reactions result from the recipient's sensitivity to plasma proteins of the donor's blood. These reactions are more common in an individual with a history of allergies. Antihistamines may be used to prevent allergic reactions. Epinephrine or corticosteroids may be used to treat a severe reaction.

Circulatory Overload. An individual with cardiac or renal insufficiency is at risk for developing circulatory overload. This is especially true if a large quantity of blood is infused in a short period of time, particularly in an elderly patient. Packed red blood cells can be split by the blood bank, allowing for one half of a unit to be given over a time frame of up to 4 hours. A fluid balance assessment, including baseline auscultation of the patient's lungs, is performed. Complaints of shortness of breath and the presence of adventitious breath sounds may indicate fluid overload in any patient.

Sepsis. Blood products can become infected from improper handling and storage. Bacterial contamination of blood products can result in bacteremia, sepsis, or septic shock.

Transfusion-Related Acute Lung Injury. Transfusion-related acute lung injury (TRALI) is characterized by the sudden development of noncardiogenic pulmonary edema (acute lung injury). It usually occurs within 2 to 6 hours after transfusion of blood products, but may occur as late as 48 hours after transfusion. With the reduction of clerical errors, leukocyte-reduced products, more effective screening, and the prevention of the transmission of infectious agents, TRALI has surpassed hemolytic reactions as the leading cause of transfusion-related death. It is thought to be due to an antibody-mediated reaction between the recipient's leukocytes and antileukocyte antibodies from donors who were sensitized during pregnancy or by previous transfusions. This causes pulmonary capillary inflammation and increased permeability, leading to respiratory distress and potentially death.[93,94]

Massive Blood Transfusion Reaction. An acute complication of transfusing large volumes of blood products is termed *massive blood transfusion reaction.* Massive blood transfusion reactions can occur when replacement of RBCs or blood exceeds the total blood volume within 24 hours. In this situation, an imbalance of normal blood elements results because clotting factors, albumin, and platelets are not found in RBC transfusions.

Additional problems such as hypothermia, citrate toxicity, hypocalcemia, and hyperkalemia may occur when massive blood transfusions are given. Hypothermia and cardiac dysrhythmias can result from rapid infusion of large quantities of cold blood. Blood-warming equipment prevents this problem. Citrate toxicity and hypocalcemia can occur from the use of large quantities of blood products, because citrate is part of the storage solution; calcium binds to the citrate. Citrate toxicity is likely to develop when blood is transfused at a rate of 1 unit in 10 minutes (or 8 to 10 units of RBCs within a few hours). Manifestations such as muscle tremors and ECG changes may be observed with hypocalcemia but can be prevented or reversed by the infusion of 10% calcium gluconate (10 ml with every liter of citrated blood). Hyperkalemia results when potassium leaks from RBCs in stored blood. Mild to severe signs and symptoms can occur, including nausea, muscle weak-

TABLE 31-33 Acute Transfusion Reactions

Reaction	Cause	Clinical Manifestations	Management	Prevention
Acute hemolytic	Infusion of ABO-incompatible whole blood, RBCs, or components containing 10 ml or more of RBCs. Antibodies in the recipient's plasma attach to antigens on transfused red blood cells causing RBC destruction.	Chills, fever, low back pain, flushing, tachycardia, dyspnea, tachypnea, hypotension, vascular collapse, hemoglobinuria, acute jaundice, dark urine, bleeding, acute renal failure, shock, cardiac arrest, death.	Treat shock and DIC if present. Draw blood samples for serologic testing slowly to avoid hemolysis from the procedure. Send urine specimen to the laboratory. Maintain BP with IV colloid solutions. Give diuretics as prescribed to maintain urine flow. Insert indwelling urinary catheter or measure voided amounts to monitor hourly urine output. Dialysis may be required if renal failure occurs. Do not transfuse additional RBC-containing components until blood bank has provided newly crossmatched units.	Meticulously verify and document patient identification from sample collection to component infusion.
Febrile, nonhemolytic (most common)	Sensitization to donor WBCs, platelets, or plasma proteins.	Sudden chills and fever (rise in temperature of $>1°$ C), headache, flushing, anxiety, vomiting, muscle pain.	Give antipyretics as prescribed—avoid aspirin in thrombocytopenic patients. *Do not restart transfusion* unless physician orders.	Consider leukocyte-poor blood products (filtered, washed, or frozen) for patients with a history of two or more such reactions.
Mild allergic	Sensitivity to foreign plasma proteins.	Flushing, itching, urticaria (hives).	Give antihistamine, corticosteroid as directed. If symptoms are mild and transient, transfusion may be restarted slowly. Do not restart transfusion if fever or pulmonary symptoms develop.	Treat prophylactically with antihistamines. Consider washed RBCs and platelets.
Anaphylactic and severe allergic	Sensitivity to donor plasma proteins. Infusion of IgA proteins to IgA-deficient recipient who has developed IgA antibody.	Anxiety, urticaria, dyspnea, wheezing, progressing to cyanosis, bronchospasm, hypotension, shock, and possible cardiac arrest.	Initiate CPR, if indicated. Have epinephrine ready for injection (0.4 ml of a 1:1000 solution SQ or 0.1 ml of 1:1000 solution diluted to 10 ml with saline for IV use). *Do not restart transfusion.*	Transfuse extensively washed RBC products, from which all plasma has been removed. Use blood from IgA-deficient donor. Use autologous components.
Circulatory overload	Fluid administered faster than the circulation can accommodate.	Cough, dyspnea, pulmonary congestion, headache, hypertension, tachycardia, distended neck veins.	Place patient upright with feet in dependent position. Administer prescribed diuretics, oxygen, morphine. Phlebotomy may be indicated.	Adjust transfusion volume and flow rate based on patient size and clinical status. Have blood bank divide unit into smaller aliquots for better spacing of fluid input.
Sepsis	Transfusion of bacterially infected blood components.	Rapid onset of chills, high fever, vomiting, diarrhea, marked hypotension, or shock.	Obtain culture of patient's blood and send bag with remaining blood and tubing to blood bank for further study. Treat septicemia as directed—antibiotics, IV fluids, vasopressors.	Collect, process, store, and transfuse blood products according to blood banking standards and infuse within 4 hr of starting time.
Transfusion-related acute lung injury (TRALI)	Reaction between transfused antileukocyte antibodies and recipient's leukocytes, causing pulmonary inflammation and capillary leak.	Fever, hypotension, tachypnea, dyspnea, decreased oxygen saturation, frothy sputum.	Send bag with remaining blood and tubing to blood bank for further study; draw blood for arterial blood gases and HLA or antileukocyte antibodies; obtain chest x-ray. Provide oxygen and administer corticosteroids (diuretics of no value). Initiate CPR if needed and provide ventilatory and blood pressure support if needed.	Provide leukocyte-reduced products. Identify donors who are implicated in TRALI reactions and do not allow them to donate.

BP, Blood pressure; *CPR,* cardiopulmonary resuscitation; *HLA,* human leukocyte antigen; *IgA,* immunoglobulin A; *IV,* intravenous; *RBC,* red blood cell; *SQ,* subcutaneous; *WBC,* white blood cell.

TABLE 31-34 Delayed Transfusion Reactions

Reaction	Clinical Manifestations
Delayed hemolytic	Fever, mild jaundice, decreased hemoglobin. Occurs as early as 3 days or as late as several months, but usually 5-10 days posttransfusion as the result of destruction of transfused RBCs by alloantibodies not detected during crossmatch. Generally, no acute treatment is required, but hemolysis may be severe enough to warrant further transfusions.
Hepatitis B*	Elevated liver enzymes (AST and ALT), anorexia, malaise, nausea and vomiting, fever, dark urine, jaundice. Usually resolves spontaneously within 4-6 wk. Chronic carrier state can develop and can result in permanent liver damage. Treat symptomatically. (See Chapter 44.)
Hepatitis C*	Similar to hepatitis B, but symptoms are usually less severe. Chronic liver disease and cirrhosis may develop. Before introduction of anti-HCV test, accounted for 90%-95% of all posttransfusion hepatitis. Treat symptomatically. (See Chapter 44.)
Iron overload	Excess iron is deposited in the heart, liver, pancreas, and joints, causing dysfunction. Heart failure, dysrhythmias, impaired thyroid and gonadal function, diabetes, arthritis, cirrhosis. Commonly occurs in patients receiving >100 units for chronic anemia (e.g., sickle cell anemia, β-thalassemia) over a period of time. Treat symptomatically. Deferoxamine (Desferal), which chelates and removes accumulated iron via the kidneys, may be administered IV or subcutaneously. Deferasirox (Exjade) is an oral agent that chelates iron.
Other	Other infectious diseases and agents may be transmitted via transfusion, including cytomegalovirus, HTLV-1, and those causing malaria.

ALT, Alanine aminotransferase; *AST,* aspartate aminotransferase; *HCV,* hepatitis C virus; *HTLV-1,* human T-cell leukemia virus, type 1; *IV,* intravenous; *RBCs,* red blood cells.
*New cases of transfusion-related hepatitis B and C are not common.

ness, diarrhea, paresthesias, flaccid paralysis of the cardiac or respiratory muscles, and cardiac arrest. Electrolyte monitoring is an important aspect of care of the patient receiving massive transfusions of blood products.[91]

Delayed Transfusion Reactions. Delayed transfusion reactions include delayed hemolytic reactions (discussed previously), infections, and iron overload (see Table 31-34).

Infection. Infectious agents transmitted by blood transfusion include hepatitis B and C viruses, HIV, human herpesvirus type 6 (HSV-6), Epstein-Barr virus (EBV), human T-cell leukemia virus, type 1 (HTLV-1), cytomegalovirus (CMV), and malaria. Hepatitis is still the most common viral infection transmitted, although its incidence has been decreasing. Hepatitis B virus can be detected in the blood by the presence of hepatitis B surface antigen (HBsAg). A test for hepatitis C antibodies in donor blood is used to exclude the use of any donated blood testing positive for hepatitis C. Therefore the risk of transmission of hepatitis C has been reduced. Leukocyte-reduced blood products drastically reduce the risk of blood transfusion–associated viral infections, including CMV.

In the past, HIV was transmitted by contaminated blood and blood products. This posed a serious problem for an individual who received infected transfusions. Patients with hemophilia who received antihemophilic factors, which had been prepared from pooled plasma of a large number of donors of which some donors were infected, have a high rate of HIV infection from transfusion sources. Presently, the use of recombinant antihemophilic factors (see Table 31-18), donor education, donor screening, and HIV antibody testing has greatly reduced the transmission of HIV by blood transfusion or factor replacement therapy.

Autotransfusion

Autotransfusion, or autologous transfusion, consists of removing whole blood from a person and transfusing that blood back into the same person. The problems of incompatibility, allergic reactions, and transmission of disease can be avoided. Methods of autotransfusion include the following:

- *Autologous donation or elective phlebotomy* (predeposit transfusion). A person donates blood before a planned surgical procedure. The blood can be frozen and stored for up to 10 years. Usually the blood is stored without being frozen and is given to the person within a few weeks of donation. This technique is especially beneficial to the patient with a rare blood type or for any patient who might be expected to require limited blood product support during a major surgical procedure (e.g., elective orthopedic surgery).
- *Autotransfusion.* A newer method for replacing blood volume involves safely and aseptically collecting, filtering, and returning the patient's own blood lost during a major surgical procedure or from a traumatic injury. This system was originally developed in response to patients' concerns about the safety of blood from blood products. However, today it provides an important way to safely replace volume and stabilize bleeding patients. Collection devices are most often used during surgeries. Some systems allow blood to be automatically and continuously reinfused; others require collection for a period of time (usually no longer than 4 hours) and then the blood is reinfused.

Drainage after the first 24 hours or drainage that is suspected to contain pathogens should not be reinfused. Anticoagulants may or may not be added before reinfusion. Development of clots after blood is filtered through the collection system can sometimes prevent reinfusion of the blood. Sometimes blood that has been collected has become depleted of its normal coagulation factors; therefore monitoring coagulation studies in the patient receiving an autotransfusion is important.[91]

CRITICAL THINKING EXERCISE

CASE STUDY

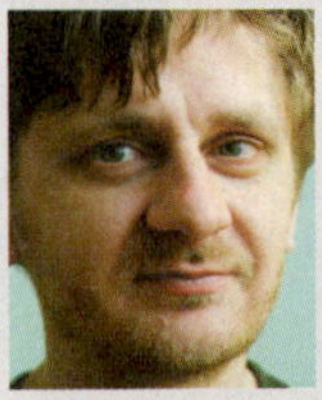

Leukemia

Patient Profile. J.J., a 35-year-old white man, went to the emergency department because of severe bruising caused by a fall while hiking.

Subjective Data

- Complains of oral pain and white patches covering his tongue
- Has had a 2-month history of fatigue, malaise, and flu symptoms
- Has taken numerous prescribed antibiotics and increased rest and sleep in the past 2 months without relief of symptoms

Objective Data

Physical Examination

- Has bruises and ecchymoses from fall
- Gingiva has petechiae and patchy white spots
- Temperature 102.2° F (39° C)
- Has splenomegaly

Laboratory Results

- Hematocrit 30%
- Hb 8.8 g/dl
- WBC count 120,000/μl (120 × 10^9/L)
- Platelet count 25,000/μl (25 × 10^9/L)

Bone Marrow Biopsy

- Multiple myeloblasts (greater than 50%)

Critical Thinking Questions

1. What components of the laboratory test results suggest acute leukemia?
2. How is acute myelogenous leukemia treated?
3. What is the prognosis for JJ?
4. What are the main priorities for patient teaching with a newly diagnosed young adult with leukemia?
5. What are the life-threatening problems that can occur as a result of this disease and treatment? How can the nurse anticipate and assess for these problems?
6. Based on the assessment data presented, write one or more nursing diagnoses. Are there any collaborative problems?

NCLEX EXAMINATION REVIEW QUESTIONS

The number of the question corresponds to the same-numbered objective at the beginning of the chapter.

1. In a severely anemic patient, the nurse would expect to find
   a. dyspnea and tachycardia.
   b. cyanosis and pulmonary edema.
   c. cardiomegaly and pulmonary fibrosis.
   d. ventricular dysrhythmias and wheezing.
2. When obtaining assessment data from a patient with a microcytic, hypochromic anemia, the nurse would question the patient about
   a. folic acid intake.
   b. dietary intake of iron.
   c. a history of gastric surgery.
   d. a history of sickle cell anemia.
3. A nursing intervention for a patient with severe anemia of chronic kidney disease includes
   a. monitoring stools for guaiac.
   b. instructions in high-iron diet.
   c. taking vital signs every 8 hours.
   d. teaching self-injection of erythropoietin.
4. The nursing management of a patient in sickle cell crisis includes
   a. bed rest and heparin therapy.
   b. blood transfusions and iron replacement.
   c. aggressive analgesic and oxygen therapy.
   d. platelet administration and monitoring of CBC.
5. A complication of the hyperviscosity of polycythemia is
   a. thrombosis.
   b. cardiomyopathy.
   c. pulmonary edema.
   d. disseminated intravascular coagulation (DIC).
6. When providing care for a patient with thrombocytopenia, the nurse instructs the patient to
   a. dab his or her nose instead of blowing.
   b. be careful when shaving with a safety razor.
   c. continue with physical activities to stimulate thrombopoiesis.
   d. avoid aspirin because it may mask the fever that occurs with thrombocytopenia.
7. The nurse would anticipate that a patient with von Willebrand's disease undergoing surgery would be treated with administration of vWF and
   a. thrombin.
   b. factor VI.
   c. factor VII.
   d. factor VIII.
8. DIC is a disorder in which
   a. the coagulation pathway is genetically altered, leading to thrombus formation in all major blood vessels.
   b. an underlying disease depletes hemolytic factors in the blood, leading to diffuse thrombotic episodes and infarcts.
   c. a disease process stimulates coagulation processes with resultant thrombosis, as well as depletion of clotting factors, leading to diffuse clotting and hemorrhage.
   d. an inherited predisposition causes a deficiency of clotting factors that leads to overstimulation of coagulation processes in the vasculature.
9. Appropriate nursing actions when caring for a hospitalized patient with severe neutropenia include
   a. perirectal care and platelet administration.
   b. oral care and red blood cell administration.
   c. monitoring lung sounds and invasive blood pressures.
   d. strict hand washing and frequent vital sign assessment.
10. Because myelodysplastic syndrome arises from the pluripotent hematopoietic stem cell in the bone marrow, laboratory results the nurse would expect to find include
    a. an excess of T cells.
    b. an excess of platelets.
    c. a deficiency of granulocytes.
    d. a deficiency of all cellular blood components.
11. The most common type of leukemia in older adults is
    a. acute myelocytic leukemia.
    b. acute lymphocytic leukemia.
    c. chronic lymphocytic leukemia.
    d. chronic myelocytic leukemia.
12. Multiple drugs are often used in combinations to treat leukemia and lymphoma because
    a. there are fewer toxic and side effects.
    b. the chance that one drug will be effective is increased.
    c. the drugs are more effective without causing side effects.
    d. the drugs can interrupt cell growth at multiple points in the cell cycle.
13. The nurse is aware that a major difference between Hodgkin's lymphoma and non-Hodgkin's lymphoma is that
    a. Hodgkin's lymphoma occurs only in young adults.
    b. Hodgkin's lymphoma is considered potentially curable.
    c. non-Hodgkin's lymphoma can present in multiple organs.
    d. non-Hodgkin's lymphoma is treated only with radiation therapy.
14. A patient with multiple myeloma becomes confused and lethargic. The nurse would expect that these clinical manifestations may be explained by diagnostic results that indicate
    a. hyperkalemia.
    b. hyperuricemia.
    c. hypercalcemia.
    d. CNS myeloma.

15. When reviewing the patient's hematologic laboratory values after a splenectomy, the nurse would expect to find
    a. leukopenia.
    b. RBC abnormalities.
    c. decreased hemoglobin.
    d. increased platelet count.
16. Complications of transfusions that can be decreased by the use of leukocyte reduction filters for red blood cells and platelets are
    a. chills and back pain.
    b. leukostasis and neutrophilia.
    c. fluid overload and pulmonary edema.
    d. transmission of cytomegalovirus and alloimmunization.

REFERENCES

1. Marks PW, Glader B: Approach to anemia in the adult and child. In Hoffman R, et al, editors: *Hematology: basic principles and practice,* ed 4, Philadelphia, 2005, Elsevier.
2. Schrier SL: Approach to the adult patient with anemia. Available at *www.UpToDate.com,* version 13.2 (accessed October 31, 2005).
3. Andres E, Loukili NH, Noel E, et al: Vitamin B_{12} (cobalamin) deficiency in elderly patients, *Can Med Assoc J* 171:251, 2004.
4. American Dietetic Association: Available at *www.eatright.org* (accessed June 20, 2006).
5. Brittenham G: Disorders of iron metabolism: iron deficiency and overload. In Hoffman R, et al, editors: *Hematology: basic principles and practice,* ed 5, Philadelphia, 2005, Elsevier.
6. Dietary Guidelines for Americans 2005: Available at *www.healthierus.gov/dietary* guidelines (accessed June 20, 2006).
7. Cohen AR, Galanello R, Pennell DJ, et al: Thalassemia, *American Society of Hematology* 1:14, 2004.
8. Martin MB, Foote D, Carson S: Help your patient meet the challenges of β-thalassemia major, *Nursing* 34:32hn1, 2004.
9. Antony AC: Megaloblastic anemias. In Hoffman R, et al, editors: *Hematology: basic principles and practice,* ed 4, Philadelphia, 2005, Elsevier.
10. Weiss G, Goodnough LT: Anemia of chronic disease, *N Engl J Med* 35:10, 2005.
11. Brodsky RA, Jones RJ: Aplastic anaemia, *Lancet* 365:1647, 2005.
12. March JC: Management of acquired aplastic anaemia, *Blood Rev* 19:143, 2005.
13. Bevans MF, Shalabi RA: Management of patients receiving antithymocyte globulin for aplastic anemia and myelodysplastic syndrome, *Clin J Oncol Nurs* 8:377, 2004.
14. Hebbel RP: Pathobiology of sickle cell disease. In Hoffman R, et al, editors: *Hematology: basic principles and practice,* ed 4, Philadelphia, 2005, Elsevier.
15. Saunthararajah Y, Vichinsky EP, Embury S: Sickle cell disease. In Hoffman R, et al, editors: *Hematology: basic principles and practice,* ed 4, Philadelphia, 2005, Elsevier.
16. Embury SH, Vichinsky E: Overview of the clinical manifestations of sickle cell disease. Available at *www.UpToDate.com,* version 13.2 (accessed June 20, 2006).
17. Johnson L: Managing acute and chronic pain in sickle cell disease, *Nursing Times* 101:40, 2005.
18. D'Arcy Y: Managing sickle-cell crisis, *Nursing* 34:24, 2004.
19. Buchanan GR, DeBaun MR, Quinn CT, et al: Sickle cell disease, *American Society of Hematology* 1:35, 2004.
20. Matthews AL, Grimes SJ, Wiesner GL, et al: Clinical consult: iron overload—hereditary hemochromatosis, *Prim Care* 31:767, 2004.
21. Tefferi A: Polycythemia vera: a comprehensive review and clinical recommendations, *Mayo Clin Proc* 78:174, 2003.
22. Munson B: About polycythemia vera, *Nursing* 35:28, 2005.
23. George JN: Drug-induced thrombocytopenia; clinical manifestations and diagnosis of idiopathic thrombocytopenic purpura in adults: treatment and prognosis of idiopathic thrombocytopenic purpura in adults. Available at *www.UpToDate.com,* version 13.2 (accessed June 20, 2006).
24. Thompson MICROMEDEX, Healthcare Series Vol. 125 (2005).
25. Drachman JG: Inherited thrombocytopenia: when a low platelet count does not mean ITP, *Blood* 103:390, 2004.
26. Rose BD, George JN: Causes of thrombotic thrombocytopenic purpura–hemolytic uremic syndrome in adults: diagnosis of thrombotic thrombocytopenic purpura–hemolytic uremic syndrome in adults. Available at *www.UpToDate.com,* version 13.2 (accessed June 20, 2006).
27. Cines DB, Bussel JB, McMillan RB, et al: Congenital and acquired thrombocytopenia, *American Society of Hematology* 1:390, 2004.
28. Coutre S: Heparin-induced thrombocytopenia. Available at *www.UpToDate.com,* version 13.2 (accessed December 31, 2005).
29. Warkentin TE: Heparin-induced thrombocytopenia, *Dis Mon* 51:141, 2005.
30. Slichter SJ: Platelet transfusion: future directions, *Vox Sanguin* 87(suppl 2):S47, 2004.
31. Rose BD, Kaplan AA, George JN: Treatment of thrombotic thrombocytopenic purpura–hemolytic uremic syndrome in adults. Available at *www.UpToDate.com,* version 13.2 (accessed June 20, 2006).
32. Greinacher A: Heparin-induced thrombocytopenia: an overview of clinical presentation, pathogenesis, diagnosis and treatment, *Thrombosis and Haemostasis, Supplement* (Symposium XIX Congress of the International Society on Thrombosis and Haemostasis), July 18, 2003.
33. Warkentin TE: Heparin-induced thrombocytopenia, *Dis Mon* 51(2-3):141, 2005.
34. Burrus N, Holz S: Managing the risks of thrombocytopenia, *Nursing* 35:32hn2, 2005.
35. Lozier JN, Kessler CM: Clinical aspects and therapy of hemophilia. In Hoffman R, et al, editors: *Hematology: basic principles and practice,* ed 4, Philadelphia, 2005, Elsevier.
36. Mannucci PM: Drug therapy: treatment of von Willebrand's disease, *N Engl J Med* 351:683, 2004.
37. Robinson P: Is surgery safe for a patient with hemophilia? *Nursing* 35:32hn1, 2005.
38. Mannucci PM, Duga S, Peyvandi F: Recessively inherited coagulation disorders, *Blood* 104:1243, 2004.
39. Wada H: Disseminated intravascular coagulation, *Clin Chim Acta* 344:13, 2004.
40. Leung LL: Clinical features, diagnosis, and treatment of disseminated intravascular coagulation. Available at *www.UpToDate.com,* version 13.2 (accessed June 20, 2006).
41. Levi M: Current understanding of disseminated intravascular coagulation, *Br J Haematol* 124:567, 2004.
42. Dempfle CE: Coagulopathy of sepsis, *Thromb Haemost* 91:213, 2004.
43. Dressler DK: DIC: coping with a coagulation crisis, *Nursing* 34:58, 2004.
44. Camp-Sorrell D: Myelosuppression. In Itano JK, Taoka KN, editors: *Core curriculum for oncology nursing,* ed 4, Philadelphia, 2005, Elsevier.
45. Crighton M: Dimensions of neutropenia in adult cancer patients: expanding conceptualizations beyond the numerical value of the absolute neutrophil count, *Cancer Nurs* 27:275, 2004.
46. Sipsas NV, Bodey GP, Kontoyiannis DP: Perspectives for the management of febrile neutropenic patients with cancer in the 21st century, *Cancer* 103:1103, 2005.
47. West F, Mitchell SA: Evidence-based guidelines for the management of neutropenia following outpatient hematopoietic stem cell transplantation, *Clin J Oncol Nurs* 8:601, 2004.
48. Baehner RL: Overview of neutropenia. Available at *www.UpToDate.com,* version 13.2 (accessed June 20, 2006).
49. Hughes WT, Armstrong D, Bodey GP, et al: 2002 guidelines for the use of antimicrobial agents in neutropenic patients with cancer, *Clin Infect Dis* 34:730, 2002.
50. Spielberger R: Palifermin for oral mucositis after intensive therapy for hematologic cancers, *N Engl J Med* 351:2590, 2004.
51. Centers for Disease Control and Prevention, Infectious Disease Society of America, and the American Society of Blood and Marrow Transplantation: Guidelines for preventing opportunistic infections among hematopoietic stem cell transplant recipients, *MMWR Morb Mortal Wkly Rep* 49: RR-10, 2000.
52. Eggenberger SK, Krumwiede N, Meiers SJ, et al: Family care strategies in neutropenia, *Clin J Oncol Nurs* 8:617, 2004.
53. Pinto A, De Filippi R, Frigeri F, et al: Aging and the hemopoietic system, *Clin Rev Oncol/Hematol* 48S:S3, 2003.
54. Hofmann WK, Lubbert M, Hoelzer D, et al: Myelodysplastic syndromes, *Hematol J* 5:1, 2004.
55. Kaminskas E, Farrell AT, Wang YC, et al: FDA drug approval summary: azacitidine (5-azacytidine, Vidaza) for injectable suspension, *Oncologist* 10:176, 2005.
56. Jemal A, Murray T, Ward E, et al: Cancer statistics, 2005, *CA Cancer J Clin* 55:10, 2005.
57. Stone RM, O'Connell MR, Sekeres MA: Acute myeloid leukemia, *American Society of Hematology* 1:98, 2004.
58. Pui CH, Relling MV, Downing JR: Acute lymphoblastic leukemia, *N Engl J Med* 350:1535, 2004.
59. Redaelli A: A systematic literature review of the clinical and epidemiological burden of acute lymphoblastic leukaemia (ALL), *Eur J Cancer Care* 14:53, 2005.
60. Erlich RB, Ghayee HK, Noga SJ: Chronic lymphocytic leukemia: will recent major advances lead to cure? *Clin Geriatr* 12:41, 2004.

61. Shanafelt TD, Call TG: Current approach to diagnosis and management of chronic lymphocytic leukemia, *Mayo Clin Proc* 79:388, 2004.
62. Zakarija A, Peterson LC, Tallman MS: Hairy cell leukemia. In Hoffman R, et al, editors: *Hematology: basic principles and practice,* ed 4, Philadelphia, 2005, Elsevier.
63. Thomas DA, O'Brien S, Bueso-Ramos C, et al: Rituximab in relapsed or refractory hairy cell leukemia, *Blood* 102:3906 2003.
64. Slavin S: Reduced-intensity conditioning or nonmyeloablative stem cell transplantation: introduction, rationale, and historic background, *Semin Oncol* 31:1, 2004.
65. Goldman JM, Melo JV: Chronic myeloid leukemia—advances in biology and new approaches to treatment, *N Engl J Med* 349:1451, 2003.
66. O'Brien S, Tefferi A, Valent P: Chronic myelogenous leukemia and myeloproliferative disease, *American Society of Hematology* 1:146, 2004.
67. Hillmen P: Advancing therapy for chronic lymphocytic leukemia—the role of rituximab, *Semin Oncol* 31(suppl 2):22, 2004.
68. Lancet JE, Karp JE: Toward more effective treatment of the elderly patient with acute myelogenous leukemia, *Clin Geriatr* 11:30, 2003.
69. Iwamoto RR: Nursing care of the client with lymphoma or multiple myeloma. In Itano JK, Taoka KN, editors: *Core curriculum for oncology nursing,* ed 4, Philadelphia, 2005, Elsevier.
70. Meyer RM, Ambiner RF, Stroobants S: Hodgkin's lymphoma: evolving concepts with implications for practice, *American Society of Hematology* 1:184, 2004.
71. Diehl V, Thomas RK, Re D: Part II: Hodgkin's lymphoma—diagnosis and treatment, *Lancet* 5:19, 2004.
72. Mauch PM, Canellos GP: Staging and selection of treatment modality in patients with Hodgkin's disease. Available at *www.UpToDate.com,* version 13.2 (accessed June 20, 2006).
73. Canellos GP: Lymphoma: present and future challenges, *Semin Hematol* 41(suppl 7):26, 2004.
74. Hennessy BT, Hanrahan EO, Daly PA: Non-Hodgkin lymphoma: an update, *Lancet* 5:341, 2004.
75. Freedman AS: Approach to the diagnosis, staging, and prognosis of non-Hodgkin's lymphoma. Available at *www.UpToDate.com,* version 13.2 (accessed June 20, 2006).
76. Coiffier B: Effective immunochemotherapy for aggressive non-Hodgkin's lymphoma, *Semin Oncol* 31(suppl 2):7, 2004.
77. Gisselbrecht C, Mounier N: Improving second-line therapy in aggressive non-Hodgkin's lymphoma, *Semin Oncol* 31(suppl 2):12, 2004.
78. Seymour JF: New treatment approaches to indolent non-Hodgkin's lymphoma, *Semin Oncol* 31(suppl 2):27, 2004.
79. Peggs KS, Mackinnon S, Linch C: The role of allogeneic transplantation in non-Hodgkin's lymphoma, *Br J Haematol* 128:153, 2004.
80. Knobler E: Current management strategies for cutaneous T-cell lymphoma, *Clin Dermatol* 12:197, 2004.
81. Walker PL, Dang NH: Denileukin diftitox as novel targeted therapy in non-Hodgkin's lymphoma, *Clin J Oncol Nurs* 8:169, 2004.
82. Vose JM: Bexxar: novel radioimmunotherapy for the treatment of low-grade and transformed low-grade non-Hodgkin's lymphoma, *Oncologist* 9:160, 2004.
83. Riley MB, Byar K: The rationale for and background of radioimmunotherapy: an emerging therapy for B-cell non-Hodgkin's lymphoma, *Semin Oncol Nurs* 20:1, 2004.
84. Hendrix D: Radiation safety guidelines for radioimmunotherapy with yttrium 90 ibritumomab tiuxetan, *Clin J Oncol Nurs* 8:31, 2004.
85. Devenney B, Erickson C: Multiple myeloma: an overview, *Clin J Oncol Nurs* 8:401, 2004.
86. Kroger N: Autologous-allogeneic tandem stem cell transplantation in patients with multiple myeloma, *Leukemia Lymphoma* 46:813, 2005.
87. Colson K, Doss DS, Swift R, et al: Bortezomib, a newly approved proteasome inhibitor for the treatment of multiple myeloma: nursing implications, *Clin J Oncol Nurs* 8:473, 2004.
88. Aster JC: Diseases of white blood cells, lymph nodes, spleen, and thymus. In Kumar V, et al, editors: *Robbins and Cotran pathologic basis of disease,* Philadelphia, 2005, Elsevier.
89. Shurin SB: The spleen and its disorders. In Hoffman R, et al, editors: *Hematology: basic principles and practice,* ed 4, Philadelphia, 2005, Elsevier.
90. Kirschman RA: Finding alternatives to blood transfusion, *Nursing* 34:58, 2004.
91. Ness PM, Kruskall MS: Principles of red blood cell transfusion. In Hoffman R, et al, editors: *Hematology: basic principles and practice,* ed 4, Philadelphia, 2005, Elsevier.
92. Brecher ME, editor: *American Association of Blood Banks technical manual,* ed 14, 2002, Bethesda, Md, American Association of Blood Banks (AABB).
93. Gajic O, Moore SB: Transfusion-related acute lung injury, *Mayo Clin Proc* 80:766, 2005.
94. Wu YY, Snyder EL: Transfusion reactions. In Hoffman R, et al, editors: *Hematology: basic principles and practice,* ed 4, Philadelphia, 2005, Elsevier.

RESOURCES

American Cancer Society
800-ACS-2345 or 866-228-4327
www.cancer.org

American Hemochromatosis Society
407-829-4488 or 407-333-1284
www.hemochromatosis.org

American Sickle Cell Anemia Association
216-229-8600
www.ascaa.org

Aplastic Anemia and MDS International Foundation, Inc.
800-747-2820 or 410-867-0242
www.aamds.org

Cooley's Anemia Foundation
800-522-7222 or 718-321-CURE (2873)
www.thalassemia.org

International Myeloma Foundation
800-452-2873 or 818-487-7455
www.myeloma.org

Leukemia and Lymphoma Society
800-955-4572
www.leukemia-lymphoma.org

National Cancer Institute
800-4-CANCER (422-6237) or 301-435-3848
http://cis.nci.nih.gov

National Heart, Lung, and Blood Institute
National Institutes of Health
NHLBI Information Center
301-592-8573
www.nhlbi.nih.gov

National Hemophilia Foundation
800-42-HANDI or 212-328-3700
www.hemophilia.org

Sickle Cell Disease Association of America, Inc.
800-421-8453 or 410-528-1555
www.sicklecelldisease.org

For additional Internet resources, see the website for this book at *http://evolve.elsevier.com/Lewis/medsurg*.

Hematology System

Section
7

Problems of Oxygenation: Perfusion

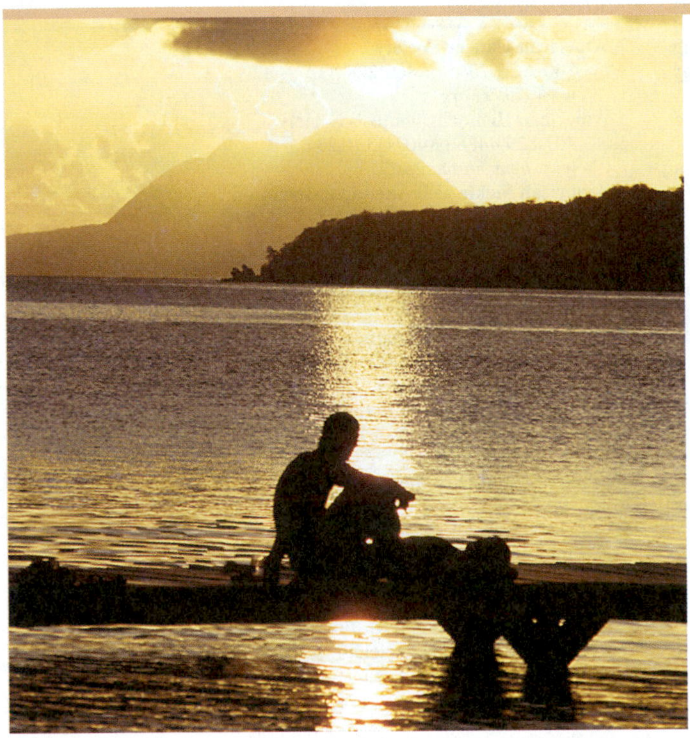

Section Outline

What matters is the condition of the heart.

Marcus J. Borg

Nursing Assessment
Cardiovascular System

32

Angela J. DiSabatino and Linda Bucher

LEARNING OBJECTIVES

1. Describe the anatomic location and function of the following cardiac structures: pericardial layers, atria, ventricles, semilunar valves, and atrioventricular valves.
2. Describe coronary circulation and the areas of heart muscle supplied by the major coronary arteries.
3. Explain the normal sequence of events involved in the conduction pathway of the heart.
4. Describe the structure and function of arteries, veins, capillaries, and endothelium.
5. Define blood pressure and the mechanisms involved in its regulation.
6. Identify the waveforms and the associated cardiac events represented on a normal electrocardiogram.
7. Identify the significant subjective and objective assessment data related to the cardiovascular system that should be obtained from a patient.
8. Describe the appropriate techniques used in the physical assessment of the cardiovascular system.
9. Differentiate normal from common abnormal findings of a physical assessment of the cardiovascular system.
10. Describe the age-related changes of the cardiovascular system and differences in assessment findings.
11. Describe the purpose, significance of results, and nursing responsibilities of diagnostic studies of the cardiovascular system.

KEY TERMS

afterload, p. 742
arterial blood pressure, p. 743
cardiac index, p. 742
cardiac output, p. 742
cardiac reserve, p. 742
diastole, p. 742
diastolic blood pressure, p. 743
ejection fraction, p. 757
mean arterial pressure, p. 744
point of maximal impulse, p. 750
preload, p. 742
pulse pressure, p. 743
systole, p. 742
systolic blood pressure, p. 743

Electronic Resources

Supplemental content related to Chapter 32 can be found . . .

Companion CD

- Stress-Busting Kit for Nursing Students
- NCLEX Examination Review Questions
- Animations:
  - Auscultation of Heart Valves
  - Blood Flow: Circulatory System
  - Cardiac Cycle During Systole and Diastole
  - Pulse Variations
- Audio Clips:
  - Diastolic Murmur
  - Fourth Heart Sound (S_4)
  - Murmurs: Blowing, Harsh or Rough, and Rumble
  - Murmurs: High, Medium, and Low
  - S_1 at Various Locations
  - S_2 at Various Locations
  - Single S_1
  - Single S_2
  - Systolic Murmur
  - Third Heart Sound (S_3)
- Video Clips:
  - Auscultation: Cardiac, with Bell
  - Auscultation: Cardiac, with Diaphragm
  - Auscultation: Cardiac, with Diaphragm and Bell
  - Auscultation: Carotid Artery
  - Inspection and Palpation: Cardiac Auscultatory Landmarks
  - Inspection and Palpation: Cardiac, Anterior Chest
  - Inspection and Palpation: Pulses, Lower Extremities
- Comprehensive Glossary

Evolve Website

http://evolve.elsevier.com/Lewis/medsurg

- Content Updates
- Key Points (Printable and CD/MP3 Download)
- Concept Map Creator
- Expanded Audio Glossary
- Key Term Flash Cards
- Electronic Calculators
- Physical Examination Video Clips:
  - Neck
  - Upper Extremities
  - Anterior Chest, Lungs, and Heart
  - Precordium and Jugular Veins
  - Breasts and Heart
- WebLinks

Reviewed by Cheryl L. Tuohy, RN, MSN, FNP-C, Certified Family Nurse Practitioner, Delaware Medical Group, Mill Creek Medical Associates, LLL (Internal Medicine), and Clinical Nursing Faculty, University of Delaware, Newark, Del.

STRUCTURES AND FUNCTIONS OF THE CARDIOVASCULAR SYSTEM

Heart

Structure. The heart is a four-chambered hollow muscular organ normally the approximate size of a fist. It lies within the thorax in the mediastinal space that separates the right and left pleural cavities (Fig. 32-1). The heart is composed of three layers: a thin inner lining, the *endocardium;* a layer of muscle, the *myocardium;* and a fibrous outer layer, the *epicardium.* The heart is surrounded by the *pericardium,* a fibroserous sac. The inner (visceral) layer of the pericardium is in contact with the epicardium, and the outer (parietal) layer is in contact with the mediastinum. A small amount of pericardial fluid (approximately 10 to 30 ml) lubricates the space between the pericardial layers *(pericardial space)* and prevents friction between the surfaces as the heart contracts.

The heart is divided vertically by the septum. This creates a right and left atrium and a right and left ventricle. The thickness of the wall of each chamber is different. The atrial myocardium is thinner than that of the ventricles, and the left ventricular wall is 2 to 3 times thicker than the right ventricular wall.[1,2] The thickness of the left ventricle is necessary to generate the force needed to pump the blood into the systemic circulation.

Blood Flow Through the Heart. The right atrium receives venous blood from the inferior and superior venae cavae and the coronary sinus. The blood then passes through the tricuspid valve into the right ventricle. With each contraction, the right ventricle pumps blood through the pulmonic valve into the pulmonary artery and to the lungs (Fig. 32-2).

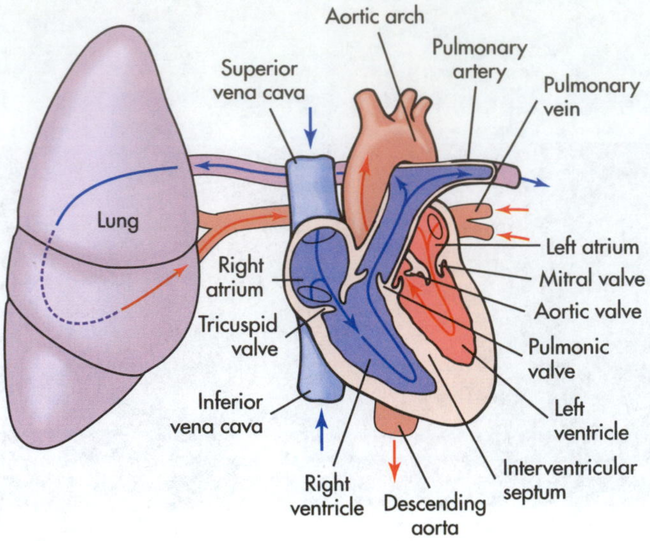

FIG. 32-2 Schematic representation of blood flow through the heart. *Arrows* indicate direction of flow.

Blood flows from the lungs to the left atrium by way of the pulmonary veins. It then passes through the mitral valve and into the left ventricle. As the heart contracts, blood is ejected through the aortic valve into the aorta and thus enters the high-pressure systemic circulation (see Fig. 32-2).

Cardiac Valves. The four valves of the heart serve to keep blood flowing in a forward direction. The cusps of the mitral and tricuspid valves are attached to thin strands of fibrous tissue termed *chordae tendineae* (Fig. 32-3). Chordae are anchored in the papillary muscles of the ventricles. This support system prevents the eversion of the leaflets into the atria during ventricular contraction. The pulmonic and aortic valves (also known as *semilunar valves*) prevent blood from regurgitating into the ventricles at the end of each ventricular contraction (see Fig. 32-3).

Blood Supply to the Myocardium. The myocardium has its own blood supply, the *coronary circulation* (Fig. 32-4). Blood flow into the two major coronary arteries occurs primarily during diastole (relaxation of the myocardium). The left coronary artery arises from the aorta and divides into two main branches: the left anterior descending artery and left circumflex artery. These arteries

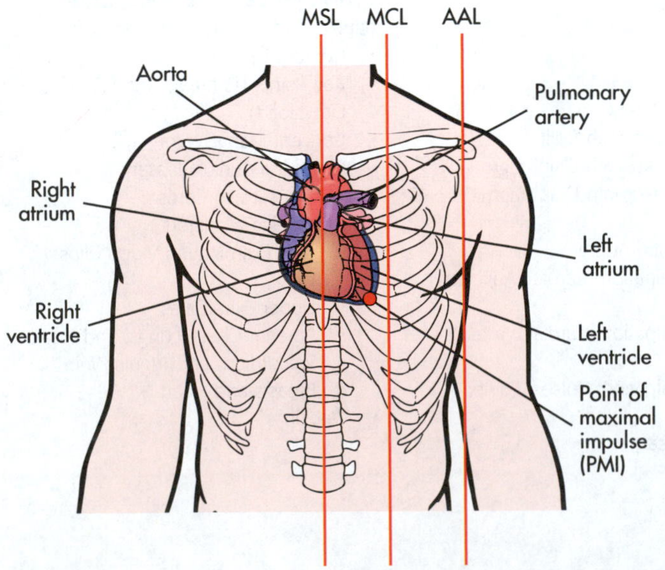

FIG. 32-1 Orientation of the heart within the thorax. *Red lines* indicate the midsternal line *(MSL),* midclavicular line *(MCL),* and anterior axillary line *(AAL).*

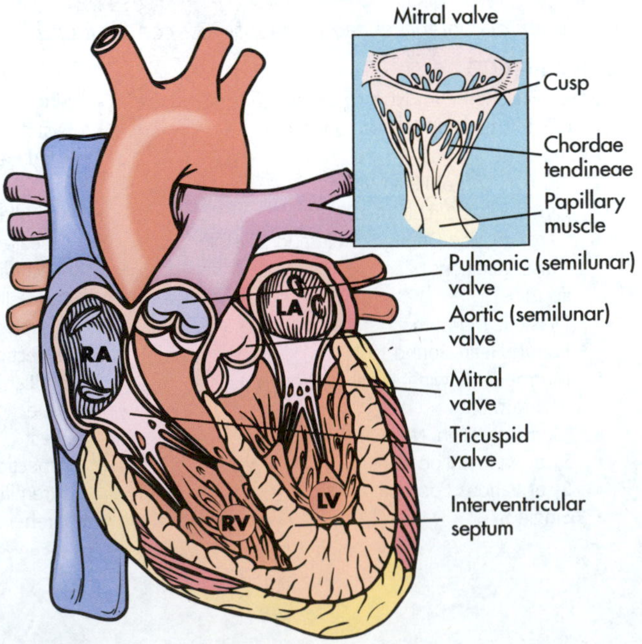

FIG. 32-3 Anatomic structures of the heart valves. *LA,* Left atrium; *LV,* left ventricle; *RA,* right atrium; *RV,* right ventricle.

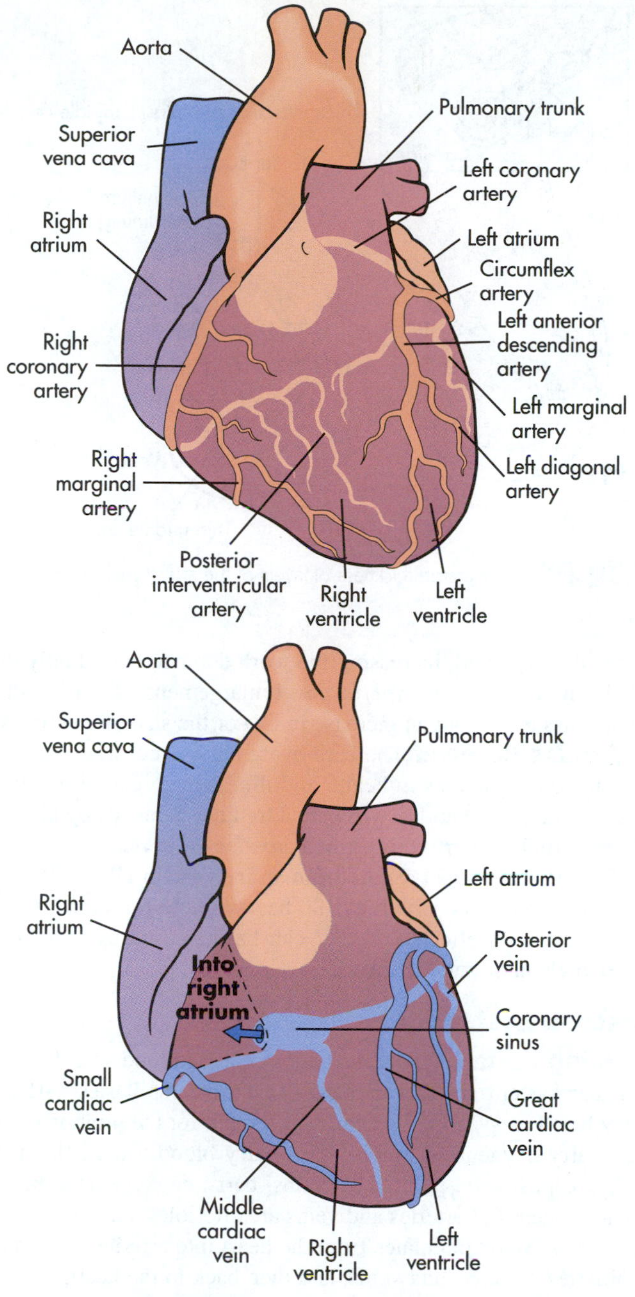

FIG. 32-4 Coronary arteries and veins.

supply the left atrium, the left ventricle, the interventricular septum, and a portion of the right ventricle. The right coronary artery also arises from the aorta, and its branches supply the right atrium, the right ventricle, and a portion of the posterior wall of the left ventricle. In 90% of people, the atrioventricular (AV) node and the bundle of His, part of the cardiac conduction system, receive blood supply from the right coronary artery. For this reason, obstruction of this artery often causes serious defects in cardiac conduction.

The divisions of coronary veins parallel the coronary arteries. Most of the blood from the coronary system drains into the coronary sinus, which empties into the right atrium near the entrance to the inferior vena cava (see Fig. 32-4).

Conduction System. The conduction system is specialized nerve tissue responsible for creating and transporting the electrical impulse, or **action potential.** This impulse initiates depolarization

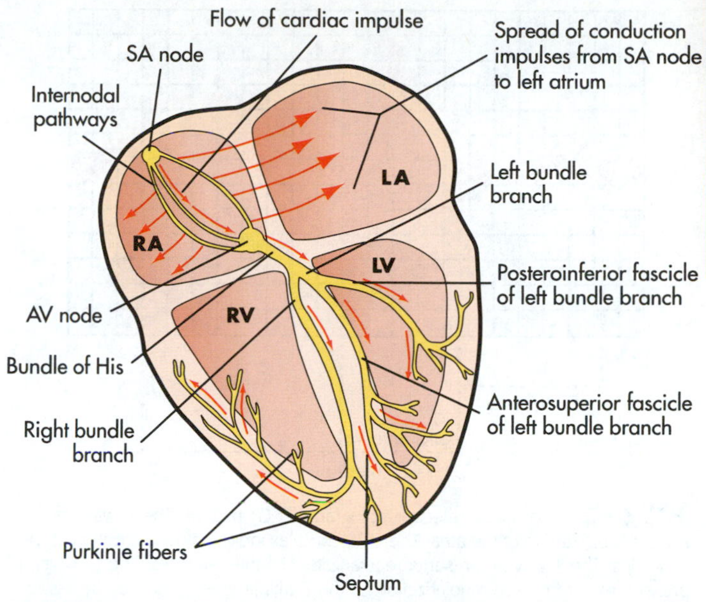

FIG. 32-5 Conduction system of the heart. *AV,* Atrioventricular; *LA,* left atrium; *LV,* left ventricle; *RA,* right atrium; *RV,* right ventricle; *SA,* sinoatrial.

and subsequently cardiac contraction. The electrical impulse is initiated by the sinoatrial (SA) node (the pacemaker of the heart) (Fig. 32-5). Each impulse generated at the SA node travels swiftly through the muscle fibers of the atria by internodal pathways and cell-to-cell conduction. Mechanical contraction of the atria follows the depolarization of the cells.

The electrical impulse travels from the atria to the AV node. The excitation then moves through the bundle of His and the left and right bundle branches. The left bundle branch has two fascicles (divisions): anterior and posterior. The action potential diffuses widely through the walls of both ventricles by means of *Purkinje fibers.* The efficient ventricular conduction system delivers the impulse within 0.12 second. This triggers a synchronized ventricular contraction.

The cardiac cycle starts with depolarization of the SA node. Its climax is ejection of blood into the pulmonary and systemic circulations. It ends with repolarization when the contractile fiber cells and the conduction pathway cells regain their resting polarized condition. Cardiac muscle cells have a compensatory mechanism that makes them unresponsive or refractory to restimulation during the action potential. During systole there is an *absolute refractory period* during which cardiac muscle does not respond to any stimuli. After this period, cardiac muscle gradually recovers its excitability and a *relative refractory period* occurs by early diastole.

Electrocardiogram. The electrical activity of the heart can be detected on the body surface through the use of electrodes and is recorded on an electrocardiogram (ECG). The letters P, QRS, T, and U are used to identify the separate waveforms (Fig. 32-6). The first wave, P, begins with the firing of the SA node and represents depolarization of the fibers of the atria. The QRS complex represents depolarization from the AV node throughout the ventricles. There is a delay of impulse transmission through the AV node that accounts for the time interval between the end of the P wave and the beginning of the QRS wave. The T wave represents repolarization of the ventricles. The U wave, if seen, may represent repolarization of the Purkinje fibers or it may be associated with hypokalemia.

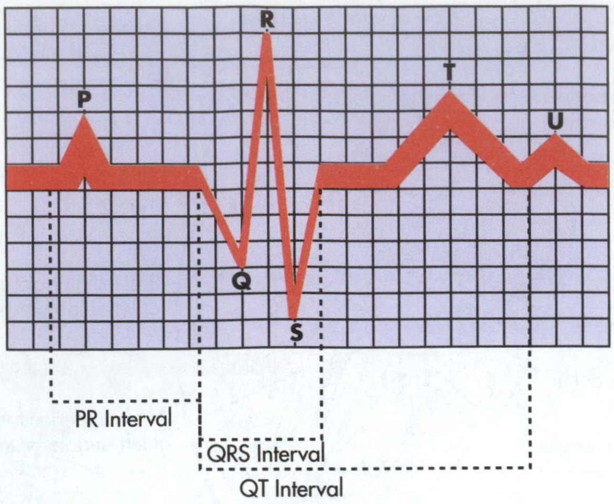

FIG. 32-6 The normal electrocardiogram (ECG) pattern. The P wave represents depolarization of the atria. The QRS complex indicates depolarization of the ventricles. The T wave represents repolarization of the ventricles. The U wave, if present, may represent repolarization of the Purkinje fibers or it may be associated with hypokalemia. The PR, QRS, and QT intervals reflect the length of time it takes for the impulse to travel from one area of the heart to another.

Intervals between these waves (PR, QRS, and QT intervals) reflect the length of time it takes for the impulse to travel from one area of the heart to another. These time intervals can be measured, and deviations from these time references often indicate pathology. See Chapter 36 for a complete discussion on ECG monitoring.

Mechanical System. *Depolarization* triggers mechanical activity. **Systole,** contraction of the myocardium, results in ejection of blood from the ventricles. Relaxation of the myocardium, **diastole,** allows for filling of the ventricles. **Cardiac output** (CO) is the amount of blood pumped by each ventricle in 1 minute. It is calculated by multiplying the amount of blood ejected from the ventricle with each heartbeat, the *stroke volume* (SV), by the heart rate (HR) per minute:

$$CO = SV \times HR$$

For the normal adult at rest, CO is maintained in the range of 4 to 8 L/min. **Cardiac index** (CI) is the CO divided by the body surface area (BSA). The CI adjusts the CO to the body size. The normal CI is 2.8 to 4.2 L per minute per meter squared (L/min/m^2).

Factors Affecting Cardiac Output. Numerous factors can affect either the HR or the SV and thus the CO. The HR is regulated primarily by the autonomic nervous system. The factors affecting the SV are preload, contractility, and afterload.[1] Increasing preload, contractility, and afterload increases the workload of the myocardium, resulting in increased oxygen demand.

Frank Starling's law states that, to a point, the more the myocardial fibers are stretched, the greater their force of contraction. The volume of blood in the ventricles at the end of diastole, before the next contraction, is called **preload.** Preload determines the amount of stretch placed on myocardial fibers.

Contractility can be increased by norepinephrine released by the sympathetic nervous system, as well as by epinephrine. Increasing contractility raises the SV by increasing ventricular emptying.

Afterload is the peripheral resistance against which the left ventricle must pump. Afterload is affected by the size of the ventricle, wall tension, and arterial blood pressure. If the arterial blood pressure is elevated, the ventricles will meet increased resistance

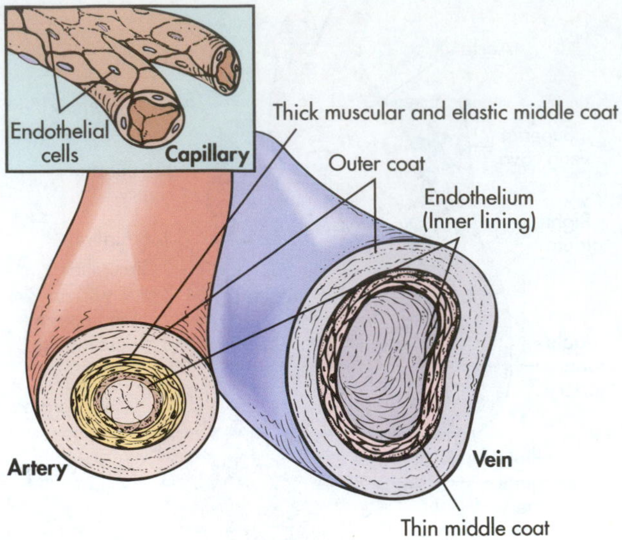

FIG. 32-7 Comparative thickness of layers of the artery, vein, and capillary.

to ejection of blood, increasing the work demand. Eventually this results in *ventricular hypertrophy* (enlargement of the cardiac muscle tissue without an increase in CO or the size of chambers).

Cardiac Reserve. The cardiovascular system must respond to numerous situations in health and illness (e.g., exercise, stress, hypovolemia). The ability to respond to these demands by altering CO threefold or fourfold is termed **cardiac reserve.**

The increase in CO results from an increase in HR or SV. The HR can increase to as high as 180 beats/minute for short periods without harmful effects. The SV can be increased by increasing either preload or contractility.

Vascular System

Blood Vessels. The three major types of blood vessels in the vascular system are the arteries, veins, and capillaries. Arteries carry blood away from the heart and, except for the pulmonary artery, carry oxygenated blood. Veins carry blood toward the heart and, except for the pulmonary veins, carry deoxygenated blood. Small branches of arteries and veins are arterioles and venules, respectively. Blood circulates from the heart into arteries, arterioles, capillaries, venules, and veins, and then back to the heart.

Arteries and Arterioles. The arterial system differs from the venous system by the amount and type of tissue that makes up arterial walls (Fig. 32-7). The large arteries have thick walls that are composed mainly of elastic tissue. This elastic property cushions the impact of the pressure created by ventricular contraction and provides recoil that propels blood forward into the circulation. Large arteries also contain some smooth muscle. Examples of large arteries are the aorta and the pulmonary artery.

Arterioles have relatively little elastic tissue and more smooth muscle. Arterioles serve as the major control of arterial blood pressure and distribution of blood flow. They respond readily to local conditions such as low O_2 and increasing levels of CO_2 by dilating or constricting.

The innermost lining of the arteries is the endothelium. The endothelium serves to maintain hemostasis, promote blood flow, and, under normal conditions, inhibit blood coagulation. When the endothelial surface is disrupted (e.g., rupture of an atherosclerotic plaque), the coagulation cascade is initiated and results in the formation of a fibrin clot.

Capillaries. The thin capillary wall is made up of endothelial cells, with no elastic or muscle tissue (see Fig. 32-7). There are many miles of capillaries in an adult. The exchange of cellular nutrients and metabolic end products takes place through these thin-walled vessels.

Veins and Venules. Veins are large-diameter, thin-walled vessels that return blood to the right atrium (see Fig. 32-7). The venous system is a low-pressure, high-volume system. The larger veins contain semilunar valves at intervals to maintain the blood flow toward the heart and to prevent backward flow. The amount of blood in the venous system is affected by a number of factors, including arterial flow, compression of veins by skeletal muscles, alterations in thoracic and abdominal pressures, and right atrial pressure.

The largest veins are the *superior vena cava,* which returns blood to the heart from the head, neck, and arms, and the *inferior vena cava,* which returns blood to the heart from the lower part of the body. These large-diameter vessels are affected by the pressure in the right side of the heart. Elevated right atrial pressure can cause distended neck veins or liver engorgement as a result of resistance to blood flow.

Venules are relatively small vessels made up of a small amount of muscle and connective tissue. Venules collect blood from various capillary beds and channel it to the larger veins.

Regulation of the Cardiovascular System

Autonomic Nervous System. The autonomic nervous system consists of the sympathetic nervous system and the parasympathetic nervous system (see Chapter 56).

Effect on the Heart. Stimulation of the sympathetic nervous system increases the HR, the speed of impulse conduction through the AV node, and the force of atrial and ventricular contractions. This effect is mediated by specific sites in the heart called beta (β)-adrenergic receptors that are receptors for norepinephrine and epinephrine.

In contrast, stimulation of the parasympathetic system (mediated by the vagus nerve) causes a decrease in HR by slowing the SA node rate and thus conduction through the AV node.

Effect on the Blood Vessels. The source of neural control of blood vessels is the sympathetic nervous system. The alpha (α)-adrenergic receptors are located in vascular smooth muscles. Stimulation of the α-adrenergic receptors results in vasoconstriction. Decreased stimulation to the α-adrenergic receptors causes vasodilation. (Sympathetic nervous system receptors that influence blood pressure are presented in Chapter 33, Table 33-1.)

The parasympathetic nerves have selective distribution in the blood vessels. Blood vessels in skeletal muscle do not receive parasympathetic input.

Baroreceptors. *Baroreceptors* in the aortic arch and carotid sinus (at the origin of the internal carotid artery) are sensitive to stretch or pressure within the arterial system. Stimulation of these receptors sends information to the vasomotor center in the brainstem. This results in temporary inhibition of the sympathetic nervous system and enhancement of the parasympathetic influence, causing a decreased HR and peripheral vasodilation. Decreased arterial pressure causes the opposite effect.

Chemoreceptors. *Chemoreceptors* are located in the aortic arch and carotid body. They are capable of initiating changes in HR and arterial pressure in response to decreased arterial O_2 pressure, increased arterial CO_2 pressure, and decreased plasma pH. When the chemoreceptor reflexes are stimulated, they subsequently stimulate the vasomotor center to increase cardiac activity.

Blood Pressure

The **arterial blood pressure** (BP) is a measure of the pressure exerted by blood against the walls of the arterial system. The **systolic blood pressure** (SBP) is the peak pressure exerted against the arteries when the heart contracts. The **diastolic blood pressure** (DBP) is the residual pressure of the arterial system during ventricular relaxation (or filling). BP is usually expressed as the ratio of systolic to diastolic pressure.

The two main factors influencing BP are cardiac output (CO) and *systemic vascular resistance* (SVR):

$$BP = CO \times SVR$$

SVR is the force opposing the movement of blood. This force is created primarily in small arteries and arterioles.

Normal blood pressure is systolic BP <120 mm Hg and diastolic BP <80 mm Hg[3] (see Chapter 33).

Measurement of Arterial Blood Pressure. BP can be measured by invasive and noninvasive techniques. The invasive technique consists of catheter insertion into an artery. The catheter is attached to a transducer, and the pressure is measured directly (see Chapter 66).

Noninvasive, indirect measurement of BP can be done with a sphygmomanometer and a stethoscope. The sphygmomanometer consists of an inflatable cuff and a pressure gauge. The BP is measured externally by auscultating for sounds of turbulent blood flow through a compressed artery (termed **Korotkoff sounds**). The brachial artery is the recommended site for taking a BP.

After placing the appropriate size cuff on the upper arm, the cuff is inflated to a pressure 20 to 30 mm Hg above the systolic pressure. This causes blood flow in the artery to cease. As the pressure in the cuff is lowered, the artery is auscultated for Korotkoff sounds. There are five phases of Korotkoff sounds. The first phase is a tapping sound caused by the spurt of blood into the constricted artery as the pressure in the cuff is gradually deflated. This sound is considered the SBP. The fifth phase occurs when the sound disappears and is known as the DBP.[3] Clinically the BP is recorded as SBP/DBP (e.g., 120/80). Occasionally an auscultatory gap is heard. An *auscultatory gap* is a loss of sound between the SBP and the DBP. Proper BP technique (e.g., correct cuff size, positioning arm at heart level) is important for accurate BP values (see Chapter 33, Table 33-13).

In addition to the auscultatory technique, another noninvasive way to measure BP indirectly is to use an automated device that uses oscillometric measurements to assess BP. Though this method does not involve auscultation of Korotkoff sounds, the same attention to proper technique is important for accuracy. Finally, SBP (and pulse) can be assessed using a Doppler ultrasonic flowmeter. The handheld transducer is positioned over the artery (identified by audible, pulsatile sounds). The cuff is applied above the artery, inflated until the sounds disappear, and then another 20 to 30 mm Hg beyond that point. The cuff is then slowly deflated until sounds return. This point is the SBP.[4]

Pulse Pressure and Mean Arterial Pressure. Pulse pressure is the difference between the SBP and DBP. It is normally about one third of the SBP. If the BP is 120/80, the pulse pressure is 40. An increased pulse pressure may occur during exercise or in individuals with atherosclerosis of the larger arteries due to increased SBP. A decreased pulse pressure may be found in cardiac failure or hypovolemia.

Another measurement related to BP is **mean arterial pressure** (MAP). The MAP is the perfusion pressure felt by organs in the body. It is not the average of the diastolic and systolic pressures because the duration of diastole exceeds that of systole at normal HRs. MAP is calculated as follows:

$$MAP = (SBP + 2\ DBP) \div 3$$

A person with a BP of 120/60 has a MAP of 80. A MAP of greater than 60 is necessary to sustain the vital organs of an average person under most conditions. If the MAP falls significantly below this number for an appreciable time, vitals organs will be underperfused and will become ischemic.

GERONTOLOGIC CONSIDERATIONS
EFFECTS OF AGING ON THE CARDIOVASCULAR SYSTEM

Cardiovascular disease is the most common cause of hospitalization and the second cause of death in adults less than age 85. It remains the leading cause of death in adults greater than age 85. The most common cardiovascular problem is coronary artery disease (CAD) secondary to atherosclerosis. It is difficult to separate normal aging changes from the pathophysiologic changes of atherosclerosis. Current thinking suggests that many of the physiologic changes in the cardiovascular system of the elderly are a result of the combined effects of the aging process, disease, environmental factors, and lifetime health behaviors rather than age alone.[4,5]

With increased age, the amount of collagen in the heart increases and elastin decreases. These changes affect the contractile and distensible properties of the myocardium. One of the major age-associated alterations in the cardiovascular response to physical or emotional stress is a decrease in CO and SV caused by decreased contractility and HR response to increased stress. The resting HR is not markedly affected by aging.

Cardiac valves become thicker and stiffer from lipid accumulation, degeneration of collagen, and fibrosis.[5] The aortic and mitral valves are most frequently affected. These changes result in either regurgitation of blood when the valve should be closed or narrowing of the orifice of the valve (stenosis) when the valve should be open. The turbulent blood flow across the affected valve results in a *murmur.*

The number of pacemaker cells in the SA node decreases with age. By age 75, a person may have only 10% of the normal number of pacemaker cells, though this is compatible with normal SA node function.[2] Similar decreases in the number of conduction cells in the AV node, the bundle of His, and the bundle branches also occur with aging. Fibrosis of the bundle branches has been shown to precipitate chronic heart block in persons 65 years and older.[2] A normal ECG of an aging patient may show small, inconspicuous increases in PR, QRS, and QT intervals.

The autonomic nervous system control of the cardiovascular system is altered with aging. The number and function of β-adrenergic receptors in the heart decrease with age. Therefore the older adult not only has a decreased response to physical and emotional stress but also is less sensitive to β-adrenergic agonist drugs.

Arterial blood vessels thicken and become less elastic with age.[6] Arteries increase their sensitivity to vasopressin (antidiuretic hormone). Both of these changes contribute to a progressive increase in SBP and a decrease or no change in DBP with age. Consequently, an increase in the pulse pressure is found. Hypertension is not considered a normal consequence of aging and should be treated.

Orthostatic hypotension is estimated to be present in >30% of patients over age 70 with systolic hypertension.[7] Despite the changes associated with aging, the heart is able to function adequately under most circumstances.

Age-related changes in the cardiovascular system and differences in assessment findings are presented in Table 32-1.

ASSESSMENT OF THE CARDIOVASCULAR SYSTEM

Subjective Data

A careful health history and physical examination should aid the nurse in differentiating symptoms that reflect a cardiovascular problem from problems of other body systems. Common chief cues that should alert the nurse to the possibility of underlying

TABLE 32-1 GERONTOLOGIC DIFFERENCES IN ASSESSMENT
Cardiovascular System

Changes	Differences in Assessment Findings
Chest Wall	
Kyphosis	Altered chest landmarks for palpation, percussion, and auscultation; distant heart sounds
Heart	
Myocardial hypertrophy, ↑ collagen and scarring, ↓ elastin	↓ Cardiac reserve, heart failure
Downward displacement	Difficulty in isolating apical pulse
↓ CO, HR, SV in response to exercise or stress	Slowed, ↓ response to exercise and stress; slowed recovery from activity
Cellular aging changes and fibrosis of conduction system	↓ Amplitude of QRS complex and slight lengthening of PR, QRS, and QT intervals; irregular cardiac rhythms, ↓ maximal HR, ↓ HR variability
Valvular rigidity from calcification, sclerosis, or fibrosis, impeding complete closure of valves	Systolic murmur (aortic or mitral) possible without being indication of cardiovascular pathology
Blood Vessels	
Arterial stiffening caused by loss of elastin in arterial walls, thickening of intima of arteries, and progressive fibrosis of media	↑ In systolic and possible ↑ or ↓ in diastolic BP; possible widened pulse pressure; pedal pulses diminished, ↑ in intermittent claudication
Venous tortuosity increased	Inflamed, painful, or cordlike varicosities

BP, Blood pressure; *CO,* cardiac output; *HR,* heart rate; *SV,* stroke volume.

cardiovascular problems should be explored and documented (Table 32-2).

Important Health Information

Past Health History. Many illnesses affect the cardiovascular system directly or indirectly. The patient should be questioned about a history of chest pain, shortness of breath, alcoholism and/or tobacco use, anemia, rheumatic fever, streptococcal sore throat, congenital heart disease, stroke, syncope, hypertension, thrombophlebitis, intermittent claudication, varicosities, and edema.

Medications. An assessment of the patient's current and past use of medications should be made. This includes over-the-counter (OTC) drugs and herbal supplements, and prescription drugs. For example, aspirin, which prolongs the blood clotting time, is contained in many drugs used to alleviate cold symptoms. A medication assessment should list the name of the drug, the dose, and the patient's understanding of its purpose and side effects. Noncardiac drugs that may adversely affect the cardiovascular system also should be assessed (Table 32-3).

Surgery or Other Treatments. The patient should also be asked about specific treatments, past surgeries, or hospital admissions related to cardiovascular problems. Any hospitalizations for diagnostic workups or cardiovascular symptoms should be explored. It should be noted whether an ECG or a chest x-ray has been done for baseline data.

Functional Health Patterns. The strong correlation between components of a patient's lifestyle and cardiovascular health supports the need to review each functional health pattern. Key questions to ask a person with a cardiovascular problem are listed in Table 32-4.

Health Perception–Health Management Pattern. The nurse should ask the patient about the presence of cardiovascular risk factors. Major risk factors include elevated serum lipids, hypertension, tobacco use, sedentary lifestyle, and obesity. Stressful lifestyle and diabetes mellitus should also be investigated.

If the patient uses tobacco, the number of pack-years of tobacco use (number of packs smoked per day multiplied by the number of years the patient has smoked) should be estimated. The patient's attitude about tobacco use, as well as attempts to stop and methods used, should be documented. Alcohol use should also be recorded. This information should include type of alcohol, amount, frequency, and any changes in the reaction to it. The use of habit-forming drugs, including recreational drugs, also should be noted. It is also important to obtain information on the patient's perception of how this illness may affect the future level of wellness and ability for self-care.

A question about the patient's allergies is appropriate. The nurse should determine whether a drug reaction or an allergic reaction was ever experienced. A specific question regarding any allergic reaction to shellfish is important as this may warn of potential dye allergies. If the patient has been treated for allergies, understanding of this therapy should be determined. The patient should also be asked whether an anaphylactic reaction has ever been experienced.

Confirmed illnesses of blood relatives can highlight any hereditary or familial tendencies toward CAD, peripheral vascular disease, hypertension, bleeding, cardiac disorders, diabetes mellitus, atherosclerosis, and stroke. Any family members who were diagnosed with cardiac disease younger than age 55 should be noted. In addition, disorders affecting the vascular system, such as intermittent claudication and varicosities, may be familial. Finally, a family health history of noncardiac conditions such as asthma, renal disease, liver disease, and obesity should be assessed because they can affect the cardiovascular system.

Nutritional-Metabolic Pattern. Being underweight or overweight may indicate potential cardiovascular problems. Thus it is important to assess the patient's weight history in relation to height and build. A typical day's diet should be examined for its adequacy in relation to the patient's lifestyle. The amount of salt, saturated fats, and triglycerides in the patient's diet should be determined. In addition to actual food habits, which may be influenced greatly by

TABLE 32-2 Cues to Cardiovascular Problems

Manifestations	Description
Fatigue	No energy, need more rest than usual, normal activities result in tiring
Fluid retention	Weight gain, bloated feeling; bilateral swelling of lower extremities; tightening of clothing; shoes no longer fitting comfortably; marks or indentations left from constricting garments
Irregular heartbeat	Sensation of heart in throat or skipped beats; palpitations
Dyspnea	Shortness of breath; air hunger, especially after exertion; uncomfortable awareness of breathing; additional pillows or upright chair necessary for sleep
Pain	Indigestion, burning, numbness, tightness, or pressure in midchest; epigastric or substernal pain radiating to shoulder, neck, arms, jaws
Tenderness in calf of leg	Inability to bear weight; swelling of the involved extremity; inflamed, warm skin over vein
	Distended, discolored, tortuous veins in calves of legs; ache in lower extremities after standing for short periods
Syncope, near syncope	Fainting; dizzy with change of position; light-headedness
Altered neurologic function	Change in sensory or motor function, temporary or permanent
Leg pain	Tight squeezing pain in thigh, calf muscles with walking, relief with rest

TABLE 32-3 Adverse Cardiovascular Effects of Common Noncardiac Drugs and Agents

Drug Classification	Examples of Drugs	Cardiovascular Effects
Tricyclic antidepressants	amitriptyline (Elavil), doxepin (Sinequan)	Dysrhythmias, orthostatic hypotension
Antipsychotics	chlorpromazine (Thorazine), haloperidol (Haldol)	Dysrhythmias, orthostatic hypotension
Hormone replacement therapy	estrogen + progestin (Ortho-Novum, Prempro)	Hypertension, myocardial infarction, thromboembolus
Anticancer agents	daunorubicin (Cerubidine), doxorubicin (Adriamycin)	Dysrhythmias, cardiomyopathy
Corticosteroids	cortisone (Cortone), prednisone (Orasone)	Hypotension, edema, potassium depletion
Psychostimulants	cocaine, amphetamines	Tachycardia, angina, hypertension, dysrhythmias
Herbal supplements	ma huang (Ephedra)	Hypertension, tachycardia, palpitations, angina

TABLE 32-4 HEALTH HISTORY
Cardiovascular System

Health Perception–Health Management Pattern
- Do you practice any preventive measures to decrease cardiovascular risk factors?*
- Have you noticed an increase in cardiovascular symptoms such as chest pain or dyspnea?*
- Does your cardiovascular problem cause you to be less able to care for yourself?*
- Do you foresee any potential self-care problems because of your cardiovascular problem?*
- Have you ever used tobacco? If yes, in what form, how much, and for how long? Have you tried to quit? If yes, what methods have you tried? Are you interested in more information about quitting?
- How often and how much alcohol do you drink?

Nutritional-Metabolic Pattern
- Describe your usual daily diet, including sodium and fluid intake.
- What is your present weight? What was your weight 1 year ago? If different, explain.
- Does eating cause fatigue or shortness of breath?*

Elimination Pattern
- Do your feet or ankles ever swell?* If yes, how far up your legs? Does it go away after sleeping all night?
- Have you ever taken medication to help you get rid of excess fluid or to relieve constipation?*
- Do you ever strain to have a bowel movement?

Activity-Exercise Pattern
- Are your activities of daily living or exercise limited because of your cardiovascular problem?*
- When were you last able to comfortably perform your usual activities or exercise?
- Do you experience any discomfort or side effects as a result of exercise or any activity?*
- Can you comfortably walk and talk at the same time?
- How often do you attend activities outside your home?
- What was your most strenuous activity in the last few months?

Sleep-Rest Pattern
- How many pillows do you sleep on at night? Has this changed recently?*
- Do you ever wake up suddenly and feel as if you cannot catch your breath?*
- Do you have a history of sleep apnea?*
- How many times a night do you awaken to urinate?

Cognitive-Perceptual Pattern
- Do you ever experience dizziness or fainting?*
- Do you ever find it difficult to verbally express yourself or to remember things?*
- Do you experience any pain (e.g., chest pain, leg pain with activity) as a result of your cardiovascular problem?*

Self-Perception–Self-Concept Pattern
- Have your perceptions of yourself changed since you were diagnosed with a cardiovascular disease?*
- How has your cardiovascular disease affected the quality of your life?

Role-Relationship Pattern
- Has this illness affected any of the roles that you play in your daily life?*
- How have your significant others been affected by your disease?

Sexuality-Reproductive Pattern
- Has your cardiovascular disease caused a change in your sexual activity?*
- Do you experience any cardiac-related symptoms during sexual activity?*
- Do any of your medications affect your ability to participate in sexual activities?*

Coping–Stress Tolerance Pattern
- Describe your normal coping mechanisms during times of stress or anxiety.
- Who or where would you turn to during a time of stress? Are these people or services helping you now?*
- Do you practice any stress reduction techniques?*
- Do you often feel anger or hostility?*
- Do you feel capable of handling your present health situation? Explain.
- Do you experience any cardiovascular symptoms (e.g., chest pain, palpitations) during times of stress, anger, or hostility?*

Values-Belief Pattern
- What influence have your values or beliefs had during your illness?
- Do you feel any conflicts between your values or beliefs and the plan of care?*
- Describe any cultural or religious beliefs that may influence the treatment of your cardiovascular problem.

*If yes, describe.

ethnicity, the patient's attitudes and plans relative to diet and weight management should be investigated.

Elimination Pattern. The patient on diuretics may report increased urinary elimination. Problems with constipation should be investigated and documented. Straining during a bowel movement (Valsalva maneuver) should be avoided in a patient with cardiovascular problems. Cardiovascular problems may impair the patient's ability to get to a toilet as quickly as necessary. The patient should be questioned about this if incontinence or constipation is problematic.

Activity-Exercise Pattern. The benefit of exercise to cardiovascular health is indisputable, with sustained aerobic exercise being most beneficial. The nurse should inquire about the types of exercise done, the duration and frequency of each, and the occurrence of any unwanted effects. The length of time the exercise program has been practiced should be recorded, along with participation in individual or group sports. Any symptoms indicative of cardiovascular problems, such as light-headedness, chest pain, palpitations, shortness of breath, or claudication, during exercise should be noted.

The patient should also be questioned about any limitations in activities of daily living (ADLs) as a result of a cardiovascular problem. Such problems are often associated with fatigue and depression, which can be symptoms of cardiac disease. The nurse should also gather information about the patient's leisure and recreational activities. Any change in previous abilities should be noted.

Sleep-Rest Pattern. Cardiovascular problems often disrupt sleep. *Paroxysmal nocturnal dyspnea* (attacks of shortness of breath especially at night that awaken the patient) and Cheyne-Stokes respiration are associated with heart failure. Many patients with heart failure may need to sleep with their head elevated on pillows. The nurse should note the number of pillows needed for comfort and if this has changed recently.

Sleep apnea has been associated with an increase risk of life-threatening dysrhythmias, especially in patients with left ventricular failure, and should be investigated. Nocturia, a common finding with cardiovascular patients, also interrupts normal sleep patterns and should be explored.

Cognitive-Perceptual Pattern. It is important that the nurse ask both the patient and significant others about cognitive-perceptual problems. Any pain associated with the cardiovascular system, such as chest pain and claudication, should be reported. Cardiovascular problems such as dysrhythmias, hypertension, and stroke may cause problems with syncope, language, and memory.

Self-Perception–Self-Concept Pattern. If a cardiovascular event has been of acute origin, the patient's self-perception may be affected. Invasive diagnostic and palliative procedures often lead to body image concerns for the patient. When the cardiovascular disease is chronic in nature, the patient may not be able to identify the cause but can often describe the inability to "keep up" previous levels of activity or accomplishments. This too may affect the patient's quality of life. Therefore it is essential to inquire about the effects of the illness on the patient.

Role-Relationship Pattern. The patient's gender, race, and age are all related to cardiovascular health and are therefore important basic information. In addition, discussing the patient's marital status, role in the household, employment status, number of children and their ages, living environment, and significant others assists the nurse in identifying strengths and support systems in the patient's life. The nurse must assess the patient's level of satisfaction or dissatisfaction in each assigned role, which may alert the health care provider to possible areas of stress or conflict.

Sexuality-Reproductive Pattern. The patient should be asked about the effect of the cardiovascular problem on sexual patterns and satisfaction. It is common for the patient to have a fear of sudden death during sexual intercourse, causing a major alteration in sexual behavior. Fatigue or shortness of breath may also curtail sexual activity. Erectile dysfunction may be a symptom of peripheral vascular disease and/or a side effect of some medications used in treating cardiovascular problems (e.g., β-adrenergic blockers, diuretics). This side effect may result in noncompliance with medical treatment (see Chapter 33, Table 33-8). Counseling of both the patient and partner may be indicated. Patients should be asked about the use of drugs for erectile dysfunction [e.g., sildenafil (Viagra)]. These drugs are contraindicated if the patient is taking a nitrate. When taken together, life-threatening hypotension can occur.[8]

Use of hormone replacement therapy (HRT) for symptoms of menopause should be elicited in females. Studies have indicated that there is no cardiac benefit with the use of HRT. There may possibly be an increased cardiac risk with the use of HRT.[8]

Coping–Stress Tolerance Pattern. The patient should be asked to identify areas that cause stress or anxiety. Potentially stressful areas include marital relationships, family, occupation, church, friends, finances, and housing. Although many persons enjoy certain activities, these activities can be stressful at the same time that they are rewarding. The usual methods of coping with stress should be investigated.

High levels of anxiety, anger, and hostility have emerged as risk factors for cardiac disease and cardiac events.[2] The patient and the family should be asked about the frequency of these types of behavior. Information about support systems such as family, extended family and friends, counselors, or religious groups may provide excellent resources for developing a plan of care.

Values-Belief Pattern. Individual values and beliefs, which are greatly affected by culture, may play a significant role in the level of real or potential conflict a patient faces when dealing with a diagnosis of cardiovascular disease. Some patients may attribute their illness to punishment from God; others may feel that a "higher power" may assist them. Information about a patient's values and beliefs will help the nurse intervene during periods of crisis. It is also important to determine if the proposed plan of care causes any conflict with the patient's value system.

Objective Data

Physical Examination

Vital Signs. After the patient's general appearance has been observed, vital signs, including BP, heart and respiratory rates, and temperature are taken. Orthostatic (postural) BPs and HRs should be measured while the patient is lying, sitting, and standing. Normally there is a reduction of up to 15 mm Hg in the SBP and 3 to 5 mm Hg in the DBP from the lying to the standing position. HR should not increase more than 20 beats/minute from supine to standing position.[4] Baseline BP measurements should be taken in

GENDER DIFFERENCES
Cardiac Assessment

Men

- Experience the onset of heart disease earlier than women.
- Often less ill on presentation.
- Have more typical angina symptoms.
- Pain is described as substernal, crushing pain.
- Standard screening for the risk of sudden cardiac death (e.g., EPS) has been noted to be more predictive in men.
- More likely to be referred for cardiac catheterization.

Women

- Experience the onset of heart disease approximately 10 yr later than men.
- Often more ill on presentation.
- Have more comorbid conditions.
- Often have angina symptoms that are not typical.
- Pain often reported in the back, jaw, arms, epigastric region.
- May report nonpain symptoms such as fatigue, diaphoresis, palpitations, nausea, or vomiting.
- Certain diagnostic tests are less predictive for women.
- Exercise ECG testing is possibly affected by hormonal factors influencing ST changes.
- Nuclear imaging is affected by artifact from breast attenuation.
- Pharmacologic echocardiography is recommended as an effective method to evaluate women.

ECG, Electrocardiogram; *EPS,* electrophysiologic study.

both arms. These readings may vary from 5 to 15 mm Hg. A greater variance indicates pathology. The arm with the highest BP should be used for subsequent BP measurements. BP in the lower extremities is expected to be about 10 mm Hg higher than in the upper extremities.

Peripheral Vascular System

Inspection. Inspection of the skin should include color, hair distribution, and venous pattern. The extremities should be inspected for conditions such as edema, thrombophlebitis, clubbing of the nail beds, varicosities, and lesions such as stasis ulcers. Edema in the extremities can be caused by gravity, interruption of venous return, or elevation of right atrial pressure.

The large veins in the neck (internal and external jugular) should be inspected while the patient is gradually elevated from a supine position to an upright (30 to 45 degrees) position. Distention and prominent pulsations of these neck veins, referred to as *jugular venous distention,* can be caused by right atrial pressure elevation.

Palpation. Palpation of the upper and lower extremities for temperature, moisture, pulses, and edema should be done bilaterally to assess for symmetry. Edema is assessed by depressing the skin over the tibia or medial malleolus for 5 seconds. Normally, there is no indentation after releasing pressure. If pitting edema is present, it often is graded from 1+ (mild pitting) to 4+ (very deep pitting).[4]

Palpation of the pulses in the neck and extremities provides information on arterial blood flow. The pulses should be palpated to assess the rhythm (e.g., regular, irregular) and pressure within each vessel. Characteristics of the arteries on the right and left sides of the body should be compared simultaneously to determine symmetry. It is important to palpate each carotid pulse separately to avoid vagal stimulation and subsequent dysrhythmias.

When palpating the arteries identified in Fig. 32-8, the pressure of the pulse wave, or how far the vessel wall distends when the pulse occurs, is assessed. This judgment often is graded using the following scale:[4]

0 = Absent
1+ = Weak
2+ = Normal
3+ = Increased
4+ = Bounding

The *rigidity* (hardness) of the vessel should also be noted. The normal pulse will feel like a tap, whereas a vessel wall that is narrowed or bulging will vibrate. The term for a palpable vibration is *thrill.*

A measure used for assessing arterial flow to the extremities is the *capillary refill.* The patient's hands are positioned near the level of the heart and the nail beds are squeezed to produce blanching and observed for the return of color. With normal peripheral perfusion and CO, the color will return in less than 3 seconds.

Auscultation. An artery that has a narrowed or bulging wall may create turbulent blood flow. This abnormal flow can create a buzzing or humming termed a *bruit.* It can be heard with a stethoscope placed over the vessel. Auscultation of major arteries such as the carotid arteries, abdominal aorta, and femoral arteries should be part of the initial cardiovascular assessment. Abnormalities of the cardiovascular system are described in Table 32-5.

Thorax

Inspection and Palpation. An overall inspection and palpation of the bony structures of the thorax is the initial step in the examination. Next, inspect and palpate the areas where the cardiac valves project their sounds by identifying the intercostal spaces (ICSs). The raised notch, the *angle of Louis,* that is created where the manubrium and the body of the sternum are joined is readily palpable in the midline of the sternum. The angle of Louis is at the level of the second rib and can therefore be used to count ICSs and locate specific auscultatory areas (Fig. 32-9).

The following auscultatory areas can be located: the aortic area in the second ICS to the right of the sternum, the pulmonic area in the second ICS to the left of the sternum, the tricuspid area in the fifth left ICS close to the sternum, and the mitral area in the left midclavicular line at the level of the fifth ICS. A fifth auscultatory area is *Erb's point,* located at the third left ICS near the sternum. Normally, no pulsations are felt in these areas unless the patient has a thin chest wall.

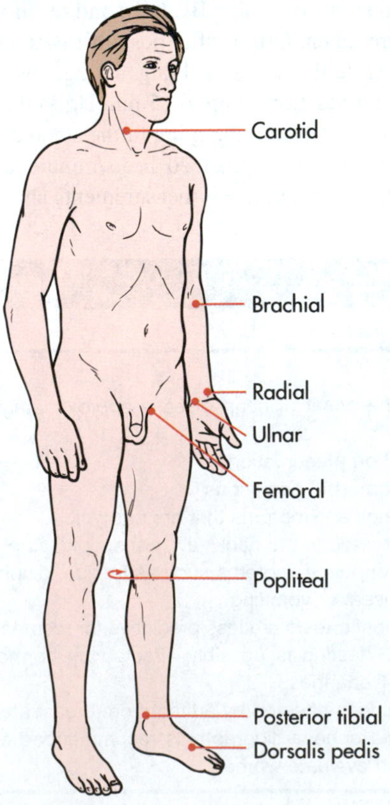

FIG. 32-8 Common sites for palpating arteries.

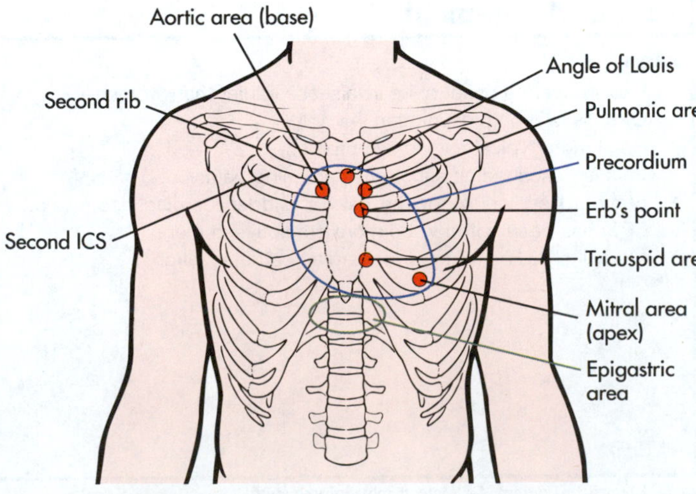

FIG. 32-9 Cardiac auscultatory areas. *ICS,* intercostal space.

TABLE 32-5 ***COMMON ASSESSMENT ABNORMALITIES*** **Cardiovascular System**

Finding	Description	Possible Etiology and Significance*
Inspection		
Distended neck veins	Vertical distance between intersection of angle of Louis and level of jugular distention greater than 3 cm with patient sitting at 30-45 degree angle	Elevated right atrial pressure; right-sided heart failure
Central cyanosis	Bluish or purplish tinge in central areas such as tongue, conjunctivae, inner surface of lips	Inadequate O_2 saturation of arterial blood due to pulmonary or cardiac disorders (e.g., congenital defects)
Peripheral cyanosis	Bluish or purplish tinge in extremities or in nose and ears	Reduced blood flow because of heart failure, vasoconstriction, cold environment
Splinter hemorrhages	Small red to black streaks under fingernails	Infective endocarditis (infection of endocardium, usually in area of cardiac valves)
Clubbing of nail beds	Obliteration of normal angle between base of nail and skin	Endocarditis, congenital defects, prolonged O_2 deficiency
Color changes in extremities with postural change	Pallor, cyanosis, mottling of skin after limb elevation; glossy skin	Chronic decreased arterial perfusion
Ulcers	*Venous:* necrotic crater-like lesion usually found on lower leg at medial malleolus; characterized by slow wound healing *Arterial:* pale ischemic base, well-defined edges usually found on toes, heels, lateral malleoli	Poor venous return, varicose veins, incompetent venous valves; arteriosclerosis, diabetes
Varicose veins	Visible dilated, tortuous vessels in lower extremities	Incompetent valves in vein
Palpation		
Pulse		
Bounding	Sharp, brisk, pounding pulse	Hyperkinetic states (anxiety, fever), anemia, hyperthyroidism
Thready	Weak, slowly rising pulse; easily obliterated by pressure	Blood loss, decreased cardiac output, aortic valve disease, peripheral arterial disease
Irregular	Regularly irregular or irregularly irregular; skipped beats	Cardiac dysrhythmias
Pulsus alternans	Regular rhythm but strength of pulse varies with each beat	Heart failure
Absent	Lack of pulse	Atherosclerosis, thrombus, trauma, embolus
Thrill	Vibration of vessel or chest wall	Aneurysm, aortic regurgitation, arteriovenous fistula
Rigidity	Stiffness or inflexibility of vessel wall	Atherosclerosis
>100 bpm	Tachycardia	Exercise, anxiety, shock, need for increased cardiac output, hyperthyroidism
<60 bpm	Bradycardia	Rest, SA or AV node damage, athletic conditioning, side effect of drugs (e.g., β-adrenergic blockers), hypothyroidism
Displaced point of maximal impulse (apical pulse)	Point of maximal impulse is palpated (or auscultated) below the fifth ICS and to the left of the MCL	Left ventricular dilation
Extremities		
Unusually warm extremities	Hands and feet warmer than normal	Possible thyrotoxicosis
Cold extremities	Hands and/or feet cold to touch, external covering necessary for comfort	Intermittent claudication, peripheral arterial obstruction, low cardiac output, severe anemia
Pitting edema of lower extremities or sacral area	Visible finger indentation after application of firm pressure	Interruption of venous return to heart, fluid in tissues
Positive Homans' sign	Presence of calf pain during sharp dorsiflexion of foot	Thrombophlebitis
Abnormal capillary filling time	Blanching of nail bed for more than 3 sec after release of pressure	Reduced arterial capillary perfusion, anemia
Asymmetry in limb circumference	Measurable swelling of involved limb	Thrombophlebitis, varicose veins, lymphedema
Percussion		
Abnormal cardiac borders	Left border of cardiac dullness extends beyond MCL in fifth ICS; right border of cardiac dullness extends beyond sternal border	Cardiac enlargement due to coronary heart disease, heart failure, cardiomyopathy

AV, Atrioventricular; *ICS,* intercostal space; *MCL,* midclavicular line; *SA,* sinoatrial.
*Limited to common etiologic factors. (Further discussion of conditions listed may be found in Chapters 33-38 and 66.)

Continued

TABLE 32-5 COMMON ASSESSMENT ABNORMALITIES
Cardiovascular System—cont'd

Finding	Description	Possible Etiology and Significance*
Auscultation		
Pulse deficit	Apical heart rate exceeds the peripheral pulse rate	Cardiac dysrhythmias
Arterial bruit	Turbulent flow sound in peripheral artery	Arterial obstruction or aneurysm
Third heart sound (S_3)	Extra heart sound, low pitched, heard in early diastole, similar to sound of a gallop	Left ventricular failure; volume overload; mitral, aortic, or tricuspid regurgitation; hypertension (possible)
Fourth heart sound (S_4)	Extra heart sound, low pitched, heard in late diastole, similar to sound of a gallop	Forceful atrial contraction from resistance to ventricular filling (e.g., in left ventricular hypertrophy, aortic stenosis, hypertension, coronary artery disease)
Cardiac murmurs	Turbulent sounds occurring between normal heart sounds; characterized by loudness, pitch, shape, quality, duration, timing	Cardiac valve disorder, abnormal blood flow patterns
Pericardial friction rub	High-pitched, scratchy sound heard during S_1 and/or S_2 at the apex. Heard best with patient sitting and leaning forward, and at the end of expiration	Pericarditis

A valvular disorder may be suspected if abnormal pulsations or thrills are felt. Next, the epigastric area, which lies on either side of the midline just below the xiphoid process, is inspected and palpated. In a thin person the pulsation of the abdominal aorta may be visible and can normally be palpated here. Next, the precordium, which is located over the heart, is inspected for heaves. **Heaves** are sustained lifts of the chest wall in the precordial area that can be seen or palpated. They may be caused by left ventricular hypertrophy. Normally no pulsations are seen or felt here.

When the patient is recumbent, the mitral valve area is inspected and palpated for the **point of maximal impulse** (PMI) (also known as the *apical pulse*), which is due to the pulsation of the apex of the heart. This pulsation or ventricular thrust lies medial to the midclavicular line in the fourth or fifth ICS. If the PMI is palpable, its position is recorded in relation to the midclavicular line and ICSs. When the PMI is below the fifth ICS and left of the midclavicular line, the heart may be enlarged.

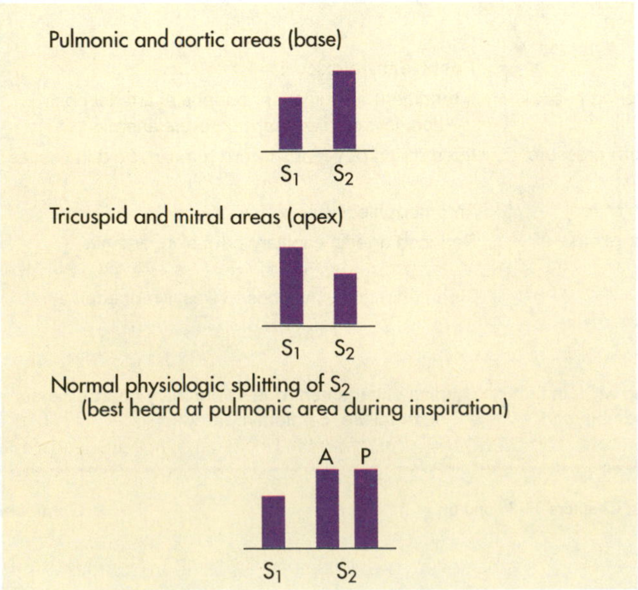

FIG. 32-10 Heart sounds. *A,* Aortic; *P,* pulmonic.

Percussion. The borders of the right and left sides of the heart can be estimated by percussion. Standing to the right of the recumbent patient, the curve of the rib in the fourth and fifth ICSs starting at the midaxillary line is percussed. The percussion note over the heart is dull in comparison with the resonance over the lung, and the location of cardiac dullness is recorded in relation to the midclavicular line.

Auscultation. The movement of the cardiac valves creates some turbulence in the blood flow resulting in normal heart sounds (Fig. 32-10). These sounds can be heard through a stethoscope placed on the chest wall. The first heart sound (S_1), which is associated with the closure of the tricuspid and mitral (AV) valves, has a soft *lub* sound. The second heart sound (S_2), which is associated with the closure of the aortic and pulmonic (semilunar) valves, has a sharp *dup* sound. S_1 signals the beginning of systole. S_2 signals the beginning of diastole (Fig. 32-11). The nurse should listen to the auscultatory areas in sequence with both the diaphragm and bell of the stethoscope.

The first and second heart sounds are heard best with the diaphragm of the stethoscope because they are high pitched. Extra heart sounds (S_3 or S_4), if present, are heard best with the bell of the stethoscope because they are low pitched. Having the patient leaning forward while sitting accentuates sounds from the second ICSs (aortic and pulmonic areas), whereas the left lateral decubitus position accentuates sounds produced at the mitral area.

The nurse listens at the apical area with the diaphragm of the stethoscope while simultaneously palpating the radial pulse. A judgment about the rhythm (regular or irregular) is also made when listening at the apex. If the apical and radial pulses are not

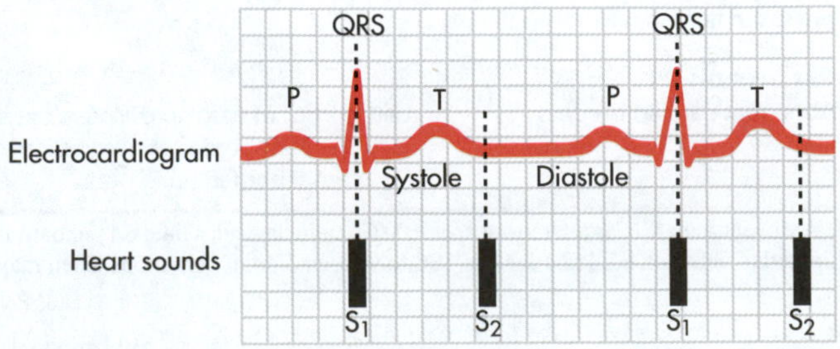

FIG. 32-11 Relationship of electrocardiogram, cardiac cycle, and heart sounds.

equivalent, one nurse should count the apical pulse while a second person is simultaneously counting the radial pulse. The difference between the two numbers is called a *pulse deficit* and can indicate cardiac dysrhythmias.

Palpating one carotid artery while auscultating at the apex allows differentiation of S_1 from S_2. Because S_1 (lub) occurs almost simultaneously with ventricular contraction (systole), it is heard when the carotid pulse is felt.

Normally no sound is heard between S_1 and S_2 during the periods of systole and diastole. Sounds that are heard during these periods may represent abnormalities and should be described. An exception to this is a normal splitting of S_2, which is best heard at the pulmonic area during inspiration (see Fig. 32-10). Splitting of this heart sound can be abnormal if it is heard during expiration or if it is constant (fixed) during the respiratory cycle.

The S_3 heart sound is a low-intensity vibration of the ventricular walls usually associated with decreased compliance of the ventricles during filling. An S_3 heart sound may be normal (physiologic) in young adults and is pathologic in patients with left ventricular failure or mitral valve regurgitation. It is heard closely after S_2 and is known as a *ventricular gallop.* The S_4 heart sound is a low-frequency vibration caused by atrial contraction. It precedes S_1 of the next cycle and is known as an *atrial gallop.* An S_4 heart sound may be normal in older adults with no evidence of heart disease and is pathologic in patients with CAD, cardiomyopathy, left ventricular hypertrophy, or aortic stenosis.[4]

Murmurs are sounds produced by turbulent blood flow through the heart or the walls of large arteries. Most murmurs are the result of cardiac abnormalities, but some occur in normal cardiac structures. Murmurs are graded on a six-point scale of loudness and recorded as a Roman numeral ratio; the numerator is the intensity of the murmur and the denominator is always VI, which indicates that the six-point scale is being used. A I/VI indicates a soft, faint murmur; a VI/VI indicates a murmur that can be heard without a stethoscope.

Pericardial friction rubs are high-pitched, scratchy sounds that may be transient or intermittent and may last several hours to days. They are caused by friction that occurs when inflamed surfaces of the pericardium, known as pericarditis, move against each other. Friction rubs are usually heard best at the apex, with the patient upright and leaning forward, and following expiration.[4]

If an abnormal sound is heard, it should be documented. This description should include the timing (during systole or diastole), location (the anatomic site on the chest where it is heard the loudest), pitch (heard best with the diaphragm or the bell of the stethoscope), position (heard best when patient is recumbent, sitting and leaning forward, or in the left lateral decubitus position), characteristics (scratchy, harsh, musical, soft), and any other abnormal findings (irregular cardiac rhythms or palpable chest wall heaves) associated with the sound.

The most common abnormal sounds and abnormal assessment findings are described in Table 32-5. A method of recording data from the cardiovascular assessment is presented in Table 32-6.

DIAGNOSTIC STUDIES OF THE CARDIOVASCULAR SYSTEM

Numerous diagnostic procedures add to the information obtained from the history and physical examination of the cardiovascular system. The most common studies used to assess the cardiovascular system are presented in Table 32-7.

TABLE 32-6 Normal Physical Assessment of the Cardiovascular System

Inspection	Normal skin color with capillary refill <3 sec; thorax symmetric, PMI not visible; no JVD with patient at 45-degree angle
Palpation	PMI palpable in fifth ICS at left MCL; no thrills or heaves; slight palpable pulsations of abdominal aorta in epigastric area; carotid and extremity pulses 2+ and equal bilaterally; no pedal edema
Percussion	Unable to distinguish right-sided heart border
Auscultation	S_1 and S_2 heard; apical-radial rate equal, 72, and regular; no murmurs or extra heart sounds

ICS, Intercostal space; *JVD,* jugular venous distention; *MCL,* midclavicular line; *PMI,* point of maximal impulse.

Blood Studies

Numerous blood studies contribute information about the cardiovascular system. For example, studies of the blood itself reflect the O_2-carrying capacity (red blood cell count and hemoglobin) and coagulation properties (clotting times). (See Chapter 30 for hematology studies.)

Cardiac Markers. When myocardial cells are injured, they release their contents, including enzymes and other proteins, into the circulation. These biochemical markers are useful in the diagnosis of myocardial injury and necrosis. The enzymes characteristic of cardiac injury are creatine kinase (CK), lactate dehydrogenase (LDH), and serum aspartate aminotransferase (AST), formerly called serum glutamic-oxaloacetic transaminase (SGOT). Because these enzymes are found in a variety of body tissues, they can be elevated as a result of injury to the muscles, liver, brain, and other organs. LDH and AST levels are no longer used as markers of myocardial injury. CK is present in heart muscle, skeletal muscle, and brain tissue. CK-MM is found primarily in the skeletal muscle, and CK-BB is found in the brain and nervous tissue. CK-MB elevation is specific for myocardial tissue injury. CK-MB levels rise 4 to 6 hours after symptom onset, peak in 18 to 24 hours, and return to baseline within 3 days after myocardial infarction (MI).[9]

Cardiac-specific troponin is a myocardial muscle protein released into circulation after injury. There are two subtypes, cardiac-specific troponin T (cTnT) and cardiac-specific troponin I (cTnI), that are specific to myocardial tissue. Normally there is no circulating troponin, so a rise in its level is diagnostic of myocardial injury. cTnT and cTnI are detectable within 1 hour of myocardial injury, have high specificity at 3 to 6 hours following the onset of symptoms, and reach peak levels within 12 hours.[9]

Myoglobin is a low-molecular-weight heme protein found in cardiac and skeletal muscle. Myoglobin elevation is a sensitive indicator of early myocardial injury, and serum elevations occur within 30 to 60 minutes after injury but decline rapidly after 7 hours. Its clinical value is limited due to the nonspecificity of myoglobin for MI and its brief presence following infarction.[9]

Correct interpretation of diagnostic tests requires consideration of the time frame from the onset of symptoms together with the time frame of the expected presence and elevated levels of the biomarkers. The additional data (patient symptoms, history, and ECG changes) complete the diagnostic picture for the patient with a suspected MI.[9]

Serum Lipids. Serum lipids consist of triglycerides, cholesterol, and phospholipids. They circulate in the blood bound to protein. Thus they are often referred to as *lipoproteins* (see Chapter 34, Fig. 34-5).

Text continued on page 756.

TABLE 32-7 ***DIAGNOSTIC STUDIES*** **Cardiovascular System**

Study	Description and Purpose	Nursing Responsibility
Blood Studies		
CK-MB	Immunochemical process using monoclonal antibodies that measures this cardiospecific enzyme. Concentrations >5% of total creatine kinase (CK) are highly indicative of MI. Serum levels increase within 4-6 hr after MI.	Explain to patient the purpose of serial sampling (every 6-8 hr ×3) in conjunction with serial ECGs.
Cardiac-specific troponins	Contractile proteins that are released following an MI. Both troponin T and troponin I are highly specific to cardiac tissue. *Normal:* Troponin T (cTnT): <0.1 ng/ml *Normal:* Troponin I (cTnI): <0.4 ng/ml cTnI 0.5-2.3 ng/ml indeterminate or suspicious for myocardial injury cTnI >2.3 ng/ml positive for myocardial injury	Rapid bedside assays are available. Serial sampling often done in conjunction with CK-MB and ECG.
Myoglobin	Low-molecular-weight protein that is 99%-100% sensitive for myocardial injury. Serum concentrations rise 30-60 min after MI. *Normal:* <92 ng/ml (men) <76 ng/ml (women)	Cleared from the circulation rapidly and most diagnostic if measured within first 12 hr of onset of chest pain.
C-reactive protein (CRP)	Marker of inflammation that can predict risk of cardiac disease and cardiac events, even in patients with normal lipid values. *Normal:* <1 mg/L *Moderate Risk:* 1-3 mg/L *High Risk:* >3 mg/L	Stable levels that can be measured nonfasting and anytime during the day. May be more predictive risk factor of cardiac disease than LDLs for women.
Homocysteine	Amino acid produced during protein catabolism that has been identified as a risk factor for cardiovascular disease. It is postulated that homocysteine causes damage to the endothelium or has a role in formation of thrombi. *Optimal:* <12 μmol/L *Moderate Risk:* 12-15 μmol/L *High Risk:* >15 μmol/L	Hyperhomocysteinemia resulting from dietary deficiencies is treated with folic acid, B_6, and B_{12} supplements.
b-Type natriuretic peptide (BNP)	Peptide that causes natriuresis. Elevation indicates presence of heart failure and distinguishes cardiac vs. respiratory cause of dyspnea. *Normal:* <100 pg/ml	Infusion of nesiritide (Natrecor) will elevate levels temporarily.
Serum Lipids		
Cholesterol	Cholesterol is a blood lipid. Elevated cholesterol is considered a risk factor for atherosclerotic heart disease. Level can be measured at any time of the day in a nonfasting state. *Normal:* 140-200 mg/dl (3.62-5.17 mmol/L) (varies with age and gender)	Cholesterol levels can be obtained in a nonfasting state, but for triglyceride levels and lipoproteins, fasting state for at least 12 hr (except for water) is necessary, and no alcohol intake is allowed for 24 hr before testing.
Triglycerides	Triglycerides are mixtures of fatty acids. Elevations are associated with cardiovascular disease. *Normal:* 40-190 mg/dl (0.45-2.15 mmol/L) (varies with age)	
Lipoproteins	Electrophoresis is done to separate lipoproteins into HDL, LDL, and VLDL and chylomicrons. There are marked day-to-day fluctuations in serum lipid levels. More than one determination is needed for accurate diagnosis and treatment. *Normal:* varies with age. Desirable LDL without CAD is <130 mg/dl (or 3.4 mmol/L). Desirable LDL level with CAD is ≤100 mg/dl (or 3.4 mmol/L) Desirable HDL is 37-70 mg/dl (0.97-1.83 mmol/L) for men; 40-88 mg/dl (1.05-2.30 mmol/L) for women.	Risk for cardiac disease is assessed by dividing the total cholesterol level by the HDL level. Target values are <5 for men and <4.4 for women.
Lipoprotein-associated phospholipase A_2 ($Lp-PLA_2$)	Enzyme immunoassay (PLAC test) is done to measure the level of $Lp-PLA_2$. Elevated levels of $Lp-PLA_2$ are associated with vascular inflammation and increased risk for CAD. *Normal:* 131-376 ng/ml (men) 120-342 ng/ml (women)	$Lp-PLA_2$ levels can be obtained in a nonfasting state.

CAD, Coronary artery disease; *ECG,* electrocardiogram; *HDL,* high-density lipoproteins; *HR,* heart rate; *IV,* intravenous(ly); *LDL,* low-density lipoproteins; *MI,* myocardial infarction; *NPO,* nothing by mouth; *VLDL,* very-low-density lipoproteins.

TABLE 32-7 DIAGNOSTIC STUDIES
Cardiovascular System—cont'd

Study	Description and Purpose	Nursing Responsibility
Chest X-Ray	Patient is placed in two upright positions to examine the lung fields and size of the heart. The two common positions are posteroanterior (PA) and lateral. Normal heart size and contour for the individual's age, gender, and size are noted.	Inquire about frequency of recent x-rays and possibility of pregnancy. Provide lead shielding to areas not being viewed. Remove any jewelry or metal objects that may obstruct the view of the heart and lungs.
ECG	Electrodes are placed on the chest and extremities, allowing the ECG machine to record cardiac electrical activity from different views. Can detect rhythm of heart, activity of pacemaker, conduction abnormalities, position of heart, size of atria and ventricles, presence of acute injury, and history of MI.	Prepare skin and apply electrodes and leads. Inform patient that no discomfort is involved. Instruct patient to avoid moving to decrease motion artifact.
Ambulatory ECG Monitoring		
Holter monitoring	Recording of ECG rhythm for 24-48 hr and then correlating rhythm changes with symptoms recorded in diary. Normal patient activity is encouraged to simulate conditions that produce symptoms. Electrodes are placed on chest and a recorder is used to store information, print it, and analyze it for any rhythm disturbance. It can be performed on an inpatient or outpatient basis.	Prepare skin and apply electrodes and leads. Explain importance of keeping an accurate diary of activities and symptoms. Tell patient that no bath or shower can be taken during monitoring. Skin irritation may develop from electrodes.
Transtelephonic event recorder	Records rhythm disturbances that are not frequent enough to be recorded in one 24-hr period. It allows more freedom than a regular Holter monitor. Some units have electrodes that are attached to the chest and have a loop of memory that captures the onset and end of an event. Other types are placed directly on patient's wrist, chest, or fingers and have no loop of memory, but record the patient's ECG in real time. Recordings are transmitted over the phone to a receiving unit, and the recordings are printed out for review. Tracings can then be erased and the unit can be reused.	Instruct in the use of equipment for recording and transmitting of transient events. Teach patient about skin preparation for lead placement or steady skin contact for units not requiring electrodes. This will ensure the reception of optimal ECG tracings for analysis.
Exercise Treadmill Test	Various protocols are used to evaluate the effect of exercise tolerance on myocardial function. A common protocol uses 3-min stages at set speeds and elevation of the treadmill belt. Continual monitoring of vital signs and ECG rhythms for ischemic changes are important in the diagnosis of left ventricular function and CAD. An exercise bike may be used if the patient is unable to walk on the treadmill.	Instruct patient to wear comfortable clothes and shoes that can be used for walking and running. Instruct patient about procedure and importance of reporting any symptoms that may occur. Monitor vital signs and obtain 12-lead ECG before exercise, during each stage of exercise, and after exercise until all vital signs and ECG changes have returned to normal. Monitor patient's response throughout procedure. Contraindications include any reasons patient is unable to reach peak exercise.
6-Minute Walk Test	Distance patient is able to walk on a flat surface in 6 min. Used to measure response to treatments and functional capacity for activities of daily living.	Instruct patient to wear comfortable shoes. Inform patient to carry or pull oxygen if used routinely. Patient should be encouraged to walk as quickly as possible.
Echocardiogram • M-mode • Two-dimensional (2-D) • Color-flow imaging or color Doppler • Real-time 3-dimensional (3-D) • Contrast	Transducer that emits and receives ultrasound waves is placed in four positions on the chest above the heart. Transducer records sound waves that are bounced off the heart. Also records direction and flow of blood through the heart and transforms it to audio and graphic data that measure valvular abnormalities, congenital cardiac defects, wall motion, ejection fraction, and cardiac function.	Place patient in a supine position on left side facing equipment. Instruct family and patient about procedure and sensations (pressure and mechanical movement from head of transducer). No contraindications to procedure exist.
Stress echocardiogram	Combination of exercise test and echocardiogram. Resting images of the heart are taken with ultrasound and then the patient exercises. Postexercise images are taken immediately after exercise (within 1 min of stopping exercise). Differences in left ventricular wall motion and thickening before and after exercise are evaluated.	Instruct and prepare patient for treadmill or exercise bicycle. Inform patient of importance of timely return to examination table for imaging after exercise. Contraindications include any reasons patient is unable to reach peak exercise.

Continued

Cardiovascular System

TABLE 32-7 DIAGNOSTIC STUDIES
Cardiovascular System—cont'd

Study	Description and Purpose	Nursing Responsibility
Echocardiogram—cont'd		
Pharmacologic echocardiogram	Used as a substitute for the exercise stress test in individuals unable to exercise. Dobutamine (a positive inotropic agent) or dipyridamole is infused IV and dosage is increased in 5-min intervals while echocardiogram is performed to detect wall motion abnormalities at each stage.	Start IV infusion. Administer medication per protocol. Monitor vital signs before, during, and after test until baseline achieved. Monitor patient for signs and symptoms of distress during procedure. Contraindications include any known allergies to medications.
Transesophageal echocardiogram (TEE)	A probe with an ultrasound transducer at the tip is swallowed. The physician controls angle and depth. As it passes down the esophagus, it sends back clear images of heart size, wall motion, valvular abnormalities, and possible source of thrombi without interference from lungs or chest ribs. A contrast medium may be injected IV for evaluating direction of blood flow if an atrial or ventricular septal defect is suspected. Doppler ultrasound and color flow imaging can also be used concurrently.	Instruct patient to be NPO for at least 6 hr before test. Remove dentures. A bite block is placed in the mouth. IV sedation is administered and throat is locally anesthetized. A designated driver is needed if done in the outpatient department. Monitor vital signs and oxygen saturation levels and perform suctioning continually during procedure. Assist patient to relax. Patient may not eat or drink until gag reflex returns. Sore throat is temporary.
Nuclear Cardiology	Study involves IV injection of radioactive isotopes. Radioactive uptake is counted over the heart by scintillation camera. It supplies information about myocardial contractility, myocardial perfusion, and acute cell injury.	Explain procedure to patient. Establish IV line for injection of isotopes. Explain that radioactive isotope used is a small, diagnostic amount and will lose most of its radioactivity in a few hours. Inform the patient that he or she will be lying still on back with arms extended overhead for 20 min. Repeat scans are performed within a few minutes to hours after the injection.
Exercise nuclear imaging	^{99m}Technetium-sestamibi or other nuclear imaging agent is injected IV and used to evaluate blood flow in different parts of the heart. Images are taken at rest and after exercise. For stress testing, the injection is given at maximum heart rate on bicycle or treadmill. Patient is then required to continue exercise for 1 min to circulate the radioactive isotope. Scanning is done 15-60 min after exercise. A resting scan may have to be performed 60-90 min after initial infusion or it may have to be done 24 hr prior. A 3-4 hr interval between rest and stress studies is required. Follow-up scan may have to be done 24 hr later.	Explain procedure to patient. Instruct patient to eat only a light meal between scans. Certain medications may need to be held for 1-2 days before the scan.
Pharmacologic nuclear imaging	Dipyridamole or adenosine is used to produce vasodilation when patients are unable to tolerate exercise. Vasodilation will increase blood flow to well-perfused coronary arteries. Scanning procedure is same.	Explain procedure to patient. Instruct patient to hold all caffeine products for 12 hr before procedure. Certain medications may need to be held for 1 day before the scan. Observe patient for side effects (e.g., bronchospasm). Aminophylline may be given to prevent or reverse side effects. Dobutamine is used if vasodilators are contraindicated. Contraindications include any known allergies to medications.
Multigated acquisition (MUGA) **scan**	^{99m}Technetium-sestamibi is mixed with a small amount of the patient's blood and reinjected (IV). Images are acquired at various points in the cardiac cycle. Indicated for patients with MI, heart failure, or valvular heart disease. It also can be used to evaluate the effect of various cardiac or cardiotoxic medications on the heart.	Explain procedure to patient. Establish IV line for removal of blood sample and reinjection of isotope. Establish ECG monitoring. Inform patient that procedure involves little or no risk.
Positron emission tomography (PET)	Uses two radionuclides. Nitrogen-13-ammonia is injected IV first and scanned to evaluate myocardial perfusion. A second radioactive isotope, fluoro-18-deoxyglucose, is then injected and scanned to show myocardial metabolic function. In the normal heart, both scans will match, but in an ischemic or damaged heart, they will differ. The patient may or may not be stressed. A baseline resting scan is usually obtained for comparison.	Instruct patient on procedure. Explain that patient will be scanned by a machine and will need to stay still for a period of time. Patient's glucose level must be between 60 and 140 mg/dl (3.3-7.8 μmol/L) for accurate glucose metabolic activity. If exercise is included as part of testing, patient will need to be NPO and refrain from tobacco and caffeine for 24 hr before test.

CAD, Coronary artery disease; *ECG,* electrocardiogram; *HDL,* high-density lipoproteins; *HR,* heart rate; *IV,* intravenous(ly); *LDL,* low-density lipoproteins; *MI,* myocardial infarction; *NPO,* nothing by mouth; *VLDL,* very-low-density lipoproteins.

TABLE 32-7 ***DIAGNOSTIC STUDIES***
Cardiovascular System—cont'd

Study	Description and Purpose	Nursing Responsibility
Magnetic Resonance Imaging (MRI)	Noninvasive imaging technique obtains information about cardiac tissue integrity, aneurysms, ejection fractions, cardiac output, and patency of proximal coronary arteries. It does not involve ionizing radiation and is an extremely safe procedure. It provides images in multiple planes with uniformly good resolution.	Explain procedure to patient. Inform patient that the small diameter of the cylinder, along with loud noise of the procedure, may cause panic or anxiety. Antianxiety drugs and music may be recommended. Patient must lie still during MRI. Contraindicated for persons with any implanted metallic devices.
Magnetic resonance angiography (MRA)	Same as MRI but with use of gadolinium as IV contrast medium to evaluate arterial disease.	Contraindications include any known allergies to contrast medium and persons with any implanted metallic devices.
Electron Beam Computed Tomography (EBCT)	Noninvasive scan used to quantify calcium deposits in coronary arteries and heart valves. May have clinical applications as a screening test for cardiac disease.	Explain procedure to patient. Inform patient that procedure is quick and involves little or no risk.
Cardiac Catheterization	Study involves insertion of catheter into heart to obtain information about O_2 saturation and pressure readings within heart chambers. Contrast medium is injected to assist in examining structure and motion of heart. Procedure is done by insertion of catheter into a vein (for right side of heart) or an artery (for left side of heart) (see text).	Before procedure, obtain written permission. Check for iodine sensitivity. Withhold food and fluids for 6-18 hr before procedure. Give sedative, if ordered. Inform patient about use of local anesthesia, insertion of catheter, and feeling of warmth when dye is injected and fluttering sensation of heart as catheter is passed. Note that patient may be instructed to cough or take a deep breath when catheter is inserted and that patient is monitored by ECG throughout procedure. After procedure, assess circulation to extremity used for catheter insertion. Check peripheral pulses, color, and sensation of extremity every 15 min for 1 hr and then with decreasing frequency. Observe puncture site for hematoma and bleeding. Place compression device over arterial site, if indicated. Monitor vital signs. Assess for abnormal HR, dysrhythmias, and signs of pulmonary emboli (respiratory difficulty).
Coronary angiography	Study involves injection of radiopaque contrast medium directly into coronary arteries by same procedure as for cardiac catheterization. It is used to evaluate patency of coronary arteries and collateral circulation.	Same as for cardiac catheterization.
Intracoronary ultrasound	Invasive study used to provide ultrasound information about the coronary arteries. A very small ultrasound probe is introduced into the coronary artery, similar to coronary angiography. Information obtained is used to assess size and consistency of plaque, arterial walls, and effectiveness of intracoronary artery treatment.	Same as for cardiac catheterization.
Electrophysiology study (EPS)	Invasive study used to record intracardiac electrical activity using catheters (with multiple electrodes) inserted via the femoral vein into the right side of heart. The catheter electrodes record the electrical activity in different cardiac structures. In addition, dysrhythmias can be induced.	Obtain written consent. Antidysrhythmic agents may be discontinued several days before study. Keep patient NPO 6-8 hr before test. Give premedication to promote relaxation and throughout the procedure if ordered. IV sedation often used during the procedure. Patient must have continuous ECG monitoring after the procedure.
Peripheral Arteriography and Venography*	Study involves injection of radiopaque contrast medium into either arteries or veins. Serial x-rays taken to detect and visualize any atherosclerotic plaques, occlusion, aneurysms, or traumatic injury.	Carefully explain procedure to patient. Check for iodine allergy. Give mild sedative, if ordered. Check extremity with puncture site for pulsation, warmth, color, and motion after procedure. Inspect insertion site for bleeding or swelling. Observe patient for allergic reactions to dye.
Hemodynamic Monitoring	Hemodynamic monitoring of arterial blood pressures, pulmonary artery pressure, pulmonary artery wedge pressure, and cardiac output is done to evaluate cardiovascular status and response to treatment.	Patients requiring hemodynamic monitoring are critically ill and are monitored in intensive care units (see Chapter 66).

*Additional peripheral vascular diagnostic studies are found in Table 38-8.

Triglycerides are the main storage form of lipids and constitute approximately 95% of fatty tissue. Cholesterol, a structural component of cell membranes and plasma lipoproteins, is a precursor of corticosteroids, sex hormones, and bile salts. In addition to being absorbed from food in the gastrointestinal tract, cholesterol can also be synthesized in the liver. Phospholipids contain glycerol, fatty acids, phosphates, and a nitrogenous compound. Although formed in most cells, phospholipids usually enter the circulation as lipoproteins synthesized by the liver. Apoproteins are water-soluble proteins that combine with most lipids to form lipoproteins.

Different classes of lipoproteins contain varying amounts of the naturally occurring lipids. These include the following:

1. *Chylomicrons:* primarily exogenous triglycerides from dietary fat
2. *Low-density lipoproteins (LDLs):* mostly cholesterol with moderate amounts of phospholipids
3. *High-density lipoproteins (HDLs):* about one half protein and one half phospholipids and cholesterol
4. *Very-low-density lipoproteins (VLDLs):* primarily endogenous triglycerides with moderate amounts of phospholipids and cholesterol

A lipid profile test usually consists of cholesterol, triglyceride, LDL, and HDL measurements. An elevation in LDL level has a strong and direct association with CAD; an increased HDL level has been associated with a decreased risk of CAD.[2] High levels of HDLs serve a protective role by mobilizing cholesterol from tissues. Increased triglyceride levels are also linked to the progression of CAD.[10] Although the association between elevated serum cholesterol levels and CAD exists, determination of total cholesterol level alone is not sufficient for an assessment of coronary risk. A risk assessment for CAD is determined by comparing the total cholesterol to HDL ratio over time.[11] An increase in the ratio indicates increased risk. This combination provides more information than either value alone. The patient must fast for 12 to 14 hours before the blood draw to eliminate the effects of a recent meal. A specimen should not be drawn if the patient is having acute stress.

Plasma levels of apolipoprotein A-1 (apo A-1) (the major HDL protein) and apolipoprotein B (apo B) (the major LDL protein) may be better predictors of CAD than HDLs or LDLs. Measurements of these lipoproteins may replace cholesterol-lipoprotein determinations in assessing the risk of CAD but typically are used for patients with known coronary artery disease, suspected familial hypercholesterolemia, or other lipid disorders.[2]

Lipoprotein (a), or Lp(a), is being assessed for its role as a risk factor for CAD.[2] Increased levels of Lp(a), especially with increased levels of LDH, have been associated with the progression of atherosclerosis. In addition, Lp(a) has been found to have thrombogenic properties that increase the risk of clot formation at the site of intravascular lesions.[12]

Lipoprotein-Associated Phospholipase A_2. Lipoprotein-associated phospholipase A_2 (Lp-PLA_2) is an enzyme made by macrophages. Lp-PLA_2 promotes vascular inflammation through the hydrolysis of oxidized LDLs within the intima of blood vessels, thus contributing directly to the development of atherosclerosis. Elevated levels of Lp-PLA_2 are indicative of the vascular inflammation that is associated with the formation of plaque within the arteries.

Serum levels of Lp-PLA_2 are measured by the PLAC test. Elevated results on the PLAC test even without an elevation in LDL cholesterol levels has been related to an increased risk of having CAD. The PLAC blood test can be included in a normal clinical evaluation to better determine a patient's risk for developing CAD.

C-Reactive Protein (CRP). CRP is a protein produced by the liver during periods of acute inflammation. It is emerging as an independent risk factor for CAD and a predictor of cardiac events. In one large study of women, it was found to be more predictive of cardiac events than LDLs.[2]

Homocysteine (Hcy). Hcy is an amino acid that is produced during protein catabolism. Elevated Hcy levels can be either hereditary or acquired from dietary deficiencies of B_6, B_{12}, or folate. Elevated levels of Hcy have been linked to an increased risk of a first cardiac event. They have also been identified as a predictor of CAD, stroke, and thromboembolism even in the presence of normal lipid levels. It is recommended that Hcy testing be performed in those patients with a familial predisposition for early cardiovascular disease.[2,13]

Cardiac Natriuretic Peptide Markers. There are three natriuretic peptides: atrial natriuretic peptide (ANP) originates in the atrium, b-type natriuretic peptide (BNP) in the ventricles, and c-type natriuretic peptide in endothelial and renal epithelial cells. BNP has emerged as the marker of choice for distinguishing a cardiac or respiratory cause of dyspnea. When ventricular DBP increases (e.g., heart failure), BNP is released and serves to increase natriuresis.[2] (ANP and BNP are also discussed in Chapter 33 on p. 765 and in Chapter 35 on pp. 824 and 832.)

Chest X-Ray

A radiographic picture can depict cardiac contours, heart size and configuration, and anatomic changes in individual chambers (Fig. 32-12). The radiographic image records any displacement or enlargement of the heart, presence of extra fluid around the heart (pericardial effusion), and pulmonary congestion.

Electrocardiogram

The basic P, QRS, and T waveforms (see Fig. 32-6) are used to assess cardiac function. Deviations from the normal sinus rhythm can indicate abnormalities in heart function. There are many types

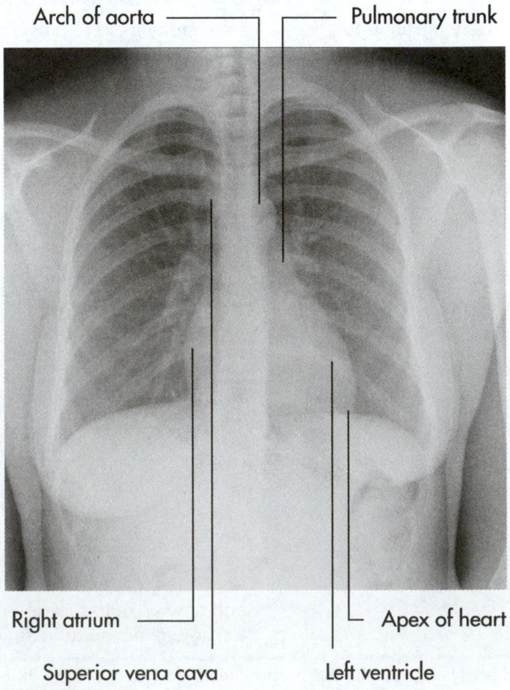

FIG. 32-12 Chest x-ray: Standard posterior-anterior view.

of electrocardiographic monitoring, including resting ECG, ambulatory ECG monitoring, and exercise or stress testing.

A resting ECG helps identify at one point in time primary conduction abnormalities, cardiac dysrhythmias, cardiac hypertrophy, pericarditis, myocardial ischemia, site and extent of MI, pacemaker performance, and effectiveness of drug therapy. It is also used to monitor recovery from an MI. (See Chapter 36 for a complete discussion on ECG monitoring.)

Ambulatory Electrocardiogram Monitoring. Continuous ambulatory ECG (Holter monitoring) can provide diagnostic information over a greater period of time than a standard resting ECG. In Holter monitoring a recorder is worn by the patient for 24 to 48 hours, and the resulting ECG information is then stored until it is played back for printing and evaluation. Holter monitoring gives the patient freedom to perform usual activities of daily living and those that may be associated with cardiovascular symptoms. The patient maintains a record of activities, symptoms, and sleep, and this record is correlated with the ECG events recorded by the device (see Table 32-7).

Transtelephonic Event Recorders. This type of recorder is helpful for monitoring less frequent ECG events. The monitor is a portable unit that uses electrodes to transmit a limited ECG over the phone to a receiving device. A disadvantage of this type of monitoring is that, if the event occurs for only a short duration, the symptoms may be over before the patient puts on the device and calls the assigned number. Likewise, if patients are extremely symptomatic (e.g., syncopal), they may not be physically able to transmit the ECG.

Exercise or Stress Testing

Cardiac symptoms frequently occur only with activity due to the demand on the coronary arteries to provide additional oxygen. Exercise testing is a method used to evaluate the cardiovascular response to physical stress. This is helpful in assessing cardiovascular disease and defining limits for exercise programs. Patient selection for exercise testing is appropriate for individuals who do not have limitations related to walking or using a bicycle and those without abnormal ECGs that limit diagnostic interpretation (e.g., pacemakers, left bundle branch block). β-Adrenergic blockers may be held 24 hours before the test as they will blunt the heart rate and not allow the patients to achieve maximal heart rate. Patients should be instructed to refrain from eating, drinking caffeine-containing drinks, smoking, or participating in strenuous exercise for 3 hours prior to the test.

The placement of electrodes is similar to a regular 12-lead placement (see Chapter 36). Resting BPs and ECGs are performed in the supine position, while standing, and after hyperventilation to provide a baseline for comparison of any changes during exercise.

As the patient exercises on a treadmill or stationary bicycle, the BP, ECG, and often the oxygen saturation level are measured and monitored. The patient exercises to either peak HR (calculated by subtracting the person's age from 220) or to peak exercise tolerance, at which time the test is terminated and the treadmill is slowed while the patient continues walking. The test is also terminated for moderate to severe chest discomfort, significant increase or decrease in BP from baseline, or significant ECG changes indicating ischemia associated with CAD. The ECG is monitored after exercise for rhythm disturbances or, if ECG changes occurred with exercise, for return to baseline.

6-Minute Walk Test. A 6-minute walk test may be used for patients with heart or peripheral arterial disease to measure response to medical interventions and determine functional capacity for daily physical activities.[14] The total distance that a patient can quickly walk on a flat surface in the 6-minute time interval is measured. This test is useful in patients who are unable to perform a treadmill or bicycle exercise test.

Echocardiogram

The echocardiogram uses ultrasound waves to record the movement of the structures of the heart. In the normal heart, ultrasonic sound waves directed at the heart are reflected back in typical configurations (Fig. 32-13). The echocardiogram provides information about abnormalities of (1) valvular structure and motion, (2) cardiac chamber size and contents, (3) ventricular muscle and septal motion and thickness, (4) pericardial sac, and (5) ascending aorta. The **ejection fraction** (EF) or the percentage of end-diastolic blood volume that is ejected during systole can also be measured. The EF provides information about the function of the left ventricle during systole.

Two commonly used types are the *M-mode* (motion-mode) and the *two-dimensional* (2-D) *echocardiogram.* In the M-mode type, a single ultrasound beam is directed toward the heart, recording the motion of the intracardiac structures, as well as detecting wall thickness and chamber size. The 2-D echocardiogram sweeps the ultrasound beam through an arc, producing a cross-sectional view, and shows correct spatial relationships among the structures.

Doppler technology allows for sound evaluation of the flow or motion of the scanned object (heart valves, ventricular walls, blood flow). Color-flow imaging (duplex) is the combination of 2-D echocardiography and Doppler technology. It uses color changes to demonstrate the velocity and direction of blood flow. Pathologic conditions, such as valvular leaks and congenital defects, can be diagnosed more effectively. Stress echocardiography, a combination of treadmill test and ultrasound images, evaluates segmental wall motion abnormalities.[7] By using a digital computer system to compare images before and after exercise, wall motion and segmental function can be clearly seen. This diagnostic test provides the information of an exercise stress test with the information gained from an echocardiogram. For those individuals unable to exercise, infusion of a pharmacologic agent—usually dobutamine (Dobutrex) or dipyridamole (Persantine)—causes pharmacologic

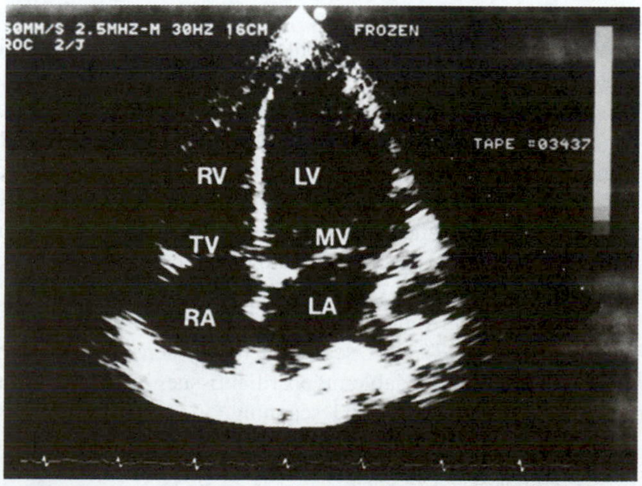

FIG. 32-13 Apical four-chamber two-dimensional echocardiographic view in a normal patient. *LA,* Left atrium; *LV,* left ventricle; *MV,* mitral valve; *RA,* right atrium; *RV,* right ventricle; *TV,* tricuspid valve.

stress on the heart while the patient is resting. The same ultrasound technology is used.

Transesophageal echocardiography (TEE) is used to provide more precise echocardiography of the heart than surface 2-D echocardiography by eliminating interference from the chest wall and lungs. The TEE uses a modified, flexible endoscope probe with an ultrasound transducer in the tip for imaging of the heart and great vessels. The probe is introduced into the esophagus to the level of the heart, and M-mode, 2-D, pulsed Doppler, and color-flow imaging can be obtained.

TEE is used frequently in an outpatient setting primarily for evaluation of mitral regurgitation, presence of thrombus prior to cardioversion, or source of cardiac emboli. In addition, TEE has application in the operating room to assess presurgical and postsurgical cardiac function and in the emergency department for suspicion of aortic dissection.

The risks of TEE are minimal. However, complications may include perforation of the esophagus, hemorrhage, dysrhythmias, vasovagal reactions, and transient hypoxemia. TEE is contraindicated if the patient has a history of esophageal disorders, dysphagia, or radiation therapy to the chest wall. Patients must have sedation during a TEE.

Contrast echocardiography uses intravenous contrast agents (e.g., albumin microbubbles, agitated saline) to assist in delineation of the images, especially in technically difficult patients.[2] When these agents are injected into the cardiac blood pool, they greatly enhance reflectivity for the ultrasound procedure.

Real-time three-dimensional (3-D) ultrasound is a new technology that uses multiple 2-D echo images with computer technology to provide a reconstruction of the heart. This technique generates precise information about the structures of the heart and how these structures change during the cardiac cycle.[2] It is useful for the detection of congenital heart defects and endocarditis as well as for the calculation of ventricular volumes.[7]

Nuclear Cardiology

One of the most common nuclear imaging tests is the multigated acquisition (MUGA) or cardiac blood pool scan. This test provides information on wall motion during systole and diastole, cardiac valves, and EF. A small amount of the patient's blood is removed, mixed with a radioactive isotope (e.g., ^{99m}technetium-sestamibi [Cardiolite]), and reinjected. Using the ECG for timing, images are acquired during the cardiac cycle.

Single-photon emission computed tomography (SPECT) is used for the evaluation of the myocardium at risk of infarction and to determine infarction size. Small amounts of a radioactive isotope (e.g., ^{99m}technetium-tetrofosmin [Myoview] or thallium-201) are injected intravenously, and recordings are made of the radioactivity emitted over a specific area of the body. The total radiation exposure is minimal. The circulation of this tagged material can be used to detect coronary artery blood flow, intracardiac shunts, motion of ventricles, EF, and size of the heart chambers.

Positron emission tomography (PET) scanning uses two isotopes (see Table 32-7). PET scans are highly sensitive in distinguishing viable and nonviable myocardial tissue. Equipment costs limit the widespread use of PET scanning.[2]

Perfusion imaging is also used with exercise testing to determine whether the coronary blood flow changes with increased activity. Stress perfusion imaging may show an abnormality even when a resting image is normal. This procedure is indicated to diagnose CAD, determine the prognosis in already diagnosed CAD, assess the physiologic significance of a known coronary lesion, and assess the effectiveness of various therapeutic modalities such as coronary artery bypass surgery or percutaneous coronary intervention (see Chapter 34). Cardiolite imaging can also provide an estimate of the magnitude of myocardial salvage at the time of acute MI. Since Cardiolite remains in the myocardium for several hours after injection, a patient can be injected prior to treatment and later scanned to obtain a picture of the potential infarct size pretreatment. A second injection later will determine the final infarct size, and the change between the two images demonstrates myocardial salvage.

Stress perfusion imaging is always preferred but, if a patient is unable to tolerate exercise, intravenous dipyridamole or adenosine (Adenocard) may be given to dilate the coronary arteries and simulate the effect of exercise. After the vasodilator takes effect, the isotope is injected and the nuclear procedure proceeds. All caffeine and theophylline products must be held 12 hours before the study as they counteract the vasodilator effects of the stress agents. Calcium channel blockers and β-adrenergic blockers should be held 24 hours before the test. Patients may be given aminophylline (Phyllocontin) either prophylactically at the end of the test or in response to symptoms as it is a specific blocker of the vasodilators and will eliminate or reduce adverse side effects (e.g., bronchospasm). Dobutamine is used as a pharmacologic adrenergic stress agent for patients who have contraindications to vasodilator stress agents. The protocol for its use is similar for the vasodilator stress tests, and adverse side effects are rare.[15]

Magnetic Resonance Imaging

Although not widely used because of equipment size and access, magnetic resonance imaging (MRI) allows detection and localization of areas of MI in a 3-D view. It is sensitive enough to gauge even small MIs not apparent with SPECT imaging and can assist in the final diagnosis of MI. It is also beginning to play a role in prediction of viability and recovery from MI. Its utility for diagnosis of presence and severity of CAD is still being studied.[15]

Magnetic resonance angiography (MRA) is used for imaging vascular occlusive disease and abdominal aortic aneurysms. The contrast material is non-iodine based and is injected through an intravenous line. The MRA images compare favorably to duplex ultrasound of arterial stenosis.[16]

Computed Tomography

Computed tomography (CT) with spiral technology is a noninvasive scan used to quantify calcium deposits in coronary arteries. It has been limited by the difficulty of imaging the constantly moving heart and the need for patients to hold their breath for each set of image acquisitions.[7] Electron beam computed tomography (EBCT), also known as ultrafast CT, uses a scanning electron beam to allow quantification of calcification in the coronary arteries and the heart valves. A calcium score can be formulated for a segment of a coronary artery, a specific coronary artery, or the entire coronary system.[2] Several studies have shown that EBCT coronary calcium scores are predictive of cardiac events.[11] The test is rapid and noninvasive and may have clinical applications for screening in patients with and without symptoms of cardiac disease (Fig. 32-14).

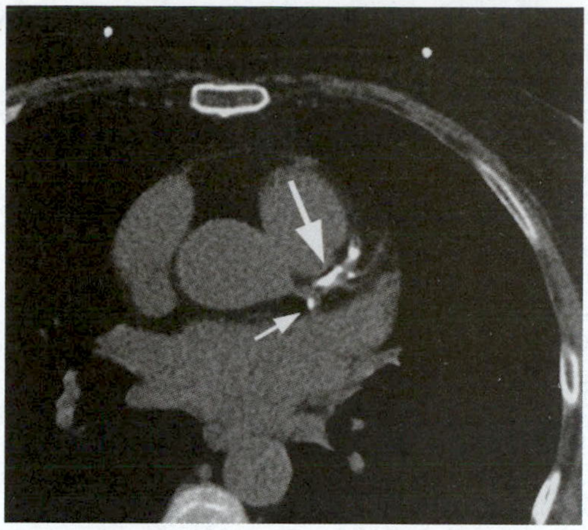

FIG. 32-14 Examples of coronary calcification of the left anterior descending coronary artery *(large arrow)* and left circumflex artery *(small arrow)* as seen on electron beam computed tomography.

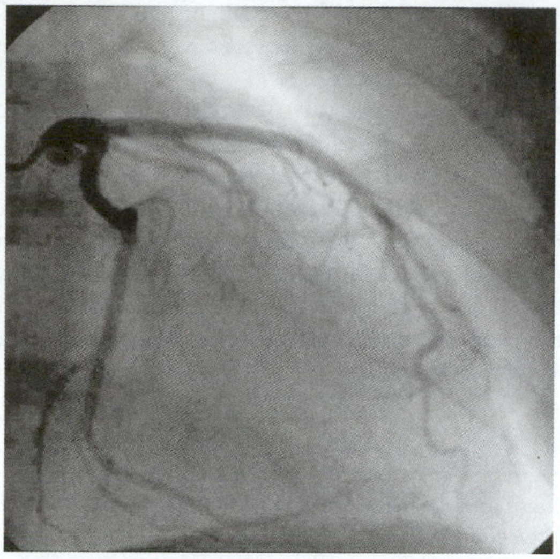

FIG. 32-15 Normal left coronary artery angiogram.

Cardiac Catheterization and Coronary Angiography

Cardiac catheterization is a common outpatient procedure. It provides a means of obtaining information about CAD, congenital heart disease, valvular heart disease, and ventricular function. Cardiac catheterization can be used to measure intracardiac pressures and O_2 levels in various parts of the heart, as well as CO and EF. With injection of contrast media and fluoroscopy, the coronary arteries can be visualized, chambers of the heart can be outlined, and wall motion can be observed.

Cardiac catheterization is performed by insertion of a radiopaque catheter into the right or left side of the heart. For the right side of the heart, a catheter is inserted through an arm vein (basilic or cephalic) or a leg vein (femoral). The catheter is advanced into the vena cava, the right atrium, and the right ventricle. The catheter is further inserted into the pulmonary artery, and pressures are recorded. The catheter is then advanced until it is wedged or lodged in position. This position is called the *pulmonary artery wedge position.* The pulmonary artery wedge position (wedge pressure) obstructs the flow and pressure from the right side of the heart and looks forward through the pulmonary capillary bed to the pressure in the left side of the heart. The wedge pressure is used to assess the function of the left side of the heart.

The left heart catheterization is performed by insertion of a catheter into a femoral or brachial artery. The catheter is passed in a retrograde manner up the aorta, across the aortic valve, and into the left ventricle. Coronary angiography can be done with a left heart catheterization (Fig. 32-15).

Patients frequently feel a temporary hot and flushed sensation with contrast media injection. (See Table 32-7 for the nursing responsibilities related to cardiac catheterization.)

Complications of cardiac catheterization include bleeding or hematoma at the puncture site; allergic reactions to the contrast media; looping, kinking, or breaking off of the catheter; infection; thrombus formation; dysrhythmias; MI; stroke; puncture of the ventricles, cardiac septum, or lung tissue; and, rarely, death.

Intracoronary Ultrasound. Intracoronary ultrasound (ICUS), also known as intravascular ultrasound (IVUS), is an invasive procedure performed in the catheterization laboratory in conjunction with coronary angiography. The 2-D or 3-D ultrasound images provide a cross-sectional view of the arterial walls of the coronary arteries. In this procedure, a miniature transducer attached to a small catheter is introduced through a peripheral artery and advanced to the artery to be studied. Once in the artery, ultrasound images are obtained. The health of the arterial layers is assessed, as is the composition, location, and thickness of any plaque.

ICUS is currently used to diagnose severity of CAD. It may also evaluate the vessel response to treatments such as stent placement and atherectomy as well as any complications that may have occurred during the procedure (see Chapter 34).

Because the patient will most often have ICUS in addition to angiography or a coronary intervention, nursing care of the patient following ICUS is similar to that following cardiac catheterization (see Table 32-7).

Electrophysiology Study. Electrophysiologic study (EPS) is the direct study and manipulation of the electrical activity of the heart using electrodes placed inside the cardiac chambers. It provides information on SA node function, AV node conduction, and ventricular conduction. It is particularly helpful in determining the source and treatment of dysrhythmias. Patients with a history of symptomatic supraventricular or ventricular tachycardias may be at risk for sudden cardiac death. Information obtained during an EPS can assist in making an accurate diagnosis and guiding appropriate treatment decisions.[17]

Catheters are inserted in a similar method as for right and left heart catheterization. These catheters are placed at specific anatomic sites within the heart to record electrical activity. Nursing care for patients after EPS includes close ECG monitoring, frequent assessment of vital signs and puncture site, and other responsibilities related to care of a patient following a cardiac catheterization.

Blood Flow and Pressure Measurements

Peripheral Vessel Blood Flow. Duplex imaging is useful in the diagnosis of occlusive disease in the peripheral blood vessels and for the diagnosis of thrombophlebitis. Peripheral vessel blood flow can be assessed by injection of contrast media into the appropriate arteries or veins (arteriography and venography). With these tests, arterial occlusions and venous abnormalities can be located. (Additional studies of peripheral blood vessels are discussed in Chapter 38 and Table 38-8.)

Hemodynamic Monitoring. Bedside hemodynamic monitoring of pressures of the cardiovascular system is frequently used to assess cardiovascular status and monitor patient response to interventions. Invasive hemodynamic monitoring using intraarterial and pulmonary artery catheters can be used to monitor arterial BP, intracardiac pressures, and CO. The central venous pressure (CVP) is a measurement of preload and can be used to monitor the pressure in the right atrium. See Chapter 66 for a complete discussion of hemodynamic monitoring.

NCLEX EXAMINATION REVIEW QUESTIONS

The number of the question corresponds to the same-numbered objective at the beginning of the chapter.

1. A patient with a tricuspid valve disorder will have impaired blood flow between the
   a. vena cava and right atrium.
   b. left atrium and left ventricle.
   c. right atrium and right ventricle.
   d. right ventricle and pulmonary artery.
2. A patient with an MI of the anterior wall of the left ventricle most likely has an occlusion of the
   a. left marginal artery.
   b. right marginal artery.
   c. right descending artery.
   d. left anterior descending artery.
3. If the Purkinje system is damaged, conduction of the electrical impulse is impaired through the
   a. atria.
   b. AV node.
   c. ventricles.
   d. bundle of His.
4. The portion of the vascular system responsible for hemostasis is the
   a. thin capillary vessels.
   b. endothelial layer of the arteries.
   c. elastic middle layer of the veins.
   d. smooth muscle of the arterial wall.
5. When a person's blood pressure rises, the homeostatic mechanism to compensate for an elevation involves stimulation of
   a. baroreceptors that inhibit the sympathetic nervous system, causing vasodilation.
   b. chemoreceptors that inhibit the sympathetic nervous system, causing vasodilation.
   c. baroreceptors that inhibit the parasympathetic nervous system, causing vasodilation.
   d. chemoreceptors that stimulate the sympathetic nervous system, causing an increased heart rate.
6. A P wave on an ECG represents an impulse
   a. arising at the SA node and repolarizing the atria.
   b. arising at the SA node and depolarizing the atria.
   c. arising at the AV node and depolarizing the atria.
   d. arising at the AV node and spreading to the bundle of His.
7. When checking the capillary filling time of a patient, the color returns in 5 seconds. The nurse recognizes this finding as indicative of
   a. a normal response.
   b. thrombus formation in the veins.
   c. lymphatic obstruction of venous return.
   d. impaired arterial flow to the extremities.
8. The auscultatory area in the left midclavicular line at the level of the fifth ICS is the
   a. aortic area.
   b. mitral area.
   c. tricuspid area.
   d. pulmonic area.
9. When assessing the patient, the nurse notes a palpable precordial thrill. This finding may be caused by
   a. heart murmurs.
   b. gallop rhythms.
   c. pulmonary edema.
   d. ventricular hypertrophy.
10. When assessing the cardiovascular system of a 79-year-old patient, the nurse expects to find
    a. a narrowed pulse pressure.
    b. diminished carotid artery pulses.
    c. difficulty in isolating the apical pulse.
    d. an increased heart rate in response to stress.
11. An important nursing responsibility for a patient recovering from a cardiac catheterization is
    a. checking the percutaneous site and distal pulses.
    b. assisting the patient to ambulate upon return to the unit.
    c. informing the patient that general anesthesia was given.
    d. instructing the patient about radioactive isotope injection.

REFERENCES

1. Drake RL, Vogl W, Mitchell AWM: *Gray's anatomy for students,* Philadelphia, 2005, Elsevier.
2. Woods SL, Froelicher ES, Motzer SU, et al: *Cardiac nursing,* ed 5, Philadelphia, 2005, Lippincott.
3. American Heart Association. *Heart and stroke statistics—2005 update,* Dallas, Tex, 2005, American Heart Association.
4. Jarvis C: *Physical examination and health assessment,* ed 4, St Louis, 2004, Saunders.
5. Ebersole P, Hess P, Luggen AS: *Toward healthy aging,* ed 6, St Louis, 2004, Mosby.
6. Huether SE, McCance KL: *Understanding pathophysiology,* ed 3, St Louis, 2004, Mosby.
7. Zipes DP, Libby P, Bonow R, et al: *Braunwald's heart disease: a textbook of cardiovascular medicine,* ed 6, Philadelphia, 2007, Elsevier.
8. Lehne R: *Pharmacology for nursing care,* ed 6, St Louis, 2007, Saunders.
9. Chernecky CC, Berger BJ: *Laboratory tests and diagnostic procedures,* ed 4, Philadelphia, 2004, Saunders.
10. Grundy SM, Cleeman JI, Merz CN, et al: Implications of recent clinical trials for the National Cholesterol Education Program, Adult Treatment Panel III Guidelines, *Circulation* 110:227, 2004.
11. American College of Cardiology and American Heart Association: Expert consensus document on electron-beam computed tomography for the diagnosis and prognosis of coronary artery disease, *Circulation* 102:126, 2002.
12. Busby-Whitehead MJ, Blackman MC: Clinical implications of abnormal lipoprotein metabolism. In Barker LR, et al, editors: *Principles of ambulatory medicine,* ed 5, Baltimore, 1999, Williams & Wilkins.
13. Malinow MR, Giles WH, Macko RF, et al: Homocysteine, diet, and cardiovascular diseases: a statement for healthcare professionals from the nutrition committee, American Heart Association, *Circulation* 99:178, 1999.
14. American Thoracic Society: ATS statement: guidelines for the six-minute walk test, *Am J Respir Crit Care Med* 166:111, 2002.
15. Wackers F, Bruni W, Zaret BL: *Nuclear cardiology: the basics,* Totowa, NJ, 2004, Humana.
16. Botnar RM, Stuber M, Danias PG, et al: Coronary magnetic resonance angiography, *Cardiol Rev* 9:77, 2001.
17. Josephson ME: *Clinical cardiac electrophysiology: techniques and interpretations,* Philadelphia, 2001, Lippincott.

RESOURCES

Resources for this chapter are listed at the end of Chapter 33 on p. 783 and at the end of Chapter 34 on p. 820.

In helping others we shall help ourselves, for whatever good we give out completes the circle and comes back to us.

Flora Edwards

Nursing Management Hypertension

33

Elisabeth G. Bradley

LEARNING OBJECTIVES

1. Describe the mechanisms involved in the regulation of blood pressure.
2. Identify the pathophysiologic mechanisms associated with primary hypertension.
3. Describe the clinical manifestations and complications of hypertension.
4. Describe strategies for the prevention of primary hypertension.
5. Describe the collaborative care for hypertension, including drug therapy and lifestyle modifications.
6. Discuss the collaborative care of the older adult with hypertension.
7. Describe the nursing management of the patient with hypertension, emphasizing patient education.
8. Describe the clinical manifestations and collaborative care of hypertensive crisis.

KEY TERMS

blood pressure, p. 762
hypertension, p. 761
hypertensive crisis, p. 781
orthostatic hypotension, p. 778
prehypertension, p. 761
primary hypertension, p. 765
secondary hypertension, p. 765
systemic vascular resistance, p. 762

Electronic Resources

Supplemental content related to Chapter 33 can be found . . .

Companion CD

- Stress-Busting Kit for Nursing Students
- Interactive Case Study: Hypertension
- NCLEX Examination Review Questions
- Comprehensive Glossary

Evolve Website evolve

http://evolve.elsevier.com/Lewis/medsurg

- Content Updates
- Key Points (Printable and CD/MP3 Download)
- Concept Map Creator
- Expanded Audio Glossary
- Key Term Flash Cards
- Electronic Calculators
- WebLinks

Hypertension, or high blood pressure (BP), is defined as a persistent systolic blood pressure (SBP) ≥140 mm Hg, diastolic blood pressure (DBP) ≥90 mm Hg, or current use of antihypertensive medication.[1] Hypertension is an important medical and public health issue. It exists worldwide at epidemic rates affecting an estimated 1 billion people. At least 65 million American adults, or nearly 1 in 3, have high BP. The prevalence of hypertension among citizens of the United States and Canada is 32% and 22%, respectively. Hypertension means that the heart is working harder than normal, putting both the heart and the blood vessels under strain. There is a direct relationship between hypertension and cardiovascular disease (CVD). There is a proportional increase in the risk of myocardial infarction, heart failure, stroke, and renal disease with higher BP.[1]

Approximately 28% of Americans, or 59 million people, have **prehypertension,** which is defined as a SBP of 120 to 139 or DBP of 80 to 89.[2] These individuals are at high risk of developing hypertension. The prevalence of hypertension increases with age; people who do not have hypertension at age 55 have a 90% chance of developing it later in life. A SBP of >140 mm Hg is a more important cardiovascular risk factor for developing hypertension than an elevated DBP in individuals older than age 50.[1]

CVD is the number one cause of death in women in the United States and in most of the developed areas of the world.[3] Unfortunately, less than half of all American women are aware that CVD is their leading killer.[4] The American Heart Association published a set of evidence-based guidelines for the prevention of CVD in women.[3] These guidelines focus on lifestyle recommendations and

Reviewed by Judy Hendricks, MS, ANP, CDE, Adult Nurse Practitioner, Christiana Care Health Systems, Newark, Del.; and Anne C. Muller, RN, MSN, CRNP, CNS, Clinical Nurse Specialist, Hospital of the University of Pennsylvania, Philadelphia, Pa.

GENDER DIFFERENCES
Hypertension

Men
- Before age 55, hypertension is more common in men than in women.
- Men with hypertension are more likely to suffer an MI than a stroke.

Women
- After age 55, hypertension is more common in women than in men.
- Part of the rise in BP in women is attributed to menopause-related factors such as estrogen withdrawal, overproduction of pituitary hormones, and weight gain.
- Women with hypertension are more likely to suffer a stroke than an MI.
- Hypertension occurs in >75% of African American women over the age of 75 years.
- ACE inhibitor-induced cough and diuretic-induced hyponatremia are more common in women.
- Oral contraceptives may cause small increases in BP in many women, and frank hypertension in a small percentage of women.
- Effects usually seen in initial period of contraceptive use and during dosage changes.

ECG, Electrocardiogram; *EPS,* electrophysiology study

CULTURAL AND ETHNIC HEALTH DISPARITIES
Hypertension

- African Americans, as compared to other ethnic groups, have the highest prevalence of hypertension in the world.
- African Americans develop hypertension at a younger age than whites.
- African American women have a higher incidence of hypertension than African American men.
- Hypertension is more aggressive in African Americans and results in more severe end-organ damage.
- African Americans have a higher mortality rate related to hypertension than whites.
- African Americans and whites living in the southeastern United States have a higher incidence of hypertension than similar ethnic groups living in other parts of the United States.
- African Americans produce less renin and do not respond as well to angiotensin inhibitors.
- African Americans and Asians have a higher risk of angioedema and have a higher incidence of cough as side effects from angiotensin-converting enzyme inhibitors than whites.
- Mexican Americans have lower levels of awareness of hypertension and its treatment than other ethnic groups.
- Mexican Americans are less likely to receive treatment for hypertension than whites and African Americans.
- Mexican Americans and Native Americans have lower rates of adequate blood pressure control than whites and African Americans.

major risk factor interventions, and can be used as an educational tool for women. Gender differences in hypertension are presented in the box at the top of the page.

Hypertension and its management among various racial and ethnic groups in the United States demand special attention from health care providers. Contributing factors to the development of high BP include cardiovascular risk factors combined with socioeconomic conditions and ethnic differences.[5] The third National Health and Nutrition Examination Survey (NHANES) intentionally oversampled Mexican Americans, African Americans, elderly, and children in an effort to provide reliable estimates of the prevalence of hypertension in these groups.[6] Cultural and Ethnic Health Disparities related to hypertension are presented in the box above.

The status of hypertension control has improved considerably over the past 20 years. Large-scale education programs provided by national organizations have increased awareness of hypertension. In the 20-year period from 1980 to 2000, the percentage of patients receiving treatment for hypertension has increased from 31% to 59%. Over the same 20-year period, the percentage of patients with hypertension on medication who have their BP controlled has also improved substantially, from 10% to 34%. However, considerable work remains for diagnosing, educating, and treating hypertension. Many people (30%) with hypertension do not know they have it because it is generally an asymptomatic condition. Two thirds of hypertensive patients do not have their BP controlled.[1] Individuals who remain undiagnosed and untreated for hypertension present the greatest challenge and opportunity for health care providers. The U.S. government has set health promotion objectives for Americans known as the *Healthy People 2010* goals. These goals include reducing the proportion of adults with hypertension to 16% and increasing the proportion of hypertensive adults whose BP is under control to 50%[7] (see Healthy People Box on p. 768).

NORMAL REGULATION OF BLOOD PRESSURE

Blood pressure is the force exerted by the blood against the walls of the blood vessel. It must be adequate to maintain tissue perfusion during activity and rest. The maintenance of normal BP and tissue perfusion requires the integration of both systemic factors and local peripheral vascular effects. Arterial BP is primarily a function of cardiac output and systemic vascular resistance. The relationship is summarized by the following equation:

$$\text{Arterial blood pressure} = \text{Cardiac output} \times \text{Systemic vascular resistance}$$

Cardiac output (CO) is the total blood flow through the systemic or pulmonary circulation per minute. CO is described as the stroke volume (amount of blood pumped out of the left ventricle per beat [approximately 70 ml]) multiplied by the heart rate (HR) for 1 minute. **Systemic vascular resistance** (SVR) is the force opposing the movement of blood within the blood vessels. The radius of the small arteries and arterioles is the principal factor determining vascular resistance. A small change in the radius of the arterioles creates a major change in the SVR. If SVR is increased and CO remains constant or increases, arterial BP will increase.

The mechanisms that regulate BP can affect either CO or SVR, or both. Regulation of BP is a complex process involving nervous, cardiovascular, renal, and endocrine functions (Fig. 33-1). BP is regulated by both short-term (seconds to hours) and long-term (days to weeks) mechanisms. Short-term mechanisms, including the sympathetic nervous system and vascular endothelium, are active within a few seconds. Long-term mechanisms include renal and hormonal processes that regulate arteriolar resistance and blood volume.

Sympathetic Nervous System

The nervous system, which reacts within seconds after a decrease in arterial pressure, increases BP primarily by activation of the sympathetic nervous system (SNS). Increased SNS activity increases HR and cardiac contractility, produces widespread vasoconstriction in the peripheral arterioles, and promotes the release of renin from the kidneys. The net effect of SNS activation is to increase arterial pressure by increasing both CO and SVR.

Changes in BP are sensed by specialized nerve cells called *baroreceptors,* located in the carotid artery and the arch of the aorta, and transmitted to the vasomotor centers in the brainstem. Information received in the brainstem is relayed throughout the brain by complex networks of interneurons exciting or inhibiting efferent nerves, thereby influencing cardiovascular function. SNS efferent nerves innervate cardiac and vascular smooth muscle cells. Under normal conditions, a low level of continuous SNS activity maintains tonic vasoconstriction. BP may be reduced by withdrawal of SNS activity or by stimulation of the parasympathetic nervous system, which decreases the HR (via the vagus nerve) and thereby decreases CO.

The neurotransmitter norepinephrine (NE) is released from SNS nerve endings. NE activates receptors located in the sinoatrial node, myocardium, and vascular smooth muscle. The response to NE depends on the type and density of receptors present. SNS receptors are classified as α_1, α_2, β_1, and β_2 (Table 33-1). α-Adrenergic receptors located in peripheral vasculature cause vasoconstriction when stimulated by NE. β_1-Adrenergic receptors in the heart respond to NE and epinephrine with increased HR *(chronotropic),* increased force of contraction *(inotropic),* and increased speed of conduction. The smooth muscle of the blood vessels has α_1-adrenergic and β_2-adrenergic receptors. β_2-Adrenergic receptors are activated primarily by epinephrine released from the adrenal medulla and cause vasodilation. Diminished responsiveness of cardiovascular cells to SNS stimulation is one of the most significant cardiovascular effects of aging.

The sympathetic vasomotor center, located in the medulla, interacts with many areas of the brain to maintain normal BP under various conditions. During exercise the motor area of the cortex is stimulated, activating the vasomotor center and the SNS through neuronal connections. This causes an appropriate increase in CO and BP to accommodate the increased oxygen demand of the exercising muscles. During postural change from lying to standing, there is a transient decrease in BP. The vasomotor center is stimulated and activates the SNS, causing peripheral vasoconstriction and increased venous return to the heart. If this response did not occur, there would be inadequate blood flow to the brain, resulting in dizziness or syncope. Cerebral cortical perceptions such as pain and stress activate the vasomotor centers through the neuronal connections.

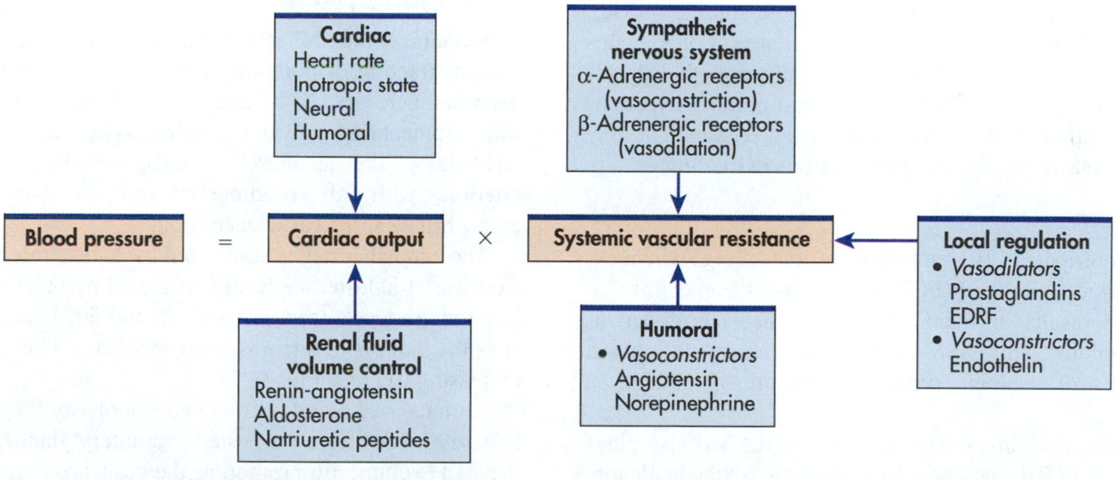

FIG. 33-1 Factors influencing blood pressure. *EDRF,* Endothelium-derived relaxing factor.

TABLE 33-1 Sympathetic Nervous System Receptors Affecting Blood Pressure

Receptor	Location	Response When Activated
α_1	Vascular smooth muscle	Vasoconstriction
	Heart	Increased contractility
α_2	Presynaptic membrane	Inhibition of norepinephrine release
	Vascular smooth muscle	Vasoconstriction
β_1	Heart	Increased contractility (positive inotropic effect)
		Increased heart rate (positive chronotropic effect)
		Increased conduction (positive dromotropic effect)
	Juxtaglomerular cells	Increased renin secretion
β_2	Smooth muscle of peripheral blood vessels in skeletal muscle and coronary arteries	Vasodilation
Dopaminergic receptors	Primarily renal and mesenteric blood vessels	Vasodilation

Baroreceptors. Baroreceptors (pressoreceptors) are specialized nerve cells located in the carotid arteries and arch of the aorta. They have an important role in the maintenance of BP stability during normal activities. They are sensitive to stretching and, when stimulated by an increase in BP, send inhibitory impulses to the sympathetic vasomotor center in the brainstem. Inhibition of sympathetic activity results in decreased heart rate, decreased force of contraction, and vasodilation in peripheral arterioles. Increased parasympathetic activity (vagus nerve) reduces HR.

A fall in BP, sensed by the baroreceptors, leads to activation of the SNS. The result is constriction of the peripheral arterioles, increased HR, and increased contractility of the heart. In the presence of long-standing hypertension, the baroreceptors become adjusted to elevated levels of BP and recognize this level as "normal." The baroreceptor reflex is less responsive in some older adults.

Vascular Endothelium

The vascular endothelium is a single cell layer that lines the blood vessels. Previously considered inert, it is now known to produce vasoactive substances and growth factors. Nitric oxide, an endothelium-derived relaxing factor (EDRF), helps maintain low arterial tone at rest, inhibits growth of the smooth muscle layer, and inhibits platelet aggregation. Other substances released by the vascular endothelium with local vasodilator effects include prostacyclin and endothelium-derived hyperpolarizing factor.

Endothelin (ET), produced by the endothelial cells, is an extremely potent vasoconstrictor. There are three subclasses of endothelins: ET-1, ET-2, and ET-3. ET-1 is the most potent endothelin in producing vasoconstriction. ET-1 also causes adhesion and aggregation of neutrophils and stimulates smooth muscle growth. Endothelial cell function and dysfunction is an area of ongoing investigation. There is some evidence that vascular endothelial dysfunction may contribute to atherosclerosis and primary hypertension. The prevention or reversal of endothelial dysfunction may become important for therapeutic interventions in the future.

Renal System

The kidneys contribute to BP regulation by controlling sodium excretion and extracellular fluid (ECF) volume (see Chapter 45). Sodium retention results in water retention, which causes an increased ECF volume. This increases the venous return to the heart, increasing the stroke volume, which elevates the BP through an increase in CO.

The renin-angiotensin-aldosterone system (RAAS) also plays an important role in BP regulation. In response to SNS stimulation, decreased blood flow through the kidneys, or decreased serum sodium concentration, renin is secreted from the juxtaglomerular apparatus in the kidney. Renin is an enzyme that converts angiotensinogen to angiotensin I. Angiotensin-converting enzyme (ACE) converts angiotensin I into angiotensin II (A-II), which can increase BP by two different mechanisms (see Chapter 45, Fig. 45-4). First, A-II is a potent vasoconstrictor and increases vascular resistance, resulting in an immediate increase in BP. Second, over a period of hours or days, A-II increases BP indirectly by stimulating the adrenal cortex to secrete aldosterone, which causes sodium and water retention by the kidneys resulting in increased blood volume and increased CO (Fig. 33-2).

Angiotensin II also functions at a local level within the heart and blood vessels. The local vasoactive effects of A-II include vasoconstriction and tissue growth that results in remodeling of the vessel walls. These changes are associated with the development of primary hypertension and also the long-term effects of hypertension (e.g., atherosclerosis, renal disease, cardiac hypertrophy).

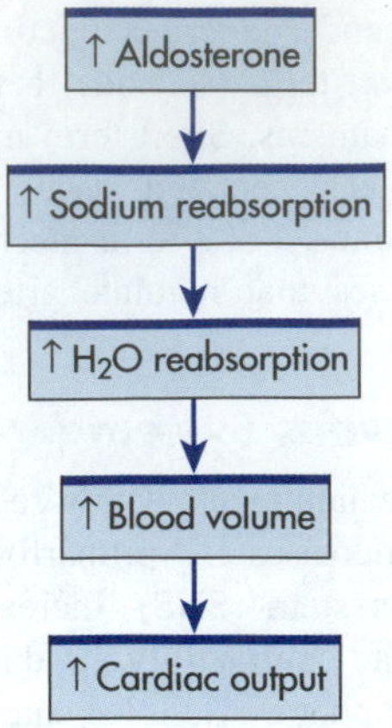

FIG. 33-2 Mechanism of action of aldosterone.

Prostaglandins (PGE_2 and PGI_2) secreted by the renal medulla have a vasodilator effect on the systemic circulation. This results in decreased SVR and lowering of BP. (Prostaglandins are discussed in Chapter 13.) The natriuretic peptides (atrial natriuretic peptide [ANP] and b-type natriuretic peptide [BNP]) secreted by cardiac cells antagonize the effects of antidiuretic hormone (ADH) and aldosterone by promoting natriuresis (excretion of sodium in urine) and diuresis resulting in reduced blood volume and a decrease in BP.

Endocrine System

Stimulation of the SNS results in release of epinephrine along with a small fraction of norepinephrine by the adrenal medulla. Epinephrine increases CO by increasing HR and myocardial contractility. Epinephrine activates β_2-adrenergic receptors in peripheral arterioles of skeletal muscle, causing vasodilation. In peripheral arterioles with only α_1-adrenergic receptors (skin and kidneys), epinephrine causes vasoconstriction.

The adrenal cortex is stimulated by A-II to release aldosterone. (Release of aldosterone is also regulated by other factors, such as low sodium levels [see Chapters 48 and 50].) Aldosterone stimulates the kidneys to retain sodium and water. This increases BP by increasing CO (see Fig. 33-2).

An increased blood sodium and osmolarity level stimulates the release of ADH from the posterior pituitary gland. ADH increases the ECF volume by promoting the reabsorption of water in the distal and collecting tubules of the kidneys. The resulting increase in blood volume can cause an elevation in BP.

In the healthy person, these regulatory mechanisms function in response to the demands of the body. When hypertension develops, one or more of the BP-regulating mechanisms are defective.

HYPERTENSION

Classification of Hypertension

Table 33-2 describes the BP classification for people 18 years of age and older. The classification of BP is based on the average of two or more properly measured, seated BP readings on each of two or more office visits. The new guidelines include the classification of prehypertension, BP 120 to 139/80 to 89 mm Hg. About 28% of Americans, or about 59 million people, have prehypertension.[2]

TABLE 33-2 Classification of Hypertension

Category	SBP (mm Hg)		DBP (mm Hg)
Normal	<120	and	<80
Prehypertension	120-139	or	80-89
Hypertension, Stage 1	140-159	or	90-99
Hypertension, Stage 2	≥160	or	≥100

From the National Institutes of Health: *Seventh Report of the Joint National Committee on Prevention, Detection, Evaluation, and Treatment of High Blood Pressure,* Washington, DC, 2003, U.S. Department of Health and Human Services.
DBP, Diastolic blood pressure; *SBP,* systolic blood pressure.

Subtypes of Hypertension

Isolated Systolic Hypertension. **Isolated systolic hypertension** (ISH) is defined as an average SBP ≥140 mm Hg coupled with an average DBP <90 mm Hg.[8] Although ISH does occur in younger adults, it is much more common in older adults. Blood pressure patterns change as part of the aging process. The SBP continues to rise with aging; the DBP rises until approximately age 55 and then declines. Older adults often have ISH caused by loss of elasticity in large arteries from atherosclerosis. An SBP greater than 140 mm Hg is a more important risk factor for cardiovascular disease than an elevated DBP in individuals older than age 50. ISH is the most common form of hypertension for this age group. Control of ISH decreases the incidence of stroke, heart failure, cardiovascular mortality, and total mortality.[1]

Pseudohypertension. *Pseudohypertension,* or false hypertension, can occur with advanced (often calcified) arteriosclerosis. Sclerotic arteries do not collapse when the cuff is fully inflated, presenting much higher cuff pressures than are actually present within the vessels. Pseudohypertension is suspected if arteries feel rigid or when few retinal or cardiac signs are found relative to the pressures obtained by cuff. *Osler's sign* (a palpable radial or brachial artery after the blood pressure cuff is fully inflated) has a low sensitivity and specificity for pseudohypertension and is not recommended. The only way to accurately measure BP in pseudohypertension is through the use of an intraarterial catheter.

Etiology

The etiology of hypertension can be classified as either primary or secondary.

Primary Hypertension. **Primary** (essential or idiopathic) **hypertension** is elevated BP without an identified cause and accounts for 90% to 95% of all cases of hypertension. Although the exact cause of primary hypertension is unknown, several contributing factors, including increased SNS activity, overproduction of sodium-retaining hormones and vasoconstrictors, increased sodium intake, greater than ideal body weight, diabetes mellitus, and excessive alcohol consumption have been identified. Primary hypertension is the focus of this chapter because of its prevalence in clinical practice and impact on health.

Secondary Hypertension. **Secondary hypertension** is elevated BP with a specific cause that often can be identified and corrected. This type of hypertension accounts for 5% to 10% of hypertension in adults and more than 80% of hypertension in children. If a person below age 20 or over age 50 suddenly develops hypertension, especially if it is severe, a secondary cause should be suspected. Clinical findings that suggest secondary hypertension include unprovoked hypokalemia; abdominal bruit heard over the renal arteries; variable BPs with a history of tachycardia, sweating and tremor; or a family history of renal disease.

Causes of secondary hypertension include the following: (1) coarctation or congenital narrowing of the aorta; (2) renal disease such as renal artery stenosis and parenchymal disease (see Chapter 46); (3) endocrine disorders such as pheochromocytoma, Cushing syndrome, and hyperaldosteronism (see Chapter 50); (4) neurologic disorders such as brain tumors, tetraplegia, and head injury; (5) sleep apnea; (6) medications such as sympathetic stimulants (including cocaine), monoamine oxidase inhibitors taken with tyramine-containing foods, estrogen replacement therapy, oral contraceptive pills, and nonsteroidal antiinflammatory drugs (NSAIDs); (7) cirrhosis; and (8) pregnancy-induced hypertension. Treatment of secondary hypertension is directed at eliminating the underlying cause. Secondary hypertension is a contributing factor to hypertensive crisis (see section at end of this chapter).

Pathophysiology of Primary Hypertension

For arterial pressure to rise, there must be an increase in either CO or SVR. Increased CO is sometimes found in the prehypertensive and borderline hypertensive person. Later in the course of hypertension, SVR rises and the CO returns to normal. The hemodynamic hallmark of hypertension is persistently increased SVR. This persistent elevation in SVR may come about in various ways. Factors that are known to be related to the development of primary hypertension or contribute to its consequences are presented in Table 33-3.

Heredity. Genetic abnormalities associated with several rare forms of hypertension have been identified. However, the contribution of genetic factors to BP levels in the general population is very small.[1] Environmental factors also have a role in contributing to the development of high blood pressure. In practice, children and siblings of persons with hypertension should be more carefully screened and strongly advised to adopt healthy lifestyles to prevent hypertension.

Water and Sodium Retention. Excessive sodium intake is considered responsible for initiation of hypertension in some people. Populations with a low sodium intake (usually primitive hunter-gatherer societies) show little or no hypertension and no progressive increase in BP with age as is found in industrialized societies. In addition, when people from these societies adopt industrialized lifestyles, the prevalence of hypertension increases. When sodium is restricted in many hypertensive people, their BP falls. A high sodium intake may activate a number of pressor mechanisms and cause water retention. Although almost everyone in Western countries consumes a high-sodium diet, only about 20% develop hypertension. This indicates that some degree of sodium sensitivity must be present for high sodium intake to trigger the development of hypertension. In clinical practice, there is not an easy or simple test to identify individuals whose BP will rise with even a small increase in salt intake (salt sensitive) versus those who can ingest large amounts of sodium without much change in BP (salt resistant).[9] Certain demographic factors such as obesity, increasing age, African American ethnicity, diabetes, and chronic kidney disease are more commonly associated with BP salt sensitivity.[9]

Altered Renin-Angiotensin Mechanism. High plasma renin activity (PRA) results in the increased conversion of angiotensinogen to angiotensin I (see Chapter 45, Fig. 45-4). Angioten-

TABLE 33-3 Risk Factors for Primary Hypertension

Age	SBP rises progressively with increasing age. After age 50, an SBP >140 mm Hg is a more important cardiovascular risk factor than DBP.
Alcohol	Excessive alcohol intake is strongly associated with hypertension. Patients with hypertension should limit their daily intake to 1 oz of alcohol.
Cigarette smoking	Smoking greatly increases the risk of cardiovascular disease. People with hypertension who smoke are at even greater risk for cardiovascular disease.
Diabetes mellitus	Hypertension is more common in diabetics. When hypertension and diabetes coexist, complications (e.g., target organ disease) are more severe.
Elevated serum lipids	Elevated levels of cholesterol and triglycerides are primary risk factors in atherosclerosis. Hyperlipidemia is more common in people with hypertension.
Excess dietary sodium	High sodium intake can contribute to hypertension in some patients and can decrease the effectiveness of certain antihypertensive medications.
Gender	Hypertension is more prevalent in men in young adulthood and early middle age (<55 yr of age). After age 55, hypertension is more prevalent in women.
Family history	History of a close blood relative (e.g., parents, sibling) with hypertension is associated with an increased risk for developing hypertension.
Obesity	Weight gain is associated with increased frequency of hypertension. The risk is greatest with central abdominal obesity.
Ethnicity	Incidence of hypertension is twice as high in African Americans as in whites.
Sedentary lifestyle	Regular physical activity can help control weight and reduce cardiovascular risk. Physical activity may decrease BP.
Socioeconomic status	Hypertension is more prevalent in lower socioeconomic groups and among the less educated.
Stress	People exposed to repeated stress may develop hypertension more frequently than others. People who develop hypertension may respond differently to stress than those who do not develop hypertension.

DBP, Diastolic blood pressure; *SBP,* systolic blood pressure.

sin II causes direct arteriolar constriction, promotes vascular hypertrophy, and induces aldosterone secretion. Thus altered renin-angiotensin mechanisms may contribute to the development and maintenance of hypertension. Any rise in BP inhibits the release of renin from the renal juxtaglomerular cells. Based on this feedback loop, low levels of PRA would be expected in patients with primary hypertension. However, only about 30% have low PRA, 50% have normal levels, and 20% have high PRA. These normal or high PRA levels may be related to excess renin secretion from ischemic nephrons.

Stress and Increased Sympathetic Nervous System Activity. It has long been recognized that arterial pressure is influenced by factors such as anger, fear, and pain. Physiologic responses to stress, which are normally protective, may persist to a pathologic degree, resulting in prolonged increase in SNS activity. Increased SNS stimulation produces increased vasoconstriction, increased HR, and increased renin release. Increased renin activates the angiotensin mechanism and increases aldosterone secretion, both leading to elevated BP. People exposed to high levels of repeated psychologic stress develop hypertension to a greater extent than those who do not experience as much stress.

TABLE 33-4 Manifestations of Target Organ Disease

Organ	Manifestations
Cardiac	Clinical, electrocardiographic, or radiologic evidence of coronary artery disease (e.g., previous myocardial infarction, coronary revascularization) Left ventricular hypertrophy or "strain" by ECG or left ventricular hypertrophy by echocardiography Left ventricular dysfunction or heart failure
Cerebrovascular	Transient ischemic attack or stroke
Peripheral vascular	One or more major pulses in the extremities (except for dorsalis pedis) reduced or absent; intermittent claudication; abdominal or carotid bruits/thrills; aneurysm
Renal	Serum creatinine ≥1.5 mg/dl (130 μmol/L) Proteinuria (1+ or greater) Microalbuminuria
Retinopathy	Generalized or focal narrowing of retinal arterioles Arteriovenous nicking Hemorrhages or exudates, with or without papilledema

From the National Institutes of Health: *Seventh Report of the Joint National Committee on Prevention, Detection, Evaluation, and Treatment of High Blood Pressure,* Washington, DC, 2003, U.S. Department of Health and Human Services.
ECG, Electrocardiography.

Insulin Resistance and Hyperinsulinemia. Abnormalities of glucose, insulin, and lipoprotein metabolism are common in primary hypertension. They are not present in secondary hypertension and do not improve when hypertension is treated. Insulin resistance is a risk factor for the development of hypertension and cardiovascular disease. High insulin concentration in the blood stimulates SNS activity and impairs nitric oxide–mediated vasodilation. Additional pressor effects of insulin include vascular hypertrophy and increased renal sodium reabsorption.

Endothelial Cell Dysfunction. Vascular endothelial cells are known to be the source of multiple vasoactive substances. Some hypertensive people have a reduced vasodilator response to nitric oxide. Endothelin produces pronounced and prolonged vasoconstriction. The role of endothelial dysfunction in the pathogenesis and treatment of hypertension is an area of ongoing investigation.

Clinical Manifestations

Hypertension is often called the "silent killer" because it is frequently asymptomatic until it becomes severe and target organ disease has occurred. A patient with severe hypertension may experience a variety of symptoms secondary to effects on blood vessels in the various organs and tissues or to the increased workload of the heart. These secondary symptoms include fatigue, reduced activity tolerance, dizziness, palpitations, angina, and dyspnea. In the past, symptoms of hypertension were thought to include headache, nosebleeds, and dizziness. However, unless BP is very high or low, these symptoms are not more frequent in people with hypertension than in the general population.[5]

Complications

The most common complications of hypertension are *target organ diseases* (Table 33-4) occurring in the heart (hypertensive heart disease), brain (cerebrovascular disease), peripheral vasculature (peripheral vascular disease), kidney (nephrosclerosis), and eyes (retinal damage).

Hypertensive Heart Disease

Coronary Artery Disease. Hypertension is a major risk factor for coronary artery disease (CAD). In people older than 50 years, systolic hypertension is a much more important risk factor for cardiovascular disease than diastolic hypertension.[1] The mechanisms by which hypertension contributes to the development of atherosclerosis are not fully known. The "response-to-injury" hypothesis of atherogenesis suggests that hypertension disrupts the coronary artery endothelium, thus exposing the intimal layer to activated white blood cells and platelets. Growth factors released by the vascular endothelium and platelets may induce smooth muscle proliferation within the lesion. These arteriolar changes result in a stiffened arterial wall and a narrowed internal lumen, and account for a high incidence of CAD and the resulting problems of angina and myocardial infarction (MI).

Left Ventricular Hypertrophy. Sustained high BP increases the cardiac workload and produces left ventricular hypertrophy (LVH) (Fig. 33-3). Initially, LVH is an adaptive or compensatory mechanism that strengthens cardiac contraction and increases cardiac output. However, increased contractility increases myocardial work and oxygen consumption. When the heart can no longer meet the demands for myocardial oxygen, heart failure develops. Progressive LVH, especially in association with CAD, is associated with the development of heart failure.

Heart Failure. Heart failure occurs when the heart's compensatory adaptations are overwhelmed and the heart can no longer pump enough blood to meet the metabolic needs of the body (see Chapter 35). Contractility is depressed, and stroke volume and cardiac output are decreased. The patient may complain of shortness of breath on exertion, paroxysmal nocturnal dyspnea, and fatigue. Signs of an enlarged heart may be present on x-ray, and an electrocardiogram (ECG) may show electrical changes indicative of LVH.

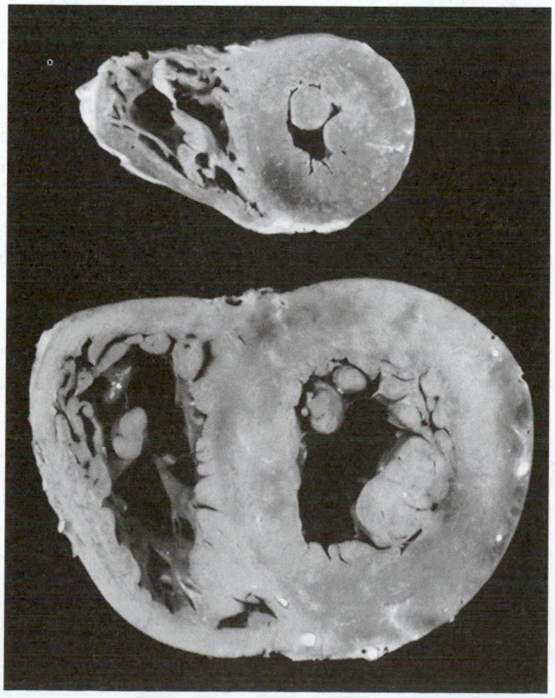

FIG. 33-3 Massively enlarged heart caused by hypertrophy of both ventricles. The normal heart weighs 335 g *(top)*. The heart with biventricular hypertrophy weighs 1100 g. The patient had suffered from severe systemic hypertension.

Cerebrovascular Disease. Atherosclerosis is the most common cause of cerebrovascular disease. Hypertension is a major risk factor for cerebral atherosclerosis and stroke. Even in mildly hypertensive people, the risk of stroke is 4 times higher than in normotensive people. Adequate control of BP diminishes the risk of stroke.

Atherosclerotic plaques are commonly distributed at the bifurcation of the common carotid artery into the internal and external carotid arteries. Portions of the atherosclerotic plaque or the blood clot that forms with disruption of the plaque may break off and travel to intracerebral vessels, producing a thromboembolism. The patient may experience transient ischemic attacks or a stroke. (These conditions are discussed in Chapter 58.)

Hypertensive encephalopathy may occur after a marked rise in BP if the cerebral blood flow is not decreased by autoregulation. Autoregulation is a physiologic process that maintains constant cerebral blood flow despite fluctuations in arterial blood pressure. Normally as pressure in the cerebral blood vessels rises, the vessels constrict to maintain constant flow. When arterial blood pressure exceeds the body's ability to autoregulate, the cerebral vessels suddenly dilate, capillary permeability increases, and cerebral edema develops, producing a rise in intracranial pressure. If left untreated, patients die quickly from brain damage. (Cerebral blood flow and autoregulation are discussed in Chapter 57.)

Peripheral Vascular Disease. As it does with other vessels, hypertension speeds up the process of atherosclerosis in the peripheral blood vessels, leading to the development of peripheral vascular disease, aortic aneurysm, and aortic dissection (see Chapter 38). *Intermittent claudication* (ischemic muscle pain precipitated by activity and relieved with rest) is a classic symptom of peripheral vascular disease involving the arteries.

Nephrosclerosis. Hypertension is one of the leading causes of end-stage renal disease, especially among African Americans. Some degree of renal dysfunction is usually present in the hypertensive patient, even one with a minimally elevated BP. Renal dysfunction is the direct result of ischemia caused by the narrowed lumen of the intrarenal blood vessels. Gradual narrowing of the arteries and arterioles leads to atrophy of the tubules, destruction of the glomeruli, and eventual death of nephrons. Initially intact nephrons can compensate, but these changes may eventually lead to renal failure. Common laboratory indications of renal dysfunction are microalbuminuria, proteinuria, microscopic hematuria, and elevated blood urea nitrogen (BUN) and serum creatinine levels. The earliest manifestation of renal dysfunction is usually nocturia (See Chapter 47).

Retinal Damage. The appearance of the retina provides important information about the severity and duration of the hypertensive process. The retina is the only place in the body where the blood vessels can be directly visualized. Therefore damage to retinal vessels provides an indication of concurrent vessel damage in the heart, brain, and kidney. An ophthalmoscope is used to visualize the blood vessels of the eye. Manifestations of severe retinal damage include blurring of vision, retinal hemorrhage, and loss of vision.

Diagnostic Studies

Measurement of BP is discussed in Chapter 32 on p. 743 and in the Nursing Management section later in this chapter.

There is some controversy as to how extensive a diagnostic workup should be in the initial evaluation of a person with hypertension. Because most hypertension is classified as primary hypertension, testing for secondary causes is not routinely done. Basic laboratory studies are performed to (1) identify or rule out causes of secondary hypertension, (2) evaluate target organ disease, (3) determine overall cardiovascular risk, or (4) establish baseline levels before initiating therapy.

Table 33-5 lists basic diagnostic studies that are performed in a person with hypertension. Routine urinalysis, BUN, and serum creatinine levels are used to screen for renal involvement and to provide baseline information about kidney function. Creatinine clearance, the rate at which creatinine is cleared from the circulation, reflects the glomerular filtration rate. Decreases in creatinine clearance indicate renal insufficiency. Creatinine clearance can be measured quantitatively in a timed urine collection. It can also be estimated from the serum creatinine level. (Serum creatinine and creatinine clearance are discussed in Chapters 45 and 47.)

Measurement of serum electrolytes, especially potassium levels, is important to detect hyperaldosteronism, a cause of secondary hypertension. Blood glucose levels should be assessed to assist in the diagnosis of diabetes mellitus. A lipid profile provides information about additional risk factors that predispose to atherosclerosis and cardiovascular disease. Uric acid levels are determined to establish a baseline, because the levels often rise with diuretic therapy. An ECG provides baseline information about the cardiac status. It is helpful in identifying the presence of LVH, cardiac ischemia, or previous MI. Because of the prognostic importance of LVH, echocardiography may also be performed. If the patient's age, history, physical examination findings, or severity of hypertension points to a secondary cause, further diagnostic testing is indicated.

TABLE 33-5 *COLLABORATIVE CARE* Hypertension

Diagnostic Studies
History and physical examination
Routine urinalysis
Basic metabolic panel (serum glucose, sodium, potassium, chloride, carbon dioxide, calcium, BUN, and creatinine)
Complete blood count
Serum lipid profile (total lipids, triglycerides, HDL and LDL cholesterol, total-to-HDL cholesterol ratio)
Serum uric acid
12-lead electrocardiogram (ECG)
Optional:
- 24-hour urinary creatinine clearance
- Echocardiography
- Liver function studies
- Serum thyroid-stimulating hormone (TSH)

Collaborative Therapy
Periodic monitoring of BP
- Home BP monitoring
- Ambulatory BP monitoring (if indicated)
- Every 3-6 months by health care provider once BP is stabilized

Nutritional therapy (see Table 33-7)
- Restrict sodium
- Reduce weight (if indicated)
- Restrict cholesterol and saturated fats
- Maintain adequate intake of potassium
- Maintain adequate intake of calcium and magnesium

Regular, moderate physical activity
Cessation of smoking (see Chapter 12, Tables 12-4, 12-5, and 12-6)
Moderation of alcohol consumption
Stress management (see Chapter 9)
Antihypertensive drugs (see Table 33-8)
Patient teaching

BP, Blood pressure; *BUN,* blood urea nitrogen; *HDL,* high-density lipoprotein; *LDL,* low-density lipoprotein.

Ambulatory Blood Pressure Monitoring (ABPM). Some patients have elevated BP readings in a clinical setting and normal readings when BP is measured elsewhere. This phenomenon is referred to as "white coat" hypertension. Self-monitoring of BP at home and at work is a practical, economical approach that may be considered prior to ABPM. ABPM is a noninvasive, fully automated system that measures BP at preset intervals over a 24-hour period. The equipment includes a BP cuff and a small microprocessing unit that fits into a pouch worn on a shoulder strap or belt. Patients are instructed to hold their arm still by their side when the device is taking a reading and asked to maintain a diary of activities that may affect BP. Medicare reimbursement is now provided for ABPM in patients with suspected white coat hypertension.[1,8] Other potential applications for ABPM include apparent drug resistance, hypotensive symptoms with hypertensive medications, episodic hypertension, or SNS dysfunction.

As with most physiologic phenomena, BP demonstrates diurnal variability expressed as sleep-wakefulness difference. For day-active people, BP is highest in the early morning, decreases during the day, and is lowest at night. BP at night (when asleep) usually drops by 10% or more from daytime (awake) BP.[8] Some patients with hypertension do not show a normal, nocturnal dip in BP and are referred to as "nondippers." The absence of diurnal variability has been associated with more target organ damage and an increased risk for cardiovascular events. The presence or absence of diurnal variability can be determined by ABPM.

Collaborative Care

Clinical guidelines for the management of hypertension have been published.[1] The goal in treating a patient with hypertension is to control BP and reduce overall cardiovascular risk. (Treatment recommendations are summarized in Tables 33-5 and 33-6, and Fig. 33-4.) Treatment goals are to lower BP to <140 mm Hg systolic and <90 mm Hg diastolic for most persons with hypertension (<130 mm Hg systolic and <80 mm Hg diastolic for those with diabetes mellitus and chronic kidney disease). Lifestyle modifications are indicated for all patients with prehypertension and hypertension.

Lifestyle Modifications. Lifestyle modifications should be used in all patients with prehypertension and hypertension.[1] These modifications are directed toward reducing BP and overall cardiovascular risk. Modifications include (1) weight reduction, (2) DASH (Dietary Approaches to Stop Hypertension) eating plan, (3) dietary sodium reduction, (4) moderation of alcohol consumption, (5) regular aerobic physical activity, and (6) avoidance of tobacco use (smoking and chewing).

Weight Reduction. Overweight individuals have an increased incidence of hypertension and increased risk for cardiovascular disease. Weight reduction has a significant effect on lowering BP

HEALTHY PEOPLE
Prevention and Control of Hypertension

- Maintain a healthy weight
- Reduce salt and sodium intake
- Increase level of physical exercise
- Limit consumption of alcohol to moderate levels
- Monitor blood pressure and know if blood pressure is high, low, normal, or borderline for hypertension
- If ordered, take medication to control blood pressure

TABLE 33-6 Classification and Management of Blood Pressure

BP Classification	SBP* mm Hg	DBP* mm Hg	Lifestyle Modification	Initial Drug Therapy: Without Compelling Indication	Initial Drug Therapy: With Compelling Indications†
Normal	<120	and <80	Encourage	No antihypertensive drug indicated	Drug(s) for compelling indications‡
Prehypertension	120-139	or 80-89	Yes	No antihypertensive drug indicated	Drug(s) for compelling indications‡
Stage 1 hypertension	140-159	or 90-99	Yes	Thiazide-type diuretics for most. May consider ACE inhibitor, ARB, BB, CCB, or combination	Drug(s) for compelling indications‡ Other antihypertensive drugs (diuretics, ACE inhibitor, ARB, BB, CCB) as needed
Stage 2 hypertension	≥160	or ≥100	Yes	Two-drug combination for most§ (usually thiazide-type diuretic and ACE inhibitor or ARB or BB or CCB).	

From the National Institutes of Health: *Seventh Report of the Joint National Committee on Prevention, Detection, Evaluation, and Treatment of High Blood Pressure,* Washington, DC, 2003, U.S. Department of Health and Human Services.

DBP, Diastolic blood pressure; *SBP,* systolic blood pressure.

Drug abbreviations: *ACE,* Angiotensin-converting enzyme; *ARB,* angiotensin II receptor blocker; *BB,* β-adrenergic blocker; *CCB,* calcium channel blocker.

*Treatment determined by highest BP category.

†Compelling indications include heart failure, previous myocardial infarction, high cardiovascular risk, diabetes mellitus, chronic kidney disease, and recurrent stroke prevention.

‡Treat patients with chronic kidney disease or diabetes to BP goal of <130/80 mm Hg.

§Initial combined therapy should be used cautiously in those at risk for orthostatic hypotension.

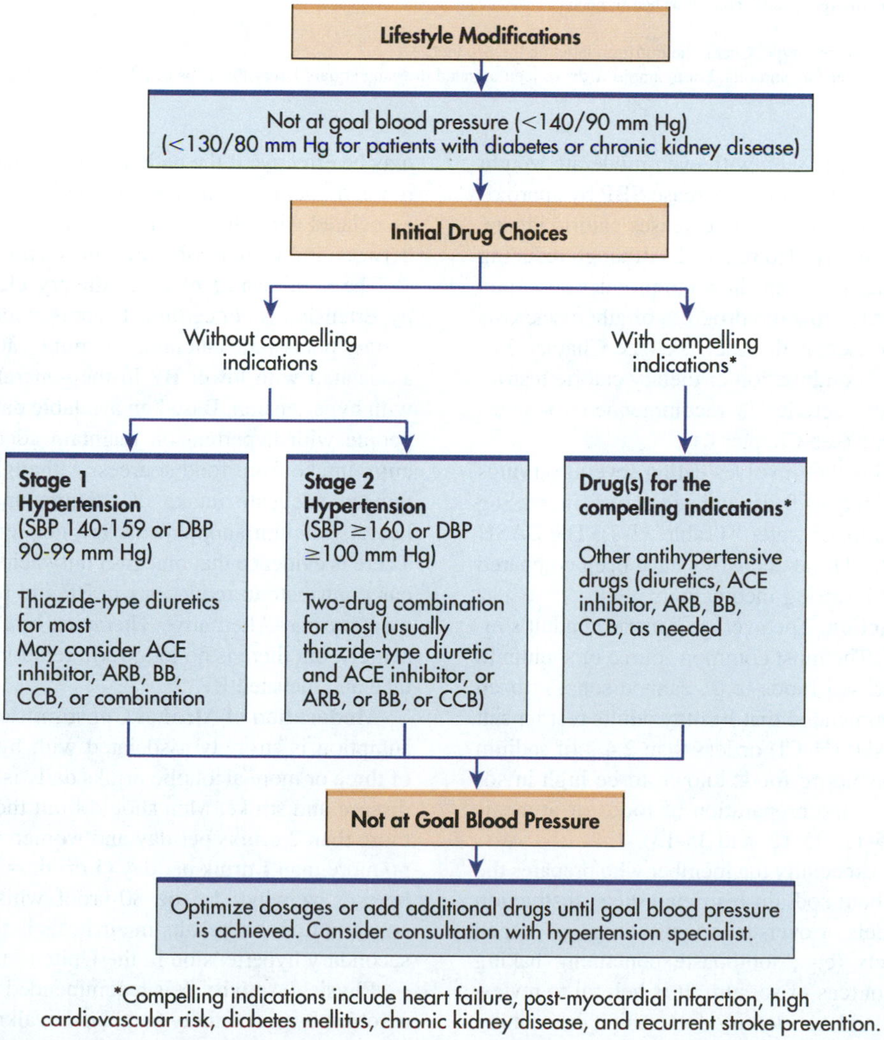

FIG. 33-4 Treatment algorithm for hypertension. *DBP,* Diastolic blood pressure; *SBP,* systolic blood pressure. Drug abbreviations: *ACE,* Angiotensin-converting enzyme; *ARB,* angiotensin II receptor blocker; *BB,* β-adrenergic blocker; *CCB,* calcium channel blocker.

Cardiovascular System

TABLE 33-7 *NUTRITIONAL THERAPY* DASH Diet for Hypertension

Food Group	Daily Servings*	Serving Sizes	Rationale
Grains and grain products	7-8	1 slice bread, 1 oz dry cereal,† ½ cup cooked rice, pasta, or cereal	Major sources of energy and fiber
Vegetables	4-5	1 cup raw leafy vegetable, ½ cup cooked vegetable, 6 oz vegetable juice	Rich sources of potassium, magnesium, and fiber
Fruits	4-5	6 oz fruit juice, 1 medium fruit, ¼ cup dried fruit, ½ cup fresh, frozen, or canned fruit	Important sources of potassium, magnesium, and fiber
Low-fat or fat-free dairy foods	2-3	8 oz milk, 1 cup yogurt, 1½ oz cheese	Major sources of calcium and protein
Meat, poultry, and fish	2 or less	3 oz cooked meats, poultry, or fish	Rich sources of protein and magnesium
Nuts, seeds, and dry beans	4-5/wk	⅓ cup or 1½ oz nuts, 2 tbs or ½ oz seeds, ½ cup cooked dry beans	Rich sources of energy, magnesium, potassium, protein, and fiber
Fats and oils‡	2-3	1 tsp soft margarine, 1 tbs low-fat mayonnaise, 2 tbs light salad dressing, 1 tsp vegetable oil	Added fat and high-fat sources should be minimal; DASH has 27% of calories as fat, including fat in or added to foods
Sweets	5/wk	1 tbs sugar, 1 tbs jelly or jam, ½ oz jelly beans, 8 oz lemonade	Sweets should be low in fat

Source: National Heart, Lung, and Blood Institute: *The DASH diet,* NIH Publication No 03-4082, Washington, DC, 2003, National Institutes of Health. Available at *www.nhlbi.nih.gov/health/public/heart/nbp/dash.*

DASH, Dietary Approaches to Stop Hypertension. The DASH eating plan above is based on approximately 2000 calories per day. The number of daily servings in a food group may vary from those listed, depending on specific caloric or health needs.

*Except as noted.

†Equals ½ to 1¼ cup, depending on cereal type. Check the nutrition label on the product.

‡Fat content changes serving counts for fats and oils. For example, 1 tbs of regular salad dressing equals 1 serving; 1 tbs of a low-fat dressing equals ½ serving; 1 tbs of a fat-free dressing equals 0 servings.

in many people, and the effect is seen with even moderate weight loss. A weight loss of 10 kg (22 lb) may decrease SBP by approximately 5 to 20 mm Hg.[1] When a person decreases caloric intake, sodium and fat intake are usually also reduced. Although reducing the fat content of the diet has not been shown to produce sustained benefits in BP control, it may slow the progress of atherosclerosis and reduce overall cardiovascular disease risk (see Chapter 34). Weight reduction through a combination of dietary calorie restriction and moderate physical activity is recommended for overweight hypertensive patients (see Chapter 41).

DASH Eating Plan. This diet involves eating several servings of fish each week, eating plenty of fruits and vegetables, increasing fiber intake, and drinking a lot of water[10] (Table 33-7). The DASH diet significantly lowers BP. These decreases have been compared to those achieved with BP-lowering medication.[1]

Dietary Sodium Reduction. The average American adult's intake of salt totals 15 g/day. The most common source of sodium in the American diet is processed foods (e.g., canned soups, frozen dinners). It has been recommended that healthy adults restrict salt intake to less than 6 g of salt (NaCl) or less than 2.4 g of sodium per day.[1,2] This involves avoiding foods known to be high in sodium and not adding salt in the preparation of foods or at meals (see Chapter 35, Tables 35-11, 35-12, and 35-13).

The patient and family, especially the member who prepares the meals, should be taught about sodium-restricted diets. Instruction should include reading labels of over-the-counter drugs, packaged foods, and health products (e.g., toothpaste containing baking soda) to identify hidden sources of sodium. It is helpful to review the patient's normal diet and to identify foods high in sodium. Analysis of a 3-day diet history will help identify foods high in sodium in the patient's usual diet.

Sodium restriction may be enough to control BP in some patients with hypertension. If drug therapy is needed, a lower dose may be effective if the patient also restricts sodium intake. Furthermore, moderate sodium restriction lessens the risk of hypokalemia associated with diuretic therapy. However, the response may differ between individuals who are salt sensitive or salt resistant.

The significance of other dietary elements for the control of hypertension is not certain. There is evidence that greater levels of dietary potassium, calcium, vitamin D, and omega-3 fatty acids are associated with lower BP in the general population and in those with hypertension. Based on available data, it is recommended that people with hypertension maintain adequate potassium and calcium intake from food sources. Although it is important to maintain an adequate intake of calcium and vitamin D for general health, calcium supplements are not recommended to lower BP. There is evidence that omega-3 fatty acids found in certain fish oils can contribute to reductions in BP and triglycerides (see Complementary and Alternative Therapies box). Caffeine may raise BP acutely, but there is no long-term relationship between caffeine intake and elevated BP.

Moderation of Alcohol Consumption. Excessive alcohol consumption is strongly associated with hypertension. Consumption of three or more alcoholic drinks daily is also a risk factor for heart disease and stroke. Men should limit their intake of alcohol to no more than 2 drinks per day and women and lighter weight men to no more than 1 drink per day (1 drink = 1.5 oz alcohol [e.g., 12 oz beer, 5 oz wine, 1.5 oz 80-proof whiskey]). Excessive alcohol consumption that results in cirrhosis is the most frequent cause of secondary hypertension in the United States.

Physical Activity. It is recommended that all adults have regular aerobic physical activity (e.g., brisk walking) at least 30 minutes per day most days of the week. Moderately intense activity such as brisk walking, jogging, and swimming can lower BP, promote relaxation, and decrease or control body weight. Regular activity of this type can reduce SBP in the hypertensive patient by approximately 4 to

COMPLEMENTARY AND ALTERNATIVE THERAPIES

Fish Oil/Omega-3 Fatty Acids

Dietary sources of omega-3 fatty acids include fish oil, which contains both docosahexaenoic acid (DHA) and eicosapentaenoic acid (EPA). Fish oil may be obtained by eating oily fish or by taking a supplement. Oily fish include anchovies, bluefish, carp, catfish, halibut, herring, lake trout, mackerel, pompano, salmon, striped sea bass, tuna (albacore), and whitefish. Potentially harmful contaminants such as dioxins, methylmercury, and polychlorinated biphenyls (PCBs) are found in some species of fish.

Omega-3 fatty acids should not be confused with omega-6 fatty acids.

Clinical Uses

- Hypertension, hypertriglyceridemia, cardiovascular disease prevention*
- Rheumatoid arthritis†

Effects

May include reduction of blood triglyceride levels and small reductions in BP. Effects appear to be dose dependent. May also reduce inflammation, reduce blood clotting, reduce buildup of atherosclerotic plaques in arteries of the heart. The American Heart Association recommends including fish in the diet of all individuals and fish oil supplements for those with history of cardiovascular disease.

Nursing Implications

Generally safe in recommended dosages for up to 2 to 3½ years. Dosages greater than 3 g/day may result in increased risk of bleeding. Use with caution in diabetic patients or patients with bleeding disorders. Use with caution in patients taking medications, herbs, or supplements that also increase the risk of bleeding. Advise patients to consult a health care provider before using fish oils at dosages greater than 3 g/day. Fish oil taken for many months may cause a deficiency of vitamin E. Vitamin E is added to many fish oil products. More research is needed to determine safety of supplements during pregnancy or lactation. Advise women who are pregnant or lactating to limit intake of oily fish and to seek the recommendation of their health care provider.

Adapted from Ulbricht CE, Basch EM: *Natural standard herb and supplement reference: evidence-based clinical reviews*, Mosby, 2005, St. Louis *(www.naturalstandard.com)*; and Agency for Healthcare Research and Quality: *Health effects of omega-3 fatty acids on cardiovascular disease,* Publication No 04-E009-2, Rockville, Md, 2004, Agency for Healthcare Research and Quality. Available at *www.ahrq.gov/clinic/tp/o3cardtp.htm.*

*Strong scientific evidence for their use.

†Good scientific evidence for their use.

9 mm Hg. Sedentary people should be advised to increase activity levels gradually. People with heart disease or other serious health problems need a thorough examination, possibly including a stress test, before beginning an exercise program.

Avoidance of Tobacco Products. Nicotine contained in tobacco causes vasoconstriction and increases BP in hypertensive people. In addition, smoking tobacco is a major risk factor for cardiovascular disease. The cardiovascular benefits of discontinuing tobacco use can be seen within 1 year in all age-groups. Everyone, especially a hypertensive patient, should be strongly advised to avoid tobacco use. The lower amounts of nicotine contained in smoking cessation aids usually will not raise BP and may be used as indicated. People who continue to use tobacco products should be advised to monitor their BP during use. (Tobacco use and smoking cessation are discussed in Chapter 12.)

Stress Management. Stress can raise BP on a short-term basis and has been implicated in the development of hypertension. Relaxation therapy, guided imagery, and biofeedback may be useful in helping patients manage stress, thus decreasing BP. Psychosocial factors such as time urgency and impatience and hostility have been associated with an increase in the long-term risk of hypertension in young adults.[11]

Drug Therapy. The general goals of drug therapy are to achieve BP <140/90 mm Hg (<130/80 mm Hg for patients with diabetes mellitus or chronic kidney disease). Drug therapy is not recommended for those persons with prehypertension unless it is required by another condition, such as diabetes mellitus or chronic kidney disease.

The drugs currently available for treating hypertension have two main actions: (1) they decrease the volume of circulating blood and (2) they reduce SVR (Table 33-8). The drugs used in the treatment of hypertension include diuretics, adrenergic (SNS) inhibitors, direct vasodilators, angiotensin inhibitors, and calcium channel blockers. The various sites and methods of action are presented in Fig. 33-5.

Although the precise action of diuretics in the reduction of BP is unclear, it is known that they promote sodium and water excretion, reduce plasma volume, decrease sodium in the arteriolar walls, and reduce the vascular response to catecholamines. Adrenergic-inhibiting agents act by diminishing the SNS effects that increase BP. Adrenergic inhibitors include drugs that act centrally on the vasomotor center and peripherally to inhibit norepinephrine release or to block the adrenergic receptors on blood vessels. Direct vasodilators decrease the BP by relaxing vascular smooth muscle and reducing SVR. Calcium channel blockers increase sodium excretion and cause arteriolar vasodilation by preventing the movement of extracellular calcium into cells.

There are two types of angiotensin inhibitors. The first type is angiotensin-converting enzyme (ACE) inhibitors, which prevent the conversion of angiotensin I to angiotensin II and thus reduce angiotensin II (A-II)–mediated vasoconstriction and sodium and water retention. The second type is A-II receptor blockers (ARBs), which prevent angiotensin II from binding to its receptors in the walls of the blood vessels.

Thiazide-type diuretics are used as initial therapy for most patients with hypertension, either alone or in combination with one of the other classes. Compelling indications requiring the use of other antihypertensive drugs as initial therapy include heart failure, previous MI, high risk for coronary artery disease, diabetes mellitus, chronic kidney disease, and recurrent stroke prevention. If a drug is not tolerated or is contraindicated, then one of the other classes (see Table 33-8) shown to reduce cardiovascular events should be used instead.

Most patients who are hypertensive will require two or more antihypertensive medications to achieve their BP goals. Addition of a second drug from a different class should be initiated when use of a single drug in adequate doses fails to achieve the BP goal. When BP is more than 20/10 mm Hg above SBP and DBP goals, consideration should be given to initiating therapy with two drugs, either as separate prescriptions or in combination therapy (Table 33-9 on p. 777).

Once antihypertensive therapy is initiated, most patients should return for follow-up and adjustment of medications at approximately monthly intervals until the BP goal is reached. More frequent visits will be necessary for patients with stage 2 hypertension or with complicating comorbid conditions. After BP is at goal

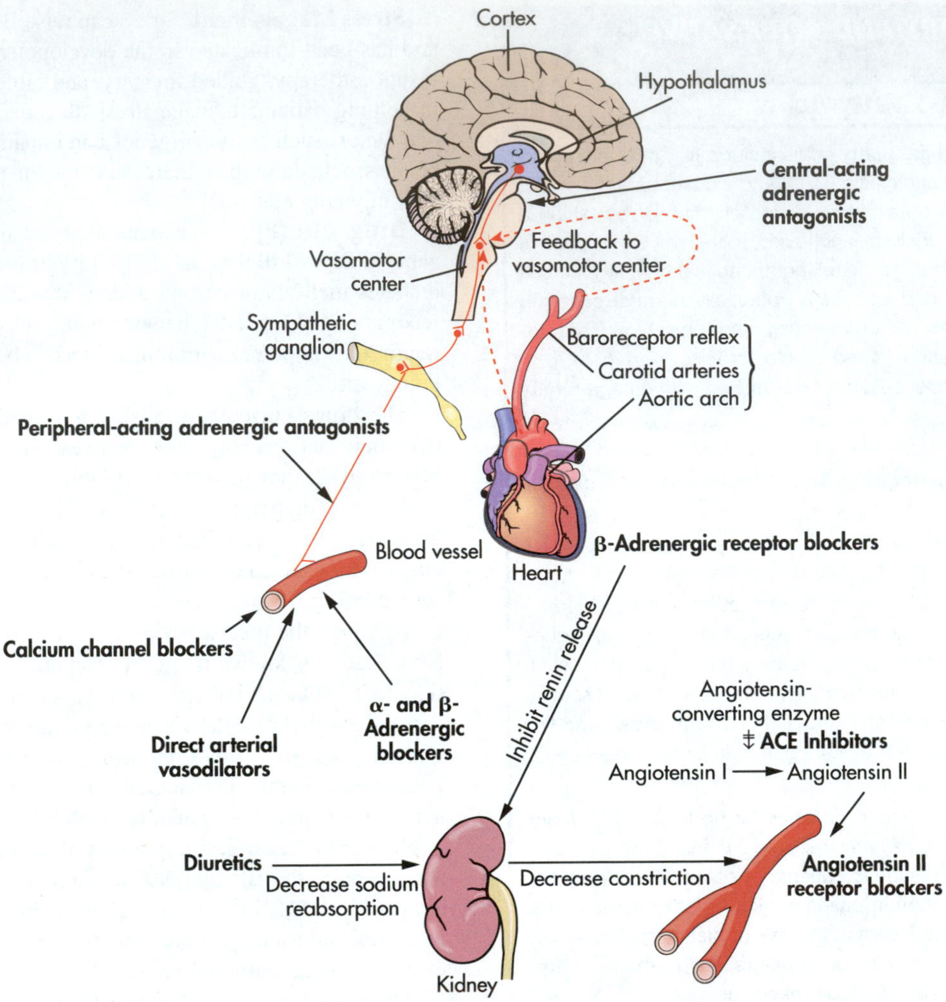

FIG. 33-5 Site and method of action of various antihypertensive drugs *(bold type). ACE,* Angiotensin-converting enzyme.

and stable, follow-up visits can usually be at 3- to 6-month intervals. Comorbidities, such as heart failure, associated diseases such as diabetes, and the need for ongoing monitoring (e.g., laboratory testing), influence the frequency of visits.

Side effects and adverse effects of antihypertensive drugs may be so severe or undesirable that the patient does not comply with therapy. Table 33-8 describes the major side effects of antihypertensive drugs. Hyperuricemia, hyperglycemia, and hypokalemia are common side effects with both thiazide and loop diuretics. ACE inhibitors lead to high levels of bradykinin, which can cause coughing. An individual who develops a cough with the use of ACE inhibitors may be switched to an ARB. Hyperkalemia can be a serious side effect of the potassium-sparing diuretics and ACE inhibitors. Sexual dysfunction may occur with some of the diuretics. Orthostatic hypotension and sexual dysfunction are two undesirable effects of adrenergic-inhibiting agents. Tachycardia and orthostatic hypotension are potential adverse effects of both vasodilators and angiotensin inhibitors.

Patient Teaching Related to Drug Therapy. Patient and family teaching related to drug therapy is needed to identify and minimize side effects and to cope with therapeutic effects. Side effects of antihypertensive drug therapy are common. Side effects may be an initial response to a drug and may decrease with continued use of the drug. Informing the patient about side effects that lessen with time may enable the individual to continue taking the drug. The number or severity of side effects may be related to the dosage, and it may be necessary to change the drug or decrease the dosage. In this case, the patient should be advised to report the side effects to the health care provider who prescribed the medication.

A common side effect of several of these drugs is orthostatic hypotension. This condition is caused by an alteration of the autonomic nervous system's mechanisms for regulating pressure, which are required for position changes. Consequently, the patient may feel dizzy, weak, and faint when assuming an upright position after sitting or lying down. (Specific measures to control or decrease orthostatic hypotension are presented in Table 33-14 later in this chapter.)

***Drug Alert** - Doxazosin (Cardura)*
- *Use caution with administration of initial dose.*
- *Syncope (sudden loss of consciousness) occasionally occurs 30-90 minutes following initial dose, a too-rapid increase in dose, or addition of another antihypertensive agent to therapy.*

Sexual dysfunction may occur with many of the antihypertensive drugs (see Table 33-8) and can be a major reason that a patient does not adhere to the treatment plan. Problems can range from decreased libido to erectile dysfunction. Rather than discussing a sexual problem with a health care professional, the patient may decide to simply stop taking the drug. The nurse should approach the patient on this sensitive subject and encourage discussion of any sexual dysfunc-

Text continued on p. 776.

TABLE 33-8 DRUG THERAPY
Hypertension

Drug	Mechanism of Action	Side Effects and Adverse Effects	Nursing Considerations
Diuretics			
Thiazide and Related Diuretics			
bendroflumethiazide (Naturetin) benzthiazide (Aquatag, Exna) chlorothiazide (Diuril) chlorthalidone (Hygroton, Apo-Chlorthalidone*) hydrochlorothiazide (Microzide, Esidrix, HydroDIURIL, Oretic, Apo-Hydro,* Novo-Hydrazide,* Urozide*) metolazone (Zaroxolyn) methyclothiazide (Enduron, Duretic*) trichlormethiazide (Metahydrin, Naqua, Trichlorex*)	Inhibit NaCl reabsorption in the distal convoluted tubule; increase excretion of Na^+ and Cl^-. Initial decrease in ECF; sustained decrease in SVR. Lower BP moderately in 2-4 wk.	Fluid and electrolyte imbalances (volume depletion, hypokalemia, hyponatremia, hypochloremia, hypomagnesemia, hypercalcemia, hyperuricemia, metabolic alkalosis); CNS effects (vertigo, headache, weakness); GI effects (anorexia, nausea, vomiting, diarrhea, constipation, pancreatitis); sexual problems (erectile dysfunction, decreased libido); blood dyscrasias; and dermatologic (photosensitivity, skin rash) effects. Decreased glucose tolerance.	Monitor for orthostatic hypotension, hypokalemia, and alkalosis. Thiazides may potentiate cardiotoxicity of digoxin by producing hypokalemia. Dietary sodium restriction reduces the risk of hypokalemia. NSAIDs can decrease diuretic and antihypertensive effect of thiazide diuretics. Advise patient to supplement with potassium-rich foods. Current doses are lower than previously recommended.
Loop Diuretics			
bumetanide (Bumex) ethacrynic acid (Edecrin) furosemide (Lasix) torsemide (Demadex)	Inhibit NaCl reabsorption in the thick ascending limb of the loop of Henle. Increase excretion of Na^+ and Cl^-. More potent diuretic effect than thiazides, but shorter duration of action. Less effective for hypertension.	Fluid and electrolyte imbalances as with thiazides, except no hypercalcemia. Ototoxicity (hearing impairment, deafness, vertigo) that is usually reversible. Metabolic effects, including hyperuricemia, hyperglycemia, increased LDL cholesterol and triglycerides with decreased HDL cholesterol.	Monitor for orthostatic hypotension and electrolyte abnormalities. Loop diuretics remain effective despite renal insufficiency. Diuretic effect of drug increases at higher doses.
Potassium-Sparing Diuretics			
amiloride (Midamor) triamterene (Dyrenium)	Reduce K^+ and Na^+ exchange in the distal and collecting tubules. Reduce excretion of K^+, H^+, Ca^+, and Mg^+.	Hyperkalemia, nausea, vomiting, diarrhea, headache, leg cramps, and dizziness.	Monitor for orthostatic hypotension and hyperkalemia. Contraindicated in patients with renal failure. Use with caution in patients on ACE inhibitors or angiotensin II blockers. Avoid potassium supplements.
Aldosterone Receptor Blockers			
spironolactone (Aldactone) eplerenone (Inspra)	Inhibit the Na^+-retaining and K^+-excreting effects of aldosterone in the distal and collecting tubules.	Same as amiloride and triamterene; may cause gynecomastia, erectile dysfunction, decreased libido, and menstrual irregularities.	Monitor for orthostatic hypotension and hyperkalemia. Do not combine with potassium-sparing diuretics or potassium supplements. Use with caution in patients on ACE inhibitors or angiotensin II blockers. These drugs are also classified as potassium-sparing diuretics.
Adrenergic Inhibitors			
Central-Acting α-Adrenergic Antagonists			
clonidine (Catapres) clonidine patch (Catapres-TTS)	Reduces sympathetic outflow from CNS. Reduces peripheral sympathetic tone, produces vasodilation, decreases SVR and BP.	Dry mouth, sedation, erectile dysfunction, nausea, dizziness, sleep disturbance, nightmares, restlessness, and depression. Symptomatic bradycardia in patients with conduction disorder.	Sudden discontinuation may cause withdrawal syndrome including rebound hypertension, tachycardia, headache, tremors, apprehension, and sweating. Chewing gum or hard candy may relieve dry mouth. Alcohol and sedatives increase sedation. Patch may be given transdermally with fewer side effects and better compliance.
guanabenz (Wytensin)	Same as clonidine.	Same as clonidine.	Same as clonidine, but not available in transdermal formulation.

ACE, Angiotensin-converting enzyme; *BP,* blood pressure; *CNS,* central nervous system; *ECF,* extracellular fluid; *GI,* gastrointestinal; *HDL,* high-density lipoprotein; *IV,* intravenous; *LDL,* low-density lipoprotein; *NSAIDs,* nonsteroidal antiinflammatory drugs; *SVR,* systemic vascular resistance.
*Canadian brand names.

Continued

TABLE 33-8 DRUG THERAPY
Hypertension—cont'd

Drug	Mechanism of Action	Side Effects and Adverse Effects	Nursing Considerations
Adrenergic Inhibitors—cont'd			
Central-Acting α-Adrenergic Antagonists—cont'd			
guanfacine (Tenex)	Same as clonidine.	Same as clonidine.	Same as clonidine, but not available in transdermal formulation.
methyldopa (Aldomet)	Same as clonidine.	Sedation, fatigue, orthostatic hypotension, decreased libido, erectile dysfunction, dry mouth, hemolytic anemia, hepatotoxicity, sodium and water retention, depression.	Instruct patient about daytime sedation and avoidance of hazardous activities. Administration of a single daily dose at bedtime minimizes sedative effect.
Peripheral-Acting α-Adrenergic Antagonists			
guanethidine (Ismelin)	Prevents peripheral release of norepinephrine, resulting in vasodilation; lowers CO and reduces SBP more than DBP.	Marked orthostatic hypotension, diarrhea, cramps, bradycardia, retrograde or delayed ejaculation, sodium and water retention.	May cause severe orthostatic hypotension; not recommended for use in patients with cerebrovascular or coronary insufficiency or in older adults; advise patient to rise slowly and wear support stockings. Hypotensive effect is delayed for 2-3 days and lasts 7-10 days after withdrawal. Once-daily dosing.
guanadrel sulfate (Hylorel)	Same as guanethidine.	Similar to guanethidine.	Must be given twice daily.
reserpine (Serpasil)	Depletes central and peripheral stores of norepinephrine; results in peripheral vasodilation (decreases SVR and BP).	Sedation and inability to concentrate, depression, nasal stuffiness.	Contraindicated in patients with history of depression. Monitor mood and mental status regularly. Advise patient to avoid barbiturates, alcohol, and opioids.
α_1-Adrenergic Blockers			
doxazosin (Cardura) prazosin (Minipress) terazosin (Hytrin)	Block α_1-adrenergic effects, producing peripheral vasodilation (decreases SVR and BP).	Variable amount of orthostatic hypotension depending on the plasma volume. May see profound orthostatic hypotension with syncope within 90 min after initial dose. Retention of salt and water.	Reduced resistance to the outflow of urine in benign prostatic hyperplasia. Taking drug at bedtime reduces risks associated with orthostatic hypotension. Beneficial effects on lipid profile.
phentolamine (Regitine)	Blocks α_1-adrenergic receptors, resulting in peripheral vasodilation (decreases SVR and BP).	Acute, prolonged hypotension, cardiac dysrhythmias, tachycardia, weakness, flushing. Abdominal pain, nausea, and exacerbation of peptic ulcer.	Used in short-term management of pheochromocytoma. Also used locally to prevent necrosis of skin and subcutaneous tissue after extravasation of adrenergic drug. No oral formulation.
β-Adrenergic Blockers			
acebutolol (Sectral) atenolol (Tenormin) betaxolol (Kerlone) bisoprolol (Zebeta) carteolol (Cartrol) metoprolol (Lopressor) nadolol (Corgard) penbutolol (Levatol) pindolol (Visken) propranolol (Inderal) timolol (Blocadren)	Reduce BP by antagonizing β-adrenergic effects. Cardioselective agents block β_1-adrenergic receptors. Nonselective agents block β_1- and β_2-adrenergic receptors. Decrease CO and reduce sympathetic vasoconstrictor tone. Decrease renin secretion by kidneys.	Hypotension, bronchospasm, atrioventricular conduction block, impaired peripheral circulation. Nightmares, depression, erectile dysfunction, weakness, reduced exercise capacity. May induce or exacerbate heart failure in susceptible patients. Sudden withdrawal of β-adrenergic blockers may cause rebound hypertension and exacerbate symptoms of ischemic heart disease.	β-Adrenergic blockers vary in lipid solubility, selectivity, and presence of partial sympathomimetic effect, which explains different therapeutic and side effect profiles of specific agents. Monitor pulse and BP regularly. Use with caution in patients with diabetes mellitus because drug may depress the tachycardia associated with hypoglycemia. Nonselective agents may cause bronchospasm, especially in patients with a history of asthma.
esmolol (Brevibloc)	Reduces BP by antagonizing β_1-adrenergic effects.		IV administration; rapid onset and very short duration of action.

BP, Blood pressure; *CO,* cardiac output; *DBP,* diastolic blood pressure; *ECG,* electrocardiogram; *IV,* intravenous; *SBP,* systolic blood pressure; *SVR,* systemic vascular resistance.

TABLE 33-8 ***DRUG THERAPY* Hypertension—cont'd**

Drug	Mechanism of Action	Side Effects and Adverse Effects	Nursing Considerations
Adrenergic Inhibitors—cont'd			
Combined α- and β-Adrenergic Blockers			
carvedilol (Coreg) labetalol (Normodyne, Trandate)	α_1-, β_1-, and β_2-adrenergic blocking properties producing peripheral vasodilation and decreased heart rate. Reduces CO, SVR, and BP.	Hypotension, bradycardia, orthostatic hypotension, dizziness, fatigue, nausea, vomiting, dyspepsia, paresthesia, nasal stuffiness, erectile dysfunction, edema. Hepatic toxicity.	Same as β-adrenergic blockers. IV form available for hypertensive crisis in hospitalized patients. Patients must be kept supine during IV administration. Assess patient tolerance of upright position (severe orthostatic hypotension) before allowing upright activities (e.g., commode).
Direct Vasodilators			
fenoldopam (Corlopam)	Activates dopamine receptors, resulting in systemic and renal vasodilation.	Tachycardia, angina, headache, nausea, flushing.	IV use only for hypertensive crisis in hospitalized patients. Use cautiously in patients with glaucoma. Patient should remain supine for 1 hr after administration.
hydralazine (Apresoline)	Reduces SVR and BP by direct arterial vasodilation.	Headache, nausea, flushing, palpitation, tachycardia, dizziness, and angina. Hemolytic anemia, vasculitis, and rapidly progressive glomerulonephritis.	IV use for hypertensive crisis in hospitalized patients. Twice-daily oral dosage. Not used as monotherapy because of side effects. Contraindicated in patients with coronary artery disease; used with caution in patients over 40 yr of age.
minoxidil (Loniten)	Reduces SVR and BP by direct arterial vasodilation.	Reflex tachycardia, marked sodium and fluid retention (may require loop diuretics for control), and hirsutism. May cause ECG changes (flattened and inverted T waves) not related to ischemia.	Reserved for treatment of severe hypertension associated with renal failure and resistant to other therapy. Once- or twice-daily dosage.
nitroglycerin (Tridil)	Relaxes arterial and venous smooth muscle, reducing preload and SVR. At low dose, venous dilation predominates; at higher dose, arterial dilation is present.	Hypotension, headache, vomiting, flushing.	IV use for hypertensive crisis in hospitalized patients with myocardial ischemia. Administered by continuous IV infusion with pump or control device.
sodium nitroprusside (Nipride)	Direct arterial vasodilation reduces SVR and BP.	Acute hypotension, nausea, vomiting, muscle twitching. Signs of thiocyanate toxicity include anorexia, nausea, fatigue, and disorientation.	IV use for hypertensive crisis in hospitalized patients. Administered by continuous IV infusion with pump or control device. Intraarterial monitoring of BP recommended. Wrap IV solutions with an opaque material to protect from light; stable for 24 hr. Metabolized to cyanide, then thiocyanate. Monitor thiocyanate levels with prolonged use (>3 days) or doses (≥4 mcg/kg/min).
Ganglionic Blockers			
trimethaphan (Arfonad)	Interrupts adrenergic control of arteries, results in vasodilation, and reduces SVR and BP.	Visual disturbance, dilated pupils, dry mouth, urinary hesitancy, subjective chilliness.	IV use for initial control of BP in patient with dissecting aortic aneurysm. Administered by continuous IV infusion with pump or control device.

Continued

Cardiovascular System

TABLE 33-8 *DRUG THERAPY* Hypertension—cont'd

Drug	Mechanism of Action	Side Effects and Adverse Effects	Nursing Considerations
Angiotensin Inhibitors			
Angiotensin-Converting Enzyme Inhibitors			
benazepril (Lotensin) captopril (Capoten) enalapril (Vasotec) fosinopril (Monopril) lisinopril (Prinivil, Zestril) moexipril (Univasc) perindopril (Aceon) quinapril (Accupril) ramipril (Altace) trandolapril (Mavik)	Inhibit angiotensin-converting enzyme, reduce conversion of angiotensin I to angiotensin II (A-II), prevent A-II–mediated vasoconstriction.	Hypotension, dizziness, loss of taste, cough, hyperkalemia, acute renal failure, skin rash, angioedema.	Aspirin and NSAIDs may reduce drug effectiveness. Addition of diuretic enhances drug effect. Should not be used with potassium-sparing diuretics. Inhibit breakdown of bradykinin, which may cause a dry, hacking cough. Angiotensin II receptor blockers are an acceptable alternative as they do not affect bradykinin levels. Can cause fetal morbidity or mortality. Captopril may be given orally for hypertensive crisis.
enalaprilat (Vasotec I.V.)	Inhibits ACE when oral agents not appropriate.	Same as oral forms.	Given IV over 5 min; may monitor BP.
Angiotensin II Receptor Blockers			
candesartan (Atacand) eprosartan (Teveten) irbesartan (Avapro) losartan (Cozaar) olmesartan (Benicar) tasosartan (Verdia) telmisartan (Micardis) valsartan (Diovan)	Prevent action of angiotensin II and produce vasodilation and increased salt and water excretion.	Hyperkalemia, decreased renal function.	Full effect on BP may not be seen for 3-6 wk.
Calcium Channel Blockers			
amlodipine (Norvasc) diltiazem extended release (Cardizem CD, Cardizem LA, Dilacor XR, Tiazac) felodipine (Plendil) isradipine (DynaCirc CR) nicardipine sustained release (Cardene SR) nifedipine long acting (Adalat CC, Procardia XL) verapamil intermediate release (Isoptin, Calan) nisoldipine (Sular) verapamil long acting (Isoptin SR, Covera-HS, Calan SR) verapamil timed release (Verelan PM)	Block movement of extracellular calcium into cells, causing vasodilation and decreased heart rate, contractility, and SVR.	Bradycardia, first-degree AV block, nausea, headache, dizziness, peripheral edema, flushing, rash, gingival hyperplasia, constipation (with verapamil).	Use with caution in patients with heart failure. Contraindicated in patients with second- or third-degree heart block. Avoid grapefruit when on nifedipine. Use of sublingual short-acting nifedipine in hypertensive emergencies is unsafe and not effective. Serious adverse events (e.g., stroke, acute MI) have been reported. IV nicardipine available for hypertensive crisis in hospitalized patients. Change peripheral IV infusion sites every 12 hr.

ACE, Angiotensin-converting enzyme; *AV,* atrioventricular; *BP,* blood pressure; *IV,* intravenous; *NSAIDs,* nonsteroidal antiinflammatory drugs; *SVR,* systemic vascular resistance.

tion that may be experienced. The sexual problems may be easier for the patient to discuss and handle once it has been explained that the drug may be the source of the problem and the side effects can be decreased or eliminated by changing to another antihypertensive drug. The patient should be encouraged to discuss side effects with the health care provider who prescribed the medication. If the patient is reluctant to do so, the nurse may offer to alert the health care provider to the sexual side effect that the patient is experiencing. There are so many options now in treating hypertension that a plan that is acceptable to the patient should be achievable.

Some unpleasant effects of drugs result from their therapeutic effect, but the impact can be minimized. For example, dry mouth and frequent voiding are unpleasant effects of diuretics. Sugarless gum or candy may relieve the dry mouth. The nurse can assist the patient to develop a medication schedule to minimize unpleasant effects. When frequent urination interrupts sleep, taking the diuretic earlier in the day may be beneficial. Side effects of vasodilators and adrenergic inhibitors decrease if the drugs are taken in the evening. It should be remembered that BP is lowest during the night and highest shortly after awakening. Therefore drugs with 24-hour duration of action should be taken as early in the morning as possible (e.g., 4 or 5 AM if the patient awakens to void).

Resistant Hypertension. *Resistant hypertension* is the failure to reach goal BP in patients who are adhering to full doses of an appropriate three-drug therapy regimen that includes a diuretic. Health care professionals need to carefully explore reasons why the patient is not at goal BP (Table 33-10).

TABLE 33-9 DRUG THERAPY
Combination Drug Therapy for Hypertension

Combinations	Trade Names
Angiotensin-Converting Enzyme Inhibitors and Diuretics	
benazepril/hydrochlorothiazide	Lotensin HCT
captopril/hydrochlorothiazide	Capozide
enalapril/hydrochlorothiazide	Vaseretic
fosinopril/hydrochlorothiazide	Monopril-HCT
lisinopril/hydrochlorothiazide	Prinzide, Zestoretic
moexipril/hydrochlorothiazide	Uniretic
quinapril/hydrochlorothiazide	Accuretic
Angiotensin II Receptor Blockers and Diuretics	
candesartan/hydrochlorothiazide	Atacand HCT
eprosartan/hydrochlorothiazide	Teveten HCT
irbesartan/hydrochlorothiazide	Avalide
losartan/hydrochlorothiazide	Hyzaar
olmesartan medoxomil/hydrochlorothiazide	Benicar HCT
telmisartan/hydrochlorothiazide	Micardis HCT
valsartan/hydrochlorothiazide	Diovan HCT
β-Adrenergic Blockers and Diuretics	
atenolol/chlorthalidone	Tenoretic
bisoprolol/hydrochlorothiazide	Ziac
metoprolol/hydrochlorothiazide	Lopressor HCT
nadolol/bendroflumethiazide	Corzide
propranolol/hydrochlorothiazide	Inderide
timolol/hydrochlorothiazide	Timolide
Centrally Acting Drugs and Diuretics	
methyldopa/hydrochlorothiazide	Aldoril
reserpine/chlorthalidone	Demi-Regroton
reserpine/hydrochlorothiazide	Hydropres
prazosin/polythiazide	Minizide
guanethidine/hydrochlorothiazide	Esimil
clonidine/chlorthalidone	Combipres
Angiotensin-Converting Enzyme Inhibitors and Calcium Channel Blockers	
amlodipine/benazepril	Lotrel
enalapril/felodipine	Lexxel
enalapril/diltiazem	Teczem
trandolapril/verapamil	Tarka
Diuretics and Diuretics	
amiloride/hydrochlorothiazide	Moduretic
spironolactone/hydrochlorothiazide	Aldactazide
triamterene/hydrochlorothiazide	Dyazide, Maxzide

NURSING MANAGEMENT
PRIMARY HYPERTENSION

Nursing Assessment

Subjective and objective data that should be obtained from a patient with hypertension are presented in Table 33-11.

Nursing Diagnoses

Nursing diagnoses and collaborative problems for the patient with hypertension include, but are not limited to, those presented in Table 33-12.

Planning

The overall goals for the patient with hypertension are that the patient will (1) achieve and maintain the individually determined goal BP; (2) understand, accept, and implement the therapeutic plan; (3) experience minimal or no unpleasant side effects of therapy; and (4) be confident of ability to manage and cope with this condition.

TABLE 33-10 Causes of Resistant Hypertension

Improper BP measurement
Volume overload
- Excess sodium intake
- Volume retention from kidney disease
- Inadequate diuretic therapy

Drug-induced or other causes
- Nonadherence
- Inadequate drug doses
- Inappropriate combinations of drug therapy
- Nonsteroidal antiinflammatory drugs
- Cocaine, amphetamines, other illicit drugs
- Sympathomimetics (decongestants, anorectics)
- Oral contraceptives
- Corticosteroids
- Cyclosporine and tacrolimus (Prograf)
- Erythropoietin
- Licorice (including some chewing tobacco)
- Selected over-the-counter dietary supplements and medicines (e.g., ephedra, ma huang, bitter orange)

Associated conditions
- Increasing obesity
- Excess alcohol consumption

Identifiable causes of secondary hypertension

From the National Institutes of Health: *Seventh Report of the Joint National Committee on Prevention, Detection, Evaluation, and Treatment of High Blood Pressure,* Washington, DC, 2003, U.S. Department of Health and Human Services.

Nursing Implementation

Health Promotion. Primary prevention of hypertension provides an attractive alternative to the costly cycle of managing hypertension and its complications. Current recommendations for primary prevention are based on lifestyle modifications that have been shown to prevent or delay the expected rise in BP in susceptible people. A diet rich in fruits, vegetables, and low-fat dairy foods, with reduced saturated and total fats, significantly lowers BP (see Table 33-7). This diet has been recommended for primary prevention in the general population. Dietary modifications that do not require active participation of the individual, such as industry reducing the amount of salt added to processed foods, may be even more effective.

To raise awareness about the dangers of high blood pressure, the National Heart, Lung, and Blood Institute has developed special web pages and educational materials for health care professionals, patients, and the public. These include an updated "Your Guide to Lowering High Blood Pressure" web page, which can be found at *www.nhlbi.nih.gov/hbp.*

Individual Patient Evaluation. The majority of cases of hypertension are identified through routine screening procedures such as insurance, preemployment, and military physical examinations. The nurse in these settings, as well as in most other practice settings, is in an ideal position to assess for the presence of hypertension, identify the risk factors for hypertension and coronary artery disease, and teach the patient about these conditions. In addition to BP determination, a complete health assessment should include such factors as age, gender, and race; diet history (including sodium and alcohol intake); weight patterns; and family history of heart disease, stroke, renal disease, and diabetes mellitus. Medications taken, both prescribed and over-the-counter, should be noted. The patient should be asked about

TABLE 33-11 NURSING ASSESSMENT
Hypertension

Subjective Data

Important Health Information

Past health history: Known duration and past workup of high BP; cardiovascular, cerebrovascular, renal, or thyroid disease; diabetes mellitus; pituitary disorders; obesity; dyslipidemia; menopause or hormone replacement status

Medications: Use of any prescription or over-the-counter, illicit, or herbal medications or products; previous use of antihypertensive drug therapy

Functional Health Patterns

Health perception–health management: Family history of hypertension or cardiovascular disease; tobacco use, alcohol use; sedentary lifestyle

Nutritional-metabolic: Usual salt and fat intake; weight gain or loss

Elimination: Nocturia

Activity-exercise: Fatigue; dyspnea on exertion, palpitations on exertion, exertional chest pain; intermittent claudication, muscle cramps

Cognitive-perceptual: Dizziness; blurred vision; paresthesias

Sexual-reproductive: Erectile dysfunction, decreased libido

Coping–stress tolerance: Stressful life events

Objective Data

Cardiovascular

BP consistently >140 mm Hg systolic or >90 mm Hg diastolic, orthostatic change in BP and pulse; abnormal heart sounds; laterally displaced, sustained, forceful apical pulse; diminished or absent peripheral pulses; carotid, renal, or femoral bruits; presence of peripheral edema

Gastrointestinal

Obesity; abnormal waist-hip ratio

Neurologic

Mental status changes

Possible Findings

Abnormal serum electrolytes (especially potassium); ↑ BUN, creatinine, glucose, cholesterol, and triglyceride levels; proteinuria, microalbuminuria, microscopic hematuria; evidence of ischemic heart disease and left ventricular hypertrophy on ECG; evidence of structural heart disease and left ventricular hypertrophy on echocardiogram; evidence of arteriovenous nicking, retinal hemorrhages, and papilledema on funduscopic examination.

BP, Blood pressure; *BUN,* blood urea nitrogen; *ECG,* electrocardiogram.

a previous history of high BP and the results of treatment (if any) (see Table 33-11).

Blood Pressure Measurement. The auscultatory method of BP measurement is recommended (Table 33-13). Initially, the BP is taken at least 2 times, at least 1 minute apart, with the average pressure recorded as the value for that visit. Waiting for at least 1 minute between readings allows the venous blood to drain from the arm and prevents inaccurate readings. Size and placement of BP cuff are important considerations for accurate measurement. Use of a cuff that is too small or too large will result in readings that are falsely high or low, respectively. The cuff is placed snugly around the patient's bare upper arm with the midline of the bladder of the cuff (usually marked on the cuff by the manufacturer) placed above the brachial artery. Use of the forearm is acceptable in patients who have upper arm circumference >20 inches (51 cm) and a thigh or extra-large cuff does not fit the upper arm. When this procedure is used, the forearm is supported at heart level and the clinician auscultates Korotkoff sounds over the radial artery, detects systolic pressure with a Doppler, or uses an oscillometric device. This method provides only a general estimate of SBP, and

TABLE 33-12 NURSING DIAGNOSES AND COLLABORATIVE PROBLEMS
Hypertension

Nursing Diagnoses

Ineffective health maintenance *related to* lack of knowledge of pathology, complications, and management of hypertension

Anxiety *related to* complexity of management regimen, possible complications, and lifestyle changes associated with hypertension

Sexual dysfunction *related to* side effects of antihypertensive medication

Ineffective therapeutic regimen management *related to*
- Lack of knowledge
- Unpleasant side effects of medication
- Return of blood pressure to normal while on medication
- High cost of some medications
- Inconvenient schedule for taking medications
- Lack of trusting relationship with health care provider

Disturbed body image *related to* diagnosis of hypertension

Ineffective tissue perfusion *related to* complications of hypertension (specify):
- Cerebral
- Cardiovascular
- Renal
- Retinal

Collaborative Problems

Potential complication: adverse effects from antihypertensive therapy

Potential complication: hypertensive crisis

Potential complication: stroke

Potential complication: myocardial infarction

DBP is largely overestimated. The accuracy of these methods has not been validated.[8]

BP measurements of both arms should be performed initially to detect any differences between arms. Atherosclerotic narrowing of the subclavian artery can cause a falsely low reading on the side where the narrowing occurs. Therefore the arm with the higher reading should be used for all subsequent BP measurements.

The patient's arm is uncovered and placed at the level of the heart for BP measurement. For BP measurements taken in the sitting position, the arm is raised to the level of the heart and supported. For measurements taken in a supine position, the arm should also be raised to heart level and supported (e.g., small pillow). If the arm is resting on the bed, it will be below heart level.

Orthostatic (or postural) changes in BP and pulse should be measured in older adults, in people taking antihypertensive drugs, and in patients who report symptoms consistent with reduced BP upon standing (e.g., light-headedness, dizziness, syncope). Serial BP and pulse are measured with the patient in the supine, sitting, and standing positions. BP and pulse are initially measured with the patient in the supine position after at least 2 to 3 minutes of rest, measured again within 1 to 2 minutes of repositioning the patient in the sitting position with legs dangling, and measured within 1 to 2 minutes of repositioning the patient to the standing position. Usually the SBP decreases slightly (<10 mm Hg) on standing, whereas the DBP and pulse increase slightly. A decrease of 20 mm Hg or more in SBP, a decrease of 10 mm Hg or more in DBP, and/or an increase of 20 beats/minute or more in pulse from supine to standing is defined as **orthostatic hypotension.** Common causes of orthostatic hypotension include intravascular volume loss and inadequate vasoconstrictor mechanisms related to disease or medications.

In the acute care setting, BP measurement is typically performed to evaluate vital signs, volume status, and effects of medications as

TABLE 33-13 Manual Blood Pressure Measurement

The patient should not have smoked, exercised, or ingested caffeine within 30 min before measurement.

1. Seat patient with legs uncrossed and back supported. Bare patient's arm and support it at heart level.
2. Begin measurement after patient has rested quietly for 5 min. Ask patient to relax as much as possible and not to talk during the measurement.
3. Measure and record BP in both arms initially.
4. Select the appropriate cuff size. The rubber bladder should nearly (at least 80%) or completely encircle the arm. Cuff width should be at least 40% of the arm circumference.
5. Measurements should be taken with a recently calibrated aneroid or mercury sphygmomanometer, or electronic oscillometric device.
6. For auscultatory measurement, estimate systolic blood pressure (SBP) by palpating the radial pulse and inflating the cuff until the pulse is obliterated. Inflate the cuff 20 to 30 mm Hg above this level.
7. Deflate the cuff at a rate of 2 to 3 mm Hg/sec.
8. Record the SBP and the diastolic blood pressure (DBP). Note the SBP when the first of two or more Korotkoff sounds is heard and the DBP when the disappearance of sound occurs.
9. Average two or more readings (taken at intervals of at least 1 min). Obtain additional readings if the first two readings differ by more than 5 mm Hg.
10. Provide the patient (verbally and in writing) with the BP reading, BP goal, and recommendations for follow-up.

From the National Institutes of Health: *Seventh Report of the Joint National Committee on Prevention, Detection, Evaluation, and Treatment of High Blood Pressure,* Washington, DC, 2003, U.S. Department of Health and Human Services.
BP, Blood pressure.

TABLE 33-14 PATIENT AND FAMILY TEACHING GUIDE Hypertension

When presenting information to the patient and/or family, the nurse should do the following:

General Instructions

1. Provide the numeric value of the patient's BP and explain what it means (e.g., high, low, normal, borderline). Encourage patient to monitor BP at home.
2. Inform the patient that hypertension is usually asymptomatic and symptoms do not reliably indicate BP levels.
3. Explain that hypertension means high blood pressure and does not relate to a "hyper" personality.
4. Explain that long-term follow-up and therapy are necessary to treat hypertension. Therapy involves lifestyle changes (e.g., weight management, sodium reduction, smoking cessation) and, in most cases, medications.
5. Explain that therapy will not cure, but should control hypertension.
6. Tell patient that controlled hypertension is usually compatible with an excellent prognosis and a normal lifestyle.
7. Explain the potential dangers of uncontrolled hypertension.

Instructions Related to Medications

1. Be specific about the names, actions, dosages, and side effects of prescribed medications.
2. Tell the patient to plan regular and convenient times for taking medications and measuring BP.
3. Tell the patient not to discontinue drugs abruptly because withdrawal may cause a severe hypertensive reaction.
4. Tell the patient not to double up on doses when a dose is missed.
5. Inform the patient that, if BP increases, the patient should not take an increased medication dosage before consulting with the health care provider.
6. Tell the patient not to take a medication belonging to someone else.
7. Tell the patient to supplement diet with foods high in potassium (e.g., citrus fruits and green leafy vegetables) if taking potassium-losing diuretics.
8. Tell the patient to avoid hot baths, excessive amounts of alcohol, and strenuous exercise within 3 hours of taking medications that promote vasodilation.
9. Many medications cause orthostatic hypotension. Explain that the effects of orthostatic hypotension can be reduced by instructing the patient to arise slowly from bed, sit on the side of the bed for a few minutes, stand slowly, not stand still for prolonged periods of time, do leg exercises to increase venous return, sleep with the head of the bed raised or on pillows, and lie or sit down when dizziness occurs.
10. Many medications cause sexual problems (e.g., erectile dysfunction, decreased libido). Encourage the patient to consult with the health care provider about changing drugs or dosages if sexual problems develop.
11. Inform the patient that the side effects of medication(s) often diminish with time.
12. Caution about potentially high-risk over-the-counter medications, such as high-sodium antacids, appetite suppressants, and cold and sinus medications. Advise patient to read warning labels and to consult with a pharmacist.

BP, Blood pressure.

opposed to the diagnosis of hypertension. Medications, acute illness, bed rest, and alterations in usual diet all have an impact on blood pressure values. The health care provider should be informed of any patient with a persistent elevation in BP. These patients should also be evaluated for hypertension after discharge.[8]

Screening Programs. Screening programs in the community are widely used to assess people's BP. At the time of the BP measurement, each person should be informed in writing of the numeric value of the reading and, if necessary, why further evaluation is important. Effort and resources should be focused on controlling BP in the person already identified as having hypertension; identifying and controlling BP in at-risk groups such as African Americans, obese people, and blood relatives of people with hypertension; and screening those with limited access to the health care system.

Cardiovascular Risk Factor Modification. Education regarding cardiovascular risk factors is appropriate for individual and targeted screening programs. Modifiable cardiovascular risk factors include hypertension, obesity, diabetes mellitus, tobacco use, and physical inactivity. Risk factors can easily be identified and modification discussed with the patient. (Health-promoting behaviors for cardiovascular risk factors are discussed in Chapter 34, Table 34-3.)

Ambulatory and Home Care. The primary nursing responsibilities for long-term management of hypertension are to assist the patient in reducing BP and complying with the treatment plan. Nursing actions include patient and family teaching (Table 33-14), detection and reporting of adverse treatment effects, compliance assessment and enhancement, and evaluation of therapeutic effectiveness. Patient and family teaching includes the following: (1) nutritional therapy, (2) drug therapy, (3) physical activity, (4) home monitoring of BP (if appropriate), and (5) tobacco cessation (if applicable).

Physical Activity. Physical activity is bodily movement produced by skeletal muscles that requires energy expenditure. Health benefits from physical activity can be achieved with moderate-intensity aerobic activities (e.g., brisk walking). The goal for all adults is at least 30 min/day, most days of the week.[1] Generally physical activity is more likely to be sustained if it is safe and enjoyable, fits easily into the daily schedule, and does not generate financial or social costs. Shopping malls in many communities are open early in the morning (before shopping hours) and provide a warm, safe, flat area for walking. In some communities, health clubs offer special "off-peak" rates to encourage physical activity among older adults. Cardiac rehabilitation programs offer supervised exercise with education about reduction of cardiovascular risk factors. Nurses can assist people with hypertension to increase their physical activity by identifying and communicating the need for increased activity, explaining the difference between physical activity and moderate-intensity aerobic exercise, assisting in initiating an exercise plan, and following up appropriately.

Home BP Monitoring. Some patients benefit from regularly monitoring their BP at home. Home BP measurement may give a more valid indication of BP because the patient is more relaxed. The patient should be instructed to take BP readings after resting quietly for 3 to 5 minutes in a comfortable chair with the upper arm at heart level. The average of three readings, separated by at least 1 minute, should be used as the BP reading.[3] The patient should be advised not to smoke, exercise, or ingest caffeine for 30 minutes prior to taking BP measurements. It is important to emphasize to the patient that a single reading is not as important as a series of readings over a period of time. The patient should be instructed to take BP readings daily when treatment is initiated or medications are adjusted and weekly once the BP has stabilized. A log of the BP measurements should be maintained by the patient and brought to office visits. Devices that have memory or printouts of the readings are recommended to facilitate accurate reporting.[8]

Home BP readings may help achieve patient compliance by reinforcing the need to remain on therapy. A patient may become excessively concerned with the BP readings when using home monitoring. Generally, however, this practice should reassure the patient that the treatment is effective.

Patient Compliance. A major problem in the long-term management of the patient with hypertension is poor compliance with the prescribed treatment plan. The reasons are many and include inadequate patient teaching, unpleasant side effects of drugs, return of BP to normal range while on medication, lack of motivation, high cost of drugs, lack of insurance, and lack of a trusting relationship between the patient and the health care provider. In addition to using BP determinations as an indicator of compliance, the nurse should also assess the patient's diet, activity level, and lifestyle.

Individual assessment to determine the reasons that the patient is not complying with the treatment plan and the development of an individualized plan with the patient's assistance are essential. The plan should be compatible with the patient's personality, habits, and lifestyle. Active patient participation increases the likelihood of adherence to the treatment plan. Measures such as involving the patient in scheduling medication convenient to a daily routine, helping the patient link pill taking with another daily activity, selecting medications that are affordable, and involving family members (if necessary) help increase patient compliance. Substituting combination tablets for multiple drugs once the BP is stabilized may also facilitate compliance, because the patient has to take fewer drugs each day and the cost may be less. It is important to help the patient and the family understand that hypertension is a chronic condition that cannot be cured but can be controlled with drug therapy, diet therapy, physical activity, periodic evaluation, and other relevant lifestyle changes.

Evaluation

The overall expected outcomes are that the patient with hypertension will

- achieve and maintain goal BP as defined for the individual
- understand, accept, and implement the therapeutic plan
- experience minimal or no unpleasant side effects of therapy

EVIDENCE-BASED PRACTICE

Does Reduction in Dietary Salt Decrease Blood Pressure?

Clinical Question

In persons with normal or elevated blood pressure (P), what is the effect of a modest reduction in salt intake (I) compared to no alteration in salt intake (C) on blood pressure (BP) reduction (O)?

Best Available Evidence

Systematic review (meta-analysis) of randomized controlled trials (RCTs)

Critical Appraisal and Synthesis of Evidence

- Meta-analysis of 11 RCTs (n = 2220) of normotensive individuals who reduced their salt intake for 4 or more wk had a median reduction in their salt intake of 4.4 g/day and an average decrease of 2 mm Hg in their systolic BP and 1 mm Hg in their diastolic BP.
- Meta-analysis of 17 RCTs (n = 734) of hypertensive patients who reduced their salt intake for 4 or more wk had a median reduction in their salt intake of 4.6 g/day and an average decrease of 5 mm Hg in their systolic BP and 3 mm Hg in their diastolic BP.

Conclusions

- Reduction of salt intake to 5 to 6 g/day for 1 mo or more will lower BP and likely decrease risk for cardiovascular disease.
- Within the daily intake range of 3 to 12 g/day, the lower the salt intake, the lower the BP.

Implications for Nursing Practice

- Include assessment of usual salt intake during nutritional assessment.
- Include in patient education that a modest reduction in salt to 5-6 g/day will decrease BP.
- Provide appropriate educational materials for how to achieve salt intake reduction (e.g., DASH eating plan [see Table 33-7]).
- Have patient consult with dietitian to assist in teaching about salt reduction in diet.

Reference for Evidence

He FJ, MacGregor GA: Effect of longer-term modest salt reduction on blood pressure. *The Cochrane Database of Systematic Reviews* 4, 2004.

PICO: P, Patient population of interest; *I*, intervention or area of interest; *C*, comparison of interest or comparison group; *O*, outcome(s) of interest (see p. 6).

GERONTOLOGIC CONSIDERATIONS
HYPERTENSION

The number of Americans age 65 and older continues to rise, and will comprise 20% of the population by the year 2030.[12] The prevalence of hypertension increases with age. In 1999 to 2000, approximately 81% of adults in the United States with hypertension were 45 years of age or older.[13] The lifetime risk of developing hypertension is approximately 90% for middle-aged (age 55 to 65) and older (age >65) normotensive men and women.[14] In industrialized countries, SBP rises throughout the life span, whereas DBP rises until approximately age 55 and then declines due to an increase in central arterial stiffness.[15] Isolated systolic hypertension (ISH) is the most common form of hypertension in individuals over 50 years of age. Additionally, older adults are more likely to have white coat hypertension.[8]

The following age-related physical changes play a role in the pathophysiology of hypertension in the older adult: (1) loss of tissue elasticity; (2) increased collagen content and stiffness of the myocardium; (3) increased peripheral vascular resistance; (4) decreased adrenergic receptor sensitivity; (5) blunting of baroreceptor reflexes; (6) decreased renal function; and (7) decreased renin response to sodium and water depletion. In the older adult taking antihypertensive medication, absorption of some drugs may be altered as a result of decreased splanchnic blood flow. Metabolism and excretion of drugs may also be prolonged.

Careful technique is important in assessing BP in older adults. In some older people, there is a wide gap between the first Korotkoff sound and subsequent beats. This is called the *auscultatory gap*. Failure to inflate the cuff high enough may result in seriously underestimating the SBP. This problem can be avoided by palpating the brachial or radial artery while inflating the cuff to a level above the disappearance of the pulse.

Older adults are sensitive to BP changes. Therefore reducing SBP to <120 mm Hg in a person with long-standing hypertension could lead to inadequate cerebral blood flow. Older adults also produce less renin and are more resistant to the effects of ACE inhibitors and angiotensin II receptor blockers.

Because of varying degrees of impaired baroreceptor reflex mechanisms, orthostatic hypotension occurs often in older adults, especially in those with ISH. Orthostatic hypotension in this age-group is often associated with volume depletion or chronic disease states, such as decreased renal and hepatic function or electrolyte imbalance. To reduce the likelihood of orthostatic hypotension, antihypertensive drugs should be started at low doses and increased cautiously. BP and pulse should be measured in the supine, sitting, and standing positions at every visit.

HYPERTENSIVE CRISIS

Hypertensive crisis is a severe and abrupt elevation in BP, arbitrarily defined as a DBP >140 mm Hg.[16] The rate of rise of BP is more important than the absolute value in determining the need for emergency treatment. Patients with chronic hypertension can tolerate much higher BP than previously normotensive people. Prompt recognition and management of hypertensive crisis is essential to decrease the threat to organ function and life.

Hypertensive crisis occurs most commonly in patients with a history of hypertension who have failed to comply with their prescribed medications or who have been undermedicated. In this setting, rising BP is thought to trigger endothelial damage and the release of vasoconstrictor substances. A vicious cycle of BP elevation ensues leading to life-threatening damage to target organs. Hypertensive crisis related to cocaine or crack use is becoming a more frequent problem. Other drugs such as amphetamines, phencyclidine (PCP), and lysergic acid diethylamide (LSD) may also precipitate hypertensive crisis that may be complicated by drug-induced seizures, stroke, MI, or encephalopathy. Table 33-15 lists causes of hypertensive crisis.

TABLE 33-15 Causes of Hypertensive Crisis

- Exacerbation of chronic hypertension
- Renovascular hypertension
- Preeclampsia, eclampsia
- Pheochromocytoma
- Drugs (cocaine, amphetamines)
- Monoamine oxidase inhibitors taken with tyramine-containing foods
- Rebound hypertension (from abrupt withdrawal of some hypertensive drugs such as clonidine [Catapres] or β-adrenergic blockers)
- Necrotizing vasculitis
- Head injury
- Acute aortic dissection

Hypertensive crisis is classified by the degree of organ damage and the rapidity with which the BP must be lowered. *Hypertensive emergency,* which develops over hours to days, is a situation in which a patient's BP is severely elevated (>180/120 mm Hg) with evidence of acute target organ damage, especially damage to the central nervous system.[1] Hypertensive emergencies can precipitate encephalopathy, intracranial or subarachnoid hemorrhage, acute left ventricular failure with pulmonary edema, MI, renal failure, dissecting aortic aneurysm, and retinopathy.[16] *Hypertensive urgency,* which develops over days to weeks, is a situation in which a patient's BP is severely elevated but there is no clinical evidence of target organ damage.

Clinical Manifestations

A hypertensive emergency is often manifested as *hypertensive encephalopathy,* a syndrome in which a sudden rise in BP is associated with headache, nausea, vomiting, seizures, confusion, stupor, and coma. The manifestations of encephalopathy are the results of increased cerebral capillary permeability leading to cerebral edema and a disruption in cerebral function.[16] Other common manifestations are blurred vision and transient blindness from papilledema and retinopathy.

Renal insufficiency ranging from minor impairment to complete renal shutdown may occur. Rapid cardiac decompensation ranging from unstable angina to infarction and pulmonary edema is also possible with patients presenting with chest pain and dyspnea. Aortic dissection causes excruciating chest and back pain often accompanied by diaphoresis and the loss of pulses in an extremity.

Patient assessment is extremely important, especially monitoring for signs of neurologic dysfunction, retinal damage, heart failure, pulmonary edema, and renal failure. The neurologic manifestations are often similar to the presentation of a stroke. However, a hypertensive crisis does not show focal or lateralizing signs often seen with a stroke.

NURSING *and* COLLABORATIVE MANAGEMENT HYPERTENSIVE CRISIS

BP level alone is a poor indicator of the seriousness of the patient's condition and is not the major factor in deciding the treatment for a hypertensive crisis. The association between elevated BP and signs of new or progressive target organ damage (e.g., cerebrovascular, cardiac, retinal, or renal involvement) determines the seriousness of the situation.

Hypertensive emergencies require hospitalization, intravenous (IV) administration of antihypertensive drugs, and intensive care monitoring. When treating hypertensive emergencies, the mean arterial pressure (MAP) is often used instead of systolic and diastolic readings to guide and evaluate therapy. MAP is calculated as follows:

$$MAP = \frac{(SBP + 2\ DBP)}{3}$$

The initial treatment goal is to decrease MAP by no more than 25% within minutes to 1 hour. If the patient is stable, the target goal for BP is 160/100 to 110 mm Hg over the next 2 to 6 hours. Lowering the BP excessively may decrease cerebral, coronary, or renal perfusion and could precipitate a stroke, acute MI, or renal failure. Additional gradual reductions toward a normal BP should be implemented over the next 24 to 48 hours if the patient is clinically stable. Special circumstances include patients with aortic dissection, who should have their SBP lowered to <100 mm Hg if tolerated. Another exception is patients with acute ischemic stroke, in whom BP may be lowered to enable the use of thrombolytic agents. Finally, an elevated BP in the immediate poststroke period may be a compensatory response to improve cerebral perfusion to ischemic brain tissue. Currently, there is no clear evidence supporting the use of antihypertensive medications in these patients[1] (see Chapter 58).

IV drugs used for hypertensive emergencies include vasodilators (e.g., sodium nitroprusside [Nitropress], nitroglycerin [Tridil], fenoldopam [Corlopam], hydralazine [Apresoline], nicardipine [Cardene]), adrenergic inhibitors (e.g., phentolamine [Regitine], labetalol [Normodyne], esmolol [Brevibloc]), and the ACE inhibitor enalaprilat (Vasotec IV).[1] Sodium nitroprusside is the most effective IV drug for the treatment of hypertensive emergencies. Fenoldopam selectively activates dopamine receptors, resulting in renal and systemic vasodilation. Oral agents may be administered in addition to IV drugs to help make an earlier transition to long-term therapy. The mechanisms of action and the adverse effects of these drugs are presented in Table 33-8.

***Drug Alert** - Labetalol (Normodyne)*

- *Instruct patient not to discontinue drug abruptly as this may precipitate angina and/or heart failure.*

Antihypertensive drugs administered IV have a rapid (within seconds to minutes) onset of action. The patient's BP and pulse should be taken every 2 to 3 minutes during the initial administration of these drugs. The use of an intraarterial line (see Chapter 66) or an automated, noninvasive BP machine to monitor the BP is required. The rate of drug administration is titrated according to the level of MAP or BP. It is important to prevent hypotension and its effects in a person whose body has adjusted to an elevated BP. An excessive reduction in BP may cause stroke, MI, or visual changes. Continual ECG monitoring is frequently done to observe for cardiac dysrhythmias. Extreme caution is needed in treating the patient with coronary artery disease or cerebrovascular insufficiency. Hourly urinary output should be measured to assess renal perfusion. Careful monitoring of vital signs and urinary output provides information regarding the effectiveness of these drugs and the patient's response to therapy. Patients receiving IV antihypertensive drugs may be restricted to bed; getting up (e.g., to use the commode) may cause severe cerebral ischemia and fainting.

Regular, ongoing assessment is essential to evaluate the patient with severe hypertension. Frequent neurologic checks, including level of consciousness, pupillary size and reaction, movement of extremities, and reactions to stimuli, help detect any changes in the patient's condition. Cardiac, pulmonary, and renal systems should be monitored for decompensation caused by the severe elevation in BP (e.g., pulmonary edema, heart failure, angina, renal failure).

Hypertensive urgencies usually do not require IV medications but can be managed with oral agents. The patient with a hypertensive urgency may not need hospitalization, but requires frequent follow-up. The oral drugs most frequently used for hypertensive urgencies are captopril (Capoten), labetalol (Normodyne), and clonidine (Catapres) (see Table 33-8). The disadvantage of oral medications is the inability to regulate the dosage moment to moment, as can be done with IV medications. If a patient with a hypertensive urgency is not hospitalized, outpatient follow-up should be arranged within 24 hours.

***Drug Alert** - Clonidine (Catapres)*

- *Instruct patient*
  - *to change positions slowly to limit orthostatic hypotension.*
  - *to avoid hazardous activities as drug may cause drowsiness.*
  - *not to discontinue abruptly to prevent rebound hypertension.*

A patient with severe elevation of BP but without target organ damage may not require emergent drug therapy or hospitalization. Allowing the patient to sit for 20 or 30 minutes in a quiet environment may significantly reduce BP. Oral drugs may then be instituted or adjusted. Additional nursing interventions include encouraging the patient to verbalize any concerns or fears, answering questions regarding hypertension, and eliminating any adverse stimuli (e.g., excess noise) in the patient's environment.

Once the hypertensive crisis is resolved, it is important to determine the cause. The patient will need appropriate management and extensive education to avoid future crises.

CRITICAL THINKING EXERCISE

CASE STUDY

Primary Hypertension

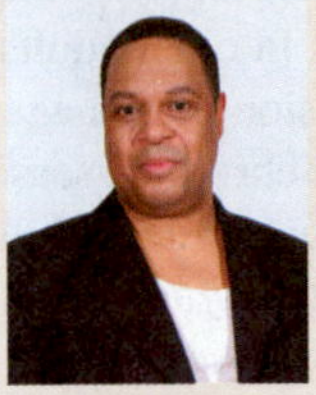
Case Study photo ©iStockphoto.com/ Matthew Gough.

Patient Profile. Roger is a 45-year-old African American man with no previous history of hypertension. At a screening clinic 1 month ago, his BP was found to be 180/120 mm Hg. He has been followed by his primary care provider for the past month. During this time he has been taking hydrochlorothiazide 12.5 mg/day.

Subjective Data

- Father died of stroke at age 60
- Mother is alive but has hypertension
- States that he feels fine and is not a "hyper" person
- Smokes one pack of cigarettes daily
- Drinks a six-pack of beer on Friday and Saturday nights
- Has been told that BP medication interferes with sexual relationships

Objective Data

Physical Examination

- Retinopathy
- Blood pressure: 166/108 mm Hg
- Sustained apical impulse palpable in the fourth intercostal space just lateral to the midclavicular line

Diagnostic Studies

- ECG: left ventricular hypertrophy
- Urinalysis: protein 30 mg/dl (0.3 g/L)
- Serum creatinine level: 1.6 mg/dl (141 mmol/L)

Collaborative Care

- Low-sodium diet
- Hydrochlorothiazide 25 mg/day
- Captopril (Capoten) 50 mg bid

Critical Thinking Questions

1. What risk factors for hypertension does Roger have?
2. What evidence of target organ damage is present?
3. What misconceptions about hypertension should be corrected?
4. Based on the assessment data presented, what are the nursing priorities for Roger? Include one or more priority nursing diagnoses. What are the collaborative problems?
5. What areas would you focus on in teaching this patient about his illness?

NCLEX EXAMINATION REVIEW QUESTIONS

The number of the question corresponds to the same-numbered objective at the beginning of the chapter.

1. If a patient has decreased cardiac output caused by fluid volume deficit and marked vasodilation, the regulatory mechanism that will increase the blood pressure by improving both of these is
   a. release of antidiuretic hormone (ADH).
   b. secretion of prostaglandins PGE_2 and PGI_2.
   c. stimulation of the sympathetic nervous system.
   d. activation of the renin-angiotensin-aldosterone system.
2. While obtaining subjective assessment data from a patient with hypertension, the nurse recognizes that a modifiable risk factor for the development of hypertension is
   a. a low-calcium diet.
   b. excessive alcohol consumption.
   c. a family history of hypertension.
   d. consumption of a high-protein diet.
3. Target organ damage that can occur from hypertension includes
   a. headache and dizziness.
   b. retinopathy and diabetes.
   c. hypercholesterolemia and renal dysfunction.
   d. renal dysfunction and left ventricular hypertrophy.
4. A high-risk population that should be targeted in the primary prevention of hypertension is
   a. overweight children.
   b. African Americans.
   c. business executives.
   d. middle-aged women.
5. In teaching a patient with hypertension about controlling the condition, the nurse recognizes that
   a. all patients with elevated BP require medication.
   b. it is not necessary to limit salt in the diet if taking a diuretic.
   c. obese persons must achieve a normal weight in order to lower BP.
   d. lifestyle modifications are indicated for all persons with elevated BP.
6. A major consideration in the management of the older adult with hypertension is to
   a. prevent pseudohypertension from converting to true hypertension.
   b. recognize that the older adult is less likely to comply with the drug therapy than a younger adult.
   c. ensure that the patient receives larger initial doses of antihypertensive drugs because of impaired absorption.
   d. use careful technique in assessing the BP of the patient because of the possible presence of an auscultatory gap.
7. A patient with newly diagnosed hypertension has a blood pressure of 158/98 after 12 months of exercise and diet modifications. The nurse advises the patient that
   a. medication may be required because the BP is still not at goal.
   b. continued BP monitoring every 3 months is all that will be necessary for treatment.
   c. because lifestyle modifications were not effective, they do not need to be continued and drugs will be used.
   d. he will have to make more vigorous changes in his lifestyle if he wants to stay off medication for his hypertension.
8. A patient is admitted to the hospital in hypertensive crisis. The nurse recognizes that hypertensive urgency differs from hypertensive emergency in that
   a. the BP is always higher in a hypertensive emergency.
   b. hypertensive emergencies always require intraarterial BP measurement.
   c. hypertensive urgency is treated with rest and tranquilizers to lower the BP.
   d. hypertensive emergencies are associated with evidence of target organ damage.

REFERENCES

1. Seventh Report of the Joint National Committee on Detection, Evaluation, and Treatment of High Blood Pressure (JNC-7), *JAMA* 289:2560, 2003. Available at *www.nhlbi.nih.gov/guidelines/hypertension/index.htm.*
2. American Heart Association: *Heart and stroke statistics—2005 update,* Dallas, 2005, American Heart Association.
3. Mosca L, Appel LJ, Benjamin EJ, et al: Evidence-based guidelines for cardiovascular disease prevention in women, *Arterioscler Thromb Vasc Biol* 24(3):e29, 2004.
4. Mosca L, Ferris A, Fabunmi R, et al: Tracking women's awareness of heart disease: an American Heart Association national study, *Circulation* 109:573, 2004.
5. Kountz DS: Hypertension in ethnic populations: tailoring treatments, *Clin Cornerstone* 6:39, 2004.
6. Hajjar I, Kotchen TA: Trends in prevalence, awareness, treatment and control of hypertension in the United States, 1988–2000, *JAMA* 290:199, 2003.
7. U.S. Department of Health and Human Services: *Healthy people 2010,* vol 1, ed 2. Objectives for improving health, Part A, focus area 12: heart disease and stroke, Washington, DC, 2001, U.S. Department of Health and Human Services. Available at *www.healthypeople.gov/Document/html/volume1/12heart.htm.*
8. Pickering TG, Hall JE, Appel LJ, et al: Recommendations for blood pressure measurement in humans and experimental animals: Part 1: Blood pressure measurement in humans, *Hypertension* 45:142, 2005.
9. Weir MR: Dietary salt, blood pressure, and microalbuminuria, *J Clin Hypertension* 6:23, 2004.
10. National Heart, Lung, and Blood Institute: *Your guide to lowering your blood pressure with DASH,* NIH Publication No 06-4082, Bethesda, Md, 2006, National Heart, Lung, and Blood Institute. Available at *www.nhlbi.nih.gov/health/public/heart/hdp/dash.*
11. Yan LL, Liu K, Matthews KA, et al: Psychosocial factors and risk of hypertension: the Coronary Artery Risk Development in Young Adults (CARDIA) study, *JAMA* 290:2138, 2003.
12. Clark AP, Baldwin K: Best practices for care of older adults: highlights and summary from the preconference, *Clin Nurse Spec* 18:288, 2004.
13. Fields LE, Burt VL, Cutler JA, et al: The burden of adult hypertension in the United States 1999 to 2000: a rising tide, *Hypertension* 44:398, 2004.
14. Vasan RS, Beiser A, Seshadri S, et al: Residual lifetime risk for developing hypertension in middle-aged women and men: the Framingham Heart Study, *JAMA* 287:1003, 2002.
15. Mitchell GF, Parise H, Benjamin EJ, et al: Changes in arterial stiffness and wave reflection with advancing age in healthy men and women: the Framingham Heart Study, *Hypertension* 43:1239, 2004.
16. Huether SE, McCance KL: *Understanding pathophysiology,* ed 3, St Louis, 2004, Mosby.

RESOURCES

American Heart Association
800-AHA-USA-1 or 800-242-8721
www.americanheart.org

American Society of Hypertension
212-696-9099
www.ash-us.org

National High Blood Pressure Education Program
301-592-8573
www.nhlbi.nih.gov/hbp/index.html

For additional Internet resources, see the website for this book at *http://evolve.elsevier.com/Lewis/medsurg.*

The thousand mysteries around us would not trouble but interest us, if only we had cheerful, healthy hearts.

Friedrich Wilhelm Nietzsche

34 *Nursing Management* Coronary Artery Disease and Acute Coronary Syndrome

Linda Griego Martinez and Linda Bucher

LEARNING OBJECTIVES

1. Describe the etiology and pathophysiology of coronary artery disease, angina, and acute coronary syndrome.
2. Identify risk factors for coronary artery disease and the nursing role in the promotion of therapeutic lifestyle changes in patients at risk.
3. Compare and contrast the precipitating factors, clinical manifestations, and collaborative care and nursing management of the patient with coronary artery disease and chronic stable angina.
4. Describe the clinical manifestations, complications, diagnostic study results, and collaborative care of the patient with acute coronary syndrome.
5. Describe the pathophysiology of myocardial infarction from the onset of injury through the healing process.
6. Identify commonly used drug therapy in treating patients with coronary artery disease and acute coronary syndrome.
7. Identify key issues to include in the rehabilitation of patients recovering from acute coronary syndrome and coronary revascularization procedures.
8. Describe the precipitating factors, clinical presentation, and collaborative care of patients who are at risk for or have experienced sudden cardiac death.

KEY TERMS

acute coronary syndrome, p. 802
angina, p. 796
atherosclerosis, p. 785
chronic stable angina, p. 796
collateral circulation, p. 786
coronary artery disease, p. 785
coronary revascularization, p. 801
metabolic equivalent (MET), p. 817
myocardial infarction, p. 803
percutaneous coronary intervention, p. 801
Prinzmetal's angina, p. 797
silent ischemia, p. 797
stent, p. 801
sudden cardiac death, p. 817
unstable angina, p. 802

Electronic Resources

Supplemental content related to Chapter 34 can be found . . .

Companion CD

- Stress-Busting Kit for Nursing Students
- Interactive Case Study: Myocardial Infarction
- NCLEX Examination Review Questions
- Comprehensive Glossary

Evolve Website

http://evolve.elsevier.com/Lewis/medsurg

- Content Updates
- Key Points (Printable and CD/MP3 Download)
- Concept Map Creator
- Expanded Audio Glossary
- Key Term Flash Cards
- Audio Lecture: Risk Factors for Coronary Artery Disease
- Customizable Nursing Care Plan: Acute Coronary Syndrome
- Patient and Family Instruction Guides in English and Spanish:
  - Decreasing Risk Factors for Coronary Artery Disease
  - FITT Physical Activity Guidelines after Acute Coronary Syndrome
- Electronic Calculators
- WebLinks

Cardiovascular disease is the major cause of death in the United States (Fig. 34-1). Coronary artery disease (CAD) is the most common type of cardiovascular disease and accounts for the majority of these deaths.[1] Patients with CAD can be asymptomatic or develop chronic stable angina. Unstable angina (UA) and myocardial infarction (MI) are more serious manifestations of CAD and are termed acute coronary syndrome (ACS). The American Heart Association (AHA) estimates that 1.2 million Americans will have an MI annually and about one fourth of these will die in an emergency department (ED) or before reaching a hospital. Although the mortality rate from MI decreased by 26.3% between 1999 and 2002 due to advances in treatment, it

Reviewed by Kelly Dodds, RN, MSN, APRN-BC, Clinical Nurse Specialist, Barnes-Jewish Hospital, St Louis, Mo; and Linda M. Hoke, RN, PhD, CCRN, Clinical Nurse Specialist, Cardiac Care Unit, Hospital of the University of Pennsylvania, Philadelphia, Pa, and Adjunct Assistant Professor in Nursing in the Associate Faculty of the School of Nursing, University of Pennsylvania School of Nursing, Philadelphia, Pa.

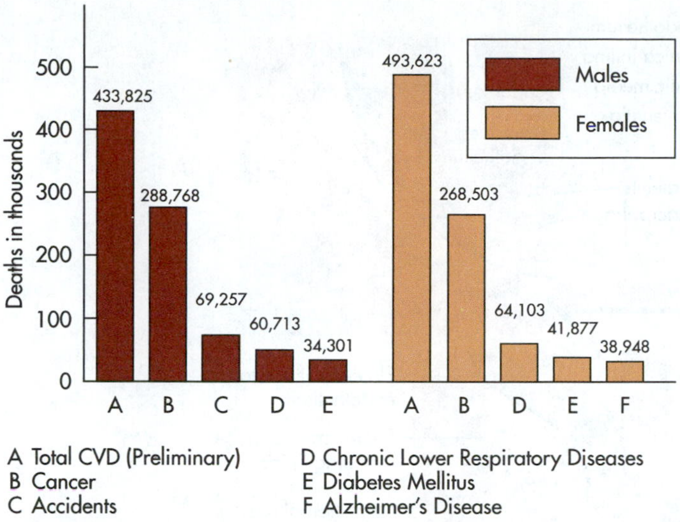

FIG. 34-1 Leading causes of death for all men and women. *CVD,* Cardiovascular disease.

remains the leading cause of all cardiovascular disease deaths and deaths in general.

CORONARY ARTERY DISEASE

Coronary artery disease is a type of blood vessel disorder that is included in the general category of atherosclerosis. The term **atherosclerosis** is derived from two Greek words: *athere,* meaning "fatty mush," and *skleros,* meaning "hard." This combination indicates that atherosclerosis begins as soft deposits of fat that harden with age. Atherosclerosis is often referred to as "hardening of the arteries." Although this condition can occur in any artery in the body, the *atheromas* (fatty deposits) have a preference for the coronary arteries. Arteriosclerotic heart disease, cardiovascular heart disease, ischemic heart disease, coronary heart disease, and CAD are all terms used to describe this disease process.

Etiology and Pathophysiology

Atherosclerosis is the major cause of CAD. It is characterized by a focal deposit of cholesterol and lipids, primarily within the intimal wall of the artery. The genesis of plaque formation is the result of complex interactions between the components of the blood and the elements forming the vascular wall.[2] Inflammation and endothelial injury play a central role in the development of atherosclerosis.

Intact normal endothelium is more than a simple barrier between the vessel wall and the lumen of the vessel. Normally, it is nonreactive to platelets and leukocytes, as well as coagulation, fibrinolytic, and complement factors. However, the endothelial lining can be injured as a result of tobacco use, hyperlipidemia, hypertension, diabetes, hyperhomocysteinemia, and infection (e.g., *Chlamydia pneumoniae,* herpes) causing a local inflammatory response[3,4] (Fig. 34-2, *A*).

C-reactive protein (CRP), a nonspecific marker of inflammation, is increased in many patients with CAD. Chronic exposure to even minor elevations of CRP can trigger the rupture of plaques and promote the oxidation of low-density lipoprotein (LDL) cholesterol, leading to increased uptake by macrophages in the endothelial lining.[5,6]

Developmental Stages. CAD is a progressive disease that takes many years to develop. When it becomes symptomatic, the disease process is usually well advanced. The stages of development in atherosclerosis are (1) fatty streak, (2) fibrous plaque resulting from smooth muscle cell proliferation, and (3) complicated lesion.

Fatty Streak. *Fatty streaks,* the earliest lesions of atherosclerosis, are characterized by lipid-filled smooth muscle cells.[2] As streaks of fat develop within the smooth muscle cells, a yellow tinge appears. Fatty streaks can be observed in the coronary arteries by age 15 and involve an increasing amount of surface area as the patient ages. It is generally believed that treatment that lowers LDL cholesterol may reverse this process[4] (Fig. 34-2, *B*).

Fibrous Plaque. The *fibrous plaque stage* is the beginning of progressive changes in the endothelium of the arterial wall. These changes can appear in the coronary arteries by age 30 and increase with age.

Normally the endothelium repairs itself immediately, but in the person with CAD the endothelium is not rapidly replaced, allowing LDLs and growth factors from platelets to stimulate smooth muscle proliferation and thickening of the arterial wall. Once endothelial injury has occurred, lipoproteins (carrier proteins within the bloodstream) transport cholesterol and other lipids into the arterial intima. The fatty streak is eventually covered by collagen forming a fibrous plaque that appears grayish or whitish.[2,4] These plaques can form on one portion of the artery or in a circular fashion involving the entire lumen. The borders can be smooth or irregular with rough, jagged edges.[2] The result is a narrowing of the vessel lumen and a reduction in blood flow to the distal tissues (Fig. 34-2, *C*).

Complicated Lesion. The final stage in the development of the atherosclerotic lesion is the most dangerous. As the fibrous plaque grows, continued inflammation can result in plaque instability, ulceration, and rupture.[4] Once the integrity of the artery's inner wall

GENDER DIFFERENCES
Coronary Artery Disease

Men	Women
• Men tend to manifest CAD 10-15 yr earlier than women. • Initial cardiac event for men is more often MI than angina. • Men have a higher incidence of left ventricular hypertrophy than women.	• CAD causes more deaths in women than in men. • Initial cardiac event for women is more often angina than MI. • Women with the long QT syndrome have an increased incidence of sudden cardiac death compared to men with the same disorder. • Before menopause, women have higher HDL cholesterol levels and lower LDL cholesterol levels than men. • After menopause, LDL levels increase. • Women complain of palpitations more frequently than men.

CAD, Coronary artery disease; *HDL,* high-density lipoprotein; *LDL,* low-density lipoprotein; *MI,* myocardial infarction.

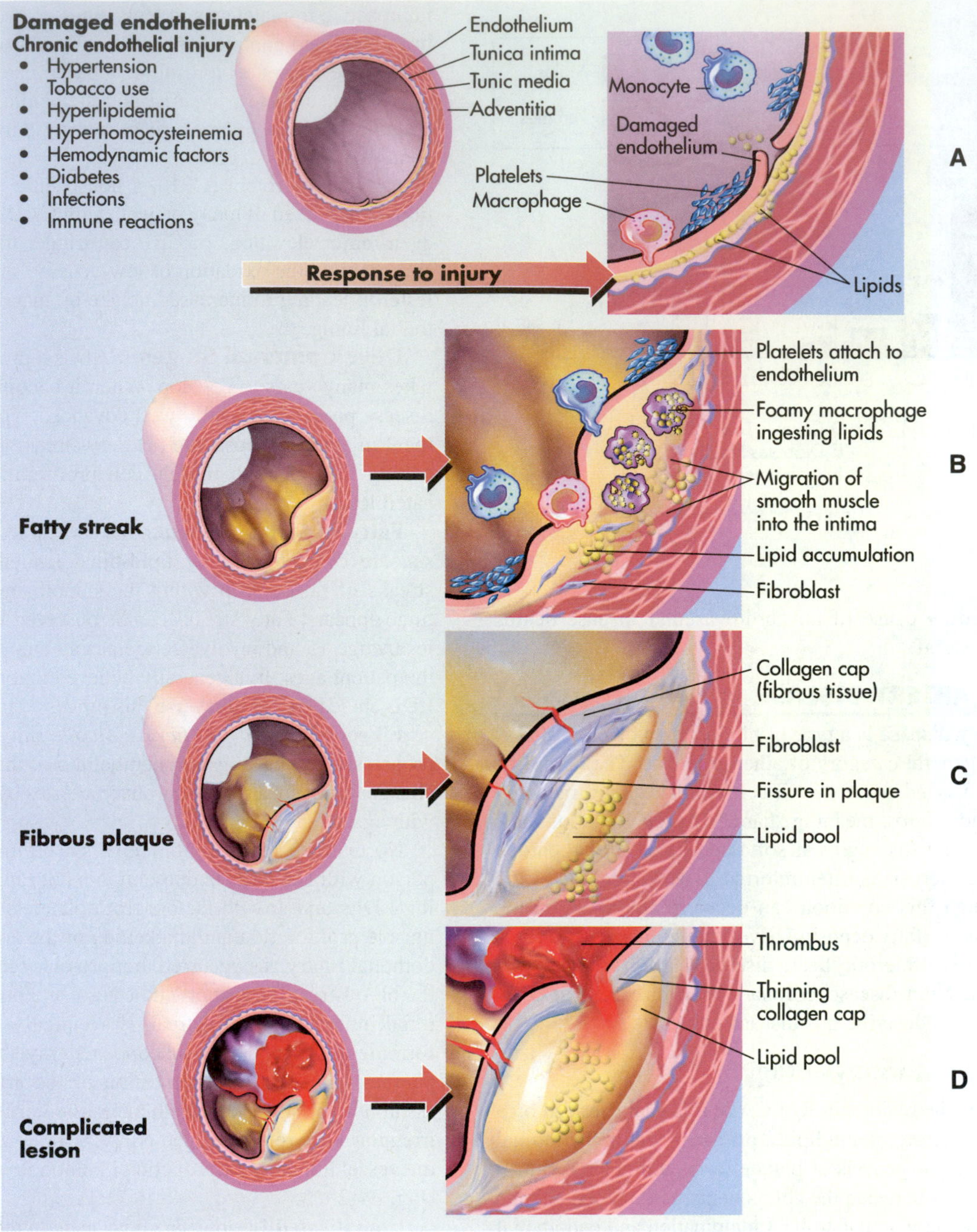

FIG. 34-2 Progression of atherosclerosis. **A,** Damaged endothelium. **B,** Diagram of fatty streak and lipid core formation. **C,** Diagram of fibrous plaque. Raised plaques are visible: some are yellow, others are white. **D,** Diagram of complicated lesion: thrombus is red, collagen is blue. Plaque is complicated by red thrombus deposition.

has become compromised, platelets accumulate in large numbers, leading to a thrombus. The thrombus may adhere to the wall of the artery, leading to further narrowing or total occlusion of the artery. Activation of the exposed platelets causes expression of glycoprotein IIb/IIIa receptors that bind fibrinogen. This, in turn, leads to further platelet aggregation and adhesion, further enlarging the thrombus. At this stage, the plaque is referred to as a *complicated lesion*[4] (Fig. 34-2, *D*).

Collateral Circulation. Normally some arterial anastomoses or connections, termed **collateral circulation,** exist within the coronary circulation. The growth and extent of collateral circulation are attributed to two factors: (1) the inherited predisposition to develop new blood vessels *(angiogenesis)* and (2) the presence of chronic ischemia. When an atherosclerotic plaque occludes the normal flow of blood through a coronary artery and the resulting *ischemia* is chronic, increased collateral circulation develops (Fig. 34-3). When occlusion of the coronary arteries occurs slowly over a long period, there is a greater chance of adequate collateral circulation developing, and the myocardium may still receive an adequate amount of blood and oxygen. However, with rapid-onset CAD (e.g., familial hypercholesterolemia) or coronary spasm, the time is inadequate for collateral development, and a diminished arterial flow results in a more severe ischemia or infarction.

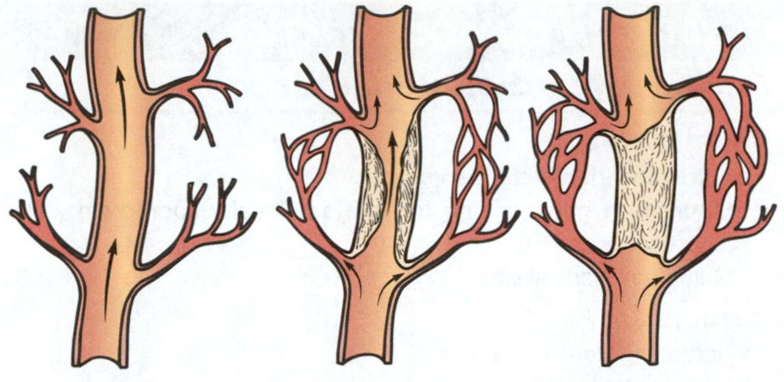

FIG. 34-3 Vessel occlusion with collateral circulation. **A,** Open, functioning coronary artery. **B,** Partial coronary artery closure with collateral circulation being established. **C,** Total coronary artery occlusion with collateral circulation bypassing the occlusion to supply blood to the myocardium.

CULTURAL AND ETHNIC HEALTH DISPARITIES
Coronary Artery Disease

- White, middle-aged men have the highest incidence of coronary artery disease.
- African Americans have an early age of onset of coronary artery disease.
- African American women have a higher incidence and death rate related to coronary artery disease than white women. African Americans have more severe coronary artery disease than whites.
- Native Americans <35 yr of age have heart disease mortality rates twice as high as other Americans. Major modifiable cardiovascular risk factors for Native Americans are obesity and diabetes mellitus.
- Hispanics have lower death rates from heart disease than non-Hispanic whites.

CAD develops over many years, and clinical manifestations will not be apparent in the early stages of the disease. Therefore it becomes extremely important to identify people at risk so that therapeutic lifestyle changes and some treatment strategies can be initiated early.

Risk Factors for Coronary Artery Disease

Risk factors are characteristics or conditions that are statistically associated with a high incidence of a disease. Many risk factors have been associated with CAD. Risk factors in different populations may vary. For example, major risk factors for CAD in the United States, such as high serum cholesterol and hypertension, are less prevalent in Japanese and Puerto Rican populations.[2,7,8]

Risk factors can be categorized as nonmodifiable and modifiable (Table 34-1). *Nonmodifiable risk factors* are age, gender, ethnicity, family history, and genetic inheritance. *Modifiable risk factors* include elevated serum lipids, hypertension, tobacco use, physical inactivity, obesity, diabetes, metabolic syndrome, psychologic states, and homocysteine level.[7,9]

Data on risk factors have been obtained in several major studies. In the Framingham study (one of the most widely known), 5209 men and women were observed for 20 years. Over time, it was noted that elevated serum cholesterol (>240 mg/dl), elevated systolic blood pressure (BP) (>160 mm Hg), and tobacco use (one or more packs a day) were positively correlated with an increased incidence of CAD.

TABLE 34-1 Risk Factors for Coronary Artery Disease

Nonmodifiable Risk Factors	Modifiable Risk Factors
Age	***Major***
Gender (men > women until 60 yr of age)	Serum lipids: elevated triglycerides, and LDL cholesterol; decreased HDL cholesterol*
Ethnicity (whites > African Americans)	Hypertension: ≥140/90 mm Hg*
Genetic predisposition and family history of heart disease	Tobacco use
	Physical inactivity
	Obesity: Waist circumference >102 cm (39.8 inches) in men and >88 cm (34.3 inches) in women or body mass index >30 kg/m²*
	Contributing
	Diabetes mellitus
	Fasting blood sugar >110 mg/dl*
	Psychologic states
	Homocysteine levels

HDL, High-density lipoprotein; *LDL,* low-density lipoprotein.
*Three or more of these risk factors meet the criteria for metabolic syndrome as defined by the National Heart, Lung, and Blood Institute and American Heart Association.

Recently, it has been shown that the degree of coronary artery calcification correlates with the severity of CAD. Calcification can be detected by noninvasive means such as electron beam computed tomography (EBCT) (see Chapter 32, Fig. 32-14). Measurement of coronary calcification may be useful for predicting adverse cardiovascular events. However, many issues need to be resolved before coronary calcium screening is routinely used in clinical practice. These issues include (1) optimal coronary calcium thresholds, which can vary according to age, gender, and race; and (2) cost-effectiveness of using this measure to improve clinical outcomes.

Although LDL cholesterol has been the focal point of risk determination for CAD, many patients who have an MI have normal LDL cholesterol. There has been recent interest in lipoprotein-associated phospholipase A2 (Lp-PLA_2), an enzyme produced by macrophages that promotes vascular inflammation. Elevations in Lp-PLA_2 have been associated with an increased risk of CAD. Lp-PLA_2 levels can be evaluated in conjunction with LDL-cholesterol levels and may be ordered as a part of the overall clinical evaluation of a patient's risk for developing CAD (see Chapter 32). The PLAC test for Lp-PLA_2 can aid in determining if a patient with non-elevated LDL cholesterol may be at increased risk for developing CAD. The PLAC blood test can be included as part of a normal clinical evaluation to better determine a patient's risk for developing CAD.

Nonmodifiable Risk Factors

Age, Gender, and Ethnicity. The incidence of CAD and MI is highest among white, middle-aged men. After age 65, the incidence in men and women equalizes although cardiovascular disease causes more deaths in women than men.[10] Additionally, CAD is present in African American women at rates higher than their white counterparts.[1] (See Cultural and Ethnic Health Disparities box for additional differences in CAD among ethnic groups of Americans.)

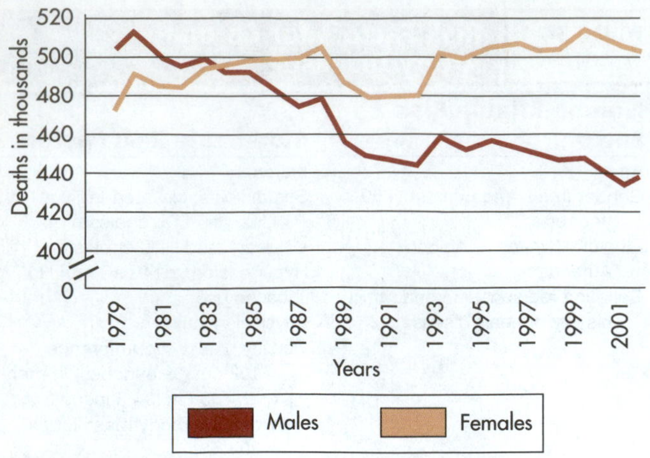

FIG. 34-4 Cardiovascular disease mortality trends for men and women. *CVD,* Cardiovascular disease.

Heart disease kills almost 10 times more women than breast cancer. Even though cardiovascular disease remains the leading cause of death in women and the mortality rate for women with CAD has remained relatively constant in recent years, only 15% of women consider CAD their greatest health risk[1,10] (Fig. 34-4). Only recently has there been research focusing on the manifestations and course of CAD in women. Women tend to manifest CAD 10 years later in life than men. This is thought to be related to the loss of the cardioprotective effects of natural estrogen with the onset of menopause. Most women have symptoms of angina rather than MI when presenting with their initial cardiac event (see Gender Differences box on p. 785).

Family History and Genetics. Genetic predisposition is an important factor in the occurrence of CAD, although the exact mechanism of inheritance is not fully understood. Some congenital defects in coronary artery walls predispose the person to the formation of plaques. Familial hypercholesterolemia, an autosomal dominant disorder, has been strongly associated with CAD at early ages (see the Genetics in Clinical Practice box). In most cases, patients presenting with angina or MI can name a parent or sibling who has died of CAD.

Modifiable Major Risk Factors

Elevated Serum Lipids. An elevated serum lipid level is one of the four most firmly established risk factors for CAD.[2,9,11] The various types of serum lipids are presented in Fig. 34-5. The risk of CAD is associated with a serum cholesterol level of more than 200 mg/dl (5.2 mmol/L) or a fasting triglyceride level of more than 150 mg/dl (3.7 mmol/L). (See Table 32-7 for normal serum lipid values.)

For lipids to be used and transported by the body, they must become soluble in blood by combining with proteins. Lipids combine with proteins to form *lipoproteins.* Lipoproteins are vehicles for fat mobilization and transport. The different types of lipoproteins vary in composition and are classified as high-density lipoproteins (HDLs), LDLs, and very-low-density lipoproteins (VLDLs).

HDLs contain more protein by weight and fewer lipids than any other lipoprotein. HDLs carry lipids away from arteries and to the liver for metabolism (Fig. 34-6). Therefore high serum HDL levels are desirable and low HDL levels are considered a risk factor for the development of CAD. This process of HDL transport prevents lipid accumulation within the arterial walls. The higher the HDL levels in the blood, the lower the risk of CAD.

There are two types of HDLs: HDL_2 and HDL_3. They are differentiated by their density and apoprotein composition. Apoproteins are found on lipoproteins and activate enzyme or receptor sites that promote the removal of fat from plasma. Several types of apoproteins exist (e.g., apoprotein A-I, apoprotein A-II, apoprotein B-100, apoprotein C-I, apoprotein E-2). Women produce more apoprotein A-I than men, and premenopausal women have HDL_2 levels approximately 3 times greater than men. This is thought to be related to the protective effects of natural estrogen. After menopause, their HDL_2 levels quickly approximate those of men.

HDL levels can be increased by physical activity, moderate alcohol consumption, and estrogen administration. In general, HDL

GENETICS IN CLINICAL PRACTICE
Familial Hypercholesterolemia

Genetic Basis
- Autosomal dominant disorder
- Mutation in gene coding for the low-density lipoprotein (LDL) receptor
- Multiple mutant alleles

Incidence
- Heterozygotes: 1 in 500
- Homozygotes: rare

Genetic Testing
- Disorder characterized by elevated serum LDLs
- Serum lipid profile can be used to measure total cholesterol, triglycerides, LDLs, and high-density lipoproteins (HDLs)
- DNA testing available

Clinical Implications
- Common genetic disease
- Leading cause of coronary artery disease
- High cholesterol levels are a result of defective function of the LDL receptors
- Plasma levels of LDLs elevated throughout life
- Develop severe atherosclerosis in early to middle years

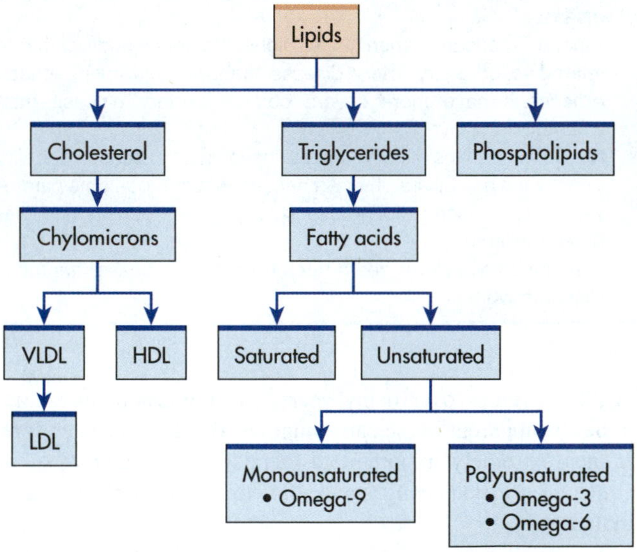

FIG. 34-5 Types of serum lipids. *HDL,* High-density lipoprotein; *LDL,* low-density lipoprotein; *VLDL,* very-low-density lipoprotein.

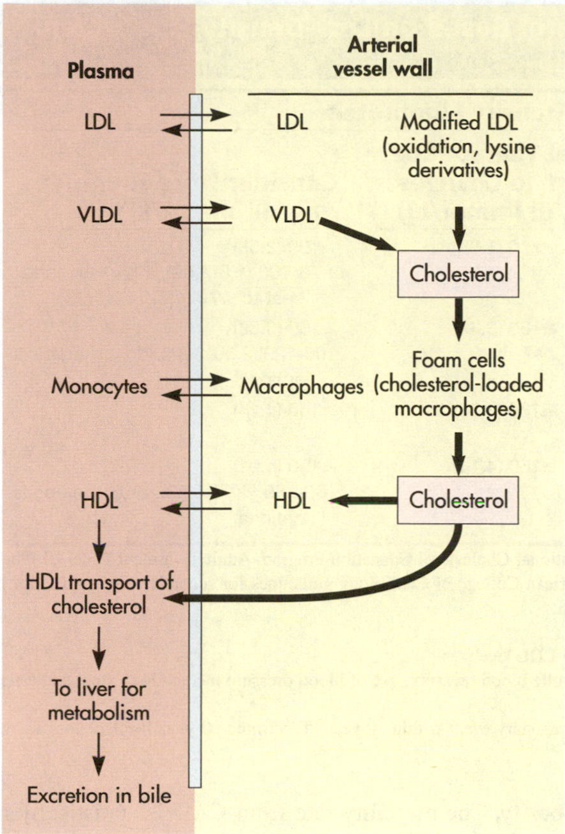

FIG. 34-6 Specific types of serum lipoproteins *(LDL* and *VLDL)* deliver cholesterol to cells of the blood vessel wall, mostly to macrophages that become cholesterol foam cells. These are predominant early features of atherosclerotic lesions. HDL is an important cholesterol-transporting carrier, delivering cholesterol to the liver to be excreted in the bile.

levels are higher in children and women, decrease with age, and are low in persons with CAD. Current research on drug and dietary therapy is focused on strategies to increase HDL levels.[7]

LDLs contain more cholesterol than any of the other lipoproteins and have an affinity for arterial walls.[2,12,13] VLDLs contain both cholesterol and triglycerides and also are thought to deposit cholesterol directly on the walls of arteries. Elevated LDL levels correlate most closely with an increased incidence of atherosclerosis and CAD. Therefore low serum LDL levels are desirable.[13,14]

Certain diseases (e.g., type 2 diabetes, chronic renal failure), drugs (e.g., corticosteroids, hormone replacement therapy), and genetic disorders have been associated with elevated triglyceride levels. Lifestyle factors that can contribute to elevated triglycerides include high alcohol consumption, high intake of refined carbohydrates and simple sugars, and physical inactivity.[8,13] When a high triglyceride level is combined with a high LDL level, a smaller, denser LDL particle is formed, which favors deposition on arterial walls. This pattern is often found in people with insulin resistance.

Lipid metabolism is not completely understood, and there is increased interest in the role of the various components of lipoproteins, such as the apoproteins, in development of CAD. A more sophisticated serum screening test can be used to diagnose various lipid disorders involving these other components.[15]

The current national guidelines for treating elevated LDL cholesterol are based on a person's 10-year risk for having a nonfatal MI or dying from a coronary event and his or her LDL levels. Risk scores are calculated based on information about the following: (1) age, (2) gender, (3) use of tobacco, (4) systolic BP, (5) use of BP medications, (6) total cholesterol, and (7) HDL cholesterol level.[11] In general, persons with no or only one risk factor are considered low risk for the development of CAD, and the LDL goal is <160 mg/dl (4.14 mmol/L). Persons at very high risk have CAD and multiple risk factors. The LDL goal for this group is <70 mg/dl (1.8 mmol/L).[11,13,15] Treatment goals and strategies are summarized in Table 34-2.

Hypertension. The second major risk factor in CAD is hypertension, which is defined as a BP ≥140/90 mm Hg. Hypertension has been identified as a major risk factor for heart disease beginning with the Framingham study.[12] In postmenopausal women, hypertension is associated with a higher incidence of CAD than in men and premenopausal women. Hypertension increases the risk of death from CAD 10-fold in all persons.

In 2003, the National Institutes of Health redefined normal BP as <120 mm Hg/80 mm Hg, prehypertension as BP of 120 to 139 mm Hg/80 to 89 mm Hg, stage 1 hypertension as 140 to 159 mm Hg/90 to 99 mm Hg, and stage 2 hypertension as BP ≥160 mm Hg/100 mm Hg.[16] The cause of hypertension in 90% of those affected is unknown, but it is usually controllable with diet and/or drugs. Therapeutic lifestyle changes should begin in people with prehypertension. Those with stage 1 or 2 hypertension often require more than one drug to reach therapeutic goals[16] (see Table 33-8).

The stress of a constantly elevated BP increases the rate of atherosclerotic development. This is related to the shearing stress that causes endothelial injury. Atherosclerosis, in turn, causes narrowed, thickened arterial walls and decreases the distensibility and elasticity of vessels. More force is required to pump blood through diseased arterial vasculature, and this increased force is reflected in a higher BP. This increased workload is also manifested by left ventricular hypertrophy and decreased stroke volume with each contraction. Salt intake is positively correlated with elevated BP, adding volume and increasing systemic vascular resistance (SVR) to the cardiac workload. (See Chapter 33 for a complete discussion of hypertension.)

Tobacco Use. A third major risk factor in CAD is tobacco use. The risk of developing CAD is 2 to 6 times higher in those who smoke tobacco than in those who do not. Further, tobacco smoking has been linked to a decrease in estrogen levels, placing premenopausal women at greater risk for CAD. Risk is proportional to the number of cigarettes smoked. Changing to lower nicotine or filtered cigarettes does not affect risk.

Studies have shown strong evidence that chronic exposure to environmental tobacco (secondhand) smoke also increases the risk of CAD.[15,17] Pipe and cigar smokers, who often do not inhale, have been found to have an increased risk of CAD similar to those exposed to environmental tobacco smoke.

Nicotine in tobacco smoke causes catecholamine (i.e., epinephrine, norepinephrine) release. These hormones cause an increased heart rate (HR), peripheral vasoconstriction, and increased BP. These changes increase the cardiac workload, necessitating greater myocardial oxygen consumption. Nicotine also increases platelet adhesion, which increases the risk of emboli formation.[8,10]

Carbon monoxide, a by-product of combustion found in tobacco smoke, affects the oxygen-carrying capacity of hemoglobin by reducing the sites available for oxygen transport. Thus the effects of an increased cardiac workload, combined with the oxygen-depleting effect of carbon monoxide, significantly decrease the oxygen available to the myocardium. There is also some indication

TABLE 34-2 Treatment Decisions for High Blood Cholesterol Based on Low-Density Lipoprotein Levels

	Low-Density Lipoprotein		
Risk Category	**Goal (mg/dl [mmol/L])**	**Initial Therapeutic Lifestyle Changes (mg/dl [mmol/L])**	**Consider Drug Therapy* (mg/dl [mmol/L])**
High risk: CAD,† peripheral vascular disease, carotid artery disease, or ACS	<100 (2.59)	≥70 (1.8)	>100 (2.59) if 70-100 (1.8-2.59), it is reasonable to treat to <70 (1.8)
Moderately high risk: ≥2 risk factors and 10-yr risk score‡ 10%-20%	<130 (3.36) <100 (2.59), optional goal	≥130 (3.36)	≥130 (3.36) 100-129 (2.59-3.34), drug therapy is optional
Moderate risk: ≥2 risk factors and 10-yr risk score‡ <10%	<130 (3.36)	≥130 (3.36)	≥160 (4.14)
Lower risk: 0-1 risk factors	<160 (4.14)	≥160 (4.14)	≥190 (4.91) 160-189 (4.14-4.89), drug therapy is optional

Source: Grundy SM, Cleeman JI, Merz MB, et al: Implications of recent clinical trials for the National Cholesterol Education Program Adult Treatment Panel III Guidelines, *Circulation* 110:227, 2004; Smith SC, Allen J, Blair SN, et al: American Heart Association/American College of Cardiology guidelines for secondary prevention for patients with coronary and other atherosclerotic vascular disease: 2006 update, *Circulation* 113:2363, 2006.

ACS, Acute coronary syndrome; *CAD,* coronary artery disease.

*When drug therapy is initiated, therapy should be sufficient to achieve a 30% to 40% decrease in LDL levels.

†CAD risk factors considered in the treatment of high LDL include age, gender, tobacco use, systolic blood pressure, use of blood pressure medications, total cholesterol, and HDL cholesterol.

‡At-risk score refers to the probability (percentage chance) of having a nonfatal MI or dying of a coronary event within 10 years. Electronic 10-yr risk calculators are available at *http://hin.nhlbi.nih.gov/atpiii/calculator.asp?usertype=prof.*

that carbon monoxide may also be a chemical irritant, thus causing injury to the endothelium.[8,12]

The benefits of smoking cessation are dramatic and almost immediate. CAD mortality rates drop to those of nonsmokers within 12 months.[8,12] However, nicotine is highly addictive and often calls for intensive intervention to assist people to quit. In one study, researchers found that time spent with follow-up calls and home counseling increased the chances of quitting over standard care of 30 minutes of counseling and an educational pamphlet. In addition, it was found that the use of nicotine replacement therapy also contributed to successful quitting. Barriers to successful quitting included multiple relapses, stress, weight gain, lack of support, and depression.[18] (See Chapter 12 and Tables 12-4, 12-5, and 12-6 for information on smoking cessation.)

Physical Inactivity. Physical inactivity is a fourth major modifiable risk factor. Physical inactivity implies a lack of adequate physical exercise on a regular basis. The current recommendation for health-promoting regular physical activity is defined as brisk walking that occurs at least 5 or more times a week for at least 30 minutes, causing perspiration and an increase in HR by 30 to 50 beats/minute.[8,15]

The mechanism by which physical inactivity predisposes to CAD is mostly still unknown. Physically active people have increased HDL levels, and exercise enhances fibrinolytic activity, thus reducing the risk of clot formation. It is also believed that exercise encourages the development of collateral circulation.

Exercise training for those who are physically inactive decreases the risk of CAD through more efficient lipid metabolism, increased HDL_2 production, and more efficient oxygen extraction by the working muscle groups, thereby decreasing the cardiac workload. Physically active persons are seldom obese and can achieve a 5- to 10-mm Hg drop in their BP, thus reducing three risk factors in CAD.[8]

Obesity. The mortality rate from CAD is statistically higher in obese individuals. Obesity is defined as a body mass index (BMI) of >30 kg/m^2. BMI is a calculation of body fat based on height and weight and can be calculated online *(http://nhlbisupport.com/bmi/bmicalc.htm).* The increased risk for CAD is proportional to the degree of obesity. Obese persons are thought to produce increased levels of LDLs and triglycerides, which are strongly implicated in atherosclerosis. Obesity is often associated with hypertension, which is 3 times more likely to develop in an obese person than in a person of normal weight. There is also evidence that individuals who tend to store fat in the abdomen (an "apple" figure) rather than in the hips and buttocks (a "pear" figure) have a higher incidence of CAD[1,8,13] (see Chapter 41, Fig. 41-5). As obesity increases, the heart size grows, causing increased myocardial oxygen consumption. In addition, there is an increase in insulin resistance in obese individuals.[19]

Modifiable Contributing Risk Factors

Diabetes Mellitus. The incidence of CAD is 2 to 4 times greater among persons who have diabetes, even those with well-controlled blood glucose levels, than the general population. The patient with diabetes manifests CAD not only more frequently but also at an earlier age. There is no age difference between male or female patients with diabetes in the onset of manifestations of CAD. Diabetes virtually eliminates the lower incidence of CAD in premenopausal women. Diabetic women have 5 to 7 times higher risk for CAD than nondiabetic women.[8,19,20] Undiagnosed diabetes is frequently discovered at the time of MI. Because the person with diabetes has an increased tendency toward connective tissue degeneration and endothelial dysfunction, it is thought that this condition may account for the tendency toward atheroma development seen in the patient with diabetes. Diabetic patients also have alterations in lipid metabolism and tend to have high cholesterol and triglyceride levels.[8,19,20]

Metabolic Syndrome. *Metabolic syndrome* refers to a cluster of risk factors for CAD whose underlying pathophysiology is thought to be related to insulin resistance. These risk factors include obesity as defined by increased waist circumference, elevated triglycerides, hypertension, abnormal serum lipids, and an elevated fasting blood glucose[21,22] (see Table 41-10). These multiple, interrelated risk factors of metabolic origin appear to promote the development of CAD. (Metabolic syndrome is discussed in Chapter 41.)

Psychologic States. The Framingham study provided early evidence that certain behaviors and lifestyles are conducive to the development of CAD.[23,24] Several behavior patterns have been correlated with CAD. However, the study of these behaviors remains controversial and complex. One type of behavior is referred to as type A and includes perfectionism and a hardworking, driving personality. The type A person often suppresses anger and hostility, has a sense of time urgency, is impatient, and often creates stress and tension. This person is more prone to MIs than a type B person, who is more easygoing, takes upsets in stride, knows personal limitations, takes time to relax, and is not an overachiever. Meta-analysis of the type A personality studies has shown that the studies that demonstrated a positive correlation between type A personality and CAD were equal in number to the studies that failed to show a correlation with CAD.[23,24]

Studies now are focusing on specific negative psychologic or behavioral states thought to increase risk of CAD, including depression, hopelessness, anxiety, hostility, and anger.[8,25,26] In one review, depression was supported as a risk factor for both the development and worsening of CAD.[27] Depressed patients have elevated levels of circulating catecholamines that may contribute to endothelial injury and inflammation, and platelet activation.[28] More research on the treatment of depression and other negative psychologic states in patients with or at risk for CAD is needed to improve the emotional and physical health of these patients.[26]

Stressful states have also been correlated with the development of CAD. Sympathetic nervous system (SNS) stimulation and its effect on the heart are generally considered to be the physiologic mechanism by which stress predisposes to the development of CAD. SNS stimulation causes an increased release of catecholamines (i.e., epinephrine, norepinephrine). This stimulation increases HR and intensifies the force of myocardial contraction, resulting in increased myocardial oxygen demand. Also, stress-induced mechanisms can cause elevated lipid and glucose levels and alterations in blood coagulation, which can lead to increased atherogenesis.[8]

Homocysteine. High blood levels of homocysteine have been linked to an increased risk for CAD and other cardiovascular diseases.[29,30] Homocysteine, a sulfur-containing amino acid, is produced by the breakdown of the essential amino acid methionine, which is found in dietary protein. High homocysteine levels (>12 to 15 μmol/L) possibly contribute to atherosclerosis by (1) damaging the inner lining of blood vessels, (2) promoting plaque buildup, and (3) altering the clotting mechanism to make clots more likely to occur.

Research is ongoing to determine if a decline in homocysteine can reduce the risk of heart disease.[29] B-complex vitamins (B_6, B_{12}, folic acid) have been shown to lower blood levels of homocysteine. Generally, a screening test for homocysteine is not recommended, but limited to those suspected of having elevated levels, such as older patients with pernicious anemia or people who develop CAD at an early age.

NURSING *and* COLLABORATIVE MANAGEMENT CORONARY ARTERY DISEASE

■ *Health Promotion*

The appropriate management of risk factors in CAD may prevent, modify, or retard the progression of the disease. In the United States during the past 30 years, there has been a gradual and persistent decline in coronary deaths, especially in men (see Fig. 34-4). The decline can be attributed to the efforts of people to become generally healthier as well as advances in pharmacology and technology to treat CAD. Prevention and early treatment of heart disease must involve a multifactorial approach and needs to be ongoing throughout the life span (see Healthy People box).

Identification of High-Risk Persons. Regardless of the health care setting, nurses are well suited to identify the person at risk for CAD. Risk screening involves obtaining personal and family health histories. The patient should be questioned about a family history of heart disease in parents and siblings. The presence of any cardiovascular symptoms should be noted (see Table 32-4). Environmental factors, such as eating habits, type of diet, and level of exercise, are assessed to elicit lifestyle patterns. A psychosocial history is included to determine tobacco use, alcohol ingestion, type A behaviors, recent life-stressing events, and the presence of any negative psychologic states (e.g., anxiety, depression, hopelessness). The place of work and the type of work can provide important information on the kind of activity performed, exposure to pollutants or noxious chemicals, and the degree of emotional stress associated with employment.

The nurse should identify the patient's attitudes and beliefs about health and illness. This information can give some indication of how disease and lifestyle changes may affect the patient and can reveal possible misconceptions about heart disease. Knowledge of the patient's educational background is helpful in deciding at what level to begin teaching. If the patient is taking medications, it is important to know what they are, when they are taken, and what the patient's compliance and attitudes are regarding the taking of medications.

Management of High-Risk Persons. Once a high-risk person is identified, preventive measures can be taken. Risk factors such as age, gender, ethnicity, and genetic inheritance cannot be modified. However, the person with any of these risk factors can still modify the risk of CAD by controlling or changing the additive effects of modifiable risk factors. For example, a young man with a family history of heart disease can decrease the risk of CAD by maintaining an ideal body weight, getting adequate physical exercise, reducing intake of saturated fats, and avoiding tobacco use.

The person who has modifiable risk factors should be encouraged and motivated to make lifestyle changes to reduce the risk of CAD. The nurse can play a major role in teaching health-promoting

HEALTHY PEOPLE

Prevention of Heart Disease

- Achieve and maintain a healthy weight
- Reduce salt and sodium intake
- Increase level of physical activity
- Avoid use of all tobacco products
- Limit alcohol intake to small to moderate amounts (12 oz beer, 4 oz wine, 1 oz hard liquor)
- Chose a diet that is low in dietary cholesterol and total and saturated fat, and high in fruits and vegetables

behaviors to the person at risk for CAD (Table 34-3). For highly motivated persons, knowing how to reduce this risk may be the only information they need to get started.

For the person who is less motivated to assume responsibility for health, the idea of risk factor reduction may be so remote that the person is unable to perceive a threat of CAD in his or her life. Few persons desire to make lifestyle changes, especially in the absence of symptoms. The nurse should first assist this person in clarifying personal values. Then, by explaining the risk factors and having the person identify the personal vulnerability to various risks, the nurse may help the person recognize the susceptibility to CAD. The nurse may also help the person set realistic goals and allow the person to choose which risk factor(s) to change first. Some persons are reluctant to change until they begin to manifest overt symptoms or actually suffer an MI. Others, having suffered an MI, may find the idea of changing lifelong habits still unacceptable. The nurse must be able to identify such attitudes and respect them.

TABLE 34-3 *PATIENT AND FAMILY TEACHING GUIDE* Decreasing Risk Factors for Coronary Artery Disease

Risk Factor	Health-Promoting Behaviors
Hypertension	• Have regular blood pressure (BP) checkups. • Take prescribed medications for BP control. • Reduce salt intake. • Stop tobacco use. • Control or reduce weight. • Perform physical activity regularly.
Elevated serum lipids	• Reduce total fat intake. • Reduce animal (saturated) fat intake. • Take prescribed medications for lipid reduction. • Adjust total caloric intake to achieve and maintain ideal body weight. • Engage in regular physical activity. • Increase amount of complex carbohydrates and vegetable proteins in diet.
Tobacco use*	• Enroll in a smoking cessation program. • Change daily routines associated with smoking to reduce desire to smoke. • Substitute other activities for smoking. • Ask family members to support efforts to stop smoking. • Avoid exposure to environmental (second-hand) smoke.
Physical inactivity	• Develop and maintain routine for physical activity 5 or more times a wk. • Increase activities to a fitness level.
Stressful lifestyle	• Increase awareness of behaviors that are detrimental to health. • Alter patterns that are conducive to stress (e.g., get up 30 min earlier so breakfast is not eaten on way to work). • Set realistic goals for self. • Reassess priorities in light of health needs. • Learn effective stress management strategies (see Chapter 9). • Seek professional help if feeling depressed, hopeless, anxious, etc. • Plan time for adequate rest and sleep.
Obesity†	• Change eating patterns and habits. • Reduce caloric intake to achieve body mass index of 18.5-24.9 kg/m^2. • Increase physical activity to increase caloric expenditure. • Avoid fad and crash diets, which are not effective in the long run. • Avoid large, heavy meals.
Diabetes‡	• Follow the recommended diet. • Reduce weight and control diet. • Take prescribed antidiabetic medications. • Monitor blood glucose levels regularly.

*Smoking cessation is discussed in Chapter 12 and Tables 12-4, 12-5, and 12-6.
†See Chapter 41 for additional health-promoting behaviors.
‡See Chapter 49 for additional health-promoting behaviors.

Physical Activity

A physical activity program should be designed to improve physical fitness by following the FITT formula: **F**requency (how often), **I**ntensity (how hard), **T**ype (isotonic), and **T**ime (how long). The current recommendation for physical activity is to perform aerobic activity of moderate intensity for at least 30 minutes 5 or more days a week. Moderate intensity and type can be defined by brisk walking, hiking, biking, and swimming. Many studies have shown the benefit of physical activity in reducing risk for CAD.[8,15] Regular physical activity contributes to weight reduction, reduction of at least 10% in systolic BP, and, in some men more than women, an increase in HDL cholesterol.[8] Type 2 diabetics experience an improvement in glucose utilization with exercise, leading to better blood glucose control.[18,19] The American Heart Association (AHA) has two programs to encourage people (Just Move—Your Personal Fitness Center at *www.justmove.org*), and especially women (Choose to Move at *www.s2mw.com/choosetomove*) to increase their daily physical activity.

Nutritional Therapy

The Adult Treatment Panel III of the National Heart, Lung, and Blood Institute has recommended *therapeutic lifestyle changes* for all people to reduce the risk of CAD by lowering LDL cholesterol. These recommendations provide guidelines that emphasize a decrease in saturated fat and cholesterol and an increase in complex carbohydrates (e.g., whole grains, fruit, vegetables)[31] (Tables 34-4 and 34-5). Fat intake should be about 30% of calories, with most coming from monounsaturated fats found in nuts and oils such as olive or canola oil.[31] Red meats, eggs, and whole milk products are major sources of saturated fat and cholesterol and should be reduced or eliminated from diets. If the serum triglyceride level is elevated, alcohol intake and simple sugars should be reduced or eliminated.

Omega-3 fatty acids have been shown to reduce the risks associated with CAD when consumed regularly. For individuals without CAD, the American Heart Association recommends eating fatty fish twice a week because fatty fish such as salmon and tuna contain two types of omega-3 fatty acids: eicosapentaenoic acid (EPA) and docosahexaenoic acid (DHA). Patients with CAD are encouraged to take EPA and DHA supplements with their diet. The American Heart Association also recommends eating tofu, other forms of soybean, canola, walnut, and flaxseed because these products contain alpha-linolenic acid, which becomes omega-3 fatty acid in the body. For more information on the American Heart Association's nutritional recommendations, see their website *www.americanheart.org*.

Several studies have demonstrated regression in coronary atherosclerosis and reduction in coronary events by lifestyle changes, including a low-saturated-fat diet, avoidance of tobacco, and increase in physical activity. Many of these studies included cholesterol-lowering drug therapy as well.[11,15,32,33]

■ Cholesterol Lowering Drug Therapy

In the United States, an estimated 107 million Americans have cholesterol levels ≥200 mg/dl (5.2 mmol/L).[1] A complete lipid profile is recommended every 5 years beginning at age 20. The person with a serum cholesterol level >200 mg/dl is at high risk for CAD and should be treated. Treatment usually begins with dietary caloric restriction (if overweight), decreased dietary fat and cholesterol intake, and increased physical activity. The guidelines for treatment of high cholesterol focus on LDL levels (see Table 34-2). Serum cholesterol levels are reassessed after 6 weeks of diet therapy. If they remain elevated, additional dietary options (see Complementary and Alternative Therapies box on p. 796) and drug therapy (Table 34-6) may be considered.[11,13-15,33]

Drugs That Restrict Lipoprotein Production. The statin drugs are the most widely used and studied lipid-lowering drugs. Examples include lovastatin (Mevacor), pravastatin (Pravachol), simvastatin (Zocor), fluvastatin (Lescol), atorvastatin (Lipitor), and rosuvastatin (Crestor). These drugs inhibit the synthesis of cholesterol in the liver by blocking hydroxymethylglutaryl coenzyme A (HMG-CoA) reductase. An unexplained result of the inhibition of cholesterol synthesis is an increase in hepatic LDL receptors. Consequently, the liver is able to remove more LDLs from the blood. In addition, a small increase in HDLs is also seen with the use of statins.[34] Serious adverse effects of these drugs are rare and include liver damage and myopathy that can progress to rhabdomyolysis (breakdown of skeletal muscle). Liver enzymes (e.g., aspartate aminotransferase, alanine aminotransferase) must be regularly monitored, and checked any time dosage is increased. Creatine kinase enzymes are assessed if symptoms of myopathy (e.g., muscle aches, weakness) occur.[13,15,34]

TABLE 34-4 NUTRITIONAL THERAPY
Therapeutic Lifestyle Changes Diet*

Nutrient	Recommended Intake as Percentage of Total Daily Calories
Total fat†	25%-35%
Saturated fat	<7%
Polyunsaturated fat	Up to 10%
Monounsaturated fat	Up to 20%
Carbohydrate	50%-60%
Protein	Approximately 15%
Cholesterol	<200 mg
Sodium	≤2400 mg
Dietary fiber	20-30 g
Total calories‡	Balance energy intake and expenditure to maintain desirable body weight and prevent weight gain.

Daily food guide is available at *www.nhlbi.nih.gov/chd/lifestyles.htm.*
*Therapeutic dietary options for further reduction in low-density lipoproteins include the addition of 2 g/day of plant sterols (e.g., margarines, nuts, seeds, legumes, vegetable oils, and other plant sources) and an additional 10 to 25 g of soluble dietary fiber.
†This recommendation allows for increased intake of unsaturated fat in place of carbohydrates in people with diabetes or metabolic syndrome.
‡Daily energy expenditure should include at least moderate physical activity.

Drug Alert - *Simvastatin (Zocor)*
- *Increased risk for rhabdomyolysis when also used with gemfibrozil (Lopid) or niacin.*
- *Signs of rhabdomyolysis: ↑ creatine kinase levels, muscle tenderness.*

TABLE 34-5 NUTRITIONAL THERAPY
Therapeutic Lifestyle Changes Diet Menu*

Breakfast

Oatmeal (1 cup)
- Fat-free milk (1 cup)
- Raisins (¼ cup)

Honeydew melon (1 cup)
Orange juice, calcium fortified (1 cup)
Coffee (1 cup) with fat-free milk (2 tbs)

Lunch

Roast beef sandwich
- Whole-wheat roll (1 medium)
- Roast beef, lean (2 oz)
- Swiss cheese, low fat (1 oz)
- Romaine lettuce (2 leaves)
- Tomato (2 slices)
- Mustard (2 tsp)

Pasta salad (½ cup)
- Pasta noodles (¼ cup)
- Mixed vegetables (¼ cup)
- Olive oil (1 tsp)

Apple (1 medium)
Iced tea, unsweetened (1 cup)

Dinner

Flounder (2 oz) cooked with olive oil (2 tsp)
- Parmesan cheese (1 tbs)

Rice (1 cup)
- Soft margarine (1 tsp)

Broccoli (½ cup)
- Soft margarine (1 tsp)

Strawberries (1 cup) topped with low-fat frozen yogurt (½ cup)
Water (1 cup)

Snack

Popcorn (2 cups) cooked with canola oil (1 tbs)
Peaches, canned in water (1 cup)
Water (1 cup)

Nutrient Analysis

Calories	1795
Cholesterol (mg)	115
Fiber (g)	28
Soluble (g)	9
Sodium (mg)	1128
Carbohydrates, % calories	57
Total fat, % calories	27
Saturated fat, % calories	6
Monounsaturated fat, % calories	14
Polyunsaturated fat, % calories	6
Trans fat (g)	2
Omega-3 fat (g)	0.4
Protein, % calories	19

Source: National Institutes of Health: *Third Report of the National Cholesterol Education Program Expert Panel. Detection, Evaluation, and Treatment of High Blood Cholesterol in Adults (Adult Treatment Panel III): final report,* Publication No 02-5215, Bethesda, Md, 2002, U.S. Department of Health and Human Services.
g, grams; *mg,* milligrams; *tbs,* tablespoon; *tsp,* teaspoon; *oz,* ounce.
*The sample menu is appropriate for a 25- to 49-year-old-female. No salt is added in recipe preparation or as seasoning. The menu meets or exceeds the Daily Reference Intake for nutrients.

EVIDENCE-BASED PRACTICE

What Is the Most Effective Cardiac Rehabilitation Program?

Clinical Question

In patients with coronary artery disease (CAD) (P), are comprehensive cardiac rehabilitation programs (I) more effective than exercise-only cardiac rehabilitation programs (C) in reducing mortality (O)?

Best Available Evidence

Systematic review of randomized controlled trials (RCTs)

Critical Appraisal and Synthesis of Evidence

- 32 RCTs ($n = 8440$)
- Reduction in all-cause mortality
  - Exercise-only cardiac rehabilitation—27%
  - Comprehensive cardiac rehabilitation (e.g., exercise in addition to psychosocial and educational interventions)—13%
- Reduction in total cardiac mortality
  - Exercise-only cardiac rehabilitation—31%
  - Comprehensive cardiac rehabilitation—26%
- Despite the reductions in mortality (cardiac and all cause), these programs did not reduce occurrence of nonfatal myocardial infarction.

Conclusions

- Exercise-based cardiac rehabilitation is effective in reducing cardiac deaths and other causes of mortality in cardiac patients.
- More research is necessary to determine whether exercise only or a comprehensive cardiac rehabilitation intervention is more beneficial.
- A broader sample is needed for subsequent studies that would include more women and is more ethnically diverse.

Implications for Nursing Practice

- Counsel patients at risk for CAD on the benefits of exercise.
- Include an exercise component in health and wellness programs for patients with CAD and/or those who have had a cardiac event.

Reference for Evidence

Jolliffe JA, Rees K, Taylor RS, et al: Exercise-based rehabilitation for coronary heart disease, Cochrane Heart Group, *Cochrane Database of Systematic Reviews 4,* 2005.

PICO: P, Patient population of interest; *I,* intervention or area of interest; *C,* comparison of interest or comparison group; *O,* outcome(s) of interest (see p. 6).

Niacin (Nicobid), a water-soluble B vitamin, is highly effective in lowering LDL and triglyceride levels by interfering with their synthesis. It has been shown to convert patients from a "pattern B," small, dense LDLs, to a "pattern A," larger, fluffier LDLs. These fluffier lipoproteins are less prone to deposition in arterial walls.[13,15] Niacin also increases HDL levels better than many other lipid-lowering drugs. Unfortunately, adverse effects of this drug are common and may include severe flushing, pruritus, gastrointestinal (GI) complaints, and orthostatic hypotension. Aspirin or a nonsteroidal antiinflammatory drug (NSAID) taken 30 minutes to 1 hour before administration may eliminate flushing.

Drug Alert - *Niacin*
- *Instruct patient that flushing (especially of face and neck) will occur within 20-30 min after taking drug and lasting for 30-60 min.*
- *After 2 wk the side effect should diminish.*

The fibric acid derivatives work by accelerating the elimination of VLDLs and increasing the production of apoproteins A-I and A-II. They are the most effective drugs for lowering triglycerides, and also increasing HDL levels. They have no effect on LDLs. Examples include fenofibrate (TriCor) and gemfibrozil (Lopid). Although most patients tolerate the drugs well, complaints may include GI irritability. These drugs should be used with caution when combined with statin medications.[13,15]

Drug Alert - *Gemfibrozil (Lopid)*
- *May increase the risk of bleeding in patients taking warfarin (Coumadin).*
- *May increase the effects of hypoglycemic drugs (e.g., insulin).*

Drugs That Increase Lipoprotein Removal. The major route of elimination of cholesterol is via conversion to bile acids in the liver. Bile-acid sequestrants increase conversion of cholesterol to bile acids and decrease hepatic cholesterol content. These nonabsorbable compounds include cholestyramine (Questran), colestipol (Colestid), and colesevelam (WelChol). The primary effect is a decrease in total cholesterol and LDLs.

Administration of these drugs can be associated with complaints related to palatability and a variety of upper and lower GI symptoms, including belching, heartburn, nausea, abdominal pain, and constipation. The bile-acid sequestrants have been known to interfere with absorption of other drugs (e.g., warfarin [Coumadin], thiazides, thyroid hormones, β-adrenergic blockers). Separating the time of administration of these drugs from other drugs may decrease this adverse effect.[13,15]

Drugs That Decrease Cholesterol Absorption. Ezetimibe (Zetia) selectively inhibits the absorption of dietary and biliary cholesterol across the intestinal wall. It is used as an adjunct to dietary changes, especially in patients with primary hypercholesterolemia. When combined with a statin (e.g., ezetimibe/simvastatin [Vytorin]), even greater reductions in LDLs were found.[34]

Drug therapy for hyperlipidemia is likely to be prolonged, perhaps continuing for a lifetime. It is essential that diet modification be used to minimize the need for drug therapy. The patient must fully understand the rationale and goals of treatment, as well as the safety and side effects of lipid-lowering drug therapy.[13,15]

Antiplatelet Therapy

Unless contraindicated (e.g., history of GI bleeding), low-dose aspirin is recommended for people at risk for CAD, especially those with a calculated 10-year CAD risk of ≥10%[1] (see Table 34-2). This recommendation is based on studies that have shown a decrease in first MIs, primarily in men, when taking aspirin. Recently, some cholesterol-lowering drugs have been co-packaged with aspirin (e.g., aspirin and pravastatin [Pravigard PAC]) to improve ease of administration and compliance.

The recent Women's Health Initiative Study demonstrated that women ages 45 to 65 did not experience the same benefit from aspirin therapy compared to men. However, the benefit was seen in women over 65. Aspirin therapy is not recommended for women with low risk for CAD before age 65. After age 65, aspirin is recommended unless contraindicated.[35] Common side effects of aspirin therapy include GI upset and bleeding. For people who are aspirin intolerant, clopidogrel (Plavix) can be considered.

TABLE 34-6 DRUG THERAPY
Hyperlipidemia

Classification and Examples	Mechanism of Action and Effects	Side Effects	Nursing Considerations
HMG-CoA Reductase Inhibitors (Statins)			
atorvastatin (Lipitor) fluvastatin (Lescol) lovastatin (Mevacor) pravastatin (Pravachol) simvastatin (Zocor) rosuvastatin (Crestor)	Block synthesis of cholesterol and increase LDL receptors in liver ↓ LDL 18%-55% ↓ Triglycerides 7%-30% ↑ HDL 5%-15%	Rash, GI disturbances, elevated liver enzymes, myopathy, rhabdomyolysis	Well tolerated with few side effects. Monitor liver enzymes and creatine kinase (if muscle weakness or pain occurs).
Niacin			
Niacin (Nicobid, Nicotinex) Nicotinic acid (Slo-Niacin, Novo-Niacin)	Inhibits synthesis and secretion of VLDL and LDL ↓ LDL 5%-25% ↓ Triglycerides 20%-50% ↑ HDL 15%-35%	Flushing and pruritus in upper torso and face, GI disturbances (e.g., nausea and vomiting, dyspepsia, diarrhea), orthostatic hypotension, can elevate homocysteine levels	Most side effects subside with time; decreased liver function may occur with high doses. Taking aspirin or NSAID 30 min to 1 hr before drug may prevent flushing; take drug with food. Treat elevated homocysteine levels with folic acid.
Fibric Acid Derivatives			
fenofibrate (TriCor) gemfibrozil (Lopid)	Decrease hepatic synthesis and secretion of VLDL; reduce triglycerides by ↓ VLDL ↓ LDL 5%-20% ↓ Triglycerides 10%-20% ↑ HDL 15%-35%	Rashes, mild GI disturbances (e.g., nausea, diarrhea), elevated liver enzymes	May ↑ effects of warfarin (Coumadin). When used in combination with statins, may increase adverse effects of statins, especially myopathy.
Bile-Acid Sequestrants			
cholestyramine (Questran) colestipol (Colestid) colesevelam (WelChol)	Bind with bile acids in intestine, forming insoluble complex and excreted in feces Binding results in removal of LDL and cholesterol ↓ LDL 20%	Unpleasant quality to taste, GI disturbances (e.g., indigestion, constipation, bloating)	Effective and safe for long-term use; side effects diminish with time. Interfere with absorption of digoxin, thiazide diuretics, warfarin, some antibiotics (e.g., vancomycin [Vancocin]).
Cholesterol Absorption Inhibitor			
ezetimibe (Zetia)	Inhibits the intestinal absorption of cholesterol ↓ LDL 19% ↑ HDL 4%	Infrequent, but may include headache and mild GI distress	When used with a statin, LDL is further reduced. Should not be used by patients with liver impairment.

GI, Gastrointestinal; *HDL*, high-density lipoprotein; *LDL*, low-density lipoprotein; *NSAID*, nonsteroidal antiinflammatory drug; *VLDL*, very-low-density lipoprotein.

GERONTOLOGIC CONSIDERATIONS
CORONARY ARTERY DISEASE

The incidence of cardiac disease is greatly increased in the elderly and is the leading cause of death in older persons.[1] In the older adult, CAD is often a result of the complex interaction of nonmodifiable risk factors (e.g., age) and lifelong modifiable risk behaviors (e.g., inactivity, tobacco use). There is evidence that strategies to reduce CAD risk are effective in this age-group but are often underprescribed.[36]

Aggressive treatment of hypertension and hyperlipidemia will stabilize plaques in the coronary arteries of older adults, and cessation of tobacco use helps decrease the risk for CAD at any age.[37] Similarly, the older patient should be encouraged to consider a planned program of physical activity. Activity performance, endurance, and ability to tolerate stress can be improved in the older adult with physical training.[37] Positive psychologic benefits can be derived from physical activity and can include increased self-esteem and emotional well-being and improved body image. For the older adult who is obese, it is recommended that making modest dietary changes and slowly increasing physical activity (e.g., walking) will result in more positive benefits than aiming for significant weight loss.

When planning a physical activity program for the older adult, the nurse should remember the following: (1) longer warm-up periods are needed, (2) longer periods of low-level activity or longer rest periods between sessions are advisable, and (3) heat intolerance may be caused by decreased ability to sweat efficiently. The patient should be taught to avoid physical activity in extremes of temperature and to maintain a moderate pace. The older adult should exercise a minimum of 30 to 40 minutes 3 or 4 times a week.

Encouraging the older patient to adopt a healthy lifestyle may increase quality of life and reduce the risk of CAD and fatal cardiac events. The older adult faces many of the same challenges when it comes to making lifestyle changes. Research has shown that there are two points when the elderly may consider change: when hospitalized and when symptoms (e.g., chest pain) are the

COMPLEMENTARY AND ALTERNATIVE THERAPIES

Natural Lipid-Lowering Agents*

Agent	Uses
Niacin (nicotinic acid)†	High cholesterol
Garlic‡	High cholesterol, high triglycerides Cardiovascular disease prevention
Omega-3 fatty acids† (found in fish oil)	High triglycerides Cardiovascular disease prevention
Psyllium (soluble fiber)†	High cholesterol
Phytosterols (plant sterols and stanols)§ (found in nuts, seeds, soybeans, and vegetable oils)	High cholesterol
Red yeast rice† (product of yeast [*Monascus purpureus*] grown on rice)	High cholesterol
Soy†	High cholesterol

Adapted from Ulbricht CE, Basch EM: *Natural standard herb and supplement reference: evidence-based clinical reviews,* St Louis, 2005, Mosby. Available at *www.naturalstandard.com.*

*Cardiovascular disease is a serious health problem. Herbal or other natural therapy should not be initiated without consultation with a health care provider. This is especially important when conventional drug therapy for cardiovascular disease is also being used.

†Strong scientific evidence for its use.

‡Good scientific evidence for its use.

§Use based on tradition, theory, or limited scientific evidence.

result of CAD and not normal aging[36] (see Table 32-1). The nurse should assess the older adult for readiness to change and then help the patient to select the lifestyle changes most likely to produce the greatest reduction in risk for CAD.

Chronic Stable Angina: Manifestation of Coronary Artery Disease

CAD is a progressive disease, and patients may be asymptomatic for many years or they may develop chronic stable chest pain syndromes.

Etiology and Pathophysiology

When the demand for myocardial oxygen exceeds the ability of the coronary arteries to supply the heart with oxygen, *myocardial ischemia* occurs. **Angina,** or chest pain, is the clinical manifestation of reversible myocardial ischemia. Either an increased demand for oxygen or a decreased supply of oxygen can lead to myocardial ischemia (Table 34-7). The primary reason for insufficient blood flow is narrowing of coronary arteries by atherosclerosis.[38] For ischemia secondary to atherosclerosis to occur, the artery is usually 75% or more obstructed (stenosed).

On the cellular level, the myocardium becomes hypoxic within the first 10 seconds of coronary occlusion. With total occlusion of the coronary arteries, contractility ceases after several minutes, depriving the myocardial cells of oxygen and glucose for aerobic metabolism. Anaerobic metabolism begins and lactic acid accumulates. Myocardial nerve fibers are irritated by the increased lactic acid and transmit a pain message to the cardiac nerves and upper thoracic posterior nerve roots. This is the reason for referred cardiac pain to the left shoulder and arm. In ischemic conditions, cardiac cells are viable for approximately 20 minutes. With restoration of blood flow, aerobic metabolism resumes, contractility is restored, and cellular repair begins.

TABLE 34-7 Factors Determining Myocardial Oxygen Needs

Decreased Oxygen Supply	Increased Oxygen Demand or Consumption
Noncardiac	
Anemia	Anxiety
Hypoxemia	Cocaine use
Pneumonia	Hypertension
Asthma	Hyperthermia
Chronic obstructive pulmonary disease	Hyperthyroidism
Low blood volume	Physical exertion
Cardiac	
Coronary artery spasm	Aortic stenosis
Coronary artery thrombosis	Cardiomyopathy
Dysrhythmias	Dysrhythmias
Heart failure	Tachycardia
Valve disorders	

TABLE 34-8 PQRST Assessment of Angina

The following can be used as a memory device to assist in obtaining information from the patient who has chest pain.

	Factor	Questions to Ask Patient
P	Precipitating events	What events or activities precipitated the pain (e.g., argument, exercise, resting)?
Q	Quality of pain	What does the pain feel like (e.g., pressure, dull, aching, tight, squeezing)?
R	Radiation of pain	Where is the pain located? Does the pain radiate to other areas (e.g., back, arms, jaw, teeth, shoulder, elbow)?
S	Severity of pain	On a scale of 0 to 10 with 10 being the most severe pain you could imagine, how would you rate the pain?
T	Timing	When did the pain begin? Has the pain changed since this time? Have you had pain like this before?

CHRONIC STABLE ANGINA

Chronic stable angina refers to chest pain that occurs intermittently over a long period with the same pattern of onset, duration, and intensity of symptoms. When questioned (Table 34-8), some patients may deny feeling pain but will describe a pressure or ache in the chest. It is an unpleasant feeling, often described as a constrictive, squeezing, heavy, choking, or suffocating sensation. Angina is rarely sharp or stabbing, and it usually does not change with position or breathing. Many people with angina complain of indigestion or a burning sensation in the epigastric region. Although most of the pain experienced by people with angina appears substernally, the sensation may occur in the neck or radiate to various locations, including the jaw, shoulders, and down the arms (Fig. 34-7). Often people will complain of pain between the shoulder blades and dismiss it as not being related to their heart.

The pain usually lasts for only a few minutes (3 to 5 minutes) and commonly subsides when the precipitating factor is relieved (Table 34-9). Pain at rest is unusual. An electrocardiogram (ECG) usually reveals transient ST segment depression, indicating ischemia (see Chapter 36).

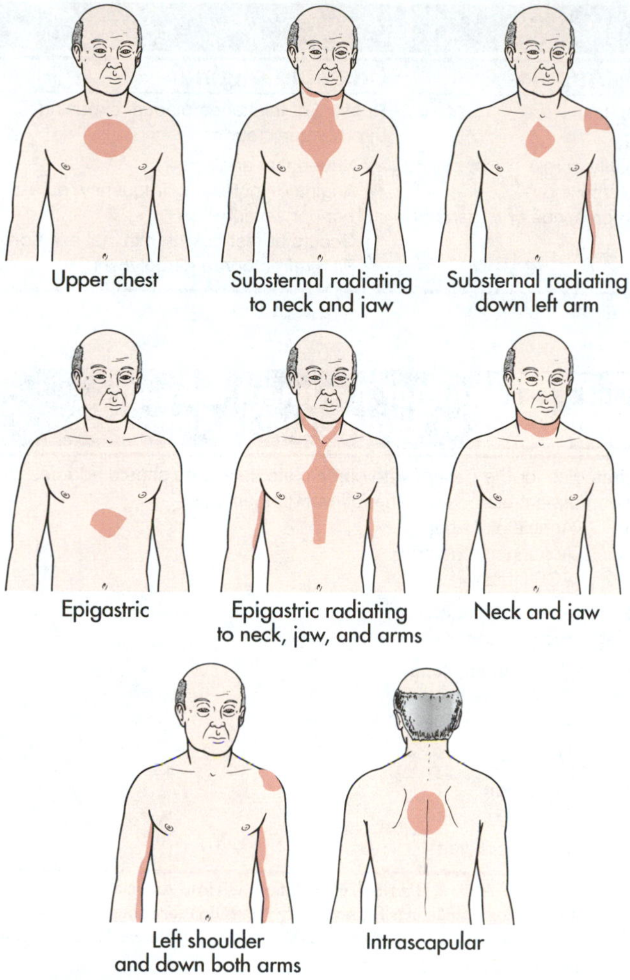

FIG. 34-7 Location of pain during angina or myocardial infarction.

Chronic stable angina can be controlled with medications on an outpatient basis. Because chronic stable angina is often predictable, medications can be timed to provide peak effects during the time of day when angina is likely to occur. For example, if angina occurs when rising, the patient can take medication as soon as awakening and wait 30 minutes to 1 hour before engaging in activity. (The different types of angina are compared in Table 34-10.)

Silent Ischemia

Silent ischemia refers to ischemia that occurs in the absence of any subjective symptoms.[38] Patients with diabetes have an increased prevalence of silent ischemia that is thought to be related to diabetic neuropathy affecting the nerves that innervate the cardiovascular system.[39] When patients are monitored (e.g., Holter monitor) and silent ischemia occurs, ECG changes are revealed. Ischemia with pain or without pain has the same prognosis.

Nocturnal Angina and Angina Decubitus. *Nocturnal angina* occurs only at night but not necessarily when the person is in the recumbent position or during sleep. *Angina decubitus* is chest pain that occurs only while the person is lying down and is usually relieved by standing or sitting.

Prinzmetal's Angina. **Prinzmetal's angina** *(variant angina)* often occurs at rest, usually in response to spasm of a major coronary artery. It is a rare form of angina and is frequently seen in patients with a history of migraine headaches and Raynaud's phenomenon. The spasm may occur in the absence of CAD, as well as with documented disease. Prinzmetal's angina is not usually precipitated by increased physical demand. Coronary spasm can be described as a strong contraction of smooth muscle in the coronary artery caused by an increase in intracellular calcium.

Factors that may precipitate coronary artery spasm include increased myocardial oxygen demand and increased levels of certain substances (e.g., histamine, angiotensin, epinephrine, norepinephrine, prostaglandins). When spasm occurs, the patient experiences angina and transient ST segment elevation (see Chapter 36). The pain may occur during rapid-eye-movement (REM) sleep when myocardial oxygen consumption increases. The pain may be relieved by moderate exercise or it may disappear spontaneously. Cyclic, short bursts of pain at a usual time each day may also occur with this type of angina. It is usually treated with calcium channel blockers and/or nitrates.

TABLE 34-9 Precipitating Factors of Angina

Physical Exertion
• Increases HR, reducing the time the heart spends in diastole (the time of greatest coronary blood flow), resulting in an increase in myocardial oxygen demand.   • Isometric exercise of the arms (e.g., raking, lifting heavy objects, or snow shoveling) can cause exertional angina.
Temperature Extremes
• Increase workload of the heart.   • Blood vessels constrict in response to a cold stimulus.   • Blood vessels dilate and blood pools in the skin in response to a hot stimulus.
Strong Emotions
• Stimulate the sympathetic nervous system.   • Increase the workload of the heart.
Consumption of Heavy Meal
• Can increase the workload of the heart.   • During the digestive process, blood is diverted to the GI system, reducing blood flow in the coronary arteries.
Tobacco Use
• Nicotine stimulates catecholamine release, causing vasoconstriction and an increased HR.   • Diminishes available oxygen by increasing the level of carbon monoxide.
Sexual Activity
• Increases the cardiac workload and sympathetic stimulation.   • In a person with CAD, the extra cardiac workload may precipitate angina.
Stimulants (e.g., cocaine, amphetamines)
• Increase HR and subsequent myocardial oxygen demand.
Circadian Rhythm Patterns
• Are related to the occurrence of chronic stable angina, Prinzmetal's angina, MI, and sudden cardiac death.   • Manifestations of CAD tend to occur in the early morning after awakening.

CAD, Coronary artery disease; *GI,* gastrointestinal; *HR,* heart rate; *MI,* myocardial infarction.

COLLABORATIVE MANAGEMENT: CHRONIC STABLE ANGINA

The treatment of chronic stable angina is aimed at decreasing oxygen demand and/or increasing oxygen supply. Continued emphasis on the reduction of risk factors is a priority and should include

TABLE 34-10 Comparison of Types of Angina

	Chronic Stable Angina	Prinzmetal's Angina	Unstable Angina
Etiology	Myocardial ischemia, usually secondary to CAD	Coronary vasospasm	Rupture of thickened plaque, exposing thrombogenic surface
Characteristics	• Episodic pain lasting 5-15 min • Provoked by exertion • Relieved by rest or nitroglycerin	• Occurs primarily at rest • Triggered by smoking • May occur in presence or absence of CAD	• New-onset angina • Angina of increasing frequency, duration, or severity • Occurs at rest or with minimal exertion • Pain refractory to nitroglycerin

CAD, Coronary artery disease.

those strategies discussed for patients with CAD (see page 791 to 796). In addition to antiplatelet and cholesterol-lowering drug therapy, the most common therapeutic intervention for the management of chronic stable angina is the use of nitrate therapy to enhance coronary blood flow[40-43] (Table 34-11 and Fig. 34-8).

TABLE 34-11 Major Treatment Elements of Chronic Stable Angina

Strategies for the patient with chronic stable angina should address all the treatment elements in the following mnemonic:

A	Antiplatelet agent Antianginal therapy ACE inhibitor*
B	β-Adrenergic blocker Blood pressure
C	Cigarette smoking Cholesterol
D	Diet Diabetes
E	Education Exercise
F	Flu vaccination*

*Source: Smith SC, Allen J, Blair SN, et al: American Heart Association/American College of Cardiology guidelines for secondary prevention for patients with coronary and other atherosclerotic vascular disease: 2006 update, *Circulation* 113:2363, 2006.
ACE, Angiotensin-converting enzyme.

Drug Therapy

Drug therapy for chronic stable angina is aimed at preventing MI and death, and reducing symptoms. Aspirin (previously discussed) is recommended in the absence of contraindications (Table 34-12).

Short-Acting Nitrates. Short-acting nitrates are first-line therapy for the treatment of angina. Nitrates produce their principal effects by the following mechanisms:

1. *Dilating peripheral blood vessels.* This results in decreased SVR, venous pooling, and decreased venous blood return to the heart. Therefore myocardial oxygen demand is decreased because of the reduced cardiac workload.
2. *Dilating coronary arteries and collateral vessels.* This may increase blood flow to the ischemic areas of the heart. However, when the coronary arteries are severely atherosclerotic, coronary dilation is difficult to achieve.

Sublingual Nitroglycerin. Nitroglycerin given sublingually (Nitrostat) or by translingual spray (Nitrolingual) will usually relieve pain in approximately 3 minutes and has a duration of approximately 30 to 60 minutes. The recommended dose is 1 tablet taken sublingually (SL) or 1 metered spray for symptoms of angina. If symptoms are unchanged or worse after 5 minutes, the patient should be instructed to contact the emergency medical services (EMS) system.[43]

***Drug Alert** - Nitroglycerin*
- *Tablet or spray needs to be administered under the tongue.*
- *Instruct patient not to combine with drugs used for erectile dysfunction (e.g., sildenafil [Viagra]).*
- *Monitor for orthostatic hypotension as it may occur after administration.*

The patient must be instructed in the proper use of nitroglycerin. It should be easily accessible to the patient at all times. For protection from degradation, tablets should be kept in a tightly closed dark glass bottle. The patient should be instructed to place a nitroglycerin tablet under the tongue and allow it to dissolve. If using the spray, it should be directed under the tongue, not inhaled. Nitroglycerin should cause a tingling sensation. If tingling is not felt and chest pain still persists, the patient should contact EMS. The patient should be warned that HR may increase and a pounding headache, dizziness, or flushing may occur. The patient should be cautioned against quickly rising to a standing position because orthostatic hypotension may occur after nitroglycerin use.

Nitroglycerin can be used prophylactically before undertaking an activity that the patient knows may precipitate an anginal attack. In these instances the patient can take a tablet 5 to 10 minutes before beginning the activity. Any changes in the usual pattern of pain, especially increasing frequency or nocturnal angina, should be reported to the health care provider.

Nitroglycerin tablets are marketed in light-resistant bottles with metal caps. Because they tend to lose potency once a bottle has been opened, the patient should be advised to purchase a new supply every 6 months.

Long-Acting Nitrates. Nitrates, such as isosorbide dinitrate (Isordil) and isosorbide mononitrate (Imdur), are longer acting than SL or translingual nitroglycerin and can be used to reduce the incidence of anginal attacks.[42] The predominant side effect of all nitrates is headache from the dilation of cerebral blood vessels. Patients can be advised to take acetaminophen (Tylenol) with their nitrate to relieve the headache. Over time, the headaches may decrease but the principal antianginal effect is still present.

Orthostatic hypotension is a complication of all nitrates. Nurses should monitor BP after the initial dose as the venous dilation that occurs may cause a drop in BP, especially in volume-depleted patients. Finally, tolerance to nitroglycerin-induced vasodilation can develop. It is recommended that patients schedule an 8-hour nitrate-free period every day, usually during the night, unless the patient experiences nocturnal angina.[34,41]

Nitroglycerin Ointment. Nitropaste is a 2% nitroglycerin topical ointment dosed by the inch. It is placed on the skin, over a flat muscular area that is free of hair and/or scars (e.g., upper arm). Once ab-

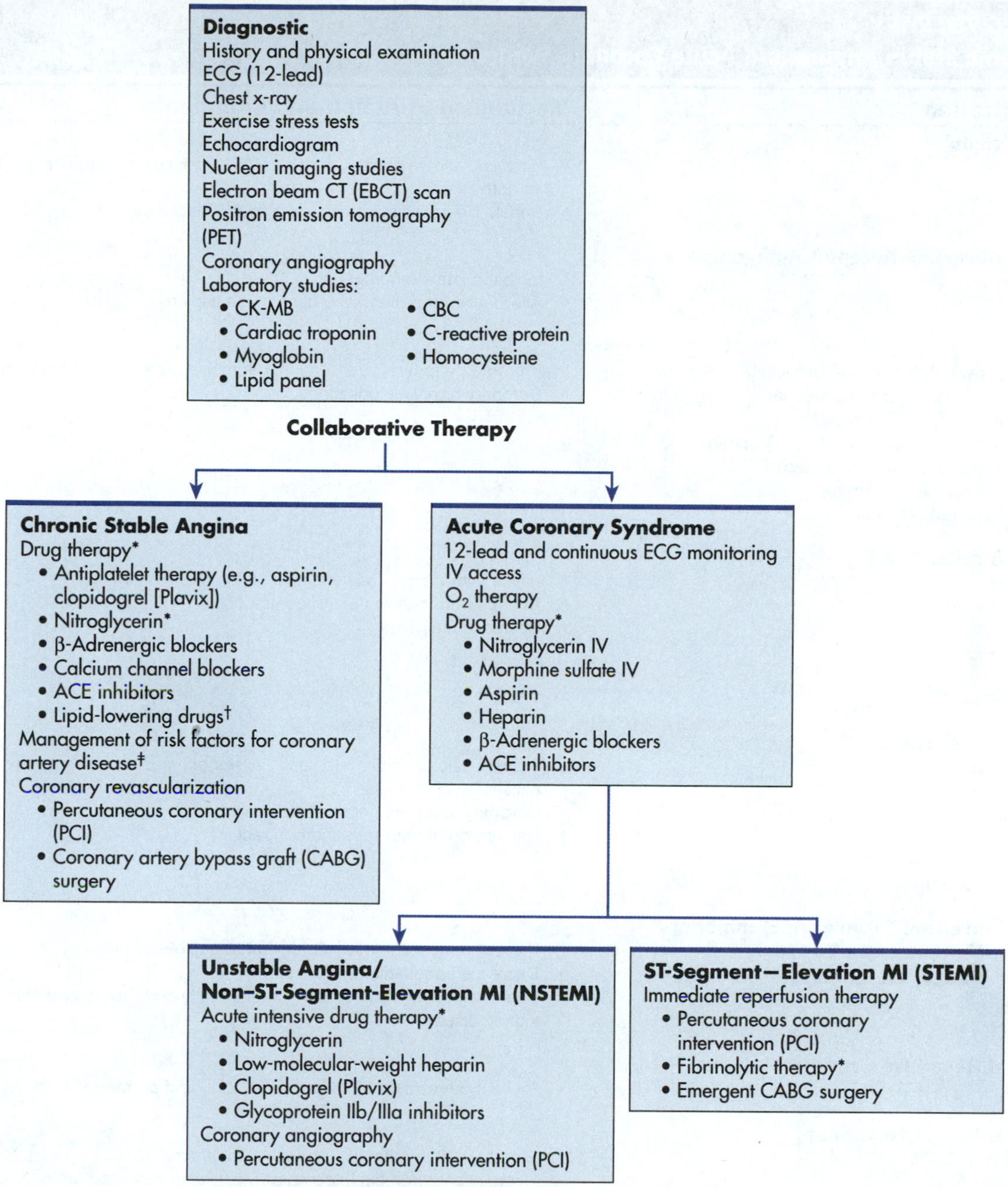

FIG. 34-8 Collaborative care: chronic stable angina and acute coronary syndrome. *ACE,* Angiotensin-converting enzyme; *CBC,* complete blood count; *CK,* creatine kinase; *ECG,* electrocardiogram.
*See Table 34-12.
†See Table 34-6.
‡See Tables 34-2, 34-3, and 34-4.

sorbed, it produces anginal prophylaxis for 3 to 6 hours. It has been found to be especially useful for nocturnal and unstable angina.

Transdermal Controlled-Release Nitrates. Currently two systems are available for transdermal nitroglycerin drug administration: reservoir and matrix. The reservoir system delivers the drug using a rate-controlled permeable membrane. The matrix system provides for a slow delivery of the drug through a polymer matrix. Both reservoir and matrix delivery systems offer the advantages of steady plasma levels within the therapeutic range during 24 hours, thus making only one application a day necessary. The reservoir system has the disadvantage of dose dumping if the reservoir seal is punctured or broken. An advantage of the matrix system is that there can be no dose dumping. Both systems achieve plasma drug level steady states by 2 hours.

β-Adrenergic Blockers. β-Adrenergic blockers are the preferred drugs for the management of chronic stable angina.[42] Examples include propranolol (Inderal), metoprolol (Lopressor), nadolol (Corgard), atenolol (Tenormin), and carvedilol (Coreg). These drugs decrease myocardial contractility, HR, SVR, and BP, all of which reduce the myocardial oxygen demand. β-Adrenergic blockers also have been shown to decrease morbidity and mortality in patients with CAD, especially following MI.[43]

TABLE 34-12 DRUG THERAPY
Chronic Stable Angina and Acute Coronary Syndrome

Drug Classification	Mechanism of Action and Comments
Antiplatelet Agents aspirin	• Inhibits cyclooxygenase, which in turn produces thromboxane A_2, a potent platelet activator • Should be administered as soon as ACS is suspected
Adenosine Diphosphate Receptor Antagonists clopidogrel (Plavix)	• Inhibits platelet aggregation • Alternative for patient who cannot use aspirin
Nitrates Sublingual nitroglycerin (Nitrostat, NitroQuick) Translingual spray nitroglycerin (Nitrolingual) Nitroglycerin ointment (Nitro-Bid, Nitrol) Transdermal nitroglycerin (Transderm-Nitro, Minitran) Extended-release buccal tablets (Nitrogard) Isosorbide dinitrate (Isordil, Sorbitrate) IV nitroglycerin (Nitro-Bid IV, Tridil)	• Promote peripheral vasodilation, decreasing preload and afterload • Coronary artery vasodilation
β-Adrenergic Blockers* atenolol (Tenormin) carvedilol (Coreg) esmolol (Brevibloc) metoprolol (Lopressor) nadolol (Corgard) propranolol (Inderal)	• Inhibit sympathetic nervous stimulation of the heart • Reduce both heart rate and contractility • Decrease afterload
Calcium Channel Blockers* amlodipine (Norvasc) diltiazem (Cardizem) felodipine (Plendil) nifedipine (Procardia) nicardipine (Cardene) verapamil (Calan, Isoptin)	• Prevent calcium entry into vascular smooth muscle cells and myocytes (cardiac cells) • Coronary and peripheral vasodilation • Reduce both heart rate and contractility
Angiotensin-Converting Enzyme (ACE) Inhibitors* captopril (Capoten) enalapril (Vasotec)	• Prevent conversion of angiotensin I to angiotensin II • Decrease endothelial dysfunction • Useful with heart failure, tachycardia, MI, hypertension, diabetes, and chronic kidney disease
Unfractionated Heparins† heparin (Hepalean, Lipo-Hepin, Calciparine)	• Prevent conversion of fibrinogen to fibrin and prothrombin to thrombin
Low-Molecular-Weight Heparins† dalteparin (Fragmin) enoxaparin (Lovenox)	• Bind to antithrombin III, enhancing its effect • Heparin–antithrombin III complex inactivates activated factor X and thrombin • Prevent conversion of fibrinogen to fibrin
Glycoprotein IIb/IIIa Inhibitors abciximab (ReoPro) eptifibatide (Integrelin) tirofiban (Aggrastat)	• Prevent the binding of fibrinogen to platelets, thereby blocking platelet aggregation • Standard antiplatelet therapy in combination with aspirin for patients at high risk for unstable angina
Opioid Analgesics Morphine (morphine sulfate; Duramorph)	• Functions as an analgesic and sedative • Acts as a vasodilator to reduce preload and myocardial O_2 consumption
Fibrinolytic Therapy recombinant plasminogen activator (rPA; reteplase [Retavase]) tissue plasminogen activator (tPA; alteplase [Activase]) TNK-tPA (tenecteplase [TNKase])	• Breaks up fibrin meshwork in clots • Used only in ST-segment-elevation MI

ACS, Acute coronary syndrome; *IV,* intravenous; *MI,* myocardial infarction.
*See Table 33-8.
†See Table 38-9.

β-Adrenergic blockers have many side effects and are sometimes poorly tolerated.[42] Side effects may include bradycardia, hypotension, wheezing, and GI complaints. Many patients also complain of weight gain, depression, and sexual dysfunction. β-Adrenergic blockers should be avoided in patients with asthma and used cautiously in patients with diabetes as they mask signs of hypoglycemia. β-Adrenergic blockers should not be discontinued abruptly without medical supervision as this may precipitate an increase in the frequency and intensity of angina attacks.[34]

Calcium Channel Blockers. If β-adrenergic blockers are contraindicated, are poorly tolerated, or do not control anginal symptoms, calcium channel blockers (e.g., nifedipine [Procardia], verapamil [Calan], diltiazem [Cardizem], nicardipine [Cardene]) are used.[42] These drugs are also used to manage Prinzmetal's angina. Most of these agents have sustained-release versions for longer action with the hope of increased patient adherence and stable blood levels of the drug. The three primary effects of calcium channel blockers are (1) systemic vasodilation with decreased SVR, (2) decreased myocardial contractility, and (3) coronary vasodilation.

Cardiac muscle and vascular smooth muscle cells are more dependent on extracellular calcium than skeletal muscles and are therefore more sensitive to calcium channel blocking agents. Calcium channel blockers cause smooth muscle relaxation and relative vasodilation of coronary and systemic arteries, thus increasing blood flow.

Calcium channel blockers potentiate the action of digoxin by increasing serum digoxin levels during the first week of therapy. Therefore serum digoxin levels should be closely monitored after starting this therapy. The patient should be taught the signs and symptoms of digoxin toxicity.

Angiotensin-Converting Enzyme Inhibitors. Certain high-risk patients with chronic stable angina may benefit from the addition of an angiotensin-converting enzyme (ACE) inhibitor (e.g., captopril [Capoten]) to the drug regimen.[42] These would include patients with diabetes, significant CAD as determined by coronary angiography (e.g., multivessel disease), and/or previous history of MI with left ventricular dysfunction. (ACE inhibitors are discussed later in the chapter and in Chapter 33 and Table 33-8.)

Ranolazine. Ranolazine (Ranexa) is used to treat chronic angina based on its antianginal and anti-ischemic effects. The exact mechanism of action is unknown. Because ranolazine prolongs the QT interval, it should only be used by patients who have not responded to other antianginal drugs. It should be used in combination with amlodipine, β blockers, or nitrates. Common side effects include dizziness, headache, constipation, and nausea.

Diagnostic Studies

When a patient has a history of CAD or CAD is suspected, the physician will order a variety of studies (see Fig. 34-8). After a detailed health history and physical examination, a chest x-ray is usually taken to look for cardiac enlargement, aortic calcifications, and pulmonary congestion. A 12-lead ECG is obtained and compared with an earlier tracing when possible. Certain laboratory tests (e.g., lipid profile) and diagnostic studies (e.g., Holter monitoring, echocardiogram) will be ordered to confirm CAD and identify specific risk factors for CAD.

For patients with known CAD and chronic stable angina, common diagnostic studies include 12-lead ECG, echocardiogram, exercise stress testing, pharmacologic nuclear imaging, and coronary angiography.[42] (See Chapter 32 and Table 32-7 for a discussion of these studies, including nursing considerations.) Two of these studies are discussed in further detail here.

Exercise Stress Testing. Treadmill exercise testing is an important diagnostic test done for the patient with chronic stable angina. ST segment and T wave changes during exercise are an indirect assessment of coronary artery perfusion. Severely abnormal ECGs on exercise testing indicate a significant disease process, and may indicate the need for coronary angiography. Unfortunately, the ECG stress test is not always conclusive for CAD. A false-positive test may be found (especially in women), and a false-negative test may be seen if the patient is exercised submaximally or if only one coronary artery is involved. Pharmacologic nuclear imaging and echocardiography can complement exercise testing, especially in people with inconclusive results on the exercise testing or who are unable to exercise.

Cardiac Catheterization. It is not uncommon for a patient with chronic stable angina to undergo a diagnostic cardiac catheterization and coronary angiography. If a coronary lesion is amenable to an intervention, **coronary revascularization** with an elective **percutaneous coronary intervention** (PCI) may be done.[40,41] During this procedure, a catheter equipped with an inflatable balloon tip is inserted into the appropriate coronary artery. When the blockage is located, the catheter is passed through it, the balloon is inflated, and the atherosclerotic plaque is compressed, resulting in vessel dilation. This procedure is called *balloon angioplasty.* Unfractionated heparin (UH) or low-molecular-weight heparin (LMWH) is given in conjunction with PCI to maintain the open vessel.

Intracoronary stents are often inserted in conjunction with balloon angioplasty. Stents are used to treat abrupt or threatened abrupt closure and restenosis following balloon angioplasty. A **stent** is an expandable meshlike structure designed to maintain vessel patency by compressing the arterial wall and resisting vasoconstriction (Figs. 34-9 and 34-10). Stents are carefully placed over the angioplasty site to hold the vessel open. Because stents are thrombogenic, the patient is also treated with oral antiplatelet

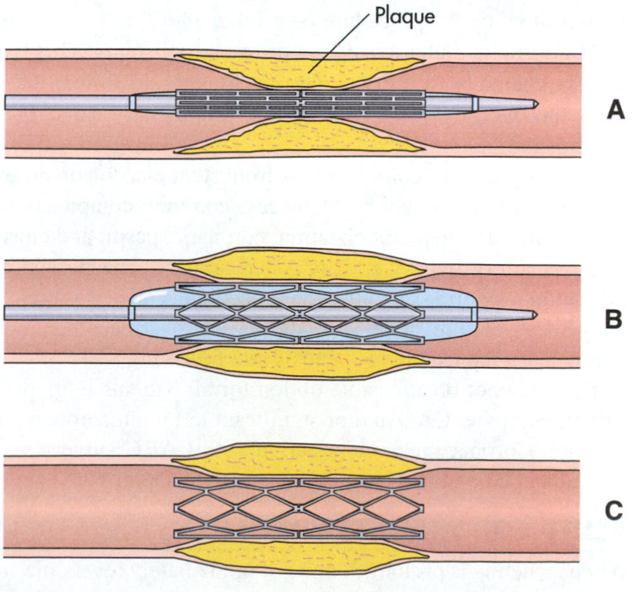

FIG. 34-9 Placement of a coronary artery stent. **A,** The stent is positioned at the site of the lesion. **B,** The balloon is inflated, expanding the stent. The balloon is then deflated and removed. **C,** The implanted stent is left in place.

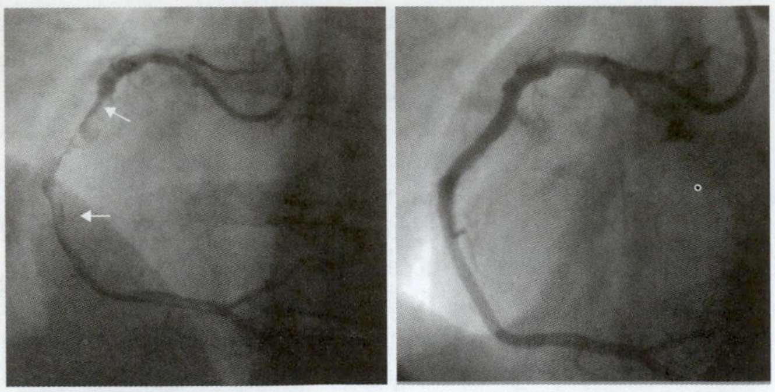

FIG. 34-10 **A,** A thrombotic occlusion of the right coronary artery is noted *(arrows)*. **B,** Right coronary artery is opened and blood flow restored following angioplasty and placement of a 4-mm stent.

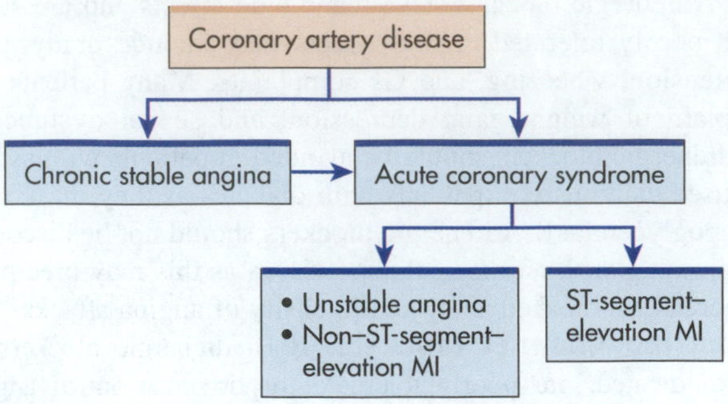

FIG. 34-11 Relationships among coronary artery disease, chronic stable angina, and acute coronary syndrome. *MI,* Myocardial infarction.

GENDER DIFFERENCES

Acute Coronary Syndrome (ACS)

Men

- Incidence of MI is highest among white, middle-aged men.
- After the age of 65, the incidence of MI in men and women equalizes.
- Men present more frequently than women with an acute MI as the first manifestation of CAD.
- Men develop greater collateral circulation than women.

Women

- Women are older than men when presenting with first MI.
- Once a women reaches menopause, her risk for an MI quadruples.
- Fewer women than men present with "classic" signs and symptoms of UA or MI.
- Fatigue is often the first symptom of ACS in women.
- Women experience more "silent" MIs compared to men.
- Among those who have an MI, women are more likely to suffer a fatal cardiac event within 1 yr than men.
- Women report more disability after a cardiac event than men.
- Women who have coronary artery bypass graft surgery have a higher mortality rate and more complications after surgery than men.

CAD, Coronary artery disease; *MI,* myocardial infarction; *UA,* unstable angina.

agents such as aspirin or clopidogrel. An intravenous (IV) infusion of a glycoprotein IIb/IIIa inhibitor (e.g., tirofiban [Aggrastat]) has been found to be beneficial for preventing abrupt closure of the stents. The infusion is initiated during PCI and maintained for 12 hours following the procedure (see Table 34-12).

Many stents that are used are drug-eluting stents. This type of stent is coated with a drug (e.g., paclitaxel, sirolimus) that prevents the overgrowth of new intima, the primary cause of stent restenosis.[44,45]

The most serious complications from stent placement are abrupt closure and vascular injury. Other less common complications include acute MI, stent embolization, coronary spasm, and emergent coronary artery bypass graft (CABG) surgery. The possibility of dysrhythmias during and after the procedure is always present. The use of drug-eluting stents and advances in pharmacotherapy have significantly reduced the restenosis rate following PCI.

PCI may not be a feasible option for all patients (e.g., patients with three-vessel CAD and/or significant left main coronary artery disease). Coronary revascularization with CABG surgery may be recommended and is discussed later in the chapter.[40]

ACUTE CORONARY SYNDROME

When ischemia is prolonged and not immediately reversible, **acute coronary syndrome** (ACS) develops and encompasses the spectrum of unstable angina (UA), *non–ST-segment-elevation myocardial infarction* (NSTEMI), and *ST-segment–elevation myocardial infarction* (STEMI) (Fig. 34-11). Although each remains a distinct diagnosis, this nomenclature (ACS) reflects the relationships among the pathophysiology, diagnosis, prognosis, and interventions for these disorders.

Etiology and Pathophysiology

ACS is associated with deterioration of a once stable atherosclerotic plaque. The once stable plaque ruptures, exposing the intima to blood and stimulating platelet aggregation and local vasoconstriction with thrombus formation. This unstable lesion may be partially occluded by a thrombus (manifesting as UA or NSTEMI) or totally occluded by a thrombus (manifesting as STEMI).[43,46] What causes a coronary plaque to suddenly become unstable is not well understood, but systemic inflammation (described earlier) is thought to play a role.[9] Patients with suspected ACS require immediate hospitalization.

Manifestations of Acute Coronary Syndrome

UNSTABLE ANGINA

Chest pain that is new in onset, occurs at rest, or has a worsening pattern is called **unstable angina.** The patient with chronic stable angina may develop UA, or UA may be the first clinical manifestation of CAD. Unlike chronic stable angina, UA is unpredictable and represents an emergency. The patient with previously diagnosed chronic stable angina will describe a significant change in the pattern of angina. It will occur with increasing frequency and is easily provoked by minimal or no exertion, during sleep, or even at rest. The patient without previously diagnosed angina will describe anginal pain that has progressed rapidly in the last few hours, days, or weeks, often culminating in pain at rest.[41]

Women seek medical attention more often with symptoms of UA than men. Studies have shown that women will have prodromal symptoms that are early manifestations of CAD, but because they are not recognized as such, many women present with UA before CAD is diagnosed.[47] These symptoms include fatigue, shortness of breath, indigestion, and anxiety. Fatigue is the most prominent symptom. Because fatigue can be a symptom of many different diseases and syndromes, a careful history of CAD risk factors should be obtained to identify these women.

MYOCARDIAL INFARCTION

A **myocardial infarction** occurs as a result of sustained ischemia, causing irreversible myocardial cell death (necrosis) (Figs. 34-12 and 34-13). Eighty percent to 90% of all acute MIs are secondary to thrombus formation.[42,46] When a thrombus develops, perfusion to the myocardium distal to the occlusion is halted, resulting in necrosis. Contractile function of the heart stops in the necrotic area(s). The degree of altered function depends on the area of the heart involved and the size of the infarction. Most MIs involve some portion of the left ventricle.

The acute MI process takes time. Cardiac cells can withstand ischemic conditions for approximately 20 minutes before cellular death begins. The earliest tissue to become ischemic is the subendocardium (the innermost layer of tissue in the cardiac muscle). If ischemia persists, it takes approximately 4 to 6 hours for the entire thickness of the heart muscle to become necrosed (Fig. 34-14).

Infarctions are usually described based on the location of damage (e.g., anterior, inferior, lateral, or posterior wall infarction). Damage can occur in more than one location (e.g., anterolateral MI, anteroseptal MI). The location of the infarction correlates with the involved coronary circulation. For example, inferior wall infarctions result from occlusions in the right coronary artery. Anterior wall infarctions result from occlusions in the left anterior descending artery. Occlusions in the left circumflex artery usually cause lateral and/or posterior wall MIs.

The degree of preestablished collateral circulation also influences the severity of infarction (see Fig. 34-3). In an individual with a history of CAD, collateral circulation may be established that provides the area surrounding the infarction site with a blood supply. This is one explanation why the younger person who has an MI is often likely to have a more serious impairment than an older person with the same degree of occlusion.

Clinical Manifestations of Myocardial Infarction

Pain. Severe, immobilizing chest pain not relieved by rest, position change, or nitrate administration is the hallmark of an MI. Persistent and unlike any other pain, it is usually described as a heaviness, pressure, tightness, burning, constriction, or crushing. Common locations are substernal, retrosternal, or epigastric areas. The pain may radiate to the neck, jaw, and arms or to the back (see Fig. 34-7). It may occur while the patient is active or at rest, or asleep or awake. However, it commonly occurs in the early morning hours. It usually

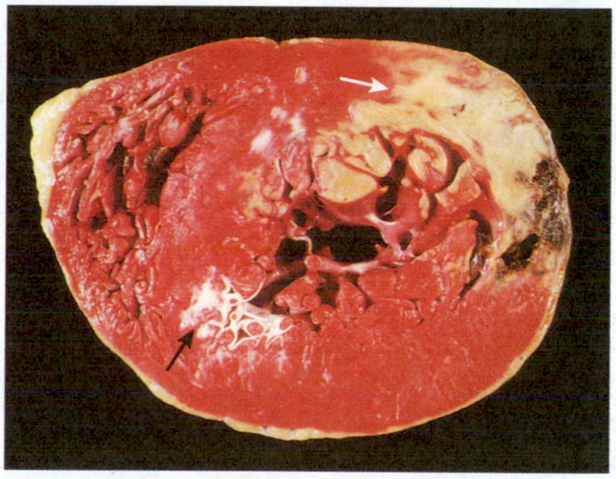

FIG. 34-13 Acute myocardial infarction in the posterolateral wall of the left ventricle. This is demonstrated by the absence of staining in the areas of necrosis *(white arrow)*. Note the scarring from a previous anterior wall myocardial infarction *(black arrow)*.

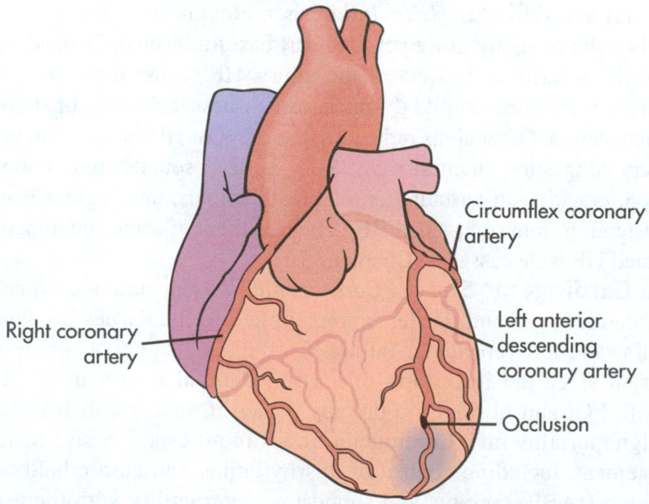

FIG. 34-12 Occlusion of the left anterior descending coronary artery, resulting in a myocardial infarction.

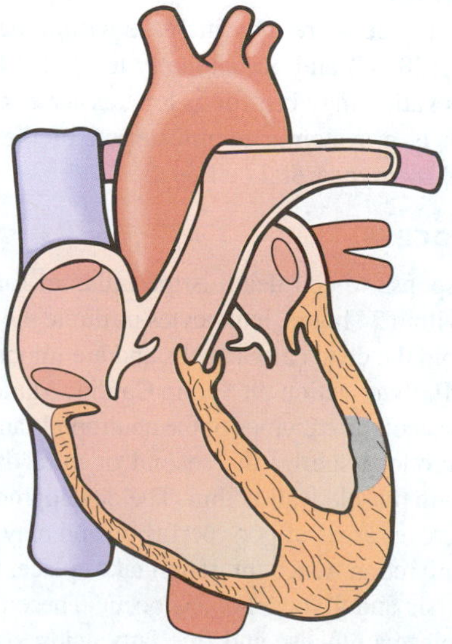

FIG. 34-14 Myocardial infarction involving the full thickness of the left ventricular wall.

lasts for 20 minutes or more and is described as more severe than usual anginal pain. When epigastric pain is present, the patient may relate it to indigestion and take antacids without relief.

Not everyone has classic symptoms. Some patients may not experience pain but may have "discomfort," weakness, or shortness of breath. Although women and men have more similarities in their symptoms of an acute MI than differences, some women may experience atypical discomfort, shortness of breath, or fatigue.[47,48] Patients with diabetes are more likely to experience silent (asymptomatic) MIs due to cardiac neuropathy and present with atypical symptoms (e.g., dyspnea). An older patient may experience a change in mental status (e.g., confusion), shortness of breath, pulmonary edema, dizziness, or a dysrhythmia.

Sympathetic Nervous System Stimulation. During the initial phase of MI, catecholamines (norepinephrine and epinephrine) are released from the ischemic myocardial cells that normally contain varying quantities of these substances. The increased sympathetic nervous system stimulation results in release of glycogen, diaphoresis, and vasoconstriction of peripheral blood vessels. On physical examination, the patient's skin may be ashen, clammy, and cool to touch.

Cardiovascular Manifestations. In response to the release of catecholamines, the BP and HR may be elevated initially. Later, the BP may drop because of decreased cardiac output (CO). If severe enough, this may result in decreased renal perfusion and urine output. Crackles may be noted in the lungs, persisting for several hours to several days, suggesting left ventricular dysfunction. Jugular venous distention, hepatic engorgement, and peripheral edema may indicate right ventricular dysfunction.

Cardiac examination may reveal abnormal heart sounds that may seem distant. Careful auscultation may reveal splitting of heart sounds. Other abnormal sounds suggesting ventricular dysfunction are S_3 and S_4. In addition, a loud holosystolic murmur may develop and may indicate a septal defect or mitral valve dysfunction.

Nausea and Vomiting. The patient may be nauseated and vomit. Nausea and vomiting can result from reflex stimulation of the vomiting center by the severe pain. These symptoms can also result from vasovagal reflexes initiated from the area of the infarcted myocardium.

Fever. The temperature may increase within the first 24 hours up to 100.4° F (38° C) and occasionally to 102.2° F (39° C). The temperature elevation may last for as long as 1 week. This increase in temperature is a systemic manifestation of the inflammatory process caused by myocardial cell death.

Healing Process

The body's response to cell death is the inflammatory process (see Chapter 13). Within 24 hours, leukocytes infiltrate the area. Enzymes are released from the dead cardiac cells and are important diagnostic indicators of MI. (See section on Serum Cardiac Markers later in this chapter.) The proteolytic enzymes of the neutrophils and macrophages remove all necrotic tissue by the second or third day. During this time, the necrotic muscle wall is thin. The development of collateral circulation improves areas of poor perfusion and may limit the zones of injury and infarction. Once infarction takes place, catecholamine-mediated lipolysis and glycogenolysis occur. These processes allow the increased plasma glucose and free fatty acids to be used by the oxygen-depleted myocardium for anaerobic metabolism. For this reason, serum glucose levels are frequently elevated after MI.[46]

The necrotic zone is identifiable by ECG changes (e.g., ST segment elevation, pathologic Q wave) and by nuclear scanning after the onset of symptoms. At this point, the neutrophils and monocytes have cleared the necrotic debris from the injured area, and the collagen matrix that will eventually form scar tissue is laid down.

At 10 to 14 days after MI, the beginning scar tissue is still weak. The myocardium is considered to be especially vulnerable to increased stress because of the unstable state of the healing heart wall. It is also at this time that the patient's activity level may be increasing, so special caution and assessment are necessary. By 6 weeks after MI, scar tissue has replaced necrotic tissue. At this time, the injured area is said to be healed. The scarred area is often less compliant than the surrounding fibers. This condition may be manifested by uncoordinated wall motion, ventricular dysfunction, or pump failure.[46]

These changes in the infarcted muscle also cause changes in the unaffected myocardium as well. In an attempt to compensate for the infarcted muscle, the normal myocardium will hypertrophy and dilate. This process is called *ventricular remodeling.* Remodeling of normal myocardium can lead to the development of late heart failure (HF), especially in the individual with atherosclerosis of other coronary arteries and/or an anterior MI.[46]

Complications of Myocardial Infarction

Dysrhythmias. The most common complication after an MI is dysrhythmias, which are present in 80% of MI patients. Dysrhythmias are the most common cause of death in patients in the prehospital period. Dysrhythmias are caused by any condition that affects the myocardial cell's sensitivity to nerve impulses, such as ischemia, electrolyte imbalances, and sympathetic nervous system stimulation. The intrinsic rhythm of the heartbeat is disrupted, causing a fast HR (tachycardia), a slow HR (bradycardia), or an irregular beat, all of which adversely affect the ischemic myocardium.

Life-threatening dysrhythmias occur most often with anterior wall infarction, HF, or shock. Complete heart block is seen in massive infarction. Ventricular fibrillation, a common cause of sudden cardiac death, is a lethal dysrhythmia that most often occurs within the first 4 hours after the onset of pain. Premature ventricular contractions may precede ventricular tachycardia and fibrillation. Life-threatening ventricular dysrhythmias must be treated immediately. (See Chapter 36 for a detailed description of dysrhythmias and their management.)

Heart Failure. *Heart failure* is a complication that occurs when the pumping power of the heart has diminished. Depending on the severity and extent of the injury, HF occurs initially with subtle signs such as mild dyspnea, restlessness, agitation, or slight tachycardia. Other signs indicating the onset of HF include pulmonary congestion on chest x-ray, S_3 or S_4 heart sounds on auscultation, crackles on auscultation of breath sounds, and jugular vein distention from right-sided HF. (The treatment of acute decompensated HF is discussed in Chapter 35.)

Cardiogenic Shock. *Cardiogenic shock* occurs when inadequate oxygen and nutrients are supplied to the tissues because of severe left ventricular failure. Cardiogenic shock occurs less often since the institution of early and rapid treatment of MI with PCI and fibrinolytic therapy. When it does occur, it has a high mortality rate. Cardiogenic shock requires aggressive management, including control of dysrhythmias, intraaortic balloon pump (IABP) therapy, and support of contractility with the use of vasoactive drugs. The goal of therapy is to maximize oxygen delivery, reduce oxygen demand, and prevent complications such as acute renal failure.[46] (Cardiogenic shock is discussed in Chapter 67.)

Papillary Muscle Dysfunction. *Papillary muscle dysfunction* may occur if the infarcted area includes or is adjacent to the papillary muscle that attaches to the mitral valve (see Fig. 32-3). Papillary muscle dysfunction causes mitral valve regurgitation, which increases the volume of blood in the left atrium. This condition aggravates an already compromised left ventricle by reducing CO even further. Papillary muscle dysfunction is detected by a systolic murmur at the cardiac apex radiating toward the axilla.

Papillary muscle rupture is a rare but life-threatening complication causing massive mitral valve regurgitation, which results in dyspnea, pulmonary edema, and decreased CO. There is rapid clinical deterioration of the patient. Treatment consists of rapid afterload reduction with nitroprusside and/or IABP therapy and immediate open heart surgery with mitral valve replacement.[46] (See Chapter 37 for discussion of valve disorders.)

Ventricular Aneurysm. *Ventricular aneurysm* results when the infarcted myocardial wall becomes thinned and bulges out during contraction. The patient with a ventricular aneurysm may experience refractory HF, dysrhythmias, and angina. Besides ventricular rupture, which is fatal, ventricular aneurysms harbor thrombi that can lead to an embolic stroke.

Pericarditis. Acute *pericarditis,* an inflammation of the visceral and/or parietal pericardium, may result in cardiac compression, decreased ventricular filling and emptying, and HF. It may occur 2 to 3 days after an acute MI as a common complication of the infarction. Pericarditis is characterized by chest pain, which may vary from mild to severe, and is aggravated by inspiration, coughing, and movement of the upper body. The pain may be relieved by sitting in a forward position. The pain is usually different from pain associated with an MI.

Assessment of the patient with pericarditis may reveal a friction rub over the pericardium. The sound may be best heard with the diaphragm of the stethoscope at the mid- to lower sternal border. It may be persistent or intermittent. Fever may also be present.

Diagnosis of pericarditis can be made with serial 12-lead ECGs. Characteristic ECG changes are diffuse and reflect the inflammation of the pericardium. Treatment may include pain relief by aspirin, corticosteroids, or NSAIDs. (Pericarditis is discussed in Chapter 37.)

Dressler Syndrome. *Dressler syndrome* is characterized by pericarditis with effusion and fever that develops 4 to 6 weeks after MI. It may also occur after open heart surgery. It is thought to be caused by an antigen-antibody reaction to the necrotic myocardium. The patient experiences pericardial pain, fever, a friction rub, pleural effusion, and arthralgia. Laboratory findings include an elevated white blood cell count and an elevated sedimentation rate. Short-term corticosteroids are used to treat this condition. (Dressler syndrome is discussed in Chapter 37.)

DIAGNOSTIC STUDIES

Unstable Angina and Myocardial Infarction

In addition to the patient's history of pain, risk factors, and health history, the primary diagnostic studies used to determine whether a person has UA or an MI include an ECG and serum cardiac markers (see Fig. 34-8).

Electrocardiogram Findings. The ECG is the primary tool to rule out or confirm UA or an MI. Changes in the QRS complex, ST segment, and T wave caused by ischemia and infarction can develop quickly with UA and MI. For diagnostic and treatment purposes, it is important to distinguish between STEMI, and UA or NSTEMI. Patients with STEMI tend to have a more extensive MI that is associated with prolonged and complete coronary occlusion, and the development of a pathologic Q wave on the ECG. Patients with UA or NSTEMI usually have transient thrombosis or incomplete coronary occlusion and usually do not develop pathologic Q waves. Areas of ischemia or infarction may be noted on the ECG. Because MI is a dynamic process that evolves with time, the ECG often reveals the time sequence of ischemia, injury, infarction, and resolution of the infarction.

The ECG may also be normal or nondiagnostic when the patient comes to the ED with a complaint of chest pain. Within a few hours, the ECG may change to reflect the infarction process. These changes take place when cellular damage has occurred, interrupting the normal electrical depolarization of the ventricles. When the initial ECG is nondiagnostic, serial ECGs are done every 2 to 4 hours.[46] (See Chapter 36 for discussion of ECG changes associated with ischemia and MI.)

Serum Cardiac Markers. Certain proteins, called *serum cardiac markers,* are released into the blood in large quantities from necrotic heart muscle after an MI. These markers, specifically serum cardiac enzymes and troponin, are important in the diagnosis of MI. When cardiac cells die, their intracellular enzymes are released into circulation. The increase in serum cardiac markers that occurs after cellular death can indicate whether cardiac damage is present and the approximate extent of the damage. Creatine kinase (CK) and troponin are typically measured to diagnose an MI. (Fig. 34-15 indicates the peak level and duration of these markers in the presence of MI.)

CK levels begin to rise approximately 3 to 12 hours after an MI, peak in 24 hours, and return to normal within 2 to 3 days. The CK enzymes may be fractionated into bands, including the MB band. The CK-MB band is specific to myocardial cells and can help quantify myocardial damage.

Cardiac-specific troponin is a myocardial muscle protein released into circulation after myocardial injury. In the heart there are two subtypes: cardiac-specific troponin T (cTnT) and cardiac-specific troponin I (cTnI). These markers are highly specific indi-

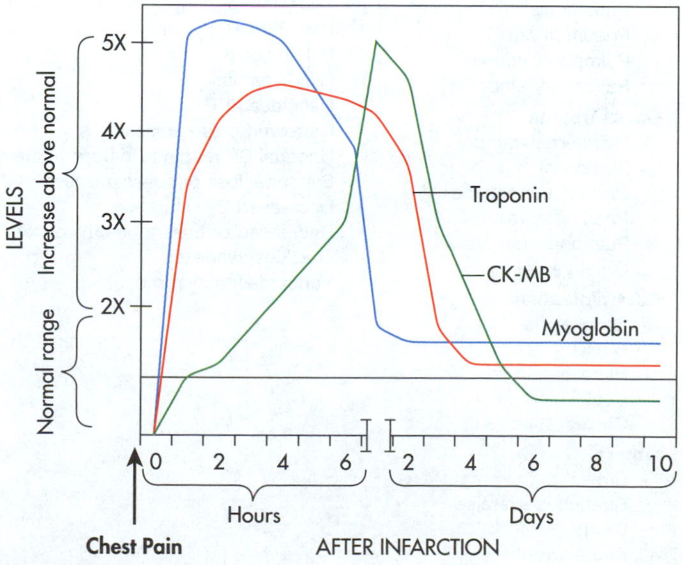

FIG. 34-15 Serum cardiac markers in the blood after myocardial infarction. *CK,* Creatine kinase.

cators of MI and have greater sensitivity and specificity for myocardial injury than CK-MB.[6,46] Troponin rises as quickly as CK. It is usually used for diagnostic purposes in conjunction with total CK and the MB fraction.[6,46] Serum levels of cTnI and cTnT increase 3 to 12 hours after the onset of MI, peak at 24 to 48 hours, and return to baseline over 5 to 14 days.

Myoglobin is released into circulation within a few hours after an MI. Although it is one of the first serum cardiac markers that increase after an MI, it lacks cardiac specificity. In addition, it is rapidly excreted in urine so that blood levels return to normal range within 24 hours after an MI (see Table 32-7).

Coronary Angiography. The patient with UA or NSTEMI may undergo coronary angiography to evaluate the extent of the disease and to determine the most appropriate therapeutic modality. If appropriate, a PCI may be performed at this time. Others may be treated with conservative medical management. It remains controversial which is the best management for UA and NSTEMI.[40,41] Coronary angiography is the only way to confirm the diagnosis of Prinzmetal's angina.

Other Measures

When the ECG and serum cardiac markers do not confirm MI, other measures for diagnosing UA may be considered (see Table 32-7). Exercise stress testing and echocardiograms may be used when a patient has an abnormal but nondiagnostic baseline ECG. A dobutamine (Dobutrex) stress echocardiogram can be performed in patients unable to exercise. (See Chapter 32 for additional information on cardiac assessment.)

COLLABORATIVE CARE

It is extremely important that a patient with ACS is rapidly diagnosed and treated to preserve cardiac muscle. Initial management of the patient with chest pain most often occurs in the ED. Emergency care of the patient with chest pain is presented in Table 34-13. An IV route is established to provide an accessible means for emergency drug therapy. Sublingual nitroglycerin and aspirin (chewable) are given if not done by emergency medical personnel prior to arrival at the ED. Morphine sulfate is given IV for pain unrelieved by nitroglycerin. Oxygen is administered by nasal cannula at a rate of 2 to 4 L/min. The patient will usually receive ongoing care in a critical care unit or telemetry unit, where continuous ECG monitoring is available. Dysrhythmias may be detected, and appropriate treatment can be instituted. The collaborative care of ACS is presented in Fig. 34-8 on p. 799.

Vital signs, including pulse oximetry, are monitored frequently during the first few hours after admission and are monitored closely thereafter. Bed rest and limitation of activity are initially ordered for 12 to 24 hours, with a gradual increase in activity unless contraindicated.

For patients with UA or NSTEMI with negative cardiac markers and ongoing angina, a combination of aspirin, heparin (UH or LMWH), and a glycoprotein IIb/IIIa inhibitor (e.g., abciximab

TABLE 34-13 *EMERGENCY MANAGEMENT* Chest Pain

Etiology

Cardiovascular
- Angina
- Myocardial infarction
- Dysrhythmia
- Pericarditis
- Aortic aneurysm
- Aortic valve disease

Respiratory
- Costochondritis
- Pleurisy
- Pneumonia
- Pneumothorax
- Pulmonary edema
- Pulmonary embolus

Chest Trauma
- Rib/sternal fracture
- Flail chest
- Cardiac tamponade
- Pneumothorax
- Pulmonary contusion
- Great vessel injury

Gastrointestinal
- Esophagitis
- GERD
- Hiatal hernia
- Peptic ulcer
- Cholecystitis

Others
- Stress
- Strenuous exercise
- Drugs
- Acute anxiety

Assessment Findings

- Pain in chest, neck, arm, or shoulder
- Cold, clammy skin
- Diaphoresis
- Nausea and vomiting
- Epigastric pain
- Indigestion/heartburn
- Dyspnea
- Weakness
- Anxiety
- Feeling of impending doom
- Tachycardia
- Irregular HR, murmurs
- Palpitations
- Dysrhythmias
- Decreased BP
- Narrowed pulse pressure
- Unequal BP readings in upper extremities
- Syncope, loss of consciousness
- Decreased O_2 saturation
- Decreased or absent breath sounds
- Crackles, wheezes
- Pericardial friction rub

Interventions

Initial
- Ensure patent airway.
- Administer O_2 by nasal cannula or non-rebreather mask.
- Obtain 12-lead ECG.
- Insert two IV catheters.
- Assess pain using PQRST mnemonic (see Table 34-8).
- Medicate for pain as ordered (e.g., morphine, nitroglycerin).
- Initiate continuous ECG monitoring and identify underlying rhythm.
- Obtain baseline blood work (e.g., cardiac markers).
- Obtain portable chest x-ray.
- Assess for antiplatelet, anticoagulation, or fibrinolytic therapy; or PCI as appropriate.
- Administer aspirin and β-adrenergic blockers for cardiac-related chest pain unless contraindicated.
- Administer antidysrhythmic drugs as indicated.

Ongoing Monitoring
- Monitor vital signs, level of consciousness, cardiac rhythm, and O_2 saturation.
- Monitor response to medications (e.g., decrease in chest pain) and remedicate or titrate medications (e.g., nitroglycerin) as needed.
- Provide reassurance and emotional support to patient and family.
- Explain all interventions/procedures to patient in simple terms.
- Anticipate need for intubation if respiratory distress is evident.
- Prepare for CPR, defibrillation, transcutaneous pacing, or cardioversion.

BP, Blood pressure; *CPR*, cardiopulmonary resuscitation; *ECG*, electrocardiogram; *GERD*, gastroesophageal reflux disease; *HR*, heart rate; *IV*, intravenous; *PCI*, percutaneous coronary intervention.

[ReoPro], eptifibatide [Integrelin], tirofiban [Aggrastat]) is recommended. PCI is considered once the patient is stabilized and angina is controlled, or if angina returns or increases in severity.[40]

For patients with STEMI or NSTEMI with positive cardiac markers, reperfusion therapy is initiated (see Fig. 34-8). *Reperfusion therapy* can include emergent PCI or fibrinolytic (thrombolytic) therapy. The goal in the treatment of MI is to salvage as much myocardial muscle as possible.

Emergent PCI

In centers performing at least 200 PCI procedures a year, and that have trained interventional cardiologists and cardiac surgical capability, emergent PCI is recommended as the first line of treatment for patients with confirmed MI (i.e., definitive ECG changes and/or positive cardiac markers).[43,46] The goal is to open the affected artery within 90 minutes of arrival to the ED. In this situation, the patient will have a cardiac catheterization to locate the blockage(s), assess the severity of the blockage(s), determine the presence of collateral circulation, and evaluate left ventricular function. With actual visualization of the coronary artery system and left ventricular function, treatment modalities most beneficial to the patient can be selected. Usually PCI with the placement of drug-eluting stent(s) will be performed. Patients with severe left ventricular dysfunction may require the addition of IABP therapy, and a small percentage of patients may require emergent CABG surgery.

The advantages of PCI are that (1) it provides an alternative to surgical intervention; (2) it is performed with local anesthesia; (3) the patient is ambulatory 24 hours after the procedure; (4) the length of hospital stay is approximately 1 to 3 days compared with the 4- to 6-day stay of someone having CABG surgery, thus reducing hospital costs; and (5) there is rapid return to work (approximately 5 to 7 days after PCI) instead of a 2- to 8-week convalescence after CABG.

Many advances have been made in PCI during the last decade. Guidewires and catheters with greater flexibility have been developed, enabling cardiologists to maneuver the catheters to distal and proximal lesions. Today PCI is more frequently performed than CABG surgery. Reduction of lesion size by greater than 50% occurs in 90% of patients.[41] Techniques have been developed to provide blood flow to the distal myocardium during balloon inflation, increasing the safety of the procedure. Dilation may also be done for stenotic grafts from a previous CABG surgery.

The most serious complication of PCI is dissection of the newly dilated coronary artery. If the damage is extensive, the coronary artery could rupture, causing cardiac tamponade, ischemia and infarction, decreased CO, and possible death. There is also danger from infarction should the lesion be calcified and a portion of the plaque dislodges and occludes the vessel distal to the catheter. Coronary spasm from the mechanical irritation of the catheter or balloon can occur as well as chemical irritation from the contrast medium injection used to visualize the artery. Abrupt closure is a complication that can occur in the first 24 hours after PCI. Restenosis after PCI can also occur, and risk is greatest in the first 30 days following the procedure. Nursing care of the patient following PCI is similar to that of cardiac catheterization (see Chapter 32, Table 32-7).

Fibrinolytic Therapy

Fibrinolytic therapy offers the advantages of availability and rapid administration in facilities that do not have an interventional cardiac catheterization lab or when one is too far away to safely transfer the patient. Treatment of MI with fibrinolytic therapy is aimed at stopping the infarction process by dissolving the thrombus in the coronary artery and reperfusing the myocardium. To be of most benefit, fibrinolytic therapy must be given as soon as possible, ideally within the first hour after onset of symptoms and preferably within the first 6 hours after the onset of symptoms. If reperfusion occurs within 6 hours, a 25% reduction in mortality rate has been shown.[43,46]

Indications and Contraindications. All fibrinolytics are given IV (see Table 34-12). The choice of a thrombolytic agent is guided by considerations of cost, efficacy, and ease of administration. Although these drugs have different mechanisms of action and different pharmacokinetics, they all produce an open artery by lysis of the thrombus in the coronary artery. The goal for the administration of a fibrinolytic is within 30 minutes of the patient's arrival to the ED. Optimal outcomes can be achieved if the fibrinolytic is administered within 60 minutes of onset of symptoms.[43]

Because all the fibrinolytics produce lysis of the pathologic clot, they may also lyse other clots (e.g., a postoperative site). Therefore patient selection is important because minor or major bleeding can be a complication of therapy.[43] Inclusion criteria for fibrinolytic therapy include (1) chest pain typical of acute MI ≤6 hours in duration, (2) 12-lead ECG findings consistent with acute MI, and (3) no absolute contraindications (Table 34-14). Although patients presenting with chest pain >6 hours in duration and ECG changes indicative of MI may be considered for fibrinolytic therapy, research on the benefit of this therapy is inconclusive.[43,46]

Procedure. Each hospital has a protocol to follow for administration of fibrinolytic therapy. However, there are several common factors. Blood for baseline labs is drawn, two to three lines for IV therapy are started, and all other invasive procedures are done before the fibrinolytic agent is given. This procedure reduces the possibility of bleeding in the patient.

Depending on the drug selected, therapy may be administered in one IV bolus or over a period of time (30 to 90 minutes). The

TABLE 34-14 Contraindications for the Use of Fibrinolytic Therapy

Absolute Contraindications
- Active internal bleeding or bleeding diathesis (excluding menstruation)
- Known history of cerebral aneurysm or arteriovenous malformation
- Known intracranial neoplasm (primary or metastatic)
- Previous cerebral hemorrhage
- Recent (within past 3 mo) ischemic stroke
- Significant closed-head or facial trauma within 3 mo
- Suspected aortic dissection

Relative Contraindications
- Active peptic ulcer disease
- Current use of anticoagulants
- Pregnancy
- Prior ischemic stroke >3 mo, dementia, or known intracranial pathology not covered in absolute contraindications
- Recent (within 3 wk) surgery (including eye laser surgery) or puncture of noncompressible vessel
- Recent (within 2-4 wk) internal bleeding
- Serious systemic disease (e.g., advanced/terminal cancer, severe liver/kidney disease)
- Severe uncontrolled hypertension (BP >180/110 mm Hg) on presentation or chronic severe poorly controlled hypertension
- Traumatic or prolonged (>10 min) cardiopulmonary resuscitation

BP, Blood pressure.

time at which therapy begins is noted, and the patient is monitored during and after the period of time that the fibrinolytic is administered. ECG, vital signs, pulse oximetry, and heart and lung assessments are completed frequently to evaluate the patient's response to therapy. When reperfusion occurs (i.e., the coronary artery that was occluded is opened, blood flow is restored to the myocardium), several clinical markers may change. The most reliable marker is the return of the ST segment to baseline on the ECG. Other markers include a resolution of chest pain, and a rapid rise of the CK-MB enzymes within 3 hours of therapy and peaking within 12 hours. The CK-MB levels increase as the necrotic myocardial cells release CK-MB enzymes into the circulation after perfusion has been restored to the area. The presence of *reperfusion dysrhythmias* (e.g., accelerated idioventricular rhythm) is a less reliable marker of reperfusion. These dysrhythmias are generally self-limiting and do not require aggressive treatment. (See Chapter 36 for management of dysrhythmias.)

A major concern with fibrinolytic therapy is reocclusion of the artery. The site of the thrombus is unstable, and another clot may form or spasm of the artery may occur. Because of this possibility, most physicians begin IV heparin therapy. If another clot develops, the patient will have similar complaints of chest pain, and ECG changes will return. The patient will be reevaluated and may receive a second dose of the fibrinolytic or be transferred to a cardiac catheterization lab for *rescue PCI*.

The major complication with fibrinolytic therapy is bleeding. Ongoing nursing assessment is essential. Minor bleeding (e.g., surface bleeding from IV sites or gingival bleeding) is expected and can be controlled by applying a pressure dressing or ice packs. If signs and symptoms of major bleeding occur (e.g., drop in BP, an increase in HR, a sudden decrease in the patient's level of consciousness, blood in the urine or stool), the physician should be notified and the therapy should be stopped.

Drug Therapy

IV nitroglycerin, aspirin, β-adrenergic blockers, and systemic anticoagulation with either LMWH given subcutaneously or IV UH are the initial drug treatments of choice for ACS.[43,46] IV antiplatelet agents (e.g., glycoprotein IIb/IIIa inhibitor) may also be used if PCI is anticipated. ACE inhibitors are added for select patients following MI (discussed below). Calcium channel blockers or long-acting nitrates can be added if the patient is already on adequate doses of β-adrenergic blockers or cannot tolerate β-adrenergic blockers, or has Prinzmetal's angina.[43,46]

Drug therapy for patients with ACS is presented in Table 34-12 and Fig. 34-8. These drugs are discussed on pp. 798 to 801. ACS-specific discussion of select drugs is presented in this section.

IV Nitroglycerin. IV nitroglycerin (Tridil) is used in the initial treatment of the patient with ACS. The goal of therapy is to reduce anginal pain and improve coronary blood flow. It has an immediate onset of action and can be titrated to prevent, treat, and stop UA.[41,49]

IV nitroglycerin is used to decrease preload and afterload while increasing the myocardial oxygen supply. IV nitroglycerin is usually titrated to relieve pain. Because hypotension is a common side effect, BP is closely monitored during this time. Patients who do become hypotensive are often volume depleted and can benefit from an IV fluid bolus.[43,46] Tolerance is another side effect of IV nitrate therapy. An effective strategy for this phenomenon is titrating the dose down at night during sleep and titrating the dose up during the day.

Morphine Sulfate. Morphine sulfate is given for chest pain that is unrelieved by nitroglycerin. As a vasodilator, it decreases cardiac workload by lowering myocardial oxygen consumption, reducing contractility, and decreasing BP and HR. In addition, morphine can help reduce anxiety and fear. In rare situations, morphine can depress respirations. Patients should be monitored for signs of bradypnea or hypoxia, a condition to be avoided in myocardial ischemia and infarction.

β-Adrenergic Blockers. β-Adrenergic blockers are used to decrease myocardial oxygen demand by reducing HR, BP, and contractility. The use of these drugs in the first hours of MI have shown to reduce the size of the infarction and incidence of complications. The continuation of β-adrenergic blockers indefinitely is recommended.[43] (See Table 34-12 and Chapter 33 and Table 33-8 for a discussion of β-adrenergic blockers.)

Angiotensin-Converting Enzyme Inhibitors. ACE inhibitors (e.g., captopril [Capoten]) are recommended following anterior wall MIs or MIs that result in decreased left ventricular function (ejection fraction [EF] <40%) or pulmonary congestion.[43,46] The use of ACE inhibitors can help prevent ventricular remodeling and prevent or slow the progression of HF. ACE inhibitors should be continued indefinitely. For patients who cannot tolerate ACE inhibitors, angiotensin receptor blockers (e.g., losartan [Cozaar]) should be considered[43] (see Tables 34-12 and 33-8).

Antidysrhythmia Drugs. Dysrhythmias are the most common complications after an MI. In general, they are not treated aggressively unless they are life threatening. (The drugs used in the treatment of dysrhythmias are discussed in Chapter 36.)

Cholesterol-Lowering Drugs. A fasting lipid panel should be obtained on all patients admitted with ACS. Cholesterol-lowering drugs are recommended for all patients with elevated LDL cholesterol (see Tables 34-2 and 34-6).

Stool Softeners. After an MI, the patient may be predisposed to constipation as a result of bed rest and opioid administration. Stool softeners such as docusate sodium (Colace) are given to facilitate and promote the comfort of bowel evacuation. This prevents straining and the resultant vagal stimulation from the Valsalva maneuver. Vagal stimulation produces bradycardia and can provoke dysrhythmias.

Nutritional Therapy

Initially, patients may be NPO (nothing by mouth) except for sips of water until stable (e.g., pain free, nausea resolved). Diet is advanced as tolerated to a low-salt, low-saturated-fat, and low-cholesterol diet (see Tables 34-4 and 34-5).

Coronary Surgical Revascularization

Coronary revascularization with CABG surgery is recommended for patients who (1) fail medical management, (2) have left main coronary artery or three-vessel disease, (3) are not candidates for PCI (e.g., lesions are long or difficult to access), or (4) have failed PCI with ongoing chest pain.[50]

Coronary Artery Bypass Graft Surgery. CABG surgery consists of the construction of new conduits (vessels to transport blood) between the aorta, or other major arteries, and the myocardium distal to the obstructed coronary artery (or arteries). The procedure involves one or more grafts using the internal mammary artery, saphenous vein, radial artery, gastroepiploic artery, and/or inferior epigastric artery.

CABG surgery requires a *sternotomy* (opening of the chest cavity) and the use of *cardiopulmonary bypass* (CPB). CPB involves diverting (bypassing) the patient's blood from the heart to the CPB machine. Here blood is oxygenated and returned (via a pump) to the patient. In this way, vital organs are perfused while the surgeon operates on a nonbeating, bloodless heart.

The internal mammary artery (IMA) is the most common artery used for bypass graft. The left and/or right IMA is left attached to its origin (the subclavian artery) and dissected from the chest wall. It is then *anastomosed* (connected with sutures) to the coronary artery distal to the stenosis. The long-term patency rate for IMA grafts is 90% after 10 years[50] (Fig. 34-16).

The saphenous vein is also used for bypass grafts. It is removed from one or both legs and sections are anastomosed proximally to the ascending aorta and to a coronary artery distal to the blockage. Saphenous vein grafts do develop diffuse intimal hyperplasia, which contributes to future stenosis and graft occlusions. The use of antiplatelet therapy and statins after surgery has improved vein graft patency. Patency rates of these grafts are 66% at 10 years. When vein grafts do become stenosed, stents have been used to open occlusions.[50]

There has been recent interest in the use of the radial artery for bypass graft. The radial artery is a thick muscular artery that is prone to spasm when mechanically stimulated. Perioperative calcium channel blockers and long-acting nitrates are used to control this complication. Early studies show patency rates at 5 years to be as high as 84%. There have been no reports of extremity complications (e.g., hand ischemia, wound infection) following the dissection of this artery.[50]

For patients with previous CABG surgery, the gastroepiploic or inferior epigastric artery can be used. These arteries are excellent conduits. However, the dissection of the arteries is extensive, increasing the length of surgery and the risk for wound complications at the harvest site, especially in an obese or diabetic patient.[50] Because of the number of patients requiring reoperation, research on the use of alternative arteries (e.g., bovine IMAs) and veins (e.g., umbilical veins), and synthetic grafts (e.g., Dacron grafts), will become increasingly more important.[50]

CABG surgery remains a palliative treatment for CAD and not a cure. Studies have demonstrated improved patient outcomes, quality of life, and survival after CABG surgery.[50] However, postoperative complications and mortality increase as a function of age. Women have higher operative mortality rates than men. This has been attributed to the late treatment of CAD in women resulting in women presenting at an older age, and more ill (e.g., decreased left ventricular function) at surgery. Other possible causes include smaller diameter coronary vessels and the less frequent use of the IMA.[50]

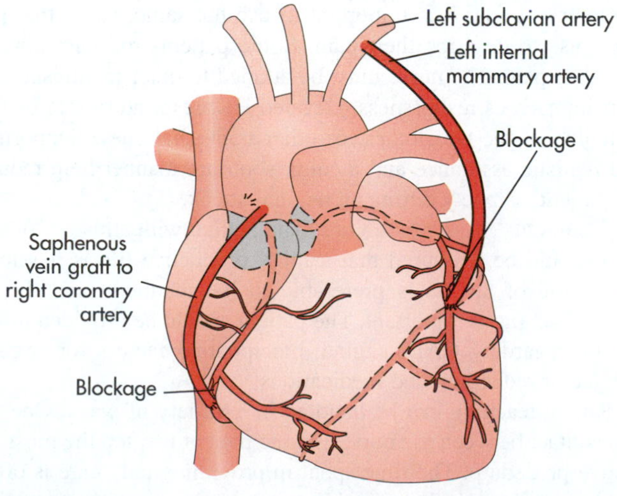

FIG. 34-16 Distal end of the left internal mammary artery is grafted below the area of blockage in the left anterior descending artery. Proximal end of the saphenous vein is grafted to the aorta and the distal end is grafted below the area of blockage in the right coronary artery.

Minimally Invasive Direct Coronary Artery Bypass. With recent efforts to reduce cost, length of hospital stay, and morbidity, newer approaches to CABG surgery have been developed. *Minimally invasive direct coronary artery bypass* (MIDCAB) is a technique that offers the patient with single-vessel disease (i.e., left anterior descending or right coronary artery disease) an approach to surgical treatment that does not involve a sternotomy and CPB.

The technique requires several small incisions between the ribs. A thoracoscope is used to dissect the IMA. The heart is slowed using a β-adrenergic blocker (e.g., esmolol [Brevibloc]) or stopped temporarily with adenosine (Adenocard), and a mechanical stabilizer is used to immobilize the anastomosis site. The IMA is then sutured to the left anterior descending or right coronary artery. A radial artery or saphenous vein graft may be used if the IMA is not available.

Off-Pump Coronary Artery Bypass. The *off-pump coronary artery bypass* (OPCAB) procedure uses full or partial sternotomy

ETHICAL DILEMMAS

Justice

Maria, who is 56 years old, was recently discharged from the hospital following a myocardial infarction and a ventricular aneurysm. She is divorced and helps take care of her two grandchildren. Until recently she was employed full time, but because of her fatigue she cannot go back to work. Therefore she has now lost her health insurance. Because of the fatigue, she can barely care for her grandchildren.

Maria needs cardiac rehabilitation but, because she has no health insurance, she cannot afford it. She has applied for disability and Medicaid, but this may take many months to obtain. She knows if she delays getting adequate health care and rehabilitation, her disease may progress to the point where she may no longer be able to care for her grandchildren.

Important Points for Consideration

- Health care coverage (access) in the United States is tied to employment. However, there are millions of people who are gainfully employed and do not have health care insurance.
- There are four types of health care entitlement programs in this country under which people obtain health access: active military, veterans, Medicare for the elderly, and Medicaid for the disadvantaged and disabled.
- Despite these programs, there remain nearly 50 million people who do not have health care coverage; this is an issue of justice and nonmaleficence.
- Lack of health care coverage often contributes to failure in accessing health care services, which in turn contributes to increased severity of illness and chronic health problems.
- Failure to seek appropriate follow-up care for a health problem can lead to inappropriate use of emergency medical services and contribute to escalating health costs in the United States.

Critical Thinking Questions

1. How can nurses assist Maria in identifying potential resources for successful cardiac rehabilitation?
2. What can nurses do to work toward a health care system where everyone has access to essential services?

to enable access to all coronary vessels. OPCAB is also performed on a beating heart using mechanical stabilizers and without CPB.

Transmyocardial Laser Revascularization. *Transmyocardial laser revascularization* (TMR) is an indirect revascularization procedure used for patients with advanced CAD who are not candidates for traditional bypass surgery and who have persistent angina after maximum medical therapy. The procedure involves the use of a high-energy laser that is triggered electrocardiographically to create channels between the left ventricular cavity and the coronary microcirculation (ventriculocoronary anastomoses). The channels allow blood to flow into ischemic areas. The procedure may be performed during cardiac catheterization as a percutaneous TMR or during surgery using a left anterior thoracotomy incision.

Complications following TMR include ventricular dysrhythmias, postoperative bleeding and cardiac tamponade, accidental perforation of the great vessels or epicardial coronary arteries, damage to the chordae tendineae, and low cardiac output. Although blood flow to the myocardium is improved immediately through the patent channels extending from the outside of the heart to the interior of the left ventricle, optimal results are not seen until the formation of new blood vessels that arise from laser channels and begin to supply the myocardium. Optimal results are seen at about 3 to 6 months.

NURSING MANAGEMENT CHRONIC STABLE ANGINA AND ACUTE CORONARY SYNDROME

Nursing Assessment

Subjective and objective data that should be obtained from a patient with ACS are presented in Table 34-15.

TABLE 34-15 NURSING ASSESSMENT Acute Coronary Syndrome

Subjective Data

Important Health Information

Past health history: Previous history of CAD, angina, MI, aortic stenosis, heart failure, or cardiomyopathy; hypertension, diabetes, anemia, lung disease; hyperlipidemia

Medications: Use of aspirin, nitrates, β-adrenergic blockers, calcium channel blockers, angiotensin-converting enzyme inhibitors; antihypertensive drugs; cholesterol-lowering drugs; vitamin and herbal supplements

Functional Health Patterns

Health perception–health management: Family history of heart disease; sedentary lifestyle; tobacco use

Nutritional-metabolic: Indigestion, heartburn, nausea, belching, vomiting

Elimination: Desire to void, straining at stool

Activity-exercise: Palpitations, dyspnea, dizziness, weakness

Cognitive-perceptual: Substernal chest pain or pressure (squeezing, constricting, aching, sharp, tingling), possible radiation to jaw, neck, shoulders, back, or arms

Coping–stress tolerance: Stressful lifestyle, depression; anger, anxiety; feeling of impending doom

Objective Data

General

Anxiety, fear, restlessness

Integumentary

Cool, clammy, pale skin

Cardiovascular

Tachycardia or bradycardia, pulsus alternans (alternating weak and strong heartbeats), dysrhythmias (especially ventricular), S_3, S_4, ↑ or ↓ BP, murmur

Possible Findings

Negative or positive serum cardiac markers, ↑ serum lipids; ↑ WBC count; positive exercise stress test and thallium scans; ST segment and T wave abnormalities on ECG; cardiac enlargement, calcifications, or pulmonary congestion on chest x-ray; abnormal wall motion with stress echocardiogram; positive coronary angiography

BP, Blood pressure; *CAD,* coronary artery disease; *ECG,* electrocardiogram; *MI,* myocardial infarction; *WBC,* white blood cell.

Nursing Diagnoses

Nursing diagnoses for the patient with ACS may include, but are not limited to, those presented in NCP 34-1.

Planning

The overall goals for a patient with ACS include (1) relief of pain, (2) preservation of myocardium, (3) immediate and appropriate treatment, (4) effective coping with illness-associated anxiety, (5) participation in a rehabilitation plan, and (6) reduction of risk factors.

Nursing Implementation: Chronic Stable Angina

Health Promotion. Behaviors to reduce the risk for CAD are presented in Table 34-3 and discussed on pp. 791 to 794.

Acute Intervention. If a nurse is present during an anginal attack, the following measures should be instituted: (1) administration of supplemental oxygen, (2) determination of vital signs, (3) 12-lead ECG, (4) prompt pain relief first with a nitrate followed by a opioid analgesic if needed, (5) auscultation of heart sounds, and (6) comfortable positioning of the patient. The patient will most likely appear distressed and have pale, cool, clammy skin. The BP and HR will probably be elevated and an atrial gallop (S_4) sound may be heard. If a ventricular gallop (S_3) is heard, it may indicate left ventricular dysfunction. A murmur may be heard during an anginal attack secondary to ischemia of a papillary muscle of the mitral valve. The murmur is likely to be transient and disappear with the cessation of symptoms.

The nurse should ask the patient to rate the pain on a scale of 0 to 10 before and after treatment to evaluate the effectiveness of the interventions. It is important to use the same words that patients use to describe their pain. Some patients may not always verbalize pain. The nurse must be attuned to other manifestations of pain, such as restlessness, elevated HR, respiratory rate or BP, clutching of the bedclothes, or other nonverbal cues. Supportive and realistic assurance and a calm, soothing manner help reduce the patient's anxiety during an anginal attack.

Ambulatory and Home Care. The patient with a history of angina should be reassured that a long, productive life is possible. Prevention of angina is preferable to its treatment, and this is where teaching is important. The patient should be provided information regarding CAD, angina, precipitating factors for angina, risk factor reduction, and medications.

Patient teaching can be handled in a variety of ways. One-to-one contact between the nurse and the patient is often the most effective procedure. The time spent in providing daily care is often an ideal teaching period. Teaching tools such as pamphlets, videotapes, heart models, and especially written information are necessary components of patient and family teaching (see Chapter 5).

NURSING CARE PLAN 34-1

Patient with Acute Coronary Syndrome

NURSING DIAGNOSIS **Acute pain** *related to* myocardial ischemia *as evidenced by* severe chest pain and tightness, radiation of pain to the neck and arms

PATIENT GOAL Reports relief of pain

OUTCOMES (NOC)	INTERVENTIONS (NIC) and *RATIONALES*
Pain Control	***Cardiac Care: Acute***
• Uses preventive measures ____ • Uses analgesics appropriately ____ • Reports uncontrolled symptoms to health care professional ____ • Reports pain controlled ____ **Measurement Scale** 1 = Never demonstrated 2 = Rarely demonstrated 3 = Sometimes demonstrated 4 = Often demonstrated 5 = Consistently demonstrated	• Evaluate chest pain (e.g., intensity, location, radiation, duration, and precipitating and alleviating factors) *in order to accurately evaluate, treat, and prevent further ischemia.* • Monitor effectiveness of oxygen therapy *to increase oxygenation of myocardial tissue and prevent further ischemia.* • Administer medications to relieve/prevent pain and ischemia *to decrease anxiety and cardiac workload.* • Obtain 12-lead ECG during pain episode *to help differentiate angina from extension of MI or pericarditis.* • Monitor cardiac rhythm and rate and trends in blood pressure and hemodynamic parameters (e.g., central venous pressure and pulmonary artery wedge pressure) *to monitor for hypotension and bradycardia, which may lead to hypoperfusion.*

NURSING DIAGNOSIS **Ineffective tissue perfusion (cardiac)** *related to* myocardial injury *as evidenced by* decrease in BP, dyspnea, dysrhythmias, peripheral edema, and pulmonary edema

PATIENT GOAL Maintains stable signs of effective cardiac perfusion

OUTCOMES (NOC)	INTERVENTIONS (NIC) and *RATIONALES*
Cardiac Pump Effectiveness	***Cardiac Care***
• Angina ____ • Peripheral edema ____ • Dyspnea ____ • Dysrhythmia ____ • Pulmonary edema ____ • Weight gain ____ **Measurement Scale** 1 = Severe 2 = Substantial 3 = Moderate 4 = Mild 5 = None	• Monitor vital signs frequently *to determine baseline and ongoing changes.* • Monitor for cardiac dysrhythmias, including disturbances of both rhythm and conduction, *to identify and treat significant dysrhythmias.* • Monitor respiratory status for symptoms of heart failure *to maintain appropriate levels of oxygenation and observe for signs of pulmonary edema.* • Monitor fluid balance (e.g., intake/output, daily weight) *to monitor renal perfusion and observe for fluid retention.* • Arrange exercise and rest periods *to avoid fatigue and decrease the oxygen demand on myocardium.*

NURSING DIAGNOSIS **Anxiety** *related to* perceived or actual threat of death, pain, possible lifestyle changes *as evidenced by* restlessness, agitation, and verbalization of concern over lifestyle changes and prognosis as substantiated by patient's statement of "What is going to happen when I die … everyone relies on me"

PATIENT GOAL Reports decreased anxiety and increased sense of self-control

OUTCOMES (NOC)	INTERVENTIONS (NIC) and *RATIONALES*
Anxiety Self-Control	***Anxiety Reduction***
• Monitors intensity of anxiety ____ • Seeks information to reduce anxiety ____ • Controls anxiety response ____ • Uses relaxation techniques to reduce anxiety ____ **Measurement Scale** 1 = Never demonstrated 2 = Rarely demonstrated 3 = Sometimes demonstrated 4 = Often demonstrated 5 = Consistently demonstrated	• Observe for verbal and nonverbal signs of anxiety. • Identify when level of anxiety changes *since anxiety increases the need for oxygen.* • Use a calm, reassuring approach *so as not to increase patient's anxiety.* • Instruct patient in use of relaxation techniques (e.g., relaxation breathing, imagery) *to enhance self-control.* • Encourage family to stay with patient *to provide comfort.* • Encourage verbalization of feelings, perceptions, and fears *to decrease anxiety and stress.* • Provide factual information concerning diagnosis, treatment, and prognosis *to decrease fear of the unknown.*

Continued

NURSING CARE PLAN 34-1
Patient with Acute Coronary Syndrome—cont'd

NURSING DIAGNOSIS **Activity intolerance** *related to* fatigue secondary to decreased cardiac output and poor lung and tissue perfusion *as evidenced by* fatigue with minimal activity, inability to care for self without dyspnea, and increased heart rate

PATIENT GOAL Achieves a realistic program of activity that balances physical activity with energy-conserving activities

OUTCOMES (NOC)

Activity Tolerance

- Oxygen saturation with activity ____
- Pulse rate with activity ____
- Ease of breathing with activity ____
- Walking pace ____
- Ease of performing ADLs ____

Measurement Scale

1 = Severely compromised
2 = Substantially compromised
3 = Moderately compromised
4 = Mildly compromised
5 = Not compromised

INTERVENTIONS (NIC) and *RATIONALES*

Cardiac Care

- Monitor patient's response to antidysrhythmic medications *since these medications will affect BP and pulse prior to activity.*
- Arrange exercise and rest periods to avoid fatigue and *to increase activity tolerance without rapidly increasing cardiac workload.*

Energy Management

- Assist patient to understand energy conservation principles (e.g., the requirement for restricted activity) *to conserve energy and promote healing.*
- Teach patient and significant other techniques of self-care that will minimize oxygen consumption (e.g., self-monitoring and pacing techniques for performance of activities of daily living) *to promote independence as well as minimize O_2 consumption.*

NURSING DIAGNOSIS **Ineffective therapeutic regimen management** *related to* lack of knowledge of risk factors, disease process, rehabilitation, home activities, and medications *as evidenced by* frequent questioning about illness, management, and care after discharge

PATIENT GOAL Describes risk factors, the disease process, and rehabilitation activities necessary to manage the therapeutic regimen

OUTCOMES (NOC)

Knowledge: Cardiac Disease Management

- Description of usual course of disease process ____
- Description of symptoms of worsening disease ____
- Description of ways to manage controllable risk factors ____
- Description of importance of completing recommended cardiac rehabilitation program ____
- Description of effects of medications ____

Measurement Scale

1 = None
2 = Limited
3 = Moderate
4 = Substantial
5 = Extensive

INTERVENTIONS (NIC) and *RATIONALES*

Teaching: Disease Process

- Appraise the patient's current level of knowledge related to myocardial infarction *to obtain information on patient's teaching needs.*
- Explain the pathophysiology of the disease and how it relates to anatomy and physiology *to individualize the information and to increase understanding.*
- Discuss lifestyle changes that may be required to prevent further complications and/or control disease process *to get the cooperation of the patient's significant support system.*
- Refer the patient to local community agencies/support groups *so that the patient and family have resources and support available.*

Teaching: Prescribed Medication

- Instruct the patient on the purpose and action of each medication.
- Instruct the patient on the dosage, route, and duration of each medication *so that patient understands the reason for taking the medication and will be less likely to refuse to take medications.*

The patient should be assisted in identifying factors that precipitate angina (see Table 34-9). The patient should be given instruction on how to avoid or control precipitating factors. For example, the patient should be taught to avoid exposure to extremes of weather and the consumption of large, heavy meals. If a heavy meal is ingested, adequate rest should be planned for 1 to 2 hours after eating because blood is shunted to the GI tract to aid digestion and absorption.

The patient should be assisted in identifying personal risk factors in CAD. Once these are known, various methods of decreasing any modifiable risk factors should be discussed (see Table 34-3).

Teaching the patient and the family about diets that are low in sodium and reduced in saturated fats may be appropriate (see Tables 34-4 and 34-5). Maintaining ideal body weight is important in controlling angina because weight above this level increases the myocardial workload.

Adhering to a regular, individualized program of physical activity that conditions the heart rather than overstresses the myocardium is important. Most patients can be advised to walk briskly on a flat surface at least 30 minutes a day, 5 or more days a week.[8]

It is important to teach the patient and the family in the proper use of nitroglycerin (see pp. 798 to 799). Nitroglycerin tablets or ointments may be used prophylactically before an emotionally stressful situation, sexual intercourse, or physical exertion (e.g., climbing a long flight of stairs).

Counseling should be provided to assess the psychologic adjustment of the patient and the family to the diagnosis of CAD and the resulting angina. Many patients feel a threat to their identity and self-esteem and may be unable to fill their usual roles in society. These emotions are normal and real.

Nursing Implementation: Acute Coronary Syndrome

Acute Intervention. Priorities for nursing interventions in the initial phase of ACS include pain assessment and relief, physiologic monitoring, promotion of rest and comfort, alleviation of stress and anxiety, and understanding of the patient's emotional and behavioral reactions. Research has shown that patients with increased anxiety levels have a greater risk for adverse outcomes such as recurrent ischemic events and dysrhythmias.[48] Proper management of these priorities decreases the oxygen needs of a compromised myocardium and reduces the risk of complications. In addition, the nurse should institute measures to avoid the hazards of immobility while encouraging rest.

Pain. Nitroglycerin, morphine sulfate, and supplemental oxygen should be provided as needed to eliminate or reduce chest pain. Ongoing evaluation and documentation of the effectiveness of the interventions is important. Once pain is relieved, the nurse may have to deal with denial in a patient who interprets the absence of pain as an absence of cardiac disease.

Monitoring. A patient has continuous ECG monitoring while in the ED and intensive care unit and usually after transfer to a stepdown or general unit. The nurse should be educated in ECG interpretation so that dysrhythmias causing further deterioration of the cardiovascular status can be identified and treated. During the initial period after MI, ventricular fibrillation is the most common lethal dysrhythmia. In many patients, this dysrhythmia is preceded by premature ventricular contractions or ventricular tachycardia. The nurse should also monitor the patient for the presence of silent ischemia by monitoring the ST segment for shifts above or below the baseline of the ECG. Silent ischemia occurs without clinical symptoms such as chest pain, but its presence places a patient at higher risk for adverse outcomes and even death.[48] If episodes of silent ischemia are seen on the monitor, the physician should be notified. (See Chapter 36 for a complete discussion of ECG monitoring.)

In addition to frequent vital signs, intake and output should be evaluated at least once a shift, and physical assessment should be carried out to detect deviations from the patient's baseline parameters. Included is an assessment of lung sounds and heart sounds and inspection for evidence of early HF (e.g., dyspnea, tachycardia, pulmonary congestion, distended neck veins).

Assessment of the patient's oxygenation status is important, especially if the patient is receiving oxygen. Also, the nares should be checked for irritation or dryness, which can cause considerable discomfort if the nasal route is used for oxygen administration.

Rest and Comfort. With a severe insult to the myocardium, as in the case of ACS, it is important for the nurse to promote rest and comfort. Bed rest may be ordered for the first few days after an MI involving a large portion of the ventricle. A patient with an uncomplicated MI (e.g., angina resolved, no signs of complications) may rest in a chair within 8 to 12 hours after the event. The use of a commode or bedpan is based on patient preference.

When sleeping or resting, the body requires less work from the heart than it does when active. It is important to plan nursing and therapeutic actions to ensure adequate rest periods free from interruption. Comfort measures that can promote rest include frequent oral care, adequate warmth, a quiet atmosphere, use of relaxation therapy (e.g., guided imagery), and assurance that personnel are nearby and responsive to the patient's needs.

It is important that the patient understand the reasons why activity is limited. However, in spite of this limitation, the patient is not completely restricted. Gradually the cardiac workload is increased through more demanding physical tasks so that the patient can achieve a discharge activity level adequate for home care. Phases of cardiac rehabilitation are outlined in Table 34-16.

Anxiety. Anxiety is present in all patients with ACS to various degrees. The nurse's role is to identify the source of anxiety and assist the patient in reducing it. If the patient is afraid of being alone, a family member should be allowed to sit quietly by the bedside or to check in with the patient frequently. If a source of anxiety is fear of the unknown, the nurse should explore these concerns with the patient and help with appropriate reality testing.

If anxiety is caused by lack of information, the nurse should provide teaching appropriate to the patient's stated need and level. The nurse should answer the patient's questions with clear, simple explanations sufficient to reduce the patient's anxiety.

It is important to start teaching at the patient's level rather than to present a prepackaged protocol. Frequently the patient is not yet ready to hear about the pathogenesis of CAD. The earliest questions usually relate to how the disease affects perceived control and independence. These questions include the following:

- When will I leave the intensive care unit?
- When can I be out of bed?
- When will I be discharged?
- When can I return to work?
- How much change will I have to make in my life?
- Will this happen again?

The nurse should advise that a more complete teaching program begins once the patient is feeling stronger. Frequently the

TABLE 34-16 Phases of Rehabilitation Following Acute Coronary Syndrome

Phase I: Hospital
- Occurs while the patient is still hospitalized.
- Activity level depends on severity of angina or MI.
- Patient may initially sit up in bed or chair, perform range-of-motion exercises and self-care (e.g., washing, shaving), and progress to ambulation in hallway and limited stair climbing.
- Attention focuses on management of pain, anxiety, dysrhythmias, and complications.

Phase II: Early Recovery
- Begins after the patient is discharged.
- Usually lasts from 2 to 12 wk and is conducted in an outpatient facility.
- Activity level is gradually increased under the supervision of the cardiac rehabilitation team and with ECG monitoring.
- Team may suggest that physical activity (e.g., walking) be initiated at home.
- Information regarding risk factor reduction is provided at this time.

Phase III: Late Recovery
- Long-term maintenance program.
- Individual physical activity programs are designed and implemented at home, a local gym, or the rehabilitation center.
- Patient and family possibly restructure lifestyles and roles.
- Lifestyle changes should become lifelong habits.
- Medical supervision is still recommended.

ECG, Electrocardiogram; *MI,* myocardial infarction.

patient may not be able to consciously examine the most pervasive concern of ACS patients: Am I going to die? Even if a patient denies this concern, it is helpful for the nurse to initiate conversation by remarking that fear of dying is a common concern reported by most patients who have experienced ACS. This gives the patient "permission" to talk about an uncomfortable and fearful topic.

Emotional and Behavioral Reactions. The emotional and behavioral reactions of a patient are varied and frequently follow a predictable response pattern (Table 34-17). The role of the nurse is to understand what the patient is currently experiencing, to assist the patient in testing reality, and to support the use of constructive coping styles. Denial may be a positive coping style in the early phase of recovery from ACS.

The nurse has an obligation to maximize and enhance the patient's social support systems. This entails assessing the support structure of the patient and family and allowing it to function. Often the patient is separated from the most significant support system at the time of hospitalization. The nurse's role can include talking with the family, informing them of the patient's progress, allowing the patient and the family to interact as necessary, and supporting the family members who will be able to provide the necessary support to the patient. Open visitation is helpful in decreasing anxiety and increasing support for the patient with ACS. Social isolation has been associated with negative outcomes following MI in both men and women.[51] It is important for the nurse to help the patient identify additional support systems (e.g., spiritual care, Mended Hearts) that can help the patient after discharge.

Coronary Revascularization. Patients with ACS may undergo coronary revascularization with PCI or CABG surgery. The major nursing responsibilities for the care of the patient following PCI involves monitoring for signs of recurrent angina; frequent assessment of vital signs, including HR and rhythm; evaluation of the groin site for signs of bleeding; and maintenance of bed rest per institution policy (see Table 32-7).

For patients having CABG surgery, care is provided in the intensive care unit for the first 24 to 36 hours. Ongoing and intensive monitoring of the patient's hemodynamic status is critical. The patient will have numerous invasive lines for monitoring cardiac status and other vital organs (see Chapter 66). These include a pulmonary artery catheter for measuring cardiac output and other hemodynamic parameters, an intraarterial line for continuous BP monitoring, pleural and mediastinal chest tubes for chest drainage, continuous ECG monitoring to detect dysrhythmias, an endotracheal tube connected to mechanical ventilation, epicardial pacing wires for emergency pacing of the heart, a urinary catheter to monitor urine output, and a nasogastric tube for gastric decompression. Most patients will be extubated within 12 hours and transferred to a step-down unit within 24 hours for continued monitoring of cardiac status.

Many of the postoperative complications that develop after CABG surgery relate to the use of CPB. Major consequences of CBP include bleeding and anemia from damage to red blood cells and platelets, fluid and electrolyte imbalances, and hypothermia as blood is cooled as it passes through the CPB machine. Nursing care is focused on assessing the patient for bleeding (e.g., chest tube drainage, incision sites), monitoring fluid status, replacing electrolytes as needed, and restoring temperature (e.g., warming blankets).

Postoperative dysrhythmias, specifically atrial dysrhythmias, are common in the first 3 days after CABG surgery. Twenty percent to 40% of patients develop postoperative atrial fibrillation. Discharge is often delayed in these patients due to the need for anticoagulation. (See Chapter 36 for information on treatment of atrial fibrillation.)

Nursing care for the patient with a CABG also involves caring for the surgical sites: the chest, arm, leg, and/or abdomen. Care of the radial artery harvest site includes careful observation of the incision site, as well as monitoring sensory and motor function of the distal thumb and fingers. The patient with radial artery harvest should be on a calcium channel blocker for approximately 3 months to decrease the incidence of arterial spasm at the arm or anastomosis site.

The care of the leg wound is similar to the postoperative care after the stripping of varicose veins (see Chapter 38). The management of the chest wound, which involves a sternotomy, is similar to that of other chest surgeries (see Chapter 28).

Elective CABG is generally well tolerated in the older patient. However, the incidence of postoperative complications is high, including dysrhythmias, stroke, and infection. The nurse caring for older adults must be aware that, although the benefits of treatment may outweigh risks in this population, complications are higher than in younger individuals.

Postoperative nursing care of the patient with a MIDCABG or OPCAB procedure is similar to that for CABG surgery patients.

TABLE 34-17 Emotional and Behavioral Responses to Acute Coronary Syndrome

Denial
- May have history of ignoring symptoms related to heart disease.
- Minimizes severity of medical condition.
- Ignores activity restrictions.
- Avoids discussing illness or its significance.

Anger
- Is commonly expressed as, "Why did this happen to me?"
- May be directed at family, staff, or medical regimen.

Anxiety and Fear
- Fears long-term disability and death.
- Overtly manifests apprehension, restlessness, insomnia, tachycardia.
- Less overtly manifests increased verbalization, projection of feelings to others, hypochondriasis.
- Fears activity.
- Fears recurrent angina, heart attacks, and sudden death.

Dependency
- Is totally reliant on staff.
- Is unwilling to perform tasks or activities unless approved by health care provider.
- Wants to be monitored by ECG at all times.
- Is hesitant to leave the intensive care unit or hospital.

Depression
- Mourns loss of health, altered body function, and changes in lifestyle.
- Realizes seriousness of situation.
- Begins to worry about future implications of health problem.
- Shows manifestations of withdrawal, crying, apathy.
- May be more evident after discharge.

Realistic Acceptance
- Focuses on optimum rehabilitation.
- Plans changes compatible with altered cardiac function.

ECG, Electrocardiogram.

Pain management is essential because patients report higher levels of pain with thoracotomy incisions than a sternotomy incision. The recovery time is somewhat shorter with these procedures, and patients often resume routine activities sooner than patients who have CABG surgery.

Ambulatory and Home Care. *Rehabilitation* may be defined as the process of helping the patient adjust to a disability by teaching integration of all resources and concentrating more on existing abilities than on permanent disabilities. *Cardiac rehabilitation* is the restoration of a person to an optimal state of function in six areas: physiologic, psychologic, mental, spiritual, economic, and vocational. Many persons recover from ACS physically, yet they may never attain psychologic well-being because of misconceptions about the illness or a need to practice illness behaviors. Returning to work and resuming all activities have long been outcome measures of cardiac rehabilitation and are important in terms of the cost-effectiveness of cardiac care and rehabilitation.

In considering rehabilitation, the nurse and patient must recognize that CAD is a chronic disease. It will not be cured, nor will it disappear by itself. Therefore basic changes in lifestyle must be made to promote recovery and health. These changes must frequently be made at a time when a person is middle-aged or older. The patient must also realize that recovery takes time. Resumption of physical activity after ACS or CABG surgery is slow and gradual. However, with appropriate and adequate supportive care, recovery is more likely to occur.

Patient Teaching. Patient teaching begins with the ED nurse and progresses through the staff nurse to the community health nurse. The purpose of teaching is to give the patient and family the tools they need to make informed decisions about attainment of health. For teaching to be meaningful, the patient must be aware of the need to learn. Careful assessment of the patient's learning needs helps the nurse set goals and objectives that are realistic.

The timing of the teaching is important. When patients or families are in crisis (either physiologic or psychologic), they may not be very interested in learning new information. It is important to remember that early questions should be answered initially in simple, brief terms, without detailed elaboration, and that the answers to these questions often require repetition and elaboration. When the shock and disbelief accompanying a crisis subside, the patient and family are better able to focus on new information.

In addition to teaching the patient and the family what they wish to know, several types of information are considered necessary in achieving optimal health. A teaching guide for the patient with ACS is presented in Table 34-18.

When medical terminology is used, its meaning should be explained in lay terms. For example, it can be explained that the heart, a four-chambered pump, is a muscle that needs oxygen like all other muscles in order to work properly. When blood vessels supplying the heart muscle with oxygen become narrowed by atherosclerosis, there is less oxygen available to the heart muscle. It is a good idea for the nurse to have a model of the heart or to use a pad and pencil to sketch what is being explained. Literature written for a nonmedical audience is available through the American Heart Association. Videotapes are also helpful tools that can be used to teach patients.

Anticipatory guidance involves preparing the patient and the family for what to expect in the course of recovery and rehabilitation. By learning what to expect during treatment and recovery, the patient gains a sense of control over life. This sense of perceived control allows the patient to consciously consider stressors and thus possibly to promote recovery.

TABLE 34-18 PATIENT AND FAMILY TEACHING GUIDE Acute Coronary Syndrome

The nurse needs to teach the following to the patient and the family:

- Signs and symptoms of angina and MI and reasons they occur*
- Anatomy and physiology of the heart and vessels
- Cause and effect of atherosclerosis
- Definition of terms (e.g., CAD, angina, MI, sudden cardiac death, HF)
- Healing after MI
- Identification of and decreasing risk factors* (see Table 34-3)
- Rationale for tests and treatments, including ECG, blood tests, and angiography, and monitoring, rest, diet, and medications*
- Appropriate expectations about recovery and rehabilitation (anticipatory guidance)
- Resumption of work, physical activity, sexual activity
- Measures to take to promote recovery and health
- Importance of the gradual, progressive resumption of activity*
- When and how to seek help (e.g., contact EMS)

CAD, Coronary artery disease; *ECG,* electrocardiogram; *EMS,* emergency medical services; *HF,* heart failure; *MI,* myocardial infarction.
*Identified by patients as most important to learn before discharge.

The idea of perceived control is operationalized as the process by which the patient exercises choice and makes decisions by cutting back. Cutting back is one way of minimizing the psychologic and physiologic losses after MI (or any other life-changing event). The patient considers what must be cut back (changed), weighs this against what should be cut back, and finally determines what will be cut back. For example, a middle-aged man who smokes two packs of cigarettes a day, is 20 pounds overweight, and gets no physical exercise has a seemingly overwhelming task. He may decide that he can live with a weight reduction diet and will get more exercise (although perhaps not daily) but that it is not possible for him to quit smoking. He reasons that, because he is modifying two of the three risk factors, he will be safe if he cuts back on tobacco use. Ideally the tobacco risk factor should be a priority for this patient, but if information regarding risks and effects of tobacco use is not accepted, the nurse must respect the patient's need for control.

Physical Activity. Physical activity is an integral part of the rehabilitation program. It is necessary for optimal physiologic functioning and psychologic well-being. It has a direct, positive effect on maximal oxygen uptake, increasing CO, decreasing blood lipids, decreasing BP, increasing blood flow through the coronary arteries, increasing muscle mass and flexibility, improving the psychologic state, and assisting in weight loss and control. A regular schedule of physical activity, even after many years of sedentary living, is beneficial.[52]

One method used to identify levels of physical activity is through **metabolic equivalent (MET)** units: 1 MET is the amount of oxygen needed by the body at rest—3.5 ml of oxygen per kilogram per minute or 1.4 cal/kg of body weight per minute. The MET is used to determine the energy costs of various exercises (Table 34-19).

In the hospital, the activity level is gradually increased so that by the time of discharge the patient can tolerate moderate-energy activities of 3 to 6 METs. Many patients with UA that has resolved or an uncomplicated MI are in the hospital for approximately 3 to 4 days. By day 2, the patient can ambulate in the hallway and begin limited stair climbing (e.g., three to four steps). Many physicians order low-level treadmill tests before discharge to assess readiness for discharge, accurate HR for an exercise prescription, and potential for

TABLE 34-19 Energy Expenditure in Metabolic Equivalents

Low-Energy Activities (<3 METs or <3 cal/min)	
Activities in Hospital	***Activities Outside Hospital***
Resting supine	Sweeping floor
Eating	Painting, seated
Washing hands, face	Driving car
	Sewing by machine
Moderate-Energy Activities (3-6 METs or 3-5 cal/min)	
Activities in Hospital	***Activities Outside Hospital***
Sitting on bedside commode	Bricklaying
Showering	Ironing, standing
Using bedpan	Cycling at 5.5 mph on level ground
Walking at 3.75 mph	Golfing
	Dancing
High-Energy Activities (6-8 METs or 6-8 cal/min)	
Walking 5 mph	
Performing carpentry	
Ascending a flight of stairs	
Mowing lawn using walking mower	
Very-High-Energy Activities (>9 METs or >9 cal/min)	
Skiing	
Heavy labor	
Running more than 6 mph	
Cycling more than 13 mph	
Shoveling heavy snow	

MET, Metabolic equivalent unit; *mph,* miles per hour.

ischemia or reinfarction. If tests are positive (i.e., ischemia at a low level of energy expenditure), the patient is evaluated for cardiac catheterization before discharge. If the test is negative, a catheterization may still be done before discharge or several weeks after discharge.[40] Because of the short hospital stay, it is critical to give the patient specific guidelines for physical activity so that overexertion will not occur. It is important to stress that the patient should "listen to what the body is saying"—the most important facet of recovery.

Teaching the patient to check the pulse rate is a nursing responsibility. The patient should be taught the parameters within which to exercise. The patient should be told the maximum HR that should be present at any point. If the HR exceeds this level or does not return to the rate of the resting pulse within a few minutes, the patient should stop and rest. The patient should also be instructed to stop exercising if angina or dyspnea occurs.

In a normal, healthy person the minimum threshold for improving cardiorespiratory fitness is 60% of the age-predicted maximum HR (which is calculated by subtracting the person's age from 220). The ideal training target HR is 80% of maximum HR. The patient who has been physically inactive and is just beginning an exercise program should do so under supervision whenever possible. The more important factor is the patient's response to physical activity in terms of symptoms rather than absolute HR, especially since many patients are on β-adrenergic

TABLE 34-20 *PATIENT AND FAMILY TEACHING GUIDE* FITT Physical Activity Guidelines After Acute Coronary Syndrome

Warm-up/Cool-down
Mild stretching for 3 to 5 min before the physical activity and 5 min after the activity is important. Activity should not be started or stopped abruptly.

Frequency
The patient should perform physical activity 5 or more times a wk.

Intensity
Activity intensity should be determined by the patient's HR. If a treadmill test has not been performed, the person recovering from an MI should not exceed 20 beats/min over the resting HR.

Type of Physical Activity
Physical activity should be regular, rhythmic, and repetitive, using large muscles to build up endurance (e.g., walking, cycling, swimming, rowing).

Time
Physical activity can be from 30 to 60 min. It is important to begin slowly at personal tolerance (perhaps only 5 to 10 min) and build up to 30 min.

HR, Heart rate; *MI,* myocardial infarction.

blockers and may not be able to reach a target HR. This is a point that cannot be overstressed. Basic physical activity guidelines for patients following ACS are based on the FITT formula and are presented in Table 34-20.

The basic categories of physical activity are static (isometric) and dynamic (isotonic). Most daily activities are a mixture of the two. *Static activities* involve the development of tension during muscular contraction but produce little or no change in muscle length or joint movement. Lifting, carrying, and pushing heavy objects are primarily isometric activities. Because the HR and BP increase rapidly during isometric work, exercise programs involving isometric exercises should be limited.

Isotonic activities involve changes in muscle length and joint movement with rhythmic contractions at relatively low muscular tension. Walking, jogging, swimming, bicycling, and jumping rope are examples of activities that are predominantly isotonic. Isotonic exercise can put a safe, steady load on the heart and lungs and may also improve the circulation in many organs.

Many patients will be referred to an outpatient cardiac rehabilitation program (see Table 34-16). These programs have been found to be beneficial to patients, but not all patients choose or are able to participate in them. Home-based cardiac rehabilitation programs have been developed as an alternative. Physical activity guidelines are developed for the patient, and staff maintain ongoing contact with the patient (e.g., telephone, exercise logs, email).[52] Maintaining contact with the patient appears to be the key to the success of these programs.

Research has shown that older women (≥65 years) who experience MI have poor adherence to a regular physical activity program.[53] Often these women describe continued fatigue post-MI that is poorly understood.[53] One study found that home-based cardiac rehabilitation programs were more successful for older women compared to traditional outpatient programs.[48]

Another factor that has been linked to poor adherence to a physical activity program after MI is depression.[53] Both men and women experience mild to moderate depression post-MI that should resolve in 1 to 4 months.[48] If depression persists after this, patients should be referred for appropriate treatment (e.g., counseling, medication).

Resumption of Sexual Activity. It is important to include sexual counseling for cardiac patients and their partners. This often-neglected area of discussion may be difficult for both patients and health care providers to approach. However, the patient's concern about resumption of sexual activity after hospitalization for ACS often produces more stress than the physiologic act itself. About one third of men and women do not resume sexual activity or have a decrease in sexual activity after MI.[48] The majority of these patients changed their sexual behavior not because of physical problems, but because they were concerned about sexual inadequacy, death during coitus, and impotence. The misconceptions held by these persons could have been clarified with specific counseling by a concerned and knowledgeable health care provider.

Before the nurse provides guidelines on resumption of sexual activity, it is important to know the physiologic status of the patient, the physiologic effects of sexual activity, and the psychologic effects of having a heart attack. Sexual activity for middle-aged men and women with their usual partners is no more strenuous than climbing two flights of stairs.

Many nurses are unsure of how and when to begin counseling about resumption of sex. It is helpful to consider sex as a physical activity and to discuss or explore feelings in this area when other physical activities are discussed. One helpful approach is, "Many people who have had a heart attack wonder when they will be able to resume sexual activity. Has this been of concern to you?" Another is, "If sexual activity has been of concern to you, this information should be helpful." This type of nonthreatening statement brings up the topic, allows the patient to explore personal feelings, and gives the patient an opportunity to raise questions with the nurse or another health care provider. Common guidelines are presented in Table 34-21.

TABLE 34-21 ***PATIENT AND FAMILY TEACHING GUIDE*** **Sexual Activity After Acute Coronary Syndrome**

- Planning of resumption of sexual activity should correspond to sexual activity before hospitalization for acute coronary syndrome.
- Physical training seems to improve the physiologic response to coitus; therefore daily physical activity during recovery should be encouraged.
- Consumption of food and alcohol should be reduced before intercourse is anticipated (e.g., waiting 3 to 4 hr after ingesting a large meal before engaging in sexual activity).
- Familiar surroundings and a familiar partner reduce anxiety.
- Masturbation may be a useful sexual outlet and may reassure the patient that sexual activity is still possible.
- Hot or cold showers should be avoided just before and just after intercourse.
- Foreplay is desirable because it allows a gradual increase in heart rate before orgasm.
- Positions during intercourse are a matter of individual choice.
- Orogenital sex places no undue strain on the heart.
- A relaxed atmosphere free of fatigue and stress is optimal.
- Prophylactic use of nitrates is effective in decreasing angina during sexual activity.
- Use of erectile agents (e.g., sildenafil [Viagra]) is contraindicated if taking nitrates in any form.
- Anal intercourse may cause undue cardiac stress because of the possibility of inducing a vasovagal response.

The patient needs to know that the inability to perform sexually after MI is common and that sexual dysfunction usually disappears after several attempts. The nurse should reinforce the idea that patience and understanding usually solve the problem. However, with the availability of drugs to correct erectile dysfunction, many male patients may be interested in using them. The nurse should caution the patient that these drugs should not be used with nitrates as severe hypotension and even death have been reported. The nurse should encourage patients to discuss the use of these drugs with their health care provider.[54]

It is not uncommon for a patient who experiences chest pain on physical exertion to have some angina during sexual stimulation or intercourse. The patient should be instructed to take nitroglycerin prophylactically. It is also helpful to have the patient avoid sex soon after a heavy meal or after excessive ingestion of alcohol, when extremely tired or stressed, or with unfamiliar partners. Anal intercourse is to be avoided because of the likelihood of eliciting a vasovagal response.

The patient should be counseled that resumption of sex depends on the patient and his or her partner's emotional readiness and on the physician's assessment of the extent of recovery. It is now known that it is safe to resume sexual activity 7 to 10 days after an uncomplicated MI.[43,46] Some physicians believe that the patient should decide when he or she is ready to resume sex. Others say that a patient must be able to climb two flights of stairs briskly without dyspnea or angina before sexual activity can be resumed.

Reading material on resumption of sexual activity may be presented to the patient to facilitate discussion. The nurse should return to clarify and explain as necessary. Calmly and matter-of-factly introducing the subject of resumption of sexual activity during teaching about physical activity has positive effects of eliciting questions and concerns that might not have otherwise surfaced. For example, the nurse might begin, "Sexual activity is like other forms of activity and should be gradually resumed after MI. If your ability to perform sexually is concerning you, the energy expenditure has been found to be no more than walking briskly or climbing two flights of stairs." This forms a factual basis for the patient to begin to seek information and explore personal feelings about resuming sex.

▪ *Evaluation*

The expected outcomes for the patient with an ACS are presented in NCP 34-1.

SUDDEN CARDIAC DEATH

Sudden cardiac death (SCD) is unexpected death from cardiac causes. SCD accounts for approximately 300,000 deaths a year in the United States and 45,000 deaths a year in Canada.[55,56] Of these deaths, 56% occur out of the hospital or in the ED. Of the patients who survive SCD, only 20% are discharged from the hospital without neurologic impairment.

CAD is the most common cause of SCD and accounts for 80% of all SCDs. The affected person may or may not have a known history of CAD, and SCD may be the first sign of illness for 25% of those who die of heart disease.[55]

Etiology and Pathophysiology

In SCD there is an abrupt disruption in cardiac function, producing an abrupt loss of cardiac output and cerebral blood flow. Death usually occurs within 1 hour of the onset of acute symptoms (e.g., angina, palpitations).

The majority of cases of SCD are caused by acute ventricular dysrhythmias (e.g., ventricular tachycardia, ventricular fibrillation). Less commonly, SCD may occur as a result of a primary left ventricular outflow obstruction (e.g., aortic stenosis, hypertrophic cardiomyopathy).

Persons who experience SCD as a result of CAD fall into two groups: (1) those who had an acute MI and (2) those who did not have an acute MI. The latter group accounts for the majority of cases of SCD.[55] In this instance, victims usually have no warning signs or symptoms. Patients who survive are at risk for another SCD event due to the continued electrical instability of the myocardium that caused the initial event to occur.

The second, smaller group of patients includes those who have had an MI and have suffered SCD. In these cases, patients usually do have prodromal symptoms, such as chest pain, palpitations, and dyspnea.

It is difficult to predict who is at risk for SCD. However, left ventricular dysfunction (EF <30%) and ventricular dysrhythmias following MI have been found to be the strongest predictors.[55] Other risk factors for SCD include (1) male gender (especially African American men), (2) family history of premature atherosclerosis, (3) tobacco use, (4) diabetes mellitus, (5) hypercholesterolemia, (6) hypertension, and (7) cardiomyopathy.

NURSING *and* COLLABORATIVE MANAGEMENT SUDDEN CARDIAC DEATH

People who have been resuscitated following an episode of SCD generally require a diagnostic workup to determine whether they have had an MI. Thus serial analysis of cardiac markers and ECGs must be obtained, and the patient must be treated accordingly. (See section on Collaborative Care of ACS.) In addition, because most persons with SCD have CAD, cardiac catheterization is indicated to determine the possible location and extent of coronary artery occlusion. PCI or CABG surgery may be indicated.

Most SCD patients have a lethal ventricular dysrhythmia that is associated with a high incidence of recurrence. Thus it is useful to know when those persons are most likely to have a recurrence and what drug therapy is the most effective treatment. Assessment of dysrhythmias in these patients includes 24-hour Holter monitoring or other type of event recorder, exercise stress testing, signal-averaged ECG, and electrophysiologic study (EPS).[55] EPS is performed under fluoroscopy, pacing electrodes are placed in selected intracardiac areas, and stimuli are selectively used to attempt to produce dysrhythmias. The patient's response to various antidysrhythmic medications can be determined and monitored in a controlled environment. (EPS is discussed in Chapters 32 and 36.)

The most common approach to preventing a recurrence is the use of an implantable cardioverter-defibrillator (ICD). Research has shown that an ICD improves survival compared to drug therapy alone.[55,56] (ICDs are discussed in Chapter 37.) Drug therapy with amiodarone (Cordarone) did not improve survival in clinical trials, but may be used in conjunction with an ICD to decrease episodes of ventricular dysrhythmias.[55]

The nurse caring for a survivor of SCD should be attuned to the patient's psychosocial adaptation to this sudden "brush with death." Many of these patients develop a "time bomb" mentality. They fear the recurrence of cardiopulmonary arrest and may become anxious, angry, and depressed. Their families are likely to experience the same feelings. This fear often interferes with resumption of normal activities such as sexual and recreational activities.[57] Patients and families also may need to deal with additional issues such as possible driving restrictions and change in occupation. The grief response varies among patients and families. The nurse should be attuned to the specific needs of the patient and the family and teach them accordingly while providing appropriate emotional support.

CRITICAL THINKING EXERCISE

CASE STUDY

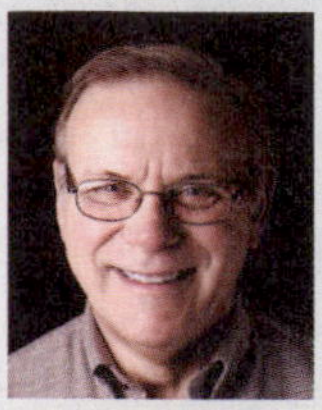

Case Study photo ©iStockphoto.com/ Floyd Anderson.

Myocardial Infarction

Patient Profile. Mr. D., a 51-year-old, white, successful businessman, was rushed to the hospital by ambulance after experiencing crushing substernal chest pain that radiated down his left arm. He also complained of dizziness and nausea.

Subjective Data

- Has a history of chronic stable angina and hypertension
- States he is "borderline diabetic"
- Overweight but recently lost 10 pounds
- Rarely exercises
- Has three teenage children who are causing "problems"
- Recently experienced loss of best friend and business partner, who died from cancer

Objective Data

Physical Examination

- Diaphoretic, short of breath, nauseous
- BP 165/100, pulse rate 120, respiratory rate 26/min

Diagnostic Studies

- ECG shows occasional premature ventricular contractions and ST elevation in leads II, III, aVF, V_5, V_6
- Cardiac-specific troponin I level elevated
- Cholesterol 350 mg/dl (9.1 mmol/L)
- Hb A1C 9.0%
- Inferolateral wall MI

Collaborative Care

Emergency Department

- Oxygen 2 L/min via nasal cannula
- aspirin 325 mg (chewable)
- reteplase IV
- nitroglycerin IV, titrate to relieve chest pain; hold for systolic BP <100 mm Hg
- morphine 2 to 4 mg IV q5min prn for chest pain unrelieved by nitroglycerin
- Weight-based heparin IV
- metoprolol (Lopressor) 5 mg IV q5min × 3 doses
- Vital signs, pulse oximetry every 10 minutes during infusion of reteplase

Critical Thinking Questions

1. Which coronary artery(ies) is/are most likely occluded in Mr. D.'s coronary circulation?
2. Explain the pathogenesis of CAD. What risk factors may contribute to its development? What risk factors were present in Mr. D.'s life?
3. What is angina? How does chronic stable angina differ from angina associated with myocardial infarction?

4. Explain the pathophysiologic basis for the clinical manifestations that Mr. D. exhibited.
5. Explain the significance of the results of the laboratory tests and ECG findings.
6. Provide a rationale for each treatment measure ordered for Mr. D.
7. Based on the assessment data presented, write one or more priority nursing diagnoses.

NCLEX EXAMINATION REVIEW QUESTIONS

The number of the question corresponds to the same-numbered objective at the beginning of the chapter.

1. In teaching a patient about coronary artery disease, the nurse explains that the changes that occur in this disorder involve
   a. formation of fibrous tissue around coronary arteries.
   b. diffuse involvement of plaque formation in coronary veins.
   c. accumulation of lipid and fibrous tissue within the coronary arteries.
   d. chronic vasoconstriction of coronary arteries leading to permanent vasospasm.
2. After teaching about ways to decrease risk factors for CAD, the nurse recognizes that additional instruction is needed when the patient says,
   a. "I would like to add weight lifting to my exercise program."
   b. "I can't keep my blood pressure normal without medication."
   c. "I can change my diet to decrease my intake of saturated fats."
   d. "I will change my lifestyle to reduce activities that increase my stress."
3. A hospitalized patient with angina tells the nurse that she is having chest pain. The nurse bases her actions on the knowledge that ischemia
   a. will always progress to myocardial infarction.
   b. will be relieved by rest, nitroglycerin, or both.
   c. indicates that irreversible myocardial damage is occurring.
   d. is frequently associated with vomiting and extreme fatigue.
4. The clinical spectrum of acute coronary syndrome includes
   a. unstable angina and STEMI.
   b. unstable angina and NSTEMI.
   c. stable angina and sudden cardiac death.
   d. unstable angina, STEMI, and NSTEMI.
5. In planning activity for the patient recovering from an MI, the nurse recognizes that the healing heart wall is most vulnerable to stress
   a. 3 weeks after the infarction.
   b. 4 to 6 days after the infarction.
   c. 10 to 14 days after the infarction.
   d. when healing is complete at 6 to 8 weeks.
6. A patient is admitted to the CCU with chest pain of 24 hours duration, ECG findings consistent with an acute MI, and rare ventricular dysrhythmias. The nurse plans care for the patient based on the expectation that the patient will be managed with
   a. fibrinolytic therapy.
   b. endotracheal intubation.
   c. intravenous nitroglycerin.
   d. intraaortic balloon pump therapy.
7. Three days after MI, a patient states that he does not understand what the alarm is about because his problem was just a case of "bad indigestion." His reaction is an example of
   a. anger.
   b. denial.
   c. projection.
   d. depression.
8. The most common pathologic finding in individuals at risk for sudden cardiac death is
   a. aortic valve disease.
   b. mitral valve disease.
   c. left ventricular dysfunction.
   d. atherosclerotic heart disease.

REFERENCES

1. American Heart Association: *2005 heart and stroke facts statistics,* Dallas, 2005, American Heart Association.
2. Libby P: The vascular biology of atherosclerosis. In Zipes DP, et al, editors: *Heart disease: a textbook of cardiovascular medicine,* ed 7, Philadelphia, 2005, Saunders.
3. Futterman G, Lemberg L: Seminal changes in the management of the acute coronary event: current concepts, *Am J Crit Care* 12:73, 2003.
4. Huether SE, McCance KL: *Understanding pathophysiology,* ed 3, St Louis, 2004, Mosby.
5. Futterman G, Lemberg L: A quick test predicts acute coronary events, *Am J Crit Care* 12:262, 2003.
6. Kaul P, Mc Acleer EP: New biomarkers for MI and unstable angina, *Clinical Advisor* January 2005.
7. Nasser SA, Flack JM: Risky business: focus on concomitant CV risks, *Clinical Advisor* December 2004.
8. Haskell WL: Cardiovascular disease prevention and lifestyle interventions: effectiveness and efficacy, *J Cardiovasc Nurs* 18:245, 2003.
9. Nissen S, Tuzcu EM, Schoenhagen P, et al: Statin therapy, LDL cholesterol, C-reactive protein, and coronary artery disease, *N Engl J Med* 352:29, 2005.
10. The American College of Obstetricians and Gynecologists Women's Health Care Physicians: Coronary artery disease, *Obstet Gynecol* 104(4 Suppl):41S, 2004.
11. Grundy SM, Cleeman JI, Merz MB, et al: Implications of recent clinical trials for the National Cholesterol Education Program Adult Treatment Panel III Guidelines, *Circulation* 110:227, 2004.
12. Ridker PM, Genest J, Libby P: Risk factors for atherosclerotic disease. In Zipes DP, et al, editors: *Heart disease: a textbook of cardiovascular medicine,* ed 7, Philadelphia, 2005, Saunders.
13. Berra K, Klieman L: National Cholesterol Education Program: adult Treatment Panel III—new recommendations for lifestyle and medical management of dyslipidemia, *J Cardiovasc Nurs* 18:85, 2003.
14. Farmer JA, Gotto AM: The heart protection study: expanding the boundaries for high-risk coronary disease prevention, *Am J Cardiol* 92:3i, 2003.
15. Smith SC, Allen J, Blair SN, et al: American Heart Association/American College of Cardiology guidelines for secondary prevention for patients with coronary and other atherosclerotic vascular disease: 2006 update, *Circulation* 113:2363, 2006.
16. National Institutes of Health: *Seventh Report of the Joint National Committee on Prevention, Detection, Evaluation, and Treatment of High Blood Pressure (JNC 7),* Publication No 03-5233, Bethesda, Md, 2003, U.S. Department of Health and Human Services.
17. He J, Vupputuri S, Allen K, et al: Passive smoking and the risk of coronary heart disease—a meta-analysis of epidemiologic studies, *N Engl J Med* 340:920, 1999.
*18. Buchanan LM, El-Banna M, White A, et al: An exploratory study of multicomponent treatment intervention for tobacco dependency, *J Nurs Scholarsh* 36:324, 2004.
19. Fritschi C, Richlin D: The metabolic syndrome: early action to decrease risks for cardiovascular disease, *AAOHN J* 52:320, 2004.
20. Kernan-Schroeder D, Cunningham M: Glycemic control and beyond: the ABCs of standards of care for type 2 diabetes and cardiovascular disease, *J Cardiovasc Nurs* 16:44, 2002.
21. Grundy SM, Brewer HB, Cleeman JI, et al, for the National Heart, Lung, and Blood Institute and American Heart Association: Definition of metabolic syndrome: Report of the National Heart, Lung, and Blood Institute/American Heart Association conference on scientific issues related to definition, *Circulation* 109:433, 2004.
22. Khan R, Buse J, Ferrannini E, et al: The metabolic syndrome: time for a critical appraisal, *Diabetes Care* 28:2289, 2005.
23. Futterman LG, Lemberg L: The Framingham heart study: a pivotal legacy of the last millennium, *Am J Crit Care* 9:147, 2000.
24. Barsky R: Psychiatric and behavioral aspects of cardiovascular disease. In Zipes DP, Libby P, Bonow R, et al: *Braunwald's heart disease: a*

*Nursing research–based reference.

textbook of cardiovascular medicine, ed 7, Philadelphia, 2005, Elsevier Saunders.

25. Berkman LF, Blumenthal J, Burg M, et al: Effects of treating depression and low perceived social support on clinical events after myocardial infarction: the Enhancing Recovery in Coronary Heart Disease Patients (ENRICHD), *JAMA* 289:3106, 2003.
26. Kubzansky LD, Davidson KW, Rozanski A: The clinical impact of negative psychological states: expanding the spectrum of risk for coronary artery disease, *Psychosom Med* 67:S10, 2005.
27. Frasure-Smith N, Lesperance F: Reflections on depression as a cardiac risk factor, *Psychosom Med* 67:S19, 2005.
28. Carney RM, Freedlan KE, Veith RC: Depression, the autonomic nervous system, and coronary artery disease, *Psychosom Med* 67:S29, 2005.
29. Coffey M, Crowder GK, Cheek DJ: Reducing coronary artery disease by decreasing homocysteine levels, *Crit Care Nurse* 23(1):25, 2003.
30. Wang G, Mao JM, Wang X, et al: Effect of homocysteine on plaque formation and oxidative stress in patients with acute coronary syndromes, *Chin Med J (Engl)* 117:1650, 2004.
31. National Institutes of Health: *Third report of the National Cholesterol Education Program Expert Panel. Detection, evaluation, and treatment of high blood cholesterol in adults (Adult Treatment Panel III): final report,* Publication No 02-5215, Bethesda, Md, 2002, U.S. Department of Health and Human Services.
32. Ornish D, Scherwitz LW, Billings JH, et al: The Lifestyle Heart Trial: intensive lifestyle changes for reversal of coronary heart disease, *JAMA* 280:2001, 1998.
33. Braun LT, Davidson MH: Cholesterol-lowering drugs bring benefits to high-risk populations even when LDL is normal, *J Cardiovasc Nurs* 18:44, 2003.
34. Lehne RA: *Pharmacology for nursing care,* ed 6, St Louis, 2007, Saunders.
35. Sayer P: The women's health study: aspirin results, *Geriatr Med* 35:73, 2005.
36. Deaton C: State of the science for the care of older adults with heart disease, *Nurs Clin North Am* 39:495, 2004.

*37. Fair JM: Cardiovascular risk factor modification: is it effective in older adults? *J Cardiovasc Nurs* 18:161, 2003.

38. Gantz P, Gantz W: Coronary blood flow and myocardial ischemia. In Zipes DP, Libby P, Bonow R, et al: *Braunwald's heart disease: a textbook of cardiovascular medicine,* ed 7, Philadelphia, 2005, Elsevier Saunders.
39. Vinik AI, Maser RE, Mitchell BD, et al: Diabetic autonomic neuropathy, *Diabetes Care* 26:1553, 2003.
40. Braunwald E, Antman EM, Beasley JW, et al, for the American College of Cardiology and American Heart Association: Management of patients with unstable angina and non-STEMI, *Circulation* 106:1893, 2002.
41. Gluckman TJ, Sachdev M, Schulman SP, et al: A simplified approach to the management of non-ST-segment elevation acute coronary syndromes, *JAMA* 293:349, 2005.
42. Gibbons RJ, Abrams J, Chatterjee K, et al: ACC/AHA 2002 guidelines update for the management of patients with chronic stable angina—summary article: a report of the ACC/AHA Task Force Practice Guidelines, *Circulation* 107:149, 2003.
43. Antman EM, Anbe DT, Armstrong PW, et al: ACC/AHA guidelines for the management of patients with ST-elevation myocardial infarction—executive summary: a report of the ACC/AHA Task Force on Practice Guidelines, *Circulation* 110:588, 2004.
44. Popma JJ, Kantz RE: Percutaneous transluminal coronary intervention. In Zipes DP, Libby P, Bonow R, et al: *Braunwald's heart disease: a textbook of cardiovascular medicine,* ed 7, Philadelphia, 2005, Elsevier Saunders.
45. Schampaert E, Cohen EA, Schluter M, et al, for the C-SIRIUS Investigators: The Canadian study of the sirolimus-eluting stent in the treatment of patients with long de novo lesions in small native coronary arteries (C-SIRIUS), *J Am Coll Cardiol* 43:1110, 2004.
46. Antman EM, Braunwald E: Acute myocardial infarction. In Zipes DP, Libby P, Bonow R, et al: *Braunwald's heart disease: a textbook of cardiovascular medicine,* ed 7, Philadelphia, 2005, Elsevier Saunders.

*47. McSweeney JC, Cody M, O'Sullivan P, et al: Women's early warning symptoms of acute myocardial infarction, *Circulation* 108:2619, 2003.

*48. Deaton C, Namasivayam S: Nursing outcomes in coronary heart disease, *J Cardiovasc Nurs* 19:308, 2004.

49. Cannon CC, Braunwald E, Lee T: Unstable angina. In Zipes DP, Libby P, Bonow R, et al: *Braunwald's heart disease: a textbook of cardiovascular medicine,* ed 7, Philadelphia, 2005, Elsevier Saunders.
50. Eagle KA, Guyton RA, Davidoff R, et al: ACC/AHA 2004 guideline update for CABG surgery: a report of the ACC/AHA Task Force on Practice Guidelines (Committee to Update 1999 CABG Guidelines), 2004. Available at *www.acc.org/clinical/guidelines/cabg/cabg.pdf* (accessed June 30, 2006).

*51. McSweeney JC, Coon S: Women's inhibitors and facilitators associated with making behavioral changes after myocardial infarction. *Medsurg Nurs* 13:49, 2004.

52. Franklin BA, Swain DP, Shephard RJ: New insights in the prescription of exercise for coronary patients. *J Cardiovasc Nurs* 18:116, 2003.

*53. Crane PB: Fatigue and physical activity in older women after myocardial infarction, *Heart Lung* 34:30, 2005.

54. Cheitlin MD: Sexual activity and cardiovascular disease, *Am J Cardiol* 92:9A, 2003.
55. Obias-Manno D, Wijetunga M: Risk stratification and primary prevention of sudden cardiac death, *AACN Clin Issues* 15:404, 2004.
56. Davis DR, Tang AL: Implantable cardioverter defibrillators: therapy against Canada's leading killer, *CMAJ* 171:1053, 2004.

*57. Shea J: Quality of life issues in patients with implantable cardioverter defibrillators, *AACN Clin Issues* 15:478, 2004.

*Nursing research–based reference.

RESOURCES

American College of Cardiology
800-253-4636 x 694 or 301-897-5400
www.acc.org

American College of Cardiovascular Nursing
813-677-8675
www.accn.net

American Heart Association
800-AHA-USA-1 or 800-242-8721
www.americanheart.org

International Society for Minimally Invasive Cardiac Surgery
www.ismics.org

The Mended Hearts
888-HEART99 (888-432-7899) or 214-706-1442
www.mendedhearts.org

National Cholesterol Education Program
301-592-8573
www.nhlbi.nih.gov/chd

National Heart, Lung, and Blood Institute of the National Institutes of Health
www.nhlbi.nih.gov/index.htm

National Heart Savers Association
www.heartsavers.org

Society for Cardiovascular Angiography and Interventions
800-992-7224 or 301-581-3450
www.scai.org

Society of Interventional Radiology
800-488-7284 or 703-691-1805
www.sirweb.org

For additional Internet resources, see the website for this book at *http://evolve.elsevier.com/Lewis/medsurg.*

It is more important to know what sort of person has a disease than to know what sort of disease a person has.

Hippocrates

Nursing Management Heart Failure

35

Mary Ann House-Fancher and Hatice Y. Foell

LEARNING OBJECTIVES

1. Compare the pathophysiology of systolic and diastolic ventricular failure.
2. Discuss the compensatory mechanisms involved in heart failure.
3. Describe the nursing and collaborative management of the patient with acute decompensated heart failure and pulmonary edema.
4. Describe the collaborative care and nursing management, including drug and nutritional therapy, of the patient with chronic heart failure.
5. Describe the indications for cardiac transplantation and the nursing management of cardiac transplant recipients.

KEY TERMS

cardiac transplantation, p. 837
diastolic failure, p. 822
heart failure, p. 821
paroxysmal nocturnal dyspnea, p. 825
pulmonary edema, p. 824
systolic failure, p. 822

Electronic Resources

Supplemental content related to Chapter 35 can be found ...

Companion CD
- Stress-Busting Kit for Nursing Students
- Interactive Case Study: Heart Failure
- NCLEX Examination Review Questions
- Comprehensive Glossary

Evolve Website
http://evolve.elsevier.com/Lewis/medsurg
- Content Updates
- Key Points (Printable and CD/MP3 Download)
- Concept Map Creator
- Expanded Audio Glossary
- Key Term Flash Cards
- Customizable Nursing Care Plan: Heart Failure
- Patient and Family Instruction Guide in English and Spanish: Heart Failure
- Electronic Calculators
- WebLinks

HEART FAILURE

Heart failure (HF) is an abnormal clinical condition involving impaired cardiac pumping. It results in the characteristic pathophysiologic changes of vasoconstriction and fluid retention. Heart failure, formerly called congestive HF, is the terminology preferred today since not all patients with HF have pulmonary congestion. HF is not a disease. It is associated with numerous types of cardiovascular diseases, particularly long-standing hypertension, coronary artery disease (CAD), and myocardial infarction (Table 35-1). HF is characterized by ventricular dysfunction, reduced exercise tolerance, diminished quality of life, and shortened life expectancy.

In most industrial nations, HF has become a major health problem. In contrast to other cardiovascular diseases, HF is increasing in incidence. This increase is due, in part, to improved survival after cardiovascular events, and in part to the increased aging population. Currently about 5 million people in the United States have HF. The American Heart Association (AHA) estimates that 470,000 new cases are diagnosed each year. HF dramatically increases with advancing age. As the elderly population increases, HF incidence and prevalence will continue to rise. Approximately 1 in every 100 older adults has HF. The incidence of HF is similar in men and women. HF is the most common reason for hospital admission in adults older than 65 years.[1]

Heart failure is associated with high rates of morbidity, mortality, and economic costs.[1] The in-hospital mortality for these patients is 4.1%, with a mean length of hospital stay of 6.5 days. Hospital readmission rates for patients with HF are 20% at 30 days

Reviewed by Kathleen K. Salati, MSN, CCRN, NP-C, Adult Nurse Practitioner/Heart Failure, Christiana Care Health System, Newark, Del; and Erlinda C. Wheeler, RN, DNS, Associate Professor, University of Delaware, Newark, Del.

and 50% at 6 to 12 months. With hospital readmission, mortality increases to 10% at 30 days and up to 20% to 40% at 12 months.[2] These statistics reflect the increasing challenge of treating patients with HF.

Etiology and Pathophysiology

CAD and advancing age are the primary risk factors for HF. Other factors, such as hypertension, diabetes, cigarette smoking, obesity, and high serum cholesterol, can also contribute to the development of HF. Hypertension is a major contributing factor, increasing the risk of HF approximately threefold. The risk of HF increases progressively with the severity of hypertension, and systolic and diastolic hypertension equally predict risk. Diabetes predisposes an individual to HF regardless of the presence of concomitant CAD or hypertension. Diabetes is more likely to predispose women than men to HF.[1]

TABLE 35-1 Causes of Heart Failure

Chronic	Acute
Coronary artery disease	Acute myocardial infarction
Hypertension	Dysrhythmias
Rheumatic heart disease	Pulmonary emboli
Congenital heart disease	Thyrotoxicosis
Cor pulmonale	Hypertensive crisis
Cardiomyopathy	Rupture of papillary muscle (e.g., mitral valve)
Anemia	Ventricular septal defect
Bacterial endocarditis	Myocarditis
Valvular disorders	

CULTURAL AND ETHNIC HEALTH DISPARITIES

Heart Failure

- African Americans have a higher incidence of HF, develop HF at an earlier age, and experience higher rates of mortality related to HF than whites.
- African Americans experience more ACE inhibitor-related angioedema than whites.
- Isosorbide dinitrate and hydralazine (BiDil) is used for the treatment of HF in African Americans; drug is only approved for use in this ethnic group.
- Asians have an extremely high risk (50%) for ACE inhibitor-related cough.

ACE, Angiotensin-converting enzyme; *HF,* heart failure.

HF may be caused by any interference with the normal mechanisms regulating cardiac output (CO). CO depends on (1) preload, (2) afterload, (3) myocardial contractility, (4) heart rate (HR), and (5) metabolic state of the individual. (Preload and afterload are discussed in Chapter 32.) Any alteration in these factors can lead to decreased ventricular function and the resultant manifestations of HF.

The major causes of HF may be divided into two subgroups: (1) primary causes (see Table 35-1) and (2) precipitating causes (Table 35-2). Precipitating causes often increase the workload of the ventricles, resulting in a decompensated condition that leads to decreased myocardial function.

Pathology of Ventricular Failure. Heart failure is classified as systolic or diastolic failure (or dysfunction).

Systolic Failure. Systolic failure, the most common cause of HF, results from an inability of the heart to pump blood. It is a defect in the ability of the ventricles to contract (pump). The left ventricle (LV) loses its ability to generate enough pressure to eject blood forward through the aorta. Over time, the LV becomes thin-walled, dilated, and hypertrophied. The hallmark of systolic dysfunction is a decrease in the left ventricular *ejection fraction* (the percentage of total ventricular filling volume that is ejected during each ventricular contraction). Normal ejection fraction (EF) is greater than 55% of the ventricular volume. Systolic failure is caused by impaired contractile function (e.g., myocardial infarction), increased afterload (e.g., hypertension), cardiomyopathy, and mechanical abnormalities (e.g., valvular heart disease).

Diastolic Failure. Diastolic failure is an impaired ability of the ventricles to relax and fill during diastole. Approximately 20% to 40% of patients with HF have diastolic failure with a normal EF and systolic function in the presence of HF symptoms.[2] Decreased filling of the ventricles will result in decreased stroke volume and CO. Diastolic failure is characterized by high filling pressures due to stiff or noncompliant ventricles and results in venous engorgement in both the pulmonary and systemic vascular systems. The diagnosis of diastolic failure is made on the basis of the presence of pulmonary congestion, pulmonary hypertension, ventricular hypertrophy, and a normal EF.[3]

Diastolic failure is usually the result of left ventricular hypertrophy from chronic systemic hypertension, aortic stenosis, or hypertrophic cardiomyopathy. Diastolic failure is commonly seen in older adults, and predominantly women, as a result of myocardial fibrosis and hypertension (see Gender Differences Box). However, the majority of patients who present with HF and normal systolic function do not have an identifiable heart disease.[2]

TABLE 35-2 Precipitating Causes of Heart Failure

Cause	Mechanism
Anemia	↓ O_2-carrying capacity of the blood stimulating ↑ in CO to meet tissue demands
Infection	↑ O_2 demand of tissues, stimulating ↑ CO
Thyrotoxicosis	Changes the tissue metabolic rate, ↑ HR and workload of the heart
Hypothyroidism	Indirectly predisposes to ↑ atherosclerosis; severe hypothyroidism decreases myocardial contractility
Dysrhythmias	May ↓ CO and ↑ workload and O_2 requirements of myocardial tissue
Bacterial endocarditis	*Infection:* ↑ metabolic demands and O_2 requirements *Valvular dysfunction:* causes stenosis and regurgitation
Pulmonary disease (e.g., pulmonary embolism)	↑ Pulmonary pressure and exerts pressure on the RV, leading to RV hypertrophy and failure
Paget's disease	↑ Workload of the heart by ↑ vascular bed in the skeletal muscle
Nutritional deficiencies	May ↓ cardiac function by ↑ myocardial muscle mass and myocardial contractility
Hypervolemia	↑ Preload causing volume overload on the RV

CO, Cardiac output; *HR,* heart rate; *RV,* right ventricle.

GENDER DIFFERENCES
Heart Failure

Men	Women
• Men experience systolic dysfunction more frequently than women. • Men with asymptomatic systolic dysfunction experience greater mortality benefit from ACE inhibitor therapy than women.	• Women experience diastolic dysfunction more frequently than men. • Women have a higher risk of ACE inhibitor-related cough than men. • Benefits of long-term use of digitalis in women may not justify the risks (e.g., drug-related death) when compared to men. • Women with heart failure experience major depression more frequently than men.

ACE, Angiotensin-converting enzyme.

Less common is isolated right ventricular diastolic failure. This results from pulmonary hypertension (chronic or acute) and causes reduced right ventricular emptying, resulting in a low left ventricular filling pressure and reduced CO. Acute right ventricular failure can cause rapid cardiac demise despite a normal LV.

Mixed Systolic and Diastolic Failure. Systolic and diastolic failure of mixed origin is seen in disease states such as dilated cardiomyopathy (DCM). DCM is a condition in which poor systolic function (weakened muscle function) is further compromised by dilated left ventricular walls that are unable to relax (see Chapter 37). These patients often have extremely poor EFs (less than 35%), high pulmonary pressures, and *biventricular failure* (both ventricles may be dilated and have poor filling and emptying capacity).

The patient with ventricular failure of any type has low systemic arterial blood pressure (BP), low CO, and poor renal perfusion. Poor exercise tolerance and ventricular dysrhythmias are also common. Whether a patient arrives at this point acutely from a myocardial infarction (MI) or chronically from worsening cardiomyopathy or hypertension, the body's response to this low CO is to mobilize its compensatory mechanisms to maintain CO and BP.

Compensatory Mechanisms. HF can have an abrupt onset as with acute MI, or it can be an insidious process resulting from slow, progressive changes. The overloaded heart resorts to compensatory mechanisms to try to maintain adequate CO. The main compensatory mechanisms include (1) sympathetic nervous system activation, (2) neurohormonal responses, (3) ventricular dilation, and (4) ventricular hypertrophy.

Sympathetic Nervous System Activation. Sympathetic nervous system (SNS) activation is often the first mechanism triggered in low-CO states. However, it is the least effective compensatory mechanism. In response to an inadequate stroke volume and CO, there is increased SNS activation, resulting in the increased release of catecholamines (epinephrine and norepinephrine). This results in an increased HR and myocardial contractility, and peripheral vasoconstriction. Initially this increase in HR and contractility improves CO. However, over time these factors act in a detrimental fashion by increasing the myocardium's need for oxygen and the workload of the already failing heart. The vasoconstriction causes an immediate increase in preload, which may initially increase CO. However, an increase in venous return to the heart, which is already volume overloaded, actually worsens ventricular performance.

Neurohormonal Response. As the CO falls, blood flow to the kidneys decreases. This is sensed by the juxtaglomerular apparatus in the kidney as decreased volume. In response, the kidneys release renin, which converts angiotensinogen to angiotensin I (see Chapter 45 and Fig. 45-4). Angiotensin I is subsequently converted to angiotensin II by a converting enzyme made in the lungs. Angiotensin II causes (1) the adrenal cortex to release aldosterone, which results in sodium and water retention, and (2) increased peripheral vasoconstriction, which increases BP. This response is known as the renin-angiotensin-aldosterone system (RAAS).

Low CO causes a decrease in cerebral perfusion pressure. The posterior pituitary then secretes antidiuretic hormone (ADH). ADH increases water reabsorption in the renal tubules, causing water retention and therefore increased blood volume. As a result, blood volume is increased in a person who is already volume overloaded.

Other factors also contribute to the development of HF. The production of *endothelin,* produced by the vascular endothelial cells, is stimulated by ADH, catecholamines, and angiotensin II. Endothelin results in further arterial vasoconstriction and an increase in cardiac contractility and hypertrophy.[4]

Locally, proinflammatory cytokines are released by cardiac myocytes in response to various forms of cardiac injury (e.g., MI). Two cytokines, tumor necrosis factor (TNF) and interleukin-1 (IL-1), further depress cardiac function by causing cardiac hypertrophy, contractile dysfunction, and myocyte cell death.[3] Over time, a systemic inflammatory response is also mounted and accounts for the cardiac wasting, muscle myopathy, and fatigue that accompany advanced HF.[4,5]

Activation of the SNS and the neurohormonal response lead to elevated levels of norepinephrine, angiotensin II, aldosterone, ADH, endothelin, and proinflammatory cytokines. Together, these factors result in an increase in cardiac workload, myocardial dysfunction, and *ventricular remodeling.* Remodeling involves hypertrophy of the cardiac myocytes, resulting in large, abnormally shaped contractile cells. This eventually leads to increased ventricular mass, changes in ventricular shape, and impaired contractility. Although the ventricles become larger, they become less effective pumps. All of these factors are overexpressed in HF and eventually perpetuate the downward spiral of progressive HF syndrome.[4,5]

Dilation. *Dilation* is an enlargement of the chambers of the heart. It occurs when pressure in the heart chambers (usually the left ventricle) is elevated over time. The muscle fibers of the heart stretch in response to the volume of blood in the heart at the end of diastole. The degree of stretch is directly related to the force of the contraction (systole) *(Frank-Starling law).* Initially this increased contraction leads to increased CO and maintenance of arterial BP and perfusion. Initially dilation is an adaptive mechanism to cope with increasing blood volume. Eventually this mechanism becomes inadequate because the elastic elements of the muscle fibers are overstretched and can no longer contract effectively, thereby decreasing the CO.[5]

Hypertrophy. In chronic HF, *hypertrophy* is an increase in the muscle mass and cardiac wall thickness in response to overwork and strain. It occurs slowly because it takes time for this increased muscle tissue to develop. Hypertrophy generally follows persistent or chronic dilation and thus further increases the contractile power of the muscle fibers. This will lead to an increase in CO and maintenance of tissue perfusion. However, hypertrophic heart muscle has poor contractility, requires more oxygen to perform work, has poor coronary artery circulation (tissue becomes more easily ischemic), and is prone to ventricular dysrhythmias.

Counterregulatory Mechanisms. The body's ability to try to maintain balance is demonstrated by several counterregulatory processes. Natriuretic peptides (atrial natriuretic peptide [ANP] and b-type natriuretic peptide [BNP]) are hormones produced by the heart muscle that promote venous and arterial vasodilation (thus reducing afterload and preload). Natriuretic peptides are endothelin and aldosterone antagonists and enhance diuresis by increasing glomerular filtration rates (thus reducing preload and volume stress) and blocking the effects of the RAAS. In addition, they inhibit the development of cardiac hypertrophy and may have antiinflammatory effects. ANP is produced by the atrium, and BNP is produced by the ventricles. ANP is primarily triggered by increases in volume. BNP is primarily triggered by increased pressure. Prolonged atrial and ventricular distention (during HF) leads to a depletion of these factors.[6] Nitric oxide (NO) is another substance released from the vascular endothelium in response to the compensatory mechanisms activated in HF. Like the natriuretic peptides, NO works to relax the arterial smooth muscle, resulting in vasodilation and decreased afterload.[4]

Cardiac compensation occurs when compensatory mechanisms succeed in maintaining an adequate CO that is needed for tissue perfusion. *Cardiac decompensation* occurs when these mechanisms can no longer maintain adequate CO and inadequate tissue perfusion results.

Types of Heart Failure

HF is usually manifested by biventricular failure, although one ventricle may precede the other in dysfunction. Normally the pumping actions of the left and right sides of the heart are synchronized, producing a continuous flow of blood. However, as a result of pathologic conditions, one side may fail while the other side continues to function normally for a period of time. Because of the prolonged strain, both sides of the heart will eventually fail, resulting in *biventricular failure.*

Left-Sided Failure. The most common form of HF is left-sided failure (Fig. 35-1). Left-sided failure results from left ventricular dysfunction, which prevents normal blood flow and causes blood to back up into the left atrium and into the pulmonary veins. The increased pulmonary pressure causes fluid extravasation from the pulmonary capillary bed into the interstitium and then the alveoli, which is manifested as pulmonary congestion and edema.

Right-Sided Failure. Right-sided failure causes a backup of blood into the right atrium and venous circulation. Venous congestion in the systemic circulation results in jugular venous distention, hepatomegaly, splenomegaly, vascular congestion of the gastrointestinal (GI) tract, and peripheral edema. The primary cause of right-sided failure is left-sided failure. In this situation, left-sided failure results in pulmonary congestion and increased pressure in the blood vessels of the lung (pulmonary hypertension). Eventually, chronic pulmonary hypertension (increased right ventricular afterload) results in right-sided hypertrophy and failure. *Cor pulmonale* (right ventricular dilation and hypertrophy caused by pulmonary disease) can also cause right-sided failure (see Chapter 28). Right ventricular infarction may also cause isolated right ventricle (RV) failure.

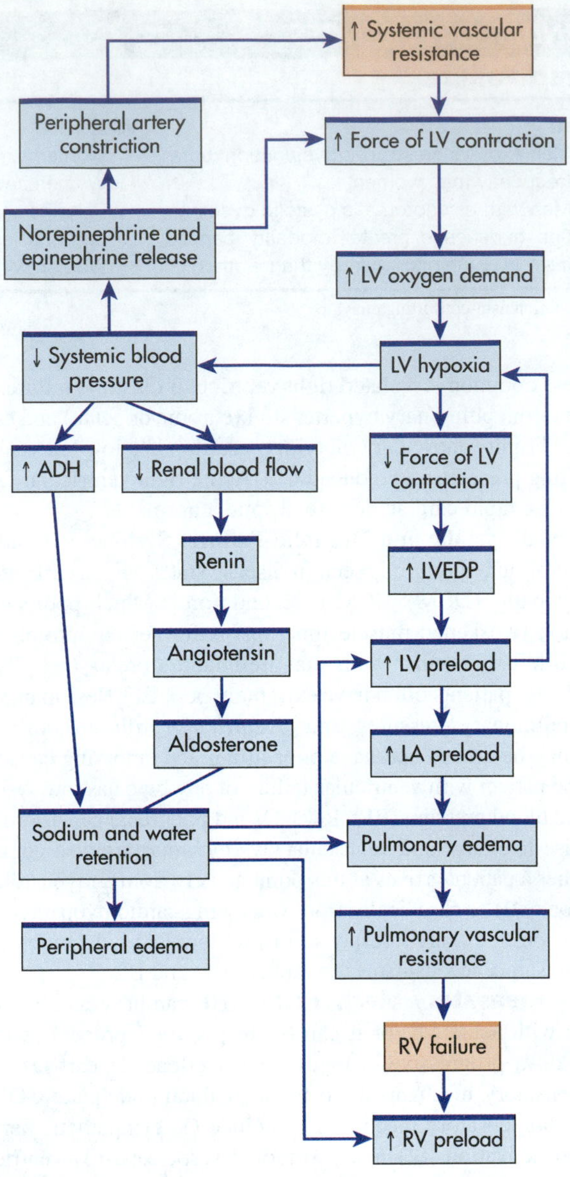

FIG. 35-1 Left-sided heart failure from elevated systemic vascular resistance. Left-sided heart failure leads to right-sided heart failure. Systemic vascular resistance and preload are exacerbated by the renin-angiotensin-aldosterone system. *ADH,* Antidiuretic hormone; *LA,* left atrium; *LV,* left ventricle; *LVEDP,* left ventricular end-diastolic pressure; *RV,* right ventricle.

Clinical Manifestations of Acute Decompensated Heart Failure

Regardless of etiology, acute decompensated heart failure (ADHF) typically manifests as **pulmonary edema,** an acute, life-threatening situation in which the lung alveoli become filled with serosanguineous fluid (Fig. 35-2). The most common cause of pulmonary edema is acute left ventricular failure secondary to CAD. (Other etiologic factors for pulmonary edema are listed in Chapter 28, Table 28-26.)

In most cases of ADHF, there is an increase in the pulmonary venous pressure caused by decreased efficiency of the LV. This results in engorgement of the pulmonary vascular system. As a result, the lungs become less compliant, and there is increased resistance in the small airways. In addition, the lymphatic system increases its flow to help maintain a constant volume of the pulmonary extravascular fluid. This early stage is clinically associated

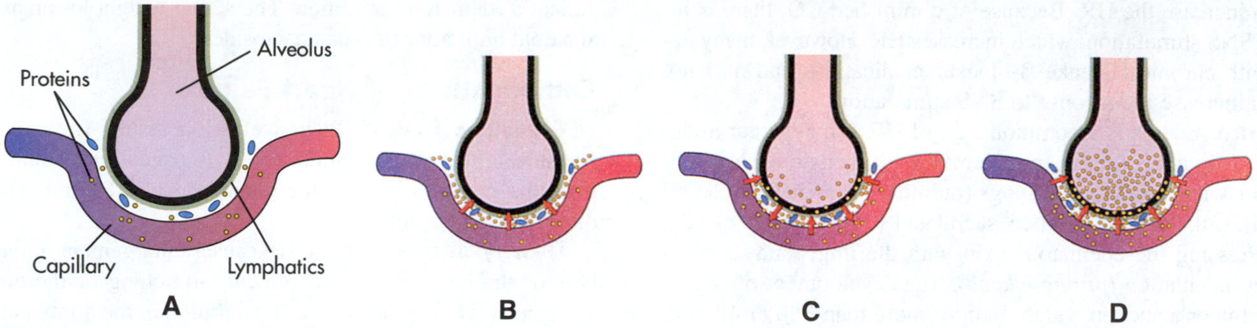

FIG. 35-2 As pulmonary edema progresses, it inhibits oxygen and carbon dioxide exchange at the alveolar-capillary interface. **A,** Normal relationship. **B,** Increased pulmonary capillary hydrostatic pressure causes fluid to move from the vascular space into the pulmonary interstitial space. **C,** Lymphatic flow increases in an attempt to pull fluid back into the vascular or lymphatic space. **D,** Failure of lymphatic flow and worsening of left heart failure result in further movement of fluid into the interstitial space and into the alveoli.

with a mild increase in the respiratory rate and a decrease in partial pressure of oxygen in arterial blood (PaO_2).

If pulmonary venous pressure continues to increase, the increase in intravascular pressure causes more fluid to move into the interstitial space than the lymphatics can drain. *Interstitial edema* occurs at this point. Tachypnea develops and the patient becomes symptomatic (short of breath out of proportion to activity level). If the pulmonary venous pressure increases further, the tight alveoli lining cells are disrupted and a fluid containing red blood cells (RBCs) moves into the alveoli (alveolar edema). As the disruption becomes worse from further increases in the pulmonary venous pressure, the alveoli and airways are flooded with fluid (see Fig. 35-2). This is accompanied by a worsening of the arterial blood gas values (i.e., lower PaO_2 and possible increased partial pressure of carbon dioxide in arterial blood [$PaCO_2$] and progressive respiratory acidemia).

Clinical manifestations of pulmonary edema are unmistakable. The patient is usually anxious, pale, and possibly cyanotic. The skin is clammy and cold from vasoconstriction caused by stimulation of the SNS. The patient has severe dyspnea, as evidenced by the use of accessory muscles of respiration, a respiratory rate greater than 30 breaths/minute, and orthopnea. There may be wheezing and coughing with the production of frothy, blood-tinged sputum. Auscultation of the lungs may reveal crackles, wheezes, and rhonchi throughout the lungs. The patient's HR is rapid, and BP may be elevated or decreased depending on the severity of the HF.

Clinical Manifestations of Chronic Heart Failure

The clinical manifestations of chronic HF depend on the patient's age, the underlying type and extent of heart disease, and which ventricle is failing to pump effectively. Table 35-3 lists the manifestations of right-sided HF and left-sided HF. The patient with chronic HF will probably have manifestations of biventricular failure.

Fatigue. Fatigue is one of the earliest symptoms of chronic HF. The patient notices fatigue after activities that normally are not tiring. The fatigue is caused by decreased CO, impaired perfusion to vital organs, decreased oxygenation of the tissues, and anemia. Anemia can result from poor nutrition, renal disease, or drug therapy (e.g., angiotensin-converting enzyme [ACE] inhibitors).

Dyspnea. *Dyspnea* (shortness of breath) is a common manifestation of chronic HF. It is caused by increased pulmonary pressures secondary to interstitial and alveolar edema. Dyspnea can occur with mild exertion or at rest. *Orthopnea* is shortness of breath that occurs when the patient is in a recumbent position. **Paroxysmal nocturnal dyspnea** (PND) occurs when the patient is asleep. It is caused by the reabsorption of fluid from dependent body areas when the patient is recumbent. The patient awakens in a panic, has feelings of suffocation, and has a strong desire to seek relief by sitting up. Careful questioning of patients often reveals adaptive behavior such as sleeping with two or more pillows to aid breathing. Because there are increased pulmonary pressures and fluid accumulation in the lung tissues, the patient may have a persistent, dry cough, unrelieved with position change or over-the-counter cough suppressants. A dry, hacking cough may be the first clinical symptom of HF.

Tachycardia. Tachycardia is an early clinical sign of HF. One of the body's first mechanisms to compensate for a failing ventri-

TABLE 35-3 Clinical Manifestations of Heart Failure

Right-Sided Heart Failure	Left-Sided Heart Failure
Signs	
RV heaves	LV heaves
Murmurs	Pulsus alternans (alternating pulses: strong, weak)
Jugular venous distention	↑ HR
Edema (e.g., anterior tibias, medial malleoli, scrotum, sacrum)	PMI displaced inferiorly and posteriorly (LV hypertrophy)
Weight gain	↓ PaO_2, slight ↑ $PaCO_2$ (poor O_2 exchange)
↑ HR	Crackles (pulmonary edema)
Ascites	S_3 and S_4 heart sounds
Anasarca (massive generalized body edema)	Pleural effusion
Hepatomegaly (liver enlargement)	Changes in mental status
	Restlessness, confusion
Symptoms	
Fatigue	Weakness, fatigue
Anxiety, depression	Anxiety, depression
Dependent, bilateral edema	Dyspnea
Right upper quadrant pain	Shallow respirations up to 32-40/min
Anorexia and GI bloating	Paroxysmal nocturnal dyspnea
Nausea	Orthopnea (shortness of breath in recumbent position)
	Dry, hacking cough
	Nocturia
	Frothy, pink-tinged sputum (advanced pulmonary edema)

GI, Gastrointestinal; *HR,* heart rate; *LV,* left ventricle; *PaO_2,* partial pressure of oxygen in arterial blood; *$PaCO_2$,* partial pressure of carbon dioxide in arterial blood; *PMI,* point of maximal impulse; *RV,* right ventricle.

cle is to increase the HR. Because of diminished CO, there is increased SNS stimulation, which increases HR. However, many patients with chronic HF take β-blocker medications and may not show an increase in response to SNS stimulation.

Edema. Edema is a common sign of HF. It may occur in dependent body areas (peripheral edema), liver (hepatomegaly), abdominal cavity (ascites), and lungs (pulmonary edema and pleural effusion). If the patient is in bed, sacral and scrotal edema may develop. Pressing the edematous skin with the finger may leave a transient indentation *(pitting edema)*. The development of dependent edema or a sudden weight gain of more than 3 lb (1.4 kg) in 2 days is often indicative of exacerbated HF.

Nocturia. A person with chronic HF who has decreased CO will also have impaired renal perfusion and decreased urinary output during the day. However, when the person lies down at night, fluid movement from interstitial spaces back into the circulatory system is enhanced. This causes increased renal blood flow and diuresis. The patient may complain of having to void 6 or 7 times during the night.

Skin Changes. Because tissue capillary oxygen extraction is increased in a person with chronic HF, the skin may appear dusky. It may also be cool and damp to the touch from diaphoresis. Often the lower extremities are shiny and swollen, with diminished or absent hair growth. Chronic swelling may result in pigment changes, causing the skin to appear brown or brawny in areas covering the ankles and lower legs.

Behavioral Changes. Cerebral circulation may be impaired with chronic HF secondary to decreased CO. The patient or family may report unusual behavior, including restlessness, confusion, and decreased attention span or memory. This may also be secondary to poor gas exchange and worsening HF.

Chest Pain. HF can precipitate chest pain due to decreased coronary perfusion from decreased CO and increased myocardial work. Angina-type pain may accompany either ADHF or chronic HF.

Weight Changes. Many factors contribute to weight changes. Initially there may be a progressive weight gain from fluid retention. However, over time the patient is often too sick to eat. Abdominal fullness from ascites and hepatomegaly frequently causes anorexia and nausea. Renal failure may also contribute to fluid retention. In many cases the muscle and fat loss is masked by the patient's edematous condition. The actual weight loss may not be apparent until after the edema subsides.

Complications of Heart Failure

Pleural Effusion. Pleural effusion results from increasing pressure in the pleural capillaries. A transudation of fluid occurs from these capillaries into the pleural space. (Pleural effusion is discussed in Chapter 28.)

Dysrhythmias. Chronic HF causes enlargement of the chambers of the heart. This enlargement (stretching of the atrial and ventricular tissues) may cause an alteration in the normal electrical pathway, especially in the atria. When numerous sites in the atria fire spontaneously and rapidly (atrial fibrillation), the organized spread of atrial depolarization (contraction or systole) no longer occurs. This loss of the atrial contraction can reduce CO by 10% to 20%. Atrial fibrillation also promotes thrombus formation within the atria, which may break loose and form emboli. Patients with atrial fibrillation are at risk for stroke and require treatment with cardioversion, antidysrhythmics, and/or anticoagulants. (Dysrhythmias are discussed in Chapter 36.)

Patients with HF and an EF less than 35% have a high risk of fatal dysrhythmias: nearly one half experience sudden cardiac death, usually due to ventricular ischemia causing ventricular tachycardia or fibrillation. (Sudden cardiac death is discussed in Chapter 34.)

Left Ventricular Thrombus. With ADHF or chronic HF, the enlarged LV and decreased CO combine to increase the chance of thrombus formation in the LV. Current guidelines of the American College of Cardiology (ACC) and American Heart Association (AHA) recommend anticoagulation in patients with HF and atrial fibrillation or very poor left ventricular function (e.g., EF <20%). Once a thrombus has formed, it may also decrease left ventricular contractility, decrease CO, and further worsen the patient's perfusion. The development of emboli from the thrombus also places the patient at risk for stroke.

Hepatomegaly. HF can lead to severe hepatomegaly, especially with RV failure. The liver lobules become congested with venous blood. The hepatic congestion leads to impaired liver function. Eventually liver cells die, fibrosis occurs, and cirrhosis can develop (see Chapter 44).

TABLE 35-4 Comparison of NYHA Functional Classification of Persons with Heart Disease and ACC/AHA Stages of Heart Failure

NYHA Functional Classification of Heart Disease	ACC/AHA Stages of Heart Failure
Class I No limitation of physical activity. Ordinary physical activity does not cause fatigue, dyspnea, palpitations, or anginal pain.	**Stage A** Patients at high risk of developing left ventricular dysfunction because of the presence of conditions that are strongly associated with the development of HF.
Class II Slight limitation of physical activity. No symptoms at rest. Ordinary physical activity results in fatigue, dyspnea, palpitations, or anginal pain.	**Stage B** Patients who developed structural heart disease that is strongly associated with the development of HF but who have never shown signs of HF.
Class III Marked limitation of physical activity. Usually comfortable at rest. Ordinary physical activity causes fatigue, dyspnea, palpitations, or anginal pain.	**Stage C** Patients who have current or prior symptoms of HF associated with underlying structural heart disease.
Class IV Inability to carry on any physical activity without discomfort. Symptoms of cardiac insufficiency or of angina may be present even at rest. If any physical activity is undertaken, discomfort is increased.	**Stage D** Patients with advanced structural heart disease and marked symptoms of HF at rest despite maximal medical therapy and who require specialized interventions.

ACC/AHA, American College of Cardiology/American Heart Association; *HF*, heart failure; *NYHA*, New York Heart Association.

TABLE 35-5 b-Type Natriuretic Peptide Levels*

BNP <100 pg/ml HF very improbable	BNP 100-500 pg/ml HF probable	BNP >500 pg/ml HF very probable

BNP, b-type natriuretic peptide; *HF,* heart failure.
*Levels will be temporarily elevated in patients receiving nesiritide (Natrecor) and may be elevated in patients with chronic, stable HF.

Renal Failure. The decreased CO that accompanies chronic HF results in decreased perfusion to the kidneys and can lead to renal insufficiency or failure (see Chapter 47).

Classification of Heart Failure

The New York Heart Association (NYHA) has developed functional guidelines for classifying people with heart disease. The classification is based on the person's tolerance to physical activity. The ACC/AHA have defined stages for people with HF beginning with people at risk for HF and progressing to people with advanced HF [7] (Table 35-4).

Diagnostic Studies

Diagnosing HF is often difficult since neither patient signs nor symptoms are highly specific, and both may mimic many other medical conditions, such as anemia or lung disease. The primary goal in diagnosis is to determine the underlying etiology of HF. Measures to assess the cause and degree of HF include a thorough history, physical examination, chest x-ray, electrocardiogram (ECG), laboratory data (cardiac enzymes, BNP, serum chemistries, liver function studies, thyroid function studies, and complete blood count), hemodynamic assessment, echocardiogram, stress testing, and cardiac catheterization. EF can be measured using echocardiography and/or nuclear imaging studies (see Table 32-7). EF can be used to differentiate between systolic and diastolic HF, an important distinction to make in the early treatment of HF. BNP levels are used to assist in the diagnosis of HF. In general, levels correlate positively with the degree of left ventricular dysfunction and can help to differentiate dyspnea caused by HF from other causes of dyspnea (e.g., exacerbation of chronic obstructive pulmonary disease)[6] (Table 35-5). Diagnostic studies used for the patient with ADHF are presented in Table 35-6, and those for the patient with chronic HF are presented in Table 35-7.

A complete history, physical, diagnostic, and laboratory assessment is necessary to identify the cause of HF, aggravating factors, potential risk factors that may influence outcomes, and current clinical status. The patient's comorbid conditions, especially active chronic conditions, may act as exacerbating factors affecting the plan of care and influencing the timing and intensity of therapies.

TABLE 35-6 COLLABORATIVE CARE Acute Decompensated Heart Failure and Pulmonary Edema

Diagnostic
- History and physical examination
- ABGs, serum chemistries, cardiac enzymes, BNP level, liver function tests
- Chest x-ray
- Hemodynamic monitoring
- 12-lead ECG
- Echocardiogram
- Nuclear imaging studies (see Table 32-7)
- Cardiac catheterization

Collaborative Therapy
- Treatment of underlying cause
- High Fowler's position
- O_2 by mask or nasal catheter; BiPAP
- BP, HR, RR, urinary output at least q1hr
- Continuous ECG and pulse oximetry monitoring
- Hemodynamic monitoring (e.g., intraarterial BP, PAWP, CO)
- Drug therapy: diuretics IV (furosemide [Lasix]); nitroglycerin IV; morphine IV; nesiritide (Natrecor); inotropic therapy (see Table 35-9)
- Daily weights
- Possible cardioversion (e.g., atrial fibrillation)
- Endotracheal intubation and mechanical ventilation
- Circulatory assist devices (e.g., intraaortic balloon pump, ventricular assist device)

ABGs, Arterial blood gases; *BiPAP,* bilevel positive airway pressure; *BNP,* b-type natriuretic peptide; *BP,* blood pressure; *CO,* cardiac output; *ECG,* electrocardiogram; *HR,* heart rate; *IV,* intravenous; *PAWP,* pulmonary artery wedge pressure; *RR,* respiratory rate.

NURSING *and* COLLABORATIVE MANAGEMENT ACUTE DECOMPENSATED HEART FAILURE AND PULMONARY EDEMA

With the addition of new pharmaceutical agents and device therapies, the management of ADHF and chronic HF has dramatically changed in the last 5 years. The goals of therapy for both ADHF and chronic HF are to decrease patient symptoms, reverse ventricular remodeling, improve quality of life, and decrease mortality and morbidity. Management therapies are similar for both clinical conditions.

The challenge of planning and providing nursing care that promotes the best possible clinical outcomes to the patient with ADHF remains a complex task. Because of the large number of patients and the high cost of care associated with hospital readmissions, acute and critical care nurses must develop and implement

TABLE 35-7 COLLABORATIVE CARE Chronic Heart Failure

Diagnostic
- History and physical examination
- Determination of underlying cause
- Serum chemistries, cardiac enzymes, BNP level, liver function tests
- Chest x-ray
- 12-lead ECG
- Echocardiography
- Exercise stress testing
- Nuclear imaging studies (see Table 32-7)
- Hemodynamic monitoring
- Cardiac catheterization

Collaborative Therapy
- Treatment of underlying cause
- Oxygen therapy at 2-6 L/min by nasal cannula
- Rest-activity periods
- Drug therapy (see Table 35-9)
- Daily weights
- Sodium-restricted diet
- Circulatory assist devices (e.g., ventricular assist device)
- Cardiac resynchronization therapy with internal cardioverter-defibrillator
- Cardiac transplantation

BNP, b-type natriuretic peptide; *ECG,* electrocardiogram.

TABLE 35-8 Core Measures for Heart Failure

- Written discharge instructions or educational material must be given to the patient or caregiver and include all of the following: activity level, diet, discharge medications, follow-up appointment, weight monitoring, and symptom management.
- Left ventricular function must be documented in the hospital record to indicate that it was assessed before or during hospitalization or will be assessed after discharge.
- Patients with known systolic dysfunction of moderate to severe impairment (ejection fraction less than 40%) and without contraindication to angiotensin-converting enzyme inhibitor will be prescribed an angiotensin-converting enzyme inhibitor at hospital discharge. An angiotensin receptor blocker is an acceptable alternative for patients with contraindication to angiotensin-converting enzyme inhibitors.
- Patients who are current smokers or former smokers who quit in the past 12 months will be given smoking cessation advice or counseling during the hospital stay.

strategies that are associated with improved outcomes. The Joint Commission on Accreditation of Healthcare Organizations recently established four core measures in the acute management of patients with HF to promote adherence to basic standards of evidence-based care[8] (Table 35-8).

The optimal treatment of ADHF remains a challenge and an important area of research today. The use of various diuretic regimens, vasoactive drugs, newer pharmacologic agents, ultrafiltration, and novel device therapy is being explored. Data from the Acute Decompensated Heart Failure National Registry (ADHERE) indicate that patients receiving early treatment with intravenous (IV) diuretics and vasoactive drugs have better outcomes and shorter hospital and intensive care unit (ICU) stays than patients who have delays in treatment. This information has led to new protocols from the ACC/AHA regarding the treatment of ADHF.[7]

Diuretics have long been the standard drugs used for decreasing preload and improving the patient's signs and symptoms. This single therapeutic approach is now under reconsideration due to the findings from the ADHERE. Thus treatment strategies should include improving left ventricular function by decreasing intravascular volume, decreasing venous return (preload), decreasing afterload, controlling HR and rhythm, improving gas exchange and oxygenation, increasing CO, reducing anxiety, preserving target organ function (e.g., kidneys), and decreasing progression of the disease.[7,9] This would include the use of oxygen therapy, diuretics, vasodilators, and possibly inotropic agents. Circulatory assist devices may also be used for the acutely ill patient to preserve heart and target organ function. Table 35-6 lists the major components of the therapeutic approach.

Decreasing Intravascular Volume

Decreasing intravascular volume with the use of diuretics reduces venous return. A loop diuretic (e.g., furosemide [Lasix], bumetanide [Bumex]) may be used to decrease volume because it may be administered by IV push and its action within the kidney occurs rapidly. By decreasing venous return to the LV and thereby reducing preload, the overfilled LV may contract more efficiently and improve CO. This increases left ventricular function, decreases pulmonary vascular pressures, and improves gas exchange.

The use of a loop diuretic may be delayed until the patient is assessed for hemodynamic and renal function and started on other vasodilator agents. The use of IV loop diuretic therapy alone has been shown to be associated with an increased risk of fatal dysrhythmias, aggravated renal dysfunction, and enhanced activation of the RAAS and SNS. Overall, the effects of loop diuretics actually increase systemic vascular resistance (afterload), decrease preload, and cause electrolyte imbalances.[10]

Ultrafiltration, or aquapheresis, is an option for the patient with volume overload. Ultrafiltration has generally been achieved through hemodialysis or central venous access. Newer technology allows removal of up to 500 ml/hr of fluid through either a peripheral or central venous line without significantly changing mean arterial pressure. When ultrafiltration is performed, volume is removed similar to hemodialysis but without hemodynamic instability. This therapeutic modality may be an appropriate adjunctive therapy for patients with HF and renal failure. Current research trials are ongoing to evaluate this modality for the patient with ADHF.[9] (Ultrafiltration is discussed in Chapter 47.)

Decreasing Venous Return

Decreasing venous return *(preload)* reduces the amount of volume returned to the LV during diastole. This can be accomplished by placing the patient in a high Fowler's position with the feet horizontal in the bed or dangling at the bedside. This position helps decrease venous return because of the pooling of blood in the extremities. This position also increases the thoracic capacity, allowing for improved ventilation. IV nitroglycerin is a vasodilator used in the treatment of ADHF. It reduces circulating volume by decreasing preload and also increases coronary artery circulation by dilating the coronary arteries. Therefore nitroglycerin reduces preload, slightly reduces afterload (in high doses), and increases myocardial oxygen supply. When titrating IV nitroglycerin, BP is monitored frequently (every 5 to 10 minutes) to avoid symptomatic hypotension.

Decreasing Afterload

Afterload is the resistance against which the LV must pump; that is, it is the amount of work the LV has to produce to eject blood into the systemic circulation. Systemic vascular resistance (SVR) is a determinant of afterload, as is left ventricular filling. If afterload is reduced, the CO of the LV improves and thereby decreases pulmonary congestion.

IV sodium nitroprusside (Nipride) is a potent vasodilator that reduces preload and afterload. Because of its rapid onset of action and potent effects on the vascular system, it is the drug of choice for the patient with ADHF and pulmonary edema. By reducing both preload and afterload (by arterial and venous dilation), myocardial contraction improves, increasing CO and reducing pulmonary congestion. Complications of IV sodium nitroprusside include (1) hypotension and (2) thiocyanate toxicity, which can develop after 48 hours of use. Patients receiving sodium nitroprusside must have their BP monitored frequently (every 5 to 10 minutes) during the titration of the drug because profound hypotension is the principal adverse effect.

Drug Alert - Nitroprusside (Nipride)
- *Too rapid rate of IV administration can reduce BP too quickly.*
- *Headache, nausea, dizziness, dyspnea, blurred vision, sweating, and restlessness can occur.*
- *Assess BP prior to administration and continuously during administration.*

Morphine sulfate also reduces preload and afterload and is frequently used in the treatment of ADHF and pulmonary edema. It dilates both the pulmonary and systemic blood vessels, a goal in decreasing pulmonary pressures and improving the gas exchange. Morphine sulfate also reduces anxiety and may assist in reducing dyspnea.

Nesiritide (Natrecor) is an IV vasoactive therapy for ADHF. It is a recombinant form of BNP and causes both arterial and venous dilation. The main hemodynamic effects of nesiritide include (1) a reduction in pulmonary artery wedge pressure (PAWP) and (2) an increase in CO without increasing myocardial oxygen consumption or the occurrence of dysrhythmias.[11] In addition, renal perfusion is enhanced, thus protecting the kidney. Nesiritide also has direct renal effects, resulting in the inhibition of the RAAS and promotion of natriuresis and diuresis.[9] Although classified as a vasodilator, nesiritide is also referred to as a neurohormonal blocking agent and is indicated for short-term treatment of ADHF. The main adverse effect of nesiritide is symptomatic hypotension, so BP should be closely monitored.

Improving Gas Exchange and Oxygenation

Gas exchange may be improved by several measures. IV morphine sulfate decreases oxygen demands, which may be raised as a result of anxiety and subsequent increased musculoskeletal and respiratory activity. Administration of oxygen helps increase the percentage of oxygen in inspired air. (Oxygen therapy is discussed in Chapter 29.) In severe pulmonary edema the patient may need noninvasive ventilatory support (e.g., bilevel positive airway pressure [BiPAP]) or intubation and mechanical ventilation. (Ventilatory support is discussed in Chapter 66.)

Improving Cardiac Function

In a patient who is or becomes hemodynamically unstable—that is, becomes progressively hypotensive, has an HR that is abnormally fast or slow, develops dysrhythmias, or becomes hypoxic with cool and clammy skin—nursing care becomes more urgent and treatment protocols may require aggressive, complex therapies. The use of diuretics, morphine sulfate, and vasodilators may not be sufficient to control symptoms. The addition of inotropic therapy may be warranted, as well as the initiation of hemodynamic monitoring to evaluate the effectiveness of interventions. Once a pulmonary artery catheter is in position, accurate measurement of CO, pulmonary artery pressure (PAP), and PAWP may be made and therapy instituted and titrated to maximize CO. A PAWP of 14 to 18 mm Hg will generally achieve the goal of increasing CO. (Hemodynamic monitoring is discussed in Chapter 66.)

Digitalis is a positive inotrope that improves left ventricular function. Digitalis increases contractility but also increases myocardial oxygen consumption. Because digitalis requires a loading dose and time to accomplish hemodynamic improvement, it is not recommended for the initial treatment of ADHF.

Other positive inotropes that can be considered include the β-adrenergic agonists (e.g., dopamine [Intropin], dobutamine [Dobutrex], epinephrine, norepinephrine [Levophed]). Stimulation of β-adrenergic receptors results in an increase in cyclic adenosine monophosphate (cAMP) within the myocardial cells and an increase in contractility (inotropic effect) and HR. The β-adrenergic agonists are typically used as a short-term treatment of ADHF in the ICU and, most recently, on step-down or intermediate care units with ECG monitoring capability. Dopamine is a β-adrenergic agonist used for treatment of severe ADHF and cardiogenic shock. In addition to increasing myocardial contractility and SVR, activation of dopamine receptors in the kidneys dilates the renal blood vessels and enhances urine output.[12] Unlike dopamine, dobutamine is a selective β-adrenergic agonist and works selectively on the receptors in the heart. Dobutamine does not increase SVR and may be preferred for short-term treatment of ADHF.[12]

Drug Alert - *Dopamine (Intropin)*
- *Extravasation with tissue sloughing may occur with IV administration.*
- *Monitor IV site for extravasation to prevent necrosis.*
- *High dosages may produce ventricular dysrhythmias.*

Potential problems related to long-term treatment with β-adrenergic agonists include tolerance, increased ventricular irritability, and increased need for oxygen by the myocardium. In addition, these drugs are only available for IV use.

Inamrinone (Inocor) and milrinone (Primacor) are two phosphodiesterase inhibitors that have been called inodilators because they increase myocardial contractility (inotropic effect) and promote peripheral vasodilation. Inhibition of phosphodiesterase increases cAMP, which enhances calcium entry into the cell and improves myocardial contractility. They increase CO and reduce arterial pressure (decrease afterload). Studies have shown inamrinone to be superior to dobutamine or dopamine in improving cardiac function.[12] Like dopamine and dobutamine, these drugs are only available for IV use. Adverse effects include dysrhythmias, thrombocytopenia, and hepatotoxicity.

Although these inotropic agents can effectively increase CO, reduce filling pressures, and lead to short-term clinical improvement, some data suggest that their use may be associated with increased overall mortality.[11] Currently, inotropic therapy is only recommended for use in the short-term management of patients with ADHF who have not responded to conventional pharmacotherapy (e.g., diuretics, vasodilators, morphine sulfate).[7]

Reducing Anxiety

Reduction of anxiety is an important nursing function, since anxiety may increase the SNS response and further increase myocardial workload. Reducing anxiety may be facilitated by a variety of nursing interventions (see NCP 35-1) and the use of sedative medications (e.g., benzodiazepines, morphine sulfate). When morphine sulfate is used, the patient often experiences relief from dyspnea and, consequently, the anxiety that is often associated with dyspnea. Though morphine-induced respiratory depression is rare, the patient's respiratory rate should be monitored.

Once the patient is more stable, determination of the cause of pulmonary edema is important. Diagnosis of systolic or diastolic failure will then determine further management protocols. Aggressive drug therapy may continue with IV forms of diuretics, vasodilators, and inotropes. Nursing care focuses on continual physical assessment, hemodynamic monitoring, and evaluating the patient's response to treatment.

Collaborative Care: Chronic Heart Failure

The main goal in the treatment of chronic HF is to treat the underlying cause and contributing factors, maximize CO, provide treatment to alleviate symptoms, improve ventricular function, improve quality of life, preserve target organ function, and improve mortality and morbidity (see Table 35-7). The management of dysrhythmias is discussed in Chapter 36, hypertension in Chapter 33, valvular disorders in Chapter 37, and coronary artery disease in Chapter 34.

In a person with HF, oxygen saturation of the blood is reduced because the blood is not adequately oxygenated in the lungs. Ad-

ETHICAL DILEMMAS

Competence

Situation

A 60-year-old man has been awaiting a heart transplantation for 6 months. He has been a patient in intensive care for 1 month as he has required a ventricular assist device for his failing heart. He recently suffered a stroke, which is a complication of the device, that left him paralyzed on his right side. He is only able to answer yes/no questions by shaking his head. He has required mechanical ventilation since his stroke. For the past 2 weeks hemodialysis has been required because of renal failure. For the past several days, when the nurses suction him, he tries to prevent the ventilator tubing from being reconnected by turning his head or by pushing it away with his left hand. Although he does not have any advance directives, his wife and daughter state that, on numerous occasions before these events, he expressed that he would not want to live if he lost his independence. His wife and daughter request to have the mechanical ventilator withdrawn.

Important Points for Consideration

- Informed consent related to treatment decisions entails four elements: (1) information provided about possible treatment options must be understandable to the patient; (2) possible outcomes of the various treatment options must be explained; (3) the patient must have the capacity to deliberate about the treatment choices and their consequences; and (4) the patient's treatment decision must be freely chosen or made without coercion.
- It may be difficult under certain circumstances, such as with impaired communication, to determine a patient's capacity to make an informed treatment decision.
- Health care providers cannot assume that a patient who does not have the capacity to make decisions in one area (e.g., hemodialysis) is incapable of making decisions related to other aspects of his or her care, such as continued mechanical ventilation.
- The wife, acting as the patient's surrogate decision maker, is using substituted judgment to indicate what the patient would want based on his previously expressed wishes.
- State statutes may vary on what is "clear and convincing evidence" of a patient's expressed wishes for end-of-life care or whether the patient meets certain "qualifying conditions" for withholding or withdrawing care, as in Illinois.

Critical Thinking Questions

1. What would you do next given the patient's behavior and the information that you have obtained from the patient's wife?
2. What are your feelings about participating in the care of a patient in whom withdrawal of treatment will result in death?

ministration of oxygen improves saturation and assists greatly in meeting tissue oxygen needs. Thus oxygen therapy helps relieve dyspnea and fatigue. Optimally either pulse oximetry or arterial blood gases (ABGs) are used to monitor the effectiveness of oxygen therapy.

Physical and emotional rest allows the patient to conserve energy and decreases the need for additional oxygen. The degree of rest recommended depends on the severity of HF. A patient with severe HF may be on bed rest with limited activity. A patient with mild to moderate HF can be ambulatory with a restriction of strenuous activity. The patient should be instructed to participate in limited activities with adequate recovery periods.

EVIDENCE-BASED PRACTICE

Does Patient Discharge Education Improve Clinical Outcomes in Chronic Heart Failure Patients?

Clinical Question

For patients with chronic heart failure (P), will a 1-hr patient education session at discharge (I) improve clinical outcomes (O) compared to patients who receive no education (C)?

Best Available Evidence

Randomized controlled trial (RCT).

Critical Appraisal and Synthesis of Evidence

- RCT ($n = 223$) of patients with chronic heart failure.
- Patients received a 1-hr one-on-one teaching session with a nurse educator upon hospital discharge.
- Patients who received the education had improved adherence to self-care, lower risk of rehospitalization and death, and lower cost of care.

Conclusion

Adding a 1-hr patient education session at time of discharge improves clinical outcomes, increases self-care adherence, and reduces cost of care for patients with heart failure.

Implications for Nursing Practice

- Planning for patient discharge is essential to improve clinical outcomes.
- Discharge education should include information about the cause of heart failure, drug therapy, dietary limitations, and importance of self-care behaviors (e.g., smoking cessation, daily weight monitoring).

Reference for Evidence

Koelling TM, Johnson ML, Cody RJ, et al: Discharge education improves clinical outcomes in patients with chronic heart failure, *Circulation* 111:179, 2005.

PICO: P, Patient population of interest; *I,* intervention or area of interest; *C,* comparison of interest or comparison group; *O,* outcome(s) of interest (see p. 6).

Nonpharmacologic therapies are now being used in the management of HF patients who are receiving maximum medical therapy, continue to have NYHA Functional Class III or IV symptoms, and have a widened QRS interval. One therapy is biventricular pacing. Traditional pacemakers pace one or two chambers (e.g., atrium and/or ventricle). *Cardiac resynchronization therapy* (CRT) coordinates right and left ventricle contractility through biventricular pacing. The ability to have normal electrical conduction within the right and left ventricles increases left ventricular performance and CO. This additional therapy allows patients to increase their exercise capacity and decrease their overall symptoms. CRT does not prolong life, but does improve quality of life in patients with NYHA Functional Class III and IV HF.[13] CRT therapy can be combined with traditional pacing capability as well as defibrillator technology. If the patient has ischemia-induced HF and an EF of <35%, the implementation and use of an implantable cardioverter-defibrillator (ICD) with CRT may be warranted.[13] Life-threatening ventricular dysrhythmias (e.g., ventricular tachycardia) are a complication of the ischemic myocardium and can cause sudden cardiac death. The addition of the ICD in these patients has reduced the overall mortality. (Pacemakers and defibrillators are discussed in Chapter 36.)

Cardiac transplantation is one form of treatment for ADHF and chronic HF. However, the lack of donor hearts and the challenges of care make it an option for only a small number of patients with

COMPLEMENTARY AND ALTERNATIVE THERAPIES

Hawthorn

Clinical Uses
- Heart failure*
- Coronary artery disease (angina)†

Effects
May improve performance of damaged myocardium, improve myocardial perfusion, prevent or reduce symptoms of mild-to-moderate heart failure.

Nursing Implications
Generally safe when used in recommended dosages under the supervision of a health care professional for treatment of heart failure. Use with caution in the elderly or in patients at risk for hypotension. Use with caution in patients taking other cardiovascular medications, herbs, or supplements due to possibility of additive effects. Contraindicated in pregnancy and lactation.

Adapted from Ulbricht CE, Basch EM: *Natural standard herb and supplement reference: evidence-based clinical reviews,* St Louis, 2005, Mosby (available at *www.naturalstandard.com*).
*Strong scientific evidence for its use.
†Unclear scientific evidence for its use.

HF. Stringent criteria are necessary to select the few patients with advanced HF who can even hope to receive a transplanted heart. (Heart transplantation is discussed later in this chapter.)

Several mechanical options are available to sustain HF patients with deteriorating conditions, especially those awaiting cardiac transplantation. The intraaortic balloon pump (IABP) is frequently employed in the setting of MI or perioperatively during cardiac surgery. The IABP can be useful in the hemodynamically unstable HF patient because it decreases SVR, PAWP, and PAP as much as 25%, leading to improved CO.[14] However, the limitations of bed rest, infection, and vascular complications preclude long-term use. (IABPs are discussed in Chapter 66.) Ventricular assist devices (VADs) provide highly effective long-term support for up to 2 years and have become standard care in many heart transplant centers. VADs are used as a bridge to transplantation, effectively increasing cardiac function until a donor heart becomes available for the patient. The use of a permanent, implantable VAD, known as destination therapy, is an option for patients with advanced NYHA Functional Class IV HF who are not candidates for heart transplantation.[15] (VADs are discussed in Chapter 66.)

Drug Therapy: Chronic Heart Failure

General therapeutic objectives for drug management of chronic HF include the following: (1) identification of the type of HF and underlying causes, (2) correction of sodium and water retention and volume overload, (3) reduction of cardiac workload, (4) improvement of myocardial contractility, and (5) control of precipitating and complicating factors. The aims of treating HF are to improve symptoms, minimize side effects of treatment, decrease morbidity, improve quality of life, and prolong survival.[16] Current therapeutic approaches stress the role of diuretics, vasodilators, β-blockers, and inotropic agents[12] (Table 35-9).

Diuretics. Diuretics are used in HF to mobilize edematous fluid, reduce pulmonary venous pressure, and reduce preload (see Table 33-8). If excess extracellular fluid is excreted, blood volume returning to the heart can be reduced and cardiac function improved.

TABLE 35-9 DRUG THERAPY Heart Failure

Diuretics (see Table 33-8)
morphine sulfate
Vasodilators
- ACE inhibitors (see Table 33-8)
- nitroprusside (Nipride)
- nitroglycerin
- b-Type natriuretic peptide: nesiritide (Natrecor)

β-Adrenergic blockers (see Table 33-8)
Positive inotropes
- Digitalis glycoside: digoxin (Lanoxin)
- β-Adrenergic agonists: dopamine (Intropin), dobutamine (Dobutrex)
- Phosphodiesterase inhibitors: inamrinone (Inocor), milrinone (Primacor)
- Calcium sensitizer: levosimendan (Simdax)*

Angiotensin II receptor blockers: losartan (Cozaar), valsartan (Diovan)
Antidysrhythmic drugs (see Table 36-8)

ACE, Angiotensin-converting enzyme.
*FDA approval is pending.

Diuretics act on the kidney by promoting excretion of sodium and water. Many varieties of diuretics are available, and some have specific indications for use. Thiazide diuretics may be the first choice in chronic HF because of their convenience, safety, low cost, and effectiveness. They are particularly useful in treating edema secondary to HF and in controlling hypertension. The thiazides inhibit sodium reabsorption in the distal tubule, thus promoting excretion of sodium and water.

Loop diuretics (e.g., furosemide [Lasix], bumetanide [Bumex], torsemide [Demadex]) are potent diuretics. These drugs act on the ascending loop of Henle to promote sodium, chloride, and water excretion. Furosemide is commonly used in ADHF and chronic HF because it is slightly more predictable in its response. Problems in using loop diuretics include reduction in serum potassium levels, ototoxicity, and possible allergic reaction in the patient who is sensitive to sulfa-type drugs.

Spironolactone (Aldactone) is an inexpensive, potassium-sparing diuretic that promotes sodium and water excretion but blocks potassium excretion by blocking receptors for aldosterone in the distal renal tubules. More important, aldosterone receptor antagonism has been shown to be effective because it blocks the harmful neurohormonal effects of aldosterone on the heart blood vessels. Spironolactone appears to add to the benefits of angiotensin-converting enzyme (ACE) inhibitors, and is appropriate to use while renal function is adequate. Spironolactone may also be used in conjunction with other diuretics, such as furosemide.[12]

***Drug Alert** - Spironolactone (Aldactone)*
- *Assess for hyperkalemia during treatment.*
- *Use with caution in patients taking digoxin as hyperkalemia may reduce the effects of digoxin.*
- *Instruct patient to avoid foods high in potassium (e.g., bananas, oranges, dried apricots).*

Vasodilators. Vasodilator drugs are a class of drugs clearly shown to improve survival in HF. The goals of vasodilator therapy in the treatment of HF include (1) increasing venous capacity, (2) improving EF through improved ventricular contraction, (3) slowing the process of ventricular dysfunction, (4) decreasing heart size, (5) avoiding stimulation of the neurohormonal responses initiated by the compensatory mechanisms of HF, and (6) enhancing neurohormonal blockade.

Angiotensin-Converting Enzyme Inhibitors. The benefits of ACE inhibitors in the treatment of all stages of HF have been well documented.[7,9] ACE inhibitors are useful in both systolic and diastolic HF, and they are the first-line therapy in the treatment of chronic HF. Examples of ACE inhibitors include captopril (Capoten), benazepril (Lotensin), and enalapril (Vasotec). Other examples of ACE inhibitors are discussed in Chapter 33 and listed in Table 33-8.

Drug Alert - *Captopril (Capoten)*
- *Excessive hypotension may occur.*
- *Monitor patient for first-dose hypotension (first-dose syncope).*
- *Skipping doses or discontinuing the drug can result in rebound hypertension.*

The conversion of angiotensin I to the potent vasoconstrictor angiotensin II requires the presence of ACE (see Chapter 45, Fig. 45-4). ACE inhibitors exert their effects by blocking this enzyme, resulting in decreased levels of angiotensin II. As a result, plasma aldosterone levels are also reduced. Thus ACE inhibitors are now regarded as neurohormonal blocking agents in the treatment of HF.

Because CO is dependent on afterload in chronic HF, the reduction in SVR seen with the use of ACE inhibitors produces a significant increase in CO. Furthermore, with the use of ACE inhibitors, although BP may be decreased, tissue perfusion is maintained or increased as a result of improved CO and diuresis is enhanced by the suppression of aldosterone. Other hemodynamic changes include a reduction in (1) PAP, (2) right arterial pressure, and (3) left ventricular filling pressure. As a neurohormonal blocker, ACE inhibitors also decrease the development of ventricular remodeling by inhibiting ventricular hypertrophy.

ACE inhibitor therapy used in combination with diuretic therapy has shown to be beneficial in decreasing mortality in patients with chronic HF.[7] ACE inhibitors counterbalance the alteration in renal mechanisms responsible for sodium and water retention in patients with chronic HF. The use of ACE inhibitor and diuretic therapy has the effect of increasing exercise tolerance, improving EF, and decreasing hospital readmissions in patients with chronic HF.[7]

Major side effects of ACE inhibitors include symptomatic hypotension, intractable cough, hyperkalemia, *angioedema* (allergic reaction involving edema of the face and airways), and renal insufficiency (when ACE inhibitors are used in high doses). Aging and baseline renal insufficiency slow the metabolism of ACE inhibitors and may therefore lead to increased serum drug levels. It is recommended that these drugs be started at the lowest dose and that BP and renal function (e.g., serum creatinine) be monitored at regular intervals. Adequate titration of ACE inhibitors to target doses that are associated with increased survival is critical.[12] Overall, ACE inhibitors are well tolerated by patients.

Nitrates. Nitrates cause vasodilation by acting directly on the smooth muscle of the vessel wall. Their effects primarily involve increasing venous capacitance, dilating the pulmonary vasculature, and improving arterial compliance. Therefore the major hemodynamic effect of nitrates is to decrease preload. Nitrates are of particular benefit in the management of myocardial ischemia related to HF because they promote vasodilation of the coronary arteries. One specific deterrent to the use of nitrates in HF is nitrate tolerance. In addition, men with HF may experience erectile dysfunction and as a result take an erectile agent [(e.g., sildenafil (Viagra)]. Erectile agents are contraindicated in patients taking nitrates as together they could precipitate profound hypotension.

Human b-Type Natriuretic Peptide. Nesiritide is a synthetic form of human BNP. Nesiritide has gained importance in the treatment of ADHF and is being studied for its use in the ongoing treatment of patients with chronic HF (see earlier discussion). Outpatient management of ADHF and chronic HF using parenteral natriuretic peptides is an emerging strategy that appears to be clinically effective, may lead to fewer hospitalizations, and may improve quality of life. When combined with the control of cardiovascular risk factors and correction of precipitating mechanisms for decompensation, it is hopeful that treatment of HF with natriuretic peptides in the outpatient setting may reduce morbidity and mortality.[2]

β-Adrenergic Blockers. The use of β-adrenergic blockers in the management of HF continues to evolve. Marked improvement in patient survival has been shown with the use of β-adrenergic blockers, specifically carvedilol (Coreg) and metoprolol (Toprol-XL).[12] β-Adrenergic blockers directly block the negative effects of the SNS on the failing heart, such as increased HR. It is recommended that they be used in combination with other therapies (e.g., ACE inhibitors, diuretics, digitalis). Because β-adrenergic blockade can reduce myocardial contractility, care must be taken to start gradually, increasing the dosage slowly every 2 weeks as tolerated by the patient. Major adverse effects include edema, worsening of HF, hypotension, fatigue, and bradycardia.[12]

Drug Alert - *Carvedilol (Coreg)*
- *Overdosage can produce profound bradycardia, hypotension, bronchospasm, and cardiogenic shock.*
- *Assess BP and pulse at beginning of treatment and q4hr.*
- *Abrupt withdrawal may result in sweating, palpitations, and headaches.*

Positive Inotropes. The use of positive inotropic agents in the patient with HF is directed at improving cardiac contractility to increase CO, decrease left ventricular diastolic pressure, and decrease SVR. Types of inotropic agents used in treating HF are listed in Table 35-9.

Digitalis Glycosides. Digitalis glycosides [e.g., digoxin (Lanoxin)] have been used for more than 200 years and remain the mainstay in the treatment of HF. However, the use of digitalis preparations has recently been questioned. While they have shown to reduce symptoms, they have not been shown to prolong life.[12] Digitalis preparations are particularly useful in the treatment of HF accompanied by atrial flutter and/or fibrillation with a rapid ventricular rate. They increase the force of cardiac contraction (inotropic action). They also decrease the conduction speed within the myocardium and slow the HR (chronotropic action). These actions allow for more complete emptying of the ventricles, thus diminishing the volume remaining in the ventricles during diastole. CO increases because of an increased stroke volume from improved contractility.

An individual receiving a digitalis preparation is prone to develop digitalis toxicity (Table 35-10). Early symptoms of toxicity include anorexia, nausea, and vomiting. Visual disturbances, such as "yellow" vision, can occur with digitalis toxicity. Dysrhythmias are a common but often late indication of digitalis toxicity. Although almost any dysrhythmia can occur, the types most frequently found are premature ventricular beats, atrial fibrillation, and first-degree heart block.[12]

Hypokalemia, secondary to the use of potassium-depleting diuretics (e.g., thiazides, loop diuretics), is one of the most common causes of digitalis toxicity. Low serum potassium enhances the ac-

TABLE 35-10 DRUG THERAPY
Manifestations of Digitalis Toxicity

Gastrointestinal System
Anorexia, nausea, vomiting

Visual System
Blurred vision, colored vision (yellow tinge to vision), visual halos around dark objects

Central Nervous System
Fatigue, drowsiness

Cardiovascular System
Dysrhythmias (e.g., atrial fibrillation, premature ventricular contractions, ventricular fibrillation, heart block); bradycardia; tachycardia; apical-radial pulse deficit; heart failure

tion of digitalis, causing a therapeutic dose to achieve toxic levels. Similarly, hyperkalemia inhibits the action of digitalis, causing a therapeutic dose to become subtherapeutic. Both hypo- and hyperkalemia also precipitate the development of dysrhythmias. Monitoring the serum potassium levels of patients receiving digitalis preparations and potassium-depleting and potassium-sparing diuretics is essential. Other electrolyte imbalances, such as hypercalcemia and hypomagnesemia, can also precipitate digitalis toxicity. (Manifestations of electrolyte imbalances are discussed in Chapter 17.)

Diseases of the kidney and liver increase the susceptibility to digitalis toxicity because most preparations are metabolized and eliminated by these organs. An older adult is especially prone to digitalis toxicity because digitalis accumulation occurs sooner with decreased liver and kidney function and slowed body metabolism, which occur with aging.

The usual treatment of toxicity consists of withholding the drug until the symptoms subside. In the case of life-threatening toxicity, digoxin immune Fab (ovine) (Digibind) is an antidote that can be given IV. The treatment of life-threatening dysrhythmias is instituted as needed (see Chapter 36).

β-Adrenergic Agonists. β-Adrenergic agonists are typically used in the short-term treatment of ADHF refractory to conventional pharmacotherapy. Their role in long-term therapy of HF is controversial. Potential problems related to long-term treatment with β-adrenergic agonists include tolerance, increased ventricular irritability, and increased need for oxygen by the myocardium.[12]

Calcium Sensitizers. Calcium sensitizers are novel positive inotropic agents in the treatment of HF. They improve cardiac performance by interacting directly with contractile proteins without affecting intracellular calcium concentrations or increasing myocardial oxygen demand. They are used in patients who need inotropic support who are also at risk for myocardial ischemia. They produce cardioprotective effects while simultaneously enhancing ventricular contractile function. Levosimendan (Simdax) is a calcium sensitizer recently available in Europe and currently undergoing clinical trials in the United States.[9]

Angiotensin II Receptor Blockers. In patients who are unable to tolerate ACE inhibitors because of angioedema or intractable cough, angiotensin II receptor blockers such as losartan (Cozaar) and valsartan (Diovan) may be used.[16,17] These agents prevent the vasoconstrictor and aldosterone-secreting effects of angiotensin II by binding to the angiotensin II receptor sites. Efficacy of these drugs is similar to ACE inhibitors except that the incidence of adverse effects (e.g., intractable cough) is lower (see Table 33-8).

BiDil. A combination drug containing isosorbide dinitrate and hydralazine (BiDil) is used for the treatment of HF in African Americans who are already being treated with standard therapy. The drug is only approved for use with this ethnic group. As an antihypertensive agent, hydralazine relaxes the arteries and decreases the work of the heart. The antianginal agent, isosorbide dinitrate, relaxes the veins as well as the arteries. Isosorbide seems to work by releasing nitric oxide at the blood vessel wall, but its effect usually wears off after half a day. Hydralazine may prevent this loss of effect. How these two drugs work together is not fully known, but studies have shown a decrease in HF symptoms, hospitalizations, and mortality in African Americans. Common side effects of BiDil are headache and dizziness.

Nutritional Therapy: Chronic Heart Failure

Diet education and weight management are critical to the patient's control of chronic HF. The nurse or dietitian should obtain a detailed diet history, determining not only what foods the patient eats and when, but also the sociocultural value of food to the patient. The nurse can use this information to assist the patient in making appropriate dietary choices when developing a diet plan. The National Heart, Lung, Blood Institute (NHLBI) provides useful dietary guidelines for heart healthy food preparation for people of various cultures (e.g., Hispanics, Native Americans, Asian Americans, African Americans). These are available online at *www.nhlbi.nih.gov/health/index.htm#recipes.* Diet and weight management recommendations must be individualized and culturally sensitive if the necessary changes are to be realized.

The edema of chronic HF is often treated by dietary restriction of sodium. The patient should be taught what foods are low and high in sodium and ways to enhance food flavors without the use of salt (e.g., substituting lemon juice and various spices). The degree of sodium restriction depends on the severity of the HF and the effectiveness of diuretic therapy. Diets that are severely restricted in sodium are rarely prescribed because they are unpalatable and patient compliance is poor. The Dietary Approaches to Stop Hypertension (DASH) diet is effective as a first-line therapy for many individuals with isolated systolic hypertension (see Chapter 33, Table 33-7). This diet is now also widely used for the patient with HF, with or without hypertension.

The average American adult's daily dietary intake of sodium ranges from 7 to 15 g. A commonly prescribed diet for a patient with mild HF is a 2.5-g sodium diet (Table 35-11). All foods high in sodium should be eliminated (Tables 35-12 and 35-13). For more severe HF, sodium intake is restricted to 500 to 1000 mg (see Table 35-11). On this diet, milk, cheese, bread, cereals, canned soups, and some canned vegetables must be severely restricted. The patient and family must be instructed on how to read labels to look for sodium context.

Fluid restrictions are not commonly prescribed for the patient with mild to moderate HF. Diuretic therapy, ACE inhibitors, and digitalis preparations act as effective diuretics to promote fluid excretion. However, in moderate to severe HF and renal insufficiency, fluid restrictions are usually implemented.

Instructing patients to weigh themselves daily is important for monitoring fluid retention, as well as weight reduction. Patients should be instructed to weigh themselves at the same time each day, using the same scale and preferably before breakfast, while

TABLE 35-11 NUTRITIONAL THERAPY
Low-Sodium Diets

General Principles

Do not add salt or seasonings containing sodium when preparing foods.*
Do not use salt at the table.*
Avoid high-sodium foods (e.g., canned soups, processed meats, cheese, frozen meals).
Limit milk products to 2 cups daily.

Sample Menu Plans for 2400-mg Sodium Diet

Breakfast	Sodium (mg)
⅔ cup bran cereal	161
(⅔ cup Shredded Wheat cereal)†	3
1 slice whole-wheat bread	149
1 medium banana	1
6 oz fruit yogurt, fat free	85
1 cup fat-free milk	126
2 tbs jelly	5
Coffee, 8 oz	5
Lunch	
Chicken breast sandwich	
2 slices (3 oz) chicken breast, skinless	65
2 slices whole wheat bread	299
1 slice (¾ oz) American cheese	328
(1 slice [¾ oz] Swiss cheese, natural)†	54
Large-leaf romaine lettuce	1
2 slices tomato	90
1 tbs mayonnaise, low fat	90
1 medium peach	7
Dinner	
¾ cup vegetarian spaghetti sauce	459
(6 oz no-salt-added tomato paste)†	260
1 cup spaghetti	1
3 tbs Parmesan cheese	349
Spinach salad	
1 cup fresh spinach leaves	24
¼ cup fresh carrots (grated)	10
¼ cup fresh mushrooms (sliced)	1
2 tbs vinaigrette dressing	0
½ cup canned pears, juice pack	4
½ cup corn, cooked from frozen	4
Snack	
⅓ cup almonds	4
¼ cup dried apricots	3
6 oz fruit yogurt, fat free	85

Modifications for Other Low-Sodium Diets

500-mg Sodium Diet

Restrict milk products to 1 cup daily.
Limit meat to 4 oz daily.
Use salt-free butter, bread, vegetables, and starches.

1000-mg Sodium Diet

Restrict milk products to 1 cup daily.
Use salt-free butter and vegetables.

*1 tsp of salt equals 2.3 g of sodium.
†Substitutes to reduce to 1500-mg sodium diet.

wearing the same type of clothing. This helps ensure valid comparisons from day to day and helps identify early signs of fluid retention. If a patient experiences a weight gain of 3 lb (1.4 kg) over 2 days or a 3- to 5-lb (2.3-kg) gain over a week, the primary care provider should be called.[18]

TABLE 35-12 Sodium Label Language

Phrase	What It Means
Sodium free or salt free	<5 mg per serving
Very low sodium	35 mg or less sodium per serving
Low sodium	140 mg or less of sodium per serving
Low-sodium meal	140 mg or less of sodium per 3.5 oz
Reduced or less sodium	At least 25% less sodium than regular
Light in sodium	50% less sodium than regular
Unsalted or no salt added	No salt added to the product during process

Use caution with products advertised as no-salt replacements—they may contain high potassium.

TABLE 35-13 NUTRITIONAL THERAPY
Sodium Content in Different Food Groups

Usually only a small amount of sodium occurs naturally in foods. Most sodium is added during processing. The following list gives examples of varying amounts of sodium that occur in foods before and after processing.

Food Groups	Sodium (mg)
Grains and Grain Products	
Cooked cereal, rice, pasta, unsalted, ½ cup	0-5
Ready-to-eat cereal, 1 cup	100-360
Bread, 1 slice	110-175
Vegetables	
Fresh or frozen, cooked without salt, ½ cup	1-70
Canned or frozen with sauce, ½ cup	140-460
Tomato juice, canned, ¾ cup	820
Fruit	
Fresh, frozen, canned, ½ cup	0-5
Low-Fat or Fat-Free Dairy Foods	
Milk, 1 cup	120
Yogurt, 8 oz	160
Natural cheeses, 1½ oz	110-450
Processed cheeses, 1½ oz	600
Nuts, Seeds, and Dry Beans	
Peanuts, salted, ⅓ cup	120
Peanuts, unsalted, ⅓ cup	0-5
Beans, cooked from dried or frozen, without salt, ½ cup	400
Meats, Fish, and Poultry	
Fresh meat, fish, poultry, 3 oz	30-90
Tuna, canned, water pack, no salt added, 3 oz	34-45
Tuna, canned, water pack, 3 oz	250-350
Ham (lean) roasted, 3 oz	1020

NURSING MANAGEMENT
CHRONIC HEART FAILURE

Nursing Assessment

Subjective and objective data that should be obtained from a patient with HF include those presented in Table 35-14.

Nursing Diagnoses

Nursing diagnoses for the patient with HF include, but are not limited to, those presented in NCP 35-1.

TABLE 35-14 NURSING ASSESSMENT Heart Failure

Subjective Data

Important Health Information

Past health history: CAD (including recent MI), hypertension, cardiomyopathy, valvular or congenital heart disease, diabetes mellitus, thyroid or lung disease, rapid or irregular heart rate

Medications: Use of and compliance with any cardiac medications; use of diuretics, estrogens, corticosteroids, nonsteroidal antiinflammatory drugs, over-the-counter drugs, herbal supplements

Functional Health Patterns

Health perception–health management: Fatigue, depression, anxiety

Nutritional-metabolic: Usual sodium intake; nausea, vomiting, anorexia, stomach bloating; weight gain, ankle swelling

Elimination: Nocturia, decreased daytime urinary output, constipation

Activity-exercise: Dyspnea, orthopnea, cough; palpitations; dizziness, fainting

Sleep-rest: Number of pillows used for sleeping; paroxysmal nocturnal dyspnea, insomnia

Cognitive-perceptual: Chest pain or heaviness; RUQ pain, abdominal discomfort; behavioral changes; visual changes

Objective Data

Integumentary

Cool, diaphoretic skin; cyanosis or pallor, peripheral edema (right-sided heart failure)

Respiratory

Tachypnea, crackles, rhonchi, wheezes; frothy, blood-tinged sputum

Cardiovascular

Tachycardia, S_3, S_4, murmurs; pulsus alternans, PMI displaced inferiorly and posteriorly, jugular vein distention

Gastrointestinal

Abdominal distention, hepatosplenomegaly, ascites

Neurologic

Restlessness, confusion, decreased attention or memory

Possible Findings

Altered serum electrolytes (especially Na^+ and K^+), ↑ BUN, creatinine, or liver function tests; chest x-ray demonstrating cardiomegaly, pulmonary congestion, and interstitial pulmonary edema; echocardiogram showing increased chamber size, decreased wall motion, decreased EF; atrial and ventricular enlargement on ECG; ↓ O_2 saturation

BUN, Blood urea nitrogen; *CAD,* coronary artery disease; *ECG,* electrocardiogram; *EF,* ejection fraction; *MI,* myocardial infarction; *PMI,* point of maximal impulse; *RUQ,* right upper quadrant.

Planning

The overall goals for the patient with HF include (1) a decrease in symptoms (e.g., shortness of breath, fatigue), (2) a decrease in peripheral edema, (3) an increase in exercise tolerance, (4) compliance with the medical regimen, and (5) no complications related to HF.

Nursing Implementation

Health Promotion. An important measure used to prevent HF is the treatment or control of the underlying heart disease. For example, in valvular disease, valve replacement should be planned before lung congestion develops. Coronary revascularization procedures should be performed in patients with CAD. Another important preventive measure concerns early and continued treatment of hypertension. Hyperlipidemic states in persons with CAD should be managed with diet, exercise, and medication. The use of antidysrhythmic agents or pacemakers is indicated for people with serious dysrhythmias or conduction disturbances. In addition, patients with HF should be counseled to obtain vaccinations against the flu and pneumonia.

When a patient is diagnosed with HF, preventive care should focus on slowing the progression of the disease. Knowledge of the importance of following the medication, diet, and exercise regimens is essential. Research has shown that exercise training (e.g., cardiac rehabilitation) does improve symptoms of chronic HF but is often underprescribed.[19] The acute care nurse may request home nursing care for the patient and family to provide for follow-up care and to monitor the patient's response to treatment. Early detection of signs and symptoms of worsening failure may help modify care and prevent an acute episode requiring future hospitalization.

Acute Intervention. Successful HF management depends on several important principles: (1) HF is a progressive disease, and treatment plans are established with quality-of-life goals; (2) symptom management is controlled by the patient with self-management tools (e.g., daily weights, drug regimens, diet and exercise plans); (3) salt and water must be restricted; (4) energy must be conserved; and (5) support systems are essential to the success of the entire treatment plan.[20,21]

Many persons with HF will experience one or more episodes of ADHF. When they do, they are usually admitted through the emergency department, initially stabilized, and then managed in an ICU. Once their condition has improved, they will be transferred to a step-down or general unit. The nursing care plan for the patient with HF applies to the patient with stabilized ADHF or chronic HF (see NCP 35-1).

Ambulatory and Home Care. HF is a chronic illness for most persons. Important nursing responsibilities are (1) teaching the patient about the physiologic changes that have occurred, (2) assisting the patient to adapt to both the physiologic and psychologic changes, and (3) integrating the patient and the patient's family or support system in the overall care plan. Research has revealed that patients with NYHA Functional Class III or IV HF have a high risk for anxiety and depression.[22] In one large study, major depression was found to be more prevalent in female patients and patients less than 60 years of age.[23] It must be emphasized to the patient that it is possible to live productively with this chronic health problem. Effective home health care can prevent or limit future hospitalization. Home nursing care will follow up with ongoing clinical assessments, monitoring vital signs, and evaluating response to therapies. Managing these patients out of the hospital is a priority of care. A patient and family teaching guide for the patient with HF is presented in Table 35-15.

Patients with HF are usually required to take medication for the rest of their lives. This often becomes difficult because a patient may be asymptomatic when HF is under control. It must be stressed that the disease is chronic and that medication must be continued to keep the HF under control.

The patient should evaluate the action of the prescribed drugs and be taught to recognize the manifestations of drug toxicity. The patient should also be taught how to take her or his pulse rate and to know under what circumstances drugs, especially digitalis and β-adrenergic blockers, should be withheld and a health care provider consulted. The pulse rate should always be taken for 1 full minute. A pulse rate lower than 50 beats/minute may be a contraindication to taking a digitalis preparation or β-adrenergic blocker unless specified otherwise by the health care provider. However, in the absence of symptoms (e.g., heart block, ventricular ectopy, syncope), a pulse rate of less than 50 beats/minute may be acceptable. It may also be appropriate to instruct patients in home BP

NURSING CARE PLAN 35-1

Patient with Heart Failure

NURSING DIAGNOSIS **Activity intolerance** *related to* fatigue secondary to cardiac insufficiency and pulmonary congestion *as evidenced by* dyspnea, shortness of breath, weakness, increase in heart rate on exertion, and patient's statement, "I feel too weak to do anything."

PATIENT GOAL Will achieve a realistic program of activity that balances physical activity with energy-conserving activities

OUTCOMES (NOC)

Activity Tolerance

- Pulse rate with activity ____
- Oxygen saturation with activity ____
- Respiratory rate with activity ____
- Systolic BP with activity ____
- Diastolic BP with activity ____
- Electrocardiogram findings ____
- Skin color ____
- Ease of performing ADLs ____

Measurement Scale

1 = Severely compromised
2 = Substantially compromised
3 = Moderately compromised
4 = Mildly compromised
5 = Not compromised

INTERVENTIONS (NIC) and *RATIONALES*

Energy Management

- Encourage alternate rest and activity periods *to reduce cardiac workload.*
- Provide calming diversionary activities to promote relaxation *to reduce O_2 consumption and to relieve dyspnea and fatigue.*
- Monitor patient's oxygen response (e.g., pulse rate, cardiac rhythm, and respiratory rate) to self-care or nursing activities *to determine level of activity that can be performed.*
- Teach patient and significant other techniques of self-care that *will minimize oxygen consumption* (e.g., self-monitoring and pacing techniques for performance of activities of daily living).

Activity Therapy

- Assist to choose activities consistent with physical, psychologic, and social capabilities *to determine level of activity that can be performed.*
- Collaborate with occupational, physical, and/or recreational therapists *to plan and monitor activity/exercise program.*
- Determine patient's commitment to ↑ frequency and/or range of activities/exercise *to provide patient with obtainable goals.*

NURSING DIAGNOSIS **Excess fluid volume** *related to* cardiac failure *as evidenced by* edema, dyspnea on exertion, increased weight gain, and patient's statement, "I'm short of breath and my ankles are so big and puffy!"

PATIENT GOAL Experiences reduced edema or absence of edema

OUTCOMES (NOC)

Fluid Balance

- Peripheral pulses ____
- Serum electrolytes ____
- BP ____
- Skin turgor ____
- Stable body weight ____
- Urine specific gravity ____

Measurement Scale

1 = Severely compromised
2 = Substantially compromised
3 = Moderately compromised
4 = Mildly compromised
5 = Not compromised

INTERVENTIONS (NIC) and *RATIONALES*

Fluid/Electrolyte Management

- Weigh patient daily and monitor trends *to evaluate fluid retention/diuresis and weight reduction.*
- Monitor for abnormal serum electrolyte levels *to assess response to treatment.*

Hypervolemia Management

- Monitor respiratory pattern for symptoms of respiratory difficulty *for early recognition of pulmonary congestion.*
- Monitor hemodynamic status, including CVP, MAP, PAWP, if available, *to evaluate effectiveness of therapy.*
- Monitor renal function and intake and output *to monitor fluid balance.*
- Monitor for therapeutic effect of diuretic (↑ urine output, ↓ CVP, ↓ adventitious breath sounds) *to assess response to treatment.*

ADLs, Activities of daily living; *BP,* blood pressure; *CVP,* central venous pressure; *HF,* heart failure; *MAP,* mean arterial pressure; *PAWP,* pulmonary artery wedge pressure.

monitoring, especially for those HF patients with hypertension. The patient should also be taught the symptoms of hypo- and hyperkalemia if diuretics that deplete or spare potassium are being taken. Frequently the patient who is taking thiazide or loop diuretics is given supplemental potassium.

The nurse, physical therapist, or occupational therapist can instruct the patient in energy-conserving and energy-efficient behaviors after an evaluation of daily activities has been done. For example, once the nurse understands the patient's daily routine, suggestions can be made for simplification of work or modification of an activity. Frequently the patient needs a prescription for rest after an activity. Many hard-driving persons need the "permission" to not feel "lazy." Sometimes an activity that the patient enjoys may need to be eliminated. In such situations the patient should be helped to explore alternative activities that cause less physical and cardiac stress. The physical environment may require modification in situations in which there is an increased cardiac workload demand (e.g., frequent climbing of stairs). The nurse can help the patient identify areas where outside assistance can be obtained.

The home health nurse is essential in the care of the HF patient and family. Frequent physical assessments, including vital signs and weight, are extremely important. Home health nurses frequently work within protocols set up with the patient's health care team. The protocols may enable the nurse and patient to identify problems, such as an increase in weight and HR as evidence of worsening HF, and institute interventions to prevent hospitaliza-

NURSING CARE PLAN 35-1
Patient with Heart Failure—cont'd

NURSING DIAGNOSIS **Impaired gas exchange** *related to* increased preload, mechanical failure, or immobility *as evidenced by* increased respiratory rate, shortness of breath, dyspnea on exertion, and patient's statement, "I just can't seem to catch my breath."

PATIENT GOAL Maintains adequate respiratory rate and rhythm for activities of daily living

OUTCOMES (NOC)

Respiratory Status: Gas Exchange

- Ease of breathing ____
- Oxygen saturation ____
- PaO_2 ____

Measurement Scale

1 = Severely compromised
2 = Substantially compromised
3 = Moderately compromised
4 = Mildly compromised
5 = Not compromised

- Dyspnea with exertion ____
- Dyspnea at rest ____

Measurement Scale

1 = Severe
2 = Substantial
3 = Moderate
4 = Mild
5 = None

INTERVENTIONS (NIC) and *RATIONALES*

Respiratory Monitoring

- Monitor rate, rhythm, depth, and effort of respirations *to evaluate changes in respiratory status.*
- Auscultate breath sounds, noting areas of decreased/absent ventilation and presence of adventitious sounds, *to assess congestion.*
- Monitor for dyspnea and events that improve and worsen it *to detect events that can influence ADLs.*

Oxygen Therapy

- Administer supplemental O_2 as ordered *to maintain O_2 levels.*
- Change O_2 delivery device from mask to nasal prongs during meals as tolerated *to sustain O_2 levels while doing ADLs.*
- Monitor the effectiveness of O_2 therapy *to identify hypoxemia and establish range of O_2 saturation.*

Positioning

- Position to alleviate dyspnea (e.g., semi-Fowler position), as appropriate, *to improve ventilation by decreasing venous return to the heart and increasing thoracic capacity.*

NURSING DIAGNOSIS **Anxiety** *related to* dyspnea or perceived threat of death *as evidenced by* restlessness, irritability, expression of feelings of life threat, and patient's statement, "Don't leave me alone, I'm afraid I might die."

PATIENT GOAL Verbalizes less anxiety about condition and prognosis

OUTCOMES (NOC)

Anxiety Self-Control

- Uses effective coping strategies ____
- Seeks information to reduce anxiety ____
- Controls anxiety response ____

Measurement Scale

1 = Never demonstrated
2 = Rarely demonstrated
3 = Sometimes demonstrated
4 = Often demonstrated
5 = Consistently demonstrated

INTERVENTIONS (NIC) and *RATIONALES*

Anxiety Reduction

- Use a calm, reassuring approach *to increase confidence in caregiver and relieve anxiety.*
- Explain all procedures, including sensations likely to be experienced during a procedure, *to promote sense of security.*
- Help patient identify situations that precipitate anxiety *to plan appropriate use of anxiety-reducing techniques.*
- Create an atmosphere to facilitate trust (e.g., answer call bell promptly and make frequent checks) *to promote sense of security.*
- Instruct patient in use of relaxation techniques (e.g., imagery) *to help alleviate anxiety.*

ADLs, Activities of daily living; *PaO_2,* partial pressure of oxygen in arterial blood.

Continued

tion. This may include altering medications and initiating fluid restrictions. Home health nursing care of HF patients is paramount in reducing the number of hospitalizations, increasing functional capacity, and increasing quality of life.

Evaluation

The expected outcomes for the patient with HF are presented in NCP 35-1.

CARDIAC TRANSPLANTATION

The first heart transplant was performed in 1967. Since that time, **cardiac transplantation** (transfer of a heart from one person to another) has become the treatment of choice for patients with refractory end-stage HF, cardiomyopathy, and inoperable CAD. Table 35-16 identifies the indications for transplantation in patients with refractory end-stage HF.[7]

Once an individual meets the criteria for cardiac transplantation, the goal of the evaluation process is to identify patients who would most benefit from a new heart. After a complete physical examination and diagnostic workup, the patient and family then undergo a comprehensive psychologic profile that includes assessing coping skills, family support systems, and motivation to follow the rigorous regimen that is essential to a successful transplantation. The complexity of the transplant process may be overwhelming to a patient with inadequate support systems and a poor understanding of the lifestyle changes required after transplant.

NURSING CARE PLAN 35-1
Patient with Heart Failure—cont'd

NURSING DIAGNOSIS **Deficient knowledge** *related to* disease process *as evidenced by* questions about the disease and patient's statement, "I don't know why I keep getting sick."

PATIENT GOAL Describes disease process and rationales for dietary and medication regimen

OUTCOMES (NOC)

Knowledge: Disease Process

- Description of specific disease process ____
- Description of complications ____
- Descriptions of precautions to prevent complications ____

Measurement Scale

1 = None
2 = Limited
3 = Moderate
4 = Substantial
5 = Extensive

INTERVENTIONS (NIC) and *RATIONALES*

Teaching: Disease Process

- Appraise the patient's current level of knowledge related to specific disease process *to identify needed areas of teaching.*
- Describe common signs and symptoms of the disease *so patient will know signs and symptoms to report to health care provider.*
- Instruct the patient on measures to prevent/minimize side effects of treatment for the disease *so patient may be able to decrease number of acute episodes of HF.*

Teaching: Prescribed Diet

- Appraise the patient's current level of knowledge about prescribed diet *to assess areas needing additional instruction.*

Teaching: Prescribed Medication

- Review patient's knowledge of medications *to determine where further teaching is needed.*
- Include the family/significant others *to provide support for the patient.*

TABLE 35-15 *PATIENT AND FAMILY TEACHING GUIDE* Heart Failure

Health Promotion
1. Obtain annual flu vaccination.
2. Obtain pneumococcal vaccine (e.g., Pneumovax) and revaccination after 5 yr (for people at high risk of infection or serious disease).
3. Consider smoking cessation and weight reduction, if appropriate.

Rest
1. Plan a regular daily rest and activity program.
2. After exertion, such as exercise and ADLs, plan a rest period.
3. Shorten working hours or schedule rest period during working hours.
4. Avoid emotional upsets. Verbalize any concerns, fears, feelings of depression, etc. to health care provider.

Drug Therapy
1. Take each drug as prescribed daily.
2. Develop a check-off system (e.g., daily chart) to ensure medications have been taken.
3. Take pulse rate each day before taking medications (if appropriate). Know the parameters that your health care provider wants for your heart rate.
4. Learn to take own BP at determined intervals (if appropriate). Know your target BP limits.
5. Know signs and symptoms of orthostatic hypotension and how to prevent them (see Table 33-14).
6. Know signs and symptoms of internal bleeding (bleeding gums, increased bruises, blood in stool or urine) and what to do if on anticoagulants.
7. Know own INR if taking warfarin (Coumadin) and how often to have blood monitored.

Dietary Therapy
1. Consult the written diet plan and list of permitted and restricted foods.
2. Examine labels to determine sodium content. Also examine the labels of over-the-counter drugs such as laxatives, cough medicines, and antacids.
3. Avoid using salt when preparing foods, or adding salt to foods.
4. Weigh yourself in the early morning after arising and emptying your bladder. Use the same scale and wear the same or similar clothes every day.
5. Report weight gain of 3 lb (1.4 kg) in 2 days, or 3-5 lb (2.3 kg) in a week.
6. Eat smaller, more frequent meals.

Activity Program
1. Increase walking and other activities gradually, provided they do not cause fatigue and dyspnea. Consider a cardiac rehabilitation program.
2. Avoid extremes of heat and cold.
3. Keep regular appointments with health care provider.

Ongoing Monitoring
1. Know the signs and symptoms of recurring or progressing heart failure.
2. Recall the symptoms experienced when illness began; reappearance of previous symptoms may indicate a recurrence.
3. Report immediately to health care provider any of the following:
   - Difficulty breathing, especially with exertion or when lying flat
   - Waking up breathless at night
   - Frequent dry, hacking cough, especially when lying down
   - Fatigue, weakness
   - Swelling of ankles, feet, or abdomen; swelling of face or difficulty breathing (if taking ACE inhibitors)
   - Nausea with abdominal swelling, pain, and tenderness
   - Dizziness or fainting
   - Weight gain of 3 lb (1.4 kg) in 2 days, or 3-5 lb (2.3 kg) in a week
4. Follow up with health care provider on regular basis.
5. Consider joining a local support group with your family members and/or support person(s).

ACE, Angiotensin-converting enzyme; *ADLs,* activities of daily living; *BP,* blood pressure; *INR,* international normalized ratio.

TABLE 35-16 Indications for Cardiac Transplantation for Patients with End-Stage Heart Failure

Absolute Indications
For hemodynamic compromise due to HF: • Refractory cardiogenic shock • Dependence on IV inotropes to maintain organ perfusion • Peak exercise oxygen consumption <50% of predicted normal
Cardiac ischemia that severely and consistently limits ADLs and is not amenable to revascularization procedures (e.g., coronary bypass surgery, percutaneous coronary intervention)
Refractory, symptomatic, life-threatening ventricular dysrhythmias (e.g., ventricular tachycardia)
Relative Indications
Peak exercise oxygen consumption <55% of predicted normal and major limitations of ADLs
Persistent unstable ischemia that is not amenable to pharmacologic or revascularization interventions
Persistent fluid overload/renal dysfunction in spite of adherence to medical regimen
Insufficient Indications
Low EF
History of NYHA Functional Class III or IV
Peak exercise oxygen consumption >55% of predicted normal

ADLs, Activities of daily living; *EF,* ejection fraction; *HF,* heart failure; *IV,* intravenous; *NYHA,* New York Heart Association.

Once an individual is accepted as a transplant candidate (this may happen rapidly during an acute illness or over a longer period), he or she is placed on a transplant list. Patients may wait at home and receive ongoing medical care if their medical condition is stable. If their condition is not stable, they may require hospitalization for more intensive therapy. Unfortunately, the overall waiting period for a transplant is long, and many patients die while waiting for a transplant (see Ethical Dilemmas box on p. 830).

Donor and recipient matching is based on body and heart size and ABO type. Negative lymphocyte crossmatch (explained in Chapter 14) and avoidance of a transplantation from a cytomegalovirus (CMV)–positive donor to a CMV-negative recipient are important.

Most donor hearts are obtained at sites distant from the institution performing the transplant. The maximum acceptable time from harvesting the donor heart to transplantation is 4 to 6 hours.

The recipient is prepared for surgery, and cardiopulmonary bypass is used. The usual surgical procedure involves removing the recipient's heart, except for the posterior right and left atrial walls and their venous connections. The recipient's heart is then replaced with the donor heart, which has been trimmed to match. Care is taken to preserve the integrity of the donor sinoatrial (SA) node so that a sinus rhythm may be achieved postoperatively.

Immunosuppressive therapy usually begins in the operating room. Regimens vary, but they usually include azathioprine (Imuran), corticosteroids, and cyclosporine. Tacrolimus (Prograf) is also used as an immunosuppressant. (The mechanisms of action and side effects of these and other immunosuppressants are discussed in Chapter 14 and Table 14-18.) Currently cyclosporine is used with corticosteroids for maintenance immunosuppression. Its use has resulted not only in reduced rejection, but also in slowing the rejection process so that early treatment can be instituted. Because of the use of immunosuppressants, infection is the primary complication following transplantation.

Endomyocardial biopsies are typically obtained from the right ventricle (via the right internal jugular vein) on a weekly basis for the first month, monthly for the following 6 months, and yearly thereafter to detect rejection. The Heartsbreath test is used along with endomyocardial biopsy to assess organ rejection in heart transplant patients. The test works by measuring the amount of methylated alkanes (natural chemicals found in the breath and air) in a patient's breath. The patient breathes into a plastic mouthpiece that is attached to a breath-collecting device. The device subtracts the amount of methylated alkanes in a patient's breath from the amount of methylated alkanes in the room air. The value generated by the device is compared with the results of a biopsy performed during the previous month to measure the probability of the transplanted heart being rejected. The Heartsbreath test is used in the first year following heart transplantation and along with the results of a heart biopsy to help guide short-term and long-term medical care of heart transplant patients. The test's greatest value may be in helping to separate less severe organ rejection (grades 0, 1, and 2) from more severe rejection (grade 3). In addition, peripheral blood T lymphocyte monitoring is done to assess the recipient's immune status.

Advances in surgical technique and postoperative care have improved early survival rates after cardiac transplantation. In the first year after transplantation, the major causes of death are acute rejection and infection. Later on, malignancy (especially lymphoma) and coronary artery vasculopathy are major causes of death. Nursing management throughout the posttransplant period focuses on promoting patient adaptation to the transplant process, monitoring cardiac function, managing lifestyle changes, and providing ongoing teaching of the patient and family.

Several devices are available as a bridge to transplantation, but only two have received Food and Drug Administration (FDA) approval for heart recovery after a life-threatening cardiac event. The AB5000™ Circulatory Support System and the BVS® 5000 Biventricular Support System provide temporary support for one or both sides of the heart in circumstances in which the heart has failed but has the potential to recover (e.g., reversible HF, myocarditis, and acute MI).[24] The Thoratec Ventricular Assist Device (VAD) system can also support one or both ventricles, and it has been approved as a bridging device for transplantation and for recovery of the heart after cardiac surgery.

Artificial Heart

The lack of available transplant hearts and the increasing number of patients in need have triggered the movement to develop artificial hearts. Two implantable artificial hearts, the CardioWest Total Artificial Heart and the AbioCor Implantable Replacement Heart, have been developed. They are both designed with materials that minimize coagulation and contain motor-driven pumping systems (artificial ventricles) that operate on both internal and external batteries (Fig. 35-3). An electronic package in the abdomen monitors the system, including adjusting the heart rate based on the patient's activity. An external battery pack allows for periods of independence from the console. The total artificial heart requires no immunosuppression and may hold promise for short-term survival in patients with end-stage HF.[9]

Ongoing Research

The use of adult and embryonic stem cells to replace myocardial cells damaged from heart disease and to establish new blood vessels to supply the regenerated heart muscle is gaining attention.

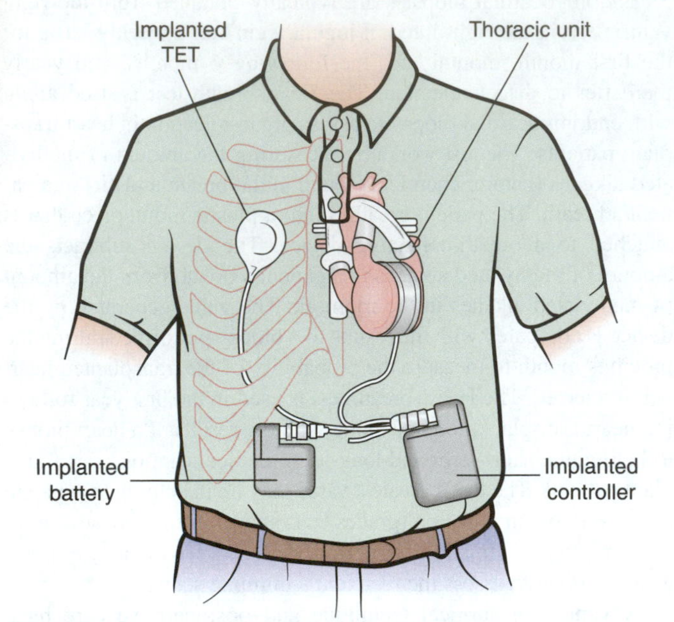

FIG. 35-3 The AbioCor Heart Replacement System has two main components: the implantable parts consisting of the thoracic unit (replacement heart), battery, controller, and transcutaneous energy transmission (TET) unit; and the external parts (not shown) consisting of the console and the Patient-Carried Electronics (PCE) such as the battery, control module, and external TET.

Research is focused on directing stem cells to become cardiomyocytes (the contractile cells of the heart), vascular endothelial cells (cells that form the inner lining of the blood vessels), and smooth muscle cells (cells that form the wall of the blood vessels). Scientists hope that providing replacement tissue for the damaged heart will have immense advantages over heart transplantation and the use of artificial hearts.[25]

CRITICAL THINKING EXERCISE

CASE STUDY

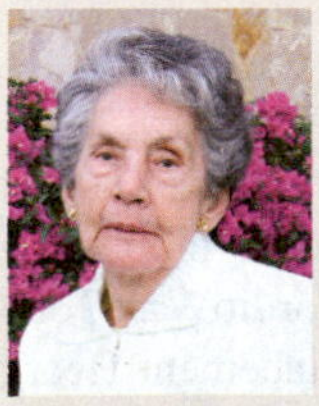

Case Study photo ©iStockphoto.com/Andresr.

Heart Failure

Patient Profile. Mrs. E., a 70-year-old Hispanic woman, was admitted to the medical unit with complaints of increasing shortness of breath.

Subjective Data

- Had a severe MI at 58 years of age
- Has experienced increasing shortness of breath during the last 2 weeks
- Recently had a respiratory tract infection; has persistent cough, and edema in legs 2 weeks ago
- Cannot climb a flight of stairs without getting short of breath
- Sleeps with head elevated on three pillows
- Does not always remember to take medication

Objective Data

Physical Examination

- In respiratory distress, use of accessory muscles, respiratory rate 36 breaths/minute
- Systolic heart murmur
- Moist crackles in both lungs
- Cyanotic lips and extremities
- Skin cool and diaphoretic

Diagnostic Studies

- Chest x-ray results: cardiomegaly with right and left ventricular hypertrophy; fluid in lower lung fields
- Echocardiogram results: EF 20%

Collaborative Care

- digoxin 0.25 mg PO daily
- furosemide (Lasix) 40 mg IV bid
- potassium 40 mEq PO bid
- enalapril (Vasotec) 5 mg PO daily
- 2-g sodium diet
- Oxygen 6 L/min by nasal catheter
- Daily weights
- Daily 12-lead ECG; serum electrolytes; cardiac enzymes q8hr × 3

Critical Thinking Questions

1. Explain the pathophysiology of Mrs. E.'s heart disease and dyspnea.
2. What clinical manifestations of HF did Mrs. E. exhibit?
3. What is the significance of the findings of the diagnostic studies?
4. How would a serum BNP be beneficial in the diagnosis of HF?
5. Explain the rationale for each of the medical orders prescribed for Mrs. E.
6. What are the priority nursing interventions for Mrs. E.?
7. Based on the assessment data presented, write one or more priority nursing diagnoses. Identify any collaborative problems.
8. What teaching measures should be instituted to prevent recurrence of ADHF?

NCLEX EXAMINATION REVIEW QUESTIONS

The number of the question corresponds to the same-numbered objective at the beginning of the chapter.

1. The nurse recognizes that primary manifestations of systolic failure include
   a. ↓ afterload and ↓ left ventricular end-diastolic pressure.
   b. ↓ ejection fraction and ↑ PAWP.
   c. ↓ PAWP and ↑ left ventricular EF.
   d. ↓ pulmonary hypertension associated with normal EF.
2. A compensatory mechanism involved in HF that leads to inappropriate fluid retention and additional workload of the heart is
   a. ventricular dilation.
   b. ventricular hypertrophy.
   c. neurohormonal response.
   d. sympathetic nervous system activation.
3. A drug used in the management of a patient with ADHF and pulmonary edema that will decrease both preload and afterload and provide relief of anxiety is
   a. amrinone.
   b. furosemide.
   c. dobutamine.
   d. morphine sulfate.
4. A patient with chronic HF and atrial fibrillation is treated with a digitalis glycoside and a loop diuretic. To prevent possible complications of this combination of drugs, the nurse needs to
   a. monitor serum potassium levels.
   b. keep an accurate measure of intake and output.

c. teach the patient about dietary restriction of potassium.
d. withhold the digitalis and notify the health care provider if the heart rate is irregular.

5. The primary causes of death in patients with heart transplants in the first year include
a. infection and dysrhythmias.
b. rejection and dysrhythmias.
c. infection and acute rejection.
d. myocardial infarction and cancer.

REFERENCES

1. American Heart Association: *Heart disease and stroke statistics—update,* Dallas, 2004, American Heart Association.
2. Yancy CW, Burnett JC Jr, Fonarow GC, et al: Decompensated heart failure: is there a role for the outpatient use of nesiritide? *Congest Heart Fail* 10:230, 2004.
3. Aurigemma GP, Zile MR, Gaasch WH: Clinical practice: diastolic failure, *N Engl J Med* 351:1097, 2004.
4. Woods SL, Froelicher ES, Motzer SU, et al: *Cardiac nursing,* ed 5, Philadelphia, 2005, Lippincott Williams & Wilkins.
5. Huether SE, McCance KL: *Understanding pathophysiology,* ed 3, St Louis, 2004, Mosby.
6. Silver MA, Maisel A, Yancy CW, et al: BNP Consensus Panel 2004: a clinical approach for the diagnostic, prognostic, screening, treatment monitoring, and therapeutic roles of natriuretic peptides in cardiovascular diseases, *Congest Heart Fail* 10(suppl 3):1, 2004.
7. Hunt SA, Baker DW, Chin MH, et al: ACC/AHA guidelines for the evaluation and management of chronic heart failure in the adult: executive summary. A report of the American College of Cardiology/American Heart Association Task Force on Practice Guidelines (Committee to revise the 1995 Guidelines for the Evaluation and Management of Heart Failure), *J Am Coll Cardiol* 38:2101, 2001.
8. Joint Commission on Accreditation of Healthcare Organizations: Specification manual for national hospital quality measures version 2.0b: implementation to begin with July 1, 2006 discharges. Available at *www.jointcommission.org/PerformanceMeasurementPerformance Measurement/Current +NHQM+Manual.htm* (accessed July 13, 2006).
9. Fedson SE: Current treatment of acute decompensated heart failure, *New Developments in Cardiovascular Diseases* 1:1, 2004.
10. Sorrentino M: News from the 2004 meeting of the Heart Failure Society of America, *New Devel Cardiovasc Dis* 1:1, 2004.
11. Burger AJ, Horton DP, LeJemtel T, et al: Effect of nesiritide (b-type natriuretic peptide) and dobutamine on ventricular arrhythmias in the treatment of patients with acutely decompensated congestive heart failure: the PRECEDENT study, *Am Heart J* 144:1102, 2002.
12. Lehne RA: *Pharmacology for nursing care,* ed 6, St Louis, 2007, Saunders.
13. Albert NM: Cardiac resynchronization therapy through biventricular pacing in patients with heart failure and ventricular dyssynchrony, *Crit Care Nurse* 23:2, 2003.
14. Sirbu H, Busch T, Aleksic I, et al: Ischemic complications with intra-aortic balloon counterpulsation: incidence and management, *Cardiovasc Surg* 8:66, 2000.
15. National Heart, Lung, and Blood Institute: Next generation ventricular assist devices for destination therapy: executive summary (last updated April 30, 2005). Available at *www.nhlbi.nih.gov/meetings/workshops/next-gen-vads.htm* (accessed June 28, 2005).
16. Richards D: Guidelines for prescribing angiotensin-receptor blockers (ARBs), *Oxford Radcliffe Hospitals* 3:1, 2003. Available at *http://static.oxfordradcliffe.net/med/mil/PDF/MILV3N9.PDF.*
17. Lee VC, Rhew DC, Dylan M, et al: Meta-analysis: angiotensin-receptor blockers in chronic heart failure and high-risk acute myocardial infarction, *Ann Intern Med* 141:693, 2004.
18. Silver MA, Cianci P, Pisano CL: *Outpatient management of heart failure,* Oak Lawn, Ill, 2004, Heart Failure Institute and Heart Failure Center.
*19. ExTraMATCH Collaborative: Exercise training meta-analysis of trials in patients with chronic heart failure, *Br Med J* 328:189, 2004.
*20. Deaton C: Outcome measurement, *J Cardiovasc Nurs* 14(4):116, 2000.
*21. Moser D, Worster PC: Effect of psychosocial factors on physiologic outcomes in patients with heart failure, *J Cardiovasc Nurs* 14(4):106, 2000.
22. Artinian NT: The psychosocial aspects of heart failure, *AJN* 103:32, 2003.
*23. Freeland KE, Rich MW, Skala JA, et al: Prevalence of depression in hospitalized patients with congestive heart failure, *Psychosom Med* 65:119, 2003.
24. DiGiorgi PL, Rao V, Naka Y, et al: Which patient, which pump?, *J Heart Lung Transplant* 22:221, 2003.
25. Wollert K, Drexler H: Clinical applications of stem cells for the heart, *Circ Res* 96:151, 2005.

RESOURCES

American Association of Cardiovascular and Pulmonary Rehabilitation (AACVPR)
312-321-5146
www.aacvpr.org

American Association of Heart Failure Nurses
888-452-2436
www.aahfn.org

American College of Cardiology
Heart House
800-253-4636, ext. 694 or 301-897-5400
www.acc.org

American Heart Association
800-AHA-USA-1 (242-8721)
www.americanheart.org

Council on Cardiovascular Nursing
American Heart Association
214-373-6300
www.americanheart.org

Heart Failure Society of America
www.hfsa.org

International Society for Heart and Lung Transplantation
972-490-9495
www.ishlt.org

National Heart, Lung, and Blood Institute
National Institutes of Health
301-592-8573
www.nhlbi.nih.gov

The Mended Hearts
888-432-7899 or 214-706-1442
www.mendedhearts.org

For additional Internet resources, see the website for this book at *http://evolve.elsevier.com/Lewis/medsurg.*

*Nursing research–based reference.

Always bear in mind that your own resolution to success is more important than any other one thing.

Abraham Lincoln

36 Nursing Management Dysrhythmias

Linda Bucher

LEARNING OBJECTIVES

1. Describe the nursing management of patients requiring continuous electrocardiographic (ECG) monitoring.
2. Identify the clinical characteristics and ECG patterns of normal sinus rhythm, common dysrhythmias, and acute coronary syndrome (ACS).
3. Describe the nursing and collaborative management of patients with common dysrhythmias and ECG changes associated with ACS.
4. Differentiate between defibrillation and cardioversion, identifying indications for their use and physiologic effects of each.
5. Describe the management of patients with temporary and permanent pacemakers.
6. Describe the management of patients with implantable cardioverter-defibrillators.
7. Explain the management of patients undergoing electrophysiologic testing and radiofrequency catheter ablation therapy.

KEY TERMS

asystole, p. 855
atrial fibrillation, p. 852
atrial flutter, p. 851
automaticity, p. 846
cardiac pacemaker, p. 858
complete heart block, p. 854
dysrhythmias, p. 842
electrocardiogram, p. 843
premature atrial contraction, p. 850
premature ventricular contraction, p. 854
ventricular fibrillation, p. 855
ventricular tachycardia, p. 854

Electronic Resources

Supplemental content related to Chapter 36 can be found . . .

Companion CD

- Stress-Busting Kit for Nursing Students
- Interactive Case Study: Atrial Fibrillation
- NCLEX Examination Review Questions
- Comprehensive Glossary

Evolve Website

http://evolve.elsevier.com/Lewis/medsurg

- Content Updates
- Key Points (Printable and CP/MP3 Download)
- Concept Map Creator
- Expanded Audio Glossary
- Key Term Flash Cards
- Algorithms for Treatment of Dysrhythmias
- Electronic Calculators
- WebLinks

RHYTHM IDENTIFICATION AND TREATMENT

The ability to recognize normal and abnormal cardiac rhythms, called **dysrhythmias,** is an essential skill for the nurse. Cardiac monitoring is now used in a wide range of hospital, clinic, and home settings. Prompt assessment of dysrhythmias and the patient's response to the rhythm is critical. This chapter describes basic principles of electrocardiographic (ECG) monitoring and recognition of common dysrhythmias as well as ECG changes that are associated with acute coronary syndrome (ACS). For more detailed information on ECG interpretation, the reader should refer to dedicated texts on this topic.[1-3]

Conduction System

Four properties of cardiac cells enable the conduction system to initiate an electrical impulse, which is transmitted through the cardiac tissue, stimulating muscle contraction (Table 36-1). The conduction system of the heart is made up of specialized neuromuscular tissue located throughout the heart (see Chapter 32, Fig. 32-5). A normal cardiac impulse begins in the sinoatrial (SA) node in the upper right atrium. It is transmitted over the atrial myocardium via Bachmann's bundle and internodal pathways, causing atrial contraction. The impulse then travels to the atrioventricular (AV) node through the bundle of His and down the left and right bundle

Reviewed by Barbara Pope, RN, MSN, CCRN, CCNS, Critical Care Clinical Educator, Albert Einstein Healthcare Network, Jefferson Health System, Philadelphia, Pa.; and Tamekia L. Thomas, RN, BSN, Cardiac Staff Development Specialist, Christiana Care Health System, Christiana Hospital, Newark, Del.

TABLE 36-1 Properties of Cardiac Cells

Automaticity	Ability to initiate an impulse spontaneously and continuously
Excitability	Ability to be electrically stimulated
Conductivity	Ability to transmit an impulse along a membrane in an orderly manner
Contractility	Ability to respond mechanically to an impulse

branches, ending in the Purkinje fibers, which transmit the impulse to the ventricles.

Conduction to the point just before the impulse leaves the Purkinje fibers takes place within the time of the PR interval of the ECG. When the impulse emerges from the Purkinje fibers, ventricular depolarization occurs, producing mechanical contraction of the ventricles and the QRS complex on the ECG. The electrical activity of the heart is illustrated in Chapter 32, Fig. 32-6.

Nervous Control of the Heart

The autonomic nervous system plays an important role in the rate of impulse formation, the speed of conduction, and the strength of cardiac contraction. The components of the autonomic nervous system that affect the heart are the right and left vagus nerve fibers of the parasympathetic nervous system and fibers of the sympathetic nervous system.

Stimulation of the vagus nerve causes a decreased rate of firing of the SA node, slowed impulse conduction of the AV node, and decreased force of cardiac muscle contraction. Stimulation of the sympathetic nerves that supply the heart has essentially the opposite effect on the heart.[4]

Electrocardiographic Monitoring

The **electrocardiogram** is a graphic tracing of the electrical impulses produced in the heart. The wave forms on the ECG are produced by the movement of charged ions across the membranes of myocardial cells, representing depolarization and repolarization.

The membrane of a cardiac cell is semipermeable, allowing it to maintain a high concentration of potassium and a low concentration of sodium inside the cell. A high concentration of sodium and a low concentration of potassium are maintained outside the cell. The inside of the cell, when at rest, or in the polarized state, is negative compared with the outside. When a cell or groups of cells are stimulated, each cell membrane changes its permeability and allows sodium to move rapidly into the cell, making the inside of the cell positive compared with the outside *(depolarization).* A slower movement of ions across the membrane restores the cell to the polarized state, which is called *repolarization.*[1,3] In Fig. 36-1, the phases of the cardiac action potential are as follows: phase 0 is the upstroke of rapid depolarization; phases 1, 2, and 3 represent repolarization; and phase 4 is a polarized state.[1] Antidysrhythmia drugs have a direct effect on the various phases of the action potential.[1] When antidysrhythmia drugs are used in a clinical setting, an understanding of the ionic shifts in the cardiac cell and the action potential mechanism is important.

Conventionally there are 12 recording leads in the ECG. Six of the 12 ECG leads measure electrical forces in the frontal plane (leads I, II, III, aVR, aVL, and aVF) (Fig. 36-2). The remaining six leads (V_1 through V_6) measure the electrical forces in the horizontal plane (precordial leads). The 12-lead ECG may show changes

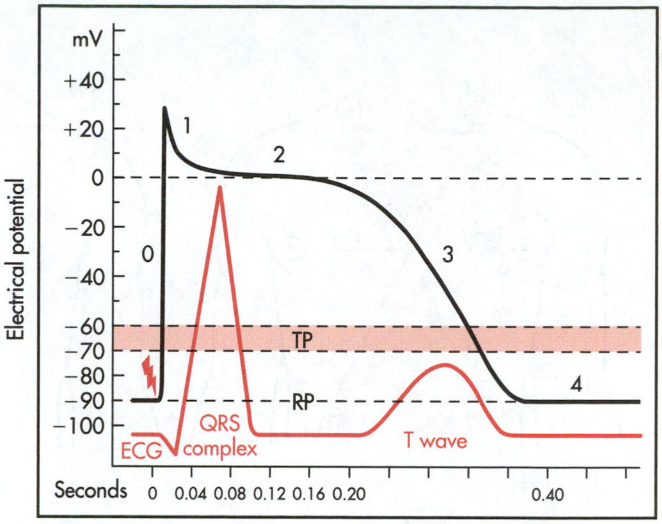

FIG. 36-1 Phases of the cardiac action potential. The electrical potential, measured in millivolts (mV), is indicated along the vertical axis of the graph. Time, measured in seconds (sec), is indicated along the horizontal axis. There are five phases of the action potential, labeled as phase 0 through phase 4. Each phase represents a particular electrical event or combination of electrical events. Phase 0 is the upstroke of rapid depolarization and corresponds with ventricular contraction. Phases 1, 2, and 3 represent repolarization. Phase 4 is known as complete repolarization (or the polarized state) and corresponds to diastole. *TP,* Threshold membrane potential; *RP,* resting membrane potential.

that are indicative of structural changes or damage such as ischemia, infarction, enlarged cardiac chambers, electrolyte imbalance, or drug toxicity.[1] Obtaining 12 ECG views of the heart is also helpful in the assessment of dysrhythmias. An example of a normal 12-lead ECG appears in Fig. 36-3.

When a patient's ECG is being continuously monitored, 1 to 12 ECG leads may be used. The most common leads selected are lead II, V_1, and MCL_1 (Fig. 36-4). MCL_1 is a modified chest lead that is similar to V_1 and is used when only three leads are available for monitoring. Current recommendations state that monitoring leads should be selected based on the patient's clinical situation.[5]

The ECG can be visualized continuously on a monitor oscilloscope. A recording of the ECG (i.e., rhythm strip) is obtained on ECG paper attached to the monitor. This provides documentation of the patient's rhythm. It also allows for measurement of complexes and intervals, and assessment of dysrhythmias.

It is essential to know how to measure time and voltage on the ECG paper to correctly interpret an ECG. ECG paper consists of large (heavy lines) and small (light lines) squares (Fig. 36-5). Each large square incorporates 25 smaller squares (five horizontal and five vertical). Each small square represents 0.04 second horizontally and 0.1 millivolt (mV) vertically. This means that the large square equals 0.20 second and that 300 large squares equal 1 minute. Vertically, one large square is equal to 0.5 mV. These squares are used to calculate the heart rate (HR) and intervals between different ECG complexes.

A variety of methods can be used to calculate the HR from an ECG. Probably the most accurate way is to count the number of QRS complexes in 1 minute. However, this method is time consuming. If the rhythm is regular, a simpler process can be used. Every 3 seconds a marker appears on the ECG paper. The nurse can count the number of R-R intervals in 6 seconds and multiply that number by 10. An R wave is the first upward (or positive) de-

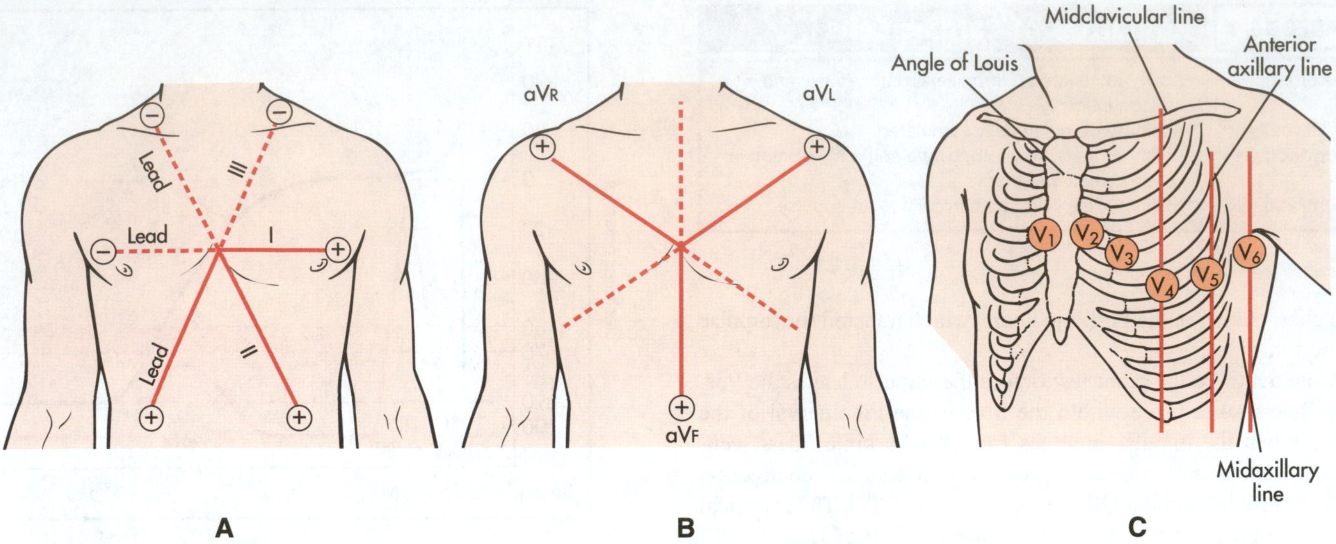

FIG. 36-2 **A,** Limb leads I, II, and III. Leads are located on the extremities. Illustrated are the angles from which these leads view the heart. **B,** Lead placement for limb leads aVR, aVL, and aVF. These unipolar leads use the center of the heart as their negative electrode. **C,** Lead placement for the chest electrodes: V_1, fourth intercostal space at the right sternal border; V_2, fourth intercostal space at the left sternal border; V_3, halfway between V_2 and V_4; V_4, fifth intercostal space at the left midclavicular line; V_5, anterior axillary line and same horizontal level as V_4; V_6, midaxillary line and same horizontal level as V_4.

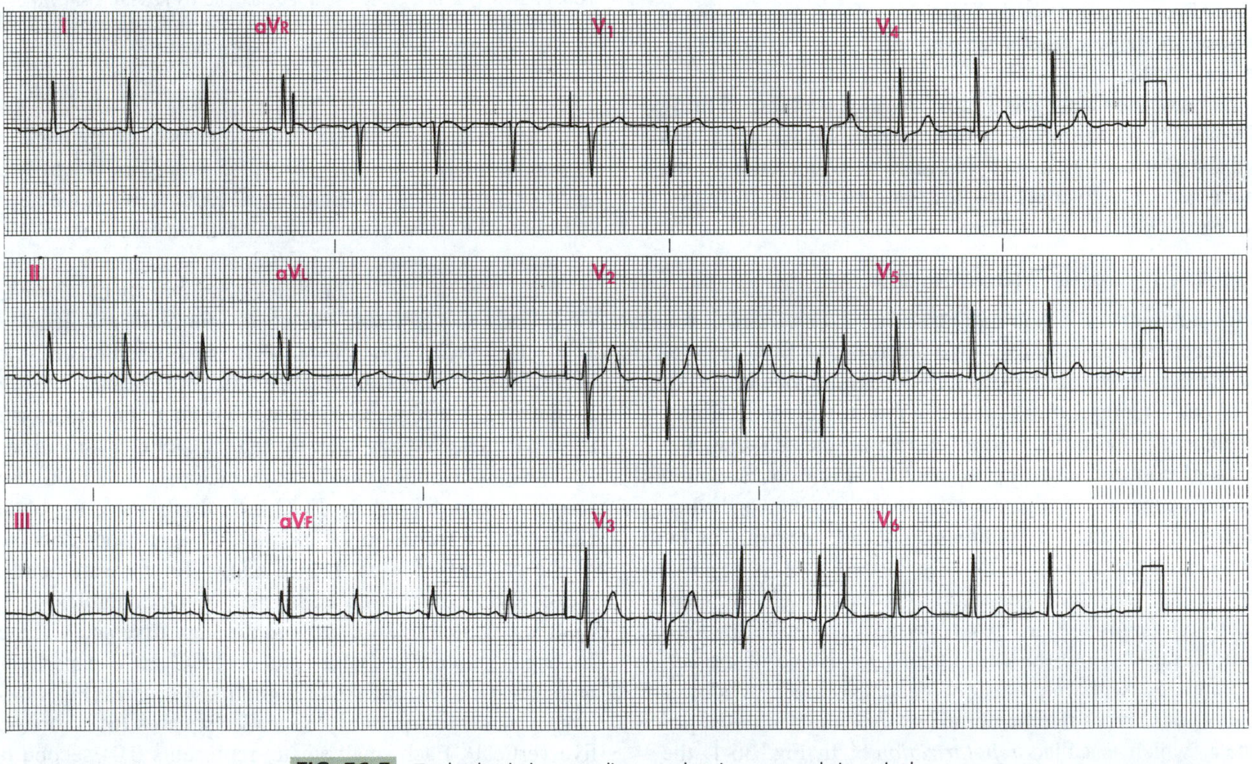

FIG. 36-3 Twelve-lead electrocardiogram showing a normal sinus rhythm.

flection of the QRS complex. This will yield the approximate number of beats per minute (Fig. 36-6).

Another rapid method for calculating the HR when the rhythm is regular is to count the number of small squares between one R-R interval. This number can be divided into 1500 to get the HR. The number of large squares between one R-R interval can also be counted and divided into 300 (see Fig. 36-6). These methods are accurate only if the rhythm is regular.

An additional way to measure distances on the ECG strip is to use calipers. Calipers are used for fine measurements, especially for points of a specific wave or interval. Many times a P or R wave will not fall directly on a light or heavy line. The fine points of the calipers can be placed exactly on the components to be measured and then moved to another part of the strip for time measurement.

ECG leads are attached to the patient's chest wall via an electrode pad fixed with electrical conductive paste. For best contact, excessive hair on the chest wall should be clipped using scissors. The skin should be prepared by rubbing gently with dry gauze until slightly pink. If the skin is oily, alcohol may be used first. In the case of a diaphoretic patient, benzoin may be applied to the skin before electrode placement. If leads and electrodes are not firmly placed, or if there is muscle activity or electrical interference from

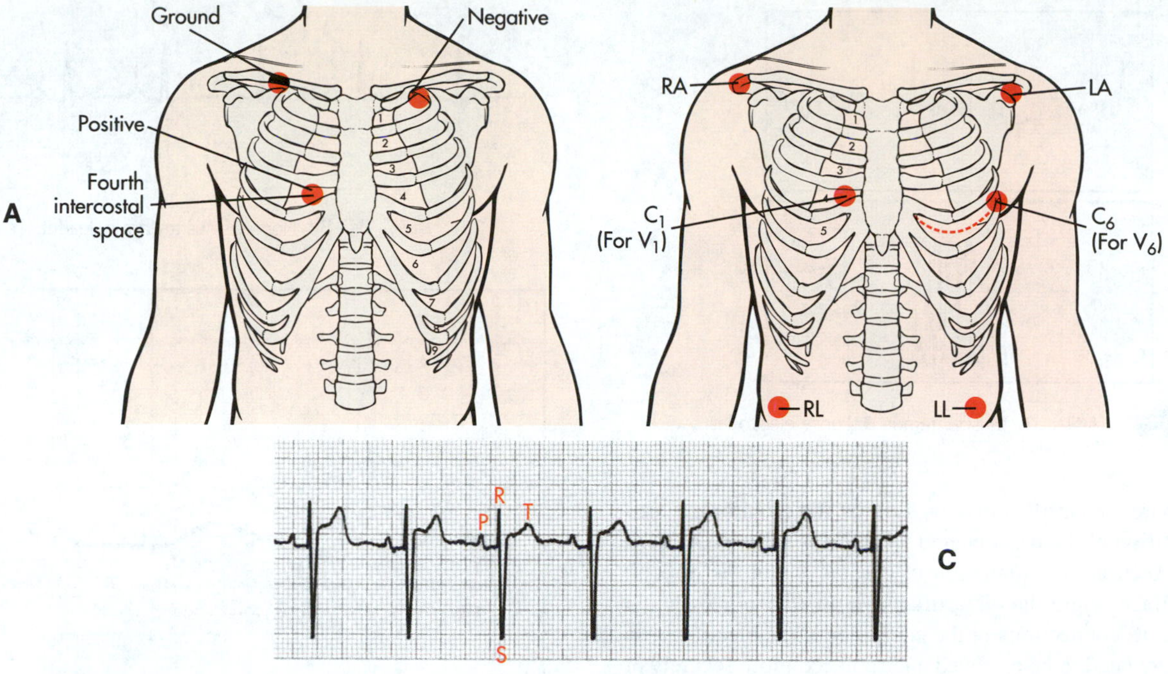

FIG. 36-4 **A,** Lead placement for MCL_1 using a three-lead system. **B,** Lead placement for V_1 or V_6 using a five-lead system. **C,** Typical electrocardiogram tracing in lead MCL_1. *C,* Chest; *LA,* left arm; *LL,* left leg; *MCL,* modified chest lead; *RA,* right arm; *RL,* right leg.

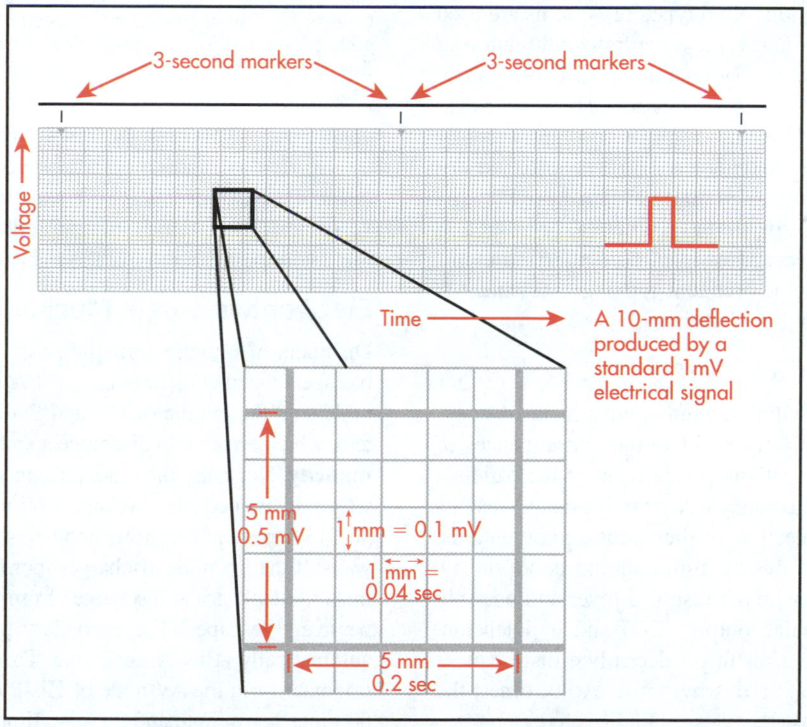

FIG. 36-5 Time and voltage on the electrocardiogram.

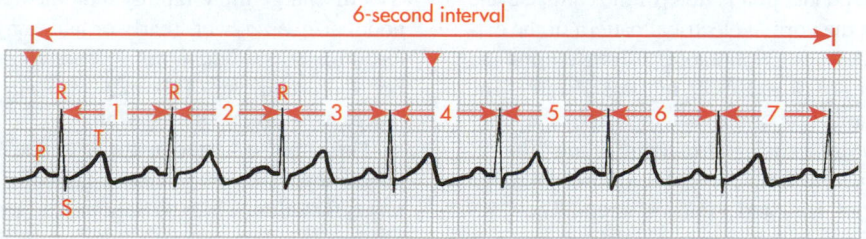

FIG. 36-6 When the rhythm is regular, heart rate can be determined at a glance. The estimated heart rate is 70.

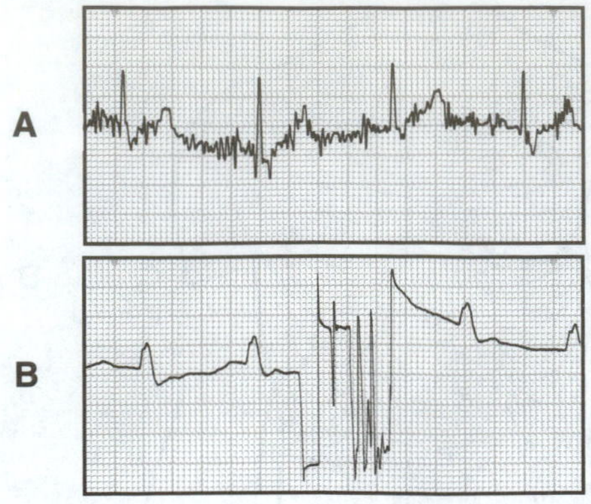

FIG. 36-7 Artifact. **A,** Muscle tremor. **B,** Loose electrodes.

an outside source, an artifact may be seen on the monitor. An artifact is a distortion of the baseline and waveforms seen on the ECG (Fig. 36-7). Accurate interpretation of cardiac rhythm is difficult when an artifact is present. If artifacts occur, the nurse should check for secure connections in the equipment. The electrodes on the patient may need to be removed and replaced more securely or in areas that are less affected by movement.[6]

Telemetry Monitoring. **Telemetry monitoring** is the observation of a patient's HR and rhythm to rapidly diagnose dysrhythmias, ischemia, or infarction.[7] Two types of systems are used for telemetry monitoring. The first type, a centralized monitoring system, requires a nurse or telemetry technician to continuously observe all patients' rhythms at a central location. The second system of telemetry monitoring does not require constant nurse or technician surveillance. These systems have the capability of detecting and storing data. Sophisticated alarm systems provide different levels of detection of dysrhythmias, ischemia, or infarction depending on the severity of each. However, computerized monitoring systems are not fail-proof. Frequent nursing assessment is important when caring for monitored patients.

Assessment of Cardiac Rhythm

When assessing the cardiac rhythm, the nurse must make an accurate interpretation and immediately evaluate the consequences of the findings for the individual patient. Assessment of the patient's hemodynamic response to any change in rhythm is essential as this information will guide the selection of therapeutic interventions. Determination of the cause of dysrhythmias should be a priority. For example, tachycardias may be the result of fever and possibly may cause a decrease in cardiac output (CO) and hypotension. Certain dysrhythmias may be a result of electrolyte disturbances and may lead to a life-threatening dysrhythmia.[7] At all times, the patient, not the "monitor," must be assessed and treated.

Normal sinus rhythm refers to a rhythm that originates in the SA node and follows the normal conduction pattern of the cardiac cycle (Fig. 36-8). Fig. 36-9 shows the normal electrical pattern of the cardiac cycle. Table 36-2 provides a description of ECG waveforms and intervals and possible sources of disturbances in these features. The P wave represents the depolarization of the atria (passage of an electrical impulse through the atria), causing atrial contraction. The PR interval represents the time period for the impulse to spread through the atria, AV node, bundle of His, and Purkinje fibers. The QRS complex represents depolarization of the ventricles (ventricular contraction) and the QRS interval represents the time it takes for depolarization. The ST segment represents the time between ventricular

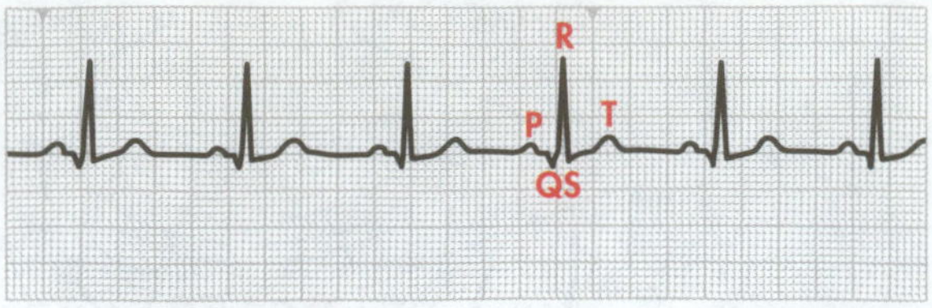

FIG. 36-8 Normal sinus rhythm in lead II.

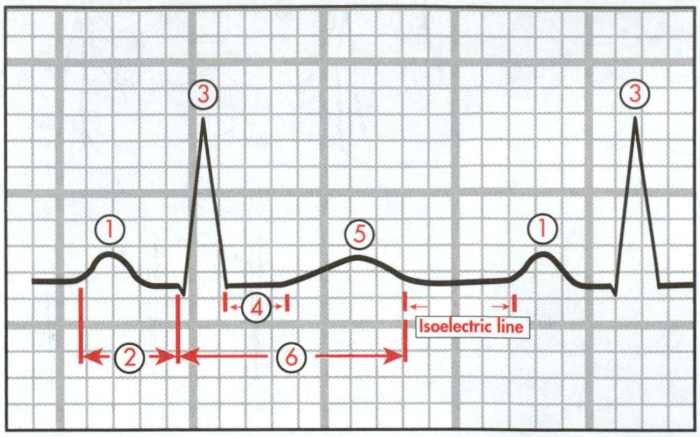

FIG. 36-9 The electrocardiogram complex as seen in a normal sinus rhythm. *1,* P wave (normal is 0.06 to 0.12 sec); *2,* PR interval (normal is 0.12 to 0.20 sec); *3,* QRS complex (normal is 0.04 to 0.12 sec); *4,* ST segment (normal is 0.12 sec); *5,* T wave (normal is 0.16 sec); *6,* QT interval (normal is 0.34 to 0.43 sec). Isoelectric (flat) line represents the absence of electrical activity in the cardiac cells.

depolarization and repolarization. This segment should be flat or *isoelectric* and represents the absence of any electrical activity between these two events. The T wave represents repolarization of the ventricles. The QT interval represents the total time for depolarization and repolarization of the ventricles.

Electrophysiologic Mechanisms of Dysrhythmias

Disorders of impulse formation can cause dysrhythmias. The heart has specialized cells found in the SA node, parts of the atria, the AV node, and the bundle of His and Purkinje fibers (His-Purkinje) system, which are able to discharge spontaneously. This is termed **automaticity.** Normally the main pacemaker of the heart is the SA node, which spontaneously discharges 60 to 100 times per minute (Table 36-3). A pacemaker from another site may be discharged in two ways. If the SA node discharges more slowly than a secondary pacemaker, the electrical discharges from the secondary pacemaker may passively "escape." The secondary pacemaker will then discharge automatically at its intrinsic rate. These secondary pacemakers may originate from the AV node or His-Purkinje system at rates of 40 to 60 times per minute and 20 to 40 times per minute, respectively.

Another way that secondary pacemakers can originate is when they discharge more rapidly than the normal pacemaker of the SA node. *Triggered beats* (early or late) may come from an *ectopic focus* (area outside the normal conduction pathway) in the atria, AV node, or ventricles. This may result in a dysrhythmia, which replaces the normal sinus rhythm.

The impulse started by the SA node or an ectopic focus must be conducted to the entire heart chamber. The property of myocardial tissue that allows it to be depolarized by a stimulus is called **excitability**. This is an important part of the transmission of the impulse from one fiber to another. The level of excitability is determined by the length of time after depolarization that the tissues can be re-

TABLE 36-2 Definition and Sources of Disturbance in Electrocardiogram Waveforms and Intervals*

Description	Duration (sec)	Source of Disturbance
P wave: Represents time for the passage of the electrical impulse through the atrium causing atrial depolarization; should be upright	0.06-0.12	Disturbance in conduction within atria
PR interval: Measured from beginning of P wave to beginning of QRS complex; represents time taken for impulse to spread through the atria, AV node and bundle of His, the bundle branches, and Purkinje fibers, to a point immediately preceding ventricular contraction	0.12-0.20	Disturbance in conduction usually in AV node, bundle of His, or bundle branches but can be in atria as well
QRS interval: Measured from beginning to end of QRS complex; represents time taken for depolarization of both ventricles	0.04-0.12	Disturbance in conduction in bundle branches or in ventricles
ST segment: Measured from the S wave of the QRS complex to the beginning of the T wave; represents the time between ventricular depolarization and repolarization; should be flat (isoelectric)	0.12	Disturbances usually caused by ischemia or infarction
T wave: Represents time for ventricular repolarization; should be upright	0.16	Disturbances usually caused by electrolyte imbalances, ischemia, or infarction
QT interval: Measured from beginning of QRS complex to end of T wave; represents time taken for entire electrical depolarization and repolarization of the ventricles	0.34-0.43	Disturbances usually affecting repolarization more than depolarization and caused by drugs, electrolyte imbalances, and changes in heart rate

AV, Atrioventricular.
*Heart rate influences the duration of these intervals, especially those of the PR and QT intervals.

TABLE 36-3 Intrinsic Rates of the Conduction System

SA node	60-100 times/minute
AV node	40-60 times/minute
Bundle of His, Purkinje fibers	20-40 times/minute

AV, Atrioventricular; *SA,* sinoatrial.

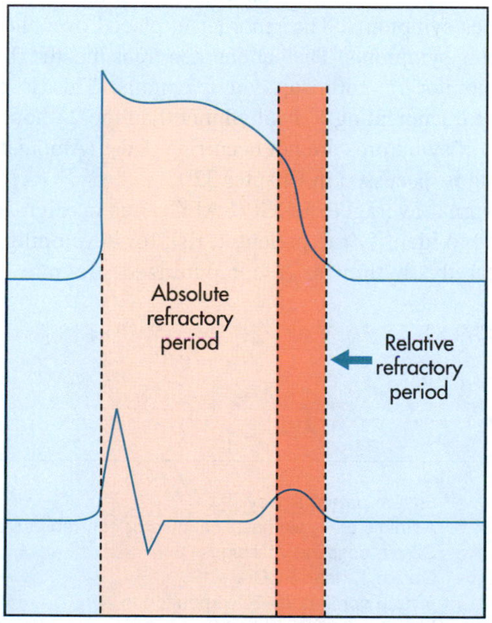

FIG. 36-10 Absolute and relative refractory periods correlated with the cardiac muscle's action potential and with an ECG tracing.

stimulated. The recovery period after stimulation is called the *refractory phase* or period. The *absolute refractory phase* or period occurs when excitability is zero and heart tissue cannot be stimulated. The *relative refractory period* occurs slightly later in the cycle, and excitability is more likely. In states of *full excitability,* the heart is completely recovered. Fig. 36-10 shows the relationship between the refractory period and the ECG.

TABLE 36-4 Common Causes of Dysrhythmias

Cardiac Conditions

- Accessory pathways
- Cardiomyopathy
- Conduction defects
- Heart failure
- Myocardial cell degeneration
- Myocardial infarction
- Valve disease

Other Conditions

- Acid-base imbalances
- Alcohol
- Caffeine, tobacco
- Connective tissue disorders
- Drug effects (e.g., antidysrhythmia drugs, stimulants, β-adrenergic blockers) or toxicity
- Electric shock
- Electrolyte imbalances (e.g., hypokalemia, hypocalcemia)
- Emotional crisis
- Herbal supplements
- Hypoxia, shock
- Metabolic conditions (e.g., thyroid dysfunction)
- Near-drowning
- Poisoning

If conduction is depressed and if some areas of the heart are blocked (e.g., by necrosis), the unblocked areas are activated earlier than the blocked areas. When the block is unidirectional, this uneven conduction may allow the initial impulse to reenter areas that were previously not excitable but have recovered. The reentering impulse may be able to depolarize the atria and ventricles, causing a premature beat. If the reentrant excitation continues, tachycardia occurs.[3]

Evaluation of Dysrhythmias

Dysrhythmias occur as the result of various abnormalities and disease states.[3,7] The cause of a dysrhythmia influences the treatment of the patient. Common causes of dysrhythmias are presented in Table 36-4. Table 36-5 presents a systematic approach to assessing a cardiac rhythm.

TABLE 36-5 Systematic Approach to Assessing Cardiac Rhythm

When assessing a cardiac rhythm, a systematic approach should be used. A recommended approach includes the following:

1. Note the P wave. Is it upright or inverted? Is there one for every QRS complex?
2. Evaluate the atrial rhythm. Is it regular or irregular?
3. Calculate the atrial rate.
4. Measure the duration of the PR interval. Is it normal duration or prolonged?
5. Evaluate the ventricular rhythm. Is it regular or irregular?
6. Calculate the ventricular rate.
7. Measure the duration of the QRS complex. Is it normal duration or prolonged?
8. Assess the ST segment. Is it isoelectric, elevated, or depressed?
9. Measure the duration of the QT interval. Is it normal duration or prolonged?
10. Note the T wave. Is it upright or inverted?

Questions to consider then include the following:

1. What is the dominant rhythm and/or dysrhythmia?
2. What is the clinical significance of the findings?
3. What is the treatment for the particular rhythm?

Dysrhythmias occurring in out-of-hospital settings present problems of management. Determination of the rhythm by cardiac monitoring is a high priority. If indicated, the emergency medical services (EMS) system is contacted after the patient has been assessed. Emergency care of the patient with a dysrhythmia is outlined in Table 36-6.

In addition to continuous ECG monitoring during hospitalization, several other methods are used to evaluate cardiac dysrhythmias and the effectiveness of antidysrhythmia drug therapy. An electrophysiologic test (an invasive method) and Holter monitoring, event recorder monitoring, exercise treadmill testing, and signal-averaged ECG (all noninvasive methods) can be performed on both an inpatient and an outpatient basis.

An *electrophysiologic study (EPS)* is performed to identify different mechanisms of tachydysrhythmias (dysrhythmias with rates $>$100), as well as heart blocks, bradydysrhythmias (dysrhythmias with rates $<$100), and causes of syncope. It can also be used to identify locations of accessory pathways and to determine the effectiveness of antidysrhythmia drugs. It involves introducing several electrode catheters transvenously through the femoral vein to the right side of the heart with fluoroscopic guidance. Electrical stimulation to various areas of the atrium and ventricle is performed to induce the dysrhythmia. Immediate cardioversion or defibrillation may be required as serious dysrhythmias can be provoked during the procedure.

Preprocedure anxiety is common for the patient undergoing EPS. Emotional support from the nurse is important. Patients should be instructed that they will be sedated but conscious during the procedure. Nursing care before and after the procedure is similar to that for cardiac catheterization (see Chapter 32). (EPS is also discussed in Chapter 32.)

The Holter monitor is a device that records the ECG while the patient is ambulatory. The device can record heart rhythm for 24 to 48 hours while the patient performs daily activities. The patient maintains a diary in which activities and any symptoms are recorded. Events in the diary can later be correlated with any dysrhythmias observed on the recording. The monitor is generally a useful device for detecting significant dysrhythmias and evaluating the effects of drugs during a patient's normal activities. It can also be used for detecting ischemia by analyzing ST segments. A limitation of the device is that the patient who has frequent ventricular dysrhythmias, some of which may be lethal, may not have these dysrhythmias during the monitored time. (Holter monitoring is also discussed in Chapter 32.)

Use of event monitors has greatly improved the evaluation of outpatient dysrhythmias. Event monitors are recorders that are activated by the patient and can be used only at the time the patient experiences symptoms. The recorder is placed over the patient's chest during symptoms. The patient then transmits the rhythm to a central monitoring company via telephone. This is an easier method of documenting a dysrhythmia than the 24-hour monitor, especially if symptoms are not occurring daily. (Ambulatory ECG monitoring is discussed in Chapter 32.)

The signal-averaged ECG (SAECG) is a high-resolution ECG used to identify the patient at risk for developing complex ventricular dysrhythmias. A computerized program and ECG

TABLE 36-6 *EMERGENCY MANAGEMENT* Dysrhythmias

Etiology	Assessment Findings	Interventions
See Table 36-4	• Irregular rate and rhythm; tachycardia, bradycardia • Decreased or increased blood pressure • Decreased O_2 saturation • Chest, neck, shoulder, back, jaw, or arm pain • Dizziness, syncope • Dyspnea • Extreme restlessness, anxiety • Decreased level of consciousness, confusion • Feeling of impending doom • Numbness, tingling of arms • Weakness and fatigue • Cold, clammy skin • Diaphoresis • Pallor • Palpitations • Nausea and vomiting	**Initial** • Ensure patent airway • Administer O_2 via nasal cannula or non-rebreather mask • Obtain baseline vital signs • Obtain 12-lead ECG • Initiate continuous ECG monitoring • Identify underlying rhythm • Identify dysrhythmia • Establish IV access **Ongoing Monitoring** • Monitor vital signs, level of consciousness, O_2 saturation, and cardiac rhythm • Anticipate need for administration of antidysrhythmia drugs • Anticipate need for intubation if respiratory distress is evident • Prepare to initiate advanced cardiac life support (e.g., CPR, defibrillation, transcutaneous pacing)

CPR, Cardiopulmonary resuscitation; *ECG*, electrocardiogram; *IV*, intravenous.

machine are used for the test. The identification of electrical activity called *late potentials* on the SAECG strongly suggests that the patient is at risk for developing serious ventricular dysrhythmias.

Exercise treadmill testing is used for evaluation of cardiac rhythm response to exercise. Exercise-induced dysrhythmias can be reproduced and analyzed, and drug therapy can be evaluated. These tests are performed with routine treadmill testing protocols.

Diagnostic procedures for assessment of the cardiovascular system are presented in Chapter 32, Table 32-7.

Types of Dysrhythmias

Examples of the ECG tracings of common dysrhythmias are presented in Figs. 36-11 through 36-19. Descriptive characteristics of common dysrhythmias are presented in Table 36-7.

Sinus Bradycardia. In *sinus bradycardia* the conduction pathway is the same as that in sinus rhythm but the SA node fires at a rate less than 60 beats/minute. This is referred to as *absolute bradycardia* (Fig. 36-11, *A*). *Relative bradycardia* refers to an HR that is less than expected for the patient's condition, causing the patient to be symptomatic.[7]

Clinical Associations. Sinus bradycardia may be a normal sinus rhythm in aerobically trained athletes and in other individuals during sleep. It also occurs in response to carotid sinus massage, Valsalva maneuver, hypothermia, increased intraocular pressure, increased vagal tone, and administration of parasympathomimetic drugs (e.g., bethanechol [Duvoid]). Disease states associated with sinus bradycardia are hypothyroidism, increased intracranial pressure, obstructive jaundice, and inferior wall myocardial infarction (MI).

TABLE 36-7 Characteristics of Common Dysrhythmias

Pattern	Rate and Rhythm	P Wave	PR Interval	QRS Complex
NSR	60-100 beats/minute and regular	Normal	Normal	Normal
Sinus bradycardia	<60 beats/minute and regular	Normal	Normal	Normal
Sinus tachycardia	>100 beats/minute and regular	Normal	Normal	Normal
PAC	Usually 60-100 beats/minute and irregular	Abnormal shape	Normal	Normal (usually)
PSVT	100-300 beats/minute and regular	Abnormal shape, may be hidden in the preceding T wave	Normal or shortened	Normal (usually)
Atrial flutter	*Atrial:* 250-350 beats/minute and regular *Ventricular:* > or <100 beats/minute and may be regular or irregular	Flutter (F) waves (saw-toothed pattern); more flutter waves than QRS complexes; may occur in a 2:1, 3:1, 4:1, etc. pattern	Not measurable	Normal (usually)
Atrial fibrillation	*Atrial:* 350-600 beats/minute and irregular *Ventricular:* > or <100 beats/minute and irregular	Fibrillatory (f) waves	Not measurable	Normal (usually)
Junctional dysrhythmias	40-140 beats/minute and regular	Inverted, may be hidden in QRS complex	Variable	Normal (usually)
First-degree AV block	Normal and regular	Normal	>0.20 sec	Normal
Second-degree AV block				
Type I (Mobitz I, Wenckebach heart block)	*Atrial:* Normal and regular *Ventricular:* Slower and irregular	Normal	Progressive lengthening	Normal QRS width, with pattern of one nonconducted (blocked) QRS complex
Type II (Mobitz II heart block)	*Atrial:* Usually normal and regular *Ventricular:* Slower and regular or irregular	More P waves than QRS complexes (e.g., 2:1, 3:1)	Normal or prolonged	Widened QRS, preceded by two or more P waves, with nonconducted (blocked) QRS complex
Third-degree AV block (complete heart block)	*Atrial:* Regular but may appear irregular due to P waves hidden in QRS complexes *Ventricular:* 20–40 beats/minute and regular	Normal, but no connection with QRS complex	Variable	Normal or widened, no relationship with P waves
PVC	Underlying rhythm can be any rate; regular or irregular rhythm; PVCs occur at variable rates	Not usually visible; hidden in the PVC	Not measurable	Wide and distorted
VT	150-250 beats/minute and regular or irregular	Not usually visible	Not measurable	Wide and distorted
Accelerated idioventricular rhythm	40-100 beats/minute and regular	Not usually visible	Not measurable	Wide and distorted
Ventricular fibrillation	Not measurable and irregular	Absent	Not measurable	Not measurable

AV, Atrioventricular; *NSR,* normal sinus rhythm; *PAC,* premature atrial contraction; *PSVT,* paroxysmal supraventricular tachycardia; *PVC,* premature ventricular contraction; *VT,* ventricular tachycardia.

A

B

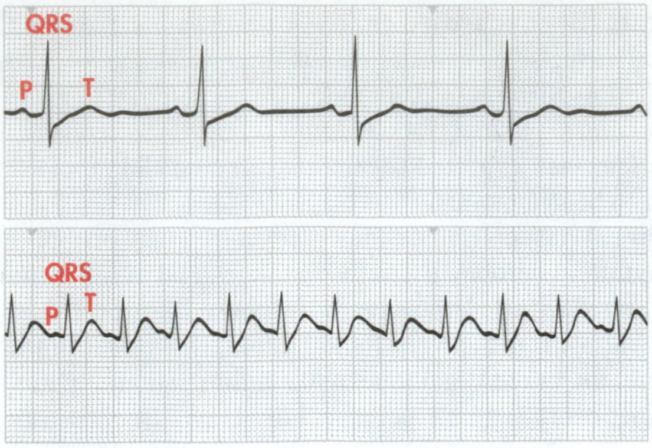

FIG. 36-11 **A,** Sinus bradycardia. **B,** Sinus tachycardia.

ECG Characteristics. In sinus bradycardia, HR is less than 60 beats/minute and the rhythm is regular. The P wave precedes each QRS complex and has a normal shape and duration. The PR interval is normal, and the QRS complex has a normal shape and duration.

Clinical Significance. The clinical significance of sinus bradycardia depends on how the patient tolerates it hemodynamically. Signs of symptomatic bradycardia can include pale, cool skin; hypotension; weakness; angina; dizziness or syncope; confusion or disorientation; and shortness of breath.

Treatment. Treatment consists of administration of atropine (an anticholinergic drug) for the patient with symptoms. Pacemaker therapy may be required.

Sinus Tachycardia. The conduction pathway is the same in *sinus tachycardia* as that in normal sinus rhythm. The discharge rate from the sinus node is increased as a result of vagal inhibition or sympathetic stimulation. The sinus rate is greater than 100 beats/minute (Fig. 36-11, *B*).

Clinical Associations. Sinus tachycardia is associated with physiologic and psychologic stressors such as exercise, fever, pain, hypotension, hypovolemia, anemia, hypoxia, hypoglycemia, myocardial ischemia, heart failure (HF), hyperthyroidism, anxiety, and fear. It can also be an effect of drugs such as epinephrine (EpiPen), norepinephrine (Levophed), atropine (AtroPen), caffeine, theophylline (Theo-Dur), nifedipine (Procardia), or hydralazine (Apresoline). In addition, many over-the-counter cold remedies have active ingredients (e.g., pseudoephedrine [Sudafed]) that can cause tachycardia.

ECG Characteristics. In sinus tachycardia, HR is greater than 100 beats/minute and the rhythm is regular. The P wave is normal, precedes each QRS complex, and has a normal shape and duration. The PR interval is normal, and the QRS complex has a normal shape and duration.

Clinical Significance. The clinical significance of sinus tachycardia depends on the patient's tolerance of the increased HR. The patient may have symptoms of dizziness, dyspnea, and hypotension. Increased myocardial oxygen consumption is associated with an increased HR. Angina or an increase in infarction size may accompany persistent sinus tachycardia in the patient with an acute MI.

Treatment. Treatment is based on the underlying cause. If the patient is experiencing tachycardia from pain, tachycardia should resolve with effective pain management. Treating hypovolemia should resolve any associated tachycardia. In certain situations, intravenous (IV) adenosine (Adenocard) and β-adrenergic blockers (e.g., metoprolol [Lopressor]) may be used to reduce HR and decrease myocardial oxygen consumption.

Drug Alert - Adenosine (Adenocard)
- *Monitor patient's ECG continuously. Brief period of asystole may be observed.*
- *Observe patient for flushing, dizziness, chest pain, or palpitations.*

Premature Atrial Contraction. A **premature atrial contraction** (PAC) is a contraction originating from an ectopic focus in the atrium in a location other than the sinus node. The ectopic signal originates in the left or right atrium and travels across the atria by an abnormal pathway, creating a distorted P wave (Fig. 36-12). At the AV node, it may be stopped (nonconducted PAC), delayed (lengthened PR interval), or conducted normally. If the signal moves through the AV node, in most cases it is conducted normally through the ventricles.

Clinical Associations. In a normal heart, a PAC can result from emotional stress or physical fatigue, or from the use of caffeine, tobacco, or alcohol. A PAC can also result from hypoxia, electrolyte imbalances, and disease states such as hyperthyroidism, chronic obstructive pulmonary disease (COPD), and heart disease including coronary artery disease (CAD) and valvular disease.

ECG Characteristics. HR varies with the underlying rate and frequency of the PAC, and the rhythm is irregular. The P wave has a different shape from that of the P wave originating from the SA node. It may be notched or have downward (or negative) deflection, or it may be hidden in the preceding T wave. The PR interval may be shorter or longer than the PR interval originating from the SA node, but it is within normal limits. The QRS complex is usually normal. If the QRS interval is 0.12 second or longer, abnormal conduction through the ventricles is present.

Clinical Significance. In persons with healthy hearts, isolated PACs are not significant. In persons with heart disease, frequent PACs may indicate enhanced automaticity of the atria, or a reentry mechanism. Such PACs may warn of or initiate more serious dysrhythmias (e.g., supraventricular tachycardia).

Treatment. Treatment depends on the patient's symptoms. Withdrawal of sources of stimulation such as caffeine or sympathomimetic drugs may be warranted. β-Adrenergic blockers may be used to decrease PACs.

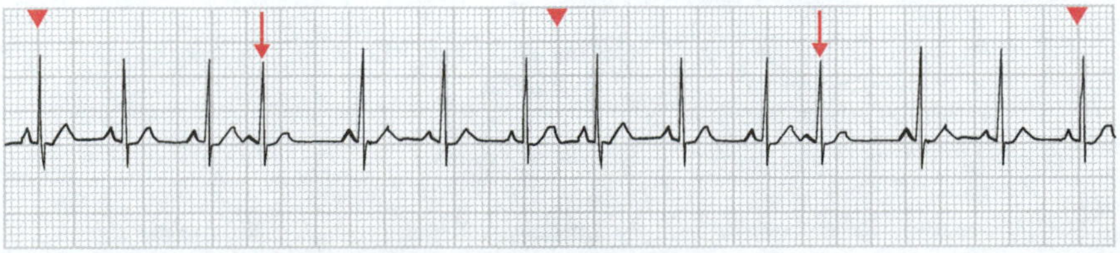

FIG. 36-12 Premature atrial contractions *(arrows)*.

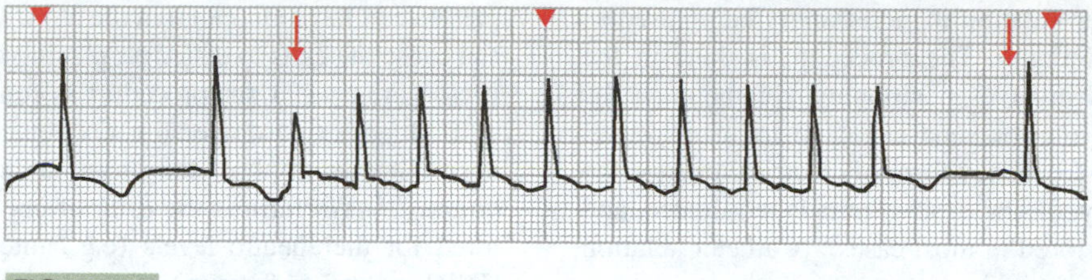

FIG. 36-13 Paroxysmal supraventricular tachycardia (PSVT). *Arrows* indicate beginning and ending of PSVT.

Paroxysmal Supraventricular Tachycardia. *Paroxysmal supraventricular tachycardia* (PSVT) is a dysrhythmia originating in an ectopic focus anywhere above the bifurcation of the bundle of His (Fig. 36-13). Identification of the ectopic focus is often difficult even with a 12-lead ECG as it requires recording the dysrhythmia as it is initiated.

PSVT occurs because of a reentrant phenomenon (reexcitation of the atria when there is a one-way block). Usually a PAC triggers a run of repeated premature beats. *Paroxysmal* refers to an abrupt onset and termination. Termination is sometimes followed by a brief period of asystole. Some degree of AV block may be present. PSVT can occur in the presence of Wolff-Parkinson-White (WPW) syndrome, or "preexcitation." In this syndrome, there are extra conduction pathways, or *accessory pathways.*

Clinical Associations. In the normal heart, PSVT is associated with overexertion, emotional stress, deep inspiration, and stimulants such as caffeine and tobacco. PSVT is also associated with rheumatic heart disease, digitalis toxicity, CAD, and cor pulmonale.

ECG Characteristics. In PSVT, HR is 100 to 300 beats/minute and rhythm is regular or slightly irregular. The P wave is often hidden in the preceding T wave, but if seen, it may have an abnormal shape. The PR interval may be shortened or normal, and the QRS complex is usually normal.

Clinical Significance. The clinical significance of PSVT depends on symptoms and HR. A prolonged episode and HR greater than 180 beats/minute may precipitate a decreased CO, resulting in hypotension, dyspnea, and angina.

Treatment. Treatment for PSVT includes vagal stimulation and drug therapy. Common vagal maneuvers include Valsalva and coughing. IV adenosine is the first drug of choice to convert PSVT to a normal sinus rhythm. This drug has a short half-life (10 seconds) and is well tolerated by most patients.[3,7] IV β-adrenergic blockers, calcium channel blockers (e.g., diltiazem [Cardizem]), digoxin (Lanoxin), and amiodarone (Cordarone) can also be used. For a patient with WPW, amiodarone should be used. If vagal stimulation and drug therapy are ineffective and the patient becomes hemodynamically unstable, direct current (DC) cardioversion may be used.[7] (Cardioversion is discussed on p. 857.)

If PSVT recurs in patients with WPW, they may ultimately be treated with radiofrequency catheter ablation of the accessory pathway.[8] (Catheter ablation therapy is discussed on p. 861.)

Atrial Flutter. **Atrial flutter** is an atrial tachydysrhythmia identified by recurring, regular, sawtooth-shaped flutter (F) waves that originate from a single ectopic focus in the right atrium[3] (Fig. 36-14, *A*).

Clinical Associations. Atrial flutter rarely occurs in a normal heart. In disease states, it is associated with CAD, hypertension, mitral valve disorders, pulmonary embolus, chronic lung disease, cor pulmonale, cardiomyopathy, hyperthyroidism, and the use of drugs such as digoxin, quinidine, and epinephrine.

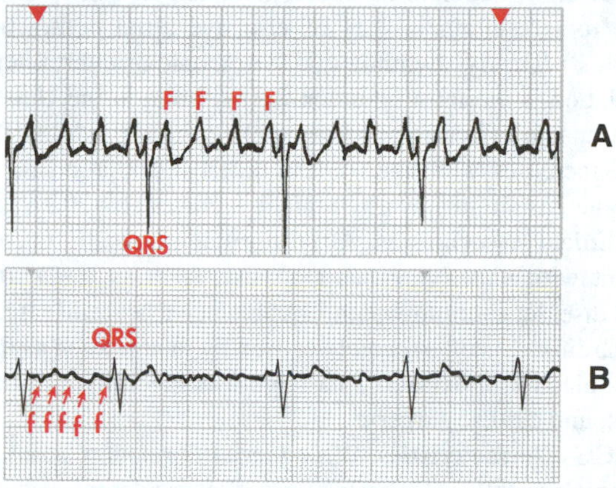

FIG. 36-14 **A,** Atrial flutter with a 4:1 conduction (four flutter *[F]* waves to each QRS complex). **B,** Atrial fibrillation. Note the chaotic fibrillatory *(f)* waves between the QRS complexes. Note: Recorded from lead V_1.

ECG Characteristics. Atrial rate is 250 to 350 beats/minute. The ventricular rate varies according to the conduction ratio. In 2:1 conduction, the ventricular rate is typically found to be approximately 150 beats/minute. Atrial rhythm is regular, and ventricular rhythm is usually regular. The atrial flutter waves represent atrial depolarization followed by repolarization. The PR interval is variable and not able to be measured. The QRS complex is usually normal. Because of the ability of the AV node to delay signals from the atria, there is usually some AV block in a fixed ratio of flutter waves to QRS complexes (e.g., 2:1, 3:1).

Clinical Significance. The high ventricular rates (>100) and loss of the atrial "kick" (atrial contraction reflected by a sinus P wave) that are associated with atrial flutter can decrease CO and cause serious consequences such as HF, especially in the patient with underlying heart disease.[8] Patients with atrial flutter are at increased risk of stroke because of the risk of thrombus formation in the atria from the stasis of blood. Warfarin (Coumadin) is used to prevent stroke in patients with atrial flutter of greater than 48 hours' duration.[7,8]

Treatment. The primary goal in treatment of atrial flutter is to slow the ventricular response by increasing AV block. Drugs used to control ventricular rate include calcium channel blockers and β-adrenergic blockers. Electrical cardioversion may be used to convert the atrial flutter to sinus rhythm in an emergency situation (i.e., the patient is hemodynamically unstable) and electively. Antidysrhythmia drugs used to convert atrial flutter to sinus rhythm or to maintain sinus rhythm include amiodarone, propafenone (Rythmol), procainamide (Pronestyl), ibutilide (Corvert), and flecainide (Tambocor).[7]

Radiofrequency catheter ablation is increasingly being used as curative therapy for atrial flutter. The procedure is done in the electrophysiology lab and involves positioning a catheter in the right atrium between the inferior vena cava and tricuspid valve. Using a low-voltage, high-frequency form of electrical energy, the tissue is ablated (or destroyed), the dysrhythmia is terminated, and normal sinus rhythm is restored in most cases.[9] (Catheter ablation in discussed on p. 861.)

Atrial Fibrillation. **Atrial fibrillation** is characterized by a total disorganization of atrial electrical activity due to multiple ectopic foci resulting in loss of effective atrial contraction (Fig. 36-14, *B*). The dysrhythmia may be chronic or intermittent. Atrial fibrillation is the most common dysrhythmia in the United States and Canada, affecting approximately 1 in 136 adults. Its prevalence increases with age. As the elderly population increases, a 60% increase in this dysrhythmia is predicted by 2020.[8]

Clinical Associations. Atrial fibrillation usually occurs in the patient with underlying heart disease, such as CAD, rheumatic heart disease, cardiomyopathy, hypertensive heart disease, HF, and pericarditis. It is often acutely caused by factors such as thyrotoxicosis, alcohol intoxication, caffeine use, electrolyte disturbances, stress, and cardiac surgery.

ECG Characteristics. During atrial fibrillation, atrial rate may be as high as 350 to 600 beats/minute. Ventricular rate can vary from as low as 50 beats/minute to as high as 180 beats/minute. Atrial fibrillation with ventricular rates greater than 100 are described as atrial fibrillation with a rapid ventricular response. When ventricular rates are less than 100, it is described as atrial fibrillation with a slow or controlled ventricular response. P waves are replaced by chaotic, fibrillatory waves in atrial fibrillation. The ventricular rhythm is usually irregular. The PR interval is not measurable, and the QRS complex usually has a normal shape and duration. At times, atrial flutter and atrial fibrillation may coexist.

Clinical Significance. Atrial fibrillation can often result in a decrease in CO because of ineffective atrial contractions or loss of atrial kick, and/or a rapid ventricular response. Thrombi may form in the atria as a result of blood stasis. An embolized clot may develop and pass to the brain, causing a stroke. Overall risk of stroke increases fivefold with atrial fibrillation. Risk of stroke is even higher in patients with structural heart disease, with hypertension, and over 65 years of age.[8]

Treatment. The goals of treatment include a decrease in ventricular response (to <100) and prevention of cerebral embolic events.[10-13] Ventricular rate control is a priority for patients with atrial fibrillation. Drugs used for rate control include calcium channel blockers (e.g., diltiazem), β-adrenergic blockers (e.g., metoprolol), and digoxin.

For some patients, conversion of atrial fibrillation to a normal sinus rhythm may be a consideration (e.g., reduced exercise tolerance with rate control drugs, contraindications to warfarin).[10,11] Antidysrhythmia drugs used for conversion to and maintenance of sinus rhythm include amiodarone, propafenone, flecainide, procainamide, and ibutilide.[7] In patients with severe left ventricular dysfunction (ejection fraction $<40\%$) or HF, amiodarone or DC cardioversion should be used.[7]

Cardioversion may be used to convert atrial fibrillation to a normal sinus rhythm. If a patient has been in atrial fibrillation for more than 48 hours, anticoagulation therapy with warfarin is recommended for 3 to 4 weeks before any attempt at cardioversion and for 4 to 6 weeks after successful cardioversion.[7] Prior to the procedure, a transesophageal echocardiogram may be performed to rule out the presence of thrombi (clots) in the atria. The cardioversion procedure can cause the clots to dislodge, placing the patient at risk for stroke. If clots are present, the procedure is contraindicated.

If drugs or cardioversion do not convert atrial fibrillation to normal sinus rhythm, long-term anticoagulation therapy is required.[10-13] Warfarin is the drug of choice, and patients are monitored for therapeutic levels (e.g., international normalized ratio [INR] in the 2 to 3 range). (See Chapter 38 for discussion of anticoagulation therapy.)

Other treatment strategies exist for patients with drug-refractory atrial fibrillation, or who cannot or choose not to have long-term anticoagulation. These include the use of radiofrequency catheter ablation (similar to procedure for atrial flutter) and the Maze procedure.[14,15] The Maze procedure is a surgical intervention that stops atrial fibrillation by interrupting the ectopic electrical signals that are responsible for this dysrhythmia. Incisions are made in both atria to stop the formation and conduction of these signals. Scar tissue generated by the incisions permanently blocks the paths of the ectopic signals that cause atrial fibrillation and restores normal sinus rhythm. Modifications to the Maze procedure include the use of cold (cryoablation) and heat (high-intensity ultrasound) rather than incisions to destroy the areas of the atria associated with the dysrhythmia.[15]

Junctional Dysrhythmias. *Junctional dysrhythmias* refer to dysrhythmias that originate in the area of the AV node, primarily because the SA node has failed to fire or the signal has been blocked. In this situation, the AV node becomes the pacemaker of the heart. The impulse from the AV node usually moves in a retrograde (backward) fashion that produces an abnormal P wave occurring just before or after the QRS complex or that is hidden in the QRS complex. The impulse usually moves normally through the ventricles. Junctional premature beats may occur, and they are treated in a manner similar to that for PACs. Other junctional dysrhythmias include junctional escape rhythm (Fig. 36-15), accelerated junctional rhythm, and junctional tachycardia. These dysrhythmias are treated according to the patient's tolerance of the rhythm and the patient's clinical condition.

Clinical Associations. Junctional dysrhythmias are often associated with CAD, HF, cardiomyopathy, electrolyte imbalances, inferior MI, and rheumatic heart disease. Certain drugs (e.g., digoxin, amphetamines, caffeine, nicotine) can also cause junctional dysrhythmias.[3]

ECG Characteristics. In junctional escape rhythm the HR is 40 to 60 beats/minute, in accelerated junctional rhythm it is 61 to 100 beats/minute, and in junctional tachycardia it is 101 to 150 beats/minute. Rhythm is regular. The P wave is abnormal in shape and inverted, or it may be hidden in the QRS complex (see Fig. 36-15). The PR interval is less than 0.12 second when the P wave precedes the QRS complex. The QRS complex is usually normal.

Clinical Significance. Junctional escape rhythms serve as a safety mechanism occurring when the SA node has not been effective. Escape rhythms such as this should not be suppressed. Accel-

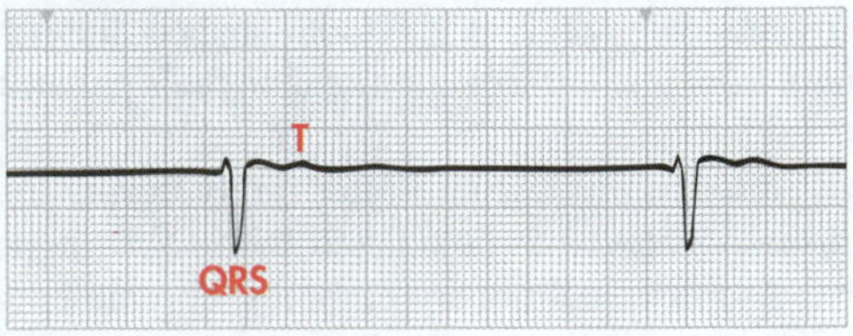

FIG. 36-15 Junctional escape rhythm. P wave is hidden in the QRS complex.

erated junctional rhythm and junctional tachycardia indicate a more serious problem with the SA node. These rhythms may result in a reduction of CO, causing the patient to become hemodynamically unstable (e.g., hypotensive).[3]

Treatment. Treatment varies according to the type of junctional dysrhythmia. If a patient has symptoms with an escape junctional rhythm, atropine can be used. In accelerated junctional rhythm and junctional tachycardia caused by digoxin toxicity, the digoxin is withheld. In the absence of digitalis toxicity, β-adrenergic blockers, calcium channel blockers, and amiodarone are used for rate control. DC cardioversion should not be used.[7]

First-Degree AV Block. *First-degree AV block* is a type of AV block in which every impulse is conducted to the ventricles but the duration of AV conduction is prolonged (Fig. 36-16, *A*). After the impulse moves through the AV node, it is usually conducted normally through the ventricles.

Clinical Associations. First-degree AV block is associated with MI, CAD, rheumatic fever, hyperthyroidism, vagal stimulation, and drugs such as digoxin, β-adrenergic blockers, calcium channel blockers, and flecainide.

ECG Characteristics. In first-degree AV block, HR is normal and rhythm is regular. The P wave is normal, the PR interval is prolonged to more than 0.20 second, and the QRS complex usually has a normal shape and duration.

Clinical Significance. First-degree AV block is usually not serious but can be a precursor of higher degrees of AV block. Patients with first-degree AV block are asymptomatic.

Treatment. There is no treatment for first-degree AV block. Modifications to causative medications may be considered. Patients should continue to be monitored for any new changes in heart rhythm.

Second-Degree AV Block, Type I. *Type I second-degree AV block (Mobitz I or Wenckebach heart block)* includes a gradual lengthening of the PR interval. It occurs because of a prolonged AV conduction time until an atrial impulse is nonconducted and a QRS complex is blocked (missing) (Fig. 36-16, *B*). Type I AV block most commonly occurs in the AV node, but it can also occur in the His-Purkinje system.

Clinical Associations. Type I AV block may result from use of drugs such as digoxin or β-adrenergic blockers. It may also be associated with CAD and other diseases that can slow AV conduction.

ECG Characteristics. Atrial rate is normal, but ventricular rate may be slower as a result of nonconducted or blocked QRS complexes. Once a ventricular beat is blocked, the cycle repeats itself with progressive lengthening of the PR intervals until another QRS complex is blocked. The rhythm appears on the ECG in a pattern of grouped beats. Ventricular rhythm is irregular. The P wave has a normal shape. The QRS complex has a normal shape and duration.

Clinical Significance. Type I AV block is usually a result of myocardial ischemia or infarction. It is almost always transient and is usually well tolerated. However, in some patients (e.g., following MI) it may be a warning signal of a more serious AV conduction disturbance.

Treatment. If the patient is symptomatic, atropine is used to increase HR, or a temporary pacemaker may be needed, especially if the patient has experienced an MI. If the patient is asymptomatic, the rhythm should be closely observed with a transcutaneous pacemaker on standby. Bradycardia is more likely to become symptomatic when one or more of the following are present: (1) hypotension, (2) HF, or (3) shock.

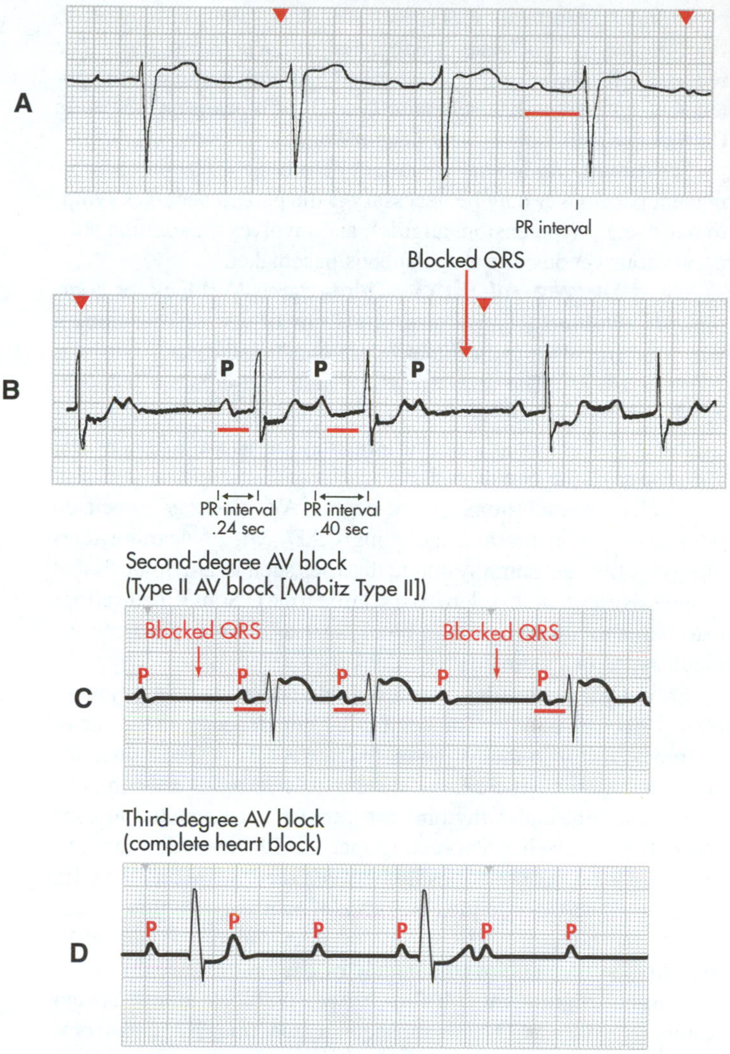

FIG. 36-16 Heart block. **A,** First-degree AV block with a PR interval of 0.40 seconds. **B,** Second-degree AV block, type I, with progressive lengthening of the PR interval until a QRS complex is blocked. **C,** Second-degree AV block, type II, with constant PR intervals and variable blocked QRS complexes. **D,** Third-degree AV block. Note that there is no relationship between P waves and QRS complexes.

Second-Degree AV Block, Type II. In *type II second-degree AV block (Mobitz II heart block),* a P wave is nonconducted without progressive antecedent PR lengthening. This almost always occurs when a block in one of the bundle branches is present (Fig. 36-16, *C*). On conducted beats, the PR interval is constant. Type II second-degree AV block is a more serious type of block in which a certain number of impulses from the SA node are not conducted to the ventricles. This occurs in ratios of 2:1, 3:1, and so on (i.e., two P waves to one QRS complex, three P waves to one QRS complex). It may occur with varying ratios. Type II AV block almost always occurs in the His-Purkinje system.

Clinical Associations. Type II AV block is associated with rheumatic heart disease, CAD, anterior MI, and digitalis toxicity.

ECG Characteristics. Atrial rate is usually normal. Ventricular rate depends on the intrinsic rate and the degree of AV block. Atrial rhythm is regular, but ventricular rhythm may be irregular. The P wave has a normal shape. The PR interval may be normal or prolonged in duration and remains constant on conducted beats. The QRS complex is usually more than 0.12 second because of bundle branch block.

Clinical Significance. Type II AV block often progresses to third-degree AV block and is associated with a poor prognosis. The reduced HR often results in decreased CO with subsequent hypotension and myocardial ischemia. Type II AV block is an indication for therapy with a permanent pacemaker.

Treatment. Temporary treatment before the insertion of a permanent pacemaker may be necessary if the patient becomes symptomatic (e.g., hypotension, angina), and involves the use of a temporary transvenous or transcutaneous pacemaker.[7,8]

Third-Degree AV Block. Third-degree AV block, or **complete heart block,** constitutes one form of AV dissociation in which no impulses from the atria are conducted to the ventricles (Fig. 36-16, *D*). The atria are stimulated and contract independently of the ventricles. The ventricular rhythm is an escape rhythm, and the ectopic pacemaker may be above or below the bifurcation of the bundle of His.

Clinical Associations. Third-degree AV block is associated with severe heart disease, including CAD, MI, myocarditis, cardiomyopathy, and some systemic diseases such as amyloidosis and progressive systemic sclerosis (scleroderma). Some medications can also cause third-degree AV block, such as digoxin, β-adrenergic blockers, and calcium channel blockers.

ECG Characteristics. The atrial rate is usually a sinus rate of 60 to 100 beats/minute. The ventricular rate depends on the site of the block. If it is in the AV node, the rate is 40 to 60 beats/minute, and if it is in the His-Purkinje system, it is 20 to 40 beats/minute. Atrial and ventricular rhythms are regular but unrelated to each other. The P wave has a normal shape. The PR interval is variable, and there is no time relationship between the P wave and the QRS complex. The QRS complex is normal if an escape rhythm is initiated at the bundle of His or above. It is widened if an escape rhythm is initiated below the bundle of His.

Clinical Significance. Third-degree AV block almost always results in reduced CO with subsequent ischemia, HF, and shock. Syncope from third-degree AV block may result from severe bradycardia or even periods of asystole.

Treatment. For symptomatic patients, a transcutaneous pacemaker is used until a temporary transvenous pacemaker can be inserted.[7] The use of drugs such as atropine, epinephrine, isoproterenol, and dopamine is a temporary measure to increase HR and support blood pressure (BP) until temporary pacing is initiated. Patients will need a permanent pacemaker as soon as possible.

Premature Ventricular Contractions. A **premature ventricular contraction** (PVC) is a contraction originating in an ectopic focus in the ventricles. It is the premature occurrence of a QRS complex, which is wide and distorted in shape compared with a QRS complex initiated from the normal conduction pathway (Fig. 36-17). PVCs that are initiated from different foci appear different in shape from each other and are called *multifocal* PVCs. PVCs that appear to have the same shape are called *unifocal* PVCs. When every other beat is a PVC, it is called *ventricular bigeminy*. When every third beat is a PVC, it is called *ventricular trigeminy*. Two consecutive PVCs are called a *couplet*.

Ventricular tachycardia occurs when there are three or more consecutive PVCs. *R-on-T phenomenon* occurs when a PVC falls on the T wave of a preceding beat. This is considered especially dangerous as the PVC is firing during the relative refractory phase of ventricular repolarization. Excitability of the cardiac cells is increased during this time, and the risk for the PVC to initiate ventricular tachycardia or ventricular fibrillation is great.

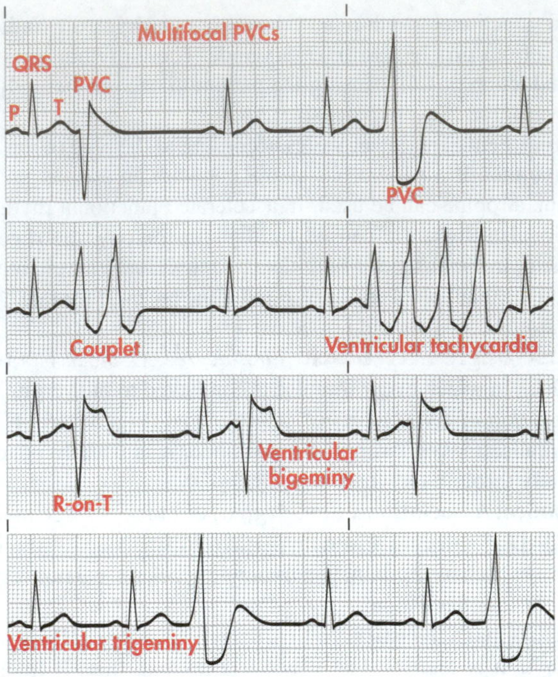

FIG. 36-17 Various forms of premature ventricular contractions (PVCs). Note: Recorded from lead II.

Clinical Associations. PVCs are associated with stimulants such as caffeine, alcohol, nicotine, aminophylline, epinephrine, isoproterenol, and digoxin. They are also associated with electrolyte imbalances, hypoxia, fever, exercise, and emotional stress. Disease states associated with PVCs include MI, mitral valve prolapse, HF, and CAD.

ECG Characteristics. HR varies according to intrinsic rate and number of PVCs. Rhythm is irregular because of premature beats. The P wave is rarely visible and is usually lost in the QRS complex of the PVC. Retrograde conduction may occur, and the P wave may be seen following the ectopic beat. The PR interval is not measurable. The QRS complex is wide and distorted in shape, lasting more than 0.12 second. The T wave is generally large and opposite in direction to the major direction of the QRS complex.

Clinical Significance. PVCs are usually a benign finding in the patient with a normal heart. In heart disease, depending on frequency, PVCs may reduce the CO and precipitate angina and HF. Because PVCs in CAD or acute MI represent ventricular irritability, the patient's physiologic response to PVCs must be monitored. It is important to assess the patient's apical-radial pulse rate as PVCs often do not generate a sufficient ventricular contraction to result in a peripheral pulse. This may lead to a pulse deficit.

Treatment. Treatment is often based on the cause of the PVCs (e.g., oxygen therapy for hypoxia, electrolyte replacement). Assessment of the patient's hemodynamic status is important to determine if treatment with drug therapy is indicated. Drugs that should be considered include β-adrenergic blockers, procainamide, amiodarone, or lidocaine (Xylocaine).

Ventricular Tachycardia. The diagnosis of **ventricular tachycardia** (VT) is made when a run of three or more PVCs occurs. It occurs when an ectopic focus or foci fire repetitively and the ventricle takes control as the pacemaker. Different forms of ventricular tachycardia exist, depending on QRS configuration. Monomorphic VT (Fig. 36-18, *A*) has QRS complexes that are the same in shape, size, and direction. Polymorphic VT occurs when

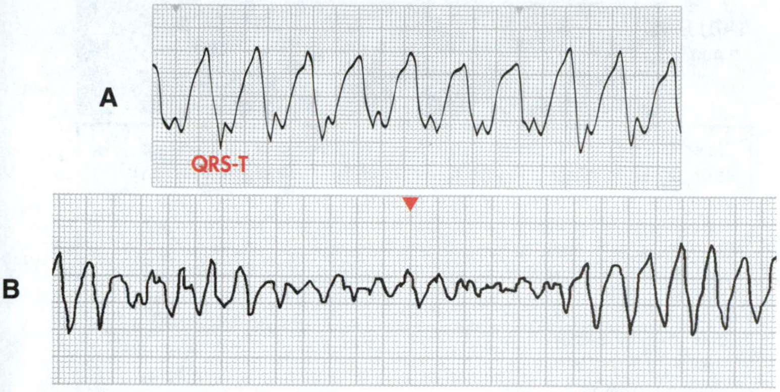

FIG. 36-18 Ventricular tachycardia. **A,** Monomorphic. **B,** Torsades de pointes (polymorphic).

the QRS complexes gradually change back and forth from one shape, size, and direction to another over a series of beats. *Torsades de pointes* (French, "twisting of the points") is polymorphic VT associated with a prolonged QT interval of the underlying rhythm (Fig. 36-18, *B*).

Ventricular tachycardia may be sustained or nonsustained. Sustained VT lasts for >30 seconds. Nonsustained VT lasts for 30 seconds or less. The development of ventricular tachycardia is an ominous sign. It is considered to be a life-threatening dysrhythmia because of decreased CO and the possibility of deterioration to ventricular fibrillation, which is a lethal dysrhythmia.

Clinical Associations. Ventricular tachycardia is associated with MI, CAD, significant electrolyte imbalances, cardiomyopathy, mitral valve prolapse, long QT syndrome, digitalis toxicity, and central nervous system disorders. The dysrhythmia has also been observed in patients who have no evidence of cardiac disease.

ECG Characteristics. Ventricular rate is 150 to 250 beats/minute. Rhythm may be regular or irregular. AV dissociation may be present, with P waves occurring independently of the QRS complex. The atria may also be depolarized by the ventricles in a retrograde fashion. The P wave is usually buried in the QRS complex and the PR interval is not measurable.

The QRS complex is distorted in appearance, with a duration exceeding 0.12 second and with the ST-T wave in the opposite direction of the QRS complex (see Fig. 36-18). The R-R interval may be irregular or regular.

Clinical Significance. Ventricular tachycardia can be stable (patient has a pulse) or unstable (patient is pulseless). Sustained ventricular tachycardia will cause a severe decrease in CO as a result of decreased ventricular diastolic filling times and loss of atrial contraction. Results include hypotension, pulmonary edema, decreased cerebral blood flow, and cardiopulmonary arrest. The dysrhythmia must be treated quickly, even if it occurs only briefly and stops abruptly. Episodes may recur if prophylactic treatment is not begun. Ventricular fibrillation may also develop.

Treatment. Precipitating causes must be identified and treated (e.g., electrolyte imbalances, ischemia). If the VT is monomorphic and the patient is hemodynamically stable (e.g., pulse is present) and has preserved left ventricular function, IV procainamide, sotalol (Betapace), amiodarone, or lidocaine is used. If the patient becomes hemodynamically unstable or has poor left ventricular function, IV amiodarone or lidocaine is given followed by cardioversion.

If the VT is polymorphic with a normal baseline QT interval, any one of the following medications is used: β-adrenergic blockers, lidocaine, amiodarone, procainamide, or sotalol. Cardioversion is used if drug therapy is ineffective.

If the VT is polymorphic with a prolonged baseline QT interval, therapies include IV magnesium, isoproterenol, phenytoin (Dilantin), lidocaine, or antitachycardia pacing (discussed later in chapter). Drugs that prolong the QT interval should be discontinued. If the rhythm is not converted, cardioversion may be needed.

VT without a pulse is a life-threatening situation and is treated in the same manner as ventricular fibrillation. Cardiopulmonary resuscitation (CPR) and rapid defibrillation are the first lines of treatment, followed by the administration of epinephrine if defibrillation is unsuccessful.[7]

An *accelerated idioventricular rhythm* (AIVR) can develop when the intrinsic pacemaker rate (SA node or AV node) becomes less than that of a ventricular ectopic pacemaker. The rate is between 40 and 100 beats/minute. It is most commonly associated with acute MI and reperfusion of the myocardium after fibrinolytic therapy or angioplasty of coronary arteries. It can be seen with digitalis toxicity. In the setting of acute MI, AIVR is usually self-limiting and well tolerated, and requires no treatment. If the patient becomes symptomatic (e.g., hypotension, angina), atropine can be considered. Temporary pacing may be required. Drugs that suppress ventricular rhythms (e.g., lidocaine) should not be used as these can terminate the ventricular rhythm and further reduce the HR.

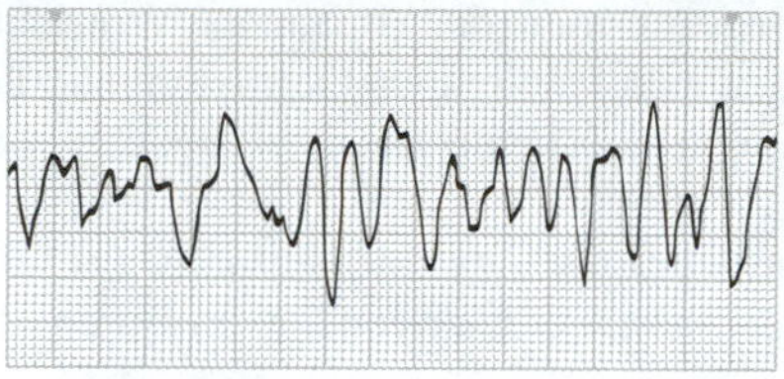

FIG. 36-19 Ventricular fibrillation.

Ventricular Fibrillation. **Ventricular fibrillation** is a severe derangement of the heart rhythm characterized on ECG by irregular undulations of varying shapes and amplitude (Fig. 36-19). This represents the firing of multiple ectopic foci in the ventricle. Mechanically the ventricle is simply "quivering," and no effective contraction, and consequently no CO, occurs.

Clinical Associations. Ventricular fibrillation occurs in acute MI and myocardial ischemia and in chronic diseases such as CAD and cardiomyopathy. It may occur during cardiac pacing or cardiac catheterization procedures as a result of catheter stimulation of the ventricle. It may also occur with coronary reperfusion after fibrinolytic therapy. Other clinical associations are accidental electric shock, hyperkalemia, hypoxemia, acidosis, and drug toxicity.

ECG Characteristics. HR is not measurable. Rhythm is irregular and chaotic. The P wave is not visible, and the PR interval and the QRS interval are not measurable.

Clinical Significance. Ventricular fibrillation results in an unresponsive, pulseless, and apneic state. If not rapidly treated, the patient will die.

Treatment. Treatment consists of immediate initiation of CPR and advanced cardiac life support (ACLS) measures with the use of defibrillation and definitive drug therapy. If a defibrillator is immediately available, there should be no delay in using it.[7]

Asystole. **Asystole** represents the total absence of ventricular electrical activity. Occasionally, P waves can be seen. No ventricular contraction occurs because depolarization does not occur. Patients are unresponsive, pulseless, and apneic. This is a lethal dysrhythmia that requires immediate treatment. Ventricular fibrillation may masquerade as asystole; thus the rhythm should be assessed in more than one lead. The prognosis of a patient with asystole is extremely poor.

Clinical Associations. Asystole is usually a result of advanced cardiac disease, a severe cardiac conduction system disturbance, or end-stage HF.

Clinical Significance. Generally the patient with asystole has end-stage cardiac disease or has a prolonged arrest and cannot be resuscitated.

Treatment. Treatment consists of CPR with initiation of ACLS measures, which include intubation, transcutaneous pacing, and IV therapy with epinephrine and atropine.

Pulseless Electrical Activity. *Pulseless electrical activity* (PEA) describes a situation in which electrical activity can be observed on the ECG, but there is no mechanical activity of the ventricles and the patient has no pulse. Prognosis is poor unless the underlying cause can be identified and quickly corrected. The most frequent causes of PEA include hypovolemia, hypoxia, metabolic acidosis, hyperkalemia or hypokalemia, hypothermia, drug overdose, cardiac tamponade, MI, tension pneumothorax, and pulmonary embolus. Treatment begins with CPR followed by intubation and IV therapy with epinephrine. Atropine is also used if the ventricular rate is slow. Treatment is directed toward correction of the underlying cause.

Sudden Cardiac Death. The term **sudden cardiac death** (SCD) refers to death from a cardiac cause. The majority of SCDs result from ventricular dysrhythmias, specifically ventricular tachycardia or fibrillation. (SCD is discussed in Chapter 34.)

Prodysrhythmia. Antidysrhythmia drugs may cause life-threatening dysrhythmias similar to those for which they are administered. This concept is termed *prodysrhythmia.* The patient who has severe left ventricular dysfunction is the most susceptible to prodysrhythmias. Digoxin and class IA, IC, and III antidysrhythmia drugs can cause a prodysrhythmic response[16] (Table 36-8). The first several days of drug therapy are the vulnerable period for developing prodysrhythmias. For this reason, many oral antidysrhythmia drug regimens are initiated in a monitored hospital setting.

Antidysrhythmia Drugs

An increasing number of antidysrhythmia drugs have become available. Table 36-8 categorizes major drug classes by primary effects on the cardiac cells.

Defibrillation

Defibrillation is the most effective method of terminating ventricular fibrillation and pulseless VT. It is most effective when the myocardial cells are not anoxic or acidotic, making rapid defibrillation critical to a successful patient outcome. Defibrillation is accomplished by the passage of a DC electric shock through the heart that is sufficient to depolarize the cells of the myocardium. The intent is that subsequent repolarization of myocardial cells will allow the SA node to resume the role of pacemaker.[7]

Defibrillators deliver energy using a monophasic or biphasic waveform. Monophasic defibrillators deliver energy in one direction and biphasic defibrillators deliver energy in two directions (Fig. 36-20). Research has shown that biphasic defibrillators deliver successful shocks at lower energies and with fewer postshock ECG abnormalities than monophasic defibrillators.[17,18]

TABLE 36-8 DRUG THERAPY
Major Classifications of Antidysrhythmic Drugs

Class I: Sodium Channel Blockers (decrease conduction velocity in the atria, ventricles, and His-Purkinje system)
IA
disopyramide (Norpace)
procainamide (Pronestyl)
quinidine
IB
lidocaine (Xylocaine)
mexiletine (Mexitil)
phenytoin (Dilantin)
tocainide (Tonocard)
IC
flecainide (Tambocor)
propafenone (Rythmol)
Other Class I
moricizine* (Ethmozine)
Class II: β-Adrenergic Blockers (decrease automaticity of the SA node, decrease conduction velocity in AV node)
acebutolol (Sectral)
atenolol (Tenormin)
esmolol (Brevibloc)
metoprolol (Lopressor)
sotalol† (Betapace)
Class III: Potassium Channel Blockers (delay repolarization)
amiodarone (Cordarone)
bretylium (Bretylol)
dofetilide (Tikosyn)
sotalol† (Betapace)
Class IV: Calcium Channel Blockers (decrease automaticity of SA node, delay AV node conduction)
diltiazem (Cardizem)
verapamil (Calan)
Other Antidysrhythmia Drugs
adenosine (Adenocard)
digoxin (Lanoxin)
ibutilide (Corvert)
magnesium

*Moricizine has both class IA and IC properties.
†Sotalol has both class II and class III properties.

The output of a defibrillator is measured in joules, or watts per second. The recommended energy for initial shocks in defibrillation depends on the type of defibrillator. Biphasic defibrillators deliver the first and any successive shocks using 150 to 200 joules. Recommendations for monophasic defibrillators include an initial shock at 360 joules. After the initial shock, CPR should be started immediately beginning with chest compressions.

Rapid defibrillation can be performed using a manual or automatic device (Fig. 36-21). Manual defibrillators require health care providers to interpret cardiac rhythms, determine the need for a shock, and deliver a shock. **Automatic external defibrillators** (AEDs) are defibrillators that have rhythm detection capability and the ability to advise the operator to deliver a shock using hands-free defibrillator pads. Proficiency in use of the AED is incorporated in the basic life support course for health care providers.[7] The nurse should be familiar with the operation of the type of defibrillator that is used in the clinical setting.

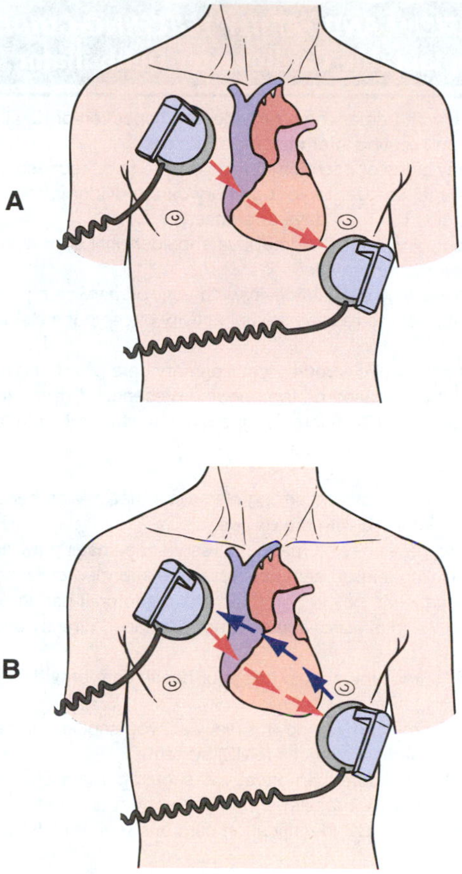

FIG. 36-20 Paddle placement and current flow in monophasic defibrillation **(A)** and biphasic defibrillation **(B).**

The following general steps are taken for defibrillation: (1) CPR should be in progress until the defibrillator is available; (2) the defibrillator should be turned on, and the proper energy level should be selected; and (3) the synchronizer switch is turned off (discussed below). Conductive materials (e.g., defibrillator gel pads) are applied to the chest, one to the right of the sternum just below the clavicle, and the other to the left of the apex. The defibrillator is charged by a button on the defibrillator or the paddles. The paddles are placed on the chest wall over the conductive material (see Fig. 36-20). The operator calls and looks to see that everyone is "all clear" to ensure that personnel are not touching the patient or the bed at the time of discharge. The charge is delivered by depressing buttons on both paddles simultaneously.

Hands-free, multifunction defibrillator pads are available and are placed on the chest as described above. Cables from the pads are connected to the defibrillator. The defibrillator is charged and discharged by the operator using buttons on the defibrillator. It is still essential that the operator assures that all personnel are clear before the defibrillator is discharged.

Synchronized Cardioversion. *Synchronized cardioversion* is the therapy of choice for the patient with hemodynamically unstable ventricular or supraventricular tachydysrhythmias. A synchronized circuit in the defibrillator is used to deliver a countershock that is programmed to occur on the R wave of the QRS complex of the ECG. The synchronizer switch must be turned on when cardioversion is planned.

The procedure for synchronized cardioversion is the same as for defibrillation with the following exceptions. If synchronized

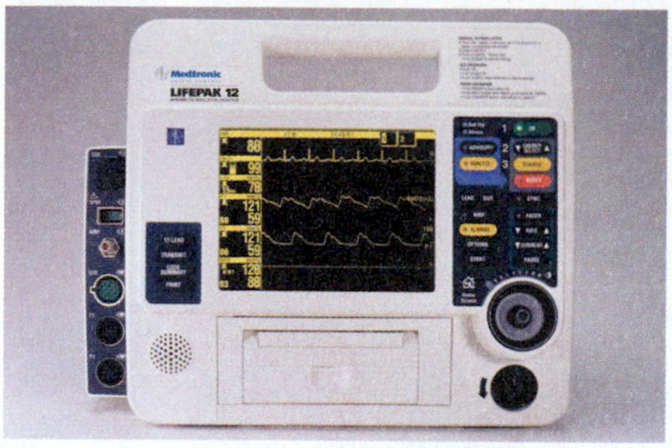

FIG. 36-21 LifePak contains a monitor, defibrillator, and transcutaneous pacemaker.

cardioversion is done on a nonemergency basis (i.e., the patient is awake and hemodynamically stable), the patient is sedated (e.g., IV midazolam [Versed]) before the procedure. Strict attention to maintenance of a patent airway is important in this situation. When a patient with supraventricular tachycardia or VT with a pulse is hemodynamically unstable, synchronized cardioversion is performed as quickly as possible. Last, the energy needed for synchronized cardioversion is generally less than the energy needed for defibrillation. Energy levels are started at 50 joules on a monophasic defibrillator and increased (e.g., 100 joules, 200 joules) if needed.

Implantable Cardioverter-Defibrillator. The *implantable cardioverter-defibrillator* (ICD) is an important technology for patients who (1) have survived SCD, (2) have spontaneous sustained VT, (3) have syncope with inducible ventricular tachycardia/fibrillation during EPS, and (4) are at high risk for future life-threatening dysrhythmias (e.g., have cardiomyopathy). Use of the ICD has significantly decreased cardiac mortality rates in these patients and has added a new dimension to the management of life-threatening dysrhythmias and the prevention of SCD.[19]

The ICD consists of a lead system placed via a subclavian vein to the endocardium. A battery-powered pulse generator is implanted subcutaneously, usually over the pectoral muscle on the patient's nondominant side. The pulse generator is similar in size to a pacemaker. The newest systems are single-lead systems instead of previous multilead or patch systems (Fig. 36-22). The ICD sensing system monitors the HR and rhythm and identifies ventricular tachycardia or ventricular fibrillation. Approximately 25 seconds after the sensing system detects a lethal dysrhythmia, the defibrillating mechanism delivers a 25-joule or less shock to the patient's heart. If the first shock is unsuccessful, the generator recycles and can continue to deliver shocks.

In addition to defibrillation capabilities, ICDs are equipped with antitachycardia and antibradycardia pacemakers. These sophisticated devices use dysrhythmia algorithms that detect dysrhythmias and determine the appropriate programmed response. These devices can initiate *overdrive pacing* of supraventricular and ventricular tachycardias, sparing the patient painful defibrillator shocks. They also provide backup pacing for bradydysrhythmias that may occur after defibrillation discharges. Preprocedure and postprocedure nursing care of the patient undergoing ICD placement is similar to the care of a patient undergoing permanent pacemaker implantation (see pp. 858 to 861).

Education of the patient who is receiving an ICD is of extreme importance. The patient experiences a variety of emotions, in-

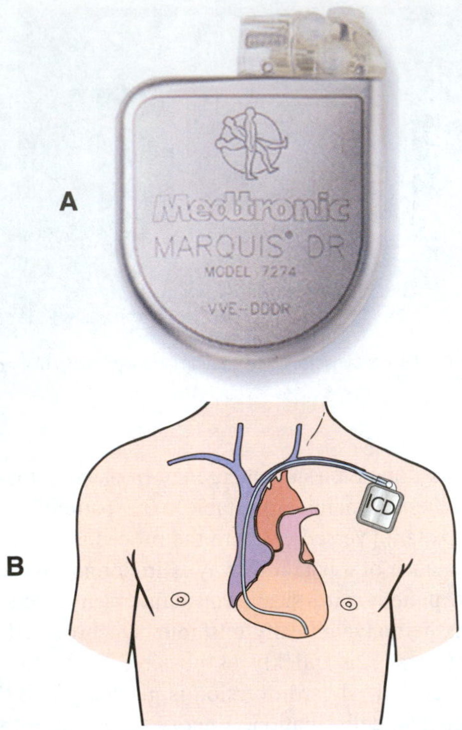

FIG. 36-22 **A,** The implantable cardioverter-defibrillator (ICD) pulse generator from Medtronic, Inc. **B,** The ICD is placed in a subcutaneous pocket over the pectoralis muscle. A single-lead system is placed transvenously from the pulse generator to the endocardium. The single lead detects dysrhythmias and delivers an electric shock to the heart muscle.

TABLE 36-9 PATIENT AND FAMILY TEACHING GUIDE Implantable Cardioverter-Defibrillator (ICD)

1. Follow up with primary care provider for inspection of ICD insertion site and routine interrogation of the ICD.
2. Report any signs of infection at incision site (e.g., redness, swelling, drainage) or fever to your primary care provider immediately.
3. Keep incision dry for 4 days after insertion.
4. Avoid lifting arm on ICD side above shoulder until approved by your primary care provider.
5. Discuss resuming sexual activity with your primary care provider. It is usually safe to resume sexual activity once your incision is healed.
6. Avoid driving until cleared by your primary care provider. This decision is usually based on the ongoing presence of dysrhythmias, the frequency of ICD firings, your overall health, and state laws regarding drivers with ICDs.
7. Avoid direct blows to ICD site.
8. Avoid large magnets and strong electromagnetic fields because these may interfere with the device.
9. You should never have a magnetic resonance imaging (MRI) scan.
10. When traveling, airport security should be informed of presence of ICD because it may set off the metal detector. If handheld screening wand is used, it should not be placed directly over the ICD.
11. If your ICD fires, you should call your health care provider immediately.
12. If your ICD fires and you do not feel well, you should contact the emergency medical services (EMS) system
13. If your ICD fires more than once, you should contact EMS.
14. A Medic Alert ID or bracelet should be worn at all times.
15. Always carry the ICD identification card and a current list of your medications.
16. Family members should learn cardiopulmonary resuscitation (CPR).

cluding fear of body image change, fear of recurrent dysrhythmias, expectation of pain with ICD discharge (described as a feeling of a blow to the chest), and anxiety about going home. Table 36-9 describes the teaching guidelines for the patient with an ICD and the patient's family. Participation in an ICD support group should be encouraged. Online resources for patients with an ICD include support groups at *www.implantable.com* and the Cardiac Arrest Survivor Network at *www.early-defib.org/survivors.asp.*

Pacemakers

The artificial **cardiac pacemaker** is an electronic device used to pace the heart when the normal conduction pathway is damaged or diseased. The basic pacing circuit consists of a power source (battery-powered pulse generator), one or more conducting leads (pacing leads), and the myocardium. The electrical signal (stimulus) travels from the pacemaker, through the leads, to the wall of the myocardium. The myocardium is "captured" and stimulated to contract (Fig. 36-23).

Recent advances in technology have been applied extensively to pacemakers. This has resulted in sophisticated, noninvasive, programmable single- and dual-chambered pacemakers with specialized circuits. Pacemakers have been developed that are more physiologically accurate, pacing the atrium and one or both of the ventricles.[19] Pacemakers were initially indicated for symptomatic bradydysrhythmias. However, advances now include antitachycardia and overdrive pacing. *Antitachycardia pacing* involves the delivery of a stimulus to the ventricle to terminate tachydysrhythmias (e.g., VT). Overdrive pacing involves pacing the atrium at rates of 200 to 500 impulses per minute in an attempt to terminate atrial

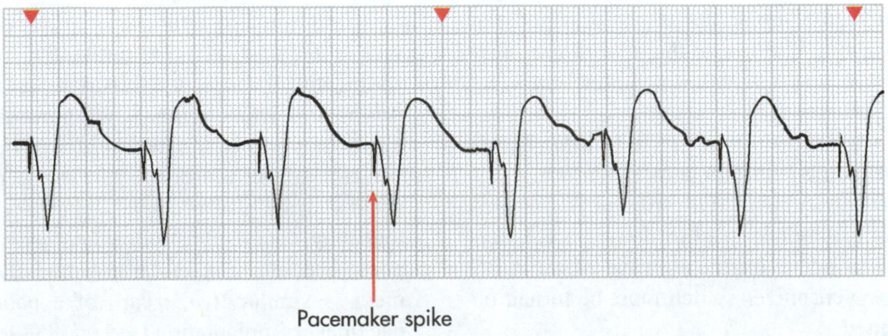

FIG. 36-23 Ventricular capture (depolarization) secondary to signal (pacemaker spike) from pacemaker lead in the right ventricle.

A

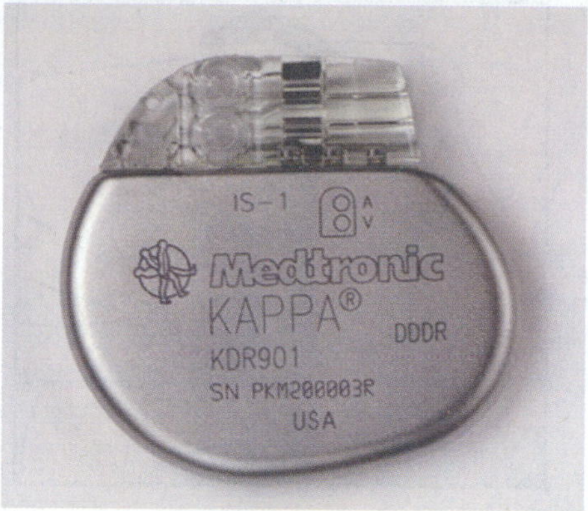

B

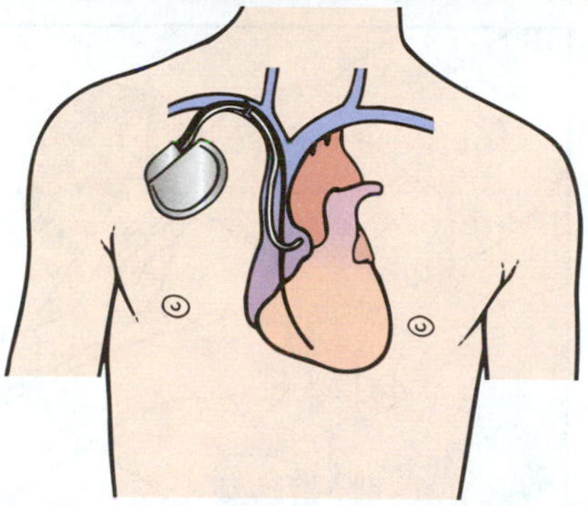

FIG. 36-24 **A,** A dual-chamber rate-responsive pacemaker from Medtronic, Inc., is designed to treat patients with chronic heart problems in which the heart beats too slowly to adequately support the body's circulation needs. **B,** Pacing leads in both the atrium and ventricle enable a dual-chamber pacemaker to sense and pace in both heart chambers.

TABLE 36-10 Indications for Permanent Pacemaker Therapy

- Acquired AV block
  - Second-degree AV block
  - Third-degree AV block
- Bundle branch block
- Cardiomyopathy
  - Dilated
  - Hypertrophic
- Heart failure
- Hypersensitive carotid sinus syndrome
- SA node dysfunction
- Tachydysrhythmias

AV, Atrioventricular; *SA,* sinoatrial.

tachycardias (e.g., atrial flutter, atrial fibrillation). Multiple other indications for pacemakers have evolved. For more detailed information on pacemaker therapy, the reader should refer to dedicated texts on this topic.[1]

A *permanent pacemaker* is one that is implanted totally within the body (Fig. 36-24). The permanent pacemaker power source is implanted subcutaneously, usually over the pectoral muscle on the patient's nondominant side. It is attached to pacing leads, which are threaded transvenously to the right atrium and one or both ventricles. Indications for insertion of permanent pacemakers are listed in Table 36-10.

A specialized type of cardiac pacing has been developed for the management of HF. More than 50% of HF patients have intraventricular conduction delays causing abnormal ventricular activation and contraction and subsequent dyssynchrony between the right

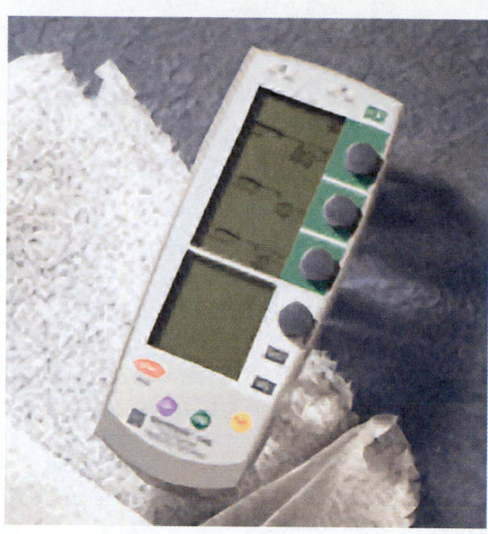

FIG. 36-25 Temporary external, dual-chamber demand pacemaker.

TABLE 36-11 Indications for Temporary Pacing*

- Maintenance of adequate HR and rhythm during special circumstances such as surgery and postoperative recovery, cardiac catheterization or coronary angioplasty, during drug therapy that may cause bradycardia, and before implantation of a permanent pacemaker
- As prophylaxis after open heart surgery
- Acute anterior MI with second-degree or third-degree AV block or bundle branch block
- Acute inferior MI with symptomatic bradycardia and AV block
- Electrophysiologic studies to evaluate patient with bradydysrhythmias and tachydysrhythmias

AV, Atrioventricular; *HR,* heart rate; *MI,* myocardial infarction.
*This table lists common indications, but is not all-inclusive.

and left ventricles. This can result in reduced systolic function, pump inefficiency, and worsened HF. *Cardiac resynchronization therapy* (CRT) is a pacing technique that resynchronizes the cardiac cycle by pacing both ventricles, thus promoting improvement in ventricular function. Several devices are available that have combined CRT with an ICD for maximum therapy. (HF is discussed in Chapter 35.)

Temporary Pacemaker. A *temporary pacemaker* is one that has the power source outside the body (Fig. 36-25). There are three types of temporary pacemakers: transvenous, epicardial, and transcutaneous. Indications for temporary pacing are listed in Table 36-11.

A *transvenous pacemaker* consists of a lead or leads that are threaded transvenously to the right atrium and/or right ventricle and attached to the external power source (Fig. 36-26). Most temporary transvenous pacemakers are inserted in critical care units in emergency situations. They are used until a permanent pacemaker can be inserted or the underlying cause of the dysrhythmia has been resolved.

Epicardial pacing is achieved by attaching an atrial and ventricular pacing lead to the epicardium during heart surgery. The leads are passed through the chest wall and attached to the external power source. Epicardial pacing leads are placed prophylactically should any bradydysrhythmias or tachydysrhythmias occur postoperatively.

A *transcutaneous pacemaker* (TCP) is used to provide adequate HR and rhythm to the patient in an emergency situation. Placement

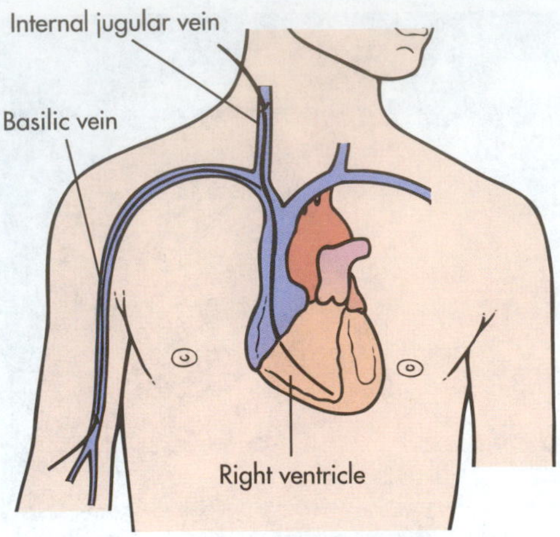

FIG. 36-26 Temporary transvenous pacemaker catheter insertion. A single lead is positioned in the right ventricle.

of the transcutaneous pacemaker is a noninvasive procedure that is used temporarily until a transvenous pacemaker can be inserted or until more definitive therapy is available.

The TCP consists of a power source and a rate- and voltage-control device that is attached to two large, multifunction electrode pads. One pad is positioned on the anterior part of the chest, usually on the V_2 or V_5 lead position, and the other pad is placed on the back between the spine and the left scapula at the level of the heart (Fig. 36-27).

Before initiating TCP therapy, it is important to tell the patient what to expect. The uncomfortable muscle contractions that the pacemaker creates when the current passes through the chest wall should be explained. The patient should be reassured that the therapy is temporary and that every effort will be made to replace the TCP with a transvenous pacemaker as soon as possible. Whenever possible, analgesia and/or sedation should be provided.

Patient Monitoring. Patients with temporary or permanent pacemakers will be ECG monitored to evaluate the status of the pacemaker. Pacemaker malfunction primarily is manifested by a failure to sense or a failure to capture. *Failure to sense* occurs when the pacemaker fails to recognize spontaneous atrial or ventricular activity, and it fires inappropriately. Failure to sense may be caused by pacer lead damage, battery failure, or dislodgement of the electrode. *Failure to capture* occurs when the electrical charge to the myocardium is insufficient to produce atrial or ventricular contraction. Failure to capture may be caused by pacer lead damage, battery failure, dislodgement of the electrode, or fibrosis at the electrode tip.

Complications of invasive temporary (i.e., transvenous) or permanent pacemaker insertion include infection and hematoma formation at the site of insertion of the pacemaker power source or leads, pneumothorax, failure to sense or capture with possible symptomatic bradycardia, perforation of the atrial or ventricular septum by the pacing lead, and appearance of "end-of-life" battery parameters on testing the pacemaker.

Several measures are taken to prevent or assess for complications and include prophylactic IV antibiotic therapy before and after insertion, postinsertion chest x-ray to check lead placement and to rule out the presence of a pneumothorax, careful observation of insertion site, and continuous ECG monitoring of the patient's rhythm. After pacemaker insertion, the patient is permitted out of bed once stable. Arm and shoulder activity is limited to prevent dislodgement of the newly implanted pacing leads. The nurse observes the insertion site for signs of bleeding and to check that the incision is intact. Any temperature elevation should be noted and pain at the insertion site should be treated. Most patients are discharged the next day if stable.

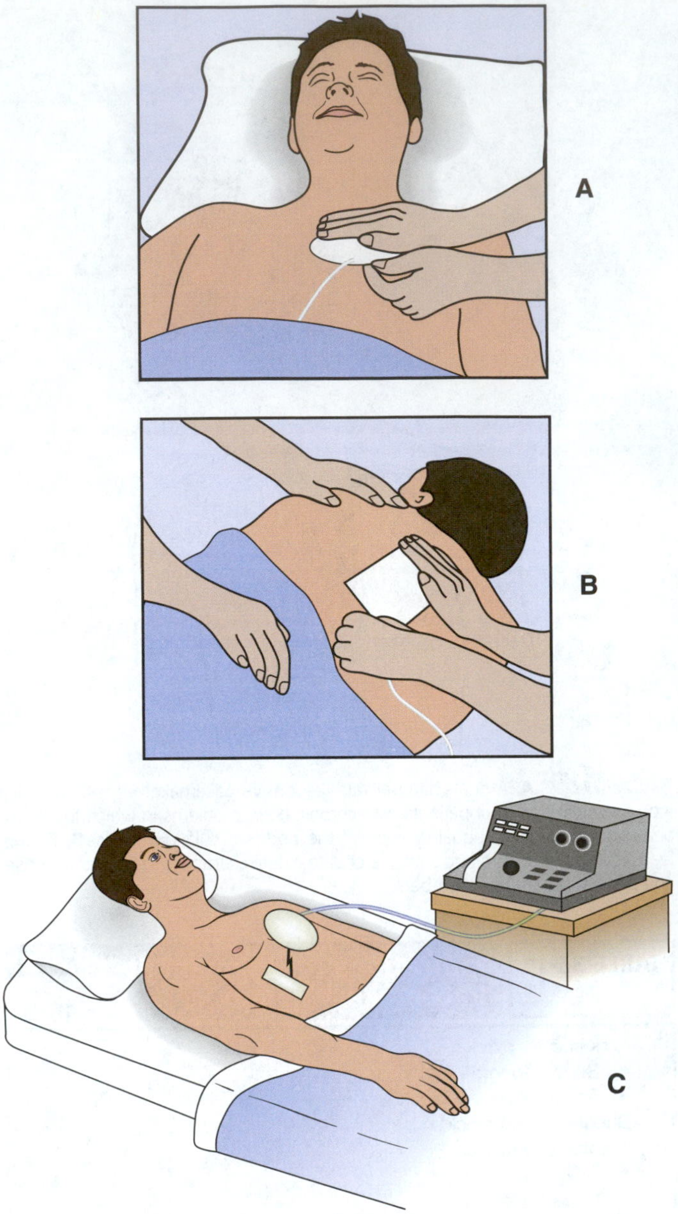

FIG. 36-27 Transcutaneous pacemaker. Pacing electrodes are placed on the patient's anterior **(A)** and posterior **(B)** chest walls and attached to an external pacing unit **(C)**.

The nurse must provide patient teaching in addition to observation for complications after pacemaker insertion. The patient with a newly implanted pacemaker may have questions about activity restrictions and fears concerning body image after the procedure. The goal of pacemaker therapy should be to enhance physiologic functioning and the quality of life. This should be emphasized to the patient, and the nurse should give specific advice on activity restrictions. Patient and family teaching for the patient with a pacemaker is outlined in Table 36-12.

TABLE 36-12 PATIENT AND FAMILY TEACHING GUIDE
Pacemaker

1. Maintain follow-up care with your primary care provider to check the pacemaker site and begin regular pacemaker function checks.
2. Report any signs of infection at incision site (e.g., redness, swelling, drainage) or fever to your primary care provider immediately.
3. Keep incision dry for 4 days after implantation.
4. Avoid lifting arm on pacemaker side above shoulder until approved by your primary care provider.
5. Avoid direct blows to pacemaker site.
6. Avoid close proximity to high-output electric generators or large magnets such as an MRI scanner. These devices can interfere with the function of the pacemaker.
7. Microwave ovens are safe to use and do not interfere with pacemaker function.
8. Travel without restrictions is allowed. The small metal case of an implanted pacemaker rarely sets off an airport security alarm.
9. Monitor pulse and inform primary care provider if it drops below predetermined rate.
10. Carry pacemaker information card at all times.
11. A Medic Alert ID or bracelet should be worn at all times.

MRI, Magnetic resonance imaging.

After discharge, pacemaker function is checked on a regular basis. This can include outpatient visits to a pacemaker interrogator/programmer, or home monitoring using telephone transmitter devices. Another method to evaluate pacemaker performance is noninvasive program stimulation. This procedure is done on an outpatient basis in the electrophysiology lab.

Radiofrequency Catheter Ablation Therapy

Radiofrequency catheter ablation therapy is a relatively new development in the area of antidysrhythmia therapy. Radiofrequency energy (produced by a low-voltage, high-frequency form of electrical energy) is used to "burn" or ablate areas of the conduction system as definitive treatment of tachydysrhythmias.

Ablation therapy is done after EPS has identified the source of the dysrhythmia. An electrode-tipped ablation catheter is used to "burn" or ablate accessory pathways or ectopic sites in the atria, AV node, and ventricles. Catheter ablation is considered the nonpharmacologic treatment of choice for AV nodal reentrant tachycardia or for reentrant tachycardia related to accessory bypass tracts, and to control the ventricular response of certain tachydysrhythmias. In some cases of uncontrolled ventricular response in atrial fibrillation or flutter that is unresponsive to medical therapy, complete ablation of the AV node or bundle of His may be performed. When this is done, the patient must have a permanent pacemaker inserted at the same time.[14]

The ablation procedure is a successful therapy with a low complication rate. Care of the patient following ablation therapy is similar to that of a patient undergoing cardiac catheterization (see Chapter 32).

ECG CHANGES ASSOCIATED WITH ACUTE CORONARY SYNDROME

The 12-lead ECG is the primary diagnostic tool used to evaluate patients presenting with ACS. Many treatment decisions are directed by the ECG changes that occur with ACS. These definitive changes are in response to ischemia, injury, or infarction of myocardial cells and will be seen in the leads that face the area of involvement (Fig. 36-28). Reciprocal (opposite) ECG changes will often be seen in the leads facing opposite the area involved in ACS. Additionally, the pattern of ECG changes will provide information on the coronary artery involved in ACS (Table 36-13).

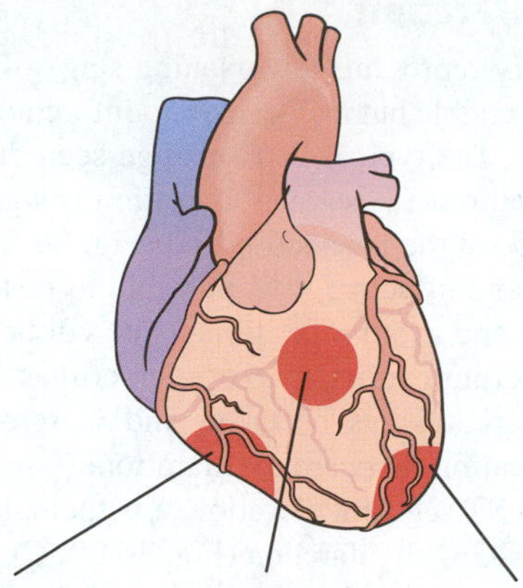

FIG. 36-28 Definitive ECG changes occur in leads that face the area of ischemia, injury, or infarction. Reciprocal changes may occur in leads facing opposite the area of ischemia, injury, or infarction.

TABLE 36-13 ECG Evidence and Associated Coronary Artery in Acute Coronary Syndrome

Area of Involvement of Left Ventricle	ECG Evidence: Leads Facing Area	ECG Evidence: Leads Opposite Area	Associated Coronary Artery
Septal wall	V_1, V_2	II, III, aVF	Left anterior descending
Anterior wall	V_2–V_4	II, III, aVF	Left anterior descending
Lateral wall, low	V_5, V_6	II, III, aVF	Left anterior descending or circumflex
Lateral wall, high	I, aVL	II, III, aVF	Circumflex
Inferior wall	II, III, aVF	I, aVL, V_5, V_6	Right coronary artery

ECG, Electrocardiographic.

Ischemia

Typical ECG changes that are seen in myocardial ischemia include ST segment depression and/or T wave inversion (Fig. 36-29, *A*). ST segment depression is significant if it is at least 1 mm (one small box) below the isoelectric line (see Fig. 36-5). The isoelectric line is flat and represents those normal times in the cardiac cycle when the ECG is not recording any electrical activity in the heart. These times are as follows: (1) from the end of the P wave to the start of the QRS complex, (2) the entire ST segment, and (3) from the end of the T wave to the start of the next P wave (see Fig. 36-9). Depression in the ST segment and/or T wave inversion occurs in response to the electrical disturbance in the myocardial cells due to an inadequate supply of blood and oxygen. Once treated (adequate blood flow is restored), the ECG changes will resolve, and the ECG will return to the patient's baseline. (See Chapter 34 for a complete discussion of ACS.)

Injury and Infarction

Myocardial injury represents a worsening stage of ischemia that is potentially reversible but may evolve to infarction (necrosis) of myocardial cells. The typical ECG change seen during injury is ST segment elevation. ST segment elevation is significant if it is at least 1 mm above the isoelectric line (Fig. 36-29, *B*). If treatment is prompt and effective, it is possible to restore oxygen to the myocardium and avoid infarction. This will be confirmed by the absence of serum cardiac markers. If serum cardiac markers are present, infarction has occurred and is referred to as an ST-segment–elevation myocardial infarction.

In addition to ST segment elevation, a pathologic Q wave may be seen on the ECG with infarction (Fig. 36-29, *C*). A physiologic Q wave is the first negative deflection (wave) following the P wave (see Fig. 36-9). It is normally very small and narrow (<0.04 second in duration). A pathologic Q wave that may develop during infarction will be deep and >0.03 second in duration. If it does appear, it indicates that at least half the thickness of the heart wall is involved, which is referred to as a Q wave MI.[8] The pathologic Q wave may be present on the ECG indefinitely.

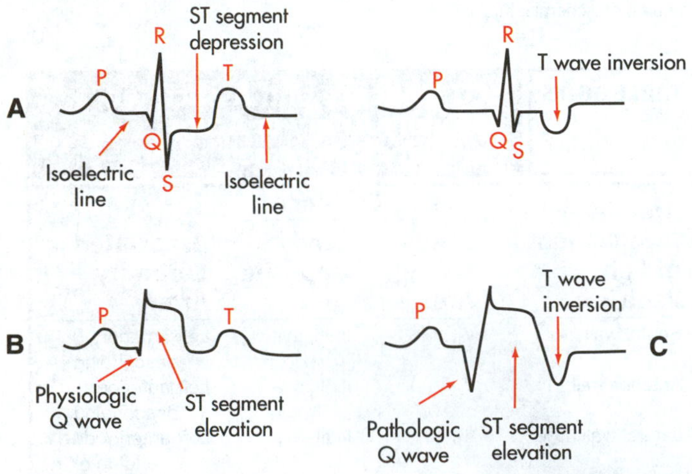

FIG. 36-29 ST segment, T wave, and Q wave changes associated with myocardial ischemia **(A),** injury **(B),** and infarction **(C).**

T wave inversion related to infarction occurs within hours following an infarction and may persist for months. The ECG changes seen in injury and infarction reflect electrical disturbances in the myocardial cells due to a prolonged lack of blood and oxygen leading to necrosis (Fig. 36-30).

Patient Monitoring

Monitoring guidelines for patients with suspected ACS include continuous, multilead ECG and ST segment monitoring.[5,6] The leads selected for monitoring should minimally include the leads that reflect the area of ischemia, injury, or infarction.

SYNCOPE

Syncope, a brief lapse in consciousness accompanied by a loss in postural tone (fainting), is a common diagnosis of patients coming into the emergency department and hospital. The causes of syncope can be categorized as cardiovascular or noncardiovascular. The most common cardiovascular causes of syncope include (1) neurocardiogenic syncope or "vasovagal" syncope (e.g., carotid sinus sensitivity) and (2) primary cardiac dysrhythmias (e.g., tachycardias, bradycardias). Others causes can be related to prosthetic valve malfunction, pulmonary emboli, aortic dissection, and hypertrophic cardiomyopathy. Noncardiovascular causes are varied and can include hypoglycemia, hysteria, unwitnessed seizure, and vertebrobasilar transient ischemic attack.[8]

A diagnostic workup for a patient with syncope from a suspected cardiac cause begins with ruling out structural and/or ischemic heart disease. This is done with echocardiography and stress testing. In the older patient, who is more likely to have ischemic and structural heart disease, EPS is used to diagnose atrial and ventricular tachydysrhythmias, as well as conduction system

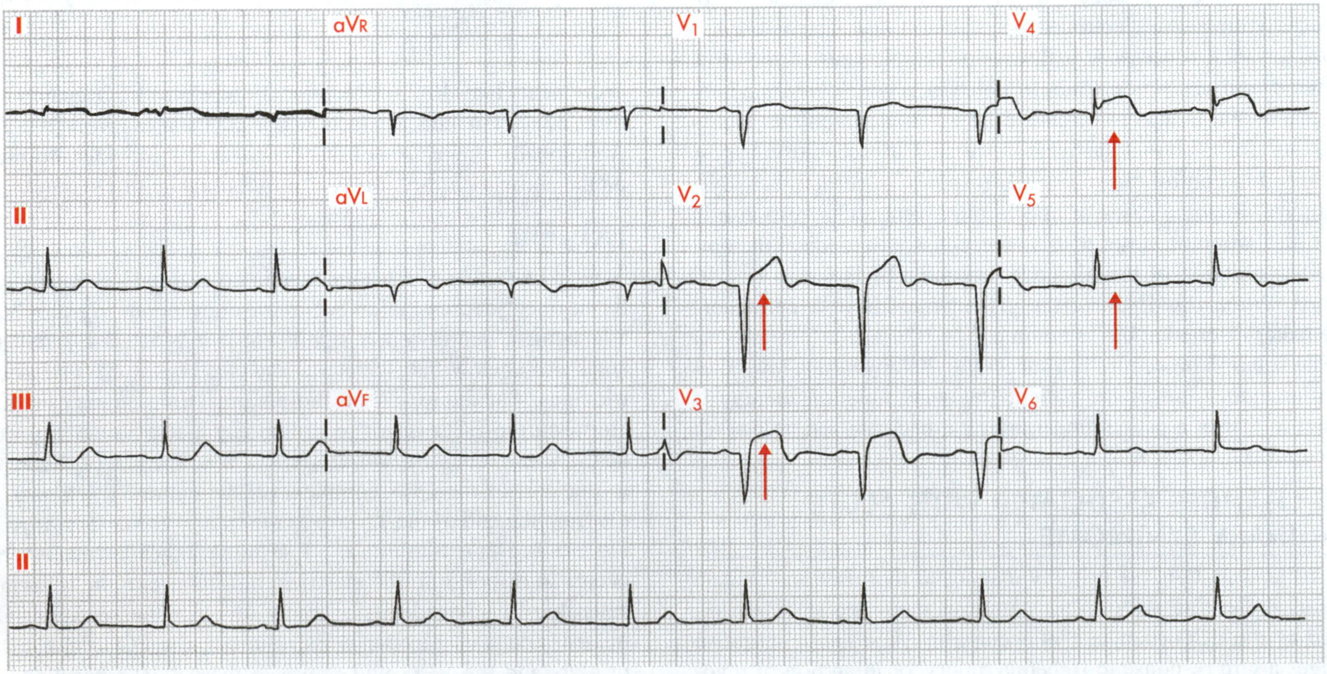

FIG. 36-30 ECG findings with anterolateral wall myocardial infarction. Note the pathologic Q waves in leads V_1 to V_3, I, and aVL, and the ST-segment–elevation in leads V_2 to V_5 *(arrows).*

disease causing bradydysrhythmias, all of which can cause syncope. These problems can be treated with antidysrhythmia drug therapy, pacemakers, ICDs, and/or catheter ablation therapy.

In patients without structural heart disease or in whom EPS testing is not diagnostic, *head-upright tilt-table testing* may be performed. Normally, an upright position results in gravity displacing 300 to 800 ml of blood to the lower extremities. Specialized nerve fibers called mechanoreceptors are located throughout the vascular system. These receptors respond to the increased blood volume by initiating a reflex increase in sympathetic stimulation and decrease in parasympathetic output. The end results are a slight increase in HR and diastolic BP, and a slight decrease in systolic BP.

In neurocardiogenic syncope, the increase in venous pooling that occurs in the upright position reduces venous return to the heart. This results in a sudden, compensatory increase in ventricular contraction. This is misinterpreted by the brain as a hypertensive state and consequently sympathetic stimulation is withdrawn. This produces a paradoxic vasodilation and bradycardia (vasovagal response). The end results are bradycardia, hypotension, cerebral hypoperfusion, and syncope.

In the head-upright tilt-table test, the patient is placed on a table supported by a belt across the torso and feet. Baseline ECG, BP, and HR are obtained in the horizontal position. Next, the table is tilted 60 to 80 degrees and the patient is maintained in this upright position 20 to 60 minutes. ECG and HR are recorded continuously and BP is measured every 3 minutes throughout the test. In healthy individuals, venous pooling activates the mechanoreceptors, resulting in the normal response described above.

If the patient's BP and HR responses are abnormal and clinical symptoms are reproduced (e.g., faintness), the test is considered positive. If after 30 minutes there is no response, the table is returned to the horizontal position and an intravenous infusion of low-dose isoproterenol may be started in an attempt to provoke a response. Neurocardiogenic syncope that recurs frequently and interferes with normal activities can be treated with a variety of drugs (e.g., metoprolol).

Other diagnostic tests for syncope include various recording devices. Holter monitors and event monitors are used, and are discussed in this chapter and Chapter 32. A subcutaneously implanted loop recording device can also be used to record the ECG during presyncopal and syncopal events. The device can be interrogated after a syncopal event in order to determine the ECG rhythm at the time to the event. For patients with a cardiovascular cause of syncope, the 1-year mortality rate can be as high as 30%.[8]

CRITICAL THINKING EXERCISE

CASE STUDY

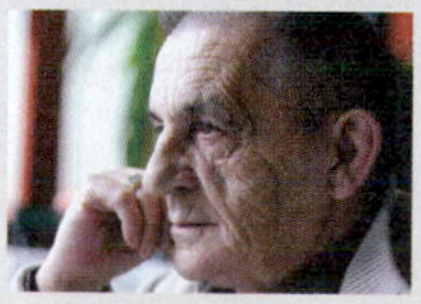

Case Study photo ©iStockphoto.com/ Joseph Jean Rolland Dubé.

Dysrhythmia

Patient Profile. J.M., a 68-year-old retired white postal worker, was admitted to the telemetry unit with a diagnosis of acute decompensated HF. He experienced a cardiac arrest (pulseless ventricular tachycardia) and was successfully defibrillated after one shock. He is transferred to the cardiac care unit. J.M. is awake but lethargic, and responds appropriately to questions.

Subjective Data
- History of two MIs and HF
- Reports shortness of breath, even in a sitting position

Objective Data

Physical Examination
- Appears weak, anxious
- BP 102/60, pulse 50/minute, respirations 26/minute
- Lungs: bilateral coarse crackles in the bases
- Heart: S_3 gallop at apex

Diagnostic Studies
- Continuous ECG monitoring

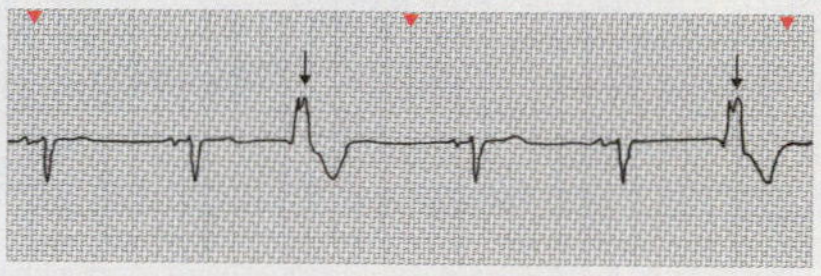

- Echocardiogram: severe left ventricular dysfunction with ejection fraction of 30%
- Serum potassium: 2.9 mEq/L (2.9 mmol/L)
- Serum cardiac markers: negative
- Serum b-type natriuretic peptide (BNP): 852 pg/ml

Collaborative Care
- amiodarone (Cordarone) infusion
- Scheduled for electrophysiologic study (EPS)

Critical Thinking Questions

1. Why is J.M. at risk for sudden cardiac death?
2. Explain the rationale for using amiodarone after cardiac arrest.
3. What methods may be used to assess the effectiveness of the antidysrhythmia therapy?
4. Interpret the rhythm strip and explain the significance of the other diagnostic studies.
5. Would J.M. be a candidate for CRT-ICD? Why or why not?
6. Based on the assessment data provided, write one or more priority nursing diagnoses.

NCLEX EXAMINATION REVIEW QUESTIONS

The number of the question corresponds to the same-numbered objective at the beginning of the chapter.

1. A patient admitted with ACS has continuous ECG monitoring. An examination of the rhythm strip reveals the following characteristics: atrial rate—74 and regular; ventricular rate—62 and irregular; P wave—normal shape; PR interval—lengthens progressively until a P wave is not conducted; QRS—normal shape. Nursing management would involve
   a. epinephrine 1 mg IV push.
   b. elective synchronized cardioversion.
   c. immediate insertion of a temporary pacemaker.
   d. careful observation for symptoms of hypotension or angina.
2. The nurse is monitoring the ECG of a patient admitted with ACS. Which of the following ECG characteristics would be most suggestive of ischemia?
   a. Sinus rhythm with a pathologic Q wave.
   b. Sinus rhythm with an elevated ST segment.
   c. Sinus rhythm with a depressed ST segment.
   d. Sinus rhythm with premature atrial contractions.
3. The ECG monitor of a patient in the cardiac care unit following an MI indicates ventricular bigeminy. The nurse anticipates
   a. performing defibrillation.
   b. treatment with IV lidocaine.
   c. insertion of a temporary pacemaker.
   d. assessing the patient's response to the dysrhythmia.

4. The nurse prepares a patient for synchronized cardioversion knowing that cardioversion differs from defibrillation in that
   a. defibrillation requires lower dose of electrical energy.
   b. cardioversion is only indicated for treatment of atrial bradydysrhythmias.
   c. defibrillation is synchronized to deliver a shock during the QRS complex.
   d. cardioversion may be done on a nonemergency basis with sedation of the patient.
5. When providing discharge instructions to a patient with a new permanent pacemaker, the nurse teaches the patient to
   a. take and record a daily pulse rate.
   b. request special hand scanning at airport and other security gates.
   c. immobilize the arm and shoulder on the side of the pacemaker insertion for 6 weeks.
   d. avoid microwave ovens because they emit radio waves that interfere with pacemaker function.
6. The nurse plans care for the patient with an implantable cardioverter-defibrillator based on the knowledge that
   a. antidysrhythmia drugs will be discontinued.
   b. all members of the patient's family should learn CPR.
   c. the patient should not drive until 1 week after the ICD has been implanted.
   d. the patient is usually relieved to have the device implanted to prevent dysrhythmias.
7. Important teaching for the patient scheduled for a diagnostic electrophysiologic study includes explaining that
   a. ventricular tachycardia may be induced and treated during the procedure.
   b. a catheter will be placed in each of the femoral arteries to allow double-catheter use.
   c. the patient will be given a general anesthetic to prevent the awareness of "sudden cardiac death" experiences.
   d. the procedure is used to "burn" or ablate areas of the conduction system that are causing bradydysrhythmias.

REFERENCES

1. Conover MB: *Understanding electrocardiography,* ed 8, St Louis, 2003, Mosby.
2. Huszar RJ: *Basic dysrhythmias: interpretation and management,* ed 3, St Louis, 2002, Mosby.
3. Atwood S, Stanton C, Storey-Davenport J: *Introduction to basic cardiac dysrhythmias,* ed 3, St Louis, 2003, MosbyJems.
4. Drake RL, Vogl W, Mitchell AWM: *Gray's anatomy for students,* Philadelphia, 2005, Elsevier.
5. Drew BJ, Califf RM, Funk M, et al: Practice standards for electrocardiographic monitoring in hospital settings, *Circulation* 110:2721, 2004.
6. Drew BJ: Celebrating the 100th birthday of the electrocardiogram: lessons learned from research in cardiac monitoring, *Am J Crit Care* 11:378, 2002.
7. American Heart Association: *Handbook of emergency cardiovascular care for healthcare providers,* Dallas, 2002, American Heart Association.
8. Woods SL, Froelicher ES, Motzer SU, et al: *Cardiac nursing,* ed 5, Philadelphia, 2005, Lippincott Williams & Wilkins.
9. Greenberg ML, Chandrakantan A: Radiofrequency catheter ablation. New York, 2006, eMedicine. Available at *www.emedicine.com/med/topic2957.htm* (accessed September 22, 2005).
10. Snow V, Weiss KB, LeFevre M, et al: Management of newly detected atrial fibrillation: a clinical practice guideline from the American Academy of Family Physicians and the American College of Physicians, *Ann Intern Med* 139:1009, 2003.
11. McNamara RL, Tamariz LJ, Segal JB, et al: Management of atrial fibrillation: review of the evidence for the role of pharmacologic therapy, electrical cardioversion, and echocardiography, *Ann Intern Med* 139:1018, 2003.
12. Zimetbaum P, Josephson ME: Is there a role for maintaining sinus rhythm in patients with atrial fibrillation? *Ann Intern Med* 141:720, 2004.
13. Bahnson TD, Grant AO: To be or not to be in normal sinus rhythm: what do we really know? *Ann Intern Med* 141:727, 2004.
14. Abramowicz M, editor: Catheter ablation of atrial fibrillation, *Med Lett* 46:59, 2004.
15. Nakajima H, Kobayashi J, Bando K, et al: Effect of cryo-maze procedure on early and intermediate term outcomes in mitral valve disease: case matched study, *Circulation* 106(suppl I):1-46, 2002.
16. Lehne RA: *Pharmacology for nursing care,* ed 6, St Louis, 2007, Saunders.
17. Bardy G, Marchlinski F, Sharma A: Multicenter comparison of truncated biphasic shocks and standard damped sine wave monophasic shocks for transthoracic ventricular defibrillation, *Circulation* 94:2507, 1996.
18. Tang W, Weil MH, Sun S, et al: The effects of biphasic waveform design on post-resuscitation myocardial function, *J Am Coll Cardiol* 43:1228, 2004.
19. Gregoratos G, Abrams J, Epstein AE, et al: ACC/AHA/NASPE 2002 guideline update for implantation of cardiac pacemakers and antiarrhythmia devices: summary article, *Circulation* 106:2145, 2002.

RESOURCES

Additional resources for this chapter are listed after Chapter 34 on page 820 and Chapter 35 on page 841.

What happens is not as important as how you react to what happens.

Thaddeus Golas

Nursing Management Inflammatory and Structural Heart Disorders

37

Nancy Stoetzner Kupper and De Ann Mitchell

LEARNING OBJECTIVES

1. Describe the etiology, pathophysiology, and clinical manifestations of infective endocarditis and pericarditis.
2. Discuss the collaborative care and nursing management of the patient with infective endocarditis and pericarditis.
3. Explain the importance of prophylactic antibiotic therapy in infective endocarditis.
4. Explain the etiology, clinical manifestations, collaborative care, and nursing management of myocarditis.
5. Describe the etiology, pathophysiology, and clinical manifestations of rheumatic fever and rheumatic heart disease.
6. Discuss the collaborative care and nursing management of the patient with rheumatic fever and rheumatic heart disease.
7. Identify the etiologies of acquired valvular heart diseases.
8. Discuss the pathophysiology, clinical manifestations, and diagnostic studies for the various types of valvular heart disease.
9. Describe the collaborative care and nursing management of the patient with valvular heart disease.
10. Describe interventions used in management of the patient with valvular heart disease.
11. Describe the pathophysiology and clinical manifestations of the different types of cardiomyopathies.
12. Discuss the nursing and collaborative management of patients with different types of cardiomyopathies.

KEY TERMS

aortic stenosis, p. 880
aortic valve regurgitation, p. 880
Aschoff's bodies, p. 876
cardiac tamponade, p. 872
cardiomyopathy, p. 885
dilated cardiomyopathy, p. 886
hypertrophic cardiomyopathy, p. 888
infective endocarditis, p. 865
Janeway's lesions, p. 867
mitral valve prolapse, p. 879
myocarditis, p. 874
Osler's nodes, p. 867
pericardial effusion, p. 872
pericardial friction rub, p. 872
pericardiocentesis, p. 873
pericarditis, p. 871
regurgitation, p. 878
rheumatic fever, p. 875
rheumatic heart disease, p. 875

Electronic Resources

Supplemental content related to Chapter 37 can be found . . .

Companion CD

- Stress-Busting Kit for Nursing Students
- Interactive Case Study: Rheumatic Fever and Heart Disease
- NCLEX Examination Review Questions
- Audio Clip: Pericardial Friction Rub
- Comprehensive Glossary

Evolve Website
http://evolve.elsevier.com/Lewis/medsurg

- Content Updates
- Key Points (Printable and CD/MP3 Download)
- Concept Map Creator
- Expanded Audio Glossary
- Key Term Flash Cards
- Customizable Nursing Care Plans:
  - Infective Endocarditis
  - Valvular Heart Disease
- Electronic Calculators
- WebLinks

Inflammatory Disorders of the Heart

INFECTIVE ENDOCARDITIS

Infective endocarditis, previously known as *bacterial endocarditis,* is an infection of the endocardial surface of the heart. The *endocardium,* the innermost layer of the heart (Fig. 37-1), is contiguous with the valves of the heart. Therefore inflammation from infective endocarditis (IE) affects the cardiac valves.

Treatment of IE with penicillin therapy has improved the prognosis of this disease. For example, the mortality rate of IE from *Streptococcus viridans* is less than 10%. In spite of the relatively uncommon nature of the disease, an estimated 15,000 new cases of

Reviewed by Angela J. DiSabatino, RN, MS, Manager, Cardiovascular Research, Christiana Care Health Services, Newark, Del; and Joyce E. Wenger, RN, MSN, CCRN, Cardiothoracic Surgery Nurse Clinician, Lancaster General Hospital, Lancaster, Pa.

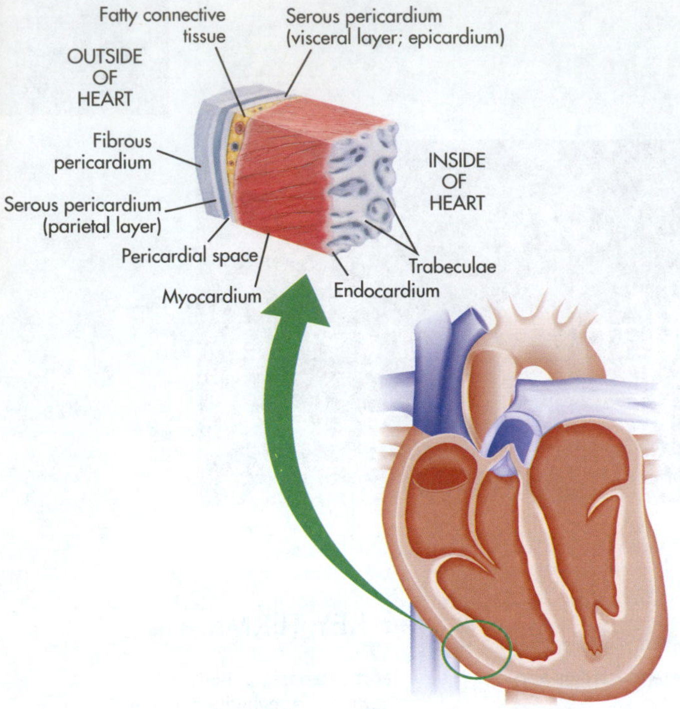

FIG. 37-1 Layers of the heart muscle and pericardium. The section of the heart wall shows the fibrous pericardium, the parietal and visceral layers of the serous pericardium (with the pericardial sac between them), the myocardium, and the endocardium.

IE are diagnosed in the United States each year, with similar numbers reported worldwide.[1]

Classification

Two forms of IE, subacute and acute, have been described. The *subacute form* typically affects those with preexisting valve disease and has a clinical course that may extend over months. In contrast, the *acute form* typically affects those with healthy valves and presents as a rapidly progressive illness. Although this classification system has been used historically, clinicians prefer to classify IE based on the cause (e.g., intravenous drug abuse IE [IVDA IE], fungal endocarditis) or site of involvement (e.g., prosthetic valve endocarditis [PVE]).

Etiology and Pathophysiology

The most common causative organisms of IE, *Staphylococcus aureus* and *Streptococcus viridans,* are bacterial (Table 37-1). Other possible pathogens include fungi and viruses. Newly identified pathogens, which are difficult to cultivate (e.g., *Bartonella, Tropheryma whipplei*), have been found to cause IE. Resistant organisms (e.g., methicillin-resistant *Staphylococcus aureus*) also cause IE and are challenging conventional antibiotic therapy.[2]

IE occurs when blood flow turbulence within the heart allows the causative organism to infect previously damaged valves or other endothelial surfaces. This can occur in individuals with a variety of underlying cardiac conditions. The principal risk factors for IE are prior endocarditis, prosthetic valves, acquired valvular disease, and cardiac lesions. Several noncardiac conditions and procedures also can allow large numbers of organisms to enter the bloodstream and initiate the infectious process (Tables 37-2 and 37-3).

TABLE 37-1 Etiologic Organisms Associated with Infective Endocarditis

Bacteria
- *Bartonella quintana*
- Chlamydiae
- Coagulase-negative staphylococci
- Enterococci
- HACEK group *(Haemophilus, Actinobacillus, Cardiobacterium, Eikenella, Kingella)*
- Methicillin-resistant *Staphylococcus aureus*
- Rickettsiae
- *Staphylococcus aureus*
- *Staphylococcus epidermidis*
- *Streptococcus bovis*
- *Streptococcus* groups A, B, and C
- *Streptococcus pneumoniae*
- *Streptococcus viridans*
- *Tropheryma whipplei*

Fungi
- Candida albicans
- Candida parapsilosis

Viruses
- Coxsackie B virus

TABLE 37-2 Predisposing Conditions for the Development of Infective Endocarditis

Cardiac Conditions
- Prior endocarditis
- Prosthetic valves
- Acquired valve disease (e.g., mitral valve prolapse with murmur, calcified aortic stenosis)
- Cardiac lesions (e.g., ventricular septal defect)
- Rheumatic heart disease (e.g., mitral valve regurgitation)
- Congenital heart disease
- Pacemakers
- Marfan syndrome
- Asymmetric septal hypertrophy
- Cardiomyopathy

Noncardiac Conditions
- Intravenous drug abuse
- Nosocomial bacteremia

Procedure-Associated Risks
- Intravascular devices (e.g., pulmonary artery catheters)
- Procedures listed in Table 37-3

Vegetations, the primary lesions of IE, consist of fibrin, leukocytes, platelets, and microbes that adhere to the valve surface or endocardium (Fig. 37-2). The loss of portions of these friable vegetations into the circulation results in *embolization.* As many as 22% to 50% of patients with IE will experience systemic embolization. This occurs from left-sided heart vegetation, progressing to various organs (particularly the brain, kidneys, and spleen) and to the extremities, causing limb infarction. Right-sided heart lesions embolize to the lungs.

The infection may spread locally to cause damage to the valves or to their supporting structures. This results in dysrhythmias, valvular incompetence, and eventual invasion of the myocardium, leading to heart failure (HF), sepsis, and heart block (Fig. 37-3).

TABLE 37-3 Procedures Requiring Antibiotic Prophylaxis to Prevent Endocarditis*

Oropharyngeal
- All dental procedures likely to produce gingival or mucosal bleeding (not simple adjustment of orthodontic appliances or shedding of deciduous teeth), including professional cleaning
- Tonsillectomy or adenoidectomy

Respiratory
- Surgical procedures or biopsy involving respiratory mucosa
- Bronchoscopy, especially with a rigid bronchoscope

Gastrointestinal
- Abdominal surgeries involving intestinal mucosa
- Esophageal dilation
- Sclerotherapy of esophageal varices
- Upper endoscopy, colonoscopy, and sigmoidoscopy

Genitourinary
- Cystoscopy
- Laparoscopy procedures
- Prostatic surgery

*This table lists selected procedures and is not all-inclusive.

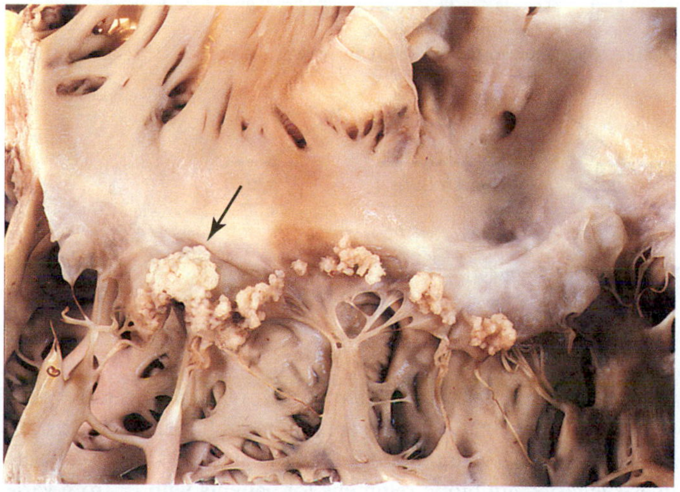

FIG. 37-2 Bacterial endocarditis of the mitral valve. The valve is covered with large, irregular vegetations *(arrow)*.

Rheumatic heart disease was, at one time, the most common cause of IE; it now accounts for <20% of cases. Currently, the main contributing factors include (1) aging (>50% of older people have calcified aortic stenosis); (2) IVDA; (3) use of prosthetic valves; (4) proliferation of intravascular device placement, resulting in nosocomial infections; and (5) renal dialysis.[3] Left-sided endocarditis is more common in patients with bacterial infections and underlying heart disease. The primary cause of right-sided endocarditis is IVDA. However, there has been an increase in left-sided valves being affected, especially with cocaine abuse. *S. aureus* is the most common etiologic organism in IVDA IE.

Clinical Manifestations

The findings in IE are nonspecific and can involve multiple organ systems. Low-grade fever occurs in more than 90% of patients. Other nonspecific manifestations include chills, weakness, malaise, fatigue, and anorexia. Arthralgias, myalgias, back pain, abdominal discomfort, weight loss, headache, and clubbing of fingers may occur in subacute forms of endocarditis.

Vascular manifestations of IE include *splinter hemorrhages* (black longitudinal streaks) that may occur in the nail beds. Petechiae may occur as a result of fragmentation and microembolization of vegetative lesions and are common in the conjunctivae, the lips, the buccal mucosa, and the palate and over the ankles, the feet, and the antecubital and popliteal areas. **Osler's nodes** (painful, tender, red or purple, pea-size lesions) may be found on the fingertips or toes. **Janeway's lesions** (flat, painless, small, red spots) may be found on the palms and soles. Funduscopic examination may reveal hemorrhagic retinal lesions called *Roth's spots*.

The onset of a new or changing murmur is noted in most patients with IE, with the aortic and mitral valves most commonly affected. The mitral murmur of endocarditis is generally a mid- to late systolic regurgitant type. The aortic murmur may be early diastolic. Murmurs are often absent in tricuspid endocarditis because right-sided heart pressures are too low to be heard. HF occurs in up to 80% of patients with aortic valve endocarditis and in approximately 50% of patients with mitral valve endocarditis.[4]

Clinical manifestations secondary to embolization in various body organs may also be present. Embolization to the spleen may result in sharp, left upper quadrant pain and splenomegaly. Local tenderness and abdominal rigidity may be present. Embolization to the kidneys may cause pain in the flank, hematuria, and azotemia. Emboli may lodge in small peripheral blood vessels of arms and legs and may cause gangrene. Embolization to the brain may cause neurologic damage resulting in hemiplegia, ataxia, aphasia, visual changes, and change in the level of consciousness. Pulmonary emboli may occur in right-sided endocarditis.

Diagnostic Studies

The patient's recent health history is important in assessing IE. Inquiry should be made regarding any recent (within the past 3 to 6 months) dental, urologic, surgical, or gynecologic procedures, including normal or abnormal obstetric delivery. Previous history of IVDA, heart disease, recent cardiac catheterization, cardiac surgery, intravascular device placement, renal dialysis, or infections (e.g., skin, respiratory, urinary tract) should be documented.

Laboratory data, especially blood cultures, should also be assessed. Two blood cultures drawn 30 minutes apart will be positive in more than 90% of patients. Culture-negative endocarditis is often associated with antibiotic usage within the previous 2 weeks, or due to a pathogen not easily detected by standard culture procedures (e.g., *Bartonella* species). Negative cultures should be kept for 3 weeks if the clinical diagnosis remains endocarditis because of the possibility of a slow-growing, causative organism.

A mild leukocytosis occurs in acute endocarditis (uncommon in subacute), with average white blood cell (WBC) counts ranging from 10,000 to 11,000/µl (10 to 11 $\times 10^9$/L). Erythrocyte sedimentation rate (ESR) and C-reactive protein (CRP) levels may be elevated.

Major criteria to diagnose IE have been established by Duke University Medical Center and include at least two of the following: positive blood cultures, new or changed cardiac murmur, or intracardiac mass or vegetation noted on echocardiography.[5] Echocardiography is valuable in the diagnostic workup for a patient with IE when the blood cultures are negative, or for the patient who is a surgical candidate and has an active infection. Trans-

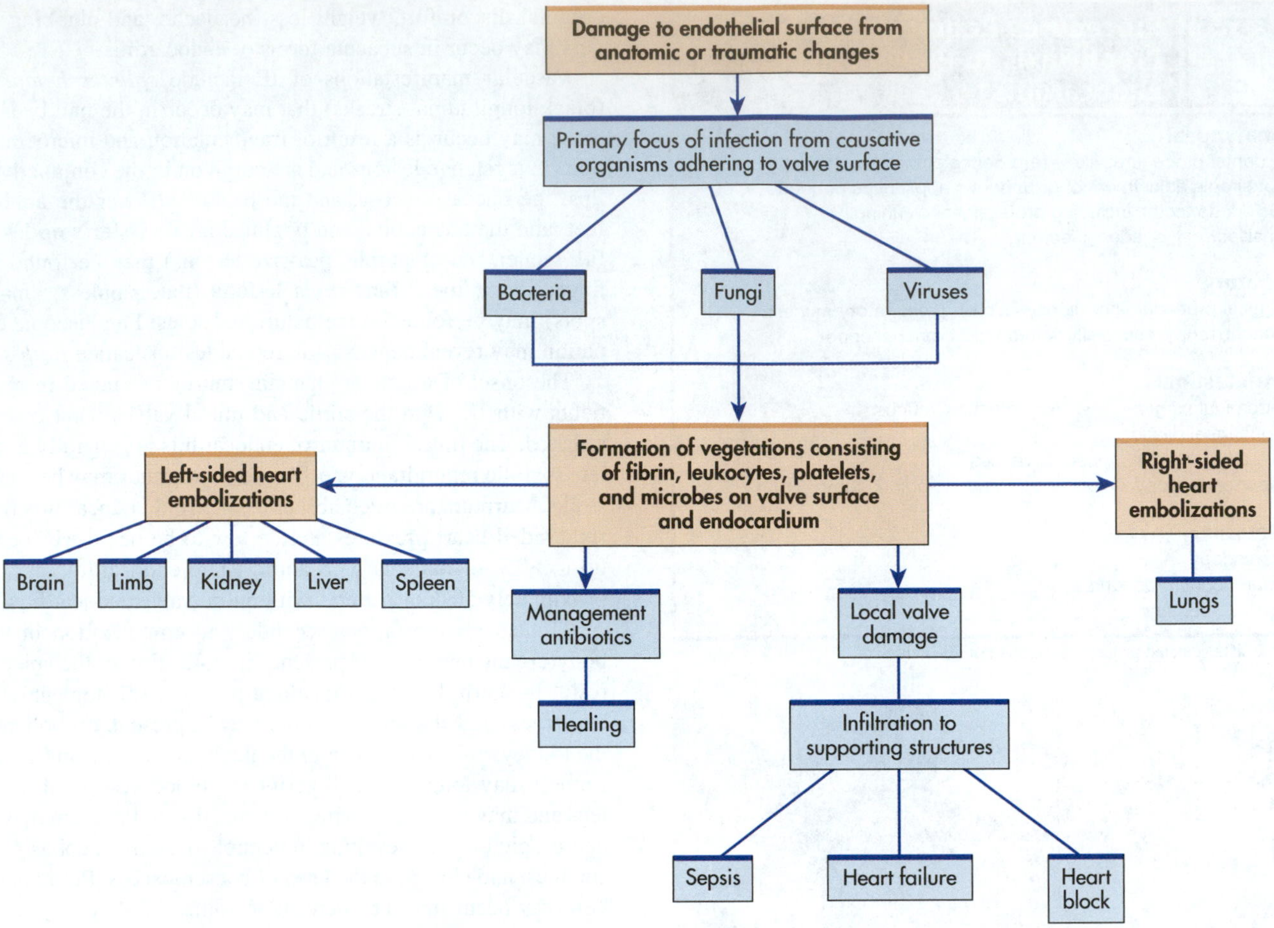

FIG. 37-3 Sequence of events in infective endocarditis.

esophageal echocardiograms and digital imaging using two- or three-dimensional transthoracic echocardiograms can detect vegetation on valves.[6]

A chest x-ray examination is done to detect the presence of *cardiomegaly* (an enlarged heart). An electrocardiogram (ECG) may show first- or second-degree atrioventricular (AV) block because the cardiac valves lie in proximity to cardiac conductive tissue, especially the AV node. Cardiac catheterization may be used to evaluate valve functioning and to assess the status of the coronary arteries when surgical intervention is being considered for patients with IE.

Collaborative Care

Prophylactic Treatment. Antibiotic prophylaxis is recommended for patients with specific cardiac conditions before they undergo certain procedures[7] (Table 37-4). Procedures that require endocarditis prophylaxis are summarized in Table 37-3. Specific antibiotic regimens are recommended for dental, respiratory tract, gastrointestinal (GI), and genitourinary (GU) procedures. Antibiotic prophylaxis should also be used for high-risk patients who (1) are to undergo removal or drainage of infected tissue, (2) receive renal dialysis, or (3) have ventriculoatrial shunts for management of hydrocephalus.[8]

Drug Therapy. Accurate identification of the infecting organism is the key to successful treatment of IE. Long-term treatment is necessary to kill dormant bacteria clustered within the valvular vegetations. Complete eradication of the organism generally takes weeks to achieve, and relapses are common. Initially, patients are hospitalized and IV antibiotic therapy is started. Table 37-5 outlines suggested antibiotic regimens for patients with IE from various organisms and with different clinical situations.[5]

Subsequent blood cultures may be performed to evaluate the effectiveness of antibiotic therapy. Blood cultures that remain positive indicate inadequate or inappropriate antibiotic administration, aortic root or myocardial abscess, or the wrong diagnosis (e.g., an infection elsewhere). Serum antibiotic drug levels are often monitored to establish therapeutic doses. Finally, renal function is monitored to establish doses for antibiotics that are nephrotoxic (e.g., vancomycin [Vancocin]) and/or for patients with poor kidney function.

Fungal infection and PVE respond poorly to antibiotic therapy alone. Early valve replacement followed by prolonged (≥6 weeks) drug therapy is recommended in these situations.[5] Valve replacement has become an important adjunct procedure in the management of IE. It is used in more than 25% of cases. (Valve replacement is discussed later in this chapter.)

Fever may persist for several days after treatment has been started and can be treated with aspirin, acetaminophen (Tylenol), ibuprofen (Motrin), fluids, and rest. Complete bed rest is usually not indicated unless the temperature remains elevated or there are signs of HF. Endocarditis coupled with HF responds poorly to both drug therapy and valve replacement and is often life threatening.

TABLE 37-4 Cardiac and Noncardiac Conditions Requiring Antibiotic Prophylaxis to Prevent Infective Endocarditis*

Conditions Associated with Risk for Infective Endocarditis

High Risk†

- Prosthetic cardiac valves
- History of endocarditis
- Surgically constructed systemic-pulmonary shunts
- Complex cyanotic congenital heart disease
- Vascular grafts (first 6 mo after implantation)

Moderate Risk†

- Acquired valvular dysfunction
- Hypertrophic cardiomyopathy
- Mitral valve prolapse with valvular regeneration or thickened valves or both

Low/Negligible Risk†

- Vascular graft material (6 mo after implantation)
- Orthopedic prosthesis
- Central nervous system ventricular shunts
- Penile prosthesis
- Intraocular lens
- Pacemakers and implantable cardiac defibrillators
- Previous coronary bypass graft surgery
- Mitral valve prolapse without valvular degeneration
- Physiologic heart murmurs
- Previous rheumatic fever without valvular dysfunction
- Coronary stents

Sources: Horstkotte D, Follath F, Gutschik E, et al: Guidelines on the prevention, diagnosis, and treatment of infective endocarditis, *Eur Heart J* 25:267, 2004; and the American Heart Association available at *www.americanheart.org.*

*This table lists common conditions but is not all-inclusive.

†Only patients in the high- or moderate-risk groups require antibiotic prophylaxis. Patients in the low-risk group should be evaluated for antibiotic prophylaxis on an individual basis.

TABLE 37-5 *DRUG THERAPY* Treatment of Infective Endocarditis with Antibiotic Therapy*

Etiologic Agent	Antibiotic Regimen Options
Streptococcal endocarditis involving native valve	Intravenous (IV) penicillin G (Pfizerpen) or IV/intramuscular (IM) ceftriaxone (Rocephin); IV penicillin G or IV/IM ceftriaxone plus IV/IM gentamicin (Garamycin); or IV vancomycin (Vancocin)
Enterococcal endocarditis involving native or prosthetic valve	IV ampicillin (Omnipen); or IV penicillin G plus IV/IM gentamicin; or IV vancomycin plus IV/IM gentamicin
Staphylococcal endocarditis in absence of prosthetic materials	IV nafcillin (Nafcil) with optional IV gentamicin; or IV vancomycin
Fungal endocarditis in native or prosthetic valves	IV amphotericin B (Fungizone)

*This table lists common drug regimens but is not all-inclusive.

NURSING MANAGEMENT INFECTIVE ENDOCARDITIS

■ *Nursing Assessment*

Subjective and objective data that should be obtained from a patient with IE are presented in Table 37-6. Heart sounds should be assessed together with vital signs to detect a murmur or a change in the character of a preexisting murmur, and the presence of extradiastolic sounds. *Arthralgia* is common and may involve multiple joints, and may be accompanied by myalgias. The patient should be assessed for joint tenderness, decreased range of motion (ROM), and muscle tenderness. The oral mucosa, conjunctivae, upper chest, and lower extremities should be examined for petechiae. A general systems assessment should be completed to facilitate recognition of hemodynamic and embolic complications.

TABLE 37-6 *NURSING ASSESSMENT* Infective Endocarditis

Subjective Data

Important Health Information

Past health history: Valvular, congenital, or syphilitic cardiac disease (including valve repair or replacement); previous endocarditis, childbirth, staphylococcal or streptococcal infections, nosocomial bacteremia

Medications: Immunosuppressive therapy

Surgery or other treatments: Recent obstetric or gynecologic procedures; invasive techniques, including catheterization, cystoscopy, intravascular procedures; recent dental or surgical procedures, GI procedures (e.g., endoscopy, colonoscopy)

Functional Health Patterns

Health perception–health management: IV drug abuse, alcohol abuse; malaise

Nutritional-metabolic: Weight gain or loss; anorexia; chills, diaphoresis

Elimination: Bloody urine

Activity-exercise: Exercise intolerance, generalized weakness, fatigue; cough, dyspnea on exertion, orthopnea; palpitations

Sleep-rest: Night sweats

Cognitive-perceptual: Chest, back, or abdominal pain; headache; joint tenderness, muscle tenderness

Objective Data

General

Fever

Integumentary

Osler's nodes on extremities; splinter hemorrhages under nail beds; Janeway's lesions on palms and soles; petechiae of skin, mucous membranes, or conjunctivae; purpura; peripheral edema, finger clubbing

Respiratory

Tachypnea, crackles

Cardiovascular

Dysrhythmia, tachycardia, new or enhanced murmurs, S_3, S_4; retinal hemorrhages

Possible Findings

Leukocytosis, anemia, ↑ ESR, ↑ CRP and cardiac enzymes; positive blood cultures; microscopic hematuria; echocardiogram showing chamber enlargement, valvular dysfunction, and vegetations; chest x-ray showing cardiomegaly and pulmonary infiltrates; ECG demonstrating ischemia and conduction defects; signs of systemic embolization or pulmonary embolism

CRP, C-reactive protein; *ECG,* electrocardiogram; *ESR,* erythrocyte sedimentation rate, *GI,* gastrointestinal; *IV,* intravenous.

■ *Nursing Diagnoses*

Nursing diagnoses for the patient with IE may include, but are not limited to, those presented in NCP 37-1.

■ *Planning*

The overall goals for the patient with IE include (1) normal or baseline cardiac function, (2) performance of activities of daily living (ADLs) without fatigue, and (3) knowledge of the therapeutic regimen to prevent recurrence of endocarditis.

NURSING CARE PLAN 37-1

Patient with Infective Endocarditis

NURSING DIAGNOSIS **Hyperthermia** *related to* infection of cardiac tissue *as evidenced by* temperature elevation, diaphoresis, chills, malaise, tachycardia, tachypnea

PATIENT GOAL Maintains normal body temperature

OUTCOMES (NOC)	INTERVENTIONS (NIC) and *RATIONALES*
Thermoregulation • Sweating when hot ____ • Shivering when cold ____ • Apical heart rate ____ • Radial pulse rate ____ • Reported thermal comfort ____ **Measurement Scale** 1 = Severely compromised 2 = Substantially compromised 3 = Moderately compromised 4 = Mildly compromised 5 = Not compromised	***Fever Treatment*** • Monitor temperature as frequently as is appropriate *to determine effectiveness of therapy.* • Administer antipyretic medication as appropriate or as ordered *to reduce fever.* • Administer medications as appropriate to *treat the cause of the fever.* • Monitor WBC *to evaluate patient's response to treatment.* • Monitor blood pressure, pulse, and respiration *to assess cardiorespiratory response to fever.* • Encourage ↑ intake of oral fluids *to replace fluids lost as result of fever.*

NURSING DIAGNOSIS **Decreased cardiac output** *related to* altered rhythm, valvular insufficiency, and fluid overload *as evidenced by* heart murmur, S_3, tachycardia, diminished peripheral pulses, adventitious breath sounds, decreased urine output, restlessness *(Outcomes and Interventions for this Nursing Diagnosis are presented in the Nursing Care Plan for Valvular Heart Disease on pp. 884 to 885.)*

NURSING DIAGNOSIS **Activity intolerance** *related to* generalized weakness, arthralgia, and alteration in O_2 transport secondary to valvular dysfunction *as evidenced by* fatigue, malaise, weakness, painful joints, dyspnea, increased or decreased respiratory rate, and BP changes

PATIENT GOAL Performs activities of living with minimal fatigue or weakness

OUTCOMES (NOC)	INTERVENTIONS (NIC) and *RATIONALES*
Activity Tolerance • Ease of breathing with activity ____ • Respiratory rate with activity ____ • Systolic BP with activity ____ • Diastolic BP with activity ____ • Ease of performing ADLs ____ **Measurement Scale** 1 = Severely compromised 2 = Substantially compromised 3 = Moderately compromised 4 = Mildly compromised 5 = Not compromised	***Energy Management*** • Monitor cardiorespiratory response to activity (e.g., tachycardia, hypertension, diaphoresis, dyspnea) *to plan or alter activities.* • Monitor patient for evidence of excess physical or emotional fatigue *to plan for changes in activity level.* • Instruct patient/significant other to recognize signs and symptoms of fatigue that require reduction in activity (e.g., pulse increases >20 bpm; no increase in activity if resting pulse >100 bpm) *since these signs indicate excessive cardiac effort.* • Encourage alternate rest and activity periods *to reduce cardiac workload.*

ADLs, Activities of daily living; *BP,* blood pressure; *WBC,* white blood cell count.

▪ *Nursing Implementation*

Health Promotion. The incidence of IE can be decreased by identifying individuals who are at risk for the development of endocarditis (see Tables 37-2 and 37-4). Assessment of the patient's history and an understanding of the disease process are crucial for planning and implementing appropriate health promotion strategies.

Teaching the patient who is at risk for or has had IE helps reduce the incidence and recurrence of the disease. Teaching is crucial for the patient's understanding of and adherence to the planned treatment regimen. The patient should understand the need to avoid persons with infection, especially upper respiratory infection, and to report cold, flu, and cough symptoms. The importance of avoiding excessive fatigue and the need to plan rest periods before and after activity should be carefully explained to the patient. Good oral hygiene, including daily care and regular dental visits, is also important. The patient must inform all health care providers performing dental, medical, or surgical procedures of the history of IE. The patient should understand the significance of the prescribed prophylactic antibiotic therapy before any invasive procedure. The patient with a history of IVDA should be referred for drug treatment.

Ambulatory and Home Care. A patient with IE has many problems that require nursing management (see NCP 37-1). IE gener-

NURSING CARE PLAN 37-1

Patient with Infective Endocarditis—cont'd

NURSING DIAGNOSIS **Deficient knowledge** *related to* lack of experience and exposure to information about disease and treatment process *as evidenced by* verbalization of misconceptions about desired or prescribed health behaviors, requests for information

PATIENT GOAL Describes disease process, appropriate treatments, and measures to prevent recurrence of disease

OUTCOMES (NOC)

Knowledge: Disease Process

- Description of specific disease process ____
- Description of effects of disease ____
- Descriptions of signs and symptoms of complications ____
- Description of precautions to prevent complications ____

Measurement Scale

1 = None
2 = Limited
3 = Moderate
4 = Substantial
5 = Extensive

INTERVENTIONS (NIC) and *RATIONALES*

Teaching: Disease Process

- Review patient's knowledge about condition *to identify teaching needs.*
- Discuss common signs and symptoms of the disease (e.g., fatigue, malaise, chills, elevated temperature, anorexia) *so health care provider can be notified and treatment initiated promptly.*
- Discuss lifestyle changes that may be required to prevent future complications and/or control the disease process (e.g., avoiding persons with infection, taking prophylactic antibiotics before dental procedures) *to reduce the risk of recurrent infective endocarditis.*

Teaching: Prescribed Medication

- Provide the patient with information about the action, purpose, and side effects of the medications *to promote safe medication therapy.*

ally requires treatment with antibiotics for 4 to 6 weeks, depending on the results of blood cultures. After initial treatment in the hospital, the patient may continue treatment in the home setting if hemodynamically stable and compliant. The adequacy of the home environment in terms of in-home support and hospital access must be determined for successful management. Patients who receive outpatient IV antibiotics will require vigilant home nursing care.

Assessment findings are often nonspecific (see Table 37-6) but can help assist with the treatment plan. Fever, chronic or intermittent, is a common early sign. The patient or family needs instructions about the importance of monitoring body temperature because persistent, prolonged temperature elevations may mean that the drug therapy is ineffective. Patients with IE are at risk for life-threatening complications, such as cerebral emboli, pulmonary edema, and HF. Patients and families must be taught to recognize signs and symptoms of these complications (e.g., change in mental status, dyspnea, chest pain).

The patient with IE needs adequate periods of physical and emotional rest. Bed rest may be necessary when fever is present or when there are complications (e.g., heart damage). Otherwise the patient may ambulate and perform moderate activity. To prevent problems because of immobility, the patient should wear elastic compression stockings, perform ROM exercises, and cough and deep breathe every 2 hours. The patient may experience anxiety and fear associated with the illness. The nurse must recognize this and implement strategies to help the patient cope with the illness.

Laboratory data should be monitored to determine the effectiveness of the antibiotic therapy. Ongoing monitoring of the patient's blood cultures is necessary to ensure eradication of the infecting organism. Intravenous (IV) lines should be monitored for patency, and antibiotics should be given when scheduled. The patient should be monitored continuously for adverse drug reactions.

During the course of therapy in either the home or the hospital setting, management will also focus on teaching the patient about the nature of the disease and on reducing the risk of reinfection. The nurse must explain to the patient the relationship of follow-up care, good nutrition, and early treatment of common infections (e.g., colds) to maintain good health. The patient should be instructed about symptoms that may indicate recurrent infection, such as fever, fatigue, malaise, and chills. If any of these symptoms occur, the patient should be aware of the importance of notifying the health care provider. Finally, the patient must be instructed about the need for and importance of prophylactic antibiotic therapy before invasive procedures (see Table 37-3).

■ *Evaluation*

Expected outcomes for the patient with infective endocarditis are presented in NCP 37-1.

ACUTE PERICARDITIS

Pericarditis is a condition caused by inflammation of the pericardial sac (the pericardium), which may occur on an acute basis. The pericardium is composed of the inner serous membrane (visceral pericardium) that closely adheres to the epicardial surface of the heart and the outer fibrous (parietal) layer (see Fig. 37-1). The pericardial space is the cavity between these two layers, and, in the normal state, it contains 10 to 30 ml of serous fluid. Although the pericardium may be congenitally absent or surgically removed, it serves a useful anchoring function, provides lubrication to decrease friction during systolic and diastolic heart movements, and assists in preventing excessive dilation of the heart during diastole.

Etiology and Pathophysiology

The common causes of acute pericarditis are listed in Table 37-7. Acute pericarditis most often is idiopathic, with a variety of suspected viral causes. The coxsackievirus B group is the most commonly identified virus. In addition to idiopathic or viral pericarditis, other causes of this condition include uremia, bacterial infection, acute myocardial infarction (MI), tuberculosis, neoplasm, and trauma.[9] Pericarditis in the acute MI patient may be described as two distinct syndromes. The first is *acute pericarditis,* which may occur within the initial 48 to 72 hours after an MI. The

TABLE 37-7 Etiologies of Pericarditis

Infectious
Viral: Coxsackievirus types A and B, echovirus, adenovirus, mumps, hepatitis, Epstein-Barr, varicella zoster, human immunodeficiency virus
Bacterial: Pneumococci, staphylococci, streptococci, *Neisseria gonorrhoeae, Legionella pneumophila,* septicemia from gram-negative organisms
Tuberculosis
Fungal: *Histoplasma, Candida* species
Infections: Toxoplasmosis, Lyme disease
Noninfectious
Uremia
Acute myocardial infarction
Neoplasms: Lung cancer, breast cancer, leukemia, Hodgkin's lymphoma, nonHodgkin's lymphoma
Trauma: Thoracic surgery, pacemaker insertion, cardiac diagnostic procedures
Radiation
Dissecting aortic aneurysm
Myxedema
Hypersensitive or Autoimmune
Post–myocardial infarction (Dressler) syndrome
Postpericardiotomy syndrome
Rheumatic fever
Drug reactions (e.g., procainamide [Pronestyl], hydralazine [Apresoline])
Rheumatologic diseases: Rheumatoid arthritis, systemic lupus erythematosus, systemic sclerosis (scleroderma), ankylosing spondylitis

second is *Dressler syndrome* (late pericarditis), which appears 4 to 6 weeks after an MI (see Chapter 34).

An inflammatory response is the characteristic pathologic finding in acute pericarditis. There is an influx of neutrophils, increased pericardial vascularity, and eventually fibrin deposition on the visceral pericardium (Fig. 37-4).

Clinical Manifestations

Clinical manifestations found in acute pericarditis include progressive, frequently severe chest pain that is sharp and pleuritic in nature. The pain is generally worse with deep inspiration and when lying supine. It is relieved by sitting. The pain may radiate to the neck, arms, or left shoulder, making it difficult to differentiate from angina. One distinction is that the pain from pericarditis can be referred to the trapezius muscle (shoulder, upper back) as the phrenic nerve innervates these two regions.[10] The dyspnea that accompanies acute pericarditis is related to the patient's need to breathe in rapid, shallow breaths to avoid chest pain and may be aggravated by fever and anxiety.

The hallmark finding in acute pericarditis is the **pericardial friction rub.** The rub is a scratching, grating, high-pitched sound believed to arise from friction between the roughened pericardial and epicardial surfaces. It is best heard with the stethoscope diaphragm firmly placed at the lower left sternal border of the chest. The pericardial friction rub does not radiate widely or vary in timing from the heartbeat, but it may require frequent auscultation to identify because it may be elusive and transient. Timing the pericardial friction rub with the pulse (and not respirations) will help distinguish it from pleural friction rub (e.g., from pleurisy).

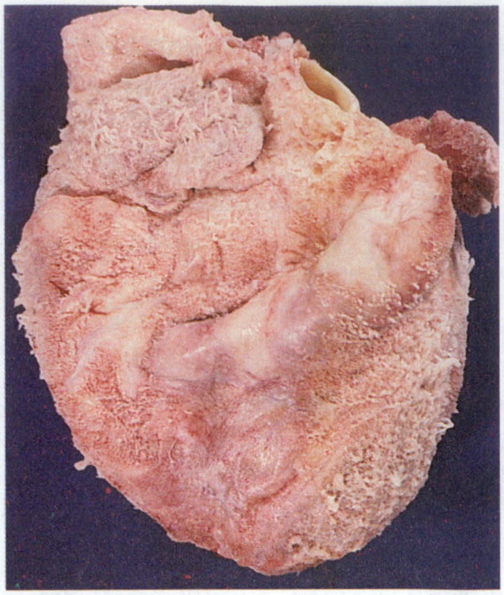

FIG. 37-4 Acute pericarditis. Note shaggy coat of fibers covering surface of heart.

Complications

Two major complications that may result from acute pericarditis are pericardial effusion and cardiac tamponade. **Pericardial effusion** is an accumulation of excess fluid in the pericardium. It can occur rapidly (e.g., chest trauma) or slowly (e.g., tuberculous pericarditis). Large effusions may compress adjoining structures. Pulmonary tissue compression can cause cough, dyspnea, and tachypnea. Phrenic nerve compression can induce hiccups, and compression of the recurrent laryngeal nerve may result in hoarseness. Heart sounds are generally distant and muffled, although blood pressure (BP) is usually maintained by compensatory mechanisms.

Cardiac tamponade develops as the pericardial effusion increases in volume, causing an increase in intrapericardial pressure. This results in compression of the heart. The speed of fluid accumulation affects the severity of clinical manifestations. Cardiac tamponade can occur acutely (e.g., rupture of heart, trauma) or subacutely (e.g., secondary to uremia, malignancy).

The patient with cardiac tamponade may report chest pain and is often confused, anxious, and restless. As the compression of the heart increases, heart sounds become muffled and the pulse pressure is narrowed. The patient will develop tachypnea, tachycardia, and a decreased cardiac output (CO). The neck veins are usually markedly distended because of jugular venous pressure elevation, and a significant pulsus paradoxus is present. *Pulsus paradoxus* is a decrease in systolic BP with inspiration that is exaggerated in cardiac tamponade. (See Table 37-8 for measurement technique.) In a patient with a slow onset of a cardiac tamponade, dyspnea may be the only clinical manifestation.

Diagnostic Studies

The ECG may be normal, or may exhibit nonspecific or specific and diffuse changes. If specific ECG changes do develop, they will evolve over a period of hours to days or weeks and can include PR segment depression, ST segment elevation, and T wave flattening and inversion. These changes are believed to be caused by superficial myocardial inflammation under the pericardium. (See Chapter 36 for more information on ECG monitoring.)

TABLE 37-8 Measurement of Pulsus Paradoxus

1. Make determination during quiet breathing with stable rhythm.
2. Determine systolic blood pressure.
3. Inflate blood pressure cuff until no sounds are heard with stethoscope.
4. Deflate cuff slowly until systolic sounds are heard on expiration, and note the pressure.
5. Deflate cuff until systolic sounds are heard throughout the respiratory cycle, and note the pressure.
6. Determine the difference between the measurements taken in steps 4 and 5. This will equal the amount of paradox:

Sounds heard on expiration at	110 mm Hg
Sounds heard throughout cycle at	82 mm Hg
Amount of paradox	28 mm Hg

The difference is normally <10 mm Hg. If the difference is >10 mm Hg, cardiac tamponade may be present.

The chest x-ray findings are generally normal, but cardiomegaly may be seen in a patient who has a large pericardial effusion (Fig. 37-5). Echocardiographic findings are more useful in determining the presence of a pericardial effusion or cardiac tamponade. Newer methods such as tissue Doppler imaging and color M-mode of early left ventricular flow help to assess diastolic function and diagnose constrictive pericarditis (discussed later in the chapter).[10] Computed tomography (CT) and magnetic resonance imaging (MRI) provide for visualization of the pericardium and pericardial space.

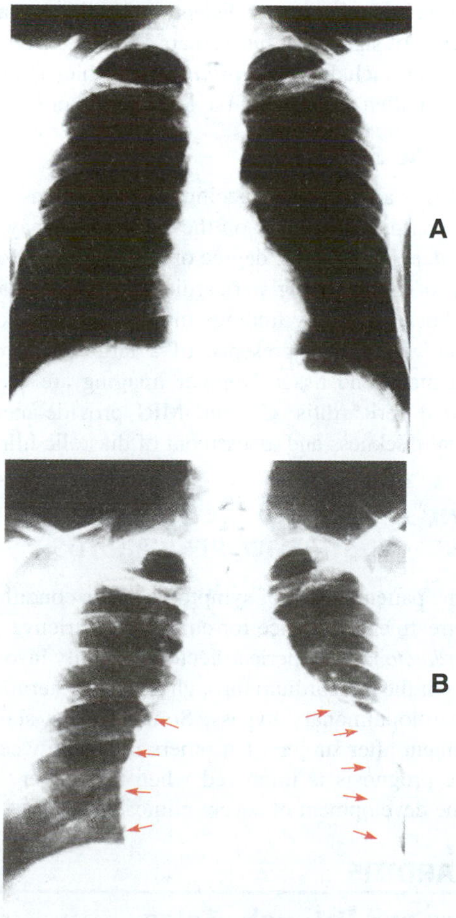

FIG. 37-5 **A,** X-ray of a normal chest. **B,** Pericardial effusion is present, and the cardiac silhouette is enlarged with a globular shape *(arrows)*.

Common laboratory findings include leukocytosis and elevation of CRP and ESR. Troponin levels may be elevated in patients with ST segment elevation and acute pericarditis, which would indicate concurrent myocardial damage. The fluid obtained during pericardiocentesis (Fig. 37-6) or the tissue from a pericardial biopsy may be analyzed to determine the cause of the pericarditis.

Collaborative Care

Management of acute pericarditis is directed toward identification and treatment of the underlying problem (Table 37-9). Antibiotics should be used to treat bacterial pericarditis. Corticosteroids are generally reserved for patients with pericarditis secondary to systemic lupus erythematosus, patients already taking corticosteroids for a rheumatologic or other immune system condition, or patients who do not respond to nonsteroidal antiinflammatory drugs (NSAIDs). When necessary, prednisone is given using a tapering dosage schedule. Corticosteroids are administered cautiously because of their numerous side effects, such as upper GI bleeding, sodium retention, hyperglycemia, hypokalemia, and Cushing syndrome (see Chapter 50).

The pain and inflammation of acute pericarditis are usually treated with NSAIDs. High-dose salicylates (e.g., aspirin) or NSAIDs (e.g., ibuprofen) are commonly used. Colchicine, an antiinflammatory agent used for gout, may be considered for patients who have recurrent pericarditis.

Pericardiocentesis is usually performed for pericardial effusion with acute cardiac tamponade, purulent pericarditis, and a high suspicion of a neoplasm (see Fig. 37-6). Hemodynamic support for the patient being prepared for the pericardiocentesis may include administration of volume expanders and inotropic agents (e.g., dopamine [Intropin]) and the discontinuation of any anticoagulants. The procedure is performed rapidly and safely using a percutaneous approach that is guided by ECG and echocardiography. If surgical drainage is necessary, a 16- to 18-gauge needle is

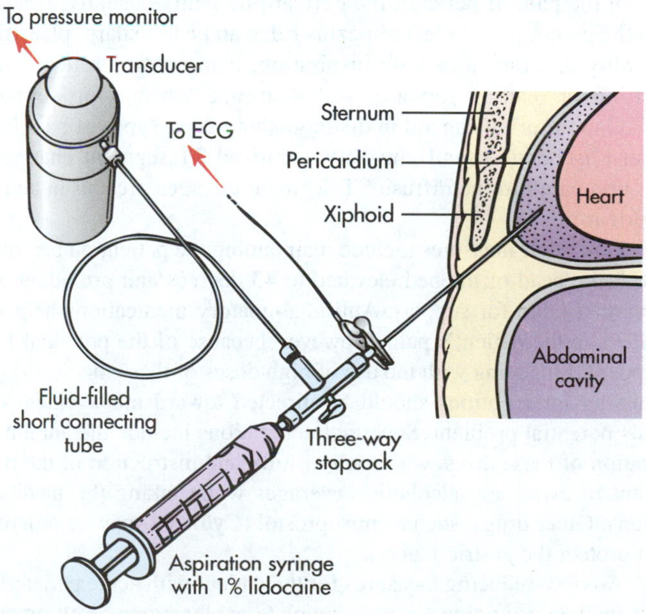

FIG. 37-6 Pericardiocentesis performed under sterile conditions in conjunction with electrocardiogram (ECG) and hemodynamic measurements.

TABLE 37-9 COLLABORATIVE CARE Acute Pericarditis

Diagnostic
History and physical examination
Auscultation of the chest (e.g., for pericardial friction rub)
Electrocardiogram
Chest x-ray
Echocardiogram
Computed tomography
Magnetic resonance imaging
Laboratory: CRP, ESR, white blood cell count
Pericardiocentesis
Pericardial biopsy
Collaborative Therapy
Treatment of underlying disease
Bed rest
Aspirin
Nonsteroidal antiinflammatory drugs
Corticosteroids
Pericardiocentesis (for large pericardial effusion or tamponade)

CRP, C-reactive protein; *ESR,* erythrocyte sedimentation rate.

inserted into the pericardial space to remove fluid for analysis and to relieve cardiac pressure. Complications from pericardiocentesis include dysrhythmias, further cardiac tamponade, pneumomediastinum, pneumothorax, myocardial laceration, and coronary artery laceration.

NURSING MANAGEMENT ACUTE PERICARDITIS

The management of the patient's pain and anxiety during acute pericarditis is a primary nursing consideration. Assessment of the amount, quality, and location of the pain is important, particularly in distinguishing the pain of myocardial ischemia (angina) from the pain of pericarditis. Pericarditic pain is usually located in the precordium or left trapezius ridge and has a sharp, pleuritic quality that increases with inspiration. Pain is often relieved by sitting or leaning forward, and worsened when lying supine. ECG monitoring can aid in distinguishing these types of pain because ischemia usually involves localized ST segment changes, as compared to the diffuse ST segment changes present in acute pericarditis.

Pain relief measures include maintaining the patient on bed rest with the head of the bed elevated to 45 degrees and providing an overbed table for support. Antiinflammatory medications help to alleviate the patient's pain. However, because of the potential for upper GI bleeding with the use of high doses of these medications, nursing interventions should be directed toward management of this potential problem. Specific interventions include the administration of these drugs with food or milk and instruction of the patient to avoid any alcoholic beverages while taking the medications. Other drugs, such as misoprostol (Cytotec), may be ordered to protect the gastric mucosa.

Anxiety-reducing measures for the patient with acute pericarditis include providing simple, complete explanations of all procedures performed and the possible cause of the pain. These explanations are particularly important for the patient whose diagnosis of acute pericarditis is being established and for the patient who has already experienced angina or an acute MI.

The potential for decreased CO exists for the patient with acute pericarditis because of the possibility of cardiac tamponade. Monitoring for the signs and symptoms of tamponade and making preparations for possible pericardiocentesis are important nursing responsibilities.

CHRONIC CONSTRICTIVE PERICARDITIS

Etiology and Pathophysiology

Chronic constrictive pericarditis results from scarring with consequent loss of elasticity of the pericardial sac. It usually begins with an initial episode of acute pericarditis (often secondary to idiopathic causes, cardiac surgery, or radiation) and is characterized by fibrin deposition with a clinically undetected pericardial effusion. Reabsorption of the effusion slowly follows, with progression toward the chronic stage of fibrous scarring, thickening of the pericardium from calcium deposition, and eventual obliteration of the pericardial space. The fibrotic, thickened, and adherent pericardium encases the heart, thereby impairing the ability of the atria and ventricles to stretch adequately during diastole.

Clinical Manifestations

Manifestations of chronic constrictive pericarditis occur over an extended time period and mimic those of HF and cor pulmonale. Many of the clinical manifestations are related to decreased CO. They include dyspnea on exertion, peripheral edema, ascites, fatigue, anorexia, and weight loss. The most prominent finding at the physical examination is jugular venous distention. Unlike cardiac tamponade, the presence of significant pulsus paradoxus is uncommon. Auscultatory findings include a *pericardial knock,* which is a loud early diastolic sound often heard along the left sternal border.

Diagnostic Studies

ECG changes are often nonspecific in chronic constrictive pericarditis. The cardiac silhouette on the chest x-ray may be normal or enlarged depending on the degree of pericardial thickening and the presence of a coexisting pericardial effusion. Two-dimensional (2-D) echocardiography findings may reveal a thickened pericardium, but without the presence of a large pericardial effusion. Color M-mode and tissue Doppler imaging are used to confirm constrictive pericarditis. CT and MRI provide measurement of pericardial thickness and assessment of diastolic filling patterns.

NURSING *and* COLLABORATIVE MANAGEMENT CHRONIC CONSTRICTIVE PERICARDITIS

Unless the patient is free of symptoms or the condition is inoperable, the treatment of choice for chronic constrictive pericarditis is a *pericardiectomy.* The pericardiectomy usually involves complete resection of the pericardium through a median sternotomy with the use of cardiopulmonary bypass. Some patients show immediate improvement after surgery, but others may take weeks. The postoperative prognosis is improved when the surgery is performed before the development of severe clinical disability.

MYOCARDITIS

Etiology and Pathophysiology

Myocarditis is a focal or diffuse inflammation of the myocardium. Possible causes include viruses, bacteria, fungi, radiation therapy, and pharmacologic and chemical factors. Viruses, particularly coxsackievirus types A and B, are the most common etiologic agents in the United States and Canada. Autoimmune disorders (e.g., polymyositis) also have been associated with the development of myocarditis. Myocarditis may also occur when no causative agent or factor can be identified (i.e., *idiopathic*). Myocarditis is frequently associated with acute pericarditis, particularly when it is caused by coxsackievirus B strains.[11]

When the myocardium becomes infected, the causative agent invades the myocytes and causes cellular damage and necrosis. The immune response is activated, and cytokines and oxygen free radicals are released. As the infection progresses, an autoimmune response is activated resulting in further destruction of myocytes. Myocarditis results in cardiac dysfunction and has been linked to the development of dilated cardiomyopathy (discussed later in chapter).

Clinical Manifestations

The clinical features of myocarditis are variable, ranging from a benign course without any overt manifestations to severe heart involvement or sudden cardiac death (SCD). Fever, fatigue, malaise, myalgias, pharyngitis, dyspnea, lymphadenopathy, and nausea and vomiting are early systemic manifestations of the viral illness.

Early cardiac manifestations appear 7 to 10 days after viral infection. These include pleuritic chest pain with a pericardial friction rub and effusion because pericarditis often accompanies myocarditis. Late cardiac signs relate to the development of HF and may include an S_3 heart sound, crackles, jugular venous distention, syncope, peripheral edema, and angina.

Diagnostic Studies

The ECG changes for a patient with myocarditis are often nonspecific but may reflect associated pericardial involvement (e.g., diffuse ST segment abnormalities). Dysrhythmias and conduction disturbances may be present. Laboratory findings are also often inconclusive. They may include mild to moderate leukocytosis and atypical lymphocytes, increased ESR and CRP levels, elevated levels of myocardial markers such as troponin, and elevated viral titers (virus is generally only present in tissue and fluid samples during the initial 8 to 10 days of illness).

Histologic confirmation of myocarditis is done through *endomyocardial biopsy* (EMB). This technique involves removing several small pieces of myocardial tissue percutaneously from the right ventricle with a special instrument called a *bioptome* and microscopically examining the samples.[12] A biopsy done during the initial 6 weeks of acute illness is most diagnostic because this is the period in which lymphocytic infiltration and myocyte damage indicative of myocarditis are present. Other studies include the use of echocardiography, nuclear scans, and MRI to evaluate cardiac function.

Collaborative Care

The specific treatment for myocarditis has yet to be established, and treatment usually consists of managing associated cardiac decompensation. Digoxin (Lanoxin) is often used to treat ventricular failure because it improves myocardial contractility and reduces ventricular rate. Digoxin should be used cautiously in patients with myocarditis because of the increased sensitivity of the heart to the adverse effects of this drug (e.g., dysrhythmias) and the potential toxicity with minimal doses. Diuretics may be used to reduce fluid volume and decrease preload. If hypotension is not present, intravenous medications such as nitroprusside (Nitropress), inamrinone (Inocor), and milrinone (Primacor) are used to reduce afterload and improve CO by decreasing systemic arterial resistance. The use of anticoagulation therapy may be considered in patients with low ejection fraction who are at risk for thrombus formation from blood stasis in the cardiac chambers.

Based on the infectious-immune theory of myocarditis, immunosuppressive therapy with agents such as prednisone, azathioprine (Imuran), and cyclosporine has been used to reduce myocardial inflammation and to prevent irreversible myocardial damage. Evidence of the success of this therapy remains inconclusive, and the use of corticosteroids for the treatment of myocarditis remains controversial.[12]

Intravenous immunoglobulin (IVIG) is being used on an experimental basis to treat myocarditis. It has been associated with improved left ventricular function and improved survival.[12] Antiviral agents (e.g., ribavirin [Virazole], α-interferon) are undergoing clinical investigation for the treatment of acute viral myocarditis.[12]

Oxygen therapy, bed rest, and restricted activity are general supportive measures used for management of myocarditis. In cases of severe HF, the use of intraaortic balloon pump therapy and ventricular assist devices may be required (see Chapters 35 and 66).

NURSING MANAGEMENT
MYOCARDITIS

Decreased CO is an ongoing nursing diagnosis in the care of the patient with myocarditis. Interventions focus on assessment for the signs and symptoms of HF. Important nursing measures to decrease cardiac workload include the use of the semi-Fowler's position, spacing of activity and rest periods, and provisions for a quiet environment. Prescribed medications that increase the heart's contractility and decrease preload, afterload, or both require careful monitoring. Ongoing evaluation of the effectiveness of these interventions is necessary.

The patient may be anxious about the diagnosis of myocarditis, recovery from myocarditis, and the therapeutic plan. Nursing measures include assessing the level of anxiety, instituting measures to decrease anxiety, and keeping the patient and family informed about therapeutic measures.

The patient who receives immunosuppressive therapy has additional problems of alterations in the immune response with the potential for infection and complications related to the therapy. Guidelines for care include monitoring for complications and providing the patient with a clean, safe environment by following proper infection control procedures.

Most patients with myocarditis recover spontaneously, although some may develop dilated cardiomyopathy. If severe HF occurs, the patient may require heart transplantation.

RHEUMATIC FEVER AND HEART DISEASE

Rheumatic fever is an inflammatory disease of the heart potentially involving all layers (endocardium, myocardium, and pericardium) of the heart. **Rheumatic heart disease** is a chronic condition resulting from rheumatic fever that is characterized by scarring and deformity of the heart valves.

Etiology and Pathophysiology

Acute rheumatic fever (ARF) is a complication that occurs as a delayed sequela (usually after 2 to 3 weeks) of a group A streptococcal pharyngitis.[13] Manifestations of ARF appear to be related to an abnormal immunologic response to group A streptococcal cell

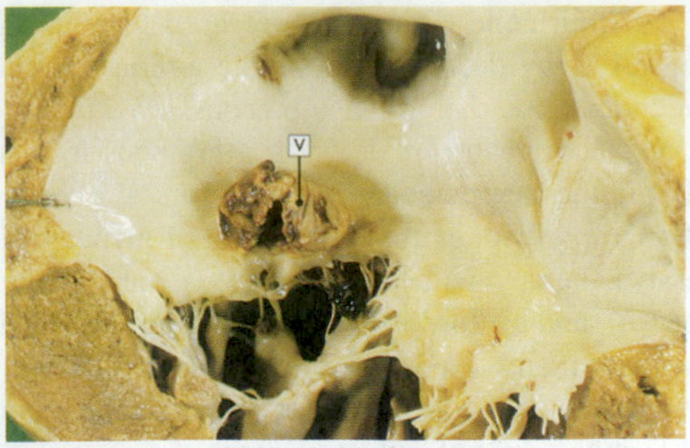

FIG. 37-7 Mitral stenosis and clumps of vegetation *(V)* containing platelets and fibrin. Mitral leaflets are thickened and fused and have clumps of vegetation containing platelets and fibrin.

membrane antigens. ARF affects the heart, joints, central nervous system (CNS), and skin.[14] ARF has declined in developed countries due to the effective use of antibiotics to treat streptococcal infections. It remains an important public health problem in developing countries. The sequela of ARF, rheumatic heart disease, is found primarily in young adults.

Cardiac Lesions and Valvular Deformities. About 40% of ARF episodes are marked by carditis, meaning that all layers of the heart (endocardium, myocardium, and pericardium) are involved. This generalized involvement gives rise to the term *rheumatic pancarditis.*

Rheumatic endocarditis is found primarily in the valves, with swelling and erosion of the valve leaflets. Vegetation forms from deposits of fibrin and blood cells in areas of erosion (Fig. 37-7). The lesions initially create fibrous thickening of the valve leaflets, fusion of commissures and chordae tendineae, and fibrosis of the papillary muscle. Valve leaflets may fuse and become thickened or even calcified, resulting in stenosis. Reduction in the mobility of valve leaflets may occur with failure of the leaflets to close properly, resulting in regurgitation. The mitral and aortic valves are most commonly affected.

Myocardial involvement is characterized by **Aschoff's bodies,** which are histologic nodules formed by a reaction to inflammation with accompanying swelling and fragmentation of collagen fibers. As the Aschoff's bodies age, they become more fibrous, and scar tissue is formed in the myocardium. In addition to Aschoff's bodies, a diffuse cellular infiltrate is present in interstitial tissues. Rheumatic pericarditis affects both layers of the pericardium, which become thickened and covered with a fibrinous exudate, and a serosanguineous pericardial effusion may develop. When healing occurs, fibrosis and adhesions develop that partially or completely obliterate the pericardial sac, but constrictive pericarditis does not occur.

These pathophysiologic changes in the heart may occur as a result of an initial attack of rheumatic fever. However, recurrent infections contribute to further structural damage.

Extracardiac Lesions. The lesions of rheumatic fever are systemic, especially involving the connective tissue. The joints, skin, and CNS can be involved in rheumatic fever.

Clinical Manifestations

The diagnosis of ARF is suggested by a clustering of signs and symptoms as well as from laboratory findings. Criteria were established by T. D. Jones in 1944, revised by the American Heart Association, and modified by the World Health Organization (WHO)

TABLE 37-10 Modified Jones Criteria for Diagnosing Acute Rheumatic Fever

Major Criteria	Minor Criteria	Evidence of Group A Streptococcal Infection
Carditis Mono- or polyarthritis Chorea Erythema marginatum Subcutaneous nodules	Clinical findings: Fever, polyarthralgia Laboratory findings: ↑ ESR, ↑ WBC count, ↑ CRP	Laboratory findings: ↑ Antistreptolysin-O titer, positive throat culture, positive rapid antigen test for group A streptococci ECG findings: Prolonged PR interval

CRP, C-reactive protein; *ECG,* electrocardiogram; *ESR,* erythrocyte sedimentation rate; *WBC,* white blood cell count.

to provide a basis for diagnosis[15] (Table 37-10). The presence of two major criteria or one major and two minor criteria plus evidence of a preceding group A streptococcal infection indicates a high probability of ARF.

Major Criteria. *Carditis* is the most important manifestation of ARF and results in three signs: (1) an organic heart murmur or murmurs of mitral or aortic regurgitation, or mitral stenosis; (2) cardiac enlargement and HF secondary to myocarditis; and (3) pericarditis resulting in muffled heart sounds, chest pain, pericardial friction rub, or signs of effusion.

Mono- or polyarthritis is the most common finding in rheumatic fever. The inflammatory process affects the synovial membranes of the joints, causing swelling, heat, redness, tenderness, and limitation of motion. The larger joints are most frequently affected, particularly the knees, ankles, elbows, and wrists.

Chorea (Sydenham's chorea) is the major CNS manifestation of ARF and often a delayed sign occurring several months after the initial infection. It is characterized by involuntary movements, especially of the face and limbs, muscle weakness, and disturbances of speech and gait.

Erythema marginatum lesions are a less common feature of ARF. The bright pink, nonpruritic, maplike macular lesions occur mainly on the trunk and proximal extremities, and may be exacerbated by heat (e.g., warm bath).

Subcutaneous nodules, usually associated with severe carditis, are firm, small, hard, painless swellings located over extensor surfaces of the joints, particularly knees, wrists, and elbows.

Minor Criteria. Minor clinical manifestations (see Table 37-10) are frequently present and are helpful in diagnosing the disease. The minor criteria are used as supplemental data to confirm the presence of rheumatic fever when only one major criterion is present.

Evidence of Infection. In addition to the major and minor criteria, there must also be evidence of a preceding group A streptococcal infection. Table 37-10 lists the various laboratory tests used to confirm evidence of infection.

Complications

A complication that can result from ARF is *chronic rheumatic carditis.* It results from changes in valvular structure that may occur months to years after an episode of ARF. Rheumatic endocarditis can result in fibrous tissue growth in valve leaflets and chordae tendineae with scarring and contractures. The mitral valve is

TABLE 37-11 COLLABORATIVE CARE
Rheumatic Fever

Diagnostic
History and physical examination
Laboratory findings*
Chest x-ray
Echocardiogram
Electrocardiogram
Collaborative Therapy
Bed rest
Antibiotics
Corticosteroids
Salicylates
Nonsteroidal antiinflammatory drugs

*See Table 37-10.

most frequently involved. Other valves that may be affected are the aortic and tricuspid valves.

Diagnostic Studies

No single diagnostic test exists for rheumatic fever (see Table 37-10). An echocardiogram may show valvular insufficiency and pericardial fluid or thickening. A chest x-ray may show an enlarged heart if HF is present. The most consistent ECG change is delayed AV conduction as evidenced by prolongation of the PR interval.

Collaborative Care

Treatment consists of drug therapy and supportive measures (Table 37-11). Antibiotic therapy does not modify the course of the acute disease or the development of carditis. It does eliminate residual group A streptococci remaining in the tonsils and pharynx and prevent the spread of organisms to close contacts. Salicylates, NSAIDs, and corticosteroids are the antiinflammatory agents most widely used in the management of ARF. All are effective in controlling the fever and joint manifestations. Salicylates or NSAIDs are used when arthritis is the main manifestation, and corticosteroids are used if severe carditis is present.

NURSING MANAGEMENT
RHEUMATIC FEVER AND HEART DISEASE

■ *Nursing Assessment*

Subjective and objective data that should be obtained from a patient with rheumatic fever and heart disease are presented in Table 37-12. It is important to note that rheumatic fever is more likely to reoccur in a person with a previous history of rheumatic fever than in the general population.

The skin of the patient should be assessed for subcutaneous nodules and erythema marginatum. The procedure involves palpation for subcutaneous nodules over all bony surfaces and along extensor tendons of the hands and feet. The nodules range in size from 1 to 4 cm and are hard, painless, and freely movable. Erythema marginatum can occur on the trunk and inner aspects of the upper arm and thigh. The erythematous maplike maculae do not itch and are not raised. The possible presence of these bright pink maculae should be assessed in good light because the rash is difficult to observe, especially if the patient is dark skinned.

TABLE 37-12 NURSING ASSESSMENT
Rheumatic Fever and Rheumatic Heart Disease

Subjective Data
Important Health Information
Past health history: Recent streptococcal infection, previous history of rheumatic fever or rheumatic heart disease
Functional Health Patterns
Health perception–health management: Family history of rheumatic fever; malaise
Nutritional-metabolic: Anorexia, weight loss
Activity-exercise: Palpitations; generalized weakness, fatigue; ataxia
Cognitive-perceptual: Chest pain; migratory joint pain and tenderness (especially large joints)
Objective Data
General
Fever
Integumentary
Subcutaneous nodules and erythema marginatum
Cardiovascular
Tachycardia, pericardial friction rub, muffled heart sounds; gallop rhythm, murmurs; peripheral edema
Neurologic
Chorea (involuntary, purposeless, rapid motions; facial grimaces)
Musculoskeletal
Signs of mono- or polyarthritis, including swelling, heat, redness, limitation of motion (especially of knees, ankles, elbows, shoulders, wrists)
Possible Findings
Cardiomegaly on chest x-ray; prolonged PR interval on ECG; valve abnormalities, chamber dilation, and pericardial effusion on echocardiogram; ↑ antistreptolysin-O titer, positive throat culture, positive rapid antigen test for group A streptococci; ↑ ESR, ↑ CRP, leukocytosis

CRP, C-reactive protein; *ECG,* electrocardiogram; *ESR,* erythrocyte sedimentation rate.

■ *Nursing Diagnoses*

Nursing diagnoses for the patient with rheumatic fever and heart disease may include, but are not limited to, the following:

- Activity intolerance *related to* arthralgia secondary to joint pain, pain from pericarditis, and HF
- Decreased cardiac output *related to* valve dysfunction or HF
- Ineffective therapeutic regimen management *related to* lack of knowledge concerning the need for long-term prophylactic antibiotic therapy and possible disease sequelae

■ *Planning*

The overall goals for a patient with rheumatic fever include (1) normal or baseline heart function, (2) resumption of daily activities without joint pain, and (3) verbalization of the ability to manage the disease.

■ *Nursing Implementation*

Health Promotion. Rheumatic fever is one of the cardiovascular diseases that is preventable. Prevention involves early detection and immediate treatment of group A streptococcal pharyngitis. Adequate treatment of streptococcal pharyngitis prevents initial attacks of rheumatic fever. Treatment consists of intramuscular

(IM) injection of penicillin G benzathine (Bicillin LA) or oral penicillin V potassium (Beepen-VK). If the patient is allergic to penicillin, erythromycin (E-Mycin) or azithromycin (Zithromax) may be substituted. Oral therapy requires faithful adherence to the full course of treatment. The nurse's role is to educate the community to seek medical attention for symptoms of streptococcal pharyngitis and to emphasize the need for adequate treatment of this infection.

Acute Intervention. The primary goals of managing a patient with ARF are to control and eradicate the infecting organism; prevent cardiac complications; and relieve joint pain, fever, and other symptoms. The nurse should administer antibiotics as ordered to treat the streptococcal infection and teach the patient that oral antibiotic therapy requires faithful adherence to the full course of therapy. Antipyretics, NSAIDs, and corticosteroids should be administered as prescribed and fluid intake monitored.

Promotion of optimal rest is essential to reduce the cardiac workload and to diminish the metabolic needs of the body. Relief of joint pain is an important nursing goal. Painful joints should be positioned for comfort and proper alignment. Heat may be applied and salicylates or NSAIDs administered to relieve joint pain.

After the acute symptoms have subsided, the patient without carditis should ambulate. If the patient has carditis with HF, bed rest restrictions should be applied (see Chapter 35 for care of a patient with HF). Nonstrenuous activities should be encouraged once recovery has begun.

Ambulatory and Home Care. Secondary prevention aims at preventing the recurrence of rheumatic fever. The patient with a previous history of rheumatic fever should be taught about the disease process, possible sequelae, and the continual need for prophylactic antibiotics.

Prior history of rheumatic fever makes the patient more susceptible to a second attack after a streptococcal infection. The best prevention is monthly injections of long-acting penicillin. Alternative treatment is administration of oral penicillin or erythromycin 1 or 2 times a day. Rheumatic fever without carditis after age 18 may require only 5 years of prophylactic antibiotic therapy, or therapy may continue indefinitely in patients with frequent exposure to group A streptococcus. Prophylactic treatment should continue for life in individuals who develop rheumatic heart disease.

The dosage of antibiotics used in maintenance prophylaxis of rheumatic fever is not adequate to prevent IE when invasive procedures are performed. Additional prophylaxis is necessary if a patient with known rheumatic heart disease has dental or surgical procedures involving the upper respiratory, GI (e.g., endoscopy), or GU tract (see Table 37-3). The nurse must explain the difference between these two prophylactic programs.

Patient teaching should encourage good nutrition, hygienic practices, and the importance of receiving adequate rest. The patient should also be cautioned about the possibility of development of valvular heart disease. The nurse should teach the patient to seek medical attention if symptoms such as excessive fatigue, dizziness, palpitations, or exertional dyspnea develop.

■ *Evaluation*

The expected outcomes for the patient with rheumatic fever and heart disease include

- ability to perform ADLs with minimal fatigue and pain
- adherence to treatment regimen
- expression of confidence in managing disease

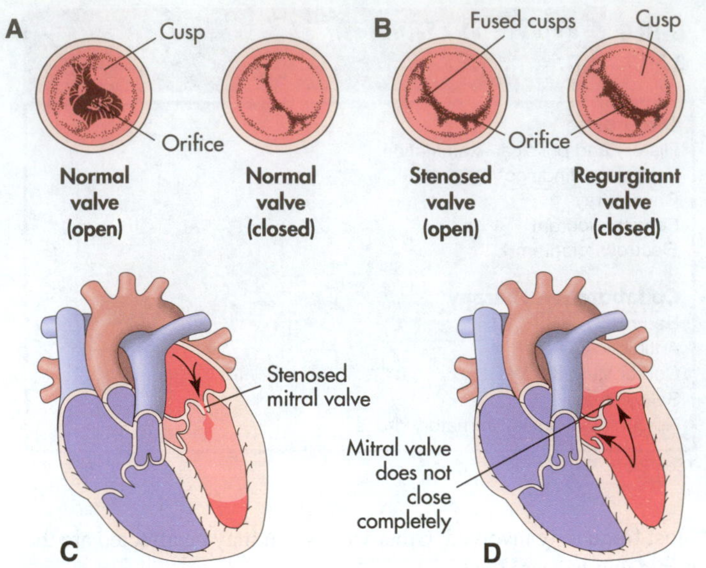

FIG. 37-8 Valvular stenosis and regurgitation. **A,** Normal position of the valve leaflets, or cusps, when the valve is open and closed. **B,** Open position of a stenosed valve *(left)* and position of closed regurgitant valve *(right)*. **C,** Hemodynamic effect of mitral stenosis. The stenosed valve is unable to open sufficiently during left atrial systole, inhibiting left ventricular filling. **D,** Hemodynamic effect of mitral regurgitation. The mitral valve does not close completely during left ventricular systole, permitting blood to reenter the left atrium.

Valvular Heart Disease

The heart contains two atrioventricular valves, the mitral and the tricuspid, and two semilunar valves, the aortic and the pulmonic, which are located in four strategic locations to control unidirectional blood flow (see Fig. 32-3). Valvular heart disease is defined according to the valve or valves affected and the type of functional alteration: stenosis or regurgitation (Fig. 37-8).

The pressure on either side of an open valve is normally equal. However, in a stenotic valve, the valve orifice is smaller, impeding the forward flow of blood and creating a pressure gradient difference across an open valve. The degree of **stenosis** (constriction or narrowing) is seen in the pressure gradient differences (i.e., the higher the gradient, the greater the stenosis). In **regurgitation** (also called *valvular incompetence* or *insufficiency*), incomplete closure of the valve leaflets results in the backward flow of blood.

Valvular disorders occur in children and adolescents primarily from congenital conditions such as tricuspid atresia, pulmonary stenosis, and aortic stenosis. Valvular heart disease has remained prevalent because of an increased number of older adults, many of whom have some form of cardiovascular disease. Aortic stenosis and mitral regurgitation are common valvular disorders in the elderly. In the last 20 years, new causes of valve disease have emerged. These include valvular disorders related to acquired immunodeficiency syndrome (AIDS) and the use of some antiparkinsonian drugs (e.g., pergolide [Permax]).[16]

MITRAL VALVE STENOSIS

Etiology and Pathophysiology

Most cases of adult mitral valve stenosis result from rheumatic heart disease; rheumatic mitral stenosis is endemic in developing countries.[17] Less common causes are congenital mitral stenosis, rheumatoid arthritis, and systemic lupus erythematosus. Rheumatic endo-

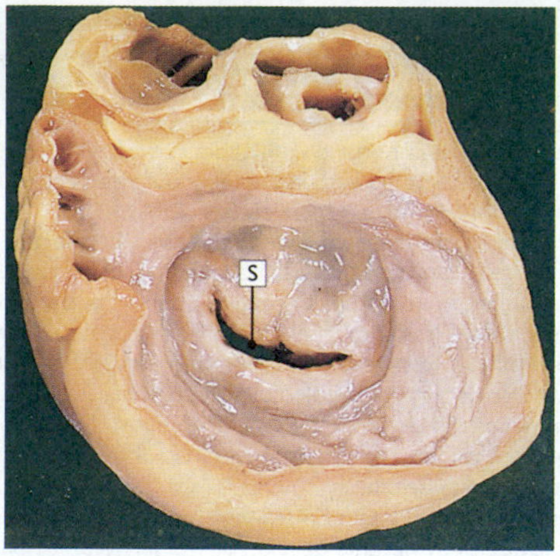

FIG. 37-9 Mitral stenosis with classic "fish mouth" orifice. *S,* Stenosis.

carditis causes scarring of the valve leaflets and the chordae tendineae. Contractures and adhesions develop between the commissures (the junctional areas). The stenotic mitral valve takes on a "fish mouth" shape because of the thickening and shortening of the mitral valve structures (Fig. 37-9). These structural deformities cause obstruction of blood flow and create a pressure difference between the left atrium and the left ventricle during diastole. Left atrial pressure and volume elevations cause increased pulmonary vasculature pressure and subsequent hypertrophy of the pulmonary vessels. In chronic mitral stenosis, pressure overload occurs in the left atrium, the pulmonary bed, and the right ventricle.

Clinical Manifestations

The primary symptom of mitral stenosis is exertional dyspnea due to reduced lung compliance (Table 37-13). Fatigue and palpitations from atrial fibrillation may also occur. Heart sounds include a loud first heart sound and a low-pitched, rumbling diastolic murmur (best heard at the apex with the stethoscope bell). Less frequently, patients may have hoarseness (from atrial enlargement pressing on the laryngeal nerve), hemoptysis (from pulmonary hypertension), chest pain (from decreased CO), and seizures or a stroke (from emboli). Emboli can arise from blood stasis in the left atrium.

MITRAL VALVE REGURGITATION

Etiology and Pathophysiology

Mitral valve function depends on intact mitral leaflets, mitral annulus, chordae tendineae, papillary muscles, left atrium, and left ventricle. Any defect in any of these structures can result in regurgitation. Most cases of mitral regurgitation (MR) are caused by MI, chronic rheumatic heart disease, mitral valve prolapse, ischemic papillary muscle dysfunction, and IE. MI with left ventricular failure increases the risk for rupture of the chordae tendineae and acute MR.

MR allows blood to flow backward from the left ventricle to the left atrium due to incomplete valve closure during systole. The left ventricle and left atrium both work harder to preserve an adequate CO. In chronic MR, the additional volume load results in atrial enlargement, ventricular dilation, and eventual ventricular hypertrophy. In acute MR, the left atrium and ventricle do not abruptly dilate. The sudden increase in pressure and volume is transmitted to the pulmonary bed, resulting in pulmonary edema and shock.

TABLE 37-13 Clinical Manifestations of Valvular Heart Diseases

	Clinical Manifestations
Mitral valve stenosis	Dyspnea on exertion, hemoptysis; fatigue; palpitations; loud, accentuated S_1; low-pitched, rumbling diastolic murmur; atrial fibrillation on ECG
Mitral valve regurgitation	*Acute*—generally poorly tolerated, with fulminating pulmonary edema and shock developing rapidly; new systolic murmur *Chronic*—weakness, fatigue, exertional dyspnea, palpitations; an S_3 gallop, holosystolic or pansystolic murmur
Mitral valve prolapse	Palpitations, dyspnea, chest pain, activity intolerance, syncope; midsystolic click, late or holosystolic murmur
Aortic valve stenosis	Angina, syncope, dyspnea on exertion, heart failure; normal or soft S_1, diminished or absent S_2, systolic crescendo-decrescendo murmur, prominent S_4
Aortic valve regurgitation	*Acute*—abrupt onset of profound dyspnea, chest pain, left ventricular failure and shock *Chronic*—fatigue, exertional dyspnea, orthopnea, PND; water-hammer pulse; heaving precordial impulse; diminished or absent S_1, S_3, or S_4; soft decrescendo high-pitched diastolic murmur, Austin-Flint murmur, systolic ejection click
Tricuspid and pulmonic stenosis	*Tricuspid*—peripheral edema, ascites, hepatomegaly; diastolic low-pitched, decrescendo murmur with increased intensity during inspiration *Pulmonic*—fatigue, loud midsystolic murmur

ECG, Electrocardiogram; *PND,* paroxysmal nocturnal dyspnea.

Clinical Manifestations

The clinical course of MR is determined by the nature of its onset (see Table 37-13). Patients with acute MR will have thready, peripheral pulses and cool, clammy extremities. A low CO may obscure a new systolic murmur. Rapid assessment (e.g., cardiac catheterization) and intervention (e.g., valve repair or replacement) are critical for a positive outcome.

Patients with chronic MR may remain asymptomatic for many years. Initial symptoms of left ventricular failure may include weakness, fatigue, palpitations, and dyspnea that gradually progress to orthopnea, paroxysmal nocturnal dyspnea, and peripheral edema. Accentuated left ventricular filling leads to an audible third heart sound (S_3), even with normal left ventricular function. The murmur is a loud holo- or pansystolic murmur at the apex radiating to the left axilla. Patients with asymptomatic MR should be monitored carefully, and surgery (valve repair or replacement) considered before significant left ventricular failure or pulmonary hypertension develops.[18]

MITRAL VALVE PROLAPSE

Etiology and Pathophysiology

Mitral valve prolapse (MVP) is an abnormality of the mitral valve leaflets and the papillary muscles or chordae that allows the leaflets to prolapse, or buckle, back into the left atrium during systole (Fig. 37-10). The etiology of MVP is unknown but is related to diverse pathogenic mechanisms of the mitral valve apparatus. The use of the term *prolapse* is unfortunate because it is used even when the valve is functionally normal. MVP is the most common

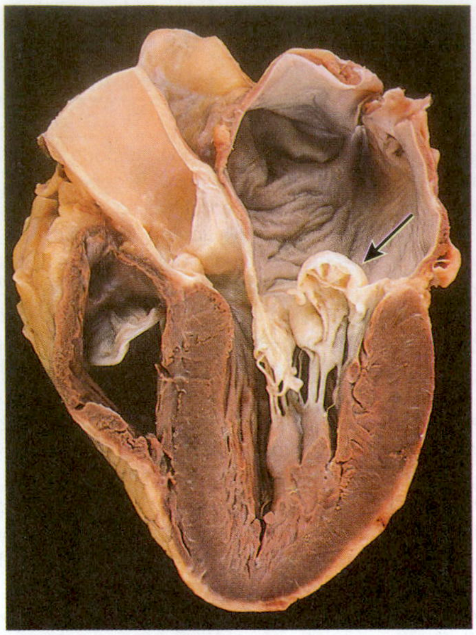

FIG. 37-10 Mitral valve prolapse. In this valvular abnormality, the mitral leaflets have prolapsed back into the left atrium. They also demonstrate hooding *(arrow)*. The left ventricle is on the right.

form of valvular heart disease in the United States, occurring 2 times more frequently in women than men.

MVP is usually benign, but serious complications can occur, including MR, IE, SCD, and cerebral ischemia. There is an increased familial incidence (autosomal dominant) in some patients. MVP in this group results from a connective tissue defect affecting only the valve, or as part of Marfan's syndrome or other hereditary conditions that affect the structure of collagen in the body. In many patients the abnormality found by echocardiography is not accompanied by any other clinical manifestations of cardiac disease, and the significance of the finding is unclear.

Clinical Manifestations

MVP covers a broad spectrum of severity. Most patients are asymptomatic and remain so for their entire lives. A characteristic of MVP is a murmur from regurgitation that gets more intense through systole. This could be a late or holosystolic murmur. Another major sign is one or more clicks usually heard in midsystole to late systole. MVP does not alter S_1 or S_2 heart sounds. Severe MR is an uncommon complication of MVP.

M-mode echocardiography confirms MVP by demonstrating late-systolic prolapse, and 2-D echocardiography reveals leaflet billowing into the left atrium. Dysrhythmias, most commonly ventricular premature contractions, paroxysmal supraventricular tachycardia, and ventricular tachycardia, may cause palpitations, light-headedness, and dizziness. IE may occur in patients with mitral regurgitation associated with MVP.

Patients may or may not have chest pain. The cause of the chest pain is not known, but it may be due to abnormal tension on the papillary muscles. If chest pain occurs, it tends to occur in clusters, especially during periods of emotional stress. Dyspnea, palpitations, and syncope may occasionally accompany the chest pain and do not respond to antianginal treatment (e.g., nitrates). β-Adrenergic blockers may be prescribed to control palpitations and chest pain.

Patients with MVP generally have a benign, manageable course unless problems associated with mitral regurgitation are present. A teaching plan for patients with MVP is presented in Table 37-14.

TABLE 37-14 PATIENT AND FAMILY TEACHING GUIDE
Mitral Valve Prolapse

1. Teach patient the importance of antibiotic prophylaxis for endocarditis before undergoing certain dental or surgical procedures if the patient has MVP with regurgitation (see Table 37-3).
2. Instruct patient to take medications as prescribed (e.g., β-adrenergic blockers to control palpitations, chest pain).
3. Advise patient to adopt healthy eating patterns and to avoid caffeine because it is a stimulant and may exacerbate symptoms.
4. Counsel patient who uses diet pills or other over-the-counter drugs to check for common ingredients that are stimulants (e.g., caffeine, ephedrine) as these will exacerbate symptoms.
5. Help patient to develop and implement an exercise program to maintain optimal health.
6. Instruct patient to contact Emergency Medical Services or health care provider if symptoms develop or worsen (e.g., palpitations, fatigue, shortness of breath, anxiety).

MVP, Mitral valve prolapse.

AORTIC VALVE STENOSIS

Etiology and Pathophysiology

Congenitally abnormal stenotic aortic valves are generally discovered in childhood, adolescence, or young adulthood. In older patients, **aortic stenosis** is a result of rheumatic fever or senile fibrocalcific degeneration that may have an etiology similar to coronary artery disease.[18,19] In rheumatic valvular disease, fusion of the commissures and secondary calcification cause the valve leaflets to stiffen and retract, resulting in stenosis. If aortic stenosis does occur due to rheumatic heart disease, mitral valve disease accompanies it. Isolated aortic valve stenosis is almost always nonrheumatic in origin. The incidence of rheumatic aortic valvular disease has been decreasing, but senile or degenerative stenosis is expected to increase as the population ages.

Aortic stenosis causes obstruction of flow from the left ventricle to the aorta during systole. The effect is left ventricular hypertrophy and increased myocardial oxygen consumption because of the increased myocardial mass. As the disease progresses and compensatory mechanisms fail, reduced CO leads to pulmonary hypertension and HF.

Clinical Manifestations

Symptoms of aortic stenosis (see Table 37-13) develop when the valve orifice becomes about one third its normal size. Symptoms include the classic triad of angina, syncope, and exertional dyspnea, reflecting left ventricular failure.[18,19] The prognosis is poor for a patient with symptoms and whose valve obstruction is not relieved. Nitroglycerin is contraindicated because it would reduce the preload necessary to help open the stiffened aortic valve. Auscultation of aortic stenosis typically reveals a normal or soft S_1; a diminished or absent S_2; a systolic, crescendo-decrescendo murmur that ends before S_2; and a prominent fourth heart sound (S_4).

AORTIC VALVE REGURGITATION

Etiology and Pathophysiology

Aortic valve regurgitation may be the result of primary disease of the aortic valve leaflets, the aortic root, or both. Acute aortic regurgitation (AR) is caused by IE, trauma, or aortic dissection and constitutes a life-threatening emergency. Chronic AR is generally the result of rheumatic heart disease, a congenital bicuspid aortic valve, syphilis, or chronic rheumatic conditions such as ankylosing spondylitis or Reiter's syndrome.

AR causes retrograde blood flow from the ascending aorta into the left ventricle during diastole, resulting in volume overload. The left ventricle initially compensates for chronic AR by dilation and hypertrophy. Myocardial contractility eventually declines and blood volumes increase in the left atrium and pulmonary bed. This results in pulmonary hypertension and right ventricular failure.

Clinical Manifestations

Patients with acute AR have sudden manifestations of cardiovascular collapse (see Table 37-13). The left ventricle is exposed to aortic pressure during diastole. The patient develops severe dyspnea, chest pain, and hypotension indicating left ventricular failure and shock that constitute a medical emergency.

Patients with chronic, severe AR develop a *water-hammer pulse* (a strong, quick beat that collapses immediately). Heart sounds may include a soft or absent S_1, presence of S_3 or S_4, and a soft, decrescendo high-pitched diastolic murmur. A systolic ejection click may also be heard, as well as a low-frequency diastolic murmur known as an *Austin-Flint murmur.*

The patient with chronic AR generally remains asymptomatic for years and is seen with exertional dyspnea, orthopnea, and paroxysmal nocturnal dyspnea only after considerable myocardial dysfunction has occurred (see Table 37-13). Angina occurs less frequently than in aortic stenosis.

TRICUSPID AND PULMONIC VALVE DISEASE

Etiology and Pathophysiology

Diseases of the tricuspid and pulmonic valves are uncommon, with stenosis occurring more frequently than regurgitation. *Tricuspid valve stenosis* occurs almost exclusively in patients with rheumatic fever, in IV drug abusers, or in patients treated with a dopamine agonist (e.g., cabergoline [Dostinex]).[16] *Pulmonary stenosis* is almost always congenital.

Tricuspid and pulmonic stenosis both result in an increase in blood volume in the right atrium and right ventricle, respectively. Tricuspid stenosis results in right atrial enlargement and elevated systemic venous pressures. Pulmonic stenosis results in right ventricular hypertension and hypertrophy (see Table 37-13).

DIAGNOSTIC STUDIES FOR VALVULAR HEART DISEASE

Diagnosis of valvular heart disease is generally based on the results of history, physical examination, echocardiogram, and cardiac catheterization (especially if surgery is considered) (Table 37-15). Chest x-ray results, ECG findings, and the clinical manifestations exhibited by the patient also aid in establishing the correct diagnosis.

An echocardiogram reveals valve structure, function, and chamber size. Transesophageal echocardiography and Doppler color-flow imaging are valuable in diagnosing and monitoring the progression of valvular heart disease. Real-time three-dimensional echocardiography may be helpful in qualitative assessments of mitral valve and congenital heart disease.[20] Cardiac catheterization detects pressure changes in the cardiac chambers, measures pressure gradients across the valves, and quantifies the size of valve openings. An ECG shows heart rate and rhythm and provides information about any ischemia or chamber enlargement. Chest x-ray reveals the heart size, alterations in pulmonary circulation, and calcification of valves.

TABLE 37-15 COLLABORATIVE CARE: Valvular Heart Disease

Diagnostic
History and physical examination
Chest x-ray
Electrocardiogram
Echocardiography
Cardiac catheterization
Collaborative Therapy
Nonsurgical
Prophylactic antibiotic therapy
• Rheumatic fever
• Infective endocarditis (see Table 37-3)
Sodium restriction
Medications to treat/control HF:
• Vasodilators (e.g., nitrates, ACE inhibitors*)
• Positive inotropes (e.g., digoxin)
• Diuretics
• β-Adrenergic blockers
Anticoagulation therapy (see Table 38-9)
Antidysrhythmic drugs
Percutaneous transluminal balloon valvuloplasty
Surgical
Commissurotomy (valvulotomy)
Valvuloplasty
Annuloplasty
Valve replacement

ACE, Angiotensin-converting enzyme; *HF,* heart failure.
*Contraindicated in aortic stenosis.

COLLABORATIVE CARE OF VALVULAR HEART DISEASE

Conservative Therapy

An important aspect of conservative management of valvular heart disease is prevention of recurrent rheumatic fever and IE (see Table 37-15). Treatment depends on the valve involved and the severity of the disease. It focuses on preventing exacerbations of HF, acute pulmonary edema, thromboembolism, and recurrent endocarditis. If manifestations of HF develop, vasodilators, positive inotropes, β-adrenergic blockers, diuretics, and a low-sodium diet are recommended (see Chapter 35).

Anticoagulant therapy is used to prevent and treat systemic or pulmonary embolization and is also used prophylactically in patients with atrial fibrillation. Dysrhythmias, especially atrial dysrhythmias, are common and are treated with digoxin, antidysrhythmic drugs, or electrical cardioversion. β-Adrenergic blockers may be used to slow the ventricular rate in patients with atrial fibrillation. (Dysrhythmias are discussed in Chapter 36.)

Percutaneous Transluminal Balloon Valvuloplasty. An alternative treatment for some patients with valvular heart disease is the *percutaneous transluminal balloon valvuloplasty* (PTBV) procedure, which splits open the fused commissures. Balloon valvuloplasty is used for mitral, tricuspid, and pulmonic stenosis, and less often for aortic stenosis. The procedure, performed in the cardiac catheterization laboratory, involves threading a balloon-tipped catheter from the femoral artery or vein to the stenotic valve so that the balloon may be inflated in an attempt to separate the valve leaflets. A single- or double-balloon technique may be used for the

PTBV procedure. Currently, the use of a single Inoue balloon with hourglass configuration allows sequential inflation. This technique is the most popular as it is easy, has good results, and has fewer complications (e.g., left ventricular perforation).[21] The PTBV procedure is generally indicated for older adult patients and for patients who are poor surgery candidates. PTBV has fewer complications than valve replacement. The long-term results of PTBV are similar to surgical commissurotomy.[21]

Surgical Therapy. The decision for surgical intervention is based on the clinical state of the patient as assessed using the New York Heart Association classification system for functional disability (see Table 35-4). The type of surgery depends on the valves involved, the valvular pathology, the severity of the disease, and the patient's clinical condition. All types of valve surgery are palliative, not curative, and patients will require lifelong health care.

Valve repair is typically the surgical procedure of choice. It is often used in mitral or tricuspid valvular heart disease and has a lower operative mortality rate than replacement. Mitral *commissurotomy* (valvulotomy) is the procedure of choice for patients with pure mitral stenosis. The less precise closed method of commissurotomy has generally been replaced by the open method in the United States, Canada, and Western Europe. The direct vision, or open, procedure requires the use of cardiopulmonary bypass, removal of thrombi from the atrium, excision of the left atrial appendage, commissure incision, and, as indicated, separation of fused chordae, splitting of underlying papillary muscle, and debriding of calcification of the valve. In contrast, the closed procedure is usually performed with the aid of a transventricular dilator inserted through the apex of the left ventricle into the ostium of the mitral valve.

Open surgical *valvuloplasty* involves repair of the valve by suturing the torn leaflets, chordae tendineae, or papillary muscles. It is primarily used to treat mitral or tricuspid regurgitation. Valve repair avoids the risks of replacement but may not establish total valve competence. Minimally invasive valvuloplasty surgery, using mini-sternotomy or parasternal approaches, has shown results comparable to the open procedure in addition to decreased length of stay, blood transfusions, and postoperative atrial fibrillation.[22]

Further repair or reconstruction of the valve may be necessary and can be achieved by annuloplasty, a procedure also used in cases of mitral or tricuspid regurgitation. *Annuloplasty* entails reconstruction of the annulus, with or without the aid of prosthetic rings (e.g., a Carpentier ring).

Prosthetic Valves. Valvular replacement may be required for mitral, aortic, tricuspid, and occasionally pulmonic valvular disease. The surgical treatment of choice for combined aortic stenosis and aortic regurgitation is valvular replacement.

A wide variety of prosthetic valves are available for use. Desirable valves are nonthrombogenic and durable and create minimal stenosis. Prosthetic valves are categorized as mechanical or biologic (tissue) valves (Table 37-16 and Fig. 37-11).

Mechanical valves are manufactured from man-made materials and consist of combinations of metal alloys, pyrolite carbon, and Dacron. *Biologic valves* are constructed from bovine, porcine, and human cardiac tissue and usually contain some man-made materials. Innovations in freezing and thawing techniques have enabled human grafts to be preserved for extensive periods while retaining viability. Mechanical prosthetic valves are more durable and last longer than biologic valves. However, they have an increased risk of thromboembolism, necessitating long-term anticoagulation therapy. The main complication of mechanical valves is hemorrhage from the use of anticoagulants.[23,24] Biologic valves do not require anticoagulation therapy due to their low thrombogenicity. However, they are less durable due to the tendency for early calcification, tissue degeneration, and stiffening of the leaflets. Problems with either type of prosthetic valves include paravalvular leaks and endocarditis.

Long-term anticoagulation is recommended for all patients with mechanical valves and for those with biologic valves who have atrial fibrillation. Some patients with biologic valves or annuloplasty with prosthetic rings may need anticoagulation the first few months after surgery until the suture lines are covered by endothelial cells (endothelialized).

The choice of valves depends on many factors. For example, if a patient cannot take an anticoagulant (e.g., women of childbearing age), a biologic valve may be considered. A mechanical valve may be best for a younger patient because it is more durable. For patients over age 65, durability is less important than the risks of hemorrhage from anticoagulants.

ETHICAL DILEMMAS
Do Not Resuscitate

Situation
A 68-year-old man has been admitted for a second mitral valve surgery and possible coronary artery bypass graft surgery. He did not adhere to the treatment plan following his original surgery 7 years ago. The nurse is worried about his future compliance with medications, diet, and exercise. His kidneys are failing and he is on dialysis, but not tolerating it well. Both the patient and family want complete therapeutic treatment and refuse to discuss Do Not Resuscitate (DNR) orders.

Important Points for Consideration
- Nonadherence with the treatment plan in the past does not always indicate the patient will not follow the plan of care in the future.
- A competent patient can decide if he wants continued treatment to be able to fight to live. This is even more important when family members support the patient's decision.
- Health care providers have an obligation to respect the patient's request for treatment unless there is no clear benefit to continued treatment. Patients' choices to continue or end treatment are based on their values and beliefs, which may not always coincide with those of the health care provider or team.
- DNR orders should reflect the patient's expressed wishes either through conversation, advance directives, or a surrogate decision maker.
- DNR orders should be reevaluated periodically with the patient and family, especially prior to major diagnostic procedures or treatments.
- If a heath care provider does not agree with a patient's treatment choice, a referral should be made to an Ethics Committee or similar group.

Critical Thinking Questions
1. What type of information should be provided to a patient and family in discussions about DNR orders? Who should provide this information?
2. What measures or strategies would be beneficial to assist the patient to better adhere to the treatment plan?

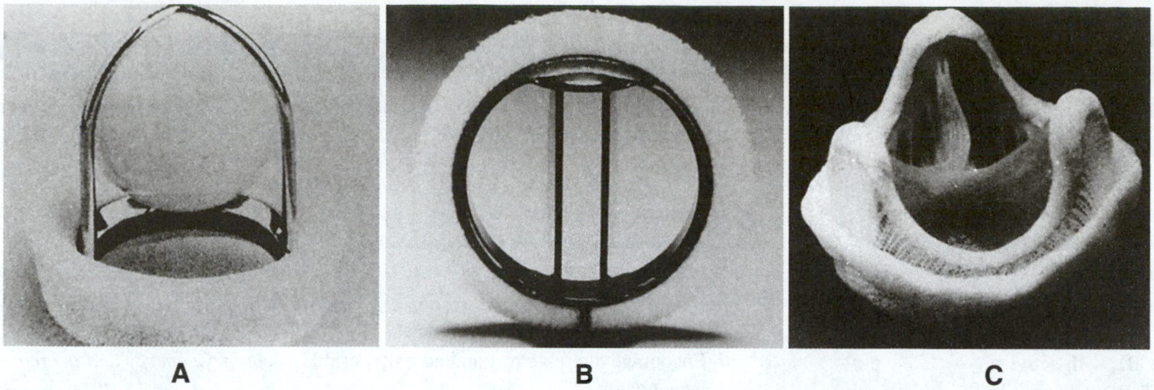

FIG. 37-11 Types of prosthetic heart valves. **A,** Starr-Edwards caged ball valve. **B,** St. Jude bi-leaflet valve. **C,** Carpentier-Edwards porcine valve.

TABLE 37-16 Types of Prosthetic Heart Valves

Type	Description
Mechanical	
Caged Ball Valve Starr-Edwards Sutter Magovern-Cromie	Metal cage with several struts mounted on a circular ring; hollow metal or plastic ball (poppett) inside of cage
Tilting-Disk Valve Lillehei-Kaster Medtronic-Hall	Mobile, lens-shaped disk attached to a circular sewing ring by two offset transverse struts; pyrolytic carbon composition
Bi-leaflet Valve St. Jude On-X CarboMedic	Two pivoting semicircular disks that open centrally, mounted directly onto a sewing ring
Biologic	
Porcine Heterograft Carpentier-Edwards Hancock Medtronic	Harvested aortic valve of pig that is preserved in glutaraldehyde and mounted on specially designed sewing ring
Pericardial Heterograft Ionescu-Shiley Carpentier-Edwards	Three leaflets composed of pericardium from 16- to 18-month-old calves that are preserved in glutaraldehyde and mounted on a Dacron-covered frame
Homograft Cadaver valve	Harvested aortic valve from human cadaver that is initially frozen until needed for valve replacement, then thawed, trimmed, and sewn into place with special mounting material

TABLE 37-17 *NURSING ASSESSMENT* Valvular Heart Disease

Subjective Data

Important Health Information

Past health history: Rheumatic fever, infective endocarditis; congenital defects, myocardial infarction, chest trauma, cardiomyopathy; syphilis, Marfan syndrome, streptococcal infections

Functional Health Patterns

Health perception–health management: IV drug abuse; fatigue

Activity-exercise: Palpitations; generalized weakness, activity intolerance; dizziness, fainting; dyspnea on exertion, cough, hemoptysis, orthopnea

Sleep-rest: Paroxysmal nocturnal dyspnea

Cognitive-perceptual: Angina or atypical chest pain

Objective Data

General

Fever

Integumentary

Diaphoresis, flushing, cyanosis, clubbing; peripheral edema

Respiratory

Crackles, wheezes, hoarseness

Cardiovascular

Abnormal heart sounds, including clicks, systolic and diastolic murmurs, S_3, and S_4; dysrhythmias, including atrial fibrillation, premature ventricular contractions; tachycardia; ↑ or ↓ in pulse pressure; hypotension, water-hammer or thready peripheral pulses

Gastrointestinal

Ascites, hepatomegaly

IV, Intravenous.

NURSING MANAGEMENT VALVULAR DISORDERS

■ Nursing Assessment

Subjective and objective data should be obtained from an individual with valvular disease and are presented in Table 37-17.

■ Nursing Diagnoses

Nursing diagnoses for the patient with valvular disease may include, but are not limited to, those presented in NCP 37-2.

■ Planning

The overall goals for the patient with valvular heart disease include (1) normal cardiac function, (2) improved activity tolerance, and (3) an understanding of the disease process and health maintenance measures.

■ Nursing Implementation

Health Promotion. Diagnosing and treating streptococcal infections and providing prophylactic antibiotics for patients with a history of rheumatic fever are critical to prevent acquired rheumatic valvular disease. The patient at risk for endocarditis and any patient with valvular heart disease must also be treated with prophylactic antibiotics (see Table 37-4).

NURSING CARE PLAN 37-2

Patient with Valvular Heart Disease

NURSING DIAGNOSIS **Activity intolerance** *related to* insufficient oxygenation secondary to decreased cardiac output and pulmonary congestion *as evidenced by* weakness, fatigue, shortness of breath, increase or decrease in pulse rate, BP changes

PATIENT GOAL Achieves optimal level of activity

OUTCOMES (NOC)

Activity Tolerance

- Pulse rate with activity ____
- Ease of breathing with activity ____
- Systolic BP with activity ____
- Diastolic BP with activity ____

Measurement Scale

1 = Severely compromised
2 = Substantially compromised
3 = Moderately compromised
4 = Mildly compromised
5 = Not compromised

INTERVENTIONS (NIC) and *RATIONALES*

Energy Management

- Monitor cardiorespiratory response to activity (e.g., pulse rate, respirations, BP) *to plan appropriate interventions.*
- Encourage alternate rest and activity periods *to conserve energy and decrease cardiac demands.*
- Encourage patient to choose activities that gradually build endurance *to increase cardiac tolerance.*
- Assist the patient/significant other to establish realistic activity goals *to promote feelings of accomplishment.*

NURSING DIAGNOSIS **Excess fluid volume** *related to* heart failure secondary to incompetent valves *as evidenced by* peripheral edema, weight gain, adventitious breath sounds, neck vein distention

PATIENT GOAL Achieves fluid and electrolyte balance

OUTCOMES (NOC)

Fluid Balance

- Adventitious breath sounds ____
- Neck vein distention ____
- Peripheral edema ____

Measurement Scale

1 = Severe
2 = Substantial
3 = Moderate
4 = Mild
5 = None

INTERVENTIONS (NIC) and *RATIONALES*

Hypervolemia Management

- Monitor changes in peripheral edema *to detect hypervolemia.*
- Monitor respiratory pattern for symptoms of difficulty (e.g., dyspnea, tachypnea) *to assess for fluid congestion in the lungs.*
- Monitor vital signs and intake and output *to assess hemodynamic response to and effectiveness of interventions.*
- Weigh patient daily and monitor trends (noting gain of >2 lb [0.9 kg]/day or >5 lb [2.3 kg]/wk) *to monitor indicators of hypervolemia.*
- Administer prescribed diuretics *to assist with removal of fluid.*

Fluid/Electrolyte Management

- Provide restricted sodium diet as ordered *to prevent fluid retention.*

NURSING DIAGNOSIS **Decreased cardiac output** *related to* valvular incompetence *as evidenced by* murmurs, dyspnea, dysrhythmias, peripheral edema

PATIENT GOALS
1. Maintains adequate tissue and organ perfusion
2. Maintains normal cardiac function

OUTCOMES (NOC)

Cardiac Pump Effectiveness

- Dysrhythmia ____
- Abnormal heart sounds ____
- Peripheral edema ____
- Dyspnea ____
- Pulmonary edema ____

Measurement Scale

1 = Severe
2 = Substantial
3 = Moderate
4 = Mild
5 = None

INTERVENTIONS (NIC) and *RATIONALES*

Cardiac Care

- Monitor vital signs, cardiovascular status, and respiratory status *to assess for manifestations of decreased cardiac output (e.g., fatigue, malaise, shortness of breath, dyspnea on exertion, palpitations, angina, widened pulse pressure).*
- Monitor for cardiac dysrhythmias, including disturbances of both rhythm and conduction, *to detect changes from baseline.*

Hemodynamic Regulation

- Administer inotropic medication as ordered *to increase myocardial contractility.*
- Elevate head of bed *to reduce venous return, reduce O_2 demand, and maximize chest excursion.*

Energy Management

- Promote bed rest/activity limitation *to decrease cardiac workload and O_2 demand.*

BP, Blood pressure.

NURSING CARE PLAN 37-2

Patient with Valvular Heart Disease—cont'd

NURSING DIAGNOSIS **Deficient knowledge** *related to* lack of experience and exposure to information about disease and treatment process *as evidenced by* verbalization of misconceptions about measures to prevent complications and requests for information

PATIENT GOAL Describes disease process and appropriate measures to prevent complications

OUTCOMES (NOC)	INTERVENTIONS (NIC) and *RATIONALES*
Knowledge: Disease Process • Description of specific disease process ____ • Description of effects of disease ____ • Description of signs and symptoms ____ • Description of measures to minimize disease progression ____ ***Knowledge: Medication*** • Description of actions of medications ____ • Description of correct administration of medication ____ **Measurement Scale** 1 = None 2 = Limited 3 = Moderate 4 = Substantial 5 = Extensive	***Teaching: Disease Process*** • Explain pathophysiology of disease process *to ensure knowledge base.* • Describe disease process and possible chronic complications (e.g., heart failure, infective endocarditis) *to ensure early reporting and treatment of complications.* • Instruct patient on measures to prevent complications (e.g., importance of notifying dentist, urologist, gynecologist, and other health care providers of valvular disease *so prophylactic antibiotic treatments can be initiated prior to invasive procedures*) and to wear Medic Alert bracelet. • Discuss lifestyle changes to prevent complications and/or control the disease (e.g., smoking cessation) *to prevent an increased cardiac workload and the oxygen-depleting effect of carbon monoxide.* • Instruct patient on signs and symptoms to report to health care provider *to assure appropriate interventions.* ***Teaching: Prescribed Medication*** • Instruct patient on purpose and action of each medication. • Provide patient with written information about action, purpose, and side effects of each medication.

The patient must adhere to recommended therapies. The individual with a history of rheumatic fever, endocarditis, and congenital heart disease should know the symptoms suggestive of valvular heart disease so that early medical treatment may be obtained.

Acute Intervention and Ambulatory and Home Care. A patient with progressive valvular heart disease may require hospitalization or outpatient care for management of HF, endocarditis, embolic disease, or dysrhythmias. HF is the most common reason for ongoing medical care.

The role of the nurse is to implement and evaluate the effectiveness of therapeutic interventions. Activity should be designed after considering the patient's limitations. An appropriate exercise plan can increase cardiac tolerance. However, activities that regularly produce fatigue and dyspnea should be restricted, and an explanation should be provided to the patient. Tobacco use should be discouraged. Strenuous physical exercise should be avoided because damaged valves may not be able to handle the demand for an increase in CO. The patient should be assisted in planning activities of daily living, with an emphasis on conserving energy, setting priorities, and taking planned rest periods. Referral to a vocational counselor may be necessary if the patient has a physically or emotionally demanding job.

Auscultation of the heart should be performed to monitor the effectiveness of digoxin, β-adrenergic blockers, and antidysrhythmic drugs. Teaching regarding the actions and side effects of drugs is important to achieve compliance. The patient must understand the importance of prophylactic antibiotic therapy to prevent IE (see Table 37-3). If the valve disease was caused by rheumatic fever, ongoing prophylaxis to prevent recurrence is necessary.

When valvular heart disease can no longer be managed medically, surgical intervention is necessary (see Chapter 34 for the care of a patient having cardiac surgery). The patient who is on anticoagulation therapy after surgery for valve replacement must have the international normalized ratio (INR) checked regularly (usually monthly) to assess the adequacy of therapy. The INR is a standardized system of reporting prothrombin time. Values of 2.5 to 3.5 are therapeutic for patients with mechanical valves.

Teaching instructions related to anticoagulation therapy are found Table 38-14. The patient must realize that valve surgery is not a cure, and that regular follow-up with a health care provider will be required. The nurse also must teach the patient about when to seek medical care. Any manifestations of infection or HF, any signs of bleeding, and any planned invasive or dental procedures require the patient to notify the health care provider. Finally, patients should be encouraged to wear a Medic Alert bracelet.

■ *Evaluation*

The expected outcomes for a patient with valvular heart disease are addressed in NCP 37-2.

Cardiomyopathy

Cardiomyopathy (CMP) constitutes a group of diseases that directly affect the structural or functional ability of the myocardium. A diagnosis of CMP is made based on the patient's clinical manifestations and noninvasive and invasive diagnostic procedures.

CMP can be classified as primary or secondary. *Primary CMP* refers to those conditions in which the etiology of the heart disease is unknown *(idiopathic)*. The heart muscle in this case is the only portion of the heart involved, and other cardiac structures are unaffected. In *secondary CMP* the cause of the myocardial disease is known and is secondary to another disease process. Common causes of secondary CMP are listed in Table 37-18.

TABLE 37-18 Causes of Secondary Cardiomyopathy

Dilated	Hypertrophic	Restrictive
Cardiotoxic agents—alcohol, cocaine, doxorubicin (Adriamycin) Genetic (autosomal dominant) or familial Hypertension Ischemia (coronary artery disease) Metabolic disorders Muscular dystrophy Myocarditis Pregnancy Valve disease	Aortic stenosis Genetic (autosomal dominant) Hypertension	Amyloidosis Endomyocardial fibrosis Neoplastic tumor Post–radiation therapy Sarcoidosis Ventricular thrombus

The World Health Organization has classified CMP conditions into three major types: dilated, hypertrophic, and restrictive.[25] Each type has its own pathogenesis, clinical presentation, and treatment protocols (Tables 37-19 and 37-20). Cardiomyopathies can lead to cardiomegaly and HF, and are the leading cause for heart transplantation.

DILATED CARDIOMYOPATHY

Etiology and Pathophysiology

Dilated cardiomyopathy is the most common type of CMP, with a prevalence of 5 to 8 cases per 100,000 people in the United States. It causes HF in 25% to 40% of cases, occurs more frequently in middle-aged African Americans and men, and has a genetic link in 30% of cases.[26] Dilated CMP is characterized by a diffuse inflammation and rapid degeneration of myocardial fibers that results in ventricular dilation, impairment of systolic function, atrial enlargement, and stasis of blood in the left ventricle. *Cardiomegaly* results from ventricular dilation (Fig. 37-12) and causes contractile dysfunction in spite of an enlarged chamber size. In contrast to HF, the walls of the ventricles do not hypertrophy (Fig. 37-13).

Dilated CMP often follows an infectious myocarditis. Other common causes of dilated CMP are listed in Table 37-18.

Clinical Manifestations

The signs and symptoms of dilated CMP may develop acutely after an infectious process or insidiously over a period of time. Most people eventually develop HF. Symptoms can include decreased exercise capacity, fatigue, dyspnea at rest, paroxysmal nocturnal dyspnea, and orthopnea. As the disease progresses the patient may experience dry cough, palpitations, abdominal bloating, nausea, vomiting, and anorexia. Signs can include an irregular heart rate with an abnormal S_3 and/or S_4, tachycardia or bradycardia, pulmonary crackles, edema, weak peripheral pulses, pallor, hepatomegaly, and jugular venous distention. Heart murmurs and dysrhythmias are common. Decreased blood flow through an enlarged heart promotes stasis and blood clot formation, and may lead to systemic embolization.

Diagnostic Studies

The diagnosis of dilated CMP is made on the basis of the patient's history and by ruling out other conditions that cause HF. Doppler echocardiography provides the basis for the diagnosis of dilated CMP in the majority of patients, and distinguishes dilated CMP from other structural abnormalities. The chest x-ray may show cardiomegaly with signs of pulmonary venous hypertension, as

TABLE 37-19 Comparison of Cardiomyopathies

	Dilated	Hypertrophic	Restrictive
Major Manifestations	Fatigue, weakness, palpitations, dyspnea	Exertional dyspnea, fatigue, angina, syncope, palpitations	Dyspnea, fatigue
Cardiomegaly	Moderate to marked	Mild to moderate	Mild
Contractility	↓	↑ or ↓	Normal or ↓
Valvular Incompetence	Atrioventricular valves, particularly mitral	Mitral valve	Atrioventricular valves
Dysrhythmias	Sinoatrial tachycardia, atrial and ventricular dysrhythmias	Atrial and ventricular dysrhythmias	Atrial and ventricular dysrhythmias
Cardiac Output	↓	Normal or ↓	Normal or ↓
Outflow Tract Obstruction	None	↑	None

TABLE 37-20 *COLLABORATIVE CARE* Cardiomyopathy

Diagnostic
History and physical examination
Electrocardiogram
Serum laboratory tests
Chest x-ray
Echocardiogram
Nuclear imaging studies
Cardiac catheterization
Endocardial biopsy

Collaborative Therapy
Treatment of underlying cause
Drug therapy
- Nitrates (except in HCM)
- β-Adrenergic blockers
- Antidysrhythmics
- ACE inhibitors
- Diuretics
- Digitalis (except in HCM with normal sinus rhythm)
- Anticoagulants (if indicated)

Ventricular assist device
Cardiac resynchronization therapy
Implantable cardioverter-defibrillator
Surgical correction
Cardiac transplant

ACE, Angiotensin-converting enzyme; *HCM,* hypertrophic cardiomyopathy.

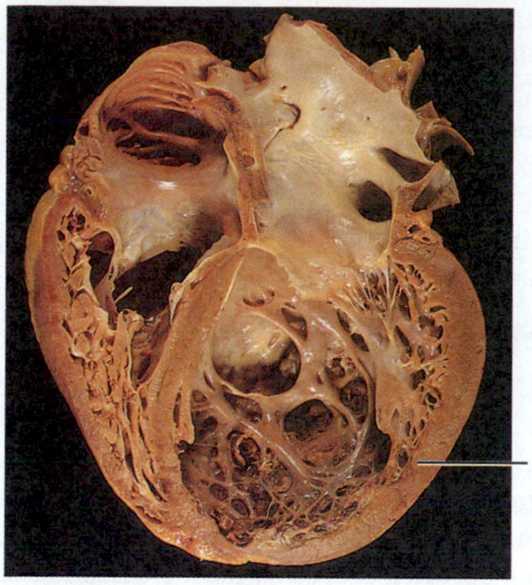

FIG. 37-12 Dilated cardiomyopathy. The dilated left ventricular wall has thinned, and the chamber size and volume are increased.

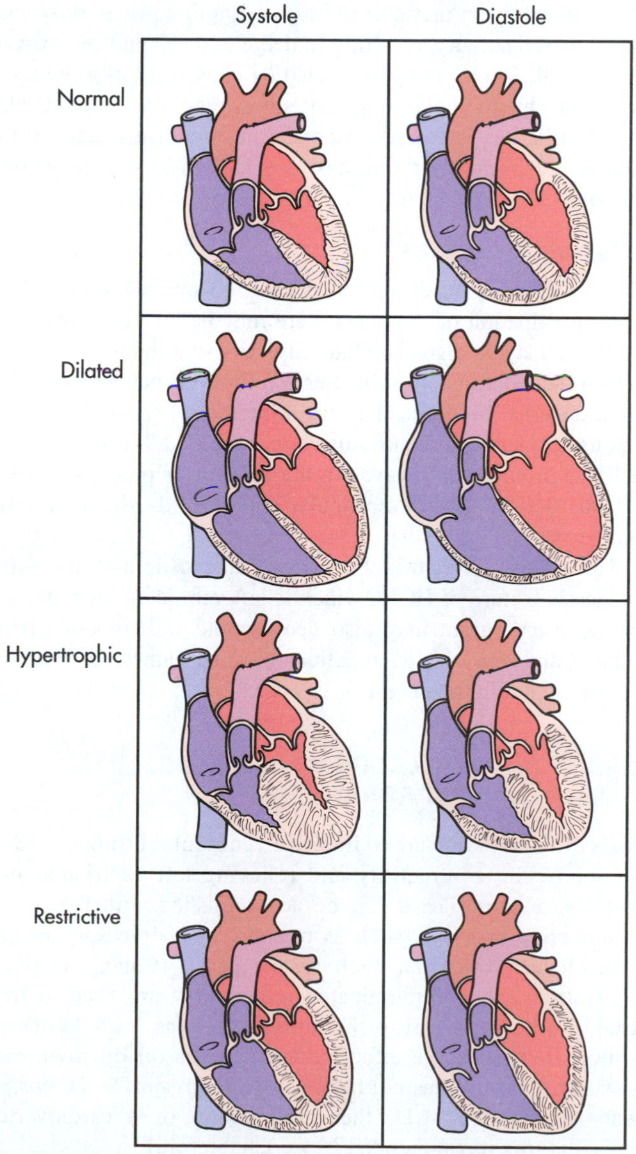

FIG. 37-13 Types of cardiomyopathies and the differences in ventricular diameter during systole and diastole, compared with a normal heart.

well as pleural effusion. The ECG may reveal tachycardia, bradycardia, and dysrhythmias with conduction disturbances. Laboratory studies may reveal elevated serum levels of b-type natriuretic peptide (BNP) in the presence of HF.

Cardiac catheterization is done to confirm or rule out coronary artery disease, and multiple gated acquisition (MUGA) radionuclide angiocardiographies are done to determine ejection fraction (EF). EFs of <20% are associated with a 50% mortality within 1 year. EMB may be done at the time of the right-sided heart catheterization to detect viral antigens in myocardial tissue.

NURSING *and* COLLABORATIVE MANAGEMENT DILATED CARDIOMYOPATHY

Interventions focus on controlling HF by enhancing myocardial contractility and decreasing afterload. This is similar to the treatment of chronic HF. Evidence-based practice guidelines from the American College of Cardiology and the American Heart Association base treatment of HF on the specific stage of disease progression[27] (see Table 35-4). Treatment of patients with class IV, stage D HF is more palliative than curative.

Several different types of drugs are used to manage HF (see Table 35-9). Nitrates (e.g., nitroglycerin [Nitrol]) and loop diuretics (e.g., furosemide [Lasix]) are used to decrease preload, and angiotensin-converting enzyme (ACE) inhibitors (e.g., captopril [Capoten]) are used to reduce afterload. β-Adrenergic blockers (e.g., metoprolol [Lopressor]) and aldosterone antagonists (e.g., spironolactone [Aldactone]) are used to control the neurohormonal stimulation that occurs in HF. Digoxin is used to treat atrial fibrillation but must be used with caution because of increased susceptibility to digoxin toxicity in these patients. Other dysrhythmias are treated with antidysrhythmics (e.g., amiodarone [Cordarone]) as indicated (see Chapter 36). Anticoagulation therapy is initiated to reduce the risk of systemic embolization from clots that may form in the heart chambers.[27]

Drug and nutritional therapy, and cardiac rehabilitation may help alleviate symptoms of HF, and improve CO and quality of life. A patient with secondary dilated CMP must be treated for the underlying disease process. For example, the patient with alcohol-related dilated CMP must abstain from all alcohol intake. (See Chapter 35 for a complete discussion of HF.)

Unfortunately, dilated CMP does not respond well to therapy, and patients may experience multiple episodes of HF. Intermittent dobutamine (Dobutrex) or milrinone (Primacor) infusions can be used. The patient is admitted to the hospital for a continuous infusion of dobutamine or milrinone followed by aggressive diuresis. Sometimes these infusions are done as an outpatient treatment or in the home under supervision of a home care nurse. After infusion, many patients experience an improvement in symptoms that lasts several weeks after therapy.

Patients also may benefit from nonpharmacologic therapies such as a ventricular assist device (VAD) to allow the heart to rest and recover from acute HF or as a bridge to heart transplantation. Additionally, cardiac resynchronization therapy and an implantable cardioverter-defibrillator may be considered in appropriate patients [28] (see Chapter 35).

The patient with terminal end-stage CMP may be considered for heart transplantation or destination therapy with a permanent or implantable VAD (see Chapter 35). Currently approximately 50%

of heart transplantations are performed for treatment of CMP. Cardiac transplant recipients have a good prognosis for survival. However, donor hearts are difficult to obtain, and many patients with dilated CMP die while awaiting heart transplantation.

Patients with dilated cardiomyopathy are very ill people with a grave prognosis who need expert nursing care. The patient's family must learn cardiopulmonary resuscitation (CPR) and how to access emergency care. The nurse should include family members and other support systems when planning a patient's care.

Home health and hospice nursing can provide the patient and the family with the continuous assessments and therapeutic interventions that are required to maximize and maintain functional status or prepare for a peaceful death. Observing for signs and symptoms of worsening HF, dysrhythmias, and embolic formation is paramount in this patient, as is monitoring drug responsiveness. The goal of therapy is to keep the patient at an optimal level of function and out of the hospital.

HYPERTROPHIC CARDIOMYOPATHY

Etiology and Pathophysiology

Hypertrophic cardiomyopathy (HCM), formerly called idiopathic hypertrophic subaortic stenosis, is asymmetric left ventricular hypertrophy without ventricular dilation. In one form of the disease, the septum between the two ventricles becomes enlarged and obstructs the blood flow from the left ventricle. It is termed *hypertrophic obstructive cardiomyopathy* (HOCM) or *asymmetric septal hypertrophy* (ASH). HCM can be idiopathic, though about one half of all cases have a genetic basis characterized by inappropriate myocardial hypertrophy (see Table 37-18). HCM occurs less commonly than dilated CMP, and is more common in men ages 30 to 40, than in women.[26] In one study, HCM occurred more frequently in young African American male athletes compared to young white male athletes.[29]

The four main characteristics of HCM are (1) massive ventricular hypertrophy; (2) rapid, forceful contraction of the left ventricle; (3) impaired relaxation (diastole); and (4) obstruction to aortic outflow (not present in all patients). Ventricular hypertrophy is associated with a thickened intraventricular septum and ventricular wall (see Figs. 37-13 and 37-14). The end result is impaired ventricular filling as the ventricle becomes noncompliant and unable to relax. The primary defect of HCM is diastolic dysfunction from left ventricular stiffness. Decreased ventricular filling and obstruction to outflow can result in decreased CO, especially during exertion. HCM is the most common cause of SCD in otherwise healthy young people. It is usually diagnosed in young adulthood and is often seen in active, athletic individuals.[29]

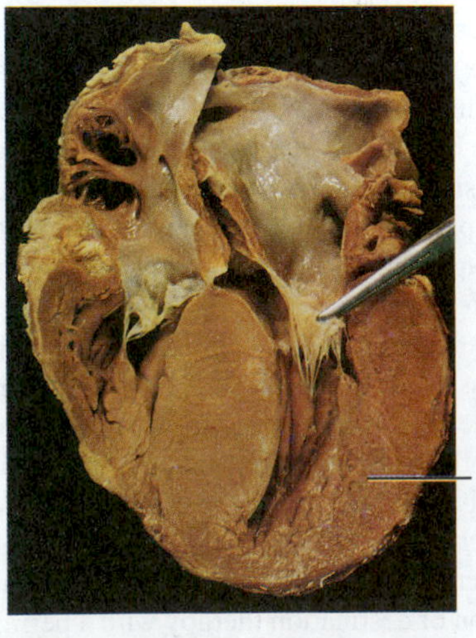

FIG. 37-14 Hypertrophic cardiomyopathy. There is marked left ventricular hypertrophy, and the chamber size and volume are decreased.

Clinical Manifestations

Patients with HCM may be asymptomatic or may have exertional dyspnea, fatigue, angina, and syncope. The most common symptom is dyspnea, which is caused by an elevated left ventricular diastolic pressure. Fatigue occurs because of the resultant decrease in CO and in exercise-induced flow obstruction. Angina can occur and is most often caused by the increased left ventricular muscle mass or compression of the small coronary arteries by the hypercontractile ventricular myocardium. The patient may also have syncope, especially during exertion. Syncope is most often caused by an increase in obstruction to aortic outflow during increased activity, resulting in decreased CO and cerebrovascular circulation. Syncope can also be caused by dysrhythmias. Common dysrhythmias include supraventricular tachycardia, atrial fibrillation, ventricular tachycardia, and ventricular fibrillation. Any of these dysrhythmias may lead to loss of consciousness or SCD (see Chapter 34).

Diagnostic Studies

Clinical findings on examination may be unremarkable. However, on palpation of the chest there may be a forced apical impulse that may be displaced laterally. Auscultation may reveal an S_4 heart sound and a systolic ejection murmur between the apex and the sternal border at the fourth intercostal space. ECG findings usually indicate ventricular hypertrophy, ST-T wave abnormalities, prominent Q waves in the inferior or precordial leads, left axis deviation, and ventricular and atrial dysrhythmias (see Chapter 36).

The echocardiogram is the primary diagnostic tool to confirm the classic feature of HCM, which is left ventricular hypertrophy. The echocardiogram may also demonstrate wall motion abnormalities and diastolic dysfunction. Cardiac catheterization may also be helpful in the diagnosis of HCM.

NURSING *and* COLLABORATIVE MANAGEMENT HYPERTROPHIC CARDIOMYOPATHY

Goals of intervention are to improve ventricular filling by reducing ventricular contractility and relieving left ventricular outflow obstruction. These can be accomplished with the use of β-adrenergic blockers, such as metoprolol (Lopressor), or calcium channel blockers, such as verapamil (Calan). Digitalis preparations are contraindicated unless they are used to treat atrial fibrillation. Antidysrhythmics, such as amiodarone or sotalol (Betapace), are effective medications for dysrhythmias. However, their use has not been shown to prevent SCD. For patients at risk for SCD, the implantation of a cardioverter-defibrillator is recommended[28] (see Chapter 36).

It has been found that atrioventricular pacing can be beneficial for patients with HCM and outflow obstruction. By pacing the ventricles from the apex of the right ventricle, septal depolarization occurs first, allowing the septum to move away from the left ventricular wall and reducing the degree of obstruction of the outflow tract.[28]

Some patients may be candidates for surgical treatment of their hypertrophied septum. The indications for surgery include severe symptoms refractory to therapy with marked obstruction to aortic outflow. The surgery is termed a *ventriculomyotomy and myectomy.* It involves incision of the hypertrophied septal muscle and resection of some of the hypertrophied ventricular muscle. Most patients have good symptomatic improvement and improved exercise tolerance after surgery.

An alternate nonsurgical procedure to reduce symptoms and the left ventricular outflow obstruction is alcohol-induced, percutaneous transluminal septal myocardial ablation (PTSMA). This procedure consists of administering alcohol into the first septal artery branching off the left anterior descending artery, which causes ischemia and septal wall myocardial infarction. Ablation of the septal wall will decrease the obstruction to flow, and the patient's symptoms will decrease. The procedure improves HF symptoms and exercise capacity 3 months after ablation.[30] Mortality rates for the procedure are approximately 1% depending on the age and condition of the patient. Information on long-term effects of PTSMA in treated patients is lacking because of the newness of the procedure. Potential complications of PTSMA include conduction disturbances (e.g., heart block) and MI beyond the intended septum.

Nursing interventions for HCM focus on relieving symptoms, observing for and preventing complications, and providing emotional and psychologic support. Teaching should focus on helping patients adjust their lifestyle to avoid strenuous activity and dehydration. Any activity or procedure that causes an increase in systemic vascular resistance (thus increasing the obstruction to forward flow) is dangerous and should be avoided. HCM patients who experience chest pain are managed by rest and elevation of the feet to improve venous return to the heart. Vasodilators such as nitroglycerin may worsen the chest pain by decreasing venous return to the heart, which would further increase obstruction of blood flow from the heart.

RESTRICTIVE CARDIOMYOPATHY

Etiology and Pathophysiology

Restrictive cardiomyopathy is the least common of the cardiomyopathic conditions. It is a disease of the heart muscle that impairs diastolic filling and stretch (see Fig. 37-13). Systolic function remains unaffected. Although the specific etiology of restrictive CMP is unknown, a number of pathologic processes may be involved in its development. Myocardial fibrosis, hypertrophy, and infiltration produce stiffness of the ventricular wall with loss of ventricular compliance. Secondary causes of restrictive CMP include amyloidosis, endocardial fibrosis, sarcoidosis, fibrosis of different etiology, and radiation to the thorax. With restrictive CMP, the ventricles are resistant to filling and therefore demand high diastolic filling pressures to maintain CO.

Clinical Manifestations

Classic symptoms of restrictive CMP are fatigue, exercise intolerance, and dyspnea because the heart cannot increase CO by increasing the heart rate without further compromising ventricular filling. Additional symptoms may include angina, orthopnea, syncope, and palpitations. The patient may have signs of HF, including dyspnea, peripheral edema, ascites, hepatomegaly, and jugular venous distention.

Diagnostic Studies

The chest x-ray may be normal, or it may show cardiomegaly from right and left atrial enlargement. Pleural effusions and pulmonary congestion may be evident in the patient with progression to HF. The ECG may reveal a mild tachycardia at rest. The most common dysrhythmias are supraventricular (atrial fibrillation) or atrioventricular block. Echocardiography may reveal a left ventricle that is normal sized with a thickened wall, slightly dilated right ventricle, and dilated atria. EMB, CT scan, and nuclear imaging may be helpful in the diagnosis.

NURSING *and* COLLABORATIVE MANAGEMENT RESTRICTIVE CARDIOMYOPATHY

Currently no specific treatment for restrictive CMP exists. Interventions are aimed at improving diastolic filling and the underlying disease process. Treatment includes conventional therapy for HF and dysrhythmias. Heart transplant may also be a consideration. Nursing care is similar to the care of a patient with HF. As in the treatment of patients with HCM, the patient should be taught to avoid situations that impair ventricular filling, such as strenuous activity, dehydration, and increases in systemic vascular resistance.

Nursing care of a patient with CMP includes individualized teaching based on the patient's clinical manifestations. All patients with CMP are at risk for IE from any procedure that may cause bacteremia and should be instructed on the need for prophylactic antibiotics (see Table 37-3). A general patient and family teaching guide is presented in Table 37-21.

TABLE 37-21 *PATIENT AND FAMILY TEACHING GUIDE* Cardiomyopathy

- Instruct patient to take all medications as prescribed and to follow up with health care provider.
- Encourage patient to use a low-sodium diet (if ordered) and to read all product labels (food and over-the-counter drugs) for sodium content.
- Unless fluids are restricted, patient should be encouraged to drink 6 to 8 glasses of water a day.
- Encourage patient to achieve and maintain a reasonable weight and avoid large meals.
- Advise patient to avoid alcohol, caffeine, diet pills, and over-the-counter cold medicines that may contain stimulants.
- Teach patient to balance activity and rest periods.
- Instruct patient to avoid heavy lifting or vigorous isometric exercises and to check with health care provider for exercise guidelines.
- Encourage the use of stress reduction activities: relaxation to relieve tension, guided imagery, diversional activities (see Chapter 9).
- Instruct patient to report any signs of heart failure to health care provider, including weight gain, edema, shortness of breath, and increased fatigue.
- Suggest that family members learn CPR because of the potential of sudden cardiac arrest (see Appendix A).
- Instruct patient to notify health care provider or dentist before any invasive medical/dental procedures as patients with cardiomyopathy are at risk for endocarditis (see Table 37-3).

CPR, Cardiopulmonary resuscitation.

CRITICAL THINKING EXERCISE

CASE STUDY

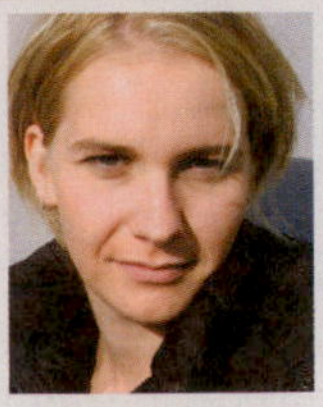

Case Study photo ©iStockphoto.com/ Kati Neudert.

Valvular Heart Disease

Patient Profile. Susan, a 35-year-old white female, is admitted to the hospital for valvular heart disease.

Subjective Data

- Reports history of IV drug use
- Prior hospital admission for infective endocarditis
- Must sleep sitting up
- Shortness of breath, even with dressing self
- Takes "water pill" for her "pressure"
- Smokes a pack of cigarettes a day

Objective Data

Physical Examination

- Third heart sound (S_3)
- Loud holosystolic murmur of mitral regurgitation
- Pitting pretibial and pedal edema
- Irregular pulse; apical pulse rate > radial pulse rate

Diagnostic Studies

- 2-D echocardiogram shows left atrial and ventricular enlargement and flail valve leaflets.
- ECG shows atrial fibrillation, enlarged left ventricle and atrium.
- Chest x-ray reveals pulmonary congestion.

Critical Thinking Questions

1. Identify the cause and course of Susan's disease based on her history and current exam.
2. Differentiate between acute and chronic mitral regurgitation.
3. What surgical procedure will Susan probably require as her condition worsens?
4. Identify three priority nursing interventions for Susan.
5. On the basis of the assessment data provided, identify at least three priority nursing diagnoses.

NCLEX EXAMINATION REVIEW QUESTIONS

The number of the question corresponds to the same-numbered objective at the beginning of the chapter.

1. A patient with a history of IV cocaine use has acute infective endocarditis. The nurse assesses the patient for
   a. weight gain.
   b. a new murmur.
   c. a distended abdomen.
   d. red spots on the chest.
2. Nursing assessment findings for acute pericarditis include
   a. wheezing and dull precordial pain.
   b. bradycardia, tachypnea, and murmur.
   c. chest pain, dyspnea, and pericardial friction rub.
   d. respiratory stridor, dull chest pain, and abdominal discomfort.
3. Prophylactic antibiotics are indicated to prevent infective endocarditis for at-risk individuals who are
   a. undergoing any dental procedure.
   b. having a viral respiratory infection.
   c. entering the third trimester of pregnancy.
   d. exposed to human immunodeficiency virus.
4. The most common underlying cause of myocarditis is
   a. heart failure.
   b. a viral infection.
   c. a bacterial infection.
   d. a myocardial infarction.
5. Teaching the patient with rheumatic fever about the disease, the nurse explains that rheumatic fever is
   a. a *Streptococcus viridans* infection.
   b. a viral infection of the endocardium and valves.
   c. a sequela of group A streptococcal infection.
   d. frequently triggered by immunosuppressive therapy.
6. A patient with rheumatic fever should be taught about the need for
   a. regular exercise.
   b. antibiotic therapy.
   c. a high-protein diet.
   d. anticoagulant therapy.
7. A common cause of aortic valve stenosis in older adults is
   a. rheumatic fever.
   b. cardiomyopathy.
   c. congenital heart disease.
   d. acute infective endocarditis.
8. Which of the following findings is indicative of left ventricular overload in a patient with chronic aortic regurgitation?
   a. Dehydration and a pericardial friction rub
   b. An audible third heart sound and a mid-systolic murmur
   c. Exertional dyspnea and a diastolic high-pitched murmur
   d. An audible third heart sound and a pansystolic or holosystolic murmur
9. A patient hospitalized with aortic stenosis has a nursing diagnosis of activity intolerance related to insufficient oxygen secondary to decreased cardiac output. An appropriate nursing intervention for this patient is to
   a. monitor ECG to assess cardiac output.
   b. maintain on bed rest to reduce tissue oxygen demands.
   c. progressively increase activity to increase cardiac tolerance.
   d. use a semi-Fowler's position to decrease venous return and increase respiratory excursion.
10. The nurse caring for a patient scheduled for a mitral valve replacement with a mechanical valve understands that this procedure
    a. is similar to a commissurotomy.
    b. requires long-term anticoagulation therapy.
    c. is the treatment of choice for an elderly patient with a history of falling.
    d. involves the insertion of a transventricular dilator into the opening of the valve.
11. Which of the following assessment findings would the nurse expect in a patient with dilated cardiomyopathy?
    a. Dyspnea and fatigue
    b. Wheezing and epigastric pain
    c. Palpitations and left lower quadrant tenderness
    d. Excessive sputum and lower abdominal cramping
12. The nurse plans care for the patient with dilated cardiomyopathy based on the knowledge that
    a. family members may be at risk because of the infectious nature of the disease.
    b. medical management of the disorder focuses on treatment of the underlying cause.
    c. the prognosis of the patient is poor, and emotional support is a high priority of care.
    d. the condition may be successfully treated with surgical ventriculomyotomy and septal ablation.

REFERENCES

1. Munson BL: Myths and facts . . . about infective endocarditis, *Nursing* 35(2):71, 2005.
2. Horstkotte D, Piper C: New aspects of infective endocarditis, *Minerva Cardioangiol* 52:273, 2004.
3. Millar BC, Moore JE: Emerging issues in infective endocarditis, *Emerg Infect Dis* 10(6), 2004. Available at *www.cdc.gov/ncidod/EID/vol10no6/03-0848.htm* (accessed April 2005).
4. Yee C: The infected heart, *Nursing Manage* 36(2):25, 2005.
5. Badour LM: Infective endocarditis: AHA Scientific Statement, *Circulation* 111:e394-e434, 2005.
6. Brusch JL: Infective endocarditis, New York, 2006, eMedicine (last updated August 15, 2005). Available at *www.emedicine.com/MED/topic671.htm* (accessed July 2006).
7. Calza L: Infective endocarditis: a review of best treatment options, *Expert Opin Pharmacother* 9:1899, 2004.
8. Hirstkotte D, et al: Guidelines on prevention, diagnosis and treatment of infective endocarditis, *Eur Hear J* 25:267, 2004.
9. Ross A: Acute pericarditis, *Postgrad Med* 115:32, 2004.
10. Throughton RW, Asher CR, Klein AL: Pericarditis seminar, *Lancet* 363:717, 2004.
11. Wisnieski A: Combating infection: muscle up your knowledge of myocarditis, *Nursing* 34:17, 2004.
12. Holcomb SS: Recognizing and managing different types of carditis, *TravelNursing* 35:6, 2005.
13. MayoClinic.com: Rheumatic fever overview, Rochester, Minn, 2005 Mayo Clinic. Available at *www.mayoclinic.com/health/rheumatic-fever/DS00250* (accessed July 20, 2006).
14. McMillin DJ, Chatwal GS: Prospects for a group A streptococcal vaccine, *Curr Opin Mol Ther* 7:11, 2005.
15. World Health Organization: Rheumatic fever and rheumatic heart disease: report of a WHO expert consultation study group (Technical Report Series No. 923), Geneva, 2004, World Health Organization.
16. Horvath J, Fross RD, Kleiner-Fisman G, et al: Severe multivalvular heart disease: a new complication of the ergot derivative dopamine agonists, *Mov Disord* 19:656, 2004.
17. Enriquez-Serano M, Avierinos JF, Messika-Zeitoun D, et al: Quantitative determinants of the outcome of asymptomatic mitral regurgitation, *N Engl J Med* 352:875, 2005.
18. Todd BA, Higgins K: Recognizing aortic and mitral valve disease, *Nursing* 35(6):58, 2005.
19. Freeman RV, Crittenden G: Acquired aortic stenosis, *Expert Rev Cardiovasc Ther* 2:107, 2004.
20. Chan KL, Liu X, Ascah KJ, et al: Comparison of real-time 3-dimensional echocardiography with conventional 2-dimensional echocardiography in the assessment of structural heart disease, *J Am Soc Echocardiogr* 17:976, 2004.
21. Vahanian A, Palacios IF: Percutaneous approaches to valvular disease, *Circulation* 109:1572, 2004.
22. Mihaljevic T, Cohn LH, Unic D, et al: One thousand minimally invasive valve operations: early and late results, *Ann Surg* 240:529, 2004.
23. Moffat-Bruce SD, Jamieson WR: Long-term performance of prostheses in mitral replacement, *J Cardiovasc Surg* 45:427, 2004.
24. Schurgers LJ, Aebert H, Vermeer C, et al: Oral anticoagulant treatment: friend or foe in cardiovascular disease? *Blood* 104:3231, 2004.
25. World Health Organization: ICD version 2006. Diseases of the circulatory system. Available at *www.who.int/icd/currentversion/fr-icd.htm* (accessed July 18, 2006).
26. Chojnowski D: Putting the pieces together of cardiomyopathy, *Nurs Made Incredibly Easy* May/June:18, 2004.
27. Hunt SA, Abraham WT, Chin MH, et al: ACC/AHA guideline update for the evaluation and management of chronic heart failure in the adult: a report of the American College of Cardiology/American Heart Association Task Force on Practice Guidelines (Writing Committee to Update the 2001 Guidelines for the Evaluation and Management of Heart Failure). *Circulation* 112:e154, 2005. Available at *http://circ.ahajournals.org/cgi/content/full/112/12/e154* (accessed July 2006).
28. Gregoratos G, Abrams J, Epstein AE, et al: ACC/AHA/NASPE 2002 guideline update for implantation of cardiac pacemakers and antiarrhythmia devices: summary article, *Circulation* 106:2145, 2002.
29. Maron BJ, Carney KP, Lever HM, et al: Relationship of race to sudden cardiac death in competitive athletes with hypertrophic cardiomyopathy, *J Am Coll Cardiol* 41:974, 2003.
30. Faber L, Meissner A, Zeimssen P, et al: Percutaneous transluminal septal myocardial ablation for hypertrophic obstructive cardiomyopathy: long term follow up of the first series of 25 patients, *Heart* 83:326, 2000.

RESOURCES

American Association of Cardiovascular and Pulmonary Rehabilitation
312-321-5146
www.aacvpr.org

American College of Cardiology
800-253-4636, ext. 694, or 301-897-5400
www.acc.org

American Heart Association
800-AHA-USA-1 (800-242-8721)
www.americanheart.org

Hypertrophic Cardiomyopathy Association
973-983-7429
www.4hcm.org

National Heart, Lung, and Blood Institute
National Institutes of Health
301-592-8563
www.nhlbi.nih.gov

The Mended Hearts
888-HEART99 (888-432-7899) or 214-706-1442
www.mendedhearts.org

For additional Internet resources, see the website for this book at *http://evolve.elsevier.com/Lewis/medsurg.*

Every good thought you think is contributing its share to the ultimate result of your life.
Grenville Kleiser

38 Nursing Management Vascular Disorders

Deirdre D. Wipke-Tevis and Kathleen Rich

LEARNING OBJECTIVES

1. Describe the etiology and pathophysiology of peripheral arterial disease.
2. Identify the major risk factors associated with peripheral arterial disease.
3. Describe the pathophysiology, clinical manifestations, and collaborative care of aortic aneurysms.
4. Discuss the perioperative nursing care of a patient having an aortic aneurysm repair.
5. Describe the pathophysiology, clinical manifestations, and collaborative care of aortic dissection.
6. Discuss the clinical manifestations, collaborative care, and surgical management of peripheral arterial disease of the lower extremities.
7. Discuss the nursing management of the patient with acute arterial insufficiency affecting the lower extremities.
8. Differentiate the pathophysiology, clinical manifestations, and collaborative care of thromboangiitis obliterans (Buerger's disease) and Raynaud's phenomenon.
9. Identify the risk factors predisposing to the development of superficial thrombophlebitis and deep vein thrombosis.
10. Differentiate between the clinical characteristics of superficial thrombophlebitis and deep vein thrombosis.
11. Describe the collaborative care and nursing management of the patient with venous thrombosis, including superficial thrombophlebitis and deep vein thrombosis.
12. Describe the nursing management of the patient receiving anticoagulation therapy.
13. Discuss the pathophysiology, clinical manifestations, and collaborative and nursing management of patients with varicose veins, venous insufficiency, or venous leg ulcers.

KEY TERMS

acute arterial ischemia, p. 907
aneurysms, p. 894
aortic dissection, p. 898
chronic venous insufficiency, p. 919
critical limb ischemia, p. 903
deep vein thrombosis, p. 909
intermittent claudication, p. 900
peripheral arterial disease, p. 893
Raynaud's phenomenon, p. 908
superficial thrombophlebitis, p. 909
thromboangiitis obliterans (Buerger's disease), p. 908
varicose veins, p. 917
venous thrombosis, p. 909
Virchow's triad, p. 909

Electronic Resources

Supplemental content related to Chapter 38 can be found . . .

Companion CD

- Stress-Busting Kit for Nursing Students
- Interactive Case Studies:
  - Abdominal Aortic Aneurysm
  - Chronic Peripheral Arterial Disease
- NCLEX Examination Review Questions
- Comprehensive Glossary

Evolve Website

http://evolve.elsevier.com/Lewis/medsurg

- Content Updates
- Key Points (Printable and CD/MP3 Download)
- Concept Map Creator
- Expanded Audio Glossary
- Key Term Flash Cards
- Customizable Nursing Care Plans:
  - Peripheral Arterial Disease of the Lower Extremities
  - Surgical Repair of the Aorta
- Patient and Family Instruction Guide in English and Spanish:
  - Anticoagulation Therapy
- Electronic Calculators
- WebLinks

Problems of the vascular system include disorders of the arteries and veins. *Peripheral arterial disease* (PAD) is a term used to describe a wide variety of conditions affecting arteries in the neck, abdomen, and extremities. PAD can be subdivided into occlusive disease, aneurysmal disease, and vasospastic phenomenon. In contrast, venous diseases primarily affect the lower extremities and can be categorized into venous thrombosis and chronic venous insufficiency.

Reviewed by Karen R. Bruni, RN, MSN, NP, CVN, Director of Nursing, Nurse Practitioner, The Vascular Group, PLLC, Albany, N.Y.; and Janet Riggs, RN, MSN, CCRN, CCNS, Research Project Manager, Penn Presbyterian Medical Center, Philadelphia, Pa.

Peripheral Arterial Disease

Peripheral arterial disease involves progressive narrowing and degeneration of the arteries of the neck, abdomen, and extremities. Regardless of the anatomic location, atherosclerosis is responsible for the majority of cases of PAD, both occlusive and aneurysmal.[1] Although PAD typically appears in the sixth to eighth decades of life, it occurs at an earlier age in persons with diabetes mellitus. Prevalence of PAD is 3 times greater in African Americans.[2] In general, between 12% and 20% of Americans age 65 and older have PAD.[3] Men in their 60s are about twice as likely (6.7%) to have PAD as are women (2.8%). However, as women age, their incidence of PAD becomes similar to or greater than that in men.[2] Thus as our population ages, PAD will become a major health care problem. It is estimated that, by 2050, PAD prevalence could affect 9.6 to 16 million Americans over the age of 65 years and 19 million overall.[3]

PAD is strongly related to other manifestations of cardiovascular disease and its risk factors. Specifically, those with PAD have 4 to 5 times the risk of dying of a cardiovascular event (e.g., myocardial infarction, stroke).[3] Therefore PAD must be thought of as a marker of advanced systemic atherosclerosis. If an individual has PAD, it is likely that she or he also has coronary artery disease and/or carotid artery disease. Unfortunately, PAD remains underdiagnosed and undertreated in a broad segment of Americans.[1,3]

Etiology and Pathophysiology

The leading cause of PAD is *atherosclerosis,* a gradual thickening of the intima and media of arteries, which leads to progressive narrowing of the vessel lumen. Although the exact cause (or causes) of atherosclerosis remain unknown, inflammation and endothelial injury have a major role (see Chapter 34). The pathologic changes that occur with atherosclerosis consist of migration and replication of smooth muscle cells, deposition of connective tissue, lymphocyte and macrophage infiltration, and accumulation of lipids.

The four most significant risk factors for PAD are cigarette smoking, hyperlipidemia, hypertension, and diabetes mellitus, with the most important being cigarette smoking. Other risk factors include obesity, hypertriglyceridemia, hyperuricemia, family history, sedentary lifestyle, and stress. Additional risk factors under investigation include serum levels of C-reactive protein (CRP), fibrinogen, ferritin, homocysteine, and lipoprotein (a).[2,4,5]

Although atherosclerosis is a diffuse process, certain segments of the arterial tree are more commonly involved, including the coronary arteries (see Chapter 34), carotid arteries (see Chapter 58), aortic bifurcation, iliac and common femoral arteries, profunda femoris artery, superficial femoral artery, and distal popliteal artery (especially in diabetics) (Fig. 38-1). The involvement is generally segmental, with normal segments interspersed between involved ones. Clinical manifestations occur when the vessel is between 60% and 75% occluded.

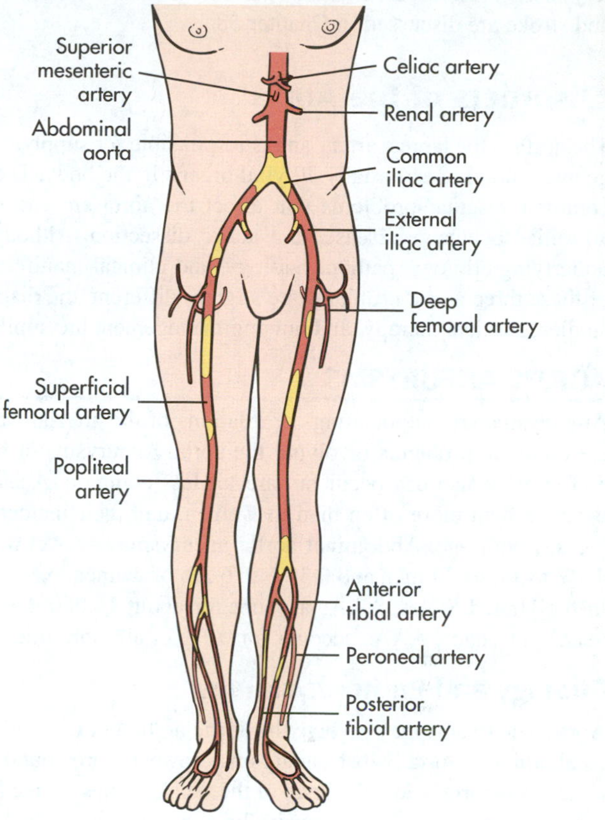

FIG. 38-1 Common anatomic locations of atherosclerotic lesions (shown in *yellow*) of the abdominal aorta and lower extremities.

CAROTID ARTERY DISEASE

Atherosclerosis is the most common cause of carotid artery disease (cerebrovascular disease) in the United States. Approximately 88% of all strokes are ischemic in nature and result from an atherothrombotic event.[3] Early identification and treatment of carotid ar-

GENDER DIFFERENCES
Vascular Disorders

Men

- Men in their 60s are almost twice as likely to have PAD as women.
- After age 85, 30% to 50% of both men and women have PAD.
- AAAs occur more frequently in men than women.
- Thromboangiitis obliterans (Buerger's disease) occurs predominantly in men <40 years of age.

Women

- As women age, the incidence of PAD is similar to or greater than that of men.
- Women with PAD have reported decreased physical functioning, more bodily pain, and greater mood disturbances than men with PAD.
- Due to anatomic differences in women (e.g., smaller femoral artery), endovascular repair of AAAs may not be an option for women.
- Raynaud's phenomenon occurs primarily in women between 15 and 40 years of age.
- Risk for DVT is greater in women over age 35 who smoke, use oral contraceptives or HRT, are pregnant or postpartum, or have a family history of DVT.
- Risk for varicose veins is greater in women who use oral contraceptives or HRT, or are pregnant.

AAAs, Abdominal aortic aneurysms; *DVT,* deep vein thrombosis; *HRT,* hormone replacement therapy; *PAD,* peripheral arterial disease.

tery disease decreases the risk of stroke. Cerebrovascular disease and stroke are discussed in Chapter 58.

Disorders of the Aorta

The aorta is the largest artery and is responsible for supplying oxygenated blood to essentially all vital organs in the body. The most common vascular problems that affect the aorta are aneurysms, aortoiliac occlusive disease, and aortic dissection. Although the underlying etiology, pathophysiology, and clinical manifestations of these three aortic problems are slightly different, the diagnostic studies, surgical therapy, and nursing management are similar.

AORTIC ANEURYSMS

Aneurysms are outpouchings or dilations of the arterial wall and are common problems involving the aorta. Aneurysms of peripheral arteries also can occur but are far less common. Aneurysms occur in men more often than in women, and their incidence increases with age. Abdominal aortic aneurysms (AAAs) occur in 4.1% to 14.2% of men and 0.35% to 6.2% of women over age 60.[6] In the United States, AAAs account for about 16,000 deaths per year.[3] In Canada, AAAs account for 0.7% of all mortalities.[7]

Etiology and Pathophysiology

Aortic aneurysms may involve the aortic arch, thoracic aorta, and/or abdominal aorta. Most aneurysms, however, are found in the abdominal aorta below the level of the renal arteries. Three fourths of true aortic aneurysms occur in the abdominal aorta (Fig. 38-2) and one fourth in the thoracic aorta. Popliteal artery aneurysms rank third in frequency. Patients may have an aneurysm in more than one location. The growth rate of aneurysms is unpredictable, but the larger the aneurysm, the greater the risk of rupture. The dilated aortic wall becomes lined with thrombi that can embolize, leading to acute ischemic symptoms in distal (downstream) branches.

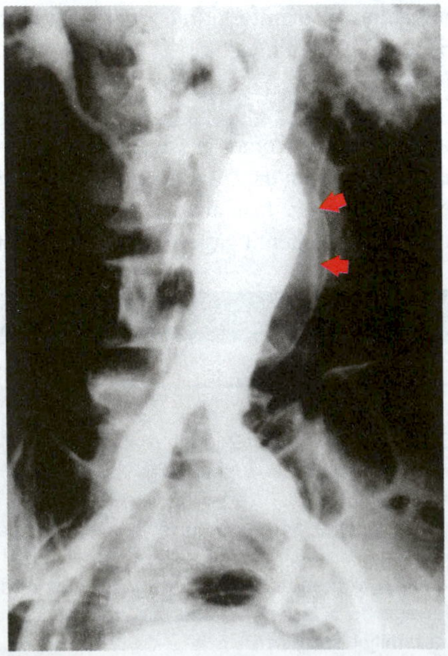

FIG. 38-2 Angiography demonstrating fusiform abdominal aortic aneurysm. Note calcification of the aortic wall *(arrows)* and extension of the aneurysm into the common iliac arteries.

A variety of disorders are associated with aortic aneurysms. However, the primary causes can be classified as degenerative, congenital, mechanical, inflammatory, or infectious. The most common etiology of aneurysms of the descending and abdominal aorta is atherosclerosis.[8] Atherosclerotic plaques deposit beneath the *intima* (the innermost layer of the arterial wall). Plaque formation is thought to cause degenerative changes in the *media* (middle layer of the arterial wall), leading to loss of elasticity, weakening, and eventual aortic dilation. Male gender and smoking appear to be stronger risk factors for AAAs of atherosclerotic origin than hypertension and diabetes.[6]

Several studies have shown a strong genetic predisposition in the development of AAAs. The familial tendency to develop aneurysms is related to a number of congenital abnormalities, including specific defects in collagen (e.g., Ehlers-Danlos syndrome) and premature degeneration of vascular elastic tissue (Marfan syndrome).[8] Less common causes of aneurysm formation include penetrating or blunt trauma from motor vehicle accidents (mechanical), inflammatory aortitis (e.g., Takayasu's or giant cell arteritis), and infectious aortitis (e.g., syphilis, *Salmonella,* human immunodeficiency virus infection).

Classification

Aneurysms generally are divided into two basic classifications: true and false aneurysms (Fig. 38-3). A *true aneurysm* is one in which the wall of the artery forms the aneurysm, with at least one vessel layer still intact. True aneurysms can be further subdivided into fusiform and saccular. A *fusiform aneurysm* is circumferential and relatively uniform in shape. A *saccular aneurysm* is

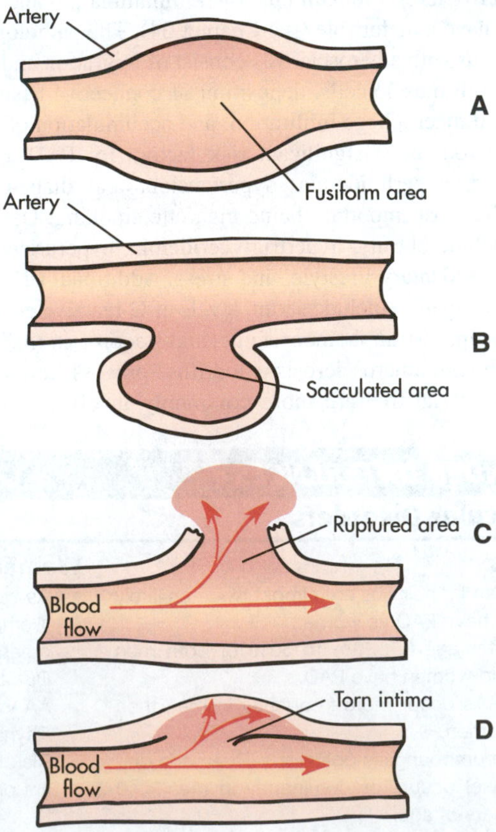

FIG. 38-3 **A,** True fusiform abdominal aortic aneurysm. **B,** True saccular aortic aneurysm. **C,** Aortic dissection. **D,** False aneurysm or pseudoaneurysm.

pouchlike with a narrow neck connecting the bulge to one side of the arterial wall.

A *false aneurysm,* or *pseudoaneurysm,* is not an aneurysm but a disruption of all layers of the arterial wall resulting in bleeding that is contained by surrounding structures. False aneurysms may result from trauma or infection, or occur after peripheral artery bypass graft surgery at the site of the graft-to-artery anastomosis. They also may result from arterial leakage after removal of cannulae such as upper or lower extremity arterial catheters and intraaortic balloon pump devices.[8]

Clinical Manifestations

Thoracic aorta aneurysms are often asymptomatic. When symptoms are present, the most common manifestation is deep, diffuse chest pain that may extend to the interscapular area. Aneurysms located in the ascending aorta and the aortic arch can produce angina from disruption of blood flow to the coronary arteries and hoarseness as a result of pressure on the recurrent laryngeal nerve. Pressure on the esophagus can cause dysphagia. If the aneurysm presses on the superior vena cava, decreased venous return can result in distended neck veins and edema of the head and arms.

AAAs also are often asymptomatic and frequently detected on routine physical examination or coincidentally when the patient is examined for an unrelated problem (e.g., abdominal x-ray, ultrasound, computed tomography [CT] scan, intravenous pyelogram, or abdominal surgery). On physical examination, a pulsatile mass in the periumbilical area slightly to the left of the midline may be detected. Bruits may be auscultated with a stethoscope placed over the aneurysm. Physical findings may be more difficult to detect in obese individuals.

Symptoms of AAAs may mimic pain associated with abdominal or back disorders. Compression of nearby anatomic structures may cause symptoms such as back pain from lumbar nerve compression or epigastric discomfort and/or altered bowel elimination from bowel compression. Occasionally, aneurysms spontaneously embolize plaque, causing "blue toe syndrome" (patchy mottling of the feet and toes in the presence of palpable pedal pulses).

Complications

The most serious complication related to an untreated aneurysm is rupture. If rupture occurs posteriorly into the retroperitoneal space, bleeding may be tamponaded by surrounding structures, preventing exsanguination and death. In this case, the patient often has severe back pain and may or may not have back or flank ecchymosis *(Grey Turner's sign).*

If rupture occurs anteriorly into the abdominal cavity, most patients do not survive long enough to get to the hospital; they die from massive hemorrhage. If the patient does reach the hospital, he or she is in hypovolemic shock with tachycardia, hypotension, pale clammy skin, decreased urine output, altered level of consciousness, and abdominal tenderness on palpation. (Shock is discussed in Chapter 67.) In this situation, simultaneous resuscitation and immediate surgical repair are necessary.

Diagnostic Studies

Chest x-rays are useful in demonstrating the mediastinal silhouette and any abnormal widening of the thoracic aorta. A plain x-ray of the abdomen may show calcification within the wall of AAAs. An electrocardiogram (ECG) may be performed to rule out evidence of myocardial infarction (MI) because some persons with thoracic aneurysms have symptoms suggestive of angina. Echocardiography assists in the diagnosis of aortic valve insufficiency related to ascending aortic dilation. Ultrasonography is useful in screening for aneurysms, and to serially monitor aneurysm size. A CT scan is the most accurate test to determine the anterior-to-posterior length, the cross-sectional diameter, and the presence of thrombus in the aneurysm.[9] Magnetic resonance imaging (MRI) also may be used to diagnose and assess the location and severity of aneurysms.

Angiography, anatomic mapping of the aortic system by contrast imaging, is not a reliable method of determining aneurysm diameter or length. It may, however, be helpful in providing the physician with accurate information about the involvement of intestinal, renal, or distal vessels. It also is useful if a suprarenal or thoracoabdominal aneurysm is suspected. (Angiography is discussed in Chapter 32.)

Collaborative Care

The goal of management is to prevent the aneurysm from rupturing. Therefore early detection and prompt treatment are imperative. Once an aneurysm is suspected, studies are performed to determine its exact size and location. A careful review of all body systems is necessary to identify any coexisting disorders, especially of the lungs, heart, or kidney, because they may influence the patient's surgical risk. If carotid and/or coronary artery obstructions are present, they may need to be corrected before the aneurysm is repaired. For individuals with small aneurysms (<4 cm), conservative therapy typically is initiated, which consists of risk factor modification, decreasing blood pressure (BP), and monitoring aneurysm size every 6 months using ultrasound, MRI, or CT scan.[8] Based upon the best available evidence, 5.5 cm is the threshold for repair in the typical patient; however, intervention at a diameter <5.5 cm is indicated in women with AAAs.[9] Surgical intervention may occur earlier in younger, low-risk patients or if the aneurysm is expanding rapidly (≥0.5-cm diameter increase over a 6-month period), in a patient who is symptomatic, or if the risk of rupture is high. In older, higher risk patients, endovascular repair of the aneurysm may be the treatment of choice.

Surgical Therapy. Preoperatively, the patient is hydrated and any electrolyte, coagulation, and hematocrit abnormalities are corrected. However, if the aneurysm has ruptured, emergent surgical intervention is required. Ruptured AAAs have a 33% to 94% mortality rate, with the lowest survival seen in women and older patients.[10-12] In the United States, elective AAA repair has a perioperative mortality rate of 3.2% to 7.0% for men and 4.5% to 10.7% for women.[11] Aneurysms repaired electively have an average 30-day mortality rate of 4.5% in Canada.[12]

The surgical technique involves (1) incising the diseased segment of the aorta; (2) removing intraluminal thrombus or plaque; (3) inserting a synthetic graft (Dacron or polytetrafluoroethylene [PTFE]), which is sutured to the normal aorta proximal and distal to the aneurysm; and (4) suturing the native aortic wall around the graft so that it will act as a protective cover (Fig. 38-4). If the iliac arteries also are aneurysmal, the entire diseased segment is replaced with a bifurcation graft. With saccular aneurysms, it may be possible to excise only the bulbous lesion, repairing the artery by primary closure (suturing the artery together) or by application of an autogenous or synthetic patch graft over the arterial defect. Use of autotransfusion, which recycles the patient's own blood, has markedly reduced the need for blood transfusions during surgery. (Autotransfusion is discussed in Chapter 31.)

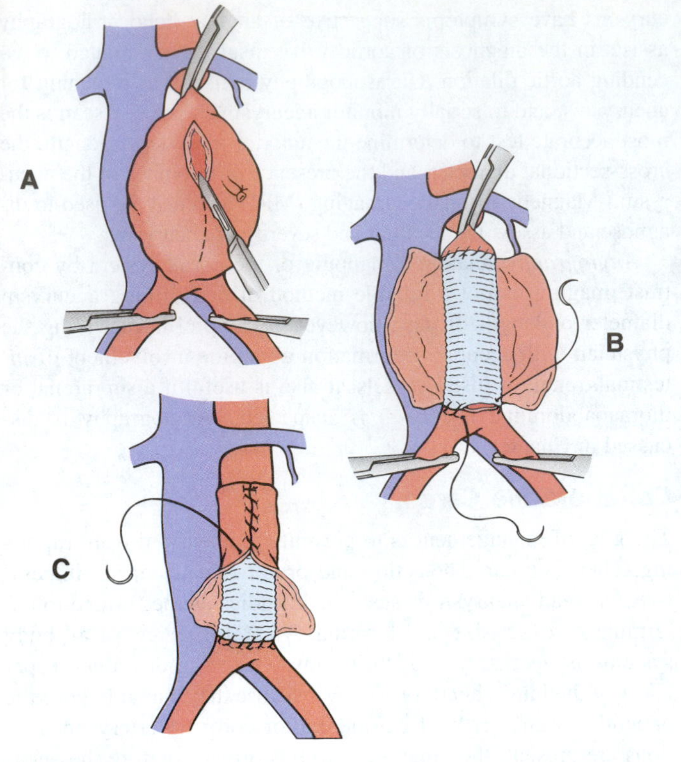

FIG. 38-4 Surgical repair of an abdominal aortic aneurysm. **A,** Incising the aneurysmal sac. **B,** Insertion of synthetic graft. **C,** Suturing native aortic wall over synthetic graft.

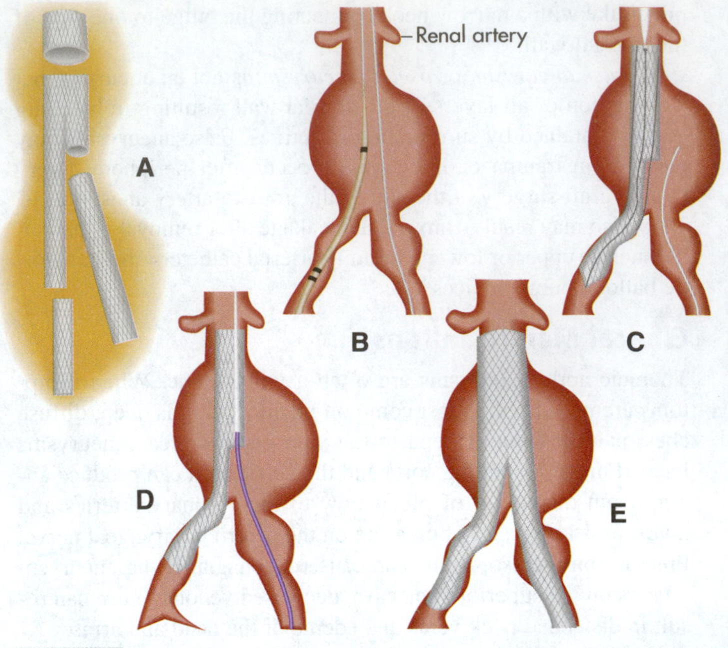

FIG. 38-5 Bifurcated (two branched) endovascular stent grafting of an aneurysm. **A,** The insertion of a woven polyester tube (graft) covered by a tubular metal web (stent). **B,** The stent graft is inserted through a large blood vessel (e.g., femoral artery) using a delivery catheter. The catheter is positioned below the renal arteries in the area of the aneurysm. **C,** The stent graft is slowly released (deployed) into the blood vessel. When the stent comes in contact with the blood vessel, it expands to a preset size. **D,** A second stent graft can be inserted in the contralateral (opposite) vessel if necessary. **E,** Fully deployed bifurcated stent graft.

All AAA resections require cross-clamping of the aorta proximal and distal to the aneurysm. Most resections can be completed in 30 to 45 minutes, after which time the clamps are removed and blood flow to the lower extremities is restored. If the AAA extends above the renal arteries or if the cross clamp must be applied above the renal arteries, adequate renal perfusion after clamp removal should be ascertained before closure of the abdominal incision. The risk of postoperative renal complications such as renal failure is increased significantly in patients who have surgical repair of AAAs above the renal arteries.

Endovascular Graft Procedure. Minimally invasive endovascular grafting is an alternative to conventional surgical repair of AAAs. The endovascular technique involves the placement of a sutureless aortic graft into the abdominal aorta inside the aneurysm via a femoral artery cutdown. The graft is constructed from a Dacron cylinder, and the surface of the graft is supported with multiple rings of extra flexible wire (Fig. 38-5). After the compactly folded graft is delivered through the sheath to the predetermined point, the graft is deployed, pressed/implanted against the vessel wall by balloon inflation (creating a circumferential seal), and anchored to the vessel by a series of small hooks. The blood then flows through the endovascular graft, thus preventing further expansion of the aneurysm due to pressure. The aneurysmal wall will begin to shrink over time because the blood is now being diverted through the endograft.

Patients must meet strict eligibility criteria to be candidates for the use of endovascular devices. Endovascular repair is most advantageous for older, higher risk patients.[13] Patients with aortoiliac occlusive disease or renal artery involvement are not suitable candidates. Due to anatomic differences in women (e.g., smaller femoral artery), endovascular repair may not be an option for many women.[11] Some of the devices are custom made for each patient using data from CT scans, angiography, and ultrasound. In other institutions, the physicians use knitted Dacron grafts combined with balloon-expandable stents.

The benefits of endovascular repair include decreased anesthesia and operative time, smaller operative blood loss, decreased morbidity and mortality, small bilateral groin incisions (instead of a large abdominal incision), more rapid resumption of physical activity, shortened length of hospital (including intensive care unit [ICU]) stays, quicker recovery, higher patient satisfaction, and reduction in overall costs.[14,15] Potential complications include aneurysm growth, aneurysm rupture, perigraft leaks (endoleaks), aortic dissection, bleeding, graft dislocation and embolization, renal artery occlusion due to graft migration, graft thrombosis, incisional site hematoma, and incisional infection. The most commonly reported complication is *perigraft leak,* which is the seeping of blood from the new endograft back into the old aneurysm site. The perigraft leak may be due to an inadequate seal at either graft end, a tear through the graft fabric, or leakage between overlapping graft segments and may require coil embolization (insertion of beads) for hemostasis.[13,14] Graft dysfunction may require conversion to a traditional surgical repair. With endovascular repair there is a higher reintervention rate and a need for long-term follow-up.[13] Although the long-term complications associated with this technique are not known, 2- and 5-year follow-up studies indicate that aneurysm rupture is rare and long-term graft patency is similar between endovascular and the standard open repair.[14,15]

A new approach to endovascular repair is percutaneous femoral access as opposed to the more traditional femoral approach via an incision (cutdown).[16] Advantages to percutaneous endograft placement include shorter operative time, shorter anesthesia time, a reduction in the use of general anesthesia, and reduced groin complications within the first 6 months after surgery.

NURSING MANAGEMENT
AORTIC ANEURYSMS AND AORTOILIAC DISEASE

■ Nursing Assessment

A thorough history and physical assessment should be performed. Because atherosclerosis is a systemic disease process, the nurse should watch for signs of cardiac, pulmonary, cerebral, and lower extremity vascular problems. The patient should be monitored for indications of aneurysm rupture, such as diaphoresis; paleness; weakness; tachycardia; hypotension; abdominal, back, groin, or periumbilical pain; changes in level of consciousness; or a pulsating abdominal mass.

Establishing baseline data is important for comparison with later postoperative assessments. In particular, the nurse should observe the patient closely for any baseline abnormalities. Special attention should be paid to the character and quality of the patient's peripheral pulses and neurologic status. Pedal pulse sites (dorsalis pedis and posterior tibial) and any skin lesions on the lower extremities should be marked and documented before surgery.

■ Planning

The overall goals for a patient undergoing aortic surgery include (1) normal tissue perfusion, (2) intact motor and sensory function, and (3) no complications related to surgical repair, such as thrombosis or infection.

■ Nursing Implementation

Health Promotion. The nurse must be aware of cardiovascular disease risk factors and be alert for opportunities to teach health promotion measures to patients and their families (see Chapter 34). Special attention should be given to the patient with a family history of aneurysm or any evidence of other cardiovascular disease.

The patient should be encouraged to reduce cardiovascular risk factors (see Chapter 34, Table 34-3), including BP control, smoking cessation (see Chapter 12), increasing physical activity, and maintaining normal body weight and serum lipid levels. These measures also are done to ensure continued graft patency following surgical repair.

Acute Intervention. The nursing role during the preoperative period includes patient and family teaching, providing support for the patient and family, and careful assessment of all body systems. Preoperative teaching should include a brief explanation of the disease process, the planned surgical procedure(s), preoperative routines, what to expect immediately after surgery (e.g., recovery room, tubes/drains), and usual postoperative timelines. Although specific preoperative routines often vary by institution and/or physician, in general, patients undergoing aortic surgery typically undergo some sort of bowel preparation (i.e., laxatives, enemas) and have a preoperative shower with an antimicrobial soap the day before surgery, receive nothing by mouth (NPO) after midnight the day before surgery, and often are given preoperative intravenous antibiotics immediately before surgery. If the patient will be going to the ICU after surgery, orientation to the ICU before surgery may be helpful to the patient and family.

Postoperatively, aortic surgery patients typically go to an ICU for close monitoring. When the patient arrives in the ICU, an endotracheal tube for mechanical ventilation, an arterial line, a central venous pressure (CVP) or pulmonary artery (PA) catheter, peripheral intravenous (IV) lines, an indwelling urinary catheter, and a nasogastric tube will likely be in place with continuous ECG and pulse oximetry monitoring. If the thorax is entered during surgery, chest tubes also will be in place. Pain medication may be administered via epidural catheter or patient-controlled analgesia.

In addition to the usual goals associated with the care of a postoperative patient (e.g., maintaining adequate respiratory function, fluid and electrolyte balance, and pain control [see Chapter 20]), the nurse must monitor graft patency and renal perfusion. The nurse also monitors for and intervenes to limit or treat dysrhythmias, infections, and neurologic complications. A nursing care plan for the patient with an aneurysm repair or other aortic surgery is available on the Evolve website *http://evolve.elsevier.com/Lewis/medsurg.*

Graft Patency. An adequate BP is important to maintain graft patency. Prolonged hypotension may result in graft thrombosis. Administration of IV fluids and blood components (as indicated) is essential for adequate blood flow to the graft. CVP readings or PA pressures and urinary output should be monitored hourly in the immediate postoperative period to help assess the patient's hydration and perfusion status.

Severe hypertension may cause undue stress on the arterial anastomoses, resulting in leakage of blood or rupture at the suture lines. Drug therapy with IV diuretics (e.g., furosemide [Lasix]) or IV antihypertensive agents (e.g., nitroprusside [Nipride], fenoldopam [Corlopam], nicardipine [Cardene]) may be indicated.[17]

Cardiovascular Status. In individuals with preexisting coronary artery disease, myocardial ischemia or infarction may occur in the perioperative period due to decreased myocardial oxygen supply or increased myocardial oxygen demands. Cardiac dysrhythmias also may occur due to electrolyte imbalances, hypoxemia, hypothermia, or myocardial ischemia. Nursing interventions include continuous ECG monitoring, frequent electrolyte and arterial blood gas (ABG) determinations, administration of oxygen and IV antidysrhythmic medications as needed, replacement of electrolytes as indicated, adequate pain control, and resumption of preoperative cardiac medications.

Infection. The development of a prosthetic vascular graft infection is a relatively rare but potentially life-threatening complication. Nursing intervention to prevent infection should include ensuring that the patient receives a broad-spectrum antibiotic as prescribed. Body temperature is assessed regularly, and elevations are promptly reported. Laboratory data are monitored for elevated white blood cell (WBC) count, which may be the first indication of an infection. In addition, the nurse should ensure adequate nutrition and observe the surgical incision for any evidence of delayed healing or signs of infection (e.g., redness, swelling, drainage).

All IV, arterial, and CVP or PA catheter insertion sites should be cared for using strict aseptic technique because they are frequent ports of entry for bacteria. Meticulous perineal care for the patient with an indwelling urinary catheter is essential to minimize the risk of urinary tract infection. Surgical incisions should be kept clean and dry.

Gastrointestinal Status. After abdominal aortic surgery, paralytic ileus may develop as a result of anesthesia and the manipulation of the bowel during surgery. The intestines may become swollen and bruised, and peristalsis ceases for variable intervals. A retroperitoneal surgical approach can be used to decrease the risk of bowel complications.

A nasogastric tube is inserted during surgery and connected to low, intermittent suction. This decompresses the stomach, prevents aspiration of stomach contents, and decreases pressure on suture lines. The nasogastric tube should be irrigated with normal saline solution as needed, and the amount and character of the drainage should be recorded. The nurse should auscultate for the return of bowel sounds. The passing of flatus is a key sign of returning bowel function and should be noted. Early ambulation will assist with the resumption of bowel functioning. It is unusual for paralytic ileus to persist beyond the fourth postoperative day.

If the blood supply to the bowel is disrupted during surgery, temporary ischemia or infarction (death) of intestinal tissue may result. Clinical manifestations of bowel ischemia include absent bowel sounds, fever, abdominal distention, diarrhea, and bloody stools. When bowel infarction does occur, reoperation is necessary as soon as possible to restore blood flow, with likely resection of the infarcted bowel. Fortunately, this serious complication is uncommon.

While the patient is NPO, meticulous mouth care should be provided every few hours. In some situations ice chips or lozenges may be given to soothe a dry or irritated throat.

Neurologic Status. Neurologic complications can occur after aortic surgery. When the ascending aorta and aortic arch are involved, nursing interventions should include assessment of level of consciousness, pupil size and response to light, facial symmetry, tongue deviation, speech, ability to move upper extremities, and quality of hand grasps (see Chapter 57). When the descending aorta is involved, nursing assessment of the ability to move lower extremities also is important. These assessments should be recorded in detail. Any alteration from the baseline assessment should be reported to the physician immediately.

Peripheral Perfusion Status. The anatomic location of the aneurysm indicates the areas of major concern related to peripheral perfusion. All peripheral pulses should be checked and recorded every hour for several hours, depending on institutional policy, and routinely thereafter at frequent intervals. When the ascending aorta and aortic arch are involved, the carotid, radial, and temporal artery pulses should be assessed. After surgery involving the descending aorta, the femoral, popliteal, posterior tibial, and dorsalis pedis pulses should be assessed (see Chapter 32, Fig. 32-8).

When checking the pulses, the nurse should mark the locations with a felt-tip pen so that others can locate them easily. Doppler ultrasound is useful in assessment of peripheral pulses. It is also important to note the skin temperature and color, capillary refill time, and sensation and movement of the extremities (see Chapter 32).

Occasionally, lower extremity pulses may be absent for a short time following surgery due to vasospasm and hypothermia. A decreased or absent pulse in conjunction with a cool, pale, mottled, or painful extremity may indicate embolization of aneurysmal thrombus or plaque, or graft occlusion. Therefore these findings should be reported to the physician immediately. Graft occlusion is treated with reoperation if identified early. In rare instances, thrombolytic therapy also may be considered. In some patients, the pulses may have been absent preoperatively because of coexistent lower extremity PAD. Comparison with the preoperative status is essential to determine the etiology of a decreased or absent pulse and the proper treatment.

Renal Perfusion Status. Postoperatively, the patient has an indwelling urinary catheter in place. In the immediate postoperative period, hourly urine outputs are recorded. An accurate record of fluid intake and urinary output should be kept until the patient resumes the preoperative diet. Daily weights also should be obtained. CVP readings and PA pressures also provide important information regarding hydration status. Daily blood urea nitrogen (BUN) and serum creatinine studies are performed to evaluate renal function. (For signs and symptoms of acute renal failure, see Chapter 47.) Irreversible renal failure may occur after aortic surgery, particularly in high-risk individuals (e.g., patients with diabetes).

One cause of decreased renal perfusion is embolization of a fragment of thrombus or plaque from the aorta that subsequently lodges in one or both of the renal arteries. This can cause ischemia of one or both kidneys. Hypotension, dehydration, prolonged aortic clamping during surgery, or blood loss also can lead to decreased renal perfusion.

Ambulatory and Home Care. The patient and family may be apprehensive about returning home after major aortic surgery. The nurse should encourage the patient to express any concerns and reassure the patient that normal activities of daily living can be resumed. The patient should be instructed to gradually increase activities. Fatigue, poor appetite, and irregular bowel habits are to be expected. Heavy lifting is avoided for at least 4 to 6 weeks following surgery. Any redness, swelling, increased pain, drainage from incisions, or fever greater than 100° F (37.8° C) should be reported to the health care provider.

The patient should be taught to observe for changes in color or warmth of the extremities. Patients can learn to palpate peripheral pulses to assess changes in their quality. The patient who has received a synthetic graft should be instructed that prophylactic antibiotics may be required before future invasive procedures, including any dental procedures.

Sexual dysfunction in male patients is not uncommon after aortic surgery. Sexual dysfunction may occur because the internal hypogastric artery is interrupted, leading to decreased arterial blood flow to the penis. In addition, the periaortic sympathetic plexus may be disrupted by the surgical procedure. Preoperatively, baseline sexual function should be documented and patient counseling is recommended. Postoperatively, a referral to a urologist may be considered if erectile dysfunction is a problem.

There are situations in which operative repair is not performed. Examples of this are the presence of a very small aneurysm (<4 cm), a patient who is not a surgical candidate (e.g., severe lung or cardiac disease), or a patient who refuses to undergo repair. The patient who does not undergo surgical repair should be urged to receive regular routine physical examinations and should be reminded that any symptom, no matter how minor, must be investigated if it persists.

■ *Evaluation*

Expected outcomes for the patient who undergoes aortic surgery include:

- patent arterial graft with adequate distal perfusion
- adequate urine output
- normal body temperature
- no signs of infection

AORTIC DISSECTION

Aortic dissection, often misnamed "dissecting aneurysm," is not a type of aneurysm. **Aortic dissection,** occurring most commonly in the thoracic aorta, is the result of a tear in the intimal (innermost) lining of the arterial wall (Figs. 38-3 and 38-6). Aortic dissection affects men more often than women and occurs most frequently

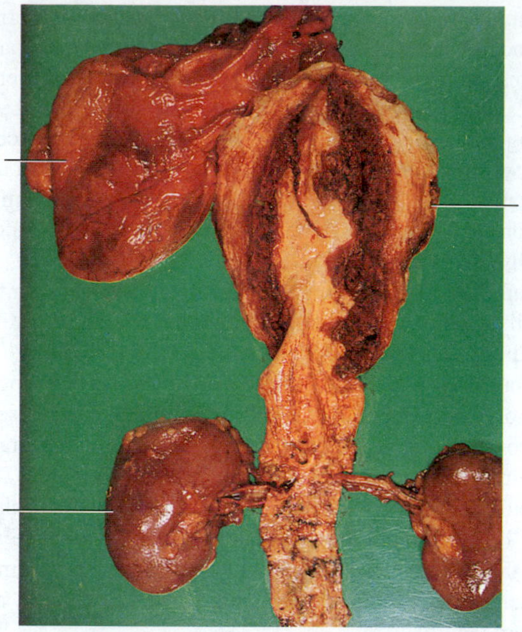

FIG. 38-6 Aortic dissection of the thoracic aorta.

between the fourth and seventh decades of life. This process usually is acute and life threatening. However, it also may be self-limiting and result in a chronic and stable process for a period of time. If patients have an acute aortic dissection and are not surgically treated, the mortality rate is 90%.[18]

Etiology and Pathophysiology

The tear in the intimal lining of the artery allows blood to "track" between the intima and media and creates a false lumen of blood flow. As the heart contracts, each systolic pulsation causes increased pressure on the damaged area, which further increases the dissection. As it extends proximally or distally, it may occlude major branches of the aorta, cutting off blood supply to areas such as the brain, abdominal organs, kidneys, spinal cord, and extremities. Occasionally a small tear develops distally and the blood flow reenters the true vessel lumen.

The exact cause of dissection is uncertain, although many experts attribute dissection to the destruction of the medial layer elastic fibers. Most people with dissection are older and have chronic hypertension. Persons with *Marfan syndrome* (a premature degeneration of vascular elastic tissue) have a high incidence of aortic dissection. Pregnancy promotes increased vascular stress because of increased total blood volume, decreased peripheral vascular resistance, and increased aortic compliance.[18] Blunt trauma also is a precipitating factor associated with aortic dissection. Areas that undergo the greatest amount of stress are most prone to dissection and include the ascending aorta, the aortic arch, and the descending aorta beyond the origin of the left subclavian artery.

Clinical Manifestations

Clinical manifestations depend on the location of the intimal tear and the extent of the dissection. The typical patient with acute aortic dissection usually has sudden, severe pain in the anterior part of the chest or intrascapular pain radiating down the spine into the abdomen or legs.[8] The pain is described as "tearing" or "ripping." The severe pain may mimic that of an MI. As the dissection progresses, pain may be located both above and below the diaphragm. Pregnant women may experience epigastric discomfort or heartburn-like symptoms.[18] Cardiovascular, neurologic, and respiratory signs also may be present.

If the aortic arch is involved, the patient may exhibit neurologic deficiencies, including an altered level of consciousness, dizziness, and weakened or absent carotid and temporal pulses. An ascending aortic dissection usually produces some degree of disruption in coronary artery blood flow and aortic valvular insufficiency. The patient may develop angina, MI, and a new high-pitched, diastolic cardiac murmur. If severe enough, these complications can result in left ventricular failure with the development of dyspnea and orthopnea caused by heart failure and pulmonary edema. When either subclavian artery is involved, radial, ulnar, and brachial pulse quality and BP readings may be significantly different between the left and right arms. As the dissection progresses down the aorta, the abdominal organs and lower extremities demonstrate evidence of altered tissue perfusion.

Complications

A severe and life-threatening complication of aortic dissection of the ascending aortic arch is *cardiac tamponade,* which occurs when blood escapes from the dissection into the pericardial sac.[8] Clinical manifestations of cardiac tamponade include hypotension, narrowed pulse pressure, distended neck veins, muffled heart sounds, and pulsus paradoxus (see Chapter 37).

Because the aorta is weakened by the medial dissection, it may rupture. Hemorrhage may occur into the mediastinal, pleural, or abdominal cavities. Rupture of a dissected aorta typically results in exsanguination and death. Dissection can lead to occlusion of the arterial supply to vital organs, such as the spinal cord, kidneys, and abdominal organs. Ischemia of the spinal cord produces symptoms varying from weakness and decreased pain sensation to complete paralysis of the lower extremities. Renal ischemia can lead to renal failure. Manifestations of abdominal ischemia include abdominal pain, decreased bowel sounds, and altered bowel elimination.

Diagnostic Studies

The diagnostic studies used to assess aortic dissection are similar to those performed for AAAs (Table 38-1). Left ventricular hypertrophy is a common finding on an echocardiogram and may be related to changes caused by systemic hypertension. A chest x-ray may show a widening of the mediastinal silhouette and left pleural effusion. A transesophageal echocardiogram (TEE) can identify dissections that are closest to the aortic root. An MRI or multi-detector row CT (MDRCT) scan are the emergency diagnostic procedures of choice. They can provide valuable information on the presence and severity of the dissection.[8,18] After the patient's condition has stabilized, angiography may be necessary to assess the extent of the dissection.

Collaborative Care

The initial goal of therapy for aortic dissection without complications is to lower the BP and myocardial contractility to diminish the pulsatile forces within the aorta (see Table 38-1). An IV β-adrenergic blocker, such as esmolol (Brevibloc), typically is used to decrease the BP and the force of myocardial contractility. Esmolol (Brevibloc) is particularly useful since it has a rapid onset and a short half-life.[18] Other antihypertensive agents such as sodium nitroprusside (Nipride), calcium channel blockers, and angiotensin-converting enzyme (ACE) inhibitors may also be used.[8,17]

TABLE 38-1 COLLABORATIVE CARE
Aortic Dissection

Diagnostic
Health history and physical examination
ECG
Chest x-ray
Multi-detector row CT scan
Transesophageal echocardiogram (TEE)
Angiogram
Magnetic resonance imaging (MRI)
Collaborative Therapy
Bed rest
Pain relief with opioids
Control of blood pressure
• Sodium nitroprusside (Nipride)
• Calcium channel blockers
• Angiotensin-converting enzyme inhibitors (see Table 33-8)
Control of myocardial contractility
• Intravenous β blockers (e.g., esmolol [Brevibloc])
• Oral β blockers (e.g., propranolol [Inderal])
Aortic resection and repair

CT, Computed tomography; *ECG,* electrocardiogram.

Conservative Therapy. The patient with aortic dissection without symptoms and complications can be treated conservatively for a period of time. Supportive treatment includes pain relief, blood transfusion (if required), and management of heart failure (if indicated). If the dissection is limited to the descending aorta, conservative therapy may be adequate. Success of the treatment is judged by relief of pain, which is an indication of stabilization of the dissection. However, if the dissection involves the ascending aorta, emergency surgery is needed.

Surgical Therapy. Surgery is indicated when drug therapy is ineffective or when complications of aortic dissection (e.g., heart failure, leaking dissection, occlusion of an artery) are present. The aorta is fragile following the dissection. Therefore surgery is delayed for as long as possible to allow time for edema in the area of the dissection to decrease and to permit clotting of the blood in the false lumen. Surgery for aortic dissection involves resection of the aortic segment containing the intimal tear and replacement with synthetic graft material. The extent of aortic replacement depends on the extent of the dissection. Even with prompt surgical intervention, 30-day mortality of acute aortic dissections remains high (10% to 28%), with causes of death related to MI, cerebral ischemia, uncontrolled bleeding, abdominal ischemia, sepsis, and multiorgan failure.[19]

NURSING MANAGEMENT
AORTIC DISSECTION

Preoperatively, nursing management includes keeping the patient in bed in a semi-Fowler position and maintaining a quiet environment. These measures assist in keeping the systolic BP at the lowest possible level that maintains vital organ perfusion (typically maintaining systolic BP between 110 and 120 mm Hg).[17] Opioids and tranquilizers should be administered as ordered. Pain and anxiety must be managed for patient comfort, especially since they may cause elevations in the systolic BP.

Continuous IV administration of antihypertensive agents requires close nursing supervision. Continuous ECG and intraarterial pressure monitoring are required (see Chapters 36 and 66). The nurse should observe for changes in the quality of peripheral pulses and for signs of increasing pain, restlessness, and anxiety. Vital signs are taken frequently, sometimes as often as every 2 to 3 minutes while obtaining control of the BP. If the blood vessels branching off the aortic arch are involved, decreased cerebral blood flow may alter the sensorium and level of consciousness. Postoperative care is similar to that after aneurysmectomy (see section on Nursing Management of Aortic Aneurysms and Aortoiliac Disease earlier in this chapter).

In preparation for discharge, the nurse should focus on patient and family teaching. The therapeutic regimen includes antihypertensive drugs. The patient needs to understand that these drugs must be taken to control BP. β-Adrenergic blockers (e.g., metoprolol [Toprol XL]) can be taken orally to continue to decrease myocardial contractility. It is important that the patient understand the drug regimen and potential side effects (e.g., dizziness). The patient should be told to discuss any side effects with the health care provider before discontinuing the drug. Finally, the nurse should instruct the patient that, if the pain returns or other symptoms progress, the patient must seek immediate help at the nearest health care facility.

PERIPHERAL ARTERIAL DISEASE OF THE LOWER EXTREMITIES

Peripheral arterial disease (PAD) of the lower extremities may affect the aortoiliac, femoral, popliteal, tibial, or peroneal arteries, or any combination of these areas (see Fig. 38-1). The femoral-popliteal area is the site most commonly affected in nondiabetic patients. The patient with diabetes mellitus tends to develop disease in the arteries below the knee, especially the anterior tibial, posterior tibial, and peroneal arteries. In advanced stages, multiple levels of occlusions are found.

Clinical Manifestations

The severity of the clinical manifestations depends on the site and extent of the obstruction and the amount of collateral circulation. The classic symptom of PAD of the lower extremities is **intermittent claudication,** ischemic muscle ache or pain that is precipitated by a consistent level of exercise, resolves within 10 minutes or less with rest, and is reproducible.[20] The ischemic pain is attributable to end products of anaerobic cellular metabolism, such as lactic acid accumulation. Once the patient stops exercising, the metabolites are cleared and the pain subsides. Disease involving the femoral or popliteal arteries causes claudication in the calf. PAD of the aortoiliac arteries produces claudication in the buttocks and the thighs. It should be noted, however, that sedentary patients with PAD may never exert themselves sufficiently to experience claudication. If PAD involves the internal iliac (hypogastric) arteries, erectile dysfunction often results. Some degree of sexual dysfunction occurs in a large portion of men with aortoiliac occlusion.[21]

Paresthesia, manifested as numbness or tingling in the toes or feet, may result from nerve tissue ischemia. True peripheral neuropathy occurs more commonly in patients with diabetes (see Chapter 49) and in those with progressive long-standing ischemia. Neuropathy produces excruciating shooting or burning pain in the extremity. It does not follow any particular nerve roots but may be present near ulcerated areas. Gradually diminishing perfusion to neurons produces loss of both pressure and deep pain sensations. Therefore injuries to the extremity often go unnoticed by the patient.

The physical appearance of the limb provides important information about the adequacy of blood flow. Trophic changes occur to the skin. The skin becomes thin, shiny, and taut. There is a loss of hair on the lower legs. Diminished or absent pedal, popliteal, or femoral pulses may be noted. Pallor or blanching of the foot is noted in response to leg elevation *(elevation pallor)*. Conversely, *reactive hyperemia* (redness of the foot) is observed when the limb is hung in a dependent position *(dependent rubor)*.

However, as the disease process advances and involves multiple arterial segments, continuous pain develops at rest. *Rest pain* most often occurs in the forefoot or toes and is aggravated by limb elevation. Rest pain occurs when there is insufficient blood flow to maintain basic metabolic requirements of the tissues and nerves of the distal extremity. Rest pain occurs more often at night because cardiac output tends to drop during sleep and the limbs are at the level of the heart. Patients often will try to achieve partial pain relief by dangling the leg over the side of the bed or sleeping in a chair to allow gravity to maximize arterial blood flow. Without revascularization, the limb may progress to ulceration and gangrene. Every attempt is made to save the limb, and typically surgery is indicated unless the patient is at high surgical risk and/or has numerous comorbid medical conditions.

Complications

PAD of the lower extremities progresses slowly. Prolonged ischemia leads to atrophy of the skin and underlying muscles. Because of the decreased arterial blood flow to the lower extremities, even minor trauma to the feet (e.g., stubbing one's toe, blister from ill-fitting shoes) may result in delayed healing, wound infection, and tissue necrosis, especially in the diabetic patient. Arterial (ischemic) ulcers most commonly occur over bony prominences on the toes, feet, and lower leg (Table 38-2). Nonhealing arterial ulcers and gangrene are the most serious complications of end-stage PAD and may result in lower extremity amputation if blood flow is not restored adequately or if severe infection occurs. If atherosclerosis has been present for an extended period, collateral circulation may prevent gangrene of the extremity.

Diagnostic Studies

Various tests have been developed to assess blood flow and to outline the vascular system (Table 38-3). Doppler ultrasound consists of a probe transducer containing a crystal that directs high-frequency sound waves toward the artery or vein being examined. The sound waves bounce off the blood cells at a rate that corresponds with the velocity (or speed) of blood flow. This emits an audible signal. When palpation of a peripheral pulse is difficult because of severe PAD, the Doppler can be useful in determining the presence of blood flow. A palpable pulse and a Doppler pulse are not equivalent, and these terms should not be used interchangeably. In addition, *segmental blood pressures* also are obtained (using Doppler ultrasound and a sphygmomanometer) at the thigh, below the knee, and at ankle level while the patient is supine. A falloff in segmental BP of more than 30 mm Hg indicates PAD.

The *ankle-brachial index* (ABI) is determined using a handheld Doppler. The ABI is calculated by dividing the ankle systolic blood pressure (SBP) by the highest brachial SBP.[20] A normal ABI is 0.91 to 1.30. An ABI between 0.71 and 0.90 indicates mild PAD, between 0.41 and 0.70 indicates moderate PAD, and <0.40 indicates severe PAD. The ABI technique also is used to follow patients postoperatively after revascularization to monitor bypass graft patency. This procedure has limited usefulness when arteries are calcified and noncompressive, as occurs in patients with diabetes mellitus. In these patients the ABI frequently is falsely elevated.

Duplex imaging, another noninvasive test, uses a bidirectional, color Doppler system to systematically map blood flow throughout the entire region of an artery. It provides anatomic and physiologic information about the blood vessels (see Chapter 32).

Angiography is used to further delineate the location and extent of the disease process. In addition, it provides information on inflow and outflow vessels to plan for surgery. Angiography is useful when an intervention (i.e., surgery, angioplasty) is indicated. Magnetic resonance angiography (MRA) is sometimes used alternatively. (Angiography and MRA are described in Chapter 32.)

Collaborative Care (see Table 38-3)

Risk Factor Modification. Due to the high risk for MI, ischemic stroke, and cardiovascular-related death in patients with PAD, the first treatment goal is to aggressively modify cardiovascular risk factors in all patients with PAD regardless of the severity of symptoms.[20,22] Smoking cessation is essential for slowing the progression of PAD to critical limb ischemia and reducing the risk of MI and death.[20,23] Smoking cessation is a complex and difficult process with a high incidence of smoking relapse.[24] (Smoking cessation is discussed in Chapter 12 and Tables 12-4, 12-5, and 12-6.)

TABLE 38-2 Comparison of Arterial and Venous Leg Ulcers

Characteristic	Arterial	Venous
Peripheral pulses	Decreased or absent	Present; may be difficult to palpate with edema
Capillary refill	>3 sec	<3 sec
Ankle-brachial index	<0.70	>0.91
Edema	Absent unless leg constantly in dependent position	Lower leg edema
Hair	Loss of hair on legs, feet, toes	Hair may be present or absent
Ulcer location	Tips of toes, foot, or lateral malleolus	Near medial malleolus
Ulcer margin	Rounded, smooth, looks "punched out"	Irregularly shaped
Ulcer drainage	Minimal	Moderate to large amount
Ulcer tissue	Black eschar or pale pink granulation	Yellow slough or dark red, "ruddy" granulation
Pain	Intermittent claudication or rest pain in foot; ulcer may or may not be painful	Dull ache or heaviness in calf or thigh; ulcer often painful
Nails	Thickened; brittle	Normal or thickened
Skin color	Dependency rubor; elevation pallor	Bronze-brown pigmentation; varicose veins may be visible
Skin texture	Thin, shiny, friable, dry	Skin thick, hardened, and indurated
Skin temperature	Cool, temperature gradient down the leg	Warm, no temperature gradient
Dermatitis	Rarely occurs	Frequently occurs
Pruritus	Rarely occurs	Frequently occurs

TABLE 38-3 COLLABORATIVE CARE
Peripheral Arterial Disease

Diagnostic
Health history and physical examination, including palpation of peripheral pulses
Doppler ultrasound studies
Segmental blood pressures
Ankle-brachial index (ABI)
Duplex imaging
Angiogram
Magnetic resonance angiography (MRA)

Collaborative Therapy
Risk factor modification
- Smoking cessation
- Regular physical exercise
- Achieve/maintain ideal body weight
- Tight glucose control in diabetics
- Tight blood pressure control
- Treatment of hyperlipidemia
- Antiplatelet agents (aspirin, ticlopidine [Ticlid], clopidogrel [Plavix])
- Angiotensin-converting enzyme inhibitors (see Table 33-8)

Treatment of claudication symptoms
- Structured walking/exercise program
- cilostazol (Pletal)
- gingko biloba
- statins (e.g., simvastatin [Zocor])
- Supplemental carnitine

Nutrition therapy
Proper foot care (see Chapter 49, Table 49-22)
Percutaneous transluminal angioplasty with or without stent
Peripheral arterial bypass surgery
Patch graft angioplasty, often in conjunction with bypass surgery
Anticoagulation therapy
Endarterectomy (for localized stenosis but rarely done)
Thrombolytic therapy
Amputation

Aggressive treatment of hyperlipidemia (low-density lipoproteins [LDLs] <100 mg/dl and triglycerides <150 mg/dl) is another goal of therapy. Research has shown that treatment of PAD patients with a lipid-lowering agent such as a statin (e.g., simvastatin [Zocor]) lowers serum cholesterol levels and reduces cardiovascular morbidity and mortality.[22] Statin use is also associated with improved walking distance and speed in patients with PAD, regardless of cholesterol levels.[25,26] Thus statins may be useful in the treatment of claudication. (Therapy to lower cholesterol is discussed in Chapter 34.)

Hypertension and diabetes mellitus are both important risk factors for PAD. However, data are not conclusive as to whether aggressive treatment will alter PAD progression.[20,22] Nonetheless, tight control of these two risk factors likely will decrease the risk of other cardiovascular events (i.e., stroke, MI, heart failure, renal failure, and death). One recent study found that careful control of BP (~128/75 mm Hg) significantly decreased the incidence of cardiovascular events in patients with PAD and diabetes.[27] BP should be maintained at <130/80 mm Hg. A glycosylated hemoglobin (A1C) <7.0% is recommended for diabetics.

Drug Therapy. Antiplatelet agents such as aspirin, ticlopidine (Ticlid), and clopidogrel (Plavix) are considered critically important for reducing the risks of MI, ischemic stroke, and cardiovascular-related death in patients with PAD.[20,22] Aspirin, however, is not tolerated by some patients because of gastrointestinal distress. Ticlopidine and clopidogrel, which inhibit platelet aggregation, also are effective in reducing the risk of MI and stroke. Ticlopidine is prescribed less frequently for patients with PAD since a number of serious side effects have been observed, including thrombocytopenia, neutropenia, and thrombotic thrombocytopenic purpura.[20] Based on the best available evidence, first-line oral antiplatelet therapy for patients with PAD should be aspirin (160 to 325 mg/day) or clopidogrel.[28] Combination antiplatelet therapy is recommended if a patient has vascular events with single-drug therapy. Antiplatelet agents have not been shown to be effective in treating claudication.[29]

A growing body of evidence supports the treatment of PAD patients with ACE inhibitors (e.g., ramipril [Altace]), regardless of whether they have hypertension or left ventricular dysfunction.[30] Benefits appear to be a decrease in cardiovascular morbidity and mortality as well as an increase in peripheral blood flow, ABI, and possibly walking distance. However, additional randomized controlled trials are needed.

In the United States, two drugs are approved to specifically treat intermittent claudication, pentoxifylline (Trental) and cilostazol (Pletal). Pentoxifylline increases erythrocyte flexibility and reduces blood viscosity.[29] Cilostazol is a phosphodiesterase inhibitor that promotes the effects of prostaglandin I_2, thus inhibiting platelet aggregation and increasing vasodilation. Cilostazol significantly increases maximal walking distance and quality of life with minimal side effects.[29,31] The most common side effects are palpitations, headache, and transient diarrhea. While cilostazol improves claudication symptoms, it does not reduce cardiovascular morbidity and mortality and is contraindicated for patients with chronic heart failure.[29] The benefit of oral anticoagulants for the treatment of intermittent claudication has not been established and, given the increased risk of bleeding, they are not recommended.[32]

PAD alters skeletal muscle metabolism.[33] One promising new approach to claudication treatment is carnitine, a naturally occurring derivative of the amino acid lysine. Supplemental carnitine is thought to improve muscle metabolism, stimulate oxidative phosphorylation, and improve exercise performance of ischemic muscles. Recent research has shown that 2 g of carnitine taken twice daily improved walking distance and quality of life in PAD patients with minimal side effects.[34] Carnitine already is available in Europe and currently is under review for approval in the United States for the treatment of PAD.[29]

Exercise Therapy. The primary nonpharmacologic treatment for claudication is a formal exercise training program.[20,22] Although exercise training has not been shown to increase collateral blood flow to the legs, it improves oxygen extraction in the legs, skeletal muscle metabolism, and vascular endothelial function.[35] Unfortunately, recent nursing research indicates that only about 50% of PAD patients participate in regular exercise.[36]

Walking is the most effective exercise for individuals with claudication. A supervised, hospital-based PAD rehabilitation program is an effective means for improving exercise performance.[35] Such programs typically include exercise for 30 to 60 minutes/day, 3 to 5 times/week, for 3 to 6 months. One advantage of a formal rehabilitation program is that patients can exercise on other equipment (e.g., exercise bicycles, rowing machines) to improve whole-body fitness and minimize boredom. However, insurance reimbursement for PAD rehabilitation programs is often problematic.[20]

A home exercise program is an alternative to a formal program. Slow, progressive physical activity should be encouraged after a warm-up period. The patient should be instructed to walk to the point of discomfort, stop and rest, and then resume walking until the discomfort recurs. Walking should be done for a prescribed time, usually 30 to 40 minutes/day, 3 to 5 times/week. An exercise therapy program also should be implemented in PAD patients after balloon angioplasty and/or peripheral arterial bypass surgery.

Nutritional Therapy. Patients with PAD should be taught to evaluate their dietary intake. Overall caloric intake should be adjusted so that the body mass index is <25 kg/m^2 and the waist circumference is <40 inches for men and <35 inches for women.[37] Within the diet, dietary cholesterol should be <200 mg/day and the saturated fat intake should be substantially reduced (see Chapter 34, Table 34-4). Soy protein products (e.g., tofu, miso) can be used in place of animal protein to help lower total cholesterol, LDL cholesterol, and triglycerides as well as increase high-density lipoprotein (HDL) cholesterol.[38] Dietary sodium should be no more than 2 g/day (see Chapter 35, Tables 35-11, 35-12, and 35-13).

Complementary and Alternative Therapies. Ginkgo biloba is effective in increasing walking distance for patients with intermittent claudication.[39] Side effects of ginkgo biloba include headache, nausea, gastric symptoms, diarrhea, and allergic skin reactions. Patients taking antiplatelet agents (e.g., aspirin), nonsteroidal antiinflammatory agents (e.g., ibuprofen [Motrin]), and anticoagulants (e.g., warfarin [Coumadin]) should consult with their health care provider before taking ginkgo biloba due to bleeding risks (see the Complementary and Alternative Therapies box). Other nutritional supplements show promising results for the treatment of PAD, but additional randomized controlled trials are needed. For example, folate, vitamin B_6, and cobalamin (vitamin B_{12}) appear to lower homocysteine levels.[40]

Care of the Leg with Critical Limb Ischemia. **Critical limb ischemia** is a chronic condition characterized by ischemic rest pain, arterial leg ulcers, and/or gangrene of the leg due to advanced PAD.[41] Conservative management goals for the patient with critical limb ischemia include protecting the extremity from trauma, decreasing vasospasm, preventing and controlling infection, and maximizing arterial perfusion. Careful inspection, cleansing, and lubrication of both feet are advised to prevent cracking of the skin and infection. Soaking of the affected foot should be avoided to prevent skin maceration (or breakdown). If ulceration is present, the affected foot should be kept clean and dry. Covering the ulcer with a dry, sterile dressing helps to maintain cleanliness and protects the limb. Ulcers with any significant depth may be treated with a variety of wound care products, but without restoration of blood flow, healing is unlikely. Footwear should be soft, roomy, and protective. Chemicals, heat, and cold should be avoided. The patient's heels should be kept free of pressure. This can be accomplished by placing a pillow under the calves so that the heels do not touch the bed. There also are many commercially available devices that provide heel elevation. In patients with critical limb ischemia not amenable to interventional or surgical procedures, the rate of primary amputation is between 10% and 40%.[41]

Several new strategies for the treatment of critical limb ischemia are under investigation. Prostaglandins have been used in Europe for the treatment of critical leg ischemia in patients who are not candidates for surgical revascularization. A recent meta-analysis indicated that patients with severe PAD treated with prostaglandin E_1 (PGE_1) had better pain relief and healing of arterial leg ulcers compared to those treated with placebo.[42] Further, patients treated with PGE_1 were more likely to be alive 6 months posttreatment. The role of prostaglandins in the treatment of intermittent claudication has not been established.[29]

Other strategies include immune modulation therapy to reduce the inflammatory response present in PAD and angiogenic gene therapy to enhance the development of collateral circulation.[41]

Interventional Radiologic Procedures. Interventional radiologic procedures are indicated when (1) intermittent claudication symptoms become incapacitating, (2) the patient experiences rest pain, or (3) severe ulceration or limb-threatening gangrene exists.

Similar to the angiography diagnostic procedure, *percutaneous transluminal balloon angioplasty* involves the insertion of a catheter through the femoral artery. However, the catheter is special and contains a cylindrical balloon. The end of the catheter is advanced to the narrowed area of the artery, the balloon is inflated, and the balloon dilates the vessel by cracking the confining atherosclerotic intimal shell while also stretching the underlying media. This procedure is used selectively in patients with localized, accessible lesions (<10 cm in length). Iliac and femoral artery lesions have responded most successfully to balloon angioplasty. It should be noted, however, that balloon angioplasty is not effective on arteries with diffuse or long segment lesions or in the majority of patients with femoral-popliteal disease.[9] Further, there is a relatively high rate of restenosis after balloon angioplasty (up to 50% restenosis at 1 year). Placement of intravascular stents during angioplasty helps relieve the problems of restenosis and arterial dissection. *Stents* are expandable metallic devices that are positioned within the artery immediately after the balloon angioplasty is performed. Stents assist in maintaining vessel patency after the procedure. Newer drug-eluting stents using paclitaxel are being studied and may help to minimize the problem of restenosis after angioplasty by reducing the amount of new tissue growth in the stent.[43] Anti-

COMPLEMENTARY AND ALTERNATIVE THERAPIES

Herbs That May Affect Clotting

Effects

Increase Anticoagulant Effects

Angelica, anise, bilberry, bromelain, celery, chamomile, devil's claw, dong quai, fenugreek, feverfew, garlic, ginger, ginkgo biloba, goldenseal, horse chestnut, licorice root, lovage root, meadowsweet, motherwort, parsley, passionflower, red clover, rue, turmeric, willow bark

Decrease Anticoagulant Effects

Coenzyme Q_{10}, ginseng, green tea, St. John's wort

Nursing Implications

- In general, these herbs should be used with caution or not at all in patients with bleeding or clotting disorders, or those patients taking medications, herbs, or supplements that affect clotting.
- Advise these patients to consult with a health care provider before using any of these herbs.
- These herbs should be discontinued at least 2 to 3 wk before surgery to avoid potential complications. If this is not possible, the herbal product in its original container should be brought to the health care provider or surgery site so the anesthesia care provider knows exactly what the patient is taking.

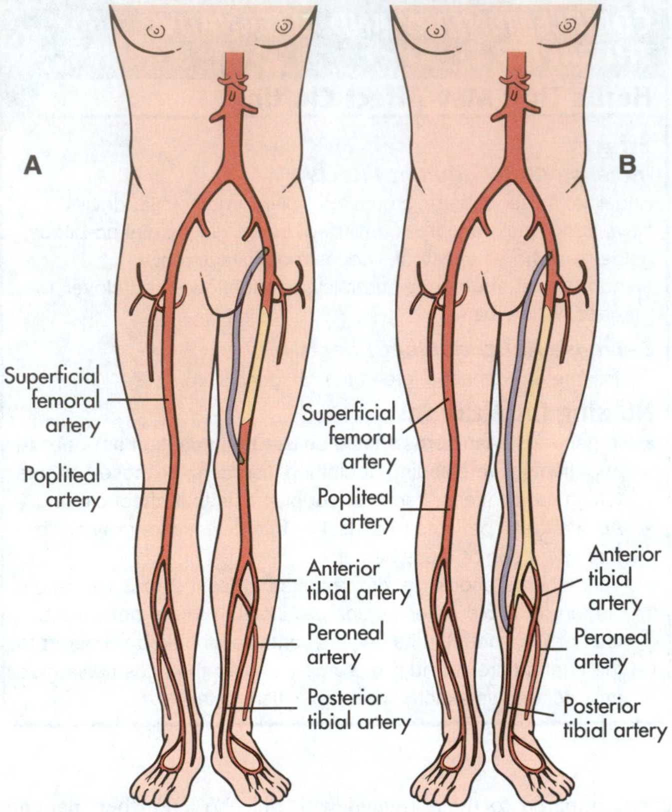

FIG. 38-7 **A,** Femoral-popliteal bypass graft around an occluded superficial femoral artery. **B,** Femoral-posterior tibial bypass graft around occluded superficial femoral, popliteal, and proximal tibial arteries.

platelet agents still are necessary after stenting procedures to reduce the risk of platelet aggregation and subsequent restenosis.

Surgical Therapy. Various surgical approaches can be used to improve arterial blood flow beyond a stenotic or occluded artery. The most common is a peripheral arterial bypass operation with autogenous (native) vein or synthetic graft material to bypass or carry blood around the lesion (Fig. 38-7). Synthetic grafts (expanded PTFE or Dacron) typically are used for long bypasses such as an axillary-femoral or axillary-popliteal bypass. When an autogenous vein is not available, human umbilical vein, cryopreserved vein, or a composite sequential bypass graft may be used.[44] Balloon angioplasty with stenting also may be used in combination with bypass surgery.

Other surgical options include *endarterectomy* (opening the artery and removing the obstructing plaque) and *patch graft angioplasty* (opening the artery, removing plaque, and sewing a patch to the opening to widen the lumen). A number of pharmacologic agents have been used postoperatively to prevent bypass graft failure, including aspirin, ticlopidine, clopidogrel, dextran, subcutaneous or intravenous unfractionated heparin (UH), low-molecular-weight heparin (LMWH) (e.g., enoxaparin [Lovenox]), and warfarin. In addition, anticoagulation with heparin in the immediate postoperative period followed by long-term warfarin therapy is sometimes used in patients with synthetic bypasses, long bypasses to small arteries, or composite bypass grafts; after reoperation of a failed bypass graft; or in patients who have a tendency to occlude grafts secondary to a thrombophilia (clotting abnormality).[32,44]

Amputation is the least desirable end-stage surgical option, but may be required if gangrene is extensive, infection is present in the bone (osteomyelitis), or all major arteries in the limb are occluded, precluding the possibility of successful peripheral arterial bypass surgery. Every effort is made to preserve as much of the limb as possible so that the potential for rehabilitation is optimized (see Chapter 63).

TABLE 38-4 NURSING ASSESSMENT Peripheral Arterial Disease

Subjective Data

Important Health Information

Past health history: Tobacco use, diabetes mellitus, hypertension, hyperlipidemia, hypertriglyceridemia, hyperuricemia, obesity; ↑ C-reactive protein, ferritin, homocysteine, or lipoprotein (a) levels; positive family history, sedentary lifestyle, stress

Functional Health Patterns

Health perception–health management: Family history of cardiovascular disease; tobacco use, including exposure to environmental smoke

Nutritional-metabolic: High saturated fat and cholesterol intake; elevated hemoglobin A1C

Activity-exercise: Exercise intolerance

Cognitive-perceptual: Buttock, thigh, or calf pain that is precipitated by exercise and that subsides with rest (intermittent claudication) or progresses to pain at rest; burning pain in forefeet and toes at rest; numbness, tingling, sensation of cold in legs or feet; progressive loss of sensation and deep pain in extremities

Sexuality-reproductive: Erectile dysfunction

Objective Data

Integumentary

Loss of hair on legs and feet; thick toenails; pallor with elevation; dependent rubor; thin, cool, shiny skin with muscle atrophy; skin breakdown and arterial ulcers, especially over bony areas; gangrene

Cardiovascular

Decreased or absent peripheral pulses; feet cool to touch; bruits may be present at pulse sites

Neurologic

Mobility or sensation impairment

Possible Findings

Arterial stenosis evident with duplex imaging, ↓ Doppler pressures, ↓ ankle-brachial index (ABI), angiography indicative of peripheral atherosclerosis

NURSING MANAGEMENT
LOWER EXTREMITY PERIPHERAL ARTERIAL DISEASE

■ Nursing Assessment

Subjective and objective data that should be obtained from a patient with PAD are presented in Table 38-4.

■ Nursing Diagnoses

Nursing diagnoses for the patient with PAD of the lower extremities (who has not undergone surgery) may include, but are not limited to, those presented in NCP 38-1.

■ Planning

The overall goals for the patient with lower extremity PAD include (1) adequate tissue perfusion, (2) relief of pain, (3) increased exercise tolerance, and (4) intact, healthy skin on extremities.

■ Nursing Implementation

Health Promotion. The patient should be assessed for risk factors and taught how to control them (see Chapter 34, Table 34-3). The nurse's role in the inpatient setting includes identifying at-risk

NURSING CARE PLAN 38-1

Patient with Peripheral Arterial Disease of the Lower Extremities

NURSING DIAGNOSIS **Ineffective tissue perfusion (peripheral)** *related to* decreased arterial blood flow *as evidenced by* intermittent claudication or rest pain, diminished or absent peripheral pulses, pallor or blanching on elevation of limb, hyperemia when limb is dependent

PATIENT GOALS
1. Identifies activities that promote and impair circulation
2. Maintains adequate peripheral tissue perfusion

OUTCOMES (NOC)

Tissue Perfusion: Peripheral

- Capillary refill toes ____
- Skin color ____
- Extremity skin temperature ____
- Right femoral pulse rate ____
- Left femoral pulse rate ____
- Right pedal pulse rate ____
- Left pedal pulse rate ____

Measurement Scale

1 = Severely compromised
2 = Substantially compromised
3 = Moderately compromised
4 = Mildly compromised
5 = Not compromised

INTERVENTIONS (NIC) and *RATIONALES*

Circulatory Care: Arterial Insufficiency

- Perform comprehensive appraisal of peripheral circulation (e.g., check peripheral pulses, edema, capillary refill, color, and temperature).
- Monitor degree of discomfort or pain with exercise, at night, or while resting *as these are indicators of worsening peripheral perfusion.*
- Provide warmth (e.g., additional bed clothes, increasing the room temperature) *to promote vasodilation and increased circulation.*
- Encourage patient to exercise *to enhance O_2 utilization in the tissues and decrease ischemic pain.*
- Instruct patient on proper foot care *to maintain skin integrity.*
- Instruct patient on factors that interfere with circulation (e.g., smoking, restrictive clothing, exposure to cold temperatures, and crossing of legs and feet) *to prevent worsening peripheral perfusion and to decrease ischemic pain.*
- Administer antiplatelet or anticoagulant medications *to promote circulation and pain-free walking.*

NURSING DIAGNOSIS **Risk for impaired skin integrity** *related to* decreased peripheral circulation, altered sensation, and increased susceptibility to infection

PATIENT GOAL Experiences intact skin, free of infection, on lower extremities

OUTCOMES (NOC)

Tissue Integrity: Skin and Mucous Membranes

- Skin temperature ____
- Sensation ____
- Tissue perfusion ____
- Skin intactness ____

Measurement Scale

1 = Severely compromised
2 = Substantially compromised
3 = Moderately compromised
4 = Mildly compromised
5 = Not compromised

INTERVENTIONS (NIC) and *RATIONALES*

Circulatory Precautions

- Instruct patient and family on protection from injury of affected area *as tissue is very fragile and wounds heal poorly due to poor circulation.*
- Instruct patient to test bath water before entering *to avoid burning skin since sensation may be diminished.*
- Instruct patient on foot and nail care *to avoid injury and infection of the extremity.*
- Maintain adequate hydration *to prevent increased blood viscosity.*
- Monitor extremities for areas of heat, redness, pain, or swelling *to detect infection.*

Skin Care: Topical Treatments

- Apply emollients to affected area *to keep skin moist and avoid cracking.*

NURSING DIAGNOSIS **Activity intolerance** *related to* imbalance between oxygen supply and demand *as evidenced by* intermittent claudication

PATIENT GOALS
1. Describes plans for a walking program
2. Demonstrates increased activity tolerance

OUTCOMES (NOC)

Activity Tolerance

- Walking pace ____
- Walking distance ____
- Ease of performing ADLs ____

Measurement Scale

1 = Severely compromised
2 = Substantially compromised
3 = Moderately compromised
4 = Mildly compromised
5 = Not compromised

INTERVENTIONS (NIC) and *RATIONALES*

Exercise Promotion

- Instruct individual about appropriate type of exercise for level of health, in collaboration with physician and/or exercise physiologist, *to provide a baseline for evaluation.*
- Instruct individual about desired frequency, duration, and intensity of the exercise program *so endurance can be increased and oxygen utilization in the tissues enhanced.*
- Assist individual to develop an appropriate exercise program to meet needs *to prevent injury during exercise.*
- Instruct individual on proper warm-up and cool-down exercises *to avoid injury.*

ADLs, Activities of daily living.

Continued

NURSING CARE PLAN 38-1

Patient with Peripheral Arterial Disease of the Lower Extremities—cont'd

NURSING DIAGNOSIS **Ineffective therapeutic regimen management** *related to* lack of knowledge of disease and self-care measures *as evidenced by* questions about disease process, wound, and treatment

PATIENT GOAL Verbalizes key elements of the therapeutic regimen, including knowledge of disease, treatment plan, reduction of risk factors, and proper ulcer/foot care

OUTCOMES (NOC)	INTERVENTIONS (NIC) and *RATIONALES*
Knowledge: Treatment Regimen • Description of specific disease process ____ • Description of self-care responsibilities for ongoing treatment ____ • Description of prescribed exercise and procedures ____ • Description of benefits of disease management ____ **Measurement Scale** 1 = None 2 = Limited 3 = Moderate 4 = Substantial 5 = Extensive	***Teaching: Individual*** • Identify factors that influence learning, such as perception of severity of illness, available support systems, cognitive ability, and physical ability, *so that teaching plan can be individualized.* ***Teaching: Disease Process*** • Appraise patient's current level of knowledge of disease related to specific disease process *to determine extent of problem and plan appropriate interventions.* • Describe disease process *to facilitate patient's understanding of illness.* • Describe common signs and symptoms *so patient can better manage illness.* • Discuss therapy/treatment options *so patient will be less anxious, be more cooperative with treatment plan, and make accurate adjustments in lifestyle.* • Discuss lifestyle changes that may be required to prevent future complications and/or control the disease process (e.g., smoking cessation, foot care) *so patient can modify risk factors related to peripheral arterial disease.*

patients. The nurse also should be involved at the community level, such as screening clinics for PAD, hyperlipidemia, hypertension, obesity, and diabetes. Young people and adults should be educated about the hazards of tobacco use and the importance of regular physical activity. The nurse also should assist in teaching diet modification to reduce the intake of cholesterol, saturated fat, and refined sugars; proper care of the feet; and the avoidance of injury to the extremities. Patients with positive family histories of cardiac, diabetic, or vascular disease should be encouraged to obtain regular follow-up care.

Acute Intervention. After surgical or radiologic intervention, the patient is placed in a recovery area for close observation. The operative extremity should be checked every 15 minutes initially and then hourly for skin color and temperature, capillary refill, presence of peripheral pulses, and sensation and movement of the extremity. Loss of palpable pulses and/or a change in the ultrasonic Doppler sound over a pulse necessitates immediate notification of the physician and/or radiologist and prompt intervention. Ankle-brachial index (ABI) measurements may be ordered, and the indices should increase from the patient's preoperative baseline. They should remain constant if the bypass (or stent) remains patent. All of these findings should be compared with the patient's preoperative baseline and with findings in the opposite limb.[44] Many patients with PAD have a history of chronic ischemic rest pain preoperatively and may be opioid tolerant. They may require aggressive pain management postoperatively.[45]

After the patient leaves the recovery area, nursing care should focus on continued circulatory assessment and monitoring for potential complications. These include bleeding, hematoma, thrombosis, embolization, and compartment syndrome. A dramatic increase in the level of pain, loss of a palpable pulse or pulses distal to the operative site, extremity pallor or cyanosis, decreasing ABIs, numbness or tingling, or a cold extremity temperature may indicate occlusion of the bypass graft and should be reported to the physician immediately.

Knee-flexed positions should be avoided except for exercise. The patient should be turned and positioned frequently with pillows to cushion the incision. Typically, by the first postoperative day, the patient should be out of bed several times daily. Short periods of different leg/body positions have not been found to impair postoperative skin oxygen levels.[46] Sitting for long periods of time should be discouraged because leg dependency may cause significant edema, resulting in discomfort and stress to suture lines, and may increase the risk of deep vein thrombosis. If significant swelling develops, a reclining position is preferred, with the edematous leg elevated above heart level. Occasionally, elastic bandages (e.g., Ace wrap) or elastic support stockings are used to help control leg edema. Walking even short distances is desirable. The use of a walker may be helpful initially, especially in the older patient.

Women with PAD have reported decreased physical functioning, more bodily pain, and greater mood disturbances than men with PAD.[47] Thus women may need require higher dosages of pain medication, greater assistance with activities of daily living, and more social support than men in the postoperative period. Although graft patency and mortality are equivalent for men and women after lower extremity revascularization, women are more likely to develop perioperative wound complications than men.[48] Careful postoperative wound assessment is important. If no complications are present, discharge from the hospital can be anticipated 3 to 5 days postoperatively.

Ambulatory and Home Care. Atherosclerosis is a systemic disease process and not just localized to the lower extremities. Therefore the overall approach to the control of atherosclerotic occlusive disease involves risk factor management (see Chapter 34, Table 34-3). Tobacco in any form is totally contraindicated, not

TABLE 38-5 PATIENT AND FAMILY TEACHING GUIDE
Peripheral Artery Bypass Surgery

The nurse should include the following in a teaching plan:

1. Reduce risk factors by stopping the use of all tobacco products, controlling blood pressure and blood glucose levels (if diabetic), lowering cholesterol and triglyceride levels, achieving/maintaining ideal body weight, and exercising regularly.
2. Know reasons for and basic mechanism of action of medications such as antiplatelets, antihypertensives, anticholesterol therapy, and pain medication and how long anticipated therapy will last.
3. Eat healthy—it is essential to recovery. Drink plenty of fluids, eat a well-balanced diet (including high-fiber foods and fresh fruits and vegetables), and eat fewer fried and high-fat foods.
4. Get a daily walk and/or participate in an exercise program. In the beginning, take several short walks a day and rest between activities. Gradually increase your walking to 30 to 40 minutes a day.
5. Care for feet and legs. Inspect feet and wash them daily. Wear clean cotton or wool socks and well-fitting shoes. File toenails straight across. Avoid sitting with legs crossed, extreme hot and cold temperatures, and prolonged standing.
6. Follow routine postoperative wound care that includes keeping incision clean and dry, not disturbing Steri-Strips (if present), and eating a well-balanced diet that includes foods high in protein, vitamins C and A, and zinc.
7. Monitor for signs and symptoms of impaired healing and/or infection of the leg incision, and notify health care provider if any of the following occur:
   - Prolonged drainage or pus from the incision
   - Increased redness, warmth, pain, or hardness along incision
   - Separation of wound edges
   - Temperature greater than 100° F (37.8° C)
8. Keep all follow-up appointments with health care provider.
9. Notify physician immediately if increased leg or foot pain or a change in the color or temperature of foot and leg is experienced.

only because of the vasoconstrictive effects of nicotine, but also because tobacco smoke impairs transport and cellular utilization of oxygen, increases blood viscosity, and increases homocysteine levels. Continuance of cigarette smoking dramatically decreases the long-term patency rates of the bypass graft, as well as increases the risk of an MI or stroke. (Smoking cessation is discussed in Chapter 12 and Tables 12-4, 12-5, and 12-6.)

All patients should be taught the importance of meticulous foot care to prevent injury. The patient should learn to inspect the legs and feet daily for skin color changes, mottling, alterations in the texture of the skin and subcutaneous fat, and reduction or absence of hair growth. Any ulceration or inflammation must be reported to the health care provider. Skin temperature and capillary refill of the toes should be evaluated. Patients may be taught to palpate pulses and report any changes to the health care provider. Thick or overgrown toenails and calluses are potentially serious and require regular attention by a skilled health care provider (e.g., podiatrist). Emphasis on foot care is especially important in the diabetic patient with PAD because diabetic neuropathy (i.e., diminished peripheral sensation) increases the susceptibility to traumatic injury and results in delay in seeking treatment (see Chapter 49, Table 49-22). Patients with poor eyesight, back problems, obesity, or arthritis may need assistance with foot care. The patient should wear clean, all-cotton or all-wool socks, and comfortable shoes with rounded (not pointed) toes and soft insoles (Table 38-5). Shoes should not be laced tightly, and new shoes should be broken in gradually.

The importance of gradual physical activity after surgery cannot be overemphasized in PAD patients. Regular physical activity has been shown to improve a number of cardiovascular risk factors, including hypertension, high cholesterol, obesity, and glucose levels. Factors that have been found to limit physical activity in PAD patients include lower levels of education, limited claudication distance, lack of social support, presence of arthritis, and increasing age.[49]

Evaluation

Expected outcomes for the patient with PAD of the lower extremities are addressed in NCP 38-1.

ACUTE ARTERIAL ISCHEMIC DISORDERS

Etiology and Pathophysiology

Acute arterial ischemia is a sudden interruption in the arterial blood supply to tissue, an organ, or an extremity that, if left untreated, can result in tissue death. It can be caused by embolism, thrombosis of a preexisting atherosclerotic artery, or trauma. Venous outflow obstruction and low-flow states also can result in acute arterial ischemia.[44] Embolization of a thrombus from the heart or an aneurysm is the most frequent cause of acute arterial occlusion. Heart conditions in which thrombi are prone to develop include infective endocarditis, MI, mitral valve disease, chronic atrial fibrillation, cardiomyopathies, and prosthetic heart valves. The thrombi become dislodged and may travel anywhere in the systemic circulation if they originate in the left side of the heart. Thrombi that originate in the right side of the heart will travel to the lungs and cause a pulmonary embolus (see Chapter 28).

Arterial emboli tend to lodge at sites of arterial branching or in areas of atherosclerotic narrowing. An acute arterial occlusion causes the oxygen and blood supply distal to the embolus to decrease suddenly. The degree and extent of symptoms depend on the size and location of the obstruction, the occurrence of clot fragmentation with embolism to smaller vessels, and the degree of PAD already present.

Sudden local thrombosis may occur at the location of an atherosclerotic plaque. Traumatic injury to the extremity itself may produce partial or total occlusion of a vessel from compression, shearing, or laceration. Acute arterial occlusion also may develop as a result of arterial dissection in the carotid artery or aorta or as a result of iatrogenic arterial injury (e.g., after angiography).

Clinical Manifestations

Signs and symptoms of an acute arterial ischemia usually have an abrupt onset. The exception is when a sudden occlusion is superimposed on preexisting PAD. In this case, the symptoms may be insidious because collateral circulation has developed.

Clinical manifestations of acute arterial ischemia include the "six Ps:" *pain, pallor, pulselessness, paresthesia, paralysis,* and *poikilothermia* (adaptation of the ischemic limb to its environmental temperature, most often cool). Without immediate intervention, ischemia may progress quickly to tissue necrosis and gangrene within a few hours. It should be noted that paralysis is a very late sign of acute arterial ischemia and signals the death of nerves supplying the extremity. Footdrop may occur as a result of nerve damage. Because nerve tissue is extremely sensitive to hypoxia, limb paralysis or ischemic neuropathy may persist after revascularization and may be permanent.

Collaborative Care

With acute arterial ischemia due to occlusion, in the absence of adequate collateral circulation, early treatment is essential to keep the affected limb viable. The treatment options are anticoagulation, thrombolysis, embolectomy, surgical revascularization, or amputation. Anticoagulant therapy is initiated immediately to prevent further enlargement of the thrombus and inhibit embolization. Continuous IV unfractionated heparin has been the traditional agent of choice (see discussion of other anticoagulant options later in this chapter).

***Drug Alert** - Anticoagulant Therapy*

- *Tell patient to avoid taking aspirin or nonsteroidal antiinflammatory drugs (NSAIDs).*
- *Instruct patient to report any signs of bleeding (e.g., melena, hematuria, epistaxis).*
- *Assess for signs of bleeding (e.g., bleeding gums, petechiae, ecchymosis).*

To restore blood flow, the embolus/thrombus should be removed as soon as possible. If the ischemic limb is stable with anticoagulation, recently formed emboli may be treated with catheter-directed thrombolysis using an intraarterial infusion of a thrombolytic agent (e.g., recombinant tissue plasminogen activator [tPA], streptokinase, or urokinase).[9,44] A percutaneous catheter is inserted into the femoral artery and threaded to the site of the clot, and the drug is infused. Unlike anticoagulants, thrombolytic agents work by directly dissolving the clot over a period of 24 to 48 hours. (Thrombolytic therapy is discussed in Chapter 34.) The catheter itself may be specialized to act as a mechanical thrombectomy device, meaning it is specifically designed to remove or fragment the thrombus.[50] Direct arteriotomy may be necessary to remove the clot. Surgical revascularization may be used in the setting of trauma (e.g., laceration of the artery) or with significant arterial occlusion. Amputation is reserved for patients in whom limb salvage is not possible. If the patient remains at risk for further embolization from a persistent source such as chronic atrial fibrillation, treatment includes long-term oral anticoagulation to prevent further acute arterial ischemic episodes (see Table 38-9 later in this chapter).

THROMBOANGIITIS OBLITERANS

Thromboangiitis obliterans (Buerger's disease) is a somewhat rare nonatherosclerotic, segmental, recurrent inflammatory vaso-occlusive disorder of the small- and medium-sized arteries, veins, and nerves of the upper and lower extremities. On very rare occasions, systemic manifestations of the disease may involve cerebral, mesenteric, and/or coronary arteries. The disorder occurs predominantly in younger men (<40 years of age). However, as many as 40% of patients with Buerger's disease are women.[51] Buerger's disease is a type of arteritis in which an inflammatory process damages the arterial wall. Lymphocytes and giant cells infiltrate the vessel wall accompanied by fibroblast proliferation.[52] Ultimately, thrombosis and fibrosis occur inside the vessel, causing tissue ischemia. Buerger's disease typically begins with ischemia of the small, distal arteries and veins, progressing to more proximal arteries. There is a very strong relationship between Buerger's disease and tobacco use.

The symptom complex of Buerger's disease often is confused with PAD and a variety of other inflammatory or autoimmune diseases. Patients may have intermittent claudication of the feet, hands, or arms. As the disease progresses, rest pain and ischemic ulcerations develop. Other signs and symptoms may include color and temperature changes in the affected limb or limbs, paresthesia, superficial thrombophlebitis, and cold sensitivity.

There are no laboratory or diagnostic tests specific to Buerger's disease. Diagnosis is made based on age of onset, history of tobacco use, clinical symptoms, involvement of distal vessels, presence of ischemic ulcerations, and exclusion of diabetes mellitus, autoimmune disease, thrombophilia, and proximal source of emboli.[51] Recent research indicates that patients with Buerger's disease have altered hemorheologic parameters (higher hematocrit, blood viscosity, and red blood cell [RBC] rigidity) compared to patients with PAD and healthy controls. This may have implications for the diagnosis and treatment of this disease.[53]

Treatment includes complete cessation of tobacco use in any form (including secondhand smoke). Nicotine replacement products should not be used. Trauma to the extremity must be avoided. Patients are told that they have a choice between their cigarettes and their affected limbs; they cannot have both. Painful ulcerations may necessitate finger or toe amputations. Amputation below the knee may be necessary in advanced cases. The amputation rate in patients who continue tobacco use is 84.3% compared to only 30.6% in patients who discontinue tobacco use.[51] The risk of amputation is eliminated by 8 years after discontinuing tobacco use. Patients with Buerger's disease have a significantly lower survival rate than age- and gender-matched controls. Although the amputation rate is lower in patients who stop using tobacco, risk of death is similar in those who continue to use tobacco and those who quit.[51]

Other therapies can be considered but have had limited success. The most commonly used medications are antiplatelet agents, followed by calcium channel blockers, α-adrenergic blockers, and anticoagulants.[51] Surgical options include revascularization and sympathectomy, with the most common being *sympathectomy* (transection of a nerve, ganglion, and/or plexus of the sympathetic nervous system). While sympathectomy is useful in improving distal blood flow and healing of ulcerations, and reducing pain, it does not alter the inflammatory process associated with Buerger's disease. Surgical bypass surgery typically is not an option because of the distal vessel involvement of the disease. However, it may be used in selected patients with severe ischemia.[54]

RAYNAUD'S PHENOMENON

Raynaud's phenomenon is an episodic vasospastic disorder of small cutaneous arteries, most frequently involving the fingers and toes. The exact etiology of Raynaud's phenomenon remains unknown. One popular theory is that the vasospasm results from an exaggerated response to sympathetic nervous system stimulation. Other contributing factors include occupationally related trauma and pressure to the fingertips as noted in typists, pianists, and those who use handheld vibrating equipment. Exposure to heavy metals (e.g., lead) may also be a contributing etiologic factor. Raynaud's phenomenon occurs primarily in young women (typically between 15 and 40 years of age). The prevalence of *primary Raynaud's phenomenon* in the United States is 11% in women and 8% in men.[55] When symptoms occur in association with autoimmune diseases such as rheumatoid arthritis, scleroderma, and systemic lupus erythematosus, it is called *secondary Raynaud's phenomenon.*

Raynaud's phenomenon is characterized by vasospasm-induced color changes of the fingers, toes, ears, and nose (white, blue, and red) (Fig. 38-8). Decreased perfusion results in pallor (white). The digits then appear cyanotic (bluish-purple). These changes are followed by rubor (red), caused by the hyperemic

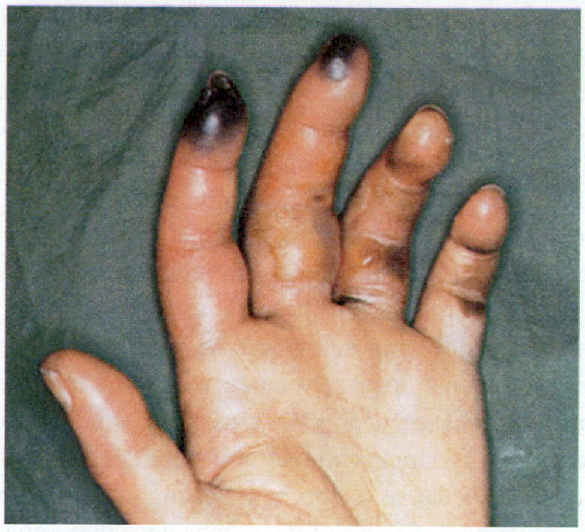

FIG. 38-8 Raynaud's phenomenon.

response that occurs when perfusion is restored. The patient usually describes coldness and numbness in the vasoconstrictive phase followed by throbbing, aching pain; tingling; and swelling in the hyperemic phase. An episode usually lasts only minutes but in severe cases may persist for several hours. Symptoms usually are precipitated by exposure to cold, emotional upsets, caffeine, and tobacco use. After frequent, prolonged attacks the skin may become thickened and the nails brittle. Occasionally, in severe forms of the phenomenon, complications include punctuate (small hole) lesions of the fingertips and superficial gangrenous ulcers in advanced stages. Similar to Buerger's disease, there is no simple diagnostic test for Raynaud's phenomenon. Diagnosis is based on persistent symptoms for at least 2 years.

Patient teaching should be directed toward prevention of recurrent episodes. Loose, warm clothing should be worn as protection from the cold, including gloves when the refrigerator or freezer is used or when cold objects are being handled. Temperature extremes should be avoided. The patient should stop using all tobacco products and avoid caffeine and other drugs with vasoconstrictive effects (e.g., amphetamines, cocaine, ergotamine, pseudoephedrine). If symptoms are exacerbated by stress, the patient needs to develop coping strategies for anxiety-producing situations. Biofeedback, relaxation training, and stress management are effective for some patients. Immersing hands in warm water often decreases the vasospasm.

When a patient's episodes are severe and other therapies are ineffective, drug therapy is considered. Currently, calcium channel blockers are the first-line drug therapy.[52] Calcium channel blockers such as nifedipine (Procardia) and diltiazem (Cardizem) relax smooth muscles of the arterioles by blocking the influx of calcium into the cells, thus reducing the number of vasospastic attacks. Nifedipine is the most commonly used calcium channel blocker for patients with Raynaud's phenomenon. A meta-analysis indicated that calcium channel blockers reduced the frequency and severity of vasospastic attacks.[56] Adverse effects of calcium channel blockers include tachycardia, headache, flushing, dizziness, and peripheral edema. Sympathectomy is considered only in advanced cases. Patients with Raynaud's phenomenon also should receive routine follow-up to monitor for development of connective tissue or autoimmune diseases. In particular, Raynaud's phenomenon may be one of the earliest manifestations of scleroderma.[57]

Disorders of the Veins

VENOUS THROMBOSIS

The most common disorder of the veins is **venous thrombosis,** the formation of a thrombus (clot) in association with inflammation of the vein. Venous thrombosis is classified as either superficial thrombophlebitis or deep vein thrombosis (Table 38-6). **Superficial thrombophlebitis** (inflammation of a superficial vein), which occurs in about 65% of all patients receiving IV therapy, is often of minor significance. **Deep vein thrombosis** (DVT) is a disorder involving a thrombus in a deep vein, most commonly the iliac and femoral veins. It occurs in at least 5% of all surgical patients. It is more serious than superficial thrombophlebitis because it can result in embolization of thrombi to the lungs.

Etiology

Three important factors (called **Virchow's triad**) in the etiology of venous thrombosis are (1) venous stasis, (2) damage of the endothelium (inner lining of the vein), and (3) hypercoagulability of the blood. The patient at risk for the development of venous thrombosis usually has predisposing conditions to these three disorders (Table 38-7).

Venous Stasis. Normal venous blood flow depends on the action of muscles in the extremities and the functional adequacy of venous valves, which allow unidirectional flow. *Venous stasis* occurs when the valves are dysfunctional or the muscles of the extremities are inactive. Venous stasis occurs more frequently in people who are obese, have chronic heart failure or atrial fibrillation, have been traveling on long trips without regular exercise, have a prolonged surgical procedure, or are immobile for long periods (e.g., spinal cord injury, fractured hip).

Endothelial Damage. Damage to the endothelium of the vein may be caused by trauma or external pressure and occurs any time a venipuncture is performed. Damaged endothelium has decreased fibrinolytic properties, predisposing to thrombus development. Increased endothelial damage is sustained when patients on IV therapy are receiving caustic substances such as antibiotics,

TABLE 38-6 Comparison of Superficial Thrombophlebitis and Deep Vein Thrombosis

	Superficial Thrombophlebitis	Deep Vein Thrombosis
Usual location	Superficial veins of arms and legs	Deep veins of arms (axillary, subclavian), legs (femoral), and pelvis (iliac, inferior or superior vena cava)
Clinical findings	Tenderness, redness, warmth, pain, inflammation and induration along the course of the superficial vein; vein appears as a palpable cord; edema rarely occurs	Tenderness to pressure over involved vein, induration of overlying muscle, venous distention; edema; may have mild to moderate pain; deep reddish color to area due to venous congestion NOTE: Some patients may have no obvious physical changes in the affected extremity.
Sequelae	Embolization rarely occurs	Embolization may occur; chronic venous insufficiency may develop

TABLE 38-7 Risk Factors for Deep Vein Thrombosis

Venous Stasis
- Advanced age
- Atrial fibrillation
- Chronic heart failure
- Obesity
- Orthopedic surgery (especially lower extremity)
- Postpartum period
- Pregnancy
- Prolonged immobility
  - Bed rest
  - Fractured leg or hip
  - Long trips without adequate exercise
  - Spinal cord injury
- Stroke
- Varicose veins

Endothelial Damage
- Abdominal and pelvic surgery (e.g., gynecologic or urologic surgery)
- Caustic or hypertonic intravenous medications
- Fractures of the pelvis, hip, or leg
- History of previous deep vein thrombosis (DVT)
- Indwelling femoral vein catheter
- Intravenous drug abuse
- Trauma

Hypercoagulability of Blood
- Antiphospholipid antibody syndrome
- Antithrombin III deficiency
- Cigarette smoking
- Dehydration or malnutrition
- Elevated lipoprotein(a) [Lp(a)]
- Factor V Leiden mutation
- High altitudes
- Hormone replacement therapy
- Hyperhomocysteinemia
- Malignancies (especially breast, brain, hepatic, pancreatic, and gastrointestinal)
- Nephrotic syndrome
- Oral contraceptives, especially in women older than 35 yr who smoke cigarettes
- Polycythemia vera
- Postpartum period
- Pregnancy
- Protein C deficiency
- Protein S deficiency
- Sepsis
- Severe anemias

potassium, chemotherapeutic agents, or hypertonic solutions such as parenteral nutrition or contrast media.

Other factors predisposing to endothelial inflammation and damage include prolonged presence (longer than 72 to 96 hours) of an IV catheter in the same site, the use of contaminated IV equipment, a fracture that causes damage to the blood vessels, diabetes mellitus, blood pooling, burns, and any unusual physical exertion that results in muscle strain.

Hypercoagulability of Blood. Hypercoagulability of blood occurs in many hematologic disorders, particularly polycythemia, severe anemias, various malignancies (especially cancers of the breast, brain, pancreas, and gastrointestinal tract), antiphospholipid antibody syndrome, antithrombin III deficiency, elevated lipoprotein(a) [Lp(a)], factor V Leiden mutation, hyperhomocysteinemia, protein C deficiency, and protein S deficiency.[58,59] A patient with sepsis is predisposed to a hypercoagulable state in response to endotoxins that are released. Some medications (e.g., corticosteroids, quinine) predispose a patient to DVT formation.

Pregnant women and women in the postpartum period are also at risk for DVT due to hypercoagulability. Inherited thrombophilias (inherited tendency to develop blood clots) further increase the risk for DVT in pregnant women and adverse pregnancy outcomes such as toxemia, placental insufficiency, and stillbirth.[60] As many as 50% of pregnant women who develop a DVT have a factor V Leiden mutation.[58]

Women of childbearing age who take estrogen-based oral contraceptives or postmenopausal women who use hormone replacement therapy (HRT) are at increased risk for venous thromboembolic disease.[59,61] Women who use oral contraceptives and smoke double their risk because of the constricting effect of nicotine on the blood vessel wall. Smoking may also cause hypercoagulability via increasing plasma fibrinogen and homocysteine levels and activating the intrinsic coagulation pathway. Women who smoke, use oral contraceptives, are over age 35, and have a family history of DVT are at an extremely high risk to develop a thrombotic event. Women with a known thrombophilia, such as factor V Leiden mutation, should not use HRT as the risk for thrombolic events may be increased as much as 15-fold.[61]

Pathophysiology

Localized platelet aggregation and fibrin entrap RBCs, WBCs, and more platelets to form a thrombus. A frequent site of thrombus formation is the valve cusps of veins, where venous stasis occurs. As the thrombus enlarges, increased numbers of blood cells and fibrin collect behind it, producing a larger clot with a "tail" that eventually occludes the lumen of the vein.

If a thrombus only partially occludes the vein, the thrombus becomes covered by endothelial cells and the thrombotic process stops. If the thrombus does not become detached, it undergoes lysis or becomes firmly organized and adherent within 5 to 7 days. The organized thrombi may detach and result in emboli. Turbulence of blood flow is a major factor contributing to detachment of the thrombus from the vein wall. The thrombus can become an embolus that flows through the venous circulation to the heart and lodges in the pulmonary circulation, becoming a pulmonary embolus.

Superficial Thrombophlebitis

Clinical Manifestations. The patient with superficial thrombophlebitis may have a palpable, firm, subcutaneous cordlike vein (see Table 38-6). The area surrounding the vein may be tender to the touch, reddened, and warm. A mild systemic temperature elevation and leukocytosis may be present. Extremity edema may or may not occur. The most common cause of superficial thrombophlebitis in the upper extremities is vein trauma caused by intraluminal cannulation of a vein or IV therapy (Fig. 38-9). Superficial thrombophlebitis in the lower extremities usually is related to trauma to the varicose veins, which is more common in older patients with long-standing venous insufficiency and in pregnant women.[62] Superficial thrombophlebitis typically is diagnosed on the basis of physical examination alone. In the legs, a venous duplex ultrasound may be used.

In rare cases, infectious or suppurative thrombophlebitis occurs at the site of an IV catheter. Unfortunately, this type of superficial thrombophlebitis often has no local signs or symptoms. A high-grade fever or septic pulmonary emboli may be the first indication of infectious thrombophlebitis.[62] An elevated WBC count and/or positive blood cultures may also be found.

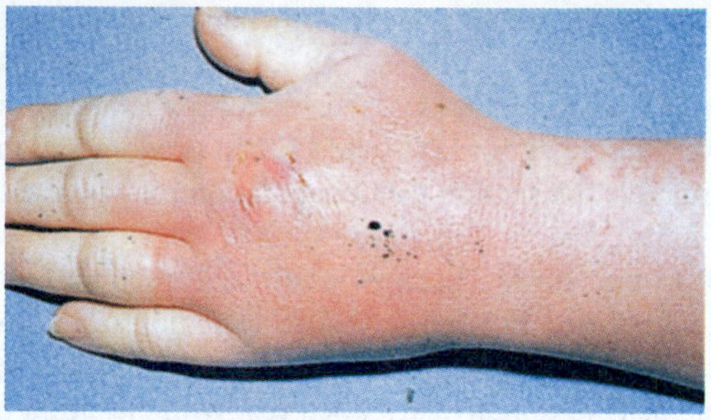

FIG. 38-9 Thrombophlebitis of the hand following IV therapy.

Collaborative Care. The treatment of superficial thrombophlebitis includes elevation of the affected extremity to promote venous return and decrease the edema and the application of warm, moist heat. Heat is used to relieve the pain and treat the inflammation. If the superficial thrombophlebitis is associated with an IV catheter or solution, the IV catheter should be removed immediately. If lower extremity superficial thrombophlebitis has occurred, elastic compression stockings are recommended once the acute thrombophlebitis has resolved. Suppurative thrombophlebitis typically requires drainage of the abscess and excision of the affected tissue.[62]

Mild oral analgesics such as acetaminophen or aspirin may be used to relieve pain. Aspirin also may be given for its antiplatelet effect. Nonsteroidal antiinflammatory drugs (NSAIDs) such as ibuprofen (Motrin) have been used to treat the inflammatory process and accompanying pain. Anticoagulant therapy is usually not indicated unless the proximal greater saphenous vein or the saphenofemoral junction is involved. Antibiotics and/or corticosteroids occasionally are used in complicated situations in which an infection or inflammation of the vein exists.[62]

Deep Vein Thrombosis

Clinical Manifestations. The patient with DVT may or may not have unilateral leg edema, extremity pain, warm skin, erythema, and a systemic temperature greater than 100.4° F (38° C). If the calf is involved, tenderness may be present on palpation. A positive Homans' sign (pain on forced dorsiflexion of the foot when the leg is raised) is a classic but very unreliable sign with frequent false positives[62] (see Table 38-6). If the inferior vena cava is involved, the lower extremities may be edematous and cyanotic. If the superior vena cava is involved, there may be symptoms in the upper extremities, neck, back, and face.

Complications. The most serious complications of DVT are pulmonary embolism (PE), chronic venous insufficiency, and phlegmasia cerulea dolens. PE is a potentially life-threatening complication of DVT (see Chapter 28).

Chronic venous insufficiency (CVI) results from valvular destruction, allowing retrograde flow of venous blood. Persistent edema, increased pigmentation, secondary varicosities, ulceration, and cyanosis of the limb when it is placed in a dependent position may develop in a person with CVI. Signs and symptoms of CVI often do not develop until several years following DVT.

Phlegmasia cerulea dolens (swollen, blue, painful leg), a very rare complication, may develop in a patient in the advanced stages of cancer. It is the result of severe lower extremity DVT(s) that involve the major lower extremity veins resulting in near-total occlusion of venous outflow. Patients typically experience sudden, massive swelling, deep pain, and intense cyanosis of the extremity. If untreated, gangrene occurs due to arterial occlusion secondary to venous obstruction, and amputation is required.

TABLE 38-8 DIAGNOSTIC STUDIES Deep Vein Thrombosis

Study	Description and Abnormal Findings
Blood Laboratory Studies	
• ACT, aPTT, bleeding time, Hb, Hct, INR, platelet count	Alterations if patient has underlying blood dyscrasia (e.g., increased Hb and Hct in patient with polycythemia)
• D-dimer testing	Fragment of fibrin formed as result of fibrin degradation and clot lysis. Elevated results suggestive of deep vein thrombosis.
Noninvasive Venous Studies	
• Venous Doppler evaluation	Determination of venous flow in deep femoral, popliteal, and posterior tibial veins; normal finding of spontaneous flow with variation transmitted by respiration cycle; abnormal finding of absence of flow augmentation with distal compression and proximal release. *Normal results:* <250 ng/ml (250 mcg/L)
• Duplex scanning	Combination of ultrasound imaging techniques and color Doppler capabilities. Vessels are examined for compressibility and intraluminal filling defects to help determine location and extent of thrombus within veins (most widely used test to diagnose deep vein thrombosis).
Venogram (Phlebogram)	X-ray determination of location and extent of clot using contrast media to outline filling defects; development of collateral circulation defined.

ACT, Activated clotting time; *aPTT,* activated partial thromboplastin time; *Hb,* hemoglobin; *Hct,* hematocrit; *INR,* international normalized ratio.

Diagnostic Studies. Various diagnostic studies are used to determine the site or location and extent of a DVT (Table 38-8).

Collaborative Care

Prevention and Prophylaxis. In patients at risk for DVT, a variety of interventions are used. Early mobilization is the easiest and most cost-effective method to decrease the risk of DVT. Patients on bed rest need to be instructed to change position, dorsiflex their feet, and rotate their ankles every 2 to 4 hours. Patients who are able to get out of bed need to be in the chair for all meals and ambulate at least 3 times per day.

Antiembolism stockings (e.g., TED hose) have long been part of DVT prevention. Studies show that these stockings (which exert about 18 mm Hg pressure) increase venous blood flow, prevent venous dilation, and stimulate endothelial fibrinolytic activity.[63] To be effective, it is essential for the nurse to measure the patient's legs, obtain the appropriate stocking size, and apply the stockings properly. Specifically, the toe hole needs to be under the toes and the heel patch needs to be over the heel, there should be no wrinkles present, and the thigh gusset needs to be on the inner thigh. Venous return is impeded by antiembolism stockings if the top elastic band is too tight or if the stockings are rolled down.[63] If a patient's thigh circumference exceeds the manufacturer's size limit, knee-length stockings are available.

EVIDENCE-BASED PRACTICE

Is Low-Molecular-Weight Heparin More Effective Than Compression Therapy in Preventing Deep Vein Thrombosis?

Clinical Question

In patients with hip fractures (P), is low-molecular-weight heparin (LMWH) (I) more effective than compression therapy (C) in prevention of deep vein thrombosis (DVT) (O)?

Best Available Evidence

- Systematic review of randomized controlled trials (RCTs)
- Randomized controlled trial (RCT)

Critical Appraisal and Synthesis of Evidence

Systematic Review

- Five RCTs (n = 487 with hip fracture) indicate mechanical compression prevents DVT but compliance is a problem.
- Five RCTs (n = 373 with hip fracture) indicate LMWH reduces the incidence of DVT.

RCT

- Surgical patients (n = 376) on a protocol of LMWH compared knee-high and thigh-high compression devices.
- No postoperative DVT occurred in 85 patients at low or moderate risk.
- Nineteen DVTs (2 with thigh-length compression devices and 11 with knee-length compression devices) occurred in the 291 high-risk patients.
- Combination of thigh-length compression devices and LMWH in surgical patients reduced rate of DVT by 2%.

Conclusions

In high-risk patients, both LMWH and thigh-high compression therapy (if applied properly and maintained) reduce DVT risk.

Implications for Nursing Practice

- Include DVT risk in initial patient assessment.
- Instruct patient and nursing staff on the appropriate application and maintenance of compression devices.
- Evaluate adherence to instruction of compression devices by tracking DVT risk and incidence.

References for Evidence

Handoll HHG, Farrar MJ, McBirnie J, et al: Heparin, low molecular weight heparin, and physical methods for preventing deep vein thrombosis and pulmonary embolism following surgery for hip fractures. Cochrane Bone, Joint and Muscle Trauma Group, *Cochrane Database of Systematic Reviews,* 3, 2006.
Zaccagnini AH, Ellis M, Williams A, et al: Randomized clinical trial of low molecular weight heparin with thigh-length or knee-length antiembolism stockings for patients undergoing surgery, *Br J Surg* 91:842, 2004.

PICO: P, Patient population of interest; *I,* intervention or area of interest; *C,* comparison of interest or comparison group; *O,* outcome(s) of interest (see p. 6).

Intermittent compression devices (ICDs) are used for hospitalized patients at moderate, high, or very high risk for DVT and PE. A variety of devices are available ranging from calf and thigh cuffs to foot pumps. They may be used in combination with antiembolism stockings. All these devices apply intermittent external pressure to the lower extremities. The compression pushes blood from the superficial veins into the deep veins, thus decreasing venous stasis. The compression also decreases venous distention, thus lowering the risk of endothelial damage. The increased blood flow velocity enhances fibrinolysis (the body's natural anticoagulation factors). ICDs will not provide effective DVT prophylaxis if the device is not applied correctly or if the patient does not wear the device continuously except during bathing, skin assessment, and ambulation.[63] ICDs are not to be worn when a patient has an active DVT due to risk of PE.

Preventive anticoagulation is used for patients at moderate, high, or very high risk for DVT and PE and is addressed in the following drug therapy section. Anticoagulation may be used in combination with ICDs.

Nonpharmacologic Therapy. The usual treatment of DVT in hospitalized patients involves bed rest, elevation of the extremity, and anticoagulation. Warm compresses also may be applied to the affected area. Traditionally, strict bed rest with elevation of the affected extremity above the level of the heart has been prescribed for 2 to 4 days until the thrombus was considered stable, therapeutic levels of anticoagulation were achieved, and the edema was resolving. It has been reported that there were no differences in the development of new PE between patients with DVT or PE on anticoagulation therapy who were placed on bed rest with those who were allowed to walk.[64]

Ideally, once the edema has resolved, the patient should be measured for specialized, custom-fit, graduated elastic compression stockings (e.g., Jobst stockings) that exert 30 to 40 mm Hg pressure at the ankle.[62,65] The use of custom-fit, graduated compression stockings (or sleeves in the case of an upper extremity) is recommended for at least 3 to 6 months to support the vein walls and valves and decrease swelling and pain on ambulation.

Since hyperhomocysteinemia is considered an independent risk factor for DVT, patients with hyperhomocysteinemia should also be treated with vitamins B_6, B_{12}, and folic acid to reduce homocysteine levels and decrease the risk of DVT.[58]

Drug Therapy. Anticoagulants are used routinely for DVT prevention and treatment. The goal of anticoagulation therapy for DVT prophylaxis is to prevent DVT formation; whereas the goals in the treatment of DVT are to prevent propagation of the clot, development of any new thrombi, and embolization. Currently, four major classes of anticoagulants, which are described in detail in this section, are available in the United States: vitamin K antagonists, indirect thrombin inhibitors, direct thrombin inhibitors, and factor Xa inhibitors[66] (Table 38-9). Anticoagulant therapy does not dissolve the clot. Lysis of the clot begins spontaneously through the body's intrinsic fibrinolytic system (see Chapter 30).

Vitamin K Antagonists. Two classes of *vitamin K antagonists* are approved in the United States, the coumarins and the indandiones. Currently, the anticoagulant of choice for long-term or extended anticoagulation is warfarin (Coumadin), a coumarin derivative. Warfarin inhibits activation of the vitamin K–dependent coagulation factors II, VII, IX, and X as well as the anticoagulant proteins C and S.[66] (Fig. 30-5 displays the clotting pathways, and clotting factors are listed in Table 30-3.) Warfarin requires 48 to 72 hours to affect prothrombin time (PT) and may take several days before maximum effect is achieved. Therefore an overlap of a parenteral anticoagulant (e.g., unfractionated heparin [UH] or low-molecular-weight heparin [LMWH]) and oral warfarin typically is required for 3 to 5 days. The level of anticoagulation is monitored daily using the international normalized ratio (INR) for warfarin. The INR is a standardized system of reporting PT based on a referenced calibration model and calculated by comparing the patient's PT with a control value. Other tests to monitor anticoagulation may be used (Table 38-10). If necessary, warfarin can be reversed with vitamin K.

A careful history of pregnancy status and medications should be taken before starting warfarin. Because warfarin is contraindi-

TABLE 38-9 ***DRUG THERAPY*** **Anticoagulant Therapy**

Anticoagulant	Drug	Route of Administration	Comments
Vitamin K Antagonists	warfarin (Coumadin, Sofarin) acenocoumarol (Sintrom)* dicumarol (bishydroxycoumarin)	PO	INR is used rather than PT for monitoring therapeutic levels. Administer at the same time each day. Antidote is vitamin K.
Unfractionated Heparin (UH)	heparin sodium Hepalean Lipo-Hepin Calciparine	Continuous IV Intermittent IV Subcutaneous	Therapeutic effects measured at regular intervals by the aPTT or ACT. Monitor complete blood counts at regular intervals. If administering subcutaneously, inject deep into subcutaneous tissue (preferably into the abdominal fatty tissue or above the iliac crest), inserting the entire length of the needle. Hold skinfold during injection but release before removing needle. Do not aspirate. Do not inject IM. Do not rub site after injection. Rotate sites. Antidote is protamine sulfate.
Low-Molecular-Weight Heparin (LMWH)	enoxaparin (Lovenox) tinzaparin (Innohep) dalteparin (Fragmin) nadroparin (Fraxiparine)* certoparin (Sandoparin†)	Subcutaneous	Routine coagulation tests typically not required. Monitor complete blood count at regular intervals. Do not expel air bubble before administering subcutaneously. Follow remaining administration guidelines as described above for unfractionated heparin. Extreme caution should be used in patients with a history of heparin-induced thrombocytopenia (risk versus benefit). Protamine sulfate partially reverses the effects of LMWH.
Direct Thrombin Inhibitors	Hirudin derivatives: lepirudin (Refludan) bivalirudin (Angiomax) desirudin (Iprivask, Revasc†)	Continuous IV	Therapeutic effect measured by ACT or aPTT ratio (1.5-2.5 times the control). Used in patients with heparin-induced thrombocytopenia when anticoagulation is still required. No antidote.
	Synthetic thrombin inhibitors: argatroban (Acova)	Continuous IV	Follow hirudin derivative guidelines.
Factor Xa Inhibitor	fondaparinux (Arixtra)	Subcutaneous	Routine coagulation tests typically not required. Monitor complete blood count at regular intervals. Do not expel air bubble before administering subcutaneously. Follow remaining administration guidelines as described for unfractionated heparin. Used in patients with heparin-induced thrombocytopenia when anticoagulation is still required. If given for DVT prophylaxis after orthopedic or abdominal surgery, the initial dose should be given no earlier than 6-8 hr after surgery.

ACT, Activated clotting time; *aPTT,* activated partial thromboplastin time; *DVT,* deep vein thrombosis; *IM,* intramuscular; *INR,* international normalized ratio; *IV,* intravenous; *PO,* oral; *PT,* prothrombin time.
*Available in Canada. Not approved by the Food and Drug Administration for use in the United States.
†Available in European Union.

TABLE 38-10 Tests of Blood Coagulation

Test	Drug Monitored	Normal Value	Therapeutic Value
International normalized ratio (INR)	Warfarin (Coumadin)	0.75-1.25	2-3
Activated partial thromboplastin time (aPTT)	Unfractionated heparin Hirudin derivatives	24-36 sec	46-70 sec
Activated clotting time (ACT)	Heparin Hirudin derivatives Argatroban (Acova)	80-135 sec	3 min

cated in pregnancy, pregnant patients requiring anticoagulation often receive subcutaneous UH or LMWH. Antiplatelet agents (e.g., aspirin) generally are contraindicated. Other drugs that interact with warfarin include NSAIDs such as ibuprofen, phenytoin (Dilantin), barbiturates (Table 38-11), and many herbal supplements[39] (see Complementary and Alternative Therapy Box on p. 903). Dietary changes also can interact with warfarin. A diet that frequently varies in vitamin K intake (e.g., green leafy vegetables) can make it difficult to achieve and maintain a therapeutic level.

Indirect Thrombin Inhibitors. *Indirect thrombin inhibitors* can be divided into two major classes: UH and LMWHs. UH (heparin) affects both the intrinsic and common pathways of blood

TABLE 38-11 Drugs, Vitamins, and Minerals That Interact with Oral Anticoagulants

Increase Anticoagulant Effects	Decrease Anticoagulant Effects
alcohol (may increase or decrease)	barbiturates (e.g., secobarbital, phenobarbital)
amiodarone (Cordarone)	carbamazepine (Tegretol)
anabolic steroids	chlordiazepoxide (Librium)
cephalosporins	cholestyramine (Questran)
chloral hydrate	estrogens
cimetidine (Tagamet)	ethchlorvynol (Placidyl)
disulfiram (Antabuse)	griseofulvin (Grifulvin V)
erythromycin	itraconazole (Sporanox)
fluconazole (Diflucan)	rifampin (Rifadin)
influenza (flu) vaccine	vitamins C and K
isoniazid (INH)	Minerals: iron, magnesium, zinc
metronidazole (Flagyl)	
miconazole (Monistat)	
neomycin	
nonsteroidal antiinflammatory drugs (NSAIDs)	
omeprazole (Prilosec)	
penicillins	
phenytoin (Dilantin)	
propafenone (Rythmol)	
quinidine	
salicylates	
sulfinpyrazone (Anturane)	
sulfonamides	
tetracycline	
thrombolytics	
thyroxine	
vitamins D and E	

coagulation by way of the plasma cofactor antithrombin. Antithrombin inhibits thrombin-mediated conversion of fibrinogen to fibrin by impacting factors II, IX, X, XI, and XII. Heparin can be administered intravenously for DVT treatment or subcutaneously for DVT prophylaxis. When given intravenously, heparin requires frequent laboratory monitoring of clotting status as measured by activated partial thromboplastin time (aPTT). If necessary, UH can be reversed with protamine sulfate.

LMWHs are derived from heparin, but the molecule size is approximately one third that of UH. While LMWHs also act via antithrombin, the shorter heparin chains have increased affinity for inhibiting factor Xa.[66] Enoxaparin (Lovenox), dalteparin (Fragmin), and tinzaparin (Innohep) are examples of LMWHs. LMWHs have a greater bioavailability, a more predictable dose response, and a longer half-life and are less costly than UH. They also have a lower incidence of bleeding complications and heparin-induced thrombocytopenia (HIT).[67,68] LMWH has the practical advantage that it does not require anticoagulant monitoring and dose adjustment.[66] LMWH is administered subcutaneously in fixed doses, once or twice daily. Duration of administration depends on the reason for use. The anticoagulant effects of LMWHs are only partially reversible with protamine sulfate.

Direct Thrombin Inhibitors. *Direct thrombin inhibitors* (DTIs) can be classified as hirudin derivatives or synthetic thrombin inhibitors. Hirudin was extracted originally from the salivary glands of the medicinal leech, *Hirudo medicinalis.* It is now manufactured through recombinant DNA technology. Hirudin binds specifically with thrombin, thereby directly inhibiting its function without causing plasma protein and platelet interactions.[66] Hirudin derivatives such as lepirudin (Refludan) and bivalirudin (Angiomax) are administered by continuous IV infusion. Desirudin (Iprivask) is administered subcutaneously and is approved for DVT prevention for hip replacement surgery.[66] Anticoagulant activity is monitored for hirudin derivatives using aPTT or activated clotting time (ACT). It should be noted, however, that as many as 60% of patients develop antihirudin antibodies. There is no antidote for hirudin derivatives if bleeding occurs.[69]

Argatroban (Acova), a synthetic direct thrombin inhibitor, inhibits thrombin. Argatroban is indicated for use in patients known to be allergic to heparin and/or hirudin derivatives or who currently are experiencing HIT who require anticoagulation.[69] Anticoagulant activity is monitored for argatroban using aPTT or ACT. Similar to hirudin derivatives, the effects of argatroban are not reversible.

Factor Xa Inhibitors. *Factor Xa inhibitors* inhibit factor Xa directly or indirectly, producing rapid anticoagulation. Fondaparinux (Arixtra) is administered subcutaneously. It is approved for DVT prevention in orthopedic patients and treatment of DVT and PE in hospitalized patients when administered in conjunction with warfarin.[66] Oral factor Xa inhibitors are under development. Similar to LMWHs, fondaparinux does not require coagulation monitoring or dose adjustment. As with direct thrombin inhibitors, factor Xa inhibitors have no antidote.

Anticoagulation Therapy for DVT Prophylaxis. For DVT prophylaxis, low-dose UH, LMWH, fondaparinux, or warfarin can be prescribed. UH typically is given subcutaneously. LMWHs have replaced heparin as the anticoagulant of choice to prevent DVT for most surgical patients. Once-daily subcutaneous dosing of LMWHs is now the standard with the exception of total knee replacement, which still requires twice-daily dosing.[70]

Fondaparinux has been studied extensively for the prevention of DVT in major hip and knee surgery patients and has superior efficacy compared to enoxaparin in this population.[71] For DVT prophylaxis, fondaparinux is administered subcutaneously once daily, with the first dose given 6 to 8 hours postoperatively to minimize bleeding. Low-dose warfarin most often is used for major hip and knee surgery patients. Regardless of the drug selected, DVT prophylaxis typically lasts the duration of the hospitalization. However, major orthopedic surgery patients may be prescribed prophylaxis for up to 1 month postdischarge.[70]

Anticoagulation Therapy for DVT Treatment. Patients with multiple comorbidities, complex medical issues, and/or a very large DVT usually are hospitalized for DVT treatment.[72] They typically receive an initial IV bolus of UH followed by continuous IV heparin infusion to maintain the target aPTT for 5 to 7 days.[73]

LMWHs now are recommended over UH for most patients with acute DVT. Furthermore, between 12% and 53% of patients with a DVT can be managed safely and effectively on an outpatient basis with LMWH.[72] Current guidelines recommend placing the patient on LMWH administered subcutaneously daily or every 12 hours.[73]

Fondaparinux can also be given for the treatment of acute DVT with a daily subcutaneous dose and may be particularly useful for patients with a history of HIT. For DVT treatment, warfarin also is prescribed and given concurrently with UH, LMWH, or fondaparinux until the warfarin is at a therapeutic level (INR 2.0 to 3.0). Warfarin then is administered for 3 to 6 months after the DVT. Recurrent episodes of DVT require lifelong anticoagulation therapy unless contraindicated.

Another treatment option currently being studied in patients with severe DVT is administration of a thrombolytic drug that directly dissolves the clot(s). Administration of streptokinase, urokinase, or recombinant tissue plasminogen activator (Alteplase) through a peripheral vein or via a catheter directly into the clot may reduce the incidence of post-phlebitic vein problems that occur after the DVT.[74] Mechanical thrombectomy catheters that use a high-speed impeller to fragment the thrombus may be used alone or in conjunction with the thrombolytic drug.[75] (Thrombolytic therapy is discussed in Chapter 34.)

Surgical Therapy. Although most patients are managed conservatively, small percentages of patients require surgical intervention. The primary indication for surgery is to prevent recurrent PE. Surgical procedures include the rarely performed open surgical venous thrombectomy and inferior vena cava interruption. Venous thrombectomy involves the removal of a DVT through an incision in the vein. Although the long-term results after a thrombectomy have been poor, improved techniques and careful patient selection have demonstrated that venous thrombectomy may have a role in treating the young patient with acute proximal short-segment DVT.[75] This procedure is done to prevent PE or to decrease the risk of the development of chronic venous insufficiency.

Vena cava interruption devices, such as the Greenfield, Simon nitinol, Vena Tech, or TrapEase filters, can be inserted percutaneously through right femoral or right internal jugular veins.[9,62] The filter device is opened and the spokes penetrate the vessel walls (Fig. 38-10). These devices result in "sieve-type" obstruction, permitting filtration of clots without interruption of blood flow.

Complications after the insertion of the intravascular filter device are rare. They include air embolism, improper placement, migration of the filter more distally into the venous system, and perforation of the vena cava with retroperitoneal bleeding.[9] Venous congestion is common and results from the accumulation of trapped clots at the filter site. Over time these clots may clog the filter and completely occlude the vena cava. Because this process is gradual, collateral vessels usually develop to maintain venous flow. However, these collateral venous pathways may also provide an alternate route for PE.

NURSING MANAGEMENT
VENOUS THROMBOSIS

■ *Nursing Assessment*

Subjective and objective data that should be obtained from a patient with venous thrombosis are presented in Table 38-12.

■ *Nursing Diagnoses*

Nursing diagnoses and collaborative problems for the patient with venous thrombosis include, but are not limited to, the following:

- Acute pain *related to* venous congestion, impaired venous return, and inflammation
- Ineffective health maintenance *related to* lack of knowledge about disorder and its treatment
- Risk for impaired skin integrity *related to* altered peripheral tissue perfusion
- Potential complication: bleeding *related to* anticoagulant therapy
- Potential complication: pulmonary embolism *related to* embolization of thrombus, dehydration, and immobility

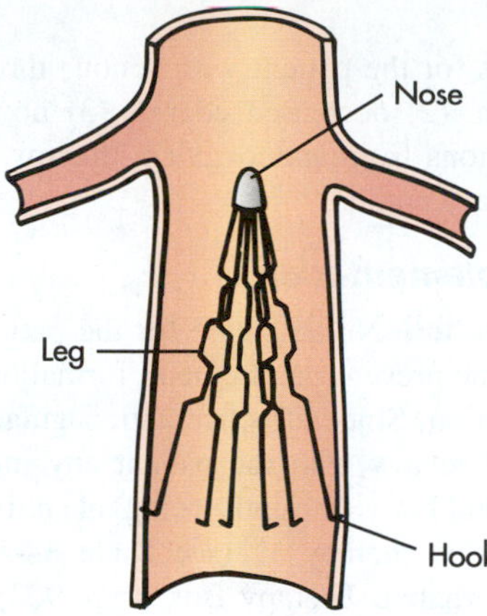

FIG. 38-10 Inferior vena caval interruption technique using Greenfield stainless steel filter to prevent pulmonary embolism.

TABLE 38-12 *NURSING ASSESSMENT* **Deep Vein Thrombosis**

Subjective Data

Important Health Information

Past health history: Trauma to vein, varicose veins, pregnancy or recent childbirth, bacteremia, obesity, prolonged bed rest, irregular heartbeat (e.g., atrial fibrillation), COPD, HF, cancer, coagulation disorders and hypercoagulable states, systemic lupus erythematosus, MI, spinal cord injury, stroke, prolonged travel

Medications: Use of estrogens (including oral contraceptives), corticosteroids, quinine, excessive amounts of vitamin E

Surgery or other treatments: Any recent surgery, especially orthopedic, gynecologic, gastric, or urologic; previous surgery involving veins; central venous catheter

Functional Health Patterns

Health perception–health management: IV drug abuse, tobacco use, obesity

Activity-exercise: Inactivity

Cognitive-perceptual: Pain in area on palpation or ambulation

Objective Data

General

Fever, anxiety, pain

Integumentary

Increased size of extremity when compared with other side; taut, shiny, warm skin, erythematous, tenderness to palpation. Some patients may have no physical changes in the affected extremity.

Cardiovascular

Distention and warmth of superficial veins; edema and cyanosis of extremities, neck, back, and face (superior vena cava involvement)

Possible Findings

Leukocytosis, abnormal coagulation, anemia or ↑ hematocrit and RBC count, ↑ D-dimer level, positive venous duplex or Doppler studies, positive venogram

COPD, Chronic obstructive pulmonary disease; *HF,* heart failure; *IV,* intravenous; *MI,* myocardial infarction; *RBC,* red blood cell.

Planning

The overall goals for the patient with venous thrombosis include (1) relief of pain, (2) decreased edema, (3) no skin ulceration, (4) no complications from anticoagulant therapy, and (5) no evidence of pulmonary emboli.

Nursing Implementation

Acute Intervention. Nursing care for the patient with DVT is directed toward the prevention of emboli formation and the reduction of inflammation. Since effective anticoagulation is essential, the nurse should review with the patient any medications, vitamins, minerals, and herbs currently being taken that may interfere with anticoagulation therapy[39,76] (see Table 38-11 and Complementary and Alternative Therapy Box on p. 903). Depending on the anticoagulant prescribed, the nurse should monitor ACT, aPTT, INR, hemoglobin, hematocrit, platelet levels, and/or liver enzymes.[66] Platelet counts are monitored for patients receiving UH or LMWH to assess for HIT. Medication doses of UH, warfarin, and direct thrombin inhibitors are titrated according to the results of clotting studies. The nurse should check the results of clotting studies before administering these drugs.

While the patient is hospitalized, nursing activities should be adjusted to monitor for and reduce the risk of bleeding that may occur with anticoagulant administration (Table 38-13). The nurse should observe closely for any signs of bleeding, including epistaxis and bleeding gingivae. Urine and stool should be examined for overt signs of blood and tested for occult blood should other signs of bleeding be present.

Particular attention should be paid to the protection of skin areas that may be traumatized. Surgical incisions should be closely observed for evidence of bleeding. Mental status changes, especially in the older patient, should be assessed as a possible indication of cerebral bleeding. Intramuscular injections should be avoided. The antidote for UH and LMWH is protamine sulfate, and the antidote for warfarin is vitamin K. These drugs must be immediately available if bleeding occurs. Fresh frozen plasma (FFP) may be administered to reverse DTIs and factor Xa inhibitors or for significant bleeding because it contains multiple clotting factors.

Ambulatory and Home Care. During all phases of care, the nurse should evaluate the patient's psychologic response to the diagnosis. Many patients are apprehensive that clots will move to the heart or lungs and cause sudden death. Every patient should be encouraged to verbalize concerns, and an attempt should be made to clarify misconceptions.

Discharge teaching should focus on elimination of modifiable risk factors for DVT, the importance of compression stockings and monitoring of laboratory values, medication instructions, and guidelines for follow-up. Modifiable risk factors for DVT include the use of tobacco, use of oral contraceptives, use of hormone replacement therapy (HRT), a sedentary lifestyle, and obesity. The patient should be taught to quit smoking and using nicotine products because nicotine increases the viscosity of the blood. Constrictive clothing, such as girdles or garters, should be avoided. Women with a history of DVT should be instructed to stop using oral contraceptives and HRT.[61] Another important preventive measure is to avoid prolonged standing or sitting in a motionless, leg-dependent position. Frequent knee flexion, ankle rotation, and active walking should be done during long periods of sitting or standing, especially on long automobile or airplane trips. Regular use of prescription, graduated compression stockings has been shown to reduce the occurrence of post-thrombotic syndrome (also known as chronic venous insufficiency).[65]

TABLE 38-13 Nursing Interventions to Prevent Bleeding Complications in Patients Receiving Anticoagulants

Assessment
- Monitor vital signs as indicated.
- Examine urine and stool for overt signs of blood.
- Inspect skin frequently, especially under any splinting devices.
- Evaluate platelet count for signs of heparin-induced thrombocytopenia.
- Evaluate appropriate laboratory coagulation tests for target therapeutic levels.
- Evaluate lower extremity for ecchymosis/hematoma development if intermittent compression device used.
- Perform assessments frequently to observe for signs and symptoms of bleeding (e.g., hypotension, tachycardia) and/or clotting.
- Notify the health care provider of any abnormalities in assessments, vital signs, or laboratory values.

Injections
- Minimize venipunctures.
- Avoid intramuscular (IM) injections.
- Use small-gauge needles for venipunctures unless replacement therapy requires a larger gauge.
- Apply manual pressure for at least 10 min (or longer if needed) on venipuncture sites.

Patient Care
- Humidify O_2 source.
- Avoid restrictive clothing.
- Apply moisturizing lotion to skin.
- Use electric razors, not straight razors.
- Perform physical care in a gentle manner.
- Instruct patient not to forcefully blow nose.
- Avoid removing/disrupting established clots.
- Lubricate tubes adequately prior to insertion.
- Use soft toothbrushes or foam swabs for oral care.
- Reposition the patient carefully at regular intervals.
- Limit tape application—use paper tape as appropriate.
- Administer stool softeners to avoid hard stools and constipation.
- Avoid restraints if possible—use only soft, padded restraints as needed.
- Use support pads, mattresses, bed cradles, and therapeutic beds as indicated.
- Apply antiembolism stockings (e.g., TED hose) or intermittent compression devices as ordered.

The patient and family should be taught about signs and symptoms of PE such as sudden onset of dyspnea, tachypnea, and pleuritic chest pain. (Pulmonary embolism is discussed in Chapter 28.) They should be instructed to contact Emergency Medical Services (EMS) should these symptoms occur.

If the patient is continuing on anticoagulant therapy, the patient and family need careful explanations of medication dosage, actions, and side effects, as well as the importance of routine blood tests and what symptoms to report to the health care provider (Table 38-14). Home monitoring devices are now available for testing of PT/INR. Patients on LMWH will need to learn how to self-administer the drug or have a friend or family member administer it. The most common problems with LMWH are bruising at the injection site. Active or younger patients need to be instructed to avoid contact sports and other high-risk activities (e.g., skiing).

TABLE 38-14 ***PATIENT AND FAMILY TEACHING GUIDE*** **Anticoagulation Therapy**

The nurse should include the following in a teaching plan:

1. Reasons for and basic mechanism of action of anticoagulant therapy and how long anticipated therapy will last.
2. Need to take medication at same time each day (preferably in afternoon or evening).
3. Need for frequent follow-up with blood tests to assess therapeutic effect of the drug and whether change in drug dosage is required.
4. Side effects and adverse effects of drug therapy requiring medical attention:
   - Any bleeding that does not stop after a reasonable amount of time (usually 10 to 15 min)
   - Blood in urine or stool; or black, tarry stools
   - Unusual bleeding from gums, throat, skin, or nose, or heavy menstrual bleeding
   - Severe headaches or stomach pains
   - Weakness, dizziness, mental status changes
   - Vomiting blood
   - Cold, blue, or painful feet
5. Avoid any trauma or injury that might cause bleeding (e.g., vigorous brushing of teeth, contact sports, in-line rollerblading, use of straight razor).
6. Avoid all aspirin-containing drugs or nonsteroidal antiinflammatory drugs.
7. Limit alcohol intake to small to moderate amount (12 oz beer, 4 oz wine, 1 oz hard liquor).
8. Wear a Medic Alert bracelet or necklace indicating what anticoagulant is being taken.
9. Avoid marked changes in eating habits, such as dramatically increasing foods high in vitamin K (e.g., broccoli, spinach, kale, greens). Do not take supplemental vitamin K.
10. Consult with health care provider before beginning or discontinuing any medication.
11. Inform all health care providers, including dentist, of anticoagulant therapy.
12. Correct dosing is essential and supervision may be required (e.g., patients experiencing confusion or cognitive impairment).
13. Avoid herbal products that may alter coagulation (see Complementary and Alternative Therapies box on p. 903).
14. Contact Emergency Medical Services immediately if chest pain, shortness of breath, palpitations (heart racing), or a feeling of passing out is experienced.

The older patient should be taught safety precautions to prevent injuries, such as falls. Should a bleeding episode occur, the patient and family should be instructed to apply pressure for 10 to 15 minutes. If the bleeding has not slowed significantly or completely resolved, they should contact EMS.

A well-balanced diet is important because calcium and vitamin E play active roles in the clotting mechanism. Patients on warfarin should be instructed to follow a consistent diet of foods containing vitamin K and to avoid any additional supplements that contain vitamin K. In addition, the patient should be instructed to avoid excessive amounts of vitamin E and alcohol. Proper hydration also is required to prevent additional hypercoagulability of the blood, which may occur in the presence of deficient fluid intake. The overweight patient needs to not only limit caloric intake but also increase physical activity levels to achieve and maintain desired weight. A balanced program of rest and exercise also improves arterial filling and venous return. Exercise programs should be developed with an emphasis on walking, swimming, and wading. Water exercise is particularly beneficial because of the gentle, even pressure of the water.

▪ *Evaluation*

The expected outcomes for the patient with venous thrombosis include

- minimal to no pain
- intact skin
- no signs of hemorrhage or occult bleeding
- no signs of respiratory distress

VARICOSE VEINS

Varicose veins, or *varicosities,* are dilated, tortuous subcutaneous veins most frequently found in the saphenous system. They may be small and innocuous or large and bulging. *Primary varicose veins* (idiopathic), which are more common in women and patients with a strong family history, are probably caused by congenital weakness of the veins. *Secondary varicose veins* typically result from a previous DVT or another identifiable obstruction. Secondary varicose veins also may occur in the esophagus (esophageal varices), in the anorectal area (hemorrhoids), and as abnormal arteriovenous (AV) connections (AV fistulas and malformations). *Reticular veins* are smaller varicose veins that appear flat, less tortuous, and blue-green in color. *Telangiectasias* (often referred to as spider veins) are very small visible vessels (generally <1 mm in diameter) that appear bluish-black, purple, or red.[77]

Etiology and Pathophysiology

The etiology of varicose veins is unknown. Superficial veins in the lower extremities become dilated and tortuous, with increased venous pressure. Risk factors for varicose veins include congenital weakness of the vein structure, female gender, use of hormones (oral contraceptives or HRT), increasing age, obesity, pregnancy, venous obstruction resulting from thrombosis or extrinsic pressure by tumors, or occupations that require prolonged standing.[62,77] As the veins enlarge, the valves are stretched and become incompetent, allowing venous blood flow to be reversed. As back pressure increases and the calf muscle pump (muscle movement that squeezes venous blood back toward the heart) fails, further venous distention results. The increased venous pressure is transmitted to the capillary bed, and edema develops.

Clinical Manifestations and Complications

Discomfort from varicose veins varies dramatically among people and tends to be worsened by superficial thrombophlebitis. In addition, many patients voice concern about cosmetic disfigurement (Fig. 38-11). The most common symptom of varicose veins is an ache or pain after prolonged standing, which is relieved by walking or by elevating the limb. Some patients feel pressure or a cramplike sensation in the legs. Swelling may accompany the discomfort. Nocturnal leg cramps in the calf may occur.

Superficial thrombophlebitis is the most frequent complication of varicose veins and may occur either spontaneously or after trauma, surgical procedures, or pregnancy. Rare complications include rupture of the varicose veins from weakening of the vessel wall and ulceration of the skin.

Diagnostic Studies and Collaborative Care

Superficial varicose veins can be diagnosed by appearance. A duplex ultrasound can detect obstruction and reflux in the venous system with considerable accuracy. It is the most widely used test to diagnose deep varicose veins.

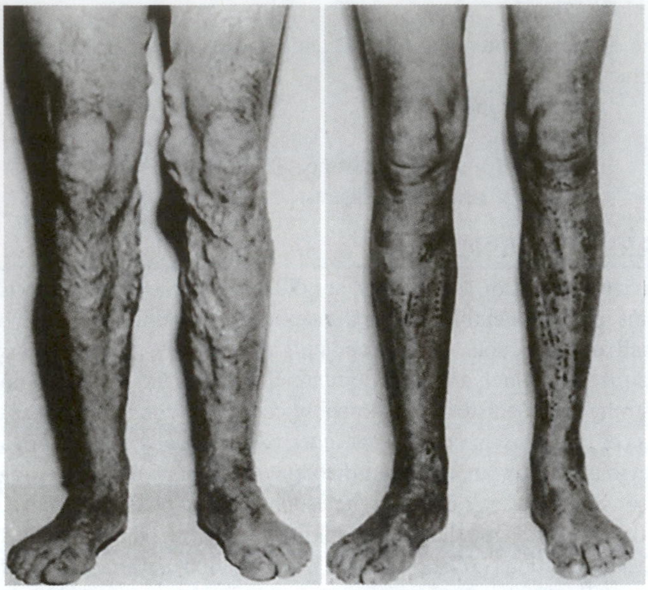

FIG. 38-11 Extensive varicosities (incompetency of the greater saphenous systems). **A,** Appearance preoperatively. **B,** Appearance 2 weeks postoperatively.

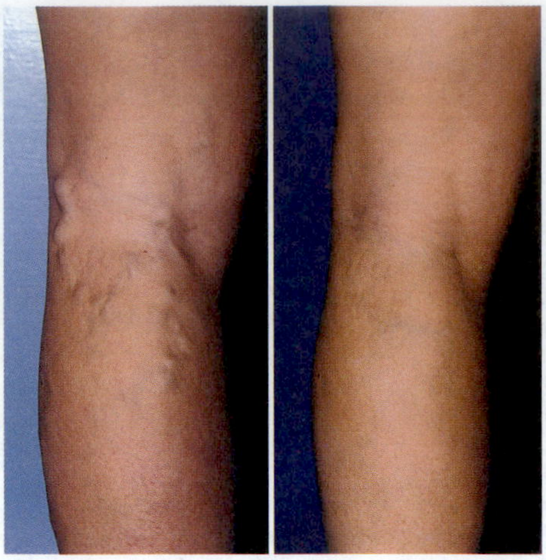

FIG. 38-12 Varicose veins and treatment with sclerotherapy. **A,** Before treatment. **B,** Clinical appearance 2½ years after treatment.

Treatment usually is not indicated if varicose veins are only a cosmetic problem. If incompetency of the venous system develops, collaborative care involves rest with the affected limb elevated, compression stockings, and exercise, such as walking. An herbal therapy used for the treatment of varicose veins is horse chestnut seed extract.[77] (See discussion of chronic venous insufficiency later in the chapter.)

Sclerotherapy involves the injection of a substance that obliterates venous telangiectasias (i.e., spider veins), reticular veins, and small, superficial varicose veins[77] (Fig. 38-12). Two sclerotherapy techniques are available: injection of a sclerosing agent alone or injection of a mixture containing a sclerosing and foaming agent. Commonly used sclerosing agents include hypertonic saline, saline plus hypertonic dextrose, morrhuate sodium, and ethanolamine oxalate. Direct IV injection of a sclerosing agent induces inflammation and results in eventual thrombosis of the vein. This procedure can be performed safely in an office setting and causes minimal discomfort. Potential complications include itching, pain, blistering, edema, hyperpigmentation, necrosis, superficial thrombophlebitis, and DVT.[77] After injection, the leg is wrapped with an elastic bandage for 24 to 72 hours to maintain pressure over the vein. After removal of the elastic bandage, compression stockings are recommended for 2 to 3 weeks to minimize complications. Long-term compression therapy is advised to help prevent the development of further varicosities.

Newer, more costly, but noninvasive options for the treatment of venous telangiectasias include laser therapy and high-intensity pulsed-light therapy.[77] Laser or light therapy is indicated for isolated small telangiectasias or for patients in whom sclerotherapy is contraindicated or has been previously ineffective. Laser treatment typically requires more than one session, scheduled at 6- to 12-week intervals. Vascular lasers work by heating the hemoglobin in the vessels, which injures the endothelium resulting in vessel sclerosis. Pulsed-light therapy is similar to laser therapy, but uses a spectrum of light rather than a single wavelength. Potential complications associated with both these therapies include pain, blistering, hyperpigmentation, and superficial erosions.

Surgical intervention is indicated for recurrent thrombophlebitis or when chronic venous insufficiency cannot be controlled with conservative therapy. The traditional surgical intervention involves ligation of the entire vein (usually the greater saphenous) and dissection and removal of its incompetent tributaries (see Fig. 38-11). An alternative, but time-consuming, technique is ambulatory phlebectomy, which involves pulling the varicosity through a "stab" incision followed by excision of the vein. Newer, less invasive procedures include endovenous occlusion using radiofrequency closure or laser, or transilluminated powered phlebectomy.[77] Both methods of endovenous occlusion involve application of local heat to obliterate the lumen of the targeted vessel. Endovenous occlusion also may be done in combination with saphenofemoral ligation. Transilluminated powered phlebectomy involves the use of a powered tissue resector to destroy the varices and removes the pieces via aspiration. Surgical treatment for varicose veins typically is done as an outpatient procedure.

NURSING MANAGEMENT
VARICOSE VEINS

Prevention is a key factor related to varicose veins. The nurse should instruct the patient to avoid sitting or standing for long periods of time, maintain ideal body weight, take precautions against injury to the extremities, avoid wearing constrictive clothing, and participate in a daily walking program.

After vein ligation surgery, the nurse should encourage deep breathing, which helps promote venous return to the right side of the heart. The extremities should be checked regularly for color, movement, sensation, temperature, presence of edema, and pedal pulses. Bruising and discoloration are considered normal. Postoperatively, the legs are elevated at a 15-degree angle to prevent edema. Compression stockings are applied and removed every 8 hours for short periods and then reapplied.

Long-term management of varicose veins is directed toward improving circulation, relieving discomfort, improving cosmetic appearance, and avoiding complications, such as superficial thrombophlebitis and ulceration. Varicose veins can recur in other veins after vein ligation. The patient should be taught proper care of the lower extremities, including cleanliness and the use of individually fitted compression stockings. The patient should be taught to put on the stockings while still lying down just before rising in the morning. The importance of periodic positioning of the legs above the heart should be stressed. The overweight patient may need assistance with weight reduction. The patient with an occupation that requires prolonged periods of standing or sitting needs to change position frequently.

CHRONIC VENOUS INSUFFICIENCY AND VENOUS LEG ULCERS

Chronic venous insufficiency (CVI), a common medical problem in the elderly, is a condition in which the valves in the veins are damaged, which results in retrograde venous blood flow, pooling of blood in the legs, and swelling. CVI, which often occurs as a result of previous episodes of DVT, can lead to *venous leg ulcers* (formerly called *venous stasis ulcers* or *varicose ulcers*). Although CVI and venous ulceration are not life-threatening diseases, they are painful, debilitating, and costly chronic conditions that can adversely affect the quality of patients' lives.[78,79]

Etiology and Pathophysiology

The causes of CVI include vein incompetence, deep vein obstruction, congenital venous malformation, AV fistula, and calf muscle failure.[80] The basic dysfunction is incompetent valves of the deep veins. As a result, hydrostatic pressure in the veins increases and serous fluid and RBCs leak from the capillaries and venules into the tissue, resulting in edema. Enzymes in the tissue eventually break down RBCs, causing the release of hemosiderin, which causes a brownish skin discoloration. Over time, the skin and subcutaneous tissue around the ankle are replaced by fibrous tissue, resulting in thick, hardened, contracted skin.

Although the causes of CVI are known, the exact pathophysiology of venous ulcers remains unknown. It is known that decreased fibrinolysis, pericapillary fibrin cuffs, and WBC trapping occur in venous ulcers.

Clinical Manifestations and Complications

In individuals with CVI, the skin of the lower leg is leathery, with a characteristic brownish or "brawny" appearance from the hemosiderin deposition. Edema usually has been persistent for a prolonged period. Eczema, or "stasis dermatitis," is often present, and pruritus is a common complaint. Patients with CVI also have a higher skin temperature in the ankle area compared to healthy adults.[81]

Venous ulcers classically are located above the medial malleolus. However, they can occur near the lateral malleolus (Fig. 38-13). The wound margins are irregularly shaped, and the tissue is typically a ruddy color (see Table 38-2). Venous ulcers are typically partial-thickness wounds that extend through the epidermis and portions of the dermis. Ulcer drainage may be extensive, especially when the leg is edematous. The ulcer is often quite painful, particularly when edema or infection is present.[82] Pain may be worse when the leg is in a dependent position.

If the venous ulcer is untreated, the lesion becomes more extensive, eroding wider and deeper, and increasing the likelihood of wound infection and cellulitis. Recurrent episodes of cellulitis may lead to destruction of the superficial lymphatics, causing a secondary lymphedema to develop. On very rare occasions, severe CVI with long-standing nonhealing venous ulceration may result in the need for amputation.

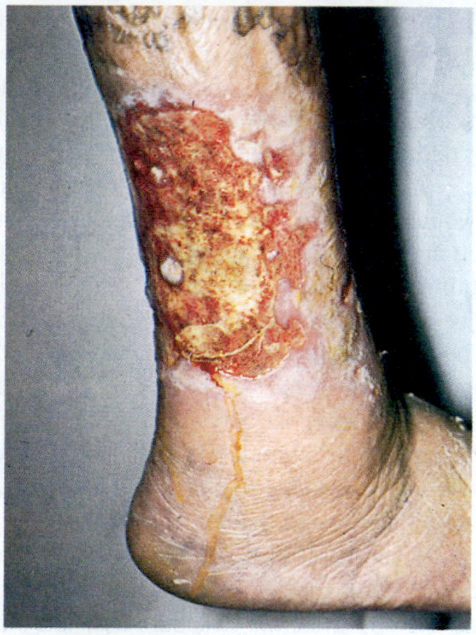

FIG. 38-13 Venous leg ulcer.

Collaborative Care

Compression is essential to the management of CVI, venous ulcer healing, and prevention of ulcer recurrence. A variety of options are available to achieve compression, including elastic wraps, custom-fitted compression stockings, elastic tubular support bandages, a Velcro wrap (Circ-Aid), intermittent compression devices, a paste bandage (Unna boot) with an elastic wrap, and multilayer (three or four) bandage systems (e.g., Profore).[80] There are benefits to each type of compression therapy, and the nurse must evaluate each patient individually when choosing an extrinsic compression method. Before instituting compression therapy, assessment of the arterial status is necessary to make sure that coexistent arterial disease is not present. An ankle-brachial index (ABI) of <0.9 suggests that the patient also has PAD and should not have high levels of compression.

Moist environment dressings are the mainstay of wound care. A variety of these dressings are available and include transparent film dressings, hydrocolloids, hydrogels, foams, calcium alginates, impregnated gauze, gauze moistened with saline, and combination dressings. When used in conjunction with extrinsic compression, moist environment dressings have proven to be more effective in hastening the healing of venous leg ulcers than dry dressings. (Hydrocolloid dressings and other dressings are discussed in Chapter 13 and Table 13-9.)

Nutritional status and intake should be evaluated in a patient with a venous leg ulcer.[83] A balanced diet with adequate protein, calories, and micronutrients is essential for healing. Nutrients most important for healing include protein, vitamins A and C, and zinc. Foods high in protein (e.g., meat, beans, cheese, tofu), vitamin A (green leafy vegetables), vitamin C (citrus fruits, tomatoes, cantaloupe), and zinc (meat, seafood) must be provided. For patients with coexistent diabetes mellitus, maintaining normal blood glucose levels facilitates the healing process.[80] For overweight individuals with CVI and no active venous ulcer, a weight reduction diet may be prescribed.

Routine prophylactic antibiotic therapy typically is not indicated. Clinical signs of infection in a venous ulcer include change in quantity, color, or odor of the drainage; presence of pus; erythema of the wound edges; change in sensation around the wound; warmth around the wound; increased local pain, edema, or both; dark-colored granulation tissue; induration around the wound; delayed healing; and cellulitis.[80] However, if signs of infection are present, a culture should be obtained and appropriate antibiotic therapy is then instituted. The usual treatment for infection is sharp debridement, wound excision, and systemic antibiotics. Nanocrystalline silver-coated dressings (e.g., Acticoat, Silvasorb) are an additional antimicrobial option for infected chronic wounds such as venous ulcers.[84]

If the ulcer fails to respond to conservative therapy, alternative treatments may be indicated. Patients at greatest risk for delayed healing are older and those with a long-standing ulcer.[85] Alternative treatments include use of a radiant heat bandage (Warm-Up active wound therapy system),[86] vacuum-assisted closure (VAC) therapy,[87] and coverage with a split-thickness skin graft, cultured epithelial autograft, allograft, or bioengineered skin such as Apligraf or Dermagraft.[88,89] Typically when a split-thickness skin graft is used, the ulcer is debrided, varicosities in the area of the lesion are removed, and veins are ligated before the tissue from a donor site is applied. (Skin grafting is discussed in Chapter 25.) While these alternative treatments may assist with venous ulcer healing, they do not replace the need for lifelong compression therapy. Hyperbaric oxygen (HBO), another alternative therapy, has not been shown to improve venous ulcer healing.[90]

An herbal therapy used for the treatment of CVI is horse chestnut seed extract (HCSE).[77] Escins, the active ingredient, are thought to act as antiexudative and antiinflammatory agents. Effects include a decrease in vascular permeability and thus a prevention of edema. A meta-analysis concluded that short-term use of oral HCSE reduced leg pain, pruritus, and swelling.[91] Minor side effects associated with HCSE included dizziness, gastrointestinal complaints, headache, and pruritus. The efficacy of HCSE in venous ulcer healing and recurrence has not been determined.

NURSING MANAGEMENT
CHRONIC VENOUS INSUFFICIENCY AND VENOUS LEG ULCERS

Long-term management of venous leg ulcers should focus on teaching the patient about self-care measures because the incidence of recurrence is high. This is particularly important because research indicates that patients with CVI lack understanding of appropriate treatments.[92] Patient and family teaching should include avoidance of trauma to the limbs, proper skin care measures, application and regular replacement of prescribed compression stockings, and appropriate activity and limb positioning.

Proper foot and leg care is essential to avoid additional trauma to the skin. In addition, because of the stasis dermatitis, patients with CVI have dry, flaky, itchy skin. Daily moisturizing of the skin decreases itching and prevents cracking. Venous dermatitis may result from contact with sensitizing products. Sensitizing products may include antibacterial agents (e.g., gentamicin, neomycin); additives in bandages/dressings (e.g., adhesives); ointments containing lanolin, parabens, alcohols, benzocaine, or balsam of Peru; and over-the-counter creams or lotions with fragrance or preservatives.[93] The wound should be assessed for signs and symptoms of infection during each dressing change.

The patient with CVI with or without a venous ulcer is instructed to avoid standing or sitting with the feet dependent for long periods. Standing or sitting with the legs in a dependent position has been shown to decrease periulcer skin blood perfusion and oxygen levels.[94] Venous ulcer patients also are instructed to elevate their legs above the level of the heart to reduce edema. Once an ulcer is healed, a daily walking program is encouraged. Prescription compression stockings should be worn daily and replaced every 4 to 6 months to reduce the occurrence of CVI.[65]

CRITICAL THINKING EXERCISE

CASE STUDY

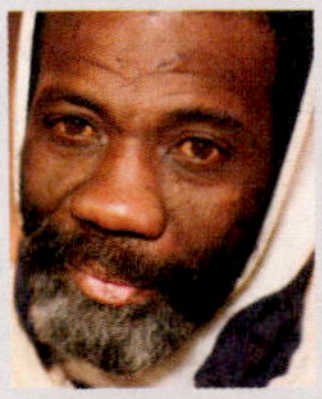

Case Study photo ©iStockphoto.com/ Kevin Russ.

Peripheral Arterial Disease

Patient Profile. Mr. J., a 76-year-old African American man, was admitted to the hospital with rest pain in both legs and a nonhealing ulcer of the big toe on the right foot.

Subjective Data

- History of a myocardial infarction, stroke, hypertension, chronic heart failure, and diabetes mellitus
- Underwent a left femoral-popliteal bypass 5 years ago
- Has a smoking history of 45 pack-years
- Has been using insulin for 30 years
- Complains of sudden, intense increase in right foot pain for past 2 hours
- Has slept in recliner with right leg in dependent position for several months

Current Medications

- furosemide 40 mg PO daily
- BiDil 1 tablet q8hr
- aspart (NovoLog) insulin with meals
- glargine insulin 50 units subcutaneously daily
- diltiazem sustained release 240 mg PO daily
- aspirin 325 mg PO daily
- St. John's wort 300 mg PO daily (self-prescribed)

Objective Data

Physical Examination

- BP 148/92; irregular apical heart rate 90/minute, respiratory rate 22/minute, oral temperature 97.9° F (36.6° C)
- Alert and oriented but anxious, no apparent physical/mental deficits from previous stroke
- Has a diminished right femoral pulse, popliteal pulse by Doppler only; posterior tibial pulse and dorsalis pedis pulse are absent (not palpable or present by Doppler)
- Right leg ABI: 0.4; left leg ABI: 0.75
- Has a 2-cm necrotic ulcer on tip of right big toe
- Has thickened toenails; shiny, thin skin on legs; and hair is absent on both feet
- Right foot is very cool, pale, and mottled in color with decreased sensation
- No peripheral edema present

- Bedside glucose measurement 298 mg/dl (last meal 4 hours prior to admission)

Critical Thinking Questions

1. What are Mr. J.'s risk factors for peripheral arterial disease?
2. Are Mr. J.'s signs and symptoms evidence of acute or chronic peripheral arterial disease? Explain your answer.
3. What is the possible cause(s) for the sudden, intense increase in right foot pain?
4. How would you interpret Mr. J.'s ABI findings?
5. What additional diagnostic tests may be performed to assess the extent of his PAD?
6. Given the physical examination data, what initial medication(s) would you expect the physician to prescribe?
7. What treatment modalities are possible for Mr. J.?
8. What are the priority nursing responsibilities in caring for Mr. J.?
9. Based on the assessment data presented, identify two priority nursing diagnoses. Are there any collaborative problems?
10. When providing patient education to Mr. J. regarding his medications, what advice should be given regarding the use of herbal supplements such as St. John's wort?

NCLEX EXAMINATION REVIEW QUESTIONS

The number of the question corresponds to the same-numbered objective at the beginning of the chapter.

1. A patient diagnosed with peripheral arterial disease is most likely to also have
   a. coronary artery disease.
   b. degenerative joint disease.
   c. a history of atrial fibrillation.
   d. a history of renal insufficiency.
2. A 62-year-old woman weighs 92 kg and has a history of daily alcohol intake, smoking, high blood pressure, high sodium intake, and sedentary lifestyle. The nurse identifies the risk factors most highly related to peripheral arterial disease in this patient as
   a. gender and age.
   b. weight and alcohol intake.
   c. cigarette smoking and hypertension.
   d. sedentary lifestyle and high sodium intake.
3. A patient is scheduled for an abdominal aortic aneurysm repair. The nurse suspects rupture of the aneurysm when
   a. the patient becomes dizzy and short of breath.
   b. the patient complains of sudden, severe back pain.
   c. a bruit and thrill are present at the site of the aneurysm.
   d. the patient develops blue, patchy mottling of the feet and toes.
4. Important nursing measures after an abdominal aortic aneurysm repair are to
   a. elevate the legs and apply TED hose.
   b. assess cranial nerves and mental status.
   c. administer IV heparin and monitor aPTT.
   d. monitor urine output, BUN, and creatinine.
5. Specific symptoms of aortic dissection vary depending on
   a. the medications that are administered.
   b. how elevated the blood pressure becomes.
   c. the aortic branches affected in the descent of the dissection.
   d. the respiratory status of the patient before dissection occurs.
6. Rest pain is a manifestation of peripheral arterial disease that occurs as a result of
   a. the beginning of a venous leg ulcer.
   b. inadequate blood flow to the nerves of the feet.
   c. inadequate blood flow to the muscles during exercise.
   d. inadequate blood flow to the skin after application of the heat.
7. A patient with infective endocarditis develops sudden left leg pain with pallor, paresthesia, and a loss of peripheral pulses. The nurse's initial action should be to
   a. notify the physician.
   b. elevate the leg to promote venous return.
   c. wrap the leg in a blanket to provide warmth.
   d. perform passive range of motion to stimulate circulation to the leg.
8. The usual medical treatment of Raynaud's phenomenon involves
   a. transluminal balloon angioplasty.
   b. amputation of the affected digits.
   c. peripheral arterial bypass surgery.
   d. administration of calcium channel blockers.
9. The patient who is most likely to have the highest risk for deep vein thrombosis is a
   a. 25-year-old obese woman who is 3 days postpartum.
   b. 25-year-old woman who smokes and uses oral contraceptives.
   c. 62-year-old man who has had a stroke with left-sided hemiparesis.
   d. 72-year-old man who had a suprapubic prostatectomy for cancer of the prostate.
10. The nurse suspects the presence of a deep vein thrombosis based on the findings of
    a. paresthesia and coolness of the leg.
    b. pain in the calf that occurs with exercise.
    c. generalized edema of the involved extremity.
    d. pallor and cyanosis of the involved extremity.
11. A priority nursing intervention in the plan of care for the patient with acute lower extremity deep vein thrombosis would include
    a. applying elastic compression stockings.
    b. administering anticoagulants as ordered.
    c. positioning the leg dependently to promote arterial circulation.
    d. encouraging walking and leg exercises to promote venous return.
12. The nurse instructs the patient discharged on anticoagulant therapy to
    a. limit intake of vitamin C.
    b. report symptoms of nausea to the physician.
    c. have blood drawn routinely to check electrolytes.
    d. be aware of and report signs or symptoms of bleeding.
13. In planning care and patient teaching for the patient with venous leg ulcers, the nurse recognizes that the most important intervention in healing and control of this condition is
    a. application of antibiotic cream to the ulcers.
    b. debridement of the ulcers with skin grafting.
    c. elevation of the extremities to increase venous return.
    d. performance of leg exercises to increase collateral circulation.

REFERENCES

1. Cheanvechai V, Harthun NL, Graham LN, et al: Incidence of peripheral vascular disease in women: is it different from that in men? *J Thorac Cardiovasc Surg* 127:314, 2004.
2. Selvin E, Erlinger TP: Prevalence of and risk factors for peripheral arterial disease in the United States: results from the National Health and Nutrition Examination Survey, 1999–2000, *Circulation* 110:738, 2004.
3. American Heart Association: *Heart disease and stroke statistics—2005 update.* Dallas, Tex., 2004, American Heart Association.

4. Taute BM, Taute R, Heins S, et al: Hyperhomocysteinemia: marker of systemic atherosclerosis in peripheral arterial disease, *Int Angiol* 23:35, 2004.
5. Zacharski LR, Chow BR, Howes PS, et al: Implementation of an iron reduction protocol in patients with peripheral vascular disease: VA cooperative study no. 410: the Iron (Fe) and Atherosclerosis Study (FeAST), *Am Heart J* 148:386, 2004.
6. Cornuz J, Sidoti Pinto C, Tevaearai H, et al: Risk factors for asymptomatic abdominal aortic aneurysm: systematic review and meta-analysis of population-based screening studies, *Eur J Public Health* 14:343, 2004.
7. Statistics Canada Health Statistics Division: *Causes of death, 1997 shelf tables* (Catalog No. 84F0209XPB), Ottawa, Canada, 1999, Statistics Canada.
8. Boyer JK, Gutierrez F, Braverman AC: Approach to the dilated aortic root, *Curr Opin Cardiol* 19:563, 2004.
9. Vogelzang RL: Percutaneous endovascular intervention and imaging techniques. In Fahey VA, editor: *Vascular nursing,* ed 4, Philadelphia, 2004, Saunders.
10. Chew HF, You CK, Brown MG, et al: Mortality, morbidity, and costs of ruptured and elective abdominal aortic aneurysm repairs in Novia Scotia, Canada, *Ann Vasc Surg* 17:171, 2003.
11. Harthun NL, Cheanvechai V, Graham LM, et al: Prevalence of abdominal aortic aneurysm and repair outcomes on the basis of patient sex: should the timing of the intervention be the same? *J Thorac Cardiovasc Surg* 127:325, 2004.
12. Dueck AD, Kucey DS, Johnston KW, et al: Survival after ruptured abdominal aortic aneurysm: effect of patient, surgeon, and hospital factors, *J Vasc Surg* 39:1253, 2004.
13. Brewster DC, Cronenwett JL, Hallett JW Jr, et al: Guidelines for the treatment of abdominal aortic aneurysms: report of a subcommittee of the Joint Council of the American Association for Vascular Surgery and Society for Vascular Surgery, *J Vasc Surg* 37:1106, 2003.
14. Matsumura JS, Brewster DC, Makaroun MS, et al: A multicenter controlled clinical trial of open versus endovascular treatment of abdominal aortic aneurysm, *J Vasc Surg* 37:262, 2003.
15. Moore WS, Matsumura JS, Makaroun MS, et al: Five-year interim comparison of the Guidant bifurcated endograft with open repair of abdominal aortic aneurysm, *J Vasc Surg* 38:46, 2003.
16. Morasch MD, Kibbe MR, Evans ME, et al: Percutaneous repair of abdominal aortic aneurysm, *J Vasc Surg* 40:12, 2004.
17. Elliott WJ: Clinical features and management of selected hypertensive emergencies, *J Clin Hypertens* 6:587, 2004.
18. Velez LL, Toal K, Goodwin SA: Two lives on the line: a case study in obstetric critical care, *Crit Care Nurse* 22(6):20, 2002.
19. Kallenbach K, Oelze T, Salcher R, et al: Evolving strategies for treatment of acute aortic dissection type A, *Circulation* 110(11 Suppl 1):II243, 2004.
20. Belch JJ, Topol EJ, Agnelli G, et al: Critical issues in peripheral arterial disease detection and management: a call to action, *Arch Intern Med* 163:884, 2003.
21. Eskandari MK, Matsumura JS, Anderson A: Surgery of the aorta. In Fahey VA, editor: *Vascular nursing,* ed 4, Philadelphia, 2004, Saunders.
22. Treat-Jacobson D, Walsh ME: Treating patients with peripheral arterial disease and claudication, *J Vasc Nurs* 21:5, 2003.
23. Willigendael EM, Teijink JA, Bartelink ML, et al: Influence of smoking on incidence and prevalence of peripheral arterial disease, *J Vasc Surg* 40:1158, 2004.
24. Cahall EJ: Assisting with tobacco cessation, *J Vasc Nurs* 22:117, 2004.
25. McDermott MM, Gurlanik JM, Greenland P, et al: Statin use and leg functioning in patients with and without lower-extremity peripheral arterial disease, *Circulation* 107:757, 2003.
26. Ebrahimi R, Saleh JR, Toggart EJ, et al: Lipid-lowering therapy in patients with peripheral arterial disease, *J Cardiovasc Pharmacol Ther* 9:271, 2004.
27. Mehler PS, Coll JR, Estacio R, et al: Intensive blood pressure control reduces the risk of cardiovascular events in patients with peripheral arterial disease and type 2 diabetes, *Circulation* 107:753, 2003.
28. Tran H, Anand SS: Oral antiplatelet therapy in cerebrovascular disease, coronary artery disease, and peripheral artery disease, *JAMA* 292:1867, 2004.
29. Hiatt WR: Treatment of disability in peripheral arterial disease: new drugs, *Curr Drug Targets Cardiovasc Haematol Disord* 4:227, 2004.
30. Hirsch AT, Duprez D: The potential role of angiotensin-converting enzyme inhibition in peripheral arterial disease, *Vasc Med* 8:273, 2003.
31. Regensteiner JG, Ware JE Jr, McCarthy WJ, et al: Effect of cilostazol on treadmill walking, community-based walking ability, and health-related quality of life in patients with intermittent claudication due to peripheral arterial disease: meta-analysis of six randomized controlled trials, *J Am Geriatr Soc* 50:1939, 2002.
32. Cosmi B, Palareti G: Is there a role for oral anticoagulant therapy in patients with peripheral arterial disease? *Curr Drug Targets Cardiovasc Haematol Disord* 4:269, 2004.
33. Bauer TA, Brass EP, Hiatt WR: Impaired muscle oxygen use at onset of exercise in peripheral arterial disease, *J Vasc Surg* 40:488, 2004.
34. Hiatt WR: Carnitine and peripheral arterial disease, *Ann N Y Acad Sci* 1033:92, 2004.
35. Falcone RA, Hirsch AT, Regensteiner JG, et al: Peripheral arterial disease rehabilitation, *J Cardiopulm Rehabil* 23:170, 2003.
*36. Oka RK, Altman M, Giacomini JC, et al: Exercise patterns and cardiovascular fitness of patients with peripheral arterial disease, *J Vasc Nurs* 22:109, 2004.
37. National Heart, Lung, and Blood Institute: *Clinical guidelines on the identification, evaluation, and treatment of overweight and obesity in adults: the evidence report* (NIH Publication No. 98-4083), Bethesda, Md., 1998, National Institutes of Health.
38. Zhan S, Ho SC: Meta-analysis of the effects of soy protein containing isoflavones on the lipid profile, *Am J Clin Nutr* 81:397, 2005.
39. De Smet PA: Herbal remedies, *N Engl J Med* 347:2046, 2002.
40. Carlsson CM, Pharo LM, Aeschlimann SE, et al: Effects of multivitamins and low-dose folic acid supplements on flow-mediated vasodilation and plasma homocysteine levels in older adults, *Am Heart J* 148:E11, 2004.
41. Novo S, Coppola G, Milio G: Critical limb ischemia: definition and natural history, *Curr Drug Targets Cardiovasc Haematol Disord* 4:219, 2004.
42. Creutzig A, Lehmacher W, Elze M: Meta-analysis of randomized controlled prostaglandin E_1 studies in peripheral arterial occlusive disease stages III and IV, *Vasa* 33:137, 2004.
43. Waugh J, Wagstaff A: The paclitaxel (TAXUS)-eluting stent: a review of its use in the management of de novo coronary artery lesions, *Am J Cardiovasc Drugs* 4:257, 2004.
44. Fahey VA, Schindler N: Arterial reconstruction of the lower extremity. In Fahey VA, editor: *Vascular nursing,* ed 4, Philadelphia, 2004, Saunders.
45. Ang P, Knight H, Matadial C, et al: Managing acute postoperative pain: is 3 hours too long? *J Perianesth Nurs* 19:312, 2004.
*46. Rich K: Effects of leg and body position on transcutaneous oxygen measurements in healthy subjects and subjects with peripheral artery disease after lower-extremity arterial revascularization: a pilot study, *J Vasc Nurs* 20:125, 2002.
47. Oka RK, Szuba A, Giacomini JC, et al: Gender differences in perception of PAD: a pilot study, *Vasc Med* 8:89, 2003.
48. Harthun NL, Cheanvechai V, Graham LM, et al: Arterial occlusive disease of the lower extremities: do women differ from men in occurrence of risk factors and response to invasive treatment? *J Thorac Cardiovasc Surg* 127:318, 2004.
*49. Oka RK, Szuba A, Giacomini JC, et al: Predictors of physical function in patients with peripheral arterial disease and claudication, *Prog Cardiovasc Nurs* 19:89, 2004.
50. Haskal Z: Mechanical thrombectomy devices for the treatment of peripheral arterial occlusions, *Rev Cardiovasc Med* 3(Suppl):S45, 2002.
51. Cooper LT, Tse TS, Mikhail MA, et al: Long-term survival and amputation risk in thromboangiitis obliterans (Buerger's disease), *J Am Coll Cardiol* 44:2410, 2004.
52. Graham LM, Ford MB: Arterial disease. In Fahey VA, editor: *Vascular nursing,* ed 4, Philadelphia, 2004, Saunders.
53. Bozkurt AK, Koksal C, Ercan M: The altered hemorheologic parameters in thromboangiitis obliterans: a new insight, *Clin Appl Thromb Hemost* 10:45, 2004.
54. Bozkurt AK, Besirli K, Koksal C, et al: Surgical treatment of Buerger's disease, *Vascular* 12:192, 2004.
55. Suter LG, Murabito JM, Felson DT, et al: The incidence and natural history of Raynaud's phenomenon in the community, *Arthritis Rheum* 52:1259, 2005.

*Nursing research–based references.

56. Thompson AE, Pope JE: Calcium channel blockers for primary Raynaud's phenomenon: a meta-analysis, *Rheumatology* 44:145, 2005.
57. Mawdsley AH, Brown SJ: Raising awareness of Raynaud's phenomenon and scleroderma, *Nurs Times* 101(8):30, 2005.
58. Caprini JA, Glase CJ, Anderson CB, et al: Laboratory markers in the diagnosis of venous thromboembolism, *Circulation* 109(12 Suppl I):I-4, 2004.
59. Marcucci R, Liotta AA, Cellai AP, et al: Increased plasma levels of lipoprotein(a) and the risk of idiopathic and recurrent venous thromboembolism, *Am J Med* 115:601, 2003.
60. Cohen SM: Factor V Leiden mutation in pregnancy, *J Obstet Gynecol Neonatal Nurs* 33:348, 2004.
61. Nguyen L, Liles DR, Lin PH, et al: Hormone replacement therapy and peripheral vascular disease in women, *Vasc Endovascular Surg* 38:547, 2004.
62. Walsh ME, Rice KL: Venous thromboembolic disease. In Fahey VA, editor: *Vascular nursing,* ed 4, Philadelphia, 2004, Saunders.
63. Bonner L: The prevention and treatment of deep vein thrombosis, *Nurs Times* 100(29):38, 2004.
64. Trujillo-Santos J, Perea-Milla E, Jimenez-Puente A, et al: Bedrest or ambulation in the initial treatment of patients with acute deep vein thrombosis or pulmonary embolism: findings from the RIETE registry, *Chest* 127:1631, 2005.
65. Kolbach DN, Sandbrink MW, Hamulyak K, et al: Non-pharmaceutical measures for prevention of post-thrombotic syndrome, *Cochrane Database Syst Rev* 1:CD004174, 2006.
66. Nutescu EA, Shapiro NL, Chevalier A, et al: A pharmacologic overview of current and emerging anticoagulants, *Cleve Clin J Med* 72(Suppl 1): S2, 2005.
67. Offord R, Lloyd AC, Anderson P, et al: Economic evaluation of enoxaparin for the prevention of venous thromboembolism in acutely ill medical patients, *Pharm World Sci* 26:214, 2004.
68. Fang, MC, Minichiello T, Auerbach AD: Cost considerations surrounding current and future anticoagulant therapies, *Cleve Clin J Med* 72(Suppl 1):S43, 2005.
69. Bartholomew JR, Begelman SM, Almahameed A: Heparin-induced thrombocytopenia: principles for early recognition and management, *Cleve Clin J Med* 72(Suppl 1):S31, 2005.
70. Kaboli PJ, Brenner A, Dunn AS: Prevention of venous thromboembolism in medical and surgical patients, *Cleve Clin J Med* 72(Suppl 1):S7, 2005.
71. Hawkins D: Clinical trials with factor Xa inhibition in the prevention of postoperative venous thromboembolism, *Am J Health Syst Pharm* 60(Suppl):S6, 2003.
72. Aujesky DA, Cornuz J, Bosson JL, et al: Uptake of new treatment strategies for deep vein thrombosis: an international audit, *Int J Qual Health Care* 16:193, 2004.
73. Jaffer AK, Brotman DJ, Michota F: Current and emerging options in the management of venous thromboembolism, *Cleve Clin J Med* 72(Suppl 1):S14, 2005.
74. Watson L, Armon M: Thrombolysis for acute deep vein thrombosis, *Cochrane Database Syst Rev* 8:CD002783, 2006.
75. Augustinos P, Ouriel K: Invasive approaches to treatment of venous thromboembolism, *Circulation* 110(Suppl I):I-27, 2004.
76. Hoblyn JC, Brooks JO: Herbal supplements in older adults: consider interactions and adverse events that may result from supplement use, *Geriatrics* 60:18, 2005.
77. Bartholomew JR, King T, Sahgal A, et al: Varicose veins: newer, better treatments available, *Cleve Clin J Med* 72:312, 2005.
78. McMullen M: The relationship between pain and leg ulcers: a critical review, *Br J Nurs* 13:S30, 2004.
79. Morgan PA, Franks PJ, Moffatt CJ, et al: Illness behavior and social support in patients with chronic venous ulcers, *Ostomy Wound Manage* 50(1):25, 2004.
80. Wipke-Tevis DD, Sae-Sia W: Caring for vascular leg ulcers: a best practices update, *Home Health Nurs* 22:237, 2004.
*81. Kelechi TJ, Haight BK, Herman J, et al: Skin temperature and chronic venous insufficiency, *J Wound Ostomy Continence Nurs* 30(1):17, 2003.
*82. Nemeth KA, Harrison MB, Graham ID, et al: Understanding venous leg ulcer pain: results of a longitudinal study, *Ostomy/Wound Manage* 50(1):34, 2004.
83. Heinen MM, van Achterberg T, op Reimer WS, et al: Venous leg ulcer patients: a review of the literature on lifestyle and pain-related interventions, *J Clin Nurs* 13:355, 2004.
84. Smith LA: Clinical experience using silver antimicrobial dressings on venous stasis ulcers, *Ostomy Wound Manage* Suppl:10, 2003.
85. Gohel MS, Taylor M, Earnshaw JJ, et al: Risk factors for delayed healing and recurrence of chronic venous leg ulcers—an analysis of 1324 legs, *Eur J Vasc Endovasc Surg* 29:74, 2005.
86. Cherry GW, Wilson J: The treatment of ambulatory venous ulcer patients with warming therapy, *Ostomy Wound Manage* 45(9):65, 1999.
87. Loree S, Dompmartin A, Penven K, et al: Is vacuum assisted closure a valid technique for debriding chronic leg ulcers? *J Wound Care* 13:249, 2004.
88. Omar AA, Mavor AI, Jones AM, et al: Treatment of venous leg ulcers with Dermagraft, *Eur J Vasc Endovasc Surg* 27:666, 2004.
89. Eisenbud D, Huang NF, Luke S, et al: Skin substitutes and wound healing: current status and challenges, *Wounds* 16:2, 2004.
90. Roeckl-Wiedmann I, Bennett M, Kranke P: Systematic review of hyperbaric oxygen in the management of chronic wounds, *Br J Surg* 92:24, 2005.
*91. Pittler MH, Ernst E: Horse chestnut seed extract for chronic venous insufficiency, *Cochrane Database Syst Rev* 2:CD003230, 2004.
92. Nunnelee JD, Spaner SD: Explanatory model of chronic venous disease in rural Midwest—a factor analysis, *J Vasc Nurs* 18:6, 2000.
*93. Hess CT: Identifying and managing venous dermatitis, *Adv Skin Wound Care* 18:242, 2005.
94. Wipke-Tevis DD, Stotts NA, Williams DA, et al: Tissue oxygenation, perfusion, and position in patients with venous leg ulcers, *Nurs Res* 50:24, 2001

RESOURCES

American Association of Cardiovascular and Pulmonary Rehabilitation (AACVPR)
312-321-5146
www.aacvpr.org

American College of Chest Physicians (ACCP)
800-343-2227 or 847-498-1400
www.chestnet.org

American Stroke Association
1-888-4-STROKE
www.strokeassociation.org

American Venous Forum
978-744-5005
www.venous-info.com

Anticoagulation Forum
617-638-7265
www.acforum.org

Canadian Cardiovascular Society (CCS)
613-569-3407
www.ccs.ca

Council on Cardiovascular Nursing
American Heart Association
800-AHA-USA-1 (800-242-8721)
www.americanheart.org

Heart and Stroke Foundation of Canada
613-569-4361
www.heartandstroke.ca

Mayo Clinic Heart and Blood Vessels Center
www.mayoclinic.com

National Heart, Lung, and Blood Institute
National Institutes of Health
301-592-8573
www.nhlbi.nih.gov

National Institute of Nursing Research
301-496-0207
www.nih.gov/ninr

Peripheral Vascular Surgical Society
831-373-0508
www.pvss.org

Society for Cardiovascular and Interventional Radiology
800-488-7284 or 703-691-1805
www.sirweb.org

*Nursing research–based references.

*Nursing research–based references.

Society for Vascular Medicine and Biology
301-581-3464
www.svmb.org

Society for Vascular Nursing (SVN)
888-536-4786
www.svnnet.org

Society for Vascular Surgery (SVS)
800-258-7188 or 312-202-5600
http://svs.vascularweb.org

Society of Vascular Technology
www.svtnet.org

Thrombosis Interest Group of Canada (TIGC)
www.tigc.org

Vascular Disease Foundation
866-PADINFO (866-723-4636) or 303-989-0500
www.vdf.org

For additional Internet resources, see the website for this book at *http://evolve.elsevier.com/Lewis/medsurg.*

Illustration Credits

Chapter 1
1-4, 1-5, from Rick Brady, Riva, Md**; 1-6,** Courtesy Elizabeth Burkhart, RN, MPH, PhD, Chicago, Ill.

Chapter 2
2-1, From McGinnis JM, Williams-Russo P, Knickman JR: The case for more active policy attention to health promotion, *Health Affairs* 21:78, 2002; **2-2,** from Health Quality Survey, Diverse Communities, Common Concerns: Assessing Health Care Quality for Minority Americans, Collins KS, Hughes DL, Doty MM et al, *The Commonwealth Fund,* March 2002; **2-3,** from Rick Brady, Riva, Md**; 2-4,** from Giger JN, Davidhizar RE: *Transcultural nursing,* ed 4, St Louis, 2004, Mosby; **Case study photo,** © 2007 JupiterImages Corporation.

Chapter 3
3-1, 3-3, 3-4, 3-6, © 2007 JupiterImages Corporation; **3-5,** from Rick Brady, Riva, Md; **Case study photo,** ©iStockphoto.com/Joseph Jean Rolland Dubé.

Chapter 4
4-1, From Wilson SF, Giddens JF: *Health assessment for nursing practice,* ed 3, St Louis, 2005, Mosby.

Chapter 5
5-1, © 2007 JupiterImages Corporation; **5-3, 5-5,** from Rick Brady, Riva, Md**; 5-6,** from Wilson SF, Giddens JF: *Health assessment for nursing practice,* ed 3, St Louis, 2005, Mosby.

Chapter 6
6-1, From Centers for Disease Control and Prevention, National Center for Health Statistics. *Health,* United States, 2004; **6-3, 6-4, 6-5, 6-6, 6-7, 6-9, 6-10,** from Rick Brady, Riva, Md**; 6-8,** from Fulmer SPICES: an overall assessment tool of older adults. Developed by Meredith Wallace and Terry Fulmer, Hartford Institute for Geriatric Nursing, New York University, New York. In Ebersole P et al: *Gerontological nursing and healthy aging,* ed 2, St Louis, 2005, Mosby; **6-11,** redrawn from Benzon J: Approaching drug regiments with a therapeutic dose of suspicion, *Geriatr Nurs* 12(4):1813, 1991.

Chapter 7
7-1, 7-3, From Potter PA, Perry AG: *Fundamentals of nursing: concepts, process, and practice,* ed 4, St. Louis, 1997, Mosby; **7-2,** from Potter PA, Perry AG: *Basic nursing, a critical thinking approach,* ed 4, St. Louis, 1999, Mosby **7-4,** from Rick Brady, Riva, Md.

Chapter 8
8-1, 8-2, From National Center for Complementary and Alternative Medicine: *The use of complementary and alternative medicine in the United States*, Bethesda, Md.; **8-4, 8-5,** courtesy Cory Shaw, San Antonio, Tex.; **8-6,** from Blake S: *Alternative remedies CD-ROM,* St Louis, 1999, Mosby; **8-7,** courtesy Effie Wood, San Antonio, Tex.; **8-8, 8-9** courtesy Lori Karhu, RMT, RN, San Antonio, Tex.; **Case study photos,** courtesy Scripps Center for Integrative Medicine, La Jolla, Calif.

Chapter 9
9-1, 9-2, 9-7, 9-8, 9-9, © 2007 JupiterImages Corporation; **Case study photo,** ©iStockphoto.com/Rosemarie Colombraro.

Chapter 10
10-1, Developed by McCaffery M, Pasero C, Paice JA. From McCaffery M, Pasero C: *Pain: clinical manual,* ed 2, St Louis, 1999, Mosby; **10-5,** from McCaffery M, Pasero C: *Pain: clinical manual,* ed 2, St Louis, 1999, Mosby; **10-6,** from Acute Pain Management Guideline Panel, 1992; **10-8,** from Salerno E, Willins J: *Pain management handbook,* St Louis, 1996, Mosby; **10-10,** from Rick Brady, Riva, Md; **Case study photo,** © 2007 JupiterImages Corporation.

Chapter 11
11-1, 11-4, 11-5, Courtesy Kathleen A. Pollard, RN, MSN, CHPN, Phoenix, Ariz.; **11-2,** from Potter PA, Perry AG: *Fundamentals of nursing: concepts, process, and practice,* ed 4, St. Louis, 1997, Mosby; **11-3, 11-6,** from Rick Brady, Riva, Md.

Chapter 12
12-1, 12-4, from Rick Brady, Riva, Md; **12-2,** From Department of Health and Human Services: *Clinical practice guideline: treating tobacco use and dependence,* Washington, DC, 2000, U.S. Public Health Service; **12-3,** © iStockphoto.com/Rebecca Ellis; **12-5,** © 2007 JupiterImages Corporation; **Case study photo,** ©iStockphoto.com/Lisa Kyle Young.

Chapter 13
13-8, Courtesy Scott Health Care—A Molnlyche Company, Philadelphia. In Potter PA, Perry AG: *Fundamentals of nursing,* ed 6, St Louis, 2005, Mosby; **13-9A,** from Habif TP: *Clinical dermatology: a color guide to diagnosis and therapy,* ed 2, St Louis, 1992, Mosby; **13-9B,** from Lemmi FO, Lemmi CAE: *Physical assessment findings CD-ROM,* Philadelphia, 2000, Saunders; **13-10,** from Morison MJ: *Prevention and treatment of pressure ulcers,*

London, 2001, Mosby; **13-11,** courtesy Robert B. Babiak, RN, BSN, CWOCN, San Antonio, Tex.; **13-12,** from Potter PA, Perry AG: *Fundamentals of nursing,* ed 6, St Louis, 2005, Mosby; **Case study photo,** ©iStockphoto.com/Gisele Gaze.

Chapter 14

14-1, From Thibodeau GA, Patton KT: *The human body in health and disease,* ed 3, St Louis, 2002, Mosby; **14-12, 14-13,** from Morison MJ: *Nursing management of chronic wounds,* Edinburgh, 2001, Mosby; **14-16,** from the U.S. Department of Health and Human Services, Washington DC; **14-18,** from McKenry L, Tessier E, Hogan M: *Mosby's pharmacology in nursing,* St Louis, 2006, Mosby.

Chapter 15

15-5, 15-6, Set of slides published in 1992 by Jon Fuller, MD and Howard Libman, MD at Boston University School of Medicine, Boston, Mass.; **15-7, 15-8,** from Grimes DE, Grimes RM: *AIDS and HIV infection,* St Louis, 1994, Mosby; **15-9,** from the Centers for Disease Control and Prevention. Courtesy Jonathan WM Gold, MD, New York, N.Y.; **Case study photo 1,** ©iStockphoto.com/Roberta Osborne; **Case study photo 2,** ©iStockphoto.com/Mike Manzano.

Chapter 16

16-1, Adapted from Kumar V, Abbas AK, and Fausto N: *Robbins and Cotran pathologic basis of disease,* ed 7, Philadelphia, 2005, Saunders; **16-4,** from Stevens A, Lowe J: *Pathology: an illustrated review in color,* ed 2, London, 2000, Mosby; **16-5,** adapted from DeVita VT, Helman S, Rosenberg SA, eds: *Cancer: principles and practice of oncology,* Philadelphia, 1997, Lippincott-Raven; **16-12,** Sauerland C, Engelking C, Wickham R, Corbi D: Vesicant extravasation part I: Mechanisms, pathogenesis, and nursing care to reduce risk, *Oncology Nursing Forum* 33(6): 1134-41, 2006.; **16-15A,** courtesy Pharmaceia Deltec, Inc, St. Paul, Minn.; **16-16B,** courtesy Strato/Infusaid, Inc, Norwood, Mass; **16-17, 16-18,** courtesy of Jormain Cady, Virginia Mason Medical Center, Seattle, Wash.; **16-23,** from Forbes CD, Jackson WF: *Color atlas and text of clinical medicine,* ed 3, London, 2003, Mosby.

Chapter 17

17-14, Redrawn from McCance KL, Huether SE: *Pathophysiology: the biologic basis for disease in adults and children,* ed 5, St Louis, 2006, Mosby; **Case study photo,** ©iStockphoto.com/Jessica Jones Photography.

Chapter 18

18-1, © 2007 JupiterImages Corporation; **Case study photo,** ©iStockphoto.com/bbear.

Chapter 19

19-1, Courtesy Greg McVicar; **19-2,** © 2007 JupiterImages Corporation; **19-4,** courtesy The Methodist Hospital, Houston, Tex. Photograph by Donna Dahms, RN, CNOR; **19-5,** from Rothrock JC: *Alexander's Care of the Patient in Surgery,* ed 13, St Louis, 2007, Mosby.

Chapter 20

Case study photo, ©iStockphoto.com/Malcolm Romain.

Chapter 21

21-1, From Thibodeau GA, Patton KT: *Anatomy and physiology,* ed 6, St Louis, 2007, Mosby; **21-5,** Adapted from Kanski J: *Clinical ophthalmology: a synopsis,* New York, 2004, Butterworth-Heinemann; **21-6,** courtesy Eye Institute, Department of Ophthalmology and Visual Services, University of Iowa Health Care, Iowa City, Iowa; **21-7,** from Thibodeau GA, Patton KT: *The human body in health and disease,* ed 4, St Louis, 2005, Mosby; **21-8,** from Seidel HM et al: *Mosby's guide to physical examination,* ed 5, St Louis, 2003, Mosby.

Chapter 22

22-2, 22-3, From Kanski J: *Clinical ophthalmology: a synopsis,* New York, 2004, Butterworth-Heinemann; **22-9,** courtesy of Siemens Hearing Solutions, Piscataway, N.J.; **22-10,** courtesy Advanced Vionics, Valencia, Calif.; **Case study photo,** © 2007 JupiterImages Corporation.

Chapter 23

23-1, From Jarvis C: *Physical examination and health assessment,* ed 4, Philadelphia, 2004, Saunders; **23-3, 23-5,** from Habif TP: *Clinical dermatology: a color guide to diagnosis and therapy,* ed 4, St Louis, 2004, Mosby; **23-4,** from Habif TP: *Clinical dermatology: a color guide to diagnosis and therapy,* ed 3, St Louis, 1996, Mosby.

Chapter 24

24-1, From Hooper BJ, Goldman NP: *Primary dermatologic care,* St Louis, 1999, Mosby; **24-2,** from Goldstein BG, Goldstein AO: *Practical dermatology,* ed 2, St Louis, 1997, Mosby. Courtesy Department of Dermatology, Medical College of Georgia, Augusta, Ga.; **24-3,** from The Skin Cancer Foundation, New York, N.Y.; **24-4, 24-5,** from Habif TP: *Clinical dermatology: a color guide to diagnosis and therapy,* ed 4, St Louis, 2004, Mosby; **24-6,** from Habif TP: *Clinical dermatology: a color guide to diagnosis and therapy,* ed 3, St Louis, 1996, Mosby; **24-7, 24-11,** from Lemmi FO, Lemmi CAE: *Physical assessment findings CD-ROM,* Philadelphia, 2000, Saunders; **24-8, 24-9, 24-10, 24-13,** from Gawkrodger D: *Dermatology: an illustrated colour text,* ed 3, Edinburgh, 2003, Churchill Livingstone; **24-14, 24-15,** from Fortunato N, McCullough SM: *Plastic and reconstructive surgery,* St Louis, 1998, Mosby; **Case study photo,** © 2007 JupiterImages Corporation.

Chapter 25

25-8, 25-10, 25-11D, Courtesy Judy A. Knighton, RegN, MScN, Toronto, Ontario, Canada; **Case study photo,** © 2007 JupiterImages Corporation.

Chapter 26

26-1, Redrawn from Price SA, Wilson LM: *Pathophysiology: clinical concepts of disease processes,* ed 6, St Louis, 2003, Mosby; **26-2, 26-3, 26-11, 26-12,** from Thompson JM et al: *Mosby's clinical nursing,* ed 5, St Louis, 2002, Mosby; **26-4A,** from Bone RC et al, editors: *Pulmonary and critical care medicine,* Vol. 1, St Louis, 1993, Mosby; **26-4B,** from Albertine KH, Williams MC, Hyde DM: Anatomy of the lungs. In Mason RJ et al (editors): *Murray and Nadel's textbook of respiratory medicine,* ed 4, Philadelphia, 2005, Saunders; **26-7A,** courtesy Nonin Medical, Inc, Plymouth, Minn.; **26-7B,** used with permission of Respironics, Inc, Murrysville, Pa.; **26-9,** modified from Wilkins RL, Stoller JK, Scanlan CL: *Egan's fundamentals of respiratory care,* ed 8, St Louis, 2003, Mosby; **26-13,** from Beare PG, Myers JL: *Adult* *health nursing*, ed 3, St Louis, 1998, Mosby; **26-14A,** courtesy Olympus America Inc, Melville, N.Y.; **26-14B,** from Meduri GU et al: Protected bronchoalveolar lavage, *Am Rev Respir Dis* 143:855, 1991; **26-15,** redrawn from Du Bois RM, Clarke SW: *Fiberoptic bronchoscopy in diagnosis and management,* Orlando, 1987, Grune & Stratton.

Chapter 27

27-4, Courtesy Robert Margulies, Miami, Fla. From Smolley LA: How to help patients with obstructive sleep apnea, *J Respir Dis* 11: 723-732, 1990; **27-8D,** Dale Medical Products, Inc, Plainville, Mass.; **27-11,** courtesy Passy-Muir, Inc, Irvine, Calif.; **27-13,** from the American Cancer Society; **27-16,** courtesy CLG Photographics, St Louis.

Chapter 28

28-2, From Damjanov I, Linder J: *Anderson's pathology*, ed 10, St Louis, 1996, Mosby; **28-8, 28-9,** from Atrium Medical Corporation, Hudson, N.H.; **28-10,** from the teaching collection of the Department of Pathology, University of Texas Southwestern Medical School, Dallas, Tex. In Kumar V, Abbas AK, and Fausto N: *Robbins and Cotran pathologic basis of disease*, ed 7, Philadelphia, 2005, Saunders; **Case Study Photo,** ©iStockphoto.com/Peeter Viisimaa.

Chapter 29

29-1, Adapted from McCance KL, Huether SE, editors: *Pathophysiology: the biologic basis for disease in adults and children,* ed 5, St Louis, 2005, Mosby; **29-3,** redrawn from Price SA, Wilson LM: *Pathophysiology: clinical concepts of disease processes*, ed 6, St Louis, 2003, Mosby; **29-5,** trom Togger DA, Brenner PS: Metered dose inhalers, *Am J Nurs* 101(10):26-32, 2001; **29-11A, 29-11B,** from Potter PA, Perry AG: *Fundamentals of nursing*, ed 5, St. Louis, 2001, Mosby; **29-14, 29-15,** courtesy Nellcor Puritan Bennett, Inc, Pleasanton, Calif; **29-18,** courtesy Axcan Scandipharm, Inc, Birmingham, Ala.; **29-19C,** from Kumar V, Abbas AK, and Fausto N: *Robbins and Cotran pathologic basis of disease,* ed 7, Philadelphia, 2005, Saunders; **Case Study Photo,** ©iStockphoto.com/Sandy Jones.

Chapter 30

30-2, From Thibodeau GA, Patton KT: *Anatomy and physiology,* ed 6, St Louis, 2007, Mosby; **30-3,** copyright Dennis Kunkel Microscopy, Inc, Kailua, Hawaii; **30-7,** from Seidel HM et al: *Mosby's guide to physical examination,* ed 6, St Louis, 2006, Mosby; **30-9,** from Herlihy B, Maebius N: *The human body in health and illness*, ed 3, Philadelphia, 2007, Saunders.

Chapter 31

31-3, Redrawn from Raven PH, Johnson GB: *Biology,* ed 2, St Louis, 1991, Mosby; **31-4,** modified from McCance KL, Huether SE: *Pathophysiology: the biologic basis for disease in adults and children,* ed 5, St Louis, 2006, Mosby; **31-6, 31-9, 31-11,** from Forbes CD, Jackson WF: *Color atlas and text of clinical medicine,* ed 3, London, 2003, Mosby; **31-8,** from Bingham BJG, Hawke M, Kwok P: *Clinical atlas of otolaryngology*, St Louis, 1992, Mosby; **31-13, 31-14, 31-17,** from Skarin AT: *Atlas of diagnostic oncology*, ed 2, London, 1996, Mosby-Wolfe; **31-16,** from Cotran RS, Kumar V, Collins T: *Robbins pathologic basis of disease*, ed 6, Philadelphia, 1999, Saunders; **Case Study Photo,** ©iStockphoto.com/Beata Pastuszek.

Chapter 32

32-1, 32-3, modified from Price SA, Wilson LM: *Pathophysiology: clinical concepts of disease processes,* ed 6, St Louis, 2003, Mosby; **32-5, 32-9,** modified from Kinney MR: *Andreoli's comprehensive cardiac care,* ed 8, St Louis, 1996, Mosby; **32-12, 32-15,** from Drake RL, Vogl W, Mitchell AWM: *Gray's anatomy for students*, Edinburgh, 2005, Churchill Livingstone; **32-13,** modified from Kinney MR: *Andreoli's comprehensive cardiac care,* ed 7, St Louis, 1991, Mosby; **32-14,** from Zipes DB et al: *Braunwald's heart disease: a textbook of cardiovascular medicine,* ed 7, St Louis, 2005, Saunders.

Chapter 33

33-1, Redrawn from West JB: *Physiological basis of medical practice,* ed 12, Baltimore, 1991, Williams & Wilkins; **33-3,** from Kissane JM: *Anderson's pathology,* ed 9, St Louis, 1990, Mosby; **33-4, 33-5,** from U.S. Department of Health and Human Services: *Seventh report of the Joint National Committee on Prevention, Detection, Evaluation, and Treatment of High Blood Pressure (JNC 7),* Washington, DC, 2003, National Institutes of Health; **Case Study Photo,** ©iStockphoto.com/Matthew Gough.

Chapter 34

34-1, 34-4, From *2005 Heart and Stroke Statistics,* American Heart Association, Dallas, Tex.; **34-2,** from Huether SE, McCance KL: *Understanding pathophysiology,* ed 3, St Louis, 2003, Mosby, **34-10,** from Zipes DB et al: *Braunwald's heart disease: a textbook of cardiovascular medicine,* ed 7, St Louis, 2005, Saunders; **34-12, 34-14,** courtesy Mayo Clinic, Rochester, Minn.; **34-13,** from Kumar V, Abbas AK, Fausto N: *Robbins and Cotran pathologic basis of disease,* ed 7, Philadelphia, 2005, Saunders; **34-16,** from Bucher L, Melander S: *Critical care nursing,* Philadelphia, 1999, Saunders; **Case Study Photo,** ©iStockphoto.com/Floyd Anderson.

Chapter 35

35-1, Modified from Huether SE, McCance KL: *Understanding pathophysiology,* ed 3, St Louis, 2004, Mosby; **35-2,** modified from Urden LD, Stacy KM, Lough ME: *Thelan's critical care nursing: diagnosis and management,* ed 5, St Louis, 2006, Mosby; **35-3,** from ABIOMED, Inc, Danvers, Mass.; **Case Study Photo,** ©iStockphoto.com/Andres Rodriguez.

Chapter 36

36-1, 36-5, 36-7, 36-8, 36-9, 36-11, 36-14B, 36-15, 36-16C, 36-16D, 36-17, 36-19, From Huszar RJ: *Basic dysrhythmias: interpretation and management,* ed 3, St Louis, 2002, Mosby; **36-2,** modified from Goldberger AL: *Clinical electrocardiography: a simplified approach,* ed 7, St Louis, 2006, Mosby; **36-4, 36-10,** modified from Urden LD, Stacy KM, Lough ME: *Thelan's critical care nursing: diagnosis and management,* ed 5, St Louis, 2006, Mosby; **36-6, 36-12, 36-13, 36-14A, 36-16A, 36-16B, 36-18, 36-23, 36-29, 36-30,** from Bucher L, Melander S: *Critical care nursing,* Philadelphia, 1999, Saunders; **36-21,** courtesy Medtronic Physio-Control, Redmond, Wash.; **36-22A, 36-24A, 36-25,** courtesy Medtronic, Inc, Minneapolis, Minn.; **36-27A, 36-27B,** from Craig, K: How to provide transcutaneous pacing, *Nursing 2005*, 35:10, 2005; **36-27C,** from Woods, et al: *Cardiac nursing*, ed 5, Philadelphia, 2005, Lippincott; **Case Study Photo,** ©iStockphoto.com/Joseph Jean Rolland Dubé.

Chapter 37

37-1, Modified from Thibodeau GA, Patton KT: *The human body in health and disease,* ed 4, St Louis, 2005, Mosby; **37-2, 37-4,** from Damjanov I, Linder J: *Pathology: a color atlas*, St Louis, 1999, Mosby; **37-5,** from Guzzetta CE, Dossey BM: *Cardiovascular nursing: holistic practice,* St Louis, 1992, Mosby; **37-6,** redrawn from Braunwald E: *Heart disease: a textbook of cardiovascular medicine,* ed 3, Philadelphia, 1988, Saunders; **37-7, 37-9,** from Stevens A, Lowe J: *Pathology: illustrated review in color,* ed 2, St Louis, 2000, Mosby; **37-8,** from McCance KL, Huether SE: *Pathophysiology: the biologic basis for disease in adults and children,* ed 5, St Louis, 2006, Mosby; **37-10, 37-12, 37-14,** from Kumar V, Abbas AK, and Fausto N: *Robbins and Cotran pathologic basis of disease,* ed 7, Philadelphia, 2005, Saunders; **37-11,** from Zipes DB et al: *Braunwald's heart disease*: *a textbook of cardiovascular medicine,* ed 7, St Louis, 2005, Saunders; **37-13,** modified from Urden LD, Stacy KM, Lough ME: *Thelan's critical care nursing: diagnosis and management,* ed 5, St Louis, 2006, Mosby; **Case Study Photo,** ©iStockphoto.com/Kati Neudert.

Chapter 38

38-2, Courtesy Jo Menzoian, Boston, MA; **38-5,** from Medtronic, Minneapolis, Minn.; **38-6,** from Damjanov I, Linder J, eds: *Anderson's pathology,* ed 10, St Louis, 1996, Mosby; **38-7,** courtesy FW LoGerfo, Boston; **38-8, 38-13,** from Kamal A, Brockelhurst JC: *Color atlas of geriatric medicine,* ed 2, 1991, Mosby-Year Book-Europe; **38-9,** from Greig JD, Garden OJ: *Color atlas of surgical diagnosis,* London, 1996, Times Mirror International Publishers; **38-11,** from Lofgren KA: Varicose veins. In Haimovici H, editor: *Vascular surgery: principles and techniques,* New York, 1976, McGraw-Hill; **Case Study Photo,** ©iStockphoto.com/Kevin Russ.

Chapter 39

39-1, 39-3, From Thibodeau GA, Patton KT: *The human body in health and disease,* ed 4, St Louis, 2005, Mosby; **39-9,** from Doughty DB, Jackson DB: *Mosby's clinical nursing series: gastrointestinal disorders,* St Louis, 1993, Mosby; **39-10, 39-11, 39-12,** from Drake RL, Vogl W, Mitchell AWM: *Gray's anatomy for students,* Edinburgh, 2005, Churchill Livingstone; **39-13,** from Given Imaging, Inc, Norcross, Ga.

Chapter 40

40-1, Modified from U.S. Department of Agriculture, Center for Nutrition Policy and Promotion, *http://www.MyPyramid.gov;* **40-2,** from Morgan SL, Weinsier RL: *Fundamentals of clinical nutrition,* ed 2, St Louis, 1998, Mosby; **40-3,** adapted with permission of the American Society for Parenteral and Enteral Nutrition [ASPEN]. ASPEN Board of Directors: Guidelines for the use of parenteral and enteral nutrition in adult and pediatric patients, *J Parenter Enteral Nutr* 26:8SA, 2002; **40-4,** modified from Mahan LK, Escott-Stump S: *Krause's food, nutrition, and diet therapy,* ed 11, Philadelphia, 2004, Saunders; **40-5, 40-6, 40-7,** redrawn from Mahan LK, Arlin M: *Krause's food, nutrition, and diet therapy,* ed 8, Philadelphia, 1992, Saunders; **Case Study Photo,** ©iStockphoto.com/Stan Rohrer.

Chapter 41

41-1, From Forbes CD, Jackson WF: *Color atlas and text of clinical medicine,* ed 3, London, 2003, Mosby.

Chapter 42

42-1, From McKenry L, Tessier E, Hogan M: *Mosby's pharmacology in nursing,* ed 22, St Louis, 2006, Mosby; **42-2,** from Kumar V, Abbas AK, and Fausto N: *Robbins and Cotran pathologic basis of disease,* ed 7, Philadelphia, 2005, Saunders; **42-3,** courtesy University of Washington, Division of Gastroenterology, St Louis; **42-4,** from Doughty DB, Jackson DB: *Mosby's clinical nursing series: gastrointestinal disorders,* St Louis, 1993, Mosby; **42-6,** courtesy Curon Medical, Inc, Sunnyvale, Calif.; **42-7, 42-9, 42-11, 42-15,** redrawn from Price SA, Wilson LM: *Pathophysiology: clinical concepts of disease processes,* ed 6, St Louis, 2003, Mosby; **42-12, 42-17,** from Kumar V, Abbas AK, and Fausto N: *Robbins and Cotran pathologic basis of disease,* ed 7, Philadelphia, 2005, Saunders; **Case Study Photo,** ©iStockphoto.com/Joseph Jean Rolland Dubé.

Chapter 43

43-2, 43-15, From Stevens A, Lowe J: *Pathology,* ed 2, London, 2000, Mosby; **43-3,** from Damjanov I, Linder J, editors: *Anderson's pathology,* ed 10, St Louis, 1996, Mosby; **43-7, 43-10,** from McCance KL, Huether SE: *Pathophysiology: the biologic basis for disease in adults and children,* ed 5, St Louis, 2006, Mosby. Courtesy David Bjorkman, MD, University of Utah School of Medicine, Department of Gastroenterology; **43-9,** from Kumar V, Abbas AK, and Fausto N: *Robbins and Cotran pathologic basis of disease,* ed 7, Philadelphia, 2005, Saunders; **43-12,** redrawn from Hampton BG, Bryant RA: *Ostomies and continent diversions,* St Louis, 1992, Mosby; **43-13,** redrawn from Meeker MH, Rothrock JC: *Alexander's care of the patient in surgery,* ed 9, St Louis, 1991; **43-17B,** from Swartz MH: *Textbook of physical diagnosis: history and examination,* ed 5, Philadelphia, 2006, Saunders; **43-19,** from Townsend CM, Beauchamp RD, Evers BM et al: *Sabiston textbook of surgery: the biological basis of modern surgical practice,* ed 17, Saunders, 2004, Philadelphia.

Chapter 44

44-1, From Kamal A, Brockelhurst JC: *Color atlas of geriatric medicine,* ed 2, St Louis, 1991, Mosby-Year Book–Europe; **44-2, 44-3, 44-5,** from McCance KL, Huether SE: *Pathophysiology: the biologic basis for disease in adults and children,* ed 5, St Louis, 2006, Mosby; **44-4, 44-13, 44-17,** from Kumar V, Abbas AK, and Fausto N: *Robbins and Cotran pathologic basis of disease,* ed 7, Philadelphia, 2005, Saunders; **44-7,** adapted from McCance KL, Huether SE: *Pathophysiology: the biologic basis for disease in adults and children,* ed 5, St Louis, 2006, Mosby; **44-11,** from LaBerge JM et al: Transjugular intrahepatic portosystemic shunts: preliminary results in 25 patients, *J Vasc Surg* 16:258, 1992; **44-15,** from Stevens A, Lowe J: *Pathology: illustrated review in color,* ed 2, London, 2000, Mosby.

Chapter 45

45-1A, 45-2, 45-5, Modified from Thibodeau GA, Patton KT: *Anatomy and physiology,* ed 6, St Louis, 2007, Mosby; **45-3,** modified from Thibodeau GA, Patton KT: *The human body in health and disease,* ed 4, St Louis, 2005, Mosby; **45-4,** adapted from Herlihy B, Maebius N: *The human body in health and disease,* ed 3, Philadelphia, 2007, Saunders; **45-6,** from Brundage DJ: *Renal disorders,* St Louis, 1992, Mosby; **45-7,** from Price SA, Wilson LM: *Pathophysiology: clinical concepts of disease processes,* ed 6, St Louis, 2003, Mosby; **45-9,** courtesy Circon Corporation, Santa Barbara, Calif.

Chapter 46

46-2, 46-4, 46-7B, 46-9, 46-10B, From Kumar V, Abbas AK, and Fausto N: *Robbins and Cotran pathologic basis of disease,* ed 7, Philadelphia, 2005, Saunders; **46-5, 46-10A,** from Stevens A, Lowe J: *Pathology: illustrated review in color,* ed 2, London, 2000, Mosby; **46-7A,** from Brundage DJ: *Renal disorders,* St Louis, 1992, Mosby. B, From Kumar V, Abbas AK, and Fausto N: *Robbins and Cotran pathologic basis of disease,* ed 7, Philadelphia, 2005, Saunders; **46-8,** from Lemmi FO, Lemmi CAE: *Physical assessment findings CD-ROM,* Philadelphia, 2000, Saunders; **46-13, 46-15, 46-16,** courtesy Lynda Brubacher, Virginia Mason Hospital, Seattle, Wash.; **Case study photo,** © 2007 JupiterImages Corporation.

Chapter 47

47-2, From Stevens A, Lowe J: *Pathology,* ed 2, Mosby, 2000, London; **47-4,** from United States Renal Data System, Minneapolis, Minn.; **47-9, 47-12,** ©1994 Baxter Healthcare Corp., Deerfield, Ill.; **47-10, 47-11,** courtesy Mary Jo Holechek, Baltimore, Md.; **47-13D, 47-17,** courtesy Vascular Access Services, LLC, St Louis; **47-14A,** courtesy Quinton Instrument Co., Seattle, Wash.; **Case Study Photo,** ©iStockphoto.com/Michael Blackburn.

Chapter 48

48-2, 48-10, Modified from Thibodeau GA, Patton KT: *Anatomy and physiology,* ed 6, St Louis, 2007, Mosby; **48-3, 48-4,** from Herlihy B, Maebius N: *The human body in health and disease,* ed 3, Philadelphia, 2007, Saunders; **48-6,** redrawn from McCance KL, Huether SE: *Pathophysiology: the biologic basis for disease in adults and children,* ed 5, St Louis, 2006, Mosby; **48-8, 48-10, 48-11,** from Thibodeau GA, Patton KT: *The human body in health and disease,* ed 4, St Louis, 2005, Mosby; **48-12,** from Thompson JM, Wilson SF: *Health assessment for nursing practice,* St Louis, 1996, Mosby.

Chapter 49

49-8A, 49-16, 49-17, From Chew SL, Leslie D: *Clinical endocrinology and diabetes: an illustrated colour text,* Edinburgh, 2006, Churchill Livingstone; **49-8B,** courtesy Medtronic MiniMed, Northridge, Calif.; **49-9,** from Medtronic Diabetes, Minneapolis, Minn.; **49-10,** from Home Diagnostics, Ft. Lauderdale, Fla.; **49-12, 49-14,** from Kumar V, Abbas AK, and Fausto N: *Robbins and Cotran pathologic basis of disease,* ed 7, Philadelphia, 2005, Saunders; **49-13,** from Urden LD, Stacy KM, Lough ME: *Thelan's critical care nursing: diagnosis and management,* ed 5, St Louis, 2006, Mosby; **Case study photo,** © 2007 JupiterImages Corporation.

Chapter 50

50-1, Courtesy Linda Haas, Seattle, Wash.; **50-3, 50-4,** redrawn from Urden LD, Stacy KM, Lough ME: *Thelan's critical care nursing: diagnosis and management,* ed 5, St Louis, 2006, Mosby; **50-6, 50-7,** from Forbes CD, Jackson WF: *Color atlas and text of clinical medicine,* ed 3, London, 2003, Mosby; **50-8, 50-12, 50-13,** from Chew SL, Leslie D: *Clinical endocrinology and diabetes: an illustrated colour text,* Edinburgh, 2006, Churchill Livingstone; **50-9,** courtesy Paul W. Ladenson, MD, The Johns Hopkins University and Hospital, Baltimore, Md. From Seidel HM et al: *Mosby's guide to physical examination,* ed 6, St Louis, 2006, Mosby; **50-10,** from Seidel HM et al: *Mosby's guide to physical examination,* ed 6, St Louis, 2006, Mosby; **Case Study Photo,** ©iStockphoto.com/Lanica Klein.

Chapter 51

51-1, From Thibodeau GA, Patton KT: *The human body in health and disease,* ed 4, St Louis, 2005, Mosby; **51-2, 51-5, 51-6, 51-9,** modified from Thibodeau GA, Patton KT: *Anatomy and physiology,* ed 6, St Louis, 2007, Mosby; **51-3, 51-4,** from Seidel HM et al: *Mosby's guide to physical examination,* ed 6, St Louis, 2006, Mosby.

Chapter 52

52-2, From Powell DE, Stilling CB: *Diagnosis and detection of breast diseases,* St Louis, 1993, Mosby; **52-4,** from Evans A et al: *Atlas of breast disease management,* Philadelphia, 1998, Saunders; **52-6,** from Swartz MH: *Textbook of physical diagnosis: history and examination,* ed 5, Philadelphia, 2006, Saunders; **52-7,** courtesy of Cytyc Corporation and affliates, Marlborough, Mass.; **52-9, 52-10B,** courtesy Brian Davies, MD. From Fortunato N, McCullough S: *Plastic and reconstructive surgery,* St Louis, 1998, Mosby; **52-10A,** from Cameron J: *Current surgical therapy,* ed 5, St Louis, 1995, Mosby; **52-11,** modified from Beare PG, Myers JL: *Adult health nursing,* ed 3, St Louis, 1998, Mosby; and Fortunato N, McCullough S: *Plastic and reconstructive surgery,* St Louis, 1998, Mosby; **Case Study Photo,** ©iStockphoto.com/Jessica Jones.

Chapter 53

53-1, 53-2, 53-3, 53-6, 53-7B, From Morse S, Moreland A, Holmes K, editors: *Atlas of sexually transmitted diseases and AIDS,* London, 1996, Mosby-Wolfe; **53-4,** courtesy USPHS, Washington DC; **53-5,** from Habif T: *Clinical dermatology: a color guide to diagnosis and therapy,* ed 4, St Louis, 2004, Mosby; **53-7A, C, 53-9C,** from the Center for Disease Control and Prevention. Courtesy of Susan Lindsley. **53-8, 53-10,** Reproduced with permission of GlaxoSmithKline, Research Triangle Park, N.C.; **53-9A,** from the Center for Disease Control and Prevention. Courtesy Joe Millar. **53-9B,** from the Center for Disease Control and Prevention. Courtesy of Dr. Wiesner. **Case Study Photo,** ©iStockphoto.com/Roberta Osborne.

Chapter 54

54-2, Courtesy Ethicon, Inc, Cornelia, Ga.; **54-3,** from Seidel HM et al: *Mosby's guide to physical examination,* ed 6, St Louis, 2006, Mosby; **54-4,** from Lowdermilk DL, Perry SE: *Maternity and women's health care,* ed 8, St Louis, 2004, Mosby; **54-6,** modified from Stenchever MA et al: *Comprehensive gynecology,* ed 4, St Louis, 2001, Mosby; **54-7,** from McCance KL, Huether SE: *Pathophysiology: the biologic basis for disease in adults and children,* ed 5, St Louis, 2006, Mosby; **54-8, 54-13B,** from Symonds EM, McPherson MBA: *Color atlas of obstetrics and gynecology,* London, 1994, Mosby; **54-9,** from Drake RL, Vogl W, Mitchell AWM: *Gray's anatomy for students,* Edinburgh, 2005, Churchill Livingstone; **54-10,** from Phipps WJ, Sands JK, and Marek JF: *Medical-surgical: nursing concepts and clinical practice,* ed 6, St Louis, 1999, Mosby; **54-12,** modified from Seidel HM et al: *Mosby's guide to physical examination,* ed 6, St Louis, 2006, Mosby; **54-14B,** from Huffman JW: *Gynecology and obstetrics,* Philadelphia, 1962, Saunders; **Case Study Photo,** ©iStockphoto.com/Brandon Clark.

Chapter 55

55-5, Modified from Iwamoto RR, Maher KE: Radiation therapy for prostate cancer, *Semin Oncol Nurs* 17(2):90-100, 2001; **55-6A,**

from Taylor PK: *Diagnostic picture tests in sexually transmitted diseases,* London, 1994, Mosby; **55-6B,** from Morse SA, Moreland AA, Holmes KK: *Atlas of sexually transmitted diseases and AIDS,* ed 2, London, 1995, Mosby-Wolfe; **55-8,** from Swartz MH: *Textbook of physical diagnosis: history and examination,* ed 5, Philadelphia, 2006, Saunders; **55-9,** from Seidel HM et al: *Mosby's guide to physical examination,* ed 6, St Louis, 2006, Mosby; **Case Study Photo,** ©iStockphoto.com/Floyd Willis.

Chapter 56

56-1, 56-5, 56-6, 56-11, 56-14, 56-15, 56-22, Modified from Thibodeau GA, Patton KT: *Anatomy and physiology,* ed 6, St Louis, 2007, Mosby; **56-4,** from Herlihy B, Maebius N: *The human body in health and illness,* ed 3, Philadelphia, 2007, Saunders; **56-9, 56-10, 56-13,** from Thibodeau GA, Patton KT: *Anatomy and physiology,* ed 6, St Louis, 2007, Mosby; **56-12,** redrawn from McCance KL, Huether SE: *Pathophysiology: the biologic basis for disease in adults and children,* ed 5, St. Louis, 2006, Mosby; **56-20A,** courtesy Hitachi Medical Systems America, Inc.; **56-20B,** from Chipps E, Clanin N, and Campbell V: *Neurologic disorders,* St Louis, 1992, Mosby.

Chapter 57

57-4, Modified from McCance KL, Huether SE: *Pathophysiology: the biologic basis for disease in adults and children,* ed 5, St Louis, 2006, Mosby; **57-6,** modified from Urden LD, Stacy KM, Lough ME: *Thelan's critical care nursing: diagnosis and management,* ed 5, St Louis, 2006, Mosby; **57-7,** from Clochesy JM et al: *Critical care nursing,* ed 2, Philadelphia, 1996, Saunders; **57-8, 57-15,** from Copstead LC, Banasik JL: *Pathophysiology,* ed 3, Philadelphia, 2005, Saunders; **57-9, 57-14,** redrawn from Barker E: *Neuroscience nursing: a spectrum of care,* ed 2, St. Louis, 2002, Mosby; **57-10,** from Wong J, Wong S, Dempster JK: Care of the unconscious patient: a problem-oriented approach, *Am Assoc Neurosci Nurses* 16:145, 1984; **57-13,** from Bingham BJG, Hawke M, Kwok P: *Clinical atlas of otolaryngology,* St Louis, 1992, Mosby; **57-16,** from Kumar V, Abbas AK, and Fausto N: *Robbins and Cotran pathologic basis of disease,* ed 7, Philadelphia, 2005, Saunders; **57-17,** from Stevens A, Lowe J: *Pathology: illustrated review in color,* ed 2, London, 2000, Mosby; **57-19,** courtesy Department of Neurological Surgery, Vanderbilt University Medical Center, Nashville, Tenn.; **Case Study Photo,** © 2007 JupiterImages Corporation.

Chapter 58

58-4, From Kumar V, Abbas AK, and Fausto N: *Robbins and Cotran pathologic basis of disease,* ed 7, Philadelphia, 2005, Saunders; **58-7,** from Abbott Vascular, Santa Clara, Calif.; **58-11,** modified from Hoeman SP: *Rehabilitation nursing,* ed 2, St Louis, 1995, Mosby; **58-12,** from Forbes CD, Jackson WF: *Color atlas and text of clinical medicine,* ed 3, London, 2003, Mosby; **58-13,** courtesy Sammons Preston, Bolingbrook, Ill.; **Case Study Photo,** ©iStockphoto.com/Roberta Osborne.

Chapter 59

59-3, From Stevens A, Lowe J: *Pathology: illustrated review in color,* ed 2, London, 2000, Mosby; **59-6,** from McCance KL, Huether SE: *Pathophysiology: the biologic basis for disease in adults and children,* ed 5, St Louis, 2006, Mosby; **59-7,** from Perkin DG: *Mosby's color atlas and text of neurology,* London, 1998, Mosby-Wolfe; **59-8,** redrawn from Rudy E: *Advanced neurological and neurosurgical nursing,* St Louis, 1984, Mosby; **59-9,** redrawn from Barker E: *Neuroscience nursing: a spectrum of care,* ed 2, St Louis, 2002, Mosby; **Case Study Photo,** ©iStockphoto.com/Bernrd Klumpp.

Chapter 60

60-1A, From Damjanov I, Linder J, editors: *Anderson's pathology,* ed 10, St Louis, 1996, Mosby; **60-3,** From Stevens A, Lowe J: *Pathology: illustrated review in color,* ed 2, London, 2000, Mosby; **60-4,** from Stuart GW, Laraia MT: *Principles and practice of psychiatric nursing,* ed 8, St Louis, 2005, Mosby; **Case Study Photo,** ©iStockphoto.com/Nancy Louie.

Chapter 61

61-1, Modified from Thibodeau GA, Patton KT: *Anatomy and physiology,* ed 6, St Louis, 2007, Mosby; **61-2,** courtesy Joe Rothrock, Media, Pa.; **61-3A,** redrawn from Chipps E, Clanin N, Campbell V: *Neurologic disorders,* St. Louis, 1992, Mosby **61-3B,** from Forbes CD, Jackson WF: *Color atlas and text of clinical medicine,* ed 3, London, 2003, Mosby; **61-4,** redrawn from Marciano FF et al: *BNI Quarterly* 11:6, 1995. In McCance KL, Huether SE: *Pathophysiology: the biologic basis for disease in adults and children,* ed 5, St Louis, 2006, Mosby; **61-5A, B, C,** from Copstead LC, Banasik JL: *Pathophysiology,* ed 3, Philadelphia, 2005, Saunders; **61-8, 61-9,** from American Spinal Injury Association/International Medical Society of Paraplegic (ASIA/IMOSP): *International standards for neurological functional classification of spinal cord injury patients* (revised), Chicago, 2002, American Spinal Cord Injury Association; **61-10, 61-13,** courtesy Michael S. Clement, MD, Mesa, Ariz.; **61-12,** courtesy Acromed Corporation, Cleveland, Ohio; **61-14,** from Barker E: *Neuroscience nursing: a spectrum of care,* ed 2, St Louis, 2002, Mosby; **Case Study Photo,** ©iStockphoto.com/Kevin Russ.

Chapter 62

62-1, From Herlihy B, Maebius N: *The human body in health and illness,* ed 3, Philadelphia, 2007, Saunders; **62-3, 62-5,** modified from Thibodeau GA, Patton KT: *Anatomy and physiology,* ed 6, St Louis, 2007, Mosby; **62-6,** from Wilson SF, Giddens JF: *Health assessment for nursing practice,* ed 3, St Louis, 2005, Mosby; **62-7,** from Lemmi FO, Lemmi CAE: *Physical assessment findings CD-ROM,* Philadelphia, 2000, Saunders; **62-8,** from Thibodeau GA, Patton KT: *Human body in health and disease,* ed 4, St Louis, 2005, Mosby.

Chapter 63

63-1, Redrawn from Price SA, Wilson LM: *Pathophysiology: clinical concepts of disease processes,* ed 6, St Louis, 2003, Mosby; **63-2,** from Thompson JM et al: *Mosby's clinical nursing,* ed 5, St Louis, 2002, Mosby; **63-3,** from *www.pinnaclesystems.com;* also in Maher AB, Salmond SW, Pellino TA: *Orthopaedic nursing,* ed 3, St Louis, 2002, Saunders; **63-4,** from Thibodeau GA, Patton KT: *Anatomy and physiology,* ed 5, St Louis, 2003, Mosby; **63-5A,** from David Lintner, MD, Houston, Tex., *www.drlintner.com;* **63-5B, C** courtesy Peter Bonner, San Antonio, Tex.; **63-9,** redrawn from Long B, Phipps W, Cassmeyer V: *Medical-surgical nursing: a nursing process approach,* St Louis, 1993, Mosby; **63-13, 63-24,** from Maher A et al, editors: *Orthopaedic nursing,* ed 3, Philadelphia, 2002, Saunders; **63-14,** courtesy Howmedica,

Inc, Allendale, Pa.; **63-15,** from Ryan DW, Park GR: *Color atlas of critical and intensive care: diagnosis and investigation,* London, 1995, Mosby-Wolfe; **63-18,** from Thompson JM et al: *Mosby's clinical nursing,* ed 4, St Louis, 1997, Mosby; **63-19,** courtesy R.A. Weinstein, Denver, Colo.; **63-21,** from Macklin EJ et al: *Hunter, Macklin, and Callahan's rehabilitation of the hand and upper extremity,* vol. 2, ed 5, St Louis, 2002, Mosby; **63-23,** from Thibodeau GA, Patton KT: *Anatomy and physiology,* ed 6, St Louis, 2007, Mosby; **63-25,** courtesy Zimmer, Inc, Warsaw, Ind.; **Case Study Photo,** ©iStockphoto.com.

Chapter 64

64-1, Redrawn from Mourad L: *Orthopedic disorders,* St Louis, 1992, Mosby; **64-2, 64-5,** from Thibodeau GA, Patton KT: *Human body in health and disease,* ed 4, St Louis, 2005, Mosby; **64-3, 64-4,** from Damjanov I, Linder J: *Anderson's pathology,* ed 10, St Louis, 1996, Mosby; **64-6,** from Eidelson SG, Spinasanta SA: *Advanced technologies to treat neck and back pain: a patient's guide,* Wheaton, Ill., 2005, SYA Press and Research; **64-7,** from DePuy Spine, Inc. Raynham, Mass.; **64-8,** from Mercier LR: *Practical orthopedics,* ed 5, St Louis, 2000, Mosby; **64-9,** from Mercier LR: *Practical orthopedics,* ed 4, St Louis, 1996, Mosby; **64-10,** from Maher A et al: *Orthopaedic nursing,* ed 3, Philadelphia, 2002, Saunders; **Case Study Photo,** ©iStockphoto.com/Roberta Osborne.

Chapter 65

65-1, 65-3, From Stevens A, Lowe J: *Pathology: an illustrated review in color,* ed 2, London, 2000, Mosby; **65-6,** from Forbes CD, Jackson WF: *Color atlas of clinical medicine,* ed 3, London, 2003, Mosby; **65-7,** from Habif TP: *Clinical dermatology: a color guide to diagnosis and therapy,* ed 4, St Louis, 2004, Mosby; **65-8,** reprinted from the Clinical Slide Collection on the Rheumatic Diseases, copyright 1991, 1995, 1997. Used by permission of the American College of Rheumatology; **65-10,** from Habif TP: *Clinical dermatology: a color guide to diagnosis and therapy,* ed 3, St Louis, 1996, Mosby; **65-12,** from Zitelli BJ, Davis HW: *Atlas of pediatric physical diagnosis,* ed 4, St Louis, 2002, Mosby; **65-13,** from Kumar V, Abbas AK, and Fausto N: *Robbins and Cotran pathologic basis of disease,* ed 7, Philadelphia, 2005, Saunders; **65-14,** redrawn from Freundlich B, Leventhal L: The fibromyalgia syndrome. In Schumacher HR Jr, Klippel JH, Koopman WJ, editors: *Primer on the rheumatic diseases,* ed 11, Atlanta, 1997, Arthritis Foundation. Reprinted with permission from The Arthritis Foundation, 1330 W. Peachtree St., Atlanta, Ga. 30309; **Case Study Photo,** ©iStockphoto.com/Jason Stitt.

Chapter 66

66-1, From Avera Health, Sioux Falls, S.Dak.; **66-2, 66-22,** courtesy Spacelabs Medical, Redmond, Wash.; **66-3,** redrawn from Gardner PE: *Hemodynamic pressure monitoring*, Redmond, Wash., 1994, Spacelabs Medical; **66-4,** redrawn from Flynn JBM, Bruce NP: *Introduction to critical care skills,* St Louis, 1993, Mosby; **66-5,** from Darovic GO, Vanriper S, Vanriper J: Fluid-filled monitoring systems. In Darovic GO: *Hemodynamic monitoring,* ed 2, Philadelphia, 1995, Saunders; **66-6, 66-8, 66-11,** modified from Urden LD, Stacy KM, Lough ME: *Thelan's critical care nursing: diagnosis and management,* ed 5, St Louis, 2006, Mosby; **66-7,** courtesy Edwards Critical Care Division, Baxter Healthcare Corporation, Santa Ana, Calif.; **66-9, 66-10,** from Lynn-McHale DJ, Carlson KK (editors): *AACN procedure manual for critical care,* ed 5, Philadelphia, 2005, Saunders; **66-13,** courtesy Datascope Corp., Fairfield, N.J.; **66-15,** from Datascope Corp., Montvale, N.J.; **66-16,** redrawn from Urden LD, Stacy KM, Lough ME: *Thelan's critical care nursing: diagnosis and management,* ed 4, St Louis, 2002, Mosby; **66-17A,** from Beare PG, Myers JL: *Adult health nursing,* ed 3, St Louis, 1998, Mosby; **66-18,** from Henneman E, Ellstrom K, St. John RE: *AACN protocols for practice: care of the mechanically ventilated patient series,* Aliso Viejo, Calif., 1999, American Association of Critical-Care Nurses; **66-19,** from Sills JR: *Respiratory care certification guide: the complete review resource for the entry level exam,* ed 2, St Louis, 1991, Mosby. In Urden LD, Stacy KM, Lough ME: *Thelan's critical care nursing: diagnosis and management,* ed 5, St Louis, 2006, Mosby; **66-20,** reprinted by permission of Nellcor Puritan Bennett Inc, Pleasanton, California; **66-21,** courtesy Lifecare, Westminster, Colo.; **66-23,** from Wiegand DL, Carlson K (editors): *AACN procedure manual for critical care,* ed 5, 2005, Saunders; **Case Study Photo,** ©iStockphoto.com/Sharon Dominick.

Chapter 67

67-2, 67-3, 67-4, 67-5, Modified from Urden LD, Stacy KM, Lough ME: *Thelan's critical care nursing: diagnosis and management,* ed 5, St Louis, 2006, Mosby; **Case Study Photo,** ©iStockphoto.com/Yvonne Chamberlain.

Chapter 68

68-6, From Richmond TS: The patient with a cervical spinal cord injury, *Focus on Critical Care* 12:27, 1985; **68-7,** courtesy Respironics, Inc, Pittsburgh, Pa.; **68-10,** from Cohen J, Powderly WG: *Infectious diseases,* ed 2, St Louis, 2004, Mosby; **68-11, 68-12,** © 2006 Hill-Rom Services, Inc. Reprinted with permission. All rights reserved; **Case Study Photo,** ©iStockphoto.com/Galina Barskaya.

Chapter 69

69-1, ©ESI Triage Research Team, 2004. Reproduced with permission; **69-3, 69-4,** courtesy Cameron Bangs, MD. From Auerbach PS, Donner HJ, Weiss EA: *Field guide to wilderness medicine,* ed, 2, St Louis, 2003, Mosby; **69-6,** from Auerbach PS, Donner HJ, Weiss EA: *Field guide to wilderness medicine,* St Louis, 1999, Mosby; **69-7,** courtesy of Centers for Disease Control, Division of Viral and Rickettsial Diseases. Available at *www.cdc.gov/ncidod/dvbid/lyme/ld_tickremoval.htm*; **69-8,** modified from Marx JA et al: *Rosen's emergency medicine: concepts and clinical practice,* vol 1, ed 6, St Louis, 2006, Mosby; **69-9,** courtesy Sherman Minton, MD. From Auerbach PS, Donner HJ, Weiss EA: *Field guide to wilderness medicine,* St Louis, 1999, Mosby; **69-10,** photo used with the permission of the American Red Cross; **Case Study Photo,** ©iStockphoto.com/Lacey Gadwill.

Index

Note: Disorder names are in **bold face.** Page numbers in **bold face** indicate main discussions. Page numbers followed by *f, t, b,* or *n* indicate figures, tables, boxed material, or notes, respectively.

Note: Disorder names are in **bold face.** Page numbers in **bold face** indicate main discussions. Page numbers followed by *f, t, b,* or *n* indicate figures, tables, boxed material, or notes, respectively.

Note: Disorder names are in **bold face.** Page numbers in **bold face** indicate main discussions. Page numbers followed by *f, t, b,* or *n* indicate figures, tables, boxed material, or notes, respectively.

Note: Disorder names are in **bold face.** Page numbers in **bold face** indicate main discussions. Page numbers followed by *f, t, b,* or *n* indicate figures, tables, boxed material, or notes, respectively.

Note: Disorder names are in **bold face.** Page numbers in **bold face** indicate main discussions. Page numbers followed by *f, t, b,* or *n* indicate figures, tables, boxed material, or notes, respectively.

Note: Disorder names are in **bold face.** Page numbers in **bold face** indicate main discussions. Page numbers followed by *f, t, b,* or *n* indicate figures, tables, boxed material, or notes, respectively.

Index

Note: Disorder names are in **bold face.** Page numbers in **bold face** indicate main discussions. Page numbers followed by *f, t, b,* or *n* indicate figures, tables, boxed material, or notes, respectively.

Note: Disorder names are in **bold face.** Page numbers in **bold face** indicate main discussions. Page numbers followed by *f, t, b,* or *n* indicate figures, tables, boxed material, or notes, respectively.

Note: Disorder names are in **bold face.** Page numbers in **bold face** indicate main discussions. Page numbers followed by *f, t, b,* or *n* indicate figures, tables, boxed material, or notes, respectively.

Note: Disorder names are in **bold face.** Page numbers in **bold face** indicate main discussions. Page numbers followed by *f, t, b,* or *n* indicate figures, tables, boxed material, or notes, respectively.

Note: Disorder names are in **bold face.** Page numbers in **bold face** indicate main discussions. Page numbers followed by *f, t, b,* or *n* indicate figures, tables, boxed material, or notes, respectively.

Note: Disorder names are in **bold face.** Page numbers in **bold face** indicate main discussions. Page numbers followed by *f, t, b,* or *n* indicate figures, tables, boxed material, or notes, respectively.

D

Note: Disorder names are in **bold face.** Page numbers in **bold face** indicate main discussions. Page numbers followed by *f, t, b,* or *n* indicate figures, tables, boxed material, or notes, respectively.

Note: Disorder names are in **bold face.** Page numbers in **bold face** indicate main discussions. Page numbers followed by *f, t, b,* or *n* indicate figures, tables, boxed material, or notes, respectively.

Note: Disorder names are in **bold face**. Page numbers in **bold face** indicate main discussions. Page numbers followed by *f*, *t*, *b*, or *n* indicate figures, tables, boxed material, or notes, respectively.

Note: Disorder names are in **bold face.** Page numbers in **bold face** indicate main discussions. Page numbers followed by *f, t, b,* or *n* indicate figures, tables, boxed material, or notes, respectively.

Note: Disorder names are in **bold face.** Page numbers in **bold face** indicate main discussions. Page numbers followed by *f, t, b,* or *n* indicate figures, tables, boxed material, or notes, respectively.

Note: Disorder names are in **bold face.** Page numbers in **bold face** indicate main discussions. Page numbers followed by *f, t, b,* or *n* indicate figures, tables, boxed material, or notes, respectively.

Note: Disorder names are in **bold face.** Page numbers in **bold face** indicate main discussions. Page numbers followed by *f, t, b,* or *n* indicate figures, tables, boxed material, or notes, respectively.

Note: Disorder names are in **bold face.** Page numbers in **bold face** indicate main discussions. Page numbers followed by *f, t, b,* or *n* indicate figures, tables, boxed material, or notes, respectively.

Note: Disorder names are in **bold face.** Page numbers in **bold face** indicate main discussions. Page numbers followed by *f, t, b,* or *n* indicate figures, tables, boxed material, or notes, respectively.

Note: Disorder names are in **bold face.** Page numbers in **bold face** indicate main discussions. Page numbers followed by *f, t, b,* or *n* indicate figures, tables, boxed material, or notes, respectively.

Note: Disorder names are in **bold face.** Page numbers in **bold face** indicate main discussions. Page numbers followed by *f*, *t*, *b*, or *n* indicate figures, tables, boxed material, or notes, respectively.

Note: Disorder names are in **bold face.** Page numbers in **bold face** indicate main discussions. Page numbers followed by *f, t, b,* or *n* indicate figures, tables, boxed material, or notes, respectively.

Note: Disorder names are in **bold face.** Page numbers in **bold face** indicate main discussions. Page numbers followed by *f, t, b,* or *n* indicate figures, tables, boxed material, or notes, respectively.

Note: Disorder names are in **bold face.** Page numbers in **bold face** indicate main discussions. Page numbers followed by *f, t, b,* or *n* indicate figures, tables, boxed material, or notes, respectively.

Note: Disorder names are in **bold face.** Page numbers in **bold face** indicate main discussions. Page numbers followed by *f, t, b,* or *n* indicate figures, tables, boxed material, or notes, respectively.

Note: Disorder names are in **bold face.** Page numbers in **bold face** indicate main discussions. Page numbers followed by *f, t, b,* or *n* indicate figures, tables, boxed material, or notes, respectively.

Note: Disorder names are in **bold face.** Page numbers in **bold face** indicate main discussions. Page numbers followed by *f, t, b,* or *n* indicate figures, tables, boxed material, or notes, respectively.

Note: Disorder names are in **bold face.** Page numbers in **bold face** indicate main discussions. Page numbers followed by *f, t, b,* or *n* indicate figures, tables, boxed material, or notes, respectively.

Note: Disorder names are in **bold face.** Page numbers in **bold face** indicate main discussions. Page numbers followed by *f, t, b,* or *n* indicate figures, tables, boxed material, or notes, respectively.

Note: Disorder names are in **bold face.** Page numbers in **bold face** indicate main discussions. Page numbers followed by *f, t, b,* or *n* indicate figures, tables, boxed material, or notes, respectively.

Note: Disorder names are in **bold face.** Page numbers in **bold face** indicate main discussions. Page numbers followed by *f, t, b,* or *n* indicate figures, tables, boxed material, or notes, respectively.

Note: Disorder names are in **bold face.** Page numbers in **bold face** indicate main discussions. Page numbers followed by *f, t, b,* or *n* indicate figures, tables, boxed material, or notes, respectively.

Index

Note: Disorder names are in **bold face.** Page numbers in **bold face** indicate main discussions. Page numbers followed by *f, t, b,* or *n* indicate figures, tables, boxed material, or notes, respectively.

Note: Disorder names are in **bold face.** Page numbers in **bold face** indicate main discussions. Page numbers followed by *f*, *t*, *b*, or *n* indicate figures, tables, boxed material, or notes, respectively.

Note: Disorder names are in **bold face.** Page numbers in **bold face** indicate main discussions. Page numbers followed by *f, t, b,* or *n* indicate figures, tables, boxed material, or notes, respectively.

Note: Disorder names are in **bold face.** Page numbers in **bold face** indicate main discussions. Page numbers followed by *f, t, b,* or *n* indicate figures, tables, boxed material, or notes, respectively.

Note: Disorder names are in **bold face.** Page numbers in **bold face** indicate main discussions. Page numbers followed by *f, t, b,* or *n* indicate figures, tables, boxed material, or notes, respectively.

Note: Disorder names are in **bold face.** Page numbers in **bold face** indicate main discussions. Page numbers followed by *f, t, b,* or *n* indicate figures, tables, boxed material, or notes, respectively.

Note: Disorder names are in **bold face.** Page numbers in **bold face** indicate main discussions. Page numbers followed by *f, t, b,* or *n* indicate figures, tables, boxed material, or notes, respectively.

Note: Disorder names are in **bold face.** Page numbers in **bold face** indicate main discussions. Page numbers followed by *f, t, b,* or *n* indicate figures, tables, boxed material, or notes, respectively.

Note: Disorder names are in **bold face.** Page numbers in **bold face** indicate main discussions. Page numbers followed by *f, t, b,* or *n* indicate figures, tables, boxed material, or notes, respectively.

Note: Disorder names are in **bold face.** Page numbers in **bold face** indicate main discussions. Page numbers followed by *f, t, b,* or *n* indicate figures, tables, boxed material, or notes, respectively.

Note: Disorder names are in **bold face.** Page numbers in **bold face** indicate main discussions. Page numbers followed by *f, t, b,* or *n* indicate figures, tables, boxed material, or notes, respectively.

Note: Disorder names are in **bold face**. Page numbers in **bold face** indicate main discussions. Page numbers followed by *f, t, b,* or *n* indicate figures, tables, boxed material, or notes, respectively.

Electronic Resources
Companion CD and Evolve

The following electronic resources are available to supplement and reinforce the content discussed in the textbook.

- Animations
- Audio and Video Clips
- Comprehensive and Chapter Glossaries with Audio Pronunciations
- Concept Map Creator
- Content Updates
- Customizable Nursing Care Plans
- Electronic Calculators
- Interactive Case Studies with Animations and Exercises
- Key Points (Printable and CD/MP3 Download)
- Key Term Flash Cards
- Patient and Family Instruction Guides in English and Spanish
- Physical Examination Videos
- Stress-Busting Kit for Nursing Students
- Additional Supplemental Information

Following is a complete listing of the specific resources available for each section and chapter in the book.

⭘ = available on Companion CD
🖱 = available on Evolve website

Section 1: Concepts in Nursing Practice (Chapters 1-12)
⭘ NCLEX Examination Review Questions (Section 1)

Chapter 1
Nursing Practice Today
⭘ Chapter Glossary with Audio Pronunciations
🖱 Key Points (Printable and CD/MP3 Download)
🖱 Key Term Flash Cards
🖱 Nursing Interventions Classification (NIC): Complete Listing
🖱 Nursing Outcomes Classification (NOC): Complete Listing
🖱 WebLinks

Chapter 2
Health Disparities
⭘ Chapter Glossary with Audio Pronunciations
🖱 Key Points (Printable and CD/MP3 Download)
🖱 Key Term Flash Cards
🖱 WebLinks

Chapter 3
Culturally Competent Care
⭘ Chapter Glossary with Audio Pronunciations
🖱 Key Points (Printable and CD/MP3 Download)
🖱 Key Term Flash Cards
🖱 WebLinks

Chapter 4
Health History and Physical Examination
⭘ Chapter Glossary with Audio Pronunciations
🖱 Key Points (Printable and CD/MP3 Download)
🖱 Key Term Flash Cards
🖱 Physical Examination Video
🖱 WebLinks

Chapter 5
Patient and Family Teaching
⭘ Chapter Glossary with Audio Pronunciations
🖱 Key Points (Printable and CD/MP3 Download)
🖱 Key Term Flash Cards
🖱 WebLinks

Chapter 6
Older Adults
⭘ Chapter Glossary with Audio Pronunciations
🖱 Key Points (Printable and CD/MP3 Download)
🖱 Key Term Flash Cards
🖱 WebLinks

Chapter 7
Community-Based Nursing and Home Care
⭘ Chapter Glossary with Audio Pronunciations
🖱 Key Points (Printable and CD/MP3 Download)
🖱 Key Term Flash Cards
🖱 WebLinks

Chapter 8
Complementary and Alternative Therapies
⭘ Chapter Glossary with Audio Pronunciations
🖱 Key Points (Printable and CD/MP3 Download)
🖱 Key Term Flash Cards
⭘ Stress-Busting Kit for Nursing Students: Take a Yoga Break
🖱 WebLinks

Chapter 9
Stress and Stress Management
🖱 Audio Lecture: *Stress*
⭘ Chapter Glossary with Audio Pronunciations
🖱 Key Points (Printable and CD/MP3 Download)
🖱 Key Term Flash Cards
⭘ Stress-Busting Kit for Nursing Students: Take a Yoga Break
🖱 WebLinks

Chapter 10
Pain
⭘ Chapter Glossary with Audio Pronunciations
⭘ Interactive Case Study: *Pain*
🖱 Key Points (Printable and CD/MP3 Download)
🖱 Key Term Flash Cards
🖱 WebLinks

Chapter 11
End-of-Life and Palliative Care
⭘ Chapter Glossary with Audio Pronunciations
🖱 Key Points (Printable and CD/MP3 Download)
🖱 Key Term Flash Cards
🖱 WebLinks

Chapter 12
Addictive Behaviors
⭘ Chapter Glossary with Audio Pronunciations
🖱 Customizable Nursing Care Plan: *Alcohol Withdrawal*
🖱 Key Points (Printable and CD/MP3 Download)
🖱 Key Term Flash Cards
🖱 Patient and Family Instruction Guide: *Smoking and Tobacco Use Cessation*
🖱 WebLinks

Section 2: Pathophysiologic Mechanisms of Disease (Chapters 13-17)

- NCLEX Examination Review Questions (Section 2)

Chapter 13
Inflammation and Wound Healing
- Chapter Glossary with Audio Pronunciations
- Customizable Nursing Care Plan: *Fever*
- Customizable Nursing Care Plan: *Pressure Ulcer*
- Interactive Case Study: *Pressure Ulcers*
- Key Points (Printable and CD/MP3 Download)
- Key Term Flash Cards
- WebLinks

Chapter 14
Genetics, Altered Immune Responses, and Transplantation
- Animation: *Function of B Cells*
- Animation: *Function of T Cytotoxic Cells*
- Chapter Glossary with Audio Pronunciations
- Key Points (Printable and CD/MP3 Download)
- Key Term Flash Cards
- WebLinks

Chapter 15
Infection and Human Immunodeficiency Virus Infection
- Chapter Glossary with Audio Pronunciations
- Interactive Case Study: *Human Immunodeficiency Syndrome and Acquired Immunodeficiency Syndrome (AIDS)*
- Key Points (Printable and CD/MP3 Download)
- Key Term Flash Cards
- Patient and Family Instruction Guide: *The Right Way to Use Antibiotics*
- Patient and Family Instruction Guide: *The Proper Use of Drug-Using Equipment*
- Patient and Family Instruction Guide: *Use of Antiretroviral Drugs*
- Patient and Family Instruction Guide: *Signs and Symptoms that HIV-Infected Patients Need to Report*
- WebLinks

Chapter 16
Cancer
- Chapter Glossary with Audio Pronunciations
- Key Points (Printable and CD/MP3 Download)
- Key Term Flash Cards
- Table: *Precautions to Minimize Risks from Neutropenia*
- Table: *Neutropenic Diet*
- WebLinks

Chapter 17
Fluid, Electrolyte, and Acid-Base Imbalances
- Chapter Glossary with Audio Pronunciations
- Fluid and Electrolyte Tutorial
- Interactive Case Study: *Hyponatremia/Fluid Volume Imbalance*
- Key Points (Printable and CD/MP3 Download)
- Key Term Flash Cards
- WebLinks

Section 3: Perioperative Care (Chapters 18-20)

- NCLEX Examination Review Questions (Section 3)

Chapter 18
Nursing Management: Preoperative Care
- Chapter Glossary with Audio Pronunciations
- Key Points (Printable and CD/MP3 Download)
- Key Term Flash Cards
- WebLinks

Chapter 19
Nursing Management: Intraoperative Care
- Chapter Glossary with Audio Pronunciations
- Key Points (Printable and CD/MP3 Download)
- Key Term Flash Cards
- WebLinks

Chapter 20
Nursing Management: Postoperative Care
- Chapter Glossary with Audio Pronunciations
- Customizable Nursing Care Plan: *Postoperative Patient*
- Interactive Case Study: *Surgery*
- Key Points (Printable and CD/MP3 Download)
- Key Term Flash Cards
- WebLinks

Section 4: Problems Related to Altered Sensory Input (Chapters 21-25)

- NCLEX Examination Review Questions (Secction 4)

Chapter 21
Nursing Assessment: Visual and Auditory Systems
- Animation: *Ears: Weber Test*
- Chapter Glossary with Audio Pronunciations
- Key Points (Printable and CD/MP3 Download)
- Key Term Flash Cards
- Physical Examination Video Clips: *Eyes*
- Physical Examination Video Clips: *Ears*
- Video Clip: *Evaluation: Central Vision and Visual Acuity*
- Video Clip: *Evaluation: Pupil Responses, Direct and Consensual*
- Video Clip: *Inspection and Palpation: External Ear*
- Video Clip: *Inspection and Palpation: External Eye*
- Video Clip: *Inspection: Ear Canal*
- WebLinks

Chapter 22
Nursing Management: Visual and Auditory Problems
- Case Study Animation: *Visual Pathway*
- Chapter Glossary with Audio Pronunciations
- Customizable Nursing Care Plan: *Patient After Eye Surgery*
- Interactive Case Study: *Cataract Surgery*
- Figure: *Refractive Errors*
- Key Points (Printable and CD/MP3 Download)
- Key Term Flash Cards
- WebLinks

Chapter 23
Nursing Assessment: Integumentary System
- Chapter Glossary with Audio Pronunciations
- Key Points (Printable and CD/MP3 Download)
- Key Term Flash Cards
- Physical Examination Video Clips: *Head and Face*
- Physical Examination Video Clips: *Back and Posterior Chest*
- Physical Examination Video Clips: *Feet, Legs, and Hips*
- WebLinks

Chapter 24
Nursing Management: Integumentary Problems
- Chapter Glossary with Audio Pronunciations
- Customizable Nursing Care Plan: *Chronic Skin Lesions*
- Key Points (Printable and CD/MP3 Download)
- Key Term Flash Cards
- WebLinks

Chapter 25
Nursing Management: Burns
- Chapter Glossary with Audio Pronunciations
- Customizable Nursing Care Plan: *Burn Patient*
- Interactive Case Study: *Burns*
- Key Points (Printable and CD/MP3 Download)
- Key Term Flash Cards
- WebLinks

Section 5: Problems of Oxygenation: Ventilation (Chapters 26-29)

- NCLEX Examination Review Questions (Section 5)

Chapter 26
Nursing Assessment: Respiratory System

- Animation: *Patterns of Respiration*
- Animation: *Percussion Tones throughout the Chest*
- Animation: *Pulmonary Circulation*
- Audio Clip: *Bronchial Breath Sounds*
- Audio Clip: *Bronchovesicular Breath Sounds*
- Audio Clip: *High Pitched Crackles*
- Audio Clip: *High Pitched Wheeze*
- Audio Clip: *Low Pitched Crackles*
- Audio Clip: *Low Pitched Wheeze*
- Audio Clip: *Pleural Friction Rub*
- Audio Clip: *Stridor*
- Audio Clip: *Vesicular Breath Sounds*
- Chapter Glossary with Audio Pronunciations
- Key Points (Printable and CD/MP3 Download)
- Key Term Flash Cards
- Physical Examination Video Clips: *Anterior Chest, Lungs, and Heart*
- Physical Examination Video Clips: *Lungs*
- Video Clip: *Inspection and Palpation: Breathing and Respiratory Excursion, Anterior Chest*
- Video Clip: *Inspection and Palpation: Respirations, Respiratory Excursion, and Tactile Fremitus, Posterior Chest*
- Video Clip: *Inspection and Percussion: Diaphragmatic Excursion*
- Video Clip: *Inspection: Nose*
- Video Clip: *Palpation: Tactile Fremitus, Posterior Chest*
- Video Clip: *Percussion: Anterior Thorax*
- WebLinks

Chapter 27
Nursing Management: Upper Respiratory Problems

- Animation: *Anatomic Location of Sinuses*
- Chapter Glossary with Audio Pronunciations
- Customizable Nursing Care Plan: *Total Laryngectomy and/or Radical Neck Surgery*
- Customizable Nursing Care Plan: *Tracheostomy*
- Interactive Case Study: *Head and Neck Cancer/Laryngectomy with Tracheostomy*
- Key Points (Printable and CD/MP3 Download)
- Key Term Flash Cards
- Patient and Family Instruction Guide: *Acute or Chronic Sinusitis*
- Patient and Family Instruction Guide: *How to Reduce Symptoms of Allergic Rhinitis*
- WebLinks

Chapter 28
Nursing Management: Lower Respiratory Problems

- Case Study Animation: *Pulmonary Embolus*
- Chapter Glossary with Audio Pronunciations
- Customizable Nursing Care Plan: *Pneumonia*
- Customizable Nursing Care Plan: *Thoracotomy*
- Interactive Case Study: *Lung Cancer*
- Interactive Case Study: *Pulmonary Embolism*
- Key Points (Printable and CD/MP3 Download)
- Key Term Flash Cards
- WebLinks

Chapter 29
Nursing Management: Obstructive Pulmonary Diseases

- Asthma Action Plan (Spanish)
- Audio Lecture: *Asthma*
- Case Study Animation: *Asthma*
- Case Study Animation: *Simple Pneumothorax and Tension Pneumothorax*
- Chapter Glossary with Audio Pronunciations
- Customizable Nursing Care Plan: *Asthma*
- Customizable Nursing Care Plan: *Chronic Obstructive Pulmonary Disease*
- Interactive Case Study: *Asthma*
- Interactive Case Study: *Chronic Obstructive Pulmonary Disease*
- Interactive Case Study: *Cystic Fibrosis*
- Key Points (Printable and CD/MP3 Download)
- Key Term Flash Cards
- Patient and Family Instruction Guide: *Home Oxygen Use*
- Patient and Family Instruction Guide: *How to Use a Dry Powder Inhaler*
- Patient and Family Instruction Guide: *How to Use Your Peak Flow Meter*
- WebLinks

Section 6: Problems of Oxygenation: Transport (Chapters 30-31)

- NCLEX Examination Review Questions (Section 6)

Chapter 30
Nursing Assessment: Hematologic System

- Chapter Glossary with Audio Pronunciations
- Key Points (Printable and CD/MP3 Download)
- Key Term Flash Cards
- Physical Examination Video Clips: *Precordium and Jugular Veins*
- Physical Examination Video Clips: *Neck*
- Physical Examination Video Clips: *Upper Extremities*
- Physical Examination Video Clips: *Anterior Chest*
- Physical Examination Video Clips: *Abdominal Reflexes, Abdominal Muscles, and Inguinal Area*
- WebLinks

Chapter 31
Nursing Management: Hematologic Problems

- Case Study Animation: *Differentiation of Blood Cells*
- Case Study Animation: *Sickle Cell Anemia*
- Chapter Glossary with Audio Pronunciations
- Customizable Nursing Care Plan: *Anemia*
- Customizable Nursing Care Plan: *Neutropenia*
- Customizable Nursing Care Plan: *Thrombocytopenia*
- Interactive Case Study: *Chronic Myelogenous Leukemia*
- Interactive Case Study: *Sickle Cell Anemia*
- Key Points (Printable and CD/MP3 Download)
- Key Term Flash Cards
- WebLinks

Section 7: Problems of Oxygenation: Perfusion (Chapters 32-38)

- NCLEX Examination Review Questions (Section 7)

Chapter 32
Nursing Assessment: Cardiovascular System

- Animation: *Auscultation of Heart Valves*
- Animation: *Blood Flow: Circulatory System*
- Animation: *Cardiac Cycle During Systole and Diastole*
- Animation: *Pulse Variations*
- Audio Clip: *Diastolic Murmur*
- Audio Clip: *Fourth Heart Sound (S_4)*
- Audio Clip: *Murmurs: Blowing, Harsh or Rough, and Rumble*
- Audio Clip: *Murmurs: High, Medium, and Low*
- Audio Clip: *S_1 at Various Locations*
- Audio Clip: *S_2 at Various Locations*
- Audio Clip: *Single S_1*
- Audio Clip: *Single S_2*
- Audio Clip: *Systolic Murmur*
- Audio Clip: *Third Heart Sound (S_3)*
- Chapter Glossary with Audio Pronunciations
- Key Points (Printable and CD/MP3 Download)
- Key Term Flash Cards
- Physical Examination Video Clips: *Neck*
- Physical Examination Video Clips: *Upper Extremities*
- Physical Examination Video Clips: *Anterior Chest, Lungs, and Heart*
- Physical Examination Video Clips: *Precordium and Jugular Veins*
- Physical Examination Video Clips: *Breasts and Heart*
- Video Clip: *Auscultation: Cardiac, with Bell*
- Video Clip: *Auscultation: Cardiac, with Diaphragm*
- Video Clip: *Auscultation: Cardiac, with Diaphragm and Bell*

- Video Clip: *Auscultation: Carotid Artery*
- Video Clip: *Inspection and Palpation: Cardiac Ausculatory Landmarks*
- Video Clip: *Inspection and Palpation: Cardiac, Anterior Chest*
- Video Clip: *Inspection and Palpation: Pulses, Lower Extremities*
- WebLinks

Chapter 33
Nursing Management: Hypertension

- Case Study Animation: *Pulmonary Hypertension*
- Chapter Glossary with Audio Pronunciations
- Interactive Case Study: *Hypertension*
- Key Points (Printable and CD/MP3 Download)
- Key Term Flash Cards
- WebLinks

Chapter 34
Nursing Management: Coronary Artery Disease and Acute Coronary Syndrome

- Audio Lecture: *Risk Factors for Coronary Artery Disease*
- Case Study Animation: *Coronary Artery Bypass Grafting*
- Case Study Animation: *Acute Myocardial Infarction*
- Chapter Glossary with Audio Pronunciations
- Customizable Nursing Care Plan: *Acute Coronary Syndrome*
- Interactive Case Study: *Myocardial Infarction*
- Key Points (Printable and CD/MP3 Download)
- Key Term Flash Cards
- Patient and Family Instruction Guide: *Decreasing Risk Factors for Coronary Artery Disease*
- Patient and Family Instruction Guide: *FITT Physical Activity Guidelines After Acute Coronary Syndrome*
- WebLinks

Chapter 35
Nursing Management: Heart Failure

- Chapter Glossary with Audio Pronunciations
- Customizable Nursing Care Plan: *Heart Failure*
- Interactive Case Study: *Heart Failure*
- Key Points (Printable and CD/MP3 Download)
- Key Term Flash Cards
- Patient and Family Instruction Guide: *Heart Failure*
- WebLinks

Chapter 36
Nursing Management: Dysrhythmias

- Algorithms for Treatment of Dysrhythmias
- Case Study Animation: *Atrial Fibrillation*
- Chapter Glossary with Audio Pronunciations
- Interactive Case Study: *Atrial Fibrillation*
- Key Points (Printable and CD/MP3 Download)
- Key Term Flash Cards
- WebLinks

Chapter 37
Nursing Management: Inflammatory and Structural Heart Disorders

- Audio Clip: *Pericardial Friction Rub*
- Chapter Glossary with Audio Pronunciations
- Customizable Nursing Care Plan: *Infective Endocarditis*
- Customizable Nursing Care Plan: *Valvular Heart Disease*
- Interactive Case Study: *Rheumatic Fever and Heart Disease*
- Key Points (Printable and CD/MP3 Download)
- Key Term Flash Cards
- WebLinks

Chapter 38
Nursing Management: Vascular Disorders

- Case Study Animation: *Abdominal Aortic Aneurysm*
- Chapter Glossary with Audio Pronunciations
- Customizable Nursing Care Plan: Peripheral Arterial Disease of the Lower Extremities
- Customizable Nursing Care Plan: Surgical Repair of the Aorta
- Interactive Case Study: *Abdominal Aortic Aneurysm*
- Interactive Case Study: *Chronic Peripheral Arterial Disease*
- Key Points (Printable and CD/MP3 Download)
- Key Term Flash Cards
- Patient and Family Instruction Guide: *Anticoagulation Therapy*
- WebLinks

Section 8: Problems of Ingestion, Digestion, Absorption, and Elimination (Chapters 39-44)

- **NCLEX Examination Review Questions (Section 8)**

Chapter 39
Nursing Assessment: Gastrointestinal System

- Animation: *Rectal Examination*
- Chapter Glossary with Audio Pronunciations
- Key Points (Printable and CD/MP3 Download)
- Key Term Flash Cards
- Physical Examination Video Clips: *Abdomen: Inspection, Auscultation, and Percussion*
- Physical Examination Video Clips: *Abdomen: Palpation*
- Video Clip: *Auscultation: Abdomen, Bowel Sounds*
- Video Clip: *Palpation: Abdomen, Superficial and Deep*
- Video Clip: *Percussion: Abdomen*
- Video Clip: *Percussion: Liver*
- Video Clip: *Percussion: Spleen*
- WebLinks

Chapter 40
Nursing Management: Nutritional Problems

- Chapter Glossary with Audio Pronunciations
- Customizable Nursing Care Plan: *Enteral Nutrition*
- Customizable Nursing Care Plan: *Parenteral Nutrition*
- Key Points (Printable and CD/MP3 Download)
- Key Term Flash Cards
- Table: Nutritional Therapy: *High-Calorie, High-Protein Diet*
- WebLinks

Chapter 41
Nursing Management: Obesity

- Chapter Glossary with Audio Pronunciations
- Interactive Case Study: *Obese Patient*
- Key Points (Printable and CD/MP3 Download)
- Key Term Flash Cards
- Table: *Nutritional therapy: 1200-Calorie-Restricted Weight-Reduction Diet*
- WebLinks

Chapter 42
Nursing Management: Upper Gastrointestinal Problems

- Case Study Animation: *Duodenal Ulcer: Pathophysiology and Symptoms*
- Chapter Glossary with Audio Pronunciations
- Customizable Nursing Care Plan: *Nausea and Vomiting*
- Customizable Nursing Care Plan: *Peptic Ulcer Disease*
- Interactive Case Study: *Oral Cancer*
- Interactive Case Study: *Peptic Ulcer Disease*
- Key Points (Printable and CD/MP3 Download)
- Key Term Flash Cards
- WebLinks

Chapter 43
Nursing Management: Lower Gastrointestinal Problems

- Audio Lecture: *Inflammatory Bowel Disease*
- Audio Lecture: *Irritable Bowel Syndrome*
- Chapter Glossary with Audio Pronunciations
- Customizable Nursing Care Plan: *Acute Infectious Diarrhea*
- Customizable Nursing Care Plan: *Colostomy/Ileostomy*
- Customizable Nursing Care Plan: *Inflammatory Bowel Disease*
- Customizable Nursing Care Plan: *Laparotomy*
- Interactive Case Study: *Ulcerative Colitis*
- Key Points (Printable and CD/MP3 Download)
- Key Term Flash Cards
- Patient and Family Instruction Guide: *Colostomy Irrigation*

- Patient and Family Instruction Guide: *Managing Constipation*
- Figure: *Intestinal Tubes*
- WebLinks

Chapter 44
Nursing Management: Liver, Pancreas, and Biliary Tract Problems
- Case Study Animation: *Laparoscopic Cholecystectomy*
- Case Study Animation: *Cholecystitis: Pathophysiology and Symptoms*
- Chapter Glossary with Audio Pronunciations
- Customizable Nursing Care Plan: *Acute Viral Hepatitis*
- Customizable Nursing Care Plan: *Cirrhosis*
- Customizable Nursing Care Plan: *Acute Pancreatitis*
- Interactive Case Study: *Acute Pancreatitis*
- Interactive Case Study: *Cholelithiasis/Cholecystitis*
- Interactive Case Study: *Hepatitis*
- Interactive Case Study: *Postnecrotic Cirrhosis*
- Key Points (Printable and CD/MP3 Download)
- Key Term Flash Cards
- WebLinks

Section 9: Problems of Urinary Function (Chapters 45-47)
- NCLEX Examination Review Questions (Section 9)

Chapter 45
Nursing Assessment: Urinary System
- Chapter Glossary with Audio Pronunciations
- Key Points (Printable and CD/MP3 Download)
- Key Term Flash Cards
- Physical Examination Video Clips: *Abdomen: Inspection, Auscultation, and Percussion*
- Physical Examination Video Clips: *Abdomen: Palpation*
- WebLinks

Chapter 46
Nursing Management: Renal and Urologic Problems
- Case Study Animation: *Nephrostomy*
- Chapter Glossary with Audio Pronunciations
- Customizable Nursing Care Plan: *Acute Renal Lithiasis*
- Customizable Nursing Care Plan: *Ileal Conduit*
- Customizable Nursing Care Plan: *Urinary Tract Infection*
- Interactive Case Study: *Bladder Cancer with Urinary Diversion*
- Interactive Case Study: *Glomerulonephritis*
- Key Points (Printable and CD/MP3 Download)
- Key Term Flash Cards
- Patient and Family Instruction Guide: *Changing Your Ileal Conduit Appliances*
- Patient and Family Instruction Guide: *Urinary Tract Infection*
- WebLinks

Chapter 47
Nursing Management: Acute Renal Failure and Chronic Kidney Disease
- Chapter Glossary with Audio Pronunciations
- Customizable Nursing Care Plan: *Chronic Kidney Disease*
- Interactive Case Study: *Kidney Transplant*
- Key Points (Printable and CD/MP3 Download)
- Key Term Flash Cards
- WebLinks

Section 10: Problems Related to Regulatory and Reproductive Mechanisms (Chapters 48-55)
- NCLEX Examination Review Questions (Section 10)

Chapter 48
Nursing Assessment: Endocrine System
- Chapter Glossary with Audio Pronunciations
- Key Points (Printable and CD/MP3 Download)
- Key Term Flash Cards
- Physical Examination Video Clips: *Abdomen: Inspection, Auscultation, and Percussion*
- Physical Examination Video Clips: *Abdomen: Palpation*
- WebLinks

Chapter 49
Nursing Management: Diabetes Mellitus
- Case Study Animation: *Insulin Function*
- Chapter Glossary with Audio Pronunciations
- Customizable Nursing Care Plan: *Diabetes Mellitus*
- Interactive Case Study: *Diabetes Ketoacidosis*
- Interactive Case Study: *Type 2 Diabetes Mellitus*
- Key Points (Printable and CD/MP3 Download)
- Key Term Flash Cards
- Patient and Family Instruction Guide: *Exercise Guidelines for Patients with Diabetes Mellitus*
- Patient and Family Instruction Guide: *Foot Care for Patients with Diabetes or Peripheral Vascular Problems*
- Patient and Family Instruction Guide: *Insulin Administration*
- Patient and Family Instruction Guide: *Management of Diabetes Mellitus*
- Patient and Family Instruction Guide: *Self-Monitoring of Blood Glucose (SMGB)*
- WebLinks

Chapter 50
Nursing Management: Endocrine Problems
- Case Study Animation: *Adrenal Function*
- Case Study Animation: *Thyroid Gland, Hormone Release*
- Chapter Glossary with Audio Pronunciations
- Customizable Nursing Care Plan: *Cushing Syndrome*
- Customizable Nursing Care Plan: *Hyperthyroidism*
- Customizable Nursing Care Plan: *Hypothyroidism*
- Interactive Case Study: *Addison's Disease*
- Interactive Case Study: *Cushing Syndrome*
- Interactive Case Study: *Hyperthyroidism*
- Key Points (Printable and CD/MP3 Download)
- Key Term Flash Cards
- Patient and Family Instruction Guide: *Corticosteroid Therapy*
- WebLinks

Chapter 51
Nursing Assessment: Reproductive System
- Animation: *Lymphatic Drainage of Breast*
- Animation: *The Menstrual Cycle*
- Chapter Glossary with Audio Pronunciations
- Key Points (Printable and CD/MP3 Download)
- Key Term Flash Cards
- Physical Examination Video Clips: *Abdominal Reflexes, Abdominal Muscles, and Inguinal Area*
- Physical Examination Video Clips: *Breasts*
- Physical Examination Video Clips: *Breasts and Heart*
- Physical Examination Video Clips: *Genitalia and Rectum (female)*
- Physical Examination Video Clips: *Rectum and Prostate Gland (male)*
- Video Clip: *Inspection and Palpation—Standing Position (Male)—1*
- Video Clip: *Inspection and Palpation—Standing Position Male)—2*
- Video Clip: *Inspection: External Genitalia (Female)*
- Video Clip: *Inspection: Female Breasts—Sitting Position*
- Video Clip: *Inspection: Speculum Examination (Female)*
- Video Clip: *Palpation: Bimanual Examination (Female)*
- Video Clip: *Palpation: Female Breasts—Supine Position*
- Video Clip: *Palpation: Inguinal Hernia Evaluation (Male)*
- WebLinks

Chapter 52
Nursing Management: Breast Disorders
- Case Study Animation: *Breast Cancer Spread*
- Chapter Glossary with Audio Pronunciations
- Customizable Nursing Care Plan: *Mastectomy or Lumpectomy*
- Interactive Case Study: *Breast Cancer*
- Key Points (Printable and CD/MP3 Download)
- Key Term Flash Cards
- WebLinks

Chapter 53
Nursing Management: Sexually Transmitted Diseases
- Chapter Glossary with Audio Pronunciations
- Key Points (Printable and CD/MP3 Download)
- Key Term Flash Cards
- WebLinks

Chapter 54
Nursing Management: Female Reproductive Problems
- Chapter Glossary with Audio Pronunciations
- Customizable Nursing Care Plan: *Abdominal Hysterectomy*
- Interactive Case Study: *Endometrial Cancer*
- Key Points (Printable and CD/MP3 Download)
- Key Term Flash Cards
- WebLinks

Chapter 55
Nursing Management: Male Reproductive Problems
- Chapter Glossary with Audio Pronunciations
- Customizable Nursing Care Plan: *Prostate Surgery*
- Interactive Case Study: *Benign Prostatic Hyperplasia (BPH)*
- Key Points (Printable and CD/MP3 Download)
- Key Term Flash Cards
- Patient and Family Instruction Guide: *Testicular Self-Examination*
- WebLinks

Section 11: Problems Related to Movement and Coordination (Chapters 56-65)
NCLEX Examination Review Questions (Section 11)

Chapter 56
Nursing Assessment: Nervous System
- Animation: *Motor Pathways and Clinical Evaluation of the Central Nervous System*
- Animation: *Reflex Arc*
- Animation: *Sensory Pathways and Clinical Evaluation of the Central Nervous System*
- Chapter Glossary with Audio Pronunciations
- Key Points (Printable and CD/MP3 Download)
- Key Term Flash Cards
- Physical Examination Video Clips: *Abdominal Reflexes, Abdominal Muscles, and Inguinal Area*
- Physical Examination Video Clips: *Ears*
- Physical Examination Video Clips: *Eyes*
- Physical Examination Video Clips: *Head and Face*
- Physical Examination Video Clips: *Neck*
- Physical Examination Video Clips: *Neurologic System: Gait and Balance*
- Physical Examination Video Clips: *Neurologic System: Motor Function and Coordination*
- Physical Examination Video Clips: *Neurologic System: Sensory Function*
- Physical Examination Video Clips: *Nose, Mouth, and Pharynx*
- Video Clip: *Evaluation: Central Vision and Visual Acuity, Cranial Nerve II—Optic Nerve*
- Video Clip: *Evaluation: Deep Tendon Reflex, Patellar Tendon*
- Video Clip: *Evaluation: Pupil Responses, Direct and Accommodation, Cranial Nerves III, IV, and VI—Oculomotor, Trochlear, and Abducens Nerves*
- Video Clip: *Evaluation: Sensory, Face, and Upper Extremities*
- Video Clip: *Evaluation: Sensory, Light Touch; Face, Upper, and Lower Extremities, Cranial Nerve V—Trigeminal Nerve*
- Video Clip: *Evaluation: Smell, Cranial Nerve I—Olfactory Nerve*
- Video Clip: *Inspection: Fine Motor Coordination, Lower Extremities*
- Video Clip: *Inspection: Fine Motor Coordination, Upper Extremities*
- WebLinks

Chapter 57
Nursing Management: Acute Intracranial Problems
- Animation: *Functional Areas of the Brain*
- Case Study Animation: *Subdural Hematoma*
- Case Study Animation: *Meningitis*
- Chapter Glossary with Audio Pronunciations
- Customizable Nursing Care Plan: *Bacterial Meningitis*
- Customizable Nursing Care Plan: *Increased Intracranial Pressure*
- Interactive Case Study: *Head Injury*
- Interactive Case Study: *Meningitis*
- Key Points (Printable and CD/MP3 Download)
- Key Term Flash Cards
- Patient and Family Instruction Guide: *Head Injury*
- WebLinks

Chapter 58
Nursing Management: Stroke
- Case Study Animation: *Blood Clot Leading to Stroke*
- Chapter Glossary with Audio Pronunciations
- Customizable Nursing Care Plan: *Stroke*
- Interactive Case Study: *Stroke*
- Key Points (Printable and CD/MP3 Download)
- Key Term Flash Cards
- Patient and Family Instruction Guide: *Warning Signs of Stroke*
- WebLinks

Chapter 59
Nursing Management: Chronic Neurologic Problems
- Case Study Animation: *Closed Reduction/Pinning of Hip Fracture*
- Case Study Animation: *Parkinson's Disease*
- Chapter Glossary with Audio Pronunciations
- Customizable Nursing Care Plan: *Headache*
- Customizable Nursing Care Plan: *Multiple Sclerosis*
- Customizable Nursing Care Plan: *Parkinson's Disease*
- Customizable Nursing Care Plan: *Seizure Disorder or Epilepsy*
- Interactive Case Study: *Parkinson's Disease and Hip Fracture*
- Interactive Case Study: *Seizures*
- Key Points (Printable and CD/MP3 Download)
- Key Term Flash Cards
- Patient and Family Instruction Guide: *Headache Management*
- WebLinks

Chapter 60
Nursing Management: Alzheimer's Disease and Dementia
- Audio Lecture: *Alzheimer's Disease*
- Case Study Animation: *Alzheimer's Disease*
- Chapter Glossary with Audio Pronunciations
- Customizable Nursing Care Plan: *Alzheimer's Disease*
- Customizable Nursing Care Plan: *Caregiver of the Patient with Alzheimer's Disease*
- Interactive Case Study: *Alzheimer's Disease*
- Key Points (Printable and CD/MP3 Download)
- Key Term Flash Cards
- Patient and Family Instruction Guide: *Early Warning Signs of Alzheimer's Disease*
- Patient and Family Instruction Guide: *Managing Alzheimer's Disease*
- WebLinks

Chapter 61
Nursing Management: Peripheral Nerve and Spinal Cord Problems
- Case Study Animation: *Spine Structure*
- Chapter Glossary with Audio Pronunciations
- Customizable Nursing Care Plan: *Spinal Cord Injury*
- Interactive Case Study: *Spinal Cord Injury*
- Key Points (Printable and CD/MP3 Download)
- Key Term Flash Cards
- Patient and Family Instruction Guide: *Autonomic Dysreflexia*
- Patient and Family Instruction Guide: *Bowel Management After Spinal Cord Injury*
- Patient and Family Instruction Guide: *Skin Care for Patient with Spinal Cord Injury*
- WebLinks

Section 8

PROBLEMS OF INGESTION, DIGESTION, ABSORPTION, AND ELIMINATION

Section 9

PROBLEMS OF URINARY FUNCTION

Section 10

PROBLEMS RELATED TO REGULATORY AND REPRODUCTIVE MECHANISMS

Section 11

PROBLEMS RELATED TO MOVEMENT AND COORDINATION

Section 12

NURSING CARE IN SPECIALIZED SETTINGS

APPENDIXES

ELSEVIER

evolve

To access your Student Resources, visit:

http://evolve.elsevier.com/Lewis/medsurg

Evolve® Student Resources for ***Lewis: Medical-Surgical Nursing: Assessment and Management of Clinical Problems,*** **Seventh Edition** offer the following features:

Student Resources

- **Audio Glossary** - an expanded version of the glossary in the book, it includes audio pronunciations for each glossary term
- **Concept Map Creator** - walks you through the process of creating individualized concept maps
- **Content Updates** - written by the textbook authors to fill you in on the latest research findings, drug information, and much more
- **Electronic Calculators** - quickly calculate body mass index, IV infusion rates, and much more
- **Fluids and Electrolytes Tutorial** - a user-friendly program to help you master this difficult material
- **Key Points** - both audio files and printable versions that you can use while on the go
- **Key Term Flash Cards** - a great study tool for mastering complex terminology
- **Nursing Care Plans** - fully customizable
- **Patient and Family Instruction Guides** - both English and Spanish
- **Online Supplements** - additional tables, care plans, illustrations, and handouts
- **Physical Examination Video Clips** - demonstrates patient assessment techniques
- **WebLinks** - regularly updated
- And don't forget about all of the exciting resources on the Companion CD: animations, NCLEX® Examination Review Questions, interactive case studies, and much more! (See listing on inside back cover.)